Massachusetts General Hospital Comprehensive Clinical Psychiatry

Second Edition

Massachusetts General Hospital
Comprehensive Clinical Psychiatry

SECOND EDITION

THEODORE A. STERN MD
Chief, Avery D. Weisman Psychiatry Consultation Service
Massachusetts General Hospital
Director, Office for Clinical Careers Massachusetts General Hospital
Ned H. Cassem Professor of Psychiatry in the field of Psychosomatic Medicine/Consultation
Harvard Medical School
Boston, MA, USA

MAURIZIO FAVA MD
Director, Clinical Research Program
Executive Vice-Chair, Department of Psychiatry
Executive Director, Clinical Trials Network and Institute, Massachusetts General Hospital
Slater Family Professor of Psychiatry, Harvard Medical School
Boston, MA, USA

TIMOTHY E. WILENS MD
Senior Staff, Child Psychiatry and Pediatric Psychopharmacology
Director of the Center for Addiction Medicine
Massachusetts General Hospital
Associate Professor of Psychiatry
Harvard Medical School
Boston, MA, USA

JERROLD F. ROSENBAUM MD
Psychiatrist-in-Chief, Massachusetts General Hospital
Chair, Executive Committee on Research
Massachusetts General Hospital
Stanley Cobb Professor of Psychiatry
Harvard Medical School
Boston, MA, USA

ELSEVIER   London, New York, Oxford, Philadelphia, St Louis, Sydney, Toronto

ELSEVIER

Notices

Knowledge and best practice in this field are constantly changing. As new research and experience broaden our understanding, changes in research methods, professional practices, or medical treatment may become necessary.

Practitioners and researchers must always rely on their own experience and knowledge in evaluating and using any information, methods, compounds, or experiments described herein. In using such information or methods they should be mindful of their own safety and the safety of others, including parties for whom they have a professional responsibility.

With respect to any drug or pharmaceutical products identified, readers are advised to check the most current information provided (i) on procedures featured or (ii) by the manufacturer of each product to be administered, to verify the recommended dose or formula, the method and duration of administration, and contraindications. It is the responsibility of practitioners, relying on their own experience and knowledge of their patients, to make diagnoses, to determine dosages and the best treatment for each individual patient, and to take all appropriate safety precautions.

To the fullest extent of the law, neither the Publisher nor the authors, contributors, or editors, assume any liability for any injury and/or damage to persons or property as a matter of products liability, negligence or otherwise, or from any use or operation of any methods, products, instructions, or ideas contained in the material herein.

ISBN: 978-0-323-29507-9
eISBN: 978-0-323-32899-9

Content Strategist: Charlotta Kryhl
Content Development Specialist: Alexandra Mortimer
Content Coordinator: Sam Crowe
Project Manager: Andrew Riley
Design: Christian Bilbow
Illustration Manager: Amy Naylor
Illustrator: MacPS
Marketing Manager: Nyasha Kapenzi

Printed in China

Last digit is the print number: 9 8 7 6 5 4 3 2 1

Working together
to grow libraries in
developing countries

www.elsevier.com • www.bookaid.org

Contents

Preface

Fortunately, the field of Psychiatry has continued to evolve. This observation led us to the realization that it was time for a new and updated comprehensive textbook of Psychiatry, written by our clinicians and researchers here at the Massachusetts General Hospital. Once again, our faculty was up to the challenge; they collaborated enthusiastically and efficiently to create this comprehensive compendium covering the diagnosis, pathophysiology, evaluation, and treatment of a wide variety of psychiatric conditions and states.

We are incredibly appreciative of the countless hours spent conceptualizing, creating, updating, and refining each chapter in this volume; yeoman's work was done by all. Without all involved pulling at the oars this endeavor would not have been possible.

To match learning styles of our readers and to solidify knowledge gained through perusal of this text, we have also included 600 board-style multiple-choice questions (MCQs) and detailed annotated answers (geared to each chapter). These MCQs are available online at https://expertconsult.inkling.com.

With the assistance of the watchful eyes of the staff at Elsevier (led by Charlotta Kryhl, Alexandra Mortimer, Andrew Riley, and Sam Crowe) our journey was completed in less than two years, enabling us to include the most up-to-date information available in each content area. In addition, Naomi Plasky (at the Massachusetts General Hospital) helped shepherd us through thousands of emails and packages among more than 175 authors who contributed to the production of 94 chapters.

On behalf of the patients we serve, we hope that this edition facilitates the conceptualization, diagnosis, understanding, and treatment of psychiatric problems and brings much-needed relief.

T.A.S.

M.F.

T.E.W.

J.F.R.

List of Contributors

Robert S. Abernethy III, MD
Psychiatrist
Massachusetts General Hospital
Assistant Professor
Department of Psychiatry
Harvard Medical School
Boston, MA, USA
Ch 10 An Overview of the Psychotherapies

Annah N. Abrams, MD
Director, Pediatric Psycho-oncology
Massachusetts General Hospital
Assistant Professor of Psychiatry
Harvard Medical School
Boston, MA, USA
Ch 5 Child, Adolescent, and Adult Development

Anne Alonso, PhD, CGP, DFAGPA†
Director, The Center for Psychoanalytic Studies and The Endowment for the Advancement of Psychotherapy
Massachusetts General Hospital
Clinical Professor of Psychology
Department of Psychiatry
Harvard Medical School
Boston, MA, USA

Menekse Alpay, MD
Clinical Assistant
Department of Psychiatry
Massachusetts General Hospital
Instructor
Department of Psychiatry
Harvard Medical School
Boston, MA, USA
Ch 79 Pathophysiology, Psychiatric Co-morbidity, and Treatment of Pain

Jonathan E. Alpert, MD, PhD
Associate Chief of Psychiatry for Clinical Services
Director, Depression Clinical and Research Program
Massachusetts General Hospital
Joyce R. Tedlow Associate Professor of Psychiatry
Harvard Medical School
Boston, MA, USA
Ch 50 Drug–Drug Interactions in Psychopharmacology

Ji Hyun Baek, MD
Research Fellow
Massachusetts General Hospital
Boston, MA, USA
Ch 44 Pharmacological Approaches to Treatment-Resistant Depression

Lee Baer, PhD
Associate Chief of Psychology
Department of Psychiatry
Massachusetts General Hospital
Clinical Professor of Psychology
Harvard Medical School
Boston, MA, USA
Ch 15 Hypnosis
Ch 62 Statistics in Psychiatric Research

Scott R. Beach, MD
Associate Training Director
MGH/McLean Adult Psychiatry Residency Program
Assistant Psychiatrist
Acute Psychiatric and Consultation-Liaison Services
Massachusetts General Hospital
Assistant Professor of Psychiatry
Harvard Medical School
Boston, MA, USA
Ch 51 Side Effects of Psychotropic Medications
Ch 55 Life-threatening Conditions in Psychiatry: Catatonia, Neuroleptic Malignant Syndrome, and Serotonin Syndrome

BJ Beck, MSN, MD
Staff, Robert B. Andrews Unit
Massachusetts General Hospital
Assistant Professor, Part-Time,
Department of Psychiatry
Harvard Medical School
Boston, MA, USA
Ch 21 Mental Disorders Due to Another Medical Condition
Ch 59 Approaches to Collaborative Care and Primary Care Psychiatry
Ch 67 Community Psychiatry
Ch 83 Intimate Partner Violence

David M. Benedek, MD
Deputy Chair
Department of Psychiatry
Uniformed Services University
Bethesda, MD, USA
Ch 90 Military Psychiatry

Eugene V. Beresin, MD
Senior Educator in Child and Adolescent Psychiatry Massachusetts General Hospital Executive Director
Massachusetts General Hospital Clay Center for Young Healthy Minds
Professor of Psychiatry
Harvard Medical School
Department of Psychiatry Massachusetts General Hospital
Boston MA, USA
Ch 01 The Doctor–Patient Relationship
Ch 02 The Psychiatric Interview
Ch 93 Psychiatry and the Media

Matt Bianchi MD
Director, Sleep Division
Massachusetts General Hospital
Assistant Professor of Neurology
Harvard Medical School
Boston, MA, USA
Ch 22 Sleep Disorders

Joseph Biederman, MD
Director of the Joint Program in Pediatric Psychopharmacology
McLean and Massachusetts General Hospital
Professor of Psychiatry
Harvard Medical School
Boston, MA, USA
Ch 49 Pharmacotherapy of Attention-Deficit/Hyperactivity Disorder across the Life Span

Mark A. Blais, PsyD
Director, Psychological Evaluation and Research Laboratory
Massachusetts General Hospital
Associate Professor of Psychology
Harvard Medical School
Boston, MA, USA
Ch 7 Understanding and Applying Psychological Assessment
Ch 11 Brief Psychotherapy: An Overview
Ch 39 Personality and Personality Disorders

Christina P.C. Borba, PhD, MPH
Director of Research
The Chester M. Pierce, M.D. Division of
 Global Psychiatry
Massachusetts General Hospital
Assistant Professor of Psychology in
 Psychiatry
Harvard Medical School
Boston, MA, USA
*Ch 94 Global Mental Health in the
 Twenty-First Century*

Jeff Q. Bostic, MD, EdD
Director, School Psychiatry
Massachusetts General Hospital
Yawkey Center for Outpatient Care
Associate Clinical Professor of
 Psychiatry
Harvard Medical School
Boston, MA, USA
*Ch 69 Child and Adolescent Psychiatric
 Disorders*

Rebecca Weintraub Brendel MD, JD
Clinical Director
Red Sox Foundation and Massachusetts
General Hospital Home Base Program
Assistant Professor of Psychiatry
Harvard Medical School
Boston, MA, USA
Ch 53 The Suicidal Patient
*Ch 60 Psychiatric and Ethical Aspects of
 Care at the End of Life*
*Ch 84 Psychiatric Correlates and
 Consequences of Abuse and Neglect*
*Ch 86 The Role of Psychiatrists in the
 Criminal Justice System*
*Ch 87 Legal and Ethical Issues in
 Psychiatry II: Malpractice and Boundary
 Violations*

Megan Moore Brennan, MD
Attending Psychiatrist
Bassett Medical Center
Assistant Clinical Professor, Columbia
 University College of Physicians and
 Surgeons
Cooperstown, NY, USA
Ch 4 Treatment Adherence

Christina A. Brezing, MD
Clinical and Research Fellow
Division of Substance Abuse
Department of Psychiatry
Columbia University College of
 Physicians and Surgeons
New York, NY, USA
Ch 53 The Suicidal Patient

Hannah E. Brown, MD
Schizophrenia Program Massachusetts
 General Hospital
Instructor in Psychiatry, Harvard
 Medical School
Boston, MA, USA
Ch 28 Psychosis and Schizophrenia

Eric Bui, MD, PhD
Center for Anxiety and Traumatic Stress
 Disorders
Massachusetts General Hospital/
 Harvard Medical School
Boston, MA, USA
Ch 32 Anxiety Disorders
*Ch 41 The Pharmacotherapy of Anxiety
 Disorders*

George Bush, MD, MMSc
Director, Massachusetts General
 Hospital Cingulate Cortex Research
 Laboratory
Assistant Director, MGH Psychiatric
 Neuroimaging Research Program
Associate Professor of Psychiatry,
 Harvard Medical School
Boston, MA, USA
*Ch 55 Life-threatening Conditions in
 Psychiatry: Catatonia, Neuroleptic
 Malignant Syndrome, and Serotonin
 Syndrome*

David C. Buxton, MD
Fellow in Child and Adolescent
 Psychiatry
Massachusetts General Hospital and
 McLean Hospital and Harvard
 Medical School
Boston, MA, USA
*Ch 69 Child and Adolescent Psychiatric
 Disorders*

Amanda W. Calkins, PhD
Center for Anxiety and Traumatic Stress
 Disorders,
Massachusetts General Hospital/
 Harvard Medical School,
Boston, MA, USA
Ch 32 Anxiety Disorders

Joan A. Camprodon, MD, MPH, PhD
Director, Laboratory for
 Neuropsychiatry and
 Neuromodulation
Director, Transcranial Magnetic
 Stimulation Clinical Service
Massachusetts General Hospital
Instructor of Psychiatry
Harvard Medical School
Boston, MA
*Ch 40 Psychiatric Neuroscience:
 Incorporating Pathophysiology into
 Clinical Case Formulation*
Ch 46 Neurotherapeutics
*Ch 72 Neuroanatomical Systems Relevant
 to Neuropsychiatric Disorders*

Jason P. Caplan, MD
Chair, Department of Psychiatry
Associate Professor of Psychiatry
Creighton University School of
 Medicine at St. Joseph's Hospital and
 Medical Center
Phoenix, AZ, USA
Ch 18 Delirium

Christopher Carter, PsyD
Director, Behavioral Medicine
Spaulding Rehabilitation Hospital
Clinical Assistant in Psychology
Clinical Psychologist
Massachusetts General Hospital
Clinical Instructor, Department of
 Psychology
Harvard Medical School
Boston, MA, USA
*Ch 82 Psychiatric Manifestations of
 Traumatic Brain Disorder*

Paolo Cassano, MD, PhD
Depression Clinical and Research
 Program (DCRP)
Massachusetts General Hospital
Instructor in Psychiatry
Harvard Medical School
Boston, MA, USA
*Ch 29 Mood Disorders: Depressive
 Disorders (Major Depressive Disorder)*

Ned H. Cassem, MA, PhL, MD, SJ, BD
Senior Psychiatrist (Retired)
Massachusetts General Hospital
Professor Emeritus of Psychiatry
Harvard Medical School
Boston, MA
Ch 18 Delirium
*Ch 60, Psychiatric and Ethical Aspects of
 Care at the End of Life*

Trina E. Chang, MD, MPH
Director of Community-Based Studies
Depression Clinical and Research
 Program
Massachusetts General Hospital
Instructor in, Department of Psychiatry
Harvard Medical School
Boston, MA , USA
Ch 61 Psychiatric Epidemiology

Marni Chanoff, MD
Clinical Associate
McLean Hospital
Instructor in Psychiatry
Harvard Medical School
Boston, MA, USA
Ch 14 Group Psychotherapy
Ch 91 Disaster Psychiatry

Lee S. Cohen, MD
Director, Center for Women's Mental
 Health
Perinatal and Reproductive Psychiatry
 Clinical Research Program
Massachusetts General Hospital
Professor of Psychiatry
Harvard Medical School
Boston, MA, USA
*Ch 31 Psychiatric Illness during Pregnancy
 and the Postpartum Period*

M. Cornelia Cremens, MD, MPH
Director, Inpatient Geriatric Psychiatry
Massachusetts General Hospital
Assistant Professor, Department of
Psychiatry
Harvard Medical School
Boston, MA, USA
Ch 71 Geriatric Psychiatry

Sharon Dekel, PhD
Research, Department of Psychiatry
Massachusetts General Hospital and
Harvard Medical School
Boston, MA, USA
*Ch 34 Trauma and Posttraumatic Stress
Disorder*

Hannah Delong, BA
Research Coordinator
Massachusetts General Hospital
Boston, MA, USA
*Ch 41 The Pharmacotherapy of Anxiety
Disorders*

Jennifer L. Derenne, MD
Clinical Associate Professor of
Psychiatry and Behavioral Sciences
Division of Child and Adolescent
Psychiatry
Stanford University School of Medicine
Stanford, CA, USA
*Ch 37 Eating Disorders: Evaluation and
Management*

Bradford C. Dickerson, MD, MMSc
Co-Director, Neuroimaging Group
Gerontology Research Unit
Department of Psychiatry
Clinical Director, Morphometry Service
Department of Neurology
Staff Behavioral Neurologist, Memory
Disorders Unit
Alzheimer's Disease Research Center
Department of Neurology
Massachusetts General Hospital
Assistant Professor, Department of
Neurology
Harvard Medical School
Boston, MA, USA
*Ch 72 Neuroanatomical Systems Relevant
to Neuropsychiatric Disorders*

Abigail L. Donovan, MD
Department of Child and Adolescent
Psychiatry
Massachusetts General Hospital
Assistant Professor of Psychiatry
Harvard Medical School
Boston, MA, USA
*Ch 17 The DSM-5: A System for
Psychiatric Diagnosis*
*Ch 92 Coping with the Rigors of
Psychiatric Practice*

Darin D. Dougherty, MD, MSc
Director, Division of Neurotherapeutics
Massachusetts General Hospital
Associate Professor of Psychiatry
Harvard Medical School
Boston, MA, USA
*Ch 33 Obsessive-compulsive Disorder and
Obsessive-compulsive and Related
Disorders*
Ch 46 Neurotherapeutics
Ch 75 Neuroimaging in Psychiatry

Simon Ducharme MD, MSc
Sidney R. Baer Fellow in Behavioral
Neurology and Neuropsychiatry
Department of Neurology
McLean Hospital
Belmont, MA, USA
Research Fellow, Department of
Psychiatry and Neurology
Massachusetts General Hospital
Harvard Medical School
Boston, MA, USA
*Ch 74 Neuropsychiatric Principles and
Differential Diagnosis*

Daniel H. Ebert, MD, PhD
Assistant in Psychiatry
Massachusetts General Hospital
Instructor in Neurobiology
Harvard Medical School
Boston, MA, USA
Ch 63 Genetics and Psychiatry

Kamryn T. Eddy, PhD
Co-Director, Eating Disorders Clinical
and Research Program
Massachusetts General Hospital
Assistant Professor of Psychiatry
(Psychology)
Harvard Medical School
Boston, MA, USA
*Ch 37 Eating Disorders: Evaluation and
Management*

Judith G. Edersheim, JD, MD
Co-Director, Center for Law
Brain & Behavior
Massachusetts General Hospital
Assistant Clinical Professor of
Psychiatry
Harvard Medical School
Boston, MA, USA
*Ch 85 Legal and Ethical Issues in
Psychiatry I: Informed Consent,
Competency, Treatment Refusal, and
Civil Commitment*

A. Evan Eyler, MD, MPH
Associate Professor, Departments of
Psychiatry and Family Medicine
University of Vermont College of
Medicine
Burlington, VT, USA
Ch 89 Rehabilitation Psychiatry

William E. Falk, MD
Director, Geriatric Psychiatry
Department of Psychiatry
Massachusetts General Hospital
Assistant Professor in Psychiatry
Harvard Medical School
Boston, MA, USA
Ch 19 Dementia

Maurizio Fava, MD
Director, Clinical Research Program
Executive Vice-Chair, Department of
Psychiatry
Executive Director, Clinical Trials
Network and Institute
Massachusetts General Hospital
Slater Family Professor of Psychiatry,
Harvard Medical School
Boston, MA, USA
*Ch 6 Diagnostic Rating Scales and
Psychiatric Instruments*
*Ch 29 Mood Disorders: Depressive
Disorders (Major Depressive Disorder)*
Ch 43 Antidepressants
*Ch 44 Pharmacological Approaches to
Treatment-Resistant Depression*

Carlos Fernandez-Robles, MD
Associate Director, Center for Psychiatry
Oncology and Behavioral Sciences
Assistant Psychiatrist, The
Avery D. Weisman
MD, Psychiatry Consultation Service
Somatic Therapies Service
Massachusetts General Hospital
Instructor, Department of Psychiatry
Harvard Medical School
Boston, MA, USA
*Ch 56 Psycho-oncology: Psychiatric
Co-morbidities and Complications of
Cancer and Cancer Treatment*

Christine T. Finn, MD
Director, Psychiatry Residency Training
Program
Director, Crises and Consultation
Service
Assistant Professor of Psychiatry
Giesel School of Medicine at
Dartmouth
Lebanon, NH, USA
Ch 63 Genetics and Psychiatry

Anne K. Fishel, PhD
Director, Family and Couples Therapy
Program
Massachusetts General Hospital
Associate Clinical Professor of
Psychology
Harvard Medical School
Boston, MA, USA
Ch 12 Couples Therapy
Ch 13 Family Therapy

Alice W. Flaherty, MD, PhD
Neurologist, Massachusetts General
Hospital
Associate Professor of Neurology and
Psychiatry
Harvard Medical School
Boston, MA, USA
Ch 81 Movement Disorders

Oliver Freudenreich, MD
Medical Director, Massachusetts
General Hospital Schizophrenia
Program
Associate Professor of Psychiatry
Harvard Medical School
Boston, MA, USA
Ch 28 Psychosis and Schizophrenia
Ch 42 Antipsychotic Drugs
*Ch 57 Psychiatric Aspects of HIV Infection
and AIDS*
Ch 64 Serious Mental Illness

Gregory L. Fricchione, MD
Associate Chief of the Department of
Psychiatry
Massachusetts General Hospital
Director, Division of Psychiatry and
Medicine
Director, Benson-Henry Institute for
Mind Body Medicine
Director, Psychosomatic Medicine
Postdoctoral Fellowship
Senior Scientist, Pierce Division of
Global Psychiatry
Professor of Psychiatry
Harvard Medical School
Boston, MA, USA
*Ch 55 Life-threatening Conditions in
Psychiatry: Catatonia, Neuroleptic
Malignant Syndrome, and Serotonin
Syndrome*
Ch 66 Culture and Psychiatry
*Ch 94 Global Mental Health in the
Twenty-First Century*

Jennifer R. Gatchel, MD PhD
Chief Resident in Psychopharmacology
Massachusetts General Hospital and
McLean Hospital Adult Psychiatry
Residency Program,Harvard Medical
School
Boston, MA, USA
Ch 19 Dementia

Anna M. Georgiopoulos, MD
Department of Child and Adolescent
Psychiatry
Massachusetts General Hospital
Assistant Professor of Psychiatry, Part
Time
Harvard Medical School
Boston, MA, USA
*Ch 17 The DSM-5: A System for
Psychiatric Diagnosis*

Adrienne T. Gerken, MD
Resident in Psychiatry
Massachusetts General Hospital and
McLean Hospital
Clinical Fellow in Psychiatry
Harvard Medical School
Boston, MA, USA
Ch 65 Aggression and Violence

Ted Avi Gerstenblith MD
Fellow in Psychosomatic Medicine
Massachusetts General Hospital
Clinical Fellow in Psychiatry
Harvard Medical School
Massachusetts General Hospital
Boston, MA, USA
Ch 22 Sleep Disorders
Ch 24 Somatic Symptom and Disorders

Mark W. Gilbertson, PhD
Psychologist, Veterans Affairs Medical
Center
Manchester, NH, USA
Instructor in Psychology, Department of
Psychiatry
Brigham and Women's Hospital and
Harvard Medical School
Boston, MA, USA
*Ch 34 Trauma and Posttraumatic Stress
Disorder*

Donald C. Goff, MD
Director, Nathan Kline Institute for
Psychiatric Research
Vice Chair of Psychiatry
NYU Langone Medical Center
Marvin Stern Professor of Psychiatry
NYU School of Medicine
New York City, NY, USA
Ch 42 Antipsychotic Drugs

Christopher Gordon, MD
Assistant Psychiatrist
Massachusetts General Hospital
Medical Director and Senior Vice
President for Clinical Services
Advocates, Inc
Associate Clinical Professor of
Psychiatry
Harvard Medical School
Boston, MA, USA
Ch 1 The Doctor–Patient Relationship
Ch 2 The Psychiatric Interview

Cathleen M. Gould, MD
Residency Training Director
Department of Psychiatry
Rush University Medical Center
Assistant Professor of Psychiatry
Rush Medical College
Chicago, IL, USA
Ch 23 Impulse-Control Disorders

Donna B. Greenberg, MD
Psychiatrist, Center for Psychiatry
Oncology and Behavioral Sciences
Massachusetts General Hospital
Associate Professor of Psychiatry
Harvard Medical School
Boston, MA, USA
*Ch 56 Psycho-oncology: Psychiatric
Co-morbidities and Complications of
Cancer and Cancer Treatment*

**David M. Greer, MD, MA, FCCM,
FAHA, FNCS, FAAN**
Professor of Neurology and
Neurosurgery
Vice Chairman of Neurology
Yale University School of Medicine
New Haven, CT, USA
*Ch 80 Psychiatric Aspects of Stroke
Syndromes*

Anne F. Gross MD
Assistant Professor of Psychiatry
Associate Residency Training Director
Oregon Health & Science University
Portland, Oregon, USA
Ch 65 Aggression and Violence

James E. Groves, MD
Psychiatry Service
Massachusetts General Hospital
Associate Clinical Professor of
Psychiatry
Harvard Medical School
Boston, MA, USA
*Ch 9 Coping with Medical Illness and
Psychotherapy of the Medically Ill*
Ch 11 Brief Psychotherapy: An Overview
*Ch 39 Personality and Personality
Disorders*

Eric P. Hazen, MD
Director, Child and Adolescent
Psychiatry Consultation-Liaison
Service
Massachusetts General Hospital
Associate Training Director
Massachusetts General Hospital/McLean
Child and Adolescent Psychiatry
Program
Instructor in Psychiatry
Harvard Medical School
Boston, MA, USA
*Ch 05 Child, Adolescent, and Adult
Development*

Sean P. Heffernan, MD
Alexander Wilson Schweizer Fellow
Department of Psychiatry and
Behavioral Sciences
Johns Hopkins Hospital
Johns Hopkins University School of
Medicine
Baltimore, MD, USA
*Ch 80 Psychiatric Aspects of Stroke
Syndromes*

David C. Henderson, MD
Director, Schizophrenia Clinical and
   Research Program
Director, Chester M. Pierce, M.D.
   Division of Global Psychiatry
Associate Professor of Psychiatry
Massachusetts General Hospital
Harvard Medical School
Boston, MA, USA
Ch 42 Antipsychotic Drugs
Ch 66 Culture and Psychiatry
*Ch 94 Global Mental Health in the
   Twenty-First Century*

John B. Herman, MD
Associate Chief of Psychiatry
Massachusetts General Hospital
Associate Professor of Psychiatry
Harvard Medical School
Boston, MA, USA
Ch 4 Treatment Adherence

José A. Hidalgo, MD
Psychiatrist at the Law and Psychiatry
   Service
Massachusetts General Hospital
Instructor of Psychiatry, Harvard
   Medical School
Boston, MA, USA
*Ch 85 Legal and Ethical Issues in
   Psychiatry I: Informed Consent,
   Competency, Treatment Refusal, and
   Civil Commitment*

John P. Hirdes, PhD
Professor, School of Public Health and
   Health Systems
University of Waterloo
Waterloo, Ontario, Canada
Ch 89 Rehabilitation Psychiatry

Charlotte Hogan, MD
Resident in Psychiatry
Massachusetts General Hospital and
   McLean Hospital
Clinical Fellow, Department of
   Psychiatry
Harvard Medical School
Boston, MA, USA
*Ch 3 Laboratory Tests and Diagnostic
   Procedures*

Daphne J. Holt, MD, PhD,
Director of Research
Massachusetts General Hospital
   Schizophrenia Program
Assistant Professor of Psychiatry
Harvard Medical School
Boston, MA, USA
Ch 28 Psychosis and Schizophrenia
*Ch 72 Neuroanatomical Systems Relevant
   to Neuropsychiatric Disorders*

Christopher J. Hopwood, PhD
Associate Professor of Clinical
   Psychology
Michigan State University
East Lansing, MI, USA
*Ch 39 Personality and Personality
   Disorders*

Honor Hsin, MD, PhD
Resident in Psychiatry
Department of Psychiatry and
   Behavioral Sciences
Stanford University School of Medicine
Stanford, CA, USA
*Ch 48 The Use of Antiepileptic Drugs in
   Psychiatry*

Jeff C. Huffman, MD
Director, Cardiac Psych Inpatient
   Program, MGH
Medical Director, Inpatient Psychiatry
Massachusetts General Hospital
Associate Professor of Psychiatry,
   Harvard Medical School
Boston, MA, USA
*Ch 51 Side Effects of Psychotropic
   Medications*
*Ch 55 Life-threatening Conditions in
   Psychiatry: Catatonia, Neuroleptic
   Malignant Syndrome, and Serotonin
   Syndrome*
*Ch 80 Psychiatric Aspects of Stroke
   Syndromes*

Lucy A. Epstein Hutner, MD
Associate Director, Psychiatry Residency
   Training Program
Assistant Professor of Psychiatry
New York University School of
   Medicine
New York, NY, USA
*Ch 60 Psychiatric and Ethical Aspects of
   Care at the End of Life*
*Ch 80 Psychiatric Aspects of Stroke
   Syndromes*

Ana Ivkovic, MD
Assistant in Psychiatry
Massachusetts General Hospital
Instructor in Psychiatry
Harvard Medical School
Boston, MA, USA
Ch 81 Movement Disorders
Ch 88 Emergency Psychiatry

Michael A. Jenike, MD
Founder, OCD Program
Massachusetts General Hospital
Founder, OCD Institute
McLean Hospital
Professor of Psychiatry
Harvard Medical School
Boston, Massachusetts, USA
*Ch 33 Obsessive-compulsive Disorder and
   Obsessive-compulsive and Related
   Disorders*

John N. Julian, MD, MS
Assistant Child Psychiatrist
McLean Hospital
Belmont
Assistant Professor, Part-Time
Department of Psychiatry
Harvard Medical School
Boston, MA, USA
Ch 20 Intellectual Disability

Jesse M. Katon
Intern, Massachusetts General Hospital
Boston, MA, USA
*Ch 94 Global Mental Health in the
   Twenty-First Century*

Navneet Kaur, BS
Clinical Research Coordinator
Laboratory for Neuropsychiatry and
   Neuromodulation
Division of Neurotherapeutics
Massachusetts General Hospital
Boston, MA, USA
Ch 46 Neurotherapeutics

John F. Kelly, PhD
Program Director, Addiction Recovery
   Management Service
Massachusetts General Hospital
Elizabeth R. Spallin Associate Professor
   of Psychiatry in Addiction Medicine
Harvard Medical School
Boston, MA, USA
Ch 26 Alcohol-Related Disorders

Alex S. Keuroghlian, MD MSc
Clinical Fellow in Psychiatry
Massachusetts General Hospital
Harvard Medical School
Boston, MA, USA
Ch 15 Hypnosis

Nancy J. Keuthen, PhD
Director, Trichotillomania Program and
   Chief Psychologist
OCD and Related Disorders Program
Department of Psychiatry
Massachusetts General Hospital
Associate Professor
Department of Psychology (Psychiatry)
Harvard Medical School
Boston, MA, USA
*Ch 33 Obsessive-compulsive Disorder and
   Obsessive-compulsive and Related
   Disorders*

Shahram Khoshbin, MD
Neurologist, Brigham and Women's
   Hospital
Associate Professor of Neurology
Harvard Medical School
Boston, MA, USA
*Ch 76 Clinical Neurophysiology and
   Electroencephalography*
*Ch 77 Psychiatric Manifestations and
   Treatment of Seizure Disorders*

Gustavo Kinrys, MD
Associate Medical Director
Clinical Trials Network and
   Institute(CTNI)
Bipolar Clinic and Research Program
   (BCRP)
Massachusetts General Hospital
Assistant Professor of Psychiatry
Harvard Medical School
Boston, MA, USA
*Ch 41 The Pharmacotherapy of Anxiety
   Disorders*

Anne Klibanski, MD
Chief, Neuroendocrine Unit
Massachusetts General Hospital
Laurie Carrol Guthart Professor of
Medicine
Harvard Medical School
Boston, MA, USA
*Ch 37 Eating Disorders: Evaluation and
Management*

Nicholas Kontos, MD
Director of Transplantation Psychiatry
Massachusetts General Hospital
Co-Associate Director
Psychosomatic Medicine Fellowship
Program
Massachusetts General Hospital
Assistant Professor of Psychiatry
Harvard Medical School
Boston, MA, USA
Ch 24 Somatic Symptom Disorders
*Ch 54 Psychiatric Consultation to Medical
and Surgical Patients*

Lawrence Kutner, PhD
Executive Director
Jack Kent Cooke Foundation
Lansdowne, VA, USA
Ch 93 Psychiatry and the Media

Daniel Lafleur, MD
Child Psychiatry Clinician Scientist
Child and Youth Mental Health
Program
British Columbia Children's Hospital
Department of Psychiatry
University of British Columbia
Vancouver, Canada
*Ch 33 Obsessive-compulsive Disorder and
Obsessive-compulsive and Related
Disorders*

Isabel T. Lagomasino, MD, MSHS
Director, Adult Psychiatry Residency
Training Program
LAC + USC Medical Center
Assistant Professor, Department of
Psychiatry and Behavioral Sciences
University of Southern California
Keck School of Medicine
Los Angeles, CA, USA
Ch 53 The Suicidal Patient

Richard T. LeBeau, PhD
Department of Psychology
University of California
Los Angeles, CA, USA
Ch 32 Anxiety Disorders

Catherine Leveroni, PhD
Psychology Assessment Center
Massachusetts General Hospital
Assistant Professor of Psychiatry
Harvard Medical School
Boston, MA, USA
Ch 8 Neuropsychological Assessment

Guy Maytal, MD
Associate Director, Ambulatory
Psychiatry
Director, Primary Care Psychiatry &
Urgent Care Psychiatry
Massachusetts General Hospital
Instructor in Psychiatry
Harvard Medical School
Boston, MA, USA
*Ch 60 Psychiatric and Ethical Aspects of
Care at the End of Life*

Jeanne McKeon, EdD
Private Practice
Marblehead
Massachusetts, USA
Ch 12 Couples Therapy

Diane W. Mickley MD, FACP, FAED
Founder and Director, Wilkins Center
for Eating Disorders
Clinical Associate Professor,
Department of Psychiatry
Yale Medical School
Greenwich, CT, USA
*Ch 37 Eating Disorders: Evaluation and
Management*

Nada Milosavljevic, MD, JD
Director, School-Based Integrative
Health Program
Massachusetts General Hospital
Instructor, Psychiatry
Harvard Medical School
Boston, MA, USA
*Ch 84 Psychiatric Correlates and
Consequences of Abuse and Neglect*

David Mischoulon, MD, PhD
Director of Research, Depression
Clinical and Research Program
Department of Psychiatry
Massachusetts General Hospital
Associate Professor of Psychiatry
Harvard Medical School
Boston, MA, USA
*Ch 6 Diagnostic Rating Scales and
Psychiatric Instruments*
Ch 52 Natural Medications in Psychiatry

Richard F. Mollica MD, MAR
Director, Harvard Program in Refugee
Trauma
Massachusetts General Hospital
Professor, Department of Psychiatry
Harvard Medical School
Boston, MA, USA
*Ch 94 Global Mental Health in the
Twenty-First Century*

Anna C. Muriel, MD, MPH
Chief, Division of Pediatric
Psychosocial Oncology
Dana-Farber/ Children's Hospital
Cancer and Blood Disorders Center
Assistant Professor of Psychiatry
Harvard Medical School
Boston, MA, USA
*Ch 5 Child, Adolescent, and Adult
Development*

Evan D. Murray, MD
Assistant in Neurology
McLean Hospital
Belmont, MA, USA
Massachusetts General Hospital
Boston, MA, USA
Director, Traumatic Brain Injury Service
Manchester VA Medical Center
Manchester, New Hampshire, USA
Instructor in Neurology
Harvard Medical School
Boston, MA, USA
Ch 73 The Neurological Examination
*Ch 74 Neuropsychiatric Principles and
Differential Diagnosis*

**George B. Murray, BS, PhL, MS, MSc,
MD†**
Senior Psychiatrist (Retired)
Massachusetts General Hospital
Associate Professor Emeritus of
Psychiatry
Harvard Medical School
Boston, MA, USA
Ch 18 Delirium

Helen B. Murray, BA
Clinical Research Coordinator
Eating Disorders Clinical and Research
Program
Massachusetts General Hospital
Boston, MA, USA
*Ch 37 Eating Disorders: Evaluation and
Management*

Shamim H. Nejad, MD
Director, Adult Burns and Trauma
Psychiatry
Division of Psychiatry and Medicine
Psychiatry Consultation Service
Massachusetts General Hospital
Assistant Professor of Psychiatry
Harvard Medical School
Boston, MA, USA
*Ch 79 Pathophysiology, Psychiatric
Co-morbidity, and Treatment of Pain*
*Ch 80 Psychiatric Aspects of Stroke
Syndromes*

Stephen E. Nicolson, MD
Director, Adult Psychiatry Consultation
  Service
Vanderbilt University Medical Center
Assistant Professor of Psychiatry
Vanderbilt School of Medicine
Nashville, Tennessee, USA
*Ch 78 Differential Diagnosis and
  Treatment of Headaches*

Andrew A. Nierenberg, MD
Associate Director, Depression Clinical
  and Research Program
Director, Bipolar Clinic and Research
  Program
Director, Clinical Research Support
  Office
Massachusetts General Hospital
Professor of Psychiatry
Harvard Medical School
Boston, MA, USA
*Ch 44 Pharmacological Approaches to
  Treatment-Resistant Depression*

Ruta M. Nonacs, MD, PhD
Assistant Psychiatrist
Massachusetts General Hospital
Instructor, Department of Psychiatry
Harvard Medical School
Boston, MA, USA
*Ch 31 Psychiatric Illness during Pregnancy
  and the Postpartum Period*
Ch 35 Dissociative Disorders

Kevin M. O'Brien, EdD, MA
Director, Disaster Mental Health
  Services
District of Columbia
Department of Behavioral Health
Washington, DC, USA
Ch 91 Disaster Psychiatry

Sheila M. O'Keefe, EdD
Director of Psychology Training
Massachusetts General Hospital
Instructor, Department of Psychology
Harvard Medical School
Boston, MA, USA
*Ch 7 Understanding and Applying
  Psychological Assessment*

Bunmi O. Olatunji, PhD
Director of Clinical Training,
  Department of Psychology,
Vanderbilt University
Associate Professor of Psychology and
  Psychiatry
Vanderbilt University
Nashville, TN, USA
*Ch 16 Cognitive-Behavioral Therapy,
  Behavioral Therapy, and Cognitive
  Therapy*

Cheryl K. Olson, MPH, ScD
Independent Public Health Researcher
Reston, VA, USA
Ch 93 Psychiatry and the Media

Dost Öngür, MD, PhD
Chief
Psychotic Disorders Division
McLean Hospital
Belmont, MA, USA
Associate Professor of Psychiatry
Harvard Medical School
Boston, MA, USA
*Ch 72 Neuroanatomical Systems Relevant
  to Neuropsychiatric Disorders*

Claire E. Oppenheim, BS
Senior Clinical Research Coordinator
Schizophrenia Clinical and Research
  Program and The Chester M. Pierce
  MD Division of Global Psychiatry
Department of Psychiatry
Massachusetts General Hospital
Boston, MA, USA
*Ch 94 Global Mental Health in the
  Twenty-First Century*

Scott P. Orr, PhD
Associate Professor of Psychology,
  Department of Psychiatry
Massachusetts General Hospital and
  Harvard Medical School
Boston, MA, USA
*Ch 34 Trauma and Posttraumatic Stress
  Disorder*

Michael J. Ostacher, MD, MPH, MMSc
Associate Director, Bipolar Disorder and
  Depression Research Program,
VAPAHCS Director, MIRECC Fellowship
  Program,
VAPAHCS Associate Professor of
  Psychiatry,
Department of Psychiatry and
  Behavioral Sciences
Stanford University School of Medicine
Palo Alto, CA, USA
Ch 30 Bipolar Disorder
Ch 47 Lithium and Its Role in Psychiatry
*Ch 48 The Use of Antiepileptic Drugs in
  Psychiatry*

Søren Dinesen Østergaard, MD, PhD
Research Fellow, Depression Clinical
  and Research Program (DCRP)
Massachusetts General Hospital
Research Fellow in Psychiatry
Harvard Medical School
Boston, MA, USA
*Ch 29 Mood Disorders: Depressive
  Disorders (Major Depressive Disorder)*

Michael W. Otto, PhD
Professor, Department of Psychology
Boston University
Boston, MA, USA
*Ch 16 Cognitive-behavioral Therapy,
  Behavioral Therapy, and Cognitive
  Therapy*

George I. Papakostas, MD
Scientific Director
Clinical Trials Network and Institute
Massachusetts General Hospital
Associate Professor of Psychiatry
Harvard Medical School
Boston, MA, USA
Ch 43 Antidepressants

Roy H. Perlis, MD, MSc
Medical Director, Bipolar Clinic and
  Research Program
Massachusetts General Hospital
Associate Professor of Psychiatry
Harvard Medical School
Boston, Massachusetts, USA
Ch 30 Bipolar Disorder
Ch 47 Lithium and Its Role in Psychiatry
Ch 53 The Suicidal Patient

William F. Pirl, MD, MPH
Director, Center for Psychiatry
  Oncology and Behavioral Sciences
Massachusetts General Hospital
Associate Professor
Department of Psychiatry
Harvard Medical School
Boston, MA, USA
*Ch 56 Psycho-oncology: Psychiatric
  Co-morbidities and Complications of
  Cancer and Cancer Treatment*

Roger K. Pitman, MD
Professor of Psychiatry
Massachusetts General Hospital and
  Harvard Medical School
Boston, MA, USA
*Ch 34 Trauma and Posttraumatic Stress
  Disorder*

Mark H. Pollack, MD
Department of Psychiatry
Rush University Medical Center
  Chicago, IL, USA
Ch 32 Anxiety Disorders
*Ch 41 The Pharmacotherapy of Anxiety
  Disorders*

Lauren Norton Pollak, PhD
Psychology Assessment Center
Massachusetts General Hospital
Boston, MA, USA
Ch 8 Neuropsychological Assessment

Alicia D. Powell, MD
Assistant Medical Director
Vinfen Corporation
Cambridge, MA, USA
*Ch 38 Grief, Bereavement, and
  Adjustment Disorders*

Laura M. Prager, MD
Psychiatrist, Lung Transplant Team
Director, Child Psychiatry Emergency
    Consult Service
Massachusetts General Hospital
Assistant Professor of Psychiatry
Harvard Medical School
Boston, MA, USA
*Ch 58 Organ Transplantation: Pre-
    transplant Assessment and Post-
    transplant Management*
Ch 88 Emergency Psychiatry

Bruce H. Price, MD
Chief of Neurology
McLean Hospital
Belmont, MA, USA
Associate Professor of Neurology
Harvard Medical School
Boston, MA, USA
Ch 73 The Neurological Examination
*Ch 74 Neuropsychiatric Principles and
    Differential Diagnosis*

Jefferson B. Prince, MD
Director of Child Psychiatry
Massachusetts General for Children at
    North Shore Medical Center and Staff
    Pediatric Psychopharmacology Clinic
Massachusetts General Hospital
Instructor in Psychiatry
Harvard Medical School
Yawkey Center for Outpatient Care
Boston, MA, USA
*Ch 49 Pharmacotherapy of Attention-
    Deficit/Hyperactivity Disorder across the
    Life Span*
*Ch 69 Child and Adolescent Psychiatric
    Disorders*

John Querques, MD
Co-Associate Director, Psychosomatic
    Medicine Fellowship Program
Massachusetts General Hospital
Assistant Professor of Psychiatry,
    Harvard Medical School
Boston, MA, USA
*Ch 54 Psychiatric Consultation to Medical
    and Surgical Patients*
*Ch 57 Psychiatric Aspects of HIV Infection
    and AIDS*

Terry Rabinowitz, MD, DDS
Medical Director
Division of Consultation Psychiatry and
    Psychosomatic Medicine
Medical Director
Telemedicine
Fletcher Allen Health Care
Professor, Departments of Psychiatry
    and Family Medicine
University of Vermont College of
    Medicine
Burlington, VT, USA
Ch 89 Rehabilitation Psychiatry

Scott L. Rauch, MD
President and Psychiatrist in Chief
McLean Hospital
Belmont, MA, USA
Chair, Partners Psychiatry and Mental
    Health
Professor of Psychiatry
Harvard Medical School
Belmont, MA, USA
*Ch 34 Trauma and Posttraumatic Stress
    Disorder*
Ch 46 Neurotherapeutics
*Ch 72 Neuroanatomical Systems Relevant
    to Neuropsychiatric Disorders*
Ch 75 Neuroimaging in Psychiatry

Hannah E. Reese, PhD
Assistant Professor
Department of Psychology
Bowdoin College
Brunswick, ME, USA
*Ch 16 Cognitive-behavioral Therapy,
    Behavioral Therapy, and Cognitive
    Therapy*

John A. Renner, Jr., MD
Associate Professor
Department of Psychiatry
Boston University School of Medicine
Clinical Instructor
Department of Psychiatry
Harvard Medical School
Associate Chief
Department of Psychiatry
Boston VA Healthcare System
Boston, Massachusetts, USA
Ch 26 Alcohol-Related Disorders
Ch 27 Drug Addiction

**Elspeth Cameron Ritchie, MD, MPH,
COL (Ret)**
Chief Medical Officer
District of Columbia
Department of Behavioral Health
Washington, DC, USA
Ch 91 Disaster Psychiatry

Rafael A. Rivas-Vazquez, PsyD, ABPP
Adjunct Associate Professor
Department of Psychology University of
    Miami
Miami, Florida, USA
*Ch 39 Personality and Personality
    Disorders*

Joshua L. Roffman, MD, MMSc
Department of Psychiatry
Massachusetts General Hospital
Assistant Professor of Psychiatry
Harvard Medical School
Boston, MA, USA
*Ch 06 Diagnostic Rating Scales and
    Psychiatric Instruments*
*Ch 40 Psychiatric Neuroscience:
    Incorporating Pathophysiology into
    Clinical Case Formulation*

Jerrold F. Rosenbaum, MD
Chief, Psychiatry Service,
Massachusetts General Hospital
Stanley Cobb Professor of Psychiatry
Harvard Medical School
Boston, MA, USA
*Ch 70 Psychiatric and Substance Use
    Disorders in Transitioning Adolescents
    and Young Adults*

Elizabeth Rosenfield, BA
Research Coordinator, Department of
    Psychiatry
Massachusetts General Hospital
Boston, MA, USA
*Ch 16 Cognitive-behavioral Therapy,
    Behavioral Therapy, and Cognitive
    Therapy*

J. Niels Rosenquist, MD, PhD
Assistant in Psychiatry
Massachusetts General Hospital
Instructor in Psychiatry
Harvard Medical School
Boston, MA, USA
Ch 68 Managed Care and Psychiatry

David Harris Rubin, MD
Director of Child and Adolescent
    Psychiatry
Residency Training
Massachusetts General Hospital and
    McLean Hospital
Associate Director
MGH Psychiatry Academy
Lecturer in Psychiatry
Harvard Medical School
Boston, MA, USA
Ch 13 Family Therapy

James R. Rundell, MD
Medical Director
Mental Health Homeless Programs
Minneapolis Veterans Administration
Health Care System
Professor of Psychiatry
University of Minnesota
Minneapolis, MN, USA
Ch 90 Military Psychiatry

Kathy M. Sanders, MD
State Medical Director
Deputy Commissioner, Clinical &
    Professional Services
Department of Mental Health
Commonwealth of Massachusetts
Assistant Professor of Psychiatry
Harvard Medical School
Boston, MA, USA
Ch 23 Impulse-Control Disorders
Ch 65 Aggression and Violence

Steven C. Schlozman, MD
Co-Director, Medical Student Education in Psychiatry
Harvard Medical School Staff Psychiatrist
Massachusetts General Hospital,
Assistant Professor of Psychiatry
Harvard Medical School
Boston, MA, USA
Ch 9 Coping with Medical Illness and Psychotherapy of the Medically Ill
Ch 10 An Overview of the Psychotherapies
Ch 35 Dissociative Disorders

Ronald Schouten, MD, JD
Director, Law & Psychiatry Service
Massachusetts General Hospital
Associate Professor of Psychiatry
Harvard Medical School
Boston, MA, USA
Ch 85 Legal and Ethical Issues in Psychiatry I: Informed Consent, Competency, Treatment Refusal, and Civil Commitment
Ch 86, The Role of Psychiatrists in the Criminal Justice System
Ch 87 Legal and Ethical Issues in Psychiatry II: Malpractice and Boundary Violations

Linda C. Shafer, MD
Psychiatrist
Massachusetts General Hospital
Wang Ambulatory Care Center
Assistant Professor of Psychiatry
Harvard Medical School
Boston, MA , USA
Ch 36 Sexual Disorders and Sexual Dysfunction

Janet Cohen Sherman, PhD,
Psychology Assessment Center
Massachusetts General Hospital
Assistant Professor of Psychiatry
Harvard Medical School
Boston, MA, USA
Ch 8 Neuropsychological Assessment

Derri Shtasel, MD, MPH
Director, Division of Public and Community Psychiatry
Massachusetts General Hospital
Associate Professor of Psychiatry
Harvard Medical School
Boston, MA, USA
Ch 64 Serious Mental Illness

Naomi M. Simon, MD, MSc
Center for Anxiety and Traumatic Stress Disorders
Massachusetts General Hospital
Chief Medical Officer
Red Sox Foundation and MGH Home Base Program
Associate Professor of Psychiatry, Harvard Medical School Director
Boston, MA, USA
Ch 32 Anxiety Disorders
Ch 41 The Pharmacotherapy of Anxiety Disorders

Samuel Justin Sinclair, PhD
Director of Research, Psychological Evaluation and Research Laboratory (The PEaRL)
Massachusetts General Hospital
Boston, MA, USA
Ch 7 Understanding and Applying Psychological Assessment

Patrick Smallwood, MD
Medical Director
Psychosomatic Medicine
Medical Director
Emergency Mental Health Services
University of Massachusetts Medical Center
Assistant Professor, Department of Psychiatry
University of Massachusetts Medical School
Worcester, MA, USA
Ch 39 Personality and Personality Disorders

Felicia A. Smith, MD
Program Director, MGH/McLean Adult Psychiatry Residency
Associate Director, MGH Division of Psychiatry and Medicine
Assistant Professor of Psychiatry
Harvard Medical School, Boston, MA, USA
Ch 3 Laboratory Tests and Diagnostic Procedures
Ch 25 Factitious Disorders and Malingering
Ch 52 Natural Medications in Psychiatry

Jordan W. Smoller, MD, ScD
Director, Psychiatric Genetics and Associate Vice-Chair
Department of Psychiatry
Massachusetts General Hospital
Professor of Psychiatry
Harvard Medical School
Boston, MA, USA
Ch 63 Genetics and Psychiatry

Thomas J. Spencer, MD
Associate Director
Pediatric Psychopharmacology Clinic
Massachusetts General Hospital
Associate Professor of Psychiatry
Harvard Medical School
Boston, MA, USA
Ch 49 Pharmacotherapy of Attention-Deficit/Hyperactivity Disorder across the Life Span

Susan E. Sprich, PhD
Director, Cognitive-Behavioral Therapy Program
Massachusetts General Hospital
Assistant Professor of Psychology in the Department of Psychiatry
Harvard Medical School
Boston, MA, USA
Ch 16 Cognitive-behavioral Therapy, Behavioral Therapy, and Cognitive Therapy

John W. Stakes, MD
Massachusetts General Hospital
Physician Director
Senior Advisor
Network Development Massachusetts General Hospital
Instructor of Neurology, Harvard Medical School Neurologist
Boston, MA, USA
Ch 22 Sleep Disorders

Theodore A. Stern, MD
Chief, Avery D. Weisman Psychiatry Consultation Service
Director, Office for Clinical Careers
Massachusetts General Hospital
Boston, MA, USA
Ned H. Cassem Professor of Psychiatry in the Field of Psychosomatic Medicine/Consultation
Harvard Medical School
Boston, MA, USA
Ch 18 Delirium
Ch 51 Side Effects of Psychotropic Medications
Ch 53 The Suicidal Patient
Ch 55 Life-threatening Conditions in Psychiatry: Catatonia, Neuroleptic Malignant Syndrome, and Serotonin Syndrome
Ch 92 Coping with the Rigors of Psychiatric Practice

S. Evelyn Stewart, MD
Director, Pediatric OCD Program
Associate Professor of Psychiatry, University of British Columbia
Senior Clinician Scientist,
Child and Family Research Institute
Vancouver, BC, Canada
Ch 33 Obsessive-compulsive and Obsessive-compulsive and Related Disorders

Samantha Andrien Stewart MD
Attending Psychiatrist
Department of Consultation-Liaison Psychiatry
Bellevue Hospital
Associate Professor, Department of Clinical Psychiatry
Columbia University and New York University
New York, NY, USA
Ch 91 Disaster Psychiatry

Thomas D. Stewart, MD
Associate Clinical Professor, Department of Psychiatry
Yale University School of Medicine
New Haven, CT, USA
Ch 89 Rehabilitation Psychiatry

Owen S. Surman, MD
Psychiatrist, Massachusetts General Hospital
Associate Professor of Psychiatry
Harvard Medical School
Boston, MA, USA
Ch 15 Hypnosis

Kaloyan S. Tanev, MD
Director of Clinical Neuropsychiatry
    Research
Massachusetts General Hospital
Instructor in Psychiatry
Harvard Medical School
Boston, MA, USA
*Ch 82 Psychiatric Manifestations of
    Traumatic Brain Disorder*

Haythum O. Tayeb, MBChB, FRCP(C)
Assistant Professor and Consultant in
    Neurology, Neuropsychiatry, and
    Clinical Neurophysiology
Division of Neurology
Department of Medicine
Faculty of Medicine
Chief, Department of Medicine
Rabigh Faculty of Medicine
King Abdulaziz University, Saudi Arabia
*Ch 76 Clinical Neurophysiology and
    Electroencephalography*

Charles T. Taylor, PhD
Department of Psychiatry
University of California
San Diego, La Jolla, CA, USA
Ch 32 Anxiety Disorders

John B. Taylor, MD, MBA
Assistant Training Director, MGH/
    McLean Adult Psychiatry Residency
    Training Program
Attending Psychiatrist, Acute Psychiatry
    Service, Psychiatry Consultation
    Service, Transplant Psychiatry
Assistant in Psychiatry
Massachusetts General Hospital
Instructor in Psychiatry
Harvard Medical School
Boston, MA, USA
Ch 11 Brief Psychotherapy: An Overview
Ch 68 Managed Care and Psychiatry
*Ch 84 Psychiatric Correlates and
    Consequences of Abuse and Neglect*

Jennifer J. Thomas, PhD
Co-Director, Eating Disorders Clinical
    and Research Program
Massachusetts General Hospital
Assistant Professor of Psychiatry
    (Psychology)
Harvard Medical School
Boston, MA, USA
*Ch 37 Eating Disorders: Evaluation and
    Management*

Kathryn J. Tompkins, MD
Resident in Psychiatry
Psychiatry
Massachusetts General Hospital/McLean
    Hospital
Clinical Fellow in Psychiatry
Psychiatry
Harvard Medical School
Boston, MA, USA
*Ch 21 Mental Disorders Due to Another
    Medical Condition*

Lara Traeger, PhD
Psychologist
Massachusetts General Hospital
Assistant Professor in Psychiatry
Harvard Medical School
Boston, MA, USA
Ch 4 Treatment Adherence

Nhi-Ha Trinh, MD, MPH
Director of Multicultural Studies,
    Depression Clinical and Research
    Program
Massachusetts General Hospital
Assistant Professor in Psychiatry
Harvard Medical School
Boston, MA, USA
Ch 19 Dementia

**Kathleen Hubbs Ulman, PhD, CGP,
FAGPA**
Director, Center for Group
    Psychotherapy
Staff Psychologist, Women's Health
    Associates
Massachusetts General Hospital
Assistant Clinical Professor in
    Psychiatry (Psychology)
Harvard Medical School
Boston, MA, USA
Ch 14 Group Psychotherapy

Débora Vasconcelos e Sá, BA, MSc
Research Coordinator
Cambridge Hospital
Harvard Medical School
Cambridge, MA, USA
*Ch 41 The Pharmacotherapy of Anxiety
    Disorders*

Adele C. Viguera, MD
Assistant Professor, Department of
    Psychiatry
Cleveland Clinic Lerner College of
    Medicine
Cleveland Clinic Neurological Institute
Cleveland, OH, USA
*Ch 31: Psychiatric Illness during Pregnancy
    and the Postpartum Period*

Brenda Vincenzi, MD
Schizophrenia Clinical and Research
    Program
Massachusetts General Hospital
Boston, MA, USA
Ch 66 Culture and Psychiatry

Mark Viron, MD
Director of Training and Education
Massachusetts Mental Health Center
Instructor in Psychiatry
Harvard Medical School
Boston, MA, USA
Ch 64 Serious mental illness

Betty Wang, MD
Assistant in Psychiatry
Department of Psychiatry
Massachusetts General Hospital
Instructor in Psychiatry
Harvard Medical School
Boston, MA, USA
*Ch 31 Psychiatric Illness during Pregnancy
    and the Postpartum Period*

E. Nalan Ward, MD
Clinical Assistant in Psychiatry
Medical Director
West End Clinic
Outpatient Addiction Services
Massachusetts General Hospital
Instructor in Psychiatry
Harvard Medical School
Boston, MA, USA
Ch 27 Drug Addiction

Ajay D. Wasan, MD, MSc
Visiting Professor of Anesthesiology
    and Psychiatry
University of Pittsburgh
Vice Chair for Pain Medicine,
    Department of Anesthesiology
UPMC Pain Medicine
Pittsburgh, PA, USA
*Ch 79 Pathophysiology, Psychiatric
    Co-morbidity, and Treatment of Pain*

Jeffrey B. Weilburg, MD
Assistant Professor of Psychiatry
Harvard Medical School
Associate Psychiatrist Associate Medical
    Director Physician Organization
Massachusetts General Hospital
Boston, MA, USA
Ch 22 Sleep Disorders

Daniel Weisholtz, MD
Instructor in Neurology
Harvard Medical School
Associate Neurologist
Brigham & Women's Hospital
Boston, MA, USA
*Ch 77 Psychiatric Manifestations and
    Treatment of Seizure Disorders*

Anna R. Weissman, MD
Resident in Psychiatry
Massachusetts General Hospital and
    McLean Hospital
Boston, MA and Belmont, MA, USA
Clinical Fellow in Psychiatry
Harvard Medical School
Boston, MA, USA
Ch 23 Impulse-Control Disorders

Charles A. Welch, MD
Psychiatrist
McLean Hospital
Belmont, MA, USA
Assistant Professor of Psychiatry
Harvard Medical School
Boston, MA, USA
Ch 45 Electroconvulsive Therapy

Timothy E. Wilens, MD
Senior Staff in Child Psychiatry and
    Pediatric Psychopharmacology
Director of the Center for Addiction
    Medicine at Massachusetts General
    Hospital
Associate Professor of Psychiatry
Harvard Medical School
Boston, MA, USA
*Ch 49 Pharmacotherapy of Attention-
    Deficit/Hyperactivity Disorder across the
    Life Span*
*Ch 70 Psychiatric and Substance Use
    Disorders in Transitioning Adolescents
    and Young Adults*

Sabine Wilhelm, PhD
Director, OCD and Related Disorders
    Program
Massachusetts General Hospital
Chief of Psychology
Massachusetts General Hospital
Professor of Psychology in the
    Department of Psychiatry
Harvard Medical School
Boston, MA, USA
*Ch 16 Cognitive-behavioral Therapy,
    Behavioral Therapy, and Cognitive
    Therapy*
*Ch 33 Obsessive-compulsive and Obsessive-
    compulsive and Related Disorders*

Nellie E. Wood, BA
Research Assistant
Massachusetts General Hospital
Boston, MA, USA
*Ch 34 Trauma and Posttraumatic Stress
    Disorder*

Christopher I. Wright, MD, PhD
Associate Neurologist
Division of Behavioral and Cognitive
    Neurology
Department of Neurology
Brigham and Women's Hospital
Boston, MA, USA
Ch 19 Dementia
*Ch 72 Neuroanatomical Systems Relevant
    to Neuropsychiatric Disorders*

Gary H. Wynn, MD
Assistant Professor
Department of Psychiatry
Uniformed Services University
Bethesda, MD, USA
Ch 90 Military Psychiatry

Albert S. Yeung, MD, ScD
Director of Primary Care Research
Depression Clinical and Research
    Program
Massachusetts General Hospital
Associate Professor of Psychiatry
Harvard Medical School
Boston, MA, USA
Ch 61 Psychiatric Epidemiology
Ch 66 Culture and Psychiatry

Courtney Zulauf, BA
Staff in Pediatric Psychopharmacology
Child Psychiatry Service,
Massachusetts General Hospital
Boston, MA, USA
*Ch 70 Psychiatric and Substance Use
    Disorders in Transitioning Adolescents
    and Young Adults*

To life-long learners everywhere, to our families, and to the memory of Drs. Thomas P. Hackett, Edward Messner, Anne Alonso, and George B. Murray... extraordinary teachers, mentors, colleagues, and friends.

T.A.S.

M.F.

T.E.W.

J.F.R.

1

The Doctor–Patient Relationship

Christopher Gordon, MD, and Eugene V. Beresin, MD

KEY POINTS

Background
- The doctor–patient relationship is a key driver of clinical outcomes—both in promoting desired results and in avoiding calamities.

Clinical and Research Challenges
- Especially in psychiatry, the physician must understand and relate to the patient as a whole person, requiring both accurate diagnosis and formulation, blending biological, social, psychological, and spiritual perspectives.

History
- Conflict is an inevitable aspect of all important relationships, and, properly managed, it can deepen and strengthen them. In the doctor–patient relationship, conflict can arise from many sources, and can either derail the relationship or provide an opportunity to improve communication, alliance, and commitment.

Practical Pointers
- An effective doctor–patient relationship involves both parties in co-creating a working relationship that is reliable, effective, and durable.
- The doctor–patient relationship accomplishes good outcomes by promoting empowered, engaged, and active partnership with patients who feel heard and accurately understood by their physicians.
- Successful doctor–patient relationships require physicians to practice a welcoming stance, participatory decision-making, and mindfulness about both the patient's and the physician's inner life.

OVERVIEW

The doctor–patient relationship—despite all the pressures of managed care, bureaucratic intrusions, and other systemic complications—remains one of the most profound partnerships in the human experience; in it, one person reveals to another his or her innermost concerns, in hope of healing.[1,2] In this deeply intimate relationship, when we earn our patients' trust, we are privileged to learn about fears and worries that our patients may not have shared—or ever will share—with another living soul; they literally put their lives and well-being in our hands. For our part, we hope to bring to this relationship technical mastery of our craft, wisdom, experience, and humility as well as our commitment to stand by and with our patient—that is, not to be driven away by any

degree of pain, suffering, ugliness, or even death itself. We foreswear our own gratification, beyond our professional satisfaction and reward, to place our patients' interests above our own. Our relationship is a moral covenant.[3] We hope to co-create a healing relationship, in which our patients can come to understand with us the sources of suffering and the options for care and healing, and partner with us in the construction of a path toward recovery.

In clinical medicine, the relationship between doctor and patient is not merely a vehicle through which to deliver care. Rather, it is one of the most important aspects of care itself. Excellent clinical outcomes—in which patients report high degrees of satisfaction, work effectively with their physicians, adhere to treatment regimens, experience improvements in the conditions of concern to them, and proactively manage their lives to promote health and wellness—are far more likely to arise from relationships with doctors that are collaborative, and in which patients feel heard, understood, respected, and included in treatment planning.[4–6] On the other hand, poor outcomes—including "non-compliance" with treatment plans, complaints to oversight boards, and malpractice actions—tend to arise when patients feel unheard, disrespected, or otherwise out of partnership with their doctors.[7–9] Collaborative care not only leads to better outcomes, but it is also more efficient than non-collaborative care in achieving good outcomes.[10,11] The relationship matters.

An effective doctor–patient relationship may be more critical to successful outcomes in psychiatry (because of the blurred boundaries between the conditions from which patients suffer and the sense of personhood of the patients themselves) than it is in other medical specialties. In psychiatry, more than in most branches of medicine, there is a sense that when the patient is ill, there is something wrong with the person as a whole, rather than what the person "has" or suffers from a discrete condition. Our language aggravates this sense of personal defectiveness or deficiency in psychiatric illness. We tend to speak of "being depressed," "I am bipolar," or "he is schizophrenic," as if these were qualities of the whole person rather than a condition to be dealt with. Even more hurtfully, we sometimes speak of people as "borderlines," or "schizophrenics," as if these labels summed up the person as a whole. This language, together with the persistent stigma attached to mental illness in our culture, amplifies the wary sense of risk of shame and humiliation that patients may experience in any doctor–patient interaction,[12] and makes it even more imperative that the physician work to create conditions of safety in the relationship.

Moreover, if we seek to co-create a healing environment in which the patient feels deeply understood (as a basis for constructing a path toward recovery), psychiatry, more than perhaps any branch of medicine, requires us to attend thoughtfully to the whole person, even to parts of the person's life that may seem remote from the person's areas of primary concern. So many psychiatric conditions from which people suffer have, in addition to important biological aspects, critically important contributions from the person's current relationships and social environment, from psychological issues from the past, and from the person's spiritual life and orientation. Much of the time, these psychological, social, or spiritual aspects of the person shed vitally important light on the nature of the person's distress, and are often crucial allies in recovery. There must be time and space in the doctor–patient relationship to know the whole person.[13] An appreciation of the person from the perspective of the person's biological ailments and vulnerabilities; the person's social connections, supports, and stressors in current time; the person's psychological issues from the past; and how the person spiritually makes sense of a life lived with the foreknowledge of death—these four models can give us a sense of the person in depth.[14]

THE OPTIMAL HEALING ENVIRONMENT: PATIENT-CENTERED CARE

Although there may be cultural factors that limit the validity of this generalization, in the main, patients strongly prefer care that centers on their own concerns; addresses their perspective on these concerns; uses language that is straightforward, is inclusive, and promotes collaboration; and respects the patient as a fully empowered partner in decision-making.[15] This model of care may be well denoted by the term *patient-centered care*[10,16] or, even better, *relationship-centered care*. In *Crossing the Quality Chasm*, the Institute of Medicine identified person-centered practice as a key to achieving high-quality care that focuses on the unique perspective, needs, values, and preferences of the individual patient.[17] Person-centered care involves a collaborative relationship in which two experts—the practitioner and the patient—attempt to blend the practitioner's knowledge and experience with the patient's unique perspective, needs, and assessment of outcome.[18]

In person-centered care, the patient's preferences and values are integral to every clinical decision, and outcomes are increasingly defined not only by evidence-based, disease-centered metrics alone, but by patient-reported and patient-defined functional outcomes.[19] One struggle for physicians is to balance the pressures to remain within the treatment path of evidence-based practice while accomplishing truly individualized care, based on the patient's perspective and values—the "quintessential skill" of modern medicine.[20]

This shift from paternalism to collaboration can be particularly challenging in situations in which the patient's competence is in question. But even in situations in which the patient is incompetent, every effort should still be made to honor the person's preferences and values, and to involve the person maximally in whatever way the patient can exercise choice.

The shift to patient-centered care in part may have been fueled by the women's movement,[21] as women have found their voice and awakened the culture to the reality of disempowering people and oppressing people through tyrannies of role and language. Moreover, the women's movement resulted in a paradigmatic shift in the healing professions, in which the perspectives of both parties have an equal claim on legitimacy and importance, and in which the relationship itself has a deep and pressing value for the outcome of any enterprise. The rise of consumerism and the wide dissemination of information on the Internet have also contributed to an emergence of more empowered patients as consumers.[21] Rapid shifts in insurance plans, have led patients to change from one practitioner to another with greater frequency, reinforcing the "informed shopper" approach to "patienthood." As Lazare and colleagues[22] presciently noted more than 30 years ago, patients increasingly view themselves as customers, and seek value, which is always in the eye of the beholder.

Quill and Brody[18] described a model of doctor–patient interaction that they termed *enhanced autonomy*. It described a relationship in which the patient's autonomous right to make critical decisions regarding his or her own care was augmented by the physician's full engagement in dialogue about these decisions (including the physician's input, recommendations, and open acknowledgment of bias, if present). Quill and Brody[18] pointed out that in purely autonomous decision-making, which they denoted as the "independent choice" model, there is a sort of perversion of patient-centeredness, in which the patient is essentially abandoned to make critical decisions without the benefit of the physician's counsel. In this model, physicians see their role as providing information, options of treatment, and odds of success; answering questions objectively; and eschewing recommendations (so as not to bias the patient or family).

In relationship-centered practice, more than patient-centered practice, the physician does not cede decision-making authority or responsibility to the patient and family, but rather enters into real dialogue about what the physician thinks is best and what the patient's and family's concerns and preferences are. Most patients and families seek a valued doctor's answer to the question (stated or not), "What would you do if this were your family member?" This transparent and candid collaboration shares power rather than cedes it, and conveys respect and concern. Enhanced autonomy involves a commitment to know the patient deeply, and to respect the patient's wishes; to share information as openly and as honestly as the patient desires; to involve others at the patient's direction; and to treat the patient as a full partner to the greatest extent possible.

In patient-centered care, the physician works to avoid inadvertently hurting, shaming, or humiliating the patient through careless use of language or other slights. When such hurt or other error occurs, the practitioner apologizes clearly and in a heartfelt way to restore the relationship.[23]

The role of the physician in patient-centered care is one of an expert who seeks to help a patient co-manage his or her health to whatever extent is most aligned with the perspective of that particular person. The role is not to cede all important decisions to the patient, whether he or she wants to participate in these decisions or not.[18]

Patient-centered care involves six processes. First, the physician endeavors to create conditions of welcome, respect, and safety, so that the patient can reveal his or her concerns and perspective. Second, the physician works to understand the patient deeply, as a whole person, listening to both the words and the "music" of what is communicated. Third, the physician confirms and demonstrates his or her understanding through direct, non-jargonistic language to the patient. Fourth, if the physician successfully establishes common ground on the nature of the problem as the patient perceives it, an attempt is made to synthesize these problems into workable diagnoses and problem lists. Fifth, using expertise, technical mastery, and experience, a path is envisioned toward healing, developed with the patient. Finally, together, the physician and patient can then negotiate about which path makes the most sense for this particular patient.

Through all of this work, the physician models and cultivates a relationship that values candor, collaboration, and authenticity; it should be able to withstand conflict—even welcoming conflict as a healthy part of human relationships.[24] In so doing, the physician–patient partnership forges a relationship that can stand the vicissitudes of the patient's illness, its treatment, and conflict as it arises in the relationship itself. In this way, the health of the physician–patient relationship takes its place as an important element on every problem list, to be actively monitored and nurtured as time passes.

Physician Practice in Patient-Centered Care

Physicians' qualities have an impact on the doctor–patient relationship. These qualities support and enhance—but are not a substitute for—technical competence and cognitive mastery. Perhaps most important is a quality of *mindfulness,*[25] a quality described by Messner[26] as one acquired through a process of constant *autognosis,* or self-awareness. Mindfulness appreciates that a person's emotional life (i.e., of both the physician and the patient) has meaning and importance and it deserves our respect and attention. Mindfulness connotes a commitment to respectful monitoring of one's own feelings, as well as to the feelings of the patient, and acceptance of feelings in both parties without judgment and with the knowledge that feelings are separate from acts.

Mindfulness, which springs from roots in Buddhism,[27] has offered much wisdom to the practice of psychotherapy (e.g., helping patients tolerate unbearable emotions without action, and helping clinicians tolerate the sometimes hideous histories their patients share with them).[28] Mindfulness helps physicians find a calm place from which to build patient relationships.[29] Mindfulness counsels us to attend to our feelings with acceptance and compassion and to those of our patients, without a compulsion to act on these feelings. Thus, the physician can be informed by the wealth of his or her inner emotional life, without being driven to act on these emotions; this can serve as a model for the relationship with the patient.

Other personal qualities in the physician that promote healthy and vibrant relationships with patients include humility, genuineness, optimism, a belief in the value of living a full life, good humor, candor, and transparency in communication.[30]

Important communication skills include the ability to elicit the patient's perspective; help the patient feel understood; explain conditions and options in clear, non-technical language; generate input and consensus about paths forward in care; acknowledge difficulty in the relationship without aggravating it; welcome input and even conflict; and work through difficulty, to mutually acceptable, win–win solutions.[31]

Practical considerations in physicians' practice include clarity on the part of the physician and the patient on mutual roles, expectations, boundaries, limitations, and contingencies (e.g., how to reach the physician or his or her coverage after hours and under what conditions, and the consequences of missed appointments).[32,33]

One of the most important ingredients of successful doctor–patient relationships (that is in terribly short supply) is time.[34] There is simply no substitute or quick alternative to sitting with a person and taking the time to get to know that person in depth, and in a private setting free from intrusions and interruptions. To physicians who practice in high-volume clinics, with beepers beeping, phones ringing, and patients scheduled every few minutes, this may seem an impossible task. However, most physicians know that what we want when we or a loved one is ill is the full and undivided attention of our doctor; patients in this regard are no different than physicians.

COLLABORATING AROUND HISTORY-TAKING

One major goal of an initial interview is to generate a database that will support a comprehensive differential diagnosis. However, there are other over-arching goals. These include demystifying and explaining the process of collaboration, finding out what is troubling and challenging the patient, co-creating a treatment path to address these problems, understanding the person as a whole, encouraging the patient's participation, welcoming feedback, and modeling a mindful appreciation of the complexity of human beings (including our inner emotional life).[35,36] At the end of the history-taking—or to use more collaborative language, after *building* a history with the patient[37]—a conversation should be feasible about paths toward healing and the patient's and doctor's mutual roles in that process (in which the patient feels heard, understood, confident in the outcome, and committed to the partnership).

Effective Clinical Interviewing

The overarching principles of effective clinical interviewing are friendliness, warmth, a capacity to help patients feel at ease in telling their stories, and an ability to engage the person in a mutual exploration of what is troubling him or her. We find that if we demystify the clinical encounter, by explaining what we are doing before we do it, and by making our thinking as transparent and collaborative as possible, we are more likely to achieve good interviews.[38] Similarly, by pausing often to ask the patient if we are understanding clearly, or seeking the patient's input and questions, we promote real conversation (rather than one-sided interrogation) that yields deeper information.[39]

We find that one useful technique is to offer to tell the patient what we know already about him or her. For example, "I wonder if it would be helpful if I told you what Dr. Smith mentioned to me when she called to refer you to me? That way, if I have any information wrong, you could straighten it out at the outset." This technique allows us to "show our cards" before we ask the patient to reveal information about himself or herself. Moreover, by inviting correction, we demonstrate right away that we honor the person's input. Last, this technique allows us to put the person's story in neighborly, non-pathological language, setting the stage for the interview to follow. For example, if the chart reveals that the person has been drinking excessively and may be depressed, we can say, "It looks like you have been having a hard time recently," leaving to the patient the opportunity to fill in details.[40]

Having opened the interview, we then try to be quiet and to make room for the person to tell his or her story, encouraging (with body language, open-ended questions, and other encouragement) the person to say more. We try to resist the temptation to jump too early to closed-ended symptom check-lists. We venture to listen deeply, to both the words and the music.

After a reasonable period of time, we summarize what we've heard, and check out whether or not we understand accurately what the patient is trying to say. Saying, "Let me see if I understand what you are saying so far," is a good way of moving to this part of the interview. In reflecting back to the patient our summary of what we have heard, it is important to use language carefully. Whenever possible, we avoid inflammatory or otherwise inadvertently hurtful language ("So, it sounds like you were hallucinating, and perhaps having other psychotic symptoms"), in favor of neighborly, neutral language ("Sounds like things were difficult—did I understand you to say you were hearing things that troubled you?"). Whenever possible, we use the exact words that the patient has used to describe his or her emotional state. For example, if the person says, "I have been feeling so tired, just so very, very tired—I feel like I have nothing left," and we say, "It sounds as if you have been exhausted," we may or may not convey to the person that we have understood them; but if we say, "You have been just so terribly tired," it is more likely that the person will feel understood.

One measure of rapport comes from getting the "nod"—that is, simply noticing if in the early stages of the interview, the patient is nodding at us in agreement and otherwise giving signs of understanding and of feeling understood.[38] If the "nod" is absent, it is a signal that something is amiss—either we have missed something important, have inadvertently offended the person, have failed to explain our process, or have otherwise derailed the relationship. A clinical interview without the "nod" is an interview in peril. Offering to say first what you know, putting the problem in neighborly language, and using the patient's own words are useful techniques for winning the "nod." Even more important is the power of simple kindness, friendliness, and neighborliness in our words, tone, and body language. Similarly, a simple apology if a person has been kept waiting, or a friendly acknowledgment of something in common ("Interesting—I grew up in Maryland, too!") can go a long, long way toward creating connection and rapport.

Having established a tone of collaboration, identified the problem, and been given the "nod," the next area of focus is the history of present illness. In eliciting the history of present illness, it is important to let the person tell his or her story. For many people, it is a deeply healing experience merely to be listened to in an empathic and attuned way.[40] We find it best to listen actively (by not interrupting and by not focusing solely on establishing the right diagnosis) and to make sure one is "getting it right" from the patient's point of view. When the physician hypothesizes that the patient's problem may be more likely to be in the psychological or interpersonal realm, it is especially important to give the patient a chance to share what is troubling him or her in an atmosphere of acceptance and empathy. For many people it is a rare and healing experience to be listened to attentively, particularly about a subject that may have been a source of private suffering for some time.

In taking the history of present illness, under the pressure of time, it can be an error to rely too quickly on symptom checklists or to ask a series of closed-ended questions to rule-in or rule-out a particular diagnosis (such as major depression). Doing this increases the risk of prematurely closing off important information that the patient might otherwise impart about the social or psychological aspects of the situation.

Having sketched in the main parameters of the person's history of the current issue, it may be wise to inquire about the last time the patient felt well with respect to this problem: the earliest symptoms recollected; associated stresses, illnesses, and changes in medications; attempts to solve the problem and their effects; and how the person elected to get help for the problem now. This may be a time to summarize, review, and request clarification.

As we move to different sections of the history, we consider explaining what we are doing and why: "I'd like now to ask some questions about your past psychiatric history, if any, to see if anything like this has happened before." This guided interviewing tends to demystify what you are doing and to elicit collaboration.[38]

The next area of focus is the past psychiatric history. The past psychiatric history can further illuminate the present illness. The interviewer should ascertain past episodes of similar or related suffering (e.g., past episodes of depression or periods of anxiety, how they were treated, and how the patient responded). The interview should establish past episodes of unrelated psychiatric illness (such as problems with anxiety, phobias, fears, and obsessions). These episodes may point the way to a diathesis toward affective or anxiety disorders that would otherwise be obscure. It may be useful to inquire about past periods of emotional difficulty as distinct from psychiatric illness *per se.*

The past medical history is a critical part of the database for every patient, regardless of the nature of the person's complaint or concern. The principal reason for this recalls the four-model method of conceptualizing psychiatric conditions.

By the end of the evaluation, it is critical that the physician be able to consider a differential diagnosis that includes hypotheses using all four models: biological, social, psychological, and spiritual. For the biological model, of course, the past medical history is essential.

If a history of substance abuse was not included in the past psychiatric history, it can be elicited here, including gross indices of abuse (such as history of detoxifications, attempts to cut down on substances, or specific substances of abuse), as well as more subtle questions, and possibly the use of structured inquiry, such as the CAGE questionnaire.[41]

The family psychiatric history can yield important clues about conditions that may have genetic significance (such as bipolar disorder, schizophrenia, mood disorders, anxiety disorders, and substance abuse). This is also a convenient time to establish a limited genogram, attending to birth order, and the current circumstances of family members.

The social and developmental history offers a rich opportunity for data-gathering in the social and psychological realms. Where the person grew up; what family life was like; how far the person advanced in school; what subjects the person preferred; and what hobbies and interests the person has, are all fertile lines of pursuit. Marital and relationship history, whether the person has been in love, whom the person admires most, and who has been most important in the person's life are even deeper probes into this aspect of the person's experience. A deep and rapid probe into a person's history can often be achieved by the simple question, "What was it like for you growing up in your family?" Spiritual orientation and practice (including whether the person ever had a spiritual practice, and if so, what happened to change it?) fit well into this section of the history.[42]

The formal mental status examination continues the line of inquiry that was begun in the history of present illness (i.e., the symptom checklists to rule-in or rule-out diagnostic possibilities and to ask more about detailed signs and symptoms to establish pertinent positives and negatives in the differential diagnosis).

An extremely important area, and one all too frequently given short shrift in diagnostic evaluations, is the area of the person's strengths and capabilities. As physicians, we are trained in the vast nosology of disease and pathology, and we admire the most learned physician as one who can detect the most subtle or obscure malady; indeed, these are important physicianly strengths. But there is, regrettably, no comparable nosology of strengths and capabilities. Yet, in the long road to recovery it is almost always the person's strengths on which the physician relies to make a partnership toward healing. It is vitally important that the physician note these strengths and let the person know that the physician sees them and appreciates them.[37]

Sometimes strengths are obvious (e.g., high intelligence in a young person with a first-break psychosis, or a committed and supportive family surrounding a person with recurrent depression). At other times, strengths are more subtle, or even counter-intuitive—for example, seeing that a woman who cuts herself repeatedly to distract herself from the agony of remembering past abuse has found a way to live with the unbearable; to some extent this is true, and this is a strength. Notable, too, may be her strength to survive, her faith to carry on, and other aspects of her life (e.g., a history of playing a musical instrument; a loving concern for children; a righteous rage to make justice in the world). Whatever the person's strengths, we must note them, acknowledge them, and remember them. An inability to find strengths and capacities to admire in a patient (alongside other attributes perhaps far, far less admirable) is almost always a sign of countertransference malice, and bears careful thought and analysis.

Finally, a clinical diagnostic interview should always include an opportunity for the patient to offer areas for discussion: "Are there areas of your life that we have not discussed that you think would be good for me to know about?" or "Are there things we have mentioned that you'd like to say more about?" or "Is there anything I haven't asked you about that I should have?"

PLANNING THE PATH FORWARD: CREATING A CLINICAL FORMULATION

Having heard the patient's story, the next challenge is to formulate an understanding of the person that can lead to a mutually-developed treatment path. A formulation is not the same thing as a diagnosis. A diagnosis describes a condition that can be reasonably delineated and described to the person and that implies a relatively foreseeable clinical course, and usually implies options of courses of treatment. As important as a diagnosis is in clinical medicine, a diagnosis alone is insufficient for effective treatment planning, and is an inadequate basis for work by the doctor–patient dyad.

In psychiatry, one method for creating a formulation is to consider each patient from a bio-socio-psycho-spiritual perspective, thinking about each patient from each of four perspectives.[14] The first of these is *biological:* Could the person's suffering be due, entirely or in part, to a biological condition of some sort (either from an acquired condition [such as hypothyroidism] or a genetic "chemical imbalance" [such as some forms of depression and bipolar disorder])? The second model is *social:* Is there something going on in the person's life that is contributing to his or her suffering, such as an abusive relationship, a stressful job, a sick child, or financial trouble? The third model is *psychological:* Although this model is more subtle, most patients will acknowledge that practically everyone has "baggage" from the past, and sometimes this baggage contributes to a person's difficulties in the present. The fourth model is *spiritual:* Although this model is not relevant for all people, sometimes it is very important. For people who at one point had faith but lost it, or for whom life feels empty and meaningless, conversation about the spiritual aspects of their suffering sometimes taps into important sources of difficulty and sometimes into resources for healing.[42]

These four models—biological "chemical imbalances," current social stressors, psychological baggage from the past, and spiritual issues—taken together provide an excellent framework for understanding most people. One of the beauties of this method is that these models are not particularly pathologizing or shame-inducing. On the contrary, they are normalizing, and emphasize that all of us are subject to these same challenges. This opens the way to collaboration.

Asking the patient whether these four models resonate with their experience, and, if they do, which ones shed light on the person's difficulties, can be a springboard to a collaborative conversation about treatment.

We also find it helpful to emphasize the very imperfect art and science of psychiatric diagnosis and prognosis—humbly acknowledging the limits of knowledge.[43] We find this tempers the sometimes stinging hurt of a stigmatized psychiatric diagnosis.

Whereas the biological, social, and spiritual models are fairly easy to conceptualize, the formulation of psychological issues can seem particularly daunting to physicians and to patients alike, since every person is dizzyingly complex. It can seem almost impossible to formulate a psychological perspective of a person's life that is neither simplistic and jargon-ridden, nor uselessly complex (and often jargon-ridden!). A useful method for making sense of the psychological aspects of the person's life is to consider whether there are recurrent patterns of difficulty, particularly in important relationships as the person looks back on his or her life.[14] To gather information to assess this model, most useful is information about the most important relationships in this person's life (in plain, non-technical terms—not only current important relationships, such as we need to assess current social function, but also who have been the most important people in the person's life over time). In this way, for example, it may become clear that the person experienced his relationship with his father as abusive and hurtful, and has not had a relationship with any other person in authority since then that has felt truly helpful and supportive. This in turn may shed light on the person's current work problems, and may illuminate some of the person's feelings of depression.

Underlying our inquiry regarding whether there may be significant recurrent patterns in the person's life that shed light on his or her current situation is the critical notion that these patterns almost always began as attempts to cope, and represent creative adaptations, or even strengths. Often these patterns—even when they involve self-injury or other clearly self-destructive behaviors—began as creative solutions to apparently insoluble problems. For example, self-injury may have represented a way of mastering unbearable feelings, and may have felt like a way of being in control, while remaining alive under unbearable circumstances. It is important that the doctor appreciate that most of the time these self-defeating behaviors began as solutions, and often continue to have adaptive value in the person's life. If we fail to appreciate the creative, adaptive side of the behavior, the person is likely to feel misunderstood, judged harshly, and possibly shamed.

Practically everyone finds the four models understandable and meaningful. Moreover, and importantly, these four models avoid language that overly pathologizes the person, and they use language that tends to universalize the patient's experience. This initial formulation can be a good platform for a more in-depth discussion of diagnostic possibilities. With this framework, the differential diagnosis can be addressed from a biological perspective, and acute social stressors can be acknowledged. The diagnosis and treatment can be framed in a manner consistent with the person's spiritual orientation. Fleshing out the psychological aspects can be more challenging, but this framework creates a way of addressing psychological patterns in a person's life and his or her interest in addressing them and their ability to address them.

TREATMENT PLANNING

Having a good formulation as a frame for a comprehensive differential diagnosis permits the doctor and the patient to look at treatment options (including different modalities, or even alternative therapies or solutions not based in traditional medicine). It is possible from this vantage point to look together at the risks and benefits of various approaches, as well as the demands of different approaches (the time and money invested in psychotherapy, for example, or the side effects that are expectable in many medication trials). The sequence of treatments, the location, the cost, and other parameters of care can all be made explicit and weighed together.

This approach also is effective in dealing with situations in which the physician's formulation and that of the patient differ, so that consultation and possibly mediation can be explored.[14] For example, the physician's formulation and differential diagnosis for a person might be that the person's heavy drinking constitutes alcohol abuse, or possibly dependence, and that cessation from drinking and the active pursuit of sobriety is a necessary part of the solution to the patient's chronic severe anxiety and depression. The patient, on the other hand, may feel that if the doctor were offering more effective treatment for his anxiety and depression, he would then be able to stop drinking. An explicit formulation enables the patient and the doctor to see where, and how, they disagree, and to explore alternatives. For example, in the case cited, the physician could offer to meet with family members with the patient, so both could get family input into the preferred solution; or the physician could offer the patient a referral for expert psychopharmacological consultation to test the patient's hypothesis.

In either case, however, the use of an explicit formulation in this way can identify problems and challenges early in the evaluation phase, and can help the physician avoid getting involved in a treatment under conditions likely to fail. Mutual expectations can be made clear (e.g., the patient must engage in a 12-step program, get a sponsor, and practice sobriety for the duration of the treatment together) and the disagreement can be used to forge a strong working relationship, or the physician and patient may agree not to work together.

The formulation and differential diagnosis are of course always in flux, as more information becomes available and the doctor and patient come to know each other more deeply. Part of the doctor's role is to welcome and nurture, to change, and to promote growth, so as to allow the relationship to grow as part of the process.[14]

OBSTACLES AND DIFFICULTIES IN THE DOCTOR–PATIENT RELATIONSHIP

Lazare and colleagues[22] pioneered the patient's perspective as a customer of the health care system. Lazare[12] subsequently addressed the importance of acknowledging the potential for shame and humiliation in the doctor–patient encounter, and, most recently, has written a profound treatise on the nature and power of true, heartfelt apology.[23] Throughout his work, Lazare has addressed the inevitable occurrence of conflict in the doctor–patient relationship (as in all important human relationships) and offered wise counsel for negotiating with the patient as a true partner to find creative solutions.[44]

Conflict and difficulty may arise from the very nature of the physician's training, language, or office environment. Physicians who use overly technical, arcane, or obtuse language distance themselves and make communication difficult. Similarly, physicians may lose sight of how intimidating, unintelligible, and forbidding medical practice—perhaps especially psychiatry—can appear to the uninitiated, unless proactive steps toward demystification occur. Similarly, over-reliance on "objective" measures, such as symptom checklists, questionnaires, tests, and other measurements, may speed diagnosis, but may alienate patients from effective collaboration. More insidious may be assumptions regarding the supposed incapacity of psychiatric patients to be full partners in their own care. Hurtful, dismissive language, or a lack of appreciation for the likelihood that a patient has previously experienced hurtful care, may damage the relationship.[15] Overly brief, symptom-focused interviews that fail to address the whole person, as well as his or her preferences, questions, and concerns, are inadequate foundations for an effective relationship.

Conflict may also arise from the nature of the problem to be addressed. In general, patients are interested in their illness—how they experience their symptoms, how their health can be restored, how to ameliorate their suffering—whereas physicians are often primarily concerned with making an accurate diagnosis of an underlying disease.[45] Moreover, physicians may erroneously believe that the patient's "chief complaint" is the one that the patient gives voice to first, whereas patients often approach their doctors warily, not leading with their main concern, which they may not voice at

all unless conditions of safety and trust are established.[46] Any inadvertent shaming of the patient makes the emergence of the real concern all the less likely.[12]

Physicians may misunderstand a patient's readiness to change and may assume that once a diagnosis or problem is identified, the patient is prepared to work to change it. In actuality, a patient may be unable or unwilling to acknowledge the problem that is obvious to the physician, or, even if able to acknowledge it, may not be prepared to take serious action to change it. Clarity about where the patient is in the cycle of change[47,48] can clarify such misunderstanding and help the physician direct his or her efforts at helping the patient become more ready to change, rather than fruitlessly urging change to which the patient is not committed. Similarly, physicians may underestimate social, psychological, or spiritual aspects of a person's suffering that complicate the person's willingness or ability to partner with the physician toward change. A deeply depressed patient, for example, whose sense of shame and worthlessness is so profound that the person feels that he or she does not deserve to recover, may be uncooperative with a treatment regimen until these ideas are examined in an accepting and supportive relationship.

Conflict may arise, too, over the goals of the work. Increasingly, mental health advocates and patients promote "recovery" as a desired outcome of treatment, even for severe psychiatric illness. Working toward recovery in schizophrenia or bipolar disorder, which most psychiatrists will regard as life-long conditions that require ongoing management, may seem unrealistic or even dishonest.[49]

It may be useful for physicians to be aware that the term *recovery* is often used in the mental health community to signify a state of being analogous to recovery from alcoholism or other substance abuse.[50] In this context, one is never construed to be a "recovered" alcoholic, but rather a "recovering" alcoholic—someone whose sobriety is solid, who understands his or her condition and vulnerabilities well, takes good care of himself or herself, and is ever alert to risks of relapse, to which the person is vulnerable for his or her entire life.

In a mental health context, "recovery" similarly connotes a process of reclaiming one's life, taking charge of one's options, and stepping out of the position of passivity and victimization that major mental illness can often involve, particularly if it involves involuntary treatment, stigmatization, or downright oppression. From this perspective, recovery means moving beyond symptomatic control of the disease to having a full life of one's own design (including work, friends, sexual relationships, recreation, political engagement, spiritual involvement, and other aspects of a full and challenging life).

Other sources of conflict in the doctor–patient relationship may include conflict over methods of treatment (a psychiatrist, perhaps, who emphasizes medication to treat depression to the exclusion of other areas of the patient's life, such as a troubled and depressing marriage), over the conditions of treatment (e.g., the frequency of appointment, length of appointment, or access to the physician after hours), or over the effectiveness of treatment (e.g., the psychiatrist believes that antipsychotic medications restore a patient's function, whereas the patient believes the same medications create a sense of being drugged and "not myself").[17]

In these examples, as in so many challenges on the journey of rendering care, an answer may lie not solely in the doctor's offered treatment, nor in the patient's "resistance" to change, but in the vitality, authenticity, and effectiveness of the relationship between them.

Access the complete reference list and multiple choice questions (MCQs) online at https://expertconsult.inkling.com

KEY REFERENCES

2. Neuberger J. Internal medicine in the 21st century: the educated patient: new challenges for the medical profession. *J Intern Med* 247:6–10, 2000.

3. Kleinman A. From illness as culture to caregiving as moral experience. *N Engl J Med* 368:1376–1377, 2013.

8. Forster HP, Schwartz J, DeRenzo E. Reducing legal risk by practicing patient-centered medicine. *Arch Intern Med* 162:1217–1219, 2002.

9. Gutheil TG, Bursztajn HJ, Brodsky A. Malpractice prevention through the sharing of uncertainty. Informed consent and the therapeutic alliance. *N Engl J Med* 311:49–51, 1984.

12. Lazare A. Shame and humiliation in the medical encounter. *Arch Intern Med* 147:1653–1658, 1987.

13. Charon R. Narrative medicine: a model for empathy, reflection, profession and trust. *JAMA* 286:1897–1902, 2001.

14. Gordon C, Riess H. The formulation as a collaborative conversation. *Harv Rev Psychiatry* 13:112–123, 2005.

16. Deegan PE, Drake RE. Shared decision making and medication management in the recovery process. *Psychiatr Serv* 57:1636–1638, 2006.

18. Quill TE, Brody H. Physician recommendations and patient autonomy: finding a balance between physician power and patient choice. *Ann Intern Med* 125:763–769, 1996.

19. Henbest RJ. Time for a change: new perspectives on the doctor-patient interaction. *S Afr Fam Pract* 10:8–15, 1989.

20. Reuben DB, Tinetti ME. Goal-oriented patient care—an alternative health outcomes paradigm. *N Engl J Med* 366(9):777–779, 2012.

21. Charles C, Whelan T, Gafni A. What do we mean by partnership in making decisions about treatment? *BMJ* 319:780–782, 1999.

22. Lazare A, Eisenthal S, Wasserman L. The customer approach to patienthood. Attending to patient requests in a walk-in clinic. *Arch Gen Psychiatry* 32:553–558, 1975.

23. Lazare A. *On apology*, Oxford, 2004, Oxford University Press.

29. Epstein RM. Mindful practice. *JAMA* 282:833–839, 1999.

30. Novack DH, Suchman AL, Clark W, et al. Calibrating the physician: personal awareness and effective patient care. *JAMA* 278:502–509, 1997.

31. Epstein RM, Alper BS, Quill TE. Communicating evidence for participatory decision making. *JAMA* 291:2359–2366, 2004.

32. Brendel RW, Brendel DH. Professionalism and the doctor-patient relationship in psychiatry. In Stern TA, editor: *The ten-minute guide to psychiatric diagnosis and treatment*, New York, 2005, Professional Publishing Group.

34. Beresin EV. The doctor-patient relationships in pediatrics. In Kaye DL, Montgomery ME, Munson SW, editors: *Child and adolescent mental health*, Philadelphia, 2002, Lippincott Williams & Wilkins.

38. Gordon C, Goroll A. Effective psychiatric interviewing in primary care medicine. In Stern TA, Herman JB, Slavin PL, editors: *The MGH guide to primary care psychiatry*, ed 2, New York, 2004, McGraw-Hill.

40. Coulehan JL, Platt FW, Egener B, et al. "Let me see if I have this right": words that help build empathy. *Arch Intern Med* 135:221–227, 2001.

43. Croskerry P. From mindless to mindful practice—cognitive bias and clinical decision making. *N Engl J Med* 368(26):2445–2450, 2013.

47. Levinson W, Cohen MS, Brady D, et al. To change or not to change: "Sounds like you have a dilemma". *Arch Intern Med* 135:386–391, 2001.

48. Prochaska J, DiClemente C. Toward a comprehensive model of change. In Miller WR, editor: *Treating addictive behaviors*, New York, 1986, Plenum Press.

50. Jacobson N, Greenley D. What is recovery: a conceptual model and explication. *Psychiatr Serv* 52:482–485, 2001.

2 The Psychiatric Interview

Eugene V. Beresin, MD, and Christopher Gordon, MD

KEY POINTS

- The purpose of the psychiatric interview is to establish a therapeutic relationship with the patient in order to collect, organize, and synthesize data that can become the basis for a formulation, differential diagnosis, and treatment plan.

- A fundamental part of establishing this relationship is fostering a secure attachment between doctor and patient, in order to facilitate mutual and open communication, to correct misunderstandings, and to help the patient create a cohesive narrative of his or her past and present situation.

- All interviews need to modify techniques in order to take into account four elements of the context: the setting, the situation, the subject, and the significance.

- Data collection should include behavioral observation, medical and psychiatric history, and a mental status examination.

- The clinician should conclude the interview by summarizing the findings and the formulation, seeking agreement with the patient, and negotiating appropriate follow-up arrangements.

- All clinicians should be aware of difficulties in the psychiatric interview, such as shameful topics and disagreements about assessment or treatment.

- Common errors in an interview include: premature closure and false assumptions about symptoms; false reassurance about a patient's condition; defensiveness around psychiatric diagnosis and treatment; maintenance of a theoretical bias about mental health and illness; inadequate explanations about psychiatric disorders and their treatment; minimization of the severity of symptoms; and inadvertent shaming of a patient without offering an apology.

OVERVIEW

The purpose of the initial psychiatric interview is to build a relationship and a therapeutic alliance with an individual or a family, in order to collect, organize, and synthesize information about present and past thoughts, feelings, and behavior. The relevant data derive from several sources: observing the patient's behavior with the examiner and with others present; attending to the emotional responses of the examiner; obtaining pertinent medical, psychiatric, social, cultural, and spiritual history (using collateral resources if possible); and performing a mental status examination. The initial evaluation should enable the practitioner to develop a clinical formulation that integrates biological, psychological, and social dimensions of a patient's life and establish provisional clinical hypotheses and questions—the differential diagnosis—that need to be tested empirically in future clinical work.

A collaborative review of the formulation and differential diagnosis can provide a platform for developing (with the patient) options and recommendations for treatment, taking into account the patient's amenability for therapeutic intervention.[1] Few medical encounters are more intimate and potentially frightening and shameful than the psychiatric examination.[2] As such, it is critical that the examiner creates a safe space for the kind of deeply personal self-revelation required.

Several methods of the psychiatric interview are examined in this chapter. These methods include the following: promoting a healthy and secure attachment between doctor and patient that promotes self-disclosure and reflection, and lends itself to the creation of a coherent narrative of the patient's life; appreciating the context of the interview that influences the interviewer's clinical technique; establishing an alliance around the task at hand and fostering effective communication; collecting data necessary for creating a formulation of the patient's strengths and weaknesses, a differential diagnosis, and recommendations for treatment if necessary; educating the patient about the nature of emotional, behavioral, and interpersonal problems and psychiatric illness (while preparing the patient for psychiatric intervention, if indicated and agreed on, and setting up arrangements for follow-up); using special techniques with children, adolescents, and families; understanding difficulties and errors in the psychiatric interview; and documenting the clinical findings for the medical record and communicating with other clinicians involved in the patient's care.

LESSONS FROM ATTACHMENT THEORY, NARRATIVE MEDICINE, AND MINDFUL PRACTICE

> *"I'm the spirit's janitor. All I do is wipe the windows a little bit so you can see for yourself."*
> **Godfrey Chips, Lakota Medicine Man**[3]

Healthy interactions with "attachment figures" in early life (e.g., parents) promote robust biological, emotional, and social development in childhood and throughout the life cycle.[4] The foundations for attachment theory are based on research findings in cognitive neuroscience, genetics, and brain development that indicate an ongoing and life-long dance between an individual's neural circuitry, genetic predisposition, brain plasticity, and environmental influences.[5] Secure attachments in childhood foster emotional resilience[6] and generate skills and habits of seeking out selected attachment figures for comfort, protection, advice, and strength. Relationships based on secure attachments lead to effective use of cognitive functions, emotional flexibility, enhancement of security, assignment of meaning to experiences, and effective self-regulation.[5] In emotional relationships of many sorts, including the student–teacher and doctor–patient relationships, there may be many features of attachment present (such as seeking proximity, or using an individual as a "safe haven" for soothing and as a secure base).[7]

What promotes secure attachment in early childhood, and how can we learn from this to understand a therapeutic doctor–patient relationship and an effective psychiatric interview? The foundations for secure attachment for children (according to Siegel) include several attributes ascribed to parents[5] (Box 2-1).

We must avoid patronizing our patients and steer clear of paternalistic power dynamics that could be implied in

---

BOX 2-1 Elements that Contribute to Secure Attachments

- Communication that is collaborative, resonant, mutual, and attuned to the cognitive and emotional state of the child.
- Dialogue that is reflective and responsive to the state of the child. This creates a sense that subjective experience can be shared, and allows for the child "being seen." It requires use of empathy, "mindsight," and an ability to "see," or be in touch with, the child's state of mind.
- Identification and repair of miscommunications and misunderstandings. When the parent corrects problems in communication, the child can make sense of painful disconnections. Repair of communication failures requires consistent, predictable, reflective, intentional, and mindful caregiving. The emphasis here is on mindfulness and reflection. Mindfulness in this instance is an example of a parent's ability for self-awareness, particularly of his or her emotional reactions to the child and the impact of his or her words and actions on the child.
- Emotional communication that involves sharing feelings that amplify the positive and mitigate the negative.
- Assistance in the child's development of coherent narratives that connect experiences in the past and present, creating an autobiographical sense of self-awareness (using language to weave together thoughts, feelings, sensations, and actions as a means of organizing and making sense of internal and external worlds).

---

analogizing the doctor–patient relationship to one between parent and child; nonetheless, if we substitute "doctor" for "parent" and similarly substitute "patient" for "child," we can immediately see the relevance to clinical practice. We can see how important each of these elements is in fostering a doctor–patient relationship that is open, honest, mutual, collaborative, respectful, trustworthy, and secure. Appreciating the dynamics of secure attachment also deepens the meaning of "patient-centered" care. The medical literature clearly indicates that good outcomes and patient satisfaction involve physician relationship techniques that involve reflection, empathy, understanding, legitimization, and support.[8,9] Patients reveal more about themselves when they trust their doctors, and trust has been found to relate primarily to behavior during clinical interviews[9] rather than to any preconceived notion of competence of the doctor or behavior outside the office.

Particularly important in the psychiatric interview is the facilitation of a patient's narrative. The practice of narrative medicine involves an ability to acknowledge, absorb, interpret, and act on the stories and struggles of others.[10] Charon[10] describes the process of listening to patients' stories as a process of following the biological, familial, cultural, and existential thread of the situation. It encompasses recognizing the multiple meanings and contradictions in words and events; attending to the silences, pauses, gestures, and non-verbal cues; and entering the world of the patient, while simultaneously arousing the doctor's own memories, associations, creativity, and emotional responses—all of which are seen in some way by the patient.[10] Narratives, like all stories, are co-created by the teller and the listener. Storytelling is an age-old part of social discourse that involves sustained attention, memory, emotional responsiveness, non-verbal responses and cues, collaborative meaning-making, and attunement to the listener's expectations. It is a vehicle for explaining behavior. Stories and

storytelling are pervasive in society as a means of conveying symbolic activity, history, communication, and teaching.[5] If a physician can assist the patient in telling his or her story effectively, reliable and valid data will be collected and the relationship solidified. Narratives are facilitated by authentic, compassionate, and genuine engagement.

A differential diagnosis detached from the patient's narrative is arid; even if it is accurate it may not lead to an effective and mutually-designed treatment path. By contrast, an accurate and comprehensive differential diagnosis that is supported by a deep appreciation of the patient's narrative is experienced by both patient and physician as more three-dimensional, and as more real, and it is more likely to lead to a mutually created and achievable plan, with which the patient is much more likely to "comply."

Creating the optimal conditions for a secure attachment and the elaboration of a coherent narrative requires mindful practice. Just as the parent must be careful to differentiate his or her emotional state and needs from the child's and be aware of conflicts and communication failures, so too must the mindful practitioner. Epstein[11] notes that mindful practitioners attend in a non-judgmental way to their own physical and mental states during the interview. Their critical self-reflection allows them to listen carefully to a patient's distress, to recognize their own errors, to make evidence-based decisions, and to stay attuned to their own values so that they may act with compassion, technical competence, and insight.[11]

Self-reflection is critical in psychiatric interviewing. Reflective practice entails observing ourselves (including our emotional reactions to patients, colleagues, and illness); our deficits in knowledge and skill; our personal styles of communicating; our responses to personal vulnerability and failure; our willingness or resistance to acknowledge error, to apologize, and to ask for forgiveness; and our reactions to stress. Self-awareness allows us to be aware of our own thinking, feelings, and actions while we are in the process of practicing. By working in this manner, a clinician enhances his or her confidence, competence, sensitivity, openness, and lack of defensiveness—all of which assist in fostering secure attachments with patients, and helping them share their innermost fears, concerns, and problems.

THE CONTEXT OF THE INTERVIEW: FACTORS INFLUENCING THE FORM AND CONTENT OF THE INTERVIEW

All interviews occur in a context. Awareness of the context may require modification of clinical interviewing techniques. There are four elements to consider: the setting, the situation, the subject, and the significance.[12]

The Setting

Patients are exquisitely sensitive to the environment in which they are evaluated. There is a vast difference between being seen in an emergency department (ED), on a medical floor, on an inpatient or partial hospital unit, in a psychiatric outpatient clinic, in a private doctor's office, in a school, or in a court clinic. Each setting has its benefits and downsides, and these must be assessed by the evaluator. For example, in the ED or on a medical or surgical floor, space for private, undisturbed interviews is usually inadequate. Such settings are filled with action, drama, and hospital personnel who race around. ED visits may require long waits, and contribute to impersonal approaches to patients and negative attitudes to psychiatric patients. For a patient with borderline traits who is in crisis, this can only create extreme frustration and possibly exacerbation of chronic fears of deprivation, betrayal, abandonment, and aloneness, and precipitation of regression.[13] For these and higher functioning patients, the public nature of the environment and the frantic pace of the emergency service may make it difficult for the patient to present very personal, private material in a calm fashion. In other public places (such as community health centers or schools), patients may feel worried about being recognized by neighbors or friends. Whatever the setting, it is always advisable to ask the patient directly how comfortable he or she feels in the examining room, and to try to ensure privacy and a quiet environment with minimal distractions.

The setting must be comfortable for the patient and the physician. If the patient is agitated, aggressive, or threatening, it is always important to calmly assert that the examination must require that everyone is safe and that we will only use words and not actions during the interview. Hostile patients should be interviewed in a setting in which the doctor is protected. An office in which an aggressive patient is blocking the door and in which there is no emergency button or access to a phone to call for help should be avoided and alternative settings should be arranged. In some instances, local security may need to be called to ensure safety.

The Situation

Many individuals seek psychiatric help because they are aware that they have a problem. This may be a second or third episode of a recurrent condition (such as a mood disorder). They may come having been to their primary care physician, who makes the referral, or they may find a doctor in other ways. Given the limitations placed on psychiatrists by some managed care panels, access to care may be severely limited. It is not unusual for a patient to have called multiple psychiatrists, only to find that their practices are all filled. Many clinics have no room for patients, or they are constrained by their contracts with specific vendors. The frustrating process of finding a psychiatrist sets the stage for some patients to either disparage the field and the health care system, or, on the other hand, to idealize the psychiatrist who has made the time for the patient. In either case, much goes on before the first visit that may significantly affect the initial interview. To complicate matters, the evaluator needs to understand previous experience with psychiatrists and psychiatric treatment. Sometimes a patient had a negative experience with another psychiatrist—perhaps a mismatch of personalities, a style that was ineffective, a treatment that did not work, or other problems. Many will wonder about a repeat performance. In all cases, in the history and relationship-building, it is propitious to ask about previous treatments, what worked, and what did not, and particularly how the patient felt about the psychiatrist. There should be reassurance that this information is totally confidential, and that the interest is in understanding that the match between doctor and patient is crucial. Even at the outset, it might be mentioned that the doctor will do his or her best to understand the patient and the problem, but that when plans are made for treatment, the patient should consider what kind of professional and setting is desired.

Other patients may come reluctantly or even with great resistance. Many arrive at the request or demand of a loved one, friend, colleague, or employer because of behaviors deemed troublesome. The patient may deny any problem, or simply be too terrified to confront a condition that is bizarre, unexplainable, or "mental." Some conditions are ego-syntonic, such as anorexia nervosa. A patient with this eating disorder typically sees the psychiatrist as the enemy—as a doctor that wants to make her "get fat." For resistant patients, it is often very useful to address the issue up front. With an anorexic patient referred by her internist and brought in by family, one could begin by saying, "Hi, Ms Jones. I know you really don't want to be here. I understand that your doctor and family are concerned about your weight. I assure you that my job is first and foremost to understand your point of view. Can you tell me why you think they wanted you to see me?" Another common situation with extreme resistance is the alcoholic individual brought in by a spouse or friend, clearly in no way ready to stop drinking. In this case you might say, "Good morning, Mr. Jones. I heard from your wife that she is really concerned about your drinking, and your safety, especially when driving. First, let me tell you that neither I nor anyone else can stop you from drinking. That is not my mission today. I do want to know what your drinking pattern is, but more, I want to get the picture of your entire life to understand your current situation." Extremely resistant patients may be brought involuntarily to an emergency service, often in restraints, by police or ambulance, because they are considered dangerous to themselves or others. It is typically terrifying, insulting, and humiliating to be physically restrained. Regardless of the reasons for admission, unknown to the psychiatrist, it is often wise to begin the interview as follows: "Hi, Ms Carter, my name is Dr. Beresin. I am terribly sorry you are strapped down, but the police and your family were very upset when you locked yourself in the car and turned on the ignition. They found a suicide note on the kitchen table. Everyone was really concerned about your safety. I would like to discuss what is going on, and see what we can do together to figure things out."

In some instances, a physician is asked to perform a psychiatric evaluation on a patient who is currently hospitalized on a medical or surgical service with symptoms arising during medical/surgical treatment. These patients may be delirious and have no idea that they are going to be seen by a psychiatrist. This was never part of their agreement when they came into the hospital for surgery, and no one may have explained the risk of delirium. Some may be resistant, others confused. Other delirious patients are quite cognizant of their altered mental status and are extremely frightened. They may wonder whether the condition is going to continue forever. For example, if we know a patient has undergone abdominal surgery for colon cancer, and has been agitated, sleepless, hallucinating, and delusional, a psychiatric consultant might begin, "Good morning, Mr. Harris. My name is Dr. Beresin. I heard about your surgery from Dr. Rand and understand you have been having some experiences that may seem kind of strange or frightening to you. Sometimes after surgery, people have a reaction to the procedure or the medications used that causes agitation, confusion, and difficulties with sleep. This is not unusual, and it is generally temporary. I would like to help you and your team figure out what is going on and what we can do about this." Other requests for psychiatric evaluation may require entirely different skills, such as when the medical team or emergency service seeks help for a family who has lost a loved one.

In each of these situations, the psychiatrist needs to understand the nature of the situation and to take this into account when planning the evaluation. In the aforementioned examples, only the introduction was addressed. However, when we see the details (discussed next) about building a relationship and modifying communication styles and questions to meet the needs of each situation, other techniques might have to be employed to make a therapeutic alliance. It is always helpful to find out as much ancillary information as possible before the interview. This may be done by talking with primary care physicians, looking in an electronic medical record, and talking with family, friends, or professionals (such as police or emergency medical technicians).

The Subject

Naturally, the clinical interview needs to take into account features of the subject, including age, developmental level, gender, and cultural background, among others. Moreover, one needs to determine "who" the patient is. In families, there may be an identified patient (e.g., a conduct-disordered child, or a child with chronic abdominal pain). However, the examiner must keep in mind that psychiatric and medical syndromes do not occur in a vacuum. While the family has determined an "identified patient," the examiner should consider that when evaluating the child, all members of the environment need to be part of the evaluation. A similar situation occurs when an adult child brings in an elderly demented parent for an evaluation. It is incumbent on the evaluator to consider the home environment and caretaking, in addition to simply evaluating the geriatric patient. In couples, one or both may identify the "other" as the "problem." An astute clinician needs to allow each person's perspective to be clarified, and the examiner will not "take sides."

Children and adolescents require special consideration. While they may, indeed, be the "identified patient," they are embedded in a home life that requires evaluation; the parent(s) or guardian(s) must help administer any prescribed treatment, psychotropic or behavioral. Furthermore, the developmental level of the child needs to be considered in the examination. Young children may not be able to articulate what they are experiencing. For example, an 8-year-old boy who has panic attacks may simply throw temper tantrums and display oppositional behavior when asked to go to a restaurant. Although he may be phobic about malls and restaurants, his parents simply see his behavior as defiance. When asked what he is experiencing, he may not be able to describe palpitations, shortness of breath, fears of impending doom, or tremulousness. However, if he is asked to draw a picture of himself at the restaurant, he may draw himself with a scared look on his face, and with jagged lines all around his body. Then when specific questions are asked, he is able to acknowledge many classic symptoms of panic disorder. For young children, the room should be equipped with toys, dollhouses, and material to create pictures.

Adolescents raise additional issues. While some may come willingly, others are dragged in against their will. In this instance, it is very important to identify and to empathize with the teenager: "Hi, Tony. I can see this is the last place you want to be. But now that you are hauled in here by your folks, we should make the best of it. Look, I have no clue what is going on, and don't even know if you are the problem! Why don't you tell me your story?" Teenagers may indeed feel like hostages. They may have *bona fide* psychiatric disorders, or may be stuck in a terrible home situation. The most important thing the examiner must convey is that the teenager's perspective is important, and that this will be looked at, as well as the parent's point of view. It is also critical to let adolescents, as all patients, know about the rules and limits of confidentiality. Many children think that whatever they say will be directly transmitted to their parents. Surely this is their experience in school. However, there are clear guidelines about adolescent confidentiality, and these should be delineated at the beginning of the clinical encounter. Confidentiality is a core part of the evaluation, and it will be honored for the adolescent; it is essential that this is communicated to them so they may feel safe in divulging very sensitive and private information without fears of repercussion. Issues such as sexuality, sexually-transmitted diseases, substance abuse, and issues in mental health are protected by state and federal statutes. There are, however, exceptions; one major exception is that if the patient or another is in danger by virtue of an adolescent's behavior, confidentiality is waived.[14]

The Significance

Psychiatric disorders are commonly stigmatized, and subsequently are often accompanied by profound shame, anxiety, denial, fear, and uncertainty. Patients generally have a poor understanding of psychiatric disorders, either from myth, lack of information, or misinformation from the media (e.g., TV, radio, and the Internet).[15] Many patients have preconceived notions of what to expect (bad or good), based on the experience of friends or family. Some patients, having talked with others or having searched on-line, may be certain or very worried that they suffer from a particular condition, and this may color the information presented to an examiner. A specific syndrome or symptom may have idiosyncratic significance to a patient, perhaps because a relative with a mood disorder was hospitalized for life, before the deinstitutionalization of mentally-disordered individuals. Hence, he or she may be extremely wary of divulging any indication of severe symptoms lest life-long hospitalization result. Obsessions or compulsions may be seen as clear evidence of losing one's mind, having a brain tumor, or becoming like Aunt Jesse with a chronic psychosis.[12] Some patients (based on cognitive limitations) may not understand their symptoms. These may be normal, such as the developmental stage in a school-age child, whereas others may be a function of congenital cognitive impairment, autism spectrum disorder, or cerebral lacunae secondary to multiple infarcts following embolic strokes.

Finally, there are significant cultural differences in the way mental health and mental illness are viewed. Culture may influence health-seeking and mental health–seeking behavior, the understanding of psychiatric symptoms, the course of psychiatric disorders, the efficacy of various treatments, or the kinds of treatments accepted.[16] Psychosis, for example, may be viewed as possession by spirits. Some cultural groups have much higher completion rates for suicide, and thus previous attempts in some individuals should be taken more seriously. Understanding the family structure may be critical to the negotiation of treatment; approval by a family elder could be crucial in the acceptance of professional help.

ESTABLISHING AN ALLIANCE AND FOSTERING EFFECTIVE COMMUNICATION

Studies of physician–patient communication have demonstrated that good outcomes flow from effective communication; developing a good patient-centered relationship is characterized by friendliness, courtesy, empathy, and partnership-building, and by the provision of information. Positive outcomes have included benefits to emotional health, symptom resolution, and physiological measures (e.g., blood pressure, blood glucose level, and pain control).[17-20]

In 1999 leaders and representatives of major medical schools and professional organizations convened at the Fetzer Institute in Kalamazoo, Michigan, to propose a model for doctor–patient communication that would lend itself to the creation of curricula for medical and graduate medical education, and for the development of standards for the profession. The goals of the Kalamazoo Consensus Statement[21] were to foster a sound doctor–patient relationship and to provide a model for the clinical interview. The key elements of this statement are summarized in Box 2-2, and are applicable to the psychiatric interview.

BOX 2-2 Building a Relationship: The Fundamental
Tasks of Communication

- Elicit the patient's story while guiding the interview by diagnostic reasoning.
- Maintain an awareness of the fact that feelings, ideas, and values of both the patient and the doctor influence the relationship.
- Develop a partnership with the patient, and form an alliance in which the patient participates in decision-making.
- Work with patients' families and support networks.

OPEN THE DISCUSSION
- Allow the patient to express his or her opening statement without interruption.
- Encourage the patient to describe a full set of concerns.
- Maintain a personal connection during the interview.

GATHER INFORMATION
- Use both open- and closed-ended questions.
- Provide structure, clarification, and a summary of the information collected.
- Listen actively, using verbal and non-verbal methods (e.g., eye contact).

UNDERSTAND THE PATIENT'S PERSPECTIVE
- Explore contextual issues (e.g., familial, cultural, spiritual, age, gender, and socioeconomic status).
- Elicit beliefs, concerns, and expectations about health and illness.
- Validate and respond appropriately to the patient's ideas, feelings, and values.

SHARE INFORMATION
- Avoid technical language and medical jargon.
- Determine if the patient understands your explanations.
- Encourage questions.

REACH AGREEMENT ON PROBLEMS AND PLANS
- Welcome participation in decision-making.
- Determine the patient's amenability to following a plan.
- Identify and enlist resources and supports.

PROVIDE CLOSURE
- Ask if the patient has questions or other concerns.
- Summarize and solidify the agreement with a plan of action.
- Review the follow-up plans.

BUILDING THE RELATIONSHIP AND THERAPEUTIC ALLIANCE

All psychiatric interviews must begin with a personal introduction, and establish the purpose of the interview; this helps create an alliance around the initial examination. The interviewer should attempt to greet the person warmly, and use words that demonstrate care, attention, and concern. Note-taking and use of computers should be minimized, and if used, should not interfere with ongoing eye contact. The interviewer should indicate that this interaction is collaborative, and that any misunderstandings on the part of patient or physician should be immediately clarified. In addition, the patient should be instructed to ask questions, interrupt, and provide corrections or additions at any time. The time frame for the interview should be announced. In general, the interviewer should acknowledge that some of the issues and questions raised will be highly personal, and that if there are issues

that the patient has real trouble with, he or she should let the examiner know. Confidentiality should be assured at the outset of the interview. These initial guidelines set the tone, quality, and style of the clinical interview. An example of a beginning is, "Hi, Mr. Smith. My name is Dr. Beresin. I am delighted you came today. I would like to discuss some of the issues or problems you are dealing with so that we can both understand them better, and figure out what kind of assistance may be available. I will need to ask you a number of questions about your life, both your past and present, and if I need some clarification about your descriptions I will ask for your help to be sure I 'get it.' If you think I have missed the boat, please chime in and correct my misunderstanding. Some of the topics may be highly personal, and I hope that you will let me know if things get a bit too much. We will have about an hour to go through this, and then we'll try to come up with a reasonable plan together. I do want you to know that everything we say is confidential. Do you have any questions about our job today?" This should be followed with an open-ended question about the reasons for the interview.

One of the most important aspects of building a therapeutic alliance is helping the patient feel safe. Demonstrating warmth and respect is essential. In addition, the psychiatrist should display genuine interest and curiosity in working with a new patient. Preconceived notions about the patient should be eschewed. If there are questions about the patient's cultural background or spiritual beliefs that may have an impact on the information provided, on the emotional response to symptoms, or on the acceptance of a treatment plan, the physician should note at the outset that if any of these areas are of central importance to the patient, he or she should feel free to speak about such beliefs or values. The patient should have the sense that both doctor and patient are exploring the history, life experience, and current symptoms together.

For many patients, the psychiatric interview is probably one of the most confusing examinations in medicine. The psychiatric interview is at once professional and profoundly intimate. We are asking patients to reveal parts of their life they may only have shared with extremely close friends, a spouse, clergy, or family, if anyone. And they are coming into a setting in which they are supposed to do this with a total stranger. Being a doctor may not be sufficient to allay the apprehension that surrounds this situation; being a trustworthy, caring human being may help a great deal. It is vital to make the interview highly personal and to use techniques that come naturally. Beyond affirming and validating the patient's story with extreme sensitivity, some clinicians may use humor and judicious self-revelation. These elements are characteristics of healers.[22]

An example should serve to demonstrate some of these principles. A 65-year-old deeply religious woman was seen for an evaluation of delirium following cardiac bypass surgery. She told the psychiatric examiner in her opening discussion that she wanted to switch from her primary care physician, whom she had seen for over 30 years. As part of her postoperative delirium, she developed the delusion that he may have raped her during one of his visits with her. She felt that she could not possibly face him, her priest, or her family, and she was stricken with deep despair. While the examiner may have recognized this as a biological consequence of her surgery and post-operative course, her personal experience spoke differently. She would not immediately accept an early interpretation or explanation that her brain was not functioning correctly. In such a situation, the examiner must verbally acknowledge her perspective, seeing the problem through her eyes, and helping her see that he or she "gets it." For the patient, this was a horrible nightmare. The interviewer might have said, "Mrs. Jones, I understand how awful you must feel.

Can you tell me how this could happened, given your long-standing and trusting relationship with your doctor?" She answered that she did not know, but that she was really confused and upset. When the examiner established a trusting relationship, completed the examination, determined delirium was present, and explained the nature of this problem, they agreed on using haloperidol to improve sleep and "nerves." Additional clarifications could be made in a subsequent session after the delirium cleared.

As noted earlier, reliable mirroring of the patient's cognitive and emotional state and self-reflection of one's affective response to patients are part and parcel of establishing secure attachments. Actively practicing self-reflection and clarifying one's understanding help to model behavior for the patient, as the doctor and patient co-create the narrative. Giving frequent summaries to "check in" on what the physician has heard may be very valuable, particularly early on in the interview, when the opening discussion or chief complaints are elicited. For example, a 22-year-old woman gradually developed obsessive-compulsive symptoms over the past 2 years that led her to be housebound. The interviewer said, "So, Ms. Thompson, let's see if I get it. You have been stuck at home and cannot get out of the house because you have to walk up and down the stairs for a number of hours. If you did not 'get it right,' something terrible would happen to one of your family members. You also noted that you were found walking the stairs in public places, and that even your friends could not understood this behavior, and they made fun of you. You mentioned that you had to 'check' on the stove and other appliances being turned off, and could not leave your car, because you were afraid it would not turn off, or that the brake was not fully on, and again, something terrible would happen to someone. And you said to me that you were really upset because you knew this behavior was 'crazy.' How awful this must be for you! Did I get it right?" The examiner should be sure to see both verbally and non-verbally that this captured the patient's problem. If positive feedback did not occur, the examiner should attempt to see if there was a misinterpretation, or if the interviewer came across as judgmental or critical. One could "normalize" the situation and reassure the patient to further solidify the alliance by saying, "Ms. Thompson, your tendency to stay home, stuck, in the effort to avoid hurting anyone is totally natural given your perception and concern for others close to you. I do agree, it does not make sense, and appreciate that it feels bizarre and unusual. I think we can better understand this behavior, and later I can suggest ways of coping and maybe even overcoming this situation through treatments that have been quite successful with others. However, I do need to get some additional information. Is that OK?" In this way, the clinician helps the patient feel understood—that anyone in that situation would feel the same way, and that there is hope. But more information is needed. This strategy demonstrates respect and understanding, and provides support and comfort, while building the alliance.

DATA COLLECTION: BEHAVIORAL OBSERVATION, THE MEDICAL AND PSYCHIATRIC HISTORY, AND THE MENTAL STATUS EXAMINATION
Behavioral Observation

There is a lot to be learned about patients by observing them before, during, and after the psychiatric interview. It is useful to see how the patient interacts with support staff of the clinic, and with family, friends, or others who accompany him or her to the appointment. In the interview one should take note of grooming, the style and state of repair of clothes, mannerisms, normal and abnormal movements, posture and gait, physical features (such as natural deformities, birth marks, or cutting marks, scratches, tattoos, or pierces), skin quality (e.g., color, texture, and hue), language (including English proficiency, the style of words used, grammar, vocabulary, and syntax), and non-verbal cues (such as eye contact and facial expressions). All these factors contribute to clinical formulation.

The Medical and Psychiatric History

Box 2-3 provides an overview of the key components of the psychiatric history.

Presenting Problems

The interviewer should begin with the presenting problem using open-ended questions. The patient should be encouraged to tell his or her story without interruptions. Many times the patient will turn to the doctor for elaboration, but it is best to let the patient know that he or she is the true expert and that only he or she has experienced this situation directly. It is best to use clarifying questions throughout the interview. For example, "I was really upset and worked up" may mean one thing to the patient and something else to an examiner. It could mean frustrated, anxious, agitated, violent, or depressed. Such a statement requires clarification. So, too, does a comment such as "I was really depressed." Depression to a psychiatrist may be very different for a patient. To some patients, depression means aggravated, angry, or sad. It might be a momentary agitated state, or a chronic state. Asking more detailed questions not only clarifies the affective state of the patient but also transmits the message that he or she knows best and that a real collaboration and dialogue is the only way we will figure out the problem. In addition, once the patient's words are clarified it is very useful to use the patient's own words throughout the interview to verify that you are listening.[23]

When taking the history, it is vital to remember that the patient's primary concerns may not be the same as the physician's. For example, while the examiner may be concerned about a bipolar disorder and escalating mania, the patient may be more concerned about her husband's unemployment and how this is making her agitated and sleepless. If this was the reason for the psychiatric visit, namely concern about coping with household finances, this should be validated. There will be ample time to get detailed history to establish a diagnosis of mania, particularly if the patient feels the clinician and she are on the same page. It is always useful to ask, "What are you most worried about?"

In discussing the presenting problems, it is best to avoid a set of checklist-type questions, but one should cover the bases to create a *Diagnostic and Statistical Manual of Mental Disorders, Fifth Edition*, differential diagnosis. It is best to focus largely on the chief complaint and present problems and to incorporate other parts of the history around this. The presenting problem is the reason for a referral, and is probably most important to the patient, even though additional questions about current function and the past medical or past psychiatric history may be more critical to the examiner. A good clinician, having established a trusting relationship, can always redirect a patient to ascertain additional information (such as symptoms not mentioned by the patient and the duration, frequency, and intensity of symptoms). Also it is important to ask how the patient has coped with the problem and what is being done personally or professionally to help him or her deal with it. One should ask if there are other problems or stressors, medical problems, or family issues that exacerbate the current complaint. Questions about extreme distress, including pain (on a scale of 0–10) must always be ascertained. After a period of open-ended questions about the

---

BOX 2-3 The Psychiatric History

IDENTIFYING INFORMATION

Name, address, phone number, and e-mail address
Insurance
Age, gender, marital status, occupation, children, ethnicity, and
  religion
For children and adolescents: primary custodians, school, and
  grade
Primary care physician
Psychiatrist, allied mental health providers
Referral source
Sources of information
Reliability

CHIEF COMPLAINT/PRESENTING PROBLEM(S)

History of Present Illness

Onset
Perceived precipitants
Signs and symptoms
Course and duration
Treatments: professional and personal
Effects on personal, social, and occupational or academic
  function
Co-morbid psychiatric or medical disorders
Psychosocial stressors: personal (psychological, medical),
  family, friends, work/school, legal, housing, and
  financial

PAST PSYCHIATRIC HISTORY

Previous Episodes of the Problem(s)

Symptoms, course, duration, and treatment (inpatient or
  outpatient)

Psychiatric Disorders

Symptoms, course, duration, and treatment (inpatient or
  outpatient)

PAST MEDICAL HISTORY

Medical problems: past and current
Surgical problems: past and current
Accidents
Allergies
Immunizations
Current medications: prescribed and over-the-counter
  medications
Other treatments: acupuncture, chiropractic, homeopathic,
  yoga, and meditation
Tobacco: present and past use
Substance use: present and past use
Pregnancy history: births, miscarriages, and abortions

Sexual history: birth control, safe sex practices, and history of,
  and screening for, sexually transmitted diseases
Past or present physical or sexual abuse
Assessment of pain (on a scale of 0–10)

REVIEW OF SYSTEMS

Family History

Family psychiatric history
Family medical history

Personal History: Developmental and Social History

Early Childhood

Developmental milestones
Family relationships

Middle Childhood

School performance
Learning or attention problems
Family relationships
Friends
Hobbies
Media use

Adolescence

School performance (include learning and attention problems)
Friends and peer relationships
Family relationships
Psychosexual history
Dating and sexual history
Work history
Substance use
Problems with the law
Media use

Early Adulthood

Education
Friends and peer relationships
Hobbies and interests
Marital and other romantic partners
Occupational history
Military experiences
Problems with the law
Media use

Mid-life and Older Adulthood

Career development
Marital and other romantic partners
Changes in the family
Media use
Losses
Aging process: psychological and physical

Adapted from Beresin EV. The psychiatric interview. In Stern TA, editor: The ten-minute guide to psychiatric diagnosis and treatment, New York, 2005, Professional Publishing Group.

---

current problem, the interviewer should ask questions about mood, anxiety, and other behavioral problems and how they affect the presenting problem. A key part of the assessment of the presenting problem should be a determination of safety. Questions about suicide, homicide, domestic violence, and abuse should not be omitted from a review of the current situation. If one is concerned about self-harm, the interviewer should ask about the possible means, including access to firearms in the home. Finally, one should ascertain why the patient came for help now, how motivated he or she is for getting help, and how the patient is faring in personal, family, social, and professional life. Without knowing more, since this is early in the interview, the examiner should avoid offering

premature reassurance, but provide support and encouragement for therapeutic assistance that will be offered in the latter part of the interview.

Past Psychiatric History

After the opening phases of the interview, open-ended questions may shift to more focused questions. In the past psychiatric history, the interviewer should inquire about previous DSM-5 diagnoses (including the symptoms of each, partial syndromes, how they were managed, and how they affected the patient's life). A full range of treatments, including outpatient, inpatient, and partial hospital, should be considered. It is most useful to ask what treatments, if any, were successful, and if so, in what ways. By the same token, the examiner should ask about treatment failures. This, of course, will contribute to the treatment recommendations provided at the close of the interview. This may be a good time in the interview to get a sense of how the patient copes under stress. What psychological, behavioral, and social means are employed in the service of maintaining equilibrium in the face of hardship? It is also wise to focus not just on coping skills, defenses, and adaptive techniques in the face of the psychiatric disorder, but also on psychosocial stressors in general (e.g., births, deaths, loss of jobs, problems in relationships, and problems with children). Discerning a patient's coping style may be highly informative and contribute to the psychiatric formulation. Does the patient rely on venting emotions, on shutting affect off and wielding cognitive controls, on using social supports, on displacing anger onto others, or on finding productive distractions (e.g., plunging into work)? Again, knowing something about a person's style of dealing with adversity uncovers defense mechanisms, reveals something about personality, and aids in the consideration of treatment options. For example, a person who avoids emotion, uses reason, and sets about to increase tasks in hard times may be an excellent candidate for a cognitive–behavioral approach to a problem. An individual who thrives through venting emotions, turning to others for support, and working to understand the historical origins of his or her problems may be a good candidate for psychodynamic psychotherapy, either individual or group.

Past Medical History

A number of psychiatric symptoms and behavioral problems are secondary to medical conditions, to the side effects of medications, and to drug–drug interactions (including those related to over-the-counter medications). The past medical history needs to be thorough, and must include past and current medical and surgical conditions, past and current use of medications (including vitamins, herbs, and non-traditional remedies), use of substances (e.g., tobacco, alcohol, and other drugs [past and present]), an immunization and travel history, pregnancies, menstrual history, a history of hospitalizations and day surgeries, accidents (including sequelae, if any), and sexual history (including use of contraception, abortions, history of sexually-transmitted diseases, and testing for the latter).

Review of Systems

By the time the examiner inquires about the past medical history and the review of systems, checklist-type questioning is adopted in lieu of the previous format of interviewing. It is useful to elicit a complete review of systems following the medical history. A number of undiagnosed medical disorders may be picked up in the course of the psychiatric interview. Many patients do not routinely see their primary care physician, and psychiatrists have a unique opportunity to consider medical conditions and their evaluation in the examination. While not a formal part of the interview, laboratory testing is a core part of the psychiatric examination. Though this chapter refers to the interview, the review of systems may alert the clinician to order additional laboratory tests and consult the primary care physician about medical investigation.

Family History

The fact that many illnesses run in families requires an examiner to ask about the family history of medical, surgical, and psychiatric illnesses, along with their treatments.

Social and Developmental History

The developmental history is important for all psychiatric patients, but especially for children and adolescents, because prevention and early detection of problems may lead to interventions that can correct deviations in development. The developmental history for early and middle childhood and adolescence should include questions about developmental milestones (e.g., motor function, speech, growth, social and moral achievements), family relationships in the past and present, school history (including grade levels reached and any history of attention or learning disabilities), friends, hobbies, jobs, interests, athletics, substance use, and any legal problems. Questions about adult development should focus on the nature and quality of intimate relationships, friendships, relationships with children (e.g., natural, adopted, products of assisted reproductive technology, stepchildren), military history, work history, hobbies and interests, legal issues, and financial problems. Questions should always be asked about domestic violence (including a history of physical or sexual abuse in the past and present).

The social history should include questions about a patient's cultural background, including the nature of this heritage, how it affects family structure and function, belief systems, values, and spiritual practices. Questions should be asked about the safety of the community and the quality of the social supports in the neighborhood, the place of worship, or other loci in the community.

An important component of the social and developmental history, particularly valuable for children and adolescents, is a media history. The overwhelming amount, availability and use of media has grown exponentially since television was introduced in the 1950s. Children 8–18 years old spend an average of 6.5 hours a day using media (if one considers the time involved with television, movies, video games, print, radio, and recorded music), much of it digital media; the time spent reaches 8 hours daily when simultaneous media are used. This takes up more time than any other activity for youth other than sleeping.[24] The impact of media, including violent media, on the growth and development of children, is under considerable debate. Studies have demonstrated that media significantly affects clinical symptoms, such as body image,[25] post-traumatic stress disorder,[26] and potentially aggressive behavior.[27] Few parents know what their children are watching or even the content of their video games.[28] Further, media is used by adults for multiple purposes, including obtaining medical and psychiatric information. Many patients will come in for an evaluation with a preconceived notion of their problem, or even ask for a specific medication based on information they have found on-line. Conversely, others will refuse treatment recommendations based on information (or misinformation) posted on-line.

Given the influence of media, both positive and negative, on the health of our youth and our adult patients, it is highly advisable to include a media history in the psychiatric interview. Beyond taking stock of what types of media are used by family members and for what purposes, clinicians, allied health professionals, and parents should become more media-literate, and understand the broad range of material and methods of transmission of information and communication.[28]

Use of Corollary Information

While many interviews of adults are conducted with just the patient in the office, it is quite useful to obtain additional information from other important people in the patient's life (such as a spouse or partner, siblings, children, parents, friends, and clergy). For example, a patient who appears para-noid and mildly psychotic in the office may deny such symp-toms or not see them as problems. In order to understand the nature of the problem, its duration and intensity, and its impact on function, others may need to be contacted (with informed consent). This applies to many other conditions, particularly substance use disorders, in which the patient may deny the quantity used and the frequency of effects of sub-stances on everyday life.

Obtaining consent to contact others in a patient's life is useful not only for information-gathering, but for the involve-ment of others in the treatment process, if needed. For chil-dren and adolescents, this is absolutely essential, as is obtaining information from teachers or other school personnel. Con-tacting the patient's primary care physician or therapist may be useful for objective assessment of the medical and psychi-atric history, as well as for corroboration of associated condi-tions, doses of medications, and past laboratory values. Finally, it is always useful to review the medical record (if accessible, and with permission).

The Mental Status Examination

The mental status examination is part and parcel of any medical and psychiatric interview. Its traditional components are indicated in Box 2-4. Most of the data needed in this model can be ascertained by asking the patient about ele-ments of the current problems. Specific questions may be needed for the evaluation of perception, thought, and cogni-tion. Most of the information in the mental status examina-tion is obtained by simply taking the psychiatric history and by observing the patient's behavior, affect, speech, mood, thought, and cognition.

Perceptual disorders include abnormalities in sensory stimuli. There may be misperceptions of sensory stimuli, known as *illusions*, for example, micropsia or macropsia (objects that appear smaller or larger, respectively, than they are). Phenomena such as this include distortions of external stimuli (affecting the size, shape, intensity, or sound of stimuli). Distortions of stimuli that are internally created are hallucinations and may occur in any one or more of the fol-lowing modalities: auditory, visual, olfactory, gustatory, or tactile.

Thought disorders may manifest with difficulties in the form or content of thought. Formal thought disorders involve the way ideas are connected. Abnormalities in form may involve the logic and coherence of thinking. Such disorders may herald neurological disorders, severe mood disorders (e.g., psychotic depression or mania), schizophreniform psy-chosis, delirium, or other disorders that impair reality testing. Examples of formal thought disorders are listed in Box 2-5.[29,30]

Disorders of the content of thought pertain to the specific ideas themselves. The examiner should always inquire about paranoid, suicidal, and homicidal thinking. Other indications of disorder of thought content include delusions, obsessions, and ideas of reference (Box 2-6).[30]

The cognitive examination includes an assessment of higher processes of thinking. This part of the examination is critical for a clinical assessment of neurological function, and is useful for differentiating focal and global disorders, delir-ium, and dementia. The traditional model assesses a variety of dimensions (Box 2-7).[31]

Alternatively, the Mini-Mental State Examination[32] may be administered (Table 2-1). It is a highly valid and reliable instrument that takes about 5 minutes to perform and is very effective in differentiating depression from dementia.

There are a number of brief, valid and reliable instruments that may be used in the history and mental status examina-tion. Since substance abuse is such a common problem, the clinician might include the CAGE examination for alcohol abuse[33,34] for adults or the CRAFFT examination for alcohol or substance abuse in teenagers aged 14–18.[35,36]

BOX 2-5 Examples of Formal Thought Disorders

- **Circumstantiality**: a disorder of association with the inclusion of unnecessary details until one arrives at the goal of the thought
- **Tangentiality**: use of oblique, irrelevant, and digressive thoughts that do not convey the central idea to be communicated
- **Loose associations**: jumping from one unconnected topic to another
- **Clang associations**: an association of speech without logical connection dictated by the sound of the words rather than by their meaning; it frequently involves using rhyming or punning
- **Perseveration**: repeating the same response to stimuli (such as the same verbal response to different questions) with an inability to change the responses
- **Neologism**: words made up; often a condensation of different words; unintelligible to the listener
- **Echolalia**: persistent repetition of words or phrases of another person
- **Thought-blocking**: an abrupt interruption in the flow of thought, in which one cannot recover what was just said

---

BOX 2-4 The Mental Status Examination

General appearance and behavior: grooming, posture, movements, mannerisms, and eye contact
Speech: rate, flow, latency, coherence, logic, and prosody
Affect: range, intensity, lability
Mood: euthymic, elevated, depressed, irritable, anxious
Perception: illusions and hallucinations
Thought (coherence and lucidity): form and content (illusions, hallucinations, and delusions)
Safety: suicidal and homicidal thoughts, self-injurious ideas, impulses, and plans
Cognition
- Level of consciousness
- Orientation
- Attention and concentration
- Memory (registration, recent and remote)
- Calculation
- Abstraction
- Judgment
- Insight

BOX 2-6 Disorders of Thought Content

- **Delusions**: fixed, false, unshakable beliefs
- **Obsessions**: persistent thought that cannot be extruded by logic or reasoning
- **Idea of reference**: misinterpretation of incidents in the external world as having special and direct personal reference to the self

BOX 2-7 Categories of the Mental Status Examination

- **Orientation**: for example, to time, place, person, and situation.
- **Attention and concentration**: for example, remembering three objects immediately, in 1 and 3 minutes; spelling "world" backward; performing digit span.
- **Memory**: registration; recent and remote memory. Registration is typically a function of attention and concentration. Recent and remote memory is evaluated by recalling events in the short and long term, for example, the names of the presidents provided backward.
- **Calculations**: evaluated typically by serially subtracting 7 from 100.
- **Abstraction**: assessed by the patient's ability to interpret proverbs or other complex ideas.
- **Judgment**: evaluated by seeing if the patient demonstrates an awareness of personal issues or problems, and provides appropriate ways of solving them.
- **Insight**: an assessment of self-reflection and an understanding of one's condition or the situation of others.

SHARING INFORMATION AND PREPARING THE PATIENT FOR TREATMENT

The conclusion of the psychiatric interview requires summarizing the symptoms and history and organizing them into a coherent narrative that can be reviewed and agreed on by the patient and the clinician. This involves recapitulating the most important findings and explaining the meaning of them to the patient. It is crucial to obtain an agreement on the clinical material and the way the story holds together for the patient. If the patient does not concur with the summary, the psychiatrist should return to the relevant portions of the interview in question and revisit the topics that are in disagreement.

This part of the interview should involve explaining one or more diagnoses (their biological, psychological, and environmental etiology) to the patient, as well as providing a formulation of the patient's strengths, weaknesses, and style of managing stress. The latter part of the summary is intended to help ensure that the patient feels understood. The next step is to delineate the kinds of approaches that the current standards of care would indicate are appropriate for treatment. If the diagnosis is uncertain, further evaluation should be recommended to elucidate the problem or co-morbid problems. This might require one or more of the following: further laboratory evaluation; medical, neurological, or pediatric referral; psychological or neuropsychological testing; use of

TABLE 2-1 Mini-Mental State Examination

MEAN SCORES			
Depression			9.7
Depression with impaired cognition			19.0
Uncomplicated depression			25.1
Normal			27.6

Maximum Score	Score		
		Orientation	
5	( )	What is the (year) (date) (day) (month)?	
5	( )	Where are we (state) (county) (town) (hospital) (floor)?	
		Registration	
3	( )	Name three objects: 1 second to say each. Then ask the patient all three after you have said them. Give 1 point for each correct answer. Then repeat them until the patient learns all three. Count trials and record.	
Trials _____			
		Attention and Calculation	
5	( )	Serial 7s: 1 point for each correct. Stop after five answers. Alternatively, spell "world" backward.	
		Recall	
3	( )	Ask for three objects repeated above. Give 1 point for each correct answer.	
		Language	
2	( )	Name a pencil and watch. (2 points)	
1	( )	Repeat the following: "No ifs, ands, or buts." (1 point)	
3	( )	Follow a three-stage command: "Take a piece of paper in your right hand, fold it in half, and put it on the floor." (3 points)	
1	( )	Read and obey the following: "Close your eyes." (1 point)	
1	( )	Write a sentence. It must contain a subject and a verb and be sensible. (1 point)	
		Visual-Motor Integrity	
1	( )	Copy design (two intersecting pentagons; all 10 angles must be present and 2 must intersect). (1 point)	
Total score _____			
Assess level of consciousness along a continuum:			
Alert	Drowsy	Stupor	Coma

Reproduced from Folstein MF, Folstein SE, McHugh PE. The Mini-Mental State Exam: a practical method for grading the cognitive state of patients for the clinician, J Psychiatr Res 1975; 12:189–198.

standardized rating scales; or consultation with a specialist (e.g., a psychopharmacologist or a sleep disorders or substance abuse specialist).

Education about treatment should include reviewing the pros and cons of various options. This is a good time to dispel myths about psychiatric treatments, either pharmacotherapy or psychotherapy. Both of these domains have significant stigma associated with them. For patients who are prone to shun pharmacotherapy (not wanting any "mind-altering" medications), it may be useful to "medicalize" the psychiatric disorder and note that common medical conditions involve attention to biopsychosocial treatment.[12] For example, few people would refuse medications for treatment of hypertension, even though it may be clear that the condition is exacerbated by stress and lifestyle. The same may be said for the treatment of asthma, migraines, diabetes, and peptic ulcers. In this light, the clinician can refer to psychiatric conditions as problems of "chemical imbalances"—a neutral term—or as problems with the brain, an organ people often forget when talking about "mental" conditions. A candid dialogue in this way, perhaps describing how depression or panic disorder involves abnormalities in brain function, may help. It should be noted that this kind of discussion should in no way be construed or interpreted as pressure—rather as an educational experience. Letting the patient know that treatment decisions are collaborative and patient-centered is absolutely essential in a discussion of this order.

A similar educational conversation should relate to the use of psychotherapies. Some patients disparage psychotherapies as "mumbo jumbo," lacking scientific evidence. In this instance, discussion can center around the fact that scientific research indicates that experience and the environment can affect biological function. An example of this involves talking about how early trauma affects child development, or how coming through an experience in war can produce post-traumatic stress disorder, a significant dysfunction of the brain. Many parents will immediately appreciate how the experiences in childhood affect a child's mood, anxiety, and behavior, though they will also point out that children are born with certain personalities and traits. This observation is wonderful as it opens a door for a discussion of the complex and ongoing interaction among brain, environment, and behavior.

THE EVALUATION OF CHILDREN AND ADOLESCENTS

Psychiatric disorders in children and adolescents will be discussed elsewhere in this book. In general, children and adolescents pose certain unique issues for the psychiatric interviewer. First, a complete developmental history is required. For younger children, most of the history is taken from the parents. Rarely are young children seen initially apart from parents. Observation of the child is critical. The examiner should notice how the child relates to the parents or caregivers. Conversely, it is important to note whether the adult's management of the child is appropriate. Does the child seem age appropriate in terms of motor function and growth? Are there any observable neurological impairments? The evaluator should determine whether speech, language, cognition, and social function are age appropriate. The office should have an ample supply of toys (including a dollhouse and puppets for fantasy play, and building blocks or similar toys), board games (for older school-age children), and drawing supplies. Collateral information from the pediatrician and schoolteachers is critical to verify or amplify parental and child-reported data.

Adolescents produce their own set of issues and problems for the interviewer.[37] A teenager may or may not be brought in by a parent. However, given the developmental processes that surround the quests for identity and separation, the interviewer must treat the teen with the same kind of respect and collaboration as with an adult. The issue and importance of ensuring confidentiality have been mentioned previously. The adolescent also needs to hear at the outset that the interviewer would need to obtain permission to speak with parents or guardians, and that any information received from them would be faithfully transmitted to the patient.

Although all the principles of attempting to establish a secure attachment noted previously apply to the adolescent, the interview of the adolescent is quite different from that of an adult. Developmentally, teenagers are capable of abstract thinking and are developmentally becoming increasingly autonomous. At the same time, they are struggling with grandiosity that alternates with extreme vulnerability and self-consciousness and managing body image, sexuality and aggression, mood lability, and occasional regression to dependency—all of which makes an interview and relationship difficult. Furthermore with incomplete myelination, particularly of their frontal lobes, incomplete until the early 20s, they are more prone to impulsivity, acting without considering consequences, and more prone to peer pressure. The interviewer must constantly consider what counts as normal adolescent behavior and what risk-taking behaviors, mood swings, and impulsivity are pathological. This is not easy, and typically teenagers need a few initial meetings for the clinician to feel capable of co-creating a narrative—albeit a narrative in progress. The stance of the clinician in working with adolescents requires moving in a facile fashion between an often-needed professional authority figure and a big brother or sister, camp counselor, and friend. The examiner must be able to know something about the particular adolescent's culture, to use humor and exaggeration, to be flexible, and to be empathic in the interview, yet not attempt to be "one of them." It is essential to validate strengths and weaknesses and to inspire self-reflection and some philosophical thinking—all attendant with the new cognitive developments since earlier childhood.

DIFFICULTIES AND ERRORS IN THE PSYCHIATRIC INTERVIEW
Dealing with Sensitive Subjects

A number of subjects are particularly shameful for patients. Such topics include sexual problems, substance abuse and other addictions, financial matters, impulsive behavior, bizarre experiences (such as obsessions and compulsions), domestic violence, histories of abuse, and symptoms of psychosis. Some patients will either deny or avoid discussing these topics. In this situation, non-threatening, gentle encouragement and acknowledgment of how difficult these matters are may help. If the issue is not potentially dangerous or life-threatening to the patient or to others, the clinician may omit some questions known to be important in the diagnosis or formulation. If it is not essential to obtain this information in the initial interview, it may be best for the alliance to let it go, knowing the examiner or another clinician may return to it as the therapeutic relationship grows.

In other situations that are dangerous (such as occurs with suicidal, homicidal, manic, or psychotic patients), in which pertinent symptoms must be ascertained, questioning is crucial no matter how distressed the patient may become. In some instances when danger seems highly likely, hospitalization may be necessary for observation and further exploration of a serious disorder. Similarly, an agitated patient who needs to be assessed for safety may need sedation or hospitalization in order to complete a comprehensive evaluation, particularly

8. Lipkin M, Frankel RM, Beckman HB, et al. Performing the medical interview. In Lipkin M Jr, Putnam SM, Lazare A, editors: *The medical interview: clinical care, education and research*, New York, 1995, Springer-Verlag.
9. Lipkin M Jr. Sisyphus or Pegasus? The physician interviewer in the era of corporatization of care. *Ann Intern Med* 124:511–513, 1996.
10. Charon R. Narrative medicine: a model for empathy, reflection, profession and trust. *JAMA* 286:1897–1902, 2001.
11. Epstein RM. Mindful practice. *JAMA* 291:2359–2366, 2004.
12. Beresin EV. The psychiatric interview. In Stern TA, editor: *The ten-minute guide to psychiatric diagnosis and treatment*, New York, 2005, Professional Publishing Group.
13. Beresin EV, Gordon C. Emergency ward management of the borderline patient. *Gen Hosp Psychiatry* 3:237–244, 1981.
14. Confidential health care for adolescents: position paper of the Society for Adolescent Medicine. Prepared by Ford C, English A, Sigman. *J Adolesc Health* 35:160–167, 2004.
15. Butler JR, Hyler S. Hollywood portrayals of child and adolescent mental health treatment: implications for clinical practice. *Child Adolesc Psychiatric Clin North Am* 14:509–522, 2005.
16. Mintzer JE, Hendrie HC, Warchal EF. Minority and sociocultural issues. In Sadock BJ, Sadock VA, editors: *Kaplan and Sadock's comprehensive textbook of psychiatry*, Philadelphia, 2005, Lippincott Williams & Wilkins.
17. Stewart MA. Effective physician–patient communication and health outcomes: a review. *CMAJ* 152:1423–1433, 1995.
18. Simpson M, Buckman R, Stewart M, et al. Doctor-patient communication: the Toronto consensus statement. *BMJ* 303:1385–1387, 1991.
21. Participants in the Bayer-Fetzer Conference on Physician-Patient Communication in Medical Education: Essential elements of communication in medical encounters: the Kalamazoo Consensus Statement. *Acad Med* 76:390–393, 2001.
22. Novack DH, Epstein RM, Paulsen RH. Toward creating physician-healers: fostering medical students' self-awareness, personal growth, and well-being. *Acad Med* 74:516–520, 1999.
23. Gordon C, Goroll A. Effective psychiatric interviewing to primary care medicine. In Stern TA, Herman JB, Slavin PL, editors: *Massachusetts General Hospital guide in primary care psychiatry*, ed 2, New York, 2004, McGraw-Hill.
24. Kaiser Family Foundation. *Generation M: media in the lives of 8–18 year olds*, Menlo Park (CA), 2005, Kaiser Family Foundation.
28. Villani SV, Olson CK, Jellinek MS. Media literacy for clinicians and parents. In Beresin EV, Olson CK editors: Child Psychiatry and the Media. *Child Adolesc Psychiat Clin N Am* 14:523–553, 2005.
29. Scheiber SC. The psychiatric interview, psychiatric history, and mental status examination. In Hales RE, Yudofsky SC, editors: *The American Psychiatric Press synopsis of psychiatry*, Washington, DC, 1996, American Psychiatric Press.
30. Sadock BJ. Signs and symptoms in psychiatry. In Sadock BJ, Sadock VA, editors: *Kaplan and Sadock's comprehensive textbook of psychiatry*, Philadelphia, 2005, Lippincott Williams & Wilkins.
31. Silberman EK, Certa K. The psychiatric interview: settings and techniques. In Tasman A, Kay J, Lieberman J, editors: *Psychiatry*, ed 2, Hoboken, NJ, 2004, John Wiley & Sons.
32. Folstein MF, Folstein SE, McHugh PE. The Mini-Mental State Exam: a practical method for grading the cognitive state of patients for the clinician. *J Psychiatr Res* 12:189–198, 1975.
33. Dhalla S, Kopec JA. The CAGE questionnaire for alcohol misuse: a review of reliability and validity studies. *Clin Invest Med* 30(1):33–41, 2007.
34. Ewing JA. Detecting alcoholism: the CAGE questionnaire. *JAMA* 252:1905–1907, 1984.
35. Knight JR, Sherritt L, Shrier LA, et al. Validity of the CRAFFT substance abuse screening test among adolescent patients. *Arch Pediatr Adolesc Med* 156(6):607–614, 2002.
36. Knight JR, Shrier LA, Bravender TD, et al. A new brief screen for adolescent substance abuse. *Arch Pediatr Adolesc Med* 153:591–596, 1999.
37. Beresin EV, Schlozman SC. Psychiatric treatment of adolescents. In Sadock BJ, Sadock VA, editors: *Kaplan and Sadock's comprehensive textbook of psychiatry*, Philadelphia, 2005, Lippincott Williams & Wilkins.

BOX 2-8 Common Errors in the Psychiatric Interview

- Premature closure and false assumptions about symptoms
- False reassurance about the patient's condition or prognosis
- Defensiveness around psychiatric diagnoses and treatment, with arrogant responses to myths and complaints about psychiatry
- Omission of significant parts of the interview, due to theoretical bias of the interview (e.g., mind–body splitting)
- Recommendations for treatment when diagnostic formulation is incomplete
- Inadequate explanation of psychiatric disorders and their treatment, particularly not giving the patient multiple options for treatment
- Minimization or denial of the severity of symptoms, due to overidentification with the patient; countertransference phenomenon (e.g., as occurs with treatment of a "very important person" [VIP] in a manner inconsistent with ordinary best practice, with a resultant failure to protect the patient or others)
- Inadvertently shaming or embarrassing a patient, and not offering an apology

---

if the cause of agitation is not known and the patient is not collaborating with the evaluative process.

Disagreements about Assessment and Treatment

There are times when a patient disagrees with a clinician's formulation, diagnosis, and treatment recommendations. In this instance, it is wise to listen to the patient and hear where there is conflict. Then the evaluator should systematically review what was said and how he or she interpreted the clinical findings. The patient should be encouraged to correct misrepresentations. Sometimes clarification will help the clinician and patient come to an agreement. At other times, the patient may deny or minimize a problem. In this case additional interviews may be necessary. It is sometimes useful to involve a close relative or friend, if the patient allows this. If the patient is a danger to self or others, however, protective measures will be needed, short of any agreement. If there is no imminent danger, explaining one's clinical opinion and respecting the right of the patient to choose treatment must be observed.

Errors in Psychiatric Interviewing

Common mistakes made in the psychiatric interview are provided in Box 2-8.

Access the complete reference list and multiple choice questions (MCQs) online at https://expertconsult.inkling.com

KEY REFERENCES

1. Gordon C, Reiss H. The formulation as a collaborative conversation. *Harv Rev Psychiatry* 13:112–123, 2005.
2. Lazare A. Shame and humiliation in the medical encounter. *Arch Intern Med* 147:1653–1658, 1987.
4. Parkes CM, Stevenson-Hinde J, Marris P, editors: *Attachment across the life cycle*, London, 1991, Routledge.
5. Siegel DJ. *The developing mind: How relationships and the brain interact to shape who we are*, ed 2, New York, 2012, Guilford Press.

3 Laboratory Tests and Diagnostic Procedures

Felicia A. Smith, MD, and Charlotte Hogan, MD

KEY POINTS

- The mainstay of psychiatric diagnosis involves a thorough history, mental status examination, and focused physical examination; however, laboratory tests and diagnostic studies are important adjuncts.
- Laboratory tests and diagnostic studies are especially useful in the diagnostic work-up of high-risk populations.
- Laboratory tests provide a clinically useful tool to monitor levels of many psychotropic drugs by guiding medication titration, preventing toxicity, and checking for compliance.
- Although neuroimaging alone rarely establishes a psychiatric diagnosis, contemporary modalities are powerful tools in both the clinical and research realms of modern psychiatry.

OVERVIEW

Modern-day psychiatrists have many tools to help make a diagnosis and to treat patients effectively. While the heart of psychiatric diagnosis remains a careful interview and mental status examination (MSE) (while paying close attention to physical findings), laboratory tests (including blood work, neuroimaging, and an electroencephalogram [EEG]) are important adjuncts. These modalities help reveal medical and neurological causes of psychiatric symptoms, as well as aid in monitoring the progression of certain diseases. They are often of particular benefit in populations (including the elderly, the chronically medically ill, substance users and abusers, and the indigent) at high risk for medical co-morbidity. Laboratory tests are also commonly used to check blood levels of psychotropic medications and to predict potential side effects. This chapter will focus on the role of a wide array of specific serum, urine, and cerebrospinal fluid (CSF) tests, as well as several diagnostic modalities (e.g., the EEG and neuroimaging), with an emphasis on the strategy and rationale for choosing when to order and how to use the data derived from particular studies. Genetic and biological markers will be discussed in subsequent chapters.

A GENERAL APPROACH TO CHOOSING LABORATORY TESTS AND DIAGNOSTIC STUDIES

Diagnoses in psychiatry are primarily made by the identification of symptom patterns, that is, by clinical phenomenology, as outlined in the *Diagnostic and Statistical Manual of Mental Disorders, Fifth Edition* (DSM-5).[1] In this light, the initial approach to psychiatric assessment consists of a thorough history, a comprehensive MSE, and a focused physical examination. Results in each of these arenas guide further testing. For example, historical data and a review of systems may reveal evidence of medical conditions, substance abuse, or a family history of heritable conditions (e.g., Huntington's disease)—each of these considerations would lead down a distinct pathway of diagnostic evaluation. An MSE that uncovers new-onset psychosis or delirium opens up a broad differential diagnosis and numerous possible diagnostic studies from which to choose. Findings from a physical examination may provide key information that suggests a specific underlying pathophysiological mechanism and helps hone testing choices. Although routine screening for new-onset psychiatric illness is often done, consensus is lacking on which studies should be included in a screening battery. In current clinical practice, tests are ordered selectively with specific clinical situations steering this choice. While information obtained in the history, the physical examination, and the MSE is always the starting point, subsequent sections in this chapter address tests involved in the diagnostic evaluation of specific presentations in further detail.

ROUTINE SCREENING

Decisions regarding routine screening for new-onset psychiatric illness involve consideration of the ease of administration, the clinical implications of abnormal results, the sensitivity and specificity, and the cost of tests. Certain presentations (such as age of onset after age 40 years, a history of chronic medical illness, or the sudden onset or rapid progression of symptoms) are especially suggestive of a medical cause of psychiatric symptoms and should prompt administration of a screening battery of tests. In clinical practice, these tests often include the complete blood cell count (CBC); serum chemistries; urine and blood toxicology; levels of vitamin B_{12}, folate, and thyroid-stimulating hormone (TSH); and rapid plasma reagent (RPR). Liver function tests (LFTs), urinalysis, and chest x-ray are often obtained, especially in patients at high risk for dysfunction in these organ systems or in the elderly. A pregnancy test is important in women of childbearing age, from both a diagnostic and treatment-guidance standpoint. Box 3-1 outlines the commonly used screening battery for new-onset psychiatric symptoms. The following sections will move from routine screening to a more tailored approach of choosing a diagnostic work-up that is based on specific signs and symptoms and a plausible differential diagnosis.

PSYCHOSIS AND DELIRIUM

New-onset psychosis or delirium merits a broad and systematic medical and neurological work-up. Table 3-1[2] outlines the wide array of potential medical causes of such psychiatric symptoms. Some etiologies include infections (both systemic and in the central nervous system [CNS]), CNS lesions (e.g., stroke, traumatic bleed, or tumors), metabolic abnormalities, medication effects, intoxication or states of withdrawal, states of low perfusion or low oxygenation, seizures, and autoimmune illnesses. Given the potential morbidity (if not mortality) associated with many of these conditions, prompt diagnosis is essential. A comprehensive, yet efficient and tailored approach to a differential diagnosis involves starting with a thorough history supplemented by both the physical examination and MSE. Particular attention should be paid to vital signs and examination of the neurological and cardiac systems. Table 3-2[3] provides an overview of selected physical findings associated with psychiatric symptoms. Based on the presence of such findings, the clinician then chooses appropriate follow-up studies to help confirm or refute the possible diagnoses. For example,

BOX 3-1 Commonly-Used Screening Battery for New-Onset Psychiatric Symptoms

SCREENING TESTS

- Complete blood count (CBC)
- Serum chemistry panel
- Thyroid-stimulating hormone (TSH)
- Vitamin B_{12} level
- Folate level
- Syphilis serologies (e.g., rapid plasma reagent [RPR], Venereal Disease Research Laboratories [VDRL])
- Toxicology (urine and serum)
- Urine or serum β-human chorionic gonadotropin (in women of childbearing age)
- Liver function tests (LFTs)

TABLE 3-1 Medical and Neurological Causes for Psychiatric Symptoms

Metabolic	Hypernatremia/hyponatremia Hypercalcemia/hypocalcemia Hyperglycemia/hypoglycemia Ketoacidosis Uremic encephalopathy Hepatic encephalopathy Hypoxemia Deficiency states (vitamin B_{12}, folate, and thiamine) Acute intermittent porphyria
Endocrine	Hyperthyroidism/hypothyroidism Hyperparathyroidism/hypoparathyroidism Adrenal insufficiency (primary or secondary) Hypercortisolism Pituitary adenoma Panhypopituitarism Pheochromocytoma
Infectious	HIV/AIDS Meningitis Encephalitis Brain abscess Sepsis Urinary tract infection Lyme disease Neurosyphilis Tuberculosis
Intoxication/ withdrawal	Acute or chronic drug or alcohol intoxication/ withdrawal Medications (side effects, toxic levels, interactions) Heavy metals (lead, mercury, arsenic, manganese) Environmental toxins (e.g., carbon monoxide)
Autoimmune	Systemic lupus erythematosus Rheumatoid arthritis
Vascular	Vasculitis Cerebrovascular accident Multi-infarct dementia Hypertensive encephalopathy
Neoplastic	Central nervous system tumors Paraneoplastic syndromes Pancreatic and endocrine tumors
Epilepsy	Post-ictal or intra-ictal states Complex partial seizures
Structural	Normal pressure hydrocephalus
Degenerative	Alzheimer's disease Parkinson's disease Pick's disease Huntington's disease Wilson's disease
Demyelinating	Multiple sclerosis
Traumatic	Intracranial haemorrhage Traumatic brain injury

Adapted from Roffman JL, Silverman BC, Stern TA. Diagnostic rating scales and laboratory tests. In Stern TA, Fricchione GL, Cassem NH et al, editors: Massachusetts General Hospital handbook of general hospital psychiatry, ed 6, Philadelphia, 2010, Saunders Elsevier.
AIDS, Acquired immunodeficiency syndrome; HIV, human immunodeficiency virus.

tachycardia in the setting of a goiter suggests possible hyperthyroidism and prompts assessment of thyroid studies (Figure 3-1).[4] On the other hand, tachycardia with diaphoresis, tremor, and palmar erythema, along with spider nevi, is suggestive of both alcohol withdrawal and stigmata of cirrhosis from chronic alcohol use (Figure 3-2).[5] The astute clinician would treat for alcohol withdrawal and order laboratory tests (including LFTs, prothrombin time [PT]/international normalized ratio [INR], and possible abdominal imaging), in addition to the screening tests already outlined in Box 3-1. Neuroimaging is indicated in the event of neurological findings, although many would suggest that brain imaging is prudent in any case of new-onset psychosis or acute mental status change (without a clear cause). An EEG may help to diagnose seizures or provide a further clue to the diagnosis of a toxic or metabolic encephalopathy. A lumbar puncture (LP) is indicated (after ruling-out an intracranial lesion or increased intracerebral pressure) in a patient who has fever, headache, photophobia, or meningeal symptoms. Depending on the clinical circumstances, routine CSF studies (e.g., the appearance, opening pressure, cell counts, levels of protein and glucose, culture results, and a Gram stain), as well as specialized markers (e.g., antigens for herpes simplex virus, cryptococcus, and Lyme disease; a cytological examination for malignancy; and acid-fast staining for tuberculosis), should be ordered. A history of risky sexual behavior or of intravenous (IV) or intranasal drug use makes testing for infection with the human immunodeficiency virus (HIV) and hepatitis C especially important. Based on clinical suspicion, other tests might include an antinuclear antibody (ANA) and an erythrocyte sedimentation rate (ESR) for autoimmune diseases (e.g., systemic lupus erythematosus [SLE], rheumatoid arthritis [RA]), ceruloplasmin (that is decreased in Wilson's disease), and levels of serum heavy metals (e.g., mercury, lead, arsenic, and manganese). Box 3-2[6] provides an initial approach to the diagnostic work-up of psychosis and delirium. Specific studies will be further discussed based on an organ-system approach to follow.

ANXIETY DISORDERS

Medical conditions associated with new-onset anxiety are associated with a host of organ systems. For anxiety, as with other psychiatric symptoms, a late onset, a precipitous course, atypical symptoms, or a history of chronic medical illness raises the suspicion of a medical rather than a primary psychiatric etiology. Table 3-3[7] lists many of the potential medical etiologies for anxiety. These include cardiac disease (including myocardial infarction [MI] and mitral valve prolapse [MVP]); respiratory compromise (e.g., chronic obstructive pulmonary disease [COPD], asthma exacerbation, pulmonary embolism, pneumonia, and obstructive sleep apnea [OSA]); endocrine dysfunction (e.g., of the thyroid or parathyroid); neurological disorders (e.g., seizures or brain injury); or use or abuse of drugs and other substances. Less common causes (e.g., pheochromocytoma, acute intermittent porphyria, and hyperadrenalism) should be investigated if warranted by the clinical

TABLE 3-2 Selected Findings on the Physical Examination Associated with Neuropsychiatric Manifestations

Elements	Possible Examples
GENERAL APPEARANCE	
Body habitus—thin	Eating disorders, nutritional deficiency states, cachexia of chronic illness
Body habitus—obese	Eating disorders, obstructive sleep apnea, metabolic syndrome (neuroleptic side effect)
VITAL SIGNS	
Fever	Infection or neuroleptic malignant syndrome (NMS)
Blood pressure or pulse abnormalities	Cardiovascular or cerebral perfusion dysfunction; intoxication or withdrawal states, thyroid disease
Tachypnea/low oxygen saturation	Hypoxemia
SKIN	
Diaphoresis	Fever; alcohol, opiate, or benzodiazepine withdrawal
Dry, flushed	Anticholinergic toxicity
Pallor	Anemia
Unkempt hair or fingernails	Poor self-care or malnutrition
Scars	Previous trauma or self-injury
Track marks/abscesses	Intravenous drug use
Characteristic stigmata	Syphilis, cirrhosis, or self-mutilation
Bruises	Physical abuse, ataxia, traumatic brain injury
Cherry red skin and mucous membranes	Carbon monoxide poisoning
Goiter	Thyroid disease
EYES	
Mydriasis	Opiate withdrawal, anticholinergic toxicity
Miosis	Opiate intoxication
Kayser–Fleischer pupillary rings	Wilson's disease
NEUROLOGICAL	
Tremors, agitation, myoclonus	Delirium, withdrawal syndromes, parkinsonism
Presence of primitive reflexes (e.g., snout, glabellar, and grasp)	Dementia, frontal lobe dysfunction
Hyperactive deep-tendon reflexes	Alcohol or benzodiazepine withdrawal, delirium
Ophthalmoplegia	Wernicke's encephalopathy, brainstem dysfunction, dystonic reaction
Papilledema	Increased intracranial pressure
Hypertonia, rigidity, catatonia, parkinsonism	Extrapyramidal symptoms (EPS) of antipsychotics, NMS, organic causes of catatonia
Abnormal movements	Parkinson's disease, Huntington's disease, EPS
Gait disturbance	Normal pressure hydrocephalus, Huntington's disease, Parkinson's disease
Loss of position and vibratory sense	Vitamin B_{12} or thiamine deficiency
Kernig or Brudzinski sign	Meningitis

Adapted from Smith FA, Querques J, Levenson JL, Stern TA. Psychiatric assessment and consultation. In Levenson JL, editor: The American Psychiatric Publishing textbook of psychosomatic medicine, Washington, DC, 2005, American Psychiatric Publishing.

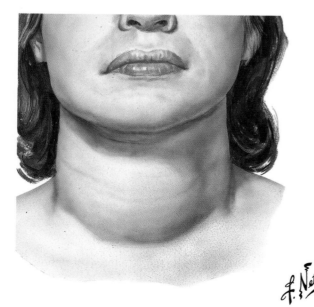

Figure 3-1. Thyroid pathology in hyperthyroidism with diffuse goiter. (From Netter Anatomy Illustration Collection, © Elsevier Inc. All rights reserved.)

presentation. See Table 3-3 for the appropriate laboratory and diagnostic tests associated with each of these diagnoses.

MOOD DISORDERS

While depression may be a primary psychiatric disorder, it is also associated with medical conditions. Clinical findings suggestive of thyroid dysfunction, Addison's disease or Cushing's disease, pituitary adenoma, neurodegenerative disorders, SLE, anemia, or pancreatic cancer should guide further testing. Work-up of these conditions is described below. The new onset of mania merits a full medical and neurological evaluation on a par with that of psychosis and delirium as previously described. While not every diagnostic test and its potential manifestation are discussed here, the following sections provide a more comprehensive system-driven approach to such a diagnostic work-up.

METABOLIC AND NUTRITIONAL

Myriad metabolic conditions and nutritional deficiencies are associated with psychiatric manifestations. Table 3-4[8] provides a list of metabolic tests with their pertinent findings associated with neuropsychiatric dysfunction. Metabolic encephalopathy should be considered in the event of abrupt changes in one's mental status or level of consciousness. The laboratory work-up

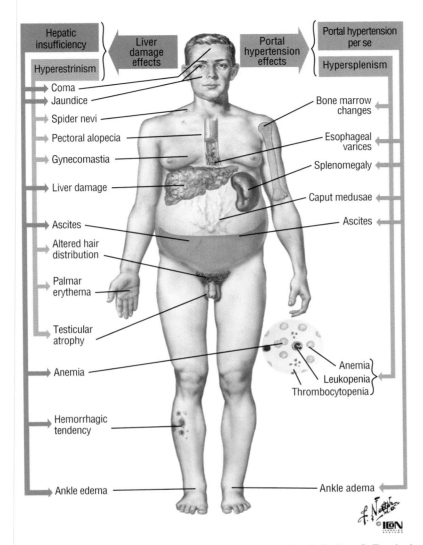

Figure 3-2. Gross features of cirrhosis of the liver. *(From Netter Anatomy Illustration Collection, © Elsevier Inc. All rights reserved.)*

BOX 3-2 Approach to the Evaluation of Psychosis and Delirium

SCREENING TESTS
- Complete blood count (CBC)
- Serum chemistry panel
- Thyroid-stimulating hormone (TSH)
- Vitamin B_{12} level
- Folate level
- Syphilis serologies
- Toxicology (urine and serum)
- Urine or serum β-human chorionic gonadotropin (in women of childbearing age)

FURTHER LABORATORY TESTS BASED ON CLINICAL SUSPICION
- Liver function tests
- Calcium
- Phosphorus
- Magnesium
- Ammonia
- Ceruloplasmin

- Urinalysis
- Blood or urine cultures
- Human immunodeficiency virus (HIV) test
- Erythrocyte sedimentation rate (ESR)
- Serum heavy metals
- Paraneoplastic studies

OTHER DIAGNOSTIC STUDIES BASED ON CLINICAL SUSPICION
- Lumbar puncture (cell count, appearance, opening pressure, Gram stain, culture, specialized markers)
- Electroencephalogram (EEG)
- Electrocardiogram (ECG)
- Chest x-ray
- Arterial blood gas

NEUROIMAGING
- Computed tomography (CT)
- Magnetic resonance imaging (MRI)
- Positron emission tomography (PET)

Adapted from Smith FA. An approach to the use of laboratory tests. In Stern TA, editor: The ten-minute guide to psychiatric diagnosis and treatment, *New York, 2005, Professional Publishing Group, Ltd, p 318.*

TABLE 3-3 Medical Etiologies of Anxiety with Diagnostic Tests

Condition	Screening Test
METABOLIC	
Hypoglycemia	Serum glucose
ENDOCRINE	
Thyroid dysfunction	Thyroid function tests
Parathyroid dysfunction	PTH, ionized calcium
Menopause	Estrogen, FSH
Hyperadrenalism	Dexamethasone suppression test or 24-hour urine cortisol
INTOXICATION/WITHDRAWAL STATES	
Alcohol, drugs, medications	Urine/serum toxicology
	Vital signs
	Specific drug levels
Environmental toxins	Heavy metal screen
	Carbon monoxide level
AUTOIMMUNE	
Porphyria	Urine porphyrins
Pheochromocytoma	Urine vanillylmandelic acid (VMA)
CARDIAC	
Myocardial infarction	ECG, troponin, CK-MB
Mitral valve prolapse	Cardiac ultrasound
PULMONARY	
COPD, asthma, pneumonia	Pulse oximetry, chest x-ray, pulmonary function tests
Sleep apnea	Pulse oximetry, polysomnography
Pulmonary embolism	D-dimer, V/Q scan, CT scan of chest
EPILEPSY	
Seizure	EEG
TRAUMA	
Intracranial bleed, traumatic brain injury	CT, MRI of brain
	Neuropsychiatric testing

Adapted from Smith FA. An approach to the use of laboratory tests. In Stern TA, editor: The ten-minute guide to psychiatric diagnosis and treatment, New York, 2005, Professional Publishing Group, Ltd, p 319.
CK-MB, Creatine phosphokinase-MB band; COPD, chronic obstructive pulmonary disease; CT, computed tomography; ECG, electrocardiogram; EEG, electroencephalogram; FSH, follicle-stimulating hormone; MRI, magnetic resonance imaging; PTH, parathyroid hormone; V/Q, ventilation/perfusion.

TABLE 3-4 Metabolic and Hematological Tests Associated with Psychiatric Manifestations

Test	Pertinent Findings
Alanine aminotransferase (ALT)	Increased in hepatitis, cirrhosis, liver metastasis Decreased with pyridoxine (vitamin B_6) deficiency
Albumin	Increased with dehydration Decreased with malnutrition, hepatic failure, burns, multiple myeloma, carcinomas
Alkaline phosphatase	Increased with hyperparathyroidism, hepatic disease/metastases, heart failure, phenothiazine use Decreased with pernicious anemia (vitamin B_{12} deficiency)
Ammonia	Increased with hepatic encephalopathy/failure, gastrointestinal bleed, severe congestive heart failure (CHF)
Amylase	Increased with pancreatic disease/cancer
Aspartate aminotransferase (SGOT/AST)	Increased with hepatic disease, pancreatitis, alcohol abuse
Bicarbonate	Increased with psychogenic vomiting Decreased with hyperventilation, panic, anabolic steroid use
Bilirubin, total	Increased with hepatic, biliary, pancreatic disease
Bilirubin, direct	Increased with hepatic, biliary, pancreatic disease
Blood urea nitrogen	Increased with renal disease, dehydration, lethargy, delirium
Calcium	Increased with hyperparathyroidism, bone metastasis, mood disorders, psychosis Decreased with hypoparathyroidism, renal failure, depression, irritability
Carbon dioxide	Decreased with hyperventilation, panic, anabolic steroid abuse
Ceruloplasmin	Decreased with Wilson's disease
Chloride	Decreased with psychogenic vomiting Increased with hyperventilation, panic

TABLE 3-4 Metabolic and Hematological Tests Associated with Psychiatric Manifestations *(Continued)*

Test	Pertinent Findings
Complete blood count (CBC) • Hemoglobin, hematocrit • White blood cell count • Platelets • Mean corpuscular volume • Reticulocyte count	Decrease associated with depression and psychosis Increase associated with lithium use and neuroleptic malignant syndrome (NMS) Decrease associated with psychotropic medications (phenothiazine, carbamazepine, and clozapine) Decrease associated with psychotropic medications (phenothiazine, carbamazepine, and clozapine) Increased with alcohol use, vitamin B_{12} or folate deficiency Decreased with certain anemias (megaloblastic, iron deficiency, chronic disease)
Creatine phosphokinase (CK, CPK)	Increased with NMS, intramuscular injection, rhabdomyolysis, restraints, dystonic reactions, antipsychotic use
Creatinine	Increased with renal disease
Erythrocyte sedimentation rate (ESR)	Increased with infection (non-specific), inflammation, autoimmune, or malignant process
Ferritin	Decreased with iron deficiency; associated with fatigue, depression
Folate	Decrease associated with fatigue, agitation, dementia, delirium, psychosis, paranoia, alcohol abuse, phenytoin use
γ-Glutamyltranspeptidase (GGT)	Increased with alcohol, cirrhosis, liver disease
Glucose	Increase associated with delirium Decrease associated with delirium, agitation, panic, anxiety, depression
Iron-binding capacity	Increased with iron deficiency anemia; associated with fatigue, depression
Iron, total	Decreased with iron deficiency anemia; associated with fatigue, depression
Lactate dehydrogenase (LDH)	Increased with myocardial infarction, pulmonary infarction, hepatic disease, renal infarction, seizures, cerebral damage, pernicious anemia; red blood cell destruction
Magnesium	Decreased with alcohol abuse; associated with agitation, delirium, seizures Increased with panhypopituitarism
Phosphorus	Decreased with renal failure, diabetic acidosis, hypoparathyroidism Decreased with cirrhosis, hyperparathyroidism, hypokalemia, panic, hyperventilation
Potassium	Increased with hyperkalemia acidosis, anxiety in cardiac arrhythmia Decreased with cirrhosis, metabolic alkalosis, psychogenic vomiting, anabolic steroid use
Protein, total	Increased with multiple myeloma, myxedema, systemic lupus erythematosus Decreased with cirrhosis, malnutrition, over-hydration (may affect protein-bound medication levels)
Sodium	Decreased with hypoadrenalism, myxedema, CHF, diarrhea, polydipsia, carbamazepine use, selective serotonin reuptake inhibitor (SSRI) use, syndrome of inappropriate antidiuretic hormone (SIADH), anabolic steroids Decrease results in increased sensitivity to lithium use
Urine aminolevulinic acid (ALA) and porphobilinogen (PBG)	Increased in acute intermittent porphyria
Vitamin A	Increased with hypervitaminosis A; associated with depression and delirium
Vitamin B_{12}	Decrease results in megaloblastic anemia, dementia, psychosis, paranoia, fatigue, agitation, dementia, delirium

Adapted from Smith FA, Alpay M, Park L. Laboratory tests and diagnostic procedures. In Stern TA, Herman JB, Gorrindo T, editors: Massachusetts General Hospital psychiatry update and board preparation, ed 3, Boston, 2012, MGH Psychiatry Academy.

of hepatic encephalopathy (which often manifests as delirium with asterixis) may reveal elevations in LFTs (e.g., aspartate aminotransferase [AST] and alanine aminotransferase [ALT]), bilirubin (direct and total), and ammonia. Likewise, the patient with uremic encephalopathy generally has an elevated blood urea nitrogen (BUN) and creatinine (consistent with renal failure). Acute intermittent porphyria (AIP) is a less common, yet still important, cause of neuropsychiatric symptoms (including anxiety, mood lability, insomnia, depression, and psychosis). This diagnosis should be considered in a patient who has psychiatric symptoms in conjunction with abdominal pain or neuropathy. When suggestive neurovisceral symptoms are present, concentration of urinary aminolevulinic acid (ALA), porphobilinogen (PBG), and porphyrin should be measured from a 24-hour urine collection. While normal excretion of ALA is less than 7 mg per 24 hours, during

an attack of AIP urinary ALA excretion is markedly elevated (sometimes to more than 10 times the upper limit of normal) as are PBG levels. In severe cases, the urine looks like port wine when exposed to sunlight due to a high concentration of porphobilin.

Nutritional deficiencies must also be considered in the patient who has depressed mood, lethargy, poor concentration, or cognitive changes. Thiamine (vitamin B_1) deficiency often starts with mood and anxiety symptoms and leads to Wernicke–Korsakoff syndrome (which is most often associated with chronic alcohol abuse) if left untreated. Severe amnestic disorders may develop with prolonged deficiencies. Cobalamin deficiency (vitamin B_{12}) is characterized by the development of a chronic macrocytic anemia (Figure 3-3) with neurological and psychiatric manifestations that include peripheral neuropathy, apathy, irritability, and depression.

Encephalopathy, with associated dementia or psychosis, may also be seen. Folate deficiency has also been associated with depression and dementia, and should be checked in malnourished patients or in those who are taking certain anticonvulsants (e.g., phenytoin, primidone, or phenobarbital), as well as oral contraceptive pills. Finally, vitamin D deficiency has been associated with mood disorders and should be considered in the depressed patient.

NEUROENDOCRINE DISORDERS

Endocrine disorders (involving thyroid, parathyroid, adrenal, and pituitary dysfunction) are associated with a vast array of psychiatric symptoms. While depression and anxiety are the most common manifestations, psychosis and delirium can arise in extreme or later-diagnosed situations. Table 3-5[9] lists diagnostic tests and pertinent laboratory findings in the work-up of suspected neuroendocrine-associated psychiatric symptoms. Approximately 8% of patients with depressive disorders have some form of thyroid dysfunction.[10] Hypothyroidism may also mimic depression (with symptoms including fatigue, lethargy, poor appetite, low mood, and cognitive dulling). Later findings can include hallucinations and paranoia—so-called "myxedema madness" (Figure 3-4).[11] Lithium therapy also causes hypothyroidism; accordingly,

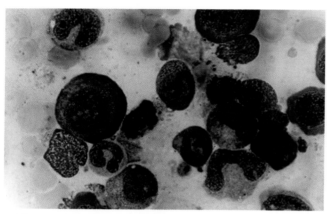

Figure 3-3. Blood smear of a patient with macrocytic anemia.

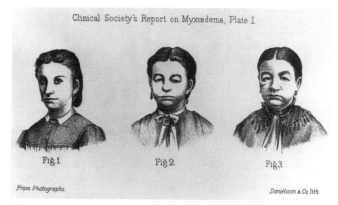

Figure 3-4. Myxedema. *(From Kim G, Davies TF: Hypothyroidism. In Besser MG, Thorner MO, editors: Comprehensive clinical endocrinology, ed 3, 2002, Elsevier Science Limited, p 139.)*

TABLE 3-5 Neuroendocrine Tests Associated with Psychiatric Manifestations

Test	Pertinent Findings
Adrenocorticotropic hormone (ACTH)	Increased in Cushing's disease, primary adrenal insufficiency, stress response, steroid use Decreased in secondary adrenal insufficiency
Alkaline phosphatase	Increased in hyperparathyroidism
Calcium	Increased in hyperparathyroidism Decreased in hypoparathyroidism
Catecholamines (urinary and plasma)	Increased in pheochromocytoma
Cortisol	Increased in Cushing's disease Decreased in adrenal insufficiency
Estrogen	Decreased in menopause and premenstrual syndrome (may be associated with depression)
Follicle-stimulating hormone (FSH)	Increased in postmenopausal women Decreased in panhypopituitarism
Gonadotropin-releasing hormone (GnRH)	Decreased in schizophrenia; variable in depression and anxiety
Growth hormone	Variable association with schizophrenia and depression
Luteinizing hormone (LH)	Decreased with panhypopituitarism; associated with depression
Parathyroid hormone	Decrease associated with anxiety Dysregulation associated with cognitive deficits
Phosphorus	Increased in hypoparathyroidism Decreased in hyperparathyroidism
Prolactin	Increased with antipsychotic use, cocaine withdrawal, acute seizure, prolactinoma
Testosterone	Increased with anabolic steroid use Decrease contributes to decreased libido, impotence
Thyroid-stimulating hormone	Increased in hypothyroidism (lithium therapy) Decreased in hyperthyroidism
Thyroxine (T_4)	Increased in hyperthyroidism Decreased in hypothyroidism (lithium therapy)

From Sadock BJ, Sadock VA. Kaplan and Sadock's synopsis of psychiatry, ed 10, Philadelphia, 2007, Lipincott Williams & Wilkins, pp 263–267.

patients taking lithium should have thyroid levels checked at least twice a year. Patients with hyperthyroidism, on the other hand, often appear restless, anxious, or labile and may appear to have an anxiety or panic disorder. Testing of TSH and thyroxine (see Table 3-5) begins the diagnostic work-up. Parathyroid disorders affect mental status largely due to perturbations in calcium and phosphate. With hyperparathyroidism, apathy, lethargy, and depression are associated with hypercalcemia. Conversely, hypoparathyroidism and concomitant hypocalcemia may manifest as a personality change or delirium.

Adrenal dysfunction can also cause psychiatric symptoms. Adrenal insufficiency may occur as a primary disease process (Addison's disease) due to autoimmune destruction of adrenal glands or as a secondary condition due to hypothalamic–pituitary disease and adrenocorticotropic hormone (ACTH) deficiency. Abrupt withdrawal of exogenous steroid therapy is a cause of secondary hypercortisolism. Psychiatric symptoms may run the gamut from apathy, negativism, depressed mood, and fatigue (an early symptom) to psychosis and delirium (a late manifestation). In primary adrenal failure a random serum cortisol level will be low, while the ACTH level will be high. Secondary adrenal failure is accompanied by low levels of both ACTH and cortisol.[12] Hypercortisolism is also problematic and may result from a variety of sources (including chronic hypersecretion of ACTH, pituitary adenoma [Cushing's disease], non-pituitary neoplasm [Cushing's syndrome], or from direct over-secretion of cortisol from an adrenal tumor or hyperplasia). Physical manifestations include the classic cushingoid stigmata (Figure 3-5)[13] of hirsutism, moon facies, truncal obesity, acne, and peripheral wasting. Psychiatric symptoms often mimic both anxiety and depression; less common manifestations include psychotic symptoms. Diagnostic evaluation involves measurement of ACTH (levels vary depending on cause of the illness) and a dexamethasone suppression test (DST) to demonstrate the impaired feedback regulation of the pituitary–adrenal axis in Cushing's syndrome from any etiology. The DST is undertaken to measure suppression of cortisol during the normal cortisol circadian rhythm, whereby dexamethasone (1 mg) is given at bedtime and cortisol levels are drawn at various times throughout the next day (generally 08:00, 16:00, and 23:00). The normal effect is suppression of cortisol release. Non-suppression is defined as a cortisol level greater than 5 mcg/dl and represents an impaired pituitary–adrenal axis feedback loop.[14,15] Severe depression (especially melancholic depression) has been associated with

non-suppression; however, sensitivity of the DST in the detection of major depression is at best moderate, making it of little benefit as a diagnostic test for primary depression.

Pituitary dysfunction disrupts multiple organ systems and, consequently, may contribute to wide-ranging psychiatric symptoms. Pituitary adenoma (Figure 3-6)[16] may cause all of the symptoms associated with Cushing's syndrome. Panhypopituitarism, as well as abnormal levels of follicle-stimulating hormone (FSH), growth hormone (GH), gonadotropin-releasing hormone (GnRH), estrogen, and testosterone, may also have neuropsychiatric effects. Levels and pertinent findings are outlined in Table 3-5.

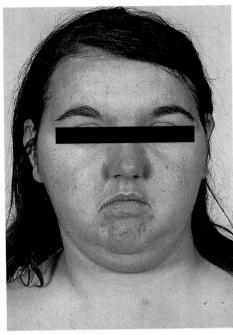

Figure 3-5. Clinical appearance of Cushing's syndrome. *(From Trainer PJ, Besser MG: Cushing's syndrome. In Besser MG, Thorner MO, editors: Comprehensive clinical endocrinology, ed 3, 2002, Elsevier Science Limited, p 194.)*

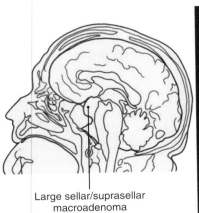

Large sellar/suprasellar macroadenoma

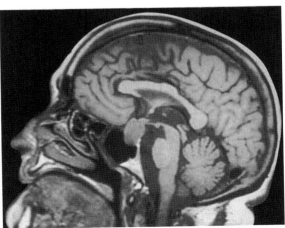

Figure 3-6. Pituitary adenoma. *(From Peebles T, Haughton VM: Neuroradiology and endocrine disease. In Besser MG, Thorner MO, editors: Comprehensive clinical endocrinology, ed 3, 2002, Elsevier Science Limited, CD-ROM.)*

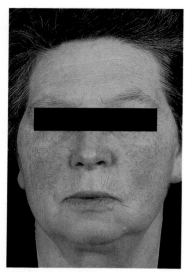

Figure 3-7. Systemic lupus erythematosus. *(Illustration used with permission from Dr. LM Buja. Originally appeared in Buja/Krueger: Netter's Illustrated Human Pathology, © 2005, Elsevier. All Rights Reserved.)*

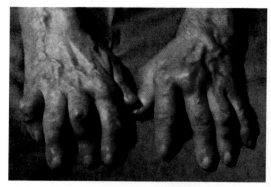

Figure 3-8. Rheumatoid arthritis. *(Illustration used with permission from Dr. LM Buja. Originally appeared in Buja/Krueger: Netter's Illustrated Human Pathology, © 2005, Elsevier. All Rights Reserved.)*

IMMUNE DISORDERS

SLE and rheumatoid arthritis (RA) are both associated with more psychiatric co-morbidity than is seen in the general population. SLE is an autoimmune disease involving inflammation of multiple organ systems; it has a high prevalence of neuropsychiatric manifestations (e.g., depression, emotional lability, anxiety, insomnia, and confusion). Mania and psychosis may also be seen—especially in patients treated with steroids. Roughly 50% of patients with SLE eventually develop neuropsychiatric manifestations.[17] Lupus usually arises in the second or third decades and is seen predominantly in women (with a female-to-male ratio of 9 : 1).[18] Physical signs of SLE include the characteristic butterfly (malar) erythema rash (Figure 3-7)[19] and acute arthritis. Laboratory work-up includes the immunofluorescence test for ANA (a test that is sensitive, but not specific), and tests for antibodies to double-stranded DNA (dsDNA) and the Smith (Sm) antigen.

RA, characterized by chronic musculoskeletal pain from inflamed joints (Figure 3-8),[19] is associated with depression in approximately 20% of individuals.[20] Co-morbid RA and depression often results in worse functional status, more painful flares, more time missed from work, and increased use of the health care system. Rheumatoid factor and acute phase reactants (such as the ESR) are often elevated in RA.

INFECTIOUS DISEASES

Infections involving the CNS appear on the differential of both acute-onset and chronic neuropsychiatric symptoms. Although fever and leukocytosis are often present, chronic infections do not cause this typical pattern. The diagnosis in this instance involves performing a careful history, physical examination, and review of systems to accompany the MSE. Particular attention should be paid to predisposing risk factors, as these significantly help guide subsequent work-up. Table 3-6[21-23] lays out the serological studies involved in the diagnosis of the human immunodeficiency virus (HIV) infection, as well as infection with herpes simplex virus (HSV), neurosyphilis, Lyme disease, and meningitis/encephalitis. Neuropsychiatric symptoms affiliated with these conditions run the gamut

from depression, anxiety, and fatigue to psychosis, mania, and dementia. Since each of these entities is fully described in Chapter 21, further description here will be deferred.

DEGENERATIVE DISORDERS

Neurodegenerative disorders are important to consider in the differential diagnosis of psychiatric symptoms. Wilson's disease is one such disorder in which the abnormal accumulation of copper leads to cirrhosis and to neuronal degeneration. It is an autosomal recessive disorder with the disease gene located on chromosome 13.[24] Wilson's disease should be considered in patients with manifestations that include speech impairment, extrapyramidal dysfunction, and new-onset psychiatric disturbance (especially in patients younger than 30 years), as well as liver disease. Diagnostic work-up includes analysis of a 24-hour urine sample for copper and plasma ceruloplasmin, as well as a slit-lamp examination for Kayser–Fleischer rings (from copper deposition in the cornea), and a liver biopsy (with measurement of liver copper). Genetic testing helps confirm the diagnosis. Figure 3-9[25] shows the multiple organ systems affected by this disorder.

Multiple sclerosis (MS), one of the most common causes of chronic neurological dysfunction in middle-aged adults,[25] may manifest with varied neurological symptoms, as well as a host of psychiatric symptoms. The primary process is one of demyelination in any CNS area (from the optic nerves to the distal spinal cord) with symptoms dependent on the area of the specific lesion. Psychiatric symptoms run the gamut from depression to anxiety to (less frequently) psychosis. From a diagnostic standpoint, neuroimaging is the most helpful adjunct to history and physical examination. Magnetic resonance imaging (MRI) of the brain characteristically shows ovoid lesions in the corpus callosum, periventricular and subcortical white matter, middle cerebellar peduncle, pons, or medulla (Figure 3-10).[25] An MRI showing spinal cord lesions helps confirm the diagnosis, while CSF studies may reveal oligoclonal bands. The variable and fluctuating symptomatology of this illness can lead to misdiagnosis as a conversion disorder—care must be taken therefore to perform an adequate diagnostic work-up. Huntington's disease, Pick's disease, and normal pressure hydrocephalus (NPH) are all disorders that often cause psychiatric symptoms. When any of these is suspected, neuroimaging is generally the mainstay of the initial diagnostic evaluation—further details are explained in detail in subsequent chapters.

TABLE 3-6 Serological Studies Associated with Conditions with Psychiatric Manifestations

Test	Pertinent Findings
Antinuclear antibody	Positive in SLE and drug-induced lupus—associated with depression, delirium, and psychosis
Epstein–Barr virus (EBV) (Monospot)	Causative agent for mononucleosis—may manifest with symptoms of depression, fatigue
Cytomegalovirus (CMV)	Positive test associated with anxiety, mood disorders
Erythrocyte sedimentation rate (ESR)	Elevated in infection, autoimmune, or malignant disease
Hepatitis A viral antigen	Positive test associated with depressive symptoms
Hepatitis B surface antigen, hepatitis B core antigen	Active hepatitis B infection linked with depressive symptoms
Hepatitis B surface antibody	Prior hepatitis B infection or vaccination
Hepatitis C antibody (screening)/hepatitis C virus RNA (confirmatory)	Chronic infection associated with neurocognitive deficits
Human immunodeficiency virus (HIV) antibody/HIV viral load	Acute infection may cause mood or psychotic symptoms; central nervous system (CNS) involvement may cause delirium, dementia, mood and psychotic symptoms, and personality change
Venereal Disease Research Laboratory (VDRL), rapid plasma reagent (RPR)	High titers in syphilis (CNS involvement with tertiary syphilis)

From Sadock BJ, Sadock VA. Kaplan and Sadock's synopsis of psychiatry, ed 10, Philadelphia, 2007, Lipincott Williams & Wilkins, pp 263–267; Sax PE, Bartlett JG. Acute and early HIV infection: Clinical manifestations and diagnosis. In UpToDate, 2013; and Chopra S, Terrault NA, Di Bisceglie AM. Screening for and diagnosis of chronic hepatitis C virus infection. In UpToDate, 2013.

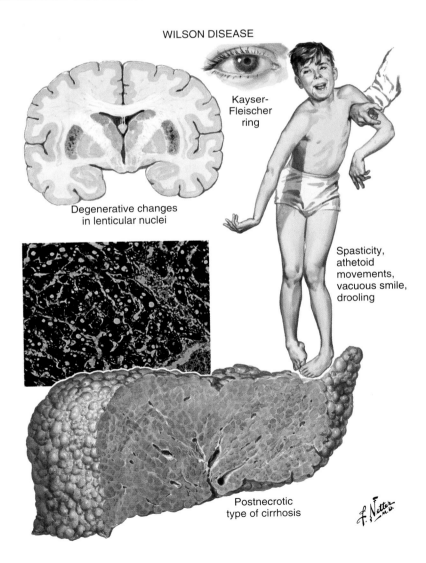

WILSON DISEASE

Kayser-Fleischer ring

Degenerative changes in lenticular nuclei

Spasticity, athetoid movements, vacuous smile, drooling

Postnecrotic type of cirrhosis

Figure 3-9. Wilson's disease. (From Netter Anatomy Illustration Collection, © Elsevier Inc. All rights reserved.)

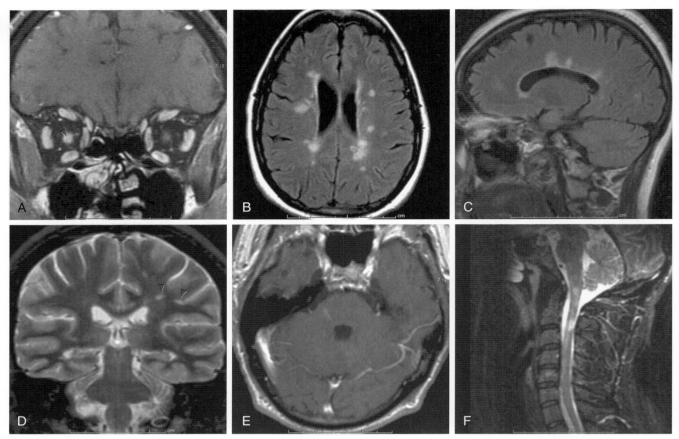

Figure 3-10. MRI findings in multiple sclerosis. *(From Netter Anatomy Illustration Collection, © Elsevier Inc. All rights reserved.)*

TABLE 3-7 Serum and Urine Toxicology Screens for Drugs of Abuse

Substance	Duration of Serum Detection	Duration of Urine Detection
Alcohol	1–2 days	1 day
Amphetamine	Variable	1–2 days
Barbiturates	Variable	3 days–3 weeks
Benzodiazepines	Variable	2–3 days
Cocaine	Hours to 1 day	2–3 days
Codeine, morphine, heroin	Variable	1–2 days
Delta-9-THC	N/A	30 days or longer (chronic use)
Methadone	15–29 hours	2–3 days
Phencyclidine	N/A	8 days
Propoxyphene	8–34 hours	1–2 days

Adapted from Roffman JL, Silverman BC, Stern TA. Diagnostic rating scales and laboratory tests. In Stern TA, Fricchione GL, Cassem NH et al, editors: Massachusetts General Hospital handbook of general hospital psychiatry, ed 6, Philadelphia, 2010, Saunders Elsevier.

SUBSTANCE USE DISORDERS

Substance abuse and withdrawal may manifest myriad psychiatric symptoms (including anxiety, depression, confusion, psychosis, and agitation). Serum and urine toxicology screens are extremely helpful whenever substance use or abuse is suspected. Table 3-7[2] summarizes substances available for testing and the estimated duration of positive results after use.

Alcohol

Alcohol levels can be quickly assessed by use of a breathalyzer, although it is important to remember that breath or serum levels of alcohol do not necessarily predict the timing of withdrawal symptoms. Those with a history of alcohol abuse should have a CBC checked to look for anemia and thrombocytopenia—both complications of chronic alcohol use. An elevated mean corpuscular volume (MCV) in the presence of anemia (typically a macrocytic anemia) should also prompt checking of vitamin B_{12} and folate levels. LFTs should be assessed to screen for hepatitis. If abnormal, it is prudent to check synthetic function with a partial thromboplastin time (PTT) and a PT/INR since chronic liver damage may lead to coagulopathy. The presence of abdominal pain or nausea and vomiting in an alcohol abuser may indicate pancreatitis—abnormal levels of amylase and lipase help to confirm this diagnosis. Chronic alcohol use may lead to a cardiomyopathy. When this is suspected (based on history and physical examination) a cardiac ultrasound can help confirm or refute the hypothesis. The presence of mental status or cognitive changes (especially with affiliated neurological signs, such as disturbance of gait or ophthalmoplegia) raises suspicion for neurological complications to which alcohol abusers are prone. These include acute events (such as subdural hematoma) or other traumatic injuries along with more chronic neurological sequelae of the illness (including Wernicke's encephalopathy) and cerebellar atrophy. Computed tomography (CT) or MRI of the brain is indicated in these situations (see the neuroimaging section later in this chapter for further details).

Cocaine and Stimulants

Abuse of cocaine and stimulants is associated with several serious risks, including cardiac, neurological, and infectious complications. Although the duration of detection of cocaine in the serum is fairly short (see Table 3-7), toxicological screening remains helpful in that a positive result confirms a clinical suspicion of use. The presence of cocaethylene in the serum indicates the combination of cocaine and alcohol use—these patients may be highly agitated. Further diagnostic work-up centers on the history and physical findings. Complaints of chest pain or abnormal vital signs are reason to check an electrocardiogram (ECG) and cardiac biomarkers (including creatine phosphokinase [CPK], troponin-t, and CPK isoenzymes), since the risk of cardiac events with acute cocaine use is significant. Likewise, the presence of neurological findings may signify acute stroke (which is high in users of cocaine)—in this situation, neuroimaging is in order. Finally, intranasal or IV cocaine use is a risk factor for HIV infection and hepatitis C—serologies for each of these should be checked in appropriate clinical settings.

Opiates

Opiate intoxication causes lethargy and pupillary constriction (Figure 3-11); opiate withdrawal, by contrast, is suspected in the setting of diaphoresis, gooseflesh, abdominal cramping, and pupillary dilation (Figure 3-12). IV and intradermal (e.g., skin popping) opiate abusers are at risk for local abscesses, as well as for systemic infections—when signs of local infection are accompanied by fever or hemodynamic instability, blood cultures should be obtained to assess for bacteremia. A heart murmur in this setting should prompt a cardiac ultrasound to rule out endocarditis. As with IV cocaine users, screening for HIV and hepatitis is also indicated in this population. Figure 3-13 summarizes the major medical consequences of opiate (IV heroin) addiction.

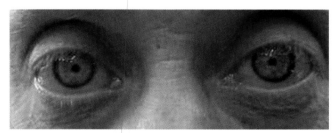

Figure 3-11. Constricted pupils of opiate intoxication.

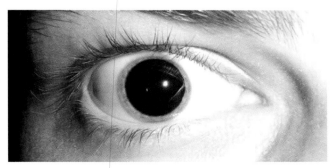

Figure 3-12. Dilated pupils of opiate withdrawal.

Steroids

Anabolic steroid abuse (embarked on to increase muscle bulk and to enhance physical performance) can have both psychiatric and medical complications. From a psychiatric perspective, users may experience euphoria, hyperactivity, anger ("roid rage"), irritability, anxiety, depression, or psychosis. If the history is unrevealing, physical stigmata (such as acne, premature balding, jaundice, and gynecomastia [males]; and deep voice, hirsutism, breast shrinkage, and menstrual irregularity [females]) may be a tip-off to use and abuse. Laboratory work-up involves determination of LFTs and levels of high-density lipoprotein (HDL) and low-density lipoprotein (LDL), which may be decreased and increased, respectively. MI and cerebrovascular diseases may also be seen.

TOXINS

In addition to substances of abuse, a variety of environmental toxins should be considered in the psychiatric setting. Table 3-8 summarizes the sources, effects, and diagnostic work-up of patients who have either accidentally or intentionally ingested heavy metals (e.g., lead, mercury, arsenic, and manganese), as well as carbon monoxide and methanol.[26-28] Neuropsychiatric manifestations range from subtle changes in personality to depression, irritability, anxiety, and delirium. Medical complications can affect a wide array of organ systems and even culminate in death. Patients at high risk of exposure (e.g., miners, in the case of arsenic) or those with a suspected suicide attempt (e.g., via carbon monoxide poisoning) should undergo further work-up as outlined in Table 3-8.

EATING DISORDERS

Like other psychiatric diagnoses, the diagnosis of eating disorders involves a comprehensive history and physical examination (see Chapter 37). In some cases, the physical manifestation may be quite suggestive, such as with cachexia in severe anorexia. Tooth decay or knuckle lesions (Russell's sign) indicate a history of self-induced vomiting. In addition to physical examination, a thorough evaluation of the patient with an eating disorder often involves diagnostic testing. The status of serum electrolytes is particularly pertinent since alterations may cause significant renal and cardiac dysfunction. An ECG should be checked in cases of severe anorexia nervosa due to the potential for bradycardia, sick sinus syndrome, and cardiac arrhythmias (and their complications). Nutritional measures (such as vitamin levels) can indicate nutritional deficiency. Interestingly, albumin levels are often normal. Patients who induce vomiting can have metabolic alkalosis (manifested by a high bicarbonate level), hypokalemia, and hypochloremia. An elevated amylase may be seen in the setting of chronic emesis, while a raised serum aldolase level is a sign of ipecac use. Further laboratory abnormalities include hypocalcemia from ongoing laxative abuse and a blunted cholecystokinin level in bulimic patients. Table 3-9 provides a summary of laboratory abnormalities in patients with eating disorders.[29]

DRUG MONITORING

Many of the commonly used psychotropic medications require laboratory monitoring. Serum levels of the drugs themselves help guide medication titration, prevent toxicity, and check for compliance. Levels may also be helpful to evaluate for slow or fast metabolism in patients who have responses out of the expected range (e.g., extreme side effects or lack of response despite high doses). In addition, the potential for

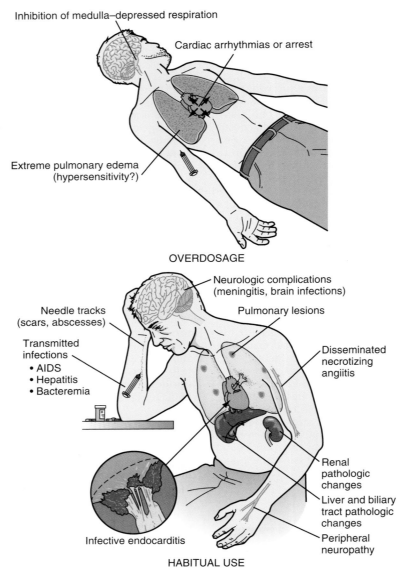

Inhibition of medulla–depressed respiration

Cardiac arrhythmias or arrest

Extreme pulmonary edema (hypersensitivity?)

OVERDOSAGE

Neurologic complications (meningitis, brain infections)

Needle tracks (scars, abscesses)

Pulmonary lesions

Transmitted infections
• AIDS
• Hepatitis
• Bacteremia

Disseminated necrotizing angiitis

Renal pathologic changes

Liver and biliary tract pathologic changes

Peripheral neuropathy

Infective endocarditis

HABITUAL USE

Figure 3-13. Consequences of heroin addiction. *(Redrawn from Cotran RS, Kumar V, Robbins SL: Robbins pathologic basis of disease, ed 5, Philadelphia, 1994, Saunders, p 396.)*

TABLE 3-8 Effects and Laboratory Work-up of Selected Toxins

Agent	Source	Effect	Work-up
Carbon monoxide	Generators, faulty heating systems, mining	Cherry red skin, headache, irritability, confusion. Subsequent hypoxic injury to brain, liver, renal tubules	Carboxyhemoglobin level
Methanol	Solvents, antifreeze	Inebriation, blindness, anion gap acidosis	Serum toxicology, arterial blood gas, electrolytes, complete blood count (CBC)
Lead	Paint, pipes	Encephalopathy, apathy, ataxia, irritability, cognitive dysfunction, delirium	Urine heavy metals, serum level (> 200 mg/ml severe encephalopathy)
Mercury	Industrial contamination, fish	"Mad hatter"—psychosis, fatigue, apathy, memory dysfunction, emotional lability. Subtle personality changes with chronic poisoning	Urine heavy metals
Manganese	Ore refineries, brick working, steel castings	"Manganese madness" (emotional lability, pathological laughter, hallucinations, aggression)—Parkinson-like syndrome	Urine heavy metals
Arsenic	Mining, insecticides, silicon-based computer chips	Fatigue, blackouts, hair loss, renal and hepatic dysfunction, encephalopathy	Urine heavy metals

TABLE 3-9 Laboratory Tests in the Work-up of Eating Disorders

Test	Pertinent Findings
Albumin	Increased with dehydration Decreased with malnutrition (often normal in anorexia)
Aldolase	Increased with ipecac abuse
Amylase	Increased with bulimia nervosa
Bicarbonate	Increased with bulimia, laxative abuse
Blood urea nitrogen	Increased with dehydration
β-human chorionic gonadotropin	Increased with pregnancy (versus amenorrhea due to anorexia)
Calcium	Decreased with chronic laxative use
Chloride	Decreased with bulimia
Cholecystokinin (CCK)	Decreased with post-prandial response in bulimia
Complete blood count (CBC)	Decreased in all blood lines associated with anorexia
Creatinine	Increased with dehydration
Glucose	Decreased with nutritional compromise
Magnesium	Decreased with nutritional compromise → cardiac arrhythmia
Potassium	Decreased with laxative abuse, diuretic abuse, bulimia → metabolic alkalosis
Protein, total	Decreased with malnutrition, over-hydration
Sodium	Decreased with water-loading, diuretic use
Thyroid-stimulating hormone	Increased with hypothyroidism
Urine specific gravity	Decreased with water-loading
Vitamin B_{12}	Decreased with nutritional compromise

organ toxicity (varies depending on the medication) makes screening for treatment-induced organ damage necessary periodically. Monitoring of mood stabilizers, antipsychotics, and antidepressants is discussed in the following subsections.

Mood Stabilizers

Table 3-10[30,31] outlines proposed monitoring of mood stabilizers (including lithium, valproic acid, and carbamazepine). Lithium has a narrow therapeutic range (generally 0.5 to 1.2 mEq/L) with steady-state levels achieved after 4 to 5 days. Levels in excess of this range put patients at acute risk for CNS, cardiac, and renal toxicity. Over the long term, lithium can also induce adverse effects on the thyroid gland, heart, and kidneys. Recommended monitoring includes baseline and follow-up measures of CBC, serum electrolytes, BUN, creatinine, thyroid function tests, and an ECG. In patients with kidney problems, a 24-hour urine sample for creatinine and protein analysis is also recommended. Finally, due to the potential teratogenic effects of lithium in the first trimester of pregnancy, serum or urine pregnancy tests should be checked in women of childbearing potential.

Recommended monitoring for those taking valproic acid or carbamazepine includes checking baseline and follow-up CBCs, electrolytes, and LFTs in addition to monitoring serum levels of the drug itself. Due to the risk of agranulocytosis with carbamazepine, a CBC should be checked every 1 to 2 weeks while titrating the medication, monthly for 4 months (once on a stable dose), and then every 6 to 12 months if the white blood cell (WBC) count is stable. Since both medications have been linked with neural tube defects, a pregnancy test should be checked at baseline and whenever pregnancy is suspected.

Antipsychotics

Clozapine is the antipsychotic medication that requires the closest monitoring. Due to the risk of agranulocytosis in approximately 1% to 2% of patients taking this medication, a CBC with a differential is required (the result of which must be provided to the pharmacy before the medication will be dispensed) on a weekly basis for the first 6 months of treatment, every other week for the next 6 months, and monthly for the remaining duration of treatment. The CBC must be checked more frequently if the WBC count drops significantly or if the WBC count is in the range of 3,000 to 3,500. Leukopenia (WBC count ≤ 2,000 to 3,000) or granulocytopenia (granulocyte count ≤ 1,000 to 2,000) prompts stoppage of the medication, checking daily CBCs, and hospitalization of the patient. Clozapine may be cautiously restarted once the blood count normalizes. If, however, agranulocytosis occurs (i.e., a WBC count of < 2,000 or a granulocyte count of < 1,000), clozapine is discontinued for life. Since seizures are associated with high-dose clozapine, a baseline EEG is helpful in a patient receiving greater than 600 mg/day of this medication.

In addition to clozapine, the atypical antipsychotic medications olanzapine and risperidone (and to a lesser extent quetiapine, aripiprazole, and ziprasidone) have been associated with weight gain, dyslipidemia, and diabetes.[32] Although there is no consensus on this matter, baseline and follow-up weights, glucose measurement, and lipid profiles are prudent for patients taking these medications. Determination of baseline and follow-up blood pressure and heart rates (to evaluate orthostasis), especially in the elderly, is also advisable. Prolactin levels are helpful for patients who develop galactorrhea while taking risperidone or typical neuroleptics. Finally, many antipsychotic medications have been associated with QTc

TABLE 3-10 Proposed Monitoring of Mood-Stabilizing Medications

Drug	Initial Tests	Blood Level Range	Warnings	Monitoring
Lithium	Electrolytes, BUN/Cr, CBC, TSH, U/A, ECG (if 35 years or older), pregnancy test	0.5–1.2 mEq/L	Lithium toxicity	Check level 8–12 hours after last dose once a week while titrating, then every 2 months with electrolytes and BUN/Cr. TSH every 6 months.
Valproic acid	CBC with differential, LFTs, pregnancy test	50–100 mEq/L	Hepatotoxicity, teratogenicity, pancreatitis	Weekly LFTs and CBC until stable dose, then monthly for 6 months, then every 6–12 months
Carbamazepine	CBC with differential, LFTs, pregnancy test	6–12 mcg/ml	Aplastic anemia, agranulocytosis, seizures, myocarditis	CBC, LFTs, drug level every 1–2 weeks while titrating, then monthly for 4 months, then every 6–12 months

Adapted from Smith FA. An approach to the use of laboratory tests. In Stern TA, editor: The ten-minute guide to psychiatric diagnosis and treatment, *New York, 2005, Professional Publishing Group, Ltd, p 324; and Hirschfeld RM, Perlis RH, Vornik LA.* Pharmacologic treatment of bipolar disorder, 2004 handbook, *New York, 2004, MBL Communications.*
BUN, Blood urea nitrogen; CBC, complete blood count; Cr, creatinine; ECG, electrocardiogram; LFTs, liver function tests; TSH, thyroid-stimulating hormone; U/A, urinalysis.

TABLE 3-11 Proposed Monitoring of Antipsychotic Medications

Drug	Initial Tests	Warnings	Monitoring
Aripiprazole	Blood pressure (orthostasis), heart rate, ECG	Black box warning for increased risk of death in elderly	Blood pressure (orthostasis), heart rate, ECG
Clozapine	CBC with differential	Agranulocytosis, seizure, myocarditis	CBC with differential every week for 6 months (or more frequently if WBC count < 3,500 cells/mm³), then every other week; weight, glucose
Olanzapine	Weight, blood pressure (orthostasis) glucose, lipid profile, ECG	Black box warning for increased risk of death in elderly	Weight, blood pressure (orthostasis), glucose, lipid profile, ECG
Risperidone	Weight, blood pressure (orthostasis), heart rate, ECG, glucose	Black box warning for increased risk of death in elderly	Weight, blood pressure (orthostasis), heart rate, ECG, glucose
Quetiapine	CBC, glucose, eye (slit-lamp) examination, ECG	Black box warning for increased risk of death in elderly	Weight, glucose, slit-lamp examination every 6 months
Ziprasidone	Serum potassium and magnesium, ECG, blood pressure, heart rate	Black box warning for increased risk of death in elderly	Serum potassium and magnesium, ECG, blood pressure, heart rate

From DrugPoint summary. In Micromedex healthcare series, 2006, Thomson Healthcare Inc.
CBC, Complete blood count; ECG, electrocardiogram; WBC, white blood cell.

prolongation and other cardiac arrhythmias. Consideration of obtaining a baseline and follow-up ECGs should be based on the patient's cardiac history, age, and use of concomitant medications in conjunction with the known cardiac effects of the medication. Table 3-11[33] describes an approach for monitoring antipsychotic medications.

Antidepressants

There are no agreed-upon guidelines for monitoring levels of antidepressant medications. Tricyclic antidepressants (TCAs) are the most frequently monitored of these since side effects that often correlate with drug levels. Steady-state levels are usually achieved in 5 days, while trough levels should be obtained 8 to 12 hours after the last dose.[34] Table 3-12 reveals proposed monitoring of tricyclic medications. An ECG is perhaps the most important test for those taking TCAs (especially in patients with a cardiac history) since cardiac conduction abnormalities are a potential complication. While other classes of antidepressants do not require routine blood monitoring, specific studies may be indicated on an individual basis to help ensure medication compliance, to check for slow or fast metabolizers, or to help adjust doses based on hepatic or renal function in the medically ill.

ELECTROENCEPHALOGRAM

The electroencephalogram (EEG) is a tool applied primarily in the evaluation of epilepsy; however, it is also often useful in the work-up of organic causes of psychiatric disorders (see Chapter 76 for a full description of the EEG). The EEG uses electrodes to measure electrical activity from neurons in the superficial cortical cell layers of the brain. The frequencies of electrical activity are divided by frequency and named with Greek letters: delta (less than 4 Hz), theta (4 to 7 Hz), alpha (8 to 12 Hz), and beta (greater than 13 Hz). Alpha waves predominate in the awake state. Figure 3-14[35] demonstrates a normal waking EEG. Normal sleep is divided into stage 1, stage 2, stages 3 and 4 (delta), and rapid eye movement (REM) sleep. Spikes and sharp waves are the most common epileptiform discharges and are often seen in combination with slow waves (Figure 3-15).[36] When looking for seizures, several methods (e.g., sleep deprivation, hyperventilation, and photic stimulation) are often used to activate seizure foci. Serial studies, nasopharyngeal leads (especially to identify deep foci), and long-term monitoring also increase the yield of the test.

An EEG (with a characteristic pattern) may be diagnostic in certain conditions (such as generalized, absence, and complex

TABLE 3-12 Proposed Monitoring of Tricyclic Medications

Drug	Initial Tests	Blood Level Range	Warnings	Monitoring
Imipramine	ECG	200–250 ng/ml (may be lower)	Dry mouth, blurred vision, constipation, urinary hesitancy, tachycardia, cardiac toxicity	Trough level 9–12 hours after last dose—symptom driven with signs of toxicity. ECG yearly or more frequently with cardiac disease
Nortriptyline	ECG	50–150 ng/ml (therapeutic window)	Dry mouth, blurred vision, constipation, urinary hesitancy, tachycardia, cardiac toxicity	Trough level 9–12 hours after last dose (5 days to reach steady state)—therapeutic window. ECG yearly and more frequent levels based on signs of toxicity
Desipramine	ECG	Unclear, >125 ng/ml correlates with higher percentage of favorable responses	Dry mouth, blurred vision, constipation, urinary hesitancy, tachycardia, cardiac toxicity	Same as imipramine
Amitriptyline	ECG	Unclear, possible range 75–175 ng/ml	Dry mouth, blurred vision, constipation, urinary hesitancy, tachycardia, cardiac toxicity	Same as imipramine

ECG, Electrocardiogram.

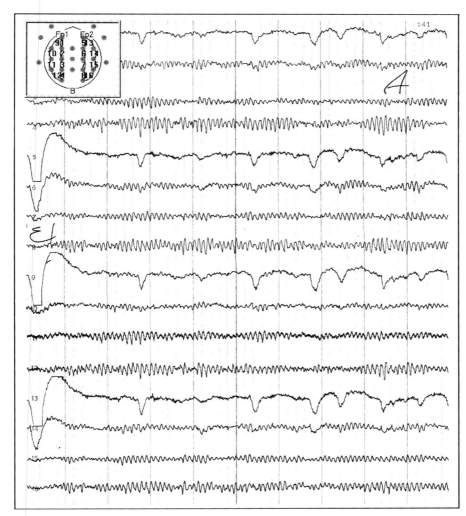

Figure 3-14. Normal waking EEG. The background is low voltage and fast. *(From Abou-Khalil B, Misulis KE: Atlas of EEG and seizure semiology, Philadelphia, 2006, Butterworth-Heinemann.)*

partial seizures). Although not diagnostic, an abnormal EEG may also help support a broader diagnosis of delirium, dementia, a focal neurological deficit, or a medication-induced mental status change. In this circumstance, the EEG must be interpreted in the context of the clinical situation. Chapter 76 provides more details on this subject. Of particular note, while a normal EEG may provide support for the diagnosis of pseudoseizures, it is not in and of itself diagnostic since a single EEG may miss true seizure activity in up to 40% of cases.[37]

NEUROIMAGING

Although neuroimaging alone rarely establishes a psychiatric diagnosis, contemporary modalities, including structural

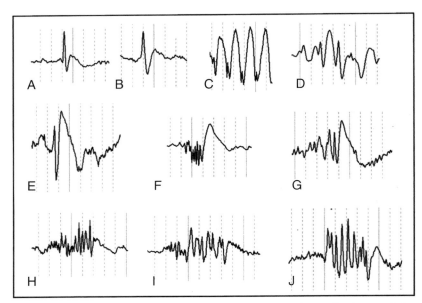

Figure 3-15. Epileptiform discharges. A, spike; B, sharp wave; C, spike-and-wave complexes; D, sharp-and-slow-wave complexes; E, slow-spike-and-wave complex; F, polyspike-and-wave complex; G, multiple-sharp-and-wave complex; H, polyspike complex; I & J, multiple sharp wave complexes. Even though spikes and sharp waves usually have after-going slow waves, the term spike-and-wave complex is usually reserved for the situation in which the slow wave is very prominent, higher in voltage than the spike. The interval between vertical lines represents 200 msec. *(From Abou-Khalil B, Misulis KE:* Atlas of EEG & seizure semiology. *Philadelphia, 2006, Butterworth-Heinemann.)*

BOX 3-3 Guidelines for Structural Neuroimaging Evaluation of the Psychiatric Patient

Acute mental status change with one or more of the following:
- Neurological abnormalities
- Head trauma
- Age 50 years or greater

New-onset psychosis
Delirium or dementia of unknown etiology
Before initial electroconvulsive therapy (ECT) treatment

Adapted from Dougherty DD, Rauch SL, Luther K. Use of neuroimaging techniques. In Stern TA, Herman JB, Slavin PL, editors: Massachusetts General Hospital guide to primary care psychiatry, *ed 2, New York, 2004, McGraw-Hill, pp 61–66.*

---

imaging (computed tomography [CT] and magnetic resonance imaging [MRI]) and functional imaging (positron emission tomography [PET] and single-photon emission computed tomography [SPECT]), are powerful tools in both the clinical and research realms of modern psychiatry. CT and MRI are particularly useful in the investigation of organic causes of psychiatric conditions; as such, their primary clinical utility at present is to rule out treatable brain lesions. A full description of neuroimaging in psychiatry can be found in Chapter 75. The following section will serve as an introduction to the role of neuroimaging in the diagnostic work-up of the patient with psychiatric symptomatology—emphasis will be placed on the structural modalities (given their greater clinical applications) while the more research-oriented functional modalities will be briefly introduced. As with all of the aforementioned tests in this chapter, consideration must be given to the indications, risks, potential benefits, cost, and limitations of any brain imaging before recommending that a patient undertake it. Box 3-3[38] outlines general guidelines to help determine the appropriateness of neuroimaging in psychiatric patients.

STRUCTURAL NEUROIMAGING
Computed Tomography

CT scanning delineates cross-sectional views of the brain by using x-rays, which attenuate differently depending on the density of the material through which they pass. Denser areas (such as bone) appear white, while less dense areas (such as gas) look black. CT is particularly good for visualizing acute bleeds (i.e., less than 72 hours old). The addition of contrast material that leaks through the blood–brain barrier often reveals tumors and abscesses. Approximately 5% of patients who receive contrast material experience an allergic reaction (with symptoms including hypotension, nausea, urticaria, and, uncommonly, anaphylaxis). A careful history regarding prior allergic reactions should therefore be obtained before the use of contrast dye. A baseline creatinine level should also be checked since chemotoxic reactions to contrast material in the kidney may cause renal insufficiency or failure. CT does not show subtle white matter lesions well, and it is contraindicated in pregnancy—women of childbearing age should have a pregnancy test before undergoing a CT scan. CT is often more readily available and less expensive than is MRI.

Magnetic Resonance Imaging

MRI uses the magnetic properties of hydrogen in water in the brain to construct images of tissue (through excitation and relaxation of nuclei). Different components of tissue do this at different rates—this is the basis of so-called T_1 and T_2 images (Figure 3-16).[39] Contrast material may be used with MRI as with CT to show areas of pathology where the blood–brain barrier or blood vessels have been compromised. The contrast used with MRI, gadolinium, is safer than is CT contrast. Ischemia is best visualized by a technique known as diffusion-weighted imaging (DWI), which tracks water movement in tissue.[40] When comparing the two, MRI is superior to CT for looking at the posterior fossa and the brainstem and in visualizing soft tissue (e.g., white matter). MRI is also

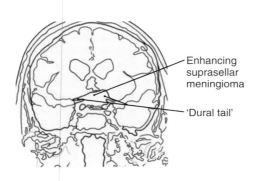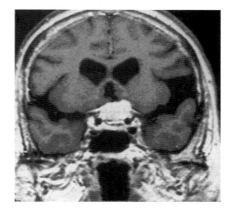

Enhancing
suprasellar
meningioma

'Dural tail'

Figure 3-16. T₁-weighted MRI showing enhancing suprasellar meningioma. *(From Peebles T, Haughton VM: Neuroradiology and endocrine disease. In Besser MG, Thorner MO, editors:* Comprehensive clinical endocrinology, *ed 3, 2002, Elsevier Science Limited, p 622.)*

TABLE 3-13 Comparison of Computed Tomography and Magnetic Resonance Imaging

Computed Tomography	Magnetic Resonance Imaging
Preferred clinical uses: • Acute hemorrhage • Acute trauma More radiation exposure Generally more economical and available	Preferred clinical uses: • Soft tissue and white matter lesions • Posterior fossa and brainstem lesions • Subacute hemorrhage Contraindicated with metallic implants Claustrophobia is an issue

preferable to CT in pregnancy, though it is still relatively contraindicated. Because of the use of a high-powered magnet, MRI is contraindicated in patients with metallic implants. Because an MRI procedure is longer, louder, and more cramped, it is often more difficult for claustrophobic patients to tolerate than is CT. Table 3-13 provides a comparison of the benefits and limitations of CT and MRI.

Positron Emission Tomography and Single-Photon Emission Computed Tomography

PET and SPECT are forms of functional neuroimaging that are chiefly used for research purposes in current practice. They both use radioactive tracers to visualize neuronal activity, cellular metabolism, and neuroreceptor profiles. PET, the "gold standard" of neuroimaging tests, uses positron emission from tracers to measure glucose metabolism or blood flow in the brain. It is very expensive and requires access to a cyclotron to produce nucleotides. SPECT, on the other hand, measures single-photon emission and is more affordable than PET (though its spatial resolution is inferior). While these modalities are mainly used in psychiatry for research purposes, a clinical role is emerging in the evaluation of dementia and seizures.[41] For example, functional neuroimaging may be beneficial in differentiating Alzheimer's disease from other forms of dementia (where it has been shown to be both sensitive and specific). As far as seizures are concerned, PET may be used to find deep seizure foci that go undetected by the EEG. In addition, PET offers the advantage of measuring both ictal and inter-ictal changes in metabolism so that diagnosis does not rely on catching the patient during seizure activity as with the routine EEG. Finally, PET may also be helpful in the clinical setting when it is used in conjunction with an EEG to provide more precise localization of seizure foci in a patient who must undergo neurosurgical intervention.

CONCLUSION

While psychiatric diagnoses rely most heavily on careful interviews and a mental status examination, laboratory tests and diagnostic modalities (such as neuroimaging and an EEG) are important adjuncts. These tests help to diagnose underlying medical and neurological causes of psychiatric symptoms and aid in the monitoring and progression of certain diseases. Populations at high risk for medical co-morbidity (such as the elderly, the chronically medically ill, substance abusers, and the indigent) may benefit in particular. Laboratory tests are also frequently used to check blood levels of psychotropic medications and to predict potential side effects. This chapter has provided an introduction to the strategy and rationale for choosing when to order a wide array of specific serum, urine, and CSF tests, as well as several diagnostic modalities (e.g., the EEG and neuroimaging). Further information with regard to specific illnesses will be addressed in subsequent chapters.

Access the complete reference list and multiple choice questions (MCQs) online at https://expertconsult.inkling.com

KEY REFERENCES

1. American Psychiatric Association. *Diagnostic and statistical manual of mental disorders*, ed 5 (DSM-5), Washington, DC, 2013, American Psychiatric Press.
2. Roffman JL, Silverman BC, Stern TA. Diagnostic rating scales and laboratory tests. In Stern TA, Fricchione GL, Cassem NH, et al., editors: *Massachusetts General Hospital handbook of general hospital psychiatry*, ed 6, Philadelphia, 2010, Saunders Elsevier.
3. Smith FA, Querques J, Levenson JL, et al. Psychiatric assessment and consultation. In Levenson JL, editor: *The American Psychiatric Publishing textbook of psychosomatic medicine*, ed 2, Washington, DC, 2011, American Psychiatric Publishing.
6. Smith FA. An approach to the use of laboratory tests. In Stern TA, editor-in-chief: *The ten-minute guide to psychiatric diagnosis and treatment*, New York, 2005, Professional Publishing Group, Ltd, pp 318.
8. Smith F, Alpay M, Park L. Laboratory tests and diagnostic procedures. In Stern TA, Herman JB, Gorrindo T, editors: *Massachusetts General Hospital psychiatry update and board preparation*, ed 3, Boston, 2012, MGH Psychiatry Academy.
9. Sadock BJ, Sadock VA. *Kaplan and Sadock's synopsis of psychiatry*, ed 10, Philadelphia, 2007, Lipincott Williams & Wilkins, pp 263–267.
15. Beck BJ. Mental disorders due to a general medical condition. In Stern TA, Herman JB, Gorrindo T, editors: *Massachusetts General Hospital psychiatry update and board preparation*, ed 3, Boston, 2012, MGH Psychiatry Academy.

22. Sax PE, Bartlett JG. Acute and early HIV infection: Clinical manifestations and diagnosis. In *UpToDate*, 2013.
23. Chopra S, Terrault NA, Di Bisceglie AM. Screening for and diagnosis of chronic hepatitis C virus infection. In *UpToDate*, 2013.
29. Becker AE, Jacobowitz Israel E. Patients with an eating disorder. In Stern TA, Fricchione GL, Cassem NH, et al., editors: *Massachusetts General Hospital handbook of general hospital psychiatry*, ed 6, Philadelphia, 2010, Saunders Elsevier.
37. Huffman JC, Smith FA, Stern TA. Patients with neurologic conditions I. Seizure disorders (including non-epileptic seizures), cerebrovascular disease, and traumatic brain injury. In Stern TA, Fricchione GL, Cassem NH, et al., editors: *Massachusetts General Hospital handbook of general hospital psychiatry*, ed 6, Philadelphia, 2010, Saunders Elsevier, p 242.
40. Hurley RA, Fisher RE, Taber KH. Clinical and functional imaging in neuropsychiatry. In Yudofsky SC, Hales RE, editors: *The American Psychiatric Publishing textbook of neuropsychiatry and behavioral neurosciences*, ed 5, Washington, DC, 2008, American Psychiatric Publishing.
41. Foster NL. Molecular imaging in neuropsychiatry. In Coffey CE, Cummings JL, editors: *The American Psychiatric Publishing textbook of geriatric neuropsychiatry*, ed 3, Washington, DC, 2011, American Psychiatric Publishing.

4 Treatment Adherence

Lara Traeger, PhD, Megan Moore Brennan, MD, and John B. Herman, MD

KEY POINTS

Background

- Among patients with a psychiatric illness, treatment adherence is associated with better treatment outcomes, a lower risk of relapse and hospitalization, and better adherence to treatments for co-morbid medical illnesses. However, barriers to adherence are common and rates of suboptimal adherence remain critically high.

History

- Over the past several decades, approaches have evolved to help patients continue treatment for chronic health problems. The term "adherence," promoted by the World Health Organization, reflects that optimal health outcomes require multi-level efforts to reduce treatment barriers encountered by patients.

Clinical and Research Challenges

- Patient adherence is a necessary component of treatment response and remission. Standardized definitions and measures of adherence are needed to support comparisons of risk factors and intervention outcomes across studies and translation to clinical work. More research also is needed to establish effective, cost-efficient ways to improve adherence in clinical settings. Adherence curricula should be included in mental health professional training and continuing education programs.

Practical Pointers

- Practitioners are encouraged to collaborate actively with patients to select and monitor psychiatric treatment regimens. Optimal patient adherence requires a complex series of behaviors. Routine assessment of both modifiable and non-modifiable barriers to adherence throughout the course of treatment will enable practitioners to tailor treatment approaches and adherence interventions for individual patients. Patient education can enhance adherence by incorporating cognitive and behavioral strategies into care plans.

OVERVIEW

Poor adherence to psychiatric treatments is a widespread clinical problem that negatively impacts rates of treatment response and remission.[1,2] While empirically-supported treatments are available for many psychiatric disorders,[3] these treatments are not universally effective. Patients commonly face difficulties in taking prescribed psychotropic medications or attending psychotherapy sessions as recommended, and therefore may not achieve optimal outcomes.[1,4] Moreover, some patients who adhere to treatment recommendations may not experience a clinically significant response, and this often leads them to remain in care and to tolerate treatment plan modifications.[5]

The World Health Organization has defined adherence as the extent to which patients' health behaviors are consistent with recommendations that they have agreed to with their practitioners.[6] This definition emphasizes that practitioners must collaborate with their patients in making decisions throughout treatment. However, researchers frequently evaluate patient adherence to psychiatric regimens in ways which do not capture the dynamics among patients, practitioners, and health care systems.[7] Common measures include the extent to which patients take their medications at the prescribed dose and timing, attend scheduled clinic appointments, and remain in care. These broad measures are discussed in this chapter (summarizing findings on the prevalence of, and the barriers to, psychiatric treatment adherence). This chapter also highlights the fact that optimal adherence is a moving target that involves complex patient behaviors and multi-factorial challenges, and may be enhanced by targeted strategies for patients, practitioners, and systems.

EPIDEMIOLOGY OF ADHERENCE

The estimated prevalence of patient adherence to the use of psychotropic medications has varied widely, due to differences in study populations, diagnoses, medication classes, and the definition of adherence. However, evidence strongly supports the notion that poor adherence is common across groups. Substantial proportions of community-dwelling patients take less than their prescribed daily doses of antipsychotics (34.6%), sedative-hypnotics (34.7%), anxiolytics (38.1%), mood stabilizers (44.9%) and antidepressants (45.9%).[8] In a retrospective study of managed care patients, approximately 57% of patients who had started a selective serotonin re-uptake inhibitor (SSRI) for depression and/or anxiety were not adherent to the medication.[7] In fact, many patients with depression (19%–28%) also do not show for scheduled clinic appointments.[9]

Reports of adherence to taking psychotropic medications further reflect problems with premature treatment discontinuation. Moreover, many patients do not inform their physician about having stopped their medication. Across studies of treatment trials for anxiety disorders (generally lasting 10–12 weeks), 18%–30% of patients discontinued their treatment prematurely.[4] Among patients with depression who were taking an SSRI, almost half (47%) had stopped filling their prescription within 2 months of treatment initiation.[10] Similarly, a pooled analysis of 1,627 patients with psychosis treated with atypical antipsychotics revealed that about half (53%) of the patients discontinued their medication soon after treatment began.[11] Researchers in the Clinical Antipsychotic Trials of Intervention Effectiveness (CATIE) reported that almost three-fourths (74%) of patients with chronic schizophrenia discontinued treatment within 4 months of its initiation.[12]

Some studies have shown that adults with depression prefer psychotherapy over antidepressants.[13] Yet, in a sample of primary care patients with depression, 74% endorsed that barriers to care made it very difficult or impossible to attend regular psychotherapy sessions.[14] Meta-analyses of cognitive-behavioral therapy (CBT) trials for anxiety disorders indicated that for patients who started CBT, between 9% and 21% discontinued the treatment early.[4]

CLINICAL AND ECONOMIC IMPACT OF NON-ADHERENCE

Poor adherence to psychiatric treatments leads to worse clinical outcomes and to excess health care utilization; these factors contribute, in turn, to the economic burden of mental illness.[1,15,16] Among patients with depression, non-adherence to antidepressants is associated with higher medical costs[7] and accounts for 5%–40% of hospital readmissions.[9] Medication non-adherence also is the most powerful predictor of relapse after a first episode of schizophrenia, independent of gender, age of onset, premorbid function, patient insight, or other key factors.[2,17] Moreover, non-adherent patients with schizophrenia are at greater risk for substance use, violence, and victimization, as well as worse overall quality of life.[18] Although little studied, patient non-adherence also may increase the risk of burnout and fatigue among psychiatric practitioners. Findings emphasize that intervening at multiple levels to enhance adherence has the potential to improve population health and well-being and to reduce excess health care utilization, beyond individual improvements in specific treatments.[6]

RISK FACTORS FOR NON-ADHERENCE

Risk factors for non-adherence are complex and varied, and remain incompletely understood. Findings are typically drawn from secondary analyses or exit interviews from randomized controlled trials (RCTs), which employ strict eligibility criteria and rigorous patient monitoring.[4] In clinical settings, practitioners must consider and address multi-factorial challenges to optimal patient adherence (Table 4-1). Key risk factors are summarized below.

Clinical Factors

Mood

Mood symptoms can increase patients' perceptions of barriers to psychiatric care and can adversely affect treatment adherence.[14] Dysphoria and hopelessness may reduce intrinsic motivation for treatment. Patients who experience psychomotor slowing, decreased energy, and poor concentration also may have difficulty engaging in self-care, attending appointments, completing cognitive-behavioral therapy (CBT) assignments, and/or taking their medications appropriately. In comparison, when patients enter a manic episode, they may experience elevated mood and energy as positive and may not want to take their medications that slow them down. Moreover, when insight and judgment are impaired, patients may not believe that they have an illness that requires treatment.

Anxiety

Anxiety disorders are associated with hyper-vigilance to internal and/or external stimuli, which may affect a patient's adherence to treatment recommendations in several ways. Some patients become too anxious to leave their home and to attend scheduled clinic appointments. Anxiety also may interfere with the optimal upward titration or tapering of medications, as patients may attribute transient physical symptoms to changes in medication dose. Among patients with obsessive-compulsive disorder (OCD), counting rituals and fears of contamination may preclude adherence to both medication and psychotherapy regimens.

Psychosis

Most reports on adherence to psychiatric treatment regimens have focused on psychotic disorders, including schizophrenia.

TABLE 4-1 Multi-factorial Influences on Treatment Adherence

Factors	Examples
Clinical	Psychiatric symptoms that may interfere with adherence
	Substance misuse
	Cognitive impairment
Treatment-related	Treatment efficacy
	Side effects
	Dose timing and frequency
	Psychotherapy modality
Patient-level	Knowledge about psychiatric symptoms and their treatments
	Attitudes, beliefs, and concerns about psychiatric symptoms/treatments
	Attitudes, beliefs, and concerns about health care systems
Practitioner-level	Knowledge, attitudes, and beliefs about psychiatric symptoms/treatments
	Knowledge, attitudes, and beliefs about barriers to patient adherence
	Use of adherence assessments and interventions throughout treatment
	Facilitation of therapeutic alliance
	Collaboration with patient in treatment decision-making
Systems-level	Mental health care coverage
	Fragmentation of patient care
	Distance from patient home to clinic/ availability of care
	Financial barriers (transportation, co-payments, child care)
	Barriers to mental health care among racial/ethnic minorities
Sociocultural	Attitudes and beliefs about psychiatric symptoms/treatments within the patient's identified communities (e.g., family, cultural, and religious)
	Mental health stigma within communities
Interactions among factors	Practitioner–patient therapeutic alliance
	Match between the patient's preferences/values and treatments
	Match between the patient's resources/ needs and prescribed treatments
	Level of a patient's trust in practitioner and health care systems
	The patient's access to/use of support for navigating barriers to adherence

Problems related to both the disorders and their treatments present significant barriers to adherence. Factors (such as positive symptoms, emotional distress, and treatment side effects [e.g., akathisia]) have predicted poor adherence.[19-23] Among patients treated with atypical antipsychotics, early discontinuation of treatment has been attributed to perceptions of poor response, to worsening of symptoms, and to an inability to tolerate the medications.[11] Notably, patients who need to change or augment their current treatment are at higher risk for its discontinuation.[24]

Substance Misuse

Misuse of substances is an important risk factor for non-adherence in patients with a variety of psychiatric disorders.[25,26] Patients who believe that mixing alcohol or illicit drugs with prescribed medications can be dangerous may eschew use of their medication in favor of alcohol or drugs. Drug intoxication and withdrawal also affect a patient's attention, memory, and mood state, which in turn, can interfere with adherence.

The financial burden of substances may also negatively affect a patients' ability to make co-payments for medications and clinic appointments.

Patient Factors: Knowledge, Attitudes, and Beliefs

Across different psychiatric diagnoses, patients' perceptions of their disorder and its treatment consistently predict adherence or the lack thereof. Patients are more likely to adhere to their medication regimen if they believe that their need for the medication is high and that risk of adverse effects related to the medication is low.[4,27,28] On the other hand, mental health stigma, denial of one's diagnosis, and lack of insight all increase the risk for treatment non-adherence.[19,20,22,23,29] Patients also may stop treatment if they believe it is unhelpful once an acute illness phase has resolved.[30] In a study of patients with bipolar I disorder, more than half were non-adherent to their medications 4 months after an episode of acute mania.[31] With regard to psychotherapy, trials of CBT for anxiety have shown that patients with a low motivation for treatment, little readiness for change, and/or low confidence in CBT in comparison to other treatments have an elevated risk for early treatment discontinuation.

Economic and Racial/Ethnic Disparities

Structural and financial barriers to taking medications and attending appointments (e.g., a lack of resources for child care, transportation, or co-payments) are important risk factors for non-adherence.[4,14] U.S. health insurance providers historically have restricted mental health services more than other medical services. Some patients may be more likely to forego psychiatric medications if they are balancing medication costs for multiple health conditions.

Racial/ethnic disparities in access to quality psychiatric care are well-documented.[32,33] However, among patients who do initiate medication or psychotherapy, evidence for differences in treatment adequacy or retention in care is more equivocal.[34] Some studies of schizophrenia and mood disorders suggests that black and Latino patients have poorer adherence to psychiatric medications, relative to white patients.[24,26,31,35] A combination of factors, such as access to psychiatric care; differences in medication metabolism, response, and side effects; and patients' beliefs and concerns about treatment, may underlie these disparities.[31] Practitioners should consider these factors during treatment selection, titration, and management.

Clinical Encounters

Poor practitioner–patient therapeutic alliances and a lack of follow-up increase the risk for treatment non-response and attrition.[4,36] Adherence and medication effects need to be monitored on an ongoing basis. Practitioners can help patients manage expectations by discussing with patients that certain treatments may cause side effects or require adjustments before they confer benefits on psychiatric symptoms and quality of life. The following sections summarize suggestions for assessing adherence and integrating adherence into all phases of treatment.

ASSESSING ADHERENCE

Currently, there is no "gold standard" measure of treatment adherence or a consensus on the adequate or optimal level of adherence among patients. Available tools for assessing patient adherence to psychotropic medications include self-report measures, daily diaries, electronic pill containers, prescription refill records, pill counts, laboratory assays, directly-observed therapy, and collateral information.[37] Practitioners should consider strengths and limitations of each method in the context of available resources and the intended purpose of assessment. Self-report measures[38] and daily diaries are inexpensive to administer, yet may be subject to the impact of social desirability or forgetting. Electronic pill containers yield detailed adherence data but may be impractical when tracking multiple medications. Having free samples and left-over pills from other prescriptions reduces the accuracy of pill-counts. Laboratory assays may identify the presence of medication classes or individual agents but cannot confirm daily administration. When appropriate, multiple measures can be used to support a more complete view of adherence.

INTEGRATING ADHERENCE INTO THE TREATMENT COURSE
Initial Consultation

Practitioners commonly underestimate patient barriers to treatment adherence.[39] Adherence must be an explicit, core element of treatment, starting with the initial consultation (Table 4-2). The practitioner begins to facilitate a therapeutic alliance early-on by transmitting a warm, non-judgmental

TABLE 4-2 Incorporation of Adherence-related Inquiries into Initial Consultation

Components	Areas of Inquiry
History of present illness	What are the patient's beliefs about symptoms and acceptable treatments?
	To what extent are barriers to adherence related to present symptoms?
	How may present symptoms affect adherence behaviors?
Past psychiatric history	To what extent were barriers to adherence related to prior psychiatric risk?
	What were the patient's attitudes about medication versus psychotherapy?
Substance abuse	Is the patient actively using alcohol or illicit drugs?
Medical history	What are the patient's beliefs about medical conditions and treatments?
Medications	What are the patient's attitudes, beliefs, and concerns about current medications?
	How does the patient cope with current medication side effects?
	What types of barriers to adherence does the patient experience?
Family history	What are familial attitudes, beliefs, and coping with psychiatric symptoms?
Social history	What are attitudes and beliefs about psychiatric symptoms and treatments within the patient's identified cultural and religious communities?
	How may non-modifiable financial concerns or living situations influence the ability to obtain, store, and take certain medications or to attend clinic?
	What role should the family play in treatment decision-making and monitoring?
Mental status examination	To what extent may insight, judgment, and/or cognitive impairments influence treatment adherence?

TABLE 4-3 Patterns of Poor Medication Adherence and Corresponding Concerns to Explore

Adherence Pattern	Potential Concerns to Explore
Takes higher dose than recommended	Are treatment recommendations understood and/or acceptable? Are symptoms inadequately managed at the lower dose? Is the patient abusing the medication?
Takes lower dose than recommended	Are treatment recommendations understood and/or acceptable? Are side effects too bothersome? Has the desired effect been achieved at the lower dose? Is the patient concerned about medication tolerance or dependence? Is the patient misusing the remaining medication?
Misses one dose per week	Are treatment recommendations understood and/or acceptable? Is the patient facing particular barriers on days in which the dose is missed? Is the patient skipping the dose or doubling the next dose?
Takes pills every other day	Are treatment recommendations understood and/or acceptable? Is the patient facing particular barriers on days in which the dose is missed? Is the patient facing difficulty with medication expenses?
Takes medications sporadically	Are treatment recommendations understood and/or acceptable? Does the patient have sufficient understanding or acceptance of the illness being treated or the treatment's mechanism of action?

stance and by demonstrating support and commitment to the patient's well-being.[40,41] Key tasks include exploring a patient's values and perspectives about symptoms and their acceptable treatment. By evaluating modifiable barriers (e.g., misinformation about medications), the practitioner may identify opportunities for intervention. The practitioner should also assess non-modifiable barriers to adherence (e.g., the patient lives far from the clinic) in order to recommend feasible treatment options.

Treatment Planning

Active collaboration will help the practitioner and the patient develop an appropriate, acceptable, and feasible treatment plan. The practitioner may present pros and cons of available treatment options to arrive at treatment recommendations. Following treatment selection, the practitioner may express belief in the treatment and thereby promote optimism that the treatment will result in positive change. As mentioned earlier, however, practitioners also should manage patients' expectations by stating that medications may require adjustments before they confer benefits. Patients are told that treatments can be discontinued if they are ineffective, cause intolerable side effects, or create other issues that are personally important. Notably, the best way for some patients to commit to a particular plan is to enhance their sense of agency to otherwise say "no".

Introduction to Adherence

As early as possible, the practitioner should explicate the role of adherence in facilitating treatment goals. This includes normalizing adherence challenges, preparing the patient for regular adherence assessments, and adopting a non-judgmental attitude toward risk of adherence lapses. Depending on a patient's barriers to adherence, practitioners may integrate specific strategies into the treatment plan, such as increasing the frequency of clinic visits,[42] using a depot injection of an antipsychotic medication,[43,44] limiting the number of daily doses,[45] and selecting medications based on tolerable side effects.[46] Authors of the 2009 Expert Consensus Guideline Series on adherence among patients with serious mental illness also emphasized the importance of services, when available, to reduce logistical barriers to care.[47]

Ongoing Assessment

Adherence can change over time, with drug over-utilization being more common during the early stages of treatment and under-utilization during its later stages.[48] The patient's initial evaluation, evolving symptom profile, and barriers to adherence will guide the nature and extent of follow-up adherence assessments (Table 4-3). Regular discussions will help the practitioner foster a treatment relationship in which a patient feels comfortable discussing adherence challenges.

The practitioner should also ask about adherence in an empathic, non-judgmental manner, using a tone of genuine curiosity (*How is it going with taking your medications?*). After introducing the topic, the practitioner may ask patients which medications they are taking and how they are taking them. Open-ended questions will identify when patients are taking medications incorrectly (with or without realizing it). Disarming inquiries are less likely to appear shaming or punitive (*Many people find it difficult to take medication—have you ever forgotten to take yours?*).

PROBLEM-SOLVING BARRIERS TO ADHERENCE

Most patients will face barriers to optimal adherence during the course of treatment. The practitioner should invest time during clinic appointments to explore non-adherence and tailor adherence strategies accordingly. A foundational approach focuses on developing and maintaining a strong therapeutic alliance with the patient. The following sections and Table 4-4 provide examples of more targeted strategies.

Education

Patients will benefit from building knowledge and insight about their condition and its treatment. Education should be provided in multiple formats (e.g., oral, written, graphic), to illustrate the rationale for the treatment dose and timing and the reason for the expected treatment duration. However, patients commonly face multiple complex challenges to managing their medication regimens. Interventions that combine patient education with cognitive and behavioral strategies are more effective than the use of education strategies alone. Across diverse health conditions, multi-component approaches have led to moderate improvements in both adherence and

TABLE 4-4 Components of Patient-focused Interventions to Enhance Adherence

Components	Sample Strategies
Education	Education on target symptoms, their treatments, and treatment side effects
	Information in multiple formats (oral, written, visual)
Motivation	Development of strong practitioner–patient therapeutic alliance
	Identification of intrinsic motivation for adherence (e.g., life goals)
	Other rewards and reinforcements for adherence
	Peer mentoring
Skills	**PROBLEM-SOLVING**
	Identification of steps involved in optimal adherence and potential barriers
	Generation and testing of potential solutions to barriers
	Use of incremental goals to reach desired level of adherence
	ADAPTIVE THINKING
	Socratic questioning to guide the patient in the discovery of problematic patterns about adherence (e.g., depressive hopelessness)
	Cognitive re-structuring to generate more realistic and helpful thoughts
	USE OF CUES
	Daily alarm (mobile phone or wrist watch)
	Pill box or electronic pill container
	Mobile phone app for adherence
	Written reminders or stickers in key areas of a patient's home
	Reminders from an informal caregiver
	Tailoring of medication schedule to daily life schedule and activities
	Telephone- or computer-based reminders for pill-taking, appointments, and/or refills
	SUPPORT
	Patient counseling/education on support-seeking skills
	Family or group-based interventions
Logistics	Case management or financial counseling to increase access to care
	Simplified dose schedule
	Adherence monitoring via diary or electronic pill cap

BOX 4-1 Adherence-related Tasks for Patients on Psychiatric Medications

- Describe psychiatric symptoms (frequency, severity, characteristics)
- Comprehend information about recommended medications
- Collaborate with the practitioner to make treatment decisions
- Obtain prescribed medications
- Safely store medications
- Follow the regimen's dose and timing (and/or make decisions about taking PRN medications)
- Identify, manage, and cope with side effects
- Obtain informal caregiver support as needed
- Attend regular follow-up clinic appointments
- Identify and raise concerns about medications
- Continue collaborating to titrate and modify the regimen as needed

clinical outcomes.[49–51] When available, some patients also may benefit from CBT or other problem-focused therapies for more intensive adherence intervention.

Motivation

Based on the transtheoretical model, readiness-to-change may fluctuate across five stages, from *pre-contemplation* (not yet committed to the need for psychiatric treatment) to *maintenance* (already adhering to treatment).[52] The practitioner should explore patients' motivations for treatment on an ongoing basis. Motivational interviewing (MI) techniques can be used as-needed to elicit intrinsic motivation and resolve ambivalence toward treatment.[53] Patients who are mandated or urged by others to start treatment are at higher risk for non-adherence relative to patients who are ready for change.[4]

Skills

Even with knowledge and motivation for treatment, many patients need to enhance their problem-solving skills to improve adherence to their prescribed regimen.[51] Adherence

comprises a complex series of tasks. Practitioners may use Box 4-1 as a starting point to help a patient break adherence into practical steps and to identify potential barriers at each step—such as obtaining medication (e.g., difficulty with co-payments), storing medication (e.g., unstable housing or desire to conceal one's psychiatric diagnosis from a housemate), taking medications on time (e.g., problems with forgetting or a co-morbid attention deficit disorder), or raising concerns with the practitioner (e.g., desire to avoid being a "bad" patient). Socratic questioning may help a patient further uncover problematic thought or behavior patterns that interfere with adherence.

Once barriers are identified, the practitioner may work with the patient to generate and test solutions for reducing them. Forgetting is one of the most common reasons that patients cite for missing or delaying use of psychiatric medications.[8] Based on an adherence intervention for patients with co-morbid depression and medical conditions,[54] patients are encouraged to identify both a plan (e.g., set up a daily alarm) and a back-up plan (e.g., stick a written reminder on one's bathroom mirror) to address each specific barrier. Moreover, the practitioner may help review the patient's daily schedule and revise medication times to match specific activities that the patient never forgets (e.g., brushing one's teeth or filling a coffee pot in the morning). Finally, patients may benefit from learning adaptive thinking strategies, such as cognitive re-structuring, to reduce severe interfering thoughts (e.g., *My need for medication is a sign that I am a weak person*). The practitioner and patient will review the success of the patient's strategies at each visit, revising them as needed and setting incremental goals for achieving optimal adherence.

Patients also may benefit from communication skills to increase social support for adherence within their family or community. Occasionally, a patient's loved ones may have concerns about the treatment or may have high expressed-emotion at home, which in turn may impede adherence. The practitioner and patient may plan to initiate an open discussion of these issues directly with loved ones, to engage them in the collaborative relationship and invite them to "walk the treatment path" with the patient. Family interventions may be needed to address problems with high expressed-emotion.[4]

Logistics

As mentioned earlier, many non-modifiable barriers, such as limitations in mental health insurance coverage and limited resources or mobility to attend clinic appointments, reduce a patient's access to care. Moreover, problems such as depression exacerbate hopelessness in navigating these types of barriers.[55] Patients with limited resources need specific, practical support to problem-solve ideas and gain access to available services. Practitioners may consider lower-cost alternatives, explore how patients pay for other medications, and refer patients to resource specialists when available.

FUTURE DIRECTIONS
Research

Standardized terminology and measures for treatment adherence are needed to compare study outcomes and translate this information into clinical practice. Prospective studies of non-adherence, including *a priori* measures of potential risk factors, multiple adherence measures, and longer follow-up periods, will increase our understanding of adherence and our ability to identify patients at risk for non-adherence or treatment attrition over time. These findings, in turn, will help researchers and clinicians to target modifiable risk factors in patients who need more intensive adherence interventions.

More research is also needed to establish effective, cost-efficient ways to improve adherence—particularly among patients who are medically complex and/or lower functioning. In stepped or collaborative care models, care managers provide patients with support in consultation with a supervising psychiatrist and each patient's primary medical provider.[56] Telephone-based care represents another model for maintaining patient engagement in care and monitoring treatment response.[57,58] Quantitative economic studies will provide leverage with privatized managed care and government agencies, by allowing researchers to demonstrate that interventions to improve adherence result in cost benefits—such as decreasing emergency department visits and hospitalizations.

Education

There are critical gaps in training for psychiatric practitioners on the assessment and management of treatment adherence. Residency training programs can provide opportunities to teach about the integration of adherence into routine clinical care. The following curricular components have been recommended: defining adherence; identifying the relationship between adherence and treatment efficacy; assessing adherence; intervening to enhance adherence; and maintaining the therapeutic alliance.[59] National conferences and continuing medical education (CME) programs provide further opportunities to disseminate state-of-the-art interventions and outcomes research.

CONCLUSION

The importance of treatment adherence among patients with psychiatric disorders cannot be over-stated. Adherence increases the likelihood that patients will experience treatment response and remission, thereby reducing the burden of mental illness for patients and health care systems. Improving adherence requires strategies that target multi-factorial barriers. In the clinic setting, practitioners should utilize a collaborative approach with patients and integrate adherence assessment and interventions into all phases of treatment. Brief strategies can be tailored to help patients increase knowledge, motivation, skills, and support for treatment adherence. Practitioner training and CME programs need to increase attention to adherence as an integral part of clinical care and an opportunity to improve patient quality-of-life and optimize health care utilization.[60]

Access the complete reference list and multiple choice questions (MCQs) online at https://expertconsult.inkling.com

KEY REFERENCES

1. Akerblad A-C, Bengtsson F, von Knorring L, et al. Response, remission and relapse in relation to adherence in primary care treatment of depression: a 2-year outcome study. *Int Clin Psychopharmacol* 21:117–124, 2006.
2. Caseiro O, Pérez-Iglesias R, Mata I, et al. Predicting relapse after a first episode of non-affective psychosis: a three-year follow-up study. *J Psychiatr Res* 46:1099–1105, 2012.
4. Taylor S, Abramowitz JS, McKay D. Non-adherence and non-response in the treatment of anxiety disorders. *J Anxiety Disord* 26:583–589, 2012.
5. Gaynes BN, Warden D, Trivedi MH, et al. What did STAR☆D teach us? Results from a large-scale, practical, clinical trial for patients with depression. *FOCUS J Lifelong Learn Psychiatry* 10:510–517, 2012.
6. World Health Organization. Adherence to long-term therapies: evidence for action. Available from: <http://www.who.int/chp/knowledge/publications/adherence_report/en/>; [Cited 2013 Jul 27].
7. Cantrell CR, Eaddy MT, Shah MB, et al. Methods for evaluating patient adherence to antidepressant therapy: a real-world comparison of adherence and economic outcomes. *Med Care* 44:300–303, 2006.
8. Bulloch AGM, Patten SB. Non-adherence with psychotropic medications in the general population. *Soc Psychiatry Psychiatr Epidemiol* 45:47–56, 2010.
11. Liu-Seifert H, Adams DH, Kinon BJ. Discontinuation of treatment of schizophrenic patients is driven by poor symptom response: a pooled post-hoc analysis of four atypical antipsychotic drugs. *BMC Med* 3:21, 2005.
14. Mohr DC, Hart SL, Howard I, et al. Barriers to psychotherapy among depressed and nondepressed primary care patients. *Ann Behav Med Publ Soc Behav Med* 32:254–258, 2006.
16. Katon W, Cantrell CR, Sokol MC, et al. Impact of antidepressant drug adherence on comorbid medication use and resource utilization. *Arch Intern Med* 165:2497–2503, 2005.
17. Alvarez-Jimenez M, Priede A, Hetrick SE, et al. Risk factors for relapse following treatment for first episode psychosis: a systematic review and meta-analysis of longitudinal studies. *Schizophr Res* 139:116–128, 2012.
19. Perkins DO, Johnson JL, Hamer RM, et al. Predictors of antipsychotic medication adherence in patients recovering from a first psychotic episode. *Schizophr Res* 83:53–63, 2006.
24. Ahn J, McCombs JS, Jung C, et al. Classifying patients by antipsychotic adherence patterns using latent class analysis: characteristics of nonadherent groups in the California Medicaid (Medi-Cal) program. *Value Heal J Int Soc Pharmacoeconomics Outcomes Res* 11:48–56, 2008.
25. Jónsdóttir H, Opjordsmoen S, Birkenaes AB, et al. Predictors of medication adherence in patients with schizophrenia and bipolar disorder. *Acta Psychiatr Scand* 127:23–33, 2013.
26. Perkins DO, Gu H, Weiden PJ, et al. Predictors of treatment discontinuation and medication nonadherence in patients recovering from a first episode of schizophrenia, schizophreniform disorder, or schizoaffective disorder: a randomized, double-blind, flexible-dose, multicenter study. *J Clin Psychiatry* 69:106–113, 2008.
30. Byrne N, Regan C, Livingston G. Adherence to treatment in mood disorders. *Curr Opin Psychiatry* 19:44–49, 2006.
34. Teh CF, Sorbero MJ, Mihalyo MJ, et al. Predictors of adequate depression treatment among Medicaid-enrolled adults. *Health Serv Res* 45:302–315, 2010.
36. Wang PS, Schneeweiss S, Brookhart MA, et al. Suboptimal antidepressant use in the elderly. *J Clin Psychopharmacol* 25:118–126, 2005.
47. Velligan DI, Weiden PJ, Sajatovic M, et al. Strategies for addressing adherence problems in patients with serious and persistent mental illness: recommendations from the expert consensus guidelines. *J Psychiatr Pr* 16:306–324, 2010.
50. Vergouwen ACM, Bakker A, Katon WJ, et al. Improving adherence to antidepressants: a systematic review of interventions. *J Clin Psychiatry* 64:1415–1420, 2003.

53. Miller WR, Rollnick S. *Motivational interviewing: helping people change*, New York, 2013, Guilford Press.
54. Safren S, Gonzalez J, Soroudi N. *Coping with chronic illness: a cognitive-behavioral approach for adherence and depression therapist guide*, ed 1, New York, 2007, Oxford University Press.
55. Mohr DC, Ho J, Duffecy J, et al. Perceived barriers to psychological treatments and their relationship to depression. *J Clin Psychol* 66:394–409, 2010.
57. Mohr DC, Ho J, Duffecy J, et al. Effect of telephone-administered vs face-to-face cognitive behavioral therapy on adherence to therapy and depression outcomes among primary care patients: a randomized trial. *JAMA* 307:2278–2285, 2012.
58. Cook PF, Emiliozzi S, Waters C, et al. Effects of telephone counseling on antipsychotic adherence and emergency department utilization. *Am J Manag Care* 14:841–846, 2008.

5   Child, Adolescent, and Adult Development

Eric P. Hazen, MD, Annah N. Abrams, MD, and Anna C. Muriel, MD, MPH

KEY POINTS

- Development is not a linear process; it proceeds unevenly throughout the life cycle with periods of great activity and periods of relative quiescence in particular areas.

- Development is a process of complex interactions between genes and the environment and between a child and his or her caregivers.

- In general, development follows a fairly predictable course, particularly in early life; however, there can be a great deal of variability between individuals that is not necessarily indicative of dysfunction.

- Theorists have identified specific stages of development, which are often based on particular developmental tasks that must be accomplished during this stage to allow for healthy function later in life.

OVERVIEW

Development is a complex process that unfolds across the life span, guided along its course by intricate interactions between powerful forces. At the level of the organism, the child and his or her caregivers participate in a sophisticated interaction that begins before birth. The child is much more than a passive recipient of knowledge and skills passed down from the parents. Rather, the child is a lively participant, actively shaping parental behavior to ensure that his or her needs are met and the developmental process may continue. On the cellular and molecular level, environmental factors influence gene expression to alter function. Current thinking about development tends to downplay models that argue for the relative influence of "nature" versus "nurture"; instead, there is a focus on the complex interplay between these factors. Neurons live or die and the synaptic connections between them wither or grow stronger depending upon experience. The results of this process will help determine the behavior of the organism and thus influence its future.

In addition to the interactions between external forces, interactions between particular realms of development are essential to the overall process. For example, increasing motor skills during toddler-hood allow a child a greater sense of autonomy and control, thus allowing the child to build a sense of himself or herself that is distinct from his or her parents.

Development is not a steady linear process. It proceeds unevenly with periods of rapid growth in particular domains, interspersed with periods of relative quiescence. An understanding of development is essential to an understanding of the individual in health or in illness at any point in the life cycle. In this chapter, we begin with a discussion of some of the major contributors to current thinking about development. We then discuss the process of development throughout the life cycle beginning in infancy.

MAJOR THEORIES OF DEVELOPMENT

Sigmund Freud

Sigmund Freud (1856–1939) created a developmental theory that was closely tied to his drive theory, which is best described in his 1905 work, *Three Essays on the Theory of Sexuality.*[1] In these essays, Freud outlined his theory of childhood sexuality and portrayed child development as a process that unfolds across discrete, universal stages. He posited that infants are born as *polymorphously perverse,* meaning that the child has the capacity to experience libidinal pleasure from various areas of the body. Freud's stages of development were based on the area of the body (oral, anal, or phallic) that is the focus of the child's libidinal drive during that phase (Table 5-1). According to Freud, healthy adult function requires successful resolution of the core tasks of each developmental stage. Failure to resolve the tasks of a particular stage leads to a specific pattern of neurosis in adult life.

The first stage of development in Freud's scheme is the *oral phase,* which begins at birth and continues through approximately 12 to 18 months of age. During this period, the infant's drives are focused on the mouth, primarily through the pleasurable sensations associated with feeding. During this phase, the infant is wholly dependent on the mother; the infant must learn to trust the mother to meet his or her basic needs. Successful resolution of the oral phase provides a basis for healthy relationships later in life and allows the individual to trust others without excessive dependency. According to Freudian theory, an infant who is orally deprived may become pessimistic, demanding, or overly dependent as an adult.

Around 18 months of age, the oral phase gives way to the *anal phase.* During this phase, the focus of the child's libidinal energy shifts to his or her increasing control of bowel function through voluntary control of the anal sphincter. Failure to successfully negotiate the tasks of the anal phase can lead to the anal-retentive character type; affected individuals are overly meticulous, miserly, stubborn, and passive-aggressive, or the anal-expulsive character type, described as reckless and messy.

Around 3 years of age, the child enters into the *phallic phase* of development, during which the child becomes aware of the genitals and they become the child's focus of pleasure.[2] The phallic phase, which was described more fully in Freud's later work, has been the subject of greater controversy (and revision by psychoanalytic theorists) than the other phases. Freud believed that the penis was the focus of interest by children of both genders during this phase. Boys in the

TABLE 5-1 Corresponding Theoretical Stages of Development

Sigmund Freud: Psychosexual Phases	Erik Erickson: Psychosocial Stages	Jean Piaget: Stages of Cognitive Development
Oral (birth–18 mo)	Trust vs. Mistrust (birth–1 yr)	Sensorimotor (birth–2 yr)
Anal (18 mo–3 yr)	Autonomy vs. Shame and Doubt (1–3 yr)	Pre-operational (2–7 yr)
Phallic (3–5 yr)	Initiative vs. Guilt (3–6 yr)	
Latency (5–12 yr)	Industry vs. Inferiority (6–12 yr)	Concrete operations (7–12 yr)
Genital (12–18 yr)	Identity vs. Role Confusion (12–20 yr)	Formal operations (11 yr–adulthood)

phallic phase demonstrate exhibitionism and masturbatory behavior, whereas girls at this phase recognize that they do not have a phallus and are subject to *penis envy.*

Late in the phallic phase, Freud believed that the child developed primarily unconscious feelings of love and desire for the parent of the opposite sex, with fantasies of having sole possession of this parent and aggressive fantasies toward the same-sex parent. These feelings are referred to as the *Oedipal complex* after the figure of Oedipus in Greek mythology, who unknowingly killed his father and married his mother. In boys, Freud posited that guilt about Oedipal fantasies gives rise to *castration anxiety,* which refers to the fear that the father will retaliate against the child's hostile impulses by cutting off his penis. The Oedipal complex is resolved when the child manages these conflicting fears and desires through identification with the same-sex parent. As part of this process, the child may seek out same-sex peers. Successful negotiation of the Oedipal complex provides the foundation for secure sexual identity later in life.[3]

At the end of the phallic phase, around 5 to 6 years of age, Freud believed that the child's libidinal drives entered a period of relative inactivity that continues until the onset of puberty. This period is referred to as *latency.* This period of calm between powerful drives allows the child to further develop a sense of mastery and ego-strength, while integrating the sex-role defined in the Oedipal period into this growing sense of self.[1]

With the onset of puberty, around 11 to 13 years of age, the child enters the final developmental stage in Freud's model, called the *genital phase,* which continues into young adulthood.[3] During this phase, powerful libidinal drives re-surface, causing a re-emergence and re-working of the conflicts experienced in earlier phases. Through this process, the adolescent develops a coherent sense of identity and is able to separate from the parents.

Erik Erikson

Erik H. Erikson (1902–1994) modified the ideas of Freud and formulated his own psychoanalytic theory based on phases of development.[4] Erikson came to the United States just before World War II. As the first child analyst in Boston, he studied children at play, as well as Harvard students, and he studied a Native American tribe in the American West. Like Freud, he presented his theory in stages and like Freud he believed that problems present in adults are largely the result of unresolved conflicts of childhood. However, Erikson's stages emphasize not the person's relationship to his or her own sexual urges and instinctual drives, but rather the relationship between a person's maturing ego and both the family and the larger social culture in which he or she lives.

Erikson proposed eight developmental stages that cover an individual's entire life.[4] Each stage is characterized by a particular challenge, or what he called a "psychosocial crisis." The resolution of the particular crisis depends on the interaction between an individual's characteristics and the surrounding environment. When the developmental task at each stage has been completed, the result is a specific ego quality that a person will carry throughout the other stages. (For example, when a baby has managed the initial stage of Trust vs. Mistrust, the resultant ego virtue is Hope.)

Erikson's stages describe a vital conflict or tension in which the "negative" pole is necessary for growth. For example, in describing the initial stage of Trust vs. Mistrust, Erikson notes that babies interact with their caregivers, and what is important is that the baby comes to find predictability, consistency, and reliability in the caretaker's actions. In turn, the baby will develop a sense of trust and dependability. However, this does not mean a baby should not experience mistrust; Erikson noted that the infant must experience distrust in order to learn trust discerningly.

It should be noted that Erikson did not believe that a person could be "stuck" at any one stage. In his theory, if we live long enough we must pass through all of the stages. The forces that push a person from stage to stage are biological maturation and social expectations. Erikson believed that success at earlier stages affected the chances of success at later ones. For example, the child who develops a firm sense of trust in his or her caretakers is able to leave them and to explore the environment, in contrast to the child who lacks trust and who is less able to develop a sense of autonomy. However, whatever the outcome of the previous stage, a person will be faced with the tasks of the subsequent stage.

Jean Piaget

Like Erikson, Jean Piaget (1896–1980) was another developmental stage theorist. Piaget was the major architect of cognitive theory and his ideas provided a comprehensive framework for an understanding of cognitive development. Piaget's first studies on how children think were conducted while he was working for a laboratory designing intelligence testing for children. He became interested not in a child's answering a question correctly, but rather, when the child's answer was wrong, understanding *why* it was wrong.[5] He concluded that younger children think differently than older children do. Through clinical interviews with children, watching children's spontaneous activity, and close observations of his own children, he developed a theory that described specific periods of cognitive development.

Piaget maintained that there are four major stages: the sensorimotor intelligence period, the pre-operational thought period, the concrete operations period, and the formal operations period (see Table 5-1).[6] Each period has specific features that enable a child to comprehend certain kinds of knowledge and understanding. Piaget believed that children pass through these stages at different rates, but maintained that they do so in sequence, and in the same order.

Characteristics of the sensorimotor intelligence period (from birth to about 2 years) are that an infant uses senses and motor skills to obtain information and an understanding about the world around him or her. There is no conceptual or reflective thought; an object is "known" in terms of what an infant can "do" to it. A significant cognitive milestone is achieved when the infant learns the concept of object permanence: that is, that an object still exists when is it not in the child's visual field. By the end of this period a child is aware of self and other, and the child understands that they are but one object among many.

From ages 2 to 7 a child uses pre-operational thought, where the child begins to develop symbolic thinking, including language. The use of symbols contributes to the growth of the child's imagination. A child might use one object to represent another in play, such as a box becoming a racecar. Piaget also described this period as a time when pre-schoolers are characterized by egocentric thinking. Egocentrism means that the child sees the world from his or her own perspective and has difficulty seeing another person's point of view. For a child of this age, everyone thinks and feels the same way as the child does. The capacity to acknowledge another's point of view develops gradually during the pre-school years; while a 2-year-old will participate in parallel play with a peer, a 4-year-old will engage in cooperative play with another child. Toward the end of this period, a child will begin to understand and to coordinate several points of view.

Just as a child in this stage fails to consider more than one perspective in personal interactions, he or she is unable to consider more than one dimension. In his famous experiment, Piaget demonstrated that a child in a pre-operational stage is unable to consider two perceptual dimensions (such as height and width). A child is shown two glasses (I and II), which are filled to the same height with water. The child agrees that the glasses have the same amount of liquid. Next, the child pours the liquid from glass I to another, shorter and wider glass (III) and is asked if the amount of liquid is still the same. The child in the pre-operational stage will answer "No," that there is more water in glass I because the water is at a higher level. By age 7, the child will understand that there is the same amount of liquid in each glass; this is termed *conservation of liquids,* and it is a concept children master when they are entering the next stage. Children also learn conservation of number, mass, and substance as they mature.

During middle childhood (ages 7 to 11), Piaget described a child's cognitive style as concrete operational. The child is able to understand and to apply logic and can interpret experiences objectively, instead of intuitively. Children are able to coordinate several perspectives and are able to use concepts, such as conservation, classification (a bead can be both green and plastic, whereas a pre-operational child would see the bead as either green or plastic), and seriation (blocks can be arranged in order of largest to smallest).

These "mental actions" enable children to think systematically and with logic; however, their use of logic is limited to mostly that which is tangible.[6] The final stage of Piaget's cognitive theory is formal operations, which occurs around age 11 and continues into adulthood. In this stage, the early adolescent and then the adult is able to consider hypothetical and abstract thought, can consider several possibilities or outcomes, and has the capacity to understand concepts as relative rather than absolute. In formal operations, a young adult is able to discern the underlying motivations or principles of something (such as an idea, a theory, or an action) and can apply them to novel situations.

Piaget conceptualized cognitive development as an active process by which children build cognitive structures based on their interactions with their environment. Similarly, he determined that moral development is a developmental process. Piaget described the earliest stages of moral reasoning as based on a strict adherence to rules, duties, and obedience to authority without questioning. Considered in parallel to his stages of cognitive development, the pre-operational child sees rules as fixed and absolute, and punishment as automatic. For the child in concrete operations, rules are mutually accepted and fair, and are to be followed to the letter without further consideration; however, as the child moves from egocentrism to perspective-taking he or she begins to see that strict adherence to the rules can be problematic. With formal operations, a child gains the ability to act from a sense of reciprocity, and is able to coordinate his or her perspective with that of others, thus basing what is "right" on solutions that are considered most fair.

Lawrence Kohlberg

Lawrence Kohlberg (1927–1987) elaborated on Piaget's work on moral reasoning and cognitive development and identified a stage theory of moral thinking that is based on the idea that cognitive maturation affects reasoning about moral dilemmas. Kohlberg described six stages of moral reasoning that are determined by a person's thought process rather than the moral conclusions the person reaches.[7] He presented a person with a moral dilemma and studied the person's response; the most famous dilemma involved Heinz, a poor man whose wife was dying of cancer. A pharmacist had the only cure, and the drug cost more money than Heinz would ever have.

Heinz went to everyone he knew to borrow the money, but he could only get together about half of what it cost. He told the druggist that his wife was dying and asked him to sell it cheaper or let him pay later. But the druggist said "No." The husband got desperate and broke into the man's store to steal the drug for his wife. Should the husband have done that? Why?[7]

How a person responds to such a dilemma places the person within three levels of moral reasoning: pre-conventional, conventional, and post-conventional. A child's answer would generally be at the first two levels, with a pre-schooler most likely at level I and an elementary school child at level II. Kohlberg stressed that moral development is dependent on a person's thought and experience, which is closely related to the person's cognitive maturation.

Kohlberg is not without his critics, who view his schema as Western, predominantly male, and hierarchical. For example, in many non-Western ethnic groups the good of the family or the well-being of the community takes moral precedence over all other considerations.[8] Such groups would not score well at Kohlberg's post-conventional level. Another critic, Carol Gilligan, sees Kohlberg's stages as biased against women. She believed that Kohlberg did not take into account the gender differences of how men and woman make moral judgments, and as such, his conception of morality leaves out the female voice.[9] She has viewed female morality as placing a higher value on interpersonal relationships, compassion, and caring for others than on rules and rights. However, despite important differences between how men and women might respond when presented with an ethical dilemma, research has shown that there is not a significant moral divide between the genders.[10]

Attachment Theory: John Bowlby and Mary Ainsworth

John Bowlby (1907–1990) was a British psychoanalyst who was interested in the role of early development in determining psychological function later in life. Bowlby particularly focused his attention on the study of *attachment,* which can be defined as the emotional bond between caregiver and infant. Bowlby's theory was grounded in his clinical work with families disrupted by World War II and with delinquent children at London's Child Guidance Clinic. Attachment theory also had its roots in evolutionary biology and studies of animal behavior, such as Harry Harlow's studies of rhesus monkeys deprived of maternal contact after birth.

Bowlby argued that human infants are born with a powerful, evolutionarily-derived drive to connect with the mother.[11] Infants exhibit *attachment behaviors* (such as smiling, sucking, and crying) that facilitate the child's connection to the mother. The child is predisposed to psychopathology if there are difficulties in forming a secure attachment, for example, in a mother with severe mental illness, or there are disruptions in attachment (such as prolonged separation from the mother). Bowlby described three stages of behavior in children who are separated from their mother for an extended period.[12] First, the child will *protest* by calling or crying out. Then the child exhibits signs of *despair,* in which he or she appears to give up hope of the mother's return. Finally, the child enters a state of *detachment,* appearing to have emotionally separated himself or herself from the mother and initially appearing indifferent to her if she returns.

Mary Ainsworth (1913–1999) studied under Bowlby and expanded on his theory of attachment. She developed a research protocol called the *strange situation,* in which an infant is left alone with a stranger in a room briefly vacated by the mother.[13] By closely observing the infant's behavior during both the separation and the reunion in this protocol, Ainsworth was able to further describe the nature of attachment in young children. Based on her observations, she categorized the attachment relationships in her subjects as secure or insecure. Insecure attachments were further divided into the categories of insecure-avoidant, insecure-resistant, and insecure-disorganized/disoriented. Trained raters can consistently and reliably classify an infant's attachments into these categories based on specific, objective patterns of behavior. Ainsworth found that approximately 65% of infants in a middle-class sample had secure attachments by 24 months of age.

Research into early attachment and its role in future psychological function is ongoing, and attachment theory continues to have a major influence in the study of child development and psychopathology. It has also influenced how the legal system approaches children, for example, by contributing to a shift toward the "best interests of the child" doctrine in determining custody decisions that began in the 1970s.

BRAIN DEVELOPMENT

Normal brain development is the result of a series of orderly events that occur both *in utero* and after birth. Recent research suggests that the brain continues to develop well into adulthood. In addition, neurodevelopment is affected by the interaction between gene expression and environmental events, which is to say that both nature and nurture play an important role.

The mature human brain is believed to have at least 100 billion cells. Neurons and glial cells derive from the neural plate, and during gestation new neurons are being generated at the rate of about 250,000 per minute.[14] Once they are made, these cells migrate, differentiate, and then establish connections to other neurons. Brain development occurs in stages, and each stage is dependent on the stage that comes before. Any disruption in this process can result in abnormal development, which may or may not have clinical relevance. It is believed that disruptions that occur in the early stages of brain development are linked to more significant pathology and those that occur later are associated with less diffuse problems.[15]

By around day 20 of gestation, primitive cell layers have organized to form the neural plate, which is a thickened mass comprised primarily of ectoderm. Cells are induced to form neural ectoderm in a complicated series of interactions between them. The neural plate continues to thicken and fold, and by the end of week 3 the neural tube (the basis of the nervous system) has formed (Figure 5-1).[16]

The neuroepithelial cells that make up the neural tube are the precursors of all central nervous system (CNS) cells, including neurons and glial cells. As the embryo continues to develop, cells of the CNS differentiate, proliferate, and migrate. Differentiation is the process whereby a primitive cell gains specific biochemical and anatomical function. Proliferation is the rapid cellular division (mitosis) that occurs near the inner edge of the neural tube wall (ventricular zone) and is followed by migration of these cells to their "correct" location. As primitive neuroblasts move out toward the external border of the thickening neural tube, this "trip" becomes longer and more complicated. This migration results in six cellular layers of cerebral cortex, and each group of migrating cells must pass through the layers that formed previously (Figure 5-2). It is believed that alterations in this process can result in abnormal neurodevelopment, such as a finding at autopsy of abnormal cortical layering in the brains of some patients with schizophrenia.[17]

Once an immature neuron arrives at its final location, it extends a single axon and up to several dendrites to establish connections to other neurons. The synapse, or the end structure of a neuron, makes contact with the dendrites of neighboring neurons. Neuronal growth and proliferation is determined by signals (such as neurotransmitters and growth factors). During subsequent stages of fetal development these connections continue to proliferate, such that at birth, a person has almost all the neurons that an individual will use in his or her lifetime.

Post-natal brain development is a period of both continued cellular growth and fine-tuning the established brain circuitry with processes of cellular regression (including apoptosis and pruning).[15] While the human brain continues to grow and to mature into the mid-twenties, the brain at birth weighs approximately 10% of the newborn's body weight, compared to the adult brain, which is about 2% of body weight. This growth is due to dendritic growth, myelination, and glial cell growth.

Apoptosis, or programmed cell death, is a normal process that improves neuronal efficiency and accuracy by eliminating cells that fail to function properly. This may include extinguishing temporary circuits that were necessary at earlier periods during development, but that are no longer required. This system of first over-growth and later pruning helps to stabilize synaptic connections and also provides the brain with the opportunity to establish plasticity in response to the environment.

There are "critical periods" of development when the brain requires certain environmental input to develop normally. For example, at age 2 to 3 months there is prominent metabolic activity in the visual and parietal cortex, which corresponds with the development of an infant's ability to integrate visual-spatial stimuli (such as the ability to follow an object with one's eyes). If the baby's visual cortex is not stimulated, this circuitry will not be well established. Synaptic growth continues rapidly during the first year of life, and is followed by pruning of un-used connections (a process that ends sometime during puberty).

Myelination of neuronal axons begins at birth, and occurs first in the spinal cord and brainstem and then in the brain. The cerebral cortex is not fully myelinated until young adulthood. Myelin acts to insulate axons and facilitates more

TRANSVERSE SECTION OF THE NEURAL PLATE

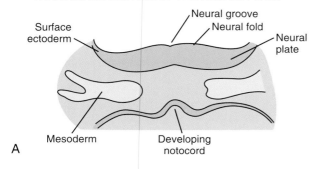

Surface ectoderm

Neural groove
Neural fold
Neural plate

Mesoderm

Developing notocord

A

FORMATION OF NEURAL GROOVE AND NEURAL CREST

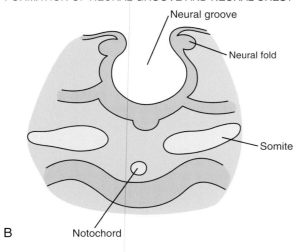

Neural groove

Neural fold

Somite

Notochord

B

DEVELOPED NEURAL TUBE

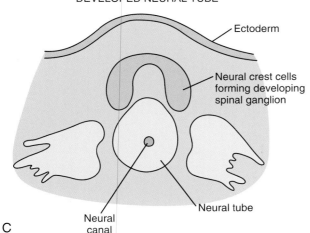

Ectoderm

Neural crest cells forming developing spinal ganglion

Neural tube

Neural canal

C

Figure 5-1. The embryonic development of the nervous system. The nervous system develops out of the outer layer of embryonic cells, called *ectoderm*. During the third week of development, the ectoderm along the midline of the embryo's dorsal surface thickens to form the *neural plate* (A). The center of the neural plate indents to form the neural groove. Over the next week, the groove deepens as the *neural folds* along each side of the neural groove curl toward each other at the midline (B). By the end of the third week of gestation, the two neural folds have joined together at the midline to form the *neural tube*, which is the basis of the entire nervous system (C). *Neural crest* cells at the dorsum of the neural tube separate to form the basis of the peripheral nervous system.

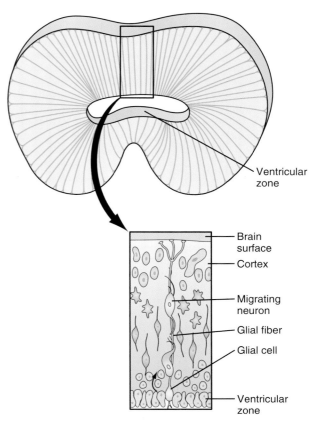

Ventricular zone

Brain surface
Cortex

Migrating neuron

Glial fiber

Glial cell

Ventricular zone

Figure 5-2. The process of neuronal migration during brain development. Neurons originate from the proliferation of primitive neuroblasts in the ventricular zone. They must then migrate outward toward the brain surface to their ultimate destination in the cortex. Glial cells are thought to assist in the migration process by providing longitudinal fibers to guide the migrating cell.

efficient information-processing; however, myelin inhibits plasticity because a myelinated axon is less able to change connections in response to a stimulus.

Newer imaging techniques have made it possible to continue to study patterns of brain development into young adulthood. In one longitudinal study of 145 children and adolescents, it was found that there is a second period of synaptogenesis (primarily in the frontal lobe) just before puberty that results in a thickening of gray matter followed by further pruning.[18] Perhaps this is related to the development of executive-function skills noted during adolescence. In another study, researchers found that white matter growth begins at the front of the brain in early childhood and moves caudally, and subsides after puberty. Spurts of growth from ages 6 to 13 were seen in the temporal and parietal lobes and then dropped off sharply, which may correlate with the critical period for language development.[19]

Social and emotional experiences help contribute to normal brain development from a young age and continue through adulthood. Environmental input can shape neuronal connections that are responsible for processes (e.g., memory, emotion, self-awareness).[20] The limbic system, hippocampus, and amygdala continue to develop during infancy, childhood, and adolescence. The final part of the brain to mature is the pre-frontal cortex, and adulthood is marked by continued refinement of knowledge and learned abilities, as well as by executive function and by abstract thinking.

Infancy (Birth to 18 Months)

Winnicott famously remarked, "There is no such thing as a baby. There is only a mother and a baby."[21] In this statement, we are reminded that infants are wholly dependent on their caretakers in meeting their physical and psychological needs. At birth, the infant's sensory systems are incompletely developed and the motor system is characterized by the dominance of primitive reflexes. Because the cerebellum is not fully formed until 1 year of age, and myelination of peripheral nerves is not complete until after 2 years of age, the newborn infant has little capacity for voluntary, purposeful movement. However, the infant is born with hard-wired mechanisms for survival that are focused on the interaction with the mother. For instance, newborns show a visual preference for faces and will turn preferentially toward familiar or female voices. The rooting reflex, in which the infant turns toward stimulation of the cheek or lips, the sucking reflex, and the coordination of sucking and swallowing allow most neonates to nurse successfully soon after birth. Though near-sighted, a focal length of 8 to 12 inches allows the neonate to gaze at the mother's face while nursing. This shared gaze between infant and mother is one of the early steps in the process of attachment.

The infant spends more than 16 hours each day sleeping in the first weeks of life. Initially, sleep occurs in irregular intervals evenly dispersed throughout the day and night. As the nervous system matures, sleep patterns shift, with a gradual decline in the total sleep time and a consolidation of this time into longer periods during the night. By 6 months of age, 70% of infants will be sleeping through the night for a period of 6 hours or more, to the relief of their weary parents, with extended naps during the day to meet their still considerable need for sleep.

Temperament

Infants demonstrate significant variability in their characteristic patterns of behavior and their ways of responding to the environment. Some of these characteristics appear to be inborn, in that they can be observed at an early age and remain fairly constant throughout the life span. The work of Stella Chess and Alexander Thomas in the New York Longitudinal Study helped capture this variability in their description of temperament.[22] Temperament, as defined by Chess and Thomas, refers to individual differences in physiological responses to the environment. Chess and Thomas described nine behavioral dimensions of temperament, as outlined in Table 5-2.

Based on these nine dimensions, Chess and Thomas found that 65% of children fit into three basic categories of temperaments. Forty percent of children in their study were categorized as "easy or flexible." The easy child tends to be calm, adaptable, easily soothed, and regular in his or her patterns of eating and sleeping. Fifteen percent of children were described as "slow to warm up or cautious." Children in this group tended to withdraw or to react negatively to new situations, but their reactions gradually become more positive with repeated exposure. Ten percent of children were categorized as "difficult, active, or feisty." These children tended to be fussy, less adaptable to changes in routine, irregular in feeding and sleeping patterns, fearful of new people and situations, and intense in their reactions. The remaining 35% of children in the study did not fit any single pattern of behavior, but rather some combination of behaviors from these categories.

Chess and Thomas hypothesized that different parenting styles would be optimal for children of different temperaments.[23] They coined the term *goodness of fit* to describe the degree to which an individual child's environment is compatible with the child's temperament in a way that allows the child to achieve his or her potential and to develop healthy self-esteem. When the child's temperament is not accommodated, there is a *poorness of fit* that may lead to negative self-evaluation and to emotional problems later in life.

Motor Development in Infancy

Primitive reflexes include the grasp reflex and the tonic neck reflex. These reflexes begin to recede between 2 and 6 months of age, allowing for increasing volitional control. The grasp reflex diminishes at 2 months of age, clearing the way for an increasing ability to voluntarily pick up objects. Voluntary grasp begins with raking hand movements that emerge at 3 to 4 months of age. By 6 months of age, an infant can reach for and grasp an object (e.g., a toy rattle) and transfer it from hand to hand. Fine pincer grasp of an object between the thumb and forefinger generally develops around 9 to 12 months of age, as exhibited when an infant is able to pick up Cheerios.

The tonic neck reflex, in which turning the newborn's head to one side produces involuntary extension of the limbs on the same side and flexion of the limbs on the opposite side, begins to fade at 4 months of age, giving way to more symmetrical posture and clearing the way for continued gross motor development. The infant begins to show increasing head control at 1 to 2 months, and increased truncal control allows the infant to roll from front to back around 4 months of age. However, in recent years, with infants spending less time on their stomachs (in large part due to the American Academy of Pediatrics recommendations that infants sleep on their backs), the typical development of rolling occurs closer to 6 months of age. The ability to sit without support develops at 6 months. Many infants begin to crawl around 8 months of age and can pull to stand around 9 months. Cruising, walking while holding onto objects (such as coffee tables and chairs), precedes independent walking, which begins around 12 months of age. Major developmental milestones are illustrated in Figure 5-3, the Denver II Developmental Assessment.[24]

TABLE 5-2 The Nine Dimensions of Temperament

ACTIVITY LEVEL	The level of motor activity demonstrated by the child and the proportion of active to inactive time
RHYTHMICITY	The regularity of timing in the child's biological functions such as eating and sleeping
APPROACH OR WITHDRAWAL	The nature of the child's initial response to a new situation or stimulus
ADAPTABILITY	The child's long-term (as opposed to initial) response to new situations
THRESHOLD OF RESPONSIVENESS	The intensity level required of a stimulus to evoke a response from the child
INTENSITY OF REACTION	The energy level of a child's response
QUALITY OF MOOD	The general emotional quality of the child's behavior, as measured by the amount of pleasant, joyful, or friendly behavior versus unpleasant, crying, or unfriendly behavior
DISTRACTIBILITY	The effect of extraneous stimuli in interfering with or changing the direction of the child's activity
ATTENTION SPAN AND PERSISTENCE	The length of time the child pursues a particular activity without interruption and the child's persistence in continuing an activity despite obstacles

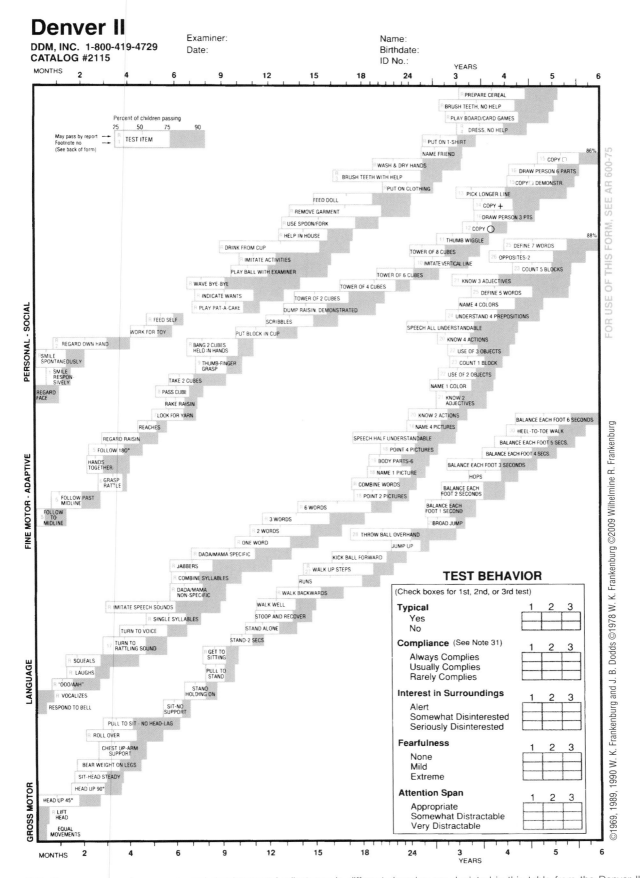

Figure 5-3. The age ranges for some normal developmental milestones in different domains are depicted in this table from the Denver II, a commonly used screening tool for developmental disorders. Items are divided into four categories: personal-social, fine motor–adaptive, language, and gross motor. Each item is depicted by a bar that corresponds to the age range, shown along the top and bottom of the chart, during which 25% to 90% of a normative sample of children is able to successfully complete that item. *(© 1969, 1989, 1990 W. K. Frankenburg and J. B. Dodds © 1978 W. K. Frankenburg © 2009 Wilhelmine R. Frankenburg.)*

Cognitive Development in Infancy

In the first 2 years of life, the infant's cognitive development follows from the infant's increased capacity to explore both the outside world and his or her own body. According to psychodynamic theories, the infant begins to develop a representation of "self" and "other" as he or she learns from early sensory and motor exploration to differentiate the self from the external world.

In Piaget's theory, described previously, the infant progresses through the sensorimotor stage in the first 2 years of life.[6] During this time, the infant learns about himself or herself and the external environment through sensory input and uses developing motor skills to learn to manipulate the environment. A major milestone during this stage is the development, between 9 and 12 months, of object permanence, in which the infant gradually realizes that objects continue to exist when they cannot be seen. Before this stage, infants will quickly give up looking for an object that has been dropped if it is not seen. Following the development of object permanence, an infant will look for a toy that had been visible to the infant and is now hidden under a blanket.

Language Development in Infancy

Communication in the first months of life is achieved through non-verbal means. However, the infant is attuned to language at birth. Newborns have been shown to preferentially attend to human voices. There is some evidence that even *in utero* the fetus shows a stronger response to the mother's voice compared to the voices of other females.[25] By 6 months infants can detect phonetic differences in speech sounds that are played to them. At 9 months, infants begin to demonstrate comprehension of individual words. By 13 months, they have a receptive vocabulary of approximately 20 to 100 words.

Expressive language development tends to lag behind receptive language and begins at age 2 months, when the infant first begins to engage in vocalizations, such as cooing. Reciprocal vocal play with the mother encourages these early vocal efforts and facilitates increasing motor control of the vocal apparatus. Infants typically begin babbling at 6 months, repeating speech sounds such as "da da da." The infant's first words are used non-specifically and often emerge around 10 to 11 months of age. At 12 months, the infant begins to use words such as "Dada" or "Mama" specifically. At 18 months, a child normally uses about 10 to 15 words.

Social and Emotional Development in Infancy

Perhaps the most significant developmental task of the infant with regard to later psychological well-being is that of attachment. The infant plays an active role in this process. The infant's early social behaviors are reflexive in nature, such as imitating the facial expressions of others, which the infant may begin to do by 4 weeks of age. Initially, the infant's smile is spontaneous and unrelated to external stimuli. With time, however, the infant smiles in response to stimuli in the environment (such as the appearance of a parent's face). This response is called the *social smile*. The social smile usually becomes distinguishable from the endogenous smile between 6 and 8 weeks. With time and social interaction with the parents, the infant smiles in response to a growing number of stimuli (such as a favorite toy).

Beginning around 3 months of age, the infant begins to show clear signs of recognizing the primary caregivers. This begins a process of narrowing the focus of attachment. *Stranger-anxiety*, in which the infant begins to show signs of distress at the approach of a stranger, may begin to emerge around 6 months and is fully present by 9 months of age. Before this, infants have an accepting and even welcoming response to unfamiliar adults. However, the 9-month-old infant generally shows a strong preference for one or both parents, and may cry, stare, or cling to the parent when others attempt to interact with the child, even those who have a close relationship with the child (such as a grandparent). Stranger-anxiety is often more intense when an infant has only one primary caregiver. It usually reaches its peak around 12 to 15 months of age. *Separation-anxiety*, as opposed to stranger-anxiety, is defined as a child's sense of discomfort on separation from the primary caretaker, and occurs when a child is between 10 and 18 months old.

Once a young child's motor skills have developed sufficiently, the child begins to use his or her new-found mobility to explore the environment. In Mahler's theory of separation-individuation, this phase of exploration is called the *practicing subphase*, which corresponds to roughly 10 to 16 months of age.[26] Early in this stage, the child experiences elation as he or she develops a sense of self and his or her abilities. However, these early explorations are characterized by the need to frequently re-establish contact with the mother, which may be achieved physically (by returning to her), visually (by seeking eye contact), or verbally (by calling out to her). This contact with the mother allows the child to regain the sense of security that he or she needs to continue explorations. The degree to which the child seeks out the mother during this phase is variable and dependent on the child's individual temperament.

As the child transitions into toddler-hood, the growing need for autonomy comes into conflict with the need to be soothed by the mother. Mahler described this stage, occurring between 16 and 24 months, as the *rapprochment subphase*. During this stage, the child is thought to become more aware of the possibility of separation from the mother. This generates anxiety that tempers the child's earlier elation and may manifest as increased clinging, whining, temper tantrums, and intense reactions to separation. Mahler theorized that the child's internal representation of the mother at this age is not sufficient to soothe the child. During the *rapprochement crisis*, the child may feel an intense need to be soothed by the mother, but is unable to accept her help. This crisis is resolved as the child builds a more stable internal representation of the mother and with it the ability to achieve gratification in doing things independently.

Many children will identify a *transitional object* to help soothe them during the process of separating from the parents. This frequently occurs around 1 year of age and generally takes the form of a soft object (such as a blanket or stuffed animal) that has some association with the mother. Winnicott hypothesized that such objects provide a physical reminder of the mother's presence before the child has fully developed an internal representation of the mother and the ability to separate without anxiety.[27] Most children will surrender their transitional object by age 5, though there is considerable variability in children's behavior in this area.

Pre-school Years (2½ to 5 Years)

The child's first clumsy steps signify more than just a motor milestone. With an increasing ability to physically navigate his or her environment, the child develops a growing sense of autonomy and control while still looking to the parents to establish the feeling of safety required in order to continue exploring. The child's experimentation in the physical world leads to an increased representational capacity and to symbolic thinking. The child's language skills explode during this time, allowing for fuller engagement in the social world.

Through both language and play, the child begins to develop an understanding of his or her own thoughts and feelings, and learns that others have thoughts and feelings distinct from his or her own.

Physical and Motor Development in the Pre-school Years

The pre-school years are a period of increased physical growth and increasing refinement of motor skills. Children typically grow 2½ to 3 inches per year between ages 2 and 5, reaching half their adult height between 2 and 3 years of age. The toddler's clumsy steps gradually give way to a more fluid and balanced gait. By 2 years of age, most children are able to run and to go up and down stairs on their own. Most children are able to ride a tricycle by age 3, and they can hop on one foot by 3½. By 4 years they can stand on one foot for several seconds, hop fairly easily, and throw a ball overhand. By 5 years, most children can skip. Over this period, fine motor skills gradually develop as well. A child can generally build a tower of 3 or 4 cubes at 18 months, 6 cubes at 2 years, and 10 cubes by 3 years. A 3-year-old child can copy a circle, a 4-year-old can copy a square, and a 5-year-old can usually copy a triangle.

Cognitive Development in the Pre-school Years

Cognitive development in the pre-school years is characterized by increasing symbolic thought. In Piaget's model, age 2 marks the end of the sensorimotor stage of development and the beginning of the pre-operational stage.[6] During this stage, children show an increase in the use of mental representations in their thinking. They learn to represent an object or idea with a symbol, such as a drawing, a mental image, or a word. The growth of symbolic thinking is evident in the pre-schooler's increased use of language, imaginary play, and drawing.

The child's thinking in the pre-school years is primarily intuitive, rather than logical. Pre-school children also demonstrate egocentricity and magical thinking. They see themselves as the center of the world and have difficulty understanding the perspectives of others. For example, they may not understand that when they are pointing to a picture in a book that they are holding (facing themselves), their parent is unable to see the picture. They also blur the distinction between fantasy and reality, as evidenced by young children's real belief in Santa Claus or in monsters.

Causal relations are also poorly understood at this age. Pre-school-age children frequently demonstrate a phenomenalistic understanding of causality, meaning that the child assumes that if two events occur together, then one event must have caused the other. This aspect of pre-school children's thinking can be important clinically in understanding how a young child interprets the events in his or her life. For instance, a pre-school-age child who has an earache from an infection might believe that he became sick from eating too many cookies or because he hit his sister. More significant changes, such as divorce or changes in caregivers, can also be attributed to their own thoughts or behavior in a particular blend of egocentrism and magical thinking, which can have more complex psychological sequelae if these misconceptions are not dispelled and guilt alleviated. Other characteristics of magical thinking at this age include *artificialism*, the belief that natural phenomena (such as thunder and lightning) are created by human beings or monsters, and *animism*, the tendency to attribute human characteristics, such as intentions and feelings, to physical objects. A child who trips on a chair leg by accident might, for example, call it a "bad chair."

Language Development in the Pre-school Years

Children's language ability explodes during the pre-school years. A child's vocabulary typically grows from 10 to 15 words at 18 months to over 50 words by 2 years of age. By age 5, the vocabulary of most children has grown to over 2,000 words. At age 2, the child begins putting two and three words together to form sentences and is able to understand multi-step commands and statements. Children's mastery of articulation typically lags behind their vocabulary. For instance, 2-year-olds frequently demonstrate errors of pronunciation (e.g., altering, shortening, or dropping speech sounds, such as "poon" for the word "spoon"). As articulation abilities mature, these errors gradually diminish. By age 4, most children make few of these errors, and their speech is mostly comprehensible to others outside their immediate circle of caregivers.

Language development in the pre-school years is highly variable, with a broad range of abilities that could be considered normal. Development is largely influenced by environmental influences, such as the amount of speech to which the child is exposed and the degree to which adults in the child's environment engage the child linguistically using questions, description, and encouragement of the child's efforts toward expressing himself or herself.[28]

Problems in language development usually occur during this time of rapid acquisition of language.[28] Stuttering affects up to 3% of pre-school-age children. While this problem usually resolves on its own, prolonged or severe stuttering may require referral to a speech therapist for treatment.[29]

As the emergence of language allows for greater connection with a child's internal world, the pre-school years are often when problems in other realms of development are first detected. Intellectual disabilities, for example, are often detected at age 2 when the child fails to attain language milestones.

Social and Emotional Development in the Pre-school Years

The growth of language skills in the pre-school years facilitates and is facilitated by a similarly explosive growth in the child's social and emotional development. Language helps organize the child's growing sense of self. The child also uses language and his or her growing mastery of symbolic thought to engage in increasingly creative play. Around age 2 to 3, play emerges as simple mimicry of daily events, such as feeding a baby. Over the next 3 years, the scenarios acted out through play become progressively more sophisticated and creative. For example, a child may progress from simply feeding the baby at age 3, to acting out the preparation of a favorite meal at age 4, to creating an elaborate domestic scene in playing "house" at age 5.

Despite being with other children (e.g., in playgroups or at a playground), play at this age is primarily solitary with minimal social interaction with other children or adults. This is described as *parallel play:* two children sitting next to each other in a pretend kitchen playing with pots and pans, but not interacting with one another. As children get older their play becomes increasingly interactive. Parallel play gives way to *associative play* around 3 years of age, in which play takes place in an increasingly overlapping space through sharing toys but remains a primarily solo endeavor with each child acting out his or her own script. In associative play, two children playing in a pretend kitchen will share the pots and pans, but cook separate meals. For most children, associative play has evolved into *cooperative play,* in which children work together on a task and can take turns with toys, by age 4. Cooperative play is seen when the children playing in the kitchen begin to work together, sharing the pots and pans to create a meal.

Cooperative play continues to evolve throughout early childhood into an increasingly structured and interactive activity in which distinct roles are assigned and acted out.

Both play and language allow the child to build an understanding of the behavior and, eventually, the inner lives of those around him or her. Between 2 and 4 years of age, children develop the ability to recognize and to label distinct emotional states, starting with the basic emotions (such as happiness, sadness, or anger). By age 3, most children are able to mimic an appropriate facial expression for these basic feelings. By age 4, most children are able to identify what emotional state would be appropriate for a particular situation. References to feelings and mental states in a child's language increase significantly beginning around age 3.

Theory of mind is a term used to indicate the child's capacity to represent and to reflect on the feelings and mental states of others. Important steps in the development of a child's theory of mind occur between 3½ and 5 years of age. At age 3, the typical child has difficulty understanding that other people have mental states that are distinct from his or her own. This can be demonstrated in a paradigm called the *false-belief task*, described by Wimmer and Perner.[30] In this paradigm, the child is presented with a story in which a character has a mistaken belief about the location of an object, and the child is asked to predict where the character will look for that object. To answer correctly on the false-belief task, a child must be able to assume the perspective of a character in the story. Between ages 3½ and 5, children's performance on this task improves as they are increasingly able to represent the mental states of others and accurately predict behavior on this basis. This capacity to appreciate the perspective of others allows for the development of more complex social interactions, empathy, and cooperation regarding the needs and feelings of others.

Moral Development in the Pre-school Years

The pre-schooler has a black-and-white view of right and wrong, and generally is motivated to follow the rules to avoid punishment. Children at this age strive to be obedient within the context of their own desires, and their behavior is governed by external validation and consequences. They gradually internalize the moral values of their world, and by age 6 have a conscience. These values are shaped by several influences, including praise, consistent parenting, limit-setting, identification with parental values, and an increasing capacity for empathy.

Gender Identity

The younger pre-schooler chooses friends without concern about gender; the younger school-age child may be aware of sexual anatomical differences between boys and girls, but gender segregation among peers has yet to occur. Sex-typed behavior develops gradually, often in concert with the development of the ability to categorize. A child's gender identity, first formed around age 2, becomes more established during early childhood. A 4-year-old child may be able to say what toys or behaviors are "for girls" or "for boys," but it is not until middle childhood that a child will adopt gender-specific behavior (as defined by cultural norms). The pre-schooler's gender identity is somewhat fluid, which might be reflected in games (such as cross-gender dress-up), or a statement from a young boy that he wants to be a mommy when he grows up.

During the pre-school years children often have an interest in their own genitals or in those of others, and they at times engage in sexual exploration, such as playing "doctor." By approximately age 6 this behavior abates, as the child is socialized and learns that in public, sexualized interests and activities are not appropriate. Exhibitionistic or compulsive sexualized behavior in public after age 6 is atypical and may warrant an evaluation.

School-age Years (5 to 12 Years)

As a child grows from pre-school-age to school-age, the developmental challenges become more varied and complex. The child's world expands beyond the primarily home-centered environment to other, more social arenas (such as nursery school and kindergarten), activities such as cub scouts or gymnastics, and play dates with peers. The pre-schooler matures from the egocentric toddler to a young child with the capacity to think logically, to empathize with others, and to exercise self-control. The child's cognitive style gradually evolves from magical thinking to one based more in logic, with an ability to understand cause and effect and to distinguish between fantasy and reality. As a child becomes more autonomous, peer relationships begin to play an increasingly important role in the young child's social and emotional development. Maturation (including increasing language acquisition, improved motor skills, continued cognitive growth, and the capacity for self-regulation) help equip the pre-school-age child for these challenges.

Middle childhood extends from approximately age 7 to the onset of puberty between ages 10 and 12. School-age children are faced with the task of integrating their newly developed and independent sense of self into a world of rules, customs, and order. Their task is more complex, but their skills—predominantly cognitive and social—are also more refined. Children may have uneven development in the following arenas with variations in skill acquisition, and may have expectable transient regressions during developmental or environmental stress or transitions.

Language Development in the School-age Years

By age 7, a child has a basic grasp of grammar and syntax. Unlike the pre-school child, whose use of language is primarily based on specific concepts and rules, the school-age child begins to comprehend variations of those rules and various constructions. The child's vocabulary continues to increase, although not as rapidly as during the pre-school years. A child in this age-group is able to understand and manipulate semantics and enjoy word play; for example, in the Amelia Bedelia series of books, Amelia throws dirt on the family couch when she is asked to "dust the furniture."[31] Language becomes an increasingly effective means of self-expression as the school-age child is able to tell a story with a beginning, a middle, and an end. This mastery of language and expression also helps young children modulate affect, as they can more readily understand and explain their frustrations.

Motor Development in the School-age Years

Steady physical growth continues into middle childhood, but at a slower rate than during early childhood. Boys are on average slightly larger than girls until around age 11, when girls are likely to have an earlier pubertal growth spurt.[32] It can be a period of uneven growth, and some children may have an awkward appearance; however, for most children of this age there is a relatively low level of concern about their physical appearance (especially for boys.) However, both peers and the media can influence how a child feels about his or her body, and even pre-pubertal girls can begin to exhibit symptoms of eating disorders and body image distortions. Gross motor skills (such as riding a bicycle) continue to improve and to develop, and by around age 9 these skills do not require specific thought or concentration, but are instead performed with ease. In this age-group mastery of specific athletic skills may emerge and can be seen by peers and family alike as a measure of competence. For the child who is less proficient at these skills, this may be a source of stress or frustration.

Hand-eye coordination and fine motor skills improve during middle childhood, and often by the fourth grade a child has skilled penmanship. During the early elementary school years, children with delayed fine motor skills may develop academic problems as this may inhibit cursive writing or copying math problems. An evaluation for the child with fine motor delay is indicated, because poor writing or copying skills may reflect an underlying learning disability.

Cognitive Development in the School-age Years

By middle childhood, a child is able to engage in logical thinking, although the child has a limited ability to extend the logic to abstract concepts. Children of this age-group tend to think in the "here and now," with a large accumulation of primarily logical, factual-based learning. They have a limited capacity for abstract or future-oriented thoughts, but they are able to comprehend rules and order.

By age 7, a child thinks more logically and less egocentrically. Gradually, a child develops cognitive flexibility, or the ability to apply learned concepts to new tasks. At this age, a child's cognitions expand because he or she is able to consider and mentally manipulate more than one variable. Piaget described the cognitive stage of middle childhood, from ages 7 to 12, as the period of concrete operations. The child is no longer limited by his or her perception, but can use logic. Children are able to apply reason as well as their own experience when they solve problems, and this is seen in the classroom as well as on the playground; a child at this level can master skills (such as reading, spelling, and mathematics) and can engage in cooperative play, sharing, and team sports.

Cognitive skills are reflected in this age-group in the types of games children play. Pre-school children tend to enjoy pretend or fantasy play more than structured games; they have not yet developed the intellectual skills to appreciate logic or strategy. By around age 7, however, children will engage in simple games with more complicated rules that may involve planning, such as Stratego or Guess Who?, while still revelling in the emotional pleasure of beating an opponent or having good luck in a game.

In middle childhood children will develop specific interests, hobbies, and skills. Children often will collect all kinds of objects, from sports cards to dolls to rocks. Hobbies might include making model cars or craft projects (such as sewing). Anna Freud suggested that hobbies are "halfway between work and play," because they involve mental skills (such as categorization or the skill to build an object), yet are also expressions of fantasy.[33]

Social and Emotional Development in the School-age Years

The task of social development is more complex for the school-age child. The school setting is more rule-bound, value-laden, and based on routine, and the child has to learn to manage relationships with adult authority figures as well as peers. Beginning at about age 6, the child is able to assimilate others' perspectives and is also learning social cues, rules, and expectations. For example, during a long graduation speech a pre-schooler might proclaim loudly, "I'm bored!" while an 8 year old might whisper to his mom, "Is this going to be over soon?"

In middle childhood, friendships and relationships with peers take on a larger significance. Children become concerned about the opinions of their classmates, and depend on their peers for companionship, as well as for validation and advice. Close bonds are often developed between same-gender peers, usually based on perceived common interests (which might include living in the same neighborhood). Children tend to pick best friends who share similar values and cultural boundaries; from ages 3 to 13, close friendships increasingly involve children of the same sex, age, ethnicity, and socioeconomic status.[34] Further, having a best friend who is not the same age or gender correlates with being rejected or ignored by one's classmates.[35]

Friendships become more intense and intimate; an 8 year old will likely describe a small circle of friends, and by age 10, children often have one "best" friend. This is more common in girls but often occurs with boys as well. Boys tend to take on a "pack" or group mentality with a sense of loyalty to the group, whereas girls often develop smaller, more intimate circles of friends and focus on maintaining their inclusion in these groups.

For the school-age child, media influences and popular culture begin to take on considerable significance. A 2010 survey demonstrated that children in the United States spend an average of 7 hours each day engaged with various forms of electronic media, with television being the most common.[36] While the specific impact of various forms of media exposure on development is often debated in the literature, there is evidence from several studies showing that children who watch more television may be at increased risk for obesity and lower school performance, and that some vulnerable children may be at increased risk of aggressive behavior when they are exposed to violent media.[37] Exposure to media is an unavoidable aspect of our society. However, caregivers who set limits on screen time and monitor their children's exposure to media may help mitigate the potentially deleterious effects of excessive or inappropriate media exposure on child development.

Moral Development in the School-age Years

Kohlberg described children of this age having achieved varying levels of moral development.[7] Children continue to internalize societal norms, but the fear of punishment or earned reward that motivates the pre-schooler gives way to hope for approval or positive feedback from adults and peers. Some middle-schoolers adopt an inflexible acceptance of rules of behavior that are to be followed. A school-age child will often become fixated on concepts of right and wrong, and lawfulness; it would be typical, for example, for a 9-year-old child to point out to her carpool driver that she was driving above the speed limit. The middle-school child assimilates the values and norms of his or her parental figures and culture, and the result is a reasonably well-formed superego and conscience. The child gains mastery of cognitive skills (such as considering two variables at one time), and he or she will begin to appreciate other points of view. In games, he or she learns that rules are mutually agreed on and, in special circumstances, can be altered. ("Since we only have three people, let's play with four outs instead of three.")

Adolescence (12 to 20 Years)

The physical, cognitive, social, sexual, and moral growth seen during adolescence is rapid and intense. There are generally three stages of adolescence, early (ages 11 to 13), middle (ages 14 to 17), and late (ages 18 to 20), although these age ranges can vary among different children. The physical changes that occur with puberty can have a profound effect on a young person's sense of self and ability to relate to others. Logical thought processes become more elaborate and are integrated with experiences. Teenagers develop the capacity to think abstractly. Peers continue to have a significant impact, and skills (such as decision-making, consideration of other's point of view, and expressing empathy) become more refined. The adolescent is able to appraise himself or herself, and in part this self-evaluation process leads toward emotional and social independence, and the making of a mature adult.

Physical Development during Adolescence

Puberty is the beginning of adolescence, and physical changes are accompanied by a heightened consciousness about one's body and sexuality. It is a time of drastic physical change. In the United States, puberty begins for girls between ages 8 and 13 years with breast bud development and continues through menarche; for boys it begins around age 14 and is marked by testicular enlargement followed by growth of the penis.[38] There are of course variations in these ages, and several factors can affect the timing of puberty and associated stages of growth, including health, weight, nutritional status, and ethnicity. For example, as a group, African American girls enter puberty earliest, followed by Mexican Americans and Caucasians.[39]

With the onset of puberty for both sexes there are periods of rapid gains in height and weight, and for boys, muscle mass. Similarly, hormonally-mediated physical changes include increased sebaceous gland activity that can result in acne. Girls often experience a growth spurt up to 2 years earlier than boys.[39] There can be an associated period of clumsiness or awkwardness, because linear limb growth may not be proportional to increased muscle mass. Furthermore, some girls experience the weight gain of puberty as problematic; in one study, 60% of adolescent girls reported that they were trying to lose weight. Physical development does not occur smoothly or at the same rate for all adolescents, and at a time when the desire to "fit in" and be "normal" is paramount, this can be a source of considerable stress.

Other physical changes that occur with early adolescence include an increased need for sleep (on average, teenagers need about $9\frac{1}{2}$ hours of nightly sleep) and a shift in the sleep-wake cycle, such that they tend to stay up later and wake up later.[40] Of course, with the demands of school and extracurricular activities, most adolescents do not get the amount of sleep they need. This can result in daytime sleepiness, which can in turn impair motor function and cognitive performance.

By age 15, most adolescents have gone through puberty and have experienced significant changes in their physical appearance. They frequently experiment with clothing or hairstyles, and may spend a significant amount of energy, time, and money on how they look. This emphasis on appearance is part of their search for a stable self. It is developmentally appropriate for a teenager to be self-absorbed at this age and somewhat obsessed with how others perceive him or her.

Late adolescence marks the transition to adulthood, and by this time most teenagers have developed a mostly adult physical appearance. As with earlier stages of adolescence, it is important to note that not all teenagers grow at a similar rate and often in late adolescence "late bloomers" catch up to their peers. Similarly, physical development is not always matched by emotional maturity; an 18-year-old young man is capable of fathering a child, but may not be ready to be a father.

Cognitive Development during Adolescence

In early adolescence, a young person is able to think logically and sometimes make rational decisions and judgments.

However, despite taking on a more mature physical appearance, a young teenager is not a "mini–grown-up." Many children in early adolescence are between Piaget's stages of concrete operation and formal operational-thinking, and they may not exhibit a consistent ability to assimilate information in a reasonable manner or think through the potential consequences of their actions. This often translates into adolescents being able to verbalize the most appropriate action, but many times not be able to make a reasoned decision in the heat of the moment.

By mid-adolescence, most teenagers have developed the capacity for abstract thinking. Piaget termed this stage as *formal operations,* where a person can evaluate and manipulate the data and emotions in his or her environment in a constructive manner, using his or her experience, as well as abstract thought.[6] The capacity to think abstractly, that is, to be able to consider an idea in a hypothetical, "what if" manner, is the hallmark of formal operations. This skill enables adolescents to navigate more complicated situations and to comprehend more complex ideas.

Despite this improved capacity for problem-solving and an ability to consider multiple possibilities or outcomes, the adolescent does not always make sound decisions. In part because of an incompletely developed pre-frontal cortex, tasks associated with executive function (such as planning, prioritizing, and controlling impulses) are not fully mastered. The adolescent may be able to think about the consequences of his or her actions, but he or she is susceptible to a variety of factors (such as emotions, peer pressure, and his or her sense of omnipotence) and as such, is vulnerable toward making poor choices. Some poor choices, such as drunk driving, have always carried significant risk. However, with the rise of social media and the omnipresence of smart phone cameras, regrettable actions that might have been forgotten after a brief embarrassment a generation ago can now be spread more widely and live in perpetuity on the Internet, often amplifying the negative consequences that teens face for their impulsive actions.

Young adults are usually thinking "like a grown-up" and are able to think abstractly, including consideration of the future. They are, in Piagetian terms, in the stage of formal operations. This does not mean they will always consider the consequences of their actions, but most late teenagers begin to formulate ideas about their future in part because they have the capacity to be introspective and reflective. However, maturation of the pre-frontal cortex continues to occur into the early twenties and with it comes improved impulse control, analytical skills, and better judgment. This cognitive maturity enables the teenager to manage the transitions that make up this developmental stage, including planning educational or vocational goals and developing more intimate relationships.

Social and Emotional Development during Adolescence

A teenager may have physical and sexual maturity that is not quite matched by his or her cognitive or emotional growth, and this can lead to behaviors that may be perceived as immature. Adolescent behavior is remarkably consistent in its lack of predictability. As the young person searches for an adult identity, there is a mix of conformity with rebellion; an adolescent may experiment with certain behaviors (including drug use or sexual activity) as a means of striving for independence. Risk-taking behaviors and limit-testing increase in this age-group, as a young teenager learns to establish his or her own boundaries and limitations. This risk-taking enhances the need for external controls (such as clear parental expectations and school rules). Such structure will provide scaffolding for a young person to establish his or her own internal controls.

Peers are a source of support as well as judgment as the teenager establishes an individual identity, and the supportive approval found in the group can influence self-confidence. At this age peers generally are same-gender friends with similar interests, and it is not uncommon for them to spend considerable time together. Social isolation is not the norm for this age, and teens who are "loners" may be more susceptible to mental health issues, such as depression.

Early adolescents compare themselves to their peers, and frequently measure themselves against others their age. There is considerable pressure to conform to the norms of the group, and teenagers will often share similar styles of clothing, haircuts, and interests with their group. This group identification is a means of establishing an identity outside of their family structure and contributes to the developmental task of separation and individuation.

Adolescents gradually expand their world outside the home, to include peers of both genders, as well as adult, nonfamily friends. Their peer group remains an important source of support, and they often engage in school-based activities, clubs, or sports. These settings provide opportunities for the teenager to safely explore a variety of relationships, some of which may develop from a friend to a romantic interest. In high school, teachers and coaches often become important figures in their lives. Some adolescents may "try on" different identities, adopting the values and styles of different groups at different times, before settling on one that feels most comfortable to them.

While romantic crushes are common during early adolescence, it is likely that dating will begin by middle adolescence. Romantic relationships tend to be short-lived, and last an average of 4 months. Expectations of dating behaviors are mediated by peers, as well as by cultural factors, and parental permission and communication play an important role.

By late adolescence, the security found in group relationships has evolved into finding security as an independent young person. A healthy young adult has less of the group mentality found in mid-adolescence and has more self-reliance and ability to tolerate other styles or point of view. Late teens establish more intimate relationships with friends of both genders; some of these relationships may be sexual and some may be emotionally intimate, and of course some may be both. They are able to separate from their parents or primary caretakers without difficulty and establish a more independent role in their family. However, there may be variation among certain groups of young adults who may have delayed independence based on extended educational pursuits or financial pressures. In some groups, the processes of late adolescence extend well into their twenties, as they search for occupational or personal roles.

Moral Development during Adolescence

An adolescent's moral principles mirror the primary developmental task of this age, namely, to separate oneself from dependence on caregivers and family. In late childhood, maintaining the rules of the group has become a value; during adolescence there is a move toward an autonomous moral code that has validity with both authority and the individual's own beliefs of what is right and wrong. Teenagers often "test" their parents' moral code. Role models are important, and while younger children might choose them for their superhuman powers, the early adolescent selects his or her heroes based on realistic and hoped-for ideals, talents, and values.

By mid-adolescence, most teenagers have a fully formed conscience and a well-developed sense of right and wrong. These values help them form a more autonomous sense of morality, where they are able to make moral decisions that are based not just on the rules but more elaborately, on their own beliefs in the context of those rules (see discussion of Kohlberg earlier in this chapter). However, despite the potential capacity for sound reasoning, it is not uncommon for teenagers' normative self-absorption, limited impulse control, and vulnerability to peer pressure to interfere with this ability. It is also important to note that not all adolescents or even adults reach this stage of moral reasoning.

As with all developmental tasks, a young adult's moral development is affected by his or her collective experience, including that with family, peers, teachers, role models, and the community. Late adolescents are able to make decisions autonomously but within a social context, using more refined cognitive skills.

Sexual Development during Adolescence

The young adolescent becomes aware of his or her physical changes and also develops sexual awareness. Most young people in this age-group are not sexually active but they are sexually curious. The middle-schooler who thought girls were "yucky" now might be interested in watching a couple kissing, or he might be interested in looking at pornographic images on the Internet. Masturbation is common in this age-group, more for boys than for girls, and this behavior should be normalized as much as possible.

Parents and caregivers help a young person develop a healthy sense of sexuality by providing information and opportunities to talk about sexual issues, and by a nonjudgmental attitude about sexual behaviors. Teenagers might rely on each other for information, or they may develop attitudes and observe behaviors based on images from movies, television, or the Internet. These sources may not be completely realistic or accurate; it is important that parents stay in tune and remain involved as a source of guidance.

The task of mid-adolescence is to manage a likely strong sexual drive with peer and cultural expectations. Sexual activity in and of itself is value-neutral and developmentally normal. In several industrialized countries, the age at first sexual intercourse has become increasingly younger over the past two decades. According to the 2011 national school-based youth risk behavior survey, 47% of American high school students have had sexual intercourse.[41] Most mid-adolescents engage in some kind of sexual activity, the extent of which depends on factors including cultural influences and socioeconomic status. For example, black and socioeconomically disadvantaged youth are more likely to be sexually active.[42]

Middle adolescents may not be engaging in sexual intercourse *per se*, but they are considering issues related to sex and sexual activity. It is important that young persons have a stable sense of self and be emotionally prepared as they make these considerations. Unstable sexual activity (such as with multiple partners, or while intoxicated) may present a myriad of problems ranging from the risk of unintended pregnancy to sexually-transmitted diseases.

In the process of developing a sexual sense of themselves, many teenagers may wonder about their sexual orientation. Sexual identity continues to develop throughout adolescence. For some young people, they are clear that they are heterosexual or homosexual; for others, sexual identity and attraction may be more fluid into adulthood. Many adolescents wonder if they are homosexual, as it is not unusual for adolescent girls to develop crushes on girlfriends or female teachers or for young men to have an erection in the company of other male peers. Some adolescents experiment with samesex sexual activity, and this may not necessarily mean they are gay. For most, sexual preference will become clearer as they mature.

Adult Development
Young Adulthood

Development does not cease with the end of adolescence. Young adulthood (generally defined as ages 20 to 30) presents challenges and responsibilities, which are not necessarily based on chronological age. Contemporary adult theorists, such as Daniel Levinson and George Vaillant, describe adult growth as periods of transition in response to mastering adult tasks, in contrast to the specific stages used to summarize child development.[43,44] The transition from adolescence to young adulthood is marked by specific developmental challenges including leaving home, re-defining the relationship with one's parents, searching for a satisfying career identity, and sustaining meaningful friendships. This is also a period when a young person develops the capacity to form more intimate relationships and will likely find a life partner.

Growth in the young adult is less a physical phenomenon and more one of a synthesis of physical, cognitive, and emotional maturity. Linear growth is replaced by adaptation and re-organization of processes that are already present. Young adulthood is described by roles and status (such as employment or parenthood), and there are a variety of developmental pathways, which are affected by factors including culture, gender, and historical trends.[45] For example, in 2010 in the United States the mean age for mothers at the birth of the first child was 25.2 years[46]; in the nineteenth century, it was common for teenagers to run a household and begin to raise a family. The trajectory of young adult growth is as much a function of the environment as continued biological growth.

Cognitive function during this stage is more sophisticated. Characteristics of adult mental processes include a sense of internal control and emotional self-regulation, greater flexibility, improved problem-solving and decision-making abilities, and an improved ability to engage in abstract thinking. Such cognitive traits enable young persons to adapt to, and shape, the environments that will in turn influence them.

There is significant variability in the transitions for young adults as they complete their high school education. Of Americans between ages 18 and 24, just under 50% are enrolled in secondary education programs or have completed college. Many young adults move away from their parents' homes as they enter the workforce or college. Such "cutting of the apron strings" can be a stressful period for the young adult, who may have yet to fully establish a stable home or social environment.

There is a period of psychological separation from one's parents that may be marked by ongoing financial or emotional dependence, but gradually young persons will establish their own home and their own community. The young adult's connection with his or her parents, too, will undergo a change from a dependent, parent–child relationship, to one that is more equitable and mutually sustaining. This growth may come full circle as the older parents age and possibly become more dependent on their now full-grown child for caretaking.

The search for a fulfilling career is a significant challenge during this period. The first major decision, such as choosing to enter the workforce or to attend college, is often made in late adolescence. In some societies, such as the United Kingdom, such a decision is often made during school-age years based primarily on intellectual aptitude. At some point during young adulthood, career choices become the primary focus and may contribute to self-esteem and a sense of fulfillment.

Young adults tend to shift their attachment from family and peer groups to a significant other. Intimacy can be sexual, emotional, or both, and young adults are capable of sustaining close interpersonal relationships with members of both genders. A young person's sexual identity is established by this period, and it is refined as the young adult strives to find a relationship that is both emotionally and sexually satisfying. Marriage, and establishing one's own home, is common and further contributes to the shift from young person to adult.

In many societies around the world, including the United States, socio-cultural changes over recent years have led many young adults to remain financially and emotionally dependent upon their parents longer and to postpone lasting decisions about their career and romantic relationships later compared with previous generations. These shifts have led to a new focus by developmental scientists on this period of life between adolescence and the greater independence of middle adulthood. This period is now sometimes referred to as "emerging adulthood."

Middle to Late Adulthood

The developmental tasks of the period from ages 30 to 60 (or retirement) include an ongoing integration of one's self with family and community. Continued development of a satisfying career, addressing the needs of one's growing children or aging parents, sustaining healthy relationships, and maintaining responsibility in one's community are characteristics of this period.

While there are no specific physical markers of moving from young adulthood to mid-life, this is a period when maturation begins to give way to aging. The human body begins to slow, and how well one functions becomes more sensitive to diet (including substance use), exercise, stress, and rest. This is often a period when chronic health problems become more problematic, or when good health may be threatened by disease or disability. Bones may lose mass and density (made more complicated by a woman's estrogen loss as she nears menopause), and vertebral compression along with loss of muscle results in a slight loss of height. After age 40, the average person loses approximately 1 cm of height every 10 years.[47] Responses to this aging process vary from person to person, but experiencing a sense of loss or sadness around these changes is not uncommon.

The physical changes associated with aging are complemented by a cognitive and psychological awareness that life will not last forever. As one approaches later life, the adolescent sense of immortality and omnipotence gives way to a realization that there are limitations to what one might accomplish or achieve. In particular, the death of one's parent often makes one irrefutably aware of one's own mortality. The development of one's own children toward independence can also change one's sense of self and one's role as caregiver and provider. Ongoing relationships, with one's spouse, children, friends, colleagues, in-laws, aging parents, or even grandchildren, are both affirming and fulfilling. Unlike relationships during adolescence or young adulthood, these friendships are not a means of establishing independence or of belonging to a particular group, but rather are a means of creating stable connections.

Late Adulthood and Senescence

The average life expectancy for a person living in the United States is 78.7 years.[48] By 2030, it is projected that half of all Americans will be over age 65. While it seems counter-intuitive to consider "old age" as part of development, there are specific developmental tasks to be achieved. These include accepting physical decline and limitations, adjusting to retirement and possibly a lower income, maintaining interests and activities, and sharing one's wisdom and experiences with families and friends. Another challenge is to accept the idea that one may become increasingly dependent on others, and that death is inevitable.

For many, work is a source of personal and social identity, pleasure, creativity, and profit. When an older person retires or stops working, he or she loses a particular role and has to establish a new identity as a non-working citizen. This may be a significant loss for some, but for others "life after work" is a period of great relief, freedom, and thriving. A healthy adjustment to this period includes finding stimulation and interest in a variety of activities, ongoing meaningful participation in their own lives and those of their loved ones, and a feeling of generativity in one's life.

Access the complete reference list and multiple choice questions (MCQs) online at https://expertconsult.inkling.com

KEY REFERENCES

1. Freud S. *Three essays on the theory of sexuality: the standard edition of the complete psychological works of Sigmund Freud*, vol. 7, London, 1905, Hogarth Press.
4. Erikson EH. *Childhood and society*, ed 2, New York, 1963, WW Norton & Company.
6. Piaget J, Inhelder B. *The psychology of the child*, New York, 1969, Basic Books.
7. Kohlberg L. Stage and sequence: the cognitive-developmental approach to socialization. In Goslin DA, editor: *Handbook of socialization theory and research*, New York, 1969, Rand McNally.
11. Bowlby J. *Attachment: attachment and loss series*, vol. 1, New York, 1969, Basic Books.
12. Bowlby J. *Separation: attachment and loss series*, vol. 2, New York, 1973, Basic Books.
13. Ainsworth MDS, Blehar MC, Waters E, et al. *Patterns of attachment: a psychological study of the strange situation*, Oxford, England, 1978, Lawrence Erlbaum.
20. Siegel DJ. *The developing mind: toward a neurobiology of interpersonal experience*, New York, 1999, Guilford.
21. Winnicott DW. *The child, the family, and the outside world*, Reading, MA, 1987, Addison-Wesley.
22. Thomas A, Chess S. *Temperament and development*, New York, 1977, Brunner/Mazel.
44. Vaillant GE. *Adaptation to life*, Boston, 1977, Little, Brown.

6 Diagnostic Rating Scales and Psychiatric Instruments

Joshua L. Roffman, MD, MMSc, David Mischoulon, MD, PhD, and Maurizio Fava, MD

KEY POINTS

Background

- Diagnostic rating scales provide validated measures of symptom severity in psychiatric disorders.
- Rating scales may be employed in both clinical and research settings.

History

- The format of psychiatric rating scales varies widely in content, length, and administration.
- Ratings can supply either global assessments of function or disorder-specific measurements.

Clinical and Research Challenges

- Clinician-rated and patient-rated scales each have advantages and disadvantages.
- It is important to select the right scale for the right condition and for the right patient.

Practical Pointers

- The information provided by diagnostic rating scales can be useful in differentiating closely-related diagnoses, selecting symptom-appropriate treatment, and monitoring treatment effects.
- Clinicians should consider using these scales in their practice in cases where the diagnosis may be in doubt, or if they wish to quantify the effect of a treatment in cases where the patient is not a good reporter of his or her state.

OVERVIEW

Unlike other medical specialties, psychiatry relies almost exclusively on patient interviews and on observation for diagnosis and treatment monitoring. With the absence of specific physical or biomarker findings in psychiatry, the mental status examination (MSE) represents our primary diagnostic instrument. The MSE provides a framework to collect the affective, behavioral, and cognitive symptoms of psychiatric disorders. Often, the MSE provides enough detail for psychiatrists to categorize symptom clusters into recognized clinical syndromes, and to initiate appropriate treatment.

However, in some settings, the MSE alone is insufficient to collect a complete inventory of patient symptoms or to yield a unifying diagnosis. For example, if a psychotic patient has symptoms of avolition, flat affect, and social withdrawal, it might be difficult to determine (from the standard diagnostic interview alone) whether this pattern reflects negative symptoms, co-morbid depression, or medication-induced akinesia.[1]

At other times, performing an MSE may not be an efficient use of time or resources to achieve the desired clinical goal: imagine how many fewer patients might be identified during depression screening days if the lengthy, full MSE were the screening instrument of choice.[2] Finally, the subjective nature of the MSE often renders it prohibitive in research studies, in which multiple clinicians may be assessing subjects; without the use of an objective, reliable diagnostic tool, subjects may be inadequately or incorrectly categorized, generating results that are difficult to interpret and from which it is difficult to generalize.[3]

By using diagnostic rating scales, clinicians can obtain objective, and sometimes quantifiable, information about a patient's symptoms in settings where the traditional MSE is either inadequate or inappropriate. Rating scales may serve as an adjunct to the diagnostic interview, or as stand-alone measures (as in research or screening milieus). These instruments are as versatile as they are varied, and can be used to aid in symptom assessment, diagnosis, treatment planning, or treatment monitoring. In this chapter, an overview of many of the psychiatric diagnostic rating scales used in clinical care and research is provided (Table 6-1). Information on how to acquire copies of the rating scales discussed in this chapter is available.

GENERAL CONSIDERATIONS IN THE SELECTION OF DIAGNOSTIC RATING SCALES

How "good" is a given diagnostic rating scale? Will it measure what the clinician wants it to measure, and will it do so consistently? How much time and expense will it require to administer? These questions are important to consider regardless of which diagnostic ratings scale is used, and in what setting. Before describing the various ratings scales in detail, several factors important to evaluating rating scale design and implementation will be considered (Table 6-2).

A first consideration concerns the psychometric measures of reliability and validity. For the psychotic patient mentioned earlier, what would happen if several different physicians watched a videotape of a diagnostic interview, and then independently scored her negative symptoms with a rating scale? The scale would be considered reliable if each of the physicians arrived at a similar rating of her negative symptoms. *Reliability* refers to the extent that an instrument produces consistent measurements across different raters and testing milieus. In this case, the negative symptom rating scale specifically demonstrates good *inter-rater reliability*, which occurs when several different observers reach similar conclusions based on the same information.

Recall that for this patient, though, negative symptoms constituted only one possible etiology for her current presentation. If the underlying problem truly reflected a co-morbid depression, and not negative symptoms, a valid negative symptom rating scale would indicate a low score, and a valid

TABLE 6-1 Diagnostic Rating Scales

GENERAL RATINGS

SCID-I and SCID-CV	Structured Clinical Interview for DSM-IV Diagnosis
MINI	Mini-International Neuropsychiatric Interview
SCAN	Schedules for Clinical Assessment in Neuropsychiatry
GAF	Global Assessment of Functioning Scale
CGI	Clinical Global Impressions Scale

MOOD DISORDERS

HAM-D	Hamilton Depression Rating Scale
MADRS	Montgomery-Asberg Depression Rating Scale
BDI	Beck Depression Inventory
IDS	Inventory of Depressive Symptomatology
QIDS-SR	Quick Inventory of Depressive Symptomatology-Self Rated
Zung SDS	Zung Self-Rating Depression Scale
HANDS	Harvard Department of Psychiatry National Depression Screening Day Scale
MSRS	Manic State Rating Scale
Y-MRS	Young Mania Rating Scale

PSYCHOTIC DISORDERS

PANSS	Positive and Negative Syndrome Scale
BPRS	Brief Psychiatric Rating Scale
SAPS	Scale for the Assessment of Positive Symptoms
SANS	Scale for the Assessment of Negative Symptoms
SDS	Schedule of the Deficit Syndrome
AIMS	Abnormal Involuntary Movement Scale
BARS	Barnes Akathisia Rating Scale
EPS	Simpson-Angus Extrapyramidal Side Effects Scale

ANXIETY DISORDERS

HAM-A	Hamilton Anxiety Rating Scale
BAI	Beck Anxiety Inventory
Y-BOCS	Yale-Brown Obsessive Compulsive Scale
BSPS	Brief Social Phobia Scale
CAPS	Clinician Administered PTSD Scale

SUBSTANCE ABUSE DISORDERS

CAGE	CAGE questionnaire
MAST	Michigan Alcoholism Screening Test
DAST	Drug Abuse Screening Test
FTND	Fagerstrom Test for Nicotine Dependence

COGNITIVE DISORDERS

MMSE	Mini-Mental State Examination
CDT	Clock-Drawing Test
DRS	Dementia Rating Scale
CPFQ	Cognitive and Physical Functioning Questionnaire

TABLE 6-2 Factors Used to Evaluate Diagnostic Rating Scales

Reliability	For a given subject, are the results consistent across different evaluators, test conditions, and test times?
Validity	Does the instrument truly measure what it is intended to measure? How well does it compare to the gold standard?
Sensitivity	If the disorder is present, how likely is it that the test is positive?
Specificity	If the disorder is absent, how likely is it that the test is negative?
Positive predictive value	If the test is positive, how likely is it that the disorder is present?
Negative predictive value	If the test is negative, how likely is it that the disorder is absent?
Cost- and time-effectiveness	Does the instrument provide accurate results in a timely and inexpensive way?
Administration	Are ratings determined by the patient or the evaluator? What are the advantages and disadvantages of this approach?
Training requirements	What degree of expertise is required for valid and reliable measurements to occur?

TABLE 6-3 Validity Calculations

	Disorder Present	Disorder Not Present
Test positive	**A** (true positive)	**B** (type 1 error)
Test negative	**C** (type 2 error)	**D** (true negative)

Sensitivity = $A/(A + C)$
Specificity = $D/(B + D)$
Positive predictive value = $A/(A + B)$
Negative predictive value = $D/(C + D)$
False-positive rate = 1 minus positive predictive value
False-negative rate = 1 minus negative predictive value

depression rating scale would yield a high score. The *validity* of a rating scale concerns whether it correctly detects the true underlying condition. In this case, the negative symptom scale produced a *true negative* result, and the depression scale produced a *true positive* result (Table 6-3). However, if the negative symptom scale had indicated a high score, a *type 1 error* would have occurred, and the patient may have been incorrectly diagnosed with negative symptoms. Conversely, if the depression scale produced a low score, a *type 2 error* will have led the clinician to miss the correct diagnosis of depression. The related measures of *sensitivity, specificity, positive predictive value,* and *negative predictive value* (defined in Table 6-2 and illustrated in Table 6-3) can provide estimates of a diagnostic rating scale's validity, especially in comparison to "gold standard" tests.

Several important logistical factors also come into play when evaluating the usefulness of a diagnostic test. Certain rating scales are freely available, whereas others may be obtained only from the author or publisher at a cost. Briefer instruments require less time to administer, which can be essential if large numbers of patients must be screened, but they may be less sensitive or specific than longer instruments and lead to more diagnostic errors. Some rating scales may be self-administered by the patient, reducing the possibility of observer bias; however, such ratings can be compromised in patients with significant behavioral or cognitive impairments. Alternatively, clinician-administered rating scales tend to be more valid and reliable than self-rated scales, but they also tend to require more time and, in some cases, specialized training for the rater. A final consideration is the cultural context of the patient (and the rater): culture-specific conceptions of psychiatric illness can profoundly influence the report and interpretation of specific symptoms and the assignment of a diagnosis. The relative importance of these factors depends on the specific clinical or research milieu, and each factor must be carefully weighed to guide the selection of an optimal rating instrument.[4,5]

GENERAL DIAGNOSTIC INSTRUMENTS

Suppose that a research study will evaluate brain differences between individuals with an anxiety disorder and healthy subjects. Anxiety is highly co-morbid with a number of psychiatric conditions, which if present among subjects in the anxiety group might confound the study results. At the same time, assurance that the "healthy" subjects are indeed free of anxiety (or of other psychiatric illnesses) would also be critical to the design of such an experiment. The use of general psychiatric diagnostic instruments, described in this section, can provide a standardized measure of psychopathology across diagnostic categories. These instruments are frequently used in research studies to assess baseline mental health and to ensure the clinical homogeneity of both patient and healthy control subjects.

BOX 6-1 Domains of the Structured Clinical Interview for DSM-IV Axis I Diagnosis (SCID)

I. Overview section
II. Mood episodes
III. Psychotic symptoms
IV. Psychotic disorders differential
V. Mood disorders differential
VI. Substance use
VII. Anxiety disorders
VIII. Somatoform disorders
IX. Eating disorders
X. Adjustment disorders

BOX 6-2 Components of the Schedules for Clinical Assessment in Neuropsychiatry (SCAN)

I. Present State Examination
   Part I: Demographic information; medical history; somatoform, dissociative, anxiety, mood, eating, alcohol and substance abuse disorders
   Part II: Psychotic and cognitive disorders, insight, functional impairment
II. Item Group Checklist
   Signs and symptoms derived from case records, other providers, other collateral sources
III. Clinical History Schedule
   Education, personality disorders, social impairment

Adapted from Skodol AE, Bender DS. Diagnostic interviews in adults. In Rush AJ, Pincus HA, First MB, et al. editors: Handbook of psychiatric measures, *Washington, DC, 2000, American Psychiatric Association.*

One of the most frequently used general instruments is the Structured Clinical Interview for DSM-IV Axis I Diagnosis (SCID-I). The SCID-I is a lengthy, semistructured survey of psychiatric illness across multiple domains (Box 6-1). An introductory segment uses open-ended questions to assess demographics, as well as medical, psychiatric, and medication use histories. The subsequent modules ask specific questions about diagnostic criteria, taken from the DSM-IV, in nine different realms of psychopathology. Within these modules, responses are generally rated as "present," "absent (or subthreshold)," or "inadequate information"; scores are tallied to determine likely diagnoses. The SCID-I can take several hours to administer, although, in some instances, raters use only portions of the SCID that relate to clinical or research areas of interest. An abbreviated version, the SCID-CV (Clinical Version), includes simplified modules and assesses the most common clinical diagnoses.

While the SCID-I is generally considered user-friendly, its length precludes its routine clinical use. An alternative general rating instrument is the Mini-International Neuropsychiatric Interview (MINI), another semi-structured interview based on DSM-IV criteria. Questions tend to be more limited with this test than with the SCID-I, and are answered in "yes/no" format; however, unlike the SCID-I, the MINI includes a module on antisocial personality disorder and has questions that focus on suicidality. Because the overall content of the MINI is more limited than the SCID-I, the MINI requires much less time to administer (15 to 30 minutes).

A third general interview, the Schedules for Clinical Assessment in Neuropsychiatry (SCAN), focuses less directly on DSM-IV categories and provides a broader assessment of psychosocial function (Box 6-2). The SCAN evolved from the older Present State Examination, which covers several categories of psychopathology, but also includes sections for collateral history, developmental issues, personality disorders, and social impairment. However, like the SCID-I, the SCAN can be time consuming, and administration requires familiarity with its format. While the SCAN provides a more complete history in certain respects, it does not lend itself to making a DSM-IV diagnosis in as linear a fashion as does the SCID-I and the MINI.

Two additional general diagnostic scales may be used to track changes in global function over time and in response to treatment. Both are clinician-rated and require only a few moments to complete. The Global Assessment of Functioning Scale (GAF) consists of a 100-point single-item rating scale that is included in Axis V of the DSM-IV diagnosis (Table 6-4). Higher scores indicate better overall psychosocial function. Ratings can be made for current function and for highest function in the past year. The Clinical Global Impressions Scale (CGI) consists of two scores, one for severity of illness (CGI-S),

TABLE 6-4 Global Assessment of Functioning Scale (GAF) Scoring

Score	Interpretation
91–100	Superior function in a wide range of activities; no symptoms
81–90	Good function in all areas; absent or minimal symptoms
71–80	Symptoms are transient and cause no more than slight impairment in functioning
61–70	Mild symptoms or some difficulty in functioning, but generally functions well
51–60	Moderate symptoms or moderate difficulty in functioning
41–50	Serious symptoms or serious difficulty in functioning
31–40	Impaired reality testing or communication, or seriously impaired functioning
21–30	Behavior considerably influenced by psychotic symptoms or inability to function in almost all areas
11–20	Some danger of hurting self or others, or occasionally fails to maintain hygiene
1–10	Persistent danger of hurting self or others, serious suicidal act, or persistent inability to maintain hygiene
0	Inadequate information

Adapted from Diagnostic and statistical manual of mental disorders DSM-IV-TR, *ed 4 (text revision), Washington, DC, 2000, American Psychiatric Association.*

and the other for degree of improvement following treatment (CGI-I). For the CGI-S, scores range from 1 (normal) to 7 (severe illness); for the CGI-I, they range from 1 (very much improved) to 7 (very much worse). A related score, the CGI Efficacy Index, reflects a composite index of both the therapeutic and adverse effects of treatment. Here, scores range from 0 (marked improvement and no side effects) to 4 (unchanged or worse and side effects outweigh therapeutic effects).

General diagnostic instruments survey a broad overview of psychopathology across many domains. They can be useful as screening tools for both patients and research subjects, and in some cases can determine whether individuals meet DSM-IV criteria for major psychiatric disorders. However, they do not provide the opportunity for detailed investigations of affective, behavioral, or cognitive symptoms, and often do not provide diagnostic clarification for individuals with atypical or complex presentations. Diagnostic rating scales that focus on specific domains (such as mood, psychotic, or anxiety symptoms) can be of greater value in these situations, as well as in research efforts that focus on symptom-specific areas. In the following sections, rating scales that are tailored to explore specific clusters of psychiatric illness and related medication side effects will be discussed.

SCALES FOR MOOD DISORDERS

The diagnosis and treatment of mood disorders present unique challenges to the psychiatrist. The cardinal features of major depressive disorder can mimic any number of other distinct neuropsychiatric illnesses, including (but not limited to) dysthymia, anxiety, bipolar-spectrum disorders, substance abuse, personality disorders, dementia, and movement disorders. In some cases, overt depressive symptoms precede the tell-tale presentation (e.g., mania) for these other disorders, and more subtle signs and symptoms of the root disorder are easily missed in standard diagnostic interviews. Moreover, because most antidepressant medications and psychotherapies take effect gradually, daily or even weekly progress can be difficult to gauge subjectively. Diagnostic rating scales can be invaluable in the clarification of the diagnosis of mood disorders and the objective measurement of incremental progress during treatment.

The Hamilton Rating Scale for Depression (HAM-D) is a clinician-administered instrument that is widely used in both clinical and research settings. Its questions focus on the severity of symptoms in the preceding week; as such, the HAM-D is a useful tool for tracking patient progress after the initiation of treatment. The scale exists in several versions, ranging from 6 to 31 items; longer versions include questions about atypical depression symptoms, psychotic symptoms, somatic symptoms, and symptoms associated with obsessive-compulsive disorder (OCD). Patient answers are scored by the rater from 0 to 2 or 0 to 4 and are tallied to obtain an overall score. Scoring for the 17-item HAM-D-17, frequently used in research studies, is summarized in Table 6-5. A decrease of 50% or more in the HAM-D score suggests a positive response to treatment. While the HAM-D is considered reliable and valid, important caveats include the necessity of training raters and the lack of inclusion of certain post-DSM-III criteria (such as anhedonia).

The Montgomery-Asberg Depression Rating Scale (MADRS), another clinician-administered instrument, also measures depressive severity, and correlates well with the HAM-D. The MADRS contains 10 items, each reflecting symptom severity from 0 to 6, with a maximum possible total score of 60. The MADRS generally covers similar symptoms to the HAM-D-17, but may be more sensitive to antidepressant-related changes than the HAM-D Scale. It is not so well suited for assessing atypical depression, since it does not examine increased appetite or sleep (see Table 6-6).

The most frequently used self-administered depression rating scale is the Beck Depression Inventory (BDI). The BDI is a 21-item scale in which patients must rate their symptoms on a scale from 0 to 3; the total score is tallied and interpreted by the clinician (Table 6-7). Like the HAM-D, the BDI may be used as a repeated measure to follow progress during a treatment trial. Although easy to administer, the BDI tends to focus more on cognitive symptoms of depression, and it excludes atypical symptoms (such as weight gain and hypersomnia).

An alternative rating scale, the Inventory of Depressive Symptomatology (IDS), provides more thorough coverage of atypical depression and symptoms of dysthymia. The IDS is available in both clinician-rated (IDS-C) and self-administered (IDS-SR) versions, and it contains 28 or 30 items. Suggested interpretation guidelines are given in Table 6-8.

The Quick Inventory of Depressive Symptomatology-Self-Report (QIDS-SR) is a 16-item self-rated instrument derived from the IDS, for measuring self-reported changes in symptom severity during antidepressant clinical trials. Each question is rated on a scale of 0 to 3 and the total score is obtained by summing the scores on most of the individual items, and summing the highest scores of 3 categories (sleep, appetite/weight, and psychomotor activity). The highest possible total score is 27. (See Table 6-9.)

Two other self-administered scales, the Zung Self-Rating Depression Scale (Zung SDS) and the Harvard Department of Psychiatry National Depression Screening Day Scale (HANDS), are frequently employed in primary care and other screening sessions due to their simplicity and ease of use. The Zung SDS contains 20 items, with 10 items keyed positively and 10 keyed negatively; subjects score each item as present from 1 or "a

TABLE 6-6 Scoring the Montgomery-Asberg Depression Rating Scale

Score	Interpretation
0–6	Not depressed
7–19	Mild depression
20–34	Moderate depression
>34	Severe depression

Adapted from Montgomery SA, Asberg M. A new depression scale designed to be sensitive to change. Br J Psychiatry 134(4):382–389, 1979.

TABLE 6-7 Scoring the Beck Depression Inventory (BDI)

Score	Interpretation
0–9	Minimal depression
10–16	Mild depression
17–29	Moderate depression
≥30	Severe depression

TABLE 6-8 Scoring the Inventory of Depressive Symptomology (IDS)

Score	Interpretation
0–13	Normal
14–25	Mildly ill
26–38	Moderately ill
39–48	Severely ill
≥49	Very severely ill

TABLE 6-9 Scoring the Quick Inventory of Depressive Symptomatology-Self-Report (QIDS-SR)

Score	Interpretation
0–5	No depression
6–10	Mild depression
11–15	Moderate depression
16–20	Severe depression
21–27	Very severe depression

Adapted from Rush AJ, Trivedi MH, Ibrahim HM, et al. The 16-item Quick Inventory of Depressive Symptomatology (QIDS), Clinician Rating (QIDS-C), and Self-Report (QIDS-SR): a psychometric evaluation in patients with chronic major depression. Biol Psychiatry 54:573–583, 2003.

TABLE 6-5 Scoring the 17-Item Hamilton Rating Scale for Depression (HAM-D-17)

Score	Interpretation
0–7	Not depressed
8–13	Mildly depressed
14–18	Moderately depressed
19–22	Severely depressed
≥23	Very severely depressed

Adapted from Kearns NP, Cruickshank CA, McGuigan KJ, et al. A comparison of depression rating scales, Br J Psychiatry 141:45–49, 1982.

TABLE 6-10 Scoring the Zung Self-Rating Depression Scale (Zung SDS)

Score	Interpretation
0–49	Normal
50–59	Minimal to mild depression
60–69	Moderate to severe depression
≥70	Severe depression

TABLE 6-11 Scoring the Harvard Department of Psychiatry National Depression Screening Day Scale (HANDS)

Score	Interpretation
0–8	Unlikely depression
9–16	Likely depression
≥17	Very likely depression

little of the time" to 4 or "most of the time." To obtain the total score, positively-keyed items are reversed and then all of the items are summed (Table 6-10). The HANDS includes 10 questions about depression symptoms, and it is scored based on the experience of symptoms from 0 or "none of the time" to 3 or "all of the time" (Table 6-11). Although the Zung SDS and HANDS take only a few minutes to administer, they are less sensitive to change than are the HAM-D and the BDI; like these other scales, the Zung SDS lacks coverage for atypical symptoms of depression.

There are fewer validated rating scales to assess manic symptoms than there are for depression. However, two clinician-administered scales, the Manic State Rating Scale (MSRS) and the Young Mania Rating Scale (Y-MRS), have both been used extensively on inpatient units to characterize the severity of manic symptoms; the Y-MRS also correlates well with length of hospital stay. The MSRS contains 26 items and is rated on a 0 to 5 scale, based on the frequency and intensity of symptoms. Particular weight is given to symptoms related to elation-grandiosity and paranoia-destructiveness. The Y-MRS consists of 11 items and is scored following a clinical interview. Four items are given extra emphasis and are scored on a 0 to 8 scale (irritability, speech, thought content, and aggressive behavior); the remaining items are scored on a 0 to 4 scale. Each of these scales may be used to detect symptoms of mania in patients with undiagnosed bipolar disorder, although their reliability to do so has not yet been formally tested.

SCALES FOR PSYCHOTIC DISORDERS

Psychotic symptoms vary widely in their presentation, from the most florid (e.g., hallucinations and delusions) to the most inert (e.g., social withdrawal and catatonia). During interviews with thought-disordered patients, it can be quite a demanding task to cover the spectrum of psychotic symptoms—not only because of their sheer heterogeneity but also because they can be extremely difficult to elicit in impaired or unco-operative individuals. Moreover, antipsychotic medications can predispose patients to movement disorders that are elusive to diagnose; for example, the overlap between negative symptoms and neuroleptic-induced akinesia can be difficult to dis-entangle during the diagnostic interview. Several diagnostic rating scales have been developed to aid clinicians in catego-rizing and monitoring psychotic symptoms, as well as move-ment disorders. Each psychotic symptom scale is administered by a clinician.

The Positive and Negative Syndrome Scale (PANSS) is a 30-item instrument that emphasizes three clusters of symp-toms: positive symptoms (e.g., hallucinations, delusions,

TABLE 6-12 Normative Data for the Positive and Negative Syndrome Scale (PANSS)

PANSS Subscale	Number of Items	Possible Score Range	50th Percentile Score
Positive symptoms	7	7–49	20
Negative symptoms	7	7–49	22
General psychopathology	16	16–112	40

Adapted from Perkins DO, Stroup TS, Lieberman JA. Psychotic disorders measures. In Rush AJ, Pincus HA, First MB, et al. editors: Handbook of psychiatric measures, Washington, DC, 2000, American Psychiatric Association.

TABLE 6-13 Domains of the Scale for the Assessment of Positive Symptoms (SAPS)

SAPS Domain	Number of Items	Possible Score Range
Hallucinations	6	0–35
Delusions	12	0–70
Bizarre behavior	4	0–20
Formal thought disorder	8	0–40

TABLE 6-14 Domains of the Scale for the Assessment of Negative Symptoms (SANS)

SANS Domain	Number of Items	Possible Score Range
Affective flattening and blunting	7	0–35
Alogia	4	0–20
Avolition-apathy	3	0–15
Anhedonia-asociality	4	0–20
Attentional impairment	2	0–10

disorganization), negative symptoms (e.g., apathy, blunted affect, social withdrawal), and general psychopathology (which includes a variety of symptoms, e.g., somatic concerns, anxiety, impulse dyscontrol, psychomotor retardation, man-nerisms, posturing). Separate scores are tallied for each of these clusters, and a total PANSS score is calculated by adding the scores of the three subscales. Each item is rated on a scale from 1 (least severe) to 7 (most severe) following a semi-structured interview (the Structured Clinical Interview for Positive and Negative Syndrome Scale, SCI-PANSS). Norma-tive data for the PANSS subscales, taken from a sample of 240 adult patients who met DSM-III criteria for schizophrenia, are given in Table 6-12.[6] Designed to organize data from a broad range of psychopathology, the PANSS provides an ideal scale for monitoring baseline symptoms and response to antipsy-chotic medications. However, it can take 30 to 40 minutes to administer and score the PANSS, and examiners must have familiarity with each of the PANSS items.

Several additional instruments are available to assess global psychopathology and positive and negative symptom severity in psychotic patients. The 18-item Brief Psychiatric Rating Scale (BPRS) evaluates a range of positive and negative symp-toms, as well as other categories (such as depressive mood, mannerisms and posturing, hostility, and tension). Each item is rated on a 7-point scale following a clinical interview. The BPRS has been used to assess psychotic symptoms in patients with both primary psychotic disorders and secondary psycho-ses, such as depression with psychotic symptoms. More detailed inventories of positive and negative symptoms are possible with the 30-item Scale for the Assessment of Positive Symptoms (SAPS) (Table 6-13) and the 20-item Scale for the Assessment of Negative Symptoms (SANS) (Table 6-14). For

---

BOX 6-3 Schedule for the Deficit Syndrome (SDS)

CRITERION 1

Negative Symptoms (Need at Least Two)

I. Restricted affect
II. Diminished emotional range
III. Poverty of speech
IV. Curbing of interests
V. Diminished sense of purpose
VI. Diminished social drive

CRITERION 2

At least two symptoms from criterion 1 must have been present for 12 months

CRITERION 3

At least two symptoms from criterion 1 are unrelated to secondary causes (i.e., anxiety, depression, adverse drug effects, psychotic symptoms, mental retardation, demoralization)

CRITERION 4

DSM-IV criteria for schizophrenia are met

Adapted from Kirkpatrick B, Buchanan RW, Mckenney PD, et al. The Schedule for the Deficit Syndrome: an instrument for research in schizophrenia, Psychiatry Res 30:119–123, 1989.

TABLE 6-15 Scoring the Beck Anxiety Inventory (BAI)

Score	Interpretation
0–9	Normal
10–18	Mild to moderate anxiety
19–29	Moderate to severe anxiety
>29	Severe anxiety

SCALES FOR ANXIETY DISORDERS

As with mood disorders and psychotic disorders, rating scales may be useful as diagnostic or adjunctive measures in the evaluation of anxiety disorders. They may also be used to track a patient's progress during trials of medications or psychotherapy. However, it is not uncommon for a patient to have anxiety symptoms that do not meet the DSM-IV threshold for any formal diagnosis. Rating scales can also help characterize and follow anxiety symptoms in these individuals.

The Hamilton Anxiety Rating Scale (HAM-A) is the most commonly used instrument for the evaluation of anxiety symptoms. The clinician-implemented HAM-A contains 14 items, with specific symptoms rated on a scale from 0 (no symptoms) to 4 (severe, grossly disabling symptoms). Covered areas include somatic complaints (cardiovascular, respiratory, gastrointestinal, genitourinary, and muscular), cognitive symptoms, fear, insomnia, anxious mood, and behavior during the interview. Administration typically requires 15 to 30 minutes. Clinically-significant anxiety is associated with total scores of 14 or greater; of note, scores in primarily depressed patients have been found in the range of 14.9 to 27.6, and those in patients with primary schizophrenia have been found to be as high as 27.5.[9]

A frequently used self-rated anxiety scale is the Beck Anxiety Inventory (BAI). In this 21-item questionnaire, patients rate somatic and affective symptoms of anxiety on a four-point Likert scale (0 = "not at all", 3 = "severely: I could barely stand it"). Guidelines for interpreting the total score are given in Table 6-15. The BAI is brief and easy to administer, but like the HAM-A, it does not identify specific anxiety diagnoses or distinguish primary anxiety from co-morbid psychiatric conditions.

Other anxiety rating scales are geared toward specific clinical syndromes. For example, the Yale-Brown Obsessive Compulsive Scale (Y-BOCS) is a clinician-administered semi-structured interview designed to measure the severity of obsessive-compulsive symptoms. The interview is preceded by an optional checklist of 64 specific obsessive and compulsive symptoms. Following the interview, the examiner rates five domains in both obsessive and compulsive subscales (Table 6-16), with a score of 0 corresponding to no symptoms and 4 corresponding to extreme symptoms. Total scores average 25 in patients with OCD, compared with less than 8 in healthy individuals.[9] The Brief Social Phobia Scale (BSPS) consists of clinician-administered ratings in 11 domains related to social phobia (Table 6-17). Severity of each symptom is rated from 0 (none) to 4 (extreme), generating three subscale scores: Fear (BSPS-F), Avoidance (BSPS-A), and Physiological (BSPS-P). These scores are summed in the Total Score (BSPS-T). A total score greater than 20 is considered clinically significant. Post-traumatic stress–associated symptoms can be measured with the Clinician Administered PTSD Scale (CAPS), which is closely matched to DSM-IV criteria. The CAPS contains 17 items that are assessed by the clinician during a diagnostic interview; each item is rated for frequency, from 0 (never experienced) to 4 (experienced daily), and for intensity, from 0 (none) to 4 (extreme). The items follow each of the four DSM-IV diagnostic criteria for post-traumatic stress disorder

each of these instruments, items are rated on a scale of 0 to 5 following a semi-structured clinical interview, such as the Comprehensive Assessment of Symptoms and History (CASH). Correlations between SAPS and SANS scores with their counterpart subscales in the PANSS are quite high.[6] Recently, it has been argued that the SANS demonstrates higher validity if attention scores are removed.[7]

An additional consideration in evaluating negative symptoms is whether they occur as a primary component of the disorder, or as a consequence of co-morbid processes, such as depression, drug effects, or positive symptoms. The Schedule for the Deficit Syndrome (SDS) uses four criteria to establish whether negative symptoms are present, enduring, and unrelated to secondary causes (Box 6-3). Each of the four criteria must be satisfied for a patient to qualify for the deficit syndrome, as defined by Carpenter and colleagues.[8]

Patients who take antipsychotic medications are at increased risk for motor disorders as a consequence of chronic dopamine blockade. Several rating scales have been designed to evaluate these motoric side effects, which can include extrapyramidal symptoms, akathisia, and tardive dyskinesia. Each scale is readily administered at baseline and then at follow-up intervals to track drug-induced movement disorders. The Abnormal Involuntary Movement Scale (AIMS) consists of 10 items that evaluate orofacial movements, limb-trunkal dyskinesias, and global severity of motor symptoms on a 5-point scale; additional items rule out contributions of dental problems or dentures. Specific instructions are provided with the scale for asking the patient certain questions or having him or her perform motor maneuvers. Both objective measures of akathisia and subjective distress related to restlessness are assessed by the Barnes Akathisia Rating Scale (BARS), which also comes with brief instructions for proper rating. Of note, this scale can also be useful in patients taking serotonin reuptake inhibitors, as such patients may also be at risk for akathisia. Finally, the Simpson-Angus Extrapyramidal Side Effects Scale (EPS) contains 10 items for rating parkinsonian and related motor symptoms. Each item is rated from 0 to 4; the score is summed and then divided by 10. A score of 0.3 was cited by the authors as the upper limit of normal.

TABLE 6-16 Domains of the Yale-Brown Obsessive Compulsive Scale (Y-BOCS)

Domain	Obsession Score Range	Compulsion Score Range
Amount of time that symptoms occupy	0–4	0–4
Interference with normal functioning	0–4	0–4
Subjective distress caused by symptoms	0–4	0–4
Degree that patient resists symptoms	0–4	0–4
Degree that patient can control symptoms	0–4	0–4

Adapted from Shear MK, Feske U, Brown C, et al. Anxiety disorders measures. In Rush AJ, Pincus HA, First MB, et al. editors: Handbook of psychiatric measures, Washington, DC, 2000, American Psychiatric Association.

TABLE 6-17 Domains of the Brief Social Phobia Scale (BSPS)

Domain: Avoidance and Fear Symptoms	Possible Avoidance Score Range	Possible Fear Score Range
Public speaking	0–4	0–4
Talking to authority figures	0–4	0–4
Talking to strangers	0–4	0–4
Being embarrassed or humiliated	0–4	0–4
Being criticized	0–4	0–4
Social gatherings	0–4	0–4
Doing something while watched	0–4	0–4
Total scores	0–28 (BSPS-A)	0–28 (BSPS-F)
PHYSIOLOGICAL SYMPTOMS		**POSSIBLE PHYSIOLOGICAL SCORE RANGE**
Blushing		0–4
Trembling		0–4
Palpitations		0–4
Sweating		0–4
Total score		0–16 (BSPS-P)

Adapted from Shear MK, Feske U, Brown C, et al. Anxiety disorders measures. In Rush AJ, Pincus HA, First MB, et al. editors: Handbook of psychiatric measures, Washington, DC, 2000, American Psychiatric Association.

TABLE 6-18 The CAGE Questionnaire

C	Have you ever felt you should *cut down* on your drinking?
A	Have people *annoyed* you by criticizing your drinking?
G	Have you ever felt bad or *guilty* about your drinking?
E	Have you ever had a drink first thing in the morning ("*eye-opener*") to steady your nerves or to get rid of a hangover?

TABLE 6-19 Scoring the Michigan Alcoholism Screening Test (MAST)

Score	Interpretation
0–2	No alcoholism
3–5	Possible alcoholism
≥6	Probable alcoholism

The CAGE questionnaire is ubiquitously used to screen for alcohol abuse and dependence. Consisting of four "yes/no" questions (organized by a mnemonic acronym) about alcohol consumption patterns and their psychosocial consequences, the CAGE takes only a few moments to administer (Table 6-18). Positive answers to at least two of the four questions signify a positive screen and the necessity of a more extended work-up; sensitivity of a positive screen has been measured at 0.78 to 0.81, and specificity at 0.76 to 0.96.[10] Further, the psychometric measures for the CAGE are significantly better than are single questions (e.g., "How much do you drink?)" or laboratory values (such as Breathalyzer or liver function tests). A slightly longer, self-administered instrument called the Michigan Alcoholism Screening Test (MAST) contains 25 "yes/no" items concerning alcohol use. The MAST also includes questions about tolerance and withdrawal, and thus it can point out longer-term problems associated with chronic alcohol abuse. While "no" answers are scored as 0, "yes" answers are weighted from 1 to 5 based on the severity of the queried symptom. Interpretation of the total MAST score is described in Table 6-19.

A readily administered screen for drug abuse or dependence, the Drug Abuse Screening Test (DAST) is a self-rated survey of 28 "yes/no" questions. As with the MAST, the DAST includes questions about tolerance and withdrawal and can therefore identify chronic drug-use problems. A briefer, 20-item version of the DAST is also available and has psychometric properties that are nearly identical to the longer version; however, each takes only a few minutes to administer and to score. A total score on the 28-item DAST of 5 or more is consistent with a probable drug abuse disorder.

Nicotine use is highly prevalent among patients with certain psychiatric disorders (e.g., schizophrenia). Smoking among psychiatric patients represents a concern not only because it places them at substantially higher risk for life-threatening medical problems but also because it can interact with hepatic enzymes and significantly alter the metabolism of psychotropic drugs. The Fagerstrom Test for Nicotine Dependence (FTND) is a six-item, self-rated scale that provides an overview of smoking habits and likelihood of nicotine dependence (Table 6-20). Although there is no recommended cutoff score for dependence, the average score in randomly selected smokers is 4 to 4.5.[10]

(PTSD), as well as several extra items related to frequently encountered co-morbid symptoms (such as survivor guilt and depression). Scores are tallied within all DSM-IV diagnostic criteria to determine whether the patient qualifies for a PTSD diagnosis.

SCALES FOR SUBSTANCE ABUSE DISORDERS

A source of considerable morbidity and mortality in their own right, substance abuse disorders are also highly co-morbid with other Axis I conditions, and, in many cases, can seriously complicate the identification, clinical course, and treatment of other psychiatric disorders. Effective screening for substance abuse in all settings in which psychiatric patients are encountered, be it the emergency department, a primary care clinic, an inpatient ward, or a non-clinical setting (such as a screening day event), can be a critical initial step in the treatment of these individuals. Diagnostic rating scales can offer a rapid and effective screen for substance abuse disorders, as well as assist with treatment planning and follow-up.

SCALES FOR COGNITIVE DISORDERS

Diagnostic rating scales can be useful in identifying primary cognitive disorders (e.g., dementia) and for screening out medical or neurological causes of psychiatric symptoms (e.g.,

TABLE 6-20 The Fagerstrom Test for Nicotine Dependence

1. How many cigarettes a day do you smoke?
   - 0: ≤10
   - 1: 11–20
   - 2: 21–30
   - 3: >31
2. Do you smoke more in the morning than during the day?
   - 0: no
   - 1: yes
3. How soon after you wake up do you smoke your first cigarette?
   - 0: >60 minutes
   - 1: 31–60 minutes
   - 2: 6–30 minutes
   - 3: ≤5 minutes
4. Which cigarette would you hate most to give up?
   - 0: not first
   - 1: first of day
5. Do you find it difficult to refrain from smoking in places where it is forbidden, for example, in church, at the library, in the cinema, and so on?
   - 0: no
   - 1: yes
6. Do you smoke even if you are so ill that you are in bed most of the day?
   - 0: no
   - 1: yes

Adapted from Heatherton TF, Kozlowski LT, Frecker RC, et al. The Fagerstrom Test for Nicotine Dependence: a revision of the Fagerstrom Tolerance Questionnaire, Br J Addiction 86: 1119–1127, 1991.

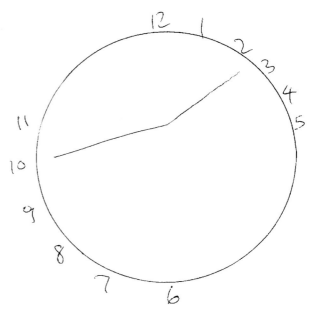

Figure 6-1. Clock-Drawing Test in a patient with a frontal lobe lesion. Draw "10 to 2."

TABLE 6-21 Scoring the Mini-Mental State Exam (MMSE)

Point Value	Task
5	Orientation to state, country, town, building, floor
5	Orientation to year, season, month, day of week, date
3	Registration of three words
3	Recall of three words after 5 minutes
5	Serial 7s or spelling "world" backward
2	Naming two items
1	Understanding a sentence
1	Writing a sentence
1	Repeating a phrase ("No ifs, ands, or buts")
3	Following a three-step command
1	Copying a design
30	Total possible score

Adapted from Folstein MF, Folstein SE, McHugh PR. Mini-Mental State. A practical method for grading the cognitive state of patients for the clinician, J Psychiatr Res 12:189–198, 1975.

stroke-related depression). A positive screen on the cognitive tests described in this section often indicates the need for a more extensive work-up, which may include laboratory tests, brain imaging, or formal neurocognitive testing. As with formal cognitive batteries (which are described in detail in Chapter 8), it is important to keep in mind that the patient's intelligence, level of education, native language, and literacy can greatly influence his or her performance on screening cognitive tests, and these factors should be carefully considered when interpreting the results.

Useful as both a baseline screening tool and an instrument to track changes in cognition over time, the Mini-Mental State Exam (MMSE) is one of the most widely used rating scales in psychiatry. The MMSE is a clinician-administered test that provides information on function across several domains: orientation to place and time, registration and recall, attention, concentration, language, and visual construction. It consists of 11 tasks, each of which is rated and summed to determine the total MMSE score (Table 6-21). A score of 24 or lower is widely considered to be indicative of possible dementia; however, early in the course of Alzheimer's disease, patients can still perform comparably with unaffected individuals. A second limitation of the MMSE is that it does not include a test of executive function, and thus might fail to detect frontal lobe pathology in an individual with otherwise intact brain function.

The Clock-Drawing Test provides an excellent screen of executive function and can be a useful adjunct to the MMSE. In the test, patients are asked to draw the face of the clock, indicating a specified time. Figure 6-1 illustrates the clock drawn by a patient with a frontal lobe lesion; the patient was asked to indicate the time "10 to 2." Note how the numbers are drawn outside the circle (which was provided by the examiner in this case) and are clustered rather than evenly spaced, indicating poor planning. The hands are joined near the top of the clock, near to the numbers 10 and 2, instead of at the center, indicating that the patient was stimulus-bound to these

numbers. The Clock-Drawing Test can also detect neglect syndromes in patients with parietal lobe lesions; in these individuals, all of the numbers may be clustered together on the right side of the circle.

The Dementia Rating Scale (DRS) presents a longer, but often more prognostically valid instrument, for dementia screening and follow-up. The DRS is a clinician-administered test that covers five cognitive domains (listed in Table 6-22), taking 30 to 40 minutes to complete. Within each domain, specific items are presented in hierarchical fashion, with the most difficult items presented first. If subjects are able to perform the difficult items correctly, many of the remaining items in the section are skipped and scored as correct. A cutoff score of 129 or 130 has been associated with 97% sensitivity and 99% specificity in diagnosing Alzheimer's disease in a large cohort of Alzheimer's patients and healthy control subjects. Repeated measures of the DRS have been demonstrated to predict the rate of cognitive decline in Alzheimer's disease; further, performance deficits in specific domains have been significantly correlated with localized brain pathology. The DRS may also have some utility in differentiating Alzheimer's disease from other causes of dementia, including Parkinson's

TABLE 6-22 Domains of the Dementia Rating Scale (DRS)

Domain	Contents	Point Value
Attention	Forward and backward digit span, one- and two-step commands, visual search, word list, matching designs	0–37
Initiation and perseveration	Verbal fluency, repetition, alternating movements, drawing alternating designs	0–37
Construction	Copying simple geometric figures	0–6
Conceptualization	Identifying conceptual and physical similarities among items, simple inductive reasoning, creating a sentence	0–39
Memory	Delayed recall of sentences, orientation, remote memory, immediate recognition of words and figures	0–25
Total score		0–144

Adapted from Salmon DP. Neuropsychiatric measures for cognitive disorders. In Rush AJ, Pincus HA, First MB, et al. editors: Handbook of psychiatric measures, Washington, DC, 2000, American Psychiatric Association.

TABLE 6-23 Scoring the Cognitive and Physical Functioning Questionnaire (CPFQ)

Score	Interpretation
7	Greater than normal functioning
8–14	Normal functioning
15–21	Minimally diminished functioning
22–28	Moderately diminished functioning
29–35	Markedly diminished functioning
36–42	Totally absent functioning

disease, progressive supranuclear palsy, and Huntington's disease.[11]

The Massachusetts General Hospital Cognitive and Physical Functioning Questionnaire (CPFQ) is a self-administered instrument with 7 items covering various cognitive symptoms (motivation, wakefulness, energy, focus, memory, word-finding, and mental acuity). Items are graded on an ordinal scale (1 = greater than normal, 2 = normal, 3 = minimally diminished, 4 = moderately diminished, 5 = markedly diminished, and 6 = totally absent). Clinicians can use the total score as an overall measure of severity. There are not yet validated cutoff points for total severity scores, as there are for some of the other instruments reviewed, but this is currently under development. A general guideline based on the range from the lowest to highest possible scores is presented on Table 6-23. This instrument is used primarily in the research setting.

CONCLUSION

In this chapter, the importance of global and disorder-specific diagnostic rating scales in psychiatry has been described. The

indications, format, and utility of some commonly used diagnostic instruments were presented, and some practical considerations surrounding their use were discussed. No diagnostic rating scale can replace a thorough interview, a carefully considered differential diagnosis, and an individualized treatment plan in psychiatry. However, rating scales can fine-tune each of these components by providing focused information in a time- and cost-efficient manner, by revealing subtle elements of psychopathology that have important treatment implications, and by supplying an objective and often sensitive means of tracking clinical changes over time. Diagnostic rating scales also provide standardized measures that ensure the integrity and homogeneity of subject cohorts in clinical investigations, improving the reliability and validity of psychiatric research studies. Thus, regardless of the setting in which they are used, diagnostic rating scales can enhance the precision of psychiatric assessment.

Access the complete reference list and multiple choice questions (MCQs) online at https://expertconsult.inkling.com

KEY REFERENCES

1. Kirkpatrick B, Buchanan RW, Ross DE, et al. A separate disease within the syndrome of schizophrenia. *Arch Gen Psychiatry* 58:165–171, 2001.
2. Bear L, Jacobs DG, Meszler-Reizes J, et al. Development of a brief screening instrument: the HANDS. *Psychother Psychosom* 69:35–41, 2000.
3. Mischoulon D, Fava M. Diagnostic rating scales and psychiatric instruments. In Stern TA, Herman JB, Gorringo TL, editors: *Massachusetts General Hospital psychiatry update and board preparation,* ed 3, Boston, Massachusetts, 2012, MGH Psychiatry Academy Publishing.
4. Roffman JL, Silverman BC, Stern TA. Diagnostic rating scales and laboratory tests. In Stern TA, Fricchione GL, Cassem NH, et al., editors: *Massachusetts General Hospital handbook of general hospital psychiatry,* ed 6, Philadelphia, 2010, Saunders/Elsevier.
5. Zarin DA. Considerations in choosing, using, and interpreting a measure for a particular clinical context. In Rush AJ, Pincus HA, First MB, et al., editors: *Handbook of psychiatric measures,* Washington, DC, 2000, American Psychiatric Association.
6. Perkins DO, Stroup TS, Lieberman JA. Psychotic disorders measures. In Rush AJ, Pincus HA, First MB, et al., editors: *Handbook of psychiatric measures,* Washington, DC, 2000, American Psychiatric Association.
7. Atbasoglu EC, Ozguven HD, Olmez S. Dissociation between inattentiveness during mental status testing and social inattentiveness in the Scale for the Assessment of Negative Symptoms attention subscale. *Psychopathology* 36:263–268, 2003.
8. Carpenter WT, Heinrichs DW, Wagman AMI. Deficit and nondeficit forms of schizophrenia: the concept. *Am J Psychiatry* 145:578–583, 1988.
9. Shear MK, Feske U, Brown C, et al. Anxiety disorders measures. In Rush AJ, Pincus HA, First MB, et al., editors: *Handbook of psychiatric measures,* Washington, DC, 2000, American Psychiatric Association.
10. Rounsaville B, Poling J. Substance use disorders measures. In Rush AJ, Pincus HA, First MB, et al., editors: *Handbook of psychiatric measures,* Washington, DC, 2000, American Psychiatric Association.
11. Salmon DP. Neuropsychiatric measures for cognitive disorders. In Rush AJ, Pincus HA, First MB, et al., editors: *Handbook of psychiatric measures,* Washington, DC, 2000, American Psychiatric Association.

7   Understanding and Applying Psychological Assessment

Mark A. Blais, PsyD, Samuel Justin Sinclair, PhD, and Sheila M. O'Keefe, EdD

KEY POINTS

Background

- Psychological assessment is a professional consultation service aimed at providing clinicians with a more complex and empirically-based picture of their patients across a number of relevant clinical domains (e.g., intellectual and neurocognitive functioning, psychopathology and clinical diagnosis, personality style).
- The evolution of psychological assessment over the last century has resulted in improved reliability and clinical validity, which in turn has enhanced patient care and clinical outcomes.

History

- Psychometrics is a broad field of study devoted to the development and application of new instruments designed to measure different psychological constructs.
- Historically, there have been multiple approaches to psychological assessment, using both rational and empirically-driven models for the development of psychological instruments.
- Psychological assessment is a complex process that incorporates a multi-method approach to data collection and integration, as a means of maximizing clinical utility.

Clinical and Research Challenges

- Psychological instruments must first undergo rigorous evaluations of reliability and validity prior to implementation, which should also be replicated across settings and populations.

Practical Pointers

- One of the benefits of psychological assessment is its ability to quantify and clarify confusing psychiatric presentations.
- It is increasingly common for patients to receive feedback about the test findings directly from the evaluating psychologist.
- Psychological assessment with patient feedback has been demonstrated to facilitate the treatment process.

OVERVIEW

Psychological assessment is a consultation service that has great potential to enhance and improve clinicians' understanding of their patients and facilitate the treatment process. In spite of this, psychological assessment consultations are underutilized in the current mental health care environment. This is unfortunate given strong evidence that psychological testing generally produces reliability and validity coefficients similar to many routine diagnostic medical tests.[1] This chapter will provide a detailed review of what a psychological assessment is comprised by and discuss the potential benefits of an assessment consultation. This will be accomplished by reviewing the methods used to construct valid psychological

instruments, the major categories of psychological tests (including detailed examples of each category), and the application and utility of these instruments in clinical assessment. Issues relating to the ordering of psychological testing and the integration of information from an assessment report into the treatment process will also be presented.

PSYCHOMETRICS: THE SCIENCE OF TEST DEVELOPMENT

Psychometrics is a broad field of study devoted to the development and application of new instruments designed to measure different psychological constructs (e.g., depression, impulsivity, personality style). Traditionally, there have been three general test development strategies employed to guide test construction: rational, empirical, and construct validation methods.

Rational test construction relies on a theory of personality or psychopathology (e.g., the cognitive theory of depression) to guide the construction of a psychological test. The process of item and scale development is conducted in a fashion to operationalize the important features of a theory. The Millon Clinical Multiaxial Inventory (MCMI) is an example of a test that was originally developed using primarily a rational test construction process.

Empirically-guided test construction, in contrast, begins with a large number of items (called an item pool) and then employs various statistical methods to determine which items differentiate known clinical groups of subjects (a process termed *empirical keying*). The items that successfully distinguish one group from another are organized to form a scale without regard to their thematic content or "face validity." The Minnesota Multiphasic Personality Inventory (MMPI) is an example of test developed using this method.

The *construct validation* method combines aspects of both the rational and the empirical test construction methodologies. Within this framework, a large pool of items is written to reflect a theoretical construct (e.g., impulsivity); then these items are empirically evaluated to determine whether they actually differentiate subjects who are expected to differ on the construct (impulsive vs. non-impulsive subjects). Items that successfully differentiate known clinical groups and that meet other psychometric criteria (i.e., they have adequate internal consistency) are retained for the scale. In addition, if theoretically-important items do not differentiate between known groups, this finding may lead to a revision in the theory. The construct validation methodology is considered the most sophisticated strategy for test development. The Personality Assessment Inventory (PAI) is an example of a test developed with a construct validation approach.

Basic Psychometric Assumptions: Reliability and Validity

To be meaningfully employed in research and/or clinical contexts, psychological tests must meet the minimum psychometric standards for reliability and validity. Reliability represents the repeatability, stability, or consistency of a subject's test score, and it is usually represented as some form of a correlation coefficient (ranging from 0 to 1.0). Research instruments can have reliability scores as low as .70, whereas clinical instruments should have reliability scores in the high .80s to low .90s. This is because research instruments are interpreted aggregately as group measures, whereas clinical instruments are interpreted for a single individual and thus require a higher level of precision. A number of reliability statistics are available for evaluating a test: *internal consistency* (the degree to which the items in a test perform in the same manner), *test-retest reliability* (the consistency of a test score over time, which typically ranges from a few days to a year), and *inter-rater reliability* (as seen on observer-judged rating scales). The kappa statistic is considered the best estimate of inter-rater reliability, because it reflects the degree of agreement between raters after accounting for chance scoring. Factors that affect reliability (the amount of error present in a test score) can be introduced by variability in the subject (subject changes over time), in the examiner (rater error, rater bias), or in the test itself (such as when given with different instructions).

Validity is a more difficult concept to understand and to demonstrate than is reliability. The validity of a test reflects the degree to which the test actually measures the construct it was designed to measure (also known as construct validity). This is often demonstrated by comparing the test in question with an already established measure (or measures). As with reliability, validity measures are usually represented as correlation coefficients (ranging from 0 to 1.0). Validity coefficients are typically squared (reported as R^2) to reflect the amount of variance shared between two or more scales. Multiple types of data are needed before a test can be considered valid. *Content validity* assesses the degree to which an instrument covers the full range of the target construct (e.g., a test of depression that does not include items covering disruptions in sleep and appetite would have limited content validity). *Predictive validity* refers to how effective a test is in predicting future occurrences of the construct, while *concurrent validity* shows how well it correlates with other existing measures of the same construct. *Convergent validity* and *divergent validity* refer to the ability of scales with different methods (interview vs. self-report) to measure the same construct (convergent validity), while also having low or negative correlations with scales that measure unrelated traits (divergent validity). Taken together, the convergent and divergent correlations indicate the specificity with which the scale measures the intended construct. It is important to realize that despite the amount of affirmative data for a given test, psychological tests are not themselves considered valid. Rather, it is the scores from tests that are valid under specific situations for making specific decisions.

Definition of a Psychological Test

There are a myriad of techniques available to facilitate making a psychiatric diagnosis and informing treatment planning, but they do not necessarily qualify as psychological tests. A psychological test is defined as a measurement tool that is made up of a series of standard stimuli (i.e., questions or visual stimuli), which are administered in a standardized manner. Responses to the stimuli are then recorded and scored according to a standardized methodology (ensuring that a given response is always scored the same way) and the patient's test results are interpreted against a representative normative sample.

MAJOR CATEGORIES OF PSYCHOLOGICAL TESTS
Intelligence Tests

Alfred Binet (1857–1911) is credited with developing the first true measure of intelligence. Binet and Theodore Simon were commissioned by the French School Board to develop a test to identify students who might benefit from special education programs. Binet's 1905 and 1908 scales form the basis of our current intelligence tests. In fact, it was the development of Binet's 1905 test that marked the beginning of modern psychological testing. His approach was practical and effective, as he developed a group of tests with sufficient breadth and depth to separate underachieving children with normal intellectual ability from those who were underachieving because of lower intellectual ability. In addition to mathematic and reading tasks, Binet also tapped into other areas (such as object identification, judgment, and social knowledge). About a decade later at Stanford University, Lewis Terman translated Binet's test into English, added additional items, and made some scoring revisions. Terman's test is still in use today and is called the Stanford-Binet Intelligence Scales.[2]

David Wechsler, to help assess recruits in World War I, combined what essentially were the Stanford-Binet verbal tasks with his own tests to form the Wechsler-Bellevue test (1939). Unlike the Stanford-Binet test, The Wechsler-Bellevue test produced a full-scale intelligence quotient (IQ) score, as well as measures of verbal and non-verbal intellectual abilities, respectively. The use of three scores for describing IQ became popular with clinicians, and the Wechsler scales were widely adopted. To this day, the Wechsler scales continue to be the dominant measure of intellectual capacity used in the United States.

Intelligence is a hard construct to define. Wechsler wrote that "intelligence, as a hypothetical construct, is the aggregate or global capacity of the individual to act purposefully, to think rationally, and to deal effectively with the environment."[3] This definition helps clarify what the modern IQ tests try to measure (i.e., adaptive functioning) and why intelligence or IQ tests can be important aids in clinical assessment and treatment planning. If an IQ score reflects aspects of effective functioning, then IQ tests measure aspects of adaptive capacity. The Wechsler series of instruments for assessing intellectual functioning cover the majority of the human age range, and begin with the Wechsler Preschool and Primary Scale of Intelligence (ages 4–6 years), followed by the Wechsler Intelligence Scale for Children-IV (6–16 years), and the Wechsler Adult Intelligence Scale-IV (16–90 years).[4,5] More recently, the Wechsler Abbreviated Scale of Intelligence-II (WASI-II; Wechsler, 2011) was also developed to provide briefer (yet reliable) measures of overall intelligence, in addition to verbal and non-verbal abilities, respectively.[6]

Over time, the Wechsler series has evolved from providing three over-arching measures of intellectual functioning (the Full Scale IQ, Verbal IQ, and Performance IQ) into a more nuanced model of cognitive functioning (Verbal Comprehension, Perceptual Reasoning, Working Memory, and Processing Speed). As with their predecessors, the current Wechsler scales are scored to have a mean of 100 and a standard deviation (SD) of 15 in the general population, which then allows for a patient to be compared against a normative standard. Additionally, this approach to scoring also allows for clinicians to note any meaningful discrepancies between verbal and non-verbal functioning, where in many cases a difference of about 15 points (or one standard deviation) can be considered both statistically significant and clinically meaningful. Table 7-1 presents an overview of IQ categories.

IQ scores do not represent a patient's innate, unchangeable intelligence. Rather, it is most accurate to view IQ scores as representing a patient's ordinal position, or percentile ranking, on the test relative to the normative sample at any given time. In other words, a score at the 50th percentile is higher than 50% of the individuals in a patient's age bracket. Clinically, IQ scores can be thought of as representing the patient's

TABLE 7-1 IQ Score Ranges with Corresponding IQ Scores and Percentile Distribution

Full-Scale IQ Score	Intelligence (IQ) Categories	Percentile in Normal Distribution
≥130	Very superior	2.2
120–129	Superior	6.7
110–119	High average	16.1
90–109	Average	50.0
80–89	Low average	16.1
70–79	Borderline	6.7
≤69	Extremely low	2.2

current level of adaptive function. Furthermore, because IQ scores contain some degree of measurement and scoring error, they should be reported with confidence intervals indicating the range of scores in which the subject's true IQ is likely to fall.

The Wechsler IQ tests are composed of 10 to 15 subtests designed to measure more discrete domains of cognitive functioning including: Verbal Comprehension (VCI: Similarities, Vocabulary, Information, Comprehension); Perceptual Reasoning (PRI: Block Design, Matrix Reasoning, Visual Puzzles, Figure Weights, Picture Completion); Working Memory (WMI: Digit Span, Arithmetic, Letter-Number Sequencing); and Processing Speed (PSI: Symbol Search, Coding, and Cancellation). Subtests are scored to have a mean of 10 and standard deviation of 3, which again allows for different interpretations to be made about someone's level of functioning based on score variability. It is also important to note here that all Wechsler scores are adjusted for age.

One of the initial strategies for interpreting a patient's WAIS performance is to review the consistency of scores. For example, an IQ of 105 falls within the average range and by itself would not raise any "red flags." However, this score may occur in situations where all composite index scores fall in the average range (reflecting minimal variability), or in cases where verbal scores are quite high and non-verbal scores are quite low (indicating a higher variability in functioning). The clinical implications in these two scenarios are quite different and would lead to very different interpretations, and thus an examination of discrepancies is essential when interpreting the profile. However, the existence of a discrepancy does not always necessitate an abnormality. In fact, the occurrence of small to medium discrepancies is not uncommon even in the general population. Typically, discrepancies of between 12 and 15 points are needed before they can be considered significant, and they should be noted in the report.

In sum, although all measures of intelligence are highly intercorrelated, intelligence is best thought of as a multifaceted phenomenon. In keeping with Binet's original intent, IQ tests should be used to assess individual strengths and weaknesses relative to a normative sample. Too often, mental health professionals become overly focused on the Full-Scale IQ score and fall into the proverbial problem of missing the trees for the forest. To counter this error, knowledge of the subtests and indexes of the WAIS-IV is essential to understanding the complexity of an IQ score.

Objective (Self-Report) Tests of Personality and Psychopathology

Modern objective personality assessment (more appropriately called self-reports) has its roots in World War I when the armed forces turned to psychology to help assess and classify new recruits. Robert Woodworth was asked to develop a self-report test to help assess the emotional stability of new recruits in the Army. Unfortunately, his test, called the Personal Data Sheet, was completed later than anticipated and it had little direct impact on the war effort. However, the methodology used by Woodworth would later influence the development of the most commonly used personality instrument, the MMPI.

Hathaway and McKinley (1943) published the original version of the MMPI at the University of Minnesota.[7] (Although the original version of the MMPI was produced in 1943, the official MMPI manual was not published until 1967.[7]) The purpose of the test was to be able to differentiate psychiatric patients from normal individuals, as well as to accurately place patients in the proper diagnostic group. A large item pool was generated, and hundreds of psychiatric patients were interviewed and asked to give their endorsement on each of the items. The same was done with a large sample of people who were not receiving psychiatric treatment. The results of this project showed that while the item pool did exceptionally well in differentiating normals from clinical groups, differentiating one psychiatric group from another was more difficult. A major confounding factor was that patients with different conditions tended to endorse the same items; this led to scales with a high degree of item overlap (i.e., items appeared on more than one scale). This method of test development, known as empirical keying (described earlier), was innovative for its time because most personality tests preceding it were based solely on items that test developers theorized would measure the construct in question (rational test development). The second innovation introduced with the MMPI was the development of validity scales that were intended to identify the response style of test takers. In response to criticisms that some items contained outdated language and that the original normative group was considered a "sample of convenience," the MMPI was revised in 1989. The MMPI-2 is the result of this revision process, and it is the version of the test currently used today.[8]

The Minnesota Multiphasic Personality Inventory–2

The Minnesota Multiphasic Personality Inventory–2 (MMPI-2) is a 567-item true/false, self-report test of psychological function.[8] As mentioned earlier, the MMPI was designed to both separate subjects into "normals" and "abnormals," and to subcategorize the abnormal group into specific classes.[9] The MMPI-2 contains 10 clinical scales that assess major categories of psychopathology and six validity scales designed to assess test-taking attitudes. MMPI raw scores are transformed into standardized T-scores where the mean is 50 and the SD is 10. A T-score of 65 or greater indicates clinically significant psychopathology on the MMPI-2. An interesting feature of the MMPI-2 is that over 300 "new" or experiential scales have been developed for the test over the years. This is made possible by the empirical keying method described earlier. Groups of items that have been shown to reliably differentiate two or more samples or populations can be added to the MMPI-2 as a clinical or supplemental scale. The addition of these scales helps sharpen and individualize the clinical interpretation of the MMPI-2 results.

The MMPI-2 validity scales are the Lie (L), Infrequency (F), correction (K), Variable Response Inventory (VRIN), True Response Inventory (TRIN), and F back (F$_B$) scales. The L scale was designed to identify respondents who attempt to minimize pathology to the extent that they deny even minor faults to which most individuals will admit. It is commonly thought of as an unsophisticated attempt to appear healthier than one might actually be (i.e., faking good). The F scale contains items of unusual or severe pathology that are infrequently endorsed by most people. Therefore, elevation of the F scale is thought of as either a "cry for help" or a more intentional attempt to appear worse off psychologically (i.e., faking bad). Like the L scale, the K scale is purported to measure defensiveness, but data have suggested that persons with a higher level of education tend to score higher on the K scale items than the L scale items.[10] A higher K scale score (more defensiveness) means that the clinical scales are likely to be lower than they should, so the MMPI-2 has a "K-corrected" formula that provides an estimation of what the clinical scales might be if the K scale were within normal limits. The K corrections were devised rationally and have not been empirically verified. The next three validity scales, VRIN, TRIN, and F(b), were added during the revision. The VRIN consists of item pairs that are expected to be answered similarly (e.g., "I feel sad most of the time" and "I consider myself to be depressed"). Too many item pairs with inconsistent answers will raise the suspicion of test invalidity. The TRIN is composed of item pairs that are not expected to be answered similarly (e.g., "I feel sad most of the time" and "I am generally a happy person"). Too many item pairs endorsed in the true direction is thought to indicate a true response bias, which can also bring the test results into question. Finally, the F(b) scale is the most recent addition and is essentially the F scale for the back half of the test. The items that make up the original F scale are all on the first half of the test, and it was observed that some patients are prone to become less invested in accurate responding as they progress through the MMPI's 567 items. An elevated F(b) scale suggests that an individual was prone to endorse less frequently rated items on the back half of the test, thus calling into question the accuracy of the results.

The MMPI-2 clinical scales include the following: (1) Hs—Hypochondriasis; (2) D—Depression; (3) Hy—Conversion Hysteria; (4) Pd—Psychopathic Deviate; (5) Mf—Masculinity-Femininity; (6) Pa—Paranoia; (7) Pt—Psychasthenia; (8) Sc—Schizophrenia; (9) Ma—Hypomania; and (0) Si—Social Introversion. The scales were named after the diagnostic groups they were attempting to identify on the original MMPI (and helps explain why terms such as "Psychasthenia" still appear on the test even though this clinical term is no longer used). To avoid confusion, most professionals who use the test currently refer to the scales by their number. Box 7-1 provides a brief description of the behaviors associated with the MMPI-2 clinical scales.

A computer-scoring program is typically used to score the MMPI-2. Raw answers are entered and scored; then the program produces a profile of the scores on all of the MMPI-2 scales. A solid line is drawn at the T = 65 level to provide an easy reference point. Scores above the line are clinically significant, and scores below the line are not clinically significant (although it should be noted that scale scores below the cutoff can still have important clinical information and are usually not ignored). A preprogrammed interpretation of the results is also provided with the scoring program, as is a list of items that may require more immediate clinical attention (e.g., "I've recently had thoughts about suicide"); these are also known as "critical items." Although the prepared report, or "canned report," provided with the scoring program can be an informative overview of the results, the exclusive use of the report is not recommended because it is not tailored to a specific patient.

The MMPI-2 is interpreted first by examining the validity scales. Scales at or above the cutoff for clinical significance (T ≥ 65) may indicate the presence of a motivated response style. However, elevation on a single validity scale does not necessarily mean that an interpretation of the clinical scales is not possible. In fact, a recent meta-analysis suggests that among the validity scales, the raw score difference between the F and K scales had the largest effect size in identifying faked

---

BOX 7-1 Behavioral Descriptions Associated with MMPI-2 Scale Elevations

VALIDITY

(L) Lie:
Unsophisticated effort to deny psychological problems
(F) Infrequency:
Excessive endorsement of infrequent symptoms—looking bad
(K) Defensiveness:
Sophisticated or subtle efforts to deny psychological problems

CLINICAL SCALES

(1) Hs—Hypochondriasis: Excessive concerns about vague physical complaints
(2) D—Depression: General sadness and depressed mood with guilt and isolation
(3) Hy—Conversion Hysteria: Lack of insight, denial of psychological problems, focus on physical complaints
(4) Pd—Psychopathic Deviate: Rebelliousness; hostility and conflicts with authority figures
(5) Mf—Masculinity-Femininity: For males, passive, aesthetic, and sensitive; for females, not interested in traditional feminine role
(6) Pa—Paranoia: Suspiciousness, hostility, and sensitivity to criticism
(7) Pt—Psychasthenia: Worried, tense, and indecisive
(8) Sc—Schizophrenia: Alienated, remote, poor concentration and logic
(9) Ma—Hypomania: Overactive, emotionally labile, racing thoughts
(0) Si—Social Introversion: Introverted, shy, lacking in social confidence

---

and real MMPI-2 profiles.[11] An MMPI-2 profile determined to be invalid essentially means that enough evidence exists to suggest that items were not answered in a consistent or straightforward manner; this calls into question the validity of the remaining items. For those valid profiles, the first phase of interpretation is to identify the *profile code type*, which is done by determining the highest two or three scales. Numerous books on MMPI-2 interpretation exist to help understand the personality characteristics of individuals who produce specific scale elevations or code types. For example, a 2-4-7 code type indicates the presence of depression (scale 2), anxiety (scale 7), and impulsivity (scale 4) and the likelihood of a personality disorder.[7] As the most researched personality instrument, what the MMPI-2 lacks in theoretical foundation, it has gained in the acquired information of the immense number of studies done with this measure. A great deal of this research has also helped to create subscales for many of the major clinical scales.

Two major products from this body of literature are the Harris-Lingoes subscales and the MMPI-2 content scales.[12-14] The Harris-Lingoes scales were based on a content analysis of the more heterogeneous clinical scales aimed at extracting factors that had highly similar items. For example, scale 2 (Depression) has five scales: Subjective Depression; Psychomotor Retardation; Physical Malfunctioning; Mental Dullness; and Brooding. Though retained in the MMPI-2 with some minor changes and included in the automated report of the MMPI-2, the data on the Harris-Lingoes scales are somewhat sparse and outdated.[8] However, examining these scales in concert with the full clinical scales can enhance the clinical richness of an MMPI-2 interpretation. The content scales underwent a more rigorous empirical process and all of the original MMPI items were used, as opposed to including items only from certain clinical scales, as was done by Harris and Lingoes.[12,13] Content scales were created by first identifying the clinically relevant areas measured by the original item pool. After an iterative process that eliminated scales and items with poor psychometric characteristics, 15 scales (with minimum item overlap) were created that measure clinically-relevant areas and were not specifically tapped by any one clinical scale. Accumulated research on the content scales suggests a stronger relationship with DSM-IV diagnoses than exists for some of the original clinical scales.

Recently, efforts have been made to reformulate the MMPI-2 clinical scales to address the unwanted impact of item overlap, while also strengthening the scales' association to the original diagnostic concept.[14] Further research will be needed to determine how successful these new scales, called the MMPI-RC scales, are in achieving these desired goals.

The Millon Clinical Multiaxial Inventory–III

The Millon Clinical Multiaxial Inventory–III (MCMI-III) is a 175-item true/false, self-report questionnaire designed to identify both symptom disorders (Axis I conditions) and personality disorders (PDs).[15] The MCMI was originally developed as a measure of Millon's comprehensive theory of psychopathology and personality.[16] Revisions of the test have reflected changes in Millon's theory along with changes in the diagnostic nomenclature. The MCMI-III is composed of three Modifier Indices (validity scales), 10 Basic Personality Scales, three Severe Personality Scales, six Clinical Syndrome Scales, and three Severe Clinical Syndrome Scales. One of the unique features of the MCMI-III is that it attempts to assess both Axis I and Axis II psychopathology simultaneously. The Axis II scales resemble, but are not identical to, the DSM-5 Axis II Disorders. Given its relatively short length (175 items vs. 567 for the MMPI-2), the MCMI-III can have advantages in the assessment of patients who are agitated, whose stamina is significantly impaired, or who are otherwise suboptimally motivated. An innovation of the MCMI continued in the MCMI-III is the use of Base Rate (BR) Scores rather than traditional T-scores for interpreting scale elevations. BR scores for each scale are set to reflect the prevalence of the condition in the standardization sample. The critical BR values are 75 and 85. A BR score of 75 on the personality scales indicates problematic traits, whereas on the symptom scales it signals the likely presence of the disorder as a secondary condition. BR scores of 85 or greater on the personality scales indicate the presence of a personality disorder. A similar elevation on the symptoms scales signals that the disorder is prominent or primary.

The Personality Assessment Inventory

The Personality Assessment Inventory (PAI) is one of the newest objective psychological tests available.[17] The PAI was developed using a construct validation framework with equal emphasis placed on theory-guided item selection and the empirical function of the scales. The PAI employs 344 items and a four-point response format (False, Slightly True, Mainly True, and Very True), which generates 22 scales with non-overlapping items. The PAI has some psychometric advantages over other self-report instruments. Unlike the MMPI-2 and MCMI, one scale elevation on the PAI will not result in a second, by proxy, scale elevation simply because those scales share items. This characteristic allows for more direct interpretation of each scale. The 22 scales of the PAI consist of four validity scales (Inconsistency [INC], Infrequency [INF], Negative Impression Management [NIM], Positive Impression Management [PIM]); 11 clinical scales (Somatic Complaints [SOM], Anxiety [ANX], Anxiety-Related Disorders [ARD], Depression [DEP], Mania [MAN], Paranoia [PAR], Schizophrenia [SCZ], Borderline [BOR], Antisocial [ANT], Alcohol [ALC], Drug [DRG]); five treatment scales (Aggression [AGG], Suicide [SUI], Stress [STR], Non-support [NON], Treatment Rejection [RXR]); and two interpersonal scales (Dominance [DOM], Warmth [WRM]). The PAI possesses outstanding psychometric features and is an excellent test for broadly assessing multiple domains of relevant psychological function.[18–20] The validity and clinical utility of the PAI is also well established.[21,22]

As was discussed with both the MMPI-2 and the MCMI, the PAI also has validity scales that were created to help detect deviant response styles. The first validity scale, INC, is a collection of item pairs that are expected to be answered in the same direction (similar to the VRIN from the MMPI-2). Typically, elevations on this scale are an indication of confusion, reading problems, or even cognitive impairment.[23] INF consists of items that are expected to be answered in a certain direction. Half of these items should be true (e.g., "Most people prefer to be happy") and half should be false (e.g., "I really enjoy paying taxes"). Elevation of the INF suggests that the respondent was overinterpreting items, was careless, or has reading difficulties. If either INC or INF is above its respective cutoff, it invalidates the test results and further interpretation of the clinical scales is not recommended. The NIM scale is designed to identify respondents who are attempting to present themselves in an overly negative light. Similar to the F scale of the MMPI-2, NIM items are rarely endorsed by most people (e.g., "I have not had a single day of happiness"). Another use for this scale, however, is to identify patients who may want their treaters to know how much psychological distress they are in (e.g., a cry for help). It is not uncommon for NIM to be elevated in clinical samples. When evaluating psychiatric inpatients, NIM scores can reach well into the 80s, which is 3 SDs above community norms. The PIM attempts to identify respondents who are trying to present themselves in an overly positive light. Research has shown that the PIM scale is highly sensitive to efforts to present oneself in an overly positive manner ("I never feel bad"); even modest elevations (T-scores ≥ 57) can raise questions about profile accuracy.

A computerized scoring program is also available for the PAI; it is similar in format to the MMPI-2 program, and it includes a canned report and a list of critical items. Like the MMPI-2, a profile is produced that shows the elevation of each scale in a T-score (recall that T-scores have a mean of 50 and an SD of 10). For the PAI, the cutoff for clinical significance is at $T \geq 70$ and a solid line is drawn at the T = 50 (mean score for community sample) and T = 70 cutoffs. An additional advantage of the PAI is the inclusion of a clinical reference group, which allows for further comparisons to be made with known clinical groups. This is represented as a "skyline" set at 2 SDs above the mean for the clinical comparison group.

Interpretation of the PAI begins with an assessment of the validity scales to see if they fall beneath the cutoffs. The clinical scales are then reviewed for elevations that lie above the cutoff for clinical significance. With the exception of the ALC and DRG scales, each clinical scale contains at least three subscales, also with non-overlapping items. The next step of interpretation includes a review of the subscales to determine which facets of the clinical syndrome are more strongly endorsed. For example, both the PAI Depression and Anxiety scales have subscales that tap the cognitive, affective, and physiological features of these disorders. Reviewing the subscales allows for more precise evaluation of where a patient feels that his or her primary difficulties lie. The treatment scales (AGG, SUI, STR, NON, RXR) measure domains that can have an impact on the course and type of treatment. For example, patients with a strong, aggressive attitude might have less capacity to participate effectively in their own treatment. The RXR scale is an estimation of a patient's willingness to engage in therapy, and it is reverse scored so that low RXR scores indicate a desire for help and an interest in receiving help. The interpersonal scales (DOM and WRM) are reviewed because they can give an estimation of how patients see themselves interacting in relationships. These scales are bipolar, which means that both high and low scores can be interpreted. After the PAI scales are reviewed and problem areas are identified, clinicians can also refer to a Goodness of Fit Index from the computer printout, which is a statistical estimation of how closely a given profile fits the profile of patients from the clinical sample that were carefully diagnosed with specific diagnoses or clinical problems (e.g., attempted suicide or faking good). As a conservative rule of thumb, coefficients of .90 or greater suggest that a given profile has a strong relationship, or "good fit."

Finally, there have also been a number of supplemental indices developed for the PAI in recent years, which among other things assess factors such as suicide and violence potential, and the need for increased level of care.[24,25] These indices have also been shown to possess strong psychometric properties and construct validity, and allow for additional information that can be useful in patient care.

Objective Tests and the DSM-5

The computer-generated reports available from objective tests frequently provide suggested DSM diagnoses. Although efforts have been made, either through the construction of scales or through research with numerous clinical populations, to validate relationships between the self-report tests and the DSM, these tests should not be used exclusively to provide any psychiatric diagnosis. That is not to say each of the self-report tests reviewed here cannot be helpful in identifying problem areas, interpersonal styles, and treatment considerations. At best, any diagnoses recommended from the results of self-report (and projective for that matter) testing are informed suggestions, and at their worst they are marketing gimmicks with little clinical validity. Psychological tests are not intended to replace competent clinicians who can integrate multiple data sources in the evaluation process. However, these tests can provide a broad range of standardized information and can assess the severity of a patient's symptoms in a precise manner.

Performance-Based Tests of Personality

The historical development of projective tests (now referred to as performance tests) is tied to psychoanalysis and to the idea of unconscious motives. Carl Jung developed the Word Association Test (1910) to measure the Freudian concept of "mental conflict"; it was one of the first attempts to standardize a projective technique. For Jung, the time it took someone to respond to a word revealed how close that subject matter was to the person's particular complex. Longer response times meant that the person was defending against the affect that was brought up by the word.

In 1921, Hermann Rorschach published his Inkblot Test. Interestingly, the idea of using inkblots was not unique to Rorschach, as Binet (1895) unsuccessfully attempted to use this method in his early testing of children in the French school system to measure visual imagination.[26] For Rorschach, a game called *Klecksographie* (Blotto) was very popular in Europe at the time when he was entering school. In this game, inkblots were used to generate artistic and colorful descriptions for entertainment. Rorschach observed that psychotic patients produced very different responses to the Blotto game than did others. After extensive systematic exploration of the diagnostic potential of having patients perceive a series of standard inkblots, he published his book *Psychodiagnostik*, which received only a lukewarm reception. Rorschach passed away within a year of the book's publication without ever realizing the impact his test would eventually have on personality assessment.

The second milestone in projective assessment came with the publication of the Thematic Apperception Test (TAT).[27] Unlike the Rorschach, which uses ambiguous inkblots, the TAT is a series of redrawn pictures of people of varying genders and ages engaged in some sort of activity. The respondent is instructed to tell a story about the picture that has a beginning, a middle, and an end and describes what the characters in the picture are thinking and feeling. The TAT stimuli were selected from pictures, magazine illustrations, and paintings. Murray, a faculty member at Harvard, had been in psychoanalysis with Carl Jung and was strongly influenced by Jung's theory. Unlike the tentative acceptance of the Rorschach during the same period, the TAT was widely accepted and used by researchers from many different theoretical orientations. This is due in part to emerging evidence in support of its construct validity and clinical utility. The TAT has sparked a wide interest, and many other tests of apperception have been developed over the years for clinical and research purposes.

Performance-based tests of psychological functioning differ substantially from objective tests. These tests are less structured and require more effort both on the part of the patient to make sense of, and to respond to, the test stimuli, and on the examiner to conduct appropriate queries into vague responses while recording each response verbatim. Even the instructions for the projective tests tend to be less specific than those of an objective test. As a result, the patient is provided with a great degree of freedom to demonstrate his or her own unique personality characteristics and psychological organizing processes. While self-report tests provide a view of the patient's "conscious" explicit motivations (what he or she wants the examiner to know), the projective tests provide insights into the patient's implicit motivations, as well as his or her typical style of perceiving, organizing, and responding to ambiguous external and internal stimuli. When combined together, data from objective and performance-based tests can provide a comprehensive multi-dimensional description of a patient's functioning.

The Rorschach Inkblot Method

The inkblot method is intended to measure the whole of one's personality functioning. It consists of inkblots on 10 cards or plates (the same inkblots produced in the original publication of the Rorschach are in use today) to which the patient is required to say what the inkblot might be. Five blots are black and white; two are black, red, and white; and three are various pastels. The Rorschach has a response phase and an inquiry phase. In the response phase, the patient is presented with the 10 inkblots one at a time and asked, "What might this be?" The responses are recorded verbatim and the examiner tries to get two responses to each of the first two cards to help the patient establish a response set. There must be at least 14 total responses with no card rejections (a card with no responses, e.g., "I don't see anything on this one") in order for the administration to be considered valid.

In the second phase, the examiner reviews the patient's responses and inquires as to where on the card the response was seen (known as "location" in Rorschach language) and what made it look that way (known as the determinants) to the patient. It is important that no additional responses are given at this point, and patients are directed as such if they report being able to see something new on second viewing of the cards. Exner's Comprehensive System (CS) for scoring the Rorschach is the mostly widely used scoring system in the United States.[26,28] The process for scoring a Rorschach response is outlined next.

For example, a patient responds to Card I with "A flying bat" in the response phase. During the inquiry, the response is first read back to the patient:

Patient: Here I used the whole card. [makes a circular motion with his hand]
Examiner: What made it look like a bat?
Patient: The color, the black made it look like a bat to me.

The examiner now has enough information to translate the response into a Rorschach score. Depending on the level of functioning of the patient, his or her willingness to participate, and the rapport between the administrator and the patient, the inquiry phase can become quite lengthy. On average, the Rorschach takes about 1 to 1.5 hours to administer.

Scoring the Rorschach can, at times, be challenging, and it requires considerable practice to master. Responses are scored on three basic tenets: where the response was located on the blot (location), the features of the blot that helped generate the response for the patient, and what the response was. The location of a blot helps the examiner to determine if what a patient sees is common and if the form of what the patient sees adheres to the actual contours of the blot. The determinants are the features that a patient uses to justify what he or she saw and can include the color, shading, texture, or features that imply active (e.g., "looks like this leaf is falling") or passive (e.g., "it's a man kneeling down and praying") movement. Each response is reviewed for the presence of scores that relate to the three tenets. A detailed review of all the individual scorable features is beyond the scope of this chapter; however, based on the inquiry outlined above, the Rorschach response would be coded as follows: Wo C'Fo A P 1.0. This code indicates that the subject used the whole blot and what he or she saw (a bat) has a commonly perceived shape (Wo), the black-and-white features of the blot were prominent in forming the percept (C'F), the percept fit the blot shape (o), and it is a popular response (P). All responses in a protocol are translated into these Rorschach codes, following the guidelines of the CS. These codes are then organized into ratios, percentages, and indexes and presented in what is known as the Structural Summary. The variables in the Structural Summary are interpreted by comparing them to a normative sample.

Combining individual Rorschach variables into indexes increases their reliability and validity. The Rorschach indexes are the Perceptual Thinking Index (PTI), the Suicide Constellation (S-CON), the Depression Index (DEPI), the Coping Deficit Index (CDI), the Hypervigilance Index (HVI), and the Obsessive Style Index (OBS). The PTI, S-CON, and DEPI have received the most empirical attention. While the validity of the DEPI has had mixed reviews, the PTI and S-CON appear to hold up well as valid measures of disordered thinking and for the identification of individuals who are at elevated risk for suicide, respectively.[29,30]

For many years, Rorschach scoring has been criticized for being too subjective. However, with Exner's creation of the Comprehensive Scoring System, the reliability and validity of the Rorschach has improved considerably.[26,28] In part due to the recent negative attention on the Rorschach, high standards of reliability have been established that must be met to publish Rorschach research.[31–33] Inter-rater kappas of .80 or better are the standard minimum for all Rorschach variables reported in published research studies. For comparison, kappas in this range are equal to, or better than, the kappas reported in many studies using structured interview DSM diagnoses. Countless numbers of studies from different research groups have been able to reach or exceed this cutoff, thus providing ample data on the reliability of scoring Rorschach data.

As with the other psychological tests reviewed in this chapter, the interpretation of a Rorschach protocol is a multiphase process. The determination of a valid protocol is the first step, and it involves a review of the number of responses (R) and a ratio known as lambda. Lambda reflects the subject's willingness to engage in the Rorschach process. Higher lambda scores are associated with patient defensiveness or lack of involvement in the process. Protocols with fewer than 14 responses and a lambda greater than 1.00 are considered invalid (a protocol is considered valid if it has at least 14 responses and a lambda ≥ 1.00). The next step in interpretation is a review of the index scores, which are a combination of many of the individual variables. For example, scores in the S-CON index provide information about a patient's level of self-destructiveness and have been shown to predict suicidal behavior. Therefore, protocols with a positive S-CON identify patients who are at an elevated risk for engaging in significant self-harm. After reviewing the indexes, Rorschach interpretation proceeds to the review of specific variable clusters, including Affective Organization; Capacity for Control and Stress Tolerance; Cognitive Mediation; Ideation; Information Processing; Interpersonal Perception; Self-Perception; and Situational Stress. Valid protocols will include scores or features that make up each of these clusters, allowing the examiner to assess the patient's function in each of these areas.

The Rorschach is also an outstanding instrument for assessing the quality of a subject's thinking and the presence of a thought disorder. The assessment of thought quality includes determining both the congruence or "fit" between what the patient saw and the contours of the blot (perceptual accuracy) and the appropriateness of the logic used to justify the response. Form Quality (FQ) reflects the fit between percept and blot and is rated on a four-point scale (superior [+], ordinary [o], unusual [u], and minus [−]). At the upper end of this scale (+, o, and to some extent u), patients use appropriate features of the blot and what they see generally corresponds to the shape of the blot where they saw the response. Poor form quality (minus responses) indicates that a patient's response does not fit the contours of the blot and represents distorted or strained perception. For example, imagine that a patient was handed an inkblot and responded as follows:

Patient: It looks like a huge spider.
Examiner (inquiry phase): What makes it look like that?
Patient: How legs come out of the top and bottom and how the big red eyes come out of the top.
Examiner: What makes it look like eyes?
Patient: They've got black dots in them.

First and foremost, the blot bears very little resemblance to a spider at a casual glance. While there may be some protrusions of black at the top left and right and, to a lesser extent, from the bottom, it is difficult to see how a common first response for most people would be spider legs. If this were an actual Rorschach card, the CS database would have a collection of many common responses taken from the normative sample to help guide the clinician's judgment. Remember, the instructions are "What might this be?" not "What does this remind you of?" The "red eyes" described by the patient are the red areas at the top center with dots in the middle. While these could easily be seen as eyes, they do not resemble spider eyes in the least. A response that more appropriately uses the contours of the blot might be as follows:

> *Patient:* The white part in the middle looks like a mushroom to me.
> *Examiner (inquiry phase):* What makes it look like that?
> *Patient:* Well. … because it's white looks like a mushroom and here's the stem and it gets wider here at the top.

This response, while not using the entire blot, is fairly easily recognizable by looking at the white area in the center of the blot. The FQ for this response would likely be scored an ordinary, or "o," and the previous response of a spider would be scored a minus, or "−." The assessment of a subject's quality of thought (associations) is based on the systematic review of his or her verbalizations for a number of specific logical violations (called Special Scores), which can include the following: improbable characteristics (e.g., "A butterfly with eyes on the back of its head"), reasoning based on position or size (e.g., "It's a claw at the top so it must be a lobster"), the inappropriate blending or merging of objects (e.g., "It looks like a spider-mushroom"), or the excessive reliance on subjective/personal knowledge to explain a perception (e.g., "I've seen a lot of spiders and this looks like one to me"). Combining measures of perceptual accuracy and association quality provide a powerful evaluation of reality contact and formal reasoning.

Thematic Apperception Test

The Thematic Apperception Test (TAT) is useful in revealing a patient's dominant motivations, emotions, and core personality conflicts.[27] The TAT consists of a series of 20 cards depicting people in various interpersonal interactions that were intentionally created to be ambiguous. The TAT is administered by presenting 8 to 10 of these cards, one at a time, with the following instructions: "Make up a story around this picture. Like all good stories it should have a beginning, a middle, and an ending. Tell me how the people feel and what they are thinking." Like the Rorschach, test examiners write each response to the card verbatim. Because the TAT cards are much less ambiguous than the Rorschach, it is very rare for an individual to be unable to generate some type of response and only one response is needed per card. Typical administration time for an eight-card set is about 30 to 45 minutes depending on the verbal ability and the motivation of the patient. Currently, no single accepted scoring method for the TAT exists, rendering it more of a "clinical technique" than a proper psychological test based on the definition provided earlier in this chapter. Nonetheless, administrations that include at least eight cards and elicit reasonably detailed stories can obtain reliable and clinically useful information.

A few standardized scoring methods have been developed for the TAT and all are limited to specific aspects of psychological function, such as the level of defense operations and the degree of psychological maturity. One method in particular that has received recent attention is the Social Cognition and Objects Relations Scale (SCORS) developed by Drew Westen for rating all types of narrative data.[34-36] The SCORS consists of eight variables scored on a seven-point Likert-type scale, where lower scores indicate greater levels of pathology. The eight SCORS variables are Complexity of Representation; Affective Quality of Representation; Emotional Investment in Relationships; Emotional Investment in Values and Moral Standards; Understanding of Social Causality; Experience and Management of Aggressive Impulses; Self-Esteem; and Identity and Coherence of Self. Each TAT response is scored based on the SCORS variables and on normative data from a variety of clinical and community populations, which allows for comparison of mean scores. The interpretation of the SCORS is based on the average score for each of the eight variables across all the responses. For example, a score of 1 or 2 on the Complexity of Representations scale suggests an individual who has little ability to see people as integrated beings (with both desirable and undesirable personality characteristics). TAT stories of these individuals tend to include people who are "all good" or "all bad." Psychologists typically assess TAT stories for emotional themes, level of emotional and cognitive integration, interpersonal relational style, and view of the world (e.g., is it seen as a helpful or hurtful place). This type of data can be particularly useful in predicting a patient's response to psychotherapy and to the psychotherapist. In many cases, information from the TAT can be discussed directly with the patient, because many themes from the TAT stories can repeat themselves in the therapeutic relationship.

Projective Drawings

Psychologists sometimes employ projective drawings (free-hand drawings of human figures or other objects; e.g., house-tree-person) as a supplemental assessment procedure. Like the TAT, projective drawings represent a clinical technique instead of a formal test, because there are no formal scoring methods. In fact, the interpretation of these drawings often draws heavily (and strictly) on psychoanalytic theory. Despite their poor psychometric properties, projective drawings can be clinically useful. For example, psychotic subjects may produce human figure drawings that are transparent with internal organs visible. Projective drawing techniques are used much more frequently with children, especially when verbal communication is limited or non-existent. It is important to remember that projective drawings are less reliable and less valid than are the other tests reviewed in this chapter.

THE ASSESSMENT CONSULTATION PROCESS AND REPORT
Obtaining the Assessment Consultation

Referring a patient for an assessment consultation is similar to referring to any professional colleague. Psychological testing cannot be done "blind." The psychologist will want to hear relevant information about the case and will explore what question (or questions) needs to be answered (this is termed the *referral question*) by the consultation. This process can be made more efficient when the clinician making the referral has given consideration to the areas of function or to clinical questions he or she would like the testing to evaluate. However, in many cases a brief discussion between the referring clinician and the assessment consultant will be sufficient to generate meaningful referral questions. Preparing a patient for psychological testing can be helpful for both the patient and the examiner by reviewing why the consultation is desired and that it will likely take a few hours to complete. An effective psychological assessment includes the timely evaluation of a patient and the provision of verbal feedback to the referral source (within a few days of the testing). A good psychological assessment also provides feedback to the patient. Unless you are thoroughly familiar with the tests used in an evaluation, it is probably best to have the test examiner provide this information. Any assessment should also include a written report sent out to the referral source and to the patient (if requested). Depending on the caseload of the examiner and the scope of the evaluation, a written report can take some time. One should not hesitate to contact the examiner if a report has not been received within a couple of weeks of the assessment. To avoid the frustration of waiting for a tardy report, one should discuss how long it will take to get a report when the case is first discussed.

Using Psychological Assessment to Enhance Care

One should consider reviewing the relevant findings with the patient even if feedback has been given both to the referring clinician and to the patient separately. This helps to confirm for the patient the value that the clinician places on the testing and the time the patient has invested in it. Many people have reservations and unfounded fears about psychological tests. Clinicians can assure patients that there are no tests for "craziness" and that the results themselves will not get the patient institutionalized. Asking questions (e.g., how the testing was for the patient, what concerns the patient has about the results, if the results coincide with how the patient sees himself or herself, and if the patient has learned anything new as a result of the testing) can actually help strengthen the therapeutic relationship and demonstrate concern for the patient's well-being.[37,38] A fair amount of theoretical and empirical writing has explored the similarities between the assessment process and therapy. This can be used to the clinician's advantage by listening to any stories the patient might provide about his or her experiences in the assessment and by seeing if they can be related to any prominent themes that have arisen in the work with the patient. In many cases, pointing out these themes can help to further outline for the patient how he or she interacts with the world. If more specific questions about the testing arise during this discussion, one should consider consulting the examiner for clarification. Finally, careful consideration should be given to the recommendations from the report. In most cases, the test examiner has either given careful thought to what would be helpful to the patient and the therapist, or has prior experience testing people with similar difficulties as the patient and could have access to resources that were previously unknown.

Understanding the Assessment Report

The report is the written statement of the psychologist's findings. It should be understandable, and plainly state and answer the referral question(s). The report should contain the following information: relevant background information; a list of the procedures used in the consultation; a statement about the validity of the test results and the confidence the psychologist has in the findings; a detailed description of the patient based on test data; and recommendations drawn from the test findings. The test findings should be presented in a logical manner that provides a rich integrated description of the patient (not a description of the individual test results). It should also contain some raw data (e.g., IQ scores) and an explanation of the measurement of the scores (e.g., The WAIS-IV index scores have a mean of 100 and an SD of 15). This will allow any follow-up testing to be meaningfully compared to the present findings. It should close with a list of recommendations. To a considerable degree, the quality of a report (and a consultation) can be judged from the recommendations provided. Many clinicians unfamiliar with psychological testing can feel compelled to read only the summary of the test findings and the recommendations. An effective report is one that should be written to include a great deal of pertinent information throughout. Just as patients are not the sum of their psychiatric symptoms, a testing report summary is only one piece of a very complex consultation process.

Access the complete reference list and multiple choice questions (MCQs) online at https://expertconsult.inkling.com

KEY REFERENCES

1. Meyer G. Psychological testing and psychological assessment. *Am Psychol* 58:128–165, 2001.
4. Wechsler D. *Wechsler Intelligence Scale for Children—Fourth Edition: Administration and Scoring Manual*, San Antonio, TX, 2003, Pearson Publishers.
5. Wechsler D. *Wechsler Adult Intelligence Scale—Fourth Edition: Administration and Scoring Manual*, San Antonio, TX, 2008, Pearson Publishers.
6. Wechsler D. *Wechsler Abbreviated Scale of Intelligence—Second Edition: Manual*, Bloomington, MN, 2011, Pearson Publishers.
17. Morey LC. *The Personality Assessment Inventory professional manual*, Odessa, 1991, Psychological Assessment Resources.
21. Slavin-Mulford J, Sinclair SJ, Blais MA. Empirical correlates of the Personality Assessment Inventory (PAI) in a clinical sample. *J Pers Assess* 94:593–600, 2012.
22. Slavin-Mulford J, Sinclair SJ, Stein MB, et al. External correlates of the Personality Assessment Inventory higher order structures. *J Pers Assess* 2013. doi:10.1080/00223891.2013.767820.
23. Blais MA, Baity MR. Exploring the psychometric properties and clinical utility of the Modified Mini-Mental State Examination (3MS) in a medical psychiatric sample. *Assessment* 12:1–7, 2005.
24. Sinclair SJ, Bello I, Nyer M, et al. The Suicide (SPI) and Violence Potential Indices (VPI) from the Personality Assessment Inventory: A preliminary exploration of validity in an outpatient psychiatric sample. *J Psychopathol Behav Assess* 34:423–431, 2012.
36. Stein MB, Slavin-Mulford J, Sinclair SJ, et al. Exploring the construct validity of the Social Cognition and Object Relations Scale through clinical assessment. *J Pers Assess* 94:533–540, 2012.
37. Ackerman SJ, Hilsenroth MJ, Baity MR, et al. Interaction of therapeutic process and alliance during psychological assessment. *J Pers Assess* 75:82–109, 2000.
38. Finn SE, Tonsager ME. Information-gathering and therapeutic models of assessment: complementary paradigms. *Psychol Assess* 9:374–385, 1997.

8 Neuropsychological Assessment

Janet Cohen Sherman, PhD, Catherine Leveroni, PhD, and Lauren Norton Pollak, PhD

KEY POINTS

- Neuropsychological assessment is a method of evaluating behavior that relies on administration of norm-referenced, standardized tests.

- A major goal of neuropsychological assessment is to determine whether, and to what extent, a patient's cognitive status has been altered. This information can provide important diagnostic information, and helps guide clinical management.

- Neuropsychological evaluations assess a broad range of cognitive functions, including intelligence, and attention, as well as executive, memory, language, visuospatial, sensory-perceptual, motor and emotional functions.

- Within each of the individual domains assessed, the neuropsychologist determines the extent and nature of the impairment in order to address questions regarding the integrity of central nervous system (CNS) function.

- The nature of a neuropsychological assessment allows for more precise observations of behavior than can be accomplished through a bedside examination.

INTRODUCTION

Neuropsychological assessment is a formalized method of observing and evaluating patients' behaviors. It distinguishes itself from other methods of inquiry regarding behavior in its goals and its methodologies. The core method that neuropsychologists utilize is the administration and interpretation of standardized tests. These tests assess a patient's level of function within different cognitive domains and provide information regarding which aspects of behavior are impaired and which are spared. Based on a patient's performance on these tests, the neuropsychological evaluation provides clinically-relevant information regarding etiologies underlying behavioral impairment, as well as information that can inform patient care and treatment. In this chapter, we present an overview of the practice of clinical neuropsychology, including its definition, goals, the types of patients referred for assessments, the domains of cognitive function assessed, and the types of measures administered.

The science of neuropsychology is dedicated to the study of brain–behavior relationships. Our understanding of how behavior is organized in the brain has been informed by observations of patients with focal brain lesions[1,2] by studies of cognitive impairment associated with different underlying disease processes,[3,4] and most recently, by neuroimaging techniques, including magnetic resonance imaging (MRI), functional MRI (fMRI), positron emission tomography (PET), and magneto-encephalography[5,6] Data from these different sources inform our understanding of the neurological underpinnings of behavior and are utilized by clinical neuropsychologists in

linking a patient's neuropsychological test performance with underlying brain dysfunction.

In assessing behavior, the clinical neuropsychologist focuses primarily on cognitive domains that include attention, executive function, language, visual perception, and memory. Examining the nature of a patient's cognitive impairment, as well as the pattern of impaired and spared behaviors, is helpful in distinguishing different underlying neurological conditions, differentiating neurological from psychiatric conditions, and discriminating normal from abnormal performance.[7] A patient's cognitive behaviors are specifically measured or quantified, allowing the neuropsychologist to determine whether a patient is performing "normally" within a particular cognitive domain and, if not, to determine the extent of impairment. The neuropsychologist utilizes the data obtained to address practical questions regarding patient care, including a patient's prognosis and ability to manage various aspects of his or her life (e.g., to live independently, to return to work, to comprehend and to follow medical instructions, and to comprehend legal documents), and to recommend possible treatments, interventions or strategies from which a patient might benefit. Finally, as the information provided is quantified, repeat neuropsychological assessments are used to track the course of a patient's disease.

Referrals for neuropsychological evaluation typically originate from a patient's treating physician (most often a neurologist, neurosurgeon, psychiatrist, or internist), but patients or their family members can also initiate a referral. Referred patients may have known neurological disease or damage, or may display or complain of cognitive dysfunction due to an unknown or unclear etiology. Patients assessed include those with acquired impairments or developmental impairments. Developmental impairments (e.g., learning disabilities, attention-deficit hyperactivity disorder [ADHD], autism spectrum disorder) arise when the brain fails to develop normally, with the cause often unknown. For children with developmental impairments, the neuropsychological evaluation can play an important role in determining diagnosis and in guiding interventions. For adults, it is often the case that a diagnosis has already been assigned, and the neuropsychologist is asked to address questions regarding the impact of the patient's impairment on his/her ability to function within a more challenging setting, for example, in higher education or work settings. This information can help determine whether specific accommodations might help address the areas of difficulty. Acquired impairments (e.g., stroke, head injury, or dementing illnesses) result from neurological disease or damage that often occurs after a period of normal development. The presentation of acquired impairments in childhood often differs from that in adulthood, with localized cerebral pathologies more common in adults and generalized insults to the central nervous system (CNS) more common in childhood.[8] Study findings differ regarding whether the recovery profiles of children are better than those of adults, due to greater brain plasticity,[9,10] or whether children's developing brains are more vulnerable to the effects of neurological insults than are adults' mature brains.[11]

Given that the goal of a neuropsychological evaluation is to determine whether behavioral function has been altered (and if so, to what extent), a critical issue that arises when characterizing the cognitive status of a patient with an acquired impairment is the determination of his or her pre-morbid level of function. The importance of baseline testing has recently received attention in determining the effects of concussive injuries. Many athletic teams, including professional and school teams, now mandate that players undergo pre-season baseline cognitive evaluations, often using a computerized cognitive screening measure.[12] Repeat testing conducted following an injury is then compared to a player's baseline performance to determine if there has been a change in cognitive functioning. This information is used to monitor a player's recovery and to guide return-to-play decisions.[13] However, in many other contexts, baseline neuropsychological data are not available, and the neuropsychologist consequently has to rely on indirect methods to estimate a patient's pre-morbid level of intellectual function. These include consideration of historical and observational data (such as level of education and occupational history, previous relevant medical history, and examination of a patient's performance on specific cognitive tests). Specifically, certain classes of learned information (for example, knowledge of word meanings, factual information, and word reading are highly correlated with pre-morbid intelligence and are generally resistant to the effects of neurological disease.[7,14] The neuropsychologist also considers the patient's pattern of performance across an array of cognitive measures, with higher scores typically reflective of pre-morbid function, and lower scores generally indicating impairment, although the role of normal variability (further discussed below) is also taken into account.[7]

While an estimation of pre-morbid level of function is necessary for the interpretation of normally-distributed behaviors (Figure 8-1), for behaviors that are more even across individuals (i.e., "species-wide" behaviors), such methods are unnecessary (with *any* behavioral dysfunction indicative of impairment).[7]

Within the class of normally-distributed behaviors, individuals display a range of abilities. For these behaviors, the neuropsychologist compares a patient's performance (i.e., raw score) to that of a normative sample. Tests that are most reliable are those for which there is a large normative sample

against which a patient's performance can be compared, and for which the normative sample is stratified according to age, level of education, and sometimes gender. Recently, increasing attention has been paid to developing test instruments and normative data that are appropriate for the specific patient's cultural background.[15,16] In interpreting a patient's test performance, the neuropsychologist converts a patient's raw scores to "standard scores," expressed according to the normative mean and standard deviation (see Figure 8-1). Scores vary in the types of standard scores expressed (e.g., standard scores, T-scores, scaled scores, or Z-scores). Scores that fall within the mean of the normative sample are considered to fall within the "average" range, while those that fall significantly above or below the mean are considered areas of strength or weakness, respectively. Scores that fall two or more standard deviations below the mean are generally considered "impaired" (see Figure 8-1). In interpreting test scores, the neuropsychologist considers how the patient's performance compares not only to the mean but also to the patient's own profile of scores. A patient who scores well above the mean on most tests, and below the mean on selective measures may be considered to exhibit "impaired" performance (*relative* to the patient's pre-morbid level of function), even though level of performance may not fall strictly in the "impaired" range on any measure. While the neuropsychologist considers differences in patient scores as a means to identify impairment, the neuropsychologist also considers normal variability. Specifically, because neuropsychological evaluations typically yield a large quantity of scores, it is important to consider the extent to which variable performances are typical vs. atypical. In fact, research on this topic finds that it is not uncommon for healthy adults to obtain some low test scores and, moreover, that individuals with higher IQ levels display greater variability among scores than do those with lower IQ levels.[17] For this reason, the neuropsychologist considers the patient's pattern of performance within the context of his/her history, behavior, and diagnosis when determining what aspects of performance are clinically relevant.[18]

Neuropsychological tests are also characterized by standardized administration, with all patients presented with test questions in the same way, and with patients' responses to

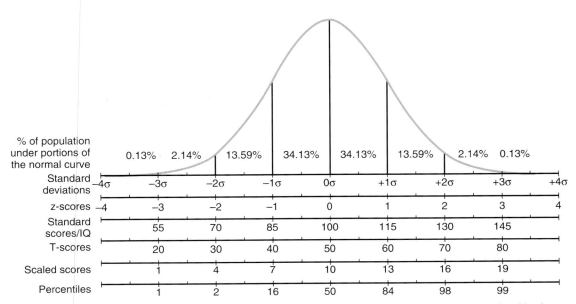

Figure 8-1 A normative curve which displays the distribution of scores around the mean. The figure shows the relationships between different normative scores, with each having a different mean and standard deviation.

stimuli scored in a standardized manner. Given that the neuropsychologist relies on normative data to interpret patients' performances, this interpretation is meaningful only if the examiner adheres to standardized test administration and scoring procedures.

While patients' performances (i.e., "scores") on a set of neuropsychological tests are the core set of data obtained from a neuropsychological evaluation, their behavior on tests can only be understood within the context of their developmental and medical history, as well as their current cognitive complaints. In addition, test data also need to be interpreted within the context of clinical (i.e., qualitative) observations regarding the patient's mood, motivation to perform, attention-to-task, and comprehension of task instructions. In interpreting test behavior, a neuropsychologist relies not only on the specific score that a patient obtains on a test, but also on the patient's response style (for example, whether it is very slow, impulsive, concrete, or perseverative in nature). This careful analysis of patient behavior provides the most meaningful information regarding a patient's level of competence, as well as how different performance variables impact a patient's ability to express that competence. These observations are of particular importance when assessing the validity of test performance (especially when assessing questions of possible malingering). In considering performance validity, the neuropsychologist relies on the administration of specific "symptom validity tests" as well as embedded measures of effort. These methods typically involve examining patterns of performances that are rarely seen in neurological or psychiatric patients (e.g., performance at or below chance on a forced-choice recognition memory measure). In cases where effort is less than optimal, test scores are interpreted cautiously, if at all.

DIMENSIONS OF BEHAVIOR ASSESSED

In the following sections, we describe the domains that are typically assessed within a neuropsychological evaluation. It should be noted that these descriptions are by no means exhaustive, but instead are presented as an overview of the types of questions and methodologies that are employed in a neuropsychological evaluation in addressing questions regarding diagnosis and patient care.

Intellectual Function

In order to interpret behavior within specific cognitive domains, a neuropsychological evaluation nearly always includes a measure of intellectual function. Intelligence can be estimated by tests that tend to correlate highly with overall intellectual function (i.e., tests of single word reading, such as the National Adult Reading Test,[19] the Wechsler Test of Adult Reading[20] or the Test of Premorbid Functioning[21]), or by administration of specific batteries of tests designed to assess intelligence (including the Wechsler Intelligence Scales,[22] and Stanford-Binet Intelligence Test[23]). An intelligence quotient ("IQ") is a derived score based on a patient's performance on a number of different subtests. The Wechsler intelligence subtests are divided into different domains that yield Index scores in the areas of Verbal Comprehension, Perceptual Reasoning, Working Memory, and Processing Speed.[22] In addition to yielding summary scores, including a Full Scale IQ and Index scores, a patient's performance on the individual subtests that comprise each of these domains can also provide important information or "clues" for the neuropsychologist as to where a patient's area of difficulty might lie, and help guide the assessment itself. However, IQ alone is not diagnostically

informative for neurologically-impaired individuals, as it is sometimes insensitive to the selective cognitive impairments that can result from focal lesions (e.g., anterograde memory impairments). Nonetheless, IQ can play an important role in understanding the nature and extent of an individual's deficits, and can be critical in understanding whether deficits are more global in nature.

Attention

The domain of "attention" is highly complex. It includes the ability to orient to a stimulus, to filter out extraneous information, and to sustain focus on a particular stimulus or activity. Its functions cannot be localized to a single anatomic brain region. Instead, attention is subserved by combinations, or "networks," of brain structures. At the most basic level, specific midbrain structures (such as the reticular activating system), play a fundamental role in alertness and arousal. Subcortical structures (such as certain thalamic nuclei), play a role in selective attention, in that they serve as a gatekeeper for both sensory input and motor output. Limbic system structures (including the amygdala), also play an important role in designating the motivational significance of a stimulus. Finally, a number of cortical regions are involved in various aspects of attention, including spatial selective attention (the inferior parietal cortex),[24] behavioral initiation and inhibition (orbital frontal region), sustained attention (anterior cingulate), task-shifting (dorsal lateral region), and visual search (frontal eye fields).[25,26]

In light of the many brain structures involved in attentional processing, it is not surprising that impairments in attention are among the most common sequelae of brain damage. Some of the more common disorders in which attentional disturbances can be significant include attention deficit hyperactivity disorder (ADHD), traumatic brain injury (TBI), stroke, dementing conditions (e.g., Alzheimer's disease or frontotemporal dementia), and hydrocephalus. In addition to various neurological disorders, diminished attentional capacity is a common secondary feature of most psychiatric conditions, including affective and psychotic disorders.

The assessment of an individual's attentional capacity is accomplished not only through the administration of standardized attentional tests, but also via clinical observation. In observing a patient's behavior within the clinical interview and the evaluation itself (i.e., test administration), the clinician obtains information regarding the patient's level of attention (for example, whether he or she is attending to examination questions or is distracted by noises outside of the examination room).

Table 8-1 provides a summary of common measures used to assess various aspects of attention within a neuropsychological evaluation. "Attentional capacity," which is also referred to as attention span, short-term memory span, or short-term memory capacity, denotes the amount of information that the individual's attentional system can process at one time. This function is typically measured by span tests, where the patient is presented with increasingly larger amounts of information and is asked to repeat back what was presented auditorily or visually. Two of the most frequently used measures include Digit Span,[22] where the patient repeats increasingly longer sequences of digits, and the visual analogue of this task, Spatial Span,[22] where the patient repeats increasingly longer tapping sequences on randomly arrayed blocks. Working memory, or the ability to manipulate information in short-term storage, is also typically assessed. For example, the patient may be asked to reverse digits or tapping sequences of increasing length, to re-arrange randomly presented sequences into a specific order,

TABLE 8-1 Assessment of Attention

Component Assessed	Measure	Example of Specific Test
Attentional capacity	Digit span forward	WAIS-IV;[22] WMS-3;[i] or RBANS Digit Span[106]
Short-term memory span	Spatial span forward	WMS-3 Spatial Span; Corsi Block Test[ii]
Working-memory	Digit span backward Spatial span backward Letter-number sequencing	WAIS-IV; WMS-3; or RBANS Digit Span WMS-3 Spatial Span; Corsi Block Test WAIS-IV or WMS-3 Letter-Number Sequencing
Complex visual search and scanning	Symbol substitution Visual search/symbol discrimination Visuomotor tracking	WAIS-IV Coding; Symbol Digit Modalities Test (SDMT)[iii] WAIS-IV Symbol Search Trail-Making Test-Part A[34]
Sensory selective attention	Cancellation Visuomotor tracking Line bisection Drawing and copying Reading	Visual Search and Attention Test;[iv] Letter and symbol cancellation tasks[v] Trail-Making Test-Part A
Sustained attention and task vigilance	Cancellation Vigilance	(see above) Conners' Continuous Performance Test (CPT-II)[vi]
Selective/divided attention	Sustained and selective serial addition Selective auditory tracking Selective attention and response inhibition	Paced Auditory Serial Addition Test (PASAT)[vii] Brief Test of Attention (BTA)[27] Stroop Color and Word Test;[40] D-KEFS Color-Word Interference Test[36]

[i]*Wechsler D.* Wechsler Memory Scale, *ed 3, The Psychological Corporation, 1997, San Antonio, TX.*
[ii]*Milner B. Interhemispheric differences in the localization of psychological processes in man.* Br Med Bulletin *27:272–277, 1971.*
[iii]*Smith A. Symbol Digit Modalities Test. Manual. Western Psychological Services, 1982, Los Angeles.*
[iv]*Trenerry MR, Crosson B, DeBoe J, et al. Visual Search and Attention Task. Psychological Assessment Resources, 1990, Odessa, FL.*
[v]*Diller L, Ben-Yishay Y, Gerstman LJ, et al. Studies in cognition and rehabilitation in hemiplegia. (Rehabilitation Monograph 50). New York University Medical Center Institute of Rehabilitation Medicine, 1974, New York, NY.*
[vi]*Conners CK. Conners' Continuous Performance Test Computer Program (version 2). Multi-Health Systems Inc., 1992, North Tonawanda, NY.*
[vii]*Gronwall DMA. Paced Auditory Serial Addition Task: A measure of recovery from concussion. Perceptual and Motor Skills 44:367–373, 1977.*

or to mentally compute solutions to orally-presented arithmetic problems. Information regarding a patient's working memory capacity can potentially shed light on an individual's deficits in other cognitive realms, such as the ability to successfully comprehend or encode complex information (e.g., an orally-conveyed story, or a written passage).

The assessment of attention also includes measures of a patient's ability to orient to stimuli around them. Patients with lateralized lesions, such as those involving the parietal or temporal lobe, may display a hemi-inattention phenomenon whereby perceptual information that is presented on the side of the body contralateral to the lesion is ignored. A parietal lobe lesion may result in a unilateral visual and/or tactile inattention phenomenon, whereas a temporal lobe lesion or lesion to the central auditory pathways may cause unilateral auditory inattention.[24,25] For example, visual hemi-inattention, also referred to as unilateral visual neglect, typically results from lesions to the right posterior cortex (although it has also been reported following frontal lesions)[7] and involves reduced awareness of visual information in the left side of space. The presence of visual inattention can be striking acutely following neurological insult. Over time, the severity of neglect diminishes, and patients are left with a more subtle deficit in the registration of information in the left side of space when the stimuli are complex or when there is competing information on the right. Within a neuropsychological assessment, the most commonly used tests of visual inattention are cancellation tasks, where the patient is asked to detect targets in an array of visually-similar stimuli. Other tests of visual neglect include line bisection tasks, drawing and copying tests (e.g., a clock face with numbers or a daisy), and reading tests

(particularly useful when the elicitation of a motor response is not possible, for example, due to hemiparesis).

Vigilance, or the patient's ability to sustain attention over time, is also assessed. Deficits in this aspect of attention are often observed in individuals with ADHD. The most commonly used testing paradigms involve the presentation of stimuli over time, with the patient instructed to respond when a pre-specified stimulus ("target") is presented. These tasks are also sensitive to impulsivity, as the patient must also inhibit a tendency to respond to non-target stimuli.

Finally, measures that assess the patient's ability to divide attention between competing stimuli are frequently given. In these tasks, the patient is typically presented with more than one type of stimulus (e.g., numbers and letters) and is asked to keep track of only one of the stimuli. For example, the Brief Test of Attention (BTA)[27] requires the patient to listen to strings of randomly-ordered numbers and letters and to only keep track of how many numbers (or letters) he or she hears.

Frontal/executive Functions

"Complex" cognitive functions, which include executive functions, social intelligence (i.e., personality, comportment, and empathy), and motivation,[28] are primarily mediated by the frontal lobes of the brain. Executive functions encompass a group of higher-order cognitive functions, including the ability to plan and initiate behavior, to both maintain and suddenly shift from a behavioral set, to organize information, to self-monitor one's responses, and to reason abstractly. Social intelligence is a term that has been used to describe such phenomena as the ability to modulate one's emotions, to inhibit various impulses (e.g., aggressive, sexual), and to feel empathy for others. Finally, motivation can be described as the emotional and behavioral "drive" to initiate, persist with, and complete a specific goal.

Disruptions of one or more of the above-described complex cognitive functions are among the most frequently encountered deficits in the typical neuropsychological practice. This is not surprising when one considers that the frontal lobes are not only the largest region of the brain, comprising more than one-third of the human cerebral cortex, but are also the most susceptible to the effects of aging and are among the most vulnerable to many causes of brain damage.[7] The frontal lobes also have extensive connections to other regions of the brain. For example, a series of parallel, anatomically-segregated neuronal circuits connect specific regions of the frontal cortex with subcortical brain structures, including the striatum, globus pallidus, substantia nigra, and the thalamus.[29,30] Three of these circuits mediate complex cognitive functions: a dorsolateral prefrontal circuit mediates executive functions, a lateral orbitofrontal circuit mediates social intelligence, and an anterior cingulate circuit mediates motivation. Thus, neurological disorders that affect subcortical structures (such as Parkinson's disease and Huntington's disease), can cause cognitive and behavioral impairments in much the same way as direct lesions to the frontal lobe. Included among the additional neurological disorders/types of neurological insults that commonly result in frontal/executive dysfunction are ADHD, TBI, stroke, and certain dementing illnesses (e.g., fronto-temporal dementia or Lewy Body disease).

The assessment measures that are utilized to evaluate dorsolateral prefrontal, or "executive," functions are somewhat different than those used to assess other cognitive domains due to the nature of this complex group of skills. Executive functions involve how a patient goes about doing a task (e.g., his or her ability to plan, to initiate behavior on a task, to organize an approach) and the extent to which the patient can be flexible in response to changing task parameters. Therefore, many of the measures that assess executive functions present stimuli that are complex, unstructured, or open-ended in format (requiring the patient to organize, shift between, or categorize the stimuli).

The ability to initiate and sustain behavior on a task is a critical executive function. Fluency tasks, where the patient is asked to generate rapid responses to a particular cue, are among the most commonly administered tests of this ability. For example, within the verbal domain, patients are given a 1-minute period to generate as many words as they can that begin with a particular letter of the alphabet. Patients can experience difficulty with this task for different reasons. These include impaired ability to "get started" (i.e., task initiation), difficulty persevering for the full minute, difficulty generating *different* responses (evidenced as perseverative tendencies, with patients getting "stuck" on a particular response), or a tendency to "lose the task set" (i.e., lose track of the cue provided by the examiner). Letter fluency tasks are most sensitive to disruptions in executive function and are often observed in patients with frontal lesions[31] or with subcortical dementing processes (such as Parkinson's disease).[32] In many cases, the patient does better when provided with structure, such as a semantic cue (e.g., where s/he is asked to list as many animals as possible). Note that tests of verbal fluency administered by the neuropsychologist differ from those given as part of physicians' mental status screens in that the neuropsychologist compares the patient's performance to age- and education-based normative data. The significance of this normative data becomes quite apparent when one considers that the mean number of words provided for the letter fluency task (F-A-S test) is 38.5 for a 20-year-old vs. 25.3 for a 75-year-old.[33] A

non-verbal analogue to measures of verbal fluency is design fluency, where the patient is asked to draw as many different designs as possible within an allotted time period.

Cognitive flexibility refers to the ability to shift to an entirely separate task or to alternate between different stimuli. One of the most commonly used and widely recognized measures of cognitive flexibility is Part B of the Trail-Making Test.[34] This task involves the rapid alternate sequencing of numbers and letters that are randomly arrayed on a page. Cognitive flexibility is also assessed on set-shifting fluency tasks (e.g., asking the patient to alternately provide items from two different categories), as well as on problem-solving measures (such as the Wisconsin Card Sorting Test[35]), where the patient needs to be responsive to changing corrective feedback in determining card-sorting strategies. A large number of perseverative errors in the face of persistent negative feedback is highly indicative of frontal system impairment.

Planning and organization also are crucial aspects of executive functions (Table 8-2). Tower tasks (e.g., DKEFS Tower Test[36]) assess spatial planning and rule-learning skills. Organizational strategies can be inferred by observing the patient's approach, particularly to tasks in which the presented stimulus is complex or unstructured in its format. For example, information regarding the patient's organizational ability is gleaned through examining the degree to which the patient clusters randomly-ordered words according to their semantic category membership on list-learning tasks (such as the California Verbal Learning Test-II).[37] A patient's approach to copying a complex figure (e.g., the Rey Osterrieth Complex Figure Test,[38] Figure 8-2) also provides information regarding organizational ability. The neuropsychologist examines the extent to which the patient appreciates and utilizes the figure's structural elements (e.g., large outer rectangle, intersecting diagonals) in copying the design, or instead, relies on a fragmented or seemingly haphazard approach (Figure 8-3).

While disruptions to conceptual thinking and reasoning can be caused by injuries to multiple brain regions outside of the frontal lobe, tests of this cognitive skill are typically placed under the heading of frontal/executive function within a neuropsychological report, as concrete tendencies in thinking are often observed in individuals with frontal lobe damage. Measures that assess the integrity of this skill include tests of proverb interpretation, tests in which the patient is asked to describe the similarity between seemingly different items (e.g., WAIS-IV Similarities[22]), and tests of pattern analysis and completion

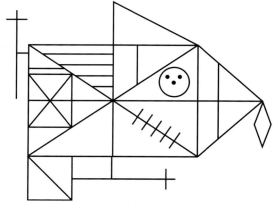

Figure 8-2 Rey-Osterrieth Complex Figure. *(From Osterrieth PA: Le test de copie d'une figure complex: contribution a l'étude de la perception et de la mémoire,* Arch Psychol *30:286–356, 1944.)*

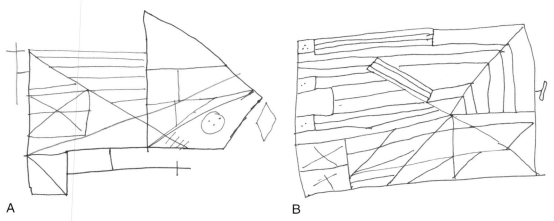

Figure 8-3 The copy of the Rey-Osterrieth Complex Figure in a) was drawn by a 67-year-old woman with a presumed diagnosis of frontotemporal dementia. The patient was given markers, in the order blue, green, purple, red, to allow for analysis of organization. The patient failed to appreciate the figure's structure, and copied the figure in a highly fragmented, piecemeal manner.The drawing in b) is a recall drawing of the Rey (drawn 30-minutes following copy) by a 73-year-old male with a question of atypical Parkinson's Disease. His recall drawing was characterized by significant perseveration as well as source-memory difficulties, with some of the elements from other figures that he had seen during the evaluation. Both of these error types are highly indicative of frontal lobe dysfunction. *(From Osterrieth PA: Le test de copie d'une figure complex: contribution a l'étude de la perception et de la mémoire,* Arch Psychol *30:286–356, 1944.)*

TABLE 8-2 Assessment of Frontal/executive Functions

Component Assessed	Measure	Example of Specific Test
Initiation and maintenance of a complex task set; generation of multiple response alternatives	Verbal fluency	Controlled Oral Word Association Test (COWAT)[33]; D-KEFS Verbal Fluency Test
	Design fluency	Ruff Figural Fluency Test[i]; Five-point Test[i]; D-KEFS Design Fluency Test
Cognitive flexibility	Visuoconceptual tracking	Trail-Making Test-part B; D-KEFS Trail-Making Test
	Card sorting	Wisconsin Card Sorting Test[35]
	Verbal fluency	(see above)
Organization/planning	Spatial organization and planning	Rey-Osterrieth Complex Figure Test[38]; D-KEFS Tower Test
	Use of semantic clustering strategies on verbal learning tasks	California Verbal Learning Test (CVLT-II)[37]
Concept formation and reasoning	Proverb interpretation	D-KEFS Proverb Test
	Verbal conceptualization	WAIS-IV Similarities; Mattis DRS Conceptualization[89]
	Non-verbal concept formation	The Category Test[i]
	Matrix reasoning	WAIS-IV Matrix Reasoning;
	Card sorting	Wisconsin Card Sorting Test (WCST); D-KEFS Sorting Test
Behavioral inhibition	Selective attention and response inhibition	Stroop Color and Word Test; D-KEFS Color-Word Interference Test
	Go/no-go	
	Behavioral ratings (self and/or family report)	Frontal Systems Behavior Scale (FrSBe)[44]
Apathy	Behavioral ratings (self and/or family report)	Frontal Systems Behavior Scale (FrSBe)

[i]*Gronwall DMA. Paced Auditory Serial Addition Task: A measure of recovery from concussion.* Perceptual and Motor Skills *44:367–373, 1977.*

(e.g., WAIS-IV Matrix Reasoning[22]). The Wisconsin Card Sorting Test (WCST) also assesses concept formation, as it assesses the patient's ability to deduce the possible sorting principles.

Rating scales that inquire about the integrity of a patient's executive functioning are also often administered. These are used by neuropsychologists to supplement information obtained from patients' test performances. One widely used scale is the Behavioral Rating Inventory of Executive Functions.[39] Items on the BRIEF inquire about such behaviors as the patient's ability to solve problems flexibly, to hold information in mind for the purpose of completing a task, to stay with an activity, to carry out tasks in a systematic manner, and to keep their workspace or living area orderly. Both patient and informant versions of this form are available.

While multiple tests of dorsolateral functions exist, there are fewer clinical measures of orbitofrontal and anterior cingulate functions. "Go/no-go" tests are frequently administered by both physicians and neuropsychologists, as they are done easily at the bedside. In one version, the patient is asked to knock twice in response to the examiner's knocking once and vice versa. In the Stroop[40] procedure, the patient is asked to name the color of ink in the face of a conflicting color word (e.g., respond "red" when the word "blue" is printed in red ink). This task requires the patient to inhibit an automatic reading response. The Iowa Gambling Test (IGT)[41] is a computer-administered measure that evaluates a patient's decision-making capacity when faced with low risk/low potential gain vs. high risk/high potential gain contingencies.

Studies have found that patients with bilateral lesions of the medial orbitofrontal and ventromedial regions of the prefrontal cortex perform poorly on this test due to a tendency to make decisions that result in a less advantageous outcome.[42,43] Despite the existence of a number of objective measures of orbitofrontal functions, the assessment of orbitofrontal (as well as anterior cingulate) functions is primarily conducted via a combination of behavioral observation and caregiver report. For example, the Frontal Systems Behavior Scale (FrSBe)[44] is a self- and family-report behavioral inventory composed of items that sample equally from the three prefrontal circuits (dorsolateral, orbital, and anterior cingulate), with the patient, and/or a family member answering questions about the patient's executive dysfunction, disinhibition, and apathy both before and after neurological injury/disease onset.

Memory

Perhaps the most common presenting complaint of patients within a neuropsychological evaluation is that of "short-term memory loss." What this means for each patient can vary greatly and the dysfunction can be related to very different etiologies. For one patient, the difficulty can be "forgetfulness" resulting from losing his/her train of thought during the course of daily activities. For a second, the memory loss could manifest itself in difficulty recalling events that have occurred in the recent past. In the first case, the disturbance may be in the area of registration, concentration, and/or working memory and the forgetfulness may be more related to a disorder of attention than memory. In contrast, the latter complaint may indicate a more primary impairment of memory. The goals of formal memory assessment are to distinguish what underlies the patient's complaint or reported symptoms, and to attempt to overlay the pattern of impairment onto the specific brain systems that may be involved, as this can be important for differential diagnosis and treatment.

The clinical neuropsychological examination focuses primarily on understanding the integrity of the patient's anterograde declarative memory functions: that is, his or her ability to form and consciously recollect facts, events, images, and episodes.[45] A limitation in a patient's ability to form new declarative memories since an injury or the onset of a disease process is, in turn, referred to as "anterograde amnesia." This disability may be accompanied by "retrograde amnesia," a more circumscribed, temporally-graded difficulty recalling facts that were learned and events that occurred prior to the injury or the onset of the illness. Non-declarative, or unconsciously mediated, memory functions (such as priming, skill learning, and conditioned responses) are typically intact in anterograde amnesia (and are generally not assessed within a neuropsychological evaluation). Anterograde amnesia results from damage to the medial temporal lobe memory system (see Chapter 72). This system includes the hippocampus and related structures (e.g., paraphippocampal gyrus, entorhinal cortex, fornix, and amygdala) as well as other brain structures with which it has rich interconnections (e.g., thalamus, basal forebrain). It is hypothesized that this system is involved in the initial binding of experience into a memory trace. The bound experience is gradually redistributed to long-term storage in the neocortex in part during slow wave sleep.[46] This process is referred to as consolidation.[47,48] The system also serves as an index system that mediates re-activation of the memory trace when the information is consciously recalled.[49] The medial temporal lobe system is thus always active, as new memories are updated and our knowledge enriched within the context of each recollection.[50] Clinically, anterograde amnesia is seen in conditions that primarily disrupt this system (such

as Alzheimer's disease), which involves degeneration in the basal forebrain and hippocampi among other structures. It also can be observed following infarction and tumors in the medial temporal lobe and associated structures, anoxic injury, temporal lobe epilepsy, trauma, and autoimmune or infections processes (e.g., herpes encephalitis). Anterograde amnesia also can result from processes involving the thalamus (such as seen in Korsakoff's disease). Typically, dense amnestic syndromes, in which the new learning deficit is severe and complete, result from bilateral disease or injury. Unilateral medial temporal lobe dysfunction or disease is more likely to result in material-specific memory deficits, with damage to the left medial temporal lobe typically resulting in difficulty learning and retaining new verbal information, and damage to the right medial temporal lobe resulting in difficulty acquiring new spatial information.[51]

The assessment of anterograde memory functions, and thereby the functional integrity of the medial temporal lobe system, typically involves presenting the patient with novel information, and testing acquisition of the information in the form of immediate recall. Consolidation and storage is measured by testing the patient's recall of the information after a delay that generally ranges from 10 to 40 minutes, depending on the measure. The neuropsychologist infers that if delayed recall is intact, the medial temporal lobe system has bound the experience, and that it is available for later recollection. The types of information presented vary, but generally include the presentation of both auditory-verbal information (e.g., word lists or stories) and visual information (e.g., designs, faces, or patterns). If there is a concern about the patient's motor skills, the neuropsychologist includes visual memory tests that do not require drawing, as difficulty with reproduction can negatively impact the patient's score, reflecting motor rather than memory impairment. In addition, visual memory tests vary in the extent to which the stimuli can be encoded verbally. If the comparative functional integrity of the medial temporal lobes is a crucial aspect of the referral question, the visual stimuli should be abstract in nature in order to provide a more pure test of memory within this modality. Examples of common standardized tests used to assess anterograde memory functions are listed in Table 8-3.

Frank anterograde amnesia accounts for only a fraction of the memory disorders that present to a neuropsychology service. In fact, many patients who present with complaints of impaired memory display deficient "strategic memory" functions that result from disruption of frontal-striatal brain systems. Strategic memory functions include the organization of incoming information at the time of encoding to enhance learning, and the initiation and activation of stored representations at the time of recollection.[52] Patients who have difficulty with strategic aspects of memory may perform well on tests of their ability to learn and recall simple or contextual material, but not on tests that require sustained effort and organization of the material for optimal performance. The patient may have difficulty freely recalling information, but will do better in a recognition format, as the information was consolidated and stored. In fact, retrieval-based memory dysfunction is the hallmark of memory disturbance associated with subcortical dementias, such as Parkinson's disease and multiple sclerosis.[53,54] A good way to elicit the difficulty is with supra-span list-learning tests: that is, lists that are longer than the normal span of attention/immediate memory. Such tests require effortful encoding, as the patient cannot simply listen and absorb the information. Several list-learning tests also embed structure into the task (e.g., semantic similarity among the words on the list). As described in the Executive Functioning section above, for these types of measures (e.g., CVLT-II[37]), the patient's performance can be examined not

TABLE 8-3 Assessment of Memory

Domain	Types of Measures	Sample Tests
Auditory-verbal Memory	Recall and recognition of unrelated words presented over multiple trials	Rey Auditory-Verbal Learning Test[i]; RBANS List Learning; Buschke Selective Reminding Test[i]
	Recall and recognition of semantically-related word presented over multiple trials	California Verbal Learning Test-II; Hopkins Verbal Learning Test-Revised[i]
	Recall and recognition of word pairs over multiple trials	WMS-III Verbal Paired Associates Learning
	Story recall	WMS-IV Logical Memory; WRAML-2 Story Memory[i]; RBANS Story Memory
Visual Memory	Recall and recognition of simple designs	WMS-IV Visual Reproduction; Benton Visual Retention Test; WRAML-2 Design Memory
	Recall and recognition of multiple designs presented over repeated trials	Brief Visuospatial Memory Test-Revised[i]
	Recall of complex visual information	Rey-Osterrieth Complex Figure Test; RBANS Figure Recall; WMS-III Family Pictures
	Learning of a spatial pattern over multiple trials	7-24 Spatial Recall Test[i]; Visual Spatial Learning Test[i]
	Face learning and recognition	WMS-III Face Recognition; Warrington Recognition Memory Test[i]
Remote/ Long-Term Memory	Recall of facts	WAIS-IV Information; WMS-III Information and Orientation
	Recall of public semantic knowledge	Famous Faces Test[58]; Transient Events Test[59]
	Autobiographical memory	Autobiographical Memory Interview[60]; WMS-III Information and Orientation

[i]Gronwall DMA. Paced Auditory Serial Addition Task: A measure of recovery from concussion. Perceptual and Motor Skills 44:367–373, 1977.

only for extent of learning and recall, but specifically for organizational strategies that can be used to enhance learning and later recall.[55] Complex figure drawing and memory tasks (e.g., Rey-Osterrieth Complex figure[38]) similarly can provide insights into strategic learning of visual information as the extent to which the individual utilizes an organized approach in the encoding (copy) phase predicts subsequent incidental and delayed recall.[56]

Dysfunction of strategic memory systems also can manifest in the person's ability to verify the accuracy of a retrieved memory, temporally-ordering information, or identifying the source of a memory. In mild cases, this can present as mild intrusions of information from one task to the next. Recognition discriminability may be impaired, especially on tests that include semantically-related distracter items. In more severe cases, deficits in source memory can present as frank confabulation, as the patient is completely unable to identify the source of, or the accuracy of, the information called into consciousness.

The majority of formalized memory measures included within a clinical neuropsychological exam assess how the brain acquires and stores new information. However, patients can also present with difficulty recollecting previously known and stored information (such as information they learned in school and through experience). For example, patients can present with semantic dementia, a variant of fronto-temporal dementia characterized by a loss of semantic and language-based associations with relative sparing of anterograde memory.[57] Cases of retrograde amnesia, or remote memory loss, are more difficult to evaluate, because the neuropsychologist does not always have a means to verify what a patient knew before the onset of a disease process or brain injury. One way to screen semantic memory is to test a patient's fund of knowledge (e.g., with the Information subtest of the WAIS-IV[22]). While it is not possible to know a person's pre-morbid knowledge base, a high degree of scatter (i.e., failing easy items while knowing more difficult items) or showing a significant mismatch between the patient's knowledge and educational/occupational background may provide clues into the degree to which semantic retrieval is intact. In addition, there are

normed tests of public/semantic knowledge (e.g., famous faces,[58] or transient events[59]). These tests include stimuli that were in the public domain for discrete periods, so it is possible to evaluate whether the remote memory loss is temporally graded.

Patients also can present with a loss of memories for episodes from their own past. For example, they may be unable to recollect significant life events (such as their wedding or the birth of a child). This can occur in association with dense anterograde amnesia or as an isolated impairment. While isolated impairments of this sort are uncommon, and in many instances deemed functional or psychiatric in origin, cases of focal retrograde amnesia have been reported following damage to the anterior temporal lobes, the basal frontal lobe, and the brainstem.[60] Assessment of personal memories can be accomplished through a semi-structured, normed interview (e.g., Autobiographical Memory Interview[61]) and a separate interview with a family member for collateral verification.

Language

In a neuropsychological assessment, a great deal about a patient's language abilities is learned simply through the interview and the clinical observation process. Based on these observations, the neuropsychologist determines if the patient's expressive language is fluent, grammatically well-formed, sensible, and whether there are obvious difficulties with articulation or word-finding. Through observational methods, the neuropsychologist also determines at a gross level whether the patient normally comprehends questions and task instructions. In cases where the patient's language is not grossly intact, the neuropsychologist not only conducts a far more in-depth assessment of language function, but also tailors the assessment of function within other cognitive domains, as the patient may not be able to comprehend, or respond to, questions in the standard format. For example, for patients who present with aphasia, the neuropsychologist may rely on a non-verbal measure of intelligence (e.g., the Test of Non-verbal Intelligence-3 [TONI-3][61]) to obtain an estimate of general cognitive ability.

For patients for whom language is not the primary complaint or impairment, formal evaluation procedures typically include measures that assess language at the single word level. For example, measures of vocabulary knowledge (which correlate quite highly with level of intellectual function) are often included on intelligence measures. For some of these measures (e.g., the WAIS-IV Vocabulary Subtest[22]), both receptive and expressive language abilities are required, as the patient is asked to provide oral word definitions. Measures that assess receptive or expressive vocabulary in isolation are also often included, with receptive measures asking the patient to perform a word-picture matching task (e.g., the Peabody Picture Vocabulary Test-IV[62]), and with expressive measures asking the patient to name pictured objects (e.g., the Boston Naming Test[63]). Deficits in naming, while quite common in patients with a primary aphasia, are also observed in patients with degraded semantic knowledge, such as patients with Alzheimer's disease (AD).[64,65] The degradation of semantic memory that is associated with the temporolimbic pathology of Alzheimer's dementia is also evident on measures of category fluency where the patient is asked to rapidly generate a list of members from a specific semantic category (e.g., animals; fruits and vegetables). Patients with subcortical dementias (e.g., frontotemporal dementia, dementia associated with Parkinson's disease, and Huntington's disease) tend to have greater difficulty on letter than category fluency tasks, with their difficulty more related to poor initiation (i.e., a deficit in executive function) rather than to a breakdown of language knowledge.[66] The difference in the difficulties experienced by these patient groups highlights the importance of distinguishing the patient's ability to access language from having a primary impairment of language knowledge itself.

Patients who present with a primary language impairment are typically those with focal lesions in the perisylvian cortex (often as the result of stroke), the region of the brain that is "specialized" for language. This includes the pars triangularis and opercularis of the inferior frontal gyrus (Broca's area), the angular gyrus, the supramarginal gyrus, and the superior temporal gyrus (Wernicke's area).[67] For most aphasic patients, the lesion is in the left perisylvian cortex, as language is lateralized to the left hemisphere in approximately 98% of right-handed individuals, and 70% of left-handed and ambidextrous individuals.[68] While a specific language impairment is most commonly the result of an acquired lesion (often as the result of stroke), isolated language impairments can also be associated with primary progressive aphasia (PPA), a form of dementia, in which language difficulties are the presenting symptom, are observed in the face of relative preservation of other cognitive and memory functions, and where the progression of the disease is characterized by a relatively specific degeneration of language function.[69] Based on current consensus criteria, PPA is divided into three clinical variants, comprising non-fluent/agrammatic variant, semantic variant, and logopenic variant, each with different aspects of language comprehension and production impaired and with particular patterns of neuroanatomic atrophy in the left frontal and temporal regions.[70]

In assessing a patient for whom language is the primary impairment, the neuropsychologist typically assesses the various components of language in greater depth. The domain of language is highly complex in nature. Within the auditory modality alone, language comprehension requires the ability to distinguish highly similar sounds (phonemes), to attribute meaning to single words, including words that denote objects, actions and abstract concepts, to associate meanings signified by word morphology (e.g., plurals and possessives) and to associate meanings conveyed through sentence grammar or

"syntax" (i.e., appreciating the different thematic relationships conveyed by an active sentence (e.g., "The boy pushed the girl.") vs. a passive sentence ("The boy was pushed by the girl."). The complexity of language is further compounded by the fact that spoken language is both produced and comprehended within "real-time," and that language is utilized within different modalities (auditory and written). There is strong evidence to indicate that highly specialized mechanisms are responsible for the operations that each of these processes requires.[71] This evidence includes the finding that patients who present with aphasia can present with an impaired ability to access different aspects of language form (e.g., semantics, but not syntax), as well as with specific impairments in their ability to utilize language (e.g., with impaired reading, but not writing, as observed in alexia without agraphia).

As it is often the case that language impairments can be highly specific in nature, characterizing a patient's language impairment requires a systematic assessment of different language functions and processes. Generally, the assessment of language in an aphasic patient includes an evaluation of a patient's expressive and receptive language within oral (spoken) and written modalities (including assessment of both reading and written expression abilities), and an assessment of a patient's abilities at the different levels of language function (e.g., phonemes, words, and sentences). Language assessments also typically include measures that assess a patient's ability to engage in different language behaviors: for example, repetition, naming, reading and writing. Evaluating a patient's language abilities at each of these levels is not only important from a clinical standpoint, specifically, in characterizing the specific nature of the deficit and how it might best be addressed, but this comprehensive approach can also be diagnostically helpful in characterizing the type of aphasia. According to "classical" views of aphasia, selective language impairments are associated with specific lesion sites, and are characterized as different clinical aphasia syndromes.[72] For example, patients with "non-fluent" (Broca's) aphasia present with speech that is halting and agrammatic (as well as with agrammatic comprehension of language[73,74] with a lesion site in the left posterior inferior frontal lobe), whereas those with "fluent" (Wernicke's) aphasia present with fluent, although non-sensical speech that includes phonemic paraphasias and neologisms as well as grossly impaired language comprehension (with lesions in the left posterior superior temporal lobe).[75] While these and other aphasia types are still commonly referred to, recent research has provided evidence for a more variable picture of the effects of a specific lesion site on language function.[67]

In assessing language functions, the neuropsychologist, and often a speech pathologist, relies on comprehensive aphasia batteries (such as the Boston Diagnostic Aphasia Examination [BDAE],[76] the Multilingual Aphasia Examination[33] [MAE, available in different languages] or the Western Aphasia Battery[77] [WAB]). The tasks included in batteries such as the BDAE assess the patient's ability to engage in different language behaviors (e.g., naming, writing, reading, and repetition), and can be utilized to determine which classical aphasia syndrome best describes the patient's preserved and impaired behaviors. More recent assessments of language function (such as the Psycholinguistic Assessment of Language Processing in Aphasia [PALPA])[71] are based on a psycholinguistic approach in which language is considered as separate processing modules that can be selectively impaired as the result of neurological damage, and in which the measures attempt to assess these individual language components in a systematic manner. Tests that are utilized to assess language within a neuropsychological evaluation are presented in Table 8-4.

TABLE 8-4 Assessment of Language

Domain	Types of Measures	Sample Tests
Receptive Language (Spoken Modality)	Word-picture matching	PPVT-IV[61]; PALPA Spoken Word-Picture Matching[70]; BDAE (3rd Edition), Word Comprehension subtest[75]
	Word definition	WAIS-IV Vocabulary
	Following commands	BDAE Commands subtest; MMSE[i]; Token Test[i]
	Sentence comprehension	BDAE Syntactic Processing subtest; PALPA Sentence-Picture Matching (Auditory)
Receptive Language (Written Modality)	Word recognition	PALPA Visual Lexical-Decision Test
	Word comprehension	BDAE Word-Identification Subtest; PALPA Written Synonym Judgments
	Sentence comprehension	PALPA Sentence-Picture matching (written version)
Expressive Language (Spoken Modality)	Confrontation naming	Boston Naming Test[63]; Expressive Vocabulary Test -2[i]
	Repetition	BDAE Repetition of Words, Non-words, Sentences
	Sentence production	BDAE Action description subtest
	Conversational speech	BDAE Picture description Test
Expressive Language (Written Modality)	Writing to dictation	PALPA Spelling to Dictation subtest
	Written picture naming	BDAE Written Picture Naming subtest
	Narrative writing	BDAE Picture Description

[i]*Gronwall DMA. Paced Auditory Serial Addition Task: A measure of recovery from concussion. Perceptual and Motor Skills 44:367–373, 1977.*

TABLE 8-5 Assessment of Visual Processing Skills

Component Assessed	Measure	Example of Specific Test
Visuoperceptual abilities	Object recognition	Benton Visual Form Discrimination[83]; Hooper Visual Organization Test[84]; BORB subtests; VOSP subtests[87]
	Face recognition	Benton Facial Recognition Test[83]
Visuospatial abilities	Spatial orientation and location	VOSP subtests
	Judgment of angular orientation	Benton Judgment of Line Orientation Test[83]
	Cancellation	Visual Search and Attention Test[110]; Letter and Symbol Cancellation Tasks[109]
	Line bi-section	
Visuoconstructional abilities	Drawing	Rey-Osterrieth Complex Figure; Clock Drawing; Mattis DRS Construction subscale
	Block design	WAIS-IV Block Design

Visuoperceptual, Visuospatial, and Visuoconstructional Functioning

In assessing visual processing skills (Table 8-5), the neuropsychologist typically focuses on the integrity of "higher-order" visual processes. Studies of both brain-damaged individuals and non-human primates[78] demonstrate not only that the neural underpinnings of higher-order visual processing skills are distinct from such "basic" visual skills as form, motion, and depth perception,[79] but also that the brain regions underlying higher-order visuospatial skills are dissociable. *Visuoperceptual abilities*, or the ability to analyze and synthesize visual information for object recognition, are subserved by an inferior occipitotemporal system, sometimes referred to as the "ventral" visual stream or the "what" system. *Visuospatial abilities*, or the processing of spatial orientation and location, are subserved by the inferior occipitoparietal system, referred to frequently as the "dorsal" visual stream or the "where" system.[80,81] *Visuoconstructional skills*, which may be defined as the ability to draw (i.e., to integrate visual and motor skills) or put together visual "parts" to form a single visual "whole," tend to be considered as a separate category. However, unlike visuoperceptual and visuospatial skills, it is difficult to localize visuoconstructional skills to one specific brain region because they require multiple spatial and motor skills and differ widely in their demands.[82] For example, performance of a block construction task likely utilizes both right and left hemisphere processing resources, as it involves the ability to accurately perceive the stimulus, analyze the relationships among its elements, and understand how to synthesize the percept from smaller parts. It also involves aspects of executive function (e.g., planning and organization) and visuomotor coordination. Deficits to the above-listed higher-order visual processes can result from a variety of neurological conditions, including focal injury (e.g., stroke) and more diffuse damage (e.g., neurodegenerative conditions as Alzheimer's disease, diffuse Lewy body disease, and Parkinson's disease).

Tests of visuoperceptual ability assess the individual's ability to analyze and synthesize visual information for successful object recognition. Included among these is the Benton Visual Form Discrimination (VFD) Test,[83] where the individual is asked to select which of four designs is an exact match for a target design, and the Hooper Visual Organization Test,[84] where patients are asked to identify objects based on drawings in which the object is presented in fragments that have been re-arranged. Measures that assess more specific abilities regarding visual form are also sometimes included in an evaluation (e.g., the Benton Facial Recognition Test[83]). Other, more comprehensive test batteries are also utilized to assess a number of different aspects of visual perception, including visual form discrimination, visual closure, figure-ground discrimination, and visuomotor integration (Motor Free Visual Perception Test-3[85]), and some of the more specific processes required for successful object recognition (e.g., perception of such basic object properties as size, orientation, and length, as well as recognition of an object across different viewpoints; Birmingham Object Recognition Battery[86]; Visual Object and Space Perception Battery VOSP[87]).

Visuospatial tests assess the individual's ability to process spatial orientation and location information. These include tests in which the patient is asked to visually scan an image, to determine the direction and specific angular orientation of stimuli, or to perceive the relative position of objects in space. Included among the most frequently administered visuospatial measures are the Benton Judgment of Line Orientation test[83] and subtests from the Visual Object and Space Perception Battery.[87]

Neuropsychologists tend to include a test of visuoconstructional ability in their test battery to a greater extent than any other measure of higher-order visual processing skills. These measures require many of the functions just described, for example, appreciating information regarding the position, orientation, and shape of a stimulus. Should the patient's ability to copy figures be impaired, then the neuropsychologist can "back-up" in order to determine where the patient's deficit might arise. At the simplest level, a patient may be asked to render copies of such figures as a circle, a diamond, or a three-dimensional cube. Such data are frequently collected to yield a rough assessment of the integrity of visuoconstructional ability and, as such, evaluation of the patient's performance is often subjective. However, various measures (e.g., WMS-IV Visual Reproduction, copy administration),[88] as well as dementia screens, including the Mattis Dementia Rating Scale (DRS),[89] include sets of simple geometric figures and additionally provide standardized scoring criteria and age-based norms. A clock-drawing test is also a useful and a widely-used tool for assessing visuospatial and visuoconstructional skills (as well as executive function, as drawing a clock requires planning as well as visuospatial and visuomotor skills, see Figure 8-4). The Rey-Osterrieth Complex Figure (ROCF)[38] is an example of a more complex drawing test. For this test, the patient is asked to render a copy of the figure (see Figure 8-2) under untimed test conditions. The accuracy of the patient's copy is assessed via the use of one of various available scoring systems.[90,91] In addition, as noted within the Frontal/Executive functions section, a qualitative analysis of the patient's *approach* to drawing the figure is also commonly conducted. Specifically, many neuropsychologists examine the extent to which the patient appreciates the figure's organizational elements and integrates these appropriately. In some cases, the patient approaches the drawing in either a piecemeal or extremely disorganized fashion, which typically serves to compromise the quality of his reproduction and also provides information regarding the integrity of the patient's executive function. Also, as described in the Memory section, subsequent to administration of the ROCF copy (i.e., immediately following and/or after a 3- or 30-minute delay period),[38] the patient's incidental

memory of the figure is frequently tested. Given that the way in which the figure was initially perceived (i.e., encoded) often impacts memory performance, these measures provide additional information regarding visuospatial functions as well as executive function to the same, if not greater, extent as they provide information regarding memory.

Other types of measures utilized to assess visuoconstruction include those in which the patient is asked to assemble blocks or puzzle pieces to form a design. Among the most commonly used tests in this category is the WAIS-IV Block Design subtest.[22] In this task, the patient is given a set of identical three-dimensional blocks, each of which includes two red, two white, and two half-red/half-white sides. The task is to arrange the blocks such that their top surface matches a presented design. The designs become increasingly more complex as test administration proceeds and the patient's final score for each design is based on both accuracy and speed. This task assesses a variety of skills including the analysis and synthesis of spatial relations, visuomotor coordination, and perceptual organization.

Emotional Functions

A common referral question within a neuropsychological evaluation is to disentangle the contribution of psychiatric processes versus brain disease to a patient's clinical presentation. However, our understanding of the function of the brain in emotional behavior and psychiatric functions is ever-increasing, and in many cases it is not possible to neatly distinguish between the two.[7] Because many neurological and psychiatric disorders share common physiological pathways, a neurological condition can induce changes in behavior, personality, emotional tone, and mood. Damage to the different parts of the brain affects emotional behavior in different ways. Diseases that affect the right frontal areas of the brain can lead to personality changes, including indifference, anosagnosia, and inappropriate euphoria.[92] Damage to the left anterior region of the brain can lead to catastrophic reactions, depression, agitation, and anxiety.[92] In fact, in many cases, the initial manifestation of neurological disease is a change in psychiatric function, mood or personality. There are many examples of this. In approximately 79% of patients with Huntington's disease, the initial symptoms of striatal degeneration are psychiatric (including depression, anxiety, or obsessive-compulsive symptoms).[93] Identification of the primary disease process is not undertaken until motor symptoms emerge later in the disease process. The hallmark early presentation of patients

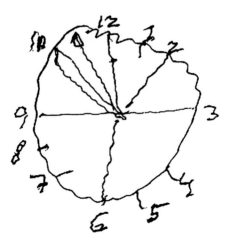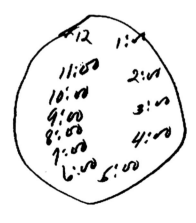

Figure 8-4 Responses to Clock-Drawing

with behavioral variant frontal temporal dementia is a change in personality and social comportment (e.g., loss of insight and awareness, loss of empathy/sympathy, disinhibition, loss of tack, loss of social graces, inertia, passivity, overactivity), rather than a change in cognitive functioning.[94]

In addition to the direct effect that neurological changes can exert on a patient's emotional and behavioral function, secondary emotional disturbances can arise due to the impact of the neurological disease process and its associated consequences on a patient's life. As with any acute or chronic illness, depressive and anxious reactions can occur as the individual reacts, adjusts, and copes with the manifestations of disease. Also, limitations placed on the patient by virtue of his or her symptoms (neurocognitive or physical) can lead to psychosocial stress that renders the patient more vulnerable to psychiatric disease. For example, stress plays a major role in the low quality of life reported by many individuals with epilepsy.[95] The relationship between the neurological process and the emotional experience can be circular. For example, diseases and conditions that affect the right hemisphere of the brain can impair the patient's perception and expression of emotion. This can have a profound impact on the patient's interpersonal and professional function, and lead to depression or social anxiety.

Depression and anxiety also can serve to exacerbate neurological symptoms (e.g., stress increases seizure frequency in individuals with epilepsy) and, in some cases, cause them (e.g., stress results in headache).[92] Depression and anxiety can also result from treatment of neurological disorders, such as medication side effects or neurosurgical procedures.

While comprehensive psychiatric assessment is beyond the scope of the typical neuropsychological examination, it is crucial for the neuropsychologist to understand the interplay between emotional functions and cognitive functions to help disentangle etiological factors and make recommendations that aim to improve the patient's quality of life. The assessment of mood begins with the clinical interview. Through interview, the neuropsychologist gains an understanding of the history and course of the emotional issues and how these relate to the disease process or cognitive symptoms. In addition, the clinician can observe the patient's affect and behavior during interview. Objective measures of psychiatric function are typically included in all exams. In fact, brief self-report measures of depression and anxiety (e.g., the Beck Depression Inventory-II,[96] Beck Anxiety Inventory,[97] Geriatric Depression Inventory[98]) are part of a neuropsychological examination whether or not an emotional component is present, as they provide a baseline for the future. As mentioned within the frontal/executive functions section, behavioral rating inventories (e.g., The Frontal Systems Behavior Scale, (FrSBe);[44] the Behavioral Rating Inventory of Executive Functions (BRIEF)[39] can provide essential insights into a patient's fronto-executive functioning. These measures can tap into critical aspects of a patient's behavioral presentation that are not always captured on cognitive tests. If the patient's insight is limited, obtaining a family member's report of the patient's behavior is helpful. In some cases, when the understanding of personality and psychiatric function is more critical to differential diagnosis or functional recommendations, the neuropsychologist will include more comprehensive objective measures, such as the Minnesota Multiphasic Personality Inventory-II (MMPI-II)[99] or the Personality Assessment Inventory (PAI).[100] For example, a common referral question is to differentiate cognitive impairment that arises from a neurological or neurodegenerative condition from that secondary to a psychiatric state, such as depression or anxiety (commonly referred to as "pseudo-dementia"). In these cases, understanding the nature and severity of the emotional symptom is paramount, because it can provide insight into the origin of the cognitive symptoms. For example, individuals with anxiety and depression may present with vigorous complaints regarding their cognitive abilities that are out of proportion to the level of dysfunction measured upon testing. In these cases, the neuropsychological examination typically reveals mild deficits in effortful processing (e.g., attention span, vigilance, encoding and retrieval-based memory loss, and slowed psychomotor speed) rather than evidence for a dense anterograde amnesia. Conversely, one would not expect severe neurocognitive impairment to result from relatively mild depressive symptoms. In these cases, the patient is more likely to display signs of a neurological condition. In fact, the psychiatric symptoms may be the manifestation of the brain disease, especially when frontal and subcortical structures are involved (commonly referred to as "pseudo-depression").[101]

Sensory-perceptual and Motor Functions

The examination of somatosensory and motor functions is a crucial part of the neurological exam. Yet, these aspects of behavior are frequently omitted in neuropsychological examinations. The neuropsychological examination focuses primarily on the assessment of cognitive processes; however, for many patients, understanding the integrity of sensory and motor skills can provide valuable insights regarding brain function. In particular, abnormal sensory-perceptual and motor findings can help the neuropsychologist lateralize neural deficits.[102] Moreover, for some patients (including those with movement disorders, and patients with certain lesions [e.g., parietal lobe lesions, cerebellar lesions]) who present for a neuropsychological evaluation, sensory and motor functions can be a crucial aspect of the patient's presenting concerns and are critical to consider in determining etiology of deficits.

One goal of a sensory-perceptual examination is to assess the patient's ability to allocate attention in a variety of sensory domains, thereby eliciting subtle signs of hemi-inattention or neglect (as described in the Visuoperception section). This is accomplished by assessing the patient's ability to experience and report simultaneous stimulation in the visual, auditory, and tactile modalities.[7,34,103] Bilateral finger agnosia, which is tested by having the patient name and identify fingers with eyes closed, is a common symptom of left parietal lobe dysfunction. Small lesions in the perisylvian area can result in focal impairments in finger gnosis. More frequently these deficits are seen in association with other indicators of left parietal and perisylvian dysfunction, such as aphasia or the constellation of symptoms comprising Gerstmann's syndrome (i.e., finger agnosia, right-left disorientation, dysgraphia, and dyscalculia).[83,102] Deficits in right–left orientation also can result from left parietal damage, and are often associated with aphasia or dementia. Impaired ability to identify right and left on another person (sitting across from the examiner) can be associated with purportedly non-dominant hemisphere functions (such as mental rotation and spatial thinking).[102] Deficits in identifying symbols written on the patients' hands or fingertips can be seen on the hand ipsilateral to a lesion, or with left parietal lobe damage.[7]

Loss of smell is associated with a variety of neurological disorders (e.g., TBI, Alzheimer's disease). For example, patients with Alzheimer's disease sometimes experience difficulty identifying smell early on in the disease process. The sensory loss can be progressive, such that later in the disease process, the patient has difficulty detecting smell altogether.[7] To test the integrity of the olfactory system, neuropsychologists sometime use the Smell Identification Test,[104] a test that assesses a patient's ability to identify a variety of common odors.

The assessment of motor functions is typically undertaken as a general measure of the integrity of the CNS. A typical motor examination includes measures of strength (e.g., hand dynamometer), speed (e.g., finger-tapping) and/or dexterity (e.g., with a grooved pegboard). These tasks are less related to IQ, educational background, and cultural factors than cognitive measures[102] and bilateral deficits in motor functions can be sensitive indicators of CNS disease or injury. Motor testing is used to gauge the comparative function of the left and right hemispheres. A large difference between the hands on a given task might implicate contralateral brain dysfunction. Patients typically exhibit a dominant hand advantage across manual motor tasks; however, depending on the study, 25%–34% of non-neurologically impaired individuals do not show this advantage.[105] In light of this, the absence of a dominant hand advantage alone does not signal neurological dysfunction, and the findings must be interpreted within the context of the rest of the neuropsychological examination. In addition, multiple factors impact motor function, and not all are neurological in nature (e.g., peripheral injury or disease, inattention, and effort[102]). It is therefore crucial to bear these factors in mind when interpreting the results of a motor examination.

BRIEF NEUROPSYCHOLOGICAL SCREENING MEASURES

While neuropsychological evaluations are often quite comprehensive, evaluating all of the aforementioned domains, this is not always feasible or necessary. Some assessments are more "focal" in nature (e.g., addressing a highly specific question regarding a patient's function), and others need to take into account various practical constraints, including the patient's level of attention or cognitive function, and the specific context in which a patient is tested (e.g., an inpatient setting). Brief screens are also sometimes helpful when the neuropsychologist is attempting to track the course of a patient's disease. For these more limited purposes, it is often more practical, as well as more useful, for the neuropsychologist to instead administer a brief "screen" in which various dimensions of cognitive behavior are assessed, but at a far more cursory level. Screening measures for such purposes include the Repeated Battery for the Assessment of Neuropsychological Status (RBANS),[106] a test that is available in two different test versions, each of which includes a brief measure of immediate and delayed memory, a brief measure of visuospatial reasoning, and a measure of visual construction, a brief measure of attention, and brief measures of language. For patients with a question of dementia, different screens are also available which similarly survey various domains of cognitive function (e.g., Mattis Dementia Rating Scale,[109] the Montreal Cognitive Assessment[107] and The Addenbrooke's Cognitive Estimation Test-R (ACE-R)[108]).

CONCLUSION

As described in this chapter, neuropsychological assessment can play an important role in diagnosis and care. Given the highly complex nature of higher-order brain functions, it can be difficult within the context of a "bedside" examination to fully appreciate the extent to which a patient may be experiencing cognitive difficulties as well as to understand the nature of the patient's deficits. The specific methodologies utilized within a neuropsychological evaluation, which involve a standardized, comprehensive, and quantifiable approach to assessing behavior, allow the neuropsychologist to obtain information that can help address questions regarding a patient's diagnosis and treatment. Moreover, communicating the findings of the evaluation to patients, as well as to those involved in their care, can help improve awareness and understanding of a patient's difficulties, and ultimately facilitate appropriate management.

ACKNOWLEDGMENTS

We gratefully acknowledge the invaluable assistance of Sarah Mayone Mancuso and Ramya Rangamannar in the preparation of this manuscript.

Access the complete reference list and multiple choice questions (MCQs) online at https://expertconsult.inkling.com

KEY REFERENCES

6. Hampton AN, Bossaerts P, O'Doherty JP. The role of the ventromedial prefrontal cortex in abstract state-based inference during decision making in humans. *J Neurosci* 26(32):8360–8367, 2006.
7. Lezak M, Howieson DB, Loring DW. *Neuropsychological Assessment*, New York, NY, 2004, Oxford University Press.
8. Anderson V, Northam E, Hendy J, et al. *Developmental Neuropsychology*, Philadelphia, PA, 2001, Psychology Press.
12. McClincy MP, Lovell MR, Pardini J, et al. Recovery from sports concussion in high school and collegiate athletes. *Brain Inj* 20(1):33–39, 2006.
14. Stebbins GT, Wilson RS. Estimation of premorbid intelligence in neurologically impaired individuals. In Snyder PJ, Nussbaum PD, editors: *Clinical Neuropsychology*, Washington, DC, 2000, American Psychological Association.
17. Binder LM, Iverson GL, Brooks BL. To err is human: "Abnormal" neuropsychological scores and variability are common in healthy adults. *Arch Clin Neuropsychol* 24(1):31–34, 2009.
18. Schretlen DJ, Munro CT, Anthony JC, et al. Examining the range of normal intraindividual variability in neuropsychological test performance. *J Int Neuropsychol Soc* 9:864–870, 2003.
22. Wechsler D. *Wechsler Adult Intelligence Scale*, ed 4, San Antonio, TX, 2008, The Psychological Corporation.
26. Mesulam MM. *Principals of Behavioral Neurology*, Philadelphia, PA, 1985, FA Davis.
30. Lichter DG, Cummings JL. *Frontal-subcortical circuits in psychiatric and neurological disorders*, New York, NY, 2001, The Guilford Press.
36. Delis DC, Kaplan E, Kramer JH. *Delis-Kaplan Executive Function System*, San Antonio, TX, 2001, The Psychological Corporation.
37. Delis DC, Kramer JH, Kaplan E, et al. *California Verbal Learning Test*, ed 2, San Antonio, TX, 2000, The Psychological Corporation.
43. Bechara A, Tranel D, Damasio H. Characterization of the decision-making deficit of patients with ventromedial prefrontal cortex lesions. *Brain* 123(11):2189–2202, 2003.
45. Tulving E, Markowitsch HJ. Episodic and declarative memory: role of the hippocampus. *Hippocampus* 8:204–1998, 1984.
48. Squire LR. Memory systems of the brain: a brief history and current perspective. *Neurobiol Learn Mem* 82(3):171–177, 2004.
49. Eichenbaum H, Otto T, Cohen NJ. Two functional components of the hippocampal memory system. *Behav Brain Sci* 17:449–518, 1994.
52. Gabrieli JD. Cognitive neuroscience of human memory. *Ann Rev Psychol* 48:87–115, 1998.
53. Gabrieli JD. Memory systems analyses of mnemonic disorders in aging and age-related diseases. *PNAS USA* 26(93):13534–13540, 1996.
65. Hodges JR, Salmon DP, Butters N. Semantic memory impairment in Alzheimer's disease: Failure of access or degraded knowledge? *Neuropsychologia* 30:301–314, 1991.
67. Caplan D. Language, Neural Basis of. In *Encyclopedia of the Human Brain*, ed 2, VS Ramachandran, The Netherlands, 2002, Amsterdam, Elsevier Science.
69. Mesulam M. Primary progressive aphasia—a language-based dementia. *N Engl J Med* 349:1535–1542, 2003.
72. Kandel ER, Schwartz JH. *Principles of Neural Science*, ed 2, New York, 1985, Elsevier.

79. Benton A, Tranel D. Visuoperceptual, visuospatial, and visuo-constructive disorders. In Heilman KM, Valenstein E, editors: *Clinical Neuropsychology*, ed 3, New York, NY, 1993, Oxford University Press.

88. Wechsler D. *Wechsler Memory Scale*, ed 4, San Antonio, TX, 2008, The Psychological Corporation.

94. Piguet O, Hornberger M, Shelley BP, et al. Sensitivity of current criteria for the diagnosis of behavioral variant frontotemporal dementia. *Neurology* 72:732–737, 2009.

102. Strauss E, Sherman EMS, Spreen O. *A Compendium of Neuropsychological Test*, ed 3, New York, NY, 2006, Oxford University Press.

9

Coping with Medical Illness and Psychotherapy of the Medically Ill

Steven C. Schlozman, MD, and James E. Groves, MD

KEY POINTS

- Physicians are constantly appraising the coping styles of their patients, and these appraisals dictate both diagnosis and treatment.
- Though there are multiple definitions of coping, *coping with chronic illness* is best defined as the behavioral style that patients use to bring quiescence and peace of mind to their medical predicament.
- There are consistent characteristics of effective and less effective coping styles, and it is essential that psychiatrists who treat medically ill patients assess their patients' particular coping mechanisms in order to deliver optimal care.

BACKGROUND

Coping with illness can be a serious problem for both the patient and the physician. Indeed, the irony of our increasing prowess in healing is our growing discomfort and our profound sense of impotence when a cure cannot be found, and when coping is the order of the day. This dilemma is both consciously realized and unconsciously experienced; both patients and staff feel the ripple effect.[1-3]

Fortunately, the psychiatrist is ideally suited to assist both the patient and the physician with the complexities of medical illness, and to pay careful attention to the complex feelings that chronic suffering engenders (in the inpatient consultative setting as well as in the outpatient clinic). In fact, there is a growing body of literature that focuses on the different mechanisms by which patients cope with chronic disease and the corresponding psychotherapeutic interventions for the patient with chronic illness. This chapter addresses the fundamentals of how patients cope, as well as the art of working psychotherapeutically with the medically ill.

HISTORY

At virtually every step of patient care, physicians and patients alike actively appraise patient coping. Though this appraisal is not always conscious, it is clear that conclusions drawn about how a patient is processing his or her illness has great bearing on therapeutic decisions, the psychological well-being of the patient, and, indeed, of the overall course of the patient's illness.[1] However, accurate appraisal of coping skills is hampered by muddled definitions of coping, by competing standardized assessments, and by a general lack of conscious consideration of how patients cope and whether their particular coping styles are effective or helpful.[4-8]

Early conceptualizations of coping centered around the "Transactional Model for Stress Management," put forth first by Lazarus and colleagues in the late 1960s.[9] This conceptualization stressed the extent to which patients interact with their environment as a means of attempting to manage the stress of illness. These interactions involve appraisals of the current medical condition, with psychological and cultural overlay that varies from patient to patient. While this definition of coping persists to this day, many have argued that though it is a useful paradigm, it is also too broad to allow for standardized assessments in patient populations. Thus, while multiple studies of patient coping exist, most clinicians favor a more open-ended evaluation of each patient, taking into consideration the unique backgrounds that patient and doctor bring to the therapeutic setting.[5] However, research to delineate a more systematic assessment of coping practices is ongoing.[10]

Coping is perhaps best defined as a problem-solving behavior that is intended to bring about relief, reward, quiescence, and equilibrium. Nothing in this definition promises permanent resolution of problems. It does imply a combination of knowing what the problems are and how to go about reaching a correct direction that will help resolution.[1,6,7]

In ordinary language, the term *coping* is used to mean only the outcome of managing a problem, and it overlooks the intermediate process of appraisal, performance, and correction that most problem-solving entails. Coping is not a simple judgment about how some difficulty worked out. It is an extensive, recursive process of self-exploration, self-instruction, self-correction, self-rehearsal, and guidance gathered from outside sources. Indeed, these assertions were central to Lazarus' initial conceptualizations.[9]

CLINICAL AND RESEARCH CHALLENGES

Coping with illness and its ramifications cannot help but be an inescapable part of medical practice. Therefore, the overall purpose of any intervention, physical or psychosocial, is to improve coping with potential problems beyond the limits of illness itself. Such interventions must take into account both the problems to be solved and the individuals most closely affected by the difficulties.

How anyone copes depends on the nature of a problem, as well as on the mental, emotional, physical, and social resources one has available for the coping process. The hospital psychiatrist is in an advantageous position to evaluate how physical illness interferes with the patient's conduct of life and to see how psychosocial issues impede the course of illness and recovery. This is accomplished largely by knowing which psychosocial problems are pertinent, which physical

---

BOX 9-1 Characteristics of Good Copers

- They are optimistic about mastering problems and, despite setbacks, generally maintain a high level of morale.
- They tend to be practical and emphasize immediate problems, issues, and obstacles that must be conquered before even visualizing a remote or ideal resolution.
- They select from a wide range of potential strategies and tactics, and their policy is not to be at a loss for fallback methods. In this respect, they are resourceful.
- They heed various possible outcomes and improve coping by being aware of consequences.
- They are generally flexible and open to suggestions, but they do not give up the final say in decisions.
- They are quite composed, and vigilant in avoiding emotional extremes that could impair judgment.

BOX 9-2 Characteristics of Poor Copers

- They tend to be excessive in self-expectation, rigid in outlook, inflexible in standards, and reluctant to compromise or to ask for help.
- Their opinion of how people should behave is narrow and absolute; they allow little room for tolerance.
- Although prone to firm adherence to preconceptions, bad copers may show unexpected compliance or be suggestible on specious grounds, with little cause.
- They are inclined to excessive denial and elaborate rationalization; in addition, they are unable to focus on salient problems.
- Because they find it difficult to weigh feasible alternatives, bad copers tend to be more passive than usual and fail to initiate action on their own behalf.
- Their rigidity occasionally lapses, and bad copers subject themselves to impulsive judgments or atypical behavior that fails to be effective.

---

symptoms are most distressing, and what interpersonal relations support or undermine coping.

Assessment of how anyone copes, especially in a clinical setting, requires an emphasis on the "here and now." Indeed, this emphasis has been borne out by the growing momentum that practices such as meditation and mindfulness have brought to the therapeutic bedside. Nevertheless, ongoing research is sorely needed to assess best practices in this growing frontier of treatment.[11,12]

More traditional, long-range forays into past history are relevant only if such investigations are likely to shed light and understanding on the present predicament. In fact, increasingly, clinicians are adopting a focused and problem-solving approach to therapy with medically ill patients. For example, supportive and behavioral therapies for medically ill children and adults in both group and individual settings have been found not only to reduce psychiatric morbidity but also to have favorable measurable effects on the course of non-psychiatric illnesses.

Few of us cope exceedingly well all of the time. For all of us, sickness imposes a personal and social burden, with accompanying significant risk and threat appraisal. Furthermore, these reactions are seldom precisely proportional to the actual dangers of the primary disease. Therefore, effective copers may be regarded as individuals with a special skill or with personal traits that enable them to master many difficulties. Characteristics of good copers are presented in Box 9-1. These are collective tendencies; they are highly unlikely to typify any specific individual. No one copes superlatively at all times, especially with problems that impose a risk and might well be overwhelming. Notably, however, effective copers seem able to choose the kind of situation in which they are most likely to prosper. In addition, effective copers often maintain enough confidence to feel resourceful enough to survive intact. Finally, it is our impression that those individuals who cope effectively do not pretend to have knowledge that they do not have; therefore, they feel comfortable turning to experts they trust. The clinical relevance of these characterizations is the extent to which we can assess how patients cope by more accurately pinpointing which traits they seem to lack.

Bad copers are not bad people, nor even incorrigibly ineffective people. In fact, it is too simplistic merely to indicate that bad copers have the opposite characteristics of effective copers. As was stressed earlier, each patient brings a unique set of cultural and psychological attributes to his or her capacity to cope. Bad copers are those who have more problems in coping with unusual, intense, and unexpected difficulties because of a variety of traits. Box 9-2 lists some characteristics of poor copers.

Indeed, structured investigations into the psychiatric symptoms of the medically ill have often yielded many of the attributes of those who do not cope well. Problems (such as demoralization, anhedonia, anxiety, pain, and overwhelming grief) all have been documented in medical patients for whom psychiatric attention was indicated.

The significance of religious or spiritual conviction in the medically ill deserves special mention. Virtually every psychiatrist works with patients as they wrestle with existential issues (such as mortality, fate, justice, and fairness). Such ruminations cannot help but invoke religious considerations in both the patient and the physician; moreover, there is a growing appreciation in the medical literature for the important role that these considerations can play.[13]

In some investigations, being at peace with oneself and with one's sense of a higher power is predictive of both physical and psychiatric recovery.[14,15] However, other studies have suggested that resentment toward God, fears of God's abandonment, and a willingness to invoke Satanic motivation for medical illness were all predictive of worsening health and an increased risk of death.[16]

Inasmuch as the role of the psychiatrist is to identify and to strengthen those attributes that are most likely to aid a patient's physical and emotional well-being, effective therapy for the medically ill involves exploring the religious convictions of patients; fostering those elements is most likely to be helpful. It is *never* the role of the physician to encourage religious conviction *de novo*. At the same time, ignoring religious content risks omitting an important element of the psychotherapeutic armamentarium.

PRACTICAL POINTERS

Coping refers to how a patient responds to, and deals with, problems that relate to *disease, sickness,* and *vulnerability.* In approaching chronically ill patients, it is helpful to conceptualize *disease* as the categorical reason for being sick, *sickness* as the individual style of illness and patienthood, and *vulnerability* as the tendency to be distressed and to develop emotional difficulties in the course of trying to cope.[1]

Given these definitions, the psychiatrist needs first to ask *why now?* What has preceded the request for consultation? How does the patient show his or her sense of futility and despair? How did the present trouble, both medical and the corresponding coping challenges, come about? Was there a time when such problems could have been thwarted? It is also important to note that often the treatment team is even more exasperated than the patient. In these instances, one must guard against the assumption that it is only the patient who is troubled by the medical predicament.

In fact, if there is any doubt about the gap between how the staff and patients differ in their cultural bias and social expectations, listen to the bedside conversation between the patient and all of the clinicians involved in his or her care. Good communication may not only reduce potential problem areas but also help patients to cope better. Good coping is a function of empathic respect between the patient and the doctor regarding the risks and points of tension in the current treatment. The psychiatrist is by no means alone in professional concern about coping, but the unique skills and mandates of psychiatric care are ideally suited to address the vicissitudes of how patients cope. As already mentioned, much of chronic disease evokes existential issues (such as death, permanent disability, low self-esteem, dependence, and alienation). These are fundamentally psychiatric considerations.

Given all of this, it is important to remember that psychiatry does not arbitrarily introduce psychosocial problems. If, for example, a patient is found to have an unspoken but vivid fear of death or is noted to suffer from an unrecognized and unresolved bereavement, fear and grief are already there, not superfluous artifacts of the evaluation procedure. Indeed, open discussion of these existential quandaries is likely to be therapeutic, and active denial of their presence is potentially detrimental, risking empathic failure and the poor compliance that accompanies the course of patients who feel misunderstood or unheard.

Being sick is, of course, much easier for some patients than for others, and for certain patients, it is preferred over trying to make it in the outside world. There is too much anxiety, fear of failure, inadequacy, pathological shyness, expectation, frustration, and social hypochondriasis to make the struggle for holding one's own appealing. At key moments of life, sickness is a solution. Although healthy people are expected to tolerate defeat and to withstand disappointments, others legitimize their low self-esteem by a variety of excuses, denial, self-pity, and symptoms, long after other patients are back to work. Such patients thrive in a complaining atmosphere and even blame their physicians. These are perverse forms of coping.

These complexities substantially complicate the role of the psychiatrist. The clinician must assess the motivation of staff and patients in asking for a psychiatric intervention. For example, the request for psychiatric consultation to treat depression and anxiety in a negativistic and passive-aggressive patient is inevitably more complicated than a simple recognition of certain key psychiatric symptoms. Such patients (through primitive defenses) can generate a profound sense of hopelessness and discomfort in their treaters. It is often an unspoken and unrecognized desire by physicians and ancillary staff that the psychiatrist shifts the focus of negativity and aggression onto himself or herself and away from the remaining treatment team. If the consulting psychiatrist is not aware of these subtleties, the intent of the consultation will be misinterpreted and the psychiatrist's efforts will ultimately fall short.

Every person needs or at least deserves a measure of support, sustenance, security, and self-esteem, even if they are not patients at all, but human beings encountered at a critical time.

In assessing problems and needs, the psychiatrist can help by identifying potential pressure points (e.g., health and well-being, family responsibility, marital and sexual roles, jobs and money, community expectations and approval, religious and cultural demands, self-image and sense of inadequacy, and existential issues) where trouble might arise.

Social support is not a hodgepodge of interventions designed to cheer up or to straighten out difficult patients. Self-image and self-esteem, for example, depend on the sense of confidence generated by various sources of social success and support. In a practical sense, social support reflects what society expects and therefore demands about health and conduct. There is in fact a burgeoning literature that addresses the necessity of support at all levels of care for patients with chronic illness.

Social support is not a "sometime" thing, to be used only for the benefit of those too weak, needy, or troubled to get along by themselves. It requires a deliberate skill, which professionals can cultivate, in order to recognize, refine, and implement what any vulnerable individual needs to feel better and to cope better. In this light, it is not an amorphous exercise in reassurance but a combination of therapeutic gambits opportunistically activated to normalize a patient's attitude and behavior. Techniques of support range from concrete assistance to extended counseling.[17,18] Their aim is to help patients get along without professional support. Social support depends on an acceptable image of the patient, not one that invariably "pathologizes." If a counselor only corrects mistakes or points out what is wrong, bad, or inadequate, insecurity increases and self-esteem inevitably suffers.

Vulnerability is present in all humans, and it shows up at times of crisis, stress, calamity, and threat to well-being and identity.[19-25]

How does a patient visualize threat? What is most feared, say, in approaching a surgical procedure? The diagnosis? Anesthesia? Possible invalidism? Failure, pain, or abandonment by the physician or family?

Coping and vulnerability have a loosely reciprocal relationship in that the better one copes, the less distress he or she experiences as a function of acknowledged vulnerability. In general, a good deal of distress often derives directly from a sense of uncertainty about how well one will cope when called on to do so. This does not mean that those who deny or disavow problems and concerns are superlative copers. The reverse may be true. Courage to cope requires anxiety confronted and dealt with, with an accurate appraisal of how much control the patient has over his or her predicament.

Table 9-1 shows 13 common types of distress. Table 9-2 describes how to find out about salient problems, the strategy used for coping, and the degree of the resolution attained.

Many interventions call on the consulting psychiatrist to ask patients to fill out forms that indicate their degree of anxiety, level of self-esteem, perceived illness, and so on. Although such queries are often sources of valuable information, these standardized inquiries are no substitute for careful and compassionate interviews. There is a strong element of social desirability present in any attempt to assess how a patient copes. How a patient deals with illness may not be the same as how he or she wishes to manage it. Vulnerability, except in extreme forms (such as depression, anger, or anxiety), is difficult to characterize, so the astute clinician must depend on a telling episode or metaphor that typifies a total reaction.

Thus far, we have discussed the following: salient characteristics of effective and less effective copers; methods by which deficits in patients can be identified and how clinicians can intervene; potential pressure points that alert clinicians to different psychosocial difficulties; types of emotional vulnerabilities; and a format for listing different coping strategies, along with questions about resolution.

The **assessment and identification** of ways in which a patient copes or fails to cope with specific problems requires both a description by the patient and an interpretation by the psychiatrist. Even so, this may not be enough. Details of descriptive importance may not be explicit or forthcoming. In

TABLE 9-1 Vulnerability

Hopelessness	Patient believes that all is lost; effort is futile; there is no chance at all; there is a passive surrender to the inevitable
Turmoil/perturbation	Patient is tense, agitated, restless, hyperalert to potential risks (real and imagined)
Frustration	Patient is angry about an inability to progress, recover, or get satisfactory answers or relief
Despondency/depression	Patient is dejected, withdrawn, apathetic, tearful, and often unable to interact verbally
Helplessness/powerlessness	Patient complains of being too weak to struggle anymore; cannot initiate action or make decisions that stick
Anxiety/fear	Patient feels on the edge of dissolution, with dread and specific fears about impending doom and disaster
Exhaustion/apathy	Patient feels too worn out and depleted to care; there is more indifference than sadness
Worthlessness/self-rebuke	Patient feels persistent self-blame and no good; he or she finds numerous causes for weakness, failure, and incompetence
Painful isolation/abandonment	Patient is lonely and feels ignored and alienated from significant others
Denial/avoidance	Patient speaks or acts as if threatening aspects of illness are minimal, almost showing a jolly interpretation of related events, or else a serious disinclination to examine potential problems
Truculence/annoyance	Patient is embittered and not openly angry; feels mistreated, victimized, and duped by forces or people
Repudiation of significant others	Patient rejects or antagonizes significant others, including family, friends, and professional sources of support
Closed time perspective	Patient may show any or all of the these symptoms, but in addition foresees an exceedingly limited future

TABLE 9-2 Coping (To Find Out How a Patient Copes)

Problem	In your opinion, what has been the most difficult for you since your illness started? How has it troubled you?
Strategy	What did you do (or are doing) about the problem?
	Get more information (rational/intellectual approach)
	Talk it over with others to relieve distress (share concern)
	Try to laugh it off; make light of it (reverse affect)
	Put it out of mind; try to forget (suppression/denial)
	Distract yourself by doing other things (displacement/dissipation)
	Take a positive step based on a present understanding (confrontation)
	Accept, but change the meaning to something easier to deal with (redefinition)
	Submit, yield, and surrender to the inevitable (passivity/fatalism)
	Do something, anything, reckless or impractical (acting out)
	Look for feasible alternatives to negotiate (if x, then y)
	Drink, eat, take drugs, and so on, to reduce tension (tension reduction)
	Withdraw, get away, and seek isolation (stimulus reduction)
	Blame someone or something (projection/disowning/externalization)
	Go along with directives from authority figures (compliance)
	Blame self for faults; sacrifice or atone (undoing self-pity)
Resolution	How has it worked out so far?
	Not at all
	Doubtful relief
	Limited relief, but better
	Much better; actual resolution

Adapted from Weisman AD. The realization of death: a guide for the psychological autopsy, Jason Aronson, 1974, New York.

these situations, the clinician must take pains to elucidate the specifics of each situation. If not, the result is only a soft approximation that generalizes where it should be precise. Indeed, the clinician should ask again and again about a topic that is unclear and re-phrase, without yielding to clichés and general impressions.

Psychiatrists have been imbued with the values of so-called empathy and intuition. Although immediate insights and inferences can be pleasing to the examiner, sometimes these conclusions can be misleading and totally wrong. It is far more empathic to respect each patient's individuality and unique slant on the world by making sure that the examiner accurately describes in detail how problems are confronted. To draw a quick inference without being sure about a highly private state of mind is distinctly unempathic. Like most individuals, patients give themselves the benefit of the doubt and claim to resolve problems in a socially desirable and potentially effective way. It takes little experience to realize that disavowal of any problem through pleasant distortions is itself a coping strategy, not necessarily an accurate description of how one coped.

Patients who adamantly deny any difficulty tend to cope poorly. Sick patients have difficult lives, and the denial of adversity usually represents a relatively primitive defense that leaves such patients unprepared to accurately assess their options. Carefully timed and empathic discussion with patients of a genuine appraisal for their current condition can help them to avoid this maladaptive approach and to address their treatment more effectively.

On the other hand, patients may attempt to disavow any role in their current illness. By seeking credit for having suffered so much, such patients reject any implication that they might have prevented, deflected, or corrected what has befallen them (see Table 9-2). Helping these patients does not necessarily require that they acknowledge their role in their particular predicament. Instead, the empathic listener identifies and provides comfort around the implicit fear that these patients harbor (i.e., that they somehow deserve their debilitation).

Suppression, isolation, and projection are common defenses. Effective copers seem to pinpoint problems clearly, whereas poor copers seem only to seek relief from further questions without attempting anything suggesting reflective analysis.

In learning how anyone copes, a measure of authentic skepticism is always appropriate, especially when it is combined with a willingness to correct later on. The key is to focus on points of ambiguity, anxiety, and ambivalence while tactfully preserving a patient's self-esteem. A tactful examiner might say, for example, "I'm really not clear about what exactly bothered you, and what you really did. ..."

The purpose of focusing is to avoid premature formulations that gloss over points of ambiguity. An overly rigid format in approaching any evaluation risks overlooking individual tactics that deny, avoid, dissemble, and blame others for difficulties. Patients, too, can be rigid, discouraging alliance, rebuffing collaboration, and preventing an effective physician–patient relationship.

Coping with illness is only one special area of human behavior. It is important to recognize that in evaluating how patients cope, examiners should learn their own coping styles and, in effect, learn from patients. Clearly, it is not enough to mean well, to have a warm heart, or to have a head filled with scientific information. Coping well requires open-ended communication and self-awareness. No technique for coping is applicable to one and all. In fact, the concept of technique may be antithetical to true understanding. A false objectivity obstructs appraisal; an exaggerated subjectivity only confuses what is being said about whom.

Psychiatrists and patients can become better copers by cultivating the characteristics of effective copers. Coping is, after all, a skill that is useful in a variety of situations, although many modifications of basic principles are called for. Confidence in being able to cope can be enhanced only through repeated attempts at self-appraisal, self-instruction, and self-correction. Coping well with illness—with any problem—does not predict invariable success, but it does provide a foundation for becoming a better coper.

Access a list of MCQs for this chapter at https://expertconsult .inkling.com

REFERENCES

1. Schlozman SC, Groves JE, Weisman AD. Coping with illness and psychotherapy of the medically ill. In: Stern TA, Fricchione GL, Cassem NH, editors: *Massachusetts General Hospital handbook of general hospital psychiatry*, ed 5, Philadelphia, 2004, Mosby.
2. Williams CM, Wilson CC, Olsen CH. Dying, death, and medical education: student voices. *J Palliative Med* 8(2):372–381, 2005.
3. Gordon GH. Care not cure: dialogues at the transition. *Patient Educ Couns* 50(1):95–98, 2003.
4. Orbach I, Mikulincer M, Sirota P, et al. Mental pain: a multidimensional operationalization and definition. *Suicide Life Threat Behav* 33(3):219–230, 2003.
5. Coyne JC, Gottlieb BH. The mismeasure of coping by checklist. *J Pers* 64(4):959–991, 1996.
6. Morling B, Evered S. Secondary control reviewed and defined. *Psychol Bull* 132(2):269–296, 2006.
7. Koch EJ, Shepperd JA. Is self-complexity linked to better coping? A review of the literature. *J Pers* 72(4):727–760, 2004.
8. Vamos M. Psychotherapy in the medically ill: a commentary. *Aust N Z J Psychiatry* 40(4):295–309, 2006.
9. Lazarus RS. *Psychological stress and the coping process*, New York, 1966, McGraw-Hill.
10. Kato T. Development of the Coping Flexibility Scale: evidence for the coping flexibility hypothesis. *J Couns Psychol* 59(2):262–267, 2012.
11. Arias AJ, Steinberg K, Banga A, et al. Systematic review of the efficacy of meditation techniques as treatments for medical illness. *J Altern Complement Med* 12(8):817–832, 2006.
12. Morone NE, Greco CM. Mind-body interventions for chronic pain in older adults: a structured review. *Pain Med* 8(4):359–375, 2007.
13. Gijsberts MJ, Echteld MA, van der Steen JT, et al. Spirituality at the end of life: conceptualization of measurable aspects—a systematic review. *J Palliat Med* 14(7):852–863, 2011.
14. Laubmeier KK, Zakowski SG, Bair JP. The role of spirituality in the psychological adjustment to cancer: a test of the transactional model of stress and coping. *Int J Behav Med* 11(1):48–55, 2004.
15. Pargament KI, Koenig HG, Tarakeshwar N, et al. Religious struggle as a predictor of mortality among medically ill patients: a 2-year longitudinal study. *Arch Intern Med* 161:1881–1885, 2001.
16. Clarke DM, Mackinnon AJ, Smith GC, et al. Dimensions of psychopathology in the medically ill: a latent trait analysis. *Psychosomatics* 41:418–425, 2000.
17. Stauffer MH. A long-term psychotherapy group for children with chronic medical illness. *Bull Menninger Clin* 62:15–32, 1998.
18. Saravay SM. Psychiatric interventions in the medically ill: outcomes and effectiveness research. *Psychiatr Clin North Am* 19:467–480, 1996.
19. Bird B. *Talking with patients*, ed 2, Philadelphia, 1973, JB Lippincott.
20. Coelho G, Hamburg D, Adams J, editors: *Coping and adaptation*, New York, 1974, Basic Books.
21. Jackson E. *Coping with crises in your life*, New York, 1974, Hawthorn Books.
22. Kessler R, Price R, Wortman C. Social factors in psychopathology: stress, social support, and coping processes. *Annu Rev Psychol* 36:531–572, 1985.
23. Moos R, editor: *Human adaptation: coping with life crises*, Lexington, MA, 1976, DC Heath.
24. Murphy L, Moriarity A. *Vulnerability, coping and growth*, New Haven, CT, 1976, Yale University Press.
25. Weisman A. *The coping capacity: on the nature of being mortal*, New York, 1984, Human Sciences.

10 An Overview of the Psychotherapies

Robert S. Abernethy III, MD, and Steven C. Schlozman, MD

KEY POINTS

- Research evidence supports the effectiveness of most psychotherapies.
- Psychotherapy training during residency includes competency in five basic psychotherapies.
- Child and adolescent psychotherapy includes more integrative strategies than does adult psychotherapy.
- All psychotherapies will require greater accountability under proposed accountable care plans.

BACKGROUND

Clinicians half-jokingly assert that the number of psychotherapies in existence might exceed the number of psychotherapists in practice. Each session, even of manual-driven psychotherapies, is unique. Many factors (e.g., patient characteristics, patient preferences, therapist's training, therapist's theoretical perspective, time in therapist's career, insurance or funds available for therapy, time available for therapy) determine how the therapist and the patient proceed.

Much psychotherapeutic activity can occur during a 20-minute psychopharmacological follow-up appointment or during the brief chat between a psychiatrist and a patient before electroconvulsive therapy (ECT), or during a visit to an empathic primary care physician (PCP). However, in this chapter, we define *psychotherapy* as the beneficial process that is embedded in the verbal interaction between a professional psychotherapist and a patient or patients.

The kinds of psychotherapy described in the literature probably number in the hundreds.[1] This overview will focus (somewhat arbitrarily) on 10 common types of psychotherapy for adults based on theory, technique, length, and patient mix. A section on psychotherapy for children and adolescents follows.

PSYCHODYNAMIC PSYCHOTHERAPY

Psychodynamic psychotherapy has the longest organized tradition of the psychotherapies. It is also known as psychoanalytic psychotherapy or expressive psychotherapy.[2] This psychotherapy can be brief or time-limited, but it is usually open-ended and long-term. Sessions are generally held once or twice per week, with the patient being encouraged to talk about "whatever comes to mind." This encouragement has been termed the *fundamental rule of psychotherapy*. The therapist, consequently, is usually non-directive but may encourage the patient to focus on feelings about "whatever comes to mind." The therapist is empathic, attentive, inquiring, non-judgmental, and more passive than in other kinds of psychotherapies. The goal of psychodynamic psychotherapy is to recognize, interpret, and work through unconscious feelings that are problematic. Often unconscious feelings are first recognized in transference phenomena. Many psychodynamic psychotherapists choose to ignore positive transference phenomena, but interpret negative phenomena. For example, the patient may express the wish to be the therapist's friend. The focus would be on the patient's disappointment and

frustration that a friendship cannot occur rather than a focus on the depth of the patient's longing for a friendship with the therapist. The psychotherapist deliberately avoids answering most questions directly or revealing personal information about himself or herself. This strategy, referred to as the *abstinent posture*, promotes the emergence of transference phenomena. The abstinent posture leaves a social void that the patient fills with his or her imagination and projections, allowing the therapist access to the patient's unconscious. The patient will get in touch with intense feelings that have been suppressed or repressed. Catharsis is the "letting go" and expression of these feelings.

At least six major theoretical systems exist under the psychodynamic model; these are summarized in Box 10-1.[3-7] Psychoanalysis is an intensive form of psychodynamic psychotherapy; several of its characteristics are summarized in Box 10-2. The time and financial cost of psychoanalysis generally put it out of range for many patients. To date, there is no persuasive evidence that psychoanalysis is more effective than psychodynamic psychotherapy. However, there is emerging evidence that psychodynamic psychotherapy is effective for a number of diagnoses.[8,9]

COGNITIVE-BEHAVIORAL THERAPY

Cognitive-behavioural therapy (CBT) is emerging as a widely-practiced psychotherapy for depression, anxiety disorders, and other psychiatric and medical diagnoses. CBT represents a merger of the pioneering work of Aaron Beck[10] (who first developed cognitive therapy for depression in the mid-1960s) and the work of Joseph Wolpe[11] (who, in 1958, described a behavior therapy, reciprocal inhibition, for anxiety disorders).

CBT is built on the assumption that conscious thoughts, feelings, and behaviors interact to create symptoms.[12] In contrast to the psychodynamic model, unconscious inner conflicts and early relationships are considered less important than here-and-now conscious awareness of thoughts, feelings, and behaviors. The therapeutic sessions are structured and collaborative. The therapist defines the goals and methodology of therapy and teaches the patient to observe the interaction of feelings, thoughts, and behaviors. Commonly used cognitive-behavioral techniques are summarized in Box 10-3. There is considerable research supporting the effectiveness of CBT for a number of disorders.[13]

SUPPORTIVE PSYCHOTHERAPY

Supportive psychotherapy has been included in the five core competencies of psychotherapy training. This "user-friendly" psychotherapy has rarely been formally taught in residency or in psychology training programs. In the heyday of psychoanalysis and psychoanalytic psychotherapy during the mid- to late-twentieth century, advice, suggestion, and encouragement were generally considered unhelpful for most patients with emotional problems. Nevertheless, Wallerstein,[14] reporting on the results of the extensive Menninger Clinic and Foundation Study of Psychoanalysis and Psychotherapy, stated that supportive psychotherapy was often as effective as psychoanalysis at relieving symptoms and achieving enduring structural change.

Supportive psychotherapy is often defined by what it is not. It does not involve analysis of the transference; it does not involve challenging defenses; it does not endeavor to change the structure of personality or character; it does not involve making the unconscious, conscious. Supportive psychotherapy is often indicated to help a patient survive a loss or to get beyond a stressful event. This therapy can be brief but often it is long term. For example, a widow may initially benefit from weekly supportive psychotherapy after the loss of her spouse. After painful grief symptoms have improved, she may see the therapist monthly for an indefinite period for maintenance supportive psychotherapy.

Supportive psychotherapy provides a safe place for the patient to express feelings, to problem-solve, and to reinforce

---

BOX 10-1 Major Theoretical Systems in the Psychodynamic Model

CLASSICAL OR STRUCTURAL THEORY

This is best represented by Sigmund Freud. Development involves oral, anal, phallic, and oedipal stages. There are dual instincts: libido and aggression. Structural theory refers to the interactions of id, ego, and superego.

EGO PSYCHOLOGY

This is best represented by Anna Freud[3]; it focuses on understanding ego defenses in order to achieve a more conflict-free ego functioning.

OBJECT RELATIONS THEORY

This is best represented by Melanie Klein[4]; it focuses on the schizoid, paranoid, and depressive positions and the tension between the true self and the false self.

SELF-PSYCHOLOGICAL THEORY

This is best represented by Heinz Kohut[5]; it addresses deficits of the self and disintegration of the self. The two self-object transference phenomena, mirroring and idealization, promote integration and are generally not interpreted.

TRANSPERSONAL PSYCHOLOGY

This is best represented by Carl Jung[6]; it focuses on archetypal phenomena from the collective unconscious.

RELATIONAL THEORY

This is best represented by Jean Baker Miller[7]; it focuses on the real relationship between patient and therapist to understand and relieve conflict and social inhibition and achieve social intimacy.

BOX 10-2 Characteristics of Psychoanalysis

- The therapist is trained in psychoanalysis at a psychoanalytic institute and has had his or her own psychoanalysis.
- The patient comes to analysis three to five times a week and usually lies on a couch; traditionally, the therapist is seated out of the patient's view.
- Transference phenomena are the focus of the analysis. The analyst's abstinent posture is considered an important catalyst for the development of transference phenomena.
- Psychoanalysis usually takes 3 or more years.
- Many psychodynamic psychotherapists seek out psychoanalysis for in-depth insight into their own unconscious.

BOX 10-3 Commonly Used Cognitive-Behavioral Techniques

PROBLEM-SOLVING

A straightforward consideration of options for the patient to solve a real-life here-and-now problem he or she is facing. Often this technique allows the therapist to help the patient recognize and correct distorted thinking.

GRADED-TASK ASSIGNMENTS

The depressed patient is encouraged to "get going" with modest tasks at first (e.g., getting out of bed and getting dressed).

ACTIVITY MONITORING AND SCHEDULING

The patient keeps a log of activities that help the therapist adjust graded-task assignments and activity scheduling.

PSYCHOEDUCATION

This involves teaching patients about their diagnoses and about how the therapy will help, what the therapist's responsibilities are, and what patients' responsibilities are for the therapy to be successful.

GIVING CREDIT

Patients are taught to give themselves credit for even modest accomplishments in order to begin to relieve the global negativism so common with depression.

FUNCTIONAL COMPARISONS OF THE SELF

Helping patients to recognize how they are improving rather than comparing themselves to others who are not depressed.

DYSFUNCTIONAL THOUGHT RECORD

Patients are taught the common cognitive distortions and encouraged to record their own examples. Common cognitive distortions include "all-or-nothing" thinking; catastrophizing; disqualifying or discounting the positive; emotional reasoning; labeling; magnification or minimization; mental filter; mind reading;

overgeneralization; personalization; "should, have to, ought to, and must" statements; and tunnel vision. Patients are encouraged to record the date and time, the situation, the automatic thought, the emotion, an alternative response, and the outcome.

COPING CARDS

The therapist helps the patient write cards that each contain a common cognitive distortion and challenges or corrections for each distortion. The patient is encouraged to read the cards often.

RELAXATION TRAINING

The patient is taught a method of relaxing (e.g., Benson's relaxation response).

ASSERTIVENESS TRAINING

The patient is taught the importance of appropriately expressing feelings, opinions, and wishes. The patient may be given a homework assignment to be assertive in an anticipated situation. The technique of "broken record" involves repeating exactly an assertion when the assertion is challenged.

RESPONSE PREVENTION

The therapist helps the patient recognize behaviors that reinforce or contribute to his or her problem (e.g., succumbing to the temptation to just get back in bed during a depressing morning).

GUIDED IMAGERY AND ROLE-PLAY

The patient is taught how to use his or her imagination to feel better. The therapist may practice with the patient taking the role of the person with whom the patient anticipates being assertive.

BIOLOGICAL INTERVENTIONS

These might include prescribing medication, reducing or stopping alcohol or coffee intake, and encouraging exercise.

BOX 10-4 Techniques Involved in the Practice of Supportive Therapy

- The therapist often makes suggestions and gives advice and responds to questions with appropriate answers.
- Transference phenomena are generally neither addressed nor interpreted. However, if negative transference threatens the therapeutic alliance, it may be addressed.
- The therapist can use clarification and confrontation but generally does not use interpretation.
- The therapist is generally active and may enhance the patient's self-esteem by direct measures (such as praise or encouragement).
- The therapist tries to allay any anxiety generated by the therapy itself.
- The therapist keeps the therapy focused in a constructive direction rather than encouraging the patient to say whatever comes to mind.
- The therapist presents himself or herself as a real person willing to direct the therapy and willing to describe how the therapy will work and what the therapist's role will be.

BOX 10-5 Criteria for Selection for Brief Psychotherapy

- **Duration**: Problems of long duration are less likely to respond to brief psychotherapy.
- **Interpersonal history**: If the patient has a history of poor interpersonal relationships, the trusting productive alliance needed for brief therapy may not occur.
- **Severity and Complexity of the patient's problem**: Is the problem too severe or complex to respond to brief psychotherapy?
- **Understanding of the problem**: Can the patient learn to understand the problem, and is the patient motivated to change?
- **Social support**: Are there supports in the patient's life that can sustain and enhance the benefits of the brief therapy?

adaptive defenses. Evidence continues to support the use of supportive psychotherapy even for challenges as complex as child and adolescent depression.[15] Techniques involved in the practice of supportive therapy are summarized in Box 10-4.

Hellerstein and colleagues[16] suggested that supportive psychotherapy be the default psychotherapy. This "user-friendly" therapy neither generates anxiety nor requires a weekly commitment for an undetermined period of time as with expressive psychodynamic psychotherapy. Research has found supportive psychotherapy to be efficacious. Hellerstein and associates[16] proposed a trial of this therapy before the more extensive, more anxiety-provoking expressive psychodynamic psychotherapy.

Several studies of psychotherapy research have found that supportive psychotherapy is effective for a variety of psychiatric diagnoses; Winston and colleagues[17] have comprehensively reviewed this literature. However, more research is needed to better understand how to integrate supportive psychotherapy with psychopharmacology and with other psychotherapy techniques for specific diagnoses.

BRIEF PSYCHOTHERAPY

Although Olfson and Pincus[18] found that the average length of psychotherapy is probably only eight visits, most of these "brief" psychotherapies represent the patient's unilateral decision to discontinue treatment. Paradoxically, Sledge and colleagues[19] found that if a brief therapy is planned with the patient, twice as many patients continue to the agreed-on endpoint than if no endpoint is agreed on. In other words, having an agreed-on limit to the number of visits reduces the dropout rate by half. Nevertheless, there is growing evidence that designated brief therapies may ultimately require longer periods of treatment.[20,21]

Brief psychotherapy is therefore defined as a psychotherapy with a pre-determined endpoint, usually 8 to 12 visits. The theory and technique of brief psychotherapy parallels the established psychotherapy "camps." Sifneos,[22] Malan,[23] Davanloo,[24] and others describe time-limited psychodynamic psychotherapy. Beck and Greenberg[25] have described time-limited cognitive therapy. Klerman's Interpersonal Psychotherapy (IPT)[26] is a time-limited therapy that focuses on here-and-now interpersonal relationships. Budman[27] described an eclectic or integrative psychotherapy that includes interpersonal, developmental, and existential issues. Hembree and co-workers[28] described a brief behavioral therapy, which includes stress inoculation training and exposure therapy.

Steenbarger[29] presented considerations for selection criteria for brief psychotherapy. These considerations form the acronym DISCUS and are presented in Box 10-5.

Perhaps the most important feature of brief psychotherapy is the activity required of the therapist. The therapist is active in the initial assessment of the patient; active in establishing, early on, the goal of the therapy and the contract for a limited number of sessions; active in keeping the therapy focused on the goals; and active in assigning homework.

There is some controversy concerning the termination of brief psychotherapy. At one extreme, Mann[30] advocated a complete termination in order to have the patient confront existentially the meaningful end of the therapy. Mann precluded contact with the patient after termination. At the other extreme is the transition of a weekly 12-session IPT into an indefinite monthly maintenance IPT. Blais and Groves[31] prescribed a re-contact after 6 months. Finally, one needs to keep in mind the possible need for longer treatments. Dogma should never trump patient need.

Research evidence for the effectiveness of brief psychotherapy is extensive.[32,33] Brief psychotherapy has been designated by the Psychiatry Residency Review Committee (RRC) as one of the five psychotherapies to be included in psychotherapy core competencies. This inclusion, plus mounting pressure from insurers to limit the length of psychotherapy, should lead to more brief psychotherapy. It is also likely that many patients, if given the option, would prefer a time-limited treatment with clear, discrete goals and an active therapist.

PSYCHIATRIC MEDICATION WITH PSYCHOTHERAPY

A patient receiving both psychotherapy and medication becomes part of a complex and multi-faceted phenomenon.[34] There are two possible approaches to mixing psychopharmacology and psychotherapy: the psychiatrist does both the psychotherapy and psychopharmacology, or the psychiatrist does the psychopharmacology and someone else does the psychotherapy. The former is referred to as integrative treatment, the latter, split treatment. There is virtually no research on whether integrative or split treatment is better for a certain diagnosis or a certain patient. However, there is some research to demonstrate that combining psychopharmacology and psychotherapy is more effective for certain diagnoses than either alone.[35] There is also some evidence that it is less expensive for a psychiatrist to provide both the psychopharmacology and the psychotherapy.[36] However, the exploration of both the benefits and challenges to this mode of treatment are ongoing. This may be more important as we move towards an accountable care system of health care delivery.[37]

The prevalence of split treatment in the United States is significantly greater than is integrative treatment for a number of reasons. First, there is a significant economic incentive for psychiatrists to do psychopharmacology exclusively, either if insurance is used or if patients self-pay. Second, many PCPs refer patients who need psychotherapy to non-medical therapists. The PCP continues to medicate the patient and a split treatment is established. A third possible reason that split treatment prevails is that recent graduates from psychiatric residency training programs may feel less competent to do psychotherapy than do residents who graduated decades earlier.

There are advantages and disadvantages to integrated care. As mentioned, research has found that integrated care is less expensive for some diagnoses. This finding may be explained by the fact that fewer visits are required with only one practitioner or that medication may be appropriately started sooner if the therapist can also prescribe. Another advantage is the efficiency if all pharmacological and psychosocial issues are known and managed by one clinician (i.e., no time is needed to communicate with another professional). The pitfalls of integrated care include the time pressure to address both psychosocial and pharmacological issues in one visit, as well as the unwitting overemphasis of one modality over the other by the psychotherapist-psychiatrist. For example, a maladaptive response to countertransference issues raised by the patient's feelings may be to focus more on medicating the feelings than on listening to, and understanding, them.

Split treatment also has advantages and disadvantages. In split treatment, the clinician can focus exclusively on his or her specific expertise. The psychotherapist does not have to re-consider dosages and side effects, and the psychopharmacologist can defer psychosocial issues to the psychotherapist. The pitfalls of split treatment are also significant. The ideal of regular communication between psychotherapist and pharmacotherapist is often hard to accomplish. The shared electronic medical record can accomplish some efficient and constructive communication, but live verbal communication can often capture important nuances that visit notes may not. Another pitfall of split treatment is the expense in terms of time and money. Some insurers will not pay for a psychotherapy visit and a psychopharmacology visit on the same day. So, if both psychotherapist and psychopharmacologist are in the same practice setting, the patient has to come in on separate days. Countertransference can also be a pitfall of split treatments. When the patient is failing, each clinician might unwittingly blame the other clinician and the other modality. Good communication and collaboration between clinicians engenders trust and respect, which will benefit the failing patient.

Another pitfall of split treatment is the fact that emergency management or hospitalization often becomes the responsibility of the psychopharmacologist, who sees the patient less frequently and is less aware of psychosocial factors. Better communication and collaboration between clinicians greatly enhances the effectiveness of the psychopharmacologist's emergency interventions.

A final pitfall of split treatment is that if a bad outcome to the psychotherapy leads to litigation, the psychopharmacologist is almost always included. This cautionary note argues for the psychopharmacologist to know the psychotherapists with whom he or she is collaborating well.

There are important considerations in the sequencing of psychotherapy and pharmacotherapy. For example, Otto and colleagues[38] found that adding CBT for a patient with a good response to benzodiazepines for panic disorder improves the success of a subsequent benzodiazepine taper. Marks and co-workers[39] found that adding a benzodiazepine early in exposure psychotherapy for phobias diminishes the effectiveness of the psychotherapy, presumably by muting the appropriate anxiety provided by graduated exposure.

Although combined medication and psychotherapy are frequently prescribed for many diagnoses, there is little evidence that the combination is more effective than either alone. Psychotherapy alone has been shown to be effective for major depression, dysthymia, obsessive-compulsive disorder (OCD), social phobia, generalized anxiety disorder (GAD), bulimia, and primary insomnia. Combined treatment may be helpful for patients in a real-life clinical setting that may be more complicated than "clean" patients suitable for randomized clinical trials (RCTs). For bipolar disorder and for schizophrenia, psychotherapy alone is contraindicated. Therefore, combined treatment for these diagnoses is standard.

INTERPERSONAL PSYCHOTHERAPY

Interpersonal psychotherapy (IPT) was developed and described by Klerman and co-workers[26] in the late 1970s. IPT is a brief therapy that is manual driven and is generally accomplished in 12 to 16 sessions. IPT was inspired by the interpersonal focus of Adolph Meyer and Harry Stack Sullivan and the attachment theory of John Bowlby. In IPT, the therapist is active and the sessions are somewhat structured. Homework is commonly encouraged by the therapy and, on occasion, a significant other may join the patient for a session. After an assessment phase, IPT includes a contract with the patient to meet for a specific number of sessions, as well as an explicit description of what the therapeutic sessions will involve and how the theoretical underpinnings of IPT relate to the goals and strategies of the therapy. IPT does not focus on transference phenomena or the unconscious. In the evaluation phase, the therapist addresses four possible interpersonal problem areas: grief or loss, interpersonal disputes, role transitions, and interpersonal deficits. One or two relevant problem areas are identified that become the focus of the therapy.

IPT has several primary goals: the reduction of depressive symptoms, the improvement of self-esteem, and the development of more effective strategies for dealing with interpersonal relationships. Having identified one or two of the four possible problem areas, the therapist proceeds with six therapy techniques described by Hirschfeld and Shea[40] (usually in order and presented in Box 10-6).

BOX 10-6 Techniques of Interpersonal Therapy

- **Exploratory techniques** to collect information about the patient's problems and symptoms
- **Encouragement of affect**, which involves helping the patient recognize, accept, and express painful feelings and to use the feelings positively in interpersonal relationships
- **Clarification**, which may involve restructuring the patient's communications
- **Communication analysis**, which involves identifying maladaptive communication patterns to help the patient communicate more effectively
- **Use of the therapeutic relationship** to examine the patient's feelings and behavior as a model of interactions in other relationships
- **Behavior-change techniques** that may involve role-playing and suggestions from the therapist for new ways of dealing with important others

A number of well-designed studies have demonstrated the effectiveness of IPT. Perhaps the largest and most often cited is the NIMH treatment of depression collaborative study by Elkin and co-workers.[41] An often-cited variant of the therapy is maintenance IPT, first described by Frank and co-workers[42] at the University of Pittsburgh. Maintenance IPT involves monthly sessions and endeavors to decrease relapse of depression after acute intensive treatment with weekly IPT or antidepressant medication.

The Pittsburgh group found that IPT was more effective than placebo and as effective as imipramine or cognitive therapy for mild to moderate depression. Maintenance IPT has also been found to decrease the relapse rate for recurrent depression,[43] but maintenance medication should accompany maintenance IPT for recurrent depression.[44]

Research also supports the use of IPT for variants of depression (such as adolescent depression, geriatric depression, dysthymia, and peri-natal depression). Two reviews of IPT research have been presented by Weissman and colleagues[45] and Stuart and Robertson.[46] The Pittsburgh group[47] has also studied a variant of IPT with social rhythm therapy for patients with bipolar disorder.

DIALECTICAL BEHAVIOR THERAPY

In the late 1980s, Marsha Linehan[48,49] at the University of Washington in Seattle developed dialectical behavior therapy (DBT) for the treatment of borderline personality disorder. DBT is a structured individual and group treatment that has four goals: mindfulness, interpersonal effectiveness, emotional regulation, and distress tolerance. These four goals are considered skills that are taught in carefully structured sessions with a skills training manual and handouts for each session. Mindfulness is the capacity to stop and to take note of thoughts and feelings. At the beginning of each session, the patients are presented with a mindfulness exercise that lasts a few minutes and encourages focus and concentration on the present, a momentary letting go of worldly cares and concerns, similar to a brief meditation or relaxation exercise. Interpersonal effectiveness describes the skill of managing relationships. For example, learning how to balance demands with priorities, learning appropriately and effectively to say no, and learning appropriately and effectively how to ask for help. Emotional regulation describes the skill of decreasing vulnerability to negative emotions and learning how to increase positive emotions. Distress tolerance is the skill of reducing the impact of painful events and emotions. Patients are taught methods of distraction and self-soothing, as well as the skill of "improving the moment."

Linehan and her fellow teachers of DBT have refused to train solo professionals. Two or more are trained together to establish a program that includes weekly staff meetings. Because borderlines are difficult to treat and manage, the required weekly meeting of staff allows for regular staff support and peer supervision regardless of the years of experience of the staff. Each weekly staff meeting begins with a mindfulness exercise.

Research comparing DBT with treatment-as-usual in the community has found four significant advantages of DBT: better treatment adherence; better quality of relationships in the patient's life; fewer self-injurious acts, such as cutting or overdoses; and fewer days in the hospital.[50] Fortunately, health insurers are beginning to fund DBT, recognizing not only the health benefits but also the benefits in terms of medical economics. In Linehan's initial research, the DBT-treated borderlines had an average of 8 days of hospitalization for the year of follow-up versus an average of 38 days of hospitalization for borderlines treated "as usual," creating a significant economic advantage for the insurer.[50]

Linehan has used the Hegelian philosophical label *dialectical* to emphasize three views of reality that are embedded in the therapy: individual parts of a system need to be related to the whole; reality is not static but always changing in response to *thesis* and *antithesis;* and the nature of reality is change and process rather than content or structure.

Partly in response to the success of DBT, a group at Cornell (Clarkin and colleagues[51]) developed a manual-driven, individual transference-focused psychotherapy for borderline personality disorder that is showing promise. DBT has also been found to be effective for women with opioid dependency.[52]

GROUP THERAPY

Group therapy is defined in this chapter as a group experience led by one or two trained professionals. Groups (e.g., Alcoholics Anonymous [AA], Overeaters Anonymous [OA], Narcotics Anonymous [NA], and Adult Children of Alcoholics [ACOA]) without a designated or trained professional leader can be highly therapeutic. Although these groups have time-tested theoretical underpinnings, we will not include the self-help group in our outline of group psychotherapies.

There are many classifications of group therapy.[53] Patients may share a common diagnosis (such as breast cancer) or a common experience (such as being a homeless Katrina victim). Groups can be open (e.g., new members may be added as others terminate) or a group may be closed (e.g., all members begin at the same time and the group terminates at one time). Open groups may continue indefinitely, and closed groups may be defined (e.g., as in a 20-session experience).

There are two common so-called boundary rules in most groups. First, all revelations in the group are considered confidential. Second, many group therapists discourage or disallow social contact between members outside of the group meetings. Exceptions to this rule might be inpatient groups on a psychiatry service.[54]

Therapy groups (e.g., DBT groups or smoking cessation groups) may have a significant psychoeducational component. Therapy groups differ in terms of theory and technique.

Psychodynamic group therapy focuses primarily on the unconscious determinants of relationships among members (e.g., group members who are in conflict or group members who are always supportive and in agreement with one another) in the group process. The group therapist may focus on unconscious phenomena of the group as a whole or may focus on a conflict between two members. Generally, in a psychodynamic group, the therapist is often silent, non-directive, and observant, which encourages the group to find a direction for itself.

Expressive, supportive, or experiential groups offer members an opportunity to share feelings around a common experience or diagnosis (e.g., a bereavement group, or patients with breast cancer). The group leader provides a focus for addressing the common experience.

Cognitive-behavioral group therapy usually provides a structured therapy for a common diagnosis (e.g., all members may have depression or all members may have post-traumatic stress disorder [PTSD]). Cognitive and behavioral principles related to the diagnosis are taught to the group. The group members do homework and report back on progress. Members learn from each other's experiences and provide each other support.

There are some classic group phenomena that might occur in any kind of group. Bion[55] described three common resistances to group work: dependency—when the group persistently looks to the therapist or one group member for direction; fight–flight—tensions arise between two or more members and then those members or others threaten to leave the group; and pairing—two members of the group dominate the conversation to the exclusion of the others or in the service of other group members too uncomfortable to get involved.

Therapy groups often have transference phenomena at work either between a patient and the therapist or between a patient and another patient. These phenomena can occur in any therapy group regardless of theoretical focus. These phenomena can be either disruptive or illuminating, but should be recognized and managed by the group therapist.

There is considerable evidence that short-term focused groups are effective,[56,57] but more research needs to be done to identify techniques or patient characteristics that promote success.

COUPLES THERAPY

Couples therapy is defined as a psychotherapy that includes both members of an established partnership. Much literature refers to marital therapy, but many couples that seek treatment are not married. The term *couples therapy* therefore includes gay partnerships, as well as heterosexual couples who choose not to be married or are not yet married. *Conjoint therapy* is another term for couples therapy.

The history of couples therapy dates back to, at least, the 1930s with so-called atheoretical marriage counseling and psychoanalytic-focused marital therapy developing independently.[58] The early psychoanalytic approach addressed the individual neurotic issues of the two patients but generally did not focus on their interaction.

In the early 1960s, family therapy began to emerge and incorporated couples therapy in its theories and techniques. In the mid-1980s, couples therapy became a discipline separate from family therapy.

There are many types of couples therapy based on different theories and techniques. Five of the most widely published and practiced therapies are presented in Box 10-7.[59–64]

There is considerable research evidence supporting the effectiveness of most of the types of couples therapies described previously.[65] Behavior marital therapy has been studied the most, especially the brief marital therapies that involve 12 to 20 sessions. Gurman,[66] in reviewing this research, found that approximately two-thirds of treated couples have a positive outcome.

Unfortunately, many clinicians who do couples therapy assume that extensive training and experience in individual therapy are adequate credentials. A cautionary quote from Prochaska[67] is, "Most therapists are about as poorly prepared for marital therapy as most spouses are for marriage."

With the high divorce rate in the United States, couples therapy will continue to have an important preventive role.

INTEGRATIVE PSYCHOTHERAPY

The tenth and final adult psychotherapy reviewed here may be the most widely practiced.[68,69] Behind the closed and confidential doors of psychotherapy offices, it is likely that psychodynamically-focused therapists occasionally use CBT or family systems techniques. Similarly, cognitive-behavioral therapists may address transference phenomena embedded in resistance to cognitive-behavioral exercises and homework. In spite of the prevalence of integrative thinking and strategies, integrative psychotherapy did not make the final list of core competencies for psychiatric residency training. An important reason for this is the prevailing opinion of psychotherapy educators that students should learn the theories and

techniques separately. This training assumption often indirectly implies that the student-therapist needs to choose one theory and technique and to focus his or her professional development in that one direction. Ultimately, many clinicians out in practice begin the process of integration, but usually well after the structured training years and well beyond supervisory oversight.

The history of psychotherapy integration may go back to the 1932 meeting of the American Psychiatric Association when Thomas French[70] presented a paper that attempted to reconcile Freud and Pavlov. In spite of this early attempt, psychoanalytic and behavioral theory and practice have persistently diverged during the subsequent 75 years. In the mid-1970s, two clinician-teachers first described integrative approaches: Paul Wachtel[71] in 1977 published *Psychoanalysis and Behavior Therapy: Toward an Integration,* and Arnold Lazarus[72] in 1976 published *Multimodal Behavior Therapy.*

BOX 10-7 Types of Couples Therapy

- **The transgenerational approaches** focus on the relationship between one's role in family of origin and the current couple difficulty. This includes Bowen's Family Systems Therapy,[59] which addresses fusion, triangulation, emotional "stuck-togetherness," and the process of family projection. The transgenerational approach also includes Object-Relations Family Therapy, described by Skynner,[60] which endeavors to get the projections in the marriage back into the individual selves. The couple with difficulty is seen as a mutual projective system.

- **The structural-strategic approach** includes Salvador Minuchin's technique[61] and Jay Haley's Mental Research Institute (MRI) Brief Strategic Therapy[62] (created in Palo Alto, where Haley and others developed the strategic method). The structural-strategic approach sees the family as a system that can be best understood by how it addresses current here-and-now issues. Problems in the family system often represent a developmental impasse in the life of the marriage. Therapist-inspired directives often help the couple get unstuck. Paradoxical directives may also be used. The therapist looks for ways to understand how the marriage is stuck—rather than how it is sick.

- **The experiential humanistic approaches** include the Satir model, named after Virginia Satir,[63] and emotionally-focused couples therapy, described by Susan Johnson.[64] These methods focus on the narrow roles that individuals play in the relationship, such as victim, blamer, placator, and rescuer. The therapist tries to help the patient get out of a persistent narrow role by encouraging connective emotional experiences in the here-and-now.

- **Behavioral approaches** use cognitive and behavioral principles to solve problems in the marriage. Behaviors that are labeled "bad" are re-examined for reinforcements in the relationship. Cognitive restructuring can occur and can relieve marital tension.

- **Postmodern couples therapy** includes solution-focused and narrative techniques. These therapies emphasize the here-and-now and embrace the fundamental assumption that problematic reality is constructed in the marriage rather than discovered. Therefore, emphasis is placed on how the couple can get out of this problem, rather than on how the couple got into the problem. In narrative couples therapy, the couple addresses their respective stories or narratives and focuses often on power and gender issues reflected in culture at large.

In 1983, a group of academic psychologists and psychiatrists formed the Society for the Exploration of Psychotherapy Integration (SEPI), which has brought together psychotherapists from all schools to seek enrichment of psychotherapy through integration. There is also now the *Journal of Psychotherapy Integration*.

An important controversy in psychotherapy integration relates to whether a comprehensive integrated theory of psychotherapy should be developed. Lazarus and Messer[73] have debated this important issue. Lazarus proposed an atheoretical technical eclecticism unique for each patient, whereas Messer proposed a theory-rich assimilative integration.

Multi-modal psychotherapy, described by Lazarus,[74] is perhaps the most widely known integrative method. Lazarus, as reflected in the debate with Messer, assumed that patients and their problems are unique and too complex to fit neatly into one theory or technique. Therefore, each patient deserves a unique integrative approach. He uses the acronym BASIC ID to promote an integrative assessment and treatment approach:

- Behavior
- Affect
- Sensation
- Imaging
- Cognitions
- Interpersonal
- Drugs—biological.

Whatever works for each unique patient should be used.

Research into integrative psychotherapy is in its infancy.[75] Because integrative psychotherapy is not manual-driven, good research would require a naturalistic focus, which has not yet been done. From their extensive analysis of RCTs in psychotherapy research, Weston and colleagues[76] concluded that in the real world of clinical practice, specific techniques demonstrated to be effective in RCTs need to be integrated into a unique approach to each complex patient.

INNOVATIVE DIRECTIONS OF PSYCHOTHERAPY RESEARCH

Although most research in psychotherapy has focused, and will continue to focus, on the demonstration of effectiveness, there are some important and innovative efforts to understand other aspects of psychotherapy. Roffman and colleagues[77] reviewed early evidence of functional neuroimaging changes with psychotherapy. Marci and Riess[78] described the use of neurophysiological measures to recognize empathic success and failure between therapist and patient. Ablon and Jones[79] described the use of the PQS, a unique measure of process in psychotherapy, to determine psychodynamic versus cognitive process in therapy sessions.

CHILD AND ADOLESCENT PSYCHOTHERAPY

As with adult psychotherapy, there are a number of different modalities by which child and adolescent psychotherapy can be practiced. However, it is likely that within child and adolescent therapy there exist even more integrative practices than in adult treatment. Therefore, in any discussion of the various modalities of psychotherapy with young people, one needs to keep in mind the fact that many of these modalities are present in all treatment endeavors.[80,81]

Also, just as with the treatment of adults, all interactions between a clinician and a child or an adolescent involve some form of psychotherapeutic action. Issues (such as patient and family compliance, patient improvement, and better communication between patient and clinician) all hinge on the realization that child–clinician interactions follow certain key

therapeutic principles that are very much part of the psychotherapeutic tradition. Attention to these issues has great bearing on the treatment of all children in virtually all settings.[82]

This section will discuss many of the same treatment modalities that have already been covered for adults. However, there are important differences among these modalities with regard to child and adolescent treatment, and these differences will therefore be stressed. To best understand these differences, a brief discussion of child and adolescent development is necessary.

Emotional, Cognitive, and Neurodevelopmental Issues for Children and Adolescents

In many ways, current neurodevelopmental research validates the empirical observations that pioneers in development (such as Erikson and Piaget) noted more than 50 years ago. Thus, at least a cursory understanding of these developmental principles is necessary to pursue psychotherapy with young people. Although a comprehensive review of their theories is beyond the scope of this chapter, it is important to note that whereas Erikson primarily discussed emotional development, Piaget focused on cognitive development.

Erik Erikson observed that humans at all stages of the life cycle progress through a series of developmental crises. These crises are often discussed as a dichotomous choice between options that will either allow the individual to either move forward developmentally, or, conversely, get "stuck", or even regress developmentally. For example, Erikson argued that the fundamental crisis for infants was one of "trust versus mistrust." In other words, infants need to learn that they can trust their world to keep them safe and healthy, and in the absence of this experience, they will not be able to manage the inherent anxiety that is naturally part of later developmental stages, such as the challenges of "initiative versus guilt," the developmental crisis that Erikson postulated characterized school-age children. Erikson called his theory the "epigenetic model," and he characterized the stages of development from infancy through adulthood (see Table 5-1 in Chapter 5).

Piaget focused instead on cognitive changes throughout the life cycle. He noted, for example, that toddlers are prone to what developmentalists call "associative logic." One idea leads to another through association rather than causality. A toddler might say, "Plates are round because the moon is full." Additionally, toddlers are prone to egocentricity (the idea that all events in the world are related to, and even caused by, their actions) and magical thinking. As children age, they progress through a concrete, rule-bound stage of thinking, ideal for learning new tools (such as reading) and for making sense of school-age games. Finally, as children enter adolescence, they become capable of abstract reasoning and recursive thinking. Abstract reasoning is necessary so that children can make sense of the more complicated concepts that they can tackle after mastering tools (such as reading), and recursive thinking allows children to imagine what others might think even if they themselves do not agree. Piaget defined a set of stages of cognitive development (see Table 5-1 in Chapter 5).

Importantly, current neurodevelopmental research shows some fascinating correlates with the theories of Erikson and Piaget, and these correlates play a large role in directing the most appropriate psychotherapeutic intervention. Briefly, as children age, their brains undergo neuronal migration and the frequency with which certain neuropathways are used changes. Younger children are more prone to tantrums and to frustration because their brains do not enjoy the same executive function for problem-solving as do older adolescents. Older adolescents use their higher cortical functions more often in solving problems, but in hotly affective settings will invoke more limbic input in making decisions. Importantly, adolescents are much more susceptible to "limbic override" in difficult situations than are adults. Current neurobiological research suggests that this is a function of under-developed executive function pathways. Therefore, one can conceptualize psychotherapy with children as playing to the neurodevelopmental strengths of the particular child.

All of this is extremely important to child therapy, because the therapist must have in mind where a child ought to be developmentally, and at the same time make an assessment of where the child currently resides along the developmental spectrum. The primary goal of any intervention with children and adolescents is to ensure that the developmental trajectory is maintained.

Child and Adolescent Psychodynamic Psychotherapy

Because the developmental trajectory is so steep during the first 18 years of life, therapists must meet young people where they live along this trajectory. For this reason, much of psychotherapy with children involves "play," and with adolescents involves the capacity to be "playful." The subject of play is what separates adult and child psychodynamic treatments.

This idea of play within therapy is somewhat controversial.[83] Critics stress that the lack of well-validated measures of treatment with dynamic therapy are even more present when examining play therapy. However, there is in fact mounting evidence for the efficacy for these techniques.[82] The most vociferous critics have described play therapy as "absurd in the light of common sense."[83] However, many clinicians feel strongly that play therapy is essential to the psychotherapeutic relationship between clinician and child, and theorists such as Anna Freud and D. W. Winnicott wrote a great deal about these ideas.[84,85] Proponents of play therapy stress that younger people make sense of their internal thoughts and feelings by expressing these ideas in their play.[84] Thus, if psychodynamic therapy is defined as helping the patient to work through unconscious conflicts, these conflicts are most easily elucidated through careful attention to the content of the child's play. For adults, the therapist encourages the patient to discuss "whatever is on his mind." For the child, the most open-ended form of therapy involves inviting the child to "play" with the clinician in a non-directed way, thus allowing for the same unconscious feelings to emerge that one uncovers in dynamic therapy with adults through talking.

While play itself is the crux of dynamic therapy with younger patients, as children age, they become less comfortable with overt play and instead move toward a more playful approach to emerging ideas. The increase in sarcasm and sexual innuendo that characterizes adolescent behavior reflects this tendency. Thus, the maintenance of alliance and the uncovering of uncomfortable and conflicted feelings with adolescents often involves a willingness to engage in playful banter that is in turn rich in psychological meaning. Additionally, the attention that adolescents pay to popular culture can be seen as an attempt to experiment with different ways of thinking about the world in the relative safety of displacement. To this end, the therapist can welcome references to popular culture as the means by which children and adolescents can displace their ideas into a more acceptable and distanced narrative.[86,87] In the end, the goals of psychodynamic therapy for adults and children are the same. However, the tools by which one arrives at these goals must correlate with the developmental strengths and capacities of the patient.

MANUAL-DRIVEN THERAPIES AND BEHAVIORAL THERAPIES

As already discussed, there are growing number of manual-driven psychotherapies that are used for both adults and children. These include CBT, IPT, and DBT. These treatments have in common clearly defined procedures with manual-documented instructions. Given these constants, these therapies have enjoyed much greater evidence of efficacy in RCTs, though this is not the same as saying that other, harder-to-study treatments are less effective.

As with adults, CBT has been used very successfully in children and adolescents for anxiety disorders, especially OCD.[88-92] Problems, such as school-refusal and depression, have also been found to respond to CBT,[89,93] and IPT has been efficacious with depression among adolescents.[94-96] There is some question, however, as to the effectiveness of IPT for suicidality in younger populations.[97]

Although borderline personality disorder is not usually diagnosed in children before age 18, there are adolescents who engage in borderline defensive structures (such as splitting, all-or-nothing thinking, and affective lability) for which DBT has been found useful.[98,99] Importantly, one might argue that all of these modalities will work best by understanding the child's developmental plight using techniques, such as humor and connection, and, as all of these therapies require a substantial commitment by the patient, none of these techniques will be effective if the child does not want to pursue treatment.

Contingency management is a form of behavioral therapy that is based on clearly defined behavioral goals, rewards for meeting these goals, and consequences for falling short of these goals.[100,101] While incentives based on rewards and consequences are potentially fundamental in parenting, enacting these criteria in a psychotherapeutic setting is tricky and works best with a strong alliance and firm "buy-in" from both patient and family. Management of impulse-related disorders (such as attention-deficit/hyperactivity disorder [ADHD]) often involves some form of contingency management.

Biofeedback is another form of behavioral therapy that involves teaching children relaxation techniques using real-time technological measurements of autonomic arousal. This form of treatment has been very effective in children and adolescents for problems such as chronic pain, as well as for severe anxiety. Because children are increasingly enamored of technology, the use of real-time measurements of variables (such as heart rate or skin conductance) often provides a special treat for children who would otherwise be recalcitrant to treatment.[102]

SYSTEMS-BASED CARE

All patients exist within complex social and environmental systems. However, the multiple environmental changes that characterize the childhood mandate that the therapist be involved with the child's world; this maximizes the therapeutic impact of the work. The most basic of these interventions involves family therapy and parent guidance.

Parent guidance is the process by which the clinician helps parents to effectively guide, connect with, and, ultimately, parent their children. This therapy requires the clinician's understanding of development, as well as the child's unique set of circumstances and the parents' particular strengths and challenges. Psychodynamic and behavioral techniques are key to this endeavor.[103,104]

Similarly, *family therapy* requires that the clinician understand the dynamics of the family itself and the role of the patient within the family system. Family therapy is discussed elsewhere in this volume, but one should note that treatment of children and adolescents often involves multiple visits with the family even in the absence of a defined family psychotherapy. In fact, all individual treatments with children necessitate some kind of parental involvement.

Similarly, group interventions are often very useful for children and adolescents who might experience social difficulties and feel uncomfortable explicating these difficulties in individual treatment. Children will often tell each other how best to handle a difficult situation, and the universality of the group experience is frequently comforting and beneficial to the child.[105] However, child dynamics can also make the group experience frightening and off-putting in the absence of a good group leader. To this end, the regression that often takes place in all forms of group therapy is perhaps especially present in child and adolescent group treatment. The clinician must be vigilant for this regression, and intervene by interpreting the regression in the context of the group process.

Finally, it is common for therapists to contact schools, camps, and other agencies where their patients might spend their time. Sometimes the most subtle office-based intervention with a child will not be nearly as effective as helping a school, for example, to better understand and appreciate the child in that particular setting. A potentially major difference between child treatment and adult psychotherapy involves this active participation in the child's external environment.

CONCLUSION

As this chapter has stressed, some forms of therapy are substantially better supported by empirically driven evidence than are others. However, this is not to say that the lack of evidence suggests an overall lack of efficacy for less-validated treatment techniques. Among the mainstream forms of psychotherapy, the constant that links all of them is the presence of trust, a solid alliance, and a sense of empathy within the caregiver. Some researchers have even suggested that these qualities are the best predictors of therapeutic success regardless of treatment modalities. To this end, all therapies must strive for connection and non-judgmental understanding. These characteristics are, in fact, the very qualities that make psychotherapy both effective and rewarding for the patient and clinician alike.

 Access the complete reference list and multiple choice questions (MCQs) online at https://expertconsult.inkling.com

KEY REFERENCES

3. Freud A. *The ego and the mechanisms of defense*, New York, 1936, International Universities Press.
8. Fonagy P, Roth A, Higgitt A. Psychodynamic psychotherapies: evidence-based practice and clinical wisdom. *Bull Menninger Clin* 69(1):1–58, 2005.
9. Leichsenring F, Hiller W, Weissberg M, et al. Cognitive-behavioral therapy and psychodynamic psychotherapy: techniques, efficacy, and indications. *Am J Psychother* 60(3):233–259, 2006.
15. Cheung AH, Kozloff N, Sacks D. Pediatric depression: an evidence-based update on treatment interventions. *Curr Psychiatry Rep* 15(8):381, 2013.
16. Hellerstein DJ, Pinsker H, Rosenthal RN, et al. Supportive therapy as the treatment model of choice. *J Psychother Practice Res* 3:300–306, 1994.

17. Winston A, Pinsker H, McCullough L. A review of supportive psychotherapy. *Hosp Comm Psychiatry* 37:1105–1114, 1986.
20. Winter SE, Barber JP. Should treatment for depression be based more on patient preference? *Patient Prefer Adherence* 9(7):1047–1057, 2013.
21. Driessen E, Van HL, Don FJ, et al. The efficacy of cognitive-behavioral therapy and psychodynamic therapy in the outpatient treatment of major depression: a randomized clinical trial. *Am J Psychiatry* 170(9):1041–1050, 2013.
24. Davanloo H. *Short-term dynamic psychotherapy*, New York, 1980, Jason Aronson.
25. Beck AT, Greenberg RL. Brief cognitive therapies. *Psychiatr Clin North Am* 2:23–37, 1979.
26. Klerman GL, Weissman MM, Rounsaville BJ, et al. *Interpersonal therapy of depression*, New York, 1984, Basic Books.
31. Blais M, Groves JE. Planned brief psychotherapy: an overview. In Stern TA, Herman JB, editors: *Psychiatry: update and board preparation*, New York, 2000, McGraw-Hill.
32. Koss MP, Shiang J. Research on brief psychotherapy. In Bergin AE, Garfield SL, editors: *Handbook of psychotherapy and behavior change*, ed 4, New York, 1994, Wiley.
36. Goldman W, McCulloch J, Cuffel B, et al. Outpatient utilization patterns of integrated and split psychotherapy and pharmacotherapy for depression. *Psychiatric Services* 49(4):477–482, 1998.
37. Meyers D. Split treatment: Coming of age. In Robert I, Hales RE, editors: *The American Psychiatric Publishing textbook of suicide assessment and management*, ed 2, Arlington, VA, 2012, American Psychiatric Publishing, Inc., pp 263–279.
40. Hirschfeld RMA, Shea MT. Mood disorders: psychosocial treatments. In Kaplan HI, Sadock BJ, editors: *Comprehensive textbook of psychiatry*, vol. 1, ed 5, New York, 1989, Williams & Wilkins.
44. Kupfer DJ, Frank E, Perel JM. Five year outcomes for maintenance therapies in recurrent depression. *Arch Gen Psychiatry* 49:769–773, 1992.
45. Weissman MM, Markowitz JW, Klerman GL. *Comprehensive guide to interpersonal psychotherapy*, New York, 2000, Basic Books.
46. Stuart S, Robinson M. *Interpersonal psychotherapy: a clinician's guide*, London, 2003, Edward Arnold.
48. Linehan MM. *Cognitive behavioral treatment of borderline personality disorder*, New York, 1993, Guilford Press.
49. Linehan MM. *Skills training manual for treating borderline personality disorder*, New York, 1993, Guilford Press.
53. Yalom ID. *The theory and practice of group psychotherapy*, New York, 2005, Basic Books.
56. Fuhrman A, Burlingame GM. Group psychotherapy research and practice. In Fuhrman A, Burlingame GM, editors: *Handbook of group psychotherapy*, New York, 1994, Wiley.
65. Baucom DH, Shoham V, Meuser KT, et al. Empirically supported couple and family interventions for marital distress and adult mental health problems. *J Consult Clin Psychol* 66:53–88, 1998.
66. Gurman AS. Marital therapies. In Gurman AS, Messer SB, editors: *Essential psychotherapies*, New York, 2005, Guilford Press.
89. Compton SN, March JS, Brent D, et al. Cognitive-behavioral psychotherapy for anxiety and depressive disorders in children and adolescents: an evidence-based medicine review. *J Am Acad Child Adolesc Psychiatry* 43(8):930–959, 2004.
92. Practice parameters for the assessment and treatment of children and adolescents with obsessive-compulsive disorder. AACAP. *J Am Acad Child Adolesc Psychiatry* 37(10 Suppl.):27S–45S, 1998.
98. 2004 APA Gold Award: using dialectical behavior therapy to help troubled adolescents return safely to their families and communities. The Grove Street Adolescent Residence of The Bridge of Central Massachusetts, Inc. *Psychiatric Services* 55(10):1168–1170, 2004.

11 Brief Psychotherapy: An Overview

James E. Groves, MD, Mark A. Blais, PsyD, and John B. Taylor, MD, MBA

KEY POINTS

- Short-term therapies typically last 12 to 36 sessions and focus on a single problem or symptom (called the focus or sector) by actively excluding less pivotal issues.

- Brief therapies differ from each other in how the focus is chosen and approached, how the therapist–patient relationship is leveraged, and whether the field of action is intrapsychic or interpersonal.

- Interpersonal psychotherapy (IPT) avoids intrapsychic interpretations and has a reputation for being the most versatile, supportive, and least invasive of the methods.

- The four main types of short-term therapy are psychodynamic, cognitive-behavioral (including dialectical behavioral [DBT]), interpersonal, and eclectic.

- Eclectic brief psychotherapy combines features of the other three and starts from the precipitating event to define a focus; it works on strengthening defenses, managing affects and addictions, and building relationship skills.

OVERVIEW

Despite the notion that psychotherapy is a long-term endeavor, most data indicate that as it is practiced in the real world it has a short course. Therefore, it is usually a "brief therapy" even if its duration is not specified as such at the outset of the treatment. Well before the nationwide impact of managed care was felt, studies consistently showed that outpatient psychotherapy typically lasted between 6 and 10 sessions. Data on national outpatient psychotherapy utilization obtained in 1987—early in the takeover of managed care—showed that 70% of psychotherapy users received 10 or fewer sessions. Only 15% of this large sample had 21 or more visits.[1]

Managed care, which increasingly dictated how psychiatrists were to be reimbursed for their care, became hostile toward open-ended psychodynamic treatments that, at the time, had little evidence on which to base their worth. Insurers pushed psychiatry to use shorter treatments that decreased the amount of physician–patient contact. A reliance on pharmacotherapy and the "med check" appointment grew from this. A confluence of factors, including an increasing evidence base, easy manualization, and restrictions placed by managed care have also led to reliance on brief, time-limited psychotherapies. Research has proven the relative efficacy of these therapies. A 2011 meta-analysis of 38 studies examining the use of interpersonal therapy (IPT) for treatment of unipolar depression confirmed its efficacy both with and without concurrent pharmacotherapy.[2]

While the literature showing the efficacy of cognitive-behavioral therapy (CBT), IPT, and other forms of brief psychotherapy is vast, the data demonstrating that its efficacy translates into cost-effectiveness is smaller but growing. A study of 707 subjects examined both the efficacy and cost-effectiveness of sertraline, IPT, and sertraline plus IPT in treating dysthymia.[3]

Two years after treatment, the two groups who received sertraline had similar clinical improvement—both of which were greater than the group that received IPT alone—but the group that received combined treatment cost, on average over two years, $480 less per person. Another study[4] examined the use of intensive short-term dynamic psychotherapy modeled from Davanloo's techniques in treating personality-disordered patients. In addition to finding the therapy effective the study estimated that, because of symptom improvement, the cost over 2 years would have amounted to a third of that of treatment-as-usual. Among patients identified as high-utilizers of health care, those enrolled in an 8-week treatment of psychodynamic-IPT showed significant reductions in health care costs for the 6 months following the psychotherapy, in comparison to those receiving treatment-as-usual.[5]

In contrast, several studies[6,7] found that brief psychotherapies were not cost-effective in comparison with treatment-as-usual. Lave and colleagues[8] found IPT to be only slightly less effective and slightly more expensive than nortriptyline in the treatment of major depression.

Because psychiatric treatment is not a one-size-fits-all endeavor, brief psychotherapies will always have their place when creating treatment plans. And, because *planned* brief psychotherapy is time-limited, its continued reimbursement by insurers is likely. However, it requires significant activation energy and time commitment from patients, as well as more manpower and upfront cost than simple psychopharmacology visits. As reductions in health care costs have become a stated goal of numerous entities—insurers, hospitals, state and federal governments—brief psychotherapy may be increasingly mandated to help control costs for high-utilizing patients, many of whom have psychiatric illness with immense medical co-morbidity. Further studies demonstrating that a reasonable initial cost will lead to significant downstream reductions in health care spending are needed.

This overview of brief psychotherapy will first focus on specific "schools" of short-term treatments. Then the "essence" of most brief treatments will be distilled: *brevity, selectivity, focus,* and specific therapist *activity*.

HISTORY OF BRIEF PSYCHOTHERAPY

Toward the end of the nineteenth century, when Breuer and Freud invented psychoanalysis, hysterical symptoms defined the focus of the work. These early treatments were brief, the therapist was active, and, basically, desperate patients selected themselves for the fledgling venture. In time, free association, exploration of the transference, and dream analysis replaced hypnosis and direct suggestion. So, as psychoanalysis evolved, the duration of treatment increased and therapist activity decreased.

Alexander's (1971) manipulation of the interval and spacing of sessions (the therapeutic "frame") explored the impact of decreased frequency, irregular spacing, therapeutic holidays, and therapist-dictated (rather than patient- or symptom-dictated) treatment schedules. All these frame changes enhanced the external reality orientation of psychotherapy. Then World War II produced large numbers of patients who needed treatment for "shell shock" and "battle fatigue." Grinker and Spiegel's (1944) treatment of soldiers ensconced *brevity* in the treatment armamentarium. Lindemann's (1944) work with survivors of the Cocoanut Grove fire—with its *focus* on grief work—also occurred during this period.

The modern era started in the 1960s when Sifneos and Malan independently developed the first theoretically coherent, short-term psychotherapies. The increased activity of Ferenczi and Rank, Lindemann's crisis work, Grinker and Spiegel's push for brevity, Alexander and French's flexible framework, and Balint's finding and holding the focus were all technical innovations, but none constituted a whole new method. Malan and Sifneos each invented ways of working that were not a grab bag of techniques but each a whole new therapy, with a coherent body of theory out of which grew an organized, specified way of proceeding.[9,10]

Over time, as therapies became briefer, they became more focused and the therapist became more active. But brevity, focus, and therapist activity are ways in which short-term therapies differ, not only from long-term therapy but also typically from one another. Patient selection makes up a fourth "essence" in the description of the short-term psychotherapies. Table 11-1 shows brevity, selectivity, focus, and therapist activity as the organizing principles for the therapies summarized in the columns below each "essence."

MODERN BRIEF PSYCHOTHERAPIES

There are four general schools of brief psychotherapy:

(1) Psychodynamic.
(2) Cognitive-behavioral.
(3) Interpersonal.
(4) Eclectic.

Each has indications and contraindications,[11-13] but it is worth acknowledging at the outset that there is no conclusive evidence that any one short-term psychotherapy is more efficacious than another.[14-17] IPT avoids intrapsychic interpretations and has a reputation for being the most versatile, supportive, and least invasive of the methods.[18] But in practice, purity of technique gets lost and most real-life therapies probably drift toward the eclectic mode.

Psychodynamic Short-term Therapies

The "interpretive" short-term therapies all feature brevity, a narrow focus, and careful patient selection, but the common feature is the nature of the therapist's activity. Psychoanalytic interpretation of defenses and appearance of unconscious conflicts in the transference appear in other short-term therapies (and are often downplayed), but only in these methods are interpretation and insight the leading edge of the method and, as in psychoanalysis, the main "curative" agents.

Sifneos's anxiety-provoking therapy (1972, 1992) is an ideal example of a brief psychodynamic psychotherapy. This treatment runs 12 to 20 sessions and focuses narrowly on issues (such as the failure to grieve, fear of success, or "triangular," futile love relationships). The therapist serves as a detached, didactic figure who holds to the focus and who challenges the patient to relinquish both dependency and intellectualization, while confronting anxiety-producing conflicts. One can think of this method as a classical oedipal-level defense analysis with all of the lull periods removed. One limiting feature is that it serves only 2%–10% of the population, the subgroup able to tolerate its unremitting anxiety without acting-out.

An illustrative contrast, Sifneos's anxiety-*suppressive* therapy, serves less healthy patients who are able to hold a job and to recognize the psychological nature of their illness, but who are unable to tolerate the anxiety of deeper levels of psychotherapy. Anxiety-provoking psychotherapy is longer, less crisis-oriented, and aimed at the production of anxiety—which then is used as a lever to get to transference material. (In psychoanalysis, transference emerges, but in short-term therapy it sometimes is elicited.)

Malan's method[19,20] is similar, but the therapist discerns and holds the focus without explicitly defining it for the patient. (In the initial trial, if the therapist has in mind the correct focus, there will be a deepening of affect and an increase in associations as the therapist tests it.) A unique feature of this treatment is that Malan sets a date to stop once the goal is in sight and the patient demonstrates the capacity to work on his or her own. A fixed date (rather than the customary set number of sessions) avoids the chore of keeping track if acting-out causes missed sessions or scheduling errors.

Malan's work is reminiscent of the British object-relations school. Like Sifneos, he sees interpretation as curative, but he aims less at defenses than at the objects they relate to. In other words, the therapist will call attention to behavior toward the therapist, but rather than asking what affect is being warded off, Malan wants to know more about the original object in the nuclear conflict who set up the transference in the first place. Malan's later work converges toward that of Davanloo's,[15,21,22] so that his and Malan's approaches are conceptually similar.

Davanloo's method can appear dramatically different from all others in terms of therapist activity. The therapist's relentless, graduated, calculated clarification, pressure, and challenge elicit the anger used to dig out the transference from behind "superego resistance." Davanloo begins by criticizing the patient's passivity, withdrawal, or vagueness, while pointing out the body language and facial expressions demonstrating them. Patients who do not decompensate or withdraw are then offered a trial interpretation: the patient's need to fail and clumsiness in the interview disguise aggression toward the therapist; the patient's need to become "a cripple," to be "amputated" and "doomed," disguises rage.

The therapist works with a "triangle of conflict"—which goes from examination of defenses to labeling affect, to impulse or behavior, in relation to the "triangle of persons." This persons triangle begins with a problematic current object, one mentioned in the first half of the initial interview. Then investigation moves to the therapist, who the patient has just been protecting from anger, and then to the parent who taught such patterns in the first place. One or two circuits around the "conflict triangle" in relation to three points of the "persons triangle" constitute the "trial therapy." This is a more elaborate version of the trial interpretations Malan and Sifneos use to test motivation and psychological-mindedness. Davanloo's patients lack the ability to distinguish between points in the "conflict [Defense/Affect/Impulse] triangle" or to experience negative affects directly. By trolling the D/A/I triangle around the "persons [Current object/Therapist/Parent] triangle," Davanloo forces the frigid patient to feel and creates a mastery experience for the patient.

These are non-psychotic, non-addicted, non-organic individuals who have a combination of retroflexed aggression and punitive superegos, but at the same time, enough observing ego to discount the apparent harshness. His patients find the seemingly harsh Davanloo method supportive; up to 35% of an average clinic's population are said to tolerate it, a range broader than either Sifneos or Malan claimed. Failures of the Davanloo "trial therapy" typically are referred to cognitive therapy.

The dynamic-existential method of James Mann[23,24] relied on a strict limit of exactly 12 sessions. Time is not just a reality, and a part of the framework, but time is an actual *tool* of treatment. Twelve sessions, which Mann chose somewhat arbitrarily, is sufficient time to do important work but short enough

TABLE 11-1 "Essences" of the Short-Term Therapies

Short-term Therapies	Brief (No. of Sessions)	Selective	Focused	Therapist Is	Active
Sifneos (anxiety provoking; analytic)	12–20	Very rigid standards: "top 2%–10% of clinic" population,* oedipal conflict, or grief; motivation essential; psychological-mindedness tested by trial interpretation	Very narrow: oedipal conflict, grief, unconscious level, transference	Teacher	Interprets transference, resistance Idealizing transference becomes ambivalent transference
Malan (analytic)	20–30 Fixed date*	Similar to Sifneos: healthy but some character pathology; able to work analytically; responds to trial interpretation with deepened affect and increased associations if focus is correct	Narrow, implicit (therapist finds it), unconscious, similar to Sifneos (anxiety-provoking)	Doctor	Similar to Sifneos; "insight" held to be curative
Davanloo (analytic)	1–40 (ca. 25)	Less healthy than Sifneos group: "top 30%–35%"—some long-standing phobic, obsessional, or masochistic personalities but must respond to "trial therapy" first session	Broader, but similar to Malan and Sifneos, plus resistance and retroflexed anger	Critic*	Confrontive of resistance, especially around anger, DAI (conflict), and CTP (persons) triangles
Mann (existential)	Exactly 12, no more, no less*	Broader patient selection, but usually not borderline; some ego strengths, especially passive-dependent patients and delayed adolescents	Broader focus (time itself*) and "central issue," termination; affective state	Empathic helper	Therapist, by being with patient through separation, helps in mastering developmental stage at which parents failed patient
Cognitive	1–14 acutely; additional 24 if chronic	Not psychotic; in crisis; coped previously; not cognitively impaired or borderline	Conscious "automatic thoughts"	Coach or director*	Therapist helps define governing slogans, refutes them, assigns homework,* mandates practice of new cognitions and behaviors
Behavioral	12–36, but highly variable	Not manic, actively psychotic, actively suicidal, or actively drug-abusing	Behaviors* in the present (e.g., of OCD); trauma symptoms (e.g., anxiety), phobias (specific and social)	Coach or doctor sometimes with site visit*	Exposure, systematic desensitization, imaging, relaxation (breathing, self-talk)
Interpersonal	12–16	Depressed patients at any level of health, with grief or interpersonal deficits and conflicts causing maladaptation or depression	Interpersonal field, not intrapsychic mechanisms	Coach or doctor (usually manual driven)	Defines interpersonal disputes, role transitions; helps reshape interpersonal behaviors*
Eclectic	Horowitz: 12 Budman: 20–40 variable spacing,* re-up option Leibovich: 36–52	Various levels of health (except organic and psychotic conditions), but progress relates to level of health	Interpersonal + cognitive Precipitating event interpersonal + developmental + existential One problematic borderline trait:* for example, low frustration tolerance	Counselor Doctor Real person	Combine all the above strategies, especially interventions aimed at shoring up defenses, repairing stress response damage

*Unique feature.

to put the patient under pressure. This set number with no reprieve is both enough time and too little. It thrusts the patient and the therapist up against the existential reality they both tend to deny: time is running out.

No other short-term therapy seems to require so much of the therapist. And even if this method does not appeal to all short-term therapists, almost every subsequent theorist in the field seems to have been influenced by Mann to some degree—even Budman and Gurman,[25] whose use of time appears so unlike Mann's. It is described somewhat in detail here because the interaction of therapist activity with phases of treatment is so clearly highlighted.

Underlying the focus the patient brings, Mann posits a "central issue" (analogous to a core conflict) in relation to the all-important issue, "time itself." The therapist is a timekeeper who existentially stays with the patient through separations, helping master the developmental stages in which parents failed the patient. Mann's theoretical point of departure (which probably *followed* the empirical finding that 12 sessions was about right) is Winnicott's[26] notion that time sense is intimately connected to reality-testing, a "capacity for concern," and unimpaired object relationships. A better sense of time and its limits is the soil for growing a better sense of objects.

During evaluation, the therapist begins to think about the "central issue" (such as problems with separation, unresolved grief, or failure to move from one developmental stage to another—delayed adolescence especially). This central issue is couched not in terms of drive or defense, but existentially, in terms of the patient's chronic suffering. If the patient is moved by this clarification, the therapist solicits the patient's agreement to work for a total of 12 sessions. The patient will at this point express some disbelief that 12 sessions is enough. But if the evaluation has been accurate and the method is suited to this patient, the therapist should look the patient in the eye and say that 12 sessions—and only 12—will be just enough.

The early sessions are marked by an outpouring of data and by the formation of a positive or idealizing transference. During this phase the therapist's job is to hold the focus on the central issue and allow the development of a sense of perfection. At about the fourth session, there is often an appearance of disillusionment and the return of a focus on symptoms. At this point the therapist makes the first interpretation that the patient is trying to avoid seeing that time is limited and avoiding feelings about separation. This sequence is repeated, and it deepens through the middle of therapy.

After the mid-point, session 6, overt resistance often occurs, perhaps lateness or absence on the part of the patient, and the emergence of negative transference. The therapist examines this in an empathic and welcoming way while inwardly examining countertransference issues that may impede the work. And finally, in the latter sessions comes a working through of the patient's pessimism and recollection of unconscious memories and previous bad separation events, along with an expectation of a repetition of the past. By the therapist's honest acceptance of the patient's anger and ambivalence over termination, the patient moves from a state of neurotic fear of separation and its attendant depression to a point where the patient is ambivalent, sad, autonomous, and realistically optimistic.

Cognitive-Behavioral Brief Therapies

The behavioral therapies have a decades-long history and a good record of achievement. The cognitive therapies are the inheritors of this earlier track record. What the two have in common is that neither addresses "root causes" of disorders of mental life, but focus almost exclusively on the patient's outward manifestations. These "non-psychological" or "non–insight oriented" styles of therapy are broadly applicable, both in terms of patients and problems. (For the cognitive-behavioral therapies, see Chapter 16.)

The method of Aaron Beck[27-29] aims at bringing the patient's "automatic" (pre-conscious) thoughts into awareness and demonstrating how these thoughts affect behavior and feelings. The basic thrust is to challenge them consciously, and to practice new behaviors that change the picture of the world and the self in it. Beck says that an individual's interpretation of events in the world is encapsulated in these fleeting thoughts, which are often cognitions at the fringes of consciousness. These "automatic thoughts" mediate between an event and the affective and behavioral response. The patient labors under a set of slogans that, by their labeling function, ossify the worldview and inhibit experimenting with new behaviors.

The therapist actively schedules the patient's day-to-day activity, and the patient is asked to list in some detail actual daily activities and to rate the degree of "mastery" and "pleasure" in each. These allow the therapist to review the week with the patient and to sculpt behaviors. Cognitive rehearsals are also used to help the patient foresee obstacles in the coming week. The therapist repeatedly explains the major premise of the cognitive model, that an intermediating slogan lies between an event and the emotional reaction. This slogan may take a verbal or pictorial form. The therapist then, using Socratic questioning, elicits from the patient statements of fact that lead to a more accurate conceptualization of the problem, while at the same time *actively interfering* with the patient's obsessive reiteration of the negative cognitive set. The patient's participation in the reasoning process provides a chance to experience the therapy before actually putting it into practice. Most of the work, however, is not done in sessions, but in homework in which the patient carries out the prescriptions of the therapist.

Interpersonal Therapy

Interpersonal psychotherapy (IPT), developed by Klerman and colleagues,[30] is a highly formalized ("manualized") treatment. It was developed primarily to treat patients with depression related to grief or loss, interpersonal disputes, role transitions, or interpersonal skill deficits, but its applicability has been broadened beyond depression to include couples' conflicts, personality disorders, and bipolar disorder, among others.

Temperamental fit between the patient and therapist plays a large role. Crits-Christoph[14] notes that "patients who have more interest in examining the subtle, complex meanings of events and interpersonal transactions are a better match" for expressive treatment, whereas those with a more concrete style may prefer cognitive therapy or IPT (p. 157). This psychotherapy de-emphasizes the transference and focuses not on mental content, but on the process of the patient's interaction with others. In IPT, behavior and communications are taken at face value. Consequently, therapists who need to find creativity in their work may dislike IPT. The strength of the method is that it poses little risk of iatrogenic harm, even to the fragile patient, and even in the hands of the inexperienced therapist.

IPT theorists acknowledge their debt to other therapies in stance and technique, but claim distinction at the level of "strategies," an orderly series of steps in evaluation and treatment. For patients with *depression related to grief,* they first review depressive symptoms, relate them to the death of the significant other, reconstruct the lost relationship, construct a narrative of the relationship, explore negative and positive feelings, and consider the patient's options for becoming involved with others.

For patients with *interpersonal disputes that cause depression,* they conduct a symptom review, relate symptom onset to the dispute, take a history of the relationship, dissect-out role expectations, and focus on correction of non-reciprocal expectations.

For patients with *role transitions,* they review the symptoms, relate the symptoms to life change, review positive and negative aspects of new and old roles, review losses, ventilate feelings, and find new role options. And finally, with patients with *interpersonal deficits that lead to depression,* they review symptoms and relate them to social isolation or unfulfillment, review past relationships, explore repetitive patterns, and (unlike the behavioral therapies) discuss the patient's *conscious* positive and negative feelings about the therapist, using them to explore the maladaptive patterns elicited earlier.

As one example of *method,* here is the algorithm for *communication analysis*: Therapists should identify:

(1) Ambiguous or non-verbal communication.
(2) Incorrect assumptions that one has indeed communicated.
(3) Incorrect assumptions that one has understood.
(4) Unnecessarily indirect verbal communication.
(5) Inappropriate silence—closing off communication.

If the therapist identifies one or more of these, this list is run through another list of therapeutic investigations of the therapeutic relationship itself to give the patient concrete examples. Then decision analysis, the major action-oriented technique of IPT, is used to help the patient diagnose and treat depressogenic interpersonal problems by finding other options.

Strupp and colleagues[31] also lay claim to the interpersonal model.[32] In it, the focus the patient brings helps the therapist to generate, recognize, and organize therapeutic data. The focus is commonly stated in terms of a cardinal symptom, a specific intrapsychic conflict or impasse, a maladaptive picture of the self, or a persistent interpersonal dilemma. It is supposed to exemplify a central pattern of interpersonal role behavior in which the patient unconsciously casts himself or herself. The method for such investigations is *narrative,* "the telling of a story to oneself and others. Hence, the focus is organized in the form of a schematic story outline" to provide a structure for "narrating the central interpersonal stories" of a patient's life (Strupp & Binder,[31] p. 68).

This narrative contains four structural elements or subplots that are the keys to the therapy:

(1) Acts of self.
(2) Expectations of others' reactions.
(3) Acts of others toward the self.
(4) Acts of self toward the self.

While learning this narrative, the therapist is expected at the same time to continually point out how these cyclic patterns cause recurrent maladaptation and pain. Co-narrating and co-editing these four subplots form the basis of the Strupp method.

The Core Conflictual Relationship Theme (CCRT) method is another formalized therapy that examines narratives. Based on Luborsky's[33–35] CCRT, it assumes that each patient has a predominant and specific transference pattern, that the pattern is based on early experience, that it is activated in important relationships, that it distorts those relationships, that it is constantly repeated in the patient's life, and that it

appears in the therapeutic relationship. A major difference in the CCRT method from examinations of the transference in the many dynamic brief therapies, however, is the systematic, active method of ferreting out the CCRT.

The focus in CCRT therapy, the "core conflictual relationship," is discovered by eliciting several *relationship episodes* (REs), descriptions of problems appearing in present and past relationships. From these RE descriptions, three components are carefully teased out—the patient's *wish* (W) in relationships, the actual or anticipated *response from others* (RO), and the patient's *response from self* (RS). In the first phase of treatment, the repeated occurrence of the CCRT is documented. In the second phase, the childhood roots of the RO are worked through. In the last phase, termination-stimulated increases in the patient's RO and RS, response from others and from self, are analyzed against the backdrop of increased conscious awareness of W, the wish.

Eclectic Therapies

The "eclectic" brief therapies[9,36] are characterized by combinations and integrations of multiple theories and techniques.

Horowitz and colleagues[37–39] owe a debt to a broad literature on stress, coping, and adaptation that spans the cognitive, behavioral, phenomenological, and ego psychological realms. The point of departure is the normal stress response: the individual perceives the event, as a loss or death. The mind then reacts with outcry ("No, no!") and then denial ("It's not true!"). These two states, denial and outcry, alternate so that the subjective experience is of unwanted intrusion of the image of the lost. Over time, "grief work" proceeds so that "working through" leads to completion.

The pathological side of this normal response to stress occurs in the stage of perception of the event when the individual is overwhelmed. In the outcry stage there is panic, confusion, or exhaustion. In the *denial* stage there is maladaptive avoidance or withdrawal by suicide, drug and alcohol abuse, dissociation, or counter-phobic frenzy. In the more complex stage of *intrusion,* the individual experiences alternation of flooded states of sadness and fear, rage and guilt, which alternate with numbness. If working through is blocked, there ensue hibernative or frozen states, constriction, or psychosomatic responses. If completion is not reached, there is ultimately an inability to work or to love.

Horowitz's therapy proceeds like the older models of Lindemann or Grinker and Spiegel, with ego psychology and information-processing theory woven in. The therapist identifies the focus—in this therapy usually a traumatic event or a loss—and tries to determine whether the patient is in the denial or the intrusion phase of maladaptation. In the *denial* phase, perception and attention are marred by a dazed state and by selective inattention. There is partial amnesia or emotional isolation. Information processing is crippled by disavowal of meanings. There is loss of a realistic sense of connection with the world. There is emotional numbness.

When the patient is stuck in the *intrusion* phase of the trauma response, perception and attention are marked by hypervigilance, overactive consciousness, and inability to concentrate. Emotional attacks or pangs of anxiety, depression, rage, or guilt intrude. Psychosomatic symptoms are common here as sequelae of the chronic flight-or-fight response.

A dozen or so sessions are used to focus on the recent stress event and work it through. In the early sessions the initial positive feelings for the therapist develop as the patient tells the story of the event. There ensues a sense of decreased pressure as trust is established. The traumatic event is related to the life of the patient as a psychiatric history is taken. In the middle phase of therapy, the patient tests the therapist and the therapist elicits associations to this stage of the relationship. There is a realignment of focus, with non-threatening surface interpretations of transference resistances. The patient is asked to understand why these resistances are currently reasonable based on past relationships. The therapeutic alliance deepens as this phase continues and the patient works on what has been avoided. There is further interpretation of defenses and warded-off contents, with linkage of these contents to the stress event. In the late middle phases, transference reactions toward the therapist are more deeply interpreted as they occur. There is continued working through of central conflicts, which emerge as termination relates them to the life of the patient. In termination there is acknowledgment of problems, as well as real gains and an adumbration of future work, for instance, anniversary mourning.

A major feature of Horowitz's work is *defensive styles*. The *hysterical* personality style has an inability to focus on detail and a tendency to be overwhelmed by the global; the *compulsive* style is the converse, with the patient unable to experience affect because of details. The therapist acts in either event to supplement the missing component and to damp out the component flooding the patient. With the global, fuzzy hysteric, the therapist asks for details; with the obsessional, the therapist pulls for affect.

In the *borderline* patient the tendency to split is damped out by anticipating that, with shame and rage, there is going to be a distortion of the patient's world into its good and bad polarities. For the patient with a *narcissistic* personality style, the tendency to exaggerate or to minimize personal actions is gently, but firmly, confronted. The *schizoid* patient is allowed interpersonal space. One of the great advantages of Horowitz's method is that it does not compete with other schools of short-term psychotherapy and it can be integrated or added in parallel.

The eclectic brief therapy of Budman and Gurman[25] rests on the interpersonal, developmental, and existential (IDE) focus. A major feature here is the belief that maximal benefit from therapy occurs early, and the optimal time for change is early in treatment. They begin with a systematic approach that begins with the individual's reason for seeking therapy *at this time*. The patient's age, date of birth, and any appropriate developmental stage-related events or anniversaries are noted. Major changes in the patient's social support are reviewed. Especially important in the Budman–Gurman system is substance abuse and its contribution to the presentation at this time.

None of these ideas is novel, but the way they are combined systematically is nicely realized with reference to eliciting the precipitating event, its relation to the focus, the relation to development, and working through with a balance of techniques. The major focus in the IDE perspective includes the following:

(1) Losses.
(2) Developmental dys-synchronies.
(3) Interpersonal conflicts.
(4) Symptomatic presentations.
(5) Personality disorders.

Budman and Gurman[25] are not snobbish about the capacity of any one course of treatment to cure the patient completely, and they welcome the patient back again in successive developmental stages at developmental crises. A particular value of this treatment is that it is non-perfectionistic, both in pulling a particular phase of therapy to an end and the lack of a feeling of failure on resuming treatment. The picture one develops of this approach is of clusters of therapies ranging along important nodal points in the individual's development.

BOX 11-1 Patient Selection Criteria for Brief Therapy

EXCLUSION CRITERIA
- Active psychosis
- Acute or severe substance abuse
- Acute risk of self-harm

INCLUSION CRITERIA
- Moderate emotional distress
- A real desire for relief
- A specific or circumscribed problem
- History of one positive relationship
- Function in one area of life
- Ability to commit to treatment

THE ESSENTIAL FEATURES OF BRIEF THERAPY
The Initial Evaluation

Patient selection begins and ends with the initial evaluation. Patients who should be excluded from short-term therapy are those with severe, chronic Axis I disorders that have not responded fully to biological treatment, chaotic acting-out personality disorders, patients specifically rejecting brief treatment, and patients for whom it is impossible to find a focus or for whom there are multiple, diffuse foci.

Some patients do well in any form of short-term treatment: for example, the high-functioning graduate student who cannot complete a dissertation. But between these extremes fall the majority. If the patient is relatively healthy, there are more options: Sifneos may be beyond the reach of the average patient, but there are Malan, Mann, and Davanloo. If the patient is less healthy, the methods of Budman and Gurman may work well, or of Horowitz, especially if there is a traumatic event to serve as a focus. If the patient is quite challenged, the Sifneos anxiety-suppressive treatment is often useful, or cognitive therapy or IPT, depending on the extent to which the focal problems are cognitive or interpersonal. Even some patients with borderline personality disorder may find help in the methods of Leibovich. The balance of this chapter presents a broadly workable algorithm for eclectic therapy.

Patient Selection

A two-session evaluation format is recommended to determine whether a patient is appropriate. The array of inclusion and exclusion criteria in Box 11-1 is fairly general, covering most forms of brief therapy. Also, they are restrictive—many patients will be screened out. For the novice brief therapist, however, the faithful use of these criteria will provide nearly ideal brief therapy patients.

Exclusion Criteria

The patient should not be actively psychotic, continuously abusing substances, or at significant risk for self-harm. The psychotic patient will not be able to make adequate use of the reality-oriented/logical aspects of the brief treatment. Substance-abusing patients should be directed to substance abuse treatment before undertaking any form of psychotherapy. Patients who are at significant risk for self-harm are not appropriate because of the difficulty of ending the treatment at a planned time. These factors should be considered categorical; the presence of any one of them should virtually rule out a patient for brief psychotherapy.

Inclusion Criteria

The candidate for brief therapy should be in moderate distress, which provides the motivation for treatment. The patient should personally want relief and not have been sent by an employer, a spouse, or some legal situation. The patient should be able to articulate a fairly specific cause of the pain or a circumscribed life problem—or be able to embrace the therapist's formulation. The patient needs to have a history of at least one positive, mutual relationship. The patient should still be functioning in at least one area of life and have the ability to commit to a treatment agreement. The candidate should be rated in all of these dimensions—the more of these qualities (degree and number) a patient has, the better he or she is as a candidate.

Developing a Focus

The focus is probably the most misunderstood aspect of brief therapy.[40] Many writers talk about "the focus" in a circular and mysterious manner, as if the whole success of the treatment rests on finding the one correct focus. What is needed, however, is a focus that both the therapist and patient can agree on and that fits the therapist's approach. For instance, the therapist can start with the "metaphoric function" of a symptom (Friedman & Fanger,[41] p. 58). The treatment is then focused around that symptom, its meaning to the patient, and its consequences. Goals are stated in a positive language, assessed as observable behavior—goals that are important to the patient and congruent with the patient's culture.

Another technique for finding a focus is the "why now?" technique used by Budman and Gurman.[25] The triggering event for therapy is often ideal, and the technique is applied by repeatedly asking the patient, "Why did you come for treatment now? Why today rather than last week, or tomorrow?" Or failing these, "Think back to the exact moment you decided to get help. What were you doing at that moment? What had just happened? What was about to happen?"

These strategies disclose four common treatment foci:

1. Losses (past, present, or pending). These can be interpersonal (such as the loss of a loved one), intrapersonal (such as the loss of a psychological ability or the loss of a support network), or functional (such as the loss of a specific ability or capacity).
2. Developmental dys-synchronies (being out of step with expected developmental stages). (This is often seen in the professional who required extensive periods of education before initiating an adult lifestyle.)
3. Interpersonal conflicts, usually repeated interpersonal disappointments, either with loved ones or employers.
4. Symptomatic manifestations—many patients attend psychotherapy simply with the desire for symptom reduction.

These foci serve as a checklist during the initial evaluation. If two of these are workable, it is important to remember that the therapist is not finding *the* focus, only a workable focus. Pick one and, if the patient agrees, stick to it.

Completing the Initial Evaluation and Setting Goals

By the completion of the second evaluation session, the therapist needs to decide whether the patient is appropriate for brief treatment, select an agreed-on focus, and have a clearly stated treatment agreement (including the number of sessions, how missed appointments will be handled, and payment plans).

The two-session evaluation format also allows the therapist to see how the patient responds to the therapist and to therapy. It can be enlightening to give the patient some kind of homework to complete between the two sessions. An initial positive response and feeling a little better in the second session bodes well, whereas a strong negative reaction conveys a worse prognosis. A more ambivalent response, such as forgetting the task, may signal problems with motivation, and this needs to be explored.

The Brief Therapy Mind-set

A certain attitude needs to be cultivated by the therapist in order to learn. There must be some open-mindedness, curiosity, and a willing suspension of disbelief about brief therapy. An example would be a willingness to consider a quick positive response as something other than a temporary "flight into health." The time-limited enterprise must be *real* for the therapist. This appears deceptively obvious, but, in practice, it is actually a difficult cognitive change to make and one that has ramifications for all treatment decisions, particularly the therapist's activity level.

The therapist must accept that some patients will return to therapy periodically across their life spans (sometimes called "intermittent brief therapy across the life cycle") and let go the notion of "cure." Setting realistic expectations needs to be a skill that the therapist has already mastered.

Being an Active Therapist

Conducting a brief, 12- to 16-session psychotherapy requires that the therapist be active—but in a certain way. Any single maneuver is useful only when utilized with a larger set of theory-based principles, especially those aimed at finding and repairing the patient's missing developmental piece, and managing resistance[42] (Box 11-2). The therapist must keep the treatment focused and the process of treatment moving forward, never forgetting that focusing *itself* pushes the therapy along. Several techniques structure and direct the therapy. These include beginning each session with a summary of the important points raised during the last session, re-stating the focus, and assignment and review of homework. Interventions that focus on the working alliance are important, as are timely interventions that limit silences and discourage deviations from the focus.

The goal of eclectic brief therapy is to restore or improve pre-morbid adaptation and function. Efforts are made by the therapist to limit and to check psychological regressions. Asking, "What did you think about that?" rather than about feelings and affect (e.g., "How did that make you feel?") can help with the exploration of potentially regressive material (e.g., sexual secrets). Limited within the session, regression is acceptable, but prolonged regressions accompanied by decreased functioning (and especially acting-out) may often be avoided by supporting high-level defenses, such as

---

BOX 11-2 Types of Therapist Activity

- Structured sessions
- Use of homework
- Development of the working alliance
- Limitation on silences
- Clarification of vague responses
- Addressing negative transference quickly
- Limitation of psychological regression

intellectualization. The therapist can ask the patient to review the therapy thus far, pick the best session and the worst session, and tell why. Such maneuvers bind anxiety and other negative affects. The patient can be urged to make lists of problems, causes, and strategies, or to keep a journal. Whenever the patient gets negative globally, he or she can be asked to break the negative perceptions down into components. Requests for clarification should be made whenever a patient produces vague or incomplete material. This would include asking for examples or for specifics, and empathically pointing out contradictions and inconsistencies.

Transference occurs in *all* treatments, including brief psychotherapy. Moreover, transference distortions strong enough to wreck a treatment occur in the beginning hours,[43] if not the opening *minutes* of therapy. Despite the fact that many aspects of brief therapy are designed to discourage the development of transference, the therapist must be ready to deal with it when it develops. Two forms are particularly important to recognize quickly: negative and erotized transferences. Transference resistance often has as its first sign some alteration in the frame (such as lateness, absence, or frequent re-scheduling) and sometimes a bid by the patient to change the focus. Negative transference can be suspected when the patient responds repeatedly with either angry or de-valuing statements, or when he or she experiences the therapy as humiliating. Early erotized transference is signaled by repeated and excessively positive comments, for example, "Oh you know me better than anyone ever has." Both of these forms of transference should be dealt with quickly from the perspective of reality. The therapist should review the patient's feelings and reasoning and relate these to the actual interaction. For example, if the therapist was inadvertently offensive, this should be admitted, while undefensively pointing out that the motive was to be helpful.

Phases of Planned Brief Therapy

The three traditional phases of psychotherapy in general apply to brief treatments as well. The *initial phase* (from the evaluation to session 2 or 3) principally includes evaluation and selection of the patient, selection of the focus, and establishment of a working alliance. This phase is ideally accompanied by some reduction in symptoms and by a low-grade positive transference, particularly as a working relationship develops. The goal is to set the frame and the structure of the therapy, while also giving the patient hope.

The *middle phase* (sessions 4 to 8 or 9) is characterized by the work getting more difficult. The patient usually becomes concerned about the time limit, feeling that the length of treatment will not be sufficient. Issues of separation and aloneness come to the fore and compete with the focus for attention. It is important for the therapist to reassure the patient (with words and a calm, understanding demeanor) that the treatment will work and direct their joint attention back to the agreed-upon focus. The patient often feels worse during this phase, and the therapist's faith in the treatment process is often tested.

The *termination phase* (sessions 8 to 12 or 16) typically is characterized by the therapy settling down, by decreased affect, and by continued work on old material, but not the introduction of new material. When the patient accepts the fact that treatment will end as planned, symptoms typically decrease. In addition to the treatment focus, post-therapy plans and the situational loss of the therapy relationship are explored. Around the termination, it is not unusual for the patient to present some new and often interesting material for discussion. While the therapist may be tempted to explore this new material, to do so is usually a mistake. A better course is

clarification of the *emergence* of new material as a healthy, understandable—but ultimately self-defeating—attempt to extend the treatment. Mild interest in the new material should be shown, but if it is not a true emergency, treatment should end as planned.

Post-treatment Contact

When therapy is completed, a patient should ideally wait 6 months before considering further therapy. It can be explained to the reluctant-to-leave patient that this allows the patient to practice newly learned psychological insights and skills in the real world. ("A very important part of your therapy is the next phase, working on your own. It would be a shame for you to give up before trying this, which is often the most interesting and helpful part of therapy.")

One should be ready to help patients with psychological troubles whenever they develop across the life span, typically at developmental milestones and role changes. Within the eclectic brief therapy framework it is not just acceptable for patients to return to therapy at multiple points during their life, it is encouraged—the door to treatment is closed, but never locked.

Access the complete reference list and multiple choice questions (MCQs) online at https://expertconsult.inkling.com

KEY REFERENCES

1. Olfson M, Pincus HA. Outpatient psychotherapy in the United States, II: patterns of utilization. *Am J Psychiatry* 151:1289–1294, 1994.
2. Cuijpers P, Geraedts AS, van Oppen P, et al. Interpersonal psychotherapy for depression: a meta-analysis. *Am J Psychiatry* 168:581–592, 2011.
3. Browne G, Steiner M, Roberts J, et al. Sertraline and/or interpersonal psychotherapy for patients with dysthymic disorder in primary care: 6-month comparison with longitudinal 2-year follow-up of effectiveness and costs. *J Affect Disord* 68:317–330, 2002.
4. Abbass A, Sheldon A, Gyra J, et al. Intensive short-term dynamic psychotherapy for DSM-IV personality disorders: a randomized controlled trial. *J Nerv Ment Dis* 196:211–216, 2008.
5. Guthrie E, Moorey J, Margison F, et al. Cost-effectiveness of brief psychodynamic-interpersonal therapy in high utilizers of psychiatric services. *Arch Gen Psychiatry* 56:519–526, 1999.
6. Hakkaart-van Roijen L, van Straten A, Al M, et al. Cost-utility of brief psychological treatment for depression and anxiety. *Br J Psychiatry* 188:323–329, 2006.
7. Bosmans JE, van Schaik DJF, Heymans MW, et al. Cost-effectiveness of interpersonal psychotherapy for elderly primary care patients with major depression. *Int J Technol Assess Health Care* 23:480–487, 2007.
8. Lave JR, Frank RG, Schulberg HC, et al. Cost-effectiveness of treatments for major depression in primary care practice. *Arch Gen Psychiatry* 55:645–651, 1998.
9. Blais MA. Planned brief therapy. In Jacobson J, Jacobson A, editors: *Psychiatric secrets*, Philadelphia, 1996, Hanley & Belfus.
10. Malone JC, Blais MA, Groves JE. Planned brief psychotherapy. In Stern TA, Herman JB, Gorrindo T, editors: *Psychiatry update and board preparation*, ed 3, Boston, 2012, MGH Psychiatry Academy.
11. Burk J, White H, Havens L. Which short-term therapy? *Arch Gen Psychiatry* 36:177–186, 1979.
12. Marmor J. Short-term dynamic psychotherapy. *Am J Psychiatry* 136:149–155, 1979.
13. Frances A, Clarkin JF. No treatment as the prescription of choice. *Arch Gen Psychiatry* 38:542–545, 1981.
14. Crits-Christoph P. The efficacy of brief dynamic psychotherapy: a meta-analysis. *Am J Psychiatry* 149:151–158, 1992.
15. Winston A, Winston B. *Handbook of integrated short-term therapy*, New York, 2002, American Psychiatric Press.

16. Leichsenring F, Rabung S, Leibling E. The efficacy of short-term psychodynamic psychotherapy in specific psychiatric disorders: a meta-analysis. *Arch Gen Psychiatry* 61:1208–1216, 2004.

17. Svartberg M, Stiles TC, Seltzer MH. Randomized, controlled trial of the effectiveness of short-term dynamic psychotherapy and cognitive therapy for cluster C personality disorders. *Am J Psychiatry* 161:810–817, 2004.

18. Weissman MM, Markowitz JC, Klerman GL. *A clinician's quick guide to interpersonal psychotherapy*, New York, 2007, Oxford University Press.

19. Malan DM. *The frontier of brief psychotherapy*, New York, 1976, Plenum.

20. Malan DM, Osimo F. *Psychodynamics, training and outcome in brief psychotherapy*, London, 1992, Butterworth-Heinemann.

21. Davanloo H. *Short-term dynamic psychotherapy*, New York, 1989, Jason Aronson.

22. Della Selva P. *Intensive short-term dynamic psychotherapy: theory and technique*, New York, 1996, John Wiley & Sons.

23. Mann J. *Time-limited psychotherapy*, Cambridge, MA, 1973, Harvard University Press.

24. Mann J. Time-limited psychotherapy. In Crits-Christoph P, Barber JP, editors: *Handbook of short-term dynamic psychotherapy*, New York, 1991, Basic Books.

25. Budman SH, Gurman AS. *Theory and practice of brief therapy*, New York, 1988, Guilford Press.

26. Winnicott DW. *Therapeutic consultations in child psychiatry*, New York, 1971, Basic Books.

27. Beck AT, Greenberg RL. Brief cognitive therapies. *Psychiatr Clin North Am* 2:23–37, 1979.

28. Groves J. *Essential papers on short-term dynamic therapy*, New York, 1996, New York University Press.

29. Dewan MJ, Steenbarger BN, Greenberg RP. *The art and science of brief psychotherapies: a practitioner's guide*, Washington, DC, 2004, American Psychiatric Publishing.

30. Klerman GL, Weissman MM, Rounsaville BJ, et al. *Interpersonal therapy of depression*, New York, 1984, Basic Books.

31. Strupp HH, Binder JL. *Psychotherapy in a new key*, New York, 1984, Basic Books.

32. Levenson H, Butler SF, Powers TA, et al. *Concise guide to brief dynamic and interpersonal therapy*, ed 2, Washington, DC, 2002, American Psychiatric Publishing.

33. Luborsky L. *Principles of psychoanalytic psychotherapy: a manual for Supportive-Expressive Treatment*, New York, 1984, Basic Books.

34. Luborsky L, Mellon J, van Ravenswaay P, et al. A verification of Freud's grandest clinical hypothesis: the transference. *Clin Psychol Rev* 5:231–246, 1985.

35. Book H. *How to practice brief psychodynamic psychotherapy: the core conflictual relationship theme method*, Washington, DC, 1998, American Psychological Association.

36. Leibovich MA. Why short-term psychotherapy for borderlines? *Psychother Psychosom* 39:1–9, 1983.

37. Horowitz M, Marmor C, Krupnick J, et al. *Personality styles and brief psychotherapy*, New York, 1984, Basic Books.

38. Stadter M, Horowitz MJ. *Object relations brief therapy: the therapeutic relationship in short-term work*, Northvale, NJ, 1996, Jason Aronson.

39. Zimmerman DJ, Groves JE. Difficult patients. In Stern TA, Fricchione GL, Cassem NH, et al., editors: *The MGH handbook of general hospital psychiatry*, ed 6, Philadelphia, 2010, Saunders/Elsevier.

40. Hall M, Arnold W, Crosby R. Back to basics: the importance of focus selection. *Psychotherapy* 27:578–584, 1990.

41. Friedman S, Fanger MT. *Expanding therapeutic possibilities: getting results in brief psychotherapy*, Lexington, MA, 1991, Lexington Books.

42. Gustafson JP. *The complex secret of brief psychotherapy*, New York, 1986, WW Norton.

43. Gill MM, Muslin HL. Early interpretation of transference. *J Am Psychoanal Assoc* 24:779–794, 1976.

12 Couples Therapy

Anne K. Fishel, PhD, and Jeanne McKeon, EdD

KEY POINTS

- Like family therapy, couples therapy is founded on systemic ideas.
- A couple's evaluation should include exploration of the presenting problem, as well as challenging and re-framing of the couple's problems.
- "The relationship" takes the role of the patient for couples therapists, who also must take into account each individual's family of origin, history of previous relationships, current stressors, and medical and psychiatric history.
- A wide variety of systemic approaches exist for treating couples; approaches that can be differentiated by their emphasis on cognition, emotion, or behavior as the focus of change.
- Most clinical approaches to working with couples aim to diminish conflict and to enhance connectedness and intimacy.

OVERVIEW

Couples therapy focuses on the pattern of interactions between two people, while allowing for the individual histories and contributions of each member. It is a treatment modality used in a variety of clinical situations—as part of a child evaluation (to assess the contribution of marital distress to a child's symptoms); in divorce mediation and child custody evaluations (to minimize the intensity of relational conflict that interferes with collaborative problem solving); in ongoing child and adolescent psychotherapy (when the parents' relationship is thought to play a part in a child's unhappiness); and as part of an ongoing family therapy (when the couple may be seen separately from the family as a whole). Couples therapy is often the treatment of choice for a range of problems: sexual dysfunction,[1] alcohol and substance abuse,[2] the disclosure of an infidelity,[3] depression and anxiety disorders,[4] infertility,[5,6] serious medical illness,[7] and parenting impasses.[8] In addition, couples therapy may be helpful in the resolution of polarized relational issues (e.g., the decision to marry or divorce, the choice to have a child or an abortion, or the decision to move to another city for one partner's career). In this chapter, the term *couples therapy* is used rather than *marital therapy* so as to include therapy with unmarried gay and lesbian couples, and unmarried heterosexual couples.

SEMINAL IDEAS IN COUPLES THERAPY

The history of couples therapy is inextricably linked to that of family therapy; the two modalities draw from the same set of concepts and techniques. However, over the past 50 years couples therapy has evolved via a systemic approach to relational difficulties. While there are many theoretical schools of couples therapy (see Chapter 13 for a sampling of different approaches), most clinicians focus on several systemic principles and constructs. In the most general terms, systemic thinking addresses the organization and pattern of a couple's interactions with one another and posits that the whole is greater than the sum of its parts. Systemic thinking leads the clinician to concentrate on several issues: on the communication between the couple and with outside figures; on the identification of relationship patterns that are dysfunctional; on ideas about the relationship as an entity that is greater than either member's version; on the impact of life cycle context and family of origin on the couple's current relational difficulties; and on some understanding about why these two people have chosen each other.

IDENTIFICATION OF DYSFUNCTIONAL RELATIONAL PATTERNS

Systemic thinkers hold that the links between partners are recursive or circular, rather than causal or linear. In other words, it makes more sense to think about relational problems as interactional sequences, rather than as one individual causing the problem in the other. Seen this way, there is little interest in assigning blame to one party or in figuring out who started the problem. Instead, the emphasis is on determining what role each member plays in maintaining the problematic relational pattern and the function that the pattern serves for the relationship.

There are two fundamental forms of relational patterns in couples (Figure 12-1): symmetrical and complementary.[9] A symmetrical relationship is characterized by each member contributing a similar behavior, so that each partner compounds and exacerbates the difficulties. A classic example is one in which both members of the couple engage in verbal abuse, so that either one's raised voice prompts an escalation of angry affect, which, in turn, triggers the other's ire. Complementarity, by contrast, refers to patterns that require each member to contribute something quite different, in a mutually-interlocking manner, to maintain the relationship. A classic example of a complementary relationship is the distancer-pursuer, in which one member does most of the asking for intimacy and connection, while the other pulls back in order to do work, take care of the children, or be alone. The circular nature of this pattern dictates that, the more one pursues, the more the other pulls back, which in turn makes the pursuer pursue more, and the distancer recoil more. Seen this way, either one could change the dance.

Over time, some therapists have questioned ideas about circularity. In particular, feminist therapists have critiqued the notion of equally-shared responsibility for a problem, particularly when this notion is applied to intimate partner violence. When a partner abuses power, particularly when a man batters a woman, circular causality runs the risk of making the woman feel equally responsible for her abuse.[10]

MATE CHOICE AND THE CONTRIBUTION OF ONE'S FAMILY OF ORIGIN

The couples therapist is curious about the nature of the initial attraction and may locate the origins of the current dilemma in the seeds of the couple's first attraction. One common explanation for early attraction is that "opposites attract," which may be understood in terms of the psychodynamic construct of projective identification.[11] This is the idea that individuals look for something in the other that is difficult for

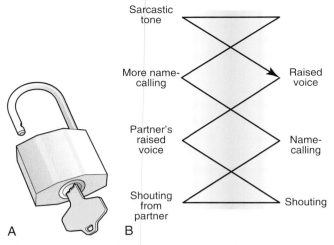

Figure 12-1. (A) Complementary and (B) symmetrical communication.

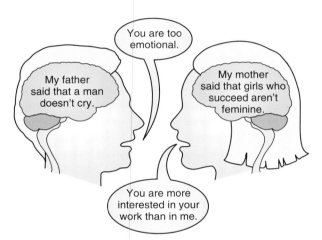

Figure 12-2. Projective identification.

them to bear or to express and then they act unconsciously to elicit the very behavior in the other that has been disavowed by the self. So, for example, a vivacious, expressive woman whose ambitions were discouraged by her family may be drawn to a cool, career-focused man whose attempts to express his feelings were ignored growing up. She may initially find his self-confidence and drive exciting, while he finds her ability to cry and to laugh invigorating. Over time, however, she may criticize him for his self-absorption, and he may criticize her for her over-emotionality. In sum, what is problematic for the self, and is the initial source of mutual attraction, over time becomes played out as conflict between the couple (Figure 12-2).[12]

Another view of mate selection is contained in the psychoanalytic notion of repetition compulsion. This is the idea that one's choice of a mate is dictated by the wish to re-create a loving relationship from childhood or to try to master an abusive relationship by re-enacting it a second time. The common observation that a man has "married his mother" is an example of this phenomenon.

COMMUNICATION

Many couples therapists stress the importance of couples developing communication skills that allow for each partner

to speak openly while the other one listens without sitting in judgment.[12,13] In addition, these same therapists encourage couples to learn how to fight fairly (i.e., without blaming, name calling, or straying from the subject at hand). However, such skill-training, with its emphasis on *how* couples talk to each other, has been transformed by social constructivists, who focus on *what* couples talk to each other about. These narrative therapists take as their starting point the idea that each partner's reality is constrained by the language that he or she uses.[14] Therefore, problems between partners occur because they lack the emotional vocabulary and narrative skills to create a dialogue that creates possibilities. Put simply, the way that a couple talks about a problem keeps the problem alive. Seen this way, communication about the problem is a critical place of intervention—the therapist looks for new language and stories, and re-frames the issues to dissolve the couple's view of the problem.

INTIMACY AND CONTROL

Systems theorists, who are interested in organization and patterns of interaction, pay attention to the rules that underlie a couple's connectedness and their decision-making. These rules are influenced by the cultural and class background of each partner, as well as by the unique contributions from their family of origin. Most relational difficulties involve differences in the degree, type, and intensity of intimacy, as well as the balance of power between them.

In assessing intimacy, the therapist asks about what activities are shared between the couple[15] and about the quality of their connection to one another. In looking at control and power, the therapist pays attention to whether decision-making is shared or mainly determined by one partner. The therapist wonders whether the control of their relationship and issues (such as children) resides within the couple, or whether the couple must answer to other family members (such as grandparents).

Systemic theorists use several constructs to describe the interplay of intimacy and control in a relationship. Boundaries are used to describe the way that a couple defines itself as a subsystem within a family and the particular rules about how they will interact with other subsystems.[16] For example, one member of a couple may wish to carve out time to vacation alone with his partner, whereas the other believes that their roles as parents always take precedence and require that the children join them. Boundaries are also described in terms of their permeability; some couples keep rigid limits on the influence others may exert on them, whereas other couples maintain very fluid boundaries with others who easily enter their relationship. Conflicts may ensue when a couple disagrees about the permeability of these boundaries or about the placement of the boundaries within the family or between the couple and the outside world.

Triangulation (Figure 12-3) is another idea that describes a common reaction to the anxiety brought by dyadic closeness.[17] Bowen[18] posited that dyadic relationships are the most vulnerable to anxiety; consequently, it is human nature to bring in a third party to try to diffuse discomfort. The third party need not even be physically present. It may be the subject of gossip between a couple, or it may be the computer that one partner retreats to every evening after dinner, or it may be the other partner's wish to be closer to his or her family. Bowen[18] maintains that the degree to which a couple engages in triangulation is determined by previous and current involvement in inter-generational triangles. Seen this way, greater relationship closeness comes from each individual becoming more differentiated, or separate from the family of origin.

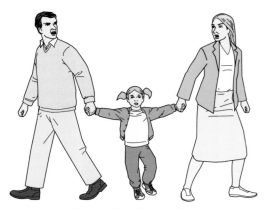

Figure 12-3. Triangulation.

TABLE 12-1 Life Cycles and Transitions

Life Cycle Stage	Emotional Task
1. Joining of families through marriage	Re-define family of origin choices to make room for new marital system
2. Becoming parents	Make room in relationship for new member Re-define relationships with extended family
3. Becoming family with adolescents	Allow for increased flexibility in boundaries for independence of children and dependence of grandparents
4. Launching stage	Re-evaluation of career and marital issues Re-assessment of parenting years
5. Retirement and on	Face loss of spouse, family, friends, health Review of life Re-focus on the couple

LIFE CYCLE CONTEXT AND TRANSITION POINTS

Many of the challenges that couples face occur in the context of the normative life cycle tasks. It is often in the transition from one developmental stage to the next that couples experience the most stress, as the requirements for flexibility and re-organization at a transition point may overwhelm the system. In general, each transition challenges the way the partners use their time[19] and the way they need to maintain established patterns while making changes in their roles and relationships.

Life cycle theorists have delineated five stages (Table 12-1) with attendant emotional tasks.[20] First comes the stage that joins families through marriage; each couple must re-define the issues and choices of their family of origin to create room for a new marital system. The next stage occurs when couples become parents. Here the main task is for the partners to make room in their relationship for new members and to re-define relationships with their extended family. The third stage is characterized by the development of the children as adolescents, when the parents must allow increased flexibility in boundaries to include adolescents' increased independence, as well as their grandparents' growing dependence. The fourth stage (the launching stage) occurs when young adults leave home: the main task for the couple is to re-evaluate their marriage and career issues as their parenting roles diminish. Finally, the fifth stage (often the longest stage) is when the partners are on their own, after the children have left home, and the couple faces aging and loss.

The timing and particular content of each stage is influenced by the couple's culture and social context. In some cultures, for example, the launching of children will coincide with their going to college, whereas in others it may not take place until the children have married and started their own

families. This stage also has been affected by the larger societal context. A century ago, the span of time from the last child leaving home until one parent died was commonly about 2 years. More recently, as a result of longer life expectancy, the end of childbearing for many women at a younger age, and the decision to have fewer children, this stage now often lasts as long as 30 years.

Couples therapists tend not to use diagnostic categories, which emphasize individual pathology and not systemic descriptions of a problem. In using the normative template of life cycle stages, the therapist can compare a particular couple's issues to the issues common to many couples at the same stage of development. For example, a therapist might say to a couple with two toddlers, "Most couples with young children experience a diminishment in their sexual lives, and they tend to fight more about issues of fairness. How do these issues affect you?" By taking what is known about large numbers of couples at a particular stage and comparing this information to an individual couple, the therapist is making use of a large body of research.

In addition to the adjustments required by the passage of time, couples are also challenged by other stresses (e.g., illnesses, moves, job losses, deaths of family members, immigration); these can complicate the normative issues of a given life cycle stage. The timing of such additional stressors will be a key factor, since events that happen "off-cycle" are hardest to absorb. For example, when an illness strikes a young couple who are trying to build a new life together, they will become more derailed than an elderly couple who have already faced several losses together. In addition, when there is generational resonance with a current challenge, the response may be more complicated. For example, a young couple expecting their first baby will feel more anxiety if there were stillbirths or other early losses in their families of origin.

CONDUCTING A COUPLES THERAPY EVALUATION

A couple's evaluation should allow the partners the opportunity to discuss their relational issues, as well as the individual contributions that each member makes (because of family of origin, current stressors, and intrapsychic difficulties). To provide an opportunity for joint and individual reflection, an evaluation is composed of four different meetings: the first is with both members of the couple, followed by individual meetings with each partner, and a final meeting, at which the clinician shares feedback and recommendations, with both members present (Box 12-1).

The evaluation should provide a balance between therapeutic empathy and therapeutic questions that challenge the partners to think differently about their problems. Throughout the evaluation the clinician looks for opportunities to offer realistic hope, to note the strengths and resources in each individual and in the couple, and to provide a place where the positions of both partners can be heard without imposing judgment. By the end of the evaluation, the therapist should have a systemic understanding of the problem, and should be able to make a recommendation for couples therapy, individual or group therapy, or no treatment at all.

The First Session with Both Members of the Couple

The initial focus of the first session rests on the provision of safety and comfort, which can be accomplished by setting clear expectations for the evaluation, by announcing that communication among the therapist and the couple will be transparent, and by showing an interest in the couple, separate from their problems. It is a good idea for the therapist to

BOX 12-1 Summary of Couples Therapy Evaluation

FIRST SESSION (BOTH MEMBERS OF THE COUPLE)

Provide a context of safety:

Go over expectation of four meetings

Set the rule that all information will be shared with both members

Summarize any contact therapist has already had during initial phone call

Ask each member to introduce himself or herself, separate from the problem

Ask about the problem:

"How did you make the decision to give me a call?"

"Each of you, tell me how you see the difficulties in your relationship?"

"Give an example."

"Have there been any other major changes in your lives over the last year?"

Expand the couple's view of the problem:

"If therapy were to be wildly successful, what would be different in your relationship?"

"What first attracted you to each other?"

"What is it like being married to you?"

"Where is the couple developmentally?"

"What can you tell me about your family of origin that is relevant to your current relationship?"

"Tell me about an instance when the problem did not occur."

THE TWO INDIVIDUAL SESSIONS

Ask open-ended questions:

"Is there anything you would like to follow up on from our initial meeting?"

"Is there anything we didn't get to that you want to make sure to broach?"

Standard questions:

"Do alcohol or drug use interfere with your function or your relationship (for yourself or with your partner)?"

"Is there any history of sexual abuse?"

"Is there previous experience with therapy or hospitalization?"

"Is there any history of suicidality, depression, anxiety, or other mental illness?"

"How is your current physical health?"

"Do you ever feel frightened of your partner?"

THE FOURTH WRAP-UP SESSION

Are there any loose ends for the couple?

Are there any loose ends for the therapist?

Provide feedback to the couple:

Comment on positive qualities of the relationship.

Comment on the level of distress in the couple, noting whether same or different for both members of the couple.

Reflect the individual points of view of each member; highlight where views overlap and diverge.

Identify the stressors and place problems in a developmental context.

Offer a systemic description of the problem.

Make recommendations for treatment

member about the other. Questions about each member's age, work, and strengths signal that the couple's resources will be part of the therapy.

The next focus of the first session is to draw out each partner's perspective on the problem. The therapist should demonstrate the capacity to empathize with each position and to hold two different views simultaneously. Many couples come to therapy with the belief that the therapist will act as a judge who decides whose point of view is correct or whose list of complaints has more merit than the other's. Early on, the therapist should sidestep such requests, by making it clear that the therapist's job is not to choose one point of view but to increase the partners' own interest in and tolerance for each other. To underscore his or her interest in hearing two different perspectives, the clinician might open with this request: "Usually in couples therapy, each member of the couple has his or her own unique perspective about the difficulties in the relationship, and his or her own hopes for change in the future. I'd like to hear from each of you how you understand your reason for seeking help." In addition, early on, the therapist might ask, "How did you make the decision to call a couples therapist?" This question is aimed at figuring out whether both partners are motivated for therapy or whether one member is a reluctant participant. During this first inquiry into the problem, the therapist is trying to convey respect and understanding for each member of the couple while remaining impartial.

In the next part of the interview, the therapist moves beyond empathic listening to asking questions that will expand each partner's understanding of their relationship. The evaluation should offer the chance for the couple to share their rehearsed, working descriptions of the problem, but it should also allow for the couple to have their beliefs challenged and stretched, creating new possibilities for change. Several questions can help move the couple's exploration of their difficulties from an individual one, focused on the faults of the other, to a more systemic, interactional definition. For example, "If you were to be in couples therapy for six months and decided at that point that the therapy had been a wild success, how would you know? What would you be talking about or doing with each other that is not happening now? What would be different about your relationship?" Such questions ask the couple to supplant their present focus on problems with a future picture of a relational goal.[21]

Another surprising question is to ask each member of the couple, "What is it like to be married to you?"[22] The expected question, of course, is "What is it like to be married to your partner?" which invites critiques of the other's personality and habits and typically elicits a fairly rehearsed response. The different question asked here invites reflection and usually elicits a pause in the conversation. When each member's version of the self matches the partner's view, the therapist knows there is agreement about some of the relational issues. When there is an incongruity between the two views, the therapist knows that he or she will have to pay attention to why there are two such different versions of the relationship. In any case, the question can also illuminate the couple's capacity for empathy and willingness to be curious in a new way about the relationship.

As part of expanding the couple's definition of the problem, the therapist may want to inquire about areas of the relationship that were not initially raised by the couple. In particular, it is important to ask about the couple's sexual relationship, since a majority of committed couples will experience sexual difficulties at some point in their relationship.[23] Discomfort with a stranger, uncertainty about the relevance of sexual problems to a couple's therapy, or anxiety and shame about the subject matter may interfere with the couple spontaneously

explain the format of the four-session consultation at the outset and to explain that information conveyed by one member during the individual session will be shared in the joint wrap-up session. Similarly, the therapist should refer to any communication he or she has already had with one member of the couple by phone. Both of these moves demonstrate the therapist's commitment to open communication and indicate his or her antipathy to keeping a secret with one bringing up sex. When the clinician does so in the first session, he or she models his or her own comfort and willingness to explore sexual issues. An opening question might be, "Is there anything you would like to change about your sexual relationship?"[24]

Each partner's family of origin is another area to ask about that may not have been part of the initial presentation. One question that asks the couple to reflect on the contribution of their history to their current relationship is, "What can you tell me about the family you grew up in that will help me understand your current dilemma?" Questions may be more finely tuned by concentrating on the current dilemma and by asking how that issue was handled by each member's parents, or in their marriage. For example, "I know that you are fighting more than you want. I wonder how disagreements were handled in each of your families?"

Another round of questions may address the couple's developmental stage and its concomitant challenges. Knowledge about common struggles associated with each stage of development will allow the clinician to probe about normative issues. For example, if a couple is having difficulties during early marriage, the therapist will inquire about the partners' separation from their own families and their capacity to make decisions jointly about dozens of issues that were once made on their own.[20] If the couple has adolescent children, the therapist may wonder about midlife career issues, changes in sexuality, and anticipation of being alone once the children leave home.[25] In addition, it is useful to ask whether there have been any changes in the last year (such as illnesses, deaths, moves, or births in their immediate or extended families). Often, a couple's difficulties will coincide with an accumulation of other stressors, and it can be helpful to point out this confluence of stressors to the couple.

In the spirit of asking about parts of the relationship that are not problem-focused, the therapist can ask about the couple's initial meeting and attraction to one another. This is a diagnostic question because most couples, no matter how angry and frustrated they are currently, will shelve these feelings in order to focus on the more idealized beginnings. When couples do not brighten and soften toward each other in discussing their early relationship, it may be an indication that the couple's capacity to tap into positive feelings, goodwill, and affection has been sorely compromised.

Other ways of asking about the couple apart from their problem are to say, "Tell me about a time when the problem did not occur, even though it seemed as though you were headed in that direction," and to ask, "What did you each do differently, or observe that the other did differently, to make this happen?" These narrative questions[14] invite the couple to stand together looking at their difficulties as outside the relationship. The questions also require each member to reflect on his or her contribution to a solution of the problem.

One thorny clinical dilemma is the handling of secrets. The therapist does not want to be in the position of asking about a secret in a couple's session, only to be lied to. Nor does the therapist want to extract a secret during an individual session that cannot be shared, only to end up colluding with one partner. Instead, it may be best to state clearly the therapeutic position of not holding any information private from the other on the grounds that keeping secrets would make the therapist untrustworthy. That said, the therapist may ask about secrets in a way that invites disclosure. For example, instead of asking, "Are either of you having a secret affair?" one might ask, "Has fidelity been a challenge for either of you to maintain?" Or, "Have either of you been concerned about the other's sexual fidelity?" Or, "What has been your understanding of what constitutes fidelity? Does it, for example, include no emotional friendships with someone from work, no use of pornography, no physical contact with another person, no cybersex?"

At the end of this first joint session, the therapist asks if the couple would like to proceed with two individual sessions, followed by a final wrap-up meeting to decide whether to proceed with couples therapy, and if so, with what agenda.

The Two Individual Meetings

These sessions offer an opportunity for the therapist to get to know each individual better and for each individual to speak without having to share the time with his or her partner. In addition, it can be a time to inquire about individual areas of function that may indicate areas of follow-up, separate from the recommendation for couples therapy. Finally, it is a chance to observe the individual alone, compared with as a member of a couple. For example, when a woman appears shy and nervous in a joint meeting but expansive and forthright in her individual meeting, it raises the question of abuse and coercion.

The following areas are important to inquire about in the individual meeting.

Alcohol and Substance Abuse

"How many drinks do you have daily? Do you use drugs recreationally? Is drinking always fun, or have you had any other experiences with it?" These questions presume usage, and therefore open the door for disclosure. If drinking and drugs are not an issue, the couple can correct the therapist. Additionally, the therapist may ask, "Does your partner think you have a problem? Do you think your partner has a problem with substance abuse?" One should listen for incongruities in perspective, with one partner, for example, minimizing a drinking problem, while the other sounds an alarm bell.

Previous Therapy

"Have you ever been in therapy before, or are you currently? What has been helpful, or not helpful, with previous therapists? Will you want me to talk to your current therapist?" Often it is best to wait until the initial consultation has been completed, so that one can keep an open mind and a systemic perspective about the couple's relationship and not be influenced by the views of an individual therapist.

History of Mental Illness

"Do you have any history of depression, anxiety, suicidality, panic attacks, or other mental illness? Have you ever been hospitalized for psychiatric reasons?" These questions may point the evaluation in the direction of a psychopharmacological assessment or a referral for individual therapy. If a patient is actively suicidal, immediate hospitalization, rather than completing the couple's evaluation, will be needed.

Sexual Abuse

"Have you ever been touched in ways that you didn't want to be, as a child or as an adult? If so, who have you told about these experiences? Have you discussed this with your partner? If so, how did he or she respond? If not, why not?" If a patient discloses a history of sexual abuse that has not previously been shared, a referral for individual therapy may be warranted. If it has not been disclosed to the partner, the therapist should discuss the possible risks and benefits of doing so in the context of couples therapy.

TABLE 13-1 The Schools of Family Therapy

School	The Theory	The Practice	The Metaphor	The Proponents
Psychodynamic	Past causes present problems Multigenerational transmission	Projective identification Transference	Lead test scientist	Normal Paul James Framo Hilda Bruch Murray Bowen Ivan Nagy
Experiential	Change through growth experiences Here-and-now focus	Small interactions Communication skills Psychodramatic techniques	Folk artist	Virginia Satir Carl Whitaker
Structural	Blueprint of healthy family Well-defined subsystems Clear boundaries Parents in charge Flexibility with outsiders	Assess formal properties Manipulate space Impose new communicational rules Re-structure the system to eliminate symptoms	Building inspector	Salvador Minuchin
Strategic	Change requires interruption of maladaptive behavior sequences Families are homeostatic First-order vs. second-order change	Paradox Inquire about behavioral sequence Introduce second-order change	Master chess player	Milton Erikson Jay Haley Paul Watzlawick John Weakland Gregory Bateson Chloe Madanes
Systemic	Change occurs as beliefs are changed No one truth Family as evolving but "stuck" Introduce new information	Circular questions Re-frame Ritual Use of team and end-of-session message	Detective	Mara Selvini Palazzoli Luigi Boscolo Gianfranco Cecchin Giulana Prata
Narrative	Power of language to transform Knowledge is inter subjective	Externalize the problem Identify exceptions to the dominant story Reflecting team	Biographer	Michael White David Epston Tom Andersen Harold Goolishian Harlene Anderson Add Jill Freedman Gene Combs

Behavioral	Family as giving its best effort to
	    maximize reward and avoid
	    negative consequences
	Maladaptive behaviors are reinforced
	    or modeled
		Functional behavioral analysis
		Positive and negative reinforcement
			Civil engineer	Robert Liberman
				Lawrence Weathers
				Gerald Patterson
				Marion Forgatch
				Ian Falloon

Psychoeducational	Deficits in skills and knowledge Family as powerful agent of change	Communication skills Problem-solving skills Coping strategies Decrease expressed emotion	Wilderness guide	Carol Anderson William McFarlane

old relationships alive by the re-enactment of conflicts that parents had with their families of origin. Thus, when Mrs. Bean projects her perfectionism onto Pam, she re-creates the conflict she had with her own mother, who lacked tolerance of impulses that were not tightly controlled.

In part, the psychodynamic family therapist gathers and analyzes multi-generational transmission of issues through the use of a genogram (Figure 13-1), a visual representation of a family that maps at least three generations of that family's history. The genogram reveals patterns (of similarity and difference) across generations—and between the two sides of the family involving many domains: parent–child and sibling roles, symptomatic behavior, triadic patterns, developmental milestones, repetitive stressors, and cut-offs of family members.[2]

In addition, the genogram allows the clinician to look for any resonance between a current developmental issue and a similar one in a previous generation. This intersection of past with present anxiety may heighten the meaning and valence of a current problem.[3] With the Bean family (including two adolescents), the developmental imperative is to work on separation; this is complicated by the catastrophic separations

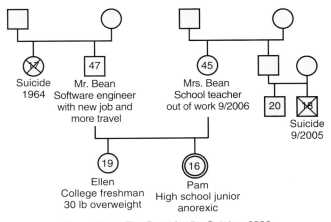

Figure 13-1. The Bean family, October 2006.

of previous adolescents. Their therapist might discover a multi-generational pattern of role reversals, where children nurture parents, as suggested by the repetition of failed attempts of adolescents to separate from their parents.

The Proponents

James Framo[4] invites parents and adult siblings to come to an adult child's session; this tactic allows the past to be re-visited in the present. This "family of origin" work is usually brief and intensive, and consists of two lengthy sessions on 2 consecutive days. The meetings may focus on unresolved issues or on disclosure of secrets; it allows the adult child to become less reactive to his or her parents.

Norman Paul[5] believes that most current symptoms in a family can be connected to a previous loss that has been insufficiently mourned. In family therapy, each member mourns an important loss while other members bear witness and consequently develop new stores of empathy.

Ivan Boszormenyi-Nagy[6] introduced the idea of the "family ledger," a multi-generational accounting system of obligations incurred and debts re-paid over time. Symptoms are understood in terms of an individual making sacrifices in his or her own life in order to re-pay an injustice from a previous generation.

Murray Bowen[7] stressed the dual importance of the individual's differentiation of self, while maintaining a connection to the family. In order to promote increased independence, Bowen coached patients to return to their family of origin and to resist the pull of triangulated relationships, by insisting that interactions remain dyadic.

The Metaphor

This therapist is like a lead-testing scientist who tests for levels of lead in one's garden to assess the legacy of toxins from previous homeowners. Only when the true condition of the soil has been revealed is the current homeowner free to make decisions about whether the soil is clean enough to plant root vegetables; somewhat contaminated, so that only fruit-bearing bushes will be safe; or so toxic that only flowers can be grown without hauling in truckloads of clean, fresh soil. Examination of the past enables the current gardener, and, by analogy, parents, to make informed choices about how the current environment needs to be adjusted and what kind of growth is allowable.

EXPERIENTIAL FAMILY THERAPY
The Theory

In contrast to the psychodynamic family therapist's focus on the past, the experiential therapist is primarily concerned with the here and now. In this model, change occurs through growth experiences that arise in the therapy session; experiences are aimed at the disruption of familiar interactions among family members. The experiential family therapist tries to make something surprising and unexpected happen, thereby amplifying affect. In general, the expression of feeling is valued over the discovery of insight. In its embrace of experience, this model is atheoretical and it can best be understood in light of its practice.

The Practice

The experiential family therapist is interested in small interactions that take place during the session. For example, the therapist might ask Pam, "Who told you about the meeting today, and what was said?" This therapist might also ask each family member, "What would you wish for right now, here today, that would make your life better?" The therapist would hope to amplify any communication that conveyed warmth and closeness and would interrupt any antagonistic communication. He or she might ask Mrs. Bean to look her husband in the eye, to hold his hand, and to ask for his help in dealing with Pam's anorexia.

This therapist uses psychodramatic, or action-oriented, techniques to create a new experience in the therapy session. She or he might "sculpt" the family, literally posing them to demonstrate the way that the family is currently organized—for example, with mother and Pam sitting very close together, with Mr. Bean with his back to them, and with Ellen outside of the circle. This therapist would hope to heighten feelings of frustration and alienation, and then to relieve those feelings with a new sculpture that places the parents together. These sculptures would serve to increase affect, to create some focus away from the identified patient, and to demonstrate the merits of the parents who are standing together to combat their daughter's anorexia.

The Proponents

Virginia Satir,[8] an early luminary in family therapy (a field that was largely founded by men), believed that good communication depends on each family member feeling self-confident and valued. She focused on what was positive in a family, and used non-verbal communication to improve connections within a family. If families learned to see, to hear, and to touch more, they would have more resources available to solve problems. She is credited with the use of family sculpting as a means to demonstrate the constraining rules and roles in a family.

Carl Whitaker[9] posited that most experience occurs outside of awareness; he practiced "therapy of the absurd," a method that accesses the unconscious by using humor, boredom, free association, metaphors, and even wrestling on the floor. Symbolic, non-verbal growth experiences followed, with an aim toward the disruption of rigid patterns of thought and behavior. As Whitaker puts it, "psychotherapy of the absurd can be a deliberate effort to break the old patterns of thought and behavior. At one point, we called this tactic the creation of process koans" (p. 11)[9]; it is a process that stirs up anxiety in family members.

The Metaphor

This type of therapist is like a folk artist who takes commonplace objects and transforms them into works of art. The viewer is surprised to find that a box of mismatched buttons could become the wings of a butterfly. Making the unfamiliar out of the familiar, and using playful techniques to do so, are key features of experiential family therapy.

STRUCTURAL FAMILY THERAPY
The Theory

The structural family therapist focuses on the structural properties of the family, rather than on affect or insight. Structure is defined by several features: by the rules of the family (e.g., what subjects can be discussed at the dinner table? What kind of affect is acceptable to express?); by boundaries within the family (e.g., do the children stay clear of marital conflict? Do siblings have their own relationship?); by boundaries between the family and the outside world (e.g., do parents easily request help from outsiders, or are they insulated?); and by the generational hierarchy (e.g., who [the parents, the adolescent, or the grandparents] is in charge of decision-making?). In this model, change occurs when the structure shifts and when symptoms are no longer needed.

This therapist approaches a family with a blueprint of what a normal family should look like, with some allowance made for cultural, ethnic, and economic variations. Most broadly stated, a high-functioning family should have well-defined parental, marital, and sibling subsystems; clear generational boundaries (with the parents firmly in charge); and flexible relationships with outsiders. The family with an eating-disordered member would be expected to have four structural fault lines: first, to be enmeshed (with little privacy and blurred boundaries between the generations so that children may be parenting parents); second, to be excessively over-protective (so that attempts by the children at autonomy are thwarted); third, to be rigid in the face of change (so that any stressor may overwhelm the family's resources); and fourth, to be relatively intolerant of individual differences (so that the family's threshold is low for individuals who voice an unpopular or maverick position).

The Practice

This therapist joins the Bean family by supporting the existing rules of the family and by making a relationship with each member. These individual relationships may later be used to re-structure the system, for example, by empowering the parents. The therapist, assessing the formal properties of the family, would earmark the shaky alliance between the parents and the lack of well-defined marital, parental, and sibling subsystems. The boundaries within the family are judged as enmeshed, with members talking about each other's feelings rather than about their own. Between the family and the outside world, the boundaries are rigid, since the Beans have not asked for any help from extended family or school personnel. This family therapist describes the family as involved in a pattern of conflict-avoidance called *triangulation*, with each parent wanting Pam to take his or her side, putting her into an impossible loyalty-bind.

As assessment becomes treatment, this therapist might challenge enmeshment by imposing a rule about communication, whereby each member should speak only for herself or himself. The therapist would try to challenge the lack of a generational hierarchy by manipulating space. For example, the therapist might ask Mr. and Mrs. Bean to sit side-by-side while also instructing Pam and Ellen to leave the room for part of the interview. To challenge the rule that conflict should be avoided, particularly regarding disagreements about how to get Pam to eat, this therapist would have the couple sit together and create a plan for the next meal while the therapist blocks any attempt to involve Pam. The family might then role-play a family meal (in a session) to illustrate Pam's role in their power struggle. Additionally, Pam and Ellen could be invited to have their own meeting to explore and to shore up their relationship.

The Proponents

Salvador Minuchin,[10,11] regarded as the founding father of structural family therapy, worked extensively while head of the Philadelphia Child Guidance Clinic with inner-city families and with families who faced delinquency and multiple somatic symptoms. Both populations had not previously been treated with family therapy. He delineated how to assess and to understand the existing structure of a family, and pioneered techniques (such as the imposition of rules of communication,

manipulation of space, and use of enactments) to modify structure.

The Metaphor

This therapist is like a building inspector who renders an opinion about the stability of a structure and guides the owner to decisions regarding a large-scale renovation or merely a cosmetic touch-up. The inspector does not care about either the furnishings or the paint colors, but is concerned with whether the walls are solid, the locks are in working order, and the wiring is functional and safe. Everything else follows smoothly if the house is solidly built.

STRATEGIC FAMILY THERAPY
The Theory

The strategic family therapist believes that change occurs when maladaptive behavioral sequences are interrupted. This therapist differentiates between two kinds of change: "first order," in which common-sense solutions to initial difficulties actually become unsolvable problems; and "second order," where random events or therapeutic interventions disrupt first-order solutions. These therapists view families as fundamentally homeostatic, or invested in maintaining the status quo even at the expense of a symptomatic family member. Consequently, this therapist anticipates a power struggle between him or her and the family and develops strategies to de-stabilize the power structure in the family. One such strategy involves the use of paradox, which is used to meet the family isomorphically at the time when they present for therapy. In essence, the position taken by the family is, "Help us get rid of the symptom, but don't make us change."

The Practice

The therapist inquires about the behavioral sequences that occur around the family's problem to understand the first-order solutions that the family has devised, solutions that themselves have become problems. The therapist is interested in the behaviors that occur when Mr. and Mrs. Bean attempt to get Pam to eat. For example, if Mr. Bean says to Pam, "Do you want to eat your sandwich?" and she says "No," he tries to reason with her. At this point, Mrs. Bean might interrupt and say, "Just eat," which annoys Mr. Bean, who says, "Let her finish eating on her own timetable." He adds, "Perhaps there is something you'd prefer to a sandwich." When Pam doesn't seem to respond, Mrs. Bean says, "Your not eating is just killing me." Pam responds by stating, "I won't eat even if you force the food down my throat." The strategic therapist notes that the more Mrs. Bean threatens, the more Pam protests; the more she protests, the more Mr. Bean tries to appease. But when he appeases, Pam still doesn't eat, and Mrs. Bean escalates her argument. Each parent feels that he or she is offering a logical solution: Mrs. Bean is insisting that Pam eat, and Mr. Bean is trying to leave the eating up to Pam. Both are first-order changes that leave Pam in an intolerable bind—to choose one parent over another.

This therapist, then, wants to introduce second-order change, by use of a paradoxical strategy (e.g., prescribing a symptom that is aimed at disrupting the current behavioral sequence). For example, the therapist could suggest, "Pam, I'd like you to resist your parents' efforts to get you to eat in order to prevent your premature compliance to parental authority." In being asked not to eat, she finds that her anorexia takes on new meaning and she is taken out of the bind of having to choose between her parents. This is a therapeutic double-bind:

that is, an intervention that mirrors the paradoxical communication in the family.

The Proponents

Milton Erikson[12] (whose focus on behavioral change relied on indirect suggestion through the use of stories, riddles, and metaphors) has heavily influenced this school. Strategic therapists have borrowed this reliance on playful storytelling techniques. The California Mental Research Institute (MRI) family therapists, including Jay Haley, Paul Wazlawick, John Weakland, and Gregory Bateson, were the earliest proponents of strategic family therapy. They encouraged therapists to look to the role of power in the therapeutic encounter, since families usually make paradoxical requests: for example, "Get us out of this mess but don't make us change."

Chloe Madanes[13] assumed that when children act out, their symptoms represent efforts to help the family. However, along with helping the family, the child's symptoms also reverse the generational hierarchy, placing the child in a position that is superior to that of his or her parents. Consequently, Madanes advocated using paradoxical techniques to re-assert the parents' authority. For example, she might invite the parent to ask the child to pretend to help out or to pretend to have the problem. In both instances, these strategies put the parents back in charge, while allowing the child a playful means of being helpful.

The Metaphor

The strategic family therapist is like a master chess player who knows from the start how he or she wants the game to turn out, and then maps out each move to get there. This therapist has a plan for each individual session and a vision for the outcome of this problem-focused therapy. In chess, as in therapy, there is a belief that a small move will set off reverberations throughout the game. This cascade of changes can similarly be planned and mapped out by the therapist.

SYSTEMIC FAMILY THERAPY
The Theory

The systemic family therapist believes that change occurs when beliefs are changed or the meaning of behavior is altered. In this view, the solutions, as well as the power to change, lie within the family. This therapist rejects the notion that the therapist holds a clear idea of what the family should look like at the end of successful treatment. The therapist does not presume to know the right truth to help a family. Instead, this therapist holds that there is no one truth; rather, some ideas are more useful than others.

The systemic therapist believes that the family is not homeostatic but instead is constantly evolving. The therapist identifies the place of "stuckness" that is marked by redundant interactional sequences, and introduces new information to the family without a plan for the family's response. This process is like seeing a mobile that has stopped moving in the wind, then pushing on it, and stepping back to watch (with surprise) how the pieces will resume movement. Movement takes place in leaps rather than in the incremental steps that are preferred by strategic family therapists.

The systemic therapist introduces new information in an effort to bring about systemic change. When Bateson[14] wrote that information is "news of a difference," he meant that we only register information that comes from making comparisons. He and other systemic therapists use circular questions, which are aimed at surfacing differences around time,

perception, ranking on a characteristic, and alliances within a family. Linear questions (e.g., "What made you depressed?") ask family members about cause and effect. Circular questions (e.g., "Who is most concerned about mother's depression? Then who? Then who?"), by contrast, take a problem and place it within the web of family relationships. Other circular questions (e.g., "Who in the family is the most concerned about Pam?" "When were things different in the family, when you weren't worried about Pam?") attempt to elicit hidden comparisons and useable information.

In addition, systemic therapists employ two additional kinds of interventions, the re-frame and the ritual. Re-framing offers interpretations of problematic behaviors that are neutral or positive and that connect everyone in the family. The therapist uses positive connotation in re-defining a problem to encourage cooperation, to introduce the idea of volition when behaviors have been regarded as outside of anyone's control, and to introduce confusion as a means to stimulate new thinking around tightly held beliefs.

A ritual is introduced, not as a behavioral directive, but as an experiment.[15] This therapist does not care if the ritual is carried out exactly as prescribed, since it is the ideas contained in the ritual that contain the power to change. When families enact two inconsistent behaviors simultaneously, a ritual can introduce time into this paradoxical system. With the Beans, the therapist might be struck by the ways that Mr. and Mrs. Bean treat Pam simultaneously as both a young girl and a young woman, undermining each other's position so that the parents are never on the same page at the same time. This therapist might suggest the following "odd-even day" ritual: "On Monday, Wednesday, and Friday, we would like you to regard Pam as a little girl who can't manage basic functions (such as eating). On Tuesday, Thursday, and Saturday, we'd like you to think about Pam as a young woman who is getting ready to leave home." The parents are given the opportunity to collaborate on a shared view of their daughter at the same time, first as a girl, then as a young woman.

Rituals and re-frames were usually introduced at the conclusion of a five-part meeting with a team of therapists and a family.[16]

The Practice

At the outset, this therapist, working either with or without a team, generates a few hypotheses to be confirmed or discounted using circular questions.[17] One hypothesis is that Pam's anorexia serves to keep her parents distracted from their own marital conflicts, which might escalate if they didn't have Pam to worry about. For example, the following circular questions could be asked: "If in five years Pam has graduated from college and is of normal weight, what would your relationship as parents be like?" "Who is most worried about Pam?" "If you weren't worried about Pam, where would that energy go?"

In trying to assess the validity of this hypothesis, the therapist pays attention to both the verbal responses of each family member and the non-verbal signs of interest in the questions. If family members seem interested in each other's responses, and if their answers are thoughtful rather than automatic, the therapist would likely craft an end-of-session intervention based on that hypothesis. The therapist might say to the Bean family, "I'm sorry that Pam feels that she has to sacrifice her well-being, health, and future to distract her parents from fighting or from being unhappy with one another. Mr. and Mrs. Bean, I think you should go out alone without informing Pam where you are going, nor when you are returning. Later, please record in a diary how she responds to this ritual." This message positively connotes Pam's anorexia and connects everyone in the family. Moreover, this is a ritual prescribed at the end that is an attempt to clarify generational boundaries.

The Proponents

Systemic family therapy was forged by a quartet of psychoanalysts (Drs. Mara Selvini Palazzoli, Luigi Boscolo, Gianfranco Cecchin, and Giulana Prata) who collaborated from 1971 to 1980 in Milan, Italy; they developed a multi-part team approach and used a one-way mirror to observe interactions. In the first part, or "presession," the team generates initial hypotheses that are based on referral information, such as "Who made the initial call?" and "What was the emotional tone on the phone?" as well as on clinical experiences of team members. In the second part of the team approach, one clinician interviews the family while the remainder of the team watches from behind a one-way mirror. The interviewing therapist seeks to confirm or refute the team's hypotheses by use of circular questions. During the third part, or "intersession," the team members create an intervention, which connects everyone in the family and offers a re-frame or ritual. Often these messages are succinct, enigmatic, hypnotic, and intended to introduce enough new information to produce change in the system.

The Milan school was also responsible for the introduction of the notions of circularity and neutrality. Circularity refers to thinking that emphasizes patterns, recursiveness, and context. Circular questions allow the therapist to be curious about the patterns of interaction in a family that are destructive to everyone, without blaming any one individual. The therapist's non-evaluative stance conveys respect and acceptance of the system, and it is synonymous with neutrality.

The Metaphor

This therapist is like the detective in a British mystery who interviews all of the suspects about a crime and then gathers them all in the parlor to tell them how the crime took place. The story he or she tells connects everyone's point of view, but is generally different from any one person's account. The experience of the reader of the story is to feel both confused and that the story makes perfect sense, even though it means re-evaluating each person's point of view. This mixture of confusion and resonance is what the systemic therapist aims for when he or she introduces a systemic opinion that alters meanings.

NARRATIVE FAMILY THERAPY
The Theory

Narrative family therapists rely on the transformative power of new language to create change. They posit that families get stuck because they have become constrained by a problem-saturated story and by constricted ways of talking among themselves about their difficulties. This therapist tries to identify the dominant stories that limit the family's possibilities, and then to amplify minor or undiscovered narratives that contain more hope for change. Dominant stories include beliefs that the family holds about itself, as well as any cultural stories (e.g., the idea that adolescents can only become adults through rebellion and rejection of their parents) that may influence the family.

These therapists use story in two significant ways: first, to de-construct, or to separate, problems from the people who experience them; and then to re-construct, or to help families re-write, the stories that they tell about their lives. These complementary processes of de-construction and re-construction

are exemplified in the technique of externalizing the problem.[18] With this technique, the therapist and the family create a name for the problem and attribute negative intentions to it so that the family can band together against the problem, rather than attack the individual who has the problem. The therapist subsequently asks about "unique outcomes," or times when the patient was free of the problem. The family is asked to wonder what made it possible at those times to find the strength to resist the pull of the problem. In time, these unusual moments of resistance are amplified and added to by more stories that feature the patient as competent and problem free.

Narrative therapists have also developed the concept known as the reflecting team, to aid in the treatment of families and the training of therapists.[19,20] With this approach a group of clinicians observe an interview through a one-way mirror, and then speak directly to the family, offering ideas, observations, questions, and suggestions.[21] These comments are offered tentatively and spontaneously so that the family can choose what is useful from among the team's offerings and reject the rest. Several narrative assumptions form the underpinning of the reflecting team[22]: the abundance of ideas generated by the team will help loosen a constricted story held by the family; the relationship between the therapist and the patient should be non-hierarchical (with an emphasis placed on sharing rather than on giving information); people change under a positive connotation; and there are no right or wrong ideas, just ones that are more or less helpful to a family.

The Practice

This therapist might begin by asking the Beans how they would know when the therapy was over. More specifically, he or she might ask the De Shazer miracle questions,[23] "If there were a miracle that took place overnight and Pam were no longer anorectic, what else would be different? How would the family be different? How would each of you be interacting with her?"

The therapist would also ask questions to de-construct the present problem by externalizing it. For example, he or she might say to Pam, "This culture helps anorexia trick young women into thinking that they will be more loveable and successful if they lose weight. What tricks has anorexia used on you?" And in an effort to construct a new story, the therapist might inquire of each of family member, "Who would be most surprised to learn that Pam has turned her back on anorexia and is taking charge of her future? When do you observe Pam saying 'no' to the tricks of anorexia and investing instead in a realistic view of herself, based on her gifts and talents?" With these questions, the narrative therapist is looking to expand and to elaborate on alternative versions of Pam that do not include her identification with an eating disorder.

Another narrative tact is to ask the Beans about the influence of culture on the problem. For example, "Do the Beans endorse the culture-based story that girls need to reject their mothers in order to grow into women?" The therapist is trying to uncover the stories that give meaning to the Beans' view of Pam's upbringing, stories that may constrain, rather than expand, possibility.

The Proponents

Michael White, in Australia, David Epston, in New Zealand and Jill Freedman and Gene Combs in Chicago are the best-known thinkers and writers of the narrative approach.[24,25] In addition to their ideas of de-constructing the problem through externalizing and re-authoring, they have emphasized the political and social context in which all clinical work occurs. Relying on the work of Foucault, they critique the professional's linkage of power and knowledge. For example, they do not make diagnoses or rely on medical records kept private from their patients. Instead, they may write a letter to a patient at the end of the session and use the same letter as the clinical note for the medical record. At the close of therapy, the record may be given to the patient or, with permission, shared with other patients who are struggling with similar difficulties.

The invention of the reflecting team is credited to Tom Andersen and his colleagues at the Tromso University in Norway in 1985. Observing the interview from behind the mirror, Andersen found that the therapist continued to follow a pessimistic view of the family, regardless of the re-framing questions that were phoned in by the team. Finally, after several attempts to re-direct the interview were thwarted, he "launched the idea to the family and the therapist that we might talk while they listened to us."[26] With the team speaking directly to the family, presenting multiple ideas in an unrehearsed way, the concept of the reflecting team took root.

The Metaphor

The narrative family therapist is like a biographer who takes the family's basic stories and transforms them with a different organization, a richer grasp of language and tone, and the addition of previously overlooked tales. The resulting story is a collaboration between therapist and family and contains story lines that hold more possibility than did the original story.

BEHAVIORAL FAMILY THERAPY
The Theory

Behavioral family therapy[27-29] derives from social learning theory, with particular attention paid to demonstrating empirical evidence for interventions. In this model, family systems represent members' best attempts to achieve personal and mutual rewards while avoiding negative consequences. In order for maladaptive behaviors to endure, they must be modeled or reinforced somewhere within the system. The therapist and the family will collaborate in an effort to identify behavioral patterns and sequences that are problematic. The therapist then employs varied, empirically-supported behavioral techniques to promote the learning of new adaptive behaviors while extinguishing their problematic predecessors.

The Practice

Behavioral family therapy relies on the ability to perform a detailed, functional behavioral analysis. The therapist begins with an assessment of the thoughts, feelings, and behaviors of each individual family member as they relate to the problem. Next, the therapist works with the family to detail representative sequences of behaviors that mark their current distress. For example, the therapist might ask the Bean family to recount with as much accuracy as possible a recent evening that culminated in an argument between Mrs. Bean and Pam over Pam's refusal to eat dinner. If dinnertime proves a particularly reliable time for conflict, the therapist might ask the family to tape record the evening events for a week (or at least make notes in a journal) to allow for more accurate observation.

The behavioral therapist will try to identify factors that both precipitate and relieve the problem. (Does Pam's refusal to eat correlate in any way with Mr. Bean's business trips? Have there been periods where the issue of Pam's eating seemed to be less of a struggle?) The consequences of the behavioral sequence are also of importance. (Do arguments between Mrs. Bean and Pam ultimately transform into arguments between Mr. and Mrs. Bean? Will Ellen typically come home from school on the weekend if she has learned of Pam having a difficult week?)

Ultimately, a hypothesis is generated as to the way each problematic behavior might be reinforced and what interventions might result in its extinction. The Bean family would be encouraged to choose specific goals. The therapist then acts as a collaborator and teacher, designing experiments that will test for behavioral changes. These will often be in the form of homework, but can also be conducted within the session. The results of these experiments will be analyzed with the same rigor of the initial assessment in order to assure all that they are proving objectively beneficial. Techniques include contingency contracting (Mr. and Mrs. Bean make reciprocal commitments to exchange positive regard for each other daily) and other operant reinforcement strategies (Mrs. Bean praises Pam's partial completion of meals, and does not comment on what is left over). Behavioral family therapy techniques have established empirical support across a broad range of conditions,[30-42] both as individual interventions and as adjuncts to other treatment modalities.

As the family collaborates experimentally with the therapist, there may be times when the stress of a crisis exceeds the family's current ability to effectively problem-solve. (Pam's medical condition declines, and Mr. and Mrs. Bean are unsuccessful in persuading Pam to consider hospitalization.) At these times, the behavioral therapist may take on a more directive role to assist in crisis management.

The Proponents

Robert Liberman[42] and Lawrence Weathers[43] have made major contributions to the field of behavioral family therapy, including their application of contingency contracting. This form of operant conditioning recognizes that families in distress tend to have an increase in aversive exchanges marked by negative affect. In the contingency contract, family members agree to undertake structured interactions designed at improving positive exchanges. Gerald Patterson,[44] along with Marion Forgatch,[45] has explored the way family systems reinforce aggressive behavior in adolescents. The reinforcement is characterized by intermittent punishment, empty threats, and parental irritability. Falloon and Liberman's[46] attention to levels of expressed emotion within families has informed both the behavioral and psychoeducational schools of family therapy.

The Metaphor

This therapist is like the civil engineer called on to re-configure well-established traffic patterns in a busy city. Congested areas must first be analyzed with respect to why drivers consistently choose these routes despite the availability of alternatives. Next, attention should be paid to how various interests (individual, government, business) might be affected by potential changes. Concerned parties would be solicited to express their concerns. Subsequently, a re-organization can be introduced in a step-wise fashion, interrupting prior patterns in an attempt to foster new ones. With each incremental change, traffic flow is measured and adjustments are made accordingly. Ultimately, the solution seeks to serve efficiency while maximizing the satisfaction of the individual, government, and business sectors.

PSYCHOEDUCATIONAL FAMILY THERAPY
The Theory

Psychoeducational family therapy[27-29] originated to assist families caring for a member with severe mental illness and functional impairment. The therapist understands family dysfunction as deficits in acquirable skills and knowledge. Through education and focused skills training, families and patients are empowered to effect their own change. The therapist anticipates deficiencies in several key domains. These include communication, problem-solving, coping, and knowledge of the illness. The therapist is also vigilant in identifying relationships that appear over-involved or hypercritical, because these are associated with an increased likelihood of relapse and exacerbations of the affected member's illness. The goal of therapy is to create an environment that is more deliberate in its fostering of mastery and recovery.

The Practice

Psychoeducational family therapy is conducted with individual families and with family groups. The treatment typically takes place in discrete phases that can be manualized for various disorders and contexts. Introduced at a time of crisis, the psychoeducational family therapist would begin with the Bean family during an inpatient hospitalization for Pam. Mrs. Bean could be allowed to mourn the loss of her healthy daughter. Ellen would be encouraged to offer happy memories of Pam before the onset of illness, illustrating family strengths in the process. During this first phase, referred to as *engagement*, the therapist seeks to establish an alliance with the family while evaluating their approach to crisis management. The therapist would seek detailed information regarding family communication styles and coping strategies while monitoring alliances and divisions. The therapist would hope to reassure the family about Pam's condition and set the stage for their participation in her treatment as effective agents of change.

Following engagement, the Bean family would be invited to an educational workshop along with a group of other families in a similar situation. Families would be provided with essential information to inform their understanding of the diagnosis, treatment, and prognosis of anorexia nervosa. Mr. and Mrs. Bean's expectation of Pam's rapid recovery following hospitalization would be challenged, along with reassurance that the expectable prolonged course does not preclude eventual recovery. Ellen's fear that Pam's amenorrhea would prevent future fertility would be dispelled. To the extent possible, the family would be encouraged to maintain regular schedules and activities. Warning signs of future relapses would be highlighted.

The next phase is marked by the process of Pam's re-entry into the community. The Bean family might meet twice weekly over the first few weeks following discharge. The therapist would offer methods designed to achieve goals important to this period. These include the maintenance of good interpersonal boundaries despite heightened anxiety and protectiveness, medication and appointment compliance, and surveillance for warning signs of impending relapse. Mr. and Mrs. Bean would receive guidance on how to effectively communicate with each other, Pam, and people outside the family as Pam begins to socialize with peers following her hospitalization.

The last phase, rehabilitation, focuses on the family's task of encouraging the slow, progressive increase of Pam's independence and responsibility for her condition. The therapist could advise the Bean family to speak with other families who have been successful in maintaining recovery from anorexia. Following months to years of cautious, gradual efforts, the Bean family would begin to anticipate the process of Pam going away to college.

The Proponents

Psychoeducational family therapy finds its origins in the treatment of schizophrenia. Carol Anderson[47] developed a psychoeducational model for schizophrenia, which she later adapted to affective disorders. William McFarlane[48] is responsible for the psychoeducational model illustrated in the previous example, which also was designed for families coping with schizophrenia. In his model, several families with schizophrenic members meet together for psychoeducation. Psychoeducational methods are finding continued empirically-supported applications for schizophrenia,[49] as well as conditions outside of the formal thought disorders,[50] and will likely continue to expand to additional diagnoses and contexts.

The Metaphor

This therapist is like a wilderness guide leading amateur enthusiasts into a state park. Before setting foot on the trails, basic myths of the forest are dispelled through basic classroom instruction. Prospective campers might learn that no snakes indigenous to the area are poisonous, while being cautioned that some innocent-looking mushrooms are. The guide then begins to lead expeditions of increasing difficulty, pointing out examples from the classroom while gradually assigning more responsibility to the campers. Finally, before letting the group explore on their own, the guide distributes flares and radios, so that help can easily be accessed should the need arise.

THE MAUDSLEY MODEL: AN EXAMPLE OF THEORY INTEGRATION

The Maudsley model of family-based treatment for anorexia nervosa in adolescents represents a powerful integration of all schools into a single, manualized, empirically-supported[33] method. This model is an example of two current trends in the field of family therapy: integration, rather than strict adherence to one theory,[51,52] and a move toward demonstrable research evidence for treatment efficacy.[53]

In general, the Maudsley model most closely resembles the psychoeducational school with its initial emphasis on education, usually at a time of crisis, followed by a multi-phase advancement toward increased independence and responsibility of the identified patient.

The first phase is single-minded in its pragmatic ultimate purpose: weight gain. In the first session, the Bean family is greeted warmly, and the therapist reviews Pam's current weight, the realities of the threat to her life, and key concepts fundamental to the illness, such as Pam's preoccupation with her body. Basic physiological effects of starvation, such as hypothermia and cardiac dysfunction, are explained in a manner understandable to the entire family. Externalization of the problem, reminiscent of the narrative school, is employed from the outset, and anorexia, rather than Pam or her family, is to be blamed for Pam's current state. The therapist models and reinforces non-critical behaviors and attitudes toward Pam and every other member of the family. High expressed emotion is discouraged.

The first phase typically includes a "family picnic" during an actual session. While there is an experiential quality to the exercise, there is a primarily structural agenda as the therapist disrupts any interactions that threaten parental control. With the therapist's assistance, Mr. and Mrs. Bean are directed to ensure that Pam eats one mouthful more than she wants to. As Pam continues to resist, Mr. Bean may give up, feeling powerless in his inability to engender a desire to eat on Pam's part. At this point, a systemic re-frame may prove helpful. Pam's resistance is analogous to the toddler who refuses penicillin in the setting of her discomfort from an infection. The penicillin must be administered nonetheless, as the toddler lacks sufficient judgment to act in her own best interest. Toddlers with serious infections must take antibiotics, and anorexics must eat. Should Pam then sabotage the session by eating well, the therapist may employ the strategic paradoxical injunction. "Pam, I want you to try to stop your parents from feeding you. I don't want you to lose your independence, just to try to find other ways to express your individuality."

Despite the pragmatism of this phase, the therapist remains vigilant for evidence of the abstract underpinnings of the dilemma. Like the psychodynamic therapist, the Maudsley model therapist respects how the past may relate to the present, and may explore Mr. Bean's sense of futility in the context of his unconscious representation of his sister's suicide.

The second phase of therapy begins as Pam establishes steady weight gain and the Beans can spontaneously express some initial relief of their anxieties. The goal is to begin to restore responsibility for eating to the adolescent. Here the emphasis on weight gain and eating becomes integrated with other adolescent issues that revolve around autonomy. Curfews and clothing styles, for example, are encouraged over eating, as areas of developing agency and individuality. Contingency contracts, such as those discussed in terms of behavioral therapy, might be employed in order for compliance with eating to be paired with parental permission for otherwise acceptable adolescent activities and interests. For example, Pam's girlfriends can stay over without too much parental intrusion so long as everyone has dinner together.

Typically, Pam's achievement of 95% of her ideal body weight would herald the final phase of this model. Here the focus is on the impact anorexia has had on Pam's identity development, while looking toward the future. Parental boundaries more typical of adolescence in the absence of anorexia become a transitional goal. Similarly, Mr. and Mrs. Bean must begin to consider their own transition, as with Pam's departure, there will be no more children living in the home year-round. Maintaining a structural stance, this element is clearly identified by the therapist as one for Mr. and Mrs. Bean to figure out, without the children's participation.

CONCLUSION

The field of family therapy has tended to value the distinctiveness of its different models[54]—the founding mothers and fathers of family therapy were typically dynamic mavericks who called attention to how different they were from individual psychotherapists and from each other. The growth of the field has not been driven by research, but rather by innovative theory and creative technique.

While there have been no studies comparing the efficacy of each of the major schools, many studies have looked at process variables and outcome measures within the behavioral[30–34,37–41] and psychoeducational[47,49] models. Shadish and colleagues,[55] summarizing their extensive meta-analysis of marital and family therapy, conclude that "no orientation is yet demonstrably superior to any other" (p. 348). The most effective approaches tend to be multi-disciplinary or integrative, such as the Maudsley model. More studies are needed to determine whether there are common factors that account for therapeutic change, regardless of the theoretical model. As with individual therapy, Wampold and colleagues[56] posit that the following

factors likely account for most of the change that transpires during family therapy: client factors, such as higher socioeconomic status, the shared cultural background between client and therapist,[57] and the family's ability to mobilize social supports; relationship factors, particularly the presence of warmth, humor, and positive regard in the therapeutic relationship[58]; and the family therapist's ability to engender hope and a sense of agency in family members. Additional common factors have been identified: client's feedback regarding progress in therapy and the quality of the therapeutic alliance.

The ability of integrative methods, such as the Maudsley model, to find empirical support speaks to the efficacy of family therapy ideology itself. To the extent that all schools and models represent a kinship by virtue of their ancestry, cause, and generativity toward future generations, it is no surprise that change and growth are spurred when new communication and collaboration between the "individuals" is achieved. This is not to suggest that the inevitable fate of family therapy is its reduction to a single, unified theory. Empirical support of efficacy for individual model-based treatments can render further efforts toward integration unnecessary and inefficient. However, when the understanding and abilities of an individual model seem "stuck," overwhelmed by a particular clinical context, it will often prove prudent to "bring in the family."

Access the complete reference list and multiple choice questions (MCQs) online at https://expertconsult.inkling.com

KEY REFERENCES

1. Fishel A. *Treating the adolescent in family therapy: a developmental and narrative approach*, Northvale, NJ, 1999, Jason Aronson.
2. Zinner J, Shapiro S. Projective identification as a mode of perception and behavior in families of adolescents. *Int J Psychoanal* 53:523–530, 1972.
3. McGoldrick M, Gerson G, Petry S. *Genograms. assessment and intervention*, ed 3, New York, 2008, Norton Professional Books.
6. Boszormenyi-Nagy I. *Invisible loyalties*, New York, 1973, Harper & Row.
7. Bowen M. *Family therapy in clinical practice*, New York, 1978, Jason Aronson.
8. Satir V. *Conjoint family therapy*, Palo Alto, CA, 1964, Science and Behavior Books.
10. Minuchin S. *Families and family therapy*, Cambridge, MA, 1974, Harvard University Press.
13. Madanes C. *Strategic family therapy*, San Francisco, 1981, Jossey-Bass.
15. Imber-Black E, Roberts J. *Rituals in families and family therapy*, New York, 1988, Norton.
17. Penn P. Circular questioning. *Fam Process* 21(3):267–280, 1982.
20. Andersen T. The reflecting team: dialogue and meta-dialogue in clinical work. *Fam Process* 26:415–428, 1987.
24. White M, Epston D. *Narrative means to therapeutic ends*, New York, 1990, Norton.
25. Freedman J, Combs G. Narrative couple therapy. In Gurman AS, editor: *Clinical handbook of couple therapy*, ed 4, New York, 2008, Guilford Press.
28. Lebow J, editor. *Handbook of clinical family therapy*, Hoboken, NJ, 2005, John Wiley & Sons.
29. Carr A. *Family therapy: concepts, process and practice*, Baffins Lane, England, 2000, John Wiley & Sons.
33. Robin AL, Siegel PT, Loepke T, et al. A controlled comparison of family versus individual therapy for adolescents with anorexia nervosa. *J Am Acad Child Adolesc Psychiatry* 38:1482–1489, 1999.
42. Liberman RL. Behavioral approaches to family and couple therapy. *Am J Orthopsychiatry* 40:106–119, 1970.
43. Weathers L, Liberman RL. Contingency contracting with families of delinquent adolescents. *Behav Ther* 6:356–366, 1975.
45. Patterson G, Forgatch M. *Parents and adolescents living together*, vol. 1, The basics, Eugene, OR, 1987, Castalia.

46. Falloon IR, Liberman RL. Behavioral therapy for families with child management problems. In Textor MR, editor: *Helping families with special problems*, New York, 1981, Jason Aronson.

51. Fraenkel P, Pinsof W. Teaching family-therapy centered integration: assimilation and beyond. *J Psychother Integration* 11(1):59–85, 2001.

52. Lebow J. The integrative revolution in couple and family therapy. *Fam Process* 36:1–18, 1997.

53. Lock J, Le Grange D, Agras WS, et al. *Treatment manual for anorexia nervosa: a family-based approach*, New York, 2001, Guilford Press.

55. Shadish WR, Ragsdale K, Glaser RR, et al. The efficacy and effectiveness of marital and family therapy: a perspective from meta-analysis. *J Marital Fam Ther* 21:345–360, 1995.

56. Sparks JA, Duncan B. Common factors in couples and family therapy. Must all have prizes? In Wampold BE, Duncan BL, Miller SD, editors: The heart and soul of change, ed 2, *Delivering what works in therapy*, Washington, DC, 2009, American Psychological Association.

13

14 Group Psychotherapy

Anne Alonso, PhD, CGP, DFAGPA†, Marni Chanoff, MD, and Kathleen Hubbs Ulman, PhD, CGP, FAGPA

KEY POINTS

Background

- Throughout history people have gathered in groups to survive and to accomplish challenging tasks. It is natural that they can heal best in groups.
- Group psychotherapy rests on the assumption that people need to move from a state of isolation to one involving contact with others who share common interests.
- Groups can vary in their length, membership, goals, techniques, and frequency of meetings.
- Group psychotherapy is an effective treatment for a wide variety of patients in outpatient or inpatient settings; it is an important aspect of treatment for the more distressed patients but it can stand alone for individuals who are more resilient and inner-directed.
- Research shows that group therapy is as effective as individual or pharmacotherapy over the course of a patient's recovery.
- The economics of group psychotherapy are a compelling argument in a climate of shrinking dollars for mental health care.

History

- Dr. Joseph Pratt is noted for conducting the first group therapy in the United States at the Massachusetts General Hospital. In 1905 he held groups for tuberculosis patients that included education, moral exhortation, sharing, and imitation as curative factors.
- In the early 1900s others in the United States experimented with using small groups (e.g., with schizophrenia, neurosis, alcoholism, children, prisoners, and, after WWII, veterans) for therapeutic purposes.
- By the 1950s modern theories of group therapy began to emerge.

Research Challenges

- Challenges to conducting research on the efficacy of group treatment rests on the difficulty in obtaining a control group, identifying and controlling the many variables that exist in a group, and creating internal validity while at the same time maintaining external validity by studying a group that reflects current clinical practice.
- Successful research on groups should include description and measurement of process variables, such as cohesion and containment.

Clinical Challenges

- Before approaching the concrete work of planning and organizing a psychotherapy group, the goals of the group must be clearly understood and be developed by the group leader. These goals will depend on the setting, the population, the time available for treatment, the treatment interventions, and the training and capacity of the leader(s). The group agreements, or contract, will be dictated by the goals.
- In outpatient settings, gathering a suitable group of patients ready to start a group is challenging.

Practical Pointers

- The greater the care taken in the designing of a group, the greater the chance of a more successful group; the more haphazard the planning, the greater the opportunity for the group to flounder around the members' resistances.
- The job of the therapist is to provide a safe context and meaning for the therapy group. This is done by designing a contract around the group's goal(s) and by carefully selecting members that are suitable for that group.
- The leader's stance in the group needs to be consistent with the goals of the group.
- Both anecdotal evidence and empirical evidence show that investment of significant amounts of time in the preparation of a patient for group therapy will improve the chances of successful entry and retention into a group.

OVERVIEW

The world of group psychotherapy has grown alongside the entire field of the many "talking therapies" during the last 75 years. Starting with Joseph Pratt in 1906 and his groups for tuberculosis (TB) patients in the early 1900s, the therapeutic use of groups expanded to specific populations, such as those with alcoholism or schizophrenia, until the 1950s saw the development of various group theories and continued expansion of its applications.[1]

Put simply, group psychotherapy rests on the assumption that people need to move from a state of isolation (that so often accompanies mental distress) and towards making contact with others who share common interests (in order to heal and to grow).[1] The presence of committed others who come together with an expert leader to explore the inner and outer workings of each member's personal dilemmas drives the process. Whether an individual suffers from serious mental illness, from conflicted life dilemmas, from medical illness, or from existential trauma, where otherwise normal people are crushed by abnormal situations (e.g., the terrorist attacks of Sept. 11, 2001; war; or natural disasters, such as Hurricane Katrina), a well-organized and well-led group can have a beneficial influence on the bio-psycho-social spectrum of the human organism.

A therapy group is a collection of patients who are selected and brought together by the leader for a shared therapeutic goal (Table 14-1). In this chapter some of the goals of a therapy group will be described. Group therapy rests on some common assumptions that apply to the entire panoply of

TABLE 14-1 Comparison of Group Psychotherapies as Currently Practiced in the United States

Group psychotherapy has developed alongside individual therapy, along dimensions that are appropriate to the patient population and to the setting in which the group is conducted. The general rule is that for the more disabled patient, who may be treated in an institutional setting, the group will need to be more supportive and aimed at reducing anxiety. For the more resilient and healthier patient in an outpatient setting, the group may be more appropriately conducted in a way that uncovers obsolete defenses and seeks to allow the individuals to find newer options around which to organize the self. The latter method is apt to increase anxiety as the syntonic becomes dystonic, on the way to a reorganization of character.

Parameters	Day Hospital/ Inpatient Group	Supportive Group Therapy	Psychodynamic Group	Cognitive-Behavioral Group
Duration	1 week to 6 months	Up to 6 months or more	1–3+ years	Up to 6 months
Indications	Acute or chronic major mental illness	Shared universal dilemmas	Neurotic disorders and borderline states	e.g., phobias, compulsive problems
Pre-group Screening	Sometimes	Usually	Always	Usually
Content Focus	Extent and impact of illness; plan for return to baseline	Symptoms, loss, life management	Present and past life situations; intra-group and extra-group relationships	Cognitive distortions, specific symptoms
Transference	Positive institutional transference encouraged	Positive transference encouraged to promote improved functioning	Positive and negative to leader and members, evoked and analyzed	Positive relationship to leader fostered; no examination of transference
Therapist Activity	Empathy and reality testing	Strengthen existing defenses by actively giving advice and support	Challenge defenses, reduce shame, interpret unconscious conflict	Create new options, active and directive
Interaction Outside of Group	Encouraged	Encouraged	Discouraged	Variable
Goals	Reconstitute defenses	Better adaptation to environment	Reconstruction of personality dynamics	Relief of specific psychiatric symptoms

Chart adapted from Stern TA, Herman JB, editors. Massachusetts General Hospital psychiatry update and board preparation, *ed 2, New York, 2004, McGraw-Hill.*

therapeutic groups. Recent psychoanalytic thinking recognizes the importance of intimate relationships at all ages and the need for others resides in all humans. The need for attachment is seen as primary by a whole host of group theorists; the press for belonging is that which yields a sense of cohesion that can help the individual tolerate the anxious moments when faced with a group of strangers.[2] For better and for worse, people who wish to belong to a cohesive community are apt to mimic and to identify with the feelings and beliefs of other members in that community.[3] At its best, this process allows for new interpersonal learning; at its worst, it raises the specter of dangerous mobs. People in distress tend to downplay and to mute their concerns to avoid facing their problems. In a group, each member is exposed to feelings, to needs, and to drives that increase the individual's awareness of his or her own passions and blind spots. There is an inevitable pull (based on the contagion and amplification that often overrides the normal shyness of individuals in a crowd of strangers) to get to know others more intimately in a group. As the members of a cohesive group move away from being strangers and get to know each other more deeply, they experience their own approaches to intimacy with others and with the self; in exchange, they receive immediate feedback on the impact they have on important others in their surroundings.

Many efforts have been made to describe the curative factors in a therapy group. Summed up into the essential elements, groups help people change and grow by allowing the individual within the group to grow and develop beyond the constrictions in life that brought that person into treatment. All group theorists have used some of the therapeutic factors identified in Table 14-2. The more common healing factors are those that act by reducing each individual's isolation, by diminishing shame (which we have come to recognize as a major pathogenic factor in mental illness), and by evoking

memories of early familial attitudes and interactions (that now can be approached differently with a new set of options in the context of support). Another healing factor is expanding one's behavioral options. The problematic interpersonal behavior patterns that developed in childhood can be reshaped into a broader emotional and behavioral repertoire that can be practiced among group members in the here and now. Provision of support and empathic confrontation can be curative as well. People often fear groups because they imagine they will be the target of harsh confrontation; they are unaware that the cohesive group is a marvellous source of concern and problem-solving. Lastly, unmourned losses are often at the root of a melancholic and depressive stance. Listening to others grieve and responding to others' awareness of our own losses can free an individual to move on.[3]

Psychotherapy groups are as good as their clarity of purpose; the group contract ensues from that clarity. Therapists form groups for a wide variety of therapeutic purposes. Many groups provide support for patients with major illnesses. People in acute and immediate distress often find support in groups that have as their main goal a re-establishment of a person's equilibrium. Patients who have suffered a breakdown of their lives and who have needed hospitalization can use groups on inpatient units or in partial hospital settings to focus on the patient's sensorium, to manage acute distress, to plan for a return to the community, to help in dealing with the shameful consequences of hospitalization and to establish outpatient treatment. Many patients who have experienced an acute medical illness find groups helpful to re-gain equilibrium, to deal with the shame inherent in losing the ability to live independently, and to prepare to re-enter the world outside of the medical environment.

Since Dr. Pratt first offered his "classes" for tubercular patients at the Massachusetts General Hospital in 1905,[4]

TABLE 14-2 Yalom's Therapeutic Factors in Group Psychotherapy

There are many attempts to categorize what is effective in group therapy. Some factors will be more or less active depending on the kind of group. For example, corrective familial experience will figure prominently in psychodynamic groups, whereas cognitive-behavioral groups will emphasize learning and reality testing. Some are universal to all groups, such as the following:

Factor	Definition
ACCEPTANCE	The feeling of being accepted by other members of the group. Differences of opinion are tolerated, and there is an absence of censure.
ALTRUISM	The act of one member helping another; putting another person's need before one's own and learning that there is value in giving to others. The term was originated by Auguste Comte (1798–1857), and Freud believed it was a major factor in establishing group cohesion and community feeling.
COHESION	The sense that the group is working together toward a common goal; also referred to as a sense of "we-ness." It is believed to be the most important factor related to positive therapeutic effects.
CONTAGION	The process in which the expression of emotion by one member stimulates the awareness of a similar emotion in another member.
CORRECTIVE FAMILIAL EXPERIENCE	The group re-creates the family of origin for some members who can work through original conflicts psychologically through group interaction (e.g., sibling rivalry, or anger toward parents).
EMPATHY	A capacity of a group member to put himself or herself into the psychological frame of reference of another group member and thereby understand his or her thinking, feeling, or behavior.
IMITATION	The conclusion of emulation or modeling of one's behavior after that of another (also called role modeling); it is also known as spectator therapy, as one patient learns from another.
INSIGHT	Conscious awareness and understanding of one's own psychodynamics and symptoms of maladaptive behavior. Most therapists distinguish two types: (1) intellectual insight—knowledge and awareness without any changes in maladaptive behavior; (2) emotional insight—awareness and understanding leading to positive changes in personality and behavior.
INSPIRATION	The process of imparting a sense of optimism to group members; the ability to recognize that one has the capacity to overcome problems; it is also known as instillation of hope.
INTERPRETATION	The process during which the group leader formulates the meaning or significance of a patient's resistance, defenses, and symbols; the result is that the patient develops a cognitive framework within which to understand his or her behavior.
LEARNING	Patients acquire knowledge about new areas, such as social skills and sexual behavior; they receive advice, obtain guidance, attempt to influence, and are influenced by other group members.
REALITY TESTING	Ability of the person to evaluate objectively the world outside the self; this includes the capacity to perceive oneself and other group members accurately.
VENTILATION	The expression of suppressed feelings, ideas, or events to other group members; sharing of personal secrets ameliorates a sense of sin or guilt (also referred to as self-disclosure).

Adapted from Yalom ID. Theory and practice of group psychotherapy, *ed 5, New York, 2005, Basic Books.*

people have come together to commiserate with one another around common problems, to share information, and to learn how to deal with the impact of those problems on their lives. These groups are often referred to as "symptom specific" or "population specific." Groups have been organized around medical illnesses (e.g., cancer, diabetes, acquired immunodeficiency syndrome [AIDS]),[5] around psychological problems (e.g., bereavement),[6] and around psychosocial sequelae of trauma (e.g., war or natural disasters).[7] The goals of such groups are to provide support and information that are embedded in a socially-accepting environment with people who are in a position to understand what the others are going through. The treatment may emerge from cognitive-behavioral principles, from psychodynamic principles, or from psychoeducational ones. Frequently, these groups tend to be time-limited; members often join at the same time and terminate together. The problems addressed in these groups are found in a broad variety of patients, from the very healthy to the more distressed, and they cut across other demographic variables (e.g., age and culture).[6]

Some psychotherapy groups seek to provide relief based on symptomatic rather than developmental diagnoses. Treatment goals include alleviation of symptoms and a change in behavior. For example, patients with eating disorders, stress, or specific phobias are clustered in groups that can promote skills for self-monitoring and replace an automatic symptom with a more adaptive set of behaviors and cognitions.[6,8,9] These groups may include members with a broad range of intrapsychic development.

Group therapy is the treatment of choice for people with chronic and habitual ways of dealing with life, even when those ways run counter to the patients' best interest.[2,10,11] Characterological problems often occur outside of the patient's awareness (often to the disbelief and the alarm of others who see the problems clearly), and are syntonic and perceived as "Who I am" when brought into awareness. Like all bad habits, such ingrained behaviors are resistant to change, even when the patient wants to make such a change. When these characterological stances occur in the group, they are often repeated and come to the attention of the other members, who respond by confrontation and with offers of alternative strategies. In current parlance the term *neurotic* implies a relatively healthy individual who contains conflict, who owns some of the responsibility, and who may be nonetheless conflicted and guilty about his or her own life related to early developmental realities. In a psychodynamic open-ended group therapy, the neurotic patient observes resistance to intimacy and ambition, and works within the multiple transferences to develop a freer access to life's options.[1,11]

A group leader must exercise authority over each of the aforementioned factors if the group is to be safe and containing for its members.[1] The privilege and burden of

clinical vignette), he was caught in a blind spot of considerable proportion having to do with his vulnerability to the contagion of affect from the members. His supervisor helped him to recognize the problem, to work out the more personal aspects of his psychological stress in his own treatment, and to learn some ways of capitalizing on the moment to his patients' advantage.

Supervision is also a way for the leader to take advantage of his or her affiliative needs and to avoid using the patient group for dealing with the loneliness of the well-functioning group leader. In addition to departmental faculty with group therapy expertise, there are professional organizations that offer ongoing training and supervision for group leaders at all levels of experience.

Access the complete reference list and multiple choice questions (MCQs) online at https://expertconsult.inkling.com

KEY REFERENCES

1. Rutan JS, Stone WS, Shay JJ, editors. *Psychodynamic group psychotherapy*, ed 4, New York, 2007, Guilford Press.
2. Kleinberg JL, editor: *The Wiley-Blackwell handbook of group psychotherapy*, Chichester, UK, 2012, Wiley-Blackwell.
3. Yalom ID. *Theory and practice of group psychotherapy*, ed 5, New York, 2005, Basic Books.
4. MacKenzie KR, editor. *Classics in group psychotherapy*, New York, 1992, Guilford Press.
5. Ulman KH. Group psychotherapy with the medically ill. In Kaplan HI, Saddock BJ, editors: *Comprehensive group psychotherapy*, ed 3, Baltimore, 1993, Williams & Wilkins.
6. Burlingame GM, Strauss B, Joyce AS. Change mechanisms and effectiveness of small group treatments. In Lambert MJ, editor: *Handbook of psychotherapy and behaviour change*, ed 6, Hoboken, New Jersey, 2013, Wiley.
7. Buchele BJ, Spitz HI. *Group interventions for the treatment of psychological trauma*, New York, NY, 2004, American Group Psychotherapy Association.
8. Ulman KH. An integrative model of stress management groups for women. *Int J Group Psychother* 50:341–361, 2000.
9. Riess H. Integrative time-limited group therapy for bulimia nervosa. *Int J Group Psychother* 52:1–26, 2002.
10. Alonso A, Swiller HI, editors. *Group therapy in clinical practice*. Washington, DC, 1993, American Psychiatric Press.
11. Kauff P. Psychoanalytic group psychotherapy: An overview. In Kleinberg JL, editor: *The Wiley-Blackwell handbook of group psychotherapy*, Chichester, UK, 2012, Wiley-Blackwell.
12. Gans JS. Broaching and exploring the question of combined group and individual therapy. *Int J Group Psychother* 40:123–137, 1990.
13. Blackford JU, Love R. Dialectical behavior therapy group skills training in a community mental health setting: a pilot study. *Int J Group Psychother* 64:645–657, 2011.
14. MacNair-Semands R. *Ethics in group psychotherapy*, New York, 2005, American Group Psychotherapy Association.
15. Greene LR. Group therapist as social scientist, with special reference to the psychodynamically oriented psychotherapist. *Am Psychologist* 67:477, 2012.
16. Burlingame GM, Strauss B, Joyce A, et al. *CORE battery-revised: An assessment tool kit for promoting optimal group selection, process and outcome*, New York, 2006, American Group Psychotherapy Association.
17. MacKenzie KR. *Time-managed group psychotherapy*, Washington, DC, 1997, American Psychiatric Press.

15 Hypnosis

Owen S. Surman, MD, Lee Baer, PhD, and Alex S. Keuroghlian, MD MSc

KEY POINTS

- Hypnosis has been used successfully for healing under various names and in varied forms for thousands of years.
- Hypnosis is most effective in the control of pain and discomfort and in the treatment of stress-related illnesses.
- Individuals differ in their responsiveness to hypnotic interventions.
- Several reliable physiological and functional neural differences have been found between individuals with high and low levels of hypnotizability.
- Multiple randomized controlled trials support the efficacy of hypnosis for a variety of psychological and physical disorders.

OVERVIEW

Hypnosis is a popular form of complementary medicine, as well as an historical antecedent and adjunct to current psychiatric practice. While definitions of hypnosis vary, it is useful to think of it as a ritualized event in which practitioner and patient(s) agree to use suggestion to promote a change in perception and behavior.

Techniques vary with the influence of social custom and an individual's professional style. Current practice typically combines specific, sometimes repetitive, spoken instruction and encouragement toward virtual experience of events with the goal of promoting adaptive expectation. Applications in psychological and medical practice are myriad, particularly in the control of pain and discomfort and in the treatment of stress-related conditions.

HISTORICAL BACKGROUND
Anton Mesmer and Mesmerism

Healers of varied traditions have used suggestive therapies throughout history. The origin of medical hypnosis is generally attributed to Anton Mesmer, a Jesuit-trained eighteenth-century physician, who believed that health was determined by a proper balance of a universally present, invisible magnetic fluid. Mesmer's early method involved application of magnets. He was an important medical figure at the Austrian court, but he fell into discredit when a scandal occurred around his care of Maria Paradise, a young harpsichordist whose blindness appears to have been a form of conversion disorder.

Mesmer re-established his practice in Paris and employed a device reminiscent of the Leyden jar, a source of significant popular interest in the Age of Enlightenment. His patients sat around a water-containing iron trough–like apparatus (a *bacquet*) with a protruding iron rod. He was a colorful figure who accompanied his invocation for restored health with the passage of a wand; there was no physical contact with his patients. Susceptible individuals convulsed and were pronounced cured. An enthusiastic public greeted Mesmer's practice and theory of "animal magnetism." However, medical colleagues were less impressed. The French Academy of Science established a committee, led by Benjamin Franklin, the American ambassador to France, who was an expert in electricity.[1] The committee found no validation for Mesmer's magnetic theories, but determined that the effects were due to the subjects' "imagination."

The work of one of Mesmer's disciples, the Marquis De Puyseguer, brought a new approach to the practice of Mesmerism. The method involved induction of a somnambulistic state associated with post-trance amnesia.

James Esdaile, a nineteenth-century Scottish physician, was the first to take advantage of this somnambulistic state induced by Mesmerism to relieve surgical pain. Esdaile served as a military officer in the British East India Company, and took care of primarily Indian patients in and around Calcutta between 1845 and 1851. Over this period, Esdaile performed more than 3,000 operations (including hundreds of major surgeries) using only Mesmerism as an anesthetic, with only a fraction of the complications and deaths that were commonplace at the time. Many of these operations were to remove scrotal tumors (scrotal hydroceles), which were endemic in India at the time, and which in extreme cases swelled to a weight greater than the rest of the individual's body. Before Esdaile's use of Mesmeric anesthesia, surgery to remove these tumors usually resulted in death, due to shock from massive blood loss during the operation.[2]

Although Esdaile's technique was clearly effective in many cases, it was controversial enough that, as in Mesmer's case a century earlier, a committee was appointed and sent to India to observe Mesmeric anesthesia first hand and to evaluate its efficacy. Esdaile performed six operations for scrotal hydroceles for the committee (which consisted of the Inspector General of hospitals, three physicians, and three judges). He carefully selected nine potential patients by attempting to induce a "Mesmeric trance" using the customary technique of passing his hands over their bodies for a period of 6 to 8 hours; as a result, three of the patients were dismissed when it was found that they could not be mesmerized even after repeated attempts over 11 days. Another three calmly faced the surgery, but when the first incision was made signaled severe pain by "twitching and writhing of their body, by facial expressions of severe pain, and by labored breathing and sighs." The remaining three patients demonstrated to the committee "no observable bodily signs of pain throughout the operation." Nevertheless, the committee dismissed Esdaile's technique as a fraud and stripped him of his medical license.

Early Applications of Hypnosis in Medical Practice

Early in the nineteenth century some surgeons advocated the use of this new procedure for pain reduction in the operating theatre. James Braid, a British surgeon, called it "hypnosis" after the Greek root for sleep. Some questioned its apparent utility, and thought it was "humbug."

The prominent French neurologist Jean Martin Charcot studied hypnosis at the Salpêtrière in Paris, where he worked with a large population of women who suffered from hysteria. Charcot linked hypnosis with hysteria and considered it an expression of neuropathology. Janet's concept of dissociation followed.

A prominent internist, Hippolyte Bernheim, studied hypnosis at a French school at Nancy. He worked with a country doctor known as "Pere Liebeault" for his *pro bono* work with patients who agreed to undergo hypnosis for therapeutic purposes. The Nancy School found hypnosis to be a normal phenomenon that operated through suggestion.

Hypnosis in Psychiatric Practice

Sigmund Freud studied with Charcot, and also at Nancy.[3] He was a skilled hypnotist, but he came to believe that it had an unwanted impact on transference and it was therefore incompatible with his psychoanalytic method. Instead, Freud substituted his method of free association.

Eriksonian hypnosis, named for its founder, Milton Erikson, is a counterpoint to Freud's earlier position. Erikson advocated strategic interactions with his patients that employed use of metaphor and indirect methods of behavior shaping. While hypnotizability is generally considered to be an individual trait, Erikson believed that the efficacy of hypnotherapy depended on the skill of the therapist.[4]

CURRENT RESEARCH AND THEORY
Theoretical Perspectives on the Hypnotic State

Theorists have debated the view of hypnosis as an altered state of consciousness. Alternatively, researchers have focused on social factors and on role-playing capacity as an explanation of the phenomena associated with hypnosis.

Martin Orne's[5] work at the University of Pennsylvania identified the demand characteristics (based on a hierarchical relationship) of interaction between the hypnotist and the subject. He used sham hypnosis as an effective research tool. Orne also addressed the memory distortion that can occur with hypnosis and exposed its lack of validity for courtroom procedures, and he defined "trance logic" as a willing suspension of belief that highly hypnotizable subjects readily experience.

Ernest Hilgard[6] and associates postulated the "neodissociation" theory of hypnosis. Hilgard saw hypnotic process as an alteration of "control and monitoring systems" as opposed to a formal alteration of conscious state. He differentiated between the unavailability of a truly unconscious process and the "split off", but subsequently retrievable material involved in dissociation.

David Spiegel[7] has pointed to absorption, dissociation, and automaticity as core components of the hypnotic experience. Absorption has been found to be the only personality trait related to an individual's ability to experience hypnosis. Box 15-1 contains several items from the Tellegen Absorption Scale to illustrate the characteristics of this trait.[8]

Effects on Physiological Function

Hypnotic suggestion has been found to produce changes in skin temperature in some subjects. Immunological change has been evident in some studies of hypnosis and allergy and in the successful treatment of warts. Changes in evoked sensory potential have also been observed with hypnotic subjects.[9] In addition, a few studies have found improved wound healing with hypnosis. However, these phenomena are not necessarily specific to the hypnotic process.

Measurement of Hypnotic Susceptibility

Reliable measurement of hypnotic susceptibility is available with several scales (including the Stanford Scales and Harvard Group Scales of Hypnotizability).[10] These scales begin with the

---

BOX 15-1 Sample Yes/No Questionnaire Items from the Tellegen Absorption Scale

- Do you often get so engrossed in music that you forget what's going on around you?
- Do you often remember experiences so vividly that you feel, in part, as if you were reliving them?
- Is it common for certain smells to trigger very vivid memories for you?
- Do you often imagine or fantasize an experience so vividly that you become engrossed in it?
- Do memories often come to you as strong physical feelings in your body that remind you of a past experience?
- Do you often become so engrossed in a good movie or book that you forget what is going on around you?
- Do your thoughts often come to you as images or pictures?

Gently close your eyes and let your body relax into the chair. Just let it support you. Keep your eyes closed and listen carefully to me and you can gradually enter a state of hypnosis. Just let your muscles relax. Begin by letting the muscles in your right foot relax. As you focus your attention on your right foot your muscles will begin to let go and relax. The muscles in your right foot and your right lower leg are relaxing. And now your right upper leg can also begin to relax. You'll feel feelings of heaviness, comfort and warmth in your right leg as it relaxes more and more. Now on the left side, focus your attention on your left foot–let the muscles in your left foot relax. Pay close attention to tingling and heavy sensations and warmth, and your left foot will relax. And as you focus on your left lower leg and calf, the muscles there will begin to relax too. Your left lower leg and now your left upper leg will begin to relax. Now I'd like you to pay attention to your right hand. Let the muscles in your right hand relax. Let the muscles go limp, and relaxed. The muscles in your lower arm will also go limp and relaxed–and in your right upper arm–your whole right arm will feel comfortable and heavy. Now on the left side–let the muscles in the fingers of the left hand go limp and relaxed. Pay close attention to the heavy, warm, comfortable feelings in your left hand and now in your left forearm. Let your left forearm and now your left upper arm begin to relax. Just let the bed or the chair support you–sink into it and let your body relax, and soon you will enter a comfortable state of hypnosis. Let the muscles in your face, your scalp, your jaws go limp and relaxed. With each breath you exhale the muscles in your stomach and chest will become more relaxed. Now to help you go deeper into hypnosis I'm going to count from 1 to 20. With each count you will feel yourself going deeper. 1-2-3-4-5 going deeper and deeper into hypnosis. 6-7-8-9-10, halfway there, always more deeply hypnotized. 11-12-13-14-15, more and more comfortable, more and more deeply hypnotized. 16-17-18-19-20. Comfortably hypnotized in a peaceful state of hypnosis. During this self-hypnosis your body and mind will relax and you can give yourself suggestions that will be helpful to your body and your mind. You will remain comfortably in this state of hypnosis until you decide that it's time to end this hypnosis and go back to your normal waking state. And when do, you will feel alert, and comfortable, and refreshed. Just remain comfortably hypnotized.

Figure 15-1. Sample hypnotic induction script used in rating hypnotizability.

---

induction of hypnosis by reading the subject a script similar to that contained in Figure 15-1.

Next, subjects are administered a series of test suggestions, graded from easy to difficult, similar to those shown in Figure 15-2, and their objective and subjective responses are scored as present or absent. Finally, a total score is computed and

Hold your left arm straight out in front of you, with your arm at shoulder height, with your palm facing downward, toward the floor.

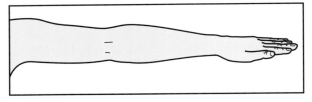

Now concentrate on your left arm, as you listen carefully to me:

- Your arm is starting to feel lighter and lighter.
- It is feeling so light that it is beginning to move up and up.
- It feels as if it doesn't have any weight at all, and it's moving up and up, more and more.
- Your arm is as light as a feather, it's weightless and rising toward the ceiling.
- It's lighter and lighter and moving up and up.
- It doesn't have any weight at all and it's moving up and up, more and more.
- It's lighter and lighter, moving up and up, more and more, higher and higher.

{Score + if arm rises at least 6 inches by end of suggestion}

Figure 15-2. Example item in a series used to assess hypnotic responsiveness.

compared with published norms for each scale. Across scales, approximately 10%–15% of subjects fall into the "high hypnotizability" range, another 15%–20% fall in the "low hypnotizability" range, and the remainder fall in an intermediate range.

Moderate levels of hypnotizability are important for clinical efficacy, although the level of hypnotic responsiveness does not ensure therapeutic success.

The Tellegen Absorption Scale correlates with hypnotic responsiveness.[8] Absorption refers to a process of concentration and a narrowing of attention. Clinical observations of absorption (e.g., in competitive sports and other forms of performance) may be a clue to a patient's hypnotizability.

Frankel and Orne[11] found that hypnotizability was generally greater among patients with monosymptomatic phobias. Patients with post-traumatic stress disorder (PTSD) and dissociative states generally have higher levels of hypnotizability. Patients with trauma early in life are typically good hypnotic responders.

Measurement of Hypnotic Depth

Measurement of hypnotic depth is a subjective process that does not correlate with clinical utility.

Functional Neuroanatomy of Hypnosis

Neuroimaging studies have found an association between high hypnotizability and mechanisms of attention (including a finding of increased volume of the anterior corpus callosum in highly hypnotizable subjects who are most adept at hypnotic anesthesia).[12,13] There is also similar activation of limbic circuits in hypnosis and in the recall of traumatic events.[14]

Hypnosis has been found to modify the perceptual response in the somatosensory system through a decrease in the amplitude of early (P100) and late (P300) waveform components of event-related potentials,[15] as well as decreasing dorsal anterior cingulate (dACC) and somatosensory cortical activity during hypnotic modulation of pain perception.[16–18] Pain

experienced through hypnotic induction is correlated with increased activity in the dACC, dorsolateral prefrontal cortex (DLPFC), parietal cortex, and thalamus.[19] High hypnotizability is associated with elevated dACC and insula activity during hypnosis used to imagine handgrip.[20] When highly hypnotizable persons were asked to perceive either color or a gray scale under hypnosis, neural activity in the fusiform and lingual regions of the brain was modulated according to these perceptual instructions regardless of whether an actual color or a gray scale was shown.[21] Moreover, hypoactivity occurs in the dACC when hypnosis is used to decrease color-word interference during the Stroop attentional test.[13,22,23]

The dACC and lateral prefrontal cortex (PFC) have been implicated in the top-down hypnotic alteration of perception, since only highly hynotizable individuals exhibit modulation of dACC and PFC activity during hypnotic analgesia, as well as during dampened Stroop interference.[16–19,23–25] When hypnosis is used to decrease the perception of pain, there is a corresponding decrease in dACC activity and elevated functional connectivity of both the anterior insula and the PFC with the primary somatosensory cortex.[26]

Hoeft and colleagues found that during neural resting states, highly hypnotizable individuals show greater activity in the DLPFC, a brain region critical for executive-control functions.[27] Additionally, highly hypnotizable individuals have increased cross-network coupling between the dACC and the DLPFC,[27] indicating greater coordination of brain regions involved in salience with those implicated in executive-control. The authors suggested that this coordinated increase in dACC and DLPFC activity may distinguish intrinsic trait hypnotizability from the acquired skill of mindfulness meditation, during which elevated neural activity is instead observed in the left frontal region.[27,28]

Genetic and Molecular Basis of Hypnosis

Trait hypnotizability has been associated with elevated cerebrospinal fluid levels of homovanillic acid, a metabolite of dopamine,[29] which figures prominently in dACC and DLPFC neurotransmission.[27] The val/met heterozygous polymorphism of the catechol-O-methyl transferase gene on chromosome 22 is correlated with higher hypnotizability, perhaps through modulation of dopamine metabolism, leading to enhanced attentional control mechanisms in the prefrontal cortex and greater absorption in tasks.[13,27,30–32]

EVIDENCE FOR THE EFFICACY OF HYPNOSIS

A number of randomized controlled trials have been conducted to assess the efficacy of hypnosis for a variety of medical and psychological conditions.[26,33,34] Box 15-2 summarizes the results of these studies, which demonstrate the strongest support for the efficacy of hypnosis in the control of pain and discomfort, usually for the more highly hypnotizable participants.

CLINICAL INDICATIONS FOR HYPNOSIS
Customary Clinical Use

Hypnotherapists commonly use direct suggestion for relaxation, followed by instruction in self-hypnosis. Sessions may be recorded for home use. Suggestion under hypnosis is commonly used for habit disorders, for reduction of a variety of somatic symptoms, and for smoking cessation. As a tool for smoking cessation it offers no general advantage over other forms of suggestion, but it may have specific appeal to some smokers.

15

BOX 15-2 Review of Current Evidence from Controlled and Partially Controlled Trials for Medical Applications of Hypnosis

EVIDENCE OF EFFICACY (SUPPORTED BY MULTIPLE RANDOMIZED CLINICAL TRIALS)

- Control of cancer pain
- Control of labor and childbirth pain
- Control of medical procedure–related pain and distress
- Reduction of symptoms of irritable bowel syndrome
- Improved post-operative outcome in wound healing, anxiety, and vomiting
- Obesity (although effects are small)

POSSIBLE EVIDENCE OF EFFICACY (SUPPORTED BY POORLY CONTROLLED TRIALS OR MIXED RESULTS)

- Control of burn pain
- Control of pain in terminally ill cancer patients
- Reduction of symptoms of asthma
- Reduction of symptoms of fibromyalgia[53]
- Smoking cessation
- Reduction of symptoms of non-ulcer dyspepsia
- Reduction of symptoms of post-traumatic stress disorder
- Reduction of symptoms of tinnitus
- Reduction of symptoms of conversion disorder

NO EVIDENCE OF EFFICACY (NEGATIVE CONTROLLED TRIALS)

- Schizophrenia
- Hayfever
- Delayed-type hypersensitivity response

Joseph Wolpe[27,35,36] applied hypnosis or progressive muscle relaxation to facilitate systematic desensitization. Arnold Lazarus[37] demonstrated the importance of patient expectation by randomizing phobic patients to one of these two techniques. There was a significant tendency of patients to respond best to their treatment of preference.

Hypnosis has continued as an adjunct to behavior therapy. Surman[38] proposed a modification of systematic desensitization termed *post-noxious desensitization,* especially applicable to performance anxiety. The approach begins with assumption of ultimate mastery about the phobic event. To date there have been no clinical trials. Hypnosis is also applicable to covert sensitization, a technique that may accompany treatment of habit disorders and tobacco dependence.

Some investigators have found that hypnosis improves the efficacy of behavior therapy for treatment of depression and other conditions. Little research has been conducted on hypnotherapy for the treatment of depression; however, Michael Yapko has suggested that hypnosis is likely to have high utility in the treatment of depression through development of positive expectancy regarding treatment, decreases in several symptoms of depression (such as ruminative thoughts and poor sleep), as well as improvement in attentional, cognitive, and perceptual styles of self-organization that can exacerbate depressive mood states.[39,40]

Assen Alladin has proposed cognitive hypnotherapy, an approach to integrating cognitive-behavioral therapy (CBT) with hypnosis, for the evidence-based treatment of depression.[41] This technique incorporates hypnosis into CBT for depression through a combination of relaxation training, somatosensory changes, demonstration of the power of the mind, expanding awareness, ego-strengthening, targeted post-hypnotic suggestions, self-hypnosis training, cognitive restructuring, use of symbolic imagery techniques, positive mood induction, behavioral activation, and social skills training.

Hypnosis for memory retrieval has sometimes provoked controversy because of the subtle influence and unintended covert suggestion of the hypnotist. For example, theoretical bias of the hypnotherapist may lead to erroneous production of traumatic memories. For similar reasons, courtroom applications of hypnotically retrieved information are of questionable validity. Skillful hypnotic recall of conscious experience can, however, be useful in helping a patient improve a sense of safety and control. Such efforts involve a cognitive-behavioral effort to facilitate a "top-down" influence for the reduction of emotional arousal.

Pain Management

A "top-down" cognitive-behavioral approach to pain management may prove helpful for adaptation to traumatic events.[42] Moreover, hypnotherapy can promote the use of imagery to modify perception of the painful experience. For example, pain may be coupled with a specific color (e.g., red) and comfort with a second color (e.g., blue or green). One can next encourage the subject to imagine a change in the color coupled with pain reduction.

Direct suggestion under hypnosis can allow for induction of "glove-hand anesthesia." The patient can be instructed to place the hand that is "asleep" over the area of perceived pain, and to experience that area becoming "anesthetized".[43] This type of approach requires a high level of hypnotic susceptibility.

Hypnotherapy is especially applicable to children because of their relatively strong capacity for imagination and for suspension of belief. It is, therefore, a useful intervention in painful conditions and medical interventions.

Surgical Care

Intra-operative use of hypnosis is of more than historical importance. Some anesthesiologists use hypnoanesthesia as an adjunct to routine intraoperative care. Hypnosis has been used as sole anesthesia for Cesarean sections, and in one report, by Marmer,[43] it was used for heart surgery (along with local anesthetic for passage of an endotracheal tube). Other obstetrical uses of hypnosis have also been described: for example, the use of hetero-hypnosis and self-hypnosis to reduce pain during labor and delivery is associated with improved infant Apgar scores and decreased duration of Stage 1 labor.[44]

Pre-operative hypnotherapy is effective for surgical phobias related to endotracheal intubation or for fear of undergoing anesthesia.

Surman[38] has used post-noxious desensitization as a routine intervention for transplant patients with pre-operative anxiety. Formal studies have found pre-operative hypnosis to be of benefit in pediatric surgery and in adults undergoing a wide range of procedures. Various studies have found improvement in post-operative nausea and vomiting,[45] in the management of pain, and in physical and psychological well-being, and some have reported reductions in post-operative recovery time.[34,46]

Medical and Dermatological Uses

Hypnosis has had successful application for anxiety reduction among general medical patients. It has proven useful in reducing the adverse effects of anxiety and airway resistance among asthmatics. Several studies have demonstrated its efficacy in irritable bowel syndrome.[47] Some claims have been made that it reduces bleeding in hemophiliacs and that the impact of Rasputin on Czar Nicholas and his wife was a product of his success with their son's episodic hemorrhages.

Dermatological applications for hypnosis abound; the technique can help reduce pruritus and scratching for some patients. The efficacy of hypnosis for the treatment of warts has been well studied, though its mechanism remains unproven.[48,49]

An excellent handbook that includes suggestions and inductions for a wide variety of clinical uses is William Kroger's *Clinical and Experimental Hypnosis in Medicine, Dentistry, and Psychology*[50]; although it was last updated in 1977, this volume still contains an unmatched wealth of information for the beginning practitioner of hypnosis.

CONTRAINDICATIONS FOR USING HYPNOSIS

Paranoia is a common-sense contraindication to hypnosis. While there may be exceptions to this rule, it would be a rare situation that would warrant its attempted use by someone lacking in extensive experience.

When coercion is at play, hypnosis should not be employed; in no case should hypnosis be used in someone who refuses to cooperate.

Hypnotherapeutic interventions in those with major psychiatric syndromes are best reserved for the well-trained or closely supervised practitioner. Nonetheless, medical professionals and psychologists have broad latitude to use hypnosis (which is, after all, a directive psychotherapeutic technique), and practitioners should feel secure in its use.

POTENTIAL COMPLICATIONS OF HYPNOSIS

Occasionally, hypnotic subjects are resistant to suggestions for the termination of hypnosis. The standard approach is to indicate that one will not be able (or willing) to work with this modality in the future if the patient does not "awaken."

Suggested imagery may be a source of anxiety (e.g., if it arouses negative meaning for the hypnotic subject). One can provide a standard approach for ending a session and instruct the patient that hypnosis can be repeated with relaxing imagery after a period of discussion.

Extensive recall of traumatic material may aggravate symptoms of PTSD, and hypnosis should therefore be used with caution in those with the condition.

Implications of past sexual abuse during hypnoanalysis can result in a false belief that proves disruptive to family relations.

HYPNOSIS AND PERFORMANCE ENHANCEMENT

There is evidence that hypnosis can enhance certain forms of athletic and cognitive performance. For example, a hypnosis intervention significantly enhanced soccer performance in collegiate athletes compared to participants in a video attention-control group, and the observed effect of hypnosis on performance was not mediated by its augmentation of self-efficacy.[51] Additionally, learning in hypnosis enhances performance in sequence learning that is dependent on the striatum, which the investigators speculate may be related to attenuation of explicit attentional processes in the frontal lobe that can interfere with striatum-based learning.[52]

TRAINING IN HYPNOTHERAPY
The Cochrane Collaborative

The University of Maryland's Center for Integrative Medicine is the site of the Cochrane Collaborative Complementary Medicine Field, which maintains a database of contacts.

The Society for Clinical and Experimental Hypnosis

The *International Journal of Clinical and Experimental Hypnosis* is a source of excellent research articles and theoretical discussion about the field of hypnosis.

The American Society of Clinical Hypnosis

The society offers training programs in several cities. The *American Journal of Clinical Hypnosis* is a valuable clinical resource for practical information related to the medical uses of hypnosis.

CONCLUSION

Hypnosis is a practical, directive, psychological treatment that has wide applicability to many traditional medical practices. It has well-established mainstream uses and can be used as an adjunct to behavior therapy. Hypnotic suggestions have been well studied and found to be beneficial in the treatment of pain, in the preparation for surgical care, and in the treatment of select medical and dermatological conditions. In several hospitals worldwide, hypnoanalgesia is routinely used as the sole method of anesthesia for minor medical and surgical procedures. Contraindications are limited to its use among paranoid individuals and to its coercive application. Inexperienced practitioners who lack supervision are wise to avoid exploratory attempts at memory retrieval or to use this modality with complex psychiatric conditions.

CURRENT CONTROVERSIES AND FUTURE CONSIDERATIONS

- Better-designed studies are needed to determine in a controlled fashion the efficacy of hypnosis in myriad conditions (e.g., asthma, dyspepsia, PTSD, and conversion disorder).
- Additional research is needed to determine the importance of pre-treatment hypnotizability in response to medical hypnosis.
- Research is needed to confirm impressions that similar methods (such as meditation and autogenic relaxation) can produce comparable results to hypnosis in appropriate patients.

Access the complete reference list and multiple choice questions (MCQs) online at https://expertconsult.inkling.com

KEY REFERENCES

1. Darnton R. *Mesmerism and the end of the Enlightenment in France*, Cambridge, 1968, Harvard University Press.
4. Haley J, editor. *Advanced techniques of hypnosis and therapy. Selected papers of Milton Erikson*, New York, 1967, Grune & Stratton.
6. Hilgard ER, Hilgard JR. *Hypnosis in the relief of pain*, Los Altos, 1975, William Kaufmann.
7. Spiegel D. Trauma, dissociation, and memory. *Ann N Y Acad Sci* 821:225–237, 1997.
8. Tellegen A, Atkinson G. Openness to absorbing and self-altering experiences ("absorption"), a trait related to hypnotic susceptibility. *J Abnorm Psychol* 83(3):268–277, 1974.
10. Weitzenhoffer AM, Hilgard ER. *Stanford Hypnotic Susceptibility Scale, forms a and b for use in research investigation in the field of hypnotic phenomena*, Palo Alto, 1959, Consult Psych Press.
11. Frankel FH, Orne MT. Hypnotizability and phobic behavior. *Arch Gen Psychiatry* 33(10):1259–1261, 1976.
13. Raz A. Attention and hypnosis: neural substrates and genetic associations of two converging processes. *Int J Clin Exp Hypn* 53(3):237–258, 2005.

14. Vermetten E, Douglas Bremner J. Functional brain imaging and the induction of traumatic recall: a cross-correlational review between neuroimaging and hypnosis. *Int J Clin Exp Hypn* 52(3): 280–312, 2004.
15. Spiegel D, Bierre P, Rootenberg J. Hypnotic alteration of somatosensory perception. *Am J Psychiatry* 146(6):749–754, 1989.
16. Rainville P, Hofbauer RK, Paus T, et al. Cerebral mechanisms of hypnotic induction and suggestion. *J Cogn Neurosci* 11(1):110–125, 1999.
19. Maquet P, Faymonville ME, Degueldre C, et al. Functional neuroanatomy of hypnotic state. *Biol Psychiatry* 45(3):327–333, 1999.
21. Kosslyn SM, Thompson WL, Costantini-Ferrando MF, et al. Hypnotic visual illusion alters color processing in the brain. *Am J Psychiatry* 157(8):1279–1284, 2000.
22. Raz A, Shapiro T, Fan J, et al. Hypnotic suggestion and the modulation of Stroop interference. *Arch Gen Psychiatry* 59(12):1155–1161, 2002.
23. Raz A, Fan J, Posner MI. Hypnotic suggestion reduces conflict in the human brain. *Proc Natl Acad Sci U S A* 102(28):9978–9983, 2005.
27. Hoeft F, Gabrieli JD, Whitfield-Gabrieli S, et al. Functional brain basis of hypnotizability. *Arch Gen Psychiatry* 69(10):1064–1072, 2012.
28. Davidson RJ, Kabat-Zinn J, Schumacher J, et al. Alterations in brain and immune function produced by mindfulness meditation. *Psychosom Med* 65(4):564–570, 2003.
30. Szekely A, Kovacs-Nagy R, Banyai EI, et al. Association between hypnotizability and the catechol-O-methyltransferase (COMT) polymorphism. *Int J Clin Exp Hypn* 58(3):301–315, 2010.
33. Covino NA, Frankel FH. Hypnosis and relaxation in the medically ill. *Psychother Psychosom* 60(2):75–90, 1993.
39. McCann BS, Landes SJ. Hypnosis in the treatment of depression: considerations in research design and methods. *Int J Clin Exp Hypn* 58(2):147–164, 2010.
40. Yapko MD, editor. Hypnosis in treating symptoms and risk factors of major depression. In *Hypnosis and treating depression: applications in clinical practice*, New York, 2006, Routledge, pp 3–24.
41. Alladin A. Evidence-based hypnotherapy for depression. *Int J Clin Exp Hypn* 58(2):165–185, 2010.
46. Fredericks L. *The use of hypnosis in surgery and anesthesiology*, Springfield, 2000, Charles C Thomas.
50. Kroger W. *Clinical and experimental hypnosis in medicine, dentistry, and psychology*, ed 2, Philadelphia, 1977, Lippincott Williams & Wilkins.
52. Nemeth D, Janacsek K, Polner B, et al. Boosting human learning by hypnosis. *Cereb Cortex* 23(4):801–805, 2013.

16 Cognitive-behavioral Therapy, Behavioral Therapy, and Cognitive Therapy

Susan E. Sprich, PhD, Bunmi O. Olatunji, PhD, Hannah E. Reese, PhD, Michael W. Otto, PhD, Elizabeth Rosenfield, BA, and Sabine Wilhelm, PhD

KEY POINTS

Background

- Cognitive-behavioral therapy (CBT) is one of the most extensively researched forms of psychotherapy that is increasingly recognized as the treatment of choice for many disorders.

History

- Cognitive-behavioral therapies represent an integration of two strong traditions within psychology: behavioral therapy (BT) and cognitive therapy (CT).

- BT employs principles of learning to change human behavior. BT techniques include exposure, relaxation, assertion training, social skills training, problem-solving training, modeling, contingency management, and behavioral activation.

- CT, initially developed as a treatment for depression, is based on the understanding that thoughts influence behavior and that maladaptive thinking styles lead to maladaptive behaviors and emotional distress. CT is now widely used for a range of disorders.

Clinical and Research Challenges

- A common concern is whether the results found in well-controlled randomized controlled trials (RCTs) of CBT translate well to routine practice in the community.

- There is an increasing focus on the dissemination of empirically-supported treatments, such that clinicians in the community are trained in the use of these treatments.

- The question of whether or not to combine pharmacotherapy and CBT may not be straightforward.

- The decision to provide combined treatment must include a careful examination of the disorder, the severity and chronicity of the disorder, the patient's treatment history, and the stage of treatment.

- There is an increasing emphasis on research that is focused on dimensions of observable behavior and on neurobiological measures, with the goal of leading to an improved understanding of psychopathology.

Practical Pointers

- CBT is a collaborative treatment.
- CBT is an active treatment.
- CBT is a structured treatment.
- CBT is evidence-based.
- CBT is a short-term treatment.

OVERVIEW

Cognitive-behavioral therapy (CBT) is one of the most extensively researched forms of psychotherapy that is increasingly recognized as the treatment of choice for many disorders.[1] Findings from randomized controlled trials (RCTs) typically suggest that CBT is better than wait-list control groups, as well as supportive treatment and other credible interventions, for specific disorders. Early implementations of CBT were largely indicated for anxiety and mood disorders.[2] However, more recent clinical research efforts have begun to develop CBT for an increasingly wider array of problems (including bipolar disorder,[3,4] eating disorders,[5] body dysmorphic disorder,[6] attention-deficit/hyperactivity disorder,[7,8] and psychotic disorders[9]).

The empirical evidence for the use of CBT for a broad range of conditions is promising.[10] However, there remains a noticeable gap between encouraging reports from clinical trials and the widespread adoption of CBT interventions among general practitioners.[11] Moreover, questions remain regarding the limits of, and indications for, the efficacy of CBT in general practice.[12] Nevertheless, it is clear that CBT represents the best of what the psychotherapy community currently has to offer in terms of evidence-supported treatment options.

CBT generally refers to a treatment that uses behavioral and cognitive interventions; it is derived from scientifically-supported theoretical models.[13,14] Thus, there exists a theoreti-cally consistent relationship between CBT techniques and the disorders that they are designed to treat.[15] Depending on the disorder, interventions may be directed toward eliminating cognitive and behavioral patterns that are directly linked to the development or maintenance of the disorder, or they may be directed toward maximizing coping skills to address the elicitation or duration of symptoms from disorders driven by other (e.g., biological) factors.

BEHAVIORAL THERAPY, COGNITIVE THERAPY, AND COGNITIVE-BEHAVIORAL THERAPY

Cognitive-behavioral therapies represent an integration of two strong traditions within psychology: behavioral therapy (BT) and cognitive therapy (CT). BT employs principles of learning to change human behavior. BT techniques include exposure, relaxation, assertion training, social skills training, problem-solving training, modeling, contingency management, and behavioral activation. Many of these interventions are a direct outgrowth of principles of operant and respondent conditioning. Operant conditioning is concerned with the modification of behaviors by manipulation of the rewards and punishments, as well as the eliciting events. For example, in the treatment of substance dependence, the use of specific contingencies between drug abstinence (as frequently confirmed by urine or saliva toxicology screens) and rewards (e.g., the chance to win a monetary reward) has proven to be a powerful strategy for achieving abstinence among chronic drug abusers.[16] Included as an operant strategy are also the myriad of interventions that use stepwise training to engender needed new skills for problem situations. For example, assertiveness training, relaxation training, and problem-solving training are all core behavioral strategies for intervening with skill deficits that may be manifest in disorders as diverse as depression, bipolar disorder, or hypochondriasis. One approach to treating depression, behavioral activation, emphasizes the return to pleasurable and productive activities, and the specific use of these activities to boost mood. Interventions involve the step-by-step programming of activities rated by patients as relevant to their personal values and likely to evoke pleasure or a sense of personal productivity. Behavioral activation will typically consist of construction of an activity hierarchy in which up to (approximately) 15 activities are rated, ranging from easiest to most difficult to accomplish. The patient then moves through the hierarchy in a systematic manner, progressing from the easiest to the most difficult activity.[17] Depending on the patient, additional interventions or skill development may be needed. For example, assertion training may include a variety of interventions, such as behavioral rehearsal, which is acting out appropriate and effective behaviors, to manage situations in which assertiveness is problematic.

Respondent conditioning refers to the changing of the meaning of a stimulus through repeated pairings with other stimuli, and respondent conditioning principles have been particularly applied to interventions for anxiety disorders. For example, influential theories such as Mowrer's[18] two-factor theory of phobic disorders emphasized the role of respondent conditioning in establishing fearful responses to phobic cues, and the role of avoidance in maintaining the fear. Accordingly, BT focuses on the role of exposure to help patients re-enter phobic situations and to eliminate (extinguish) learned fears about these phobic stimuli through repeated exposure to them under safe conditions. Exposure treatments may include any number of modalities or procedures. For example, a patient with social phobia may be exposed to a series of social situations that elicit anxiety, including *in vivo* exposure (e.g., talking on the phone, talking with strangers, giving a speech), imaginal exposure (e.g., imagining themselves in a social situation), exposure to feared sensations (termed *interoceptive exposure* because exposure involves the elicitation of feared somatic sensations, typically sensations similar to those of anxiety and panic), and exposure to feared cognitions (e.g., exposure to feared concepts using imaginal techniques). Exposure is generally conducted in a graduated fashion, in contrast to *flooding*, in which the person is thrust into the most threatening situation at the start. Exposure is designed to help patients learn alternative responses to a variety of situations by allowing fear to dissipate (become extinguished) while remaining in the feared situation. Once regarded as a passive weakening of learned exposures, extinction is now considered an active process of learning an alternative meaning to a stimulus (e.g., relearning a sense of "safety" with a once-feared stimulus),[19] and ongoing research on the principles, procedures, and limits of extinction as informed by both animal and human studies has the potential for helping clinicians further hone in on the efficacy of their exposure-based treatments. For example, there is increasing evidence that the therapeutic effects of exposure are maximized when patients are actively engaged in, and attentive to, exposure-based learning; when exposure is conducted in multiple, realistic contexts; and when patients are provided with multiple cues for safety learning.[20] Therapists should also ensure that the learning that occurs during exposure is independent of contexts that will not be present in the future (e.g., the presence of the therapist). Effective application of exposure therapy also requires prevention of safety behaviors that may undermine what is learned from exposure. Safety behaviors refer to those behaviors that individuals may use to reassure themselves in a phobic situation. For example, a patient with panic disorder may carry a cell phone or a water bottle for help or perceived support during a panic attack. These safety behaviors, while providing reassurance to patients, appear to block the full learning of true safety.[21,22] That is, when such safety behaviors are made unavailable, better extinction (safety) learning appears to result.[23,24]

CT was initially developed as a treatment for depression with the understanding that thoughts influence behavior and it is largely maladaptive thinking styles that lead to maladaptive behavior and emotional distress.[25,26] Currently, however, CT includes approaches to a wider range of disorders.[27,28]

As applied to depression, the cognitive model posits that intrusive cognitions associated with depression arise from a synthesis of previous life experiences. The synthesis of such experiences is also described as a schema, a form of semantic memory that describes self-relevant characteristics. For example, the cognitive model of depression posits that negative "schemas" about the self that contain absolute beliefs (e.g., "I am unlovable" or "I am incompetent") may result in dysfunctional appraisals of the self, the world, and the future. On exposure to negative life events, negative schemas and dysfunctional attitudes are activated that may produce symptoms of depression. Thus, maladaptive cognitive patterns and negative thoughts may also be considered risk or maintaining factors for depression.[29] Negative automatic thoughts can be categorized into a number of common patterns of thought referred to as *cognitive distortions*. As outlined in Table 16-1, cognitive distortions often occur automatically and may manifest as irrational thoughts or as maladaptive interpretations of relatively ambiguous life events.

CT,[30] and a similar approach known as rational-emotive therapy,[31] provides techniques that correct distorted thinking and offer a means by which patients can respond to maladaptive thoughts more adaptively. In addition to examining cognitive distortions (see Hollon and Garber[32] and Table 16-1), CT focuses on more pervasive core beliefs (e.g., "I am unlovable" or "I am incompetent") by assessing the themes that lie behind recurrent patterns of cognitive distortions. Those themes may be evaluated with regard to a patient's learning history (to assess the etiology of the beliefs with the goal of logically evaluating and altering the maladaptive beliefs).

A commonly used cognitive technique is cognitive restructuring. Cognitive restructuring begins by teaching a patient about the cognitive model and by providing a patient with tools to recognize (negative) automatic thoughts that occur "on-line". Most therapists use a daily log or a diary to monitor negative automatic thoughts. Some patients find it convenient to do this work using an "app" on their smart phone or using their tablet or laptop computer. The next step in cognitive restructuring is to provide the patient with opportunities to evaluate his or her thoughts with respect to their usefulness, as well as their validity. Through the process of logically analyzing thoughts, a patient is provided with a unique context for replacing distorted thoughts with more accurate and realistic thoughts. One method for helping a patient engage in critical analysis of thinking patterns is to consider the objective evidence for and against the patient's maladaptive thoughts. Thus, questions such as, "What is the evidence that I am a bad mother? What is the evidence against it?" might be asked. Another useful technique places the patient in the role of adviser.[30] In the role of adviser, a patient is asked what advice he or she might give a family member or friend in the same situation. By distancing the patient from his or her own

TABLE 16-1 Examples of Cognitive Distortions

Distortion	Description
All-or-nothing thinking	Looking at things in absolute, black-and-white categories
Mental filter	Dwelling on the negatives and ignoring the positives
Discounting the positives	Insisting that accomplishments or positive qualities "don't count"
Mind reading	Assuming that people are reacting negatively to you when there is no evidence to support the assumptions
Over-generalization	Making a negative conclusion that goes far beyond the current situation
Fortune-telling	Arbitrarily predicting that things will turn out badly
Magnification or minimization	Blowing things out of proportion or shrinking their importance inappropriately
Emotional reasoning	Reasoning from how you feel ("I feel stupid, so I must really be stupid")
"Should" statements	Criticizing yourself (or others) with "shoulds" or "shouldn'ts," "musts," "oughts," and "have-tos"
Labeling	Identifying with shortcomings ("I'm a loser")
Personalization and blame	Blaming yourself for something you weren't responsible for (and not considering more plausible explanations)

Adapted from Beck JS. Cognitive behavior therapy: basics and beyond, ed 2, New York, 2011, Guilford Press.[30]

TABLE 16-2 Examples of Well-Established Cognitive, Behavioral, and Cognitive-Behavioral Treatments for Specific Disorders

Treatment	Condition/Disorder
Cognitive	Depression
Behavioral	Agoraphobia
	Depression
	Social phobia
	Specific phobia
	Obsessive-compulsive disorder
	Headache
	Oppositional behavior
	Enuresis
	Marital dysfunction
	Female orgasmic dysfunction
	Male erectile dysfunction
	Developmental disabilities
Cognitive-behavioral	Panic, with and without agoraphobia
	Generalized anxiety disorder
	Social phobia
	Irritable bowel syndrome
	Chronic pain
	Bulimia

Adapted from Chambless DL, Baker MJ, Baucom DH, et al. Update on empirically validated therapies: II, Clin Psychol 51:3–16, 1998.[41]

maladaptive thinking, the patient is given the opportunity to engage in a more rational analysis of the issue. These techniques allow patients to test the validity and utility of their thoughts; as they evaluate their thinking and see things more rationally, they are able to function better. In addition to techniques for changing negative thinking patterns, CT also incorporates behavioral experiments. Behavioral tasks and experiments are employed in CT to provide corrective data that will challenge beliefs and underlying negative assumptions.

Concerning the mechanism of relapse prevention in CT, there is growing attention to the importance of the processing and form of negative thoughts, not just their content.[33,34] Studies suggest that cognitive interventions may be useful for helping patients gain perspective on their negative thoughts and feelings so that these events are not seen as "necessarily valid reflections of reality" (Teasdale et al.,[33] p. 285). Indeed, there is evidence that changes in meta-cognitive awareness may mediate the relapse prevention effects of CT.[33,35] Accordingly, shifting an individual's emotional response to cognitions may be an important element of the strong relapse prevention effects associated with CT.[36]

Although CT was initially developed to focus on challenging depressive distortions, basic maladaptive assumptions are also observed in a wide range of other conditions, with the development of CT approaches ranging from panic disorder,[37] post-traumatic stress disorder (PTSD),[38] social phobia,[39] and hypochondriasis,[28] to personality disorders[27] and the prevention of suicide.[40]

PUTTING BEHAVIORAL THERAPY AND COGNITIVE THERAPY TOGETHER

As a functional unification of cognitive and behavioral interventions, CBT relies heavily on functional analysis of interrelated chains of thoughts, emotions, and behavior. Thus, the principles that underlie CBT are easily exportable to a wide

range of behavioral deficits. As outlined in Table 16-2,[41] CT, BT, and their combination have garnered empirical support for the treatment of a wide range of disorders. CBT has become increasingly specialized in the last decade, and advances in the conceptualization of various disorders have brought a refinement of CBT interventions to target core features and dominant behavior patterns that characterize various disorders.

Basic Principles of Cognitive-behavioral Therapy

As outlined in Table 16-3, contemporary CBT is a collaborative, structured, and goal-oriented intervention.[1] The current forms of CBT target core components of a given disorder. For example, CBT interventions for panic disorder target catastrophic misinterpretations of somatic sensations of panic and their perceived consequences, while exposure procedures focus directly on the fear of somatic sensations. Likewise, CBT for social phobia focuses on the modification of fears of a negative evaluation by others and exposure treatments emphasize the completion of feared activities and interactions with others. For generalized anxiety disorder (GAD), CBT treatment focuses on the worry process itself, with the substitution of cognitive restructuring and problem-solving for self-perpetuating worry patterns, and the use of imaginal exposure for worries and fears. In the case of depression, CBT targets negative thoughts about the self, the world, and the future, as well as incorporating behavioral activation to provide more opportunities for positive reinforcement. Symptom management strategies (e.g., breathing re-training or muscle relaxation) or social skills training (e.g., assertiveness training) are also valuable adjuncts to exposure and to cognitive restructuring interventions.

The Basic Practice of Cognitive-behavioral Therapy

CBT is typically targeted toward short-term treatment, often in the range of 12 to 20 sessions, although even shorter treatments, emphasizing the core mechanisms of change, have

TABLE 16-3 Characteristic Features of Cognitive-behavioral Therapy

Feature	Description
CBT is *short term*	The length of therapy in CBT is largely dependent on the time needed to help the patient develop more adaptive patters of responding. However, CBT treatments generally involve approximately 8 to 20 sessions.
CBT is *active*	CBT provides a context for learning adaptive behavior. It is the therapist's role to provide the patient with the information, skills, and *opportunity* to develop more adaptive coping mechanisms. Thus, homework is a central feature of CBT.
CBT is *structured*	CBT is agenda-driven such that portions of sessions are dedicated to specific goals. Specific techniques or concepts are taught during each session. However, each session should strike a balance between material introduced by the patient and the predetermined session agenda.
CBT is *collaborative*	The therapeutic relationship is generally less of a focus in CBT. However, it is important that the therapist and patient have a good collaborative working relationship in order to reduce symptoms by developing alternative adaptive skills.

CBT, Cognitive-behavioral therapy.

been developed.[42] Treatment begins with a thorough evaluation of the problem for which the patient is seeking treatment. This generally consists of a very detailed functional analysis of the patient's symptoms and the contexts in which they occur. This assessment requires extensive history-taking, a diagnostic interview, analysis of current function (e.g., social, occupational, relational, and family), and assessment of social support. Although the assessment may require some consideration of past events, such information is generally gathered if it is directly relevant to the solution of here-and-now problems.

A key feature of CBT involves the establishment of a strong, collaborative working alliance with the patient. This is often initiated in the context of educating the patient about the nature of his or her disorder, explaining the CBT model of the etiology and maintenance of the disorder, and the intervention that is derived from the model. Educating the patient serves the function of normalizing aspects of the disorder; this can help to reduce self-blame. Psychoeducation (including information on the course of treatment) may also enhance patient motivation for change. The therapist and patient also work together to develop clear, realistic treatment goals.

To gather information on the patient's symptoms, the patient is taught early on how to monitor his or her thoughts and behaviors. This usually requires that the patient document his or her symptoms, as well as the time, date, and the level of distress and the precursors and consequences of symptoms. Self-monitoring helps a patient become aware of the timing and occurrence of target symptoms, and provides additional information on opportunities for intervention. Self-monitoring procedures are vital to help a patient identify the content of his or her thoughts; once these thoughts have been identified, they can be challenged for their accuracy and utility. The accuracy of thoughts and beliefs is often examined in the context of behavioral experiments, where patients have the opportunity to test out predictions (e.g., "I will pass out," "I will not be able to cope").

CBT also emphasizes systematic monitoring of symptom change. This may take the form of asking a patient how he or she is feeling as compared to when in previous sessions. However, more standard CBT practice consists of having a patient fill out questionnaires about his or her symptoms. Periodic assessment of symptoms provides an objective look at the nature of a patient's symptoms relative to established norms, at which symptoms have improved, and at which symptoms require more attention. Essentially, objective assessment during CBT helps inform both the patient and the therapist about the efficacy of treatment and highlights further issues that require emphasis during the treatment. Monitoring outcomes can also guide the clinician with regard to case formulation or consideration of alternative CBT interventions, if expected treatment goals are not achieved.

In many approaches to CBT, patient and therapist collaboratively set an agenda for topics to be discussed in each session. Particular attention is given to events that occurred since the previous session that are relevant to the patient's goals for treatment. Part of the agenda for treatment sessions should focus on the anticipation of difficulties that may occur before the next treatment session. These problems should then be discussed in the context of problem-solving and the implementation of necessary cognitive and behavioral skills. This may require training in skills that readily facilitate the reduction of distress. Skills, such as training in diaphragmatic breathing and progressive muscle relaxation, can be particularly useful in this regard. Although the specific interventions used during CBT may vary, the decision about which interventions to use should be informed by cognitive and learning theories that view disorders as understandable within a framework of reciprocally-connected behaviors, thoughts, and emotions that are activated and influenced by environmental and interpersonal events.

As indicated in Table 16-3, CBT is also an active treatment with an emphasis on home practice of interventions. Thus, review of homework is a major component of the CBT session. In reviewing the patient's homework, emphasis should be placed on what the patient learned, and what the patient wants to continue doing during the coming week for homework. The homework assignment, which is collaboratively set, should follow naturally from the problem-solving process in the treatment session. The use of homework in CBT draws from the understanding of therapy as a learning experience in which the patient acquires new skills. At the end of each CBT treatment session, a patient should be provided with an opportunity to summarize useful interventions from the session. This should also consist of asking the patient for feedback on the session, and efforts to enhance memories of and the subsequent home application of useful interventions.[43]

Relapse prevention skills are central to CBT as well. By emphasizing a problem-solving approach in treatment, a patient is trained to recognize the early warning signs of relapse and is taught to be "his or her own therapist." Even after termination, a patient often schedules "booster sessions" to review the skills learned in treatment. In addition, novel approaches to relapse prevention, as well as treatment of residual symptoms, emphasize the application of CBT to the promotion of well-being rather than simply the reduction of pathology.[44,45]

The Practice of Cognitive-behavioral Therapy: The Case of Panic Disorder

CBT for panic disorder generally consists of 12 to 15 sessions; it begins with an introduction of the CBT model of panic disorder (Figure 16-1).[46] The therapist begins by discussing the symptoms of panic with the patient. The symptoms of panic

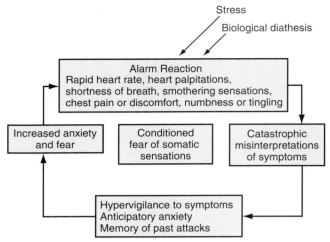

Figure 16-1. Cognitive-behavioral model of panic disorder. *(Adapted from Otto MW, Pollack MH, Meltzer-Brody S, Rosenbaum JF. Cognitive-behavioral therapy for benzodiazepine discontinuation in panic disorder patients,* Psychopharmacol Bull *28:123–130, 1992.)*

(e.g., rapid heart rate, shortness of breath, and trembling) are explained as part of our body's natural defense system that prepares us for fight or flight in the presence of a real threat. When these symptoms occur in the presence of a real danger, the response helps us survive. When the symptoms occur in the absence of a real danger, the response is a panic attack. Often when a person experiences a panic attack "out of the blue," he or she fears that something is terribly wrong. The person fears that he or she may be having a heart attack, may be seriously ill, or may be "going crazy." Patients are told that these catastrophic misinterpretations of the symptoms of panic disorder serve to maintain the disorder. Such interpretations cause the individual to fear another attack; as a consequence, the person becomes hypervigilant for any somatic sensations that may signal the onset of an attack. This hypervigilance, in turn, heightens the individual's awareness of his or her body and increases somatic sensations that lead to more anxiety. This cycle continues, culminating in a panic attack.

Over the course of treatment, the therapist works with the patient to examine the accuracy of catastrophic misinterpretations through Socratic questioning and provision of corrective information. For example, the patient may be asked to evaluate the evidence for all of the likely consequences of a panic attack. Additionally, the patient is gradually exposed to the somatic sensations that he or she fears (a process called *interoceptive exposure*). Interoceptive exposure consists of a wide variety of procedures (such as hyperventilation, exercise, or spinning in a chair[47]) meant to expose a patient to feared internal bodily experiences (e.g., tachycardia, numbness, or tingling) in a controlled fashion. Through repeated exposure to these sensations, a patient habituates to the sensations, which results in a decrease in fear and anxiety linked to internal stimuli. With repeated exposure, a patient learns that the sensations are not harmful.

Cognitive restructuring is combined with interoceptive exposure to aid the patient in reinterpreting the somatic sensations and reducing fear. For a patient with agoraphobia, gradual situational exposure is also conducted to eliminate avoidance of situations that have been associated with panic. In all exposure exercises, special attention must be paid to the elimination of safety behaviors that may interfere with habituation to the fear and extinction learning. Safety behaviors include anything that the patient may do to avoid experiencing

anxiety. This could include carrying a bottle of pills in the patient's pocket or having a cell phone with the patient to call for help. To maximize the exposure exercises, these behaviors must be gradually eliminated. The patient must learn that he or she will be okay even in the absence of such behaviors. The use of relaxation techniques for the treatment of panic may also be beneficial. However, Barlow and associates[48] found that adding relaxation to the treatment (emphasizing cognitive restructuring and interoceptive exposure) appeared to reduce the efficacy of the treatment over time (see also Schmidt et al.[49]). This suggests that, in some cases, a patient may engage in relaxation as a safety technique (i.e., a patient may rely too much on relaxation as a panic management technique at the expense of learning not to be afraid of anxiety-related sensations). Although relaxation techniques may come to serve the function of avoidance for some patients with panic disorder, studies have shown that relaxation strategies offer some benefit to patients with a wide range of anxiety disorders.[50] Thus, the decision to offer relaxation techniques in CBT for patients with panic disorder should be informed by the context in which the patient will apply such techniques.

THE EFFICACY OF COGNITIVE-BEHAVIORAL THERAPY

As outlined in Table 16-1, cognitive and behavioral techniques and their combination (CBT) are generally considered to be empirically-supported interventions for a wide range of disorders. In fact, numerous outcome trials have demonstrated that CBT is effective for a host of psychiatric disorders, as well as for medical disorders with psychological components.[51] However, diagnostic co-morbidity, personality disorders, or complex medical problems may complicate CBT treatment. Such complications do not imply that a patient will not respond well to CBT, but rather that the patient might have a slower response to treatment.

In an attempt to integrate findings from RCTs, multiple meta-analytic studies (which allow researchers to synthesize quantitatively the results from multiple studies in an effort to characterize the general effectiveness of various interventions) have been conducted. Two recent reviews of the most comprehensive meta-analyses conducted for the efficacy of CBT have nicely summarized the treatment outcome effect sizes for adult unipolar depression, adolescent depression, GAD, panic disorder with or without agoraphobia, social phobia, obsessive-compulsive disorder (OCD), PTSD, schizophrenia, marital distress, anger, bulimia, internalizing childhood disorders, sexual offending, and chronic pain (excluding headache).[10,15,52] A review of these meta-analyses and other relevant findings is presented next and summarized in Tables 16-4 to 16-10.

Adult Unipolar Depression

CT has been most extensively studied in adult unipolar depression (Table 16-4). In a comprehensive review of the treatment outcomes, Gloaguen and colleagues[53] found CT to be better than (1) being on a wait-list or being placed on a placebo, (2) antidepressant medications, and (3) other miscellaneous therapies. It was also as efficacious as BT. With regard to effectiveness, a recent meta-analysis revealed that outpatient CBT was effective in diminishing depressive symptoms in both completer (d = 1.13) and intention-to-treat (ITT) samples (d = 1.06).[54] Although a change in cognitive schemas and automatic negative thoughts has long been thought of as the central mechanism through which CT results in improvement, this has been called into question by the success of behavioral treatments of depression. In an investigation of the relative

interpersonal support, and skill-building interventions might be combined).[16,104] Despite the success of these approaches, treatment of drug dependence is an area in great need of additional strategies for boosting treatment response and the maintenance of treatment gains.

Other Psychological Conditions

CBT has been studied for numerous other psychological conditions (see Table 16-10). When compared to no treatment, CBT has been found to be effective in reducing marital distress ($d = .71$), although it was not significantly more effective than behavioral marital therapy or interpersonally oriented marital therapy.[105] A similar effect size has been reported for CBT for anger and aggression when compared to no treatment in adults ($d = .70$)[106] and children ($d = .67$).[107] In a meta-analysis examining the efficacy of CBT for childhood internalizing disorders, Grossman and Hughes[108] found that CBT, when compared to no treatment or to psychological placebo, resulted in significant improvements in anxiety ($d = .93$), depression ($d = .87$), and somatic symptoms ($d = .47$). More modest treatment effects have been reported for CBT for other psychological conditions. For example, in a review of CBT for sexual offending, Nagayama Hall[109] found an overall effect size of .35 on measures of recidivism when compared with no treatment. A meta-analysis of CBT for pain revealed effect sizes that ranged from .06 on measures of mood to .61 on measures of social role functioning, and on direct measures of the experience of pain, CBT was found to have an effect size of .33.[110]

The Effectiveness of Cognitive-behavioral Therapy

A common concern is whether the results found in well-controlled RCTs of CBT translate well to routine practice in the community.[111] Relative to this concern, Westbrook and Kirk[112] recently published a large outcome study examining the effectiveness of CBT in a free mental health clinic. They found that of 1,276 patients who started treatment, 370 dropped out before the agreed-on end of treatment. This is a higher dropout rate than is usually reported in clinical trials of CBT; however, the authors did not provide information regarding reason for dropout, which makes interpretation of this finding difficult. Because the patients in the clinic were not reliably diagnosed using a structured clinical interview, the authors relied on two measures as their outcome variables for all patients: the Beck Anxiety Inventory (BAI) and the Beck Depression Inventory (BDI). For treatment completers, the overall effect size for pre-treatment-to-post-treatment improvement was .52 on the BAI and .67 on the BDI. When the authors examined only those individuals who entered treatment with a score in the clinical range on either of these measures, the pre-treatment-to-post-treatment effect sizes rose to .94 and 1.15, respectively. These findings are consistent with indications that clinical practice frequently encounters patients who are less severe than those in clinical trials[113] and supports the efficacy of CBT in the community setting for a wide range of psychiatric disorders. Additionally, these results are very similar to other effectiveness and bench-marking trials,[114–117] suggesting that these are fairly reliable and representative outcomes for care in the community.

COMBINING COGNITIVE-BEHAVIORAL THERAPY WITH MEDICATION

Psychiatric medications are commonly considered the first line of treatment for a wide range of psychiatric disorders.

However, pharmacotherapy may not produce a complete remission of symptoms and at times may be associated with a delayed effectiveness. CBT can complement, if not replace, pharmacotherapy for various disorders. CBT can be offered to patients to control symptoms while awaiting a response to medications and to supplement or strengthen treatment response. Indeed, CBT has also been shown to be an effective treatment in addition to medication for chronic mental illnesses (such as bipolar disorder and schizophrenia).[118] These findings seem to support the notion that two treatments (CBT plus pharmacotherapy) must be better than one. However, a recent examination of the treatment outcome literature has revealed that the question of whether or not to combine pharmacotherapy and CBT may not be straightforward.[119] The decision to provide combined treatment must include a careful examination of the disorder, the severity and chronicity of the disorder, the patient's treatment history, and the stage of treatment.

For unipolar depression it appears that combining medication and CBT results in a slight advantage over either treatment alone.[58,119] However, the advantage of combined treatment is most pronounced for individuals with severe or chronic depression. CBT has been effective at preventing relapse in individuals who have already responded to antidepressants and wish to discontinue the medication. In this case, medication and CBT would be delivered in a sequential rather than simultaneous manner. Hollon and colleagues[58] suggest that CBT and pharmacotherapy may complement each other due to their different rates of change. Pharmacotherapy is typically associated with a more rapid initial change, whereas CBT has been associated with improvements slightly later, after the initiation of treatment. Thus, individuals receiving both types of treatment benefit from the early boost of medication and the later improvements associated with CBT. CBT and medication for depression may also complement each other in their mechanisms of change in the brain. Treatment of depression with CBT operates through the medial frontal and cingulate cortices to effect change in the prefrontal hippocampal pathways.[120] Treatment with paroxetine (a selective serotonin reuptake inhibitor [SSRI]) also produced changes in the prefrontal hippocampal pathways, but through the brainstem, insula, and subgenual cingulate. Thus, CBT and medication may operate through different pathways to reach the same result. However, some of the unique advantages of CBT compared to medication for depression are as follows[121]: consistent evidence for equal efficacy in patients with mild to moderate depression, without exposure to medication risks or side effects; evidence for lower relapse rates than pharmacotherapy when treatment is discontinued; evidence for long-term effectiveness equal to that of maintenance pharmacotherapy; greater tolerability than many pharmacological agents; and avoidance of long-term medication effects, including potential effects on chronicity and pregnancy-related health outcomes.

The decision to provide combined treatment for anxiety disorders involves even more complicating factors. A recent review of the treatment for panic disorder suggests that combined treatment is associated with modest short-term gains over each modality alone for panic disorder. However, in analysis of long-term outcome, combined treatment remained superior to medication alone, but was not more effective than CBT alone.[122] The results of a multi-center study investigating combination treatments for social anxiety disorder (CBT alone, fluoxetine alone, the combination of these treatments, or placebo) revealed that there was less than a 3% improvement in response rates for the addition of fluoxetine to CBT; patients treated with CBT plus fluoxetine demonstrated a response rate of 54.2% relative to a response rate of 51.7% for

CBT alone, and a response rate of 50.8% for fluoxetine alone.[123] Similar findings were reported in a multi-center study of combination treatment for adults with OCD. Outcomes for patients who received combined CBT (exposure and response prevention) and clomipramine were not significantly better than for patients who received CBT alone, and both of these groups achieved a better outcome than those treated with clomipramine alone.[124] However, in the Pediatric OCD Treatment Study (POTS), combined treatment proved superior to CBT alone and to sertraline alone which did not differ from each other.[125]

Thus, it appears that combining medication and CBT for anxiety disorders may not result in treatment gains substantially greater than those achieved through CBT alone. Considering that CBT is a more cost-effective treatment than is use of medication,[126] practitioners should consider CBT as a first-line treatment for the anxiety disorders, with pharmacotherapy as an alternative treatment for CBT non-responders. The addition of CBT to medication, however, is beneficial. There is also evidence that the addition of CBT during and after medication discontinuation enables patients to maintain treatment gains.[127]

More recent developments in combination treatment have examined a very different strategy for combination treatments: rather than combining antidepressant or anxiolytic agents with CBT, this new strategy seeks to strengthen the retention of therapeutic learning from CBT. To date, the most successful strategy of this kind has been augmenting CBT with the glutamatergic N-methyl-D-aspartate (NMDA) agonist, D-cycloserine.[128–131] This approach stems from animal research that has implicated NMDA receptors in extinction-learning. Extinction-learning appears to be enhanced by NMDA partial agonists, such as D-cycloserine.[132,133] This basic animal laboratory research has been repeatedly applied to patients with anxiety disorders, and preliminary evidence suggests that D-cycloserine may enhance the effectiveness of exposure-based CBT for acrophobia,[134] social phobia,[135] OCD,[130,136–138] and panic disorder.[139] In this application, the medication is given in individual dosages only in the context of (before or after) exposure therapy sessions, with recently emerging evidence that D-cycloserine augmentation effects are stronger when applied to exposure sessions resulting in low fear.[140,141]

RECENT DEVELOPMENTS AND FUTURE DIRECTIONS

In the past several decades, there has been an increasing focus on treatments that incorporate concepts such as mindfulness into CBT. Notably, dialectical behavior therapy (DBT) was developed by Marsha Linehan.[142,143] DBT was originally developed to treat borderline personality disorder, but has been used with various different disorders including treatment-resistant depression,[144] binge eating disorder,[145] opioid dependence,[146] and trichotillomania.[147] Along somewhat similar lines, Acceptance and Commitment Therapy (ACT) was developed by Steven Hayes and colleagues. ACT has acceptance as a major focus of treatment and also incorporates mindfulness and values work.[148] Hayes and others have referred to these new treatments as the "third wave" of cognitive and behavioral therapies, implying that they are fundamentally different than older CBT treatments (e.g., Hayes).[149] However, other authors contend that these treatments are fundamentally related to CBT and should not be classified separately.[150]

Another issue in the field of cognitive-behavioral psychology is that there are two seemingly contradictory movements in the field—one towards developing more and more specialized treatments for specific disorders (e.g., Wilhelm, et al.,[6] Safren, et al.,[7] Wilhelm et al.,[151] Piacentini, et al.,[152]) and the other towards developing treatments that are more broadly applicable across multiple different diagnostic categories, such as the "unified protocol for transdiagnostic treatment of emotional disorders".[153,154] The unified protocol is consistent with a component of the strategic plan outlined by the National Institute of Mental Health (NIMH) that is known as the Research Domain Criteria (RDoC).[155] The RDoC calls for the development of new ways of classifying psychopathology based on dimensions of observable behavior and neurobiological measures.[155] The RDoC is encouraging researchers towards conceptualizing psychopathology in more dimensional ways. As outlined above, there is much more existing research on protocols designed for specific categorical disorders; however, preliminary studies on the unified protocol are promising.[156] In the future, it is likely that more treatments will be developed for broader dimensions of psychopathology.

CONCLUSION

CBT consists of challenging and modifying irrational thoughts and behaviors. CBT interventions have been well articulated in the form of treatment manuals and their efficacy has been tested in numerous RCTs. CBT is an empirically-supported intervention and is the treatment of choice for a wide variety of conditions.[1] Despite such findings, CBT has not been widely adopted by community practitioners, primary care settings, and pharmacotherapists. Researchers are actively trying to identify and address the factors that may be contributing to this gap between science and practice. Indeed, dissemination and implementation research is a major funding priority of the National Institutes of Mental Health and the topic of intense academic debate and research. We are hopeful that with increasing funding and attention to this important topic, CBT will become widely available to patients in need.[157]

Access the complete reference list and multiple choice questions (MCQs) online at https://expertconsult.inkling.com

KEY REFERENCES

1. Hollon SD, Beck AT. Cognitive and cognitive-behavioral therapies. In Lambert MJ, editor: *Bergin and Garfield's handbook of psychotherapy and behavior change*, ed 5, New York, 2003, Wiley.
10. Butler AC, Chapman JE, Forman EM. The empirical status of cognitive-behavioral therapy: a review of meta-analyses. *Clin Psychol Rev* 26:17–31, 2006.
13. Barlow DH. *Anxiety and its disorders: the nature and treatment of anxiety and panic*, New York, 2001, Guilford Press.
18. Mowrer OH. On the dual nature of learning: a reinterpretation of "conditioning" and "problem solving". *Harv Educ Rev* 17:102–148, 1947.
25. Beck AT, Rush AJ, Shaw BF, et al. *Cognitive therapy of depression*, New York, 1979, Wiley.
26. Beck AT. Cognitive therapy of depression: new perspectives. In Clayton PJ, Barrett JE, editors: *Treatment of depression: old controversies and new approaches*, New York, 1983, Raven.
30. Beck JS. *Cognitive behavior therapy: basics and beyond*, ed 2, New York, 2011, Guilford Press.
31. Ellis A. Reflections on rational-emotive therapy. *J Consult Clin Psychol* 61:199–201, 1993.
41. Chambless DL, Baker MJ, Baucom DH, et al. Update on empirically validated therapies: II. *Clin Psychol* 51:3–16, 1998.
46. Otto MW, Pollack MH, Meltzer-Brody S, et al. Cognitive-behavioral therapy for benzodiazepine discontinuation in panic disorder patients. *Psychopharmacol Bull* 28:123–130, 1992.
52. Hofmann SG, Asnaani A, Vonk IJ, et al. The efficacy of cognitive behavioral therapy: A review of meta-analyses. *Cognit Ther Res* 36:427–440, 2012.
53. Gloaguen V, Cottraux J, Cucherat M, et al. A meta-analysis of the effects of cognitive therapy in depressed patients. *J Affect Disord* 49:59–72, 1998.

66. Gould RA, Otto MW, Pollack MH. Cognitive behavioral and pharmacological treatment of generalized anxiety disorder: a preliminary meta-analysis. *Behav Ther* 28:285–305, 1997.

70. van Balkom AJLM, Bakker A, Spinhoven P, et al. A meta-analysis of the treatment of panic disorder with or without agoraphobia: a comparison of psychopharmacological, cognitive-behavioral, and combination treatments. *J Nerv Ment Dis* 185:510–516, 1997.

75. Hofmann SG, Smits JJ. Cognitive-behavioral therapy for adult anxiety disorders: A meta-analysis of randomized placebo-controlled trials. *J Clin Psychiatry* 69:621–632, 2008.

82. Abramowitz JS, Franklin ME, Foa EB. Empirical status of cognitive-behavioral therapy for obsessive-compulsive disorder: a meta-analytic review. *Rom J Cogn Behav Psychother* 2:89–104, 2002.

89. Ballenger JC, Davidson JR, Lecrubier Y, et al. Consensus statement on posttraumatic stress disorder from the International Consensus Group on Depression and Anxiety. *J Clin Psychiatry* 61(Suppl. 5):60–66, 2000.

95. Bradley R, Greene J, Russ E. A multidimensional meta-analysis of psychotherapy for PTSD. *Am J Psychiatry* 162:214–227, 2005.

111. Westen D, Novotny C, Thompson-Brenner H. The empirical status of empirically supported therapies: assumptions, methods, and findings. *Psychol Bull* 130:631–663, 2004.

116. Elkin I, Shea M, Tracie W, et al. National Institute of Mental Health Treatment of Depression Collaborative Research Program: general effectiveness of treatments. *Arch Gen Psychiatry* 46:971–982, 1989.

125. Pediatric OCD Treatment Study (POTS) Team. Cognitive-behavior therapy, sertraline, and their combination for children and adolescents with obsessive-compulsive disorder: the Pediatric OCD Treatment Study (POTS) randomized controlled trial. *JAMA* 292:1969–1976, 2004. PubMed PMID: 15507582.

134. Ressler KJ, Rothbaum BO, Tannenbaum L, et al. Cognitive enhancers as adjuncts to psychotherapy: use of D-cycloserine in phobics to facilitate extinction of fear. *Arch Gen Psychiatry* 61:1136–1145, 2004.

142. Linehan MM. *Cognitive-behavioral treatment of borderline personality disorder*, New York, 1993, Guilford Press.

148. Hayes SC, Strosahl KD, Wilson KG. *Acceptance and Commitment Therapy: An experiential approach to behavior change*, ed 1, New York, 2003, Guilford Press.

153. Barlow DH, Farchione T, Fairholme CP, et al. *The unified protocol for the transdiagnostic treatment of emotional disorders: Therapist guide*, New York, 2011, Oxford University Press.

157. McHugh RK, Barlow DH, editors. *Dissemination and implementation of evidence-based psychological interventions*, New York, 2012, Oxford University Press.

16

Depressive Disorders

Two new depressive disorders have been added to DSM-5. The disruptive mood dysregulation disorder (DMDD) diagnosis was added to address controversy regarding the diagnosis of children with bipolar disorder. The disorder describes children who exhibit chronic irritability and frequent episodes of extreme behavioral dysregulation. The symptoms are present nearly every day, for a year or more. Thus, DSM-5 makes the distinction between chronic irritability and long-standing outbursts of extreme dysregulation, consistent with DMDD, and clearly episodic and intermittent mood symptoms, representing a change from baseline, consistent with bipolar disorder. Premenstrual dysphoric disorder is the second addition, having been elevated from the DSM-IV-TR appendix into Section II of DSM-5 due to increased scientific support for its diagnostic stability and reliability.

DSM-5 also combines the diagnoses of dysthymia and chronic major depressive disorder (MDD) into a single diagnosis: persistent depressive disorder (dysthymia). The diagnostic criteria for MDD remain largely unchanged in DSM-5, with the exception of the removal of the bereavement exclusion, the prior restriction that MDD could not be diagnosed in a patient grieving the death of a loved one within the preceding 2 months. A note is included in the text to assist clinicians in distinguishing between normal grieving and a depressive disorder.

Anxiety Disorders

The anxiety and related disorders have been re-organized within the manual. Separation anxiety disorder and selective mutism are now included within the anxiety disorders chapter, as all disorders previously grouped together as occurring in infancy, childhood or adolescence have been moved into categories with the related adult diagnoses. In addition, obsessive-compulsive disorder (OCD), post-traumatic stress disorders (PTSD), and acute stress disorder are now separate chapters, occurring sequentially with anxiety disorders in order to reflect their close relationship. Finally, panic disorder and agoraphobia are now considered as separate diagnoses, and panic attack can now be listed as a specifier for a variety of disorders as well.

Obsessive-compulsive and Related Disorders

Obsessive-compulsive and related disorders comprise a new, separate, chapter in DSM-5, reflecting recent advances that indicate that these disorders are related to each other, and distinct from other anxiety disorders. This chapter includes OCD, as well as several new disorders, including hoarding disorder and excoriation (skin picking) disorder. Hoarding disorder has been removed as a subtype of OCD due to current understanding that it is a distinct disorder with different treatments and outcomes. Trichotillomania (hair-pulling disorder) has been moved into this chapter, from the impulse-control disorders chapter. Specifiers have been added for OCD, body dysmorphic disorder, and hoarding disorder to signal that absent insight or delusional beliefs should trigger the diagnosis of the particular obsessive-compulsive or related disorder, rather than a psychotic disorder. A tic-related specifier has also been added due to recognition that a co-morbid tic disorder has important clinical implications.

Trauma- and Stressor-related Disorders

A new chapter on trauma- and stressor-related disorders has been added to DSM-5. This chapter contains reactive attachment disorder, disinhibited social engagement disorder, PTSD, acute stress disorder, and adjustment disorders.

Diagnostic criteria for PTSD and acute stress disorder have been modified. The definition of traumatic exposure has been expanded, to include direct and indirect experience, as well as repeated exposure (as in the case of first-responders). The symptom clusters have also been expanded to include new symptoms, such as persistent negative emotional states.

The diagnosis of reactive attachment disorder (RAD) has also undergone revision. The two previously described subtypes (emotionally withdrawn/inhibited and indiscriminately social/disinhibited) are now distinct disorders: reactive attachment disorder and disinhibited social engagement disorder. The separation was made based on the recognition that the two subtypes have sufficiently different correlates, courses, and responses to interventions.

Somatic Symptom and Related Disorders

DSM-5 eliminated the diagnoses of somatization disorder, hypochondriasis, pain disorder, and undifferentiated somatoform disorder. Instead, somatization disorder and undifferentiated somatoform disorder are combined into somatic symptom disorder (SSD). This disorder now includes somatic symptoms that are either distressing or disruptive to daily life, in addition to excessive thoughts, feelings and behaviors related to the somatic symptoms or health concerns. The requirement for a specific number of symptoms from four organ groups has also been eliminated, as has the requirement that symptoms be "medically unexplained."

Eating Disorders

The existing eating disorders underwent minor revisions. The criteria for anorexia nervosa no longer include the amenorrhea requirement, which could not be applied to males, or to pre-menarchal or post-menopausal women. The required frequency of binge eating for the diagnosis of bulimia has been decreased to once a week (from twice a week). Binge eating disorder, now supported by extensive scientific research, is a new diagnosis in this chapter. Finally, pica, rumination, and avoidant/restrictive food-intake disorder have all been moved into this chapter, as all childhood disorders are now grouped with their adult counterparts.

Gender Dysphoria

Gender dysphoria is a new diagnostic category in DSM-5. It replaces gender identity disorder, and emphasizes distress about gender incongruence, rather than cross-gender identification, as in DSM-IV-TR. This gender incongruence and resulting dysphoria can manifest in a variety of presentations, and separate criteria are listed for children and adolescents and adults, based on developmental stage. The term "disorder" was replaced with "dysphoria" in order to reduce stigma and to become more consistent with clinical terminology. Finally, sexual dysfunction and paraphilias have been moved to separate chapters, given the lack of relationship between these disorders and gender dysphoria.

Disruptive, Impulse Control, and Conduct Disorders

This chapter is new to the DSM-5. It combines disorders that were previously in "Disorders Usually First Diagnosed in Infancy, Childhood or Adolescence," including oppositional defiant disorder (ODD), conduct disorder, disruptive behavior disorder, with disorders from "Impulse Control Disorders Not Otherwise Specified," including intermittent explosive disorder (IED), pyromania, and kleptomania. These disorders are now grouped together due to the recognition that they are all characterized by challenges with emotional and behavioral self-regulation.

Several disorders in this section have undergone revision. For example, symptoms of ODD are now grouped in three categories (angry/irritable mood, argumentative/defiant behavior, and vindictiveness) in order to reflect the presence of both emotional and behavioral symptoms. The exclusion criterion for conduct disorder has now been removed and specific duration criteria have been added, in order to distinguish between normal child or adolescent behavior and pathology. Criteria for IED have also been expanded to include verbal aggression, as well as physical aggression, and a minimum age of 6 years is now required, to distinguish it from developmentally-normal tantrums.

Substance-related and Addictive Disorders

The diagnoses of substance abuse and dependence are no longer separate in DSM-5. Rather, a new diagnosis of substance use disorder combines the prior DSM-IV-TR diagnostic criteria. Previously, substance abuse was thought to be a milder form of a substance-related disorder; however, there is now recognition that substance abuse can present with severe symptomatology, and thus the removal of these diagnostic boundaries.

DSM-5 also adds the new category of behavioral addictions. The sole diagnosis in this category is gambling disorder. The inclusion of this disorder in the substance-related disorders chapter is a reflection of the similarity between substance and behavioral addictions in presentation, co-morbidity, physiology, and treatment.

Neurocognitive Disorders

Dementia is now replaced by the diagnosis of "neurocognitive disorder." Mild neurocognitive disorder was included in order to encourage early diagnosis and proactive treatment before the onset of more incapacitating symptoms. Subtypes are determined by specific criteria for each etiology, and the term "dementia" can still be used to specify etiologic subtype.

CRITIQUES AND LIMITATIONS OF DSM-5

Even before its release, critiques of DSM-5 began to emerge.[28-31] Some felt that normative experiences were pathologized in DSM-5.[32,33] Others noted that diagnostic criteria were more restrictive for some disorders,[34] with potential real-world ramifications for service delivery, as in the case of autism spectrum disorder.[35] Additional authors voiced dissent around decisions made regarding aspects of specific diagnoses.[36-39] Concern regarding diagnostic reliability in field trials[40] and the implementation of new dimensional approaches to personality disorders were also expressed.[41,42]

More fundamentally, efforts have been made over the years to challenge the "atheoretical" basis of the DSM and to re-introduce explicitly theoretically-driven diagnostic schemata. Some researchers have suggested the need for an explicitly biologically-based model resulting in major re-classification of disorders on the basis of underlying pathophysiology.[32] This change has remained difficult to implement with the current state of scientific knowledge. The National Institute of Mental Health's Research Domain Criteria (RDoC) project[43] is a major effort conceived "to create a framework for research on pathophysiology, especially for genomics and neuroscience, which ultimately will inform future classification schemes."[44] The RDoC can be seen as a strategy "complementary" to current diagnostic systems whose emerging findings, as they become more directly clinically relevant, could ultimately be incorporated into future versions of the DSM.[28,45]

Other writers express ambivalence about the idea of psychiatric diagnosis and the "medical model" altogether, objecting, for example, to potentially counter-therapeutic legal, ethical, social, and economic uses and misuses of diagnostic information.[28,46,47] DSM-5 recognizes the need to incorporate information sensitive to patients' experience of illness,[48] as well as sociocultural,[30,49] gender-based,[24] and developmental/life-span perspectives.[50-52] Processes for incorporating these perspectives in more sophisticated ways should continue to evolve. Some additional critiques of DSM from specific theoretical orientations are described next.

Psychodynamic Approaches

One criticism of psychiatric evaluation focused solely on determining DSM-based diagnoses is that psychodynamic formulation may be neglected. Some have suggested that psychodynamic principles be returned to the DSM. Meanwhile, a coalition of psychoanalytically-oriented organizations has developed its own diagnostic manual separate from the DSM.[53]

Behavioral Approaches

Behaviorally-oriented clinicians argue that describing a behavior divorced from its context and function is meaningless, and that behavioral functional analysis should be incorporated into diagnostic classification.[54,55] For example, it may be more helpful in behavioral treatment-planning to create categories that account for what is reinforcing rule-breaking behavior in a child, rather than listing the types or numbers of rules broken, to create a category such as "Conduct Disorder."[56]

Family/Systems Theory

The DSM-5 identifies mental disorders as occurring solely "in an individual."[5] Critics operating from a family therapy or systems orientation have questioned this fundamental assumption, particularly for children. The DSM-5 notes the clinical relevance of problematic relationship patterns but does not recognize them as mental disorders. This may result in the practical problem of difficulty receiving third-party reimbursement for treatment, no matter how impairing the relational difficulties may be for the individuals involved.[4]

CONCLUSION

A variety of arguments have been made for improving—or even discarding—the DSM diagnostic system. Given the complexity of the human brain and behavior and the variety of natural and social environments in which people live, it is likely that any future psychiatric diagnostic system will need to be considered provisional: subject to change on the basis of empirical evidence and clinical utility. Nonetheless, the DSM-5 can be used powerfully by clinicians who are attentive to its limitations and who maintain a pragmatic focus on what benefits their individual patients. The DSM-5 provides a framework that can help clinicians to gather and synthesize information systematically and to communicate clearly. A careful assessment allows the clinical psychiatrist to proceed beyond the diagnostic purview of the DSM, toward effective treatment.

Access the complete reference list and multiple choice questions (MCQs) online at https://expertconsult.inkling.com

KEY REFERENCES

1. Wakefield JC, First MB. Clarifying the distinction between disorder and non-disorder: confronting the overdiagnosis (false-positives) problem in DSM-V. In Phillips KA, First MB, Pincus HA, editors: *Advancing DSM: dilemmas in psychiatric diagnosis*, Washington, DC, 2003, American Psychiatric Association.
2. First MB, Pincus HA, Levine JB, et al. Clinical utility as a criterion for revising psychiatric diagnoses. *Am J Psychiatry* 161:946–954, 2004.
5. American Psychiatric Association. *Diagnostic and statistical manual of mental disorders*, ed 5, Arlington, VA, 2013, American Psychiatric Association.
6. World Health Organization. *International statistical classification of diseases and related health problems, tenth revision*, Geneva, 1992, World Health Organization.
7. World Health Organization. *International classification of diseases, ninth revision, clinical modification*, Ann Arbor, MI, 1978, Commission on Professional and Hospital Activities.
9. Kupfer DJ, First MB, Regier DA, editors: *A research agenda for DSM-V*, Washington, DC, 2002, American Psychiatric Association.
16. Klerman GL, Vaillant GE, Spitzer RL, et al. A debate on DSM-III. *Am J Psychiatry* 141:539–553, 1984.
17. Robins E, Guze SB. Establishment of diagnostic validity in psychiatric illness: its application to schizophrenia. *Am J Psychiatry* 126:983–987, 1970.
21. Moran M. *DSM-5* offers creative teaching opportunity. *Psychiatr News* 48(11):18–25, 2013.
22. Clarke DE, Narrow WE, Regier DA, et al. DSM-5 field trials in the United States and Canada, Part I: study design, sampling strategy, implementation, and analytic approaches. *Am J Psychiatry* 170(1):43–58, 2013.
23. Kendler KS. A history of the DSM-5 scientific review committee. *Psychol Med* 3:1–8, 2013. [Epub ahead of print].
24. Regier DA, Kuhl EA, Kupfer DJ. The DSM-5: Classification and criteria changes. *World Psychiatry* 12(2):92–98, 2013.
25. Kupfer DJ, Kuhl EA, Regier DA. DSM-5—the future arrived. *JAMA* 309(16):1691–1692, 2013.
27. Gore WL, Widiger TA. The DSM-5 Dimensional Trait Model and Five-Factor Models of General Personality. *J Abnorm Psychol* 122(3):816–821, 2013. [Epub ahead of print].
30. Jacob KS, Kallivayalil RA, Mallik AK, et al. Diagnostic and statistical manual-5: Position paper of the Indian Psychiatric Society. *Indian J Psychiatry* 55(1):12–30, 2013.
35. McPartland JC, Reichow B, Volkmar FR. Sensitivity and specificity of proposed DSM-5 diagnostic criteria for autism spectrum disorder. *J Am Acad Child Adolesc Psychiatry* 51(4):368–383, 2012. [Epub 2012 Mar 14].
37. Koukopoulos A, Sani G, Ghaemi SN. Mixed features of depression: why DSM-5 is wrong (and so was DSM-IV). *Br J Psychiatry* J203:3–5, 2013.
38. Bisson JI. What happened to harmonization of the PTSD diagnosis? The divergence of ICD11 and DSM5. *Epidemiol Psychiatr Sci* 22(3):205–207, 2013. [Epub ahead of print].
39. Birgegård A, Norring C, Clinton D. DSM-IV versus DSM-5: implementation of proposed DSM-5 criteria in a large naturalistic database. *Int J Eat Disord* 45(3):353–361, 2012.
40. Freedman R, Lewis DA, Michels R, et al. The initial field trials of DSM-5: new blooms and old thorns. *Am J Psychiatry* 170(1):1–5, 2013.
41. Livesley J. The DSM-5 personality disorder proposal and future directions in the diagnostic classification of personality disorder. *Psychopathology* 46(4):207–216, 2013. [Epub 2013 May 4].
42. Lynam DR, Vachon DD. Antisocial personality disorder in DSM-5: missteps and missed opportunities. *Personal Disord* 3(4):483–495, 2012.
43. Cuthbert BN, Insel TR. Toward the future of psychiatric diagnosis: the seven pillars of RDoC. *BMC Med* 11:126, 2013.
44. Insel T, Cuthbert B, Garvey M, et al. Research domain criteria (RDoC): toward a new classification framework for research on mental disorders. *Am J Psychiatry* 167(7):748–751, 2010.
48. Stein DJ, Phillips KA. Patient advocacy and DSM-5. *BMC Med* 11:133, 2013.
49. Lewis-Fernández R, Aggarwal NK. Culture and psychiatric diagnosis. *Adv Psychosom Med* 33:15–30, 2013. [Epub 2013 Jun 25].
50. Knapp P, Jensen PS. Recommendations for DSM-V. In Jensen PS, Knapp P, Mrazek DA, editors: *Toward a new diagnostic system for child psychopathology: moving beyond the DSM*, New York, 2006, Guilford Press.
51. Bryant C, Mohlman J, Gum A, et al. Anxiety disorders in older adults: Looking to DSM5 and beyond… *Am J Geriatr Psychiatry* 21(9):872–876, 2013. [Epub ahead of print].
52. Bögels SM, Knappe S, Clark LA. Adult separation anxiety disorder in DSM-5. *Clin Psychol Rev* 33(5):663–674, 2013. [Epub 2013 Apr 2].
53. PDM Task Force. *Psychodynamic diagnostic manual*, Silver Spring, MD, 2006, Alliance of Psychoanalytic Organizations.

18   Delirium

Jason P. Caplan, MD, Ned H. Cassem, MA, PhL, MD, SJ, BD,
George B. Murray, BS, PhL, MS, MSc, MD†, and Theodore A. Stern, MD

KEY POINTS

Incidence

- Delirium is a syndrome caused by an underlying physiological disturbance. Of patients admitted to intensive care units, delirium may develop in more than half.

Pathophysiology

- The pathophysiology of delirium remains unclear, but the current leading theory cites an excess release of endogenous dopamine and loss of acetylcholine due to conditions of oxidative stress.

Clinical Findings

- Delirium is marked by a fluctuating course of impairments in consciousness, attention, and perception. Both hypermotoric and hypomotoric variants have been described.

Differential Diagnoses

- The differential diagnosis for causes of delirium covers the entire breadth of medical practice. An important, but rare, clinical mimic of delirium is delirious mania.

Treatment Options

- Various medications can be employed in the management of delirium, with the most evidence supporting the use of neuroleptics, especially haloperidol.

Complications

- The most concerning complications of delirium are those of an unidentified and untreated underlying somatic cause. The manifestations of delirium may add further complexity by agitation resulting in injury to the patient or their caregivers. The primary concern in the use of neuroleptics in the management of delirium is prolongation of the corrected QT interval and resulting cardiac arrhythmias.

Prognosis

- If the underlying cause of delirium can be identified and treated, prognosis is generally good; however, some studies have shown persisting mild cognitive impairment following delirium, especially in cases that are not diagnosed and managed in a timely fashion.

OVERVIEW

Delirium has likely replaced syphilis as "the great imitator," as its varied presentations have led to misdiagnoses among almost every major category of mental illness. A syndrome, caused by an underlying physiological disturbance (and marked by a fluctuating course with impairments in consciousness, attention, and perception), delirium is often mistaken for depression (with a "withdrawn" or "flat" affect), for mania (with agitation and confusion), for psychosis (with hallucinations and paranoia), for anxiety (with restlessness and hypervigilance), for dementia (with cognitive impairments), and for substance abuse (with impairment in consciousness). With so diverse an array of symptoms, delirium assumes a position of diagnostic privilege in the *Diagnostic and Statistical Manual of Mental Disorders, Fifth Edition* (DSM-5), in that almost no other diagnosis can be made *de novo* in its presence.

Perhaps even more noteworthy is that delirium is a signifier of (often serious) somatic illness.[1] Delirium has been associated with increased length of stay in hospitals[2] and with an increased cost of care.[3,4] Among intensive care unit (ICU) patients prospective studies have noted that delirium occurs in 31% of admissions[5]; when intubation and mechanical ventilation are required the incidence soars to 81.7%.[1]

Sometimes, delirium is referred to as an acute confusional state, a toxic-metabolic encephalopathy, or acute brain failure; unquestionably, it is the most frequent cause of agitation in the general hospital. Delirium ranks second only to depression on the list of all psychiatric consultation requests. Given its prevalence and its importance (morbidity and mortality), the American Psychiatric Association issued practice guidelines for the treatment of delirium in 1999.[6]

Placed in this context, the consequences of misdiagnosis of delirium can be severe; prompt and accurate recognition of this syndrome is paramount for all clinicians.

DIAGNOSIS

The essential features of delirium, according to the DSM-5, are disturbances of attention, awareness, and cognition developing over a short period of time that cannot be accounted for by past or evolving dementia and present in the context of evidence that they are due to an underlying medical condition (Box 18-1).[7] The ICD-10 includes disturbances in psychomotor activity, sleep, and emotion in its diagnostic guidelines (Box 18-2).[8]

Disturbance of the sleep–wake cycle is also common, sometimes with nocturnal worsening ("sundowning") or even by a complete reversal of the night–day cycle, though it should

BOX 18-1 DSM-5 Diagnostic Criteria: Delirium

A. A disturbance in attention (i.e. reduced ability to direct, focus, sustain, and shift attention) and awareness (reduced orientation to the environment).

B. The disturbance develops over a short period of time (usually hours to a few days), represents a change from baseline attention and awareness, and tends to fluctuate in severity during the course of a day.

C. An additional disturbance in cognition (e.g., memory deficit, disorientation, language, visuospatial ability, or perception).

D. The disturbances in Criteria A and C are not better explained by another pre-existing, established, or evolving neurocognitive disorder and do not occur in the context of a severely reduced level of arousal, such as coma.

E. There is evidence from the history, physical examination, or laboratory findings that the disturbance is a direct physiological consequence of another medical condition, substance intoxication or withdrawal (i.e., due to a drug of abuse or to a medication), or exposure to a toxin, or is due to multiple etiologies.

Specify whether:

Substance intoxication delirium: This diagnosis should be made instead of substance intoxication when the symptoms in

Criteria A and C predominate in the clinical picture and when they are sufficiently severe to warrant clinical attention.

• **Coding note:** The ICD-9-CM and ICD-10-CM codes for the [specific substance] intoxication delirium are indicated in the table below. Note that the ICD-10-CM code depends on whether or not there is a comorbid substance use disorder present for the same class of substance. If a mild substance use disorder is co-morbid with the substance intoxication delirium, the 4th position character is "1," and the clinician should record "mild [substance] use disorder," before the substance intoxication delirium (e.g., "mild cocaine use disorder is co-morbid with the substance intoxication delirium"). If a moderate or severe substance use disorder is co-morbid with the substance intoxication delirium, the 4th position character is "2," and the clinician should record "moderate [substance] use disorder" or "severe [substance] use disorder," depending on the severity of the comorbid substance use disorder. If there is no co-morbid substance use disorder (e.g., after a one-time heavy use of the substance), then the 4th position character is "9,"and the clinician should record only the substance intoxication delirium.

	ICD-9-CM	ICD-10-CM		
		With use disorder, mild	With use disorder, moderate or severe	Without use disorder
Alcohol	291.0	F10.121	F10.221	F10.921
Cannabis	292.81	F12.121	F12.221	F12.921
Phencyclidine	292.81	F16.121	F16.221	F16.921
Other hallucinogen	292.81	F16.121	F16.221	F16.921
Inhalant	292.81	F18.221	F18.221	F18.921
Opioid	292.81	F11.121	F11.221	F11.921
Sedative, hypnotic, or anxiolytic	292.81	F13.121	F13.221	F13.921
Amphetamine (or other stimulant)	292.81	F15.121	F15.221	F15.921
Cocaine	292.81	F14.121	F14.221	F14.921
Other (or unknown) substance	292.81	F19.221	F19.221	F19.921

Substance withdrawal delirium: This diagnosis should be made instead of substance withdrawal when the symptoms in Criteria A and C predominate in the clinical picture and when they are sufficiently severe to warrant clinical attention.

• **Coding note** [specific substance] withdrawal delirium: **291.0 (F10.231)** alcohol; **292.0 (F11.23)** opioid; 292.0 (F13.231) sedative, hypnotic, or anxiolytic; **292.0 (F19.231)** other (or unknown) substance/medication.

Medication-induced delirium: This diagnosis applies when the symptoms in Criteria A and C arise as a side effect of a medication taken as prescribed.

• **Coding note:** The ICD-9-CM code for [specific medication]-induced delirium is **292.81.** The ICD-10-CM code depends on the type of medication. If the medication is an opioid taken as prescribed, the code is **F11.921.** If the medication is a sedative, hypnotic, or anxiolytic taken as prescribed, the code is **F13.921.** If the medication is an amphetamine-type or other stimulant taken as prescribed, the code is **F15.921.** For medications that do not fit into any of the classes (e.g., dexamethasone) and in cases in which a substance is judged to be an etiological factor but the specific class of substance is unknown, the code is **F19.921.**

293.0 (F05) Delirium due to another medical condition: There is evidence from the history, physical examination, or laboratory findings that the disturbance is attributable to the physiological consequences of another medical condition.

• **Coding note:** Use multiple spate codes reflecting specific delirium etiologies (e.g., 572.2 [K72.90] hepatic encephalopathy, 293.0 [F05] delirium due to hepatic encephalopathy). The other medical condition should also be coded and listed separately immediately before the delirium due to another medical condition (e.g., 572.2 [K72.90] hepatic encephalopathy; 293.0 [F05] delirium due to hepatic encephalopathy).

293.0 (F05) Delirium due to multiple etiologies: There is evidence from the history, physical examination, or laboratory findings that the delirium has more than one etiology (e.g., more than one etiological medical condition; another medical condition plus substance intoxication or medication side effect).

• **Coding note:** Use multiple separate codes reflecting specific delirium etiologies (e.g., 572.2 [K72.90] hepatic encephalopathy, 293.0 [F05] delirium due to hepatic failure; 291/0 [F10.231] alcohol withdrawal delirium). Note that the etiological medical condition both appears as a separate code that precedes the delirium code and is substituted into the delirium due to another medical condition rubric.

Specify if:

Acute: Lasting a few hours or days
Persistent: Lasting weeks or months.

BOX 18-1 DSM-5 Diagnostic Criteria: Delirium (*Continued*)

Specify if:

Hyperactive: The individual has a hyperactive level of psychomotor activity that may be accompanied by mood lability, agitation, and/or refusal to cooperate with medical care.

Hypoactive: The individual has a hypoactive level of psychomotor activity that may be accompanied by sluggishness and lethargy that approaches stupor.

Mixed level of activity: The individual has a normal level of psychomotor activity even though attention and awareness are disturbed. Also includes individuals whose activity level rapidly fluctuates.

BOX 18-2 ICD-10 Diagnostic Guidelines for Delirium

Impairment of consciousness and attention (on a continuum from clouding to coma; reduced ability to direct, focus, sustain, and shift attention)

Global disturbance of cognition (perceptual distortions, illusions, and hallucinations—most often visual; impairment of abstract thinking and comprehension, with or without transient delusions, but typically with some degree of incoherence; impairment of immediate recall and of recent memory but with relatively intact remote memory; disorientation for time, as well as, in more severe cases, for place and person)

Psychomotor disturbances (hypoactivity or hyperactivity and unpredictable shifts from one to the other; increased reaction time; increased or decreased flow of speech; enhanced startle reaction)

Disturbance of the sleep–wake cycle (insomnia or, in severe cases, total sleep loss or reversal of the sleep–wake cycle; daytime drowsiness; nocturnal worsening of symptoms; disturbing dreams or nightmares, which may continue as hallucinations after awakening)

Emotional disturbances (e.g., depression, anxiety or fear, irritability, euphoria, apathy, or wondering perplexity)

be emphasized that (despite previous postulation) sleep disturbance alone does not cause delirium.[9] Similarly, the term "ICU psychosis" has entered the medical lexicon; this is an unfortunate misnomer because it is predicated on the beliefs that the environment of the ICU alone is capable of inducing delirium and that the symptomatology of delirium is limited to psychosis.[9,10]

Despite wide variation in the presentation of the delirious patient, the hallmarks of delirium (although perhaps less immediately apparent) remain quite consistent from case to case. Inattention can be regarded as the *sine qua non* of delirium in that it serves to differentiate the syndrome from any other psychiatric diagnosis. This inattention (along with an acute onset, waxing and waning course, and overall disturbance of consciousness) forms the core of delirium, while other related symptoms (e.g., withdrawn affect, agitation, hallucinations, and paranoia) serve as a "frame" that can sometimes be so prominent as to detract from the picture itself.

Psychotic symptoms (such as visual or auditory hallucinations and delusions) are common among patients with delirium.[11] Sometimes the psychiatric symptoms are so bizarre or so offensive (e.g., an enraged and paranoid patient shouts that pornographic movies are being made in the ICU) that diagnostic efforts are distracted. The hypoglycemia of a man with diabetes can be missed in the emergency department (ED) if

the accompanying behavior is threatening, uncooperative, and resembling that of an intoxicated person.

While agitation may distract practitioners from making an accurate diagnosis of delirium, disruptive behavior alone will almost certainly garner some attention. The DSM-5 includes motoric specifiers for the diagnosis of delirium (i.e., hyperactive, hypoactive, or mixed). The "hypoactive" presentation of delirium is more insidious, since the patient is often thought to be depressed or anxious because of his or her medical illness. Studies of quietly delirious patients show the experience to be equally as disturbing as the agitated variant[12]; quiet delirium is still a harbinger of serious medical pathology.[13,14]

The core similarities found in cases of delirium have led to postulation of a final common neurological pathway for its symptoms. Current understanding of the neurophysiological basis of delirium is one of hyperdopaminergia and hypocholinergia, likely as a result of increased oxidative stress.[15,16] The ascending reticular activating system (RAS) and its bilateral thalamic projections regulate alertness, with neocortical and limbic inputs to this system controlling attention. Since acetylcholine is the primary neurotransmitter of the RAS, medications with anticholinergic activity can interfere with its function, resulting in the deficits in alertness and attention that are the heralds of delirium. Similarly, it is thought that loss of cholinergic neuronal activity in the elderly (e.g., due to microvascular disease or atrophy) is the basis for their heightened risk of delirium. Release of endogenous dopamine due to oxidative stress is thought to be responsible for the perceptual disturbances and paranoia that so often lead to the delirious patient being mislabeled as "psychotic." Moreover, dopamine can exacerbate agitation by potentiating the neuroexcitatory action of glutamate. As we shall discuss later, both cholinergic agents (e.g., physostigmine) and dopamine blockers (e.g., haloperidol) have proven efficacious in the management of delirium.

DIFFERENTIAL DIAGNOSIS

Treatment relies on a careful diagnostic evaluation; there is no substitute for a systematic search for the specific cause of delirium. The temporal relationship to clinical events often gives the best clues to potential causes. For example, a patient who extubated himself was almost certainly in trouble before self-extubation. When did his mental state actually change? Nursing notes should be studied to help discern the first indication of an abnormality (e.g., restlessness, mild confusion, or anxiety). If a time of onset can be established as a marker, other events can be examined for a possible causal relationship to the change in mental state. Initiation or discontinuation of a drug, the onset of fever or hypotension, or the acute worsening of renal function, if in proximity to the time of mental status changes, become more likely culprits. A number of screening instruments that can be administered by nursing staff at the bedside on a recurring basis allow for early identification of delirium. Of these, the Confusion Assessment

Method–ICU (CAM-ICU) is probably the most broadly validated and used (and is available on-line at www .icudelirium.org).[17,18] These screening instruments can serve as a trigger to initiate psychiatric consultation and timely verification of the diagnosis and search for an underlying cause.

Without a convincing temporal connection, the cause of delirium may be discovered by its likelihood in the unique clinical situation of the patient. In critical care settings, as in EDs, there are several (life-threatening) states that the clinician can consider routinely. These are states in which intervention needs to be especially prompt because failure to make the diagnosis may result in permanent central nervous system (CNS) damage. These conditions are (1) Wernicke's disease; (2) hypoxia; (3) hypoglycemia; (4) hypertensive encephalopathy; (5) hyperthermia or hypothermia; (6) intracerebral hemorrhage; (7) meningitis/encephalitis; (8) poisoning (whether exogenous or iatrogenic); and (9) status epilepticus. These conditions are usefully recalled by the mnemonic device WHHH-HIMPS (Box 18-3). Other, less urgent but still acute conditions that require intervention include subdural hematoma, septicemia, subacute bacterial endocarditis, hepatic or renal failure, thyrotoxicosis/myxedema, delirium tremens, anticholinergic psychosis, and complex partial seizures. If not already ruled out, when present, these conditions are easy to verify. A broad review of conditions frequently associated with delirium is provided by the mnemonic I WATCH DEATH (Table 18-1).

In the elderly, regardless of the setting, the onset of confusion should trigger concern about infection, with urinary tract infections (UTIs) or pneumonias as the most likely candidates.

BOX 18-3   Life-Threatening Causes of Delirium as Recalled by Use of the Mnemonic *WHHHHIMPS*

Wernicke's disease
Hypoxia
Hypoglycemia
Hypertensive encephalopathy
Hyperthermia or hypothermia
Intracerebral hemorrhage
Meningitis/encephalitis
Poisoning (whether exogenous or iatrogenic)
Status epilepticus

TABLE 18-1   Conditions Frequently Associated with Delirium, Recalled by the Mnemonic *I WATCH DEATH*

Infectious	Encephalitis, meningitis, syphilis, pneumonia, urinary tract infection
Withdrawal	Alcohol, sedative-hypnotics
Acute metabolic	Acidosis, alkalosis, electrolyte disturbances, hepatic or renal failure
Trauma	Heat stroke, burns, post-operative
CNS pathology	Abscesses, hemorrhage, seizures, stroke, tumors, vasculitis, normal pressure hydrocephalus
Hypoxia	Anemia, carbon monoxide poisoning, hypotension, pulmonary embolus, pulmonary or cardiac failure
Deficiencies	Vitamin B$_{12}$, niacin, thiamine
Endocrinopathies	Hyperglycemia or hypoglycemia, hyperadrenocorticism or hypoadrenocorticism, hyperthyroidism or hypothyroidism, hyperparathyroidism or hypoparathyroidism
Acute vascular	Hypertensive encephalopathy, shock
Toxins or drugs	Medications, pesticides, solvents
Heavy metals	Lead, manganese, mercury

In one study of elderly women with UTIs, almost half (44.8%) were found to be actively delirious or to have experienced symptoms of delirium in the prior month.[19] Once a consultant has eliminated these basic conditions as possible causes of a patient's disturbed brain function, there is time enough for a more systematic approach to the differential diagnosis. While the long-used medical admonition to think of horses when one hears hoofbeats remains true, once the consultant has ruled-out "horses" (i.e., common diagnoses), attention should turn to "zebras" (uncommon diagnoses) and potentially "unicorns" (diagnoses read about in textbooks but not usually seen in practice). Indeed, the potential causes of oxidative stress (and thus, potential causes of delirium) stretch across the entire breadth of medical practice (Table 18-2). To understand the acute reaction of the individual patient, one should begin by completely reviewing the medical record. Vital signs may reveal periods of hypotension or fever. Operative procedures and the use of anesthetics may also induce a sustained period of hypotension or reveal unusually large blood loss and its replacement. Laboratory values should be scanned for abnormalities that could be related to an encephalopathic state.

The old chart, no matter how thick, cannot be overlooked without risk. Some patients have had psychiatric consultations for similar difficulties on prior admissions. Others, in the absence of psychiatric consultations, have caused considerable trouble for their caregivers. Similar to a patient's psychiatric history, the family's psychiatric history can help make a diagnosis, especially if a major mood or anxiety disorder, alcoholism, schizophrenia, or epilepsy is present.

Examination of current and past medications is essential because pharmacological agents (in therapeutic doses, in overdose, or with withdrawal) can produce psychiatric symptoms. Moreover, these considerations must be routinely reviewed, especially in patients whose drugs have been stopped because of surgery or hospitalization or whose drug orders have not been transmitted during transfer between services. Of all causes of an altered mental status, use of drugs and withdrawal from drugs are probably the most common. Some agents are commonly known to have neuropsychiatric effects (e.g., corticosteroids), others are less well-known to precipitate delirium (e.g., fluoroquinolone antibiotics); thus it may be advisable to review the current literature using an online search engine for reports of deliriogenesis related to agents on the patients' medication list.[20] In the face of an ever-expanding list of medications associated with delirium, inclusion of a comprehensive list of these agents would be far beyond the scope of this volume.

The list of drugs that can be deliriogenic either directly or indirectly (e.g., because of drug interactions) is extensive. Although physicians are usually aware of these hazards, a common drug, such as meperidine, when used in doses above 300 mg/day for several days, causes CNS symptoms because of the accumulation of its excitatory metabolite, normeperidine, which has a half-life of 30 hours and causes myoclonus (the best clue of normeperidine toxicity), anxiety, and ultimately seizures.[21] The usual treatment is to stop the offending drug or to reduce the dose; however, at times this is not possible. Elderly patients and those with intellectual disability or a history of traumatic brain injury are more susceptible to the toxic actions of many of these drugs.

Psychiatric symptoms in medical illness can have other causes. Besides the abnormalities that may arise from the effect of the patient's medical illness (or its treatment) on the CNS (e.g., the abnormalities produced by systemic lupus erythematosus or use of high-dose steroids), the disturbance may be the effect of the medical illness on the patient's mind (the subjective CNS), as in the patient who thinks he is "washed up" after a myocardial infarction, quits, and withdraws into

TABLE 18-2 Differential Diagnoses of Delirium

General Cause	Specific Cause
Vascular	Hypertensive encephalopathy; cerebral arteriosclerosis; intracranial hemorrhage or thromboses; emboli from atrial fibrillation, patent foramen ovale, or endocarditic valve; circulatory collapse (shock); systemic lupus erythematosus; polyarteritis nodosa; thrombotic thrombocytopenic purpura; hyperviscosity syndrome; sarcoid
Infectious	Encephalitis, bacterial or viral meningitis, fungal meningitis (cryptococcal, coccidioidal, *Histoplasma*), sepsis, general paresis, brain/epidural/subdural abscess, malaria, human immunodeficiency virus, Lyme disease, typhoid fever, parasitic (toxoplasma, trichinosis, cysticercosis, echinococcosis), Behçet's syndrome, mumps
Neoplastic	Space-occupying lesions, such as gliomas, meningiomas, abscesses; paraneoplastic syndromes; carcinomatous meningitis
Degenerative	Senile and presenile dementias, such as Alzheimer's or Pick's dementia, Huntington's chorea, Creutzfeldt–Jakob disease, Wilson's disease
Intoxication	Chronic intoxication or withdrawal effect of sedative-hypnotic drugs, such as bromides, opiates, tranquilizers, anticholinergics, dissociative anesthetics, anticonvulsants, carbon monoxide from burn inhalation
Congenital	Epilepsy, post-ictal states, complex partial status epilepticus, aneurysm
Traumatic	Subdural and epidural hematomas, contusion, laceration, post-operative trauma, heat stroke, fat emboli syndrome
Intraventricular	Normal pressure hydrocephalus
Vitamin deficiency	Deficiencies of thiamine (Wernicke–Korsakoff syndrome), niacin (pellagra), vitamin B_{12} (pernicious anemia)
Endocrine-metabolic	Diabetic coma and shock; uremia; myxedema; hyperthyroidism, parathyroid dysfunction; hypoglycemia; hepatic or renal failure; porphyria; severe electrolyte or acid/base disturbances; paraneoplastic syndrome; Cushing's/Addison's syndrome; sleep apnea; carcinoid; Whipple's disease
Metals	Heavy metals (lead, manganese, mercury); other toxins
Anoxia	Hypoxia and anoxia secondary to pulmonary or cardiac failure, anesthesia, anemia
Depression—other	Depressive pseudodementia, hysteria, catatonia

Modified from Ludwig AM. Principles of clinical psychiatry, New York, 1980, Free Press.

hopelessness. The disturbance may also arise from the mind, as a conversion symptom or as malingering to get more narcotics. Finally, the abnormality may be the result of interactions between the sick patient and his or her environment or family (e.g., the patient who is without complaints until his family arrives, at which time he promptly looks acutely distressed and begins to whimper continuously). Nurses are commonly aware of these sorts of abnormalities, although they may go undocumented in the medical record.

EXAMINATION OF THE PATIENT

Appearance, level of consciousness, thought, speech, orientation, memory, mood, judgment, and behavior should all be assessed. In the formal mental status examination (MSE), one begins with the examination of consciousness. If the patient does not speak, a handy common-sense test is to ask oneself, "Do the eyes look back at me?" One could formally rate consciousness by using the Glasgow Coma Scale (see Chapter 81, Table 81-3), a measure that is readily understood by consultees from other specialties.[22]

If the patient can cooperate with an examination, attention should be examined first because if this is disturbed, other parts of the examination may be invalid. One can ask the patient to repeat those letters of the alphabet that rhyme with "tree." (If the patient is intubated, ask that a hand or finger be raised whenever the letter of the recited alphabet rhymes with tree.) Then the rest of the MSE can be performed. The Folstein Mini-Mental State Examination (MMSE),[23] which is presented in Chapter 2, Table 2-1, may be used, as may the Montreal Cognitive Assessment (MoCA) which may be more sensitive in identifying milder forms of cognitive dysfunction (the MoCA can be found on-line in a variety of languages at www.mocatest.org).[24] Specific defects are more important than is the total score. Included in the MoCA is perhaps the most dramatic (though difficult to score objectively) test of

cognition, the clock-drawing test, which can provide a broad survey of the patient's cognitive state (Figure 18-1).[25]

The patient's problem may involve serious neurological syndromes as well; however, the clinical presentation of the patient should direct the examination. In general, the less responsive and more impaired the patient is, the more one should look for "hard" signs. A directed search for an abnormality of the eyes and pupils, nuchal rigidity, hyperreflexia (withdrawal), "hung-up" reflexes (myxedema), one-sided weakness or asymmetry, gait (normal pressure hydrocephalus), Babinski's reflexes, tetany, absent vibratory and position senses, hyperventilation (acidosis, hypoxia, or pontine disease), or other specific clues can help to verify or refute hypotheses about causality that are stimulated by the abnormalities in the examination.

Frontal lobe function deserves specific attention. Grasp, snout, palmomental, suck, and glabellar responses are helpful when present.[26] Hand movements thought to be related to the pre-motor area (Brodmann's area 8) can identify subtle deficiencies. The patient is asked to imitate, with each hand separately, specific movements. The hand is held upright, a circle formed by thumb and first finger ("okay" sign), then the fist is closed and lowered to the surface on which the elbow rests (Figure 18-2 A, B). In the Luria sequence (Figure 18-3 A-C), one hand is brought down on a surface (a table or one's own leg) in three successive positions: extended with all five digits parallel ("cut"), then as a fist, and then flat on the surface ("slap"). Finally, both hands are placed on a flat surface in front of the patient, one flat on the surface, the other resting as a fist. Then the positions are alternated between right and left hands, and the patient is instructed to do likewise.

For verbally responsive patients, their response to the "Frank Jones story" can be gauged (i.e., "I have a friend, Frank Jones, whose feet are so big he has to put his pants on over his head. How does that strike you?"). Three general responses are given. Type 1 is normal: the patient sees the incongruity and

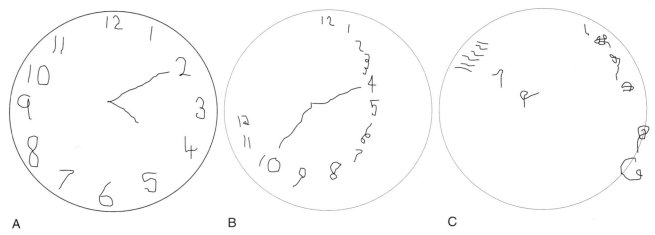

Figure 18-1. The clock-drawing test. The patient is provided with a circular outline and asked to draw the numbers as they appear on the face of a clock. Once that is complete, the patient is asked to set the hands to a particular time (often "ten past" the hour to test if the patient can suppress the impulse to include the number 10). Example A demonstrates good planning and use of space. Example B features some impulsiveness as the numbers are drawn without regard for actual location, and the time "ten past four" is represented by hands pointing to the digits 10 and 4. Note the perseveration indicated by the extra loops on the digits 3 and 6. Impulsiveness and perseveration are indicative of frontal lobe dysfunction. Example C demonstrates gross disorganization, although the patient took several minutes to draw the clock, and believed it to be a good representation.

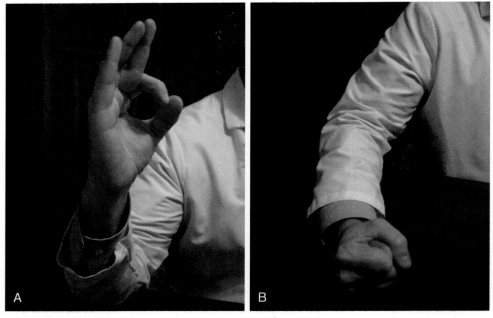

Figure 18-2. Testing of the pre-motor area.

smiles (a limbic response) and can explain (a neocortical function) why it cannot be done. Type 2 is abnormal: the patient smiles at the incongruity (a limbic connection), but cannot explain why it cannot be done. Type 3 is abnormal: the patient neither gets the incongruity nor can explain its impossibility. If the patient is too impaired to engage in a verbal interview, more direct attempts to gauge limbic and neocortical functioning may be employed. Under the guise of vision testing, the patient can be asked to count the number of fingers displayed by the examiner. If the display of a solitary middle digit provokes a different reaction (whether it be a knowing smirk or a look of shock) than the display of an index finger, the examiner can be assured of a relatively intact limbic circuit.

Laboratory studies should be carefully reviewed, with special attention paid to indicators of infection or metabolic disturbance. Toxicological screens are also frequently helpful in allowing the inclusion or exclusion of substance intoxication or withdrawal from the differential. Although less common, an increasing number of reports have documented autoimmune encephalitides as a cause of delirium.[27,28] If a basic work-up effectively rules out more common causes of delirium, markers for these autoimmune processes may be included in the next stage of investigation (Table 18-3). Neuroimaging may prove useful in the detection of intracranial processes that can result in altered mental status. Of all the diagnostic studies available, the electroencephalogram (EEG) may be the most useful tool in the diagnosis of delirium. Engel and Romano[29] reported in 1959 their (now classic) findings on the EEG in delirium, namely, generalized slowing to the theta-delta range in the delirious patient, the consistency of

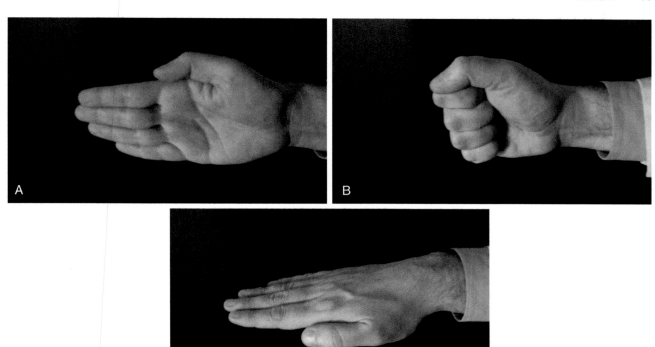

Figure 18-3. The Luria sequence.

TABLE 18-3 Antibodies Found in Autoimmune Encephalitides and their Associated Conditions

Anti-Hu	Small cell lung cancer (SCLC)
	Colon adenocarcinoma
	Thymoma
	Non-small cell lung cancer
	Prostate cancer
	Neuroblastoma
	Rhabdosarcoma
Anti-amphiphysin	SCLC
	Breast cancer
Anti-Ma2	Testicular cancer
	Breast cancer
	Non-small cell lung cancer
Anti-CV2	SCLC
	Thymoma
	Breast cancer
Anti-Ri	Endobronchial carcinoid
	Ovarian teratoma
	Breast cancer
	SCLC
Anti-VGKC complex	Thymoma
(including Anti-LGI1	Prostate cancer
and Anti-CASPR2)	Morvan's syndrome (anti-CASPR2 specific)
Anti-NMDAr	Ovarian teratoma
Anti-mGluR5	Hodgkin's lymphoma
Anti-GABA(B)	SCLC
Anti-thyroperoxidase	Steroid-responsive encephalopathy associated with thyroiditis (Hashimoto's encephalopathy)
Anti-thyroglobulin	Steroid-responsive encephalopathy associated with thyroiditis (Hashimoto's encephalopathy)

Modified from Foster AR, Caplan JP. Paraneoplastic limbic encephalitis, Psychosomatics *50(2):108–113, 2009.*

this finding despite wide-ranging underlying conditions, and resolution of this slowing with effective treatment of the delirium. EEG findings may even clarify the etiology of a delirium, since delirium tremens is associated with low-voltage fast activity superimposed on slow waves, sedative-hypnotic toxicity produces fast beta activity (>12 Hz), and hepatic encephalopathy is classically associated with triphasic waves.[30] A characteristic EEG finding called extreme delta brush has been associated with anti-NMDA receptor autoimmune encephalitis.[31]

SPECIFIC MANAGEMENT STRATEGIES FOR DELIRIUM

Psychosocial or environmental measures are rarely effective in the treatment of a *bona fide* delirium of uncertain or unknown cause. Nevertheless, it is commendable to have hospital rooms with windows, calendars, clocks, and a few mementos from home on the walls; soft and low lighting at night helps "sundowners"; and, most of all, a loving family in attendance reassures and re-orients the patient. The psychiatric consultant is often summoned because psychosocial measures have failed to prevent or to treat the patient's delirium. Restraints (e.g., geriatric chairs, "vests," helmets, locked leather restraints) are also available and quite useful to protect patients from inflicting harm on themselves or staff. One or several of these is often in place when the consultant arrives. One hoped-for outcome of the consultation is that the use of these devices can be reduced or eliminated. The unfortunate misnomer *chemical restraint* is frequently applied to the most helpful class of drugs for delirium (i.e., neuroleptics). However, physicians do not use chemical restraints (i.e., tear gas, pepper spray, mace, or nerve gas) in the treatment of agitated patients.

When the cause of the delirium seems straightforward, the treatment revolves around resolution or reversal of the underlying cause. A discovered deficiency can be replaced (e.g., of blood, oxygen, thiamine, vitamin B$_{12}$, synthroid, or glucose). Pathological conditions can be treated (e.g., diuretics for pulmonary edema, antibiotics for infection, or dialysis for acute lithium toxicity). Implicated drugs (such as meperidine) can be stopped or reduced.

Specific antidotes can reverse the delirium caused by some drugs. Flumazenil and naloxone reverse the effects of benzodiazepines and opioid analgesics, respectively. However, caution is required because use of flumazenil may precipitate seizures in a benzodiazepine-dependent patient, and naloxone can also precipitate narcotic withdrawal in a narcotic-dependent patient.

Anticholinergic delirium can be reversed by intravenous (IV) physostigmine (in doses starting at 0.5 to 2 mg). Caution is essential with use of this agent as the autonomic nervous system of the medically ill is generally less stable than it is in a healthy patient who has developed an anticholinergic delirium as a result of a voluntary or accidental overdose. Thus, routine use of physostigmine is typically limited to these cases of poisoning. Moreover, if there is a reasonably high amount of an anticholinergic drug on board that is clearing from the system slowly, the therapeutic effect of physostigmine, although sometimes quite dramatic, is usually short-lived. The cholinergic reaction to intravenously-administered physostigmine can cause profound bradycardia and hypotension, thereby multiplying the complications.[32,33] It should also be noted that a continuous IV infusion of physostigmine has been successfully used to manage a case of anticholinergic poisoning.[34] Because of the diagnostic value of physostigmine, one may wish to use it even though its effects will be short-lived. If one uses an IV injection of 1 mg of physostigmine, protection against excessive cholinergic reaction can be provided by preceding this injection with an IV injection of 0.2 mg of glycopyrrolate. This anticholinergic agent does not cross the blood–brain barrier and should protect the patient from the peripheral cholinergic actions of physostigmine.

While some anecdotal accounts and small studies have suggested benefit from the use of the oral cholinesterase inhibitors indicated for Alzheimer's dementia (i.e., donepezil, rivastigmine, galantamine),[35,36] one randomized, multicenter, double-blind, placebo-controlled trial of rivastigmine in delirium had to be abruptly halted due to significantly increased mortality in the group receiving the cholinesterase inhibitor.[37] The mechanism for this increased mortality remains obscure. Based on the data obtained before the trial was halted, rivastigmine did not decrease the duration of delirium. In the absence of evidence of any clinical utility and with the suggestion that they may increase mortality, these agents are not recommended for use in delirium.

DRUG TREATMENT

All too often, the cause of delirium is not readily identified or treated. These situations call for management of the symptoms of delirium while a more specific and effective treatment can be initiated. Opioids, benzodiazepines, neuroleptics, barbiturates, neuromuscular blocking agents, inhalant anesthetics, and assorted other agents (such as propofol, ketamine, isoflurane, chloral hydrate, and clonidine) are available (alone or in creative combinations).

Benzodiazepines (e.g., 2.5 mg of IV diazepam or 0.5 to 1 mg of midazolam) are often effective in mild agitation in the setting of withdrawal from drugs that work at the alcohol, benzodiazepine, and barbiturate receptor. Morphine is also used frequently as it calms agitation and is easily reversed if hypotension or respiratory depression ensues. Especially in higher doses, these agents can cause or exacerbate confusion in older patients.

Neuroleptics are the agent of choice for delirium. Haloperidol is probably the agent most commonly used to treat agitated delirium in the critical care setting; its effects on blood pressure, pulmonary artery pressure, heart rate, and respiration are milder than those of the benzodiazepines, making it an excellent agent for delirious patients with impaired cardiorespiratory status.[38]

Although haloperidol can be administered orally or parenterally, acute delirium with extreme agitation typically requires use of parenteral medication. IV administration is preferable to intramuscular (IM) administration because drug absorption may be poor in distal muscles if delirium is associated with circulatory compromise or with borderline shock. The deltoid is probably a better IM injection site than the gluteus muscle, but neither is as reliable as is the IV route. Second, as the agitated patient is commonly paranoid, repeated painful IM injections may increase the patient's sense of being attacked by enemy forces. Third, IM injections can complicate interpretations of muscle enzyme studies if enzyme fractionation is not readily available. Fourth, and most important, haloperidol is less likely to produce extrapyramidal symptoms (EPS) when given IV than when given IM or by mouth (PO), at least for patients without a prior serious psychiatric disorder.[39]

In contrast to the immediately-observable sedation produced by IV benzodiazepines, IV haloperidol has a mean distribution time of 11 minutes in normal volunteers[40]; this may be even longer in critically ill patients. The mean half-life of IV haloperidol's subsequent, slower phase is 14 hours. This is still a more rapid metabolic rate than the overall mean half-lives of 21 and 24 hours for IM and PO doses.

Haloperidol has not been approved by the Food and Drug Administration (FDA) for IV administration. Nonetheless, haloperidol given IV has been the standard of care for delirium for several decades and is included in practice guidelines from a variety of professional organizations.[6,41,42] Moreover, any approved drug can be used for a non-approved indication or route within the general hospital if justified as "innovative therapy."

Use of haloperidol has been associated with few adverse effects on blood pressure, heart rate, respiratory rate, or urinary output and has been linked with few EPS. The reason for the latter is not known. Studies of the use of IV haloperidol in psychiatric patients have not shown that these side effects were fewer. The reason for their rare appearance after IV administration in medically ill patients may be due to the fact that many of the medically ill patients have other medications in their system, especially benzodiazepines (that are protective against EPS) or that patients with psychiatric disorders are more susceptible to EPS.[39]

Before administration of IV haloperidol, the IV line should be flushed with 2 ml of normal saline. Phenytoin precipitates with haloperidol, and mixing the two in the same line must be avoided. Occasionally, haloperidol may also precipitate with heparin, and because many lines in critical care units are heparinized, the 2 ml flush is advised. The initial bolus dose of haloperidol usually varies from 0.5 to 20 mg; usually 0.5 mg (for an elderly person) to 2 mg is used for mild agitation, 5 mg is used for moderate agitation, and 10 mg for severe agitation. The only time when a higher initial dose should be used is when the patient has already been unsuccessfully treated with reasonable doses of haloperidol. To adjust for haloperidol's lag time, doses are usually staggered by at least a 30-minute interval. If one dose (e.g., a 5 mg dose) fails to calm an agitated patient after 30 minutes, the next higher dose, 10 mg, should be administered. Calm is the desired outcome. Partial control of agitation is usually inadequate, and settling for this only prolongs the delirium or guarantees that even higher total doses of haloperidol will be used over the prolonged course.

Haloperidol can be combined every 30 minutes with simultaneous parenteral lorazepam doses (starting with 1 to 2 mg). Because the effects of lorazepam are noticeable within 5 to 10 minutes, each dose can precede the haloperidol dose, observed for its impact on agitation, and increased if it is more effective. At least one randomized double-blind study has shown that the combination leads to more rapid efficacy and a lower overall dose of each drug.[43]

After calm is achieved, agitation should be the sign for a repeat dose. Ideally, the total dose of haloperidol on the second day should be a fraction of that used on day 1. After complete lucidity has been achieved, the patient needs to be protected from delirium only at night, by small doses of haloperidol (1 to 3 mg), which can be given PO. As in the treatment of delirium tremens, the consultant is advised to stop the agitation quickly and completely at the outset rather than barely keep up with it over several days. The maximum total dose of IV haloperidol to be used as an upper limit has not been established, although IV administration of single bolus doses of 200 mg have been used, and up to 1,600 mg has been used in a 24-hour period.[44] A continuous infusion of haloperidol has also been used to treat severe, refractory delirium.[45]

When delirium does not respond and agitation is unabated, one may wonder if the neuroleptic is producing akathisia. The best indication as to whether the treatment is causing agitation is the patient's description of an irresistible urge to move—usually the limbs, lower more often than upper. If dialogue is possible, even nodding yes or no (provided that the patient understands the question) can confirm or exclude this symptom. If the patient cannot communicate, limited options remain: to decrease the dose or to increase it and judge by the response. In our experience, it is far more common for the patient to receive more haloperidol and to improve.

Hypotensive episodes following the administration of IV haloperidol are rare and almost invariably result from hypovolemia. Ordinarily, this is easily checked in ICU patients who have indwelling pulmonary artery catheters, but because agitation is likely to return, volume replacement is necessary before one administers further doses. Local caustic effects on veins do not arise. IV haloperidol is generally safe for patients with epilepsy and traumatic brain injury, unless psychotropic drugs are contraindicated because the patient needs careful neurological monitoring. Although IV haloperidol may be used without mishap in patients receiving epinephrine (adrenaline) drips, after large doses of haloperidol a pressor other than epinephrine (e.g., norepinephrine [noradrenaline]) should be used to avoid unopposed β-adrenergic activity. IV haloperidol does not block a dopamine-mediated increase in renal blood flow. It also appears to be the safest agent for patients with chronic obstructive pulmonary disease.

Haloperidol has been associated with prolongation of the corrected QT interval (QTc) and the development of torsades de pointes (TDP).[46-48] Similar effects have been noted with all neuroleptics due to their binding at the delayed-rectifier potassium channel on cardiac muscle. The QTc should be monitored when haloperidol is used, and particular caution is urged when levels of potassium and magnesium are low, when hepatic compromise is present, or when a specific cardiac abnormality (e.g., mitral valve prolapse or a dilated ventricle) exists. Pre-menopausal women are most at risk for TDP due to the QTc prolonging effects of estrogen. Progressive QT widening after haloperidol administration should alert one to the danger, however infrequent it may be in practice (4 of 1,100 cases in one unit).[47] Delirious patients who are candidates for IV haloperidol require careful screening. Serum potassium and magnesium should be within normal range and a baseline

TABLE 18-4 Mean Neuroleptic-induced Change in QTc at Steady State

Drug	Change in QTc (msec)
Haloperidol	4.7
Olanzapine	6.8
Risperidone	11.6
Quetiapine	14.5
Ziprasidone	20.3
Thioridazine	35.6

Modified from Glassman AH, Bigger JT Jr. Antipsychotic drugs: prolonged QTc interval, torsade de pointes, and sudden death, Am J Psychiatry 158(11):1774–1782, 2001.

electrocardiogram (EKG) checked for the pretreatment QTc. QTc prolongation occurs in some patients with alcoholic liver disease; this finding is associated with adverse outcomes (e.g., sudden cardiac death).[49] It should be noted that of available neuroleptics, haloperidol has been found to have the lowest per-dose-equivalent prolongation of the QTc (Table 18-4).[50,51]

Beyond the anti-dopaminergic qualities of haloperidol, recent findings have suggested another potential mechanism by which it may exert a therapeutic effect in states of delirium. The sigma$_1$ receptor was first identified in the 1970s and was, at that time, thought to be an opioid receptor.[52] Investigations in the past decade have demonstrated that antagonism of the sigma$_1$ receptor serves to stabilize neuronal membrane in conditions of oxidative stress. Unlike other neuroleptic agents, the butyrophenone neurolpetics (i.e., haloperidol and droperidol) have been shown to be antagonists at the sigma$_1$ receptor.[53] One animal model study successfully demonstrated that haloperidol could significantly diminish ischemic lesion volume due to induction of a standardized stroke when compared to an inactive agent.[54] This ability to limit neuronal death, and thus prevent further release of dopamine or loss of cholinergic activity, may be an essential factor in the utility of haloperidol in delirium.

The availability of injectable formulations of both olanzapine and ziprasidone has prompted a growing interest in the use of the second-generation antipsychotics in the management of delirium.[55] Risperidone has the most available data supporting its use, with multiple studies showing it to be efficacious and safe for the treatment of delirium,[56-58] and one small randomized double-blind comparative study finding no significant difference in efficacy when compared with haloperidol.[59] The other members of this class (olanzapine, ziprasidone, quetiapine, clozapine, and aripiprazole) have far less supporting data, though some small studies seem to indicate some promise for management of delirium.[60-64] Agranulocytosis associated with clozapine and the resultant regulation of its use effectively eliminates any routine application of it in the management of delirium. All drugs in this class feature an FDA black box warning indicating an increased risk of death when used to treat behavioral problems in elderly patients with dementia. Similar warnings regarding a potential increased risk of cerebrovascular events are reported for risperidone, olanzapine, and aripiprazole. With decades of clinical experience in the use of haloperidol, and a dearth of available data on these newer agents, haloperidol remains the neuroleptic agent of choice for the treatment of delirium.

Dexmedetomidine is a selective α$_2$-adrenergic agonist used for sedation and analgesia in the ICU setting. Its action on receptors in the locus ceruleus results in anxiolysis and sedation while agonsim of spinal cord receptors produces analgesia. This unique mechanism of action allows effective management of agitation without the risks of respiratory depression, dependence, and deliriogenesis attendant to the benzodiazepines that have traditionally been utilized in the ICU.[65] Several randomized controlled trials have indicated a significantly lower incidence of delirium when dexmedetomidine was used for sedation when compared with midazolam, lorazepam, or propofol.[65-67] Another randomized open-label study comparing dexmedetomidine to haloperidol for the management of delirium in intubated patients demonstrated a significant reduction in time to extubation and discharge from the ICU when dexmedetomidine was used.[68] The high cost of the drug may limit its routine use for delirium, but two studies have supported its cost-effectiveness citing reduction in costs associated with prolonged stays in the ICUs as offsetting the cost of the agent itself.[65,69]

To date, there are few data to support pharmacological prophylaxis of delirium for the critically ill, although a small group of randomized, double-blind, placebo-controlled trials have demonstrated some efficacy of neuroleptics in limiting delirium. One study examining the pre-operative use of haloperidol in elderly patients undergoing hip surgery indicated decreases in the severity and duration of delirium, as well as the length of hospital stay, but no statistically significant decrease in the actual incidence of delirium.[70] Another examined the prophylactic administration of olanzapine to elderly patients undergoing joint-replacement surgery and demonstrated a decreased incidence of delirium and more frequent discharge to home (rather than to a skilled nursing facility) in the group receiving the active agent.[71] An investigation of risperidone following cardiac surgery demonstrated significant reduction in the incidence of delirium when compared to placebo.[72]

A long-held belief about the course of delirium was that once symptoms were controlled and the underlying cause identified and treated, cognition returned to normal. In short, delirium was regarded as a time-limited reversible syndrome. More recent data indicate that this view may be overly optimistic in that follow-up cognitive testing of patients that experienced a delirium revealed a far greater likelihood of subsequent diagnosis of persistent mild cognitive impairment or dementia than matched controls who did not experience a delirium.[73,74] It is unclear as to whether delirium caused these lasting cognitive changes or patients with previously undiagnosed cognitive impairments were more prone to develop delirium.

DELIRIUM IN SPECIFIC DISEASES

Critically ill patients with human immunodeficiency virus (HIV) infection may be more susceptible to the EPS of haloperidol, and to neuroleptic malignant syndrome (NMS),[75-77] leading an experienced group to recommend use of molindone.[78] The latter is associated with fewer of such effects; while it is available only as an oral agent, it can be prescribed from 5 to 25 mg at appropriate intervals or, in a more acute situation, 25 mg every hour until calm is achieved. Risperidone (0.5 to 1 mg per dose) is another recommended PO agent. If parenteral medication is required, 10 mg of chlorpromazine has been effective. Perphenazine is readily available for parenteral use as well, and 2 mg doses can be used effectively.

Patients with Parkinson's disease pose a special problem because dopamine blockade aggravates their condition. If PO treatment of delirium or psychosis is possible, clozapine, starting with a small dose of 6.25 or 12.5 mg, is probably the most effective agent available that does not exacerbate the disease. With the risk of agranulocytosis attendant to the use of clozapine, quetiapine may play a valuable role in this population, since its very low affinity for dopamine receptors is less likely to exacerbate this disorder.[79]

IV benzodiazepines (particularly diazepam, chlordiazepoxide, and lorazepam) are routinely used to treat agitated states, particularly delirium tremens, and alcohol withdrawal.[80] Neuroleptics have also been used successfully, and both have been combined with clonidine. IV alcohol is also extremely effective in the treatment of alcohol withdrawal states, particularly if the patient does not seem to respond as rapidly as expected to higher doses of benzodiazepines. The inherent disadvantage is that alcohol is toxic to both liver and brain, although its use can be quite safe if these organs do not show extensive damage (and sometimes quite safe even when they do). Nonetheless, use of IV alcohol should be reserved for extreme cases of alcohol withdrawal when other, less toxic measures have failed. A 5% solution of alcohol mixed with 5% dextrose in water run at 1 ml per minute often achieves calm quickly. Use of oral alcohol (i.e., beer, wine, and spirits) to forestall agitation due to alcohol withdrawal is to be avoided due to the toxicity of the substance, the difficulty inherent in titrating the dose, and the practical implications of providing sufficient volume to match a patient's typical outpatient consumption (which may run to a case of more of beer or a gallon of more of spirits daily).[81]

If a delirium proves resistant to usual management strategies and no underlying somatic etiology can be identified, one important mimic of delirium to consider is delirious mania or Bell's mania. This syndrome may improve with the use of mood stabilizers combined with benzodiazepines. If symptoms remain refractory to treatment, electroconvulsive therapy may be considered.[82]

CONCLUSIONS

Of all psychiatric diagnoses, delirium demands the most immediate attention since delay in identification and treatment might allow the progression of serious and irreversible pathophysiological changes. Unfortunately, delirium is all too often underemphasized, misdiagnosed, or altogether missed in the general hospital setting.[83-85] Indeed, it was not until their most recent editions that major medical and surgical texts corrected chapters indicating that delirium was the result of anxiety or depression, rather than an underlying somatic cause that required prompt investigation. In the face of this tradition of misinformation, it often falls to the psychiatric consultant to identify and manage delirium, while alerting and educating others to its significance.

Access the complete reference list and multiple choice questions (MCQs) online at https://expertconsult.inkling.com

KEY REFERENCES

1. Ely EW, Shintani A, Truman B, et al. Delirium as a predictor of mortality in mechanically ventilated patients in the intensive care unit. *JAMA* 291:1753–1762, 2004.
3. Milbrandt EB, Deppen S, Harrison PL, et al. Costs associated with delirium in mechanically ventilated patients. *Crit Care Med* 32:955–962, 2004.
4. Franco K, Litaker D, Locala J, et al. The cost of delirium in the surgical patient. *Psychosomatics* 42:68–73, 2001.
13. Stagno D, Gibson C, Breitbart W. The delirium subtypes: a review of prevalence, phenomenology, pathophysiology, and treatment response. *Palliat Support Care* 2(2):171–179, 2004.
15. Trzepacz PT. Is there a final common neural pathway in delirium? Focus on acetylcholine and dopamine. *Semin Clin Neuropsychiatry* 5(2):132–148, 2000.
16. Seaman JS, Schillerstrom J, Carroll D, et al. Impaired oxidative metabolism precipitates delirium: a study of 101 ICU patients. *Psychosomatics* 47(1):56–61, 2006.
17. Ely EW, Margolin R, Francis J, et al. Evaluation of delirium in critically ill patients: validation of the Confusion Assessment

Method for the Intensive Care Unit (CAM-ICU). *Crit Care Med* 29(7):1370–1379, 2001.

25. Matsuoka T, Narumoto J, Okamura A, et al. Neural correlates of the components of the clock drawing test. *Int Psychogeriatr* 16:1–7, 2013.

26. Nicolson SE, Chabon B, Larsen KA, et al. Primitive reflexes associated with delirium: a prospective trial. *Psychosomatics* 52(6):507–512, 2011.

27. Foster AR, Caplan JP. Paraneoplastic limbic encephalitis. *Psychosomatics* 50(2):108–113, 2009.

28. Lee SW, Donlon S, Caplan JP. Steroid responsive encephalopathy associated with autoimmune thyroiditis (SREAT) or Hashimoto's encephalopathy: A case and review. *Psychosomatics* 52(2):99–108, 2011.

29. Engel GL, Romano J. Delirium, a syndrome of cerebral insufficiency. *J Chronic Dis* 9:260–277, 1959.

30. Jacobson S, Jerrier H. EEG in delirium. *Semin Clin Neuropsychiatry* 5:86–92, 2000.

34. Stern TA. Continuous infusion of physostigmine in anticholinergic delirium: case report. *J Clin Psychiatry* 44:463–464, 1983.

37. van Eijk MM, Roes KC, Honing ML, et al. Effect of rivastigmine as an adjunct to usual care with haloperidol on duration of delirium and mortality in critically ill patients: a multicentre, double-blind, placebo-controlled randomised trial. *Lancet* 376(9755):1829–1837, 2010.

39. Menza MA, Murray GB, Holmes VF, et al. Decreased extrapyramidal symptoms with intravenous haloperidol. *J Clin Psychiatry* 48:278–280, 1987.

44. Tesar GE, Murray GB, Cassem NH. Use of high-dose intravenous haloperidol in the treatment of agitated cardiac patients. *J Clin Psychopharmacol* 5:344–347, 1985.

50. Glassman AH, Bigger JT Jr. Antipsychotic drugs: prolonged QTc interval, torsade de pointes, and sudden death. *Am J Psychiatry* 158(11):1774–1782, 2001.

51. Beach SR, Celano CM, Noseworthy PA, et al. QTc prolongation, torsades de pointes, and psychotropic medications. *Psychosomatics* 54(1):1–13, 2013.

54. Schetz JA, Perez E, Liu R, et al. A prototypical sigma-1 receptor antagonist protects against brain ischemia. *Brain Res* 1181:1–9, 2007.

55. Schwartz TL, Masand PS. The role of atypical antipsychotics in the treatment of delirium. *Psychosomatics* 43:171–174, 2002.

65. Maldonado JR, Wysong A, van der Starre PJ, et al. Dexmedetomidine and the reduction of postoperative delirium after cardiac surgery. *Psychosomatics* 50(3):206–217, 2009.

66. Pandharipande PP, Pun BT, Herr DL, et al. Effect of sedation with dexmedetomidine vs lorazepam on acute brain dysfunction in mechanically ventilated patients: the MENDS randomized controlled trial. *JAMA* 298(22):2644–2653, 2007.

70. Kalisvaart KJ, de Jonghe JF, Bogaards MJ, et al. Haloperidol prophylaxis for elderly hip-surgery patients at risk for delirium: a randomized placebo-controlled study. *J Am Geriatr Soc* 53:1658–1666, 2005.

71. Larsen KA, Kelly SE, Stern TA, et al. Administration of olanzapine to prevent postoperative delirium in elderly joint-replacement patients: a randomized, controlled trial. *Psychosomatics* 51(5):409–418, 2010.

80. Awissi DK, Lebrun G, Coursin DB, et al. Alcohol withdrawal and delirium tremens in the critically ill: a systematic review and commentary. *Intensive Care Med* 39(1):16–30, 2013.

82. Jacobowski NL, Heckers S, Bobo WV. Delirious mania: detection, diagnosis, and clinical management in the acute setting. *J Psychiatr Pract* 19(1):15–28, 2013.

85. Ely EW, Siegel MD, Inouye SK. Delirium in the intensive care unit: an under-recognized syndrome of organ dysfunction. *Semin Respir Crit Care Med* 22:115–126, 2001.

19 Dementia

Jennifer R. Gatchel, MD, PhD, Christopher I. Wright, MD, PhD, William E. Falk, MD, and
Nhi-Ha Trinh, MD, MPH

KEY POINTS

Clinical Findings

- In the DSM-IV, dementia was defined as a syndrome with multiple etiologies and characterized by a disabling decline in memory as well as an impairment in at least one other higher cortical activity (e.g., with aphasia, apraxia, agnosia, or executive dysfunction).
- In the DSM-5, cognitive disorders are classified as "neurocognitive disorders" and exist on a spectrum of cognitive and functional impairment: delirium, mild neurocognitive disorder, major neurocognitive disorder, and their etiological subtypes.
- The term "dementia" is used to refer to certain etiological subtypes (e.g., Alzheimer's disease [AD], frontotemporal lobar dementia).

Differential Diagnoses

- An evaluation of a suspected dementia or major neurocognitive disorder must include a complete history; physical, neurological, and psychiatric examinations; evaluation of cognitive function; and appropriate laboratory testing.

Epidemiology

- AD accounts for 60%–80% of all dementias and afflicts at least 5 million Americans; however, other etiologies,

both common (e.g., vascular dementia, Lewy body dementia) and rare (e.g., frontotemporal dementia, progressive supranuclear palsy), must be considered during a comprehensive evaluation.
- Longevity is the greatest risk factor for AD, as well as for most other dementing disorders, but additional factors, such as genetic propensity (particularly in the rare cases of early-onset AD) and vascular pathology, as well as modifiable lifestyle factors can contribute to its prevalence.

Pathophysiology

- Animal models, structural and functional imaging studies, and recent advances in imaging and in biomarkers have led to a new working model of a continuum of neuropathological changes in dementing disorders and AD in particular, with increasing evidence of the pre-clinical or asymptomatic stage, when neuropathological changes may already be present.

Treatment Options

- With AD in particular, attention often focuses on primary and secondary prevention and on potential curative approaches that are based on our expanding knowledge.

OVERVIEW

The *Diagnostic and Statistical Manual of Mental Disorders, Fifth Edition* (DSM-5)[1] designates cognitive disorders on a spectrum of cognitive and functional decline: delirium, mild and major neurocognitive disorders, and their etiological subtypes. The term dementia is retained for consistency; it was used in the fourth edition (DSM-IV)[2] to describe a syndrome with a decline in memory, as well as an impairment of at least one other domain of higher cognitive function (e.g., aphasia [a difficulty with any aspect of language]; apraxia [the impaired ability to perform motor tasks despite intact motor function]; agnosia [an impairment in object recognition despite intact sensory function]; or executive dysfunction [such as difficulty in planning, organizing, sequencing, or abstracting]).

While dementia is encompassed by the term major neurocognitive disorder (MNCD), for a diagnosis of MNCD to be made there must be evidence of significant cognitive decline in one or more cognitive domains (complex attention, executive function, learning and memory, language, perceptual motor, or social cognition) based on concern of the individual, a knowledgeable informant, or the clinician, as well as by objective measures of substantial cognitive impairment on standardized neuropsychological testing or quantified clinical assessment. Several important qualifiers are included in the definition: i.e., the condition must represent a change from baseline, social or occupational function must be significantly impaired, and the impairment does not occur exclusively during an episode of delirium, or cannot be accounted for by another Axis I disorder, such as major depression.[2]

Many elderly adults complain of difficulties with their memory (e.g., with learning new information or names, or finding words). In most circumstances, such lapses are normal. The term *mild cognitive impairment* (MCI) was coined to recognize an intermediate category between the normal cognitive losses associated with aging and with dementia. While MCI was subsumed under cognitive disorder not otherwise specified in DSM-IV, this less severe level of cognitive impairment most closely corresponds with "mild neurocognitive disorder" in DSM-5.[2] Diagnostic criteria include evidence for a *modest* decline in cognition from a previous level of performance in one or more cognitive domains based on concern of the individual, a knowledgeable informant, or clinician, and based on objective evidence of cognitive decline. Important qualifiers include lack of interference with independence in everyday activities, and not exclusively occurring during an episode of delirium, and not accounted for by another Axis I disorder. MCI is characterized by a notable decline in memory or other cognitive functions as compared with age-matched controls. MCI is common among the elderly, although estimates vary widely depending on the diagnostic criteria used and the assessment methods employed; some, but not all, individuals with MCI progress to dementia. According to some studies, individuals with MCI may progress to Alzheimer's disease (AD) at a rate of 10%–15% per year. Risk factors for conversion from MCI to AD include carrier status of the E4 allele of the apolipoprotein E (*APOE*) gene, clinical severity, brain atrophy, specific patterns of CSF biomarkers and cerebral glucose metabolism, and AB deposition. Further identification of factors that place people at risk for progression of cognitive decline is an active area of research.[3]

EPIDEMIOLOGY OF DEMENTIA

The most common type of dementia (accounting for 60% to 80%) is AD.[4] Among the neurodegenerative dementias, Lewy body dementia is the next most common, followed by frontotemporal dementia (FTD). Vascular dementia (formerly known as multi-infarct dementia) can have a number of different etiologies; it can exist separately from AD, but the two frequently co-occur. Indeed, there is increasing awareness that AD is often mixed with other dementia causes. Dementias associated with Parkinson's disease (PD) and Creutzfeldt–Jakob disease (CJD) are much less common. Given the challenges of making an accurate diagnosis of dementia subtypes in epidemiological studies, and in light of neuropathological data suggesting that mixed pathologies are more common than discrete subtypes, the proportion of dementias attributed to different subtypes must be interpreted with caution.[5]

THE ROLE OF AGE OF ONSET

The onset of dementia is most common in the seventies and eighties, and is quite rare before age 40. Both the incidence (the number of new cases per year in the population) and the prevalence (the fraction of the population that has the disorder) rise steeply with age. This general pattern has been observed both for dementia overall, and for AD in particular, with the prevalence increasing exponentially with age, increasing from 3% among people age 65–74 years to nearly 50% in those >85 years.[6] Estimates of the prevalence of dementia vary to some extent depending on which diagnostic criteria are used. The incidence of dementia of almost all types increases with age such that it may affect 15% of all individuals over the age of 65 years, and up to 45% of those over age 80. However, the peak age of onset varies somewhat among the dementias, with FTD and vascular dementia tending to begin earlier (e.g., in the sixties) and AD somewhat later.

Dementia is the main cause of disability among older adults and not surprisingly the economic burden of dementia is enormous. Moreover, it is expected to rise steeply with anticipated demographic shifts. A substantial fraction of the increased burden will fall on developing countries, as a larger fraction of the population survives to old age. Indeed by one estimate, while there were 36.5 million people world-wide with dementia in 2010, the number of people living with dementia is expected to double every 20 years, with most of those living in low and middle income countries.[5] Because AD and many other neurodegenerative disorders have an insidious onset, the precise age of onset is indeterminate. However, the approximate age of onset (i.e., within 2 to 5 years) is critical from both the personal and the public health points of view. It may offer an important leverage on disease risk and morbidity. A sufficient delay in onset can be equivalent to prevention with a late-onset disorder. Later onset can also decrease the burden of disease by pushing it later into the life span. From the research perspective, age of onset shows a robust relationship to genetic risk factors, and may have value as an outcome in genetic and other causal models.

EVALUATION OF THE PATIENT WITH SUSPECTED DEMENTIA

The diagnostic criteria for dementia require that a number of confounding disorders have been ruled out, particularly delirium and depression. Of note, an underlying diagnosis of dementia may predispose a patient to delirium; thus, further evaluation of cognitive deficits is required once delirium has been treated successfully. Delirium may be differentiated from dementia in several important ways; the onset of delirium

---

> **BOX 19-1** Etiologies of Dementia, and of Mild and Major Neurocognitive Disorders
>
> **VASCULAR**
> Stroke, chronic subdural hemorrhages, post-anoxic injury, diffuse white matter disease
>
> **INFECTIOUS**
> Human immunodeficiency virus (HIV) infection, neurosyphilis, progressive multi-focal leukoencephalopathy (PMLE), Creutzfeldt–Jakob disease (CJD), tuberculosis (TB), sarcoidosis, Whipple's disease
>
> **NEOPLASTIC**
> Primary versus metastatic carcinoma, paraneoplastic syndrome
>
> **DEGENERATIVE**
> Alzheimer's disease (AD), frontotemporal dementia (FTD), dementia with Lewy bodies (DLB), Parkinson's disease (PD), progressive supranuclear palsy (PSP), multi-system degeneration, amyotrophic lateral sclerosis (ALS), corticobasal degeneration (CBD), multiple sclerosis (MS)
>
> **INFLAMMATORY**
> Vasculitis
>
> **ENDOCRINE**
> Hypothyroidism, adrenal insufficiency, Cushing's syndrome, hypoparathyroidism/hyperparathyroidism, renal failure, liver failure
>
> **METABOLIC**
> Thiamine deficiency (Wernicke's encephalopathy), vitamin B_{12} deficiency, inherited enzyme defects
>
> **TOXINS**
> Chronic alcoholism, drugs/medication effects, heavy metals, dialysis dementia (aluminum)
>
> **TRAUMA**
> Dementia pugilistica
>
> **OTHER**
> Normal pressure hydrocephalus (NPH), obstructive hydrocephalus

---

is typically acute or subacute, the course often has marked fluctuations, and level of consciousness and attention are impaired.

Depression also may be difficult to distinguish from dementia, particularly as the two diagnoses are often co-morbid. Further, depression alone may cause some cognitive impairment; in such cases it may precede AD by several years. Certain features (such as a more acute onset, poor motivation, prominent negativity, and a strong family history of a mood disorder) favor a diagnosis of depression.

Establishing a precise etiology of dementia (Box 19-1) whenever possible allows for more focused treatment and for an accurate assessment of prognosis. Although reversible causes will be found in less than 15% of new cases, a diagnosis may help a patient and his or her family to understand what the future holds for them and to make appropriate personal, medical, and financial plans.

History should never be obtained from the patient alone; family members or others who have observed the patient are essential informants for an accurate history. The patient often fails to report deficits, usually because the patient is unaware of them (anosognosia). Ideally, family members should be interviewed separately from the patient so that they can be as candid as possible.

When obtaining a history one should determine the nature of the initial presentation, the course of the illness, and the associated signs and symptoms (including those that are psychiatric or behavioral). These areas are important in determining disease etiology (e.g., recognizing the characteristic abrupt onset of vascular dementia as opposed to the gradual onset of AD).

Review of systems should be extensive and must include inquiry about gait and sleep disturbance, falls, sensory deficits, head trauma, and incontinence. Obtaining the full medical history may reveal risk factors for stroke or for other general medical or neurological causes of cognitive difficulties. The psychiatric history may suggest co-morbid illnesses (such as depression or alcohol abuse), particularly if prior episodes of psychiatric illness are elicited.

Up to one-third of cases of cognitive impairment may be at least partially caused by medication effects; common offenders include anticholinergics, antihypertensive agents, various psychotropics, sedative-hypnotics, and narcotics. Any drug is suspect if its first prescription and the onset of symptoms are temporally related.

Family history can be helpful in determining the type of dementia, as discussed later. A social and occupational history is useful when assessing pre-morbid intelligence and education, changes in the patient's level of function, and any environmental risk factors.

A general physical examination is essential with particular focus paid to the cardiovascular system. Physical findings can also suggest endocrine, inflammatory, and infectious causes. A complete neurological examination (including assessment of cranial nerves, sensory and motor functions, deep tendon reflexes, and cerebellar function) may reveal focal findings that suggest vascular dementia or another degenerative disorder, such as PD. Screening for acuity of vision and hearing is important because it may reveal losses that can masquerade as, or exacerbate, cognitive decline.

Psychiatric examination may reveal evidence of delirium, depression, or psychosis. On formal mental status testing, such as with the Folstein Mini-Mental State Examination (MMSE; see Table 2-1),[7] and other cognitive tests (Table 19-1), documentation of particular findings, in addition to the overall score, allows cognitive functions to be followed over time.

Laboratory evaluation should include a complete blood count (CBC) and levels of vitamin B_{12} and folate, a sedimentation rate, electrolytes, glucose, homocysteine, blood urea nitrogen (BUN), and creatinine, as well as tests of thyroid function and liver function (see Chapter 3). Screening for cholesterol and triglyceride levels is also useful. Syphilis serology should also be included on an initial panel. A computed tomography (CT) scan of the brain, without contrast, can also be useful in identifying a subdural hematoma, hydrocephalus, stroke, or tumor.

Additional studies are indicated if the initial work-up is uninformative, if a particular diagnosis is suspected, or if the presentation is atypical (Table 19-2). Such investigations are particularly important in young patients with rapid progression of dementia or an unusual presentation. Neuropsychological testing may be quite useful, and is essential in cases where a patient's deficits are mild or difficult to characterize. Briefer screening tools, such as the MMSE, have poor sensitivity and specificity for dementia, particularly in highly educated or intelligent patients. Such tests also generally fail to assess executive function and praxis.

Other diagnostic tests can supplement initial assessment when indicated. Magnetic resonance imaging (MRI) of the brain is more sensitive for recent stroke and should be considered when focal findings are detected on the neurological examination; in addition, MRI scans can identify lesions not

TABLE 19-1 Supplemental Mental State Testing for Patients with Dementia

Area	Test
Memory	Recall name and address: "John Brown, 42 Market Street, Chicago"
	Recall three unusual words: "tulip, umbrella, fear"
Language	Naming parts: "lab coat: lapel, sleeve, cuff; watch: band, face, crystal"
	Complex commands: "Before pointing to the door, point to the ceiling"
	Word-list: "In one minute, name all the animals you can think of"
Praxis	"Show me how you would slice a loaf of bread"
	"Show me how you brush your teeth"
Visuospatial	"Draw a clock face with numbers, and mark the hands to ten after eleven"
Abstraction	"How is an apple like a banana?"
	"How is a canal different from a river?"
	Proverb interpretation

TABLE 19-2 Supplemental Laboratory Investigations

What	When	Why
Neuropsychological testing	Patient's deficits are mild or difficult to characterize	The sensitivity of the MMSE for dementia is poor, particularly in highly educated or intelligent patients (who can compensate for deficits)
Lumbar puncture (including routine studies and cytology)	Known or suspected cancer, immunosuppression, suspected CNS infection or vasculitis, hydrocephalus by CT, rapid or atypical courses	Look for infection, elevated pressure, abnormal proteins
MRI with gadolinium; EEG	Any atypical findings on neurological examination; suspected toxic-metabolic encephalopathy, complex partial seizures, Creutzfeldt–Jakob disease (CJD)	More sensitive than CT for tumor, stroke Look for diffuse slowing (encephalopathy) vs. focal seizure activity
HIV testing	Risk factors or opportunistic infections	Up to 20% of patients with HIV infection develop dementia, although it is unusual for dementia to be the initial sign
Heavy metal screening, screening for Wilson's disease or autoimmune disease	Suggested by history, physical examination, laboratory findings	May be reversible

CNS, Central nervous system; CT, computed tomography; EEG, electroencephalogram; MMSE, Mini-Mental State Examination; MRI, magnetic resonance imaging.

apparent on physical examination, so it should always be considered when the diagnosis is unclear. An electroencephalogram (EEG) may be used to identify toxic-metabolic encephalopathy, complex partial seizures, or CJD. A lumbar puncture (LP) may be indicated when cancer, infection of the central nervous system (CNS), hydrocephalus, or vasculitis is suspected. Testing for the human immunodeficiency virus (HIV) is indicated in a patient with appropriate risk factors, because up to 20% of patients with HIV infection develop dementia, although dementia is uncommon as an initial sign. Heavy metal screening, as well as tests for Lyme disease, Wilson's disease, and autoimmune diseases, should be reserved for patients in whom these etiologies are suspected.

ALZHEIMER'S DISEASE
Brief Description

AD is a progressive, irreversible brain disorder that robs those who have it of memory and overall mental and physical function; it eventually leads to death.

Epidemiology of Alzheimer's Disease

AD is the most common cause of dementia, affecting at least 5.3 million Americans and about 33.9 million people worldwide.[8,9] The prevalence of the disorder is expected to triple in the next 40 years given increases in life expectancies, and by 2050 the prevalence may reach more than 13.5 million cases in the US alone.[8] Currently, AD is the sixth leading cause of death for adults in the US. In 2013, the direct costs of caring for those with AD in the US is estimated to be $203 billion, and is projected to increase to $1.2 trillion in 2050 (in current dollars).[9] Female gender carries an increased risk, even when accounting for differences in longevity, but some of the difference is offset by a greater risk of vascular dementias in men. Many risk factors (except for male gender), including diabetes, atherosclerosis, hypertension, smoking, atrial fibrillation, and elevated cholesterol, increase the risk of AD, as well as vascular dementia, although the mechanisms are unclear.[10] A history of head trauma (severe, with loss of consciousness) also increases the risk of AD, while education, complexity of occupation, engaged lifestyle, and exercise have protective effects.[11] Indeed, many modifiable lifestyle factors may contribute to the development of AD and other dementias. Barnes and Yaffe,[8] in calculating the population-attributable risk of seven lifestyle factors, found that in the US, physical inactivity, depression, smoking, and mid-life hypertension had the highest correlation with AD risk. An additional modifiable risk factor is the effect of sleep-disordered breathing; women with sleep-disordered breathing have twice the risk of developing dementia as those without disordered breathing. The effect of diet, meanwhile, is more controversial; there is insufficient evidence to support the association of adherence to a particular diet and development of AD.[11]

Pathophysiology

In his initial 1907 case, Alois Alzheimer identified abnormal nerve cells and fiber clusters at autopsy in the cerebral cortex using what was then a new silver-staining method. These findings, considered to be the hallmark neuropathological lesions of AD, are known as neurofibrillary tangles (NFTs) and neuritic plaques (NPs) (Figure 19-1). Beta-amyloid protein, present in soluble form in the brain, but also a major component of plaques, is thought to play a central pathophysiological role in the disease, perhaps via direct neurotoxicity.[12] NFTs are found in neurons and are primarily composed of anomalous cytoskeletal proteins (such as hyperphosphorylated tau),

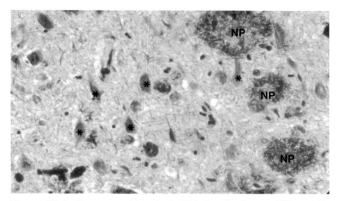

Figure 19-1. Plaques and tangles in Alzheimer's disease. NP, neuritic plaques; *, neurofibrillary tangles.

which may also be toxic to neurons and contribute to AD pathophysiology.[13,14]

However, the mechanisms by which changes in tau and beta-amyloid mediate neuronal death and dysfunction remain important unanswered questions and active areas of research. Two proposed methods of tau-mediated toxicity include NFT toxicity and conformational abnormalities of tangles, including a spreading process through multiple brain regions, in which abnormal tau can catalyze formation of abnormal tau in other cells through a prion-like process.[11] Soluble and diffusible beta-amyloid may cause cytotoxicity and synaptotoxicity, with amyloid plaques serving as reservoirs for sequestration of soluble oligmers.[11]

Genetics of Alzheimer's Disease

Before trying to identify specific genes, epidemiological approaches are used to look for evidence that genetic factors are involved in disease etiology. For AD, multiple lines of evidence support a role for genetic factors. First-degree relatives of AD patients have a twofold to threefold increased risk of developing AD, and often at a similar age, which can be reassuring for middle-aged individuals who care for elderly parents with AD. Examination of AD families generally reveals no clear pattern of inheritance, although some rare families—typically with an early onset—have an autosomal dominant inheritance, in which the disease is observed in approximately half the children in each generation, and an affected child typically has an affected parent. Twin studies are used to examine whether the increased risk in families is due to genetic factors. For AD, monozygotic twins (who share all their genes) typically show greater concordance than dizygotic twins (who share only half, like ordinary siblings). However, monozygotic twins do not uniformly share an AD diagnosis, and their age of onset may differ by 10 or more years.

In the context of genetic research, early-onset AD and late-onset AD are usually considered separately, divided by age of onset at 60 or sometimes 65 years. Early-onset AD is more likely to be familial; most autosomal dominant families have an early onset. However, late-onset AD also runs in families, and family and twin studies also support a role for genes in late-onset AD.[15] These family and twin findings hold, despite controlling for the known late-onset AD gene *APOE*.

Three genes have been identified as leading to early-onset AD in an autosomal dominant fashion. Although these genes have limited public health impact, they are devastating for affected families. These early-onset genes probably account for half of the cases of AD that occur before age 60. More critically, they have made a large contribution to our understanding of the pathophysiology of AD, and to the development of promising therapeutic strategies. Amyloid precursor protein (APP) on chromosome 21 was recognized first; there are 26 mutations that affect 72 families. The age of onset for these APP mutations varies, and it is modified by *APOE* genotype. Next discovered was presenilin 1 *(PSEN1)* on chromosome 14. There are 156 *PSEN1* mutations affecting 342 families; many have been found in a single family, often referred to as "genetically private." *PSEN1* mutations are associated with an age of onset in the forties and fifties; these mutations are not modified by the *APOE* genotype. Although overall quite rare, *PSEN1* accounts for the great majority of autosomal dominant early-onset AD. *PSEN1* mutations have also been observed in non-familial early-onset AD cases. The last early-onset gene is presenilin 2 *(PSEN2)* on chromosome 1. *PSEN2* has 10 reported mutations affecting 18 families. The age of onset is quite variable, extending into the late-onset AD range, and it is modified by *APOE* genotype.[16]

In addition to these genes, genetic factors that confer increased risk have been identified; the most powerful common risk gene is apolipoprotein E *(APOE)*. Rather than a deterministic gene like the other three, *APOE* is a susceptibility gene that increases the risk for AD without causing the disease and contributes to 40%–60% of cases. *APOE* has three alleles, 2, 3, and 4, which have a complex relationship to risk for both AD and cardiovascular disease, with the 2 allele decreasing risk of both disorders and increasing longevity, and the 4 allele increasing risk and decreasing longevity. The effect of *APOE-4* varies with age; it is most marked in the sixties, and falls substantially beyond age 80 or 90 years. *APOE* seems to act principally by modifying the age of onset, which is lowest in those with two copies of the risk allele, and intermediate in those with one. The *APOE* effect appears to be stronger in women and in Caucasians, which may relate to their lower risk of cardiovascular disease.

While APOE-4 remains the most important risk polymorphism, ten additional risk genes have been confirmed, including *PICALM* and *BIN1* (involved in protein sorting), *CLU* (the amyloid binding protein apolipoprotein J), *CR1* (a complement receptor), *CD2AP* (an adaptor gene) *TOMM40* (an outer mitochondrial membrane translocase) among others.[17] Future work utilizing whole genome exome sequencing as well as induced pluripotent stem cells derived from patients with familial or sporadic AD has promise in providing further insight into the molecular pathogenesis of AD.[17]

Patients frequently ask about their risk of AD based on their family history. Those with an autosomal dominant history are best referred for genetic counseling, ideally from an Alzheimer's Disease Research Center or a local genetic counselor. Genetic testing is commercially available for *PSEN1*, which is likely to be involved when there is an autosomal dominant family history and the age of onset is 50 or lower. It can be used both for confirmation of diagnosis and for the prediction of disease onset, but there are complex logistical and ethical issues.[18] Currently, genetic testing is only available for the remaining early-onset genes in research settings. Patients without such a history can be advised that there is an increased risk of AD in first-degree relatives. However, they should be made aware that this increase is modest and that age of onset tends to be correlated in families. Genetic testing for *APOE* can be used as an adjunct to diagnosis, but it contributes minimally. It is not recommended for the assessment of future risk because it lacks sufficient predictive value at the individual level. Many normal elderly carry an *APOE-4* allele, and many AD patients do not.

Clinical Features and Diagnosis

The typical clinical profile of AD is one of progressive memory loss. Other common cognitive clinical features include impairment of language, visuospatial ability, and executive function. Patients may be unaware of their cognitive deficits, but this is not uniformly the case. There may be evidence of forgetting conversations, having difficulty with household finances, being disoriented to time and place, and misplacing items frequently. In addition to its cognitive features, a number of neuropsychiatric symptoms are common in AD, even in its mildest clinical phases.[19] In particular, irritability, apathy, and depression are common early features, with psychosis (delusions and hallucinations) occurring more frequently later in the course of the disease.

According to original diagnostic criteria for AD, a definitive diagnosis required evidence of dementia and also rested on post-mortem findings of a specific distribution and number of its characteristic brain lesions (NFTs and NPs). Detailed clinical assessments (by psychiatry, neurology, and neuropsychology) in combination with structural and functional neuroimaging methods had a high concordance rate with autopsy-proven disease. Structural neuroimaging studies (such as MRI or CT) typically show atrophy in the medial temporal lobes, as well as in the parietal convexities bilaterally (Figure 19-2). Functional imaging studies of resting brain function or blood flow (i.e., positron emission tomography [PET] or single-photon emission computed tomography [SPECT]) display parietotemporal hypoperfusion or hypoactivity (Figure 19-3).

However, recent research advances in the areas of brain imaging and biomarkers have led to re-conceptualization of AD as existing on a continuum, with a progressive series of biological changes corresponding to pre-clinical and increasingly severe clinical stages of the disorder.[20] These changes,

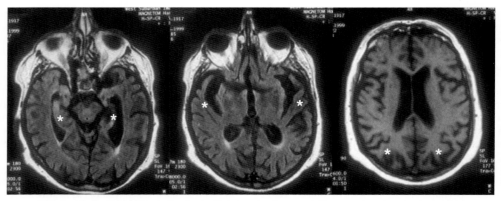

Figure 19-2. Axial MRI of atrophy in Alzheimer's disease. *, Temporal and parietal atrophy.

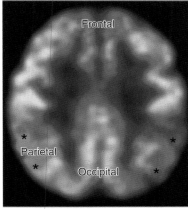

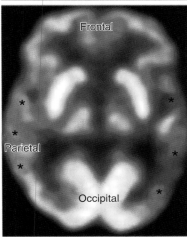

Figure 19-3. Parietotemporal hypoactivity in Alzheimer's disease. *, Regions of hypoactivity.

TABLE 19-3 FDA-Approved Pharmacotherapy for Alzheimer's Disease

Acetylcholinesterase inhibitors	Donepezil (Aricept) Rivastigmine (Exelon) Galantamine (Razadyne, formerly Reminyl)
Normalizes glutamate	Memantine (Namenda)

FDA, Food and Drug Administration.

some of which can be measured by AD biomarkers, begin in individuals who are cognitively normal, progress in those with MCI, and accumulate in dementia. Advances in CSF assays, neuroimaging, and other biomarkers now provide the ability to detect evidence of AD pathophysiology process *in vivo.*[21] Some promising biomarkers include MRI measurement of atrophy in the hippocampus and other AD-affected brain regions, PET measurements of glucose hypometabolism in AD-affected brain regions, PET measurements of fibrillar beta-amyloid deposition, and CSF measurements of beta-amyloid in combination with total tau and phosphorylated tau.[21] Indeed, increasing evidence from both genetically at-risk cohorts and clinically normal older adults suggests that the pathophysiology of AD begins years, if not decades before the diagnosis of clinical dementia.[20]

Based on these advances, the National Institute on Aging (NIA) International Working Group and Alzheimer's Association in 2011 proposed updated criteria for the diagnosis of AD and MCI, in addition to research criteria aimed at clarifying the pre-clinical stages of AD.[20] These new criteria reflect increasing knowledge of clinical course and pathophysiology: they take into account that memory impairment may not be a key clinical feature, other potential etiologies (dementia with Lewy bodies, vascular dementia, and frontotemporal dementia) as well as mixed pathology.[20] The new research criteria meanwhile focus on defining pre-clinical stages of disease based on biomarkers and genetic testing. The goals of research criteria are to provide insight into factors influencing

progression to the clinical stages of AD while also evaluating promising AD treatment in pre-clinical stages when they may be most effective. Importantly, these research criteria as well as amyloid imaging and other AD biomarkers are not recommended for use in the clinical setting as of yet[20,21]; this may lie on the horizon, as these biomarkers are further evaluated in different populations over time.

Differential Diagnosis

For AD, like other dementias, it is important to exclude potentially arrestable or reversible causes of cognitive dysfunction, or of other brain diseases that could manifest as a dementia (see Box 19-1). Beyond this, the key features are insidious onset, gradual progression, and a characteristic pattern of deficits, particularly early prominent deficits in short-term memory.

Treatments

Behavioral strategies, including environmental cues, such as re-orientation to the environment with the addition of a clock and a calendar, can be reassuring to the patient. In addition, clear communication should be emphasized in this population, including keeping the content of communication simple and to the point, and speaking clearly and loudly enough, given that decreased hearing acuity is common in the elderly. For those patients who are easily distressed or are psychotic, reassurance and distraction are strategies that can be calming.

The re-conceptualization of AD on a continuum of neuropathological and clinical impairment and identification of pre-clinical AD through biomarker studies has led to a shift in focus toward intervention with potential disease-modifying treatments in the early stages of AD.[21] Such early intervention among asymptomatic individuals before clinical or biomarker changes develop is termed *primary prevention*, and has been effective for other chronic diseases.[22] Along these lines, general types of intervention include risk reduction for the general public, prevention in those with mutation or pre-clinical disease, and treatment aimed at delaying the progression of clinical signs and symptoms.[22] Possible preventive measures include weight control and exercise, as well as normalizing blood pressure, blood sugar, and cholesterol, which have been associated with risk for not only AD but also other major neurocognitive disorders.[10] Thus far, AD trials based on lowering specific risk factors, such as cholesterol, did not slow progression in the symptomatic stage of disease. However, this remains an active area of investigation.

Current pharmacotherapy in AD (Table 19-3) addresses both the symptoms and the pathogenesis of AD, and involves primarily cholinesterase inhibitors and NMDA receptor antagonists. AD has been linked to a deficiency of acetylcholine (ACh). Three of the four medications approved by the Food and Drug Administration (FDA) now in use for treatment of AD are designed to prevent the breakdown of ACh, thereby increasing concentrations of ACh in the hippocampus and neocortex, areas of the brain important for memory and for other cognitive symptoms. These cholinesterase inhibitors include donepezil (Aricept), rivastigmine (Exelon), and galantamine (Razadyne). All have been shown to slow the progression of AD by stabilizing cognition and behavior, participation in activities of daily living (ADLs), and global function in mild-to-moderate AD, by improving cognition and behavior in moderate-to-severe patients with AD, by delaying nursing home placement, and by reducing both health care expenditures and caregiver burden for patients with AD.[23] However, the effects are modest, and they are not apparent in some individuals.

Certain pharmacokinetic properties should be kept in mind while prescribing these medications: donepezil and extended-release galantamine are given once daily, while both galantamine and rivastigmine are given twice daily; in particular, rivastigmine should be administered with meals to reduce gastrointestinal side effects. Common side effects include nausea, vomiting, diarrhea, insomnia or vivid dreams, fatigue, muscle cramps, incontinence, bradycardia, and syncope. Data also suggest that a cholinesterase inhibitor should be initiated as soon as a diagnosis of AD becomes apparent, and that treatment should be continued into the severe stages of the disease, provided that the medication is well tolerated.[24] Increasing numbers of studies are investigating the potential efficacy of introducing treatment at the stage of MCI; although studies to date have not been positive, interventions with these and other agents in pre-clinical AD and MCI remain active areas of investigation.

Another medication, memantine (Namenda), has been proven effective in patients with more severe forms of AD. Memantine normalizes levels of glutamate, a neurotransmitter involved in learning and memory, which in excessive quantities is thought to contribute to neurodegeneration. Memantine has been used in combination with cholinesterase inhibitors for greater effectiveness in slowing the progression of AD. Common side effects include dizziness, agitation, headache, and confusion. In patients with moderate-to-severe AD receiving donepezil, those assigned to continue donepezil had less cognitive decline than those assigned to discontinue the medication, and the combination of donepezil and memantine did not confer additional benefits above donepezil alone.[25]

Before the initiation of pharmacotherapy for behavioral and psychological symptoms of dementia (apathy, depression, anxiety, aggression/agitation, psychosis, sleep disturbance and disinhibition/perseveration), possible exacerbating medical (e.g., urinary infection) or environmental triggers should be carefully investigated and resolved. However, irritability and depressive symptoms have been treated effectively with antidepressant therapy (e.g., selective serotonin reuptake inhibitors [SSRIs]). The choice of agent is based principally on the side effects each particular medication produces.

There are no medications specifically FDA-approved for the neuropsychiatric manifestations of AD. However, in the course of the illness, neuropsychiatric symptoms (such as agitation, aggression, and psychosis) arise commonly and may require treatments with antipsychotic agents or mood stabilizers. Clinical experience suggests that second-generation (atypical) antipsychotics (such as olanzapine, quetiapine, risperidone, and aripiprazole) are preferred over the older conventional antipsychotics that are more likely to produce extrapyramidal side effects (EPS) (such as parkinsonism and dystonias). One recent review compared trials of atypical antipsychotics used for the treatment of neuropsychiatric symptoms in dementia and concluded that olanzapine and risperidone had the best evidence for efficacy, though effects were modest.[26] On the other hand, a recent clinical trial suggested that these and other atypical antipsychotics may be little better than placebo.[27]

Although these agents may work well if used judiciously, reports of a small but statistically significant increase in risk of cerebrovascular adverse events and death have led to an FDA warning for use of atypical antipsychotics in elderly with dementia. The potential for an increased risk of serious adverse events is of concern, and the risk/benefit ratio of antipsychotic medication use remains controversial; clinicians must weigh the risks against the potential benefits of these medications with patients and their families.

In general, such agents should be used only when necessary. Psychosis in particular does not require treatment unless it leads to dangerous behavior, causes distress to the patient, or is disruptive to the family or other caregivers. When such agents are used, choosing lower doses and titrating upward slowly is advised in this population. Once the target symptoms are controlled, it is then prudent to consider tapering off the medications after 2–3 months to determine whether longer-term treatment is necessary. Indeed, with longer-term treatment, benefits are less clear-cut and risks of severe adverse outcomes increase. Other treatment considerations involve optimizing behavioral interventions, removing deleterious medications, reducing excessive alcohol intake, and promoting restorative sleep by diagnosing and treating underlying sleep apnea.

Supportive and Long-term Care

Because AD is a chronic, progressive illness without an available disease-modifying therapy or cure, like all of the dementias described below, it creates significant burdens for the patient, his or her family, and the health care system. Giving early consideration for caregiving at home provides essential support to the patient and family. This may include a home health aide, meals-on-wheels, or a visiting nurse. Structured activities outside of the home, such as adult day care or exercise programs, are also important. Though difficult for the patient and family, it is crucial to think through the future care requirements while the patient is in early stages of the disease. This includes consideration of in-home and external care arrangements (e.g., assisted living, or a skilled nursing facility).[24]

Prognosis

Patients who live through the full course of the disease may survive for 10 to 20 years. However, many patients die in the early or middle stages of the illness.

Current AD treatments have not been found to increase survival or to definitively halt disease progression. However, several promising therapies for AD are on the horizon. These potential treatments involve targeting oxidative stress as well inhibiting enzymes (such as gamma secretase that produces beta-amyloid), or removing beta-amyloid from the brain (using immunological agents, such as beta-amyloid vaccinations or antibody infusions). Secretase inhibitors, in the initial stages of development, target secretase enzymes that are implicated in the creation of beta-amyloids.[28]

A vaccine that targets beta-amyloid protein has been in development for a number of years. Immunotherapy with the vaccine AN-1792 in an AD transgenic mouse model reduced amyloid plaques.[29] The clinical trial of this vaccine in patients with mild-to-moderate AD was halted when 6% of patients developed subacute meningoencephalitis.[30] Many passive immunization clinical trials involving anti-AB antibodies as well as IV Ig are currently underway, in addition to study of DNA-based vaccines. Ongoing antibody studies in AD include solanezumab in mild AD, crenezumab in mild-to-moderate AD, and BAN 2401 in MCI and mild AD.

Memory-consolidation compounds in development are designed to facilitate the creation of long-term memories. One approach increases levels of cyclic adenosine monophosphate (cAMP), which helps to establish long-term memories by carrying signals to proteins within brain cells. Another combats age-related forgetfulness through boosting levels of CRB, another protein that helps to establish long-term memories. Ampakines, now in phase II trials, have shown promise in normalizing the activity of glutamate by attaching to AMPA receptors, thus ramping up the voltage of electrical signals traveling between brain cells. In addition, they increase production of nerve growth factor (NGF), a naturally-occurring protein that is hypothesized to prevent brain cell death and to stimulate cell function in areas of the brain involved in memory. Additional strategies for anti-dementia drug development include nutraceuticals/medical foods, neurotransmitter-based therapies (as above), glial modulating drugs, metabolic and mitochondrial targets (antioxidants: vitamins E and C, coenzyme Q10), and tau-modulating, anti-tangle approaches (microtubule stabilizers, kinase inhibitors, and immunotherapies).

DEMENTIA WITH LEWY BODIES
Definition

Dementia with Lewy bodies (DLB) is a progressive brain disease that involves cognitive, behavioral, and motor system deterioration similar to that seen in PD.

Epidemiology and Risk Factors

DLB is arguably the second-leading cause of dementia in the elderly. Some researchers estimate that it accounts for up to 20% of dementia in the United States, afflicting 800,000 individuals. Slightly more men than women are affected. As with most dementias of adult-onset, advanced age is a main risk factor for DLB. Disease onset is usually in the seventh decade of life or later. DLB may cluster in families.

Pathophysiology

The main pathological features of DLB are proteinaceous deposits called Lewy bodies (Figure 19-4), named for Frederic H. Lewy, who first described them in the early 1900s. Among other proteins, Lewy bodies are composed of alpha-synuclein in the cortex and brainstem.[31] In PD, Lewy bodies are primarily restricted to the brainstem and dopaminergic cells of the substantia nigra. In DLB, Lewy bodies are found in the cortex and amygdala, as well as the brainstem. Triplication or mutations of the alpha-synuclein gene are rare causes of DLB. The mechanisms by which Lewy bodies cause neuronal dysfunction and eventual death are uncertain, but it is clear that both

the cholinergic and dopaminergic neurotransmitter systems are severely disrupted. Of note, Lewy body and AD pathology frequently co-occur.

Clinical Features and Diagnosis

The clinical features of DLB are similar to those of AD, and the diagnosis is challenging to make. DLB typically presents with cortical and subcortical cognitive impairments, and with visuospatial and executive dysfunction that is worse than that found in AD, with relatively spared language and memory function. A recent international consortium on DLB resulted in revised criteria for clinical and pathological diagnosis of DLB.[32] Core clinical features include fluctuating attention, recurrent visual hallucinations, and parkinsonism. Parkinsonian symptoms are also necessary for the diagnosis of DLB, with the motor symptoms occurring in most cases within about 1 year of the cognitive problems. Suggestive clinical features meanwhile include rapid eye movement (REM) behavior disorder, extreme sensitivity to neuroleptic medications, disorientation, and low dopamine transporter uptake on neuroimaging.[32] Other manifestations (such as apathy, irritability, depression, and agitation), repeated falls and syncope, autonomic dysfunction, delusions, hallucinations in other modalities, prominent slowing on electroencephalogram, and low uptake on MIBG myocardial scintography are considered supportive of the diagnosis, but not as specific.[32] While clinical features of the disease (e.g., hallucinations, fluctuations, visuospatial deficits, and REM behavior disorder) are helpful in the identification of possible cases of this disease, clinical-pathological concordance has not been great, and postmortem pathological findings of Lewy bodies in the cerebral cortex, amygdala, and brainstem are necessary to confirm the diagnosis.[33]

Structural imaging is typically not particularly helpful as atrophy may not be apparent early on in DLB (Figure 19-5, *left*). Sometimes pallor of the substantia nigra can be identified on MRI; as the disease progresses, there may be atrophy with a frontotemporal, insular, and visual cortex predominance. PET and SPECT may show evidence of decreased activity or perfusion in the occipitotemporal cortices (Figure 19-5, *right*) in early clinical disease stages. In later stages only the primary sensorimotor cortex may be spared.

Differential Diagnosis

As with AD, metabolic, inflammatory, infectious, vascular, medication-related, and structural causes for cognitive decline in the setting of parkinsonism should be excluded with testing. If the clinical picture is not highly consistent with DLB, other dementias with parkinsonism should be considered, including corticobasal degeneration (CBD), progressive supranuclear palsy (PSP), the "Parkinson's-plus" syndromes (e.g., multiple-system atrophy), and vascular parkinsonism with dementia. It is also sometimes difficult to distinguish between PD with dementia and DLB depending on the characteristics, severity, and presentation sequence of the cognitive and motor symptoms. This distinction is primarily based on whether or not parkinsonism precedes dementia for more than a year, as occurs in PD with dementia. Further, the motor symptoms of PD tend to respond better to dopaminergic therapies than they do in DLB.

Treatment

There are currently no FDA-approved treatments specific for DLB. Given the severe cholinergic losses that occur in DLB, the frequent co-occurrence of AD pathology, and several small

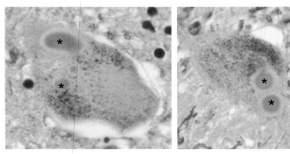

Figure 19-4. Lewy body pathology. *, Lewy bodies.

MRI   SPECT

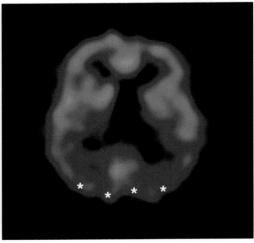

Figure 19-5. Lewy body dementia neuroimaging.

trials that suggest their effectiveness, cholinesterase inhibitors have been the off-label treatment of choice. Rivastigmine has been effective for cognitive deficits and behavioral problems in DLB as compared to placebo.[33] However, in a recent Cochrane Review summarizing the evidence from six trials investigating cholinesterase inhibitors in PD dementia, DLB, and MCI associated with PD, the authors concluded that efficacy of cholinesterase inhibitors in DLB remained unclear in contrast to their use in PDD.[34] While memantine may also be a logical choice because it enhances cognition in disorders with cholinergic deficits and it has dopaminergic effects that could benefit the parkinsonism in DLB, its efficacy has thus far been modest in two recent controlled trials.[35,36] Low dosages of levodopa/carbidopa (dopamine replacement) are sometimes helpful for the motor symptoms of DLB, although higher dosages of dopamine replacement therapy and direct dopamine agonists may exacerbate neuropsychiatric symptoms (e.g., hallucinations). Given that patients with DLB are sensitive to neuroleptics, typical antipsychotics and risperidone should be strictly avoided in patients with DLB, because even a single dose can lead to prolonged drug-induced akinesia and rigidity. Other atypical antipsychotics (such as quetiapine) may be very useful for management of DLB's behavioral symptoms, with fewer untoward motor side effects than typical antipsychotics. However, these agents pose other potential side effects (e.g., metabolic syndrome, weight gain, increased mortality risk). Tricyclic antidepressants or benzodiazepines may help with REM behavior disorder in DLB, but given their anticholinergic and sedative properties, they should be used with caution in the elderly with dementia.

Supportive Care and Long-term Management

These issues are similar as for AD, except that the neuropsychiatric features of DLB may be more severe than in AD, requiring additional supportive care. Greater levels of depression may occur in caregivers of patients with DLB versus caregivers of patients with AD; thus, early support for the patient and family is important.

Prognosis

The average duration of the disease is 5 to 7 years, though there may be substantial variability in the outcome of DLB.

The frequency of co-occurring AD and DLB pathologies in the same individual is greater than is anticipated by chance. Clinical syndromes with overlapping AD and DLB symptoms and the pathological findings have led to several diagnostic categories, such as AD with Lewy bodies or the Lewy body variant of AD. Future research in this area may elucidate the relationship and pathophysiology of both AD and DLB.

FRONTOTEMPORAL DEMENTIAS
Definition

Definitions of frontotemporal dementias (FTDs) are currently in flux. FTDs may be understood as a genetically and pathologically heterogenous group of neurodegenerative disorders that involve degeneration of different regions of the frontal and temporal lobes to differing extents. The clinical pictures and underlying pathologies are also heterogeneous. Currently subsumed under the term FTDs are Pick's disease, frontotemporal lobar degeneration, primary progressive aphasia, and semantic dementia.[37] Additionally, there can be significant overlap between FTD and motor amytrophic lateral sclerosis (FTD-ALS) as well as the atypical parkinsonian syndromes, PSP and corticobasal syndrome (CBS).[38]

Epidemiology and Genetic Risk Factors

FTD tends to manifest at younger ages than typical AD, with the majority of cases occurring in people under age 65, and it is the most common form of dementia with onset before 60 years of age, with most cases presenting between 45 and 64 years of age.[38] Unlike AD, onset after 75 years of age is rare. FTD sometimes runs in families. In fact, 25%–50% of patients with FTD have a first-degree relative with the disease, and autosomal dominant inheritance is frequently observed. Many of these families are found to harbor a mutation in *MATP*, the gene encoding the tau protein, which is found in neurofibrillary tangles. Patients with *MATP* mutations often have a motor syndrome, such as PD or PSP, along with their FTD. A total of 40 tau mutations have been reported across 113 families. In addition, FTD can sometimes be associated with mutations in *GRN*, *VCP*, *TARDBP PSEN1* and *CHMP2B*,[38,39] along with a recently identified C9ORF72 hexanucleotide repeat expansion.[39]

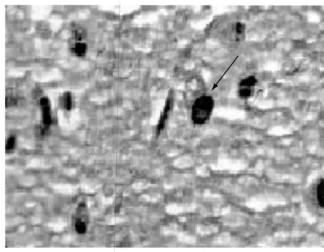

Figure 19-6. Neuropathology of frontotemporal disease: Pick's bodies.

Pathophysiology

The pathophysiology of FTD is poorly understood, and it likely represents a constellation of syndromes with different underlying causes. This notion is reflected in the variable pathologies that underlie the disease and somehow all lead to neuronal dysfunction and to death. Individuals with clinically-defined FTD may exhibit variable combinations of abnormal tau protein deposits, including tangles and Pick's bodies (as in Pick's disease, Figure 19-6); ubiquitin-positive inclusions; gliosis; non-specific spongiform degeneration; and prion-related spongiform changes. In some cases AD pathology distributed in the frontotemporal cortex can cause an FTD-like syndrome. Further, transactive response DNA-binding protein 43 (TDP-43) was identified in 2006 as the major inclusion protein in the majority of patients with amyotrophic lateral sclerosis (ALS) and in the most common subtype of FTD, frontotemporal lobar degeneration with TDP-43 pathology (FTLD-TDP).[39] Indeed, FTLD can be classified into three general categories based on the predominant neuropathological protein: microtubule-associated tau (FTLD-TAU); TAR DNA-binding protein 43 (FTLD-TDP), and fused in sarcoma protein (FTLD-FUS). Recently, the clinicopathologic overlap between ALS and FTD was supported by discovery of C9ORF72 repeat expansions, a GGGGCC hexanucleotide repeat in a non-coding region of C9ORF72 (chromosome 9 open reading frame 72), encoding an unknown C9ORF72 protein.[39] While genetic causes of FTD include tau mutations on chromosome 17 (FTD-17) (these cases often have associated symptoms of parkinsonism), currently repeat expansions in C9ORF72 are the most important genetic cause of familial ALS and FTD.[39]

Clinical Features, Diagnosis, and Differential Diagnosis

The classic hallmarks of FTD are behavioral and compartmental features out of proportion to amnesia. There is a generally slow onset followed by progressive loss of judgment, disinhibition, impulsivity, social misconduct, loss of awareness, and withdrawal. Other typical symptoms are stereotypies, excessive oral/manual exploration, hyperphagia, wanderlust, excessive joviality, sexually-provocative behaviors, and inappropriate words/actions.

In some cases, language is initially or primarily affected, and can remain as the relatively isolated deficit for years. In

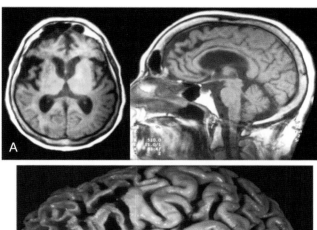
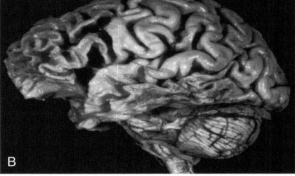

Figure 19-7. Frontotemporal atrophy (A) on MRI and (B) at autopsy.

these cases there is often primarily left hemisphere pathology selectively involving the frontal or temporal lobes, or the perisylvian cortex. Depending on the localization of left hemisphere pathology, patients may exhibit different degrees of impairment of word-finding, object-naming, syntax, or word-comprehension abilities. Primary progressive aphasia (PPA) usually refers to symptomatic involvement of the frontal (or other perisylvian) language areas leading to a dysfluent aphasia with relatively preserved comprehension.[40] Semantic dementia is characterized by significant loss of word meaning (i.e., semantic losses) with relatively preserved fluency, which results from left anterior temporal lobe involvement. However, the definitions of these syndromes are in flux, and the clinicopathological correlates are not uniform.[41]

Clinical presentations of FTD vary based on the relative involvement of the hemisphere (right or left) or lobe (frontal or temporal) involved. Patients may initially have right greater than left temporal lobe involvement and exhibit primarily a behavioral syndrome with emotional distance, irritability, and disruption of sleep, appetite, and libido. With greater initial left than right temporal lobe involvement, patients exhibit more language-related problems, including anomia, word-finding difficulties, repetitive speech, and loss of semantic information (e.g., semantic dementia).[42] In some cases of FTD the frontal lobes may be involved to a greater extent than the temporal lobes. In these instances, patients exhibit symptoms of elation, disinhibition, apathy, and aberrant motor behavior. Depending on the combination of regions involved, patients with FTD exhibit specific cognitive and neuropsychiatric symptoms. As the disease progresses to involve greater expanses of the frontotemporal cortex, the clinical features become similar. The presumption is that the atrophy and underlying pathology that accompanies FTD is regionally specific, but it becomes more generalized as the disease progresses.

The evaluation and diagnosis of FTD is similar to that of the other dementias and should include clinical evaluation, laboratory studies, neuropsychological testing, and brain imaging (structural and functional imaging). Findings on CT or MRI

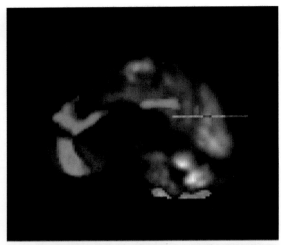

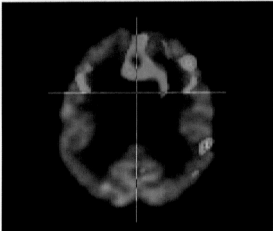

Figure 19-8. Regional hypoactivity in frontotemporal disease. Colored areas in sagittal (A) and horizontal (B) brain sections indicate activity 2 SD below the population mean. *(Courtesy of Keith Johnson.)*

scans may show frontotemporal atrophy (Figure 19-7, *A*), which can be quite striking at autopsy (Figure 19-7, *B*). Clinical findings of motor system or brainstem abnormalities should be investigated when considering the various diagnoses. For example, some cases of FTD are associated with parkinsonism (FTD-17) or motor neuron disease (e.g., amyotrophic lateral sclerosis [ALS]), with increasing evidence, as above, that ALS and FTD may be on a disease continuum with shared underlying pathogenesis. Other clinically-defined disorders may have features of FTD, but be distinguished by eye movement, sensory, or gait abnormalities (e.g., PSP, CBD, and NPH). Brain imaging studies of FTD may show focal atrophy in the frontotemporal cortices along with frontotemporal hypoperfusion or hypoactivity (Figure 19-8).

Treatment

There are no specific treatments or cures for FTD. The behavioral features are sometimes helped by SSRIs, and these are probably the best-studied treatments for these disorders. Cholinesterase inhibitors and memantine may exacerbate the neuropsychiatric symptoms. Antipsychotics (preferably atypical ones), mood stabilizers, and benzodiazepines are sometimes necessary to treat aggression and agitation, but they should be used sparingly.

Supportive Care and Long-term Management

As in the other dementias, supportive, long-term care is crucial for FTD, because it is often accompanied by loss of insight, lack of judgment, and severe behavioral symptoms.

Prognosis

There are no specific medical treatments for FTD. Across the disorders, the time between illness and death is typically about 7 years.

Although not all cases of FTD have the same underlying pathology, there is a developing notion that there is a group of associated dementias (including some instances clinically consistent with FTD) based on the presence of abnormal forms of the tau protein and TDP-43. These disorders cut across the regional neuroanatomic boundaries that typically characterize FTD and may exhibit features atypical for frontotemporal lobar degeneration. In particular, not only do some cases of clinically-defined FTD have tau pathology but also certain characteristic motor, sensory, and brainstem-related clinical features, as found in PSP, CBD, and FTD with parkinsonism or motor neuron disease. Other focal atrophies outside of the frontotemporal lobes may also reflect underlying tau pathology (such as progressive visuospatial and language dysfunction) that can occur in posterior (parietal) cortical atrophy.

VASCULAR DEMENTIA
Definition

Vascular dementia has become an overarching term that encompasses a variety of vascular-related causes of dementia, including multi-infarct dementia (MID) and small vessel disease. More recently the term "vascular cognitive impairment" has been used to take into account all forms of cognitive dysfunction caused by vascular disease, ranging from prodromal stages and mild cognitive dysfunction to dementia, or major neurocognitive impairment.

Epidemiology and Risk Factors

Various types of vascular dementia account for approximately 20% of all dementia cases, making it the second or third most common form of dementia. It is equally prevalent in males and females, but the frequency may be higher in males and in African Americans. Risk factors are similar to those for cardiovascular illness (including diabetes, hypercholesterolemia, hyperhomocysteinemia, hypertension, cigarette smoking, and physical inactivity). To the extent that these factors have familial or genetic bases, so does vascular dementia. Not all genetic risk factors have the same relevance for the different forms of vascular dementia. For example, it is uncertain whether an elevated cholesterol level is as crucial a risk factor as is hypertension for microvascular ischemic white matter disease; several large studies have failed to show a clinical benefit of decreased cholesterol for cognitive impairments even when rates of stroke and transient ischemic attacks (TIAs) are reduced.

Pathophysiology

There are several underlying causes of vascular dementia. Recurrent or specifically-localized embolic strokes (from sources such as the heart or carotid artery, or local thromboses of larger-caliber intracranial vessels) can lead to vascular dementia. These causes are most closely associated with the clinical entity of MID. Smaller subcortical strokes (e.g., lacunar

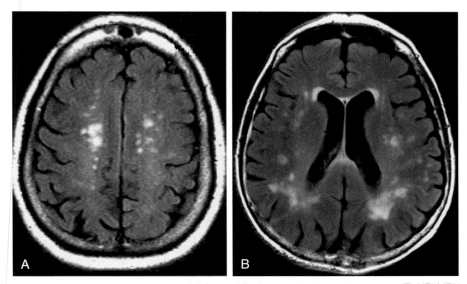

Figure 19-9. MRI of vascular dementia: small-vessel disease. (A) Coronal fluid attenuation inversion recovery (FLAIR) MRI image showing centrum semiovale ischemic white matter disease. (B) Coronal FLAIR MRI showing periventricular ischemic white matter disease.

infarctions) in gray and white matter structures may also lead to a form of vascular dementia.

White matter disease without clearly symptomatic strokes or gross tissue damage may cause insidiously-progressive cognitive decline (Figure 19-9). It is important to keep in mind that cerebral hemorrhages due to hypertension or amyloid angiopathy are possible mechanisms of vascular-induced cognitive impairment, but they require a different type of clinical management than does typical vascular occlusive disease. There are specific gene mutations (e.g., *notch 3*) that cause particular forms of vascular dementia (e.g., cerebral autosomal dominant arteriopathy with subcortical infarcts and leukoencephalopathy [CADASIL]), but these are extremely rare.

Clinical Features and Diagnosis

Vascular dementia has variable clinical features that are dependent on the localization of the vascular lesions. Overall, left hemisphere lesions tend to cause language problems, and right hemisphere lesions tend to cause visuospatial problems. Both the type of cognitive deficits and the time course of the cognitive changes are variable. Embolic or large-vessel stroke-related dementia may progress in a characteristic step-wise pattern, with intervening periods of stability punctuated by abrupt declines in cognitive function; the type of cognitive symptoms will be affected by the brain areas affected over time. This might be considered the classic presentation for vascular dementia associated with multiple infarcts, but may not be the most common presentation of vascular dementia.[43]

Multiple small subcortical infarcts may cause a more insidious decline, even in the absence of recognized stroke symptoms. However, small cortical infarcts at specific locations (e.g., the thalamus or caudate) can cause significant cognitive and motor symptoms. So-called small-vessel or microvascular ischemic disease preferentially involves the white matter, particularly in the centrum semiovale and periventricular regions (see Figure 19-9), and is also a common cause of vascular dementia. This has been called "leukoaraiosis." Symptoms in this case tend to develop in a gradual and insidious fashion and can be difficult to distinguish from AD. Memory or mood complaints are usually a presenting feature. Sometimes the memory disorder can be distinguished from that in AD.

Spontaneous recall is affected in both disorders, but recognition memory is often preserved in vascular dementia, which is not the case for AD. Presentations involving relatively isolated psychotic symptoms in the setting of preserved memory should also raise the possibility of vascular dementia. Likewise, apathy, executive dysfunction, and a relatively intact memory are suggestive of a small-vessel ischemic process. Vascular dementia is also often referable to altered frontal systems dysfunction by which there is disconnection or damage to white matter tracts that relay information to and from the region.

Differential Diagnosis

The main difficulty in diagnosing vascular dementia is distinguishing it from AD. Classically, vascular dementia is distinguished from AD based on an abrupt onset and a step-wise course. In addition, prominent executive dysfunction and preserved recognition memory are also suggestive of vascular dementia. However, in many cases the symptoms of vascular dementia overlap with those of AD. Further, autopsy studies show that the co-occurrence of AD and CNS vascular pathology is not infrequent; the interaction may cause cognitive impairment that might not otherwise occur if the same level of AD or vascular dementia pathology was present alone.

In addition, since the clinical features of vascular cognitive impairment may be variable, specific vascular lesions can mimic a variety of different dementias and even PD. The finding of focal features on examination or CNS vascular disease on structural imaging studies helps to determine the correct diagnosis.

Treatment

Treatment for vascular dementia involves control of vascular risk factors (e.g., hypercholesterolemia, hypertension, inactivity, diabetes, excess alcohol use, cigarette smoking, hyperhomocysteinemia). If strokes are found on brain imaging studies, a stroke work-up should be initiated to determine if surgery (e.g., for carotid stenosis), anticoagulation (for atrial fibrillation), or antiplatelet agents (e.g., for small-vessel strokes) are indicated. Such an evaluation may show hemorrhages from amyloid angiopathy or hypertension, in which case avoidance of anticoagulant or antiplatelet therapies may be prudent. In addition to treating these causes of CNS vascular disease, some literature indicates that symptomatic treatments (such as cholinesterase inhibitors or memantine) may be helpful for cognition.[44] However, there are no FDA-approved treatments for vascular dementia. Neuropsychiatric features (e.g., depression or psychosis) are common in vascular dementia and should be treated accordingly.

Recent work has highlighted a significant incidence of vascular-related cognitive impairment that does not reach clinical criteria for dementia. This is akin to the notion of MCI or prodromal AD. Although definitions for vascular-related cognitive impairment are currently under development, the idea highlights the importance of recognizing cognitive difficulties due to CNS vascular disease in their earliest stages so that vascular risk factors can be identified and treated.[45]

CORTICOBASAL DEGENERATION

Corticobasal degeneration (CBD) is a rare form of dementia that is related to FTD and typically involves specific motor and cognitive deficits. It usually occurs between ages 45 and 70 years, and may have a slight female predominance. It rarely runs in families, but may be associated with a specific tau gene haplotype. Pathologically, there are abnormal neuronal and glial tau accumulations in the cortex and basal ganglia, including the substantia nigra. Swollen, achromatic neurons are typical. The pathophysiology is unknown, and although thought to primarily relate to the toxic effects of the tau protein, it has been increasingly recognized to involve Tar-DNA binding protein-43 (TDP-43) positive inclusions as well as AD pathology.[46] Clinically, CBD is typically characterized by asymmetric sensorimotor symptoms involving one hemibody to a greater degree than the other, with features of cortical and basal ganglionic dysfunction. Patients tend to have problems performing complex sequenced movements and movements on command (i.e., apraxia). Dystonia and action- or stimulus-induced myoclonus are also not uncommon. One classic sensorimotor feature of CBD is the alien hand or limb phenomenon, in which a part of the body feels as if it is not one's own or like it is being moved by an external/alien force. Parkinsonian rigidity and walking problems may also develop in addition to these sensorimotor problems, as well as problems with language and memory, personality changes, and inappropriate behavior.

Structural imaging studies may show frontotemporal atrophy, asymmetric parietal atrophy, or both. Functional imaging studies may demonstrate asymmetric hypometabolism and hypoperfusion in the parietal cortex and basal ganglia with or without frontotemporal hypometabolism and hypoperfusion. In the setting of mild motor symptoms with more prominent cognitive or behavioral manifestations, CBD can be confused for AD or FTD or vascular dementia with vascular parkinsonism. Some studies indicate that up to 20% of clinically-diagnosed FTDs turn out to have the pathology of CBD. Because of the significant clinicopathologic heterogeneity, the term corticobasal syndrome (CBS) is sometimes used for patients with characteristic clinical features, while CBD is reserved for diagnosis based on neuropathological analysis.

There are no FDA-approved or other treatments specific for CBD. Treatment is therefore supportive or symptomatic based on the individual patient's specific disease manifestations.

PROGRESSIVE SUPRANUCLEAR PALSY

Progressive supranuclear palsy (PSP) is another dementia characterized by the presence of cognitive and behavioral features along with specific motor abnormalities. PSP tends to

occur in middle age and is slightly more common in men than women. It is a rare and sporadic disease, but, like CBD, it has been associated with specific tau gene haplotypes. The pathology of PSP involves (usually) abnormal tau-reactive deposits in neurons and glia that are typically concentrated in various brainstem nuclei (including the substantia nigra), but sometimes also in the cortex. In addition to involvement of systems that coordinate somatic movement, the supranuclear systems that govern the cranial nerves are also affected.

The classic clinical features of the disease are progressive difficulties with balance and gait, resulting in frequent falls early in the disease, progressive loss of voluntary control of eye movements, and progressive cognitive and behavioral difficulties. Patients with PSP often have difficulties with the coordination of eyelid opening and closing, dysarthria, dysphagia, and fixed facial expression akin to surprise. Symptoms similar to those of PD are also present, particularly akinesia and axial rigidity. The cognitive and behavioral features are usually referable to frontal lobe dysfunction and may closely resemble those of FTD (such as executive dysfunction, apathy, and reduced processing speed). CT or MRI scans may show an atrophic brainstem with frontotemporal atrophy as the disease progresses.

There are no approved therapies or cures for PSP, and management is supportive or symptomatic. It is important to assess safety issues to reduce the risk of falls and injury. Swallowing evaluations help to determine diet modifications that delay aspiration from dysphagia.

NORMAL PRESSURE HYDROCEPHALUS

Normal pressure hydrocephalus (NPH) is a condition that involves enlargement of the ventricles leading to cognitive and motor difficulties. About 250,000 people in the United States suffer from this disease; it usually occurs in adults 55 years old or older. Intermittent pressure increases are thought to cause ventricular expansion over time, with damage to the adjacent white matter tracts that connect the frontal lobes. The main clinical features are gait disturbance, frontal systems dysfunction, and urinary incontinence.[47] Patients need not have all three symptoms to have NPH. There are no clear genetic causes. The main risk factors relate to conditions that adversely affect the function of the ventricular system for cerebrospinal fluid (CSF) egress, which include history of head trauma, intracranial hemorrhage, meningitis, or any inflammatory or structural process that might damage the meninges.

Evaluation usually includes structural brain imaging (MRI or CT) demonstrating the presence of ventricular enlargement out of proportion to atrophy. Reversal of CSF flow in the cerebral aqueduct or the presence of transependymal fluid on MRI may suggest NPH.

If NPH is suspected, it is prudent to remove CSF and to measure the CSF pressure, which can be done by a variety of techniques. It is most important to perform cognitive and motor testing before and after the removal of a large volume of CSF. LP, lumbar catheter insertion or CSF pressure, and outflow-resistance monitoring in combination with pre-procedure and post-procedure neuropsychological and motor testing can be very helpful in making a diagnosis and in estimating the likelihood of treatment success.[48] Placement of a CSF shunt is the treatment of choice and can arrest or even significantly improve a patient's condition.[49]

CREUTZFELDT–JAKOB DISEASE

Creutzfeldt–Jakob disease (CJD) is a rare disorder that causes a characteristic triad of progressive dementia, myoclonus, and distinctive periodic EEG complexes; cerebellar, pyramidal and extrapyramidal findings are also characteristic, as are psychiatric symptoms, which may be among the first signs of the disease. The typical age of onset is around 60 years. CJD is caused by prions, novel proteinaceous infective agents. Prion protein, PrP, an amyloid protein encoded on chromosome 20, is the major constituent of prions. PrP normally exists in a PrPc isoform; in a pathological state, it is transformed to the PrPSc isoform, which condenses in neurons and causes their death. As prion-induced changes accumulate, the cerebral cortex takes on the distinctive microscopic, vacuolar appearance of spongiform encephalopathy. The CSF in almost 90% of CJD cases contains traces of prion proteins detected by a routine LP. CJD is transmissible and can occur as three general forms: sporadic, familial or acquired, including a variant form of CJD. Treatment in these unfortunate cases is supportive, as it follows a characteristically rapid and fatal course over an average of 6 months.[50]

CONCLUSIONS

As the population ages, the number of people with dementing disorders is increasing dramatically; most have AD, vascular dementia, DLB or a combination of these disorders. Although none are curable, all have treatable components—whether they are reversible, static, or progressive. Further, the increasing recognition of the spectrum of cognitive impairment, in mild and major neurocognitive disorders and in pre-clinical stages of AD, has potential for identifying people at earlier stages of impairment and preventing progression. The role of a psychiatrist in the diagnosis and treatment of dementing disorders is extremely important, particularly in the identification of treatable psychiatric and behavioral symptoms, which are common sources of caregiver distress and institutionalization.

Family members are additional victims of all progressive dementias. They particularly appreciate the psychiatrist who communicates with them about the diagnosis and the expected course of the disorder. They can benefit from advice on how best to relate to the patient, how to restructure the home environment for safety and comfort, and how to seek out legal and financial guidance when appropriate. Family members should also be made aware of the assistance available to them through organizations such as the Alzheimer's Association.

Great advances have been made in our understanding of the pathophysiology, epidemiology, and genetics of various dementing disorders. The likelihood of having measures for early detection, prevention, and intervention in the near future is very promising.

Access the complete reference list and multiple choice questions (MCQs) online at https://expertconsult.inkling.com

KEY REFERENCES

3. Petersen RC. Mild cognitive impairment ten years later. *Arch Neurol* 66:1447–1455, 2009.
4. Mayeux R, Stern Y. Epidemiology of Alzheimer Disease. *Cold Spring Harbor Perspect Med* 2, 2012.
5. Sosa-Ortiz AL, Acosta-Castillo I, Prince MJ. Epidemiology of Alzheimer's Disease. *Arch Med Res* 43:600–608, 2012.
8. Barnes DE, Yaffee K. The projected effect of risk factor reduction on Alzheimer's disease prevalence. *Lancet Neurol* 10:819–828, 2011.

10. Reitz C, Brayne C, Mayeux R. Epidemiology of Alzheimer Disease. *Nat Rev Neurol* 7:137–152, 2011.
11. Carillo MC, Brashear HR, Logovinsky V, et al. Can we prevent Alzheimer's disease? secondary "prevention" trials. *Alzheimers Dement* 9:123–131, 2013.
17. Gandy S, DeKosky ST. Toward the treatment and prevention of Alzheimer's disease: rational strategies and recent progress. *Ann Rev Med* 64:367–383, 2013.
20. Sperling RA, Aisen PS, Beckett LA, et al. Toward defining the preclinical stages of Alzheimer's disease: recommendations from the National Institute on Aging-Alzheimer's Association workgroups on diagnostic guidelines for Alzheimer's disease. *Alzheimers Dement* 7:280–292, 2011.
21. Alzheimer's Disease. Implications of the updated diagnostic and research criteria. *J Clin Psychiatry* 72(9):1190–1196, 2011.
22. Pillai JA, Cummings JL. Clinical trials in predementia stages of Alzheimer Disease. *Med Clin North Am* 97(3):439–457, 2013.
25. Howard R, McShane R, Lindesay J, et al. Donepezil and memantine for moderate-to-severe Alzheimer's Disease. *N Engl J Med* 366(10):893–903, 2012.
26. Carson S, McDonagh MS, Peterson K. A systematic review of the efficacy and safety of atypical antipsychotics in patients with psychological and behavioral symptoms of dementia. *J Am Geriatr Soc* 54:354–361, 2006.
28. Selkoe DJ. Defining molecular targets to prevent Alzheimer disease. *Arch Neurol* 62(2):192–195, 2005.
30. Gilman S, Koller M, Black RS, et al. Clinical effects of Abeta immunization (AN1792) in patients with AD in an interrupted trial. *Neurology* 64(9):1553–1562, 2005.
31. Jellinger KA. Alpha-synuclein pathology in Parkinson's and Alzheimer's disease brain: incidence and topographic distribution—a pilot study. *Acta Neuropathol (Berl)* 106:191–201, 2003.
32. Weisman D, McKeith I. Dementia with Lewy bodies. *Semin Neurol* 27(1):42–47, 2007.
33. McKeith IG, Dickson DW, Lowe J, et al. Diagnosis and management of dementia with Lewy bodies: third report of the DLB consortium. *Neurology* 65:1863–1872, 2005.
34. Rolinski M, Fox C, Maidment I, et al. Cholinesterase inhibitors for dementia with Lewy bodies, Parkinson's disease dementia and cognitive impairment in Parkinson's disease. *Cochrane Database Syst Rev* 14(3):CD006504, 2012.
37. Forman MS, Farmer J, Johnson JK, et al. Frontotemporal dementia: clinicopathological correlations. *Ann Neurol* 59:952–962, 2006.
38. Seltman RE, Matthews BR. Frontotemporal lobar degeneration: epidemiology, pathology, diagnosis and management. *CNS Drugs* 26(10):841–870, 2012.
39. Van Blitterswijk M, DeJesus-Hernandez M, Rademakers R. How do C9ORF72 repeat expansions cause amyotrophic lateral sclerosis and frontotemporal dementia: can we learn from other non-coding repeat expansions disorders? *Curr Opin Neurol* 25(6):689–700, 2012.
40. Mesulam MM. Primary progressive aphasia—a language-based dementia. *N Engl J Med* 349:1535–1542, 2003.
44. Bowler JV. Acetylcholinesterase inhibitors for vascular dementia and Alzheimer's disease combined with cerebrovascular disease. *Stroke* 34:584–586, 2003.
45. Bowler JV. Vascular cognitive impairment. *J Neurol Neurosurg Psychiatry* 76(Suppl. 5):v35–v44, 2005.
46. Shelley BP, Hodges JR, Kipps CM, et al. Is the pathology of corticobasal syndrome predictable in life? *Mov Disord* 24(11):1593–1599, 2009.
48. Relkin N, Marmarou A, Klinge P, et al. Diagnosing idiopathic normal-pressure hydrocephalus. *Neurosurgery* 57:S4–S16, discussion ii–v, 2005.
50. Gencer AG, Pelin Z, Kucukali C, et al. Creutzfeldt-Jakob disease. *Psychogeriatrics* 11(2):119–124, 2011.

KEY POINTS

Epidemiology

- Intellectual disability is a prevalent condition that affects 1% of the population and has multiple etiologies.

Clinical Features

- The full range of psychopathology occurs in individuals with intellectual disability and often it occurs at rates higher than in the general population.

Differential Diagnosis

- The evaluation of a person with an intellectual disability should include a current cognitive profile, an assessment of the person's developmental level, and an appreciation of the possible functional nature of the individual's behavior.

- Co-morbid medical and neurological conditions that affect behavior should always be considered in the differential diagnosis.

Treatment Options

- Treatment should be tailored to each individual's unique presentation; clear objective outcome measures should be established to assess the efficacy of treatment.

OVERVIEW

Treatment of psychiatric and behavioral disorders in individuals with an intellectual disability is both challenging and rewarding. Although it is unlikely that most psychiatrists will be called on to make a diagnosis of intellectual disability, knowledge about what defines intellectual disability, and about the clinical features of the most common syndromes related to the development of an intellectual disability, is crucial for the optimal treatment of individuals with this condition. Key questions to consider when evaluating a person with an intellectual disability include the following: How was the diagnosis made? Was the work-up complete? How severe is the cognitive impairment? What is the current developmental level of the patient? Are there any current or co-morbid medical issues that may be causing or contributing to aberrant behavior? Is there a functional aspect to accompanying problematic behavior? Which psychiatric disorders are prevalent in patients with an intellectual disability or commonly occur with identified syndromes?

Historically, those with an intellectual disability and those with severe psychiatric illness have shared the burden of a chronic illness, as well as the experience of stigmatization and alienation from society. However, individuals with an intellectual disability were initially thought to stand apart from others with brain disorders. The English Court of Wards and Liveries in the sixteenth century differentiated "idiots" from "lunatics." Kraeplin, in his initial diagnostic schema, identified intellectual disability as a separate form of psychiatric illness. It was not until 1888 when the *American Journal of Insanity* used the phrase "imbecility with insanity" that

intellectual disability and psychiatric illness were identified as potentially co-occurring conditions.

EPIDEMIOLOGY

Prevalence

The prevalence of intellectual disabilities is approximately 1%.[1-3] Prevalence rates have varied between 1% and 3% depending on the populations sampled, the criteria used, and the sampling methods applied.

Currently, there are more than 750 known causes of intellectual disability. Categories include: pre-natal/genetic disorders, neurological malformations, external/pre-natal causes (such as prematurity and toxin exposure), peri-natal causes (such as hypoxia), and post-natal causes (such as infection and neglect). In up to 25% of cases no clear etiology is found.[2-6] This can be disheartening for patients, parents, families, and caregivers, as they search for an understanding of a condition that will profoundly affect their lives. This aspect of a patient's history should be addressed at the start of treatment.

The three most common identified causes of intellectual disability are Down syndrome, fragile X syndrome, and fetal alcohol syndrome. Facial features of these conditions are provided in Figures 20-1 to 20-3; knowledge of the dysmorphic features associated with clinical syndromes aids in their identification. Down syndrome is the most common genetic cause of intellectual disability; it involves trisomy of chromosome 21. Fragile X syndrome is the most common inherited cause of intellectual disability with the *FMR1* gene located on the X chromosome. Fetal alcohol syndrome, the most common "acquired" cause of intellectual disability, has no identified chromosomal abnormality, as it is a toxin-based insult. These three etiologies account for approximately one-third of cases of intellectual disability.

CO-MORBID PSYCHOPATHOLOGY

Individuals with intellectual disability experience the full range of psychopathology, in addition to some unique behavioral conditions.[2,4,7-9] The rates of psychopathology in this population are roughly three to four times higher than in the general population[2,6]; exact determination is difficult as data collection in this area is confounded by methodological issues (including how to obtain an accurate assessment in the absence of self-report and determining how appropriate certain standardized measures might be in this population). In institutional settings up to 10% of individuals with intellectual disability also have some form of psychopathology or behavioral disorder.

Although it is generally accepted that the rates of psychopathology are higher in the intellectually disabled, there is less agreement as to why this is so. One theory posits that intellectual disability is a brain disorder with an as-yet unidentified damage to cortical and subcortical substrates. This damage confers heightened vulnerability to psychiatric disorders. Another theory holds that individuals with intellectual disability are chronically exposed to stressful and confusing environments, but they lack the cognitive capacity to successfully cope with this stress or to resolve affective conflicts. This

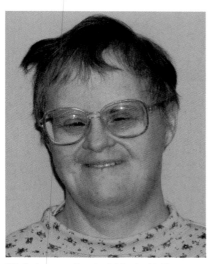

Figure 20-1. Image of an individual with Down syndrome.

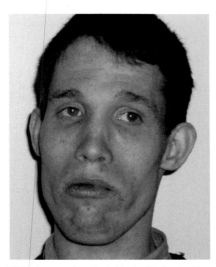

Figure 20-2. Image of an individual with fragile X syndrome.

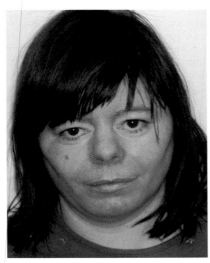

Figure 20-3. Image of an individual with fetal alcohol syndrome.

eventually wears them down and makes them more vulnerable to psychiatric disorders. Still another theory points to the paucity of good psychological care they receive, which leads to inadequate preventive measures and to delays in diagnosis and treatment.

In the past there was unwillingness on the part of the psychiatric community to aggressively diagnose and to treat what historically has been a difficult-to-diagnose population. This was superimposed on a movement in the field of intellectual disability not to "over-pathologize" behavior. Related to this has been the problem of under-diagnosis, based on the concept of diagnostic overshadowing: the attribution of all behavioral disturbances to "being intellectually disabled."[10-12] In today's treatment climate, however, one must be on guard against over-treatment in the form of misguided polypharmacy. What is needed is a thoughtful approach to diagnosis with an understanding of functional behavior that leads to optimum treatment of both psychiatric and behavioral disorders.

CLINICAL FEATURES AND DIAGNOSIS
Clinical Features

Familiarity with the diagnostic criteria of intellectual disability and its clinical manifestations will aid in the assessment of the functional strengths and weaknesses of a patient with intellectual disability who presents for diagnosis and treatment. Box 20-1 presents the *Diagnostic and Statistical Manual of Mental Disorders, Fifth Edition* criteria for intellectual disability. It should be noted that the term intellectual disability replaces the previous diagnosis of mental retardation and it is the equivalent term for the International Classification of Disorders (ICD) 11 diagnosis of intellectual developmental disorder.[1] These criteria have been adapted from work done by the American Association on Intellectual and Developmental Disabilities (AAIDD). Several changes from the previous diagnostic criteria reflect the need for clinical assessment as well as for standardized testing. Key criteria include: (1) below-average intellectual function (as defined by standard intelligence quotient [IQ] testing results that are at least 2 standard deviations below the mean [i.e., an IQ ≤ 70]), in conjunction with clinical assessment of impairment in areas such as reasoning, problem-solving, planning, judgment, and learning from experience; (2) deficits in adaptive function (compared to peers of the same age and culture) including communication, social skills, and independent living skills that restrict independent functioning in activities of daily life; and (3) onset of these deficits during the developmental period (meaning it has its onset in childhood and adolescence). It should be noted that symptoms of intellectual disability can occur outside of the developmental period, as in the case of acquired brain injury in adulthood, but this would be considered a neurocognitive disorder and not a neurodevelopmental disorder. The practical clinical assessment and care, however, might be very similar.

When reviewing the adaptive areas of function that are assessed when one considers a diagnosis of intellectual disability, one should be aware that these domains have not been empirically tested and no "gold standard" exists in terms of assessment of level of function or deficits. Multiple instruments are available to assist in the assessment; their use varies widely from state to state and from agency to agency. In addition, one can see individuals who may have been diagnosed as intellectually disabled, but who do not meet its strict IQ criteria. IQ testing can have a standard error of measurement of approximately 5 points. Conversely, there are individuals who may have had a diagnosis of intellectual disability, but

BOX 20-1 DSM-5 Diagnosis Criteria: Intellectual Disability (Intellectual Developmental Disorder)

Intellectual disability (intellectual developmental disorder) is a disorder with onset during the developmental period that includes both intellectual and adaptive functioning deficits in conceptual, social, and practical domains. The following three criteria must be met:

A. Deficits in intellectual functions, such as reasoning, problem solving, planning, abstract thinking, judgement, academic learning, and learning from experience, confirmed by both clinical assessment and individualized, standardized intelligence testing.

B. Deficits in adaptive functioning that result in failure to meet developmental and socio-cultural standards for personal independence and social responsibility. Without ongoing support, the adaptive deficits limit functioning in one or more activities of daily life, such as communication, social participation, and independent living, across multiple environmenets, such as home, school, work, and community.

C. Onset of intellectual and adaptive deficits during the developmental period.

Note: the diagnostic term *intellectual disability* is the equivalent term for the ICD-11 diagnosis of *intellectual development disorders.* Although the term *intellectual disability* is used throughout this manual, both terms are used in the title to clarify relationships with other classification systems. Moreover, a federal statute in the United States (Public Law 1110256, Rosa's Law) replaces the term *mental retardation* with *intellectual disability,* and research journals use the term *intellectual disability.* Thus, *intellectual disability* is the term in common use by medical, educational, and other professions and by the lay public advocacy groups.

• **Coding note:** The ICD-9-CM code for intellectual disability (intellectual developmental disorder) is **319**, which is assigned regardless of the severity specifier. The ICD-10-CM code depends on the severity specifier (see below).

Specify current severity:

(F70) Mild
(F71) Moderate
(F72) Severe
(F73) Profound

Reprinted with permission from the Diagnostic and statistical manual of mental disorders, ed 5, (Copyright 2013), American Psychiatric Association.

TABLE 20-1 Classification of Severity and Approximate Percentages of Intellectual Disability

Severity	IQ Range	Percentage of Intellectually Disabled Population
Mild	50–55 to 70	85
Moderate	35–40 to 50–55	10
Severe	20–25 to 35–40	3–4
Profound	Below 20–25	1–2

individuals with intellectual disability fall in the mild-to-moderate category and are the ones most likely to present for community treatment. Individuals with severe to profound intellectual disability are more commonly seen in institutional settings, but this can vary greatly from state to state and from region to region.

Diagnosis

Familiarity with a standard evaluation for intellectual disability is helpful to ensure that a patient with a diagnosis of intellectual disability has had a thorough work-up and that the diagnosis is accurate.[15,16] In addition, certain syndromes causing intellectual disability are associated with specific behaviors and psychiatric disorders. Thus, it is often helpful to identify these syndromes to aid in the clinical assessment.[17,18]

A developmental history (of early milestones and academic and adaptive function) is a good place to begin. This involves primarily ancillary sources of information (such as parents or primary caregivers) as patient accounts are often limited. The presence of a developmental disability should not discourage a psychiatrist from directly addressing this issue with the patient and the family, just as one would ask how a physical or medical disability has affected a patient's life. Most patients with an intellectual disability know that they are facing unique challenges and are "different" in some way. Addressing this directly with the patient is often appreciated, as it conveys an openness and respect for the patient as an adult. Conversely, if there is a level of uncertainty or an outright denial around the issue, this may provide important diagnostic information related to the current clinical situation.

Obtaining information from school, vocational placements, or day programs also helps to establish the accuracy of the diagnosis of intellectual disability and to assess the current clinical problem. Further corroboration of the diagnosis should be sought by reviewing the most recent evaluations of adaptive function and neuropsychiatric testing. Neuropsychiatric testing can quantify one's clinical assessment of a patient's cognitive strengths and deficits. The cause of psychopathology can sometimes be elucidated if a patient's cognitive profile does not match up well with his or her environmental situation.

Patients need thorough medical and neurological evaluations related to the diagnosis of intellectual disability and before being given a diagnosis of a psychiatric or behavioral disorder. One should consider correctable causes (including impairments of hearing and vision, a seizure disorder, or a recent head injury) of both cognitive impairments and behavioral disturbances. For example, there is a high rate of thyroid abnormalities in individuals with Down syndrome.

Although there are no laboratory findings that specifically identify intellectual disability, there are multiple causes (including metabolic disturbances, toxin exposure, and chromosomal abnormalities) of intellectual disability that can be identified via laboratory analysis.[17] If a patient with a diagnosis of an intellectual disability has never had a chromosomal

whose functional level and family support system have allowed them to live and work in society without the need for services or supervision. Psychiatrists should be aware of the general cognitive level of their patients and assess how cognitive ability may affect their clinical presentation, as well as their compliance and response to treatment.

Table 20-1 presents a classification system (based on severity) for intellectual disability along with estimates of associated IQ ranges and approximate prevalence rates within the intellectually disabled population.[2,3,13,14] DSM-5 has attempted to elaborate these categories to help the psychiatrist better appreciate a given individual's capabilities in conceptual, social, and practical domains of adaptive function.[1] These categories of severity should be used by the psychiatrist to get an approximation of how an individual with such an IQ might be expected to present. The overwhelming majority of

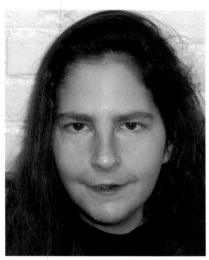

Figure 20-4. Image of an individual with Prader–Willi syndrome.

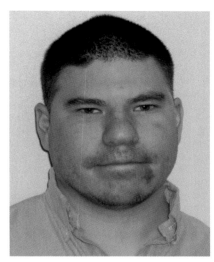

Figure 20-6. Image of an individual with 22q11 deletion syndrome.

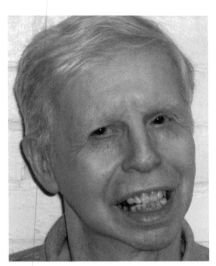

Figure 20-5. Image of an individual with Williams syndrome.

analysis, a genetics consultation is recommended. This can sometimes shed light on a previously unidentified syndrome in an adult patient that may then help to make a psychiatric diagnosis or to inform family members of potential medical issues that require monitoring. In addition, a genetics consultation can educate the psychiatrist about dysmorphic features in a patient with a given syndrome. The psychiatrist can then use this information to help identify other patients in the future. Figures 20-1 to 20-6 show individuals with some of the more commonly presenting syndromes.

The differential diagnosis for intellectual disability includes specific learning disorders, communication disorders, and neurocognitive disorders. Physical disabilities must also be considered in the differential. The presence of a physical disability should not be equated with a cognitive deficiency. Autistic spectrum disorder is considered in the differential diagnosis, but is a separate diagnostic category. However, approximately 50% of individuals with autistic spectrum disorder also have an intellectual disability but this can vary depending on the type of testing used and when in the course of development testing was done.

TREATMENT CONSIDERATIONS
Overview

Once the psychiatrist has determined that the diagnosis of intellectual disability is accurate, that the work-up is complete, and that there are no underlying medical or neurological issues affecting behavior, the patient should be assessed for behavioral or psychiatric disorders that may impact adaptive function.[19,20] The psychiatrist should begin with a basic understanding of the patient's developmental level and how this might affect the expression of psychiatric symptoms. As previously stated, the full range of psychopathology is seen in the intellectually-disabled population. In addition there are unique behavioral disorders and pathobehavioral syndromes or behavioral phenotypes to consider.[18]

The next step in the assessment of an individual with an intellectual disability involves a functional behavioral assessment that seeks to determine if the patient's behavior is "functional" in nature, that is, whether the behavior serves a purpose for the individual (not always with direct conscious awareness), such that it is reinforced and continues.[19,20] Examples include self-injury for the communication of pain, discomfort, or dislike; agitation or loud vocalizations to gain attention of staff or parents; or aggression to "get out of doing something" (i.e., escape-avoidance behavior). In each case, the observed behavior is not part of an underlying psychiatric disorder *per se*, yet it serves a purpose. If functional behavior is suspected, a referral to a certified behavior analyst should then be initiated before further assessment or treatment.

A functional behavior assessment may lead the patient back to the psychiatrist. The behavior analyst may suspect that an underlying psychiatric condition may be driving functional behavior. Examples include depression leading to a desire for increased isolation and subsequent antisocial behavior that accomplishes this goal; increased irritability (related to a mood disorder) that makes previously tolerated stimulating environments now intolerable; or the presence of a paranoid delusion that leads to aggressive behavior out of fear of harm.

Behavioral Disorders

Once a behavior appears to lack an obvious functional utility and cannot be related to an underlying medical or psychiatric condition, it falls in the realm of a behavioral disorder. Non-specific behavioral disorders (such as aggression and self-injury), as well as more specific disorders (such as stereotypy, pica, copraxia, and rumination), occur in the intellectually-disabled population.

Aggressive behavior is the main reason for psychiatric consultation and for institutionalization in the intellectually-disabled population. Once a thorough assessment has been completed and no clear etiology found, the problem falls into the realm of an impulse-control disorder. Behavioral treatment is usually the first-line treatment. Subsequent psychopharmacological interventions can be attempted if behavioral treatment proves inadequate. Typically, agents used to treat impulsive aggression are tried; these include alpha-agonists, beta-blockers, lithium, other mood stabilizers/anti-epileptic drugs, and antipsychotics.[18,19]

Self-injurious behavior (SIB) refers to behavior that potentially or actually causes physical damage to an individual's body. This should not be confused with self-mutilation or para-suicidal behavior that is more obviously volitional and seen in individuals with personality disorders. SIB in the intellectually-disabled population usually manifests as idiosyncratic, repetitive acts that occur in a stereotypic form. Behavioral therapy is the first-line treatment. Subsequent treatment includes use of selective serotonin reuptake inhibitors (SSRIs) (due to the apparent compulsive nature of the behavior) and neuroleptics in severe and refractory cases.[21,22]

Stereotypy, given the repetitive nature of the behavior, is sometimes related to SIB. Stereotypies are invariant, pathological motor behaviors or action sequences without obvious reinforcement. They often cause no real harm or dysfunction, but may be upsetting to caregivers or staff who may believe that they interfere with the patient's quality of life. These behaviors are often seen in institutionalized adults with severe to profound intellectual disability; however, they can also be seen as a normal variant in children without cognitive delay. These behaviors are often seen in circumstances of extreme stimulation or deprivation. First-line treatment for these stereotypies is behavioral. It is up to the patient or to the patient's guardian (in conjunction with the psychiatrist) to determine whether to engage in more aggressive medication treatments based on the level of dysfunction these behaviors represent. SSRIs should be considered for the initial psychopharmacological treatment because of the compulsive nature of these behaviors.[10,11,21,22]

Pica involves the eating of inedibles (including dirt, paper clips, and cigarette butts). Although usually seen in those with more severe intellectual disability, this behavior also can be seen as a normal variant in regularly-developing children. One must be aware of the potential medical hazards of ingested items; fortunately, major medical sequelae from this behavior are usually rare. Behavioral therapy (such as environmental control with limited access to preferred items and response-blocking) are the mainstays of treatment. There is minimal evidence that psychopharmacological treatments are useful, and dietary supplements have not been shown to be effective.

Copraxia involves rectal digging, feces smearing, and coprophagia. It is a rare disorder usually seen in the profoundly intellectually disabled. Once medical issues are ruled out, sensory issues can be assessed by a trained occupational therapist. Application of appropriate substitute materials can sometimes be helpful. Behavioral therapy again is a first-line treatment. Despite treatment, if the behavior persists, a compulsive or psychotic component should be considered.

Rumination refers to repeated acts of vomiting, chewing, and re-ingestion of the vomitus. It is seen in those with severe to profound intellectual disability, and it can be associated with both gastrointestinal pathology and with behavioral issues (e.g., over-feeding). Self-stimulation also must be considered, as this behavior has been seen in cases of severe sensory deprivation. Conversely, over-stimulation (with anxiety) has also been associated with this behavior. Once gastrointestinal issues are ruled out, behavioral therapy is the mainstay of treatment. If behavioral or gastrointestinal interventions are less than successful, treatment of rumination with medication (as if it were a compulsive behavior or an anxiety disorder) could be attempted; however, it should be viewed as an empiric trial.

Traditional Psychiatric Disorders

Presentations in those with intellectual disability can vary (given the decreased ability to self-report and actions that often replace words) from classic descriptions of syndromes. Conversely, individuals with intellectual disability who can provide self-reports are often motivated to be liked; they will often tell the psychiatrist what they think he or she wishes to hear. Given these limitations, the psychiatrist must rely more on ancillary sources of information; to this end the treater must help the patient, the parents, and the caregivers to structure their reporting in such a way that data are recorded and presented in as objective a way as possible. Too often data are collected unsystematically; this leaves the psychiatrist in the difficult position of gathering information from a limited number of subjective accounts. It then becomes extremely difficult to assess accurately a clinical situation or the efficacy of various interventions. This leads to less than optimal care for the patient, and to liability issues for the psychiatrist (as clinical decisions are based on less-than-accurate information).

Affective disorders are good examples where objective reporting of symptoms are necessary. Given the limitations of self-reporting for many patients with intellectual disability, the psychiatrist should initiate his or her assessment by documentation of observable mood and behavior changes from the patient's previous baseline. Mood charts kept by parents or by other caregivers are extremely useful in this regard, especially if a cyclical mood disorder is suspected. Sometimes it is only through observation of the long-term course and longitudinal care that a more definitive diagnosis will be possible. In addition, quantifiable measures (such as sleep logs, calorie counts, and weekly weights) of neurovegetative symptoms can aid in diagnosis. If behavioral changes are the primary presenting problem and there are no other clear symptoms or a family history that might clarify a diagnosis of a mood disorder, reliance on prevalence data of psychiatric disorders may be the psychiatrist's last hope. He or she may need to initiate an empiric treatment for those disorders that are more common (such as depression or anxiety).

Treatment may involve both talking therapies and medication. The type of therapy recommended should be based on the patient's strengths and developmental level and should be carried out by a therapist who has experience with the intellectually disabled. Therapy options run the gamut from grief work (especially around transitional times in development), to more concrete cognitive-behavioral therapy (CBT) coping strategies, to non-verbal techniques (such as art, music, or play therapy). Use of medications in intellectually disabled patients is the same as it is in the general population. However, in this already compromised population, whenever possible, more potent anticholinergic medications should be avoided to lessen the risk of cognitive blunting.

Anxiety disorders are common in the intellectually disabled, and observable signs and symptoms of anxiety are often more helpful than are self-reports of anxiety. Those anxiety disorders that manifest with more somatically-based symptoms are easier to diagnose, as staff can measure symptoms (such as elevated pulse and blood pressure in panic disorder), whereas chronic worry (in generalized anxiety disorder [GAD]) may be harder to measure. Anxiety rating scales, both verbal and non-verbal, can be very useful.

Anxiety issues around transitions (daily transitions and around life stages) are commonly seen. The possibility of trauma and related post-traumatic stress must always be considered, especially if there is an acute change from baseline. The intellectually disabled are a vulnerable population that is frequently exploited. Obsessive-compulsive disorder (OCD) can be difficult to distinguish from stereotypy. This is due to the difficulty eliciting self-reported ego-dystonic feelings around the behavior in question. Often, however, if a response-blocking intervention is attempted, individuals with OCD may have increased anxiety, whereas individuals with stereotypy do not. Treatment options for anxiety disorders include relaxation training and other behavioral therapy techniques. Sensory integration interventions can be tried under the guidance of a qualified occupational therapist. A variety of approved psychotropics (including benzodiazepines) should be considered for the relief of anxiety.[10,21,22]

Psychotic disorders, including schizophrenia, have been noted in the intellectually disabled since the days of Kraepelin and Bleuler. However, making an accurate diagnosis remains a challenge. Diminished and, at times, confabulatory self-reporting makes it difficult to establish accurate symptoms. In addition, talking to oneself, not related to psychosis, is observed in many individuals with intellectual disabilities, especially those with Down syndrome. Finally, given the spectrum of psychological development seen in the population, some adults may be developmentally closer to pre-schoolers than to their chronological age. Having an imaginary friend and talking to a stuffed animal would not be considered psychotic behavior in a pre-schooler, but this behavior may be misinterpreted in an adult with intellectual disability when his or her level of psychological/emotional development is not taken into consideration. In making a diagnosis of a psychotic disorder, noting an observable change from one's baseline level of function (e.g., changes in one's level of organization, activities of daily living [ADLs], and patterns of interaction with peers and staff) is key. At times there can be observable signs of responding to internal stimuli, but these should be witnessed across multiple settings. Particularly bizarre behavior is noteworthy, yet it should be considered relative to the patient's history and developmental level (with the knowledge of behaviors unique to this population). In addition, knowledge of the onset and longitudinal course of the illness (e.g., schizophrenia being more likely to manifest in younger age ranges) is useful. Obviously, family history also can provide helpful information. Treatment consists of antipsychotics, both first and second generation. It is not clear if extrapyramidal symptoms are more common in the intellectually-disabled population. However, monitoring for the presence of medication-induced movement disorders, including akathisia, should be done routinely. Target symptoms of psychosis should be clarified as much as possible so that clear outcome measures are available to monitor and assess the efficacy of medication interventions.

Other types of psychiatric disorders occur in the intellectually disabled. Substance-related disorders and personality disorders present particular challenges, as they do in the general population. These disorders usually occur in higher-functioning individuals, and their treatment (e.g., 12-step groups and more cognitive-behavioral interventions, such as modified dialectical behavior therapy [DBT] programs) is similar to that in the general population. Treatment for all other diagnostic categories depends on the psychiatrist's assessment of the patient's ability to participate in standard-of-care treatment. Adaptation of the standard of care requires experience working with the population and with teams that can individualize treatment as necessary. Target behaviors for treatment should be identified and quantified to the extent possible, so that the psychiatrist can better assess all interventions.

Syndrome-associated Disorders

Syndrome-associated disorders are specific psychiatric or behavioral disorders (e.g., self-injury and Lesch-Nyhan syndrome or dementia of the Alzheimer's type and Down syndrome) that appear to have a higher probability of occurring in individuals with a diagnosed syndrome. *Pathobehavioral syndromes* and *behavioral phenotypes*[18] are other terms that have been used to conceptualize this phenomenon. Several common syndromes are encountered in clinical practice; their salient features are provided below.

Individuals with Down syndrome (see Figure 20-1) or trisomy 21 have the classic physical features of round face, a flat nasal bridge, and short stature. Their level of intellectual disability is variable.[23] Depression is a common psychiatric co-morbidity, but perhaps better known is dementia of the Alzheimer's type.[17] However, symptoms of dementia often occur in the patient's forties and fifties. Symptomatic treatment for the accompanying behaviors can be helpful, but it is still unclear what role treatment (e.g., with anticholinesterase inhibitors or NMDA receptor antagonists) of the underlying dementia plays. Standard treatments often seek to preserve autonomous and independent function and to delay institutional placement, issues that may already have been addressed due to the patient's baseline cognitive function. Thus, the risk/benefit ratio for the treatment of the underlying dementia and the clarity of outcome measures may be less well defined for this population and should be discussed in detail with a guardian or family member prior to potential treatment.

Individuals with fragile X syndrome (see Figure 20-2) have an abnormality on the long arm of the X chromosome at the q27 site (*FMR1* gene) which leads to a trinucleotide repeat expansion. Common physical features include an elongated face, prominent ears, and macro-orchidism. The majority of affected individuals are males, but females can also be affected. Level of intellectual disability varies.[23] Of note, a percentage of female carriers can also display cognitive disabilities. The most prominent co-morbidities are attention-deficit/hyperactivity disorder and social anxiety disorder.[17] In addition, autistic features have been noted in a large percentage of individuals with fragile X syndrome.

Individuals with the Prader–Willi syndrome (see Figure 20-4) typically have short stature, hypogonadism, and marked obesity with hyperphagia. In approximately 70% of cases the syndrome results from a chromosome 15 deletion. The level of intellectual disability can vary.[23] Although the patient can have stubbornness, cognitive rigidity, and rage, the most common psychiatric co-morbidity is OCD.[17] The level of insight with regard to the excessiveness of the obsessions or compulsions can vary, but there can be an ego-dystonic aspect and verbalizations for help.

Williams syndrome (see Figure 20-5) results from a deletion on chromosome 7. These individuals have elfin-like faces and a classic starburst (or stellate) pattern of the iris. They can have supravalvular aortic stenosis, as well as renal artery stenosis and hypertension. Their level of intellectual disability varies.[23] Behaviorally, they can be loquacious communicators, a phenomenon referred to as "cocktail party speech" (often attributable to a higher verbal than performance IQ). This can be clinically deceiving, as individuals with greater verbal skills can appear to have higher functioning than they actually have. Common co-morbidities include anxiety disorders (such as GAD) and depression.[17]

Twenty-two q-eleven (22q11) deletion syndrome (including velo-cardio-facial syndrome and DiGeorge syndrome) is an autosomal dominant condition manifested by a medical history of mid-line malformations (such as cleft palate, velopharyngeal insufficiency, and cardiac malformations [such as a ventricular septal defect]) (Figure 20-6). Patients have small stature, a prominent tubular nose with bulbous tip, and a squared nasal root. There is often a history of speech delay with hypernasal speech. Their level of cognitive impairment varies from learning disabilities and mild intellectual impairment to more severe levels of intellectual disability.[23] The reason 22q11 deletion syndrome is of interest to psychiatrists is its high co-morbidity with psychosis (prevalence rates of up to 30% have been reported).[24] It has been proposed as a genetic model for understanding schizophrenia and bipolar spectrum disorders.[24]

CONCLUSION

Assessment and treatment of individuals with intellectual disability and co-occurring psychiatric and behavioral disorders remains a challenge. Intellectual disability is a prevalent condition with multiple etiologies and a rate of co-occurring psychiatric and behavioral disorders that is higher than that seen in the general population. A basic knowledge of what defines intellectual disability and its appropriate evaluation is crucial to an understanding of a very complex and underserved population. Knowledge of behavioral disorders and certain pathobehavioral syndromes unique to the population, along with an appreciation for individual differences in both developmental level and in psychiatric symptom presentation, can also help in the assessment of a given clinical situation. A psychiatrist must use his or her medical knowledge to rule out causal or contributing physical factors for a given behavior or disorder, as well as his or her understanding of the possible functional aspect that any behavior may provide. An understanding of the need for objective measures of both symptoms and outcomes in a population that cannot always speak for itself is crucial if quality care is to be delivered. Longitudinal care should be the rule, not the exception, as it is often only over time and in the context of a long-term relationship that improved understanding of the behavior occurs. In conclusion, working with intellectually disabled patients requires that the psychiatrist rely on multiple skill sets and have an open reliance on members of the treatment team. Although the clinical care of the intellectually disabled can be humbling, it can also be a most rewarding experience.

Access a list of MCQs for this chapter at https://expertconsult.inkling.com

REFERENCES

1. American Psychiatric Association. *Diagnostic and statistical manual of mental disorders*, ed 5, Washington, DC, 2013, American Psychiatric Press.
2. King BH, Hodapp RM, Dykens EM. Mental retardation. In Sadock BJ, Sadock VA, editors: *Kaplan and Sadock's comprehensive textbook of psychiatry*, ed 7, vol. 2, Philadelphia, 2000, Lippincott Williams & Wilkins.
3. Curry C, Stevenson R, Aughton D, et al. Evaluation of mental retardation: recommendations of a consensus conference: American College of Medical Genetics. *Am J Med Genet* 72:468–477, 1997.
4. King BH, State MW, Shah B, et al. Mental retardation: a review of the past 10 years. Part I. *J Am Acad Child Adolesc Psychiatry* 36:1656–1663, 1997.
5. Nurnberger J, Berrettini W. Psychiatric genetics. In Ebert M, Loosen P, Nurcombe B, editors: *Current diagnosis and treatment in psychiatry*, New York, 2000, McGraw-Hill.
6. Volkmar FR, Dykens E. Mental retardation. In Lewis M, editor: *Child and adolescent psychiatry: a comprehensive textbook*, ed 3, Philadelphia, 2002, Lippincott Williams & Wilkins.
7. Bouras N, editor: *Psychiatric and behavioral disorders in developmental disabilities and mental retardation*, New York, 1999, Cambridge University Press.
8. Gualtieri CT. *Neuropsychiatry and behavioral pharmacology*, New York, 1990, Springer-Verlag.
9. Madrid AL, State MW, King BW. Pharmacologic management of psychiatric and behavioral symptoms in mental retardation. *Child Adolesc Psychiatr Clin N Am* 9(1):225–243, 2000.
10. AACAP official action. Summary of the practice parameters for the assessment and treatment of children, adolescents, and adults with mental retardation and co-morbid mental disorders. *J Am Acad Child Adolesc Psychiatry* 38(12, Suppl.):5s–31s, 1999.
11. State MW, King BH, Dykens E. Mental retardation: a review of the past 10 years. Part II. *J Am Acad Child Adolesc Psychiatry* 36:1664–1671, 1997.
12. Szymanski LS, Wilska M. Mental retardation. In Tasman A, Kay J, Lieberman JA, editors: *Psychiatry*, vol. 1, ed 2, West Sussex, England, 2003, John Wiley & Sons.
13. American Psychiatric Association. *Diagnostic and statistical manual of mental disorders*, ed 4, text revision, Washington, DC, 2000, American Psychiatric Press.
14. McLearen J, Bryson SE. Review of recent epidemiological studies of mental retardation: prevalence, associated disorders, and etiology. *Am J Ment Retard* 92(3):243–254, 1987.
15. Jacobson JW, Mulick JA, editors: *Manual of diagnosis and professional practice in mental retardation*, Washington, DC, 1996, American Psychological Association.
16. Luckasson R, Borthwick-Duffy S, Buntinx WH, et al. *Mental retardation: definition, classification, and systems of supports*, Washington, DC, 2002, American Association on Mental Retardation.
17. Volkmar FR, editor. Mental retardation. *Child Adolesc Psychiatr Clin N Am* 5(4), 1996.
18. Moldavsky M, Lev D, Lerman-Sagie T. Behavioral phenotypes of genetic syndromes: a reference guide for psychiatrists. *J Am Acad Child Adolesc Psychiatry* 40(7):749–761, 2001.
19. Paclawskyj TR, Kurtz PF, O'Connor JT. Functional assessment of problem behaviors in adults with mental retardation. *Behav Modif* 28(5):649–667, 2004.
20. Wieseler NA, Hanson RH, editors: *Challenging behavior of persons with mental health disorders and severe developmental disabilities*, Washington DC, 1999, American Association on Mental Retardation.
21. Matlon JL, Bamburg JW, Mayville EA, et al. Psychopharmacology and mental retardation: a 10-year review (1990–1999). *Res Develop Disabl* 21(4):263–296, 2000.
22. Reiss S, Aman MG, editors: *Psychotropic medication and developmental disabilities: the international consensus handbook*, 1998, Ohio State University Nisonger Center.
23. Jones KL. *Smith's recognizable patterns of human malformation*, ed 5, Philadelphia, 1997, WB Saunders.
24. Williams NM, Owen MJ. Genetic abnormalities of chromosome 22 and the development of psychosis. *Curr Psychiatry Rep* 4:176–182, 2004.

21   Mental Disorders Due to Another Medical Condition

BJ Beck, MSN, MD, and Kathryn J. Tompkins, MD

KEY POINTS

- Mental disorders due to another medical condition should be in the differential diagnosis for every psychiatric evaluation.

- A high degree of medical suspicion and familiarity with the categories of causative medical conditions will aid in the diagnosis.

- Psychiatric symptoms may precede, coincide with, or lag behind the physical manifestation of a medical condition.

- Psychiatric symptoms may resolve, lessen, or continue after appropriate treatment of the underlying medical cause, and they may require specific treatment.

- The course of some medical conditions may not be alterable, but rigorous treatment of psychiatric distress is part of palliation.

OVERVIEW

Mental disorders due to a general medical condition (DTGMC) were defined by the *Diagnostic and Statistical Manual of Mental Disorders, Fourth Edition* (DSM-IV) as psychiatric symptoms severe enough to merit treatment, and determined to be the direct, physiological effect of a (non-psychiatric) medical condition.[1] This conceptual language substituted for previously less useful, more dichotomous terms (e.g., organic versus functional) that minimized the psychosocial, environmental influences on physical symptoms and implied that psychiatric symptoms were without physiological cause. The *Diagnostic and Statistical Manual of Mental Disorders, Fifth Edition* (DSM-5)[2] attempts to further minimize this dualism, and it makes the organic nature of the brain and its symptomatic disorders and responses more explicit by changing the terminology to "Due to *Another* Medical Condition (DTAMC)."[3] The mental disorder must be deemed the direct pathophysiological consequence of the medical condition, and not merely co-existent, or an adjustment reaction to the psychosocial consequences of the medical condition. Symptoms that are present only during delirium (i.e., with fluctuations in the level of consciousness and cognitive deficits) are not considered DTAMC. Similarly, the presence of a neurocognitive disorder (NCD) (e.g., dementia with memory impairment, aphasia, apraxia, agnosia, or disturbance of executive function) takes precedence over a diagnosis of DTAMC. Symptoms that are clearly substance-induced (e.g., alcohol intoxication or withdrawal) do not meet criteria for DTAMC.[2]

DISORDERS

Because affective, behavioral, cognitive, and perceptual disturbances are indistinguishable by etiology, every psychiatric evaluation should include mental disorders DTAMC in the differential diagnosis. With this rationale, the individual disorders are listed in DSM-5 with phenotypically similar disorders. Box 21-1 lists the various disorders under the chapter titles in which they appear in DSM-5.

PSYCHIATRIC DIFFERENTIAL DIAGNOSIS
Primary Mental Disorders

The determination of direct physiological causality is a complex issue. Box 21-2 summarizes features that should raise the clinician's suspicion of medical causation of psychiatric symptoms. The onset of psychiatric symptoms that coincides with the onset (or increased severity) of the medical condition is suggestive, but correlation does not prove causation. Mental and other medical disorders may merely co-exist. The initial presentation of a medical condition may be psychiatric (e.g., depression that manifests before the diagnostic awareness of pancreatic carcinoma), or the psychiatric symptoms may be disproportionate to the medical severity (e.g., irritability in patients with negligible sensorimotor symptoms of multiple sclerosis [MS]). It also happens that psychiatric symptoms may occur long after the onset of medical illness (e.g., psychosis that develops after years of epilepsy). Psychiatric improvement that coincides with treatment of the medical condition supports a causal relationship, although psychiatric symptoms that do not clear with resolution of the medical condition do not rule out causation (e.g., depression that persists beyond normalization of hypothyroidism). There are also mental disorders DTAMC that respond to, and require, direct treatment (e.g., inter-ictal depression), which should not be interpreted as evidence of a primary mental disorder.

Psychiatric presentations uncharacteristic of primary mental disorders should raise the suspicion of a direct physiological effect of a medical condition. Features to consider include the age of onset (e.g., new-onset panic disorder in an elderly man), the usual time course (e.g., abrupt onset of depression), and exaggerated or unusual features of related symptoms (e.g., severe cognitive dysfunction with otherwise mild depressive symptoms). On the other hand, the typical features of a psychiatric syndrome support the likelihood that medical and mental disorders are co-morbid, but not causative. Such typical features include a history of similar episodes without the co-occurrence of the medical condition, as well as a family history of the mental disorder.

Scientific standards in medical literature have established probable medical causality for certain psychiatric symptoms

---

BOX 21-1 Mental Disorders DTAMC Listed by Chapter of DSM-5

SCHIZOPHRENIA SPECTRUM AND OTHER PSYCHOTIC DISORDERS
Psychotic Disorder DTAMC
Catatonia DTAMC

BIPOLAR AND RELATED DISORDERS
Bipolar and Related Disorder DTAMC

DEPRESSIVE DISORDERS
Depressive Disorder DTAMC

ANXIETY DISORDERS
Anxiety Disorder DTAMC

OBSESSIVE-COMPULSIVE AND RELATED DISORDERS
Obsessive-Compulsive and Related Disorder DTAMC

NEUROCOGNITIVE DISORDERS
Delirium DTAMC
Major Neurocognitive Disorder DTAMC
Mild Neurocognitive Disorder DTAMC

PERSONALITY DISORDERS
Personality Change DTAMC

OTHER MENTAL DISORDERS
Other Specified Mental Disorders DTAMC
Other Unspecified Mental Disorders DTAMC

DTAMC, Due to another medical condition.

BOX 21-2 Features Suggestive of Physiological Causation of Psychiatric Symptoms

- Onset of psychiatric symptoms that coincides with onset, or increased severity, of a medical condition
- Psychiatric symptoms that improve with treatment of medical condition
- Features of syndrome uncharacteristic of primary mental disorders
- Pathophysiological explanations for psychiatric symptoms that are based on the medical condition
- Rigorous scientific literature supports medical causality for psychiatric symptoms that are more prevalent in certain medical conditions than in appropriate control groups
- Historically-accepted connections (e.g., case reports and small case series)

BOX 21-3 Categories for Another Medical Condition

ANotherMEDICalCONDITion
Autoimmune
Nutritional deficit
Metabolic encephalopathy
Endocrine disorders
Demyelination
Immune
Convulsions
Cerebrovascular disease
Offensive toxins
Neoplasm
Degeneration
Infection
Trauma

---

clinicians should think in broad terms, and they should ask specifically about over-the-counter medications, herbal (natural or dietary) supplements, prescription medications (not necessarily prescribed for the patient), and alcohol and recreational (i.e., illegal) drugs. This detail should be routine in every evaluation, with the more selective use of blood or urine toxicology, as indicated. Symptoms may derive from substance use, intoxication, or withdrawal, and such mental symptoms may persist for several weeks after the patient's last use of the substance.[4] Substance-induced mental symptoms are not necessarily evidence of misuse or abuse. Some medications may cause symptoms when used in therapeutic doses. When such symptoms resemble concomitant disease symptoms (e.g., when a patient with systemic lupus erythematosus [SLE] develops mood lability and is on steroids), it is possible that the symptoms are both substance-induced and DTAMC, in which case the clinician should code both conditions.

The "unspecified" categories in DSM-5 are reserved for symptoms characteristic of the given mental disorder (e.g., unspecified depressive disorder, unspecified neurocognitive disorder) "that cause clinically-significant distress or impairment in social, occupational or other important areas of functioning predominate but do not meet the full criteria" for any of the disorders in the identified diagnostic class,[2] and where there is etiological uncertainty or insufficient information to make a more specific diagnosis.

Another Medical Condition

ANotherMEDICalCONDITion (Box 21-3) is a mnemonic for the wide range of medical conditions that may result in psychiatric syndromes.

Infectious Diseases

The increased prevalence of immune suppression (e.g., from acquired immunodeficiency syndrome [AIDS], or from therapeutic suppression in cancer treatment or organ transplantation) has been associated with a concomitant increase in the chronic meningitides and other central nervous system (CNS) infections.

Herpes Simplex Virus (Figure 21-1[5])

Herpes simplex virus (HSV) is the most frequent etiology of focal encephalopathy, and may cause either simple or complex partial seizures.[6] With a predilection for the temporal and inferomedial frontal lobes, as illustrated in Figure 21-2,[7] HSV is well known to cause gustatory or olfactory hallucinations,

that are more prevalent in certain medical conditions than the base rate experienced by an appropriate control group. There may also be a pathophysiological explanation for the psychiatric symptoms, based on the medical disorder, metabolic perturbation, or location of brain pathology (e.g., disinhibition or decreased executive function with frontal lobe damage). Such connections should be considered suggestive, but not definitive. Every patient's symptoms should be individually scrutinized. In the absence of large studies or historically-accepted connections, case studies or small series may support a causal relationship. While mildly helpful, these less stringent reports should be met with some skepticism.

Substance-induced Disorders

Many types of substances have the potential for use, misuse, or abuse. In considering the possible role of substances,

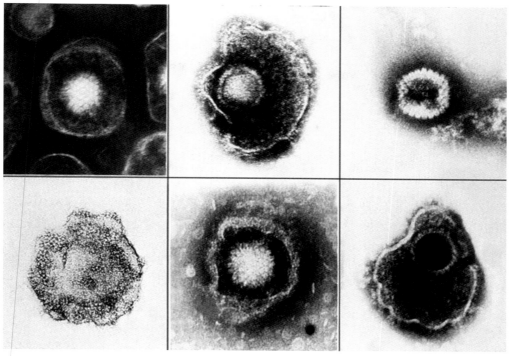

Figure 21-1. Electrograph of herpes simplex virus. *(Courtesy of the Center for Disease Control and Prevention/E.L. Palmer.)*

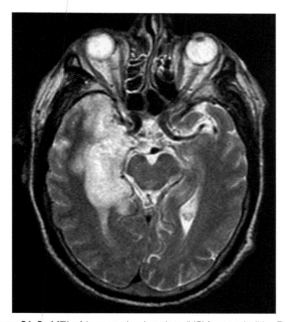

Figure 21-2. MRI of herpes simplex virus (HSV) encephalitis. Bright signal corresponds to active viral leptomeningeal and brain tissue infection of the patient's right medial temporal lobe. The temporal horn of the lateral ventricle is obliterated by hippocampal swelling. HSV tends to attack limbic structures responsible for the integration of emotion, memory, and complex behavior. *(From www.med.harvard .edu/AANLIB/cases/case25/mr1/012.html.)*

or anosmia (loss of the sense of smell).[8] This concentration in limbic structures may also explain the personality change, bizarre behavior, and psychotic symptoms that some affected patients exhibit. Such personality changes, cognitive difficulties, and affective lability may be persistent.[9] HSV-1 is responsible for most non-neonatal cases of HSV encephalitis, which does not appear to be more prevalent in the immunosuppressed population.[10] However, HSV-2, which more commonly causes aseptic meningitis in adults, can cause encephalitis during the course of disseminated disease in immunocompromised adults.[9]

Human Immunodeficiency Virus (Figure 21-3[11,12])

Patients with human immunodeficiency virus (HIV) infection experience a broad range of neuropsychiatric symptoms, collectively referred to as HIV-associated neurocognitive disorders (HAND).[13] For descriptive purposes, these disorders have been further broken down into three recognizable conditions: HIV-associated dementia (HAD); HIV-associated mild neurocognitive disorder (MND); and asymptomatic neurocognitive impairment (ANI).[13] Early cognitive and motor deficits involve attention, concentration, visuospatial performance, fine motor control, coordination, and speed.[14] The subcortical type of dementia, characterized by short-term memory problems, word-finding difficulty, and executive dysfunction, is now rare (2%) in the US.[15] Problems with sleep[16] and anxiety[17,18] are prevalent in the HIV-infected population. This is thought to be the result of wide-spread antiretroviral therapy, although some antiretrovirals have themselves been implicated as neurotoxins (e.g., efavirenz).[14] There may also be depressed mood[19] and an array of associated symptoms that resemble the neurovegetative symptoms of depression (e.g., apathy, fatigue, social withdrawal, and a lack of motivation or spontaneity). Mania and hypomania occur, though less frequently.[20] New-onset psychosis is uncommon and generally seen only

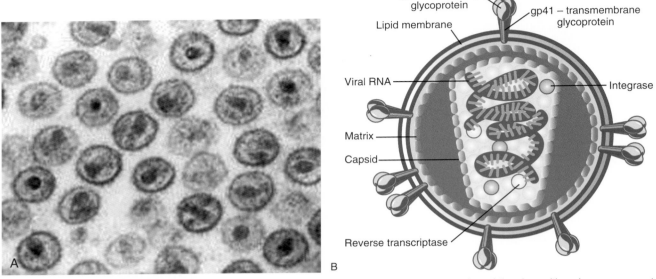

Figure 21-3. Human immunodeficiency virus (HIV). (A) Micrograph of HIV. (B) Schematic representation of the virus with various components labeled. *(A, Courtesy of the Center for Disease Control and Prevention/Dr. Edwin P. Ewing, Jr. B, From the National Institute of Allergy and Infectious Diseases, http://www.niaid.nih.gov/topics/HIVAIDS/Understanding/Biology/pages/structure.aspx.)*

in advanced stages of disease,[21] at which point patients may also develop seizures, agitation, severe disinhibition, and mutism.

The causes of HIV-related neuropsychiatric symptoms are as varied as the manifestations. Direct CNS infection, metabolic perturbations, endocrine abnormalities, malignancies, opportunistic infections, and the side effects of medications may all contribute. A consistent correlation has not been shown between the presence, severity, or location of CNS pathology and symptomatology.[22] New onset and a CD4 count of less than 600 increase the likelihood that psychiatric symptoms may be due to HIV infection (Figure 21-4),[23] or to some other (HIV-related) cause (i.e., not due to a primary mental disorder).[24]

Rabies

Generally transmitted by the infected saliva of an animal bite, rabies is a viral infection of the CNS in mammals. Human cases in the US are now so uncommon (one to two fatal cases per year since 1980[25]) that most occur after domesticated animal bites received during travel outside of this country. By the 1970s, endemic rabies sources in the US moved from domesticated animals (mostly dogs) to wild animals because of vaccination programs begun in the 1950s. While major wild reservoirs in the US are raccoons, foxes, skunks, and bats, variant bat rabies forms are now responsible for most fatal, indigenous human rabies cases.[26] This is significant because the variant forms may have a different course, require minimal inoculum, and cause infection in non-neural tissues. This results in a less classic, and thus unrecognized, presentation. In 2004, this difficulty in pre-morbid diagnosis became evident when four organ transplant recipients diagnosed with variant rabies encephalitis were traced back to single donor with a history of a bat bite.[27] Since more effective vaccines for post-exposure prophylaxis were introduced in 1979, there have been no deaths following their timely use.[28]

The average incubation time (for the more classic form of human rabies) is 4 to 8 weeks, but it is highly variable, with reports of periods as short as 10 days to as long as 1 year. The bite location, magnitude of the inoculum, and extent of host

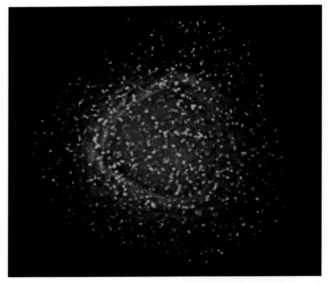

Figure 21-4. HIV infecting a cell. *(From Jouvenet N, Neil SJ, Bess C, et al. Plasma membrane is the site of productive HIV-1 particle assembly.* PLoS Biol *4(12):e435, 2006.)*

defenses are the likely determinants of the delay from contact to onset of symptoms, as the virus travels along peripheral nerves centripetally to the CNS.[29] This variable time course and presentation are summarized in Figure 21-5. Paresthesias or fasciculations at the bite location are characteristic aspects that distinguish rabies from viral syndromes with otherwise similar prodromes. Physical agitation and excitation give way to episodic confusion, psychosis, and combativeness. These episodes, possibly interspersed with lucid intervals, are the harbinger of acute encephalitis, brainstem dysfunction, and coma. Death generally occurs within 4 to 20 days. Autonomic dysfunction, cranial nerve involvement, upper motor neuron weakness and paralysis, and often vocal cord paralysis occur.

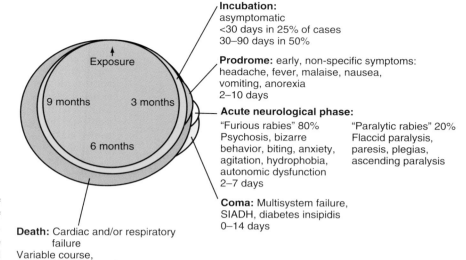

Incubation:
asymptomatic
<30 days in 25% of cases
30–90 days in 50%

Prodrome: early, non-specific symptoms:
headache, fever, malaise, nausea,
vomiting, anorexia
2–10 days

Acute neurological phase:

"Furious rabies" 80%	"Paralytic rabies" 20%
Psychosis, bizarre	Flaccid paralysis,
behavior, biting, anxiety,	paresis, plegias,
agitation, hydrophobia,	ascending paralysis
autonomic dysfunction	
2–7 days	

Coma: Multisystem failure,
SIADH, diabetes insipidis
0–14 days

Death: Cardiac and/or respiratory
        failure
Variable course,
            or
Recovery: Exceedingly rare

Figure 21-5. Time course progression of rabies infection. Bite location, magnitude of exposure, and degree of host defenses contribute to the highly variable time course as the virus travels along peripheral nerves toward the central nervous system. SIADH, Syndrome of inappropriate antidiuretic hormone.

Approximately half of rabies-infected humans experience the classic "hydrophobia"[29] (i.e., violent and severely painful spasms of the diaphragm, laryngeal, pharyngeal, and accessory respiratory muscles, triggered by attempts to swallow liquids).

Lyme Disease

Borrelia burgdorferi is the tick-borne (specifically, *Ixodes scapularis*–borne [Figure 21-6[30]]) spirochete responsible for Lyme disease, most commonly seen in the US (northeast, upper midwest, and [to a lesser extent] Pacific coastal states[31]), as well as parts of Europe. The neuropsychiatric sequelae of Lyme disease require clinicians in all areas to have a raised level of consciousness and suspicion because the symptoms are non-specific, highly variable, often delayed, and recurrent.[32] Even when suspected, the diagnosis is difficult because of the confusing array of unreliable serologic tests (e.g., Lyme enzyme-linked immunosorbent assay [ELISA], Lyme Western blot, polymerase chain reaction [PCR] assay, or culture).[33]

After the offending tick bite, ticks must stay attached for close to 36 hours to transmit the spirochete.[34] Patients may experience a mild, flu-like syndrome, and some develop a characteristic rash (erythema migrans, shown in Figure 21-7[35]), most frequently (75%–80% of US cases with rash) a single lesion surrounding the bite. However, a more disseminated rash is thought to correspond to hematogenous spread that occurs over several days to weeks. The target sites for the spirochete include the heart, eyes, joints, muscles, peripheral nervous system, or CNS, where it may lie dormant for so long (e.g., months to years) that memory of the initial bite has long since faded.[33,36] Rapid diagnosis and aggressive antibiotic treatment are the preferred course, but some patients may still experience the onset or recurrence of symptoms months to years later.[33] Controversy exists as to whether this truly constitutes a "chronic Lyme" syndrome. Some researchers believe other psychiatric conditions or "chronic multi-system illness" better accounts for these prolonged symptomatic presentations,[37,38] while others point to similarities in the science behind other chronic spirochetal syndromes (e.g. neurosyphilis) as evidentiary support.[39]

Fatigue, irritability, confusion, labile mood, and disturbed sleep may herald Lyme encephalitis. The much less common presentation of Lyme encephalomyelitis may be confused with

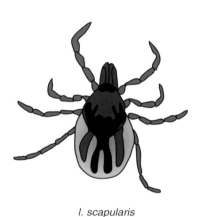

I. scapularis

Unengorged   Engorged

I. scapularis nymph

Figure 21-6. *Ixodes scapularis:* tick that causes Lyme disease. The deer tick life cycle, from egg to adult to egg, is 2 years; that accounts for the year-round presence of ticks. *(Redrawn from Haynes EB, Piesman J: How can we prevent Lyme disease?* N Engl J Med 348:2424–2430, 2003.)

multiple sclerosis. Some patients go on to develop chronic encephalopathy,[33] a broad scope of persistent disturbances in personality, behavior (e.g., disorganized, distractible, catatonic, mute, or violent), cognition (e.g., short-term memory, memory retrieval, verbal fluency, concentration, attention, orientation, and processing speed), mood (e.g., depressed, manic, or labile), and thought or perception (e.g., paranoia, hallucinations, depersonalization, hyperacusis, or photophobia). Although extremely rare, more severe sequelae may include dementia, seizures, or stroke.[36]

Neurosyphilis

Historically, less than 10% of patients with untreated syphilis develop a symptomatic form of parenchymatous neurosyphilis known as general paresis, 10 to 20 years after their initial infection.[40] After the advent of penicillin, but before the onset of AIDS, neurosyphilis was even less prevalent. Now, there is a resurgence of a less classic form of neurosyphilis, as the use of antibiotics has altered the characteristic features.[40] This more subtle presentation may be especially difficult to recognize by the generation of clinicians raised and educated in the relative absence of the disease. The signs and symptoms listed in Box 21-4, with the mnemonic PARESIS,[41] suggest the frontal

and more diffuse nature of the syndrome associated with the diffuse frontal and temporal lobe findings seen on imaging studies (Figure 21-8[42]). Personality change may be striking, and can involve apathy, poor judgment, lack of insight, irritability, and (new onset of) poor personal hygiene and grooming. Patients may also have difficulty with calculations and short-term memory. Later signs include mood lability, delusions of grandeur, hallucinations, disorientation, and dementia.[43] It is during this late stage that the classic neurological signs may appear (e.g., tremor, dysarthria, hyperreflexia, hypotonia, ataxia, and Argyll Robertson pupils [small, irregular, unequal pupils able to accommodate, but not react to light]).

The diagnostic paradigm has been to use non-treponemal serologic tests for screening (e.g., the rapid plasma reagin [RPR]) confirmed by cerebrospinal fluid (CSF) with elevated protein and lymphocytes and a positive (CSF) Venereal Disease Research Laboratory (VDRL) slide test for treponemal antibodies.[44] However, sensitive and specific treponemal serologic tests are becoming available for screening. Because they cannot distinguish between recent or remote infection, or between treated or untreated infection, they must be confirmed with non-treponemal tests, a pattern reversal, or diagnostic paradigm shift.[45]

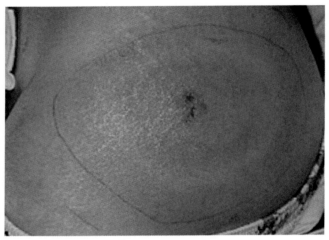

Figure 21-7. Typical erythema migrans rash in a patient with Lyme disease. *(From DePietropaolo DL, Powers JH, Gill JM, Foy AJ. Diagnosis of Lyme disease, Am Fam Physician 72:297–304, 2005, Figure 2.)*

BOX 21-4 Manifestations of General Paresis

PARESIS
- Personality
- Affect
- Reflexes (hyperactive)
- Eye (Argyll Robertson pupils)
- Sensorium (illusions, delusions, hallucinations)
- Intellect (decreased recent memory, orientation, calculation, judgment, and insight)
- Speech

From Lukehart SA, Holmes KK. Syphilis. In Fauci AS, Braunwald E, Isselbacher KJ, et al., editors: Harrison's principles of internal medicine, ed 14, New York, 1998, McGraw-Hill.

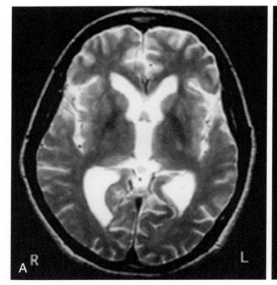
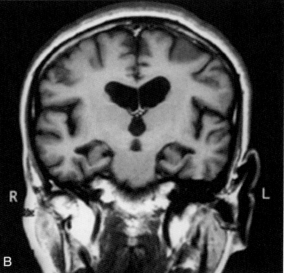

Figure 21-8. Non-specific MRI findings in general paresis. (A) Axial T$_2$-weighted image shows primarily frontal atrophy and dilated third and lateral ventricles. (B) Coronal T$_1$-weighted image demonstrates bilateral medial temporal lobe and hippocampal atrophy. *(From Kodama K, Okada S, Komatsu N, et al. Relationship between MRI findings and prognosis for patients with general paresis, J Neuropsychiatry Clin Neurosci 12:246–250, 2000, Figure 2.)*

TABLE 21-1 Common CSF Findings in Different Types of Meningitis

Condition	Pressure (mm/H₂O)	Cells/μl	Predominant Cell Type	Glucose (mg/dl)	Protein (mg/dl)	Examples	Microbiology
Normal	80–200	0–5	Lymphs	50–75	15–40	—	—
Purulent	200–300	100–5,000	> 80% PMNs	< 40	> 100	Acute bacterial, fulminant fungal, fulminant amebic meningoencephalitis	Specific pathologic bacterium identified in 60% of Gram stains, 80% of cultures
Aseptic	N or ↑	10–300	Lymphs (sometimes some PMNs)	N (Reduced in LCM and mumps))	N or ↑ (< 100)	Infectious: bacterial, partially-treated bacterial, viral, post-infectious, fungi, early listerial Non-infectious: drugs, meningeal disease, parameningeal disease, neoplasm, reaction to intrathecal injections, vaccine reactions	Viral Isolation, PCR assays Negative findings on work-up
Chronic	N or ↑ (180–300)	10–500	Lymphs	↓ < 40	↑ or ↑↑ 50–200	TB, atypical tuberculi, cryptococci, coccidioides, other fungi, sarcoidosis, Lyme disease, syphilis, cysticercosis, tumor	Acid-fast bacillus stain, culture, PCR, India Ink, cryptococcal antigen, culture

Adapted from Medscape: *http://emedicine.medscape.com/article/232915-differential, accessed on 9/21/2013.*
CSF, Cerebrospinal fluid; Lymphs, lymphocytes; N, normal; PMNs, polymorphonuclear lymphocytes; LCM, lymphocytic choriomeningitis, TB, tuberculosis; ↑, increased; ↑↑, greatly increased; ↓, decreased.

Chronic Meningitis

Although *Mycobacterium tuberculosis* is the most common cause, the fungal pathogens *Cryptococcus* and *Coccidioides* (and others endemic to specific localities) may also produce this subtle, non-specific syndrome,[46] which may be ascribed to a primary, predisposing illness, such as AIDS. The old, young, homeless, and alcoholic are also at increased risk. The chronic meningitides are treatable if recognized, but they often go undetected because they cause minimal signs (e.g., low-grade fever) and symptoms (e.g., mild headache), particularly in immunocompromised patients. The equally non-specific neuropsychiatric manifestations include confusion and problems of behavior, cognition, and memory. Characteristic CSF findings, summarized in Table 21-1,[47] include a primarily lymphocytic pleocytosis with decreased glucose and elevated protein.

Chronic, Persistent Viral or Prion Diseases

These CNS infections are exceedingly rare and invariably fatal within months to years of onset of symptoms. Even though the psychiatric symptoms may precede the severe neurological manifestations, the course is so acutely devastating as to preclude misattribution as a primary mental disorder. For completeness, this brief overview provides the clinician a passing familiarity with these historically more important entities.

Subacute sclerosing panencephalitis (SSPE) is a disease primarily of children and adolescents (usually less than age 11), in boys about twice as often as girls, after previous measles (rubeola) infection, with early primary infection (especially before age 2) posing a significantly greater risk.[48] Previously thought to occur, though rarely, after measles vaccination,[49] the vaccination is now known to be protective, and not causative, in children not already infected with the etiologic mutated measles virus (i.e., the SSPE virus).[48] Since the advent of more pervasive vaccination, the incidence of SSPE has progressively decreased. The initial manifestations, which may occur 2–10 years after the primary measles infection (mean time is 6 years[50]), may be mistaken for behavioral problems, with worsening school performance, distractibility, oppositional behavior, or temper tantrums. Ocular changes and visual symptoms

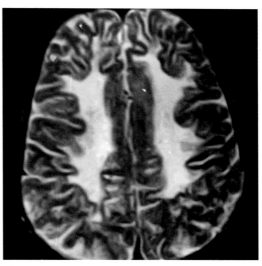

Figure 21-9. Diffuse MRI findings in subacute sclerosing panencephalitis (SSPE). T₂-weighted MRI of a child's brain with SSPE demonstrates diffuse demyelination of the white matter. *(From Garg RK. Subacute sclerosing panencephalitis, Postgrad Med J 78:63–70, 2002, Figure 2.)*

(e.g., cortical blindness) occur in about half of cases, with destructive involvement of the retina, optic nerve, and the visual cortex. Early imaging of the brain may be normal,[48] followed by obliterated sulci and small ventricles from cerebral edema, then T₂-weighted hyperintensity predominantly in the occipital lobe and subcortical white matter with relative frontal sparing, as seen in Figure 21-9.[49] Within a few months, affected children may experience myoclonic jerks, ataxia, seizures, and further intellectual decline. A characteristic electroencephalograph (EEG) pattern, which corresponds to the myoclonic jerks,[51] consists of bilateral, symmetric, high-voltage, synchronous bursts of polyphasic, stereotyped delta waves (Figure 21-10[49]). By 6 months most patients are bedridden, followed by death within 1–3 years. Despite some meager

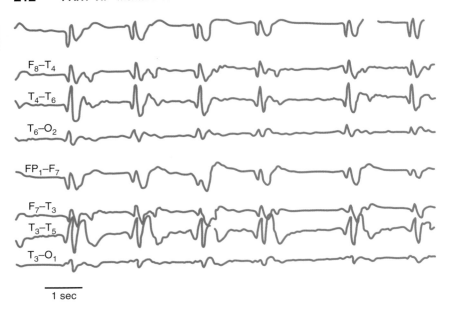

$F_8–T_4$

$T_4–T_6$

$T_6–O_2$

$FP_1–F_7$

$F_7–T_3$

$T_3–T_5$

$T_3–O_1$

1 sec

Figure 21-10. Characteristic EEG tracing in subacute sclerosing panencephalitis (SSPE). EEG demonstrates 4- to 6-second recurrences of slow-wave complexes, identical in all leads, as is common in SSPE. *(From Garg RK. Subacute sclerosing panencephalitis*, Postgrad Med J *78:63–70, 2002, Figure 1.)*

response to trials of intrathecal interferon-alpha and isoprinosine, SSPE remains highly lethal, with a reported spontaneous remission rate of 5%.[50]

Creutzfeldt-Jakob disease (CJD), in contrast, is a disease primarily of 55–75 year olds. This rapidly progressive and fatal prion disease is exceedingly rare, with most cases thought to be sporadic (sCJD). Approximately 5% to 15% appear to be familial, or genetic (gCJD).[52] Iatrogenic, person-to-person infection (iCJD) has also occurred following therapeutic use of cadaveric human growth hormone, dura mater grafts, and, in less significant numbers, corneal transplantation, cadaveric gonadotropins, and surgical instrument contamination. A variant form of CJD (vCJD), caused by infection with the etiological prion of bovine spongiform encephalopathy (BSE; also known as "mad cow disease"), tends to affect younger adults and is also implicated in person-to-person infection through blood product transfusion.[53] The initial non-specific symptoms of CJD include problems of cognition (memory or judgment), mood (lability), perception (illusions or distortions), or sensorimotor function (ataxic gait, vertigo, or dizziness). In vCJD, the early symptoms are more prominently psychiatric, behavioral, or both.[54] More ominous signs of psychosis and confusion herald the dementia and myoclonus considered the hallmarks of CJD. Patients generally die within a year, becoming spastic, mute, and finally stuporous. Suggestive diagnostic findings late in the clinical course include cerebellar atrophy on head computed tomography (CT) scan and typical EEG changes (Figure 21-11[55]). Magnetic resonance imaging (MRI) has also been found to be a reasonably sensitive and highly specific diagnostic aid,[56] although finding 14-3-3 protein in the CSF may be the most discriminating evidence for the disease.[57]

Kuru, which translates as "to shiver with fear," was endemic among Papua New Guinea highlanders of a particular tribe who ate the brains of their dead ("transumption"). The incidence of kuru—a fatal, dementing, transmissible spongiform encephalitis (TSE) with progressive extrapyramidal signs—declined along with the incidence of ritual cannibalism.[58]

Epilepsy

Epilepsy affects approximately 2 million Americans, and has a life-time prevalence of 3%.[59] A prime example of the need

for healthy skepticism in the dichotomous view of functional versus organic epilepsy continues to beg the mind/brain question. This common neurological (i.e., brain) disorder is now attributed to indiscriminate, haphazard, electrical misfiring of impulses in the brain cortex. However, before the use of the EEG (Figure 21-12) could correlate these disorganized electrical episodes with the resultant (motor, affective, behavioral, cognitive, memory, or perceptual) phenomena, seizures were considered to be moral, emotional, or mental (i.e., mind) infirmities.[60,61] Seizure manifestations, including altered or loss of consciousness, correlate with the location of abnormal brain impulses, but these manifestations are the same, non-specific responses that occur in response to stimulation (in the same anatomic area) from any input source. While generalized tonic-clonic motor activity is a syndrome readily recognized as a seizure, seizure-induced fear, depression,[62] anxiety, or psychotic symptoms[63] are indistinguishable from those of primary mental disorders. The EEG may be suggestive of seizure, but the clinical diagnosis of seizures cannot be ruled out by the lack of EEG evidence[64] (Figure 21-13).

Although a number of detailed classification systems exist, and get revised with the advent of new technology or understanding, there remains more controversy than consensus.[65] Table 21-2 presents a simplified and useful framework for this discussion. Partial seizures have focal onset, but may secondarily generalize. They may, or may not, cause motor or autonomic signs, as well as somatosensory or psychic symptoms. Generalized seizures include absence seizures (which may or may not include motor signs), as well as the more readily recognized convulsive seizures.[66]

Complex Partial Seizures

A highly underdiagnosed condition, partial seizures are responsible for most of the non-convulsive seizures experienced by an estimated 60% of epileptics in the US.[67] These seizures, largely (62%) of unknown etiology,[68] often derive from deep, limbic brain structures, commonly the temporal lobe, where abnormal impulses do not transmit to the surface electrodes of the EEG in up to 40% of patients.[64,69] This is further support for seizures remaining a clinical diagnosis, inferred, but never dismissed, by EEG interpretation.

Patients with epilepsy come to psychiatric attention because they have a high prevalence of psychiatric symptoms that are

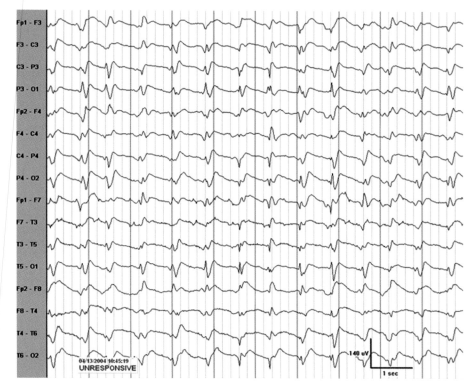

Figure 21-11. Typical EEG patterns in CJD. EEG tracing demonstrates generalized periodic triphasic sharp wave complexes (PSWC), at a rate of approximately 1 per second, typical findings late in the disease. *(From Weiser HG, Schindler K, Zumsteg D. EEG in Creutzfeldt-Jakob disease, Clin Neurophysiol 117:935–951, 2006.)*

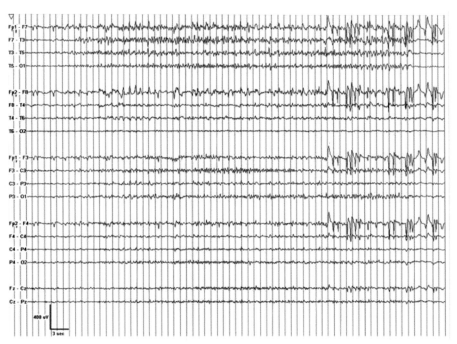

Figure 21-12. Scalp electrode EEG recording during left temporal lobe seizure. *(Courtesy of Sydney S. Cash, MD, PhD, Department of Neurology, Massachusetts General Hospital and Harvard Medical School.)*

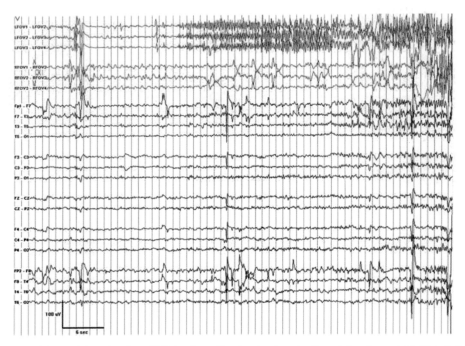

Figure 21-13. Simultaneous intracranial and surface EEG tracings. The top tracings (red) are taken from electrodes that have passed through the foramen ovale, where the onset of seizure activity in the left temporal lobe appears earlier and more dramatically than it does on the scalp electrode tracings. The surface tracings remain subtle until quite late in the seizure. *(Courtesy of Sydney S. Cash, MD, PhD, Department of Neurology, Massachusetts General Hospital and Harvard Medical School.)*

TABLE 21-2 Classification of Seizure Disorders

	Onset		Consciousness	
Term	**Focal**	**General**	**Unimpaired**	**Impaired**
Partial	X			
Simple	X		X	
Complex	X			X
Generalized		X		X

indistinguishable from those of primary mental disorders. Over half of epileptics experience depression, with higher rates for patients with complex partial seizures and those with seizure foci in the left hemisphere.[70] In contrast, the incidence of depression in matched medical and neurological control groups is only 30%. This implies that depression may be seizure-induced limbic dysfunction, and may also explain the fivefold increase in the suicide rate for epileptic patients as compared to those in the general public. Even when controlling for psychiatric disease, demographic and socioeconomic factors, epileptic patients were found to have a threefold higher rate of suicide.[71] That risk may be as much as 25 times higher for patients with temporal lobe epilepsy (TLE),[72] although this has not been consistently replicated.[73] Patients with partial seizures also experience more anxiety than those in the general public and in patients with other types of seizures.[63] In fact, partial seizures bear many of the hallmarks of panic attacks, and the two may be difficult to distinguish. Seizure-related panic may be peri-ictal (i.e., pre-ictal, ictal or post-ictal) or inter-ictal (i.e., between and independent of seizure activity). Panic attacks and seizure-related panic may occur "out of the blue," with hyperarousal, intense fear, perceptual distortion, and dissociative symptoms (e.g., depersonalization or derealization).[74] Hyperventilation, a common symptom of panic, also lowers the seizure threshold, and may appear to initiate

either event. Benzodiazepines may improve both conditions. There are features, however, that aid in the differentiation.[75] Although the fear of fainting is common in panic attacks, the actual loss or alteration of consciousness is much more common in partial seizures. Mild visual or auditory distortions may occur during panic attacks, but true hallucinations (especially olfactory or gustatory) are more suggestive of seizure activity. Similarly, automatisms (chewing or lip-smacking movements) and a confusional state after the episode strongly support a diagnosis of seizure. Another helpful difference is the vivid memory of the event in panic attacks, which leads to the "fear of fear" that is classic for panic disorder and predisposes to agoraphobia and avoidance. In contrast, following a seizure, patients often have lack of awareness or partial memory of the event, and rarely develop agoraphobia. The time course is generally more defined for panic, lasting 10 to 20 minutes, whereas ictal panic may last less than 30 seconds.[75] Complex partial seizures tend to begin with cognitive (e.g., *déjà vu, jamais vu,* or forced thinking), affective (e.g., fear, depression, or pleasure), or perceptual (e.g., illusions or olfactory or gustatory hallucinations) auras, then a brief cessation of activity, a minute or less of unresponsiveness and automatismic behavior, and, finally, a short (e.g., lasting seconds to half an hour) period of decreased or lack of awareness.

Psychotic symptoms are seen 6 to 12 times as often in epileptics than in the general population. These include, but are not limited to, the brief hallucinatory, affective, or cognitive auras, which are themselves the result of abnormal electrical impulses (i.e., seizure activity). Seizures may also be followed by post-ictal delirium of relatively short duration. However, after years of epilepsy, some patients develop an episodic or more chronic, unremitting psychosis with hallucinations, paranoia, and a circumstantial thought pattern[63] (rather than the common schizophrenic formal thought disorders of tangentiality, derailment, and thought-blocking). The epileptic's preserved affective warmth is in sharp contrast to the affective flattening more commonly seen in schizophrenia. This chronic psychosis, thought to be caused by sub-ictal, temporal lobe dysrhythmias, is often heralded by personality change and remits with relatively lower neuroleptic doses.[76] Inter-ictal personality traits commonly ascribed to TLE include obsessionality, dependence, hyperreligiosity, hypergraphia, hyposexuality, and humorlessness.[77] However, such traits remain unsubstantiated by research with structured, diagnostic instruments.[78] Less controversial is the recognized difficulty to disengage from the TLE patient's viscous, sticky, conversational style.

There are many explanations for violence, but in the rare event that it occurs during a seizure, it is never purposeful or organized, though occasionally reflexive or defensive.[79] There is controversy about a syndrome of episodic dyscontrol being more common in patients with early-onset temporal or frontal lobe epilepsy. However, such eruptions of uncontrollable rage, out of proportion to the minor infractions that set them off, are also more common in psychotic or traumatized patients, and those intellectually, educationally, socioeconomically, and psychosocially challenged. Most likely, when perpetrated by patients with epilepsy, such outbursts are the result of psychopathology (primary or inter-ictal) or brain pathology (e.g., brain injury that might also be the cause of seizures). Ictal events are, after all, the result of random firing, and not the root of focused, violent acts.

The neuropsychiatric presentation does not fully define the psychiatric challenge of epilepsy. The psychosocial consequences of living with a seizure disorder; the difficulty of substantiating partial seizures; the affective, cognitive, and physical side effects of common anti-seizure medications; and the seizure threshold-lowering effect of common psychiatric medications are among the clinical issues. The co-morbidity of seizures and inter-ictal mood symptoms does not confirm the diagnosis of mood disorder due to epilepsy, nor does that diagnosis negate the need to treat the mood disorder directly. Thus, when mood or other psychiatric syndromes seem atypical or recalcitrant to usual therapies, the lack of definitive confirmation of the clinical diagnosis of epilepsy should not dissuade the psychiatrist from starting a trial of an appropriate anti-seizure medication.

Nutritional Deficits

Given the highly processed and fortified nature of the American diet, nutritional deficits are relatively rare in this country, although they still occur in select populations. Table 21-3 summarizes the physical and neuropsychiatric manifestations of the more common deficiency states.

The physical, psychiatric, neurological, and behavioral consequences of pellagra are the result of niacin (nicotinic acid) deficiency and deficiency of the niacin precursor, tryptophan. When untreated, pellagra progresses to encephalopathy, peripheral neuropathy, diarrhea, and chronic wasting. Typical dermatological findings include angular stomatitis, glossitis, and, less often, a scaly, erythematous rash in sun-exposed skin areas ("Casal's necklace," see Figure 21-14).[80] However, the initial, non-specific manifestations (e.g., insomnia, fatigue, irritability, anxiety, and depressed mood) may be understandably misattributed to depression.[81] In the absence of niacin repletion, these progress to more ominous mental slowing, confusion, psychosis, and dementia. Leg weakness may follow as part of a spastic spinal syndrome that includes hyperreflexia, clonus, and extensor plantar responses. Rare in the US since cereal products have been niacin fortified,[82] pellagra still occurs in certain groups (e.g., alcoholics,[80] anorexics,[81] vegetarians in less developed countries, refugee populations, and recipients of bariatric surgery). Pellagrous delirium, with confusion and psychosis, is more common than frank dementia, and may be overlooked diagnostically in the setting of alcohol withdrawal.[80] Dementia is indicative of prolonged, severe deficiency, and it may not respond as quickly, or as completely, to niacin replacement as do other features.

TABLE 21-3 Clinical Manifestations of Vitamin Deficiency States

Vitamin	Deficiency State	Clinical Manifestations		Population at Risk
		Physical	*Neuropsychiatric*	
Niacin* (nicotinic acid)	Pellagra	Angular stomatitis, glossitis, rash in sun-exposed areas, peripheral neuropathy, diarrhea, chronic wasting, hyper-reflexia, clonus, extensor plantar response	Insomnia, fatigue, irritability, anxiety, depressed mood; if still untreated: mental slowing, confusion, psychosis, dementia	Alcoholics Refugees Vegetarians in less developed countries
Thiamine (vitamin B₁)	Wernicke-Korsakoff syndrome	Wernicke's encephalopathy: vomiting, horizontal nystagmus, ophthalmoplegia, fever, ataxia	Korsakoff's syndrome: retrograde amnesia, poor concentration, apathy, agitation, depressed mood, confusion, confabulation	Alcoholics (may be precipitated in asymptomatic alcoholics when glucose is administered before thiamine repletion)
	Beriberi	Cardiovascular (wet beriberi): tachycardia, high output, peripheral dilation, edema, biventricular failure Neurological (dry beriberi): peripheral neuropathy, weakness, ↓ deep tendon reflexes, sensory neuropathy	As above: poor memory and learning, apathy, confusion, confabulation	Victims of famine, or extreme poverty Patients with cancer, AIDS, hyperemesis Patients on dialysis
Cobalamin (vitamin B₁₂)	Megaloblastic anemia	↓ Position and vibratory sense, abnormal reflexes, sphincter dyscontrol, peripheral numbness and paresthesias	Apathy, irritability, depressed mood or mood lability; if prolonged and untreated: delirium (megaloblastic madness), hallucinations, paranoia, worsening cognition	Malabsorption Pernicious anemia S/p gastric bypass Inadequate intake Vegetarians

*And deficiency of the niacin precursor, tryptophan.
AIDS, Acquired immunodeficiency syndrome; S/p, status post.

In famine or extreme poverty, thiamine (vitamin B_1) deficiency causes beriberi, but in the US, the alcoholism-associated Wernicke-Korsakoff syndrome is more common. A sign of the twenty-first century may be the recent reports of etiologic starvation as a sequelae to bariatric surgery.[83-85] Prolonged malignancy[86] and hyperemesis gravidarum[87] have also (infrequently) caused the syndrome. Figure 21-15[88] demonstrates the MRI findings associated with Wernicke's encephalopathy. Factors such as total caloric intake, activity, and genetics[89] seem to mediate the presentation, because most with malnutrition or alcoholism do not exhibit symptoms. Although

single-system involvement occurs, most commonly a blend of cerebral, neuropathic, and cardiovascular signs and symptoms occurs. As with niacin deficiency, the initial symptoms tend to be non-specific (e.g., poor concentration, apathy, mild agitation, or depressed mood), but are followed by more disabling signs (e.g., confusion, amnesia, or confabulation) of prolonged, severe deficiency. Iatrogenic conversion of asymptomatic thiamine deficiency to Wernicke-Korsakoff syndrome has been reported when glucose is given before thiamine repletion.[90] However, an extensive recent literature review found no evidence above case report/series to support this long-held medical adage.[91] The authors conclude that prolonged glucose administration without thiamine repletion may be a risk factor, but that glucose administration in a hypoglycemic patient should not be delayed; thiamine may be co-administered, or given soon after the start of glucose replacement. The role of thiamine in glucose metabolism is shown in Figure 21-16.[92]

Megaloblastic macrocytic anemia, the hallmark of vitamin B_{12} (cobalamin) deficiency, is associated with neurodegenerative changes of the central and peripheral nervous systems, which manifest as decreased position and vibratory sensation, reflex abnormalities, sphincter dyscontrol, and peripheral neuropathy (e.g., numbness and paresthesias).[93] The result of malabsorption (e.g., from lack of intrinsic factor [pernicious anemia, Figure 21-17[94]], following gastric surgery, nitrous oxide, "whippit" abuse[95]) or inadequate intake (e.g., vegetarian diet), the initial, non-specific symptoms may be psychiatric (e.g., apathy, irritability, depression, or labile mood), rather than neurological or hematological. If untreated, more prolonged disease may manifest as the less frequent delirium syndrome (i.e., megaloblastic madness) of prominent hallucinations, paranoia, and worsening cognition. Early in the course, symptoms may be reversible with treatment.[96] However, more prolonged disease leads to demyelination, degenerative changes, and ultimately cell death that precludes full resolution of neurological manifestations.

Metabolic Encephalopathy

Acute changes in mental status (e.g., disorientation, disturbances of affect, behavior, cognition, or level of consciousness) are indicative of metabolic, rather than primary psychiatric, disturbances. Agitated delirium and marked

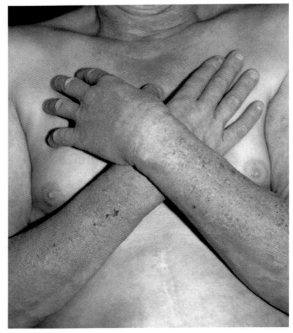

Figure 21-14. Erythematous, scaly rash in sun-exposed areas caused by pellagra (i.e., niacin deficiency); the involved neck region has been called "Casal's necklace," after Don Gaspar Casal who first described pellagra in 1735.

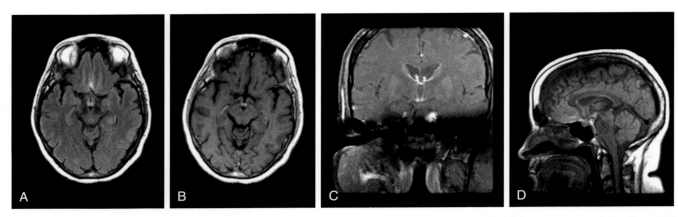

Figure 21-15. Brain MRI demonstrating isolated T2/FLAIR (A) hyperintense signal changes and Gadolinium-enhancement (B, C and D) of both mammillary bodies. Also note the anterior vermal atrophy, a common finding in patients with chronic excessive alcohol consumption. (From Beh SC, Frohman TC, Frohman EM. Isolated mammillary body involvement on MRI in Wernicke's encephalopathy. J Neurol Sci 334: 1–2, 2013.)

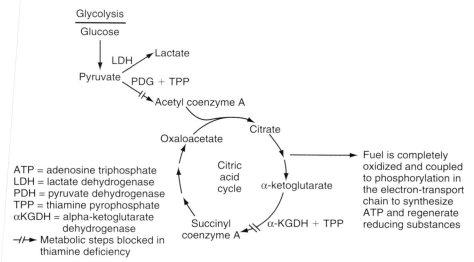

Figure 21-16. The role of thiamine in aerobic metabolism. A glucose load administered in the absence of thiamine increases the metabolic demand for thiamine, which may precipitate or worsen lactic acidosis and trigger fulminant Wernicke-Korsakoff syndrome or wet or dry beriberi. *(From Romanski S, McMahon M. Metabolic acidosis and thiamine deficiency,* Mayo Clin Proc *74:259–263, 1999.)*

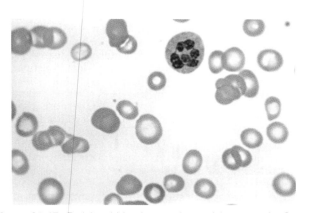

Figure 21-17. Peripheral blood smear in pernicious anemia. Smear demonstrates anisocytosis, macrocytosis, and one hypersegmented neutrophil. *(From Page Green R. Macrocytic Anemia. In: Porwit A, McCullough J, Erber WN. Blood and Bone Marrow Pathology, ed 2, 2011.)*

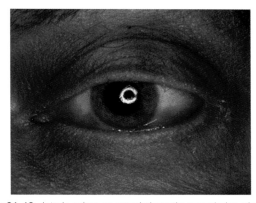

Figure 21-18. Icteric sclera as seen in hepatic encephalopathy. Jaundice, or icterus, a yellowish discoloration from increased bile pigments in the serum, may be readily identified in the sclera while skin and mucous membrane findings remain more subtle. *(From the University of Utah, Spencer S. Eccles Health Sciences Library. http://library.med.utah.edu/WebPath/CINJHTML/CINJ049.html.)*

fluctuations of consciousness are generally recognized, but quiet delirium (e.g., withdrawal, mild memory or cognitive impairment, passivity) or anxiety may be overlooked, considered to be the patient's "baseline," or erroneously ascribed to a primary mental disorder.

Hepatic Encephalopathy

Hepatocellular failure, whether acute, subacute, or chronic, may lead to an encephalopathic syndrome that spans the neuropsychiatric gamut from minimal personality change to coma.[97] The earliest signs of mild intellectual deficits often precede the classic findings of asterixis and jaundice (Figure 21-18),[98] and may be so subtle that only those most familiar with the patient will notice, and the patient's conversational ability may even limit family awareness. Other early signs include confusion, slowed cognition, poor concentration, sleep–wake reversal, poor personal grooming, and depressed, labile, or irritable mood. Episodic disorientation, rage, or inappropriate behavior may precede the progressive decline in cognition, memory, speech, and consciousness as the patient

becomes confused, disoriented, amnestic, incoherent, somnolent, and finally comatose.[99] Focal neurological signs may be more common than previously appreciated. When recognized, they appear to be more common in cirrhotic women, clear with resolution of the encephalopathy, and are not prognostically significant.[100]

Renal Insufficiency

Bizarre visual hallucinations are commonly seen in the delirium of acute renal failure, but the neuropsychiatric symptoms of chronic renal insufficiency (CRI) may be less extreme and more varied, ranging from mild cognitive slowing (e.g., difficulties in concentration, problem-solving, calculation), to severe cognitive impairment and lethargy.[101] Although appropriate dialysis may reverse some of the cognitive deficits, dialysis itself is associated with cognitive slowing, memory problems, and concentration problems (though rarely dementia since the elimination of aluminum from dialysis solutions). Depression is more common in both CRI and patients undergoing dialysis,[102] with the probable additive effects of related neurotransmission and endocrine dysfunction (e.g., hyperparathyroidism[101]). Dialysis patients with depression are twice as likely to be hospitalized or to die within 12 months as those without depression.[103]

Uremic patients are also at risk for partial (and convulsive) seizures that are often unrecognized, but associated with all of the aberrations of affect, behavior, cognition, perception, and consciousness discussed previously.

Hypoglycemic Encephalopathy

Disorientation, confusion, bizarre behavior, and hallucinations, manifestations of hypoglycemia of any cause, may be heralded by apprehension or restlessness. There may be physical signs (e.g., tachycardia or diaphoresis) or symptoms (e.g., hunger or nausea). Without treatment, patients progress to a stuporous state, followed by coma.[104] The hippocampus is particularly sensitive to repeated hypoglycemic insult, which may result in permanent amnesia.[105] In critically ill patients, hypoglycemia (as well as hyperglycemia and fluctuations in blood glucose) significantly aggravates the critical illness-induced neurocognitive dysfunction.[106]

Diabetic Ketoacidosis

Before the onset of the well-recognized "three Ps" (polyphagia, polydipsia, and polyuria), poorly controlled diabetic patients may experience vague, non-descript symptoms, such as lethargy or fatigue, followed by headache, nausea, and vomiting. The elderly are at particular risk of cognitive dysfunction from prolonged delirium caused by osmotic fluid shifts. Atypical neuroleptics, used to treat patients with mood or psychotic disorders (or agitation from delirium or dementia in elderly patients), increase the risk of insulin-resistance and associated complications (e.g., dyslipidemias, metabolic syndrome).[107]

Acute Intermittent Porphyria

This rare, autosomal dominant enzyme deficiency, with a predilection for women, interferes with heme biosynthesis and causes porphyrin rings to accumulate.[108] Symptomatic disease, with an onset between ages 20 and 50, may manifest as the classic triad (i.e., episodic, acute, colicky abdominal pain, motor polyneuropathy, and psychosis), or it may cause purely psychiatric symptoms (e.g., anxiety, insomnia, depression, mood lability, or psychosis).[109] Some previously undiagnosed chronic psychiatric patients have been found to have acute intermittent porphyria (AIP). AIP predisposes to seizures, from both the neurological effects of the disease and from electrolyte disturbances (e.g. hyponatremia) caused by hypothalamic involvement and SIADH, as well as vomiting and diarrhea.[110] Meprobamate, sulfonamide antibiotics, ergot derivatives, and many anti-seizure medications promote porphyrin synthesis that can promote attacks. Medicines known to be safe include the phenothiazines, glucocorticoids, narcotic analgesics, penicillin derivatives, insulin, gabapentin, aspirin, acetaminophen, and bromides. Besides drugs, alcohol, caloric restriction, and gonadal steroids (endogenous or exogenous) are also known to precipitate episodes.[111]

Endocrine Disorders

Because endocrine disorders are now recognized earlier in their clinical course, the psychiatric manifestations are generally depression and anxiety, rather than delirium or dementia associated with more advanced disease.

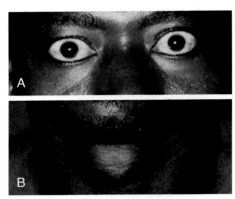

Figure 21-19. Stigmata of Graves' disease. (A) demonstrates the goiter. (B) demonstrates the exophthalmos common in Graves' disease.

Thyroid Dysfunction

Like depression, hypothyroidism is more prevalent (4:1) in women. Mild (or "subclinical") hypothyroidism shares many of the same, non-specific signs and symptoms of depression (e.g., fatigue, lethargy, weight gain, decreased appetite, depressed mood, and slowed mental and motor activity).[112-114] These features, along with cold intolerance, may be attributed to depression, aging, dementia, or Parkinson's disease. Physical findings (e.g., thin and dry hair, dry skin, constipation, stiffness, coarse voice, facial puffiness, carpal tunnel syndrome, lateral eyebrow loss, hearing loss, and delayed relaxation phase of deep tendon reflexes) aid in the diagnosis of more prolonged disease. Myxedema madness, a syndrome of hallucinations and paranoia, is a manifestation of late disease.[115] Depressed patients who are found to be hypothyroid may require both thyroid hormone replacement and antidepressant treatment, as the depressive symptoms persist after hormone replacement in about 10% of patients.

Hyperthyroidism, on the other hand, may manifest much like generalized anxiety or panic, before any of the more classic signs of Graves' disease appear (Figure 21-19).[116] Patients may complain of feeling anxious, or they may be labile, restless, and fidgety. They may have difficulties with memory, attention, planning, and productivity.[117] Other common, non-specific features include palpitations, tachycardia, diaphoresis, irritability, tremulousness, insomnia, weakness, and fatigue. Thyrotoxicosis psychosis has also been described as a primarily affective psychosis with mania and depression equally represented.[118] Despite voracious appetite, patients lose weight. In the elderly, however, this hyperactive state may be replaced by apathy, psychomotor retardation, loss of appetite, and depression.[114,119] Such patients may also experience more prominent proximal muscle wasting, heart failure, or atrial arrhythmias.[120]

Parathyroid Dysfunction

Despite the lack of conclusive correlation with absolute serum calcium levels, symptoms of parathyroid dysfunction are thought to be associated with disturbances in calcium, phosphate, and bone metabolism.[121] Primary hyperparathyroidism, associated with hypercalcemia and more common in women in their 50s and 60s, may be asymptomatic for years, and then manifest as non-specific symptoms (e.g., fatigue, abdominal pain, mental slowing, attentional or memory problems, depressed mood, anxiety, personality change, apathy, lethargy). More advanced disease has serious medical implications (e.g., hypertension, fractures, peptic ulcers, pancreatitis, kidney stones) as well as possible delirium, coma and death.[122] Parathyroidectomy has been advocated for improved quality of life in symptomatic patients, but remains controversial in those without symptoms.[122,123] Hypoparathyroidism, associated with a gradual decline in serum calcium, can also cause delirium or personality change.[124] More acute calcemic depletion results in tetany.

Adrenal Dysfunction

Adrenal insufficiency, or hypocortisolism, may be primary (e.g., autoimmune Addison's disease) or secondary (e.g., from prolonged exogenous glucocorticoids). The initial manifestation may be largely psychiatric (e.g., apathy, negativism, social withdrawal, poverty of thought, fatigue, depressed mood, irritability, and loss of appetite, interest, and enjoyment), and misattributed to depression.[124] Nausea, vomiting, weakness, hypotension, and hypoglycemia may develop, followed by delirium and coma, if glucocorticoids are not administered. Even with appropriate replacement, however, residual psychiatric symptoms may need more specific treatment, with careful consideration not to worsen hypotension. Several factors may contribute to the development and persistence of psychiatric symptoms (e.g., glucocorticoid deficit, the associated elevations of adrenocorticotropic hormone [ACTH] and corticotropin-releasing factor [CRF], dehydroepiandrosterone [DHEA] deficiency,[125] or the lack of normal diurnal and stress modulation in glucocorticoid replacement).

Hypercortisolism may also occur in several ways. It may be ACTH dependent (e.g., hypersecretion of ACTH) either from a pituitary adenoma (Cushing's disease) or a non-pituitary malignancy (Cushing's syndrome). A less common cause is ACTH-independent Cushing's syndrome (e.g., adrenal hypersecretion of cortisol from hyperplasia or tumor). Despite the classic cushingoid presentation (truncal obesity, peripheral wasting, hirsutism, moon facies, acne, and striae [Figure 21-20[126,127]]), diagnosis is frequently delayed because this usually incomplete syndrome is often preceded by psychiatric symptoms (e.g., anxiety, panic, depression, extreme irritability, crying, pronounced suicidality, and, rarely, psychosis).[128] Exogenous steroids may produce a comparable clinical picture. Some patients on prolonged steroid therapy are (psychiatrically) exquisitely sensitive to small dose alterations. High doses of steroids may trigger mania in some patients, and when such patients require episodic steroid treatment, they should receive mood-stabilizing medication as prophylaxis.[129,130]

Pituitary Dysfunction

Because of its regulatory role in multiple body systems, pituitary perturbations are associated with the full spectrum of psychiatric symptoms. Decreased pituitary function (e.g., Sheehan's syndrome: post-partum hemorrhagic pituitary destruction) results in mental slowing and depressed or labile mood. Increased pituitary function (e.g., from a pituitary adenoma or a functioning tumor) may result in a variety of syndromes (e.g., Cushing's syndrome from adrenal hyperplasia), depending on the hormonal target or system affected.[124]

Demyelinating Disorders

Although relatively uncommon, disorders of myelination come to psychiatric attention not only because the neuropsychiatric symptoms may precede physical findings but also because the nature of the sensory and motor manifestations (i.e., intermittent, subjective, and variable) may suggest psychiatric causation (e.g., somatization, anxiety, depression, or malingering). The non-specific initial symptoms may include mild changes in personality, mood, behavior, or cognition.

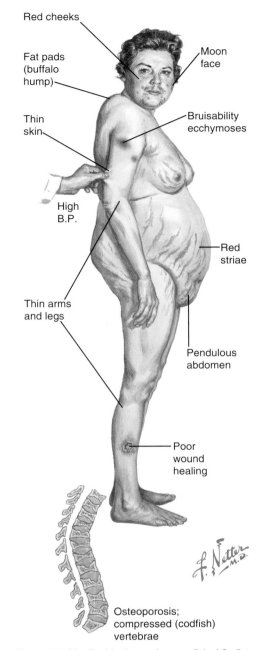

Figure 21-20. Cushing's syndrome: clinical findings.

The most common of the demyelinating disorders, multiple sclerosis (MS) has significant psychiatric symptomatology and occurs in 50 to 60 individuals per 100,000, and historically as many as 160 per 100,000 white American women raised in northern latitudes.[131] However, the latitude differential appears to be decreasing,[132] while the female-to-male ratio is increasing.[133] Amyotrophic lateral sclerosis (ALS) is a distant second, with an annual incidence of 1.6 per 100,000.[134] Metachromatic leukodystrophy, adrenoleukodystrophy, gangliosidoses, and SSPE are other, even less prevalent, disorders.

Multiple Sclerosis

Of uncertain (probably genetic and environmental) etiology, MS is an episodic, multi-focal, inflammatory cause of demyelination, more prevalent in women (female:male

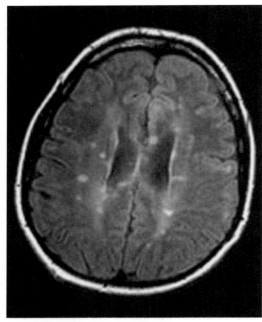

Figure 21-21. Brain MRI of patient with MS. White spots are the multiple T_2-weighted hyperintensities characteristic of MS. *(From Michigan State University College of Osteopathic Medicine.)*

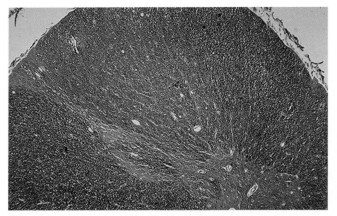

Figure 21-22. Spinal cord in a patient with ALS. Luxol-fast-blue stain demonstrates lateral column degeneration with gliosis. *(From the WebPath educational program at http://library.med.utah.edu/WebPath/CNSHTML/CNS105.html.)*

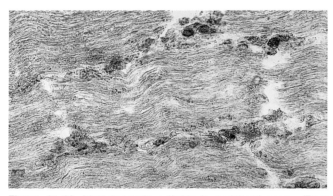

Figure 21-23. Metachromatic sulfatide in peripheral nerve. *(From Ellison D. et al. Neuropathology: A Reference Text of CNS Pathology, ed 3. Edinburgh, Mosby Elsevier, 2013.)*

incidence of 3.6 : 2.0) and in cold and temperate climates, with a typical onset between ages 20 and 40. There is involvement of the spinal cord, brainstem, cerebellum, cerebral hemispheres, and optic nerves. Psychiatric symptoms are prevalent (95%) in patients at all stages of MS, and such symptoms correlate poorly with markers of disease severity (e.g., MRI findings [Figure 21-21[135]], physical symptoms, and length of illness). Psychiatric symptoms may not resolve with remission of physical symptoms.[136] Irritability tends to be the earliest symptom.

Over three-quarters of patients will have episodes of depressed mood,[136] accompanied by a high risk of suicidality, especially in the first year of diagnosis.[137] Unlike primary depression, there is no gender or age bias for depression in MS patients. However, men with MS have a higher rate of suicide than do women. The newly diagnosed, and those diagnosed before age 30,[138,139] also have an increased risk of suicide. Other common neuropsychiatric symptoms include agitation, anxiety, apathy, disinhibition, hallucinations, or delusions. Persistent euphoria, historically associated with MS, occurs in less than 10% of patients, generally in the setting of diffuse cerebral disease. Although about 25% may experience some episode of mild mood elevation, this should not be confused with mania, which is exceedingly rare. An incongruous, upbeat nature, out of step with either the patient's condition or previous personality style, is common, and may be what was previously termed *euphoria*. Over 50% of MS patients experience some cognitive decline; approximately 20% to 30% have more serious deficits. While memory problems are common, severe dementia is not.[140] Steroids and interferon preparations used to ameliorate the effects of MS may also be iatrogenic causes of psychiatric symptoms.

Amyotrophic Lateral Sclerosis

The second most common demyelinating disorder, and the most common degenerative motor neuron disease (Figure 21-22[141]), ALS has a relentless course (i.e., death occurs within 3 to 5 years of symptom onset[142]), and fewer psychiatric manifestations (e.g., uncontrollable, or pseudobulbar, laughing and crying from degeneration in the cortical bulbar projections to the brainstem). Despite the common practice of prescribing antidepressants, only about 11% of ALS patients meet criteria for depression.[143] However, as many as one-third of patients with ALS may show frontotemporal cognitive deficits that do not correlate with site of onset; these deficits have not been shown to limit survival (when controlling for disease severity).[144]

Lipid Storage Disorders

These rare causes of demyelination are autosomal recessive, enzyme deficiency states that can occur in adulthood with both psychiatric and neuromuscular manifestations. Metachromatic leukodystrophy (Figure 21-23[145]), despite a swift, terminal course in infancy, may manifest with more insidious, progressive, cognitive decline (e.g., forgetfulness, deterioration of work or school performance) and with personality changes in adolescents or adults. Cerebellar signs (e.g., gait disturbances, masked facies, or strange postures) precede the eventual (subcortical type) dementia and psychosis, after which patients become mute and bedridden.[146] Adrenoleukodystrophy (an x-linked, recessive disorder of males) causes adrenal insufficiency and it may present with the psychiatric manifestations of primary Addison's disease, or with asymmetric myelopathic findings (e.g., homonymous hemianopsia and hemiparesis), aphasia, or dementia. Becoming more symmetric with spastic paraparesis or demyelinating polyneuropathy, the disease is progressive and generally untreatable (except for allogeneic hematopoietic cell transplantation, if provided at a very early stage of brain involvement;[147] glucocorticoids may be used to treat the adrenal deficit).[148] The adult form of Tay-Sachs disease (a lysosomal storage disease known as a gangliosidosis) may cause psychotic symptoms and seizures, whereas the neuromuscular effects (e.g., clumsiness or weakness from spinocerebellar and lower motor neuron involvement) are still mild. The cranial nerves (and therefore vision) are spared.[149] However, cognition and intelligence are more commonly affected than previously recognized.[150]

Mitochondrial Disease

These maternally-inherited disorders of mitochondrial metabolic dysfunction usually present in children, but may become apparent in adulthood with a wide range of multi-system disease. Organs and tissues especially vulnerable are those heavily reliant on aerobic metabolism (e.g., CNS [include visual and auditory pathways], heart, liver, kidneys, skeletal muscles). Psychiatric symptoms are more prevalent among those with mitochondrial disorders (e.g., depression, anxiety, mania, psychosis, cognitive impairment).[151] There is also evidence for dysfunctional mitochondrial involvement in certain psychiatric disorders (e.g., schizophrenia, bipolar disorder, major depression), as well as neurodegenerative disorders.[152]

The acronym MELAS (mitochrondrial myopathy, encephalopathy, lactic acidosis, and stroke-like episodes) refers to a syndrome of stroke-like episodes, migraines, diabetes, seizures, sensorineuronal hearing loss, short stature, and cardiomyopathy that usually presents in adolescence or early adulthood, but with rare cases of onset after the age of 40.[153] MELAS has a relapsing–remitting pattern with the hallmark transient stroke-like episodes. Serum and CSF lactate are commonly elevated. Imaging reflects white matter involvement, as well as characteristic, transient, cerebrocortical lesions that defy vascular territory (Figure 21-24).[154]

Cerebrovascular Disease

Stroke has decreased to the fourth leading cause of death in the US, behind heart disease, cancer, and chronic lower respiratory disease.[155] Although stroke risk doubles with each decade of adult age, the increasing incidence of vascular events in the younger populations is a concerning trend.[156,157] Ischemic events account for about 80% of strokes,[134] with atherosclerotic thrombosis and cerebral embolism responsible for about one-third of these. Hemorrhagic stroke is usually the result of essential hypertension, with spontaneous aneurysmal rupture and arteriovenous malformation relatively rare etiologies.

By far the most common post-stroke psychiatric manifestation, occurring in approximately 40% of patients,[158] is depression (i.e., major or minor depression), either in the immediate post-stroke period (65%) or at about 6 months following stroke. Approximately 25% of patients experience post-stroke anxiety, and three-quarters of those patients had co-morbid depressive disorders, which suggests that post-stroke anxiety in the absence of depression is rare.[159] Mania, also rare, is associated with right-sided lesions[160] of the orbitofrontal, basotemporal, basal ganglia, and thalamic areas. There is suggestive,[161] but controversial,[158,162] evidence for a correlation between depression and stroke location (left hemisphere

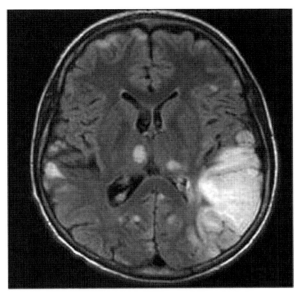

Figure 21-24. MRI of MELAS. Axial FLAIR shows hyperintense foci in a young boy with MELAS that defy vascular territory. *(From Saneto RP, Friedman SD, Shaw DW. Neuroimaging of mitochondrial disease,* Mitochondrion *8:396–413, 2008.)*

frontal, prefrontal, or basal ganglia). Other likely risk factors for depression or secondary mania include subcortical atrophy and a personal or family history of mood disorder. Previous stroke may also predispose to post-stroke depression. Besides the contribution of functional and potential psychosocial losses, post-stroke depression is likely mediated by pro-inflammatory factors and effects on neurotransmitters[158] (just as the pro-inflammatory and neuroendocrine effects of depression are independent risk factors for stroke[163]). Untreated post-stroke depression lasts about a year; minor depression is less predictable and may have a more protracted course. Depression is predictive of worse stroke recovery and it is associated with greater mortality, not because of a correlation with initial stroke severity, but because depression is associated with poor rehabilitative effort. Since post-stroke depression responds to the usual antidepressant therapies, early recognition and intervention are essential for optimal stroke outcome.[158]

Two other post-stroke syndromes give the *appearance* of mood disorders (or mood dysregulation), but they are actually disorders of affective expression, rather than mood. Patients with pseudobulbar palsy have outbursts of uncontrollable laughter or crying (and lack less intense expression, such as smiling) out of proportion to their emotional experience. This affective incontinence (the effect of multiple lacunar infarcts on the descending corticobulbar and frontopontine pathways)[164,165] is associated with dysarthria, dysphagia, and bifacial weakness. The other syndrome, aprosodia, is the inability to affectively modulate speech and gestures (motor aprosodia) or the inability to perceive the emotional content of others' speech or gestures (sensory aprosodia). Careful scrutiny is necessary to distinguish the affective blunting of aprosodia from true depression in post-stroke patients.[166]

Toxins

There is insufficient research to support the existence of environmental illness or multiple chemical sensitivity, but there are environmental toxins (e.g., carbon monoxide [CO] or lead) known to cause recognizable syndromes that may, nonetheless, be misattributed to primary physical or mental disorders. CO poisoning, from defective heating or exhaust ventilation, can manifest as a non-descript flu-like syndrome (e.g., malaise, cough, and nausea). Low-level exposure of a more chronic nature causes depressive symptoms and cognitive decline. More severe poisoning may cause delayed neuropsychiatric syndrome (DNS), characterized by a range of symptoms from subtle cognitive effects that self-resolve with time, to memory dysfunction, visual problems, parkinsonism, confabulation, and hallucinations (in severe exposures, imaging demonstrates atrophic changes in the basal ganglia and corpus callosum).[167] Low-level lead exposure, not solely a concern of young children (although children are particularly vulnerable to the neurotoxicity[168]), also manifests with non-descript psychiatric symptoms suggestive of depression (e.g., fatigue, sleepiness, depressed mood, and apathy). Adults and adolescents are at risk for excessive lead exposure from environmental, recreational, and occupational sources.[169] Besides the well-known risk of lead-based paint, running or biking in heavily trafficked areas, doing home repairs or remodeling, and even drinking from leaded crystal increases one's exposure. Artists of various crafts are at risk (e.g., stained glass, ceramic, and lead-figure artisans), as are art conservators. Those who use firearms for work or recreation should monitor their lead levels. Gasoline, solvents, and cleaning fluids are sources of organic lead exposure, associated with nightmares, restlessness, and psychotic symptoms. Extreme levels produce seizures and coma.[170] There is evidence that cumulative lead exposure earlier in life may be correlated with cognitive decline, worsening executive function, and poor dexterity later in life.[171,172]

Mercury is associated with two distinct syndromes of toxicity. If the exposure is from the organic form (e.g., methylated mercury from contaminated fish), neurological symptoms predominate (e.g., motor-sensory neuropathy, cerebellar ataxia, slurred speech, paresthesias, and visual field defects), with less dramatic psychiatric manifestations (e.g., depression, irritability, or mild dementia).[173] Toxic inorganic mercury exposure, however, has an initial psychiatric presentation (i.e., the "Mad Hatter" syndrome) of depression, irritability, and psychosis, followed by less striking neurological findings (e.g., tremor, weakness, and headache).[174] Although occupational exposure

and mercury thermometers have been largely eliminated, mercury continues to pose a threat because of its availability in folk medicines, botanical preparations, and breakable capsules (used by certain cultural or religious sects to sprinkle mercury in the home or car).[175]

Drugs of any sort (e.g., prescribed, over-the-counter, herbal, or recreational), in therapeutic or overdose proportions, are potential toxins to consider whenever there are alterations in behavior, cognition, consciousness, or personality. (If drugs are causative, however, the diagnosis would be substance-related disorder, covered in other chapters.)

Neoplasm

Every possible manifestation of CNS pathology can be produced by unfettered, local or diffuse, neoplastic growth inside the rigid cranial vault. Tumors tend to be less symptomatic than ischemic strokes affecting comparable brain volume. In adults, brain metastases of non-CNS malignancies are more common than primary brain tumors.[176] There may be clinical features that hint at the location, type, and nature (i.e., metastatic versus primary) of the tumor. Psychiatric manifestations, however, may also be related to paraneoplastic syndromes of non-brain primary malignancies.[177]

Approximately 50% to 60% of primary brain tumors are gliomas (Figure 21-25[176]), with gradual, pancortical dissemination that results in equally diffuse symptomatology (e.g., cognitive decline). A similar, non-specific pattern occurs with lymphoma or multiple metastases. In contrast, the extrinsic growth with localized brain compression of meningiomas (Figure 21-26[176]) (approximately 25% of primary brain tumors) presents a more focal, progressive pattern. Intracranial lesions can also cause seizures, either from random excitation or lack of the usual inhibitory control. Seizures are rarely from subcortical lesions, and generally correlate with diffuse cortical infiltration or (even minor) compression from meningiomas. Metastases are more likely than primary brain tumors to cause constitutional symptoms (e.g., fever, weight loss, or fatigue).

Brain tumors in adults are associated with psychiatric symptoms in 50% of patients, most of whom (80%) have frontal or limbic tumors. Frontal tumors cause incontinence

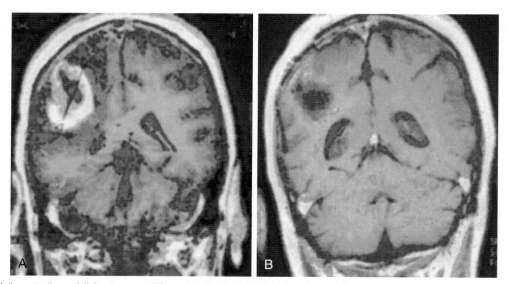

Figure 21-25. Malignant glioma (gliobastoma multiforme) in the right frontal lobe. Coronal T1-weighted magnetic resonance imaging scan with gadolinium before (A) and after (B) surgery. *(From Stevens GHJ. Brain Tumors: Meningiomas and Gliomas. In: Cleveland Clinic: Current Clinical Medicine, ed 2, 2010, Saunders.)*

of bowel and bladder, as well as personality change and depression. Tumors of the temporal lobe can cause a range of psychiatric symptoms (e.g., depression, personality change, memory dysfunction, aphasia, or Korsakoff syndrome), and they are particularly prone to cause seizures,[177] commonly associated with ictal or inter-ictal psychotic symptoms. Tumors in the upper brainstem are associated with akinetic mutism (i.e., an alert but immobile state).

Another extrinsic cancer-related source of psychiatric symptoms, paraneoplastic syndromes, may not be recognized when they occur months (or years) before other symptoms lead to tumor detection.[178] A variety of non-CNS tumors (e.g., breast, uterus, ovary, testicle, kidney, thyroid, stomach, colon) can cause these syndromes, but they are most frequently associated

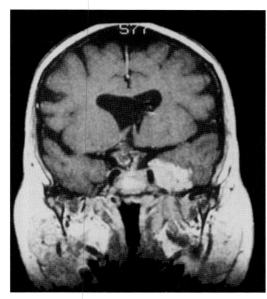

Figure 21-26. Meningioma. This coronal MRI with gadolinium demonstrates a large meningioma extending from the middle fossa into the cavernous sinus, but with notable absence of edema in the adjacent brain tissue. *(From Winn, HR. Youman's Neurological Surgery, ed 6, 2011, Saunders)*

with small cell carcinoma of the lung. Tumor production of hormones, or hormone-like substances, can give rise to the syndrome of inappropriate antidiuretic hormone secretion (SIADH), as well as to hypercortisolism, hypercalcemia, or hyperparathyroidism, and all of the concomitant neuropsychiatric manifestations. However, neurological syndromes of paraneoplastic origin are largely immune-mediated. Antibodies may be directed against onconeural antigens (intra-cellular) or cell-surface antigens. Paraneoplastic syndromes with onconeural antigens are relatively rare (although their presence is highly predictive of underlying neoplasm), with the initial presentation of ataxia (from cerebellar degeneration), dysarthria and nystagmus, followed by limbic encephalitis or encephalomyelitis. However, paraneoplastic-type syndromes involving cell-surface antigens (targeting neuronal receptors [e.g., NMDA receptors], channels, or synaptic proteins) are both more common and less predictive of underlying tumor. Nonetheless, in certain populations, up to 30%–50% of patients with anti-NMDAR encephalitis will have underlying cancer (e.g., ovarian teratoma, lymphoma).[179,180] Limbic encephalitis can present with psychiatric symptoms (e.g., depression, anxiety, irritability, personality changes, psychosis, catatonia) as well as seizures, memory loss, cognitive changes, decreased consciousness, hypoventilation and autonomic instability. Clinical findings may include mild-to-moderate lymphocytic pleocytosis, oligoclonal bands, mild protein elevation, as well as specific antibodies in CSF and serum. EEG abnormalities are generalized slowing, possible epileptic activity, as well as the classic "extreme delta brush," as in anti-NMDAR encephalitis (Figure 21-27).[181] Although there may be mesiotemporal enhancement in limbic encephalitis (and later atrophy), normal imaging does not exclude the diagnosis. Paraneoplastic neurologic syndromes to onconeural antigens do not respond well to treatment, whereas encephalitis involving cell-surface antigens appear to respond more favorably to immunotherapy and tumor removal.[179]

Colloid cysts are an example of "benign" pathology causing symptoms (e.g., depression, mood lability, psychosis, personality change, position-dependent or intermittent headache) because they take up space in a confined area and thereby compress adjacent structures. These lesions of the third ventricle press on diencephalic structures and may further increase intracranial pressure by obstructing the ventricle.[182]

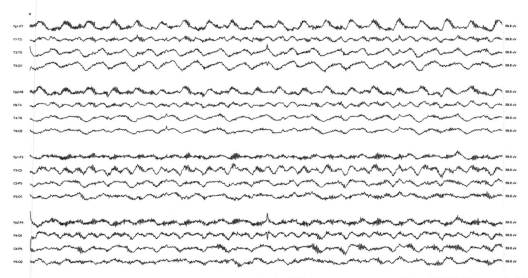

Figure 21-27. Extreme delta brush EEG pattern in anti-NMDAR encephalitis. EEG in a young woman with anti-NMDAR encephalitis demonstrates generalized rhythmic delta frequency activity at 2–2.5 Hz with superimposed rhythmic beta frequency activity. *(From Schmitt SE, Pargeon K, Frechette ES, et al. Extreme delta brush: a unique EEG pattern in adults with anti-NMDA receptor encephalitis, Neurology 79:1094–1100, 2012.)*

Degenerative Disorders

The association between movement and emotion is nowhere more apparent than in the function and dysfunction of the basal ganglia, mediated by limbic and cortical inputs, and the shared neurotransmitter systems (i.e., dopamine, γ-aminobutyric acid [GABA], serotonin, norepinephrine [noradrenaline]). Degenerative disorders in this area span motor, sensory, and psychiatric (e.g., depression, psychosis, dementia) manifestations.[183] Movement symptoms may fluctuate in proportion to the severity of emotional distress.

Parkinson's disease affects at least 1% of the population over age 60, and the prevalence may be on the rise.[184] Caused by degeneration primarily in the pars compacta of the substantia nigra, the well-defined syndrome of bradykinesia, rigidity, tremor, and characteristic gait and posture disorders are further complicated by depression in an estimated 40% (4% to 70%) of patients,[185] as well as by dementia in some (with a higher prevalence than in age-matched controls). The depression may be the result of dopamine, and to a lesser extent norepinephrine, depletion. Antidepressants, such as SSRI and SNRIs, appear to be effective without worsening motor symptoms.[186] Psychosis, which can be part of the disease, is worsened by anticholinergic and dopaminergic medications used to treat it.[185]

The major pathology of Huntington's chorea, an autosomal dominant disorder, includes striatal destruction, GABA depletion, atrophy of the caudate and putamen, and mild wasting of frontal and temporal lobes. With a prevalence of 10 per 100,000 population,[187] it manifests most commonly in the fourth or fifth decades, although the variable onset may occur in childhood, associated with a more aggressive course (with a survival time that is approximately half that of adults). Psychiatric symptoms are prominent throughout the disease progression, and they may precede the classic choreiform movements.[183,188] Initial signs may be significant attentional deficits, poor judgment, and executive dysfunction, followed by depression, apathy, social withdrawal, and poor personal hygiene. In some individuals, the manifestation may be suggestive of obsessive-compulsive disorder (OCD)[189] or schizophrenia. Patients tend to be irritable and impulsive.[183,188,190] Although the depression benefits from antidepressant pharmacotherapy, the cognitive decline (like the movement disorder) is relentless, and it progresses to dementia.

A genetic deficiency of ceruloplasmin affecting 1 to 2 per 100,000 population,[191] Wilson's disease (also called hepatolenticular degeneration)[183] is an autosomal recessive defect in copper excretion, associated with copper deposition in the liver, brain, cornea, and kidney. Rarely symptomatic before age 6, onset of symptoms frequently occurs in adolescence, but may manifest later in adulthood. About half of patients have liver manifestations (e.g., hepatitis, parenchymal disease, or cirrhosis). The other half primarily have neuropsychiatric symptoms, virtually always accompanied by the pathognomonic Kayser-Fleischer rings[191] (i.e., gold or green-brown copper deposits surrounding the cornea [Figure 21-28]).[192] The lenticular nuclei and, to lesser extents, the pons, medulla, thalamus, cerebellum, and cerebral cortex, are the brain targets of copper toxicity. Despite common neurological features (e.g., tremor, chorea, spasticity, rigidity, dysphagia, dysarthria), cognition is generally unaffected (although the dysarthria may be mistaken for intellectual disability). Patients with neurological symptoms tend to have psychiatric symptoms as well, but approximately 10% to 25% of patients have purely psychiatric symptoms.[191] Bizarre, probably frontal behavior is most common, but patients also have schizophrenia-like syndromes, as well as bipolar and more typical depressive syndromes. Psychiatric symptoms may respond to successful removal of

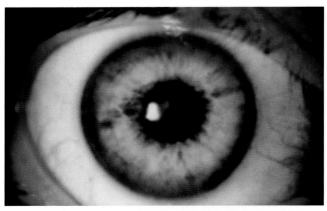

Figure 21-28. Kayser-Fleischer rings in Wilson's disease. These gold or green-brown copper deposits surrounding the cornea are almost always present when patients have neuropsychiatric symptoms. *(From Sullivan CA, Chopdar A, Shun-Shin GA. Dense Kayser-Fleischer ring in asymptomatic Wilson's disease (hepatolenticular degeneration), Br J Ophthalmol 86:114, 2002, Figure 1.)*

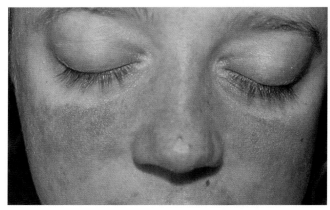

Figure 21-29. Malar rash of systemic lupus erythematosus. *(From On-line Archives of Rheumatology at www.archrheumatol .net/atlas/case68.html. Copyright 1996-2006 On-line Archives of Rheumatology.)*

excess copper; residual psychiatric symptoms, however, should be treated with standard pharmacotherapies.

Immune Diseases

Systemic lupus erythematosus (SLE) is an inflammatory, autoimmune disease with multi-system involvement (Figure 21-29[193] shows the characteristic "butterfly" rash), unknown cause, variable symptoms and time course, inconclusive diagnostic studies, and female predilection (9 : 1),[194] all of which conspire to misattribute the non-specific manifestations to primary mental disorder (e.g., major depression or somatization). Approximately half of patients initially have depression, sleep disturbance, mood lability, mild cognitive dysfunction, or psychosis. Onset of symptoms is usually between ages 20 and 50. SLE may be treated with steroids, with possible worsening of psychiatric symptoms.[195]

Acquired immunodeficiency syndrome (AIDS) is discussed earlier in the chapter and in other chapters of this book (see Chapter 57).

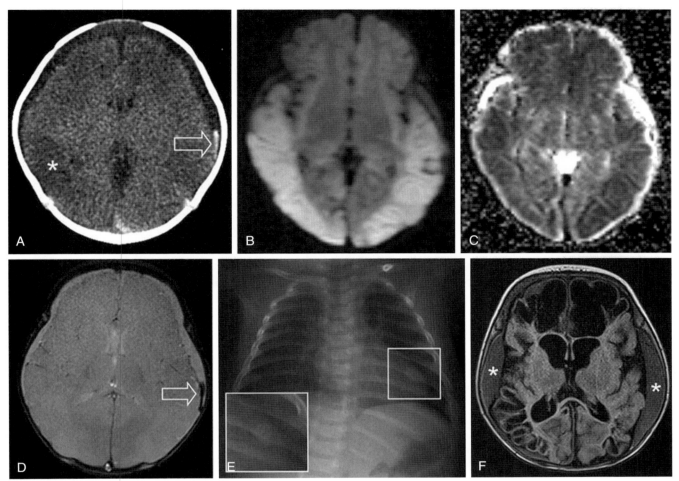

Figure 21-30. Radiographic documentation of the injuries sustained to a 2-year-old child. (A) Left subdural hematoma. (B) Temporoparietal edema on MRI. (C) Deceased signal intensity on diffusion-weighted MRI. (D) Blood clot in subdural space on FLAIR. (E) Posterior radiograph of chest. (F) MRI obtained 2 months post-injury showing multicystic encephalomalacia and bilateral subdural hygromas. *(From Sieswerda-Hoogendoorn T, Boos S, Spivack B, et al. Abusive head trauma Part II: radiological aspects,* Eur J Pediatr *171:617–623, 2012.)*

Trauma

There are 1.7 million traumatic brain injuries (see Chapter 82) yearly in the US,[196] with the highest incidence in young men. Falls are the leading cause, particularly in the elderly, followed by motor vehicle accidents, violence, and sports. Head injuries due to combat is also receiving more attention.[197] Abusive head trauma is the leading cause of traumatic death in infants, as well as the most common cause of childhood death from abuse.[198] Figure 21-30[199] depicts the serious brain injury sustained in abusive head trauma to children. Despite the drama of penetrating head injuries (e.g., gunshot wounds), the symptoms are generally focal and related to the size and location of directly involved brain tissue.

Closed head injury, on the other hand, is both much more common and much more complex, as demonstrated in Figure 21-31.[200] Neither the diffuse presentation nor the prolonged sequelae may correlate with the apparent extent of the initial insult, possibly because of the several mechanisms of injury that may occur with blunt trauma. Brain contusion and neuronal damage, frequently followed by bleeding and edema, may be the result of direct impact, parenchymal stretching, acceleration/deceleration and shearing forces, and microscopic tears.[201] The cognitive, emotional, and somatic symptoms of neurobehavioral dysfunction can last from months to years.

Limbic structures (e.g., anterior temporal lobes and the inferior frontal lobes) are at particular risk of damage from blunt trauma, which may manifest as cognitive slowing (e.g., inattention, distractibility, memory difficulties, perseveration, poor planning), personality change (e.g., irritability or impulsivity), or mood disturbance (e.g., depression, lability, anxiety).[201] Vague somatic complaints (e.g., headache, dizziness, fatigue, insomnia) may be attributed to depression. Patients also experience bothersome sensory symptoms (e.g., photophobia, blurred vision, hyperacusis, tinnitus). Multiple head injuries, advanced age, and use of drugs or alcohol predispose to post-concussive syndrome (PCS),[202] the prolonged cognitive, emotional, and somatic impairment following "head trauma that caused significant cerebral concussion."[203] There is also research evidence that victims of traumatic brain injury (TBI) have an increased prevalence of Axis I and II pathology diagnosable decades after the initial insult.[204] Because brain-injured patients tend to be exquisitely sensitive to psychotropic medication, small (i.e., "geriatric") doses should be used.

EVALUATION

Although the DSM-5 diagnosis of mental disorder DTAMC should always be on the short list of possibilities, a high degree of medical suspicion serves to guide the evaluation

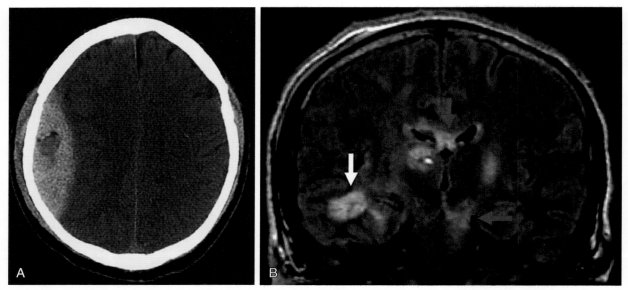

Figure 21-31. (A) Right frontoparietal epidural hematoma w/ characteristic "swirl sign" involving laceration to middle meningeal artery on non-contrast CT scan. (B) Multifocal T2 hyperintense foci reflective of traumatic axonal injury. *(From Gean AD, Fischbein NJ. Head trauma, Neuroimaging Clin N Am 20:527–556, 2010.)*

process to include the findings required to make the diagnosis or to rule it out. This should be the case for any thorough psychiatric evaluation.

History

History should be obtained from the patient and, as appropriate, any other pertinent sources (e.g., medical records, caregivers, current or past health or mental health care providers). Especially when the patient may be a questionable or limited historian, family, close friends, or partners may be valuable sources, preferably with the patient's permission (or not, in the case of emergent situations). The usual historical topics (i.e., medical, psychiatric, family, and psychosocial) should be covered with sufficient detail to hone in on possible medical causes, and to correlate the onset of physical and psychiatric symptoms. The medical history includes not only past and present illnesses, procedures, and all medications but also questions about travel, possible exposures, recent or remote head injury, seizures, and use of substances (e.g., caffeine, tobacco, alcohol, recreational drugs). Non-prescription drugs, herbal or natural supplements, folk remedies, or unusual dietary practices may also be of concern. The psychiatric history should focus on distinguishing typical from atypical features of primary mental disorder (e.g., onset, course, response to treatment, past episodes). Family history of similar symptoms, other psychiatric disorders, medical illnesses that "run" in the family or early, unexplained deaths may provide clues. The social history provides a wealth of information about the patient's life (e.g., education, occupation or work history, and living situation) and possible risk factors (e.g., recreational activities, intimate contacts, sexuality, violence, incarceration).

Examination

The Mental Status Examination (MSE) is the standard clinical survey to assess consciousness, affect, behavior, cognition, speech, thought, judgment, and insight. Clusters or patterns of findings, or deficits, may direct the examiner to seek more

detail or clarification to support a medical diagnosis, but the initial screening examination is the same as in any evaluation. Laboratory, imaging, or other specialized tests should be focused to confirm or rule out suspected diagnoses (e.g., a sleep-deprived EEG in suspected case of complex partial seizures). The overly inclusive approach to tests and procedures carries a greater risk of iatrogenic harm than warranted by the unlikely possibility of discovering unsuspected disease. Brain imaging is recommended in the case of sudden onset, focal signs, rapid progression, infectious disease, or trauma.

TREATMENT CONSIDERATIONS/STRATEGIES

To know the etiology does not imply that the mental disorder is "normal" in that situation. Despite the unalterable course of some stable, chronic, or progressive medical conditions (e.g., previous stroke or toxic exposures, degenerative or demyelinating diseases), the accompanying psychiatric symptoms should be aggressively treated. When it is possible to reverse, mitigate, or control the offending medical condition, however, appropriate medical treatment should be initiated. After correction of the underlying medical condition, some mental disorders will resolve, some may lessen, and others will continue a course similar to the primary mental disorder. Even those psychiatric symptoms that will resolve with treatment of the underlying medical condition (e.g., panic attacks with hyperthyroidism) deserve comfort measures (e.g., benzodiazepine therapy for panic symptoms) while waiting for medical resolution. Depression may lag behind the correction of hypothyroidism and may require a longer course of antidepressant therapy. Some medical conditions and the associated psychiatric symptoms may need chronic treatment, as is often the case with epilepsy and inter-ictal depression. Other considerations in treating patients with mental disorders DTAMC include the psychosocial stress of living with an acute or chronic medical condition and pre-existing primary mental or personality disorders that may exacerbate the psychiatric symptoms, interfere with the medical treatment, and generally complicate or compromise the clinical outcome.

CONCLUSIONS

The DSM-5 diagnosis of mental disorder DTAMC should be part of the differential diagnosis of every patient. Medical suspicion and a working knowledge of the general categories of medical conditions are important to making the diagnosis, because neuropsychiatric symptoms may precede, coincide with, or lag behind the medical presentation. Selective tests and procedures should be used to confirm or rule out suspected diagnoses. Some mental disorders will resolve with treatment of the underlying medical condition, some will require temporary comfort measures, and others may need ongoing aggressive treatment. Regardless of the underlying medical cause or its course, psychiatric distress should be alleviated to the fullest extent possible.

Access the complete reference list and multiple choice questions (MCQs) online at https://expertconsult.inkling.com

KEY REFERENCES

14. Spudich S. HIV and neurocognitive dysfunction. *Curr HIV/AIDS Rep* 10:235–243, 2013.
28. Feder HM Jr, Petersen BW, Robertson KL, et al. Rabies: Still a uniformly fatal disease? Historical occurrence, epidemiological trends, and paradigm shifts. *Curr Infect Dis Rep* 14:408–422, 2012.
29. Hemachudha T, Ugolini G, Wacharapluesadee S, et al. Human rabies: neuropathogenesis, diagnosis, and management. *Lancet Neurol* 12:498–513, 2013.
33. Fallon BA, Vaccaro BJ, Romano M, et al. Lyme borreliosis: neuropsychiatric aspects and neuropathology. *Psychiatr Ann* 36:120–128, 2006.
39. Miklossy J. Chronic or late Lyme neuroborreliosis: analysis of evidence compared to chronic or late neurosyphilis. *Open Neurol J* 6(Suppl. 1–M9):146–157, 2012.
45. Seña AC, White BL, Sparling PF. Novel *Treponema pallidum* serologic tests: a paradigm shift in syphilis screening for the 21st century. *Clin Infect Dis* 51:700–708, 2010.
46. Cho TA, Venna N. Management of acute, recurrent, and chronic meningitides in adults. *Neurol Clin* 28:1061–1088, 2010.
50. Gutierrez J, Issacson RS, Koppel BS. Subacute sclerosing panencephalitis: an update. *Dev Med Child Neurol* 52:901–907, 2010.
53. Brown P, Brandel JP, Sato T, et al. Iatrogenic Creutzfeldt-Jakob disease, final assessment. *Emerging Infect Dis* 18:901–907, 2012.
62. Kanner AM, Schachter SC, Barry JJ, et al. Depression and epilepsy: epidemiologic and neurobiologic perspectives that may explain their high comorbid occurrence. *Epilepsy Behav* 24:156–168, 2012.
75. Kanner AM. Ictal panic and interictal panic attacks: diagnostic and therapeutic principles. *Neurol Clin* 29:163–175, 2011.
80. Oldham MA, Ivkovic A. Pellagrous encephalopathy presenting as alcohol withdrawal delirium: a case series and literature review. *Addict Sci Clin Pract* 7:12, 2012.
85. Becker DA, Ingala EE, Martinez-lage M, et al. Dry Beriberi and Wernicke's encephalopathy following gastric lap band surgery. *J Clin Neurosci* 19:1050–1052, 2012.
91. Schabelman E, Kuo D. Glucose before thiamine for Wernicke encephalopathy: a literature review. *J Emerg Med* 42:488–494, 2012.
97. Bajaj JS, Wade JB, Sanyal AJ. Spectrum of neurocognitive impairment in cirrhosis: implications for the assessment of hepatic encephalopathy. *Hepatology* 50:2014–2021, 2009.
101. McQuillan R, Jassal SV. Neuropsychiatric complications of chronic kidney disease. *Nat Rev Nephrol* 6:471–479, 2010.
106. Duning T, van den Heuvel I, Dickmann A, et al. Hypoglycemia aggravates critical illness-induced neurocognitive dysfunction. *Diabetes Care* 33:639–644, 2010.
130. Nishimura K, Omori M, Sato E, et al. Risperidone in the treatment of corticosteroid-induced mood disorders, manic/mixed episodes, in systemic lupus erythematosus: a case series. *Psychosomatics* 53:289–293, 2012.
132. Koch-Henriksen N, Sorensen PS. Why does the north-south gradient of incidence of multiple sclerosis seem to have disappeared on the northern hemisphere? *J Neurol Sci* 311:58–63, 2011.
139. Pompili M, Forte A, Palermo M, et al. Suicide risk in multiple sclerosis: a systematic review of current literature. *J Psychosom Res* 73:411–417, 2012.
151. Mancuso M, Orsucci D, Ienco EC, et al. Psychiatric involvement in adult patients with mitochondrial disease. *Neurol Sci* 3471–3474, 2013.
158. Robinson RG, Spalletta G. Poststroke depression: a review. *Can J Psychiatry* 55:341–349, 2013.
163. Pan A, Sun Q, Okereke OI, et al. Depression and risk of stroke morbidity and mortality: a meta-analysis and systematic review. *JAMA* 306:1241–1249, 2011.
179. Leypoldt F, Wandinger KP. Paraneoplastic neurological syndromes. *Clin Exp Immunol* 175:336–348, 2014.
186. Richard IH, McDermott MP, Kurlan R, et al. A randomized, double-blind, placebo-controlled trial of antidepressants in Parkinson disease. *Neurology* 78:1229–1236, 2012.

22   Sleep Disorders

Jeffrey B. Weilburg, MD, John W. Stakes, MD, Matt Bianchi, MD, and Ted Avi Gerstenblith, MD

KEY POINTS

- Insomnia, once regarded largely as the consequence of an underlying primary problem, is now regarded as a condition in its own right.
- Insomnia and depression are linked; the presence of one predicts the occurrence of the other. Treatment of insomnia co-morbid with depression produces better outcomes for depression.
- Excessive sleepiness is a common problem that often results from sleep apnea.
- Antidepressants and stimulants may provoke or exacerbate symptoms of insomnia, periodic limb movements of sleep, or restless legs syndrome.

OVERVIEW

Sleep physiology and the diagnosis and treatment of sleep disorders are important to the practice of psychiatry. The brain regions and neurotransmitters that regulate sleep are similar to those that regulate mood and cognition, and the medications (e.g., stimulants, sedative hypnotics) used to modulate these neurotransmitters are commonly used by patients. Patients with disturbances of mood or anxiety, or with other psychiatric symptoms, often experience disturbed sleep; in addition, those with insomnia, sleep apnea, narcolepsy, and other sleep disorders often have psychiatric symptoms. There is a bi-directional association between depression and sleep.[1] Insomnia may predict the development of depression[2] and when present may worsen depression outcomes.[3] Patients with depression have physiological sleep abnormalities, including reduced amounts of deep (delta) sleep; disturbances in the overall continuity and maintenance of sleep; and alterations in the timing, amount, and composition of rapid eye movement (REM) sleep.[4] Sleep loss may also precipitate affective dysregulation (e.g., mania).[5,6]

In recognition of the importance of sleep disorders to psychiatry, each version of the *Diagnostic and Statistical Manual of Mental Disorders* (DSM) since the third edition has included a section on sleep disorders. Sleep disorder centers in the United States are routinely staffed by psychiatrists and by psychologists, who play leading roles in the research efforts on sleep and its disorders.

THE HISTORY OF SLEEP RELATED TO PSYCHIATRY

Our modern understanding of the pathophysiology of sleep began in the early part of the twentieth century, with von Economo's autopsy observation of damage to the junction between the rostral brainstem and the basal forebrain in patients with *encephalitis lethargica*. He suggested that these areas were necessary for the maintenance of wakefulness and sleep. Since then, our understanding of the wakefulness centers in the posterior hypothalamus, of the "sleep center" in the anterior hypothalamus (the ventrolateral pre-optic area [VLPO]), and of their inter-dependence has advanced dramatically.[7]

The electroencephalogram (EEG), developed in the late 1920s by Berger, a German psychiatrist, has become an important tool for understanding sleep physiology. Current classification of sleep stages is in large part based on all-night EEG monitoring that was standardized by Rechstaffen and Kales in 1968. Rapid eye movement (REM) sleep was first observed in 1953, and the link between REM sleep and dreaming began to emerge several years later. This was the first definitive association between a mental process (dreaming) and a physiological process (REM sleep). The promise of gaining insight into the relation of normal and abnormal physiological processes was a key factor that attracted psychiatrists and psychologists to the study of sleep and its disorders.

In 1956 Burwell[8] noted abnormalities of sleep during respiration in obese patients and in 1965 Gastaut and colleagues[9] in France (and Jung and Kuhlo[10] in Germany) described the syndrome of sleep apnea. New disorders, such as REM sleep behavior disorder and nocturnal eating disorder, have been recognized within the past 25 years, underscoring the fact that the field of *sleep disorders* is relatively young and growing.

SLEEP PHYSIOLOGY

All-night sleep EEGs reveal a typical pattern of sleep ("the sleep architecture") that in normal humans involves an approximately 90-minute cycling between non–rapid eye movement (NREM) sleep and REM sleep (Figure 22-1). NREM sleep is now divided into stages N1 through N3 on the basis of the EEG, electromyogram (EMG), and eye movements. Stage N1 sleep is the "light" stage of sleep; individuals often deny being asleep if awakened from this stage. Stage N3 combines the previous NREM 3 and NREM 4 and is called *"delta sleep"* or *"slow wave sleep"* because of the presence of slow, high-voltage delta waves on the EEG. Delta sleep tends to predominate during the first part of the night, and diminishes with successive cycles of REM and NREM sleep. It is associated with: lowered blood pressure (BP), muscle tone, and temperature; growth hormone (GH) secretion; and increased arousal thresholds, and slow respiratory and heart rates. It may be a time of deep rest and tissue restoration.

REM sleep is a time of physiological activation. Pulse and BP are increased and variable during REM sleep. The EEG during this stage resembles the waking EEG. However, muscle

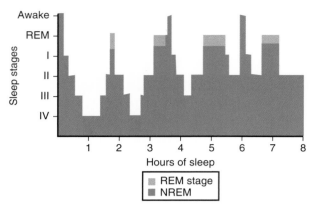

Figure 22-1. Normal adult sleep architecture. A schematic view of the REM and NREM sleep cycle through the night in a normal adult. Stage I makes up approximately 1.5% of the total sleep time, stage II about 50%, stages III and IV (together called delta sleep) about 20%, and REM between 20% and 25%. *(Adapted from Berger RJL. The sleep and dream cycle. In Kales A, editor: Sleep physiology and pathology: a symposium, Philadelphia, 1996, JB Lippincott.)*

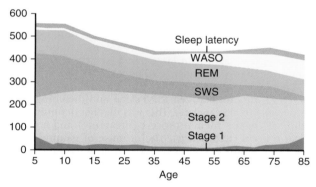

Figure 22-2. Sleep architecture: changes over the life cycle. REM, Rapid eye movement sleep; SWS, slow wave sleep; WASO, wake after sleep onset. *(From Ohayon MM, Carskadon MA, Guilleminault C, Vitiello MV. Meta-analysis of quantitative sleep parameters from childhood to old age in healthy individuals: developing normative sleep values across the human lifespan, Sleep 2004; 27:1255–1273.)*

tone is suppressed by the activation of cholinergic cells in the brainstem, producing inhibition of spinal motor neurons, which prevents the sleeper from acting out REM-related mental activity.

Sleep architecture changes throughout the normal life cycle (Figure 22-2).[11] Normal elders have somewhat less delta sleep, slightly less REM sleep, and lower sleep efficiency (i.e., more nocturnal awakenings and arousals) than normal middle-aged people.

The prevalence of sleep disorders of all types is increased in those over the age of 65 years. Complaints of insomnia (i.e., an inability to fall asleep or to stay asleep) are seen in up to 30% of the elderly, especially in women. Rates of restless legs syndrome (RLS) and periodic limb movements of sleep (PLMS) also are increased, as are rates of sleep-disordered breathing.[12,13] While age-related changes in sleep architecture may be related to loss of cells in the ventro-lateral pre-optic nucleus (VLPO), it is important to recognize that aging *per se* does not produce unsatisfactory sleep.

Circadian rhythms are regulated by the suprachiasmatic nuclei (SCN), a group of small nuclei (50,000 cells) in the anterior hypothalamus. The SCN generate their own rhythms that vary slightly from the 24-hour day based on a transcription–translation feedback system. The SCN also integrate photic and non-photic stimuli to keep the wake–sleep cycle properly and flexibly entrained with the demands of our environment. Photic stimuli arrive at the SCN via the retino-hypothalamic tract from the light-sensitive retinal cells of the eye (the melanopsin neurons, as well as the rods and cones). The SCN has outputs to the thalamus and the hypothalamus, which in turn drives cycling throughout the brain. In this way the SCN are critical to the regulation of melatonin synthesis and corticosteroid secretion. Melatonin production is greatest at night, during the dark, and is suppressed by exposure to light. Melatonin may be more associated with the absence of light than with sleep *per se*, as it is elevated during the night in both diurnal and nocturnal mammals. The primary function of melatonin appears to be the suppression of the alerting output of the SCN, but the role of melatonin in the regulation of sleep, and an understanding of the use of exogenous melatonin or melatonin receptor agonists as therapeutic agents, continues to evolve.

The control of sleep–wake function has historically been viewed as the result of two distinct processes: a homeostatic process and a circadian process.[14,15] In this model homeostatic sleep drive accumulates across periods of wakefulness. The pressure to sleep produced by the homeostatic drive is directly proportional to the duration of wakefulness (time since last sleep) and the duration of this prior sleep. Slow-wave activity when sleep eventually occurs is a marker of the degree of homeostatic drive. Although the neurobiological substrate of sleep drive is not fully understood, adenosine, an inhibitory neurotransmitter in the central nervous system (CNS), probably plays a role in the accumulation of sleep drive. Circadian factors may offset or augment the homeostatic drive, depending on clock time. During the daylight hours, and most powerfully in the early morning, the SCN emits an alerting pulse that opposes the drive for sleep. This normally allows for waking in the morning and maintenance of wakefulness across the day. Lesions to the SCN may produce increased sleep time over the 24-hour period, as well as an inability to sustain prolonged periods of wakefulness. Timing mismatches between the homeostatic drive to sleep and the alerting pulse of the circadian processes may produce difficulty sleeping during the day for people who work at night, and these are probably related to the pathogenesis of shift-work sleep disorder,[16,17] as well as some of the sleep disturbances experienced by the blind.[18]

EXAMINATION OF SLEEP AND SLEEP-RELATED COMPLAINTS
Polysomnography

Objective measurement of nocturnal sleep is obtained in the clinical sleep laboratory by the use of an all-night sleep study, or polysomnogram (PSG). Patients typically arrive in the sleep laboratory in the evening, between 8:00 and 10:00 PM. Trained technicians apply electrodes and other sensors to facilitate data collection. A limited number of EEG are applied with paste to the head; more may be used if nocturnal seizures are suspected. Electrodes on the skin near the orbits record eye movements. EMG electrodes, used to measure muscle tone and to observe muscle twitches, are applied to the legs and the chin. Electrocardiogram (ECG) electrodes are placed on the chest. A thermistor or nasal pressure gauge is placed at the nares, and strain gauge or other device is placed around the chest and the abdomen, to measure respiration rate, airflow, and respiratory effort. A pulse oximeter to measure blood hemoglobin oxygenation is placed on the earlobe or on the finger. Video monitoring allows nocturnal behaviors to be correlated with the EEG waveforms and other measures.

Patients can usually be desensitized to use of a mask before the study begins in cases where apnea is suspected.

The amount, time-to-onset (latency), and distribution of REM sleep, as well as the relative distribution of stages N1–N3 sleep, are manually scored by sleep technicians, as are EEG arousals, limb motor twitches, ECG changes, and various interruptions of breathing and their consequences (such as oxygen desaturation). All of these metrics contribute to the physician interpretation.

Home apnea test are becoming increasingly available, but this approach has strengths and limitations. The American Academy of Sleep Medicine guidelines recommend against using home kits for general screening or low-risk patients, for patients with significant medical co-morbidities, or for those with sleep disorders, such as insomnia or parasomnia, and suggest standard (in-lab) study when home-testing is negative.[19-21]

Multiple Sleep Latency Test

Patients being evaluated for narcolepsy or other forms of hypersomnolence may undergo a multiple sleep latency test (MSLT). This test is also done in the sleep laboratory, after completing a PSG the night prior. The procedure involves five nap opportunities spread throughout the day. Patients are awakened after napping for 20 minutes, and then kept awake (without stimulants) between nap opportunities. The average sleep latency is recorded, with values below 5–6 minutes regarded as consistent with significant physiological pathological sleepiness. REM latency (i.e., the time from sleep onset to REM onset) is also recorded; the presence of two or more sleep-onset REM (SOREM) periods, along with pathological sleepiness in the appropriate clinical setting, is considered diagnostic of narcolepsy.

In contrast to the overnight PSG, in which the usual medications are typically continued, the MSLT results can be confounded by certain medications. Most antidepressants suppress REM sleep, and patients who use stimulants (whether caffeine or a prescription agent) can exhibit rebound sleepiness with abrupt discontinuation. For these reasons, if it is clinically safe and appropriate to wean these drugs, it is usually recommended to do so at least 2 weeks before testing.

Patient-completed Rating Scales

A number of patient- and clinician-rated scales have been used to measure sleepiness and the symptoms of insomnia, such as the Epworth Sleepiness Scale (ESS) (Table 22-1), the Insomnia Severity Index and the Pittsburgh Sleep Quality Index. While such scales can help clinicians evaluate a patient's sleep-related complaints and sleep habits, no scale by itself can establish or rule out any diagnosis.

CLASSIFICATION OF SLEEP DISORDERS

There are three major current classification systems for sleep disorders: the *Diagnostic and Statistical Manual of Mental Disorders, Fifth Edition* (DSM-5),[22] created by the American Psychiatric Association, The *International Classification of Sleep Disorders, Second edition* (ICSD-2),[23] created by the American Academy of Sleep Medicine, and the *International Statistical Classification of Diseases and Related Health Problems, Tenth edition*[24] created by the World Health Organization. DSM-5 is intended for use by psychiatrists and general medical practitioners. It tends to drop the etiologic assumptions of DSM-IV (e.g., it does not include "primary insomnia" or "insomnia secondary to a general medical condition") and it "lumps" various insomnia sub-types ("psychophysiologic" and "paradoxical" insomnia) that are "split" in ISCD-2 and DSM-IV. ICSD-2 is intended for use primarily by sleep disorders experts. It provides more detail about each condition, and tends to "split" conditions into sub-types. This chapter is guided by the DSM-5 approach, but it also uses the ICSD, in some sections, such as insomnia. Outlines of the DSM and ICSD-2 classifications are found in Tables 22-2 and Box 22-1, along with a table showing how DSM-IV maps to DSM-5.

INSOMNIA

DSM-5 defines insomnia as "dissatisfaction with sleep quantity or quality with complaints of difficulty initiating or maintaining sleep" that is "accompanied by clinically significant distress or impairment in social, occupational, or other important areas of functioning." (see Box 22-2). Insomnia may be co-morbid with other psychiatric or medical conditions. DSM-5 specifies that the sleep difficulty occurs on 3 or more nights for 3 or more months, despite an adequate opportunity for sleep, and the absence of another primary sleep disorder (such as sleep apnea) or substance use; in addition, it cannot be explained by a co-existing medical or psychiatric problem (such as mania or hyperthyroidism). An alternative, but related, definition of insomnia is provided by ICSD-2, which regards insomnia as a repeated difficulty with sleep initiation, duration, consolidation, or quality of sleep that occurs despite

TABLE 22-1 The Epworth Sleepiness Scale (ESS)

How likely are you to doze off or fall asleep in the following situations, in contrast to just feeling tired? This refers to your usual way of life in recent times. Even if you have not done some of these things recently, try to work out how they would have affected you. Use the following scale to choose the *most appropriate number* for each situation:

1 = *low* chance of dozing
2 = *moderate* chance of dozing
3 = *high* chance of dozing

Situations	Score
Sitting and reading	___
Watching TV	___
Sitting, inactive, in a public place (e.g., a movie theater or a meeting)	___
As a passenger in a car for an hour without a break	___
Lying down to rest in the afternoon when circumstances permit	___
Sitting and talking to someone	___
Sitting quietly after lunch without alcohol	___
In a car, while stopped for a few minutes in the traffic	___
TOTAL SCORE:	___

Score ≥ 10 suggests need for evaluation for excessive sleepiness.

TABLE 22-2 Outlines of Sleep Disorders as Classified by DSM-IV and DSM-5

DSM-IV Classification	DSM-5 Classification

Primary sleep disorders
Dyssomnias
  Primary insomnia
  Primary hypersomnia
	Insomnia disorder (see Box 22-3)
	  With mental co-morbidity
	  With other medical co-morbidity
	  With other sleep disorder
	Hypersomnolence disorder (see Box 22-4)
	  With mental co-morbidity
	  With medical condition
	  With another sleep disorder

Narcolepsy	Narcolepsy (see Box 22-5)

Breathing-related sleep disorder	Breathing-related sleep disorders (see Boxes 22-6, 22-7, and 22-8)
	  Obstructive sleep apnea hypopnea
	  Central sleep apnea
	  Sleep-related hypoventilation

Circadian rhythm sleep disorder	Circadian rhythm sleep–wake disorders (see Box 22-9)
	  Delayed sleep phase type
	  Advanced sleep phase type
	  Irregular sleep–wake type
	  Non-24-hour sleep–wake type
	  Shift-work type

Dyssomnia NOS	

Parasomnias
  Nightmare disorder
  Sleep terror disorder
  Sleepwalking disorder
Parasomnia NOS
Sleep disorders related to another mental condition
Other sleep disorders
  Due to general medical condition
  Substance-induced sleep disorder
	Parasomnias (see Boxes 22-10, 22-11, and 22-12)
	  Nightmare disorder
	  REM sleep behavior disorder
	  NREM sleep arousal disorders
	Restless legs syndrome (see Box 22-13)
	Substance/medication-induced sleep disorder (see Box 22-14)

an adequate opportunity for sleep that produces daytime impairment.

DSM-5 describes sleep-onset insomnia (or initial insomnia) as involving difficulty falling asleep, sleep maintenance insomnia (or middle insomnia) as involving frequent or prolonged awakenings throughout the night, and late insomnia as involving early-morning awakening with an inability to return to sleep. It defines difficulty falling asleep as a subjective sleep latency for ≥ 20–30 minutes, and difficulty maintaining sleep as waking after 20–30 minutes. Early morning awakening involves spontaneous waking 30 minutes or more before the desired wake time, and before total sleep time reaches 6.5 hours.

Surveys find that 10%–15% of the general population has chronic insomnia. The prevalence of insomnia is higher for those seen in general medical and psychiatric settings, where approximately 25%–35% of patients have at least transient insomnia.[5]

The basis of chronic insomnia is incompletely understood. Polysomnography and other objective measures of sleep disruption often fail to establish the etiology of insomnia. However, data from other sources suggest that patients with insomnia suffer excessive levels of arousal, which may produce the perception of not sleeping. Evidence of excessive arousal has been found on analysis of EEG spectra,[25] on positron emission tomography (PET) scans,[26] and on markers of metabolic rate.[27]

Insomnia is associated with significant health care costs. It has been estimated that $12 billion is spent each year in the United States for health care services, and $2 billion is spent on medications to treat insomnia.[28] Insomnia also has a significant impact on quality of life (QOL); patients with insomnia have as much dysfunction as do patients with major depression or congestive heart failure (CHF).[29,30] Finally,

patients with insomnia may be at increased risk of sustaining a motor vehicle or other type of accident.[31]

A strong bi-directional relationship exists between insomnia and depression. Insomnia is one of the core symptoms of depression listed in DSM-5, and patients with depression commonly experience one or more symptoms of insomnia. Depressed outpatients experience similar trouble falling asleep and staying asleep. Insomnia may be an early symptom or perhaps even a predictor of depression for some patients.[32]

Insomnia may have an impact on depression-related outcomes. Depressed patients with insomnia tend to have worse outcomes for depression, as evidenced by higher rates of recurrence of depression, and higher rates of suicide than those without insomnia.[1,2] Insomnia may persist as a separate condition when the symptoms of depression remit or fully resolve[33,34]; the presence of insomnia despite treatment for depression may predict return of the depression.[35]

ICSD-2 includes several sub-types of insomnia. Habitual short-sleepers have no sleep-related symptoms, and do not have insomnia. Adjustment ("acute") insomnia occurs in response to a known stressor. In contrast, idiopathic insomnia, also known as chronic or primary insomnia, begins in childhood, without a known stressor, and continues throughout adulthood. The percentage of delta sleep may be reduced. However, some patients may have normal or relatively normal PSGs, and there are no known biological markers of this disorder.

The term "paradoxical insomnia" may be used to describe "sleep state misperception", or "subjective complaint of sleep initiation and maintenance without objective findings"; it is diagnosed when a patient complains of severe difficulty falling or staying asleep, despite a normal or relatively normal PSG, MSLT, bed partner report, and relatively normal daytime performance. These patients may be hypervigilant, and may worry

BOX 22-1 ICSD-2 Classification of Sleep Disorders

I. INSOMNIA

Insomnia (acute insomnia)
Psychophysiological insomnia
Paradoxical insomnia
Idiopathic insomnia
Insomnia due to a mental disorder
Inadequate sleep hygiene
Behavioral insomnia of childhood
Insomnia due to a drug or substance
Insomnia due to a medical condition
Insomnia not due to a substance or known physiological condition, unspecified (non-organic insomnia NOS)
Physiological (organic) insomnia, unspecified

II. SLEEP-RELATED BREATHING DISORDERS

Central sleep apnea syndromes
- Primary central sleep apnea
- Central sleep apnea due to high-altitude periodic breathing
- Central sleep apnea due to a medical condition (not Cheyne-Stokes)
- Central sleep apnea due to a drug or substance
- Primary sleep apnea of infancy (formerly primary sleep apnea of newborn)

Obstructive sleep apnea syndromes
- Obstructive sleep apnea, adult
- Obstructive sleep apnea, pediatric

III. SLEEP-RELATED HYPOVENTILATION/HYPOXEMIC SYNDROMES

Sleep-related non-obstructive alveolar hypoventilation, idiopathic
Congenital central alveolar hypoventilation syndrome
Sleep-related hypoventilation/hypoxemia due to a medical condition
- Sleep-related hypoventilation/hypoxemia due to pulmonary parenchymal or vascular pathology
- Sleep-related hypoventilation/hypoxemia due to lower airway obstruction
- Sleep-related hypoventilation/hypoxemia due to neuromuscular and chest wall disorders

Other sleep-related breathing disorder
Sleep apnea/sleep-related breathing disorder, unspecified

IV. HYPERSOMNIAS OF CENTRAL ORIGIN NOT DUE TO A CIRCADIAN RHYTHM SLEEP DISORDER, SLEEP-RELATED BREATHING DISORDER, OR OTHER CAUSE OF DISTURBED NOCTURNAL SLEEP

Narcolepsy with cataplexy
Narcolepsy without cataplexy
Narcolepsy due to a medical condition
Narcolepsy, unspecified
Recurrent hypersomnia
- Kleine-Levin syndrome
- Menstrual-related hypersomnia
- Idiopathic hypersomnia with long sleep time
- Idiopathic hypersomnia without long sleep time
- Behaviorally-induced insufficient sleep syndrome
- Hypersomnia due to a medical condition
- Hypersomnia due to a drug or substance
- Hypersomnia not due to a substance or known physiological condition (non-organic hypersomnia NOS)
- Physiological (organic) hypersomnia, unspecified (organic hypersomnia NOS)

V. CIRCADIAN RHYTHM SLEEP DISORDERS

Circadian rhythm sleep disorder, delayed sleep phase type (delayed sleep phase disorder)
Circadian rhythm sleep disorder, advanced sleep phase type (advanced sleep phase disorder)
Circadian rhythm sleep disorder, irregular sleep–wake type (irregular sleep–wake rhythm)
Circadian rhythm sleep disorder, free-running type (non-entrained type)
Circadian rhythm sleep disorder, jet lag type (jet lag disorder)
Circadian rhythm sleep disorder, shift-work type (shift-work disorder)
Circadian rhythm sleep disorder due to a medical condition
Other circadian rhythm sleep disorder (circadian rhythm disorder NOS)
Other circadian rhythm sleep disorder due to a drug or substance

VI. PARASOMNIAS

Disorders of arousal (from NREM sleep)
- Confusional arousals
- Sleepwalking
- Sleep terrors

Parasomnias usually associated with REM sleep
- REM sleep behavior disorder (including parasomnia overlap disorder and status dissociatus)
- Recurrent isolated sleep paralysis
- Nightmare disorder

Other parasomnias
- Sleep-related dissociative disorders
- Sleep-related groaning (catathrenia)
- Exploding head syndrome
- Sleep-related hallucinations
- Sleep-related eating disorder
- Parasomnia, unspecified
- Parasomnia due to a drug or substance
- Parasomnia due to a medical condition

VII. SLEEP-RELATED MOVEMENT DISORDERS

Restless legs syndrome
Periodic limb movement disorder
Sleep-related leg cramps
Sleep-related bruxism
Sleep-related rhythm movement disorder
Sleep-related movement disorder, unspecified
Sleep-related movement disorder due to a drug or substance
Sleep-related movement disorder due to a medical condition

VIII. OTHER SLEEP DISORDERS

Other physiological (organic) sleep disorder
Other sleep disorder not due to a substance or known physiological condition
Environmental sleep disorder

IX. SLEEP DISORDERS ASSOCIATED WITH CONDITIONS CLASSIFIABLE ELSEWHERE

Fatal familial insomnia
Fibromyalgia
Sleep-related epilepsy
Sleep-related headaches
Sleep-related gastroesophageal reflux disease
Sleep-related coronary artery ischemia
Sleep-related abnormal swallowing, choking, and laryngospasm

NOS, Not otherwise specified; NREM, non-rapid eye movement; REM, rapid eye movement.

TABLE 22-3 Medications and Substances That Induce Insomnia

Substance Type	Notes
Stimulants	Used as medications and as substances of abuse (including caffeine found in coffee, tea, chocolate, and cola)
Antihypertensives	Including alpha- and beta-blockers, calcium channel blockers, methyldopa, and reserpine
Asthma agents and bronchodilators	Including theophylline and albuterol
Corticosteroids	
Decongestants	Including pseudoephedrine, phenylpropanolamine, and phenylephrine
Antidepressants	Including fluoxetine, bupropion, venlafaxine, phenelzine, and Parnate (tranylcypromine)
Tobacco/nicotine	In cigarettes, cigars, and pipes
Alcohol	

TABLE 22-4 Medical Problems That Produce Insomnia

Medical Problem	Examples
Pain, acute or chronic	Arthritis, low back pain, cancer pain of any type, headache, fibromyalgia, burns, facial or dental pain, neuropathies
Cardiac/vascular disorders	Paroxysmal nocturnal dyspnea, peripheral vascular disease with cramps in extremities, congestive heart failure with orthopnea
Endocrine disorders	Menopause (with hot flashes and mood changes), hyperthyroidism or hypothyroidism (especially if associated with sleep apnea); diabetes (if associated with polyuria, nocturnal hypoglycemia or hyperglycemia and associated autonomic changes, neuropathic pain)
Gastrointestinal disorders	Gastroesophageal reflux disease of any cause, ulcers
Neurological disorders	Dementia of any type; strokes, Parkinson's and other neuromuscular degenerative diseases
Pulmonary disorders	Chronic obstructive pulmonary disease, nocturnal asthma, sleep-related laryngospasm, and rhinitis/sinusitis
Urological disorders	Uremia, nocturia, and dysuria

Insomnia may be produced by a wide range of medications and substances (Table 22-3) and medical problems (Table 22-4).

Principles of Management

Polysomnography is not routinely recommended as part of the work-up, but it can be considered for chronic or refractory cases, in part because patients with insomnia have a higher prevalence of obstructive sleep apnea (OSA), and some sedative hypnotics may have the potential to worsen OSA. In addition, a PSG may reveal periodic limb movements of sleep. Finally, a PSG can be enlightening regarding the issue of sleep misperception.

The treatment for insomnia is often multi-modal, including both medications and cognitive-behavioral measures (self-help strategies, e.g., improvements in sleep hygiene) to improve the subjective quality of sleep, relieve distress related to sleep, and to improve daytime functioning. Treatment of *transient insomnia* may simply require an explanation of the impact of stress on life, and supportive counseling to reduce anxiety. When hypnotic medications are used, their course should be of short duration. When behavioral methods do not

excessively about the impact of perceived loss of sleep on their longevity. Many patients with insomnia overestimate the degree of their sleep disturbance. This observation is critically important since the diagnosis and management of insomnia are based entirely on self-report.[36]

ICSD-2 lists the sub-type, "Psychophysiological insomnia" (formerly known as" learned or conditioned insomnia") as a patient who shows an obsessional focus on, and anxiety about, falling asleep; it produces arousal, and becomes associated with sleep initiation. Patients report that they sleep well when on vacation or away from their bedroom, but become stirred up when they try to fall asleep in their usual sleep setting. Some patients may even sleep better in the lab setting, a phenomenon known as the reverse first-night effect, perhaps due to the absence of negative associations linked with their home environment.

suffice for chronic insomnia, and/or the goal is short-term reduction of sleep-related dissatisfaction, pharmacologic therapy is a reasonable approach while remaining mindful of the potential adverse effects.

Medications for Insomnia

Over-the-counter (OTC) sleep aids, which usually contain a sedating antihistamine as the active component, are widely used by the general population.[37] However, sedating antihistamines may not reduce sleep latency, increase sleep duration, or improve daytime function.[38] They may also produce delirium and disturbances of gait and memory, especially in the elderly. The use of these agents remains controversial.

Hypnotics should be used with caution, and in the lowest effective dose; their use should be re-evaluated frequently, and attempts to wean them should be made. Older patients, their families, and caregivers (e.g., nurses and aids in nursing homes) should be warned of the risks, and fall precautions should be used.

Patients who engage in substance use and/or abuse need to achieve abstinence from alcohol and "recreational" stimulants, including caffeine and tobacco as a first step, before hypnotic and related agents are used. Patients with current or past histories of abuse of alcohol or other drugs or substances should generally not receive a benzodiazepine or related agent. Patients without a personal or family history of current or past substance abuse are at low risk for addiction to hypnotics when these agents are appropriately prescribed.

Trazodone appears to be the agent most frequently used for insomnia, but the dose-related safety and efficacy of trazodone as a hypnotic has not been formally established.[39] There is evidence that 50 mg of trazodone is as effective as 10 mg of zolpidem during the first, but not the second, week of use for a group of patients with insomnia.[40]

Tricyclic antidepressants (TCAs) are also frequently used for insomnia, as they improve sleep continuity, reduce sleep latency, increase total sleep time, and improve daytime function. Data on the optimal dosing for TCAs for insomnia are also limited, but low doses appear to be free of adverse anticholinergic side effects (which would otherwise make tricyclic agents ill-advised for use, especially in the elderly). TCAs (e.g., doxepin, amitriptyline) are toxic in overdose and have potent anticholinergic and antihistaminic effects; they may produce delirium, as well as cause problems with gait and cognition, especially in the elderly.[41,42]

Quetiapine and other atypical antipsychotics should not be considered first-line treatment for insomnia. These agents may be chosen by some clinicians for patients at risk for addiction, in the presence of agitation or psychosis, or for cases of resistant insomnia; however, caution is advised. When these agents are used to manage insomnia, doses far lower than doses for primary indications are typically provided.

Table 22-5 lists the agents approved by the Food and Drug Administration (FDA) for the treatment of insomnia. Among these, the older agents (triazolam, quazepam, temazepam, and flurazepam) are benzodiazepines. The newer agents (zolpidem [Ambien], eszopiclone [Lunesta], and zaleplon [Sonata]) work at the benzodiazepine receptor complex, and they are often called benzodiazepine receptor agonists (BZRAs). The newer agents may stimulate only a subset of benzodiazepine receptors (e.g., the benzodiazepine alpha$_1$ receptor), whereas the older agents may be less selective at these sites.[43] The clinical significance of the stimulation of a subset of receptors remains undetermined. The newer agents have been shown to be safe and effective for long-term (i.e., 6 months) use in insomnia and may have some subjective advantages compared to the older agents.[44,45] The labeling of these agents does not specifically state that these agents are approved only for short-term use. The BZRAs appear to have a low potential for abuse and dependence, but like the typical benzodiazepines are labeled as Class IV agents by the FDA. Most important, all of the classic benzodiazepines (with the exception of triazolam) have long or relatively long elimination half-lives, and may thus produce daytime sedation, and

TABLE 22-5 Agents Approved by the US Food and Drug Administration for the Treatment of Insomnia

Medication*	Duration of Action	Half-life (hrs)	Adult Dose (mg)	Indication	Comments
Temazepam (Restoril)	Intermediate	8–15	7.5–30	SMI	
Estazolam (Prosom)	Intermediate	10–24	0.5–2	SMI	
Triazolam (Halcion)	Short	2–5	0.125–0.25	SII	Potential interaction with nefazodone, ketoconazole, or other inducers of CYP3A4
Flurazepam (Dalmane)	Very long	48–120	15–30	SMI	
Quazepam (Doral)	Very long	48–120	15–30	SMI	
Eszopiclone (Lunesta)	Intermediate	5–7	1–3	SMI	Potential interaction with nefazodone, ketoconazole, or other inducers of CYP3A4
Zolpidem (Ambien, Ambien CR)	Intermediate	3	5–10	SII	Possible interaction with CYP3A4-inducing drugs; may produce next am sedation especially in women
	Intermediate	7	6.12–12.5	SII, SMI	
Zaleplon (Sonata)	Ultrashort	1	5–20	SII, SMI	Possible interaction with CYP3A4-inducing drugs; may be given for awakenings occurring during the night
Ramelteon (Rozerem)	Short	2–5	8 mg	SII	Potential interaction with fluvoxamine and other agents metabolized by CYP1A2

*Quazepam, flurazepam, estazolam, temazepam, and triazolam are all "classic" benzodiazepines. Zolpidem, zaleplon, and eszopiclone are benzodiazepine receptor agonists.
SII, Sleep initiation insomnia; SMI, sleep maintenance insomnia.

in some cases daytime impairment. Zaleplon is shorter-acting (2–3 hours), making it useful for difficultly limited to falling asleep or if the patient awakens in the middle of the night; it is less likely to cause residual sedation but may not prevent premature awakening. A sub-lingual zolpidem preparation, zolpidem tartrate (Intermezzo), is also approved for middle-of-the-night awakening. Anterograde amnesia, sleepwalking, sleep-related eating disorder, and sleep-driving without conscious awareness have all been reported with use of these agents. Use in frail elderly nursing-home residents is associated with increased risk of hip fracture.

Choice of agent can be based on cost and desired onset, duration of action, and route of metabolism. The short-acting drugs are best prescribed for those whose primary problem is *falling* asleep. The *intermediate-acting* agents may be useful for those patients who complain of problems staying asleep. *Long-acting agents* are considered when daytime anxiety compounds discomfort.

Barbiturates and chloral hydrate, while they are sedating, are not included here because they pose greater risks for lethal overdose, for dependence, and for addiction than the other agents listed.

Ramelteon is a specific agonist of melatonin receptors in the SCN. Ramelteon reduces sleep latency, but it does not improve sleep maintenance. Doses of 8 mg/day are effective; higher doses provide no additional benefit. Some patients' sleep begins to improve after several weeks of nightly use, so ramelteon may be continued if there are no adverse effects, even if there is no immediate improvement in sleep. Ramelteon does not seem to produce rebound and may be used several times a week for more than 3 months. Abuse potential appears very low; it is not a controlled substance.

Melatonin is available OTC in immediate and sustained-release formulations in a variety of doses. Clinical trials of melatonin have been mixed in part because of variation in dosing and timing. The best evidence exists for delayed sleep phase syndrome, and the combination of properly timed melatonin and light therapy is the cornerstone of chrono-therapy strategies. In general, the timing for delayed sleep phase patients is 2–3 hours before habitual bedtime, while for patients with insomnia not related to circadian delay, administration closer to bedtime is more appropriate.[46,47] Other supplements (including valerian, tryptophan, kava, chamomile, passion flower) make anecdotal claims for insomnia. Despite the wide availability of herbals and supplements, they are not well-studied, with the exception of valerian, which did not show significant benefit in a meta-analysis. Although it is not unreasonable for the willing patient to try these options, careful attention to drug interactions is necessary. For example, melatonin may alter warfarin levels.[48]

Although many patients treat their insomnia (self-medicate) with alcohol, it produces fragmented sleep. Alcohol should be avoided in patients with insomnia, especially in those who use hypnotics, as it increases the potential for hypnotic toxicity.

POTENTIAL ADVERSE EFFECTS OF HYPNOTICS
Rebound Insomnia

Rebound insomnia is a worsening of sleep beyond the level of sleep disturbance seen prior to treatment and should be differentiated from a return to pre-treatment status. Long-acting medications do not produce rebound as their blood level gradually declines across several nights. The potential for rebound can be reduced when short-acting agents are tapered, and when they are used on alternative nights, rather than being abruptly discontinued.[49,50]

Falls

Some studies suggest that the BZRAs may increase the risk of falls, especially in the elderly. Subsequent fractures are a serious and potentially life-threatening concern. Increased fall risk may extend to the day after hypnotic use. Controversy continues regarding the relative contributions to fall risk of sedative hypnotics and insomnia itself. Multi-modal treatment designed to reduce the severity of insomnia is especially important in the elderly and others at risk for falls (e.g., patients with balance or gait disturbance, lower limb neurological problems, or hypotension). Alternatives to hypnotic agents, including CBT, should be used wherever possible.[51–54]

Cognitive and Performance Disturbances

All BZRAs interfere with cognitive performance and impair motor performance. Patients may be at greatest risk for falls if they awaken and ambulate while these agents are at peak levels. Some patients cannot recall events in the hours or day following the use of BZRAs (especially the high-potency short-duration agents), even though their behavior may appear normal; others have abnormal nocturnal behaviors (such as nocturnal binge eating and driving) following the use of hypnotics. The FDA noted that all sleeping aids confer risks regarding next-morning impairment, and has reduced the recommended zolpidem dosing for women for immediate-release from 10 mg to 5 mg, and for extended-release from 12.5 mg to 6.25 mg.

Behavior Management

Pharmacological treatment can provide immediate relief of insomnia, but may be insufficient to change the habits, beliefs, and behaviors developed by patients, especially those with chronic insomnia. Behavioral approaches may address these issues and may provide effective, long-lasting relief from insomnia for many patients. Behavioral approaches can also provide relief for insomnia (Table 22-6). Formal cognitive-behavioral therapy for insomnia (CBTi) is a well-developed, structured approach that integrates sleep education and sleep hygiene with various behavioral techniques (e.g., stimulus control techniques, sleep restriction therapy, cognitive therapy, and relaxation). CBTi has an efficacy at least equal to hypnotic medication in comparative trials. It may be especially well suited as a first-line of therapy for patients with chronic insomnia, current or past histories of substance abuse, and for

TABLE 22-6 Behavioral Approaches to Insomnia

Approach	Explanation
Cognitive-behavioral therapy (CBT)	Can be used to identify and change maladaptive beliefs, behaviors, and affects around sleep
Progressive muscle relaxation	Can help reduce some of the excess stimulation experience by some patients with insomnia
Stimulus-control therapy	Can help break the association between bed and sleeplessness, and its associated frustrations that can develop in patients with insomnia
Sleep-restriction therapy	Helps patients limit the time spent in bed to the time they actually sleep
Attention to good sleep hygiene	Helps patients wind down, find a suitable sleep environment, get reasonable amounts of well-timed exercise, and avoid substances (such as caffeine) that may interfere with sleep

many patients with anxiety and character disorders. CBTi may be implemented concurrently with medication, or, in some cases, after medication has produced acute improvement and is then weaned. There is some evidence that continuation of CBTi after discontinuation of medication has better long-term outcomes than either CBTi or medication alone.

CBTi is typically provided by specially-trained psychologists, access to whom may be limited. Nonetheless, elements of CBTi can be implemented in most primary care settings with good results. The strategies employed include: education regarding good sleep hygiene, reassurance that one does not need 8 hours of sleep every night, avoidance of trying too hard to fall asleep, relaxation techniques, stimulus control to break associations among anxiety and sleep-onset-related problems, and sleep restriction therapy. Sleep restriction may be especially important for older adults who experience reduced sleep capacity. On-line versions of CBTi have been developed as well.

HYPERSOMNIA AND EXCESSIVE SLEEPINESS

Hypersomnolence includes symptoms of excessive sleep (e.g., extended nocturnal sleep or involuntary daytime sleep), deteriorated quality of wakefulness (e.g., difficulty awakening) and sleep inertia (i.e., a period of impaired performance and reduced vigilance following awakening). Sleep inertia is also known as sleep drunkenness; it may last for minutes to hours, and be associated with inappropriate, at times aggressive behaviors, confusion and ataxia. Patients with hypersomnolence may have "non-restorative sleep", which describes excess sleepiness and associated complaints of fatigue and functional impairment that appear despite the main sleep period lasting for > 9 hours. Such patients may take long (> 1 hour) daytime naps, which are also un-restorative.

Complaints of excessive daytime sleepiness (EDS) are common (found on surveys in up to 20% of the adult population). Men and women are equally affected. Onset tends to be in late adolescence or early adulthood; the course tends to be slow and progressive over several months, and persistent. Patients who sleep > 9 hours/night but with no daytime symptoms may be normal "long sleepers".

Hypersomnia may be due to various medical conditions (such as Parkinson's disease, hypothyroidism, liver or renal failure, adrenal insufficiency, head trauma, Prader–Willi syndrome, myotonic dystrophy, fragile X syndrome, Niemann–Pick type C, and Norrie disease), and various CNS lesions, often involving the hypothalamus. Drugs or substances (such as benzodiazepines, opiates, and anti-parkinsonian medications) may produce EDS, as can use of OTC medications, dietary supplements, and exposure to toxins (such as organic solvents).

In rare instances, hypersomnia (sleep duration between 16 and 18 hours per day) may be related to Kleine–Levin syndrome. Episodes of recurrent hypersomnia, which can last several weeks, alternate with normal sleep. During an episode, patients may be confused while awake and may binge eat or become hypersexual, aggressive, or irritable. DSM-5 Criteria for Hypersomnolence Disorder can be located in Box 22-3.

NARCOLEPSY

The core features of narcolepsy are an inability to maintain wakefulness during the day and to maintain sleep at night. The intrusion of sleep into wakefulness produces EDS and sleep attacks. Left untreated, those with narcolepsy tend to fall asleep several times each day. The tendency to fall asleep may be highest during periods of quiet or boredom, but may occur even during activity (such as driving, walking, or working),

> **BOX 22-3** DSM-5 Diagnostic Criteria: Hypersomnolence Disorder (780.54 (G47.10))
>
> - Self-reported excessive sleepiness (hypersomnolence) despite a main sleep period lasting at least 7 hours, with at least one of the following symptoms:
>   1. Recurrent periods of sleep or lapses into sleep within the same day
>   2. A prolonged main sleep episode of more than 9 hours per day that is non-restorative (i.e., unrefreshing)
>   3. Difficulty being fully awake after abrupt awakening.
> - The hypersomnolence occurs at least three times per week, for at least 3 months.
> - The hypersomnolence is accompanied by significant distress or impairment in cognitive, social, occupational, or other important areas of functioning.
> - The hypersomnolence is not better explained by and does not occur exclusively during the course of another sleep disorder (e.g., narcolepsy, breathing-related sleep disorder, circadian rhythm sleepwalk disorder, or a parasomnia).
> - The hypersomnolence is not attributable to the physiological effects of a substance (e.g., a drug abuse, a medication).
> - Co-existing mental and medical disorders do not adequately explain the predominant complaint of hypersomnolence.
>
>   *Specify* if:
>
> **With mental disorder**, including substance use disorders
> **With medical condition**
> **With another sleep disorder.**
> - **Coding note:** The code 780.54 (G47.10) applies to all three specifiers. Code also the relevant associated mental disorder, medical condition, or other sleep disorder immediately after the code for hypersomnolence disorder in order to indicate the association.
>
>   *Specify* if:
>
> **Acute:** Duration of less than 1 month
> **Subacute:** Duration of 1–3 months
> **Persistent:** Duration of more than 3 months.
>
>   *Specify* current severity:
>   Specify severity based on degree of difficulty maintaining daytime alertness as manifested by the occurrence of multiple attacks of irresistible sleepiness within any given day occurring, for example, while sedentary, driving, visiting with friends, or working:
>
> **Mild:** Difficulty maintaining daytime alertness 1–2 days/week
> **Moderate:** Difficulty maintaining daytime alertness 3–4 days/week
> **Severe:** Difficulty maintaining daytime alertness 5–7 days/week.
>
> *Reprinted with permission from the* Diagnostic and statistical manual of mental disorders, *ed 5, (Copyright 2013). American Psychiatric Association.*

when falling asleep is highly inappropriate, even life-threatening. The sudden onset of irresistible sleep produces a sleep attack. Sleep attacks are usually brief (less than 1 hour), and leave patients feeling refreshed. Their sleepiness, however, recurs within several hours, so planned napping may be helpful; however, by itself it is not typically a sufficient treatment.

Individuals with narcolepsy tend to sleep a normal amount during each 24-hour day. Improvement of their disturbed nocturnal sleep may reduce, but not completely resolve, EDS.[55,56]

Narcolepsy occurs with cataplexy (a sudden, brief decrease in or loss of muscle tone triggered by emotion) in at least 50% of narcoleptics. Patients may report feeling the weakness begin gradually over seconds and may try to resist. Tone may be lost in selected muscles (e.g., droop of an eyelid or jaw), or it may be widely distributed (producing collapse). The diaphragm is unaffected, so patients continue to breathe even during a severe attack. Importantly, consciousness is preserved, which distinguishes the attacks from syncope or seizure. Muscle tone begins to return after a few seconds to a few minutes, and recovery is complete. Prolonged cataplexy may occur, especially if agents (such as antidepressants) used to manage cataplexy are suddenly withdrawn. If an episode of cataplexy is prolonged, a REM-onset sleep episode may arise. The frequency of cataplexy is variable, and may decrease with age. Cataplexy may occur with, or several years after, the onset of the other symptoms of narcolepsy. The emotional triggers of cataplectic attacks often involve "positive" emotions (such as laughter), but attacks may also be triggered by "negative" emotions such as anger, fear, or sadness.[57]

Patients with narcolepsy, especially those with cataplexy, often experience hypnagogic or hypnopompic hallucinations, and sleep paralysis. Hypnagogic and hypnopompic hallucinations occur, respectively, at sleep onset and while awakening, are complex, and involve visual, auditory, and somatesthetic phenomena. Sleep paralysis is a brief (less than 60 seconds) period of an inability to move skeletal muscles on awakening. Hypnopompic hallucinations and sleep paralysis may occur together, and are often frightening, especially during initial episodes. Isolated hypnagogic or hypnopompic hallucinations or episodes of sleep paralysis may occur in normals, especially after sleep deprivation, and by themselves are not pathognomonic of narcolepsy.

Those with narcolepsy have a tendency toward elevated body mass index (BMI), and many become formally obese.[58] Disorders that are related to obesity, such as sleep apnea and diabetes, thus appear with a higher frequency in those with narcolepsy than in the general population. Patients who have narcolepsy with cataplexy have been shown to have low or undetectable levels of orexin, also called hypocretin, in their cerebrospinal fluid (CSF). Orexin is a neuropeptide produced by cells in the posterior hypothalamus, and the reduced level of orexin is believed to be correlated with loss of the cells in the posterior and lateral hypothalamus that produce it.[59]

Orexin is secreted during the waking hours; in ways that are incompletely understood, it suppresses activity of the VLPO and other brain areas, which in turn promotes wakefulness and suppresses REM. The absence of orexin causes the VLPO and wake areas to activate and deactivate in an unstable manner, producing intrusion of sleep into wake and wake into sleep.

The reason why orexin-producing cells are lost in patients with narcolepsy plus cataplexy remains unknown; genetic and autoimmune factors may play a role, but genetic and immune testing is still of uncertain clinical value. Further, factors beyond orexin loss alone may be involved, as patients with narcolepsy without cataplexy may have reduced or normal levels of CSF orexin. Secondary narcolepsy (due to trauma, infection, CNS malignancy, or a paraneoplastic symptom) is rare.

The onset of narcolepsy with cataplexy often occurs around puberty, with a peak incidence between 15 and 25 years of age, but it may appear as early as age 2. Another peak of incidence occurs around 35 to 45 years, or around menopause.

The diagnosis of narcolepsy is established using the multiple sleep latency test (MSLT), which consists of a series of five scheduled naps at 2-hour intervals, beginning 90–180 minutes after awakening from the overnight PSG aligned with the patient's habitual sleep time. Each nap opportunity is meant to be conducive to sleep and patients are instructed to close their eyes and attempt to sleep. Each opportunity is 20 minutes

long, but patients who achieve sleep at any time during this window are allowed to continue sleeping for 15 minutes to determine if REM sleep is achieved. Patients who have not aroused from the nap spontaneously are awakened at this time. Ideally, the MSLT is performed in patients who have kept a regular nocturnal sleep schedule in the week preceding the test, which can be confirmed by diary or by actigraphy. Importantly, patients should be free of medications that can influence the results, such as antidepressants (especially those that may suppress REM sleep) or stimulants. A PSG is typically done the night before the MSLT, to rule out occult primary sleep disorders and to ensure that patients obtain at least 6 hours of sleep before the MSLT begins. MSLT findings of short-sleep latency (less than 5 to 8 minutes on average across naps) and two or more sleep-onset REM periods (SOREMS) are consistent with narcolepsy. DSM-5 Criteria for Narcolepsy can be located in Box 22-4.

TREATMENT
Excessive Daytime Sleepiness

Fifteen-minute naps at lunchtime and at 5:30 PM, regular timing of nocturnal sleep, and avoidance of big meals and alcohol may produce partial relief of sleepiness for some patients, but naps alone are rarely sufficient to treat narcolepsy.

Modafinil (100 to 200 mg in the morning and before lunch) is an effective treatment for EDS in some patients. The safety and efficacy of doses above 400 mg/day have not been established, and the FDA has not approved the agent for use in larger doses, though some centers are using modafinil in doses above 400 mg for patients who have had a partial response and no adverse effects to standard, approved doses.

Methylphenidate (starting with 10 mg in the morning, 5 mg before lunch, and 5 mg around mid-afternoon, and going up to 60 mg [total] per day) is also effective for EDS in some patients. The extended-release form (20 mg SR) may be given in the morning, with the remainder of the dose provided in the afternoon, for some patients. Dextroamphetamine, in doses up to 60 mg/day, is an alternative, as is methylphenidate (10 mg of the extended-release formulation may be given in the morning, with the remainder provided in the afternoon). Lisdexamphetamine is another longer-acting option dosed typically in the morning, starting at the lower end of its approved range (20–70 mg daily). This compound is metabolized to the active agent, dextroamphetamine.

Gamma hydroxybutyrate (GHB) (sodium oxybate) is a metabolite of GABA. Its mechanism of action is unknown, but it may improve the disturbed nocturnal sleep and EDS, as well as cataplexy, for patients with narcolepsy. GHB has a short half-life, and must be given at night, in divided doses at bedtime and 3 to 4 hours later. This can be cumbersome, and patients can be confused and ataxic when they are awakened. Treatment usually starts with 1.5 g at bedtime, with doses gradually increasing to 6 to 9 g/day. Higher doses may be more effective, but may produce nausea, dizziness, and urinary incontinence. GHB is a tasteless, clear liquid, and has become notorious as a "date rape" agent. It appears to have a significant potential for abuse. It must be obtained through a carefully controlled "Xyrem distribution network." Given the toxicity and potential for abuse, great caution is required when prescribing this agent.

Cataplexy

Fluoxetine (20 to 60 mg), venlafaxine (150 to 300 mg), clomipramine (75 to 125 mg), and imipramine (75 to 125 mg) are

BOX 22-4 DSM-5 Diagnostic Criteria: Narcolepsy (347.00)

A. Recurrent periods of an irrepressible need to sleep, lapsing into sleep, or napping occurring within the same day. These must have been occurring at least three times per week over the past 3 months.

B. The presence of at least one of the following:
   1. Episodes of cataplexy, defined as either (a) or (b), occurring at least a few times per month:
      a. In individuals with long-standing disease, brief (seconds to minutes) episodes of sudden bilateral loss of muscle tone with maintained consciousness that are precipitated by laughter or joking.
      b. In children or in individuals within 6 months of onset, spontaneous grimaces or jaw-opening episodes with tongue thrusting or a global hypotonia, without any obvious emotional triggers.
   2. Hypocretin deficiency, as measured using cerebrospinal fluid (CSF) hypocretin-1 immunoreactivity values (less than or equal to one-third of values obtained in healthy subjects tested using the same assay, or less than or equal to 110 pg/mL). Low CSF levels of hypocretin-1 must not be observed in the context of acute brain injury, inflammation, or infection.
   3. Nocturnal sleep polysomnography showing rapid eye movement (REM) sleep latency less than or equal to 15 minutes, or a multiple sleep latency test showing a mean sleep latency less than or equal to 8 minutes and two or more sleep-onset REM periods.

Specify whether:

347.00 (G47.419) Narcolepsy without cataplexy but with hypocretin deficiency: Criterion B requirements of low CSF hypocretin-1 levels and positive polysomnography/multiple sleep latency test are met, but no cataplexy is present (Criterion B1 not met).

347.01 (G47.411) Narcolepsy with cataplexy but without hypocretin deficiency: In this rare subtype (less than 5% of narcolepsy cases), Criterion B requirements of cataplexy and positive polysomnography/multiple sleep latency test are met, but CSF hypocretin-1 levels are normal (Criterion B2 not met).

347.00 (G47.419) Autosomal dominant cerebellar ataxia, deafness, and narcolepsy: This subtype is caused by exon 21 DNA (cytosine-5)-methyltransferase-1 mutations and is characterized by late-onset (age 30–40 years) narcolepsy (with low or intermediate CSF hypocretin-1 levels), deafness, cerebellar ataxia, and eventually dementia. Narcolepsy Subtypes—Diagnostic Criteria

347.00 (G47.419) Autosomal dominant narcolepsy, obesity, and type 2 diabetes: Narcolepsy, obesity, and type 2 diabetes and low CSF hypocretin-1 levels have been described in rare cases and are associated with a mutation in the myelin oligodendrocyte glycoprotein gene.

347.10 (G47.429) Narcolepsy secondary to another medical condition: This subtype is for narcolepsy that develops secondary to medical conditions that cause infectious (e.g., Whipple's disease, sarcoidosis), traumatic, or tumoral destruction of hypocretin neurons.

Specify current severity:

Mild: Infrequent cataplexy (less than once per week), need for naps only once or twice per day, and less disturbed nocturnal sleep

Moderate: Cataplexy once daily or every few days, disturbed nocturnal sleep, and need for multiple naps daily

Severe: Drug-resistant cataplexy with multiple attacks daily, nearly constant sleepiness, and disturbed nocturnal sleep (i.e., movements, insomnia, and vivid dreaming).

Reprinted with permission from the Diagnostic and statistical manual of mental disorders, *ed 5, (Copyright 2013). American Psychiatric Association.*

---

all potent REM suppressors, and are all effective in the treatment of cataplexy. If there is need for discontinuation, these agents should be tapered rather than stopped suddenly so as not to produce rebound. They may precipitate the development of PLMS and of REM sleep behavior disorder, especially in older individuals with narcolepsy. Monoamine oxidase inhibitors may also be considered due to their strong REM inhibitory actions, with careful attention to adverse effect profiles.

GHB in divided doses up to 9 g/day may treat cataplexy, but the same cautions about the use of the agent mentioned previously apply.

Idiopathic hypersomnia may overlap with narcolepsy without cataplexy. Patients with this condition may routinely sleep more than 10 hours per night, but remain excessively sleepy. They may experience extreme difficulty waking up with external stimuli, such as an alarm, and have periods of "sleep drunkenness" on arousal. They may have long, non-restorative daytime naps. MSLT confirms objective sleepiness, but afflicted patients do not have two or more SOREMs.

BREATHING-RELATED SLEEP DISORDERS: OBSTRUCTIVE SLEEP APNEA, CENTRAL SLEEP APNEA, AND SLEEP-RELATED HYPOVENTILATION

Apnea may be obstructive, central, or mixed. An episode of obstructive apnea is defined as the complete cessation of airflow at the nose and mouth for at least 10 seconds despite ongoing respiratory effort. Hypopnea is defined as a reduction of airflow (greater than 30%) despite ongoing respiratory effort accompanied by a significant ($\geq$3%–4%) oxygen desaturation. Respiratory event-related arousals (RERAs) are flow limitations > 10 seconds accompanied by EEG-defined arousal. Central sleep apnea is defined as absence of airflow with concurrent absence of respiration effort as measured by strain gauge belts around the chest and/or abdomen. Mixed apnea events have a combination of central and obstructive features.

OSA is a disorder of breathing associated with recurrent transient upper airway obstruction during sleep. The presence and severity of OSA is determined by overnight PSG testing. The PSG generates a measure called the apnea-hypopnea index (AHI), which is the average number of apneas and hypopneas observed per hour of sleep, and the respiratory disturbance index (RDI) which includes apneas, hyponeas, and RERA events.[60,61]

The severity of sleep apnea is generally denoted by the AHI,[62] but DSM-5 notes that the overall severity is also informed by levels of nocturnal desaturation and sleep fragmentation. For DSM-5 diagnostic criteria for obstructive sleep apnea, central sleep apnea, and sleep-related hypoventilation please see Boxes 22-5, 22-6 and 22-7.

When the severity is mild, treatment is warranted if there is associated symptomatology, such as daytime sleepiness, or if there is a significant co-morbid condition that might be

---

BOX 22-5 DSM-5 Diagnostic Criteria: Obstructive Sleep
Apnea Hypopnea (327.23 (G47.33))

1. Evidence by polysomnography of at least five obstructive
   apneas or hypopneas per hour of sleep and either of the
   following sleep symptoms:
   A. Nocturnal breathing disturbances: snoring, snorting/
      gasping, or breathing pauses during sleep
   B. Daytime sleepiness, fatigue, or unrefreshing sleep despite
      sufficient opportunities to sleep.
2. Evidence by polysomnography of 15 or more obstructive
   apneas and/or hypopneas per hour of sleep regardless of
   accompanying symptoms.

   Specify current severity:

Mild: Apnea hypopnea index is less than 15
Moderate: Apnea hypopnea index is 15–30
Severe: Apnea hypopnea index is 15–30.

Reprinted with permission from the Diagnostic and statistical manual of
mental disorders, *ed 5, (Copyright 2013). American Psychiatric
Association.*

BOX 22-6 DSM-5 Diagnostic Criteria: Central
Sleep Apnea

A. Evidence by polysomnography of five or more central apneas
   per hour of sleep.
B. The disorder is not better explained by another current sleep
   disorder.

   Specify whether:

327.21 (G47.31) Idiopathic central sleep apnea:
   Characterized by repeated episodes of apneas and
   hypopneas during sleep caused by variability in respiratory
   effort but without evidence of airway obstruction.
786.04 (R06.3) Cheyne–Stokes breathing: A pattern of
   periodic crescendo-decrescendo variation in tidal volume that
   results in central apneas and hypopneas at a frequency of at
   least five events per hour, accompanied by frequent arousal.
**780.57 (G47.37) Central sleep apnea comorbid with opioid
   use:** The pathogenesis of this subtype is attributed to the
   effects of opioids on the respiratory rhythm generators in the
   medulla as well as the differential effects on hypoxic versus
   hypercapnic respiratory drive.

   Specify current severity:
Severity of central sleep apnea is graded according to the
   frequency of the breathing disturbances as well as the extent
   of associated oxygen desaturation and sleep fragmentation
   that occur as a consequence of repetitive respiratory
   disturbances.

Reprinted with permission from the Diagnostic and statistical manual of
mental disorders, *ed 5, (Copyright 2013). American Psychiatric
Association.*

BOX 22-7 DSM-5 Diagnostic Criteria: Sleep-Related
Hypoventilation

A. Polysomnography demonstrates episodes of decreased
   respiration associated with elevated CO_2 levels. (**Note:** In the
   absence of objective measurement of CO_2, persistent low
   levels of hemoglobin oxygen saturation associated with
   apneic/hypopneic events may indicate hypoventilation.)
B. The disturbance is not better explained by another current
   sleep disorder.

   Specify whether:

327.24 (G47.34) Idiopathic hypoventilation: This subtype is
   not attributable to any readily identified condition.
**327.25 (G47.35) Congenital central alveolar
   hypoventilation:** This subtype is a rare congenital disorder in
   which the individual typically presents in the perinatal period
   with shallow breathing, or cyanosis and apnea during sleep.
327.26 (G47.36) Comorbid sleep-related hypoventilation:
   This subtype occurs as a consequence of a medical
   condition, such as a pulmonary disorder (e.g., interstitial lung
   disease, chronic obstructive pulmonary disease) or a
   neuromuscular or chest wall disorder (e.g. muscular
   dystrophies, post-polio syndrome, cervical spinal cord injury,
   kyphoscoliosis), or medications (e.g., benzodiazepines,
   opiates). It also occurs with obesity (obesity hypoventilation
   disorder), where it reflects a combination of increased work of
   breathing due to reduced chest wall compliance and
   ventilation–perfusion mis-match and variably reduced
   ventilator drive. Such individuals usually are characterized by
   body mass index of greater than 30 and hypercapnia during
   wakefulness (with a pCO_2 of greater than 45), without other
   evidence of hypoventilation.

   Specify current severity:
Severity is graded according to the degree of hypoxemia and
   hypercarbia present during sleep and evidence of end organ
   impairment due to these abnormalities (e.g., right-sided heart
   failure). The presence of blood gas abnormalities during
   wakefulness is an indicator of greater severity.

Reprinted with permission from the Diagnostic and statistical manual of
mental disorders, *ed 5, (Copyright 2013). American Psychiatric
Association.*

---

impacted by untreated OSA. However, when the severity is moderate or higher (at least 15 obstructions per hour of sleep or an AHI > 15), treatment is warranted even if there are no daytime symptoms or co-morbidities. The AHI does not take into account the severity of oxygen desaturation, the presence of cardiac arrhythmias, or the amount of sleepiness or functional impairment, all of which may influence the necessity for treatment.

The classic signs and symptoms of OSA include snoring, gasping arousals, and witnessed apneas, but these are in fact neither sensitive nor specific for predicting the diagnosis or severity. Even EDS is not a reliable feature: over half of patients with even severe OSA do not complain of EDS and have normal Epworth Sleepiness scores, and EDS may occur without significant OSA.[63]

The symptoms associated with OSA are protean and include morning headaches, dry mouth, nocturia, decreased libido, poor concentration, and acid reflux. Some patients with OSA are depressed and become cognitively impaired, but the relationship among OSA, depression, and cognitive status is incompletely understood.[64]

Hypertension is an important correlate of OSA and may predispose patients to developing congestive heart failure (CHF).[65] Levels of C-reactive protein, and other markers of inflammation, may be elevated in patients with OSA; this may relate to cardiovascular disease in patients with OSA.[66]

Obesity is another important correlate of OSA. An increase of 10% in body weight for patients who already suffer from mild OSA is associated with a sixfold increase in the development of moderate to severe OSA.[67] This may be mediated by a critical increase in the soft tissues of the neck and throat that predisposes to airway collapse. Indeed, males with a neck diameter of 17 inches or above are at higher risk for OSA.[68]

BOX 22-8 Treatment of Obstructive Sleep Apnea

Weight loss helps but may not cure. Some patients sustain significant weight loss that may obviate the need for continuous positive airway pressure (CPAP)

CPAP helps patients with hypersomnolence

Surgical approaches include uvuloplasty and related procedures, though these may lose their benefit over time

Stimulatory agents (e.g., modafinil) help those with excessive daytime sleepiness (even when the symptom persists after treatment with CPAP)

Sedatives should be used with caution, as they may reduce arousal thresholds, thereby delaying arousal and lengthening apneic spells; this may worsen oxygen desaturation and the other negative consequences of apnea. Excessive alcohol is known to decrease upper airway muscle tone, so it may worsen both snoring and sleep apnea

---

Finally, patients with OSA may have an increased propensity for adult-onset diabetes mellitus (AODM), due to apnea-mediated insulin-resistance, and leptin response. Insulin resistance worsens with increasing weight, but it may be moderated by CPAP.[69]

It is worth noting that it is not uncommon for patients with an initially normal PSG to demonstrate OSA on a second PSG. If there is a high clinical suspicion, based on the history, physical exam, and co-morbid conditions, that OSA is present, a PSG may be repeated.

Children with OSA may be noted by parents to snore, to have agitated arousals, or unusual sleep postures (sleeping on hands and knees), or to develop enuresis. Some, but not all, children have EDS, behavioral and learning problems, or "failure to thrive".

OSA affects 1%–2% of children (onset peaks between ages 3 and 8), 2%–15% of middle-aged adults, and 20% of older adults. No gender differences in rates of occurrence are noted in children or older adults (which include post-menopausal women), whereas there is a 2–4:1 male to female predominance in middle-aged adults. Onset is typically slow, and course tends to be persistent.

Treatments for OSA are provided in Box 22-8.

Central Sleep Apnea

DSM-5 includes three sub-types of central sleep apnea (CSA): idiopathic, Cheyne–Stokes breathing, and CSA co-morbid with opioid use. The first two are associated with "periodic breathing" (hyperventilation alternating with hypoventilation) driven by abnormalities in the way the ventilatory control system responds to blood pCO_2. CSA co-morbid with opioid use appears to be associated with the effects of opioids on the respiratory rhythm generators in the medulla. Symptoms are similar to those present in OSA (Box 22-5).

Complex sleep apnea, or treatment-emergent central apnea, most commonly occurs in patients with CHF, neurological disorders, or narcotic use (including partial agonists used to treat addiction), but it can be idiopathic as well. This process is thought to be driven by carotid chemoreceptor dysfunction rather than obstruction, although both processes may be present. For example, increasing the pressure sufficiently to keep the airway open may drive CO_2 levels below the apnea threshold, resulting in provoked central pauses.

Some patients exhibit primarily central apnea on PSG testing, whereas others with seemingly obstructive apnea on diagnostic testing develop mixed or central apnea upon administration of CPAP or BiPAP. A pressure delivery system called adaptive servoventilation (ASV) is approved to treat patients for whom central apnea emerges or persists on CPAP or BiPAP.

Idiopathic CSA is probably rare. In contrast, > 20% of patients with severe CHF may be at risk for the Cheyne–Stokes sub-type. This type may appear in patients after stroke and/or renal failure as well. Up to 30% of patients using chronic opioids for non-malignant pain or on methadone maintenance may be at risk for the opioid use sub-type.

CIRCADIAN RHYTHM SLEEP–WAKE DISORDERS

Delayed Sleep Phase Disorder

This is defined by falling asleep at night and waking in the morning > 2 hours after the time required to optimize the individual's social or occupational function. It is present in approximately 7% of adolescents, and may accompany or follow another mental disorder such as depression. Patients may experience sleep inertia, sleep-onset insomnia, and EDS.

Advanced Sleep Phase Disorder

This is defined by falling asleep at night and waking up > 2 hours earlier than desired. Sleep duration is usually normal; some patients experience early morning insomnia and EDS. A family history of advanced sleep phase is often present, and when present may be associated with early onset and worsening over time.

Irregular Sleep–Wake Cycle Disorder

This is related to a disruption of the normal circadian rhythm. Sleep is fragmented, with three relatively brief sleep periods/24 hours, rather than the normal nocturnal dominant period. Patients may complain of insomnia or EDS. The disorder may be seen in children with neurodevelopmental disorders, and may develop in adults with neurodegenerative diseases.

Non-24 hour Sleep–Wake Disorder

This is rare in sighted persons, but is present in 50% of blind patients. A failure of the patient's endogenous circadian rhythm to be synchronized with the day–night cycle may produce intermittent episodes of insomnia and EDS.

Shift-work Sleep Disorder

This occurs when the circadian rhythms that regulate sleep–wake behavior are misaligned by night-shift work to the degree that patients experience clinically-significant excessive sleepiness during night work or insomnia when trying to sleep the following day. Between 5% and 10% of night-shift workers (nearly 6 million Americans) cannot adapt their circadian rhythms and their drive for sleep and, as a result, experience levels of excessive sleepiness and daytime insomnia that meet the criteria for diagnosis of SWSD. The burden of illness associate with SWSD is substantial, with profound impact on a patient's health (increased rate of ulcers and depression), job (impaired work performance and absenteeism), and safety (increased risk for accidents on the job and during commute). Additionally, the excessive sleepiness related to SWSD is associated with impaired social relationships, marital disharmony, and irritability. Treatment entails both the management of daytime sleep and night-time alertness. Clearly a first step is to maximize nocturnal sleep with behavioral and pharmacological approaches outlined in the section on insomnia management. In terms of the sleepiness during work and especially during the commute home, many workers self-medicate with caffeine. Recently, modafinil was shown to enhance alertness and decrease commute accidents. An alternative approach to

SWSD is to move the circadian rhythms closer to that of the work schedule. The appropriate exposure to light and the use of melatonin have been shown to be effective in moving the clock. However, the intrusion of light during the day and the behavioral choice of sleep pattern on non-work days limits the utility of these approaches.[70–72]

DSM-5 criteria for circadian rhythm sleep–wake disorders can be located in Box 22-9.

BOX 22-9 DSM-5 Diagnostic Criteria: Circadian Rhythm Sleep–Wake Disorders

A. A persistent or recurrent pattern of sleep disruption that is primarily due to an alteration of the circadian system or to a misalignment between the endogenous circadian rhythm and the sleep–wake schedule required by an individual's physical environment or social or professional schedule.
B. The sleep disruption leads to excessive sleepiness or insomnia, or both.
C. The sleep disturbance causes clinically significant distress or impairment in social, occupational, and other important areas of functioning.
  • Coding note: For ICD-9-CM, code **307.45** for all subtypes For ICD-10-CM, code is based on subtype.

Specify whether:

307.45 (G47.21) Delayed sleep phase type: A pattern of delayed sleep onset and awakening times, with an inability to fall asleep and awaken at a desired or conventionally acceptable earlier time.

Specify if:

Familial: a family history of delayed sleep phase is present.

Specify if:

Overlapping with non-24-hour sleep–wake type: Delayed sleep phase type may overlap with another circadian rhythm sleep–wake disorder, non-24-hour sleep–wake type.

307.45 (G47.22) Advanced sleep phase type: A pattern of advanced sleep onset and awakening times, with an inability to remain awake or asleep until the desired or conventionally acceptable later sleep or wake times.

Specify if:

Familial: a family history of advanced sleep phase is present.

307.45 (G47.23) Irregular sleep–wake type: A temporally disorganized sleep–wake pattern, such that the timing of sleep and wake periods is variable throughout the 24-hour period.

307.45 (G47.24) Non-24-hour sleep–wake type: A pattern of sleep–wake cycles that is not synchronized to the 24-hour environment, with a consistent daily drift (usually to later and later times) of sleep onset and wake times.

307.45 (G47.26) Shift work type: Insomnia during the major sleep period and/or excessive sleepiness (including inadvertent sleep) during the major awake period associated with a shift work schedule (i.e., requiring unconventional work hours).

Specify if:

Episodic: Symptoms last at least 1 month but less than 3 months
Persistent: Symptoms last 3 months or longer
Recurrent: Two or more episodes occur within the space of 1 year.

Reprinted with permission from the Diagnostic and statistical manual of mental disorders, *ed 5, (Copyright 2013). American Psychiatric Association.*

PARASOMNIAS NREM SLEEP AROUSAL DISORDER

Sleepwalking or Somnambulism

This usually occurs during slow-wave sleep, so it often is seen during the first third of the night. Patients remain asleep during the episode and have a blank, glassy stare. They are typically unresponsive to efforts of others to communicate with them. They are awakened only with difficulty and may be confused when awakened. Adults may appear to be acting-out dreams during sleepwalking, and may remember fragments of dream-like experiences, but most patients are amnestic regarding the event.

Behaviors may be complex, inappropriate, and at times violent or dangerous. Patients may move furniture in their house, and may go outside. They may urinate in a closet, or open the refrigerator and binge; they may talk or shout. They may become violent when waking is attempted. Episodes may terminate spontaneously, with some patients returning to bed, and others lying down and sleeping wherever they happen to be at the moment. Up to 4% of adults sleepwalk. In most cases, the onset of sleepwalking is during childhood, with a peak in onset between 8 and 12 years of age. Many children with sleepwalking have an early history of confusional arousals. There are cases of adult-onset sleepwalking.

The etiology of sleepwalking is unknown. There appears to be a strong familial pattern, suggesting that genetic factors play a role. Sleep deprivation and sleep apnea appear to be the most common precipitants. Patients with adult-onset sleepwalking may have a history of psychological trauma, and may be undergoing periods of life stress or anxiety. Hyperthyroidism, migraine, head injury, stroke, and encephalitis may also precipitate sleepwalking.[73]

Sleep Terrors (previously known as *pavor nocturnus*)

These are arousals from slow-wave sleep heralded by a scream or loud cry, and accompanied by fear and intense autonomic arousal (e.g., tachycardia, hyperventilation, sweating, increased muscle tone). Episodes usually occur during the first third of the night, with a scream. Patients remain asleep, or are awakened with difficulty and remain confused. Amnesia for the event is common, though some patients may recall frightening dream-like mentation. Patients may get out of bed and run about the room, and in some cases may injure themselves or others.

Sleep terrors often emerge during childhood, between ages 4 and 12, though some cases may have an adult onset. Approximately 2% of adults are affected. The etiology of sleep terrors is unknown, but genetic factors may play a role.[74]

Sleep-related Eating Disorder, or Nocturnal Binge-eating Disorder

This is characterized by recurrent episodes of eating and drinking during arousal from sleep. The arousal may be partial, with only partial recall of the event, or may be full, with substantial recall. In all cases eating and drinking behavior is experienced as out of control or involuntary. Episodes often occur nightly, in some cases several times a night. Patients may consume a variety of materials, often high-calorie food, but at times eat materials that are non-foods (such as coffee grounds, cigarette butts, or cleaning fluids). Food handling is typically sloppy; alcohol is almost never involved or consumed.

The incidence of sleep-related eating disorders is unknown, but it appears to occur most often in women (with a history of sleepwalking) between 22 and 29 years old. Sleep-related eating disorder has been reported among users of zolpidem, triazolam, lithium, and anticholinergic agents, and may be precipitated by cessation of drugs, alcohol, and cigarette use. It can also occur following life stresses (such as separations), during daytime dieting, or with the onset of narcolepsy.[75]

Nightmare Disorder, or Dream Anxiety Disorder

This is characterized by recurrent nightmares during REM sleep that produce awakenings with detailed recall of frightening dreams. Patients may remain anxious and have difficulty returning to sleep. Nightmares often appear during the second half of the night (Box 22-10).

Between 50% and 85% of the population has occasional nightmares; 2% to 8% of the adult population has recurrent

---

BOX 22-10 DSM-5 Diagnostic Criteria: Nightmare Disorder (307.47 (F51.5))

A. Repeated occurrences of extended, extremely dysphoric and well-remembered dreams that usually involve efforts to avoid threats to survival, security, or physical integrity and that generally occur during the second half of the major sleep episode.
B. On awakening from the dysphoric dreams, the individual rapidly becomes oriented and alert.
C. The sleep disturbance causes clinically significant distress or impairment in social, occupational, or other important areas of functioning.
D. The nightmare symptoms are not attributable to the physiological effects of a substance (e.g., a drug of abuse, a medication).
E. Coexisting mental and medical disorders do not adequately explain the predominant complaint of dysphoric dreams.
   Specify if:

During sleep onset
   Specify if:

With associated non-sleep disorder, including substance use disorders
With associated other medical condition
With associated other sleep disorder.
   • **Coding note:** The code 307.47 (F51.5) applies to all three specifiers. Code also the relevant associated mental disorder, medical condition, or other sleep disorder immediately after the code for nightmare disorder in order to indicate the association.
   Specify if:

Acute: Duration of period of nightmares is 1 month or less
Subacute: Duration of period of nightmares is greater than 1 month but less than 6 months
Persistent: Duration of period of nightmares is 6 months or greater.
   Specify current severity:
   Severity can be rated by the frequency with which the nightmares occur:

Mild: Less than one episode per week on average
Moderate: One or more episodes per week but less than nightly
Severe: Episodes nightly.

Reprinted with permission from the Diagnostic and statistical manual of mental disorders, *ed 5, (Copyright 2013). American Psychiatric Association.*

---

nightmares. Nightmares are common after traumatic events; nightmares continuing for more than 4 weeks after the trauma may predict the appearance of post-traumatic stress disorder (PTSD). Nightmares usually start in children ages 3 to 6 years, and are most frequent in children ages 6 to 10 years. While nightmares usually abate with adolescence, they may persist in some patients into adulthood.[76]

REM Sleep Behavior Disorder

REM sleep behavior disorder is characterized by the appearance of behaviors during REM sleep that cause injury to the self or bed partner, or disrupt sleep. Patients keep their eyes closed during the episode, and may crawl or leap up and run for a short distance. They may shout, swear, laugh, gesture, punch, kick, or flail. They appear to be acting-out violent, frightening, action-filled dreams. The patient usually awakens and is fully alert at the end of the episode, and can recall and report the events of the dream.

REM sleep behavior disorder is often long-standing and progressive, with variable frequency of reported episodes. Many patients with REM sleep behavior disorder go on to have neurodegenerative disorders (such as Parkinson's disease, Lewy body dementia, Alzheimer's disease, and multiple-system atrophy) in the decade following the onset of REM sleep behavior disorder.

The prevalence of REM sleep behavior disorder is unknown, but it appears to occur mostly in men over age 50 years, and may be common in patients with new-onset Parkinson's disease or multiple-system atrophy. REM sleep behavior disorder may be precipitated by antidepressants (except bupropion), in particular venlafaxine and mirtazapine. REM sleep behavior disorder may be a manifestation of the REM sleep abnormalities associated with narcolepsy, and may be precipitated or worsened by medications used in the treatment of narcolepsy.

The etiology of REM sleep behavior disorder is not known, but animal models of REM sleep behavior disorder suggest that it involves interference with the pathways that produce atonia during REM, disinhibition of brainstem motor pathway generators, or both.[77]

Clonazepam, with or without melatonin adjunctively, may reduce injurious nocturnal activity in patients with REM sleep behavior disorder, and has been used without the development of tolerance or dependence in many patients.

Restless Legs Syndrome

Restless legs syndrome is diagnosed when patients experience a distressing, hard-to-describe sensation mostly in their legs (but sometimes in their arms), along with an urge to stretch or move, that occurs in the late afternoon or in the evening before bedtime. Some patients may report aches, pains, or tingling, while others describe only restlessness or an abnormal sensation, and some patients report both. These symptoms typically appear intermittently, and may vary in intensity and character on different nights, but may be present nightly in 25% of cases. The symptoms of restless legs syndrome interfere with getting to sleep because patients feel they must get out of bed and move around. The discomfort may be relieved by walking or by stretching, but it returns when patients are again motionless. Although often mild, the interference with falling asleep reduces total sleep time, and can produce EDS, increased incidence of anxiety and depression, elevation in blood pressure, and impaired quality of life.

Restless legs syndrome appears in approximately 10% of the general population and in up to 24% of primary care patients. Primary, or idiopathic, restless legs syndrome has a female predominance and is often familial. Secondary restless legs syndrome appears when medical, neurological, or metabolic conditions produce iron deficiency. While the complex role of iron is incompletely understood, it probably is advisable to measure serum ferritin levels and to obtain a complete blood count (CBC) looking for the signs of iron deficiency anemia in patients with restless legs syndrome, especially if the patients have renal disease or are pregnant. Note that iron repletion may be beneficial for those in whom serum ferritin is < 50, which is in the normal range from a hematology standpoint.

Restless legs syndrome typically first appears during middle age, but the onset before age 30 in patients with a family history of restless legs syndrome may occur, and it may at times be seen in children. Diagnosis is clinical, based on a careful history addressing the cardinal features that define the condition. The drug history should be reviewed for medications that may affect dopaminergic transmission (e.g., antidepressants, neuroleptics, some calcium channel blockers). There are no diagnostic physical findings. Checking serum chemistries for purported contributing factors (e.g., creatinine, ferritin, folate) is reasonable.

Restless legs syndrome needs to be distinguished from nocturnal leg cramps which cause frank calf pain and a knot in the muscle relieved by stretching. Paresthesias from prolonged sitting and akathisia in persons with peripheral neuropathy may worsen with sitting and mimic restless legs syndrome. In persons with PLMS, other etiologies may be considered in the correct clinical context, including sleep apnea, use of neuroleptics and antidepressants, spinal cord lesions, stroke, narcolepsy, and neurodegenerative disease.

Restless legs syndrome is often co-morbid with PLMS, which may contribute to further sleep disruption and to EDS. Patients with restless legs syndrome have an increased incidence of depression, and many antidepressant medications, in particular selective serotonin reuptake inhibitors (SSRIs), can produce restless legs syndrome and PLMS. Table 22-7 and Box 22-11 show the diagnostic criteria of restless legs syndrome. Because patients often present complaining of difficulty sleeping and not symptoms of RLS, it is important to inquire about the condition as part of the work-up for insomnia.[78]

For DSM-5 diagnostic criteria for parasomnias, see Boxes 22-12, 22-13 and 22-14; for restless legs syndrome, see Box 22-11.

Restless Leg Syndrome Treatment

In many instances, symptoms are mild and sufficiently self-limited to require no treatment. In the cases where a purported etiologic factor is identified (e.g., iron deficiency), treatment should be directed at correcting it. Avoidance of alcohol (particularly wine) and caffeine and the performance of moderate exercise can also help. When restless legs syndrome is caused by antidepressants or by the taper of opiates, switching to another antidepressant or revising a tapering schedule of opiates can be useful. Acupuncture may help some patients.

When medication is required, long-acting dopamine agonists are the first choice.[79] Pramipexole, starting at 0.125 mg orally (PO) every day at bedtime (qHS), titrating up to 1.5 mg/day, can be effective, although the manufacturer's recommended maximum dose is 0.5 mg (lower than the doses used daily for parkinsonism). Ropinirole, starting at 0.25 mg PO qHS and titrating at weekly intervals up to the maximum recommended dose of 4 mg/day, is an effective alternative. Although effective, these agents have a high rate of discontinuation (up to 25%) not only for inadequate response or bothersome side effects but also because of augmentation of symptoms (e.g., onset of symptoms earlier in the day with

TABLE 22-7 Restless Legs Syndrome

Criteria Type	Description
Essential criteria	Urge to move the legs, usually accompanied by uncomfortable or unpleasant sensations in legs. Arms and other body parts may be involved. Cognitively impaired elderly may rub legs, pace, fidget, kick, tap, or toss and turn in bed
	Urge to move or unpleasant sensation begins or worsens during rest or inactivity
	Urge to move or unpleasant sensation is relieved by movement while movement continues
	Urge to move or unpleasant sensation is worse in the evening or at night than during the day, or only during evening or at night. In very severe cases, worsening at night may not be noticeable but must have been previously present
Supportive clinical features	Positive family history
	Response to dopaminergic treatment
	PLMS (during wakefulness or sleep)
Associated features	Natural clinical course
	Sleep disturbance
	Generally normal medical and physical examination

Adapted from Allen RP, Picchietti D, Hening WA, et al: Restless legs syndrome: diagnostic criteria, special considerations, and epidemiology. A report from the restless legs syndrome diagnosis and epidemiology workshop at the National Institutes of Health, Sleep Med 2003; 4:101–119.
PLMS, Periodic limb movements of sleep.

BOX 22-11 DSM-5 Diagnostic Criteria: Restless Legs Syndrome (333.94 (G25.81))

A. An urge to move the legs, usually accompanied by or in response to uncomfortable and unpleasant sensations in the legs, characterized by all of the following:
   1. The urge to move the legs begins or worsens during periods of rest or inactivity
   2. The urge to move the legs is partially or totally relieved by movement
   3. The urge to move the legs is worse in the evening or at night than during the day, or occurs only in the evening or at night
B. The symptoms in Criterion A occur at least 3 times per week and have persisted for at least 3 months
C. The symptoms are accompanied by significant distress or impairment in social, occupational, educational, academic, behavioral or other important areas of functioning
D. The symptoms are not attributable to another medical disorder or medical condition (e.g., arthritis, leg edema, peripheral ischemia, leg cramps) and are not better explained by a behavioral condition
E. The symptoms are not attributable to the physiological effects of a drug of abuse or medication (e.g., akathisia).

Reprinted with permission from the Diagnostic and statistical manual of mental disorders, ed 5, (Copyright 2013). American Psychiatric Association.

---

greater severity and possibly spread to upper extremities). Impulse control disorders (e.g., compulsive shopping, gambling, eating, and hypersexuality) may occur, mainly in those with an underlying neurodegenerative disorder and/or with higher doses. The risk of sudden sleep attacks has been reported with patients taking pramipexole or ropinirole, so patients should be cautioned about driving. Levodopa has

BOX 22-12 DSM-5 Diagnostic Criteria: Non-Rapid Eye Movement Sleep Arousal Disorders

A. Recurrent episodes of incomplete awakening from sleep, usually occurring during the first third of the major sleep episode, accompanied by either one of the following:
   1. Sleepwalking: Repeated episodes of rising from bed during sleep and walking about. While sleepwalking, the individual has a blank, staring face; is relatively unresponsive to the efforts of others to communicate with him or her; and can be awakened only with great effort.
   2. Sleep terrors: Recurrent episodes of abrupt terror arousals from sleep, usually beginning with a panicky scream. There is intense fear and signs of autonomic arousal, such as mydriasis, tachycardia, rapid breathing, and sweating, during each episode. There is relative unresponsiveness to efforts of others to comfort the individual during the episodes.
B. No or little (e.g., only a single visual scene) dream imagery is recalled.

C. Amnesia for the episodes is present.
D. The episodes cause clinically significant distress or impairment in social, occupational, or other important areas of functioning.
E. The disturbance is not attributable to the physiological effects of a substance (e.g., a drug of abuse, a medication).
F. Coexisting mental and medical disorders do not explain the episodes of sleepwalking or sleep terrors.

Specify whether:

307.46 (F51.3) Sleepwalking type.

Specify if:

With sleep-related eating
With sleep-related sexual behavior (sexsomnia)
307.46 (F51.4) Sleep terror type.

Reprinted with permission from the Diagnostic and statistical manual of mental disorders, *ed 5, (Copyright 2013). American Psychiatric Association.*

BOX 22-13 DSM-5 Diagnostic Criteria: Rapid Eye Movement Sleep Behaviour Disorder (327.42 (G47.52))

A. Repeated episodes of arousal during sleep associated with vocalization and/or complex motor behaviors.
B. These behaviors arise during rapid eye movement (REM) sleep and therefore usually occur greater than 90 minutes after sleep onset, are more frequent during the later portions of the sleep period, and uncommonly occur during daytime naps.
C. Upon awakening, the individual is completely awake, alert, and not confused or disoriented.
D. Either of the following:
   1. REM sleep without atonia on polysomnographic recording.
   2. A history suggestive of REM sleep behaviour disorder and an established synucleinopathy diagnosis (e.g., Parkinson's disease, multiple system atrophy).

E. The behaviors cause clinically significant distress or impairment in social, occupational, or other important areas of functioning (which may include injury to self or the bed partner).
F. The disturbance is not attributable to the physiological effects of a substance (e.g., a drug of abuse, a medication) or another medical condition.
G. Coexisting mental and medical disorders do not explain the episodes.

Reprinted with permission from the Diagnostic and statistical manual of mental disorders, *ed 5, (Copyright 2013). American Psychiatric Association.*

BOX 22-14 DSM-5 Diagnostic Criteria: Substance/Medication-Induced Sleep Disorder

A. A prominent disturbance in sleep that is sufficiently severe to warrant independent clinical attention.
B. There is evidence from the history, physical examination, or laboratory findings of either (1) or (2):
   1. The symptoms in Criterion A developed during or soon after substance intoxication or after withdrawal from or exposure to a medication.
   2. The involved substance/medication is capable of producing the symptoms in Criterion A.

The disturbance is not better explained by a sleep disorder that is not substance/medication-induced. Such evidence of an independent sleep disorder could include the following:

The symptoms preceded the onset of the substance/medication use; the symptoms persist for a substantial period of time (e.g., about 1 month) after the cessation of acute withdrawal or severe intoxication; or there is other evidence suggesting the existence of an independent non-substance/medication-induced sleep disorder (e.g., a history of recurrent non-substance/medication-related episodes).

The disturbance does not occur exclusively during the course of a delirium.

The sleep disturbance causes clinically significant distress or impairment in social, occupational, or other important areas of functioning.

Specify whether:

Insomnia type: Characterized by difficulty falling asleep or maintaining sleep, frequent nocturnal awakenings, or non-restorative sleep

Daytime sleepiness type: Characterized by predominant complaint of excessive sleepiness/fatigue during waking hours or, less commonly, a long sleep period

Parasomnia type: Characterized by abnormal behavioral events during sleep

Mixed type: Characterized by a substance/medication-induced sleep problem characterized by multiple types of sleep symptoms, but no symptom clearly predominates.

Specify if:

With onset during intoxications: This specifier should be used if criteria are met for intoxication with the substance/medication and symptoms developed during the intoxication period.

With onset during discontinuation/withdrawal: This specifier should be used if criteria are met for discontinuation/withdrawal from the substance/medication and symptoms developed during, or shortly after, discontinuation of the substance/medication.

Reprinted with permission from the Diagnostic and statistical manual of mental disorders, *ed 5, (Copyright 2013). American Psychiatric Association.*

been used but is shorter-acting and associated with a higher frequency of augmentation. A formulation of gabapentin was recently FDA-approved for restless legs syndrome, and off-label use of gabapentin is commonly attempted (starting at 300 mg PO qHS). Off-label use of clonazepam may be helpful, starting at 0.25 mg PO qHS and titrating up to 2 mg PO qHS, can help, but as with any benzodiazepine the risk–benefit balance should be considered. Opioids are sometimes used in the treatment of refractory or incapacitating disease that fails to respond to other therapeutic modalities, but dependence is a concern and the evidence for efficacy is based mostly on clinical experience rather than on controlled studies.[70]

Periodic Limb Movements of Sleep (in ICSD-2, Periodic Limb Movement Disorder, formerly called *nocturnal myoclonus*)

PLMS is characterized by the presence of a series of more than four rhythmic twitches of the toes and ankles, or of the knee or hip, occurring during sleep. Some patients may show similar twitching of the arms. Each burst of twitches lasts for 0.5 to 5 seconds, and is followed by a quiet period, where no twitches appear for the subsequent 4 to 90 seconds. PLMS is diagnosed when the average of twitch bursts across the night exceeds 5–10 per hour. There is considerable variability in the frequency of twitching across different nights. The twitches are associated with cortical and autonomic arousals (manifested by a change in heart rate or BP), which interrupt the continuity of sleep. The arousals may precede, coincide with, or follow the twitches, suggesting that a similar process may produce arousals and twitches. Patients may awaken during an arousal, but often simply shift into lighter sleep without actually waking. Patients may therefore be unaware of such arousals, and, indeed, of the twitching itself, so report of bed partners and obtaining a PSG may be required to make the diagnosis. Rather, patients with PLMS complain of EDS.

Patients with RLS often have PLMS, but most patients with PLMS do not have RLS symptoms, and the need to treat inci-dentally-observed PLMS remains uncertain. Approximately 70% of patients with REM sleep behavior disorder, and 45%–65% of patients with narcolepsy, have PLMS. The incidence of clinically-significant PLMS in the population is unknown, but rates of PLMS increase with age, appearing in 34% of patients over age 60, equally distributed between men and women.

The etiology of PLMS is unknown, but abnormalities in dopaminergic systems are suspected. Treatment primarily involves use of benzodiazepines, such as clonazepam, which may not stop the twitching but may blunt twitch-induced arousals.[80,81]

Access the complete reference list and multiple choice questions (MCQs) online at https://expertconsult.inkling.com

KEY REFERENCES

1. Sivertsen B, Salo P, Mykletun A, et al. The bi-directional associa-tion between depression and insomnia: The HUNT Study. *Psychosom Med* 74:758, 2012.
5. Buysse DJ. Insomnia can have a significant impact on health and overall functional capacity. *Insomnia JAMA* 309(7):706–716, 2013.
7. Saper CB, Scammell TE, Lu J. Hypothalamic regulation of sleep and circadian rhythms. *Nature* 437:1257–1263, 2004.
11. Ohayon M, Carskadon MA, Guilleminault C, et al. Meta-analysis of quantitative sleep parameters from childhood to old age in healthy individuals: developing normative sleep values across the human lifespan. *Sleep* 27:1255–1273, 2004.
15. Borbely AA, Achermann P. Sleep homeostasis and models of sleep regulation. *J Biol Rhythms* 14:557–568, 1999.
19. Collop NA, Anderson WM, Boehlecke B, et al. Clinical guidelines for the use of unattended portable monitors in the diagnosis of obstructive sleep apnea in adult patients. *J Clin Sleep Med* 3(7):737–747, 2007.
23. *The International Classification of Sleep Disorders, second edition (ICSD-2)*, 2005, American Academy of Sleep Medicine.
30. Katz DA, McHorney CA. The relationship between insomnia and health related quality of life in patients with chronic illness. *J Fam Pract* 51:229–235, 2002.
36. Harvey AG, Tang NH. Misperception of sleep in insomnia. A puzzle and a resolution. *Psychol Bull* 138:77–101, 2012.
52. Wolcott JC, Richardson KJ, Wiens MO, et al. Meta-analysis of the impact of 9 medication classes on falls in elderly person. *Arch Int Med* 169:1952–1960, 2009.
53. Berry SD, Lee Y, Cai S, et al. Nonbenzodiazepine sleep medication use and hip fractures in nursing home residents. *JAMA Intern Med* 173:754, 2013.
54. Briesacher BA, Soumerai SB, Field TS, et al. Medicare Part D's exclusion of benzodiazepines and fracture risk in nursing homes. *Arch Intern Med* 170:693, 2010.
55. Scammell TE. The neurobiology, diagnosis, and treatment of nar-colepsy. *Ann Neurol* 53:154–166, 2003.
60. Flemons WW. Clinical practice. Obstructive sleep apnea. *N Engl J Med* 347:498–505, 2002.
70. Drake CL, Roehrs T, Richardson G, et al. Shift work sleep disorder: prevalence and consequences beyond that of symptomatic day workers. *Sleep* 27:1453–1462, 2004.
73. Pilon M, Montplaisir J, Zadra A. Precipitating factors of somnam-bulism: impact of sleep deprivation and forced arousals. *Neurology* 70:2284–2290, 2008.
74. Pressman MR, Mahowald MW, Schenck CH. Sleep terrors/sleepwalking not REM behaviour disorder. *Sleep* 28:278–279, 2005.
75. Winkelman JW. Sleep-related eating disorder or night eating syn-drome: Sleep disorders, eating disorders, or both? *Sleep* 29:949–954, 2006.
79. Garcia-Borreguero D, Kohnen R, Silber MH, et al. The long term treatment of restless legs syndrome/Willis-Ekbom disease: evidence-based guidelines and clinical consensus best practice guidance: a report from the International Restless Legs Syndrome Study Group. *Sleep Med* 14:675–684, 2013.

23 Impulse-Control Disorders

Anna R. Weissman, MD, Cathleen M. Gould, MD, and Kathy M. Sanders, MD

KEY POINTS

Incidence and Epidemiology
- Impulsivity is common but diagnosed disorders range from rare to close to 10% of the population.

Pathophysiology
- Disturbances in the reward system (dopamine) as well as in the serotonergic neurocircuitry help us understand these disorders.
- Other neurotransmitters are implicated, as well as genetic linkages and vulnerabilities.

Clinical Findings
- The urge to behave in a dysfunctional manner in spite of consequences underlies most of these disorders.
- The urge to continue the behavior persists until the act is contrived.

Differential Diagnosis
- These disorders are co-morbid with psychotic, affective, personality, and addictive disorders and their differential must include these disorders.
- Medical conditions that may manifest these behaviors must be considered.

Treatment Options
- Both pharmacologic and psychosocial interventions are proven to be helpful in the treatment of impulse disorders.
- A combination of medication and therapies is most efficacious.

Prognosis
- Little is known about the prognosis of these disorders.
- Ongoing monitoring and treatment is recommended.
- Enhancing self-monitoring skills and behavioral choice through a variety of interventions offer the best outcomes.

OVERVIEW

The impulse-control disorders defined by the *Diagnostic and Statistical Manual of Mental Disorders*, ed 4, Text Revision (DSM-IV-TR)[1] (intermittent explosive disorder, kleptomania, pyromania, pathological gambling, and trichotillomania) will be the subject of this chapter. Impulsivity is the symptom common to each of these disorders. The pathological aspect of impulsivity is the inability to resist an action that could be harmful to oneself or to others. Hallmarks of this disorder include a building of tension around the desire to carry out any impulsive act that is relieved or gratified by engaging in the activity. There may be guilt, remorse, or self-reproach after the act. Other Axis I and II disorders are related to the impulse-control disorders in a complex manner, in that they are part of the differential diagnosis of impulsivity, as well as co-morbid conditions. Patients with impulse-control disorders are also likely to suffer from affective disorders, anxiety disorders, substance abuse, personality disorders, and eating disorders, as well as from paraphilias and attention-deficit disorder.[2-5] Our understanding of these disorders from neurobiological studies and evidence-based treatment studies varies from disorder to disorder; nonetheless, they share many common features.[6-9] However, DSM-5 made changes in the categorization of trichotillomania and gambling.[10] Trichotillomania is included with Obsessive-Compulsive and Related Disorders and gambling is classified with Substance-Related and Addictive Disorders. This chapter will focus on the DSM-IV-TR impulse-control disorders that include trichotillomania and gambling (Box 23-1).

INTERMITTENT EXPLOSIVE DISORDER

Intermittent explosive disorder is a diagnosis that characterizes individuals with episodes of dyscontrol, assaultive acts, and extreme aggression out of proportion to the precipitating event and not due to another Axis I, II, or III diagnosis.[1,11-14]

Epidemiology and Risk Factors

Intermittent explosive disorder is more common than previously considered, with a lifetime prevalence of 7%.[15] Men account for approximately 80% of the cases. Intermittent explosive disorder and personality change due to a general medical condition, aggressive type, are the diagnoses most often given to a patient with episodic violent behavior.[16] Risk factors include physical abuse in childhood, a chaotic family environment, substance abuse, and psychiatric disorders in the patient or his or her relatives.[8,9,13] The most common co-morbid disorders are mood disorders, anxiety disorders, and substance use disorders.

Pathophysiology

This disorder represents a complex convergence of psychosocial and neurobiological factors.[17,18] Some studies implicate serotonin neurotransmission, as evidenced by lower cerebrospinal fluid (CSF) levels and by platelet serotonin receptor expression[19] and re-uptake.[6] An elevated testosterone level may play a role in episodic violence.[17] An inverse relationship between aggression and CSF levels of oxytocin has also been reported.[20] Imaging studies have suggested a dysfunctional cortico-limbic network, with exaggerated amygdala reactivity and diminished orbito-frontal cortex and anterior cingulated activation.[21,22] Soft neurological signs may be present and reflect either trauma from earlier life experiences or genetic underpinnings of the violent behavior.[7,23] Family members frequently have similar violent outbursts, as well as a host of psychiatric diagnoses, supporting both an environmental and a genetic etiology, with genes for the serotonin transporter and monoamine oxidase (MAO) type A (MAO$_A$) interacting with childhood maltreatment and adversity to predispose to violence.[22,24]

Clinical Features and Diagnosis

Intermittent explosive disorder commonly arises in childhood and adolescence, with the mean age of onset ranging from 13 to 21 years. An episode of violence may arise in the setting of increased anger and emotional arousal before the loss of control that is out of proportion to the precipitating stressor. Aggressive outbursts in this disorder are characterized by their rapid onset, with little to no warning and that typically last less than 30 minutes.[25]

These patients may have a baseline of anger and irritability. Their lifestyle can be marginal; the disorder may make maintaining a job and stable relationships difficult. The presence of substance abuse further complicates both the diagnosis and the course. The most important feature of this disorder is that numerous other diagnoses must be ruled out before it can be diagnosed.

Most violent behavior can be accounted for by a variety of psychiatric and medical conditions, including seizures, head trauma, neurological abnormalities, dementia, delirium, and personality disorders (of the borderline or antisocial type). Anger attacks associated with major depression must also be ruled out.[26] Further, psychosis from schizophrenia or a manic episode may cause episodic violence. Aggressive outbursts while intoxicated or while withdrawing from a substance of abuse would prevent making the diagnosis of intermittent explosive disorder (Box 23-1). Intermittent explosive disorder carries significant morbidity, with 180 related injuries per 100 lifetime cases.[15]

Treatment

Psychopharmacology (e.g., anticonvulsants, lithium, beta-blockers, anxiolytics, neuroleptics, antidepressants [both serotonergic agents and polycyclics], and psychostimulants) can effectively control the chronic manifestations of this disorder.[14,27] Randomized control trials have shown benefit of fluoxetine as well as group and individual cognitive-behavior therapy (CBT).[28,29] The evidence for antiepileptic drugs in treating aggression is less robust, with four antiepileptics (valproate/divalproex, carbamazepine, oxcarbazepine, and phenytoin) showing efficacy in at least one study, but with other studies of three of those drugs showing no significant benefit.[30] The acute management of aggressive and violent behavior may also require use of physical restraints and rapid use of parenterally-administered neuroleptics and benzodiazepines (see Chapter 65).[31,32]

Supportive Care and Long-term Management

The use of CBT in both group and individual settings helps patients improve self-monitoring of behavior and learn about environmental triggers that are likely to lead to aggressive outbursts. The use of relaxation and flooding techniques may also facilitate better self-control. Psychopharmacological interventions can raise the threshold to impulsive violence and serve as an important part of long-term management. Long-term outpatient management of intermittent explosive disorder also requires attention to the therapeutic alliance between the clinician and the patient.

KLEPTOMANIA

More than 150 years ago, kleptomania was first recognized as behavior of "nonsensical pilfering," in which worthless items were stolen; such behavior was deemed outside the person's usual character.[33] Afflicted individuals were not known to have a pattern of stealing or of premeditated thievery. This disorder is characterized by an increased sense of tension before the act of stealing that is relieved by the act of stealing. It is a complex disorder with significant co-morbidities, family histories, and similarities with other affective and addictive spectrum disorders.[34-36] Since the initial documentation in the 1800s, few systematic or scientifically-rigorous studies have been conducted.

Epidemiology and Risk Factors

Although little is known about kleptomania, the prevalence within the general population has been estimated at 6 per 1,000.[37] Less than 5% of shoplifters meet criteria for kleptomania.[33] Women are more likely than are men to be diagnosed with kleptomania. Typically, there is a lag of many years between the onset of the behavior and the presentation for treatment. On average, women with the disorder seek treatment in their thirties and men seek treatment in their fifties.[33] This may be associated with disclosure when seeking treatment for another mental illness or for other factors that involve legal problems linked with stealing. Co-morbidity with other psychiatric illnesses, substance abuse, and personality disorders is high, ranging from 50% to 100%, depending on the study.[33,34,36–39]

Pathophysiology

A complex interplay of neurotransmitters (including serotonin, dopamine, and opiates), hormones, and genetic expression are implicated in impulse-control disorders, especially when the behavior is part of the motivation and reward cycle. Deficiency of serotonin in the brain facilitates impulsive behavior. Dopamine release has been associated with a "go" signal in the modulation of risk-taking behaviors. The opioid system has been associated with craving and reward, and may be implicated in the release of tension that surrounds the completion of impulsive acts. Brain regions that play important roles in the processing of motivation and reward include all the structures within the limbic system (e.g., the hypothalamus, amygdala, hippocampus, and cingulum), the prefrontal and frontal cortex, and the association cortices. From a developmental perspective, impulsive stealing may act to lift a depression by creating an over-riding stimulation and distraction. While numerous psychodynamic theories have been offered as an explanation for kleptomania, none of them has been confirmed or refuted. The exact delineation of these biological and psychological factors for the development of kleptomania has not been well established.[6,8,37,40,41]

Clinical Features and Diagnosis

Kleptomania typically has an onset in late adolescence and a chronic course of intermittent episodes of stealing over many years. Patients generally come to professional attention via court referrals or through disclosure during treatment for a related psychiatric disorder. Ego-dystonic reactions to the behavior and the lack of a premeditated nature of the stealing episodes should prompt further review. Additionally, co-morbid psychiatric conditions (including affective disorders, anxiety disorders, other impulse-control disorders, substance use disorders, eating disorders, and personality disorders) are common.[34,36–39]

Differential Diagnosis

The differential diagnosis includes criminal acts of shoplifting or stealing, malingering to avoid prosecution, antisocial personality disorder, conduct disorder, a manic episode, schizophrenia, and dementia. Based on DSM-4-TR criteria, the diagnosis is made by the degree of impulsivity, tension, and relief, as well as by guilt, remorse, and shame, attendant with the stealing behavior.

Treatment

Much of the literature about the pharmacotherapy of kleptomania has been based on case series and anecdotal reports; findings vary.[37] Monotherapy with tricyclic antidepressants (TCAs), selective serotonin reuptake inhibitors (SSRIs), anticonvulsants (such as topiramate), or anxiolytics, or combinations of these medications, have been tried with benefit in some patients.[42–44]

Case series, as well as one open-label and one double-blinded, placebo-controlled study, have shown that naltrexone reduces stealing urges and behaviors.[45,46] A pilot study using the NMDA receptor antagonist memantine had positive results in reducing stealing behaviors as well as improving mood and functioning.[47] One treatment-resistant case of kleptomania showed complete remission using the catechol O-methyltransferase (COMT) inhibitor, tolcapone, which was thought to improve executive functioning.

Psychotherapy (including insight-oriented psychotherapy and CBT that uses covert and aversive sensitization) may be helpful, especially in combination with psychopharmacotherapy.[48]

PYROMANIA

Problematic fire-setting occurs on a continuum, from children who play with matches to arsonists who set fires with the intention of destroying life or property. The phenomenon of fire-setting without any apparent motive and in the absence of any condition that would impair judgment or the ability to know right from wrong, has been described in the forensic and psychiatric literature since the 1800s.[49] Pyromania was named by Henri Marc, who described it as one of the "monomanias", conditions in which people have no apparent illness besides their inability to stop a behavior that injures themselves or others.[49] What is known about pyromania is limited by its rarity, and by the fact that most of the research in the area has considered the broader spectrum of fire-setting behaviors, from juvenile fire-setting to adult arson.

Incidence and Epidemiology

An analysis of the National Epidemiologic Survey on Alcohol and Related Conditions (NESARC) found that 1.1% of the US population had set a fire sometime during their life.[50] When subjects with antisocial personality disorder (ASPD) were excluded, the overall prevalence was 0.55%. Subjects who had set fires were more likely to be unmarried, male, and between the ages of 18 and 29 years. They were more likely to have had a history of other mental disorders, especially ASPD, alcohol use disorders, pathological gambling, or bipolar disorder, and they were three times more likely to have had some psychiatric treatment. They were more likely to have displayed other antisocial behaviors, whether or not they met criteria for ASPD.

Studies of persons who had committed arson showed varying incidences within this population, most likely due to the variety of criteria used for pyromania. A classic study by Lewis and Yarnell in 1951 showed no apparent motive for arson in 40% of case files from the National Board of Fire Underwriters.[51] Other studies of arson offenders found that 1%–3% of repeat arsonists met criteria for pyromania.[52–54]

Additional studies have looked at the incidence of pyromania in psychiatric populations. One study of adolescent inpatients found that 6.9% met criteria for pyromania.[55] Consistent with the NESARC findings that fire-setting behaviors tended to decrease after age 15,[50] a study of adult psychiatric inpatients found that 3.4% currently met criteria for pyromania, with a lifetime prevalence of 5.9%.[56] A sample of adult inpatients admitted for depression found an incidence of 2.8%; patients with pyromania had had a higher number of prior episodes of depression.[57]

Adolescents who set fires are more likely to have experienced sexual or physical abuse, and to have come from dysfunctional families. They are more likely to have suicidal thoughts, suicide attempts, and self-injurious behavior, and to express depression and hopelessness.[58]

Pathophysiology

Knowledge of the pathophysiology of pyromania is very limited. Differences in serotonergic functioning, between genders or in individuals, have been associated with impulsive behavior.[59] Studies in arsonists show lower than normal CSF concentrations of 5-HIAA, a primary metabolite of serotonin.[60] Since the prefrontal cortex is responsible for executive functioning, including the ability to control behavior, knowing that the PFC matures relatively late suggests an explanation for the reduced prevalence of pyromania and other impulse-control disorders with increasing age.[59] One case report showed that a left inferior frontal perfusion defect resolved with treatment of pyromania[61]; another case report showed measurable improvements in attention and executive control with treatment.[62]

Fire-setting has also been associated with illnesses that alter brain function (such as Klinefelter's syndrome,[63] epilepsy,[64,65] XYY syndrome, AIDS, and late luteal phase dysphoric disorder).[66]

Clinical Features and Diagnosis

Grant and Kim's 2007 study of 21 patients with pyromania found that patients reported that they set fires when they were stressed or bored, when feeling inadequate or sad, or when they were having interpersonal conflict.[67] Most patients took care to set fires in "controlled" settings where the fire would not spread easily or cause damage. Most reported that they had urges to set fires. All patients described a "rush" when they set fires; most described distress afterwards.

Differential Diagnosis

Pyromania is a diagnosis of exclusion; the differential diagnosis of fire-setting behavior is broad.

Treatment

No randomized controlled trials of pharmacotherapy for pyromania or for fire-setting have been conducted. Individual case reports describe successful treatment with clomipramine,[68] CBT and topiramate,[61] and olanzapine and valproic acid.[62] In Grant and Kim's study, two-thirds of the patients had had previous psychopharmacologic treatment, most for other conditions.[67] Topiramate has also been helpful. Escitalopram, sertraline, fluoxetine, and lithium have helped some patients, while valproic acid, citalopram, and clonazepam were not helpful to patients in this sample. Apparently psychopharmacologic treatment of co-morbid conditions has some potential for being helpful with pyromania. One patient who had told his therapist about his pyromania was helped by CBT.

CBT treatments, including chain analysis or graphing of the behavior, relaxation training, and social skills training, have been used successfully in children with fire-setting behaviors.[69]

Complications and Prognosis

Grant and Kim's study showed that patients were at risk for an increase in the frequency and severity of their behaviors over time, and for a negative impact on their work and relationships.[67] Afflicted individuals are at risk for escalation to arson, and for the development of additional impulse-control or addiction disorders. Nearly 40% of affected patients had considered suicide as a way of stopping fire-setting.

Little is known about the prognosis of adults who are treated for pyromania. CBT treatments for children and

adolescents who set fires have shown recidivism rates as low as 0.8%.[70]

GAMBLING DISORDER

The growing body of scientific literature on gambling disorder has shown elements in common with substance use disorders. Diagnostic criteria revealed an escalating pattern of a preoccupation with gambling, increased time and money spent to achieve the same effect, failures of efforts to cut down or to stop, and an escalating pattern of losses and adverse personal consequences.

Epidemiology and Risk Factors

The National Comorbidity Survey Replication estimated the prevalence of pathological gambling in the US (by DSM-IV criteria) to be 0.6%.[71] This study found a significant association with being young, male, and non-Hispanic Black with a typical onset in the mid-20s. The Gambling Impact and Behavior Study[72] interviewed a total of 2,947 adults and 534 adolescents in the US, and reviewed a database from 100 communities and 10 case studies on the effects of casino openings. The study estimated that 2.5 million Americans had a gambling disorder at the time of the survey, and that another 3 million should be considered "problem gamblers." The segment of the population with the highest and growing rate is comprised by those over the age of 65.[72]

Gambling disorder is more likely if there is a family history of alcohol or other substance dependence, mood disorders, gambling disorder, or antisocial personality disorder.[73,74] Twin studies have shown an increased incidence in the twins of affected individuals.[75] There is also an increased incidence of alcohol dependence and of major depressive disorder in co-twins, suggesting a common genetic vulnerability for both disorders.[76,77] Gambling disorder is highly co-morbid with alcohol dependence or abuse, other substance dependence or abuse, and mood, anxiety, or personality disorders; in women, it is also highly co-morbid with nicotine dependence.[78,79]

Pathophysiology

Gambling disorder, like other substance use disorders, appears to be a disorder of the brain's reward system. Neuroimaging studies have implicated meso-cortico-limbic neurocircuitry, a dopamine pathway important in reward processing, in gambling disorder. Functional magnetic resonance imaging (MRI) has demonstrated increased connectivity in pathological gambling between regions of the reward system and the prefrontal cortex, similar to those reported in substance use disorders; this suggests an imbalance between prefrontal function and the meso-limbic reward system.[80] Another recent study showed decreased activity in the ventromedial prefrontal cortex, insula, and ventral striatum in gambling disorder during multiple phases of reward processing, correlating with increased levels of impulsivity.

In keeping with these findings, persistent decision-making leading to negative consequences is also found in patients with damage to the ventromedial prefrontal cortex. This has led to the somatic marker hypothesis of decision-making, a hypothesis that has been proposed for impaired decision-making in gambling disorder and other addictive disorders. Somatic markers are the physiological changes that occur in response to primary inducers (which are stimuli associated with high-emotion states present in the environment), or to secondary inducers (which are thoughts or memories that have attached emotions and also produce change in the physiological state). The ventromedial cortex activates somatic states from thoughts or memories. Decision-making involves summation of all of the inducers, from the lights and sounds of the slot machine to the memory of the losses associated with one's last trip to the casino. Failure to include the negative states associated with thoughts and memories of losses in one's decision-making calculus biases the behavior choice toward continuing disadvantageous behavior.[81]

Multiple neurotransmitters, including dopamine, norepinephrine (noradrenaline), and serotonin have been implicated in gambling disorder.[79,82] Although one study of dopamine levels in CSF, urine, and plasma found no difference between those with gambling disorder and controls,[83] another study found lower levels of dopamine, and higher levels of dopamine metabolites, in the CSF of those with gambling disorder.[84] These results suggest higher turnover of dopamine in this disease. Moreover, it is well documented that patients with Parkinson's disease treated with dopamine agonists can develop gambling disorders.[85]

Studies of CSF levels of serotonin metabolites have shown mixed results, but there is other evidence of low serotonin availability, including decreased platelet MAO_B activity.[86] Other studies have found a blunted prolactin response after intravenous administration of clomipramine,[87] and a higher than normal prolactin release after administration of a serotonin agonist, suggesting decreased activity or availability of serotonin.[88,89] CSF levels of norepinephrine, associated with arousal and sensation-seeking, and its metabolite 3-methoxy-4-hydroxyphenylglycol (MHPG) are higher in individuals with gambling disorder.[83] Growth hormone is released in greater amounts after administration of clonidine compared to normal controls; this response suggests abnormal reactivity of the alpha-$_2$ post-synaptic norepinephrine receptors.[87]

Candidate gene associate studies had suggested that the Taq-A1 allele of the D_2 dopamine receptor, associated with other impulsive and addictive disorders, is more frequent in gambling disorder; however, subsequent studies controlling for race and ethnicity did not replicate this.[90] Other studies have connected D_1 receptor polymorphisms and co-morbid gambling disorder and alcohol dependence.[91] A less functional seven-repeat allele of the D_4 dopamine receptor has a higher incidence in women with gambling disorder. A three-repeat allele of an MAO_A promoter with lower transcriptional activity has higher incidence in men with gambling disorder; this gene has lower transcriptional activity and is located on the X chromosome, making sex differences in expression more likely. Men with this disorder also have a higher incidence of a short variant of a serotonin transporter with reduced promoter activity.[79,82]

Clinical Features and Diagnosis

The DSM-5 describes individuals with gambling disorder as having persistent and recurrent maladaptive gambling behavior that is addictive in nature (Boxes 23-2 and 23-3).

Differential Diagnosis

Differential diagnoses for gambling disorder are listed in Table 23-1.

Treatment

As with the other substance use disorders, multiple treatment modalities have been considered. Participation in Gamblers Anonymous is frequently recommended, and the combination of Gamblers Anonymous and professional treatment improves outcomes.[92]

BOX 23-2 DSM-5 Diagnostic Criteria: Gambling Disorder (312.31 (F63.0))

A. Persistent and recurrent problematic gambling behavior leading to clinically significant impairment or distress, as indicated by the individual exhibiting four (or more) of the following in a 12-month period:
1. Needs to gamble with increasing amounts of money in order to achieve the desired excitement.
2. Is restless or irritable when attempting to cut down or stop gambling.
3. Has made repeated unsuccessful efforts to control, cut back, or stop gambling.
4. Is often preoccupied with gambling (e.g., having persistent thoughts of reliving past gambling experiences, handicapping or planning the next venture, thinking of ways to get money with which to gamble).
5. Often gambles when feeling distressed (e.g., helpless, guilty, anxious, depressed).
6. After losing money gambling, often returns another day to get even ("chasing" one's losses).
7. Lies to conceal the extent of involvement in gambling.
8. Has jeopardized or lost a significant relationship, job, or educational or career opportunity because of gambling.
9. Relies on others to provide money to relieve desperate financial situations caused by gambling.
B. The gambling behavior is not better explained by a manic episode.

Reprinted with permission from the Diagnostic and statistical manual of mental disorders, *ed 5, (Copyright 2013). American Psychiatric Association.*

BOX 23-3 Gambling Disorder: Treatment Strategies

No specific treatment modality has been shown to work predictably; the following are used:
- Psychodynamic psychotherapy
- Behavioral therapy
- Cognitive therapy
- Psychotropic medications
- Naltrexone
- Memantine
- *N*-acetylcysteine
- Electroconvulsive therapy
- Gamblers Anonymous and the 12-step programs, Gam-Anon, and Gam-a-Teen are important resources.

Use of clomipramine and SSRIs has reduced or eliminated gambling behaviors in the short term. As with obsessive-compulsive disorder (OCD), patients may require higher doses of these medications than are typically required to treat depression. Naltrexone moderates activity of the meso-limbic dopamine pathway, is approved for use in opiate and alcohol use disorders, and has been shown to reduce urges and thoughts of gambling, as well as gambling behavior, with a positive response associated with a positive family history of alcoholism.[93] Mood stabilizers (e.g., lithium, valproate, and carbamazepine) have helped reduce the symptoms of gambling disorder, especially in gamblers with co-morbid bipolar disorder.[79,94,95] In a double-blind, randomized, controlled

TABLE 23-1 Differential Diagnoses for Gambling Disorder

Conditions	Characteristics
Non-disordered gambling	Typically occurs with friends or colleagues. Lasts for a limited period of time, with acceptable losses. Some individuals can experience problems with gambling that do not meet the full criteria for gambling disorder.
Professional gambling	Considers gambling a business. Risks are limited and discipline is central. Able to endure periods of loss without changing gambling behavior.
Manic episode	The patient has to meet criteria for pathological gambling at times other than during a manic episode.
Personality disorders	Problems with gambling may occur in individuals with antisocial personality disorder and other personality disorders. If the criteria are met for both disorders, both can be diagnosed.
Other medical conditions	Some patients taking dopaminergic medications (e.g., for Parkinson's disease) may experience urges to gamble. If such symptoms dissipate when dopaminergic medications are reduced in dosage or ceased, then a diagnosis of gambling disorder would not be indicated.

pilot study, N-acetylcysteine caused significant symptomatic improvement, thought to be due to restoration of extracellular glutamate concentration in the nucleus accumbens (part of the reward center).[96] In an open-label trial, memantine, another drug that targets the glutamatergic system, was associated with diminished gambling and improved cognitive flexibility.[97]

CBT is also effective in the treatment of gambling disorder.[79,98,99] Imaginal desensitization, electric aversion therapy, and imaginal relaxation have been studied. Exposure and response prevention, in which participants are exposed to gambling situations without engaging in the behavior, have also been used. Cognitive re-structuring involves the intervention in the false beliefs about gambling, including an illusion of control, and of memory biases, in which the gambler only remembers winnings. Training in problem-solving and social skills is used to reduce the dysphoric states and stress that may trigger gambling behaviors. Self-help approaches include the use of a workbook for self-monitoring and for functional analysis. A meta-analysis of 21 studies that used these behavioral treatments showed an effect size of 2.01; therefore, patients who receive CBT had outcome measures averaging 2 standard deviations above controls.[100]

Prognosis

Although the DSM-5 describes gambling disorder as a chronic and persistent disorder, Slutske's 2006 analysis[101] of the Gambling Impact and Behavior Study (GIBS)[72] suggests that some may be able to recover naturally from the disease. Slutske's[101] conclusion that individuals with gambling disorder may have the possibility of natural recovery is controversial.[102]

TRICHOTILLOMANIA

Trichotillomania is a condition of repeated urges to pull out hair, with tension before the behavior and pleasure or relief after the behavior. Patients are unable to stop pulling out their own hair even after developing visible consequences, shame, or significant impact on their daily lives. Individuals with trichotillomania report interference with function at work or at school, avoidance of intimate relationships and social activities, and low self-esteem and emotional distress.[103,104]

Epidemiology and Risk Factors

Prevalence of this condition may be underestimated due to shame and denial of the behavior. A survey of college students showed that 0.6% of men and women had met full DSM-III-R criteria for trichotillomania at some point in their lives. In this same study, 1.5% of men and 3.4% of women reported hair-pulling with visible hair loss, but without the tension and relief needed to meet diagnostic criteria.[105] Approximately 10% to 13% of college freshmen reported regular hair-pulling in another study, with 1% to 2% having bald patches sometime in their lifetime, and 1% to 2% reporting distress or tension related to the behavior.[106]

The average age of onset is between 11 and 13 years, with female patients far outnumbering male patients in adults.[107,108] In a pediatric case series of all clinic patients diagnosed with trichotillomania, 10 children between 9 and 13 years of age were identified; half were male.[109] It is not known if the female-to-male ratio changes in adult patients, or if adult men are less likely to seek treatment. Twin studies have suggested putative genetic underpinnings to trichotillomania. In one recent study, respective concordance rates for monozygotic and dizygotic twin pairs were significantly different (at 38.1% and 0%) for DSM-IV trichotillomania criteria, 39.1% and 0% using modified DSM criteria, and 58.3% and 20% for noticeable non-cosmetic hair-pulling.[110]

Trichotillomania is highly co-morbid with mood disorders, anxiety disorders, substance abuse disorders, and eating disorders.[109] Evaluated according to the DSM-III-R, two-thirds of patients in one study met criteria for an anxiety or mood disorder; one-half met criteria for an Axis II disorder.[111]

Pathophysiology

Serotonin has been studied in trichotillomania because of the association between impulsivity and serotonergic dysfunction. A study of CSF concentrations of 5-HIAA showed no significant difference between patients with trichotillomania and normal controls. However, the study demonstrated that the lower the concentration of 5-HIAA at baseline, the higher the degree of improvement after treatment with a serotonergic drug.[112]

Patients with trichotillomania have smaller left putamen volumes, implicating the striatum in this disease. Symptoms involving repetitive behaviors or thoughts may involve dysfunction in corticostriatal pathways.[113] Positron emission tomography (PET) studies have shown increased metabolic activity in the right and left cerebellum and in the right superior parietal area.[114] Morphometric magnetic resonance imaging (MRI) analysis has demonstrated lower total, right, and left cerebellar cortex volumes. There is a significant inverse relationship between severity and the volume of the left primary sensorimotor cluster of the cerebellum.[115] Diffusion tensor imaging has shown disorganization of white matter tracts involved in motor habit generation and suppression, along with affective regulation.[116]

Studies of cognitive differences between patients with trichotillomania and normal controls have shown conflicting results. Some studies show impaired non-verbal memory and executive function.[117] Another study shows no deficits in visual-spatial or executive function, but does show impairment in the Object Alternation Task, which shows an ability to establish and to maintain an alternating set,[118] and another showed deficits in tasks of divided attention.[119] One interpretation of this deficit is a problem in response flexibility; the trichotillomania patient may have difficulty switching to

TABLE 23-2 Differential Diagnosis for Trichotillomania

Normative hair removal/ manipulation	Hair removal is performed solely for cosmetic reasons. Many individuals twist and play with their hair, but this behavior does not usually qualify for a diagnosis of trichotillomania. Some may bite rather than pull hair; again, this does not qualify for a diagnosis of trichotillomania.
Psychosis	Hair removal in response to a delusion or hallucination.
Other obsessive-compulsive and related disorders	Individuals with OCD and symmetry concerns may pull out hairs as part of their symmetry rituals, and individuals with body dysmorphic disorder may remove body hair that they perceive as ugly, asymmetrical, or abnormal.
Neurodevelopmental disorders	Hair-pulling may meet the definition of stereotypies (e.g., in stereotypic movement disorder). Tics (in tic disorders) rarely lead to hair-pulling.
Another medical condition	Other causes of scarring alopecia (e.g., alopecia areata, androgenic alopecia, telogen effluvium) or non-scarring alopecia (e.g., chronic discoid lupus erythematosus, lichen planopilaris, central centrifugal cicatricial alopecia, pseudopelade, folliculitis decalvans, dissecting folliculitis, acne keloidalis nuchae). Skin biopsy or dermascopy can be used to differentiate.
Substance-related disorders	Hair-pulling symptoms may be exacerbated by certain substances—for example, stimulants—but it is less likely that substances are the primary cause of persistent hair-pulling.
Non–rapid eye movement (non-REM) parasomnia	There is one case report of repeated hair extraction occurring during non-REM sleep. The prevalence of this phenomenon is unknown; diagnosis requires polysomnography.

another behavior once the behavior has started.[119] Studies have also shown impaired inhibition of motor responses in patients with trichotillomania.[120] Genetic studies have identified multiple genes that confer biologic vulnerability to trichotillomania. These include multiple rare *SAPAP3* missense variants (a post-synaptic scaffolding protein at excitatory synapses that is highly expressed in the striatum)[121] and *SLITRK1* mutations (integral membrane proteins thought to be involved in cortex development and neuronal growth).[122] Mutations at these loci are associated with susceptibility, but are not by themselves disease-causing. They are also associated with a wider spectrum of OCD disorders.

Several primate species, mice, parrots, cats, dogs, and rabbits, develop excessive grooming behaviors when stressed. Excessive grooming has been induced experimentally in some rat pups by injection of an adrenocorticotropic hormone or hypothalamic stimulation, suggesting that grooming is an innate response.[123,124]

Clinical Features and Diagnosis

Not all patients will admit to pulling out their own hair, and some may have sought treatment for alopecia before referral to a psychiatrist. Patients may have an itching or burning sensation that precedes the behavior. Patients may start hair-pulling in response to having negative thoughts or feelings about themselves, or in response to negatively experienced interactions with others. On the other hand, patients may pull hair when they are relaxed and inattentive to their own behavior. Hairs are pulled out one by one, but some patients will pull quickly and others will select hairs carefully by differences in texture. Some patients report particular satisfaction if the root is retrieved. Some patients inspect the hair, others just discard it. Some may separate the root from the hair, and eat the root or the entire hair. Patients are ashamed of the behavior and of the resulting bald areas. They will typically camouflage the affected areas with scarves, hats, wigs, clothing, or makeup. Patients may avoid friendships, social events, athletic activity, sexual intimacy, or even work that involves opportunities for time alone to pull hair.[125-127]

On physical examination, patients will have areas of hair loss, ranging from thinned hair to complete denudement. Patients may pull hair from the scalp, eyebrows and eyelashes, face, arms, or legs; axillary, pubic, or peri-anal hair may be also involved. Patients typically have a preferred area. Areas will vary in size; on the scalp, the areas may be coin size to "tonsure

trichotillomania," in which all of the hair on the scalp has been pulled out except for a thin fringe at the scalp.

Differential Diagnosis

Differential diagnoses for trichotillomania can be reviewed in Table 23-2.

Treatment

The Massachusetts General Hospital (MGH) Hair-pulling Scale can be used to measure the clinical severity and response to treatment. Patients report the frequency of urges, the intensity of urges, and the ability to control the urges; the frequency of hair-pulling; attempts to resist hair-pulling; control over hair-pulling; and distress associated with the behavior.[128,129] Both pharmacological and behavioral treatments are used in trichotillomania. Combination treatment has been shown to be superior to either modality used alone.[130,131]

Serotonergic medications (such as clomipramine) have reduced hair-pulling behavior in controlled studies[132-134]; however, SSRIs have not been found to be efficacious, and are not considered first-line treatment.[135-138] Olanzapine, studied in open-label and randomized control trials, has been helpful[139,140]; case reports have shown the benefits of risperidone[141] and quetiapine[142] and of augmentation of serotonergic drugs with atypical antipsychotics. Topiramate has been helpful in open-label trials.[143] The glutamatergic agent *N*-acetylcysteine has also demonstrated statistically-significant reductions in trichotillomania symptoms.[144] Naltrexone has also been suggested to reduce hair-pulling behaviors, but there is not sufficient evidence for it at this time.[138]

Habit-reversal therapy for trichotillomania involves developing an awareness of the habit using self-monitoring sheets, training in muscle relaxation and diaphragmatic breathing, and then using a competing response. This technique has reduced trichotillomania symptoms with relatively large effect size.[137,145] Stimulus-control approaches can also be used. Acceptance and commitment therapy, in which patients are helped to reduce their avoidance of unpleasant internal states, has been successfully combined with habit-reversal therapy.[146]

Prognosis

Patients can significantly improve hair-pulling, depression, anxiety, self-esteem, and psychosocial function with treatment.[147] Over the longer term, patients may develop irreversible damage to the hair follicles with permanent areas of baldness or thinned hair, infections, and repetitive hand-use injuries.[138,148] Patients who eat the hair (e.g., with trichophagia) may develop trichobezoars, which are deposits of the hair within the stomach that do not pass through to the rest of the digestive system. Complications of trichobezoars include malabsorption, anemia, pancreatitis, peritonitis, small or large bowel perforation, and acute appendicitis.[149]

CONCLUSION

The impulse-control disorders are a heterogeneous group of mental illnesses that have similarities in underlying psychopathology, neuropathology, diagnosis, and treatment. The current controversy in the field surrounding these disorders is whether they are truly distinct disorders or part of a spectrum of disorders of affect, anxiety, or addiction. The co-morbidity with other major mental disorders is staggeringly high (over 70%). The impulsive and compulsive behaviors characteristically involved are destructive acts toward self or others. These destructive impulses have immediate or delayed negative consequences, yet patients persist in the face of such grave consequences. Understanding their etiology, pathophysiology, and treatment will result in significant relief from distress for many patients and their families, as well as for our society.

Access the complete reference list and multiple choice questions (MCQs) online at https://expertconsult.inkling.com

KEY REFERENCES

9. Hollander E, Stein DJ. *Clinical manual of impulse-control disorders*, Washington, DC, 2006, American Psychiatric Publishing.
10. American Psychiatric Association. *Diagnostic and statistical manual of mental disorders*, ed 5 (DSM-5), Washington, DC, 2013, American Psychiatric Publishing.
15. Kessler RC, Coccaro EF, Fava M, et al. The prevalence and correlates of DSM-IV intermittent explosive disorder in the National Comorbidity Survey Replication. *Arch Gen Psychiatry* 63:669–678, 2006.
18. Renfrew JW. *Aggression and its causes: a biopsychosocial approach*, New York, 2002, Oxford University Press.
20. Lee R, Ferris C, Van de Kar LD, et al. Cerebrospinal fluid oxytocin, life history of aggression, and personality disorder. *Psychoneuroendocrinology* 34:1567–1573, 2009.
21. Coccaro EF, McCloskey MS, Fitzgerald DA, et al. Amygdala and orbitofrontal reactivity to social threat in individuals with impulsive aggression. *Biol Psychiatry* 62:168–178, 2007.
22. Siever LJ. Neurobiology of aggression and violence. *Am J Psychiatry* 165:429–442, 2008.
25. Coccaro EF. Intermittent explosive disorder as a disorder of impulsive aggression for DSM-5. *Am J Psychiatry* 169:577–588, 2012.
28. Coccaro EF, Lee RJ, Kavoussi RJ. A double-blind, randomized, placebo-controlled trial of fluoxetine in patients with intermittent explosive disorder. *J Clin Psychiatry* 70:653–662, 2009.
29. McCloskey MS, Noblett KL, Deffenbacher JL, et al. Cognitive-behavioral therapy for intermittent explosive disorder: a pilot randomized clinical trial. *J Consult Clin Psychol* 76:876–886, 2008.
32. Maytal G, Sanders K. Aggressive and impulsive patients. In Stern TA, Fricchione G, Cassem E, et al., editors: *The MGH handbook of general hospital psychiatry*, ed 6, Philadelphia, 2010, Mosby/Elsevier Science.
37. Grant JE. Kleptomania. In Hollander E, Stein DJ, editors: *Clinical manual of impulse-control disorders*, Washington, DC, 2006, American Psychiatric Publishing.
46. Grant JE, Kim SW. Odlaug BL. A double-blind, placebo-controlled study of the opiate antagonist, naltrexone, in the treatment of kleptomania. *Biol Psychiatry* 65:600–606, 2009.
47. Grant JE, Odlaug BL, Schreiber LRN, et al. Memantine reduces stealing behaviour and impulsivity in kleptomania: a pilot study. *Int Clin Psychopharmacology* 28:106–111, 2013.
48. Grant JE, Odlaug BL, Kim SW. Assessment and treatment of kleptomania. In Grant JE, Potenza MC, editors: *The Oxford handbook of impulse control disorders*, New York, 2012, Oxford University Press.
49. Andrews J. From stack-firing to pyromania: medico-legal concepts of insane arson in British, US, and European contexts, c.1800-1913 Part I. *Hist Psychiat* 21(3):243–260, 2010.
50. Blanco C, Alegria AA, Petry NM, et al. Prevalence and correlates of firesetting in the US: Results from the National Epidemiologic Survey on Alcohol and Related Conditions (NESARC). *J Clin Psychiatry* 71(9):1218–1225, 2010.
59. Chamorro J, Bernardi S, Potenza MN, et al. Impulsivity in the general population: A national study. *J Psychiatric Res* 46(8):994–1001, 2012.
67. Grant JE, Kim SW. Clinical characteristics and psychiatric comorbidity of pyromania. *J Clin Psychiatry* 68(11):1717–1722, 2007.
71. Lobo DS, Kennedy JL. Genetic aspects of pathological gambling: a complex disorder with shared genetic vulnerabilities. *Addiction* 104:1454–1465, 2009.
79. Pallanti S, Rossi NB, Hollander E. Pathological gambling. In Hollander E, Stein DJ, editors: *Clinical manual of impulse control disorders*, Arlington, VA, 2006, American Psychiatric Publishing.
80. Koehler S, Ovadia-Caro S, van der Meer E, et al. Increased functional connectivity between prefrontal cortex and reward system in pathological gambling. *PLoS ONE* 8:e84565, 2013.
91. Lobo DS, Kennedy JL. Genetic aspects of pathological gambling: a complex disorder with shared genetic vulnerabilities. *Addiction* 104:1454–1465, 2009.
92. Petry NM. Gamblers Anonymous and cognitive-behavioral therapies for pathological gamblers. *J Gambl Stud* 21:27–33, 2005.
93. Grant JE, Kim SW, Hollander E, et al. Predicting response to opiate antagonists and placebo in the treatment of pathological gambling. *Psychopharmacology (Berl)* 200:521–527, 2008.
97. Grant JE, Chamberlain SR, Odlaug BL, et al. Memantine shows promise in reducing gambling severity and cognitive inflexibility in pathological gambling: a pilot study. *Psychopharmacology (Berl)* 212:603–612, 2010.
98. Petry NM, Ammerman Y, Bohl J, et al. Cognitive behavioral therapy for pathological gamblers. *J Consult Clin Psychol* 74:555–567, 2006.
110. Novak CE, Keuthen NJ, Stewart SE, et al. A twin concordance study of trichotillomania. *Am J Med Genet Part B* 50B:944–949, 2009.
116. Chamberlain SR, Hampshire A, Menzies LA, et al. Reduced brain white matter integrity in trichotillomania: a diffusion tensor imaging study. *Arch Gen Psychiatry* 67:965–971, 2010.
121. Züchner S, Wendland JR, Ashley-Koch AE, et al. Multiple rare SAPAP3 missense variants in trichotillomania and OCD. *Mol Psychiatry* 14:6–9, 2009.
130. Dougherty DD, Loh R, Jenike MA, et al. Single modality versus dual modality treatment for trichotillomania: sertraline, behavioral therapy, or both? *J Clin Psychiatry* 67:1086–1092, 2006.
137. Bloch MH, Landeros-Weisenberger A, Dombrowski P, et al. Systematic review: pharmacological and behavioral treatment for trichotillomania. *Biol Psychiatry* 62:839–846, 2007.
138. Franklin ME, Zagrabbe K, Benavides KL. Trichotillomania and its treatment: a review and recommendations. *Expert Rev Neurother* 11:1165–1174, 2011.
140. Van Ameringen M, Mancini C, Patterson B, et al. A randomized, double-blind, placebo-controlled trial of olanzapine in the treatment of trichotillomania. *J Clin Psychiatry* 71:1336–1343, 2010.
144. Grant JE, Odlaug BL, Kim SW. N-acetylcysteine, a glutamate modulator, in the treatment of trichotillomania: a double-blind, placebo-controlled study. *Arch Gen Psychiatry* 66:756–763, 2009.

24 Somatic Symptom Disorders

Ted Avi Gerstenblith, MD, and Nicholas Kontos, MD

KEY POINTS

Incidence

- Medically-unexplained symptoms (MUS) are ubiquitous in inpatients and outpatients.

Epidemiology

- Patients with MUS that suffer from somatoform disorders may represent the largest group with psychopathology within primary care populations (at 10%–24%).

Pathophysiology

- While the etiology of somatic symptom disorder is poorly understood and insufficiently studied epidemiologically, limited data extrapolated from other conditions suggest that a combination of factors (e.g., physiology, personality, life experiences, health cognitions, and the degree to which people experience sensations regardless of whether they have a disease) influence the development of the disorder.

Clinical Findings

- The key features of somatic symptom disorder involve persistent (i.e., more than 6 months) and excessive or disproportionate *thoughts* (about the seriousness of one's symptoms), *feelings* (high level of anxiety about health), or *behaviors* (excessive time and energy devoted to the health concern) associated with somatic concerns to the point that the symptoms cause a significant disruption in one's daily life.

- Common symptoms of conversion disorder include reduced or absent skin sensation, tunnel vision, blindness, aphonia, weakness, paralysis, tremor, dystonic movements, gait abnormalities, or abnormal limb posturing.

Differential Diagnoses

- Somatically-focused syndromes include true medical illnesses as well as somatic symptom disorder, illness anxiety disorder, functional somatic syndromes, conversion disorder, factitious disorder, and malingering.

Treatment Options

- The treatment of somatic symptom and related disorders, and, to an extent, problematic MUS in general, begins with the recognition that these conditions involve a maladaptive goal-directed behavior that specifically involves symptoms or signs of a medical illness. It can be helpful to think of most of these conditions as *abnormal illness behaviors* rather than disease entities.

- Two goals play important roles in the treatment process: (1) avoiding unnecessary diagnostic tests and thereby obviating overly aggressive medical and surgical intervention; and, (2) helping the patient tolerate and maximize functioning in the presence of symptoms rather than striving to eliminate them.

- Conducting a follow-up visit is probably more important than is any prescribed treatment.

Prognosis

- Careful, conservative medication use, especially that which targets co-morbid mood and anxiety disorders, is also important in reducing suffering, though is unlikely to reduce the somatic focus of patients with somatic symptom and related disorders.

OVERVIEW

Medically unexplained symptoms (MUS) are ubiquitous in inpatients and outpatients. With 60%–80% of the American population experiencing a somatic symptom in any given week,[1] MUS as a whole must be considered an ordinary, even normal, part of human experience. While the medical literature often suggests that dealing with MUS is a major concern, the issue actually involves a subset of patients with clinically and functionally problematic MUS.

The subset of patients with MUS that suffers from DSM IV-TR[2] somatoform disorders (the DSM-5[3] classification has been insufficiently studied epidemiologically), may represent the largest group with psychopathology within primary care populations (at 10%–24%).[4–6] Patients with MUS in the general population probably account for a disproportionate amount of medical system utilization/cost,[7] iatrogenic complications,[8] and physician and patient consternation.[9,10]

Terms used to identify patients with problematic MUS have varied. In a historical review, Berrios and Mumford[11] note that "to make sense of the evolution of all these clinical categories,

the history of the *words* (etymology) will have to be distinguished from that of the *clinical phenomena* involved (behavioral paleontology) and from that of the *concepts* periodically formulated to explain them." At different times, users of terms such as "hysteria" and "hypochondriasis" have placed greater emphasis on these words' anatomic rather than diagnostic or etiologic elements. Likewise, "somatization" and "conversion," even in the post-DSM II "atheoretical" era[12] have implied etiologic mechanisms that those who invoke these terms diagnostically may not uphold.

At least partially due to confusion in terminology, psychiatric classifications of patients with problematic MUS have not caught on in the places where they are arguably most needed—primary care and other non-psychiatric medical settings.[13] DSM-5's classification of the "Somatic Symptom and Related Disorders" is the latest attempt to simultaneously sort through problems of clinical utility, scientifically-informed validity, and etiologic neutrality.[14–17] This chapter first focuses on classification, including the DSM-IV and DSM-5 codifications, the functional somatic syndromes (FSS), and a broader conceptual scheme that is compatible with standard diagnoses. Important co-morbidities of these conditions are discussed, followed by a review of treatment principles and interventions.

Cross-walking DSM-IV to DSM-5

The DSM-5 category, Somatic Symptom and Related Disorders, corresponds to the Somatoform Disorders category in DSM-IV. The somatoform disorders were composed of somatization disorder, undifferentiated somatoform disorder, conversion disorder, pain disorder, hypochondriasis, body dysmorphic disorder, and somatoform disorder not otherwise specified. Overlapping symptoms and unclear treatment implications, among other things, made these diagnostic labels confusing and they were rarely used in non-psychiatric clinical practice. In an effort to facilitate a more user-friendly categorization, DSM-5 renamed the somatoform disorders as somatic symptom and related disorders, and lumped four disorders (somatization disorder, undifferentiated somatoform disorder, pain disorder, and, partially, hypochondriasis) under the new heading, somatic symptom disorder. Conversion disorder remains a discrete diagnostic entity, although some have suggested that it is better categorized as a

dissociative disorder given the high rates of dissociative symptoms reported in several studies of patients with conversion disorder.[18] Figure 24-1 delineates the transition of DSM-IV-TR categories to those found in DSM-5.

The core diagnosis in this class, somatic symptom disorder, de-emphasizes the previous focus on somatic symptoms that are medically unexplained. For many, perhaps most, patients appropriately assigned this diagnosis, MUS will, indeed, be present, but this is not required, and the emphasis is placed more so upon patients' excessive and maladaptive experiences of, and responses to, symptoms, whether they be explained or not. Some commentators fear that this modification might do more harm than good by pathologizing a large majority of the population as well as potentially missing more underlying medical etiologies of unexplained symptoms. DSM-5 field trials suggested that somatic symptom disorder would capture 26% of patients with irritable bowel syndrome or fibromyalgia, 15% of patients with cancer or heart disease, and that there would be a false-positive rate of roughly 7% among healthy people in the general population.[19] MUS remain key features of pseudocyesis and conversion disorder, as one must demonstrate that the symptoms are not consistent with known medical pathophysiology.

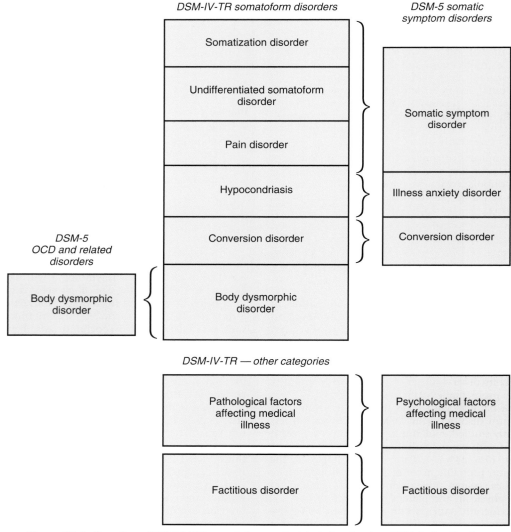

Figure 24-1. Transition of DSM-IV-TR somatoform and related disorders into DSM-5 classification.

Somatic Symptom Disorder

The key features of somatic symptom disorder involve persistent (i.e., more than 6 months) and excessive or disproportionate *thoughts* (about the seriousness of one's symptoms), *feelings* (high level of anxiety about health), or *behaviors* (excessive time and energy devoted to the health concern) associated with somatic concerns to the point that the symptoms cause a significant disruption in one's daily life.[3] These symptoms revolve around the patient's assumption that their somatic symptoms indicate underlying illness states that have been insufficiently addressed medically. While the distinction is sometimes difficult to make, the diagnosing clinician is expected to have determined that the patient's illness beliefs lack the fixed quality of the delusions, as in delusional disorder, somatic type. If an individual lacks somatic symptoms, yet still has persistent disproportionate thoughts, feelings, behaviors, and preoccupations that he or she might be sick, that person should be assessed for illness anxiety disorder (see next heading).

While the etiology of somatic symptom disorder is poorly understood and insufficiently studied epidemiologically, limited data extrapolated from other conditions suggest that a combination of factors (e.g., physiology, personality, life experiences, health cognitions, and the degree to which people experience sensations regardless of whether they have a disease) influence the development of the disorder. Risk factors include the personality trait of neuroticism, low education and socioeconomic status, recent stressful life events, female gender, older age, unemployment, and concurrent chronic physical or psychiatric illness. The prevalence of somatic symptom disorder is likely to be higher in women than men since women report more somatic symptoms.[3,20]

Illness Anxiety Disorder

While somatic symptom disorder is meant or expected to classify most individuals (~75%) who would have met criteria for the DSM-IV's category called "hypochondriasis," illness anxiety disorder accounts for the remainder. These patients are preoccupied with the idea that they are ill or that they may acquire a serious as of yet undiagnosed medical condition. The anxiety associated with the cause, meaning, or significance of the concern (rather than the somatic symptom itself) distinguishes this disorder from somatic symptom disorder, where the concern is more about distress or disability. Reassurance, negative diagnostic work-ups, and a benign somatic course do little to alleviate the anxiety of illness anxiety disorder. Fear of illness ultimately becomes a part of the identity of the afflicted. Importantly, one can have a medical condition and have co-existing illness anxiety that is disproportionate to the severity of the condition.

Although anxiety in response to serious illness can be a normal part of human experience, disproportionate and significant severity and persistence (greater than 6 months) are felt by the authors of DSM-5 to mark it as disordered. Other specific factors include the focus of worry on one's health and/or the lack thereof (as opposed to these concerns being expressions of the more global nervous preoccupation found in generalized anxiety disorder). Likewise, any given health concern is more flexible and plausible than is generally noted in patients with somatic delusions.

Since this is a newly classified disorder, its co-morbidities, risk factors, prevalence, and clinical course remain unclear. It is thought, however, to be a chronic condition that begins in early and middle adulthood. Both genes and upbringing may serve as predisposing factors. Major life stressors, threats to one's health, and a history of abuse or serious illness in childhood may serve as triggers for development of this disorder. As with the other disorders described in this chapter, one should consider cultural beliefs that can be congruent with one's mindset before making a diagnosis.

Conversion Disorder

Conversion disorder involves a loss or change in sensory or motor function that is suggestive of a physical disorder, but that lacks evidence for a known neurological or medical condition. The diagnosis can be specified by symptom type, persistence (acute and self-limiting versus chronic), and whether it occurs with or without a psychological stressor. DSM-5 eliminates the previously held criterion that one should identify an association between symptom onset and psychologically meaningful precipitants that may have led to the disorder.

Common symptoms include reduced or absent skin sensation, tunnel vision, blindness, aphonia, weakness, paralysis, tremor, dystonic movements, gait abnormalities, or abnormal limb posturing. Conversion symptoms are not under voluntary control and are usually sustained, but the patient may be able to modulate their severity. A patient with a functional gait disturbance or a weak arm, for example, may, with intense concentration, be able to demonstrate slightly better control or strength.

The diagnosis is based not on one single finding, but on the overall clinical picture. Work-ups and investigations that reveal normal findings are not sufficient to make the diagnosis. Inconsistent neurological examinations (e.g., eliciting physical signs that become positive or negative when tested in a different way) and the occasional demonstration of normal function in the supposedly disabled body part are more specific. For example, one might observe a patient crossing a leg that he subjectively cannot lift over his good one during a conversation. In the "semi-comatose" patient, deviation of the eyes toward the ground, regardless of which side the patient lies on, can sometimes demonstrate lack of an organic disorder.[21] The patient with functional blindness can be led around obstacles whereas the patient with conversion usually avoids them (a malingerer is more likely to bump into them). Another way to assess vision is to carefully watch the "blind" patient's eyes while taking out a roll of money or making a face at the patient. A malingerer is more likely to become oppositional or uncooperative during the examination.

Factors that support a diagnosis of conversion disorder include having a history of multiple similar somatic symptoms, an onset at a time of psychological or physical stress or trauma, and an association of dissociative symptoms (e.g., depersonalization, derealization, dissociative amnesia) at time of symptom onset. A prior medical illness is a common source of the symptom. The illness may bring secondary benefits of attention and support from loved ones. Those with seizures, for example, especially complex partial seizures (in which consciousness is preserved), are repeatedly exposed to a phenomenon that removes them from responsibility, evokes sympathy, and brings help from a loved one.

Conversion disorder can co-exist with non-idiopathic neurologic disease. Psychogenic non-epileptic seizures (PNES), for example, commonly co-exist with electrographically-confirmed epilepsy and can be difficult to discriminate. Epileptic and psychogenic non-epileptic seizures can be temporally related and brain changes resulting from repeated seizures may also facilitate the development of conversion symptoms.[22]

In adults, the disorder is more common in women, and its onset can occur throughout life, although the onset of non-epileptic attacks may peak in the third decade and motor symptoms may peak in the fourth decade.[3] Symptoms can be persistent or transient. While the rate of misdiagnosing conversion disorder has declined, one should proceed with caution in diagnosing conversion symptoms, since some patients will develop an organic condition that in retrospect is related to the original symptom.[23,24] At the same time, an extensive review of published cases suggests that fewer than 5% of individuals diagnosed with conversion disorder are found to eventually have a medical or neurologic condition that explained their initial presentation.[24]

The literature supports a mixed prognosis for these patients, at least in the first few years. Folks and co-workers[25] recorded a complete remission rate of 50% by discharge from the general hospital. However, the long-term course is less favorable because many patients develop recurrent conversion symptoms (20% to 25% within 1 year). Unilateral functional weakness or sensory disturbance diagnosed in hospitalized neurological patients persisted in more than 80% (of 42 patients over a median of 12.5 years).[26] Neurologists working in specialty clinics frequently encounter individuals with chronic movements and motor symptoms; in a recent review, more than one-third of patients had the same or worse symptoms at follow-up visits and when there was improvement, there was often incomplete resolution.[27] Likewise, with non-epileptic attacks, the majority of studies show that 60% or more of patients continue to have non-epileptic attacks at follow-up.[28]

Modern imaging techniques used to investigate conversion disorder have demonstrated functional neuroanatomical abnormalities in patients with conversion disorder.[29] Some studies have suggested that conversion results from dynamic reorganization of neural circuits that link volition, movement, and perception.[30] Disruption of these networks may occur at the stage of pre-conscious motor planning, modality-specific attention, or right fronto-parietal networks subserving self-recognition and the affective correlate of self-hood. Overall, however, the number of individuals studied has been small and no distinct pattern of functional brain activity has emerged.

Psychological Factors Affecting Other Medical Conditions

This diagnosis should be considered when an individual displays psychological traits or behaviors that adversely affect the course (by precipitating or exacerbating symptoms) or treatment of a medical condition. Examples of these "psychological factors" involve the impact of stressful life events, relationship style, personality traits, coping styles, and depressive symptoms. These qualities and phenomena should not constitute a psychiatric disorder in and of themselves, and it is only through their interaction with somatic illness that their adverse effects come to clinical attention. It is sufficient for there to be an association between the abnormal psychological symptom and the medical condition, as direct causality is difficult and unnecessary to demonstrate. Distinguishing between this diagnosis and adjustment disorder is frequently arbitrary, although we point out that the word "disorder" is conspicuously absent from psychological factors affecting medical illness. As with the other conditions described in this chapter, one should be careful to differentiate them from culturally-specific behaviors (e.g., using spiritual healers to manage illness).

Factitious Disorders

The factitious disorders include versions imposed on the self and imposed on another (formerly, "by proxy") in DSM-5.

Previously occupying a category of their own in DSM-IV, the factitious disorders are now subsumed within the somatic symptom and related disorders category, presumably because they were considered to be primarily "characterized by the prominent focus on somatic concerns and their initial presentation mainly in medical rather than mental health care settings."[3] Putting aside the unproductive separation of "medical" and psychiatric practice inherent in this general rationale, we note that despite this re-categorization of factitious disorder, its possible exclusive presentation with psychological features remains part of the diagnostic criteria (albeit not the subtype it formerly was). Our chapter largely treats deception syndromes (factitious disorder and malingering) as warranting separate attention from the somatic symptom and related disorders. This chapter compares and contrasts intentional and unintentional signs and symptoms below, but detailed discussions of factitious disorder and malingering can be found in Chapter 25.

Other Specified Somatic Symptom and Related Disorder

Individuals who have some symptoms characteristic of a somatic symptom and related disorder, but who do not meet full criteria, can be diagnosed with an "unspecified somatic symptom and related disorder." In addition, there are "other specified somatic symptom disorders" that include brief somatic symptom disorder, brief illness anxiety disorder (duration less than 6 months), and pseudocyesis (false belief of being pregnant associated with symptoms of pregnancy and objective signs).

Functional Somatic Syndromes

Time will tell whether the DSM-5 category, "Somatic Symptom and Related Disorders" will be considered as useful by other medical specialties and will productively supplant non-specific conceptualizations of patients with MUS—a major goal of the re-formulated diagnoses.[31] Even if this goal is achieved, several functional somatic syndromes (FSS) will remain extant as discrete entities. The FSS vary from those with relatively more academic penetration/credibility (e.g., irritable bowel syndrome, fibromyalgia) to those of more recent and lay prominence (e.g., chronic Lyme disease, "electrosensitives"). Others straddle the line between the medical mainstream and the "fringe," partly depending on where and how they are discussed and managed (e.g., chronic fatigue syndrome, multiple chemical sensitivity).

The FSS are characterized by their respective cores of MUS, with associated features, required to "rule-in" those that have established diagnostic criteria.[32-34] A psychiatrist is unlikely to be called upon to make one of these diagnoses. However, given their conceptual similarities to psychopathology, phenomenologic similarities to somatic symptom disorder, and significant co-morbidities with affective and anxiety disorders, it behooves one to have some passing familiarity with them. Table 24-1 outlines salient features of four of the better-characterized FSS. These criteria undergo revisions of their own, much as DSM does. Irritable bowel syndrome is found within the eight categories, 30 diagnoses, and 20 subtypes that make up the functional gastrointestinal disorders codified within the Rome III classification scheme.[35] Fibromyalgia and chronic fatigue syndrome are in the midst of re-framing and/or objectification of their criteria.[36,37]

While each of the FSS has its own features, literature, and adherents, there is an argument to be made that there are more commonalities than distinguishing features between them.[38] Wessely and co-workers in particular have suggested that

TABLE 24-1 Comparison of Four Functional Somatic Syndromes

	Chronic Fatigue Syndrome[a]	Irritable Bowel Syndrome[b]	Fibromyalgia[c]	Multiple Chemical Sensitivities[d]
EXCLUSION OF OTHER SOMATIC/PSYCHIATRIC CAUSE	Required	Unnecessary	Unnecessary (specifically accommodates)	Unnecessary
DURATION	≥ 6 months	≥ 6 months + 3 days per month in last 3 months	≥ 3 months	"Chronic"
SEVERITY CRITERIA	Must be met	Unspecified "pain and discomfort"	Based on pain elicitation on examination	Non-specific
REPRODUCIBILITY/RELIEF OF SYMPTOMS	Unnecessary	Relief with defecation	Based on pain elicitation on examination at 11/18 "tender point sites"	Reproducible with exposure, relief with removal of irritants
ANCILLARY SYMPTOMS	≥ 4 of the following: Cognitive impairment Sore throat Tender lymph nodes Muscle pain Multi-joint pain New headaches Unrefreshing sleep Post-exertion malaise	Onset associated with changes in frequency and form of stool	History of the following: Bilateral pain Pain above and below waist Axial skeletal pain	"Low levels" of irritant produce symptoms Multiple irritants Symptoms in multiple organ systems

Adapted from [a]Fukada K, Straus SE, Hickie I, et al. The chronic fatigue syndrome: a comprehensive approach to its definition and study, Ann Intern Med 121:953–959, 1994; [b]Longstreth GF, Thompson WG, Chey WD, et al. Functional bowel disorders, Gastroenterology 130:1480–1491, 2006; [c]Wolfe F, Smythe HA, Yunus MB, et al. The American College of Rheumatology 1990 criteria for the classification of fibromyalgia: report of the multicenter committee, Arthritis Rheum 33:160–172, 1990; and [d]Bartha RP, Baumzweiger W, Buscher DS, et al. Multiple chemical sensitivity: a 1999 consensus, Arch Env Health 54:147–149, 1999.

BOX 24-1 Supportive Evidence for a Single Functional Somatic Syndrome

- Significant epidemiological overlap among the syndromes
- Preponderance of women
- Shared links to depressive and anxiety disorders
- Shift toward central nervous system etiological explanations for most
- Shared (usually poor) prognoses and ineffectiveness of conventional treatments
- Overlapping treatment strategies
- Cognitive-behavioral therapy
- Antidepressants
- Focus on the doctor–patient relationship
- Emphasis on rehabilitation

Adapted from Wessely S, Nimnuan C, Sharpe M. Functional somatic syndromes: one or many, Lancet 354:936–939, 1999; and Wessley S. There is only one functional somatic syndrome ("for"), Br J Psychiatry185:95–96, 2004.

"there is only one functional somatic syndrome."[39,40] Supportive points for this claim are summarized in Box 24-1. Co-morbidities within and among the FSS are worth pointing out regardless of one's opinion on the "one FSS" claim. Depending on the rigor of the diagnosis (for example, use of chronic fatigue syndrome's exclusion criterion for other fatigue-causing conditions), the FSS carry across-the-board co-morbidity with depressive and anxiety disorders,[41–46] a characteristic, of course, shared by the somatic symptom disorders (albeit also with many other medical conditions).

Patients with one FSS, when subjected to diagnostic investigation for another, are found generally to have both illnesses 30%–70% of the time, with co-morbidities of >70% found in multiple studies.[45–47] In fact, the greatest risk factor for "getting"

an FSS may be prior affliction with another one.[48] A sort of inverse, seemingly shared characteristic of the FSS is the presence of high rates of undiagnosed members of the general population who do not present themselves to the health care system or consider themselves markedly disabled, yet nonetheless "meet criteria" for these illnesses.[43,49,50] Whether considered etiologic or simply characteristic, these findings reiterate the hypothesis that important features of FSS may invoke a low threshold of symptom detection and the tendency to medically interpret somatic cues. If this is the case, then these core features are shared by FSS and some of the somatic symptom disorders.[51]

Shared Parameters of Somatically-Oriented Conditions

In Table 24-2, the somatic symptom and related disorders (excluding psychological factors affecting medical illness, where MUS are not necessarily manifested), FSS, and malingering are organized according to how they fall along three parameters that are discussed individually below. Breaking down these presentations in this manner offers some coherence to disparate categories that otherwise only share the fairly vague quality of having a somatic focus.

The table and corresponding discussion is not a diagnostic schema; rather, it is a way of thinking about what is going on in these complex situations. As will be discussed, each parameter is non-binary, existing on a continuum that gets progressively murkier as one moves away from its extremes.

Manifestations

Medical problems manifest clinically via symptoms and/or signs. The conventional definition of *symptoms* refers to "any morbid phenomenon ... *experienced by the patient* and indicative of disease."[52] A *sign*, on the other hand, is "*discoverable on examination of the patient.*"[52] According to DSM-5, the entities

TABLE 24-2 Three Parameters of the Major Somatically-Focused Syndromes, with Prototypical Presentations

	Manifestations	Production	Gratification
Somatic symptom disorder, illness anxiety disorder, functional somatic syndromes	Symptoms	Unintentional	Intangible
Conversion disorder	Signs	Unintentional	Intangible
Factitious disorder	Signs	Intentional	Intangible
Malingering	Symptoms	Intentional	Tangible

collected within the category Somatic Symptom and Related Disorders "share a common feature: the prominence of somatic *symptoms* associated with significant distress and impairment."[3]

Many diseases are discoverable only by their signs, either by virtue of their physiologic nature (e.g., early stages of hypertension), or by virtue of a given patient's temperament and culture (e.g., a thigh melanoma brought before an allopathic physician only once it interfered with walking).[53] Most patients that are the subject of this chapter are not known for their stoicism, and thus DSM-5 is technically correct about the prominence of symptoms in their disorders. Somatic symptom disorder, illness anxiety disorder, and the FSS are all marked by the presence of symptoms insufficiently associated with signs and diagnostic test results—i.e., MUS.

In conversion disorder, symptoms may be prominent; however, "organically" inexplicable neurological signs are characteristic. The patient with conversion disorder does not merely complain of blindness, or weakness, or convulsions; he or she "has" them, and while these signs may not come "as advertised" (e.g., are inconsistent across time or circumstance, lack an anatomically-coherent distribution), they can be discerned on exam or observation in the absence of patient commentary.

Most instances of diagnosed factitious disorder are striking by virtue of the overt damage these people do to themselves. As such, factitious disorder is usually manifest by signs of disease, such as sepsis, hypoglycemia, and anemia. However, some authors note that while factitious disorder is almost always detected once the patient is inducing disease and manifesting signs, this stage is likely preceded and/or coincides with phases of elaboration and fabrication of symptoms without actual physical morbidity.[54] The opposite seems to be the case in malingering, with symptom fabrication being seen more often than sign induction.

Production

Psychodynamic theory has figured heavily in modern thought regarding the etiology in MUS. Hence, we have terms like "somatizing" and "conversion" that imply transformations of psychological states into physical ones. These transformations are said to occur unconsciously. Cognitive-behavioral models behind MUS also involve automatic, if not frankly unconscious, psychological processes. It is more encompassing to describe the manifestations of somatically-focused conditions as either *intentional* or *unintentional*. Even these seemingly opposite qualifiers blur into one another. Any one of us is capable of intentionally exaggerating an unintentionally incurred symptom in situations where we want to make sure that a provider or caregiver "gets" our suffering. The original production of the symptom (or sign) itself, however, is either intentional or unintentional.

Patients with somatic symptom disorder, illness anxiety disorder, and the FSS are genuine in their reports and their experiences of the symptoms of which they complain. That these symptoms seem to portray in an exaggerated fashion might speak to their perceived severity, to their desperation or fear that doctors will not take them seriously, or to

their intentional exaggeration of actual distress. The signs of conversion disorder are likewise unintentionally produced. DSM-5 has removed the "not intentionally produced or feigned" criterion from conversion disorder. However, the associated text twists itself into a pretzel by saying that this criterion was removed because of the difficulty of ruling out intentionality, yet that when intentionality is established, conversion disorder is ruled out. Criteria notwithstanding, when conversion disorder is diagnosed, the signs are presumed, even if not proven, to be unintentionally produced.

By definition, intentionality and lying are at the heart of symptom and sign production in factitious disorder and malingering. It is important to note, however, that the volitional falsification causes biological correlates of signs. For example, sepsis is sepsis, regardless of how it occurred, and must be treated as such; but the intentional deception of factitious disorder rests in *how* the patient became septic (e.g., through clandestine self-inoculation). When mere symptoms are falsified intentionally, the patient's untrue medical statements are also known, simply, as lying.

Gratification

The terms *primary and secondary gain* are sometimes used to describe ways that MUS and deception syndromes are presumed to satisfy patients' needs. Secondary gain refers to gratification derived from material items (e.g., for food, shelter, money, illicit substances) or to the items themselves. Primary gain refers to gratification derived from the relief of intrapsychic tension[55] or to the means used to relieve that tension; in the somatic domain, that means is sometimes vaguely referred to as the assumption of the "sick role."

The sick role is actually a specific term used by the sociologist Talcott Parsons in the 1950s to delineate the social functions of doctor and patient in managing disease.[56] For our purposes, we confine this discussion to the privileges and duties of doctor and patient, with special attention to those of the patient. The privileges of the sick role are purported to be: blamelessness for the products of sickness, relief from duties incompatible with the sickness, and entitlement to care. Taking some liberties with Parsons' ideas, we expand the latter to include not just medical care but nurturing from people in the patient's life. When thinking about the relationship between primary gain and the sick role, the psychological benefits of blamelessness, relief, and care for those feeling unworthy, beleaguered, and unloved becomes more clear than the vague "primary gain" would have it.

Of course, blamelessness and legal culpability, relief and disability payments, and care and shelter all can blur into one another, reminding us that the idea of distinguishing between primary and secondary gain is unsubstantiated received wisdom.[52] Our division of "immaterial" and "material" gratification is also an artificial distinction. Nonetheless, we use it to approximate convention and to minimize some of the primary/secondary gain confusion by confining ourselves to different *sources* of gratification without addressing the intrapsychic experiences associated with them.

When it comes to gratification, somatic symptom disorder, illness anxiety disorder, and FSS cluster together, with immaterial sick-role patient privileges being the source of gratification for which these patients unwittingly exchange suffering. Sick-role status depends on social acceptability of one's sickness. Hence connecting their distress to sick-role gains may partially explain the desperate, sometimes hostile, way that these patients pursue or cling to the legitimacy of their distress or FSS diagnoses. These efforts to legitimize distress can overtly or covertly eclipse patients' stated desires for relief; this may explain findings such as diminished placebo responses and the powerful negative prognostic effect of support group participation for patients with chronic fatigue syndrome.[57,58]

Patients with FSS, somatic symptom disorder, or illness anxiety disorder may eventually bring before their doctors disability paperwork or other requests for medical excuses, but these are secondary pursuits. They can, however, straddle the types of gratification delineated here (i.e., is disability purely a financial, material gain, or a symbol of the sick role). Likewise, depending on one's belief in and "discovery" of a trigger (e.g., an impending divorce hearing, an unacceptable revenge fantasy), it can be difficult to determine what type of gratification the signs of conversion disorder aim to achieve.

The similarities between somatic symptom disorder, illness anxiety disorder, FSS, and conversion disorder provide a rationale for shared elements of treatment. Sick-role privileges come with a duty to at least pursue health.[59] The discrepancy between these patients' laying claim to privileges without accepting this duty may be the real factor that makes them "heartsink patients."[60] The idea of bringing patient duty into the picture provides a topic for direct or indirect communication and limit-setting that embraces rather than challenges the patient's sick-role status, hinges it to healthier behavior, and reigns in what patients can expect from physicians (and others) while clinging to invalidism.[61] In this light the shift of focus from cure (and validation of sickness) to function gains more conceptual backing.

For the deception syndromes, of course, this treatment rationale falls apart, since these patients lack a belief in their own sick-role status and pursue it disingenuously. Note that if (in a given case, or categorically) there really is no difference between immaterial/primary and material/secondary gain, and if this is the main distinguishing characteristic between factitious disorder and malingering, then there are two possibilities. One extends the disorder status of factitious disorder to malingering; the other extends the quasi-criminal status of malingering to factitious disorder. Either way, both conditions might be better understood as behavior patterns arising and distracting from broader problems that ought to be targeted. For example, malingering might be seen in many cases as part of broader patterns of non-pathological criminality, sociopathy, or desperation; factitious disorder as a manifestation of separation avoidance in patients with borderline or other character disorders.[62,63]

TREATMENT

The treatment of somatic symptom and related disorders, and, to an extent, problematic MUS in general, begins with the recognition that these conditions involve a maladaptive goal-directed behavior that specifically involves symptoms or signs of a medical illness. It can be helpful, therefore, to think of most of these conditions as *abnormal illness behaviors* rather than disease entities.[64] Thought of in this way, treatment addresses the behavior itself.

Patients with somatic symptom and related disorders tax the general physician. Such patients are difficult to reassure; their care is both time-consuming and expensive; and they often provoke strong negative reactions in their frustrated

---

BOX 24-2 Fostering a Therapeutic Relationship with the "Somatizing" Patient

- Minimize the patient's need to legitimize symptoms/syndromes
- Gather history in a non-directive, non-judgmental fashion
- Encourage the patient to maintain a symptom diary
- Emphasize what you know the patient does *not* have
- Validate distress while avoiding unwarranted diagnostic labels
- Deflect debates over symptom etiology
- Avoid unrealistic expectations
- Focus on restoration of function rather than on cure
- Focus on symptom reduction and coping rather than on elimination of symptoms
- Avoid confusion
- Insist on being the "gatekeeper" for all of the patient's medical contacts
- Emphasize the patient's legitimate need for a long-term doctor–patient relationship
- Be willing to end the relationship if the patient repeatedly pursues outside interventions
- Avoid oversights
- Be alert to the patient's life stressors
- Be alert to co-morbid psychopathology
- Be alert to uncharacteristic changes in health status
- Do not forget about routine health maintenance

Adapted from Barsky AJ, Borus JF. Functional somatic syndromes, Ann Intern Med *130:910–921, 1999; Meador CK.* Symptoms of unknown origin, *Nashville, 2005, Vanderbilt University Press; and Drossman DA.* The functional gastrointestinal disorders and the Rome III process, Gastroenterology *130:1377–1390, 2006.*

---

providers.[65] Management of patients with these disorders begins with building a durable therapeutic doctor–patient relationship based on the physician's reliable interest in the patient as a person who is suffering and presumably wants not to suffer. Important elements in establishing this kind of a relationship with the "somatizing" patient are summarized in Box 24-2.

Once this relationship is established, two goals play important roles in the treatment process: (1) avoiding unnecessary diagnostic tests and thereby obviating overly aggressive medical and surgical intervention; and, (2) helping the patient tolerate and maximize functioning in the presence of symptoms rather than striving to eliminate them. The former is achieved through assigning a treatment team leader, developing a treatment plan, and bringing the patient on board with that plan. The latter is achieved by promoting positive reinforcement, considering and treating potential co-morbid conditions, and, in some cases, referring to psychiatric specialists. The physician helps the patient work within a treatment model that is at worst considered palliative, and at best considered the same as chronic disease management, as with conditions such as rheumatoid arthritis. It might be pointed out to some patients that the only medical conditions that can truly be "cured" are certain infections, surgical problems, and cancers. A desired side effect of this sort of treatment model is that the patient might loosen his or her grip on symptoms since they are neither necessary nor sufficient for securing a validating doctor–patient relationship.

Assigning a Leader to Develop a Treatment Plan

One physician (usually the outpatient primary care physician) should be chosen as the leader of a multi-disciplinary team (that may include consultant physicians, nurses, social workers, and other parties as needed). Even though individual team members may have opinions that vary, all involved should ultimately agree on the diagnosis. If disagreement persists, one can have all specialists submit their desired diagnostic testing (with the understanding that if the test comes back negative, the work-up will be considered complete and the patient will be informed). The leader should oversee the ordering of all tests and consultations, as well as review the results. Clear and consistent communication between all team members helps minimize staff splitting and facilitates agreement about what the patient should be told regarding the need for further work-up. Use of a systematic approach (that considers each of the pertinent medical and psychiatric diagnoses) will decrease the chance of overlooking a condition with a primarily physiologic source that could be responsible for the somatic symptom(s).

Informing the Patient about the Treatment Plan

Informing the patient about the treatment plan requires a therapeutic alliance with the patient. Some patients will be grateful that a diagnosis has been established while others will become defensive, angry, and flee from treatment. Regardless of whether one uses the actual diagnostic label, patients can benefit from an understanding of how their condition affects their life and realize that their distress can be addressed. Again, a chronic disease approach can be helpful here as the physician need not be disingenuous in presenting to the patient the impact of factors, such as genetics, temperament, family/illness experiences, life stressors, on manifestations of symptoms (whether explained or not). Further, many of these factors become viable avenues of intervention for the patient who accepts this illness model. Explaining to the patient that he or she may be more attuned to benign visceral and somatic sensations can also be beneficial within this approach while still hewing to the physician's understanding of the patient's problem. The patient's psychological strengths and the absence of other psychopathology are more important for the outcome than is the actual somatic symptom, though one must be careful here since some patients will perceive any "praise" of their strength or comment on their well-being in any domain as invalidating of their distress.

Confrontation of certain patients' approaches to health and illness is sometimes warranted,[57] but confrontation over the validity of their symptoms almost never is. Patients are particularly sensitive to the idea that an authoritative person has dismissed their suffering; their anger and sensitivity may be based on a history of abuse or neglect. The best context for discussion of the diagnosis of PNES, for example, may come after the patient and family have agreed that key representative events have been captured by video EEG monitoring.[66] Some patients sense that there is a relationship between stressful psychosocial conditions and their symptoms.

The physician must, particularly with the FSS, take pains not to excessively challenge the patient's conception of the problem. Unless the patient is being harmed by interventions or examinations they are seeking in connection with that diagnosis, this approach is seldom warranted. Remember also, that while physicians need to keep abreast of hundreds of diagnoses and even more treatments, some of these patients have, unfortunately devoted their lives to their "diagnosis." One should not engage in an argument you are likely to lose by surrender.

Frequent, Scheduled Visits

Conducting a follow-up visit is probably more important than is any prescribed treatment. In fact, the management

---

BOX 24-3 General Advice for Providers of "Somatizing" Patients

- Schedule frequent brief appointments, thereby relieving the patient of the perceived need to have symptoms to maintain the relationship with the physician
- Perform a brief, targeted physical examination at each visit
- Avoid all unnecessary interventions, both diagnostic and therapeutic
- Avoid invocation of psychological etiologies for somatic experiences

Adapted from Smith RC, Gardiner JC, Lyles JS, et al. Exploration of DSM-IV criteria in primary care patients with medically unexplained symptoms, Psychosom Med 67:123–129, 2005.

---

recommendations outlined in this section purposefully provided to consultee primary care physicians were found to reduce quarterly health care charges by 53% due to decreases in hospitalization.[67] Neither the health of the patients nor their satisfaction with their care was adversely affected by implementation of the advice. While more a containment than treatment strategy, these recommendations remain one of the few evidence-based interventions for patients with problematic MUS. These recommendations are summarized in Box 24-3.

Regular, brief (non-symptom-contingent) visits should be scheduled, every week or two (and gradually reduced to every 4–6 weeks, as tolerated) to assuage the patient's perceived need to have symptoms that maintain the relationship with a physician. If the patient calls between scheduled visits, the physician can return to more frequent visits. The patient will hopefully learn that seeing a physician is not contingent upon having symptoms. Early in the visit, the physician should pay particular attention to setting goals for each appointment, with a particular focus placed on the patient's emotional concerns. One should perform a targeted physical examination at each visit, particularly when new symptoms are articulated by the patient; during this examination the physician can inquire (in a supportive manner) about the areas of stress in the patient's life, without inference to stress as a cause for the increase in somatic concerns.

Physicians should also consider teaching patients how to manage life stress rather than putting important activities on hold until their chronic somatic symptoms are resolved. Not going to work can reinforce illness behavior. For those not chronically disabled by their condition, vocational counselors can assist in finding a less stressful job that can help provide meaning and structure.

Consideration and Treatment of Co-morbid Conditions

Individuals diagnosed with somatic symptom and related disorders are not immune to the development of new medical illnesses. A systematic differential diagnostic approach is required. Whenever someone presents with somatic symptoms, it is especially important to consider medical conditions that affect multiple organ systems or produce variable presentations (e.g., multiple sclerosis, acute intermittent porphyria, HIV infection, scleroderma, rheumatoid arthritis, systemic lupus erythematosus). In the case of conversion disorder presenting as PNES, for example, other medical conditions (e.g., convulsive syncope, paroxysmal dyskinesias, transient ischemic attacks, and limbic encephalitis) should be considered, as they can present with symptoms and signs suggestive of seizures but without epileptiform changes noted on EEG.[68]

Likewise, it is important to screen for co-morbid affective, anxiety, personality, and substance-related disorders that might better account for the patient's presentation. These disorders are likely easier to treat and their resolution may diminish somatic symptom and related disorders (although the latter disorders seldom completely resolve with treatment of their psychiatric co-morbidities, and if they do, then one should consider revisiting the initial diagnosis). Tests, such as the Minnesota Multi-phasic Personality Inventory (MMPI) and full neuropsychological test batteries can also help in refining the diagnosis.

It should be recalled that the vegetative symptoms (e.g., insomnia, fatigue, anorexia, weight loss) of major depressive disorder, and symptoms of panic (e.g., dyspnea, palpitations, chest pain, choking, dizziness, paresthesias, hot and cold flashes, sweating, faintness, trembling) are somatic. It has been reported that 25% of patients presenting with chest pain to the emergency department meet criteria for panic disorder based on DSM-IV criteria, yet the diagnosis is not made 98% of the time.[69] Older patients with major depressive disorder are also more preoccupied with somatic symptoms. Cross-culturally, the majority of patients with major depressive disorder have only somatic symptoms.[70]

Substance use disorders should likewise be considered in patients with persistent unexplained somatic symptoms, particularly pain; with pain complaints, one is often faced with the question of whether an exaggerated pain complaint is an etiologic factor in substance use or is used as a means of obtaining prescription analgesics. Psychotic disorders are both easily missed (e.g., the non-bizarre somatic delusions found in delusional disorder) and easily used to dismiss the somatic complaints of patients afflicted with these diagnoses. Personality disorders may lead patients to use somatic symptoms as a means to an end (e.g., functional weakness gains the attention and nurturance of others; somatic symptoms can be exaggerated by those with a histrionic personality).

The Role of Psychiatrists

The role for the psychiatrist in the care of patients with somatic symptom disorders and other problematic MUS is usually as a consultant who can clarify the diagnosis, the work-up, and the management of the patient. Most patients with abnormal illness behavior do not accept a referral to a psychiatric consultant and, when scheduled, many fail to appear for their appointment. Nevertheless, early involvement of a psychiatrist can facilitate diagnosis and mitigate iatrogenesis. Conversely, the psychiatrist may ultimately catalyze the diagnosis of somatic illness by noting when a patient is thought to be "somatizing" does not fit the expected symptomatic patterns of the mentally ill, or when a patient's known psychopathology leads to inappropriate application of Occam's razor to their somatic complaints.[71]

Furthermore, individuals with somatic symptom disorders induce intense affective reactions, behavioral responses, and cognitive challenges that can distract a primary physician from making an accurate diagnosis or presenting and dealing with it in a productive manner. The physicians' mindset (of being caring, trusting, and eager to help) can be challenged by dealing with patients who deceive, lie, or eagerly undergo diagnostic and surgical procedures for no apparent reason. Not purely confined to deception syndromes, the impact of these behaviors is probably more often seen in patients with MUS whose stated desire for health belies a far greater focus on illness and its associated gains. Physicians' reactions to these feelings can lead to errors of omission (such as

dismissing patients' concerns) or commission (taking the path of least resistance, or acting on aversive feelings by ordering unnecessary procedures or prescribing unwarranted medications. Psychiatrists can sometimes play a role in helping other physicians make sense of these understandable reactions and keep them from unduly interfering with care.

Finally, psychiatric consultants can take an active role in the management of patients, whether through treatment of psychiatric co-morbidities, or through direct attempts at treatment (or referral for specialized treatment) of the somatic symptom problem itself. Emerging data suggest that cognitive-behavioral therapy (CBT), particularly when delivered in the primary care setting, can help to identify and re-structure cognitive distortions, unrealistic dysfunctional beliefs, worry, and behaviors that drive many of these disorders. CBT can be helpful in reducing symptoms and lowering health care costs. Short-term psychodynamic psychotherapy has a moderate empirical base to support its use in somatic symptom syndromes and multiple studies demonstrate significant and sustained benefits, including several studies suggesting that treated patients may have fewer physician visits and hospital use.[72]

Suggestibility for Conversion Disorder

While the treatment for most of the somatic symptom and related disorders share common management themes discussed above, treatment for conversion disorder sometimes attempts to capitalize on the suggestibility that some believe underlies this disorder. It is important to remember, however, that there are no systematic, well-controlled, trials supporting the efficacy of any treatment for conversion disorder.[73]

The most common form of treatment for conversion disorder is to simply suggest that the conversion symptom will gradually improve. It is thought that this intervention is face-saving as well as optimistic.

It is helpful to confidently convey with supportive optimism that recovery is certain, yet may be gradual. Specific suggestions may be offered as well (e.g., for the "blind" patient, suggesting that vague shapes will become visible first; for the patient with lower paresis, that weight bearing will be possible and then steps with a walker and so on, or that strength in squeezing a tennis ball will be followed by strength at the wrist and then elbow joints). When patients are not given information about their diagnosis and treatment, they show no improvement or do worse after work-up.[74] Some suggest that the psychiatrist discuss the patient's life stresses and try to detect painful affects to assess the non-verbal interpersonal communication embodied by the symptom.[25]

Further intervention may not be necessary. However, if the conversion symptom persists, if the precipitating stress is chronic, or if there is massive gain, resolution of the situation becomes a target of the intervention. Because the stressors are often social, couples or family therapy may be instrumental in achieving a final resolution. Behavioral interventions, physical therapy, and reassurance are crucial, particularly for less verbal patients.[66] In general, a favorable outcome depends more on the individuals' psychological strengths and on the absence of other psychopathology than on the specific nature of the conversion symptom itself.

CONCLUSIONS

MUS are a nearly universal experience. They are a major problem for a large subset of patients and for the physicians who attempt to understand and to treat them. DSM-5 has reorganized many of these presentations within the category of Somatic Symptom and Related Disorders, which also encompasses the deception syndrome, factitious disorder (but not malingering, which is not considered a psychiatric disorder). To date, the rest of medicine has typically not used psychiatric classifications of MUS, and many of these patients end up being captured by functional somatic syndrome categories, such as fibromyalgia and chronic fatigue syndrome.

Ultimately, unexplained symptoms themselves may be less important than the illness behaviors[75] with which patients deal with them. Addressing abnormal illness behaviors[76,77] through strategic primary care approaches, psychotherapies, and/or better navigation of the privileges and duties of the patient's sick-role status can be beneficial in the effective management of these patients. Careful, conservative medication use, especially that which targets co-morbid mood and anxiety disorders, is also important in reducing suffering, though is unlikely to reduce the somatic focus of patients with somatic symptom and related disorders.

Access the complete reference list and multiple choice questions (MCQs) online at https://expertconsult.inkling.com

KEY REFERENCES

4. DeWaal MWM, Arnold IA, Eekhof JAH, et al. Somatoform disorders in general practice: prevalence, functional impairment and comorbidity with anxiety and depressive disorders. *Br J Psychiatry* 184:470–474, 2004.
7. Barsky AJ, Orav EJ, Bates DW. Somatization increases medical utilization and costs independent of psychiatric and medical comorbidity. *Arch Gen Psychiatry* 62:903–910, 2005.
9. Hahn SR. Physical symptoms and physician-experienced difficulty in the physician–patient relationship. *Ann Intern Med* 134:897–904, 2001.
13. Smith RC, Lein C, Collins C, et al. Treating patients with medically unexplained symptoms in primary care. *J Gen Intern Med* 18:478–489, 2003.
14. Mayou R, Kirmayer LJ, Simon G, et al. Somatoform disorders: time for a new approach in DSM-V. *Am J Psychiatry* 162:847–855, 2005.
16. Noyes R Jr, Stuart SP, Watson DB. A reconceptualization of the somatoform disorders. *Psychosomatics* 49:14–22, 2008.
17. McFarlane AC, Ellis N, Barton C, et al. The conundrum of medically unexplained symptoms: questions to consider. *Psychosomatics* 49:369–377, 2008.
18. Bell V, Oakley DA, Halligan PW, et al. Dissociation in hysteria and hypnosis: evidence from cognitive neuroscience. *J Neurol Neurosurg Psychiatry* 82:332–339, 2011.
24. Stone J, Smyth R, Carson A, et al. Systematic review of misdiagnosis of conversion symptoms and "hysteria." *BMJ* 331:989, 2005.
26. Stone J, Sharpe M, Rothwell PM, et al. The 12 year prognosis of unilateral functional weakness and sensory disturbance. *J Neurol Neurosurg Psychiatry* 74:591–596, 2003.
27. Gelauff J, Stone J, Edwards M, et al. The prognosis of functional (psychogenic) motor symptoms: a systemic review. *J Neurol Neurosurg Psychiary* 2013. doi:10.11365/jnnp.
28. Durrant J, Rickards H, Cavanna AE. Prognosis and outcome predictors in psychogenic nonepileptic seizures. *Epilepsy Research and Treatment* 274736, 2011.
31. Smith RC, Gardier JC, Lyles JS, et al. Exploration of DSM-IV criteria in primary care patients with medically unexplained patients. *Psychosom Med* 67:123–129, 2005.
36. Wolfe F, Clauw DJ, Fitzcharles M-A, et al. The American College of Rheumatology preliminary diagnostic criteria for fibromyalgia and measurement of symptom severity. *Arthritis Care Res* 62:600–610, 2010.
38. Fink P, Schroder A. One single diagnosis, bodily distress syndrome, succeeded to capture ten diagnostic categories of functional somatic syndromes and somatoform disorders. *J Psychosom Res* 68:415–426, 2010.
40. Wessely S, White PD. There is only one functional somatic syndrome. *Br J Psychiatry* 185:95–96, 2004.
47. Kaanaan RA, Lepine JP, Wessely SC. The association or otherwise of the functional somatic syndromes. *Psychosom Med* 69:855–859, 2007.
54. Hamilton JC, Feldman MD, Cunnien AJ. Factitious disorder in medical and clinical practices. In Rogers R, editor: *Clinical Assessment of Malingering and Deception, Third Edition*, New York, 2008, Guilford Press.
55. Taylor MA, Vaidya NA. *Descriptive Psychopathology: The Signs and Symptoms of Behavioral Disorders*, New York, 2009, Cambridge University Press.
57. Cho HJ, Hotoff M, Wessely S. The placebo response in the treatment of chronic fatigue syndrome: a systematic review and meta-analysis. *Psychosom Med* 67:301–313, 2005.
58. Huibers MJ, Wessely S. The act of diagnosis: pros and cons of labeling chronic fatigue syndrome. *Psychol Med* 36:895–900, 2006.
59. Kontos N, Querques J, Freudenreich O. Fighting the good fight: responsibility and rationale in the confrontation of patients. *Mayo Clin Proc* 87:63–66, 2012.
66. Stonnington CM, Barry JJ, Fisher RS. Conversion disorder. *Am J Psychiatry* 163(9):1510–1517, 2006.
73. Ruddy R, House A. Psychosocial interventions for conversion disorder. *Cochrane Database Syst Rev* 4:CD005331, 2005.

25 Factitious Disorders and Malingering

Felicia A. Smith, MD

KEY POINTS

Incidence

- Factitious disorder and malingering are uncommon syndromes that involve voluntary symptom production and deception of medical providers.

Pathophysiology

- Factitious disorder involves the conscious production of symptoms with the primary motivation of assuming the sick role.

Clinical findings

- Factitious disorder may manifest with predominantly physical symptoms, predominantly psychological symptoms, or a combination of the two.
- Factitious disorder imposed on another (previously referred to as factitious disorder by proxy or Münchausen by proxy) involves the intentional production of symptoms in another person (often in a child) in order to indirectly assume the sick role.

Differential Diagnosis

- Malingering is characterized by the intentional production of symptoms with clear secondary gain as the motivation.

Treatment Options

- Many treaters avoid angry confrontations, as these can increase defensiveness and elusiveness, and provoke fleeing from the hospital.

Prognosis

- These conditions are notoriously difficult to treat. Placing an emphasis on management over cure is a helpful way to re-frame the treatment goals.
- Supportive psychotherapy that fosters a relationship that isn't contingent on the development of symptoms may be useful in reducing factitious behavior.

OVERVIEW

Factitious disorders and malingering both involve voluntary symptom production and deception of medical providers. In this light, Ford has combined these two disorders under the heading of *deception syndromes*.[1] The deceptive nature often angers medical providers, making these patients some of the most memorable seen in our careers. The thought of a patient with an infection that requires multiple diagnostic studies and broad-spectrum antibiotics, only to be seen self-injecting feces into various body parts, seems incredulous to most. The motivation is often difficult to comprehend, but it separates the two diagnoses. In factitious disorder the motivation centers around assuming the sick role, while obvious external rewards are absent. Malingerers, on the other hand, are motivated by a clear-cut secondary gain (often legal or financial). The deceptive nature and the difficulty confirming the diagnosis make each of these difficult to study; thus, prevalence rates are less

than reliable. The potential subjective nature of determining the motivation (which is often murky at best) further complicates matters. It seems clear, however, that the disruption caused by these patients to themselves, to family members, and to the larger medical system is significant and merits further discussion in this chapter.

FACTITIOUS DISORDERS

Factitious illness is a complicated disorder that is marked by the conscious production of symptoms without clear secondary gain. Unlike malingering, where there is obvious secondary gain, those with factitious disorder are driven to feign or simulate illness without obtaining obvious direct benefit (except to assume the sick role); in fact, such individuals often put their health at considerable risk. They may fake, exaggerate, intentionally worsen, or simply create symptoms. They do not admit to self-harm, but rather hide it from their physicians; herein lies the paradox—those with factitious illness come to health care providers requesting help, but intentionally hide the self-induced cause of their illness. Box 25-1 lists the *Diagnostic and Statistical Manual of Mental Disorders*, ed 5, (DSM-5) criteria for factitious disorder.[2] The DSM-5 has simplified the diagnosis of factitious disorder (which previously consisted of three discrete subtypes) and now simply distinguishes between *factitious disorder imposed on self* and *factitious disorder imposed on another* (previously known as factitious disorder by proxy), and places them within the new category, somatic symptom disorders.[2] Manifestations may include physical or psychological signs or symptoms (or both). Each of these types will be further discussed in the following sections.

FACTITIOUS DISORDER IMPOSED ON SELF

In *factitious disorder imposed on self*, the medical or psychological signs or symptoms are falsified by the patient to deceive caregivers. Physical illness is more frequently feigned than is psychological illness. Examples of faked clinical problems include fever, bleeding, hypoglycemia, and seizures, as well as more elaborate productions that simulate cancers and infection with the human immunodeficiency virus (HIV).[3-6] While the term *Münchausen syndrome* is commonly used interchangeably with the physical type of factitious disorder, the classic Münchausen syndrome is reserved for the most severe and chronic form of the disorder, which is marked by the following three components: recurrent hospitalizations, travel from hospital to hospital (peregrination), and *pseudologia fantastica*.[7] *Pseudologia fantastica* is the production of intricate and colorful stories or fantasies associated with the patient's presentation. It is a form of pathological lying characterized by overlapping fact and fiction, with a repetitive quality, and often with grandiosity or an assumption of the victim role by the storyteller.[1] In some cases, it may be difficult to determine whether these fabrications are actually delusions or conscious deceptions. Patients with Münchausen syndrome often make a career out of their illness. Serial hospitalizations make employment or sustained interpersonal relationships impossible. Moreover, patients who produce significant self-trauma or develop untoward complications from medical or surgical interventions become further incapacitated. The prognosis for

BOX 25-1 DSM-5 Criteria: Factitious Disorder Imposed on Self (300.19 (F68.10))

A. Falsification of physical or psychological signs or symptoms, or induction of injury or disease, associated with identified deception.
B. The individual presents himself or herself to others as ill, impaired, or injured.
C. The deceptive behavior is evident even in the absence of obvious external rewards.
D. The behavior is not better explained by another mental disorder, such as delusional disorder or another psychotic disorder.

Specify:

Single episode
Recurrent episodes (two or more events of falsification of illness and/or induction of injury).

Reprinted with permission from the Diagnostic and statistical manual of mental disorders, *ed 5, (Copyright 2013). American Psychiatric Association.*

TABLE 25-1 Typical Clinical Presentations of Factitious Disorder

Type	Clinical Findings or Symptoms
Acute abdominal type (*laparotomaphilia migrans*)	Abdominal pain—multiple surgeries may result in true adhesions and subsequent bowel obstruction
Neurological type (*neurologica diabolica*)	Headache, loss of consciousness, or seizure
Hematological type	Anemia from blood-letting or anticoagulant use
Endocrinological type	Hypoglycemia (from exogenous insulin) Hyperthyroidism (from exogenous thyroid hormone) Hyperglycemia (from withholding of insulin)
Cardiac type	Chest pain or arrhythmia
Dermatological type (*dermatitis autogenica*)	Self-inflicted wounds or chemical abrasions
Febrile type (*hyperpyrexia figmentatica*)	Manipulation of thermometer to produce fever
Infectious type	Wounds infected with multiple organisms (often fecal material)

Adapted from Beach SR, Viguera AC, Stern TA. Factitious disorders. In Stern TA, Herman JB, Gorrindo T, editors: Massachusetts General Hospital psychiatry update and board preparation, ed 3, Boston, 2012, MGH Psychiatry Academy, pp. 161–164.

these cases is generally poor, and affected individuals may die prematurely from complications of their own self-injurious behavior or from iatrogenesis.

Clinical Features

While Münchausen syndrome is the most dramatic form of factitious illness, *common factitious disorder* is more frequently encountered.[1] As opposed to those with Münchausen syndrome, these patients do not typically use aliases or travel from hospital to hospital, but rather visit with the same physician. They are well known in their health care system due to numerous hospitalizations. While they misrepresent symptoms and feign illness, they are not as prone to pseudologia fantastica. Although conflicting data exist with regard to whether factitious disorders are more common in men or women, some suggest that common factitious disorder is more prevalent among women. Other risk factors include being unmarried, being aged 30–40, being in the health care profession, and having a cluster B personality disorder. Münchausen syndrome, on the other hand, may be more frequently seen in men in their 40s who are single and who have antisocial traits.[1] The co-morbidity with personality disorders may be a result of rigid defensive structure, poor identity formation, and prominent dependency needs.[8]

A typical hospitalization for those who feign medical illness has a number of common characteristics. The patient uses medical jargon and generally knows what diagnoses or conditions will merit hospitalization. The history is often quite dramatic and convincing, and the patient persuades the physician to provide care by appealing to narcissistic qualities, such as omnipotence. Once hospitalized, the treatment is marked by demands for specific interventions (e.g., surgery or particular medications) and by an increasing need for attention. When these are not delivered, the patient becomes angry and may accuse staff of mistreatment or misdiagnosis. If medical personnel uncover the deception, strong countertransference feelings of hatred ensue—the patient is then rapidly discharged or elopes from the hospital only to seek "treatment" at another facility soon thereafter.

The types of physical symptoms and diseases that have been faked are limited only by the imagination of those who feign them. Table 25-1 lists some common categories.

Modern-day laboratory tests and diagnostic modalities may be particularly useful in distinguishing factitious symptoms from true medical illness. For example, in the case of suspicious infection, polymicrobial culture results that indicate an uncommon source (e.g., from urine or feces) is highly suggestive. Those who inject insulin to produce hypoglycemia will have a low C-peptide on laboratory analysis, while glyburide can be measured in the urine of those suspected of taking oral hypoglycemics. Laxative abuse to cause ongoing diarrhea can be confirmed by testing for phenolphthalein in the stool.[9] Finally, diagnostic studies in cases of suspected thyrotoxicosis (from surreptitious ingestion of thyroid hormone) reveal elevated serum total or free thyroid hormone levels, undetectable serum thyrotropin levels, low serum thyroglobulin concentration, absence of goiter, and absence of circulating antithyroid antibodies.[10]

Detection of other types of physical factitious illness may require more astute physical examination or observational skills (not to mention catching the patient "in the act"). For example, fever of unknown origin may be caused by warming thermometers on light bulbs, radiators, or with a flame (though this is more difficult with the advent of the electronic thermometer). Hematuria may be produced by blood-letting from another body area (commonly from a finger prick) into the urine sample. While finding suspicious cuts may be suggestive, direct observation may be the only way to prove factitious disorder in this instance. Likewise, with non-healing wounds where self-excoriation or "picking" behavior is suspected, witnessing the act either directly or with the use of video monitoring is diagnostic. Of note, the latter brings up ethical considerations unless done with the consent of the patient. Finally, among the numerous other possible physical manifestations, those that rely on more subjective report (including joint or muscle pain, headache, renal colic, or abdominal pain) may be present for months or years before a factitious etiology is even considered, much less proven.

While the majority of those diagnosed with factitious disorder manifest physical symptoms, some patients primarily feign psychological symptoms. Psychological complaints (like physical ones) occur on a spectrum, and include depression, anxiety, psychosis, bereavement, dissociation, post-traumatic stress, and even homicidal ideation.[11-15] As with primarily physical symptomatology, separating the motive from that of playing the sick role versus one of clear and understood secondary gain (malingering) is difficult and often imperfect. In the case of factitious bereavement, for example, the patient may report a dramatic or recent loss of a child or another loved one, with a display of emotion that evokes significant sympathy in medical treaters. When the truth is discovered, the so-called deceased person may either be still alive, have died long ago, or perhaps did not really play a major role in the patient's life. Ganser's syndrome, characterized by the provision of approximate answers to questions (as well as by having amnesia, disorientation, and perceptual disturbances), may be related to factitious disorder with psychological symptoms.[1] While it was originally described as a form of malingering (mostly by prisoners), Ganser-like syndromes may be seen in medical populations as well. Finally, both physical and psychological factitious symptoms may be present in the same patient.

Diagnostic Approach

As previously alluded to, making the diagnosis of factitious illness is often difficult. However, there are several elements of a general strategic approach that may be helpful. First, when factitious illness is suspected, it is essential to obtain information from all pertinent collateral sources. These may include previous or current treaters, family members, current and old medical records, and laboratory and diagnostic studies. Verification of the "facts" presented by the patient is key. Next, one looks for historical elements that are often suggestive of factitious disease. Some of these are outlined in Box 25-2.[8] Recognition of typical presentations (including all of those outlined in Table 25-1) may provide further clues. When one is lucky enough to find medical paraphernalia or to observe the patient intentionally self-inflicting symptoms, the diagnosis is made. Of note, searching the patient's room and personal belongings without the patient's permission are controversial and, in many cases, considered an invasion of privacy. Before embarking on such an endeavor, it is prudent to consider the potential ramifications carefully and to speak with legal counsel. There is no doubt, however, that in most cases the diagnosis relies on significant detective work based on a high level of suspicion.

Differential Diagnosis

True physical disorders (especially rare or unusual diseases with few objective findings) must be considered before

---

BOX 25-2 Historical Elements Suggestive of Factitious Disorder

- Multiple hospital admissions—"hospital shopping" or peregrination
- Many forms of identification or hospital numbers under various names
- Ease with medical jargon
- Current or prior employment in a medically-related field
- Lack of verifiable history
- Few interpersonal relationships
- Early history of chronic illness
- Unexplained physical findings/multiple scars
- Failure to respond to typical treatments
- Co-morbid personality or substance abuse disorders

---

prematurely diagnosing factitious illness. Somatic symptom disorder and conversion disorder may also be mistaken for factitious disorder. The principal difference here is that the former are distinguished by symptoms not being under voluntary control, and provoked by unconscious conflicts. Moreover, these patients are typically not as savvy about medical diagnoses and they do not seek out secondary gain. This is in contrast to those who are malingering and who intentionally feign symptoms for obvious secondary gain (often financial, legal, or drug-seeking). Psychotic disorders (especially delusional disorder) and self-injurious behavior associated with personality disorders should also be distinguished from factitious illness. In the case of the latter, intentional deception is associated with factitious disorders.

Treatment Approach

Factitious disorders are notoriously difficult to treat; no single size fits all treatment. There are, however, several principles that prove helpful. The first is to avoid confrontation—especially when making the diagnosis. Direct confrontation or accusation often results in defensiveness, increased elusiveness, or flight from the hospital. Moreover, confrontation appears to be ineffective in most patients, with few of them actually admitting their behavior.[5] Interventions that allow the patient to "save face" (which requires significant skill to carry out) may be more helpful and effective.[16] Being aware of negative countertransference is also essential if one is to avoid becoming judgmental or acting on the feelings of hostility so often evoked by these patients. In this regard, it is crucial to keep documentation factual rather than affect-laden. Making an early diagnosis is one of the most important interventions, since an undiscovered diagnosis of factitious disorder exposes the patient to more potentially harmful interventions—however, avoiding iatrogenesis is a key element to treatment, such that one must strike a balance between conducting an appropriate diagnostic work-up and avoiding unnecessary invasive procedures. Finally, since this illness is often highly treatment-resistant, placing an emphasis on management over cure is a helpful way of re-framing the treatment goals. Clear and open communication between the psychiatrist and medical/surgical colleagues is essential in this regard. Since these patients often create legal and ethical issues, consultation with legal experts or hospital ethics committees is sometimes prudent. Finally, supportive psychotherapy, with the underlying goal of fostering a relationship with a health care provider that isn't contingent on the development of symptoms, may be useful in reducing factitious behavior.

FACTITIOUS DISORDER IMPOSED ON ANOTHER

Factitious disorder imposed on another involves the intentional production or feigning of physical or psychological signs or symptoms in another person for the purpose of indirectly assuming the sick role. The perpetrator in this case is most often the biological mother of a young child, although the elderly, pets, and those under the medical care of others are also at risk. The perpetrator deceives medical personnel by altering records, falsifying medical history, contaminating laboratory samples, or directly inducing injury or illness on the victim.[17] This severe form of this disorder was previously known as Münchausen by proxy. In a review of 451 cases of Münchausen by proxy, Sheridan[17] found that victims are typically 4 years old or younger, with equal percentages of men and women. She further discovered that an average of 21.8 months elapsed between the onset of symptoms and the diagnosis, and 6% of the victims died. Perhaps even more alarming is her finding that 61% of siblings had illnesses similar to those of the victims, and 25% of the victims' known siblings were dead.[18]

Clinical Features

Much like *factitious disorder imposed on self*, the symptoms in *factitious disorder imposed on another* are more commonly physical than psychological, and may run the gamut of any symptom imaginable. Common presentations involve apnea, anorexia/feeding problems, diarrhea, and seizures.[18] These may be induced in a variety of ways, from smothering the child to feeding the child laxatives or ipecac. Perpetrators often have some medical training or exposure to the illness affecting the child (e.g., a mother who has a seizure disorder). Other clinical indicators or "red flags" include the following: a patient who does not respond to appropriate treatments; symptoms that improve when the mother does not have access to the child; unexplained illnesses with other children in the family; a mother who becomes anxious when her child improves; or a mother who encourages invasive tests.[17]

Diagnostic Approach

As with all factitious illness, diagnosis may prove difficult unless the perpetrator is directly witnessed harming the victim. Box 25-3 outlines a practical approach to confirm the diagnosis when factitious disorder by proxy is suspected.[1] This may involve significant detective work, as in all cases of suspected factitious illness—the principal difference here is that when the victim is a child or is elderly, both legal obligations and privacy rights may differ from those of a typical adult patient. This is particularly pertinent with regard to mandated reporting (which varies state by state), as well as when video surveillance is proposed as a mechanism to uncover intentional harm. In general, any time that diagnostic or treatment strategies outside the usual standard of care are considered, it is best to consult with both professional medical and legal colleagues before undertaking them.

Treatment Approach

The first consideration once a diagnosis of *factitious disorder imposed on another* is made is that of protecting the victim. In many cases this means placing the child in a foster care situation (at least temporarily). Treatment then addresses both the victim and perpetrator. Although no effective treatment for victims has been established, it is generally thought that therapy to address often co-morbid psychiatric diagnoses is a good place to start. Therapy for perpetrators is generally the mainstay of treatment; however, since many perpetrators never admit to wrongdoing, this often proves difficult.

MALINGERING

The essential feature of malingering is the intentional production of false or grossly exaggerated physical or psychological symptoms, motivated by external incentives (where there is an anticipated external gain). It is important to note that malingering is not classified as a psychiatric illness.[2] Examples of tangible personal gain include avoiding military duty, avoiding work, evading criminal prosecution, obtaining drugs, or obtaining financial compensation. Box 25-4 outlines clinical indicators suggestive of possible malingering. Patients always have a clearly definable goal or external motivation for their behavior—this differentiates malingering from factitious disorders. While the prevalence of malingering is unknown, it is thought to be more common in men than women and is often co-morbid with antisocial personality disorder. Settings where these conditions intersect (e.g., prisons) likely see a higher incidence.

Clinical Features

Malingerers most often pick symptoms that are highly subjective and difficult to prove (or disprove). Vague pains (such as headache, tooth pain, or back pain) are common. The goal may be to obtain narcotics or to be placed on disability from work (among others). The presence of a lawsuit after a reported injury should also raise suspicion that the patient is malingering. As with factitious disorders, the primary symptomatology with malingering may also be psychological in nature. Malingerers may report symptoms of anxiety or depression, and try to convince the examiner of how much their function is impaired and how much they are bothered by the symptoms. The malingerer may say something like: "My panic attacks come back every time I go to work. All I want to do is to be able to work, but the panic won't allow me to. Please help me, doc."

Diagnostic and Management Approach

The presence of clearly identified secondary gain is not absolute evidence of malingering—one must be careful not to miss the diagnosis of a true medical condition in this population. When malingering is suspected, however, objective tests are crucial. When these are normal, psychological testing may be in order. The Minnesota Multiphasic Personality Inventory—2 (MMPI-2) may pick up distortions or exaggerations in both physical and psychological symptoms.[19] Direct confrontation is not advised since this often results in the patient becoming angry and fleeing from treatment. Strategies that allow the patient to save face (e.g., suggesting that the illness will improve soon) are generally more successful in that they allow the patient a way out. Avoiding iatrogenesis and remaining aware of one's own anger toward the patient (so as not to act on it) are also keys to appropriate treatment. Given that there is often overlap with legal issues in those who malinger, consultation with legal experts is frequently advisable.

CONCLUSION

Factitious disorders and malingering both share the common feature of the intentional production of symptoms that are either of a physical or psychological nature. The motivation differs from assuming the sick role in the former to obtaining external secondary gain in the latter. *Factitious disorder imposed on another* is further complicated by inflicting harm on someone else (often a young child) to assume the sick role indirectly. Each of these is tricky to diagnose and difficult to treat once the diagnosis is made. Ethical and legal considerations are also quite pertinent, as are those of avoiding iatrogenesis, which may further harm the patient. The deceptive nature of these illnesses often induces a negative countertransference (including anger and hatred toward the patient). Understanding the illnesses (including their clinical presentations, diagnostic approaches, and treatment options) brings clinicians one step closer to providing better care for this difficult population.

 Access a list of MCQs for this chapter at https://expertconsult .inkling.com

REFERENCES

1. Ford CV. Deception syndromes; factitious disorders and malingering. In Levenson JL, editor: *The American Psychiatric Publishing textbook of psychosomatic medicine*, ed 2, Arlington, VA, 2011, American Psychiatric Publishing.
2. American Psychiatric Association. *Diagnostic and statistical manual of mental disorders*, ed 5, (DSM-5), Arlington, VA, 2013, American Psychiatric Press.
3. Sutherland AJ, Rodin GM. Factitious disorders in a general hospital setting: clinical features and a review of the literature. *Psychosomatics* 31:392–399, 1990.
4. Craven DE, Steger KA, La Chapelle R, et al. Factitious HIV infection: the importance of documenting infection. *Ann Intern Med* 121:763–766, 1994.
5. Krahn LE, Li H, O'Connor MK. Patients who strive to be ill: factitious disorder with physical symptoms. *Am J Psychiatry* 160:1163–1168, 2003.
6. Fliege H, Grimm A, Eckhardt-Henn A, et al. Frequency of ICD-10 factitious disorder: survey of senior hospital consultants and physicians in private practice. *Psychosomatics* 48:60–64, 2007.
7. Asher R. Münchausen's syndrome. *Lancet* 1:339–341, 1951.
8. Beach SR, Viguera AC, Stern TA. Factitious disorders. In Stern TA, Herman JB, Gorrindo T, editors: *Massachusetts General Hospital psychiatry update and board preparation*, ed 3, Boston, 2012, MGH Psychiatry Academy.
9. Bogazzi F, Bartalena L, Scarcello G, et al. The age of patients with thyrotoxicosis factitia in Italy from 1973–1996. *J Endocrinol Invest* 22(2):128–133, 1999.
10. Thompson CR, Beckson M. A case of factitious homicidal ideation. *J Am Acad Psychiatry Law* 32(3):277–281, 2004.
11. Mitchell D, Francis JP. A case of factitious disorder presenting as alcohol dependence. *Subst Abus* 24(3):187–189, 2003.
12. Phillips MR, Ward NG, Ries RK. Factitious mourning: painless patienthood. *Am J Psychiatry* 140(4):420–425, 1983.
13. Sparr L, Pankratz LD. Factitious posttraumatic stress disorder. *Am J Psychiatry* 140(8):1016–1019, 1983.
14. Friedl MC, Draijer N. Dissociative disorders in Dutch psychiatric inpatients. *Am J Psychiatry* 157(6):1012–1013, 2000.
15. Eisendrath SJ. Factitious physical disorders: treatment without confrontation. *Psychosomatics* 30:383–387, 1989.
16. Sadock BJ, Sadock VA. Factitious disorders. In *Kaplan and Sadock's synopsis of psychiatry*, ed 9, Philadelphia, 2004, Lippincott Williams & Wilkins, pp 668–675.
17. Sheridan MS. The deceit continues: an updated literature review of Münchausen syndrome by proxy. *Child Abuse Negl* 27(4):431–451, 2003.
18. Rosenberg DA. Web of deceit: a literature review of Münchausen syndrome by proxy. *Child Abuse Negl* 11(4):547–563, 1987.
19. Lees-Haley PR, Fox DD. MMPI subtle-obvious scales and malingering: clinical versus simulated scores. *Psychol Rep* 66(3 Pt 1):907–911, 1990.

SUGGESTED READING

Barsky AJ, Stern TA, Greenberg DB, et al. Functional somatic symptoms and somatoform disorders. In Stern TA, Fricchione GL, Cassem NH, et al., editors: *Massachusetts General Hospital handbook of general hospital psychiatry*, ed 5, Philadelphia, 2004, Mosby.

26 Alcohol-Related Disorders

John F. Kelly, PhD, and John A. Renner Jr., MD

KEY POINTS

Incidence

- Alcohol misuse is one of the leading causes of morbidity and mortality in the US.

Epidemiology

- The highest rates of alcohol use, heavy binge use, and alcohol use disorders occur between the ages of 18 and 29 years.

Pathophysiology

- Alcohol causes harm through three distinct, but related pathways: intoxication, toxicity, and alcohol use disorder.

Clinical Findings

- Alcohol use disorders are heterogeneous disorders that require assessment and an individualized clinical approach.
- It is possible to screen effectively and efficiently for the presence of an alcohol use disorder using brief, validated measures.

Differential Diagnoses

- Presentation of an alcohol use disorder is often complicated by the presence of co-morbid psychiatric symptoms and disorders that require assessment and monitoring, as well as an integrated treatment approach.

Treatment Options

- A number of effective pharmacological and psychosocial treatment approaches exist for alcohol use disorders that produce outcomes similar to, or better than, outcomes for other chronic illnesses.

Complications

- Heavy drinking can lead to accidents, violence, unwanted pregnancies, and overdoses.

OVERVIEW

Alcohol is an ambiguous molecule[1] often referred to as "man's oldest friend and oldest enemy".[2] Compared to more structurally complicated substances, such as cannabis ($C_{21}H_{30}O_2$), cocaine ($C_{17}H_{21}NO_4$), or heroin ($C_{21}H_{23}NO_5$), beverage alcohol (ethanol) possesses a simple chemical structure (C_2H_5OH) that belies the complexities of its medical, psychological, and social impact (Figure 26-1).

When the alcohol molecule reaches the human brain it is generally perceived as good news; pleasant subjective experiences of euphoria, disinhibition, anxiety reduction, and sedation, are the most likely outcomes. These are often encouraged and enhanced by social contexts and by culture-bound customs. If too high a dose is imbibed too rapidly, however, acute intoxication occurs, leading to a predictable sequence of behavioral disinhibition and cognitive and motor impairments. If a large quantity of alcohol is consumed, especially

if it is done rapidly,[3] alcohol-induced amnesia ("blackouts"), coma, and death, can occur.

Like several other drugs, alcohol causes harm in three distinct, but related, ways: through intoxication, toxicity, and alcohol use disorder.[4] As depicted in Figure 26-2, the acute intoxicating effects of alcohol produce physical and psychological impairments (e.g., ataxia, poor judgment, visuo-spatial deficits, sensory distortions) and disinhibition can lead to aggression, that can result in accidents and injuries (e.g., from car crashes, falls, fights). The toxic effects of alcohol, on the other hand, produce harm through the chronic deleterious action of alcohol on the human body that can result in liver damage, including cirrhosis, as well as damage to the brain, heart, and kidneys.[5] Because of the toxicity pathway to harm, it is possible for individuals who infrequently become intoxicated to, nevertheless, develop a variety of diseases associated with alcohol's *toxic* effects, such as cirrhosis of the liver or a variety of cancers (e.g., of the colon, rectum, breast, larynx, liver, esophagus, oral cavity, pharynx[6]; Figure 26-2). Somewhat paradoxically, cirrhosis is more common among individuals *without* alcohol addiction, since more florid manifestations of dependence are likely to result in more rapid remission, incarceration, or death, preventing the chronic damaging toxic effects associated with prolonged use of alcohol.[7] Alcohol use disorder (AUD) is the third pathway through which alcohol use causes harm. AUD contributes to a range of changes in the brain that often result in alcohol addiction. This can take a heavy toll on individuals' lives (with serious domestic and social problems, family disintegration, loss of employment and increased risk of mortality). Related to these pathways is the volume and frequency at which alcohol is consumed. Low-risk consumption is, for men, no more than 14 drinks per week and, for women, no more than 7 drinks in any given week. The *pattern* of consumption is also critical, however, for obvious reasons; 14 drinks in one sitting for some could constitute a lethal dose. Thus, to minimize harm from intoxication, and to reduce the risk from AUDs, no more than 2 drinks on any given day for men and no more than 1 for women is recommended[8] (Figure 26-3). It should be emphasized, however, that this pattern of consumption is "*low* risk" and *not* "*no* risk"; meta-analyses reveal even less than 1 drink a day is associated with an increased risk for a number of cancers (including breast cancer in women).[6] It is estimated that alcohol is responsible for about 20%–30% of esophageal cancers, liver cancer, cirrhosis of the liver, homicide, epileptic seizures, and motor vehicle accidents worldwide.[9] Excessive or risky alcohol consumption is the third leading cause of death in the US, accounting for approximately 100,000 deaths annually.[10] In terms of disability-adjusted life years (DALYs) lost, alcohol accounts for more disease, disability, and mortality combined in the United States than tobacco use, even though tobacco use accounts for a higher death rate. This is because alcohol causes more illness, impairment during the prime of individuals' lives, and death (e.g., alcohol is the leading risk factor for death among men 15–59 worldwide).[11] The economic burden attributed to alcohol-related problems in the US approaches $224 billion annually.[12,13]

Alcohol-related disorders are common in the general population, are prevalent among general medical patients, and are endemic among psychiatric patients. An awareness of the substantial roles that alcohol use, misuse, and associated disorders play in medicine and psychiatry will enhance the detection of these problems and lead to more efficient and effective targeting of clinical resources.

In this chapter we review pertinent clinical manifestations of heavy alcohol use and outline strategies for effective management of alcohol-related problems. The nature, etiology, epidemiology, and typologies of alcohol-related disorders are described, and optimal screening and assessment methods (to facilitate detection and appropriate intervention) are outlined. In the final sections, details of current knowledge regarding the mechanisms of action of heavy alcohol use are provided and effective psychosocial and pharmacological treatment approaches are reviewed.

DESCRIPTION AND DEFINITION

Alcohol-related disorders can be divided into two main groups: alcohol-induced disorders (such as alcohol intoxication, delirium, alcohol withdrawal, persisting alcohol-induced amnestic disorders, and fetal alcohol spectrum disorders), and alcohol use disorder (DSM-5[14], Box 26-1).

Heavy, chronic, alcohol use may also induce psychiatric symptoms and syndromes that mimic psychotic disorder, mood disorders, and anxiety disorders. Such syndromes most often remit with abstinence, but the diagnosis of an

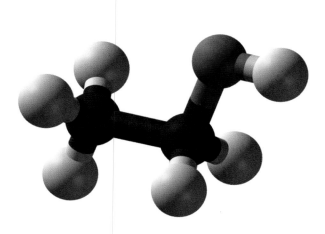

Figure 26-1. Molecular structure of beverage ethyl alcohol. *(From UCLA Chemistry,* http://www.chem.ucla.edu/harding/IGOC/E/ethanol .html*)*

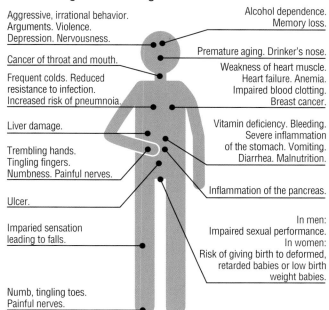

Figure 26-2. Alcohol-related disorders associated with high-risk drinking. *(From Rehm J, Room R, Monteiro M, et al. Alcohol use. In Ezzati M, Lopez AD, Rodgers A, Murray CJL, editors:* Comparative quantification of health risks: global and regional burden of disease attributable to selected major risk factors. *Geneva, 2004, World Health Organization.)*

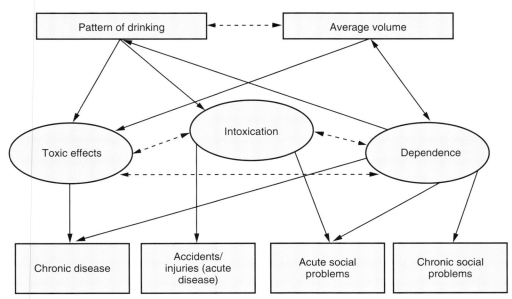

Figure 26-3. Patterns of drinking and pathways to harm. *(From Babor TF, Caetano R, Casswell S, et al.* Alcohol: no ordinary commodity-research and public policy. *ed 2. Oxford, UK, 2010, Oxford University Press.)*

BOX 26-1 The DSM-5 Diagnostic Criteria: Alcohol Use Disorder[14]

A. A problematic pattern of alcohol use leading to clinically significant impairment or distress, as manifested by at least two of the following, occurring within a 12-month period:
 1. Alcohol is often taken in larger amounts or over a longer period than was intended.
 2. There is a persistent desire or unsuccessful efforts to cut down or control alcohol use.
 3. A great deal of time is spent in activities necessary to obtain alcohol, use alcohol, or recovery from its effects.
 4. Craving, or a strong desire or urge to use alcohol.
 5. Recurrent alcohol use resulting in a failure to fulfill major role obligations at work, school, or home.
 6. Continued alcohol use despite having persistent or recurrent social or interpersonal problems caused or exacerbated by the effects of alcohol
 7. Important social, occupational, or recreational activities are given up or reduced because of alcohol use.
 8. Recurrent alcohol use in situations in which it is physically hazardous.
 9. Alcohol use is continued despite knowledge of having a persistent or recurrent physical or psychological problem that is likely to have been caused or exacerbated by alcohol.
 10. Tolerance, as defined by either of the following:
  a. A need for markedly increased amounts of alcohol to achieve intoxication or desired effect.
  b. A markedly diminished effect with continued use of the same amount of alcohol.
 11. Withdrawal, as manifested by either of the following:
  a. The characteristic withdrawal syndrome for alcohol
  b. Alcohol (or a closely related substance, such as a benzodiazepine) is taken to relieve or avoid withdrawal symptoms.

Specify if:

In early remission: After full criteria for alcohol use disorder were previously met, none of the criteria for alcohol use disorder have been met for at least 3 months but for less than 12 months (with the exception that Criterion A4, "Craving, or a strong desire or urge to use alcohol," may be met).

In sustained remission: After full criteria for alcohol use disorder were previously met, none of the criteria for alcohol use disorder have been met at any time during a period of 12 months or longer (with the exception that Criterion A4, "Craving, or a strong desire or urge to use alcohol," may be met).

Specify if:

In a controlled environment: This additional specifier is used if the individual is in an environment where access to alcohol is restricted.
 • **Coding note** based on current severity, for ICD-10-CM codes: If an alcohol intoxication, alcohol withdrawal, or another alcohol-induced mental disorder is also present, do not use the codes below for alcohol use disorder. Instead, the comorbid alcohol use disorder is indicated in the 4th character of the alcohol-induced disorder code (see the coding note for alcohol intoxication, alcohol withdrawal, or a specific alcohol-induced mental disorder). For example, if there is comorbid alcohol intoxication and alcohol use disorder, only the alcohol intoxication code is given, with the 4th character indicating whether the comorbid alcohol use disorder is mild, moderate, or severe: F10.129 for mild alcohol use disorder with alcohol intoxication or F10.229 for a moderate or severe alcohol use disorder with alcohol intoxication.

Specify current severity:

305.00 (F10.10) Mild: Presence of 2–3 symptoms.
303.90 (F10.20) Moderate: Presence of 4–5 symptoms.
303.90 (F10.20) Severe: Presence of 6 or more symptoms.

Reprinted with permission from the Diagnostic and statistical manual of mental disorders, *ed 5, (Copyright 2013). American Psychiatric Association.*

---

independent co-occurring psychiatric disorder is difficult to discern in an individual who is actively drinking. At least 4 weeks of sobriety is recommended to establish the diagnosis of an independent psychiatric disorder. The next sections describe alcohol-induced disorders and AUDs.

ALCOHOL-INDUCED DISORDERS
Alcohol Intoxication

The action of alcohol on the brain is complex. Low blood alcohol concentrations (BACs) produce activation and disinhibition, whereas higher BACs produce sedation. Behavioral disinhibition is mediated by alcohol's action as a γ-aminobutyric acid (GABA) agonist, and its interactions with the serotonin system may account for its association with violent behavior. The GABA, N-methyl-D-aspartate (NMDA), and serotonin systems have all been implicated in the escalation to violence.[15,16] Blood alcohol concentrations (BACs, measured as the percentage of alcohol in the blood) from 0.19% to 29% may impair memory or lead to an alcoholic blackout, with argumentativeness or assaultiveness developing at levels of 0.10%–0.19% and coma or death occurring at 0.40%–0.50%. Yet, chronic alcoholics may be fully alert with a BAC of more than 0.40%, owing to tolerance. Resolution of intoxication follows steady-state kinetics, so that a 70-kg man metabolizes approximately 10 ml of absolute ethanol (or 1.5 to 2 drink equivalents; 1 standard drink = 0.5 oz of whiskey, 4 oz of wine, or 12 oz of beer) per hour (Figure 26-4).

Treatment

If it becomes necessary to sedate an intoxicated individual, one should begin with a smaller-than-usual dose of a benzodiazepine to avoid cumulative effects of alcohol and other sedative-hypnotics. Once the individual's tolerance has been established, a specific dose can be safely determined. Lorazepam (Ativan) (1 to 2 mg) is effectively absorbed via oral (PO), intramuscular (IM), or intravenous (IV) administration. Diazepam (Valium) and chlordiazepoxide (Librium) are erratically and slowly absorbed after IM administration unless they are given in large, well-perfused sites. When incoordination suggests that the additive effect of a benzodiazepine has produced excessive sedation, it may be advantageous to use haloperidol 5 to 10 mg PO or IM. The initial dose should be followed by a delay of 0.5 to 1 hour before the next dose. If there is no risk of withdrawal, the patient can safely be referred to an outpatient program. Inpatient detoxification is preferable to outpatient care if the patient is psychosocially unstable; has serious medical, neurological, or psychiatric co-morbidity; has previously suffered from complications of withdrawal (such as seizures or delirium tremens [DTs]); or is undergoing

As BAC increases, so does impairment

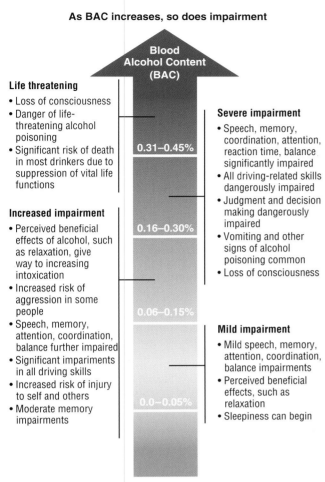

Blood Alcohol Content (BAC)

Life threatening
- Loss of consciousness
- Danger of life-threatening alcohol poisoning
- Significant risk of death in most drinkers due to suppression of vital life functions

0.31–0.45%

Increased impairment
- Perceived beneficial effects of alcohol, such as relaxation, give way to increasing intoxication
- Increased risk of aggression in some people
- Speech, memory, attention, coordination, balance further impaired
- Significant impairments in all driving skills
- Increased risk of injury to self and others
- Moderate memory impairments

0.16–0.30%

0.06–0.15%

0.0–0.05%

Severe impairment
- Speech, memory, coordination, attention, reaction time, balance significantly impaired
- All driving-related skills dangerously impaired
- Judgment and decision making dangerously impaired
- Vomiting and other signs of alcohol poisoning common
- Loss of consciousness

Mild impairment
- Mild speech, memory, attention, coordination, balance impairments
- Perceived beneficial effects, such as relaxation
- Sleepiness can begin

Figure 26-4. Impairment as a result of increased blood alcohol content (BAC). *(From National Institute on Alcohol Abuse and Alcoholism (NIAAA). Alcohol overdose: the dangers of drinking too much. NIAAA Brochures and Fact Sheets, 2013. http://pubs.niaaa.nih.gov/publications/AlcoholOverdoseFactsheet/Overdosefact.htm)*

his or her first episode of treatment.[17] Repeatedly undertreated withdrawal may place the patient at subsequent risk for withdrawal seizures and for other neurological sequelae through "kindling," an electrophysiological effect[18] that may be mediated, similar to other neurodegenerative effects of ethanol, via the glutamate excitatory neurotransmitter system.[19]

Alcohol-induced Coma

Alcohol-induced coma, although rare, is a medical emergency. It occurs when extraordinary amounts of alcohol are consumed, and it can occur in conjunction with use of other drugs. Young adults/college-age youth may be particularly susceptible when goaded into drinking contests. This age group is also at significantly higher risk for alcohol-related injuries. A 2002 study by the federally supported Task Force on College Drinking estimated that 1,400 college students in the US are killed each year in alcohol-related accidents.

Alcohol Withdrawal Syndrome

The syndrome of alcohol withdrawal can range from mild discomfort (that requires no medication) to multi-organ failure (that requires intensive care). Uncomplicated

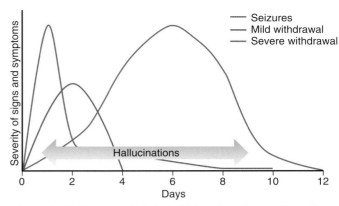

Figure 26-5. Progress of alcohol withdrawal syndrome. *(From Frank L, Pead J. New concepts in drug withdrawal: a resource handbook. Melbourne, 1995, University of Melbourne.)*

withdrawal is surprisingly common and is frequently missed. Although more than 90% of alcoholics in withdrawal need nothing more than supportive treatment, those hospitalized with co-morbid medical conditions have a higher rate of complications.[20] The most common features of uncomplicated alcohol withdrawal emerge within hours and resolve after 3 to 5 days. Early features (loss of appetite, irritability, and tremor) of uncomplicated withdrawal symptoms are predictable. A hallmark of alcohol withdrawal is generalized tremor (fast in frequency and more pronounced when the patient is under stress). This tremor may involve the tongue to such an extent that the patient cannot talk. The lower extremities may tremble so much that the patient cannot walk. The hands and arms may shake so violently that a drinking glass cannot be held without spilling the contents. Typically, the patient is hypervigilant, has a pronounced startle response, and complains of insomnia.

Less commonly, patients experience hallucinations (without delirium) or seizures associated with alcohol withdrawal. Illusions and hallucinations may appear and produce vague uneasiness. These symptoms may persist for as long as 2 weeks and then clear without the development of delirium. Grand mal seizures ("rum fits") may occur, usually within the first 2 days. More than one out of every three patients who suffer seizures develops subsequent DTs (Figure 26-5).

Treatment

Rigid adherence to a single protocol for all cases of alcohol withdrawal is unrealistic. Symptom-triggered dosing, in which dosages are individualized and only administered on the appearance of early symptoms, is often recommended. Assessment of the severity of alcohol withdrawal's signs and symptoms is best accomplished with the use of standardized alcohol withdrawal scales, such as the CIWA-Ar.[21] This reduces use of medication doses by a factor of four, substantially shortens the length of treatment, and shortens symptom duration by a factor of six,[17,22] although the benefits may be less dramatic in medically ill inpatients.[23] Chlordiazepoxide (50 to 100 mg PO) can be given initially, and be followed by 50 to 100 mg every 1 to 2 hours until the patient is sedated and the vital signs are within normal limits. Alternatively, diazepam (10 to 20 mg) may be given initially, and then repeated every 1 to 2 hours until sedation is achieved. Often a first day's dose of a long-acting benzodiazepine is sufficient for the entire detoxification process because of the self-tapering effect and slow elimination.[24] Patients with impaired liver function, the elderly, or individuals with co-occurring medical or psychiatric conditions are often better managed with a shorter-acting agent, such as lorazepam 1 to 4 mg PO or IM, or 0.5 mg/min slow IV infusion in severe withdrawal, repeated after 1 to 2 hours, with dose tapering by 25% per day over the subsequent 3 to 6 days.

The α2-agonist dexmedetomidine is sometimes used in cases of alcohol withdrawal, especially when patients require escalating doses of benzodiazepines and additional intubation and mechanical ventilation to protect airways, which can lead to complications and prolonged hospital stays.[25] Similarly, phenobarbital is used to augment benzodiazepine-assisted alcohol withdrawal to prevent the need for intubation and ICU admission. A prospective, randomized, double-blind, placebo-controlled study with 102 patients, half of whom received either a single dose of IV phenobarbital (10 mg/kg in 100 ml of normal saline) or placebo (100 ml of normal saline) in addition to a symptom-guided lorazepam-based alcohol withdrawal protocol, found that patients who received phenobarbital had fewer ICU admissions (8% vs. 25%), and there were no differences in adverse events.[26]

Alcohol Withdrawal Seizures

Withdrawal seizures occur in roughly 1% of unmedicated alcoholics undergoing withdrawal, although the prevalence is increased in individuals with inadequately treated prior episodes of alcohol withdrawal, prior alcohol withdrawal seizures, seizure disorders, and previous brain injuries. Although brain imaging may not be necessary in patients with their first episode,[27] seizures during alcohol withdrawal require careful evaluation for other causes. Indications for imaging include neurological and other physical findings suggestive of focal lesions, meningitis, or subarachnoid hemorrhage—all of which may occur in a patient with a history of alcohol withdrawal seizures. Multiple prior detoxifications predispose patients to withdrawal seizures more than the quantity or duration of a drinking history, implying a kindling cause.[28] Seizures may occur following a rapid drop in the BAC or during the 6 to 24 hours after drinking cessation. Generalized seizures typically occur (i.e., in 75% of cases) in the absence of focal findings, and in individuals with otherwise unremarkable electroencephalogram (EEG) findings. Repeated seizures may occur over a 24-hour period; however, status epilepticus occurs in less than 10% of those who seize.

Treatment

In patients without a prior seizure disorder, diphenylhydantoin offers no benefit over placebo, and given the potential for side effects, diphenylhydantoin is therefore not recommended.[28] Also, given that loading with carbamazepine or valproate may not address the rapid time course of withdrawal seizures, the most parsimonious approach remains effective treatment with benzodiazepines. Prompt treatment of early withdrawal symptoms, as described below, is the most effective measure to prevent the development of seizures. In cases where there is a known seizure disorder, however, conventional management with an anticonvulsant is in order.

Alcohol Withdrawal Delirium

Delirium tremens, or "DTs," the major acute complication of alcohol withdrawal, was renamed "alcohol withdrawal delirium" in the *Diagnostic and Statistical Manual of Mental Disorders*, ed 4 (DSM-IV).[29] Until open-heart procedures spawned new postoperative deliria, DTs were by far the most frequently encountered delirium in general hospitals, reportedly occurring in 5% of hospitalized alcoholics. Although it was first described in the medical literature more than 150 years ago and it has been frequently observed ever since, DTs still go undiagnosed in a large number of cases. It is missed because physicians tend to forget that alcoholism is rampant among people of all backgrounds and appearances.[30] Because deaths have occurred in 10% of patients with untreated alcohol withdrawal delirium and in 25% of those patients with medical or concomitant surgical complications, it is imperative to be on the alert for this life-threatening condition.

It is difficult to predict who will develop DTs. Until a decade ago, DTs rarely developed in patients younger than 30 years of age. This is no longer true. Today the condition is frequently observed in young patients who may have had a decade or more of chronic heavy alcohol consumption. The mechanisms may involve NMDA-glutamate receptor supersensitivity.[18] Although delirium is regarded as a withdrawal syndrome, some heavy drinkers fail to develop delirium after sudden withdrawal of ethanol. Infection, head trauma, and poor nutrition are potentially contributing factors to delirium. A history of DTs is the most obvious predictor of future DTs.[31]

The incidence of DTs is approximately 5% among hospitalized alcoholics and about 33% in patients with alcohol withdrawal seizures. If DTs do occur, they generally do so between 24 and 72 hours after abstinence begins. There have been reports, however, of cases in which the clinical picture of DTs did not emerge until 7 days after the last drink. The principal features are disorientation (to time, place, or person), tremor, hyperactivity, marked wakefulness, fever, increased autonomic tone, and hallucinations. Hallucinations are generally visual, but they may be tactile (in which case they are probably associated with a peripheral neuritis), olfactory, or auditory. Vestibular disturbances are common and often hallucinatory. The patient may complain of the floor moving or of being on an elevator. The hallucinatory experience is almost always frightening, such as seeing spiders and snakes that may have additional characteristics (e.g., more vivid colors and mice or insects sensed on the skin). Once the condition manifests itself, DTs usually last 2 to 3 days, often resolving suddenly after a night of sound sleep. Should it persist, an infection or subdural hematoma may be the cause. There are, however, a small number of individuals whose course is characterized by relapses with intervals of complete lucidity. These patients offer the clinician the most challenging diagnostic opportunities. As a rule of thumb, it is always wise to include DTs in the list of diagnoses considered whenever delirium appears. Even skilled clinicians are apt to miss the diagnosis of DTs when the patient's manner, social position, or reputation belies a preconceived and distorted stereotype of an "alcoholic." The clinician is also frequently misled when the delirium is intermittent and the patient is examined during a lucid stage. Although a course of intermittent episodes is highly atypical for DTs, it can occur.

The prognosis for DTs is reasonably good if the patient is aggressively medicated, but death can occur as the syndrome progresses through convulsions to coma and death. Death can also result from heart failure, an infection (chiefly pneumonia), or injuries sustained during the restless period. In a small proportion of patients the delirium may merge into Wernicke–Korsakoff syndrome, in which case the patient may not regain full mentation. This is more apt to happen in those with closely spaced episodes of DTs and in the elderly, but it should be assessed and continually monitored.[32]

Treatment

Prevention is the key. Symptom-triggered dosing for alcohol withdrawal has been shown to reduce DTs more than use of standing doses of benzodiazepine in medically ill inpatients.[23]

As in the treatment of any delirium, the prime concern must be round-the-clock monitoring so that the patient cannot harm himself or herself or others. Although not necessarily suicidal, delirious patients take unpremeditated risks. Falling out of windows, slipping down stairs, and walking into objects are common examples. Restraints should be used only when necessary. When four-point restraint is used, the patient must be closely observed, and relief must be provided every hour. Usually, use of physical restraints can be avoided with aggressive pharmacotherapy.

The delayed onset of this hyperarousal may reflect alcohol's broad effects across multiple neurotransmitter systems, chief among which may be the NMDA-glutamate system.[19] Adrenergic hyperarousal alone appears to be an insufficient explanation, so that α-adrenergic agonists (e.g., clonidine, lofexidine) alone are not sufficient. Benzodiazepines alone may not suffice. In rare cases, doses of diazepam in excess of 500 mg/day may prove insufficient. Haloperidol 5 to 10 mg PO or IM may be added and repeated after 1 to 2 hours when psychosis or agitation is present. Propofol may be used in those cases of severe DTs unresponsive to other medications.[33]

Because the B vitamins are known to help prevent peripheral neuropathy and the Wernicke–Korsakoff syndrome, their use is *vital*. Thiamine (100 mg IV) should be given immediately, and 100 mg should be given IM for at least 3 days until a normal diet is resumed. A smaller amount of thiamine may be added to infusions for IV use. Folic acid 1 to 5 mg PO or IM each day should be included to prevent megaloblastic anemia and peripheral neuropathy. A high-carbohydrate soft diet containing 3,000 to 4,000 calories a day should be given with multivitamins.

Wernicke–Korsakoff Syndrome

Victor and colleagues,[34] in their classic monograph *The Wernicke–Korsakoff Syndrome*, state that "Wernicke's encephalopathy and Korsakoff's syndrome in the alcoholic, nutritionally deprived patient may be regarded as two facets of the same disease. Patients evidence specific central nervous system pathology with resultant profound mental changes." Although perhaps 5% of alcoholics have this disorder, in 80% of these cases, the diagnosis is missed.[32] In all of the cases reported by Victor and colleagues,[34] alcoholism was a serious problem and was almost invariably accompanied by malnutrition. Malnutrition, particularly thiamine deficiency, has been shown to be the essential factor.

Wernicke's Encephalopathy

Wernicke's encephalopathy appears suddenly and is characterized by ophthalmoplegia and ataxia followed by mental disturbance. The ocular disturbance, which occurs in only 17% of cases, consists of paresis or paralysis of the external recti, with nystagmus, and a disturbance in conjugate gaze. A globally confused state consists of disorientation, unresponsiveness, and derangement of perception and memory. Exhaustion, apathy, dehydration, and profound lethargy are also part of the picture. The patient is apt to be somnolent, confused, and slow to reply, and may fall asleep in mid-sentence. Once treatment with thiamine is started for Wernicke's encephalopathy, improvement is often evident in the ocular palsies within hours. Recovery from ocular muscle paralysis is complete within days or weeks. According to Victor and colleagues,[34] approximately one-third recovered from the state of global confusion within 6 days of treatment, another third within 1 month, and the remainder within 2 months. The state of global confusion is almost always reversible, in marked contrast to the memory impairment of Korsakoff's psychosis.

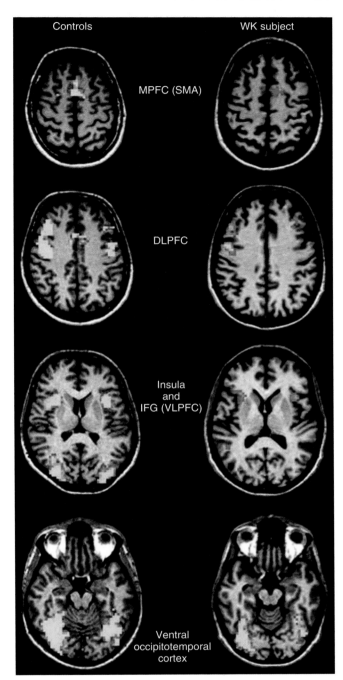

Figure 26-6. Brain activation in Wernicke–Korsakoff (WK) patients compared to controls. VLPFC, ventro lateral pre-frontal cortex; IFG, inferior frontal gyrus. *(From Caulo M, Van Hecke J, Toma L, et al. Functional MRI study of diencephalic amnesia in Wernicke–Korsakoff syndrome.* Brain *128(Pt 7):1584–1594, 2005.)*

Functional magnetic resonance imaging (fMRI) studies show substantially diminished global activation in the brain among Wernicke–Korsakoff's patients compared to normal controls (Figure 26-6).

Treatment

Administration of the B vitamin thiamine (IM or IV) should be routine for *all* suspected cases of alcohol intoxication and dependence.[35] The treatment for Wernicke's encephalopathy and Korsakoff's psychosis is identical, and both are *medical emergencies*. Because subclinical cognitive impairments can occur even in apparently well-nourished patients, routine management should include thiamine, folic acid, and multivitamins with minerals, particularly zinc. Prompt use of vitamins, particularly thiamine, prevents advancement of the disease and reverses at least a portion of the lesions where permanent damage has not yet been done. The response to treatment is therefore an important diagnostic aid. In patients who show only ocular and ataxic signs, the prompt administration of thiamine is crucial in preventing the development of an irreversible and incapacitating amnestic disorder. Treatment consists of 100 mg of thiamine and 1 mg of folic acid (given IV) immediately and 100 mg IM of thiamine each day until a normal diet is resumed, followed by oral doses for 30 days. Parenteral feedings and the administration of B-complex vitamins become necessary if the patient cannot eat. If a rapid heart rate, feeble heart sounds, pulmonary edema, or other signs of myocardial weakness appear, the patient may require digitalis. Because these patients have impaired mental function, nursing personnel should be alerted to the patient's tendency to wander, to be forgetful, and to become obstreperously psychotic.

Korsakoff's Psychosis (Alcohol-induced Persisting Amnestic Disorder)

Korsakoff's psychosis, also referred to as confabulatory psychosis and alcohol-induced persisting amnestic disorder,[29] is characterized by impaired memory in an otherwise alert and responsive individual. This condition is slow to start and may be the end stage of a lengthy alcohol-dependence process. Hallucinations and delusions are rarely encountered. Curiously, confabulation, long regarded as the hallmark of Korsakoff's psychosis, was exhibited in only a limited number of cases in the large series collected and studied by Victor and colleagues.[34] Most of these patients have diminished spontaneous verbal output, have a limited understanding of the extent of their memory loss, and lack insight into the nature of their illness.

The memory loss is bipartite. The retrograde component is the inability to recall the past, and the anterograde component is the lack of capacity for retention of new information. In the acute stage of Korsakoff's psychosis, the memory gap is so blatant that the patient cannot recall simple items (such as the examiner's name, the day, or the time) even though the patient is given this information several times. As memory improves, usually within weeks to months, simple problems can be solved, limited always by the patient's span of recall.

Patients with Korsakoff's psychosis tend to improve with time.[36] Among Victor and colleagues' patients,[34] 21% recovered more or less completely, 26% showed no recovery, and the rest recovered partially.[29] During the acute stage, however, there is no way of predicting who will improve and who will not. The EEG may be unremarkable or may show diffuse slowing, and magnetic resonance imaging (MRI) may show changes in the periaqueductal area and medial thalamus.[18] The specific memory structures affected in Korsakoff's psychosis are the medial dorsal nucleus of the thalamus and the hippocampal formations.

Fetal Alcohol Spectrum Disorder

Fetal alcohol spectrum disorder (FASD) is an umbrella term that describes the range of effects that can occur in an individual whose mother drank alcohol during pregnancy. These effects may include physical, mental, behavioral, or learning disabilities with possible life-long implications.[37] Formerly

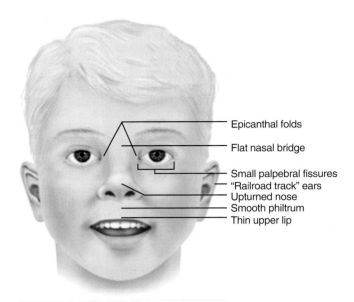

Figure 26-7. Characteristics of fetal alcohol spectrum disorder. *(From Wattendorf DJ, Muenke M. Fetal alcohol spectrum disorders.* Am Fam Physician *72(2):279–282, 285, 2005.)*

known as "fetal alcohol syndrome," these disorders can include a set of birth defects caused by alcohol during pregnancy.[38] Children with this condition typically have facial deformities, a mis-proportioned head, mental retardation, and behavioral problems (Figure 26-7).

However, even when these abnormalities are not evident, brain damage may still have occurred. Approximately 30%–40% of all women who drink heavily during pregnancy will have a baby with some degree of FASD. It is the leading cause of preventable mental retardation in the Western Hemisphere. Studies using MRI to view the brains of children with FASD show that brain areas that regulate movement and cognitive processes related to attention, perception, thinking, and memory are particularly sensitive to pre-natal alcohol exposure, and that brain size is reduced.[39]

The minimum amount of alcohol needed to produce harmful effects in exposed children is not known. Thus, the safest approach is to completely avoid alcohol during pregnancy. People with pre-natal alcohol exposure have a high risk of learning and mental disabilities, school dropout, delinquency, alcohol and other drug use disorders, mental illness, and poor psychosocial function. Education, screening, and early intervention are critical.

ALCOHOL USE DISORDERS

Alcohol use disorder has been re-classified in DSM-5 into a single, 11-item, category of "alcohol use disorder" which was constructed by combining three of the four former "abuse" criteria (repeated legal consequences was dropped) with the seven "alcohol dependence" criteria specified in DSM-IV, and by adding a new "craving" criterion. The other major classification system, the International Classification of Diseases, Version 10 (ICD-10), however, has maintained its distinction between "alcohol dependence" and "harmful use". Importantly, both systems delineate "polythetic" classifications of AUD, since only two from a list of 11 symptoms are required to meet a diagnostic threshold in DSM-5 and three in ICD-10 for a "dependence" diagnosis. This highlights a degree of heterogeneity within the syndrome that has typological and clinical implications for detecting and treating the disorder. The DSM-5 criteria can be seen in Box 26-1.

The alcohol dependence syndrome was first described in the 1970s[40] and has since been validated and generalized to describe the dependence syndrome (also often referred to as "addiction") across all psychoactive substances. Edwards and Gross[40] noted that the dependence syndrome may be recognized by the clustering of certain elements. Not all elements need be present or present to the same degree, but with increasing intensity the syndrome is likely to show logical consistency. It is conceptualized as an integration of physiological and psychological processes that leads to a pattern of heavy alcohol use that is increasingly unresponsive to external circumstances or to adverse consequences. Furthermore, they viewed the syndrome not as an all-or-nothing dichotomy, but as occurring with graded intensity, and its presentation as being influenced by personality, as well as by social and cultural contexts. Their conceptualization also introduced a "bi-axial" model with the dependence syndrome constituting one axis and alcohol-related problems the other.

In the US before DSM-III[41] there was only a single descriptive category, "alcoholism," which hitherto had been viewed as a personality disorder. DSM-III was influenced by the syndrome and bi-axial concepts of Edwards and Gross[40] and, consequently, introduced a distinction between "dependence" and "abuse." DSM-III was the first diagnostic manual of mental disorders in the US to introduce actual itemized criteria, increasing the reliability of these diagnoses.[42]

The term *alcoholism* was originally coined to describe alcohol dependence/addiction and is often still used as an alternative to *dependence*. However, it is often used more broadly to describe alcohol dependence as well as harmful/hazardous use, sometimes without explicit mention of the fact. "Dependence" has also been used to differentiate physiological dependence on a drug (e.g., on opiates following pain management after surgery) from "addiction", which may or may not include physiological dependence, but is a syndrome that involves drug-seeking behavior and a great deal of time seeking, using, and getting over the effects of the drug. These variations in usage can be confusing.[43] It may also lead to errors in clinical and scientific communication as it has implications for inferences that are drawn from clinical data and may ultimately affect treatment policy decisions.[43] Thus, we believe care should be taken in choosing descriptive terms and in using them accurately and consistently.[44-46]

As described in Box 26-1, AUD is characterized by the broad elements of neuroadaptation (tolerance and withdrawal) and an impaired ability to alter or to stop alcohol consumption for very long, despite the personal suffering it causes (impaired control over use). As a construct, assessment of AUD has been shown to be reliable and to possess good construct and predictive validity. Furthermore, The AUD construct has demonstrated construct and predictive validity and can be reliably measured.

ETIOLOGY AND EPIDEMIOLOGY
Etiology

Knowledge about the onset and course of AUDs provides valuable information for the tailoring and timing of assessments, as well as for prevention and intervention strategies. Alcohol dependence is considered a *complex* disorder with many pathways that lead to its development. Genetic and other biological factors, along with temperament, cognitive, behavioral, psychological, and sociocultural factors, are involved in the emergence of AUD.[47] Genes confer at least four separate domains of risk: alcohol metabolizing enzymes (e.g., the

functional genetic variants of alcohol dehydrogenase that demonstrate high alcohol oxidizing activity, and the genetic variant of aldehyde dehydrogenase that has low acetaldehyde oxidizing activity, protect against heavy drinking and alcoholism[48]); impulsivity and disinhibition (e.g., dopinergic *DRD2* genes[49]), psychiatric disorders (e.g., the miRNA biogenesis pathway[50] and individuals' level of response to alcohol[47,51]), although the latter be reflect differences in alcohol-metabolizing genes.

The relative contributions of genetic and environmental factors to the manifestation of AUDs can be expressed as the population-attributable risk percent, meaning the percentage of disease incidence that would be eliminated if the risk factor were removed. A genetic heritability estimate for alcohol dependence is sometimes estimated at approximately 50%, with the other 50% (equaling "100%") attributable to "environmental causes." However, these estimates are misleading since the attributable risks for a complex disease, such as alcohol dependence, can add to well over 100% because the disorder can be avoided in many different ways and can be increased by many different genetic variants. These additional percentages can be described as interactions among the various risk factors (e.g., gene–environment interactions). For example, a genetic abnormality may be necessary for a disease to occur, but the disease will not occur without the presence of an environmental risk factor. Thus, the attributable risks for the genetic aberration and the environmental factor would both be 100%. Phenylketonuria is an example of this: the disease can be avoided either by not having the genetic abnormality or by eliminating phenylalanine from the diet.[52] Similarly, regardless of an individual's high genetic risk for AUD, the disorder can be completely avoided if the individual chooses to abstain, or if there is no access to alcohol in the environment. AUDs are heterogeneous disorders. Heritable genetic factors increase the risk for developing alcohol dependence, but it should be remembered that many individuals without any family history of AUDs may still meet criteria for alcohol dependence.

Factors that influence the initiation of alcohol consumption should be distinguished from those that affect patterns of consumption once drinking is initiated. Studies of adolescent twins have demonstrated that initiation of drinking is primarily influenced by the drinking status of parents, siblings, and friends as well as by environmental variation across geographical regions where adolescent twins reside. Several cross-national studies, including studies in the US, indicate that initiation of alcohol use during adolescence is influenced chiefly by cultural rather than genetic factors.[53-55] The influence of genetic factors is negligible. Conversely, once initiated, alcohol use topography is strongly influenced by genetic factors. However, these influences are modulated also by sibling and peer-context effects (e.g., college settings) and by regional environmental variation.[56]

Pedigree, twin, and adoption studies all point to an increased risk for alcohol dependence in offspring when there is a history of such disorders in the family.[57] For example, family studies indicate a four-fold increased risk for dependence among relatives of individuals with alcohol dependence, with higher vulnerabilities for those with a greater number (higher density) of alcohol-dependent close relatives.[58] These genes influence a variety of characteristics or endophenotypes (such as impulsivity, disinhibition, and sensation seeking), enzymes (such as alcohol and aldehyde dehydrogenases), and a low level of response to alcohol's effects. These characteristics then correlate with and interact with environmental events to increase the risk for the condition.[58-60] Hence, genetic predispositions are not deterministic. AUDs are caused by a combination of interacting factors. These consist of genetic, biological, and environmental factors.

Epidemiology

Rates of alcohol use and AUD vary along several dimensions. Some of the most important among these are gender, life-stage, ethnicity, geographic location, and psychiatric co-morbidity.

In general, just over half of all Americans report alcohol consumption in the prior month.[61] Among drinkers, the lifetime prevalence for an AUD is about 14.6%. Surveys assessing past-year prevalence of these disorders indicate that nearly 8.5% (18 million) of American adults meet standard diagnostic criteria for DSM-5 AUD.[14,62] The rates of AUD in the general population vary by gender, with men having higher rates (12.4%) than women (4.9%). Highest rates of past year AUD occur among 18–29 year olds (16.2%) and the lowest among individuals age 65 years and older (1.5%). When translated into the impact AUDs have on families in the US, surveys show that more than half of all families report at least one close relative as having a drinking problem. As alluded to above, rates of heavy alcohol use and AUD among adolescents, young adults, and adults vary by geographic location, due to subcultural differences across regions. The differences may be reflected in varying proscriptions against intoxication and/or differences in alcohol policy (Figures 26-8–26-10).[63]

The highest rates of alcohol use, heavy/binge use, and AUDs occur between the ages 18 and 29.[61] Under-age drinking is a major public health problem in its own right, with about 11 million under-age persons aged 12 to 20 years (28.7%) reporting alcohol use in the past month, with the vast majority of these (10 million) drinking heavily or binging on alcohol. More males than females aged 12 to 20 years report binge drinking (22.1% versus 17.0%) and heavy drinking (8.2%

versus 4.3%). Heavy drinking in this age group can lead to accidents, violence, unwanted pregnancies, and overdosing. Among populations seen in specialty psychiatric settings, rates of heavy use are likely to be even more prevalent and screening for alcohol use should be routine.[63,64] Early exposure to alcohol is also a significant independent risk factor for developing DSM-IV alcohol dependence. In the National Epidemiologic Survey on Alcohol and Related Conditions (NESARC), among individuals who began drinking before age 14, 47% were alcohol-dependent at some point in their life, and 13% were dependent in the prior year, compared to just 9% and 2%, respectively, who began drinking after age 20.[65]

In the US, there are differences among racial groups in the use of alcohol. Caucasians and persons reporting two or more races are typically more likely than are other racial/ethnic groups to report current use.[61] An estimated 55% of Caucasians and 52% of persons reporting two or more races used alcohol in the past month, whereas the rates were 40% for Hispanics, 37% for Asians, 37% for African Americans, and 36% for American Indians or Alaska Natives. Young non–African American males are almost twice as likely as young African American males to have an AUD. While disorders generally decline with age, they increase among African American women aged 30–44 years. In terms of AUD, there are marked differences across ethnic groups in the US. Among 12–17 year olds, for example, rates are highest for Hispanics (6%) and Native Americans and Alaskans (5.7%) relative to Whites (5%), African Americans (1.8%), and Asian and Pacific Islanders (1.6%). Among adults, the 12-month prevalence of AUD is greatest among Native Americans and Alaska Natives (12.1%) than among Whites (8.9%), Hispanics (7.9%), African Americans (6.9%), and Asian and Pacific Islanders (4.5%) (Figure 26-11).

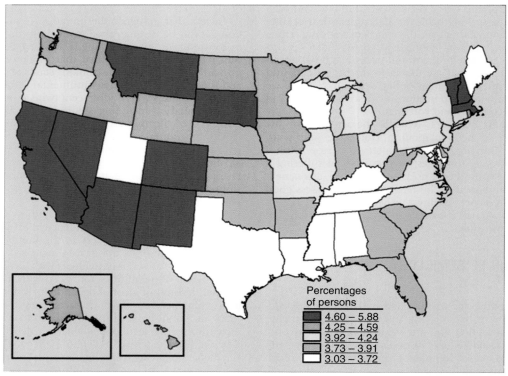

Percentages
of persons

■	4.60 – 5.88
▨	4.25 – 4.59
□	3.92 – 4.24
▨	3.73 – 3.91
□	3.03 – 3.72

Figure 26-8. Prevalence of alcohol use disorders among adolescents (ages 12–17) in the US, 2010–2011. *(From Substance Abuse and Mental Health Services Administration. Results from the 2010 National Survey on Drug Use and Health: Summary of National Findings. Rockville, MD, 2011, Substance Abuse and Mental Health Services Administration.)*

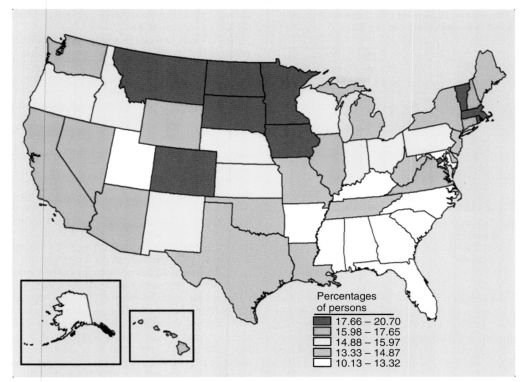

Figure 26-9. Prevalence of alcohol use disorder among young adults (ages 18–25) in the US, 2010–2011. *(From Addiction Treatment Strategies. Finger tapping study shows alcoholics may recruit other brain regions. 2012; http://www.addictionts.com/2012/08/17/finger-tapping-study-shows-alcoholics-may-recruit-other-brain-regions/, 2013.)*

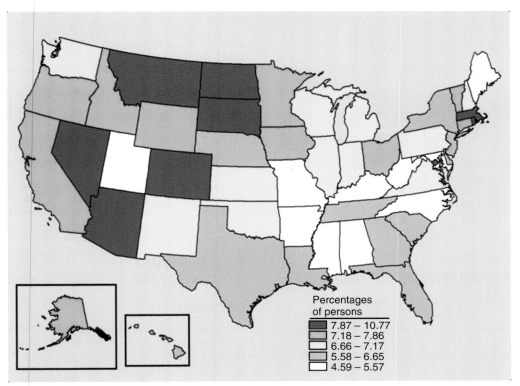

Figure 26-10. Prevalence of alcohol use disorder among persons aged 12 and older and in the United States, 2010–2011. *(From Substance Abuse and Mental Health Services Administration. Results from the 2010 National Survey on Drug Use and Health: Summary of National Findings. Rockville, MD, 2011, Substance Abuse and Mental Health Services Administration.)*

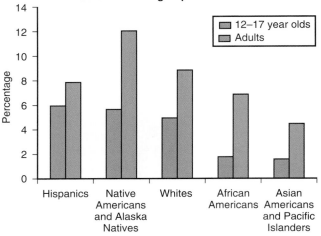

Figure 26-11. Twelve-month prevalence of alcohol use disorders across race/ethnic subgroups of the US. *(From Substance Abuse and Mental Health Services Administration. Results from the 2010 National Survey on Drug Use and Health: Summary of National Findings. Rockville, MD, 2011, Substance Abuse and Mental Health Services Administration.)*

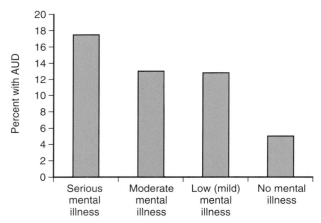

Figure 26-12. Past year alcohol use disorder among adults aged 18 or older, by level of mental illness: 2011. *(From Substance Abuse and Mental Health Services Administration. Results from the 2010 National Survey on Drug Use and Health: Summary of National Findings. Rockville, MD, 2011, Substance Abuse and Mental Health Services Administration.)*

ALCOHOL USE DISORDERS AND CO-OCCURRING PSYCHIATRIC ILLNESS

The co-occurrence of AUDs with other psychiatric disorders has been widely recognized.[66] Large-scale epidemiological surveys on co-morbidity in the US have been completed in the general household population. The most common life-time occurrences of psychiatric disorders for individuals with alcohol dependence are anxiety disorders (47%), other drug use disorders (43%), and affective disorders (41%); these are followed by conduct (32%) and antisocial personality disorder (13%). As shown in Figure 26-12, there is a moderately

strong correlation between the severity of mental illness and the prevalence of AUD.[66]

There are several possible explanations for these co-occurrences. Both conditions may be due to a common pathway (e.g., a genetic predisposition). One disorder may substantially influence the onset of the other, such as when an individual begins to use alcohol to cope with psychiatric distress (e.g., social anxiety), or when there are methodological determinants (e.g., unmeasured common causes or selection biases in some clinical studies).

These co-morbidities can be regarded clinically in two ways: a patient may present with an AUD, perhaps in an addiction-treatment setting, and also a co-occurring psychiatric illness; and a patient may present with a psychiatric disorder, perhaps in a mental health clinic, and an additional AUD. Among patients with AUDs seen in addiction-treatment settings, more than half will have at least a life-time history of another co-occurring DSM psychiatric disorder, and many will have a continuing psychiatric disturbance in one of these other areas in addition to their alcohol use. The job of the discerning clinician will be to patiently and carefully determine the presence of non–substance-induced syndromes that may persist perniciously with abstinence. The "dual diagnosis" patient can be challenging as he or she may not respond as well to standard addiction treatment, and may have greater rates of relapse, attrition, and re-admissions. However, if a co-morbid psychiatric disorder is observed or detected, determining the relative onset of the two disorders may have clinical significance, since primary disorders (i.e., those emerging first) tend to be of greater long-term clinical significance. For instance, patients whose bipolar disorder precedes the onset of their alcohol dependence tend to have better alcohol outcomes (and worse bipolar outcomes) than those whose alcohol dependence occurred first; these patients tend to have worse alcohol outcomes and better bipolar outcomes.[67] Nevertheless, both disorders will need to be attended to simultaneously for optimum results.[68,69]

For patients entering primary mental health settings, AUDs often go undetected. Left unnoticed, these disorders can undermine the salutary effects of psychotropic and psychosocial interventions aimed at ameliorating the symptoms of psychiatric illness. It is important to note that any generalizations about "dual diagnosis" patients should be made with caution. The term obviously covers an immense amount of clinical territory, since it not only covers the presence of an alcohol or other drug use disorder, which in themselves are heterogeneous and vary greatly in severity, but also a vast array of psychopathological disturbances, each with its own sub-variations and degrees of severity. Thus, the specific type, severity, and relative clinical significance of the co-morbid psychiatric disorder on the patient's presentation and future function should always be considered when approaching these dual problems. If a generalization can be made it is that both types of disorders should always be assessed and psychiatric symptoms monitored for continued and independent influence in the context of sustained abstinence from alcohol (or another drug).[70,71] If present, these conditions should be treated in an integrated fashion.[69]

Typologies

AUDs are complex and heterogeneous. Hence, attempts have been made to try to identify more homogeneous subtypes. Various typologies, some formal and others less formal, have been proposed during the past 50 years. Early typologies relied more on theoretically-framed, clinical observations. More recently, data-driven, multi-variate sub-classifications have been derived that have etiological significance and predictive validity, and may have clinical utility.

One of the first and most well-known was Jellinek's typology consisting of five subspecies of alcoholism simply labeled using the first five letters of the Greek alphabet: alpha, beta, delta, gamma, epsilon.[72] Jellinek's very broad definition of alcoholism as any use that causes harm yielded a similarly broad typology. Jellinek's typology was not successfully validated, but it did highlight the important topic of heterogeneity and it sparked further interest and efforts to identify particular subtypes of individuals suffering from alcoholism for the purposes of tailoring treatments.

During the past 25 years, multi-variate typologies have been investigated with the use of more complex data extraction methods (e.g., cluster and factor analysis). Cloninger's Type I or Type II and Babor's Type A or B were the first of these. Cloninger and colleagues[73] identified two separate forms of alcoholism based on differences in alcohol-related symptoms, patterns of transmission, and personality characteristics using data derived from a cross-fostering study of Swedish adoptees. Type I was characterized by either mild or severe alcohol use in the probands and no criminality in the fathers. These Type I alcoholics came from relatively high socioeconomic backgrounds and were frequently associated with maternal alcohol use. Type I alcoholics were thought to be more responsive to environmental influence, to have relatively mild alcohol-related problems, and to have a late age of onset (older than 25 years). On the other hand, Cloninger's Type II alcoholism is characterized as being associated with a family history, having severe alcohol problems, having other drug use, and having an early onset (before age 25). Although multi-variate statistical methods were used to identify subtypes, Cloninger's types of alcoholism have been criticized due to the small sample sizes (less than 200), sample selection methods, and indirect assessment of family variables.[74]

A second typology was proposed by Babor and colleagues[75] based on a sample of 321 alcoholic inpatients. Babor's Type A resembled Cloninger's Type 1, and was characterized by a later age of onset, fewer childhood behavior problems, and less psychopathology. Type B resembled Type II alcoholism and was defined by a high prevalence of childhood behavior problems, familial alcoholism, early onset of alcohol problems, more psychopathology, more life stress, and a more chronic treatment history.

A broad distinction of early-onset versus late-onset alcohol dependence may have some clinical matching utility, although evidence is limited. For example, use of selective serotonin reuptake inhibitors (SSRIs) has produced modest drinking reductions that may be more apparent in men with depression and late-onset type alcoholism.[76,77] Also, double-blind placebo-controlled studies of anti-craving medications (e.g., ondansetron) have shown efficacy for early-onset alcoholics, as have others (e.g., topiramate) for a broad range of unselected alcoholic patients.

Later studies examining typologies have found more than two subtypes that have clinical and etiological significance, particularly regarding gender, and internalizing/externalizing disorders, in addition to family history and age of onset. For example, several multi-variate, multi-dimensional analyses have revealed that there may be as many as four general, homogeneous subtypes of alcohol dependence[78,79]: chronic/severe, depressed/anxious, mildly affected, and antisocial.[80] These four subtypes of alcohol dependence are found within both genders and across different ethnic subgroups, but more prospective research is needed to examine their relative clinical course and responsiveness to various pharmacological and psychosocial interventions. These approaches to AUD typologies have employed either empirical or clinical/observational strategies using data derived principally from treatment samples. However, only about one-fourth of those who meet criteria for alcohol addiction actually receive treatment.[81] Thus, the majority of individuals suffering from alcohol addiction are missed, biasing our knowledge to only those alcohol-dependent cases that seek treatment—a phenomenon known as "Berkson' bias." Consequently, using data from the National Epidemiological Survey on Alcohol and Related Conditions (NESARC), Moss, Chen, and Yi[82] discovered five subtypes of alcohol dependence, distinguished by family history, age of dependence onset, endorsement of DSM-IV AUD criteria, and the presence of co-morbid psychiatric and substance use disorders. These general population-derived subtypes await further study, but they may enhance our understanding of the etiology and natural history of AUD, and lead to improved and more targeted treatment interventions.

PATHOPHYSIOLOGY AND IMAGING

The deleterious effect of alcohol is diffuse. However, the impact on the brain is central to the development of AUDs and related conditions. Of the approximately 18 million individuals with an AUD in the US, approximately one-half to two-thirds develop some sort of impairment in cognitive and/or motor processes and up to 2 million people suffer enough alcohol-induced damage to require life-long care.[83] These conditions, such as alcohol-induced persisting amnestic disorder (i.e., Wernicke–Korsakoff syndrome) and dementia, seriously affect memory, reasoning, language, and problem-solving abilities.

Importantly, many individuals with a history of alcohol dependence and neuropsychological impairments show some improvement in function within a year of abstinence, but others take considerably longer.[84–87] Unfortunately, little is known about the rate and extent to which people recover specific structures and functions once abstinence has been achieved, but the rate of recovery will likely co-vary with the topography and chronicity of alcohol use, dietary factors, and individual variables related to family history and biological vulnerability. The cerebral cortex (dorsolateral and orbitofrontal cortex),[88] and subcortical areas, such as the limbic system (e.g., amygdala), the thalamus (involved with communications within the brain), the hypothalamus (involved with hormones that affect sexual function and behavior, as well as reproduction), and the basal forebrain (involved with learning and memory) are the key brain regions susceptible to alcohol-related damage.[89] Areas that influence posture and movement, such as the cerebellum, also seem to be affected.[86] MRI and diffusion tensor imaging (DTI) can be used in combination to assess a patient's brain when he or she first stops drinking and again after long periods of sobriety, to monitor brain changes and to detect correlates of relapse.

MRI and DTI studies reveal a loss of brain tissue, and neuropsychological tests show cognitive impairments in individuals who either have an AUD or are heavy drinkers.[90] Abnormalities on scans have been reported in 50% or more of individuals with chronic alcohol dependence. These abnormalities can occur in individuals in whom there is neither clinical nor neuropsychological test evidence of cognitive defects. In individuals with binge drinking and chronic alcohol dependence, MRI has demonstrated accelerated gray matter loss,[91] which is to some extent reversible with abstinence, suggesting that some of these changes are secondary to changes in brain tissue hydration.[92]

The frontal areas of the brain are particularly susceptible to alcohol-related damage despite the fact that alcohol has diffuse bilateral cortical effects.[86,89,93] The prefrontal cortex has been shown to be important in cognitive and emotional function and interpersonal behavior. Because the prefrontal cortex is necessary for planning and for regulation of behavior, good judgment, and problem-solving, damage in these brain regions may relate to impulsivity and susceptibility to alcohol relapse and may be particularly negatively affected by alcohol.[94-96]

Positron emission tomography (PET) has been used to analyze alcohol's effects on various neurotransmitter systems, as well as on brain cell metabolism and blood flow within the brain. These studies in alcoholics have detected deficits, particularly in the frontal lobes (which are responsible for numerous functions associated with learning and memory), as well as in the cerebellum (which controls movement and coordination).[97-99]

Effects on Neurotransmitters

The typical subjective effects from alcohol include euphoria, disinhibition, anxiety reduction, sedation, and sleep. These effects are mediated by a variety of neurotransmitters including GABA, glutamate, serotonin, endorphins, and dopamine. Alcohol effects neurotransmitter systems by causing either neuronal excitation or inhibition.[100] If alcohol is consumed over extended periods (e.g., several days or weeks), receptors adapt to its presence, producing neurotransmitter imbalances that can result in sedation, agitation, depression, and other mood and behavior disorders, as well as seizures.

The results of neuropsychological testing reveal that short-term memory, performance on complex memory tasks, visual-motor coordination, visual-spatial performance, abstract reasoning, and psychomotor dexterity are the areas most seriously damaged. Intelligence scores often do not change, and verbal skills and long-term memory often remain intact. As a consequence, it is possible for individuals to appear cognitively intact unless they are administered neuropsychological tests.

Glutamate is the major excitatory neurotransmitter in the brain and it is significantly effected by alcohol. Alcohol influences the action of glutamate, and research has shown that chronic, heavy alcohol consumption increases glutamate receptor sites in the hippocampus that can effect the consolidation of memory and may account for "blackout" phenomena. Contrary to popular belief, blackouts are much more common among social drinkers than previously assumed. In a large sample of college student drinkers, more than half (51%) reported blacking out at some point in their lives, and 40% reported experiencing a blackout in the prior year.[101] Hence, blackouts should be viewed as a potential consequence of acute intoxication and not specific to alcohol dependence.

Glutamate receptors adapt to the presence of alcohol and thus become overactive during alcohol withdrawal; this process can lead to stroke and seizure.[102] Deficiencies of thiamine caused by malnutrition, common among individuals with alcohol dependence, may exacerbate this potentially destructive overactivity.[103]

GABA is also affected by alcohol use. It is the major inhibitory neurotransmitter in the brain, and alcohol appears to increase GABA's effects (i.e., increases inhibition and sedation). However, chronic, intense alcohol use leads to a gradual reduction of GABA receptors. Thus, when an individual suddenly ceases alcohol use, the decrease in inhibitory effects in combination with fewer GABA receptors and increased glutamatergic discharge contributes to over-excitation and possible withdrawal seizures. It is likely that both GABA and glutamate systems interact in this process.[104] The effects of chronic alcohol use are influenced by adaptations in $GABA_A$ receptor function and expression, and subcellular localization that contribute to tolerance, dependence, and withdrawal hyperexcitability (Figure 26-13).[105] Patients with alcohol dependence should be assessed and monitored for signs of alcohol withdrawal and signs of other associated problems.

Alcohol also directly stimulates release of other neurotransmitters, such as serotonin,[106,107] as well as endorphins[108] and dopamine (DA),[109] which contribute to the subjective euphoria and rewarding effects associated with alcohol.[100] Research findings regarding acetylcholine and other neurotransmitters are mixed and effects are currently not as well understood.

Intense, chronic use of alcohol has wide-ranging deleterious effects on the brain. These can lead to lasting, sometimes life-long, impairments in function that result in prodigious familial, social, and fiscal costs. Consequently, education, prevention, and early detection and intervention are keys to minimizing the impact on individuals and their loved ones.

SCREENING AND ASSESSMENT

Given the regrettable impact that a failure to detect and intervene with alcohol problems can have, routine screening for alcohol misuse should be standard in all clinical settings. There are brief and effective screening measures that can yield

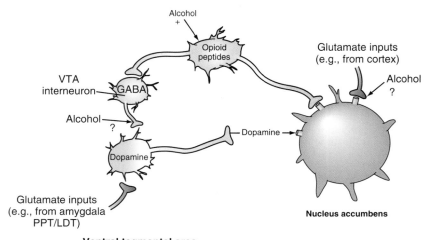

Figure 26-13. Alcohol's effect on neurotransmitter systems. VTA, ventral tegmental area; PPT, pedunculopontine tegmental nucleus; LDT, laterodorsal tegmental nucleus *(From Gilpin NW, Koob GF. Neurobiology of alcohol dependence: focus on motivational mechanisms. National Institute on Alcohol Abuse and Alcoholism (NIAAA).)*

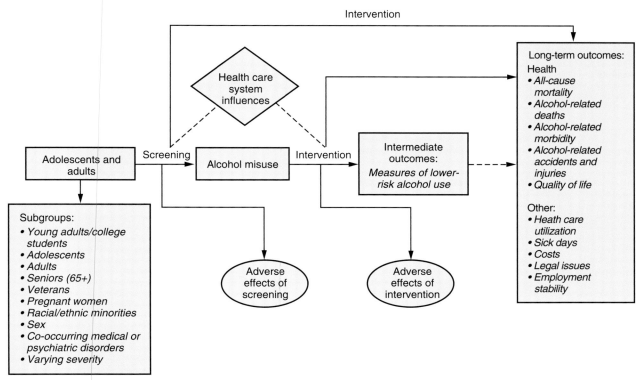

Figure 26-14. Screening and assessment process. *(From Jonas DE, Garbutt JC, Brown JM, et al. Screening, behavioral counseling, and referral in primary care to reduce alcohol use. Rockville, 2012, Agency for Health Research and Quality.)*

high rates of detection of these pervasive and debilitating disorders. Controlled studies reveal that even a brief, detailed discussion by a clinician can yield measurable reductions in the consequences from alcohol misuse (Figure 26-14).[110,111]

The National Institute on Alcohol Abuse and Alcoholism (NIAAA) has recommended either the use of a single alcohol screening question (SASQ) or administration of the Alcohol Use Disorders Identification Test (AUDIT) self-report questionnaire as standard screening procedures for the detection of alcohol-related problems. The AUDIT (Table 26-1) and manual are available for free, in English and in Spanish; the AUDIT has been validated across a variety of cultural and ethnic groups. When using the SASQ clinicians are advised to ask if an individual has consumed five or more standard drinks (for a man) on one occasion during the last year (four drinks for women). A positive response may indicate an alcohol-related problem and requires more detailed assessment.[63] A more traditional alternative screening interview is captured by the CAGE acronym,[112] although this has less sensitivity to detect harmful and hazardous patterns of alcohol use, and has not been validated in adolescents, the elderly, and women. When even more brevity is required due to time constraints, such as in busy clinical settings, a shorter 3-item version of the AUDIT called the AUDIT-C, includes only the first three AUDIT items (i.e., the three "Consumption" items; hence the "C"). This shorter version has been shown to possess about as much sensitivity and specificity as the full 10-item AUDIT[113] and can be used efficiently in primary care settings with a cut-off score of 4 or more for a man and 3 or more for a woman.[114] In psychiatric settings, a cut-off score 4 or more is recommended.

Compared to the SASQ or the AUDIT and AUDIT-C, the CAGE lacks sensitivity to detect hazardous/problem drinking. Similar to the CAGE interview, the TWEAK interview (i.e., "Tolerance," others "Worried" about your drinking, "Eye-opener,"

"Amnesia," ever wanted to/tried to "Cut down"), is brief and has good psychometric properties, but similar to the CAGE is a "life-time" measure and lacks sensitivity to detect hazardous drinking. The Michigan Alcoholism Screening Test (MAST) is another self-report measure with good psychometric properties, but is longer than the AUDIT.

For adolescents the CRAFFT screen is recommended, which is the acronym for having ever ridden in a CAR driven by someone (including yourself) who was "high" or had been using alcohol or drugs; ever used alcohol or drugs to RELAX, feel better about yourself, or fit in; ever use alcohol or drugs while ALONE; ever FORGOT things while using alcohol or drugs; FAMILY or FRIENDS ever recommend cutting down on drinking or drug use; ever gotten into TROUBLE while using alcohol or drugs. These questions have excellent sensitivity and specificity.[115] One point is given for each positively endorsed item and a score of 2 or more is indicative of a potential AUD that requires further assessment. Figure 26-15 shows the probability of an AUD based on derived screening score.

Medical biomarker screens may also be useful. Screening for recent alcohol use can be a carried out with a Breathalyzer or a sample of urine or saliva. For more chronic use, laboratory markers, such as the serum γ-glutamyl transpeptidase (GGT), the mean corpuscular volume (MCV),[20] and the percent carbohydrate-deficient transferrin (% CDT) can be used. CDT is the newest alcohol biomarker approved by the Food and Drug Administration (FDA) in 2001.[116] It is the only laboratory test approved specifically for the detection of heavy drinking.[117] An average daily consumption of 60 g of alcohol or more (i.e., approximately 5 standard drinks in the US) for at least the previous 2 weeks causes a higher percentage of transferrin. CDT, quantified as a percent of total serum transferring, rather than the absolute level of CDT, is recommended as it corrects for individual variations in transferrin levels. Laboratory test results of more than 2.5% suggest heavy

TABLE 26-1 The AUDIT/AUDIT-C (IN BOX) for Alcohol Screening[113,114]

PATIENT: Because alcohol use can affect your health and can interfere with certain medications and treatments, it is important that we ask some questions about your use of alcohol. Your answers will remain confidential so please be honest. Place an X in one box that best describes your answer to each question.

Questions	0	1	2	3	4	Score
How often do you have a drink containing alcohol?	Never	Monthly or less	2 to 4 times a month	2 to 3 times a week	4 or more times a week	
How many drinks containing alcohol do you have on a typical day when you are drinking?	1 or 2	3 or 4	5 or 6	7 to 9	10 or more	
How often do you have five or more drinks on one occasion?	Never	Less than monthly	Monthly	Weekly	Daily or almost daily	
How often during the last year have you found that you were not able to stop drinking once you had started?	Never	Less than monthly	Monthly	Weekly	Daily or almost daily	
How often during the last year have you failed to do what was normally expected of you because of drinking?	Never	Less than monthly	Monthly	Weekly	Daily or almost daily	
How often during the last year have you needed a first drink in the morning to get yourself going after a heavy drinking session?	Never	Less than monthly	Monthly	Weekly	Daily or almost daily	
How often during the last year have you had a feeling of guilt or remorse after drinking?	Never	Less than monthly	Monthly	Weekly	Daily or almost daily	
How often during the last year have you been unable to remember what happened the night before because of your drinking?	Never	Less than monthly	Monthly	Weekly	Daily or almost daily	
Have you or someone else been injured because of your drinking?	No		Yes, but not in the last year		Yes, during the last year	
Has a relative, friend, doctor, or other health care worker been concerned about your drinking or suggested you cut down?	No		Yes, but not in the last year		Yes, during the last year	
Total:						

NOTE: This self-report questionnaire (the Alcohol Use Disorders Identification Test [AUDIT]) is from the World Health Organization. To reflect standard drink sizes in the United States, the number of drinks in question 3 was changed from 6 to 5. A free AUDIT manual with guidelines for use in primary care is available online at http://www.who.org.

Information from Reinert DF, Allen JP. The alcohol use disorders identification test: an update of research findings. Alcohol Clin Exp Res 31(2):185–199, 2007, and Bradley KA, DeBenedetti AF, Volk RJ, Williams EC, Frank D, Kivlahan DR. AUDIT-C as a brief screen for alcohol misuse in primary care. Alcohol Clin Exp Res 31(7):1208–1217, 2007.

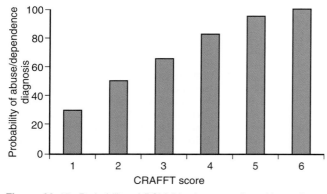

Figure 26-15. Probability of DSM-IV substance abuse/dependence diagnosis based on CRAFFT adolescent screening score. (From Center for Adolescent Substance Abuse Research. The CRAFFT Screening Interview. Boston, 2009, Children's Hospital Boston.)

drinking. Regarding specificity, other than heavy alcohol use, only end-stage liver disease, biliary cirrhosis, and a rare genetic variability will elevate CDT. Ethyl glucuronide (EtG) is a newer biomarker and is a direct metabolite of alcohol. It has been evaluated as a biomarker test for alcohol use and to monitor abstinence (e.g., among health care professionals, attorneys, airline pilots in recovery from addiction). EtG can be detected in urine up to 7 days and in hair for months after alcohol has left the body.[118] A disadvantage of EtG is that it can yield false positives from incidental exposure, from things such as mouthwash, foods, and over-the-counter medications.

Many of these biomarker measures lack sensitivity, but can be helpful if used in combination (e.g., CDT and GGT) and especially when used with other screening measures, such as the AUDIT. Screening for alcohol problems has been shown to be very cost-effective.[119]

Screening for alcohol withdrawal is also critical since, as mentioned previously, alcohol withdrawal can be life-threatening. The Clinical Institute Withdrawal Assessment for Alcohol Revised (CIWA-Ar)[21] is a semi-structured, 5-minute interview used to assess and quantify severity of withdrawal from alcohol. It is easy to administer and possesses very good psychometric properties. It is thus an efficient and reliable method that can prevent serious or life-threatening problems and is useful to help clinicians determine levels of care.[21] Recent evidence suggests, however, that this scale may underestimate symptoms of alcohol withdrawal in certain ethnic groups, such as Native Americans.[120]

There are several measures that can be employed to assess the presence of an AUD and the degree of dependence and impairment. The choice of each may depend on the time demands and specialization of the clinical setting. For clinical diagnostic purposes, the Structured Clinical Interview for Diagnosis (SCID), Substance Use Disorders module, can be used. This is a valid and reliable, semi-structured, assessment tool that will give life-time and current diagnoses for AUD and can be completed in approximately 20 minutes.[121] Also, as detailed more below in the section on Brief Interventions, the Alcohol Use Disorders Identification Test (AUDIT)[122] can be used as a screening tool and to help determine treatment recommendations.

The Addiction Severity Index (ASI) is a semi-structured interview that assesses multiple domains of function (e.g., legal, work, and psychiatric, as well as alcohol and drug use) and is widely used in clinical and research settings. It has adequate psychometrics and can be completed in approximately 30 to 40 minutes. The Alcohol Dependence Scale (ADS) is a self-report measure that focuses on the core dependence syndrome. It contains 25 items and takes approximately 5 minutes to complete. It assesses past-year symptoms, with a score of 9 or more indicative of alcohol dependence. The Leeds Dependence Questionnaire (LDQ)[123,124] is a brief 10-item self-report measure that measures severity of addiction across multiple substances, including alcohol. The Drinker Inventory of Consequences (DRINC) is a 50-item, multi-dimensional self-report that takes about 5 minutes to complete. It is a validated measure of drinking consequences with good psychometric properties. There are a variety of other assessment tools available that assess drinking topography, chronicity, and impact.[125,126] Many of these measures have clinical utility as they can elucidate the drinking topography, chronicity, addiction severity, and degree of impairment that can inform the type and level of treatment intensity.[127] Also, these may become increasingly important as health systems move to performance-based payments.[128]

TREATMENT FOR ALCOHOL USE DISORDERS

As with most difficulties that individuals encounter during their lives, individuals suffering from AUDs first try to resolve their problems without help. They may mobilize their own skills and, through a process of trial and error, learn ways to minimize or resolve these problems. Successful resolution of an alcohol problem without formal intervention is often called "natural recovery".[129] Others use informal resources, such as a member of the clergy, a friend, or a family member, or access Alcoholics Anonymous (AA) or another mutual-help group. When these resources are realized to be insufficient to cope with the magnitude of the problem, individuals often seek formal treatment, although informal resources (e.g., AA) may continue to be used as effective adjuncts.[130,131]

Given the variability in the demographic and drinking patterns of patients, and the addiction severity and impact that alcohol use has had in their lives, a number of treatment options should be available to help patients.[2] The National Institute of Alcohol Abuse and Alcoholism (NIAAA) was founded in 1970. This began a federally supported public health initiative that increased research efforts to develop, test, and implement effective interventions for risky alcohol use, as well as for abuse and dependence. Numerous reviews of the treatment literature[132-135] indicate that a wide array of empirically-based, effective treatments can be brought to bear on these problems. These range from brief interventions to more intensive and extensive individual and group-based psychosocial interventions and, increasingly, pharmacological interventions.[134]

Brief Intervention

A concerned and focused assessment with brief advice by a health care provider can make a positive difference to drinking problems. Brief interventions are generally recommended for those who drink to excess, but are generally not showing signs of addiction. Thus, its goal may be moderate drinking rather than abstinence.[135-137] Brief interventions are generally restricted to four or fewer sessions, lasting from a few minutes to 1 hour each, designed to be conducted by clinicians, not necessarily specialized in addiction.[138]

Research indicates that brief interventions for alcohol problems are more effective than no intervention[139-142] and, in some cases, can be as effective as more extensive intervention.[135,143] Capitalizing on these findings, and in order to expand access to treatment for alcohol-related problems, the Center for Substance Abuse Treatment (CSAT) has devised an initiative known as "Screening, Brief Intervention, Referral, and Treatment" (SBIRT). The goal of the initiative is intended to shift the emphasis to alcohol users whom the traditional system has largely ignored—the large number of individuals who consume more than the medically-accepted limits but are not yet dependent. Rejecting the notion that only people with very heavy alcohol use levels or who are alcohol dependent need targeted interventions, SBIRT assumes that everyone, regardless of current level of alcohol consumption, can benefit from learning the facts about safe alcohol consumption and knowing how their own usage compares to accepted limits. Using the AUDIT/AUDIT-C as a screening device, front-line clinicians in any setting can assess for alcohol-related problems quickly and easily. SBIRT triage guidelines provide recommendations along the lines of an individual's alcohol involvement. Simple clinical advice to cut down or stop is recommended if someone scores between 7 and 16 on the AUDIT; multiple sessions of brief treatment and monitoring are recommended if an individual scores between 16 and 19 (or has consumed alcohol to intoxication five or more days per month, as disclosed on screening interview); and if an individual has an AUDIT score of 20 or more a referral for more intensive assessment and treatment is recommended.[144]

What is it about brief interventions that make them effective? After reviewing the key ingredients in a variety of brief intervention protocols, Miller and Sanchez[145] proposed six critical elements that they summarized with the acronym FRAMES: Feedback, Responsibility, Advice, Menu, Empathy, and Self-efficacy. The clinician completes some assessment and provides Feedback on the patient's alcohol-related problems ("Your results show. ..."), stresses the patient's Responsibility to address the problem ("It's your choice. ..."), gives clear Advice to change drinking behavior ("I would recommend that you cut down or stop. ..."), provides a Menu of treatment strategies ("There a number of different things you might do. ..."), expresses Empathy for the patient's problem ("This can be difficult to hear and making changes is not always easy, but. ..."), and stresses Self-efficacy ("However, it is quite possible for you to achieve this. ...")—the expectation is that the patient has the skills needed to successfully resolve his or her drinking problems. Additional components of goal-setting, follow-up, and timing also have been identified as important to the effectiveness of brief interventions.[136,146] Even brief contact with an addiction specialist has been shown to yield improvement in 30% to 50% of patients. However, brief interventions are more effective with those who have no prior psychiatric illness or history of addiction treatment and good social function and resources.[147] Although non-specialist clinicians, such as primary care providers, can have an impact on heavy or at-risk drinking through appropriate brief intervention, patients with alcohol dependence tend to experience better outcomes when seen by addiction specialists (e.g., counselors, social workers, and addiction-trained nurses, or physicians with specialized addiction training) than general practitioners,[148,149] perhaps due to their more specific education and training on addiction. For example, compared with general consultation psychiatrists, specialist addiction nurse consultants were found to double the rate of patient follow-through and completion in rehabilitation.[150]

Intensive-Extensive Interventions

Three broad elements are important in recovery from AUDs: deconditioning, skills training, and cognitive re-structuring.[151] There is a broad array of evidence-based interventions for AUDs that address these critical elements.[132,133,152] Some of these include Twelve-Step Facilitation (TSF), a professional therapy designed to engage patients and support long-term involvement in the fellowship of AA; motivational enhancement therapy (MET), an intervention based on the principles of motivational interviewing[146,153]; a variety of cognitive-behavioral approaches, such as the Community Reinforcement Approach (CRA), designed to engage multiple therapeutic elements in the community; interpersonal system-based interventions, such as behavioral marital therapy (BMT) and family therapies; and pharmacotherapies (e.g., naltrexone/depot natrexone, acamprosate, or disulfiram).

Although most interventions are directly focused on the primary sufferer (the individual with the AUD), it is clear that loved ones also suffer greatly as a result of the AUD. Community Reinforcement and Family Training (CRAFT) is a validated approach based on the concept that a supportive environment "community" will help the alcohol-dependent person achieve recovery. CRAFT targets individuals who refuse to participate in treatment through their loved ones. It provides specific, contingency-based strategies that support family members and friends in their efforts to help their loved one become engaged in treatment. It has been shown also to substantially reduce psychological distress and symptoms among the family members themselves.[154]

Despite vastly differing theoretical assumptions regarding the specifics of treatment content, and for how long, at what intensity, and by whom the treatment should be delivered, comparisons of the relative efficacy of active treatments reveal surprisingly similar effects, suggesting that they may all mobilize common change processes.[155] However, it seems clear that it is the *duration and continuity* of care that is linked to treatment outcome rather than amount or intensity.[46,155-157] Consequently, there have been recent shifts from intensive inpatient services to "extensive" outpatient models of addiction recovery management and ongoing assessment and re-intervention that match the chronic relapse-prone nature of addictive disorders (e.g., telephone case monitoring and long-term outpatient treatment).[158-160]

In recent years, there has tended to be an almost exclusive focus on high-fidelity delivery of manualized treatment content rather than a focus on the characteristics of the clinician who delivers the content and how it is delivered. The issue of therapeutic alliance and successfully gaining the patient's trust is often fundamental to the success of treatment, yet is seldom specifically addressed. A respectful, empathic, patient-centered approach appears to be most helpful, and a harsh, confrontational approach may increase the patient's resistance.[132] The principles and practices of motivational

TABLE 26-2 Motivational Interviewing Processes

Engaging	Establishing a helpful connection and working relationship
Focusing	Developing and maintaining specific direction in the conversation about change
Evoking	Eliciting the patients' own motives about change
Planning	Developing commitment to change and forming a specific action plan to change

From Miller WR, Rollnick S. Motivational interviewing: helping people change, ed 3. New York, 2012, Guilford Press.

interviewing[153] are a particularly useful framework in this regard and have strong empirical support for use among individuals with AUDs (Table 26-2). The main principles here are to avoid arguing with a patient, to "roll with resistance" (e.g., try to understand the patients' frame of reference), to develop discrepancies between the patient's values and his or her behavior, to support the patient's self-efficacy/confidence to achieve the desired outcome, and to be empathic. There are four main processes of MI: engaging (establishing a helpful connection and working relationship), focusing (developing and maintaining specific direction in the conversation about change), evoking (eliciting the patients' own motives about change), and planning (developing commitment to change and forming a specific action plan to change).[146]

Emanating from the brief intervention literature and humanistic psychology, motivational interviewing has been shown to be an important and effective way to interact with patients with a range of alcohol problems, including dependence. It has been defined as a patient-centered, yet directive, method for enhancing intrinsic motivation to change by exploring and resolving patient ambivalence.[153] This approach has been shown to be helpful for many patients.[161-163] It can be used as a stand-alone intervention but can also be an effective way to communicate with patients while providing other interventions.

Studies of treatment outcome show that patients treated for addiction have similar rates of improvement as patients treated for other chronic medical diseases.[164] For example, between 40% and 60% of patients treated for addiction to alcohol remain abstinent after a year and another 15% maintain clinically meaningful improvement in their alcohol use problems. Similarly, during the course of a year, 60% of patients with high blood pressure or asthma and 70% of diabetics maintain improvements in their symptoms.[39,165] While full remission and recovery can take many years to achieve following initial attempts to stop,[166] full sustained remission is the most likely ultimate outcome.[167] Consequently, AUD can be considered a good prognosis disorder with adequate extensive monitoring, management, and re-intervention when necessary.[46]

Engaging and retaining individuals in treatment for at least 90 days is associated with better long-term treatment outcomes.[168] Individual or group counseling and other behavioral therapies are critical components of effective treatment for alcohol addiction. Behavioral therapy also facilitates interpersonal relationships and the individual's ability to function in the family and community contexts. In therapy, issues of motivation can be addressed, and assertiveness, goal-setting skills, and problem-solving strategies can be learned along with new ways to replace alcohol-related activities with other constructive and rewarding activities.

Pharmacological Interventions

Three medications have been approved by the FDA for the treatment of alcohol dependence: disulfiram (approved in 1947), intended to prevent any drinking through the

TABLE 26-3 Pharmacological Treatments for Alcoholism

Drug (Trade Name)	Pharmacokinetics/Pharmacodynamics	Effects
Disulfiram (Antabuse)	Inhibits acetaldehyde dehydrogenase, leading to a build-up of acetaldehyde	Produces undesirable consequences when alcohol is consumed, including flushing, palpitations, nausea, vomiting, and headache
Naltrexone (ReVia, Long acting = Vivitrol)	μ-opioid receptor antagonist	Reduces the reinforcement/euphoria produced by alcohol
Acamprosate	Antagonist at glutamatergic N-methyl-D-aspartate (NMDA) receptors and agonist at gamma-aminobutyric acid (GABA) type A receptors	Reduces alcohol cravings

anticipated threat of the very unpleasant reaction caused by the alcohol–disulfiram interaction; naltrexone (approved as an oral formulation in 1994 with the long-acting injectable formulation approved in 2006), intended to reduce the reinforcing effect of alcohol and to reduce the severity of relapse and the extent of heavy drinking; and acamprosate (approved in 2004), intended to reduce the probability of any drinking by reducing symptoms associated with postacute withdrawal/craving following initial detoxification (Table 26-3).

Disulfiram inhibits acetaldehyde dehydrogenase, leading to a build-up of the ethanol metabolite acetaldehyde. It has been shown to reduce drinking days in alcohol-dependent persons by approximately 50%.[169] If a patient drinks alcohol after taking disulfiram, the build-up of acetaldehyde produces flushing, hypotension, headache, nausea, and vomiting (Table 26-3). Treatment of severe disulfiram–ethanol reactions may require a modified Trendelenburg position, an anticholinergic agent for bradycardia, and ascorbic acid 1 mg IV every 1 to 2 hours. The effectiveness of disulfiram is compromised by poor compliance. However, if a spouse or significant other is willing to participate and to observe and monitor the compliance with the medication, effectiveness increases substantially. A written contract in this regard between spouse and partner, which is often done in behavioral marital therapy (BMT), enhances compliance and outcomes.[170-172]

The opiate antagonist naltrexone which has no specific adverse reaction with alcohol has produced reductions in drinking-days presumably through diminished reward from alcohol secondary to actions on central brain reward pathways.[173,174] The recent FDA-approval for a long-acting IM formulation of naltrexone in April 2006 significantly expands pharmacotherapy options. Best results have been reported in patients able to sustain a week of abstinence before their first injection. Naltrexone also appears to be most effective in patients with a strong family history of alcoholism. Because both naltrexone and disulfiram have a slight risk for hepatotoxicity, liver function studies are recommended at baseline and then at 1, 3, and every 6 months thereafter. Also, pharmacogenetic research suggests that individuals with the OPRM1 genotype may respond particularly well to naltrexone.[175]

Acamprosate is another drug that has been approved for relapse-prevention among individuals suffering from alcohol addiction. It is thought to act primarily at glutamate-NMDA receptors by moderating symptoms related to prolonged alcohol withdrawal (i.e., post-acute withdrawal), and is thus most effective in patients who have recently completed detoxification. It is preferred for patients with liver damage since acamprosate is metabolized through the kidneys and not the liver. Meta-analyses suggest that, in keeping with the purported mechanisms of action of naltrexone and acamprosate, naltrexone has stronger effects on reducing heavy drinking (presumably through diminishing alcohol's mu opioid receptor-mediated rewarding effects), while acamprosate is better at increasing complete abstinence (presumably through attenuating rebound glutamate-NMDA mediated excitation).

SSRIs have produced only modest drinking reductions—independent of antidepressant effects—through an anti-craving effect. This effect may be more apparent in men with depression and late-onset alcoholism.[76,77] The SSRIs do not appear to have any relapse-prevention effect in women. Recent double-blind placebo-controlled studies have shown efficacy for ondansetron in early-onset alcoholics and topiramate has shown promise as an effective pharmacotherapy for alcohol dependence in a broad range of alcohol-dependent individuals.[176,177] All of these agents are gaining renewed interest as adjuncts to a comprehensive psychosocial recovery program and should be considered in the treatment of all individuals with AUD.

Substance-induced psychiatric symptoms are common before admission for detoxification and may persist for 2–4 weeks after detoxification.[70,71] If symptoms continue for longer than 4 weeks, it suggests the existence of an independent co-occurring psychiatric disorder. In these situations, a specific psychiatric treatment plan is required to address the co-occurring disorder. Studies support initiation of an SSRI for co-occurring major depression, mood stabilizers for bipolar illness, buspirone for generalized anxiety, and second-generation antipsychotics for a psychotic illness.[178] The best outcomes are seen when treatment for any co-occurring psychiatric disorder is integrated into the addiction recovery program.[69,179]

Alcoholics Anonymous and Long-term Support

As with other chronic illnesses, relapses to alcohol use can occur during or after successful treatment episodes. Hence, addicted individuals often require prolonged treatment and multiple episodes of care to achieve long-term abstinence and fully restored function. Participation in mutual-help organizations, such as AA, during and following treatment is often also helpful and cost-effective in helping patients achieve and maintain recovery.[180-186] Other organizations such as SMART Recovery, Secular Organization for Sobriety, and Women for Sobriety are also likely to be helpful to many patients, but are less available and little is known about their effectiveness.[181,184,185,187] A recent randomized comparative trial, however, found benefit for problem-drinkers who were randomized to receive either an on-line cognitive-behavioral intervention featuring the elements of SMART Recovery, attendance at SMART Recovery meetings, or both, and found that all groups improved significantly across the 3-month follow-up.[188]

AA possesses several elements that make it attractive as an ongoing adjunct to formal AUD treatment. It is accessible and flexible, with meetings held several times a day in many communities, and patients can self-select meetings that seem like a good fit. AA members also often make themselves available "on demand" (e.g., by telephone), providing a degree of flexibility not available in professional settings. This degree of availability means that AA is self-adaptive: patients can access these resources at times of high relapse risk (e.g., unstructured

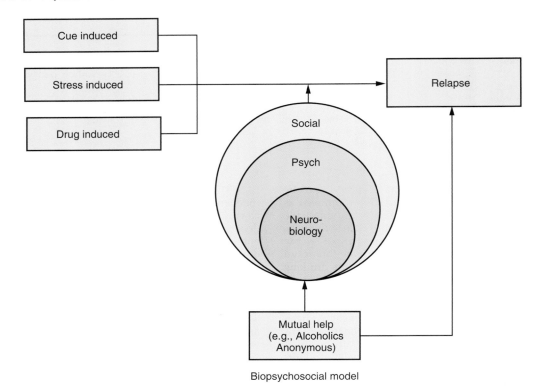

Biopsychosocial model

Figure 26-16. Biopsychosocial model of how mutual help organizations, such as Alcoholics Anonymous may attenuate relapse risk over time. *(From Kelly JF, Yeterian JD. Mutual-help groups for alcohol and other substance use disorders. In McCrady BS, Epstein EE, editors:* Addictions: a comprehensive guidebook. *ed 2. New York, 2013, Oxford University Press.)*[131]

time; evenings/weekends) or whenever they feel they need it. Furthermore, it provides recovery-specific experience and support, with members serving as role models. AA meeting formats also provide continuing reminders of past negative experiences and the positive benefits of staying sober that help maintain and enhance recovery momentum.[189] AA also possesses a low threshold for entry, with no paperwork or third-party insurance approval, and AA can be attended free of charge for as long as individuals desire, making it a highly cost-effective public health resource.[185] Studies with adults[182,183] and adolescents[190] reveal that participation in AA can enhance recovery outcomes and remission rates while simultaneously and substantially reducing health care costs.

In theory, the influence of common precursors to alcohol relapse (i.e., stress-related, cue-related, and drug-related) may be attenuated by participation in groups like AA through AA's ability to mobilize salutary changes in individuals' social networks as well in several psychological domains. Figure 26-16 illustrates the relationship between common high-risk precursors to relapse and how mutual-help organizations (MHOs), like AA might attenuate this risk through facilitating changes in social networks, psychological factors (e.g., enhancing coping, abstinence self-efficacy, motivation for abstinence), and bio/neurobiological factors.[131,191]

Empirically, there has now been rigorous scientific studies conducted on how exactly MHOs, like AA, confer recovery benefits. These studies suggest that the main ways that AA aids remission and recovery is through facilitating changes in the social networks of attendees and by boosting abstinence self-efficacy, coping, and by maintaining abstinence motivation.[192,193] Evidence suggests too that these broad benefits may depend on severity of dependence[191] and also gender,[194] whereby for more severely addicted individuals, in addition to facilitating important social network changes, AA may also

aid recovery by reducing negative affect and increasing spiritual practices.

AA and similar approaches that examine broader character, lifestyle, and spiritual issues are popular in the US and in many other countries.[195] In the US, AA is the most commonly sought-after source of help for an alcohol problem,[196] with 1.3 million members, and 60,000 meetings held weekly,[197] and it has been shown empirically to be helpful in achieving and maintaining abstinence for many different types of patients (including men and women, those with religious/spiritual and non-religious/non-spiritual backgrounds, and those who are dually diagnosed).[185,198-202]

When encouraging AA participation and making AA referrals, greatest success is achieved if clinicians use empirically-supported methods. For example, Twelve-Step Facilitation (TSF)[203] is an empirically-supported therapy for helping patients become actively involved in AA, and manuals can be obtained free of charge through the NIAAA website (www.niaaa.nih.gov). TSF approaches involve educating patients about the content, format, and structure of mutual-help groups early during treatment, and then continuing to monitor patients' reactions and responses to meeting attendance.[189] Also, substantially more effective referrals to AA can be made if clinicians assist patients in making personal contact with existing members whenever possible to facilitate fellowship integration.[201,204-210] Interventions that incorporate or employ TSF have been shown to enhance patients' outcomes by approximately 10%–20% over and above outcomes achieved with standard CBT.[208]

CONCLUSIONS

Alcohol misuse and related disorders permeate virtually every aspect of psychiatry and medicine. Preventing early exposure to alcohol among youth, minimizing heavy use, and screening for the presence of alcohol-induced, and alcohol use, disorders can help prevent an array of acute and chronic debilitating morbidities and loss of life. An enhanced sensitivity for, and appreciation of, the magnitude and pervasiveness of alcohol's effects on mental and physical function should advance the use of routine assessment and appropriate intervention that can lead to similarly widespread individual, family, and societal benefits.

Access the complete reference list and multiple choice questions (MCQs) online at https://expertconsult.inkling.com

KEY REFERENCES

4. Babor TF, Caetano R, Casswell S, et al. *Alcohol: no ordinary commodity-research and public policy*, ed 2, Oxford, UK, 2010, Oxford University Press.

6. Bagnardi V, Rota M, Botteri E, et al. Light alcohol drinking and cancer: a meta-analysis. *Ann Oncol* 24(2):301–308, 2013.

8. U.S. Department of Health and Human Services and U.S. Department of Agriculture. *Dietary Guidelines for Americans*, 2005, Washington, DC, 2005, HHS and USDA.

11. World Health Organization. *Global status report on alcohol and health*, Geneva, Switzerland, 2011, World Health Organization.

12. Bouchery EE, Harwood HJ, Sacks JJ, et al. Economic costs of excessive alcohol consumption in the U.S. 2006. *Am J Prev Med* 41(5):516–524, 2011.

26. Rosenson J, Clements C, Simon B, et al. Phenobarbital for acute alcohol withdrawal: a prospective randomized double-blind placebo-controlled study. *J Emerg Med* 44(3):592–598, e592, 2013.

32. Isenberg-Grzeda E, Kutner HE, Nicolson SE. Wernicke–Korsakoff syndrome: under-recognized and under-treated. *Psychosomatics* 53(6):507–516, 2012.

45. Kelly JF, Westerhoff CM. Does it matter how we refer to individuals with substance-related conditions? A randomized study of two commonly used terms. *Int J Drug Policy* 21:202–207, 2010.

46. Kelly JF, White WL, eds. Addiction Recovery Management. In Rosenbaum JF, editor: *Current clinical psychiatry*, New York, 2011, Springer.

47. Schuckit MA. An overview of genetic influences in alcoholism. *J Subst Abuse Treat* 36(1):S5–S14, 2009.

57. Urbanoski KA, Kelly JF. Understanding genetic risk for substance use and addiction: a guide for non-geneticists. *Clin Psychol Rev* 32(1):60–70, 2012.

58. Schuckit MA. *Vulnerability factors for alcoholism*, Baltimore, 2002, Lippincott Williams & Wilkins.

63. National Institute on Alcohol Abuse and Alcoholism (NIAAA). *Helping patients who drink too much: a clinician's guide and related professional support services: National Institute on Alcohol and Alcoholism*, Washington, DC, 2005, USDHHS.

81. Dawson DA, Grant BF, Stinson FS, et al. Recovery from DSM-IV alcohol dependence: United States, 2001–2002. *Addiction* 100(3):281–292, 2005.

94. Everitt BJ, Robbins TW. Neural systems of reinforcement for drug addiction: from actions to habits to compulsion. *Nature Neurosci* 8(11):1481–1489, 2005.

110. Fleming MF. Brief interventions and the treatment of alcohol use disorders: current evidence. *Rec Dev Alcohol* 16:375–390, 2003.

130. Kelly JF, Yeterian JD. Empirical awakening: the new science on mutual help and implications for cost containment under health care reform. *Subst Abus* 33(2):85–91, 2012.

131. Kelly JF, Yeterian JD. Mutual-help groups for alcohol and other substance use disorders. In McCrady BS, Epstein EE, editors: *Addictions: A comprehensive guidebook*, ed 2, New York, 2013, Oxford University Press.

133. Moyer A, Finney JW, Swearingen CE, et al. Brief interventions for alcohol problems: a meta-analytic review of controlled investigations in treatment-seeking and non-treatment-seeking populations. *Addiction* 97(3):279–292, 2002.

134. Maisel NC, Blodgett JC, Wilbourne PL, et al. Meta-analysis of naltrexone and acamprosate for treating alcohol use disorders: when are these medications most helpful? *Addiction* 108(2):275–293, 2013.

138. Madras BK, Compton WM, Avula D, et al. Screening, brief interventions, referral to treatment (SBIRT) for illicit drug and alcohol use at multiple healthcare sites: comparison at intake and 6 months later. *Drug Alcohol Depend* 99(1–3):280–295, 2009.

157. White WL. *Recovery management and recovery-oriented systems of care: scientific rationale and promising practices*, 2008, Northeast Addiction Technology Transfer Center, Great Lakes Addiction Technology Transfer Center, Philadelphia Department of Behavioral Health/Mental Retardation Services.

158. Dennis ML, Scott CK. Four-year outcomes from the Early Re-Intervention (ERI) experiment using Recovery Management Checkups (RMCs). *Drug Alcohol Depend* 121(1–2):10–17, 2012.

164. McClellan A, Lewis D, O'Brien C, et al. Drug dependence, a chronic medical illness: implications for treatment, insurance, and outcomes evaluation. *JAMA* 284(13):1689–1695, 2000.

167. White WL. *Recovery/remission from substance use disorders: An analysis of reported outcomes in 415 scientific reports, 1868–2011*, 2012, Philadelphia Department of Behavioral Health and Intellectual disability Services, Great Lakes Addiction Technology Transfer Center.

181. Humphreys K. *Circles of recovery: self-help organizations for addictions*, Cambridge, UK, 2004, Cambridge University Press.

187. Kelly JF, White W. Broadening the base of addiction recovery mutual aid. *J Groups Addict Recover* 7(2–4):82–101, 2012.

192. Kelly JF, Magill M, Stout RL. How do people recover from alcohol dependence? A systematic review of the research on mechanisms of behavior change in Alcoholics Anonymous. *Addict Res Theory* 17(3):236–259, 2009.

194. Kelly JF, Hoeppner B. Does Alcoholics Anonymous work differently for men and women? A moderated multiple-mediation analysis in a large clinical sample. *Drug Alcohol Depend* 130(1–3):186–193, 2013.

27 Drug Addiction

John A. Renner, Jr., MD, and E. Nalan Ward, MD

KEY POINTS

Incidence

- Depending on the drug used and the clinical setting, up to 50% of patients in mental-health treatment will have a co-occurring substance-use disorder.

Epidemiology

- Substance abuse is a major public health problem that affects a large number of psychiatric patients.
- Screening for substance use and abuse should be a routine part of all mental-health evaluations.
- The problem is particularly severe in public sector treatment settings.

Prognosis

- Research has demonstrated that integrated treatment delivered in settings that are skilled in the management of both mental-health and substance-use disorders will significantly improve outcome.

Treatment Options

- Brief interventions, motivational-enhancement therapy, cognitive-behavioral therapy, and pharmacotherapy with methadone and buprenorphine are each efficacious for addictions.
- Psychiatrists need to become adept in the use of evidence-based treatment for substance-use disorders.
- The availability of effective psychotherapies and pharmacotherapies for addictive disorders makes it possible to successfully manage patients (in outpatient settings) who are addicted to opiates and cocaine.

Complications

- Unrecognized and untreated substance-use disorders are associated with poor outcomes and treatment failure for co-occurring mental health disorders.

OVERVIEW

The chronic, relapsing nature of substance abuse is inappropriately thought to imply that substance-abuse treatment is not helpful. This leads clinicians to ignore multiple opportunities to intervene in the disease process. Most clinicians fail to appreciate that the relapse rate of other common chronic medical disorders (e.g., diabetes, hypertension, asthma) exceeds that for substance-use disorders.[1] Problems related to substance abuse should always be addressed with the same degree of compassion and persistence that is directed to other common relapsing medical disorders.

Among individuals who abuse drugs, 53% have a co-occurring psychiatric disorder. Successful treatment of this expanding group of patients requires that clinicians improve their skills in the management of patients with substance-use disorders and co-occurring psychiatric disorders.

The National Survey on Drug Use and Health (NSDUH) findings in 2011 showed that 22.5 million Americans, or 8.7% of the population ≥ age 12, used an illicit drug in the past month.[2] Marijuana continues to be the most commonly-abused illicit drug, followed by non-medical use of prescribed or over-the-counter (OTC) medication abuse (Figure 27-1).

During the last decade, the number of patients treated for substance abuse–related problems in the US has grown steadily. Between 2004 and 2011, the number of emergency department (ED) visits for drug-related events increased by 100%.[3] In the same period, the number of drug-related suicide attempts rose by 41%. Adolescents and young adults were the most vulnerable to the adverse effects of drug use. The majority of ED visits for those in these age groups were the result of medical emergencies related to drug misuse/abuse (Figure 27-2).

In 2011, cocaine and marijuana were the most commonly-used illicit drugs that led to ED visits.[3] Non-medical use of prescription drug or OTC medication–related ED visits increased by 132% between 2004 and 2011, with opiate/opioid involvement rising by 183%.[3]

These results are not surprising in that they reflect the extent of the prescription pain-reliever addiction epidemic in the US. About 4.5 million individuals reported current non-medical use of pain relievers in 2011.[2]

In recent years, the liberal prescription of potent opioid medications, as well as their increased availability and diversion in communities, have played a significant role in the development of this public health problem.[4] More than half of those who use illicit pain relievers reported that they had obtained the pain relievers from family or friends[2] (Figure 27-3).

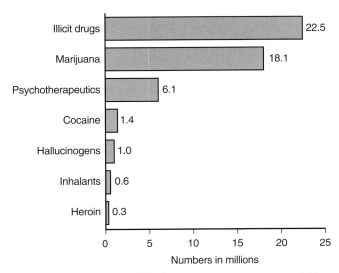

Figure 27-1. Past month illicit drug use among persons aged 12 or older: 2011. *(Findings from National Survey on Drug Use and Health, 2011: Summary of National Findings, NSDUH Series H-44, HHS Publication No. (SMA) 12-4713. Rockville, MD: Substance Abuse and Mental Health Services Administration, 2012.)*

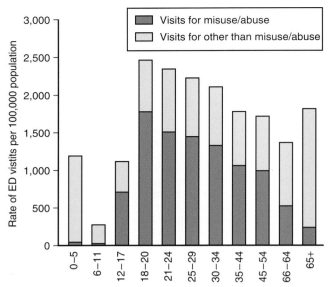

Figure 27-2. Rates of drug-related ED visits per 100,000 population, by age group, 2011. *(From Substance Abuse and Mental Health Services Administration, Center for Behavioral Health Statistics and Quality. Drug Abuse Warning Network, 2008: National Estimates of Drug-Related Emergency Department Visits. HHS Publication No. SMA 11-4618. Rockville, MD, 2011, HHS.)*

THE NEUROBIOLOGY OF ADDICTION

Disruption of the endogenous reward systems in the brain is a common feature of drug abuse; most addictive drugs act by disrupting central nervous system (CNS) dopamine circuits. Acutely, synaptic dopamine increases and circuits that mediate motivation and drive, conditioned learning, and inhibitory controls are disrupted (Figure 27-4). This enhancement of synaptic dopamine is particularly rewarding for individuals with abnormally low density of the D_2 dopamine receptor (D_2DR). Normal individuals (with normal D_2DR levels) find this experience too intense and aversive and thus may be shielded from the risk of addiction. Low D_2DR availability is associated with an increased risk for abuse of cocaine, heroin, methamphetamine, alcohol, and methylphenidate. Chronic drug use produces long-lasting and significant decreases in dopamine brain function, manifested by decreases in both the D_2DR and dopamine cell activity. These decreases are also associated with dysfunction in the prefrontal cortex, including the orbitofrontal cortex (which is involved in salience attribution) and the cingulated gyrus (which is involved in inhibitory control and mood regulation). Low baseline levels of beta-plasma endorphins are associated with a higher endorphin response to alcohol and an increased risk for alcohol dependence; it is less clear whether this abnormality also increases the risk for opiate dependence. Table 27-1 lists the major drugs of abuse and the associated disruption of CNS neurotransmitter systems.

COCAINE
Abuse

The percent of persons with cocaine dependence or abuse decreased between 2006 and 2011 from 0.7 to 0.3 %.[2] In 2011,

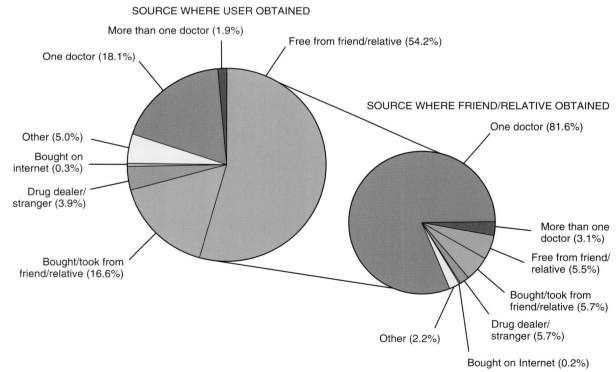

Figure 27-3. Source where pain relievers were obtained for most recent non-medical use among past year users aged 12 or older: 2010–2011. The Other category includes the sources "Wrote Fake Prescription," "Stole from Doctor's Office/Clinic/Hospital/Pharmacy," and "Some Other Way." *(Findings from National Survey on Drug Use and Health: Summary of National Findings, NSDUH Series H-44, HHS Publication No. (SMA) 12-4713. Rockville, MD: Substance Abuse and Mental Health Services Administration, 2012.)*

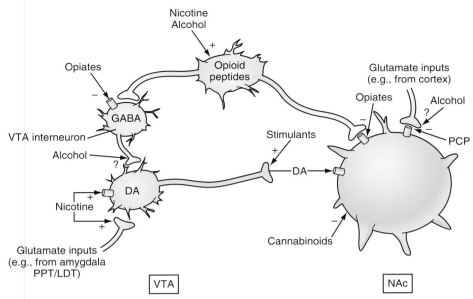

Figure 27-4. Converging acute actions of drugs of abuse on the ventral tegmental area and nucleus accumbens. DA, dopamine; GABA, γ-aminobutyric acid; LDT, laterodorsal tegmentum; NAc, nucleus accumbens; PCP, phencyclidine; PPT, pedunculopontine tegmentum; VTA, ventral tegmental area. *(Redrawn from Nestler EJ. Is there a common molecular pathway for addiction? Nat Neurosci 8(11):1445–1449, 2005.)*

TABLE 27-1 Neurobiology of Drug Reinforcement

Drug Type	Mechanism of Reinforcement
Cocaine	Mesolimbic dopamine system
Amphetamines	
Nicotine	
Opioids	Mesolimbic dopamine system
Alcohol	GABA and glutamate
	Dopamine and serotonin
	Opioid peptide systems
Cannabinoids	Dopamine in the nucleus accumbens

GABA, γ-aminobutyric acid.

the number of persons with cocaine dependence or abuse was roughly 821,000. Despite the downward trend, cocaine, after alcohol, remained the leading substance of abuse related to frequent ED contacts, general hospital admissions, family violence, and other social problems.[3] Cocaine use resulted in 40% of all illicit drug-related ED visits in 2011. Even individuals with normal psychological profiles are vulnerable to compulsive cocaine use. Acute use leads to intense euphoria that is often associated with increased sexual desire and with improved sexual function. These rewards are often followed by a moderate-to-severe post–cocaine use depression that stimulates a strong incentive for further cocaine use. These responses are primarily mediated by disruptions of synaptic dopamine. The initial cocaine response is a function of elevated dopamine generated by blockade of the dopamine reuptake transporter (DAT) and the inhibition of the reuptake of synaptic dopamine. Chronic cocaine use leads to down-regulation of dopamine receptors and ultimately to depletion of synaptic dopamine, which is thought to be the cause of post–cocaine use depression (Figure 27-5). Like other stimulants, cocaine also disrupts the synthesis and reuptake of serotonin. Other receptors affected include norepinephrine, N-methyl-D-aspartate (NMDA), gamma-aminobutyric acid (GABA), and opioid receptors. Plasma cholinesterases rapidly convert cocaine into benzoylecognine (BE), an inactive metabolite that can be detected in the urine for 3 days. When alcohol is taken in conjunction with cocaine, liver esterases produce

cocaethylene, an active metabolite that has a longer half-life (2–4-hours) and is more cardiotoxic than cocaine. The combination of cocaine and marijuana also produces more intense euphoria, higher plasma levels, and more cardiotoxicity than does cocaine alone.

The signs and the symptoms of acute cocaine intoxication are similar to those of amphetamine abuse. Typical complaints associated with intoxication include anorexia, insomnia, anxiety, hyperactivity, and rapid speech and thought processes ("speeding"). Signs of adrenergic hyperactivity (such as hyperreflexia, tachycardia, diaphoresis, and dilated pupils responsive to light) may also be seen. More severe symptoms (e.g., hyperpyrexia, hypertension, cocaine-induced vasospastic events [e.g., stroke or myocardial infarction]) are relatively rare among users, but are fairly common in those seen in hospital EDs. Patients may also manifest stereotyped movements of the mouth, face, or extremities. Snorting the drug may produce rhinitis or sinusitis and, rarely, perforations of the nasal septum. Free-basing (inhalation of cocaine alkaloid vapors) may produce bronchitis. Grand mal seizures are another infrequent complication. Patients also describe "snowlights" (i.e., flashes of light usually seen at the periphery of the visual field). Crack is a highly addictive free-base form of cocaine that is sold in crystals and can be smoked.

The most serious psychiatric problem associated with chronic cocaine use is a cocaine-induced psychosis (manifest by visual and auditory hallucinations and paranoid delusions often associated with violent behavior). Tactile hallucinations (called "coke bugs") involve the perception that something is crawling under the skin. A cocaine psychosis may be indistinguishable from an amphetamine psychosis, but it usually does not last as long. High doses of stimulants can also cause a state of excitation and mental confusion known as "stimulant delirium."

Management

Cocaine abuse became common among affluent young people in the early to mid-1980s, but with the availability of packaged smokable cocaine, or crack, in low-cost doses, all classes and racial groups have become potential users. Occasional cocaine

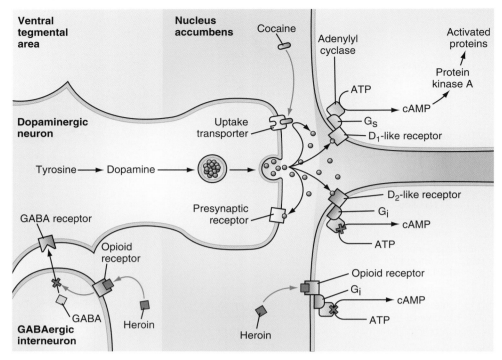

Figure 27-5. Schematic of the effects of cocaine and heroin in the synapse. *(Redrawn and adapted from Leshner A and the US National Institute on Drug Abuse. New understandings of drug addiction, Hospital Practice Special Report, 1997. New York, 1997, McGraw-Hill.)*

use does not require specific treatment except in the case of a life-threatening overdose. Most potentially lethal doses are metabolized within 1 hour. In the interim, intubation and assisted breathing with oxygen may be necessary. Stroke has been reported, and death can be caused by ventricular fibrillation or myocardial infarction. The cardiac status should therefore be monitored closely. High doses of benzodiazepines are recommended for management of stimulant-induced delirium and agitation. Neuroleptics should be avoided because of the risk of potentially fatal hyperthermia. Intravenous (IV) diazepam should be used to control convulsions.

Chronic cocaine use produces tolerance, severe psychological dependency, and physiological dependence (marked by irritability, anhedonia, low mood, insomnia or hypersomnia, and anxiety).[5] Dependent users typically follow a cyclical pattern of 2 or 3 days of heavy binge use, followed by a withdrawal "crash." Use is resumed again in 3 to 4 days, depending on the availability of cash and the drug. A gradual reduction in use of the drug is almost never possible. Detoxification is accomplished by the abrupt cessation of all cocaine use, usually through restricted access (e.g., a loss of funds or contacts, or incarceration). Symptoms of withdrawal begin to resolve within 7 days; the value of medication treatment for withdrawal symptoms has yet to be confirmed. Drugs that enhance CNS catecholamine function may reduce craving, although they are of limited clinical benefit and they have not been proven effective in double-blind placebo-controlled trials. There is some indication that amantadine (an indirect dopamine agonist) and propranolol may be helpful to individuals with severe withdrawal symptoms. The major complication of withdrawal is a severe depression with suicidal ideation.[6] If this occurs, the patient typically requires psychiatric hospitalization. The need for inpatient care may be time-limited, since suicidal ideation usually clears promptly with the cessation of cocaine use. A less severe anhedonic state may persist for 2 to 3 months and is thought to reflect a more persistent state of dopamine depletion.

For the cocaine addict, the compulsion to use is overwhelming. For this reason, a hospitalized, cocaine-dependent patient should be monitored closely and should have a drug screen performed after behavioral change, particularly after departures from the floor or receiving visitors. Urine should be examined for cocaine metabolites and, preferably, for all drugs of abuse.

Once compulsive cocaine use has begun, it is almost impossible for the user to return to a pattern of occasional, controlled use. Such individuals are also likely to develop problems with alcohol and other drugs. For that reason, the goal of treatment should be abstinence from cocaine and all other drugs. All cocaine abusers should be referred for individual or group counseling, and participation in 12-step self-help programs should be strongly recommended. Manual-guided cognitive-behavioral therapy (CBT) has been efficacious in the treatment of cocaine dependence.[7] Twelve-step facilitation and CBT appear to be helpful, particularly in individuals with more severe dependence and in those with co-morbid disorders.[8] Family members or significant others should be referred separately to Al-Anon because they will gain insights that may help them eliminate systemic support for the patient's drug use. There is no Food and Drug Administration (FDA)–approved pharmacotherapy for cocaine dependence. Trials with desipramine, fluoxetine, bupropion, amantadine, and carbamazepine have had inconsistent results. Positive responses have been reported in trials with topiramate, baclofen, and modafinil, but these drugs require further investigation. Several trials with disulfiram have shown benefit, with reduced craving and use, and a reported increase in the aversive effects of cocaine should the patient relapse. These reactions are thought to be mediated by the inhibitory effect of disulfiram on dopamine beta-hydroxylase. This action will elevate depleted plasma dopamine levels in chronic users and will produce abnormally high dopamine levels if cocaine is ingested; this results in a dysphoric experience for most users.

AMPHETAMINES
Abuse

In 2011, roughly 970,000 persons ≥ 12 years were active non-medical users of prescription stimulants.[2] Between 2004 and 2011, prescription CNS stimulants led to a striking 307% increase in ED visits. Among these agents, the ADHD drug amphetamine-dextroamphetamine (e.g., Adderall®) showed a 650% increase during that period.[3]

Illicitly-produced methamphetamine fueled an epidemic of abuse on the West Coast and in much of the Midwest in the 1990s. Since then, the number of methamphetamine abusers had declined as a result of stricter federal controls on the production and distribution of certain medications.

The primary action of these drugs is an increase in synaptic dopamine via the release of dopamine into the synapse; methamphetamine also blocks the DAT. This produces a dopamine "high" that is both more intense and longer lasting than results from cocaine, lasting anywhere from 8 to 24 hours. Methamphetamine, invented for military use by the Japanese in World War I, is currently a schedule II drug, that can be taken orally ("speed"), taken anally, smoked ("crystal"), snorted, or injected. It has been approved for the treatment of ADHD and obesity. Long-term use of amphetamines can cause cognitive impairment (including dulled awareness, decreased intellectual capacity, memory impairment, and motor retardation). Positive positron emission tomography (PET) scans show loss of DAT in the caudate and the putamen, and magnetic resonance imaging (MRI) studies show decreased perfusion in the putaman and the frontal cortex as well as loss of volume in both the amygdala and the hippocampus. Routine medical evaluation may uncover the most common type of amphetamine abuse seen in clinical settings (involving use of amphetamines to control obesity and that later led to chronic amphetamine abuse). Amphetamine abusers quickly develop tolerance and may use 100 mg each day in an unsuccessful effort to control weight. This type of amphetamine abuse can be treated by abruptly discontinuing the drug or by gradually tapering the dose. In either case, the patient should be given a more appropriate program for weight control.

A more serious problem involves the patient who develops a severe psychological dependence on amphetamines and who may have the same symptoms seen in younger street-drug users and abusers. Illicit amphetamine and methamphetamine (speed) use accounted for 12.8 % of all illicit-drug-use-related ED visits in 2011.[3]

The signs and symptoms of acute amphetamine intoxication are similar to those of cocaine abuse. Long-term effects include depression, brain dysfunction, and weight loss. In addition, either with acute or chronic amphetamine intoxication a paranoid psychosis without delirium can develop. Although typically seen in young people who use IV methamphetamine hydrochloride, paranoia can also occur in chronic users of dextroamphetamine or other amphetamines. A paranoid psychosis may also occur with or without other manifestations of amphetamine intoxication. The absence of disorientation distinguishes this condition from most other toxic psychoses. This syndrome is clinically indistinguishable from an acute schizophrenic episode of the paranoid type, and the correct diagnosis is often made in retrospect, based on a history of amphetamine use and a urine test that is positive for amphetamines. Use of haloperidol or low-dose atypical antipsychotics is often effective in the acute management of this type of substance-induced psychosis.

Other distinctive features of chronic stimulant abuse include dental problems (e.g., caries, missing teeth, bleeding and infected gums), muscle cramps (related to dehydration and low levels of magnesium and potassium), constipation (due to dehydration), nasal perforations, and excoriated skin lesions (speed bumps) (Figure 27-6). The urine may have a stale smell due to ammonia constituents used in the illicit manufacture of methamphetamine.

Treatment

Amphetamines can be withdrawn abruptly. If the intoxication is mild, the patient's agitation can be handled by reassurance alone. The patient can be "talked down," much as one might handle an adverse D-lysergic acid diethylamide (LSD) reaction. If sedation is necessary, benzodiazepines are the drugs of choice. Phenothiazines should be avoided because they may heighten dysphoria and increase the patient's agitation. Hypertension will usually respond to sedation with benzodiazepines. When severe hypertension arises, phentolamine is recommended for vasodilation. Beta- or mixed alpha- and beta-adrenergic blockers (such as propranolol or labetalol) are to

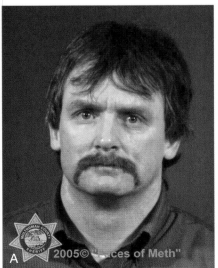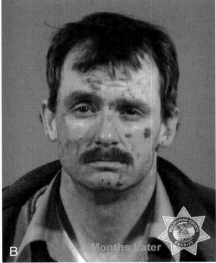

Figure 27-6. Face of a patient with chronic methamphetamine abuse. Before use (A) and after 3 months of use (B). *(From the Faces of Meth educational program. Copyright 2005 Multnomah County [Oregon] Sheriff's Office, Portland, Oregon.)*

be avoided because they may exacerbate stimulant-induced cardiovascular toxicity.

Most signs of intoxication clear in 2 to 4 days. The major problem is management of depression upon discontinuation of amphetamine use. In mild cases, this depression can be manifest by lethargy, as well as by the temptation to use amphetamines for energy. In more serious cases, the patient may become suicidal and require inpatient psychiatric treatment. The efficacy of antidepressants in such cases has not been adequately documented. Even with support and psychotherapy, most patients experience symptoms of depression for 3 to 6 months following the cessation of chronic amphetamine abuse. CBT has been helpful, but it may need to be adapted to allow for the cognitive impairment associated with long-term methamphetamine use.

CLUB DRUGS

During the 1990s the abuse of "club drugs," primarily 3,4-methylenedioxy-methamphetamine (MDMA, or "ecstasy"), γ-hydroxybutyrate (GHB), and ketamine steadily increased. This trend was reversed between 1998 and 2001 when the Monitoring the Future Survey (MFS) reported a steep decline in the use of ecstasy. The drop has been attributed to a general recognition of the dangers associated with the use of this drug. In 2012, MFS reported a 1.5% past-year use of club drugs among 12th graders.[9]

MDMA has both amphetamine-like and hallucinogenic effects. Its primary mechanism of action is via indirect serotonin agonism, but it also affects dopamine and other neurotransmitter systems. These club drugs increase synaptic dopamine and alter serotonergic neurotransmission. MDMA was initially used experimentally to facilitate psychotherapy, but its use was banned after it was found to be neurotoxic to animals. The intense feelings of empathy experienced by users may be a result of the flooding of the serotonin system. In toxic amounts, it produces distorted perceptions, confusion, hypertension, hyperactivity, and potentially fatal hyperthermia. With chronic use, serotonin stores are depleted and subsequent doses produce a less robust high and more unpleasant side effects (such as teeth gnashing and restlessness). Frequent users learn to anticipate these effects and tend to limit their long-term consumption of the drug.

GHB (sodium oxybate) is structurally similar to GABA and it acts as a CNS depressant. It has been approved by the FDA as a schedule III controlled substance for the treatment of narcolepsy. GHB has a relatively low therapeutic index; as little as twice the dose that produces euphoria can cause CNS depression. In overdose it can produce a potentially fatal coma; it has also been identified as a "date rape" drug. Ketamine ("Special K," "Super K," or "K") is a non-competitive NMDA antagonist that is classified as a dissociative anesthetic. It is currently used as a veterinary anesthetic and it can produce delirium, amnesia, and respiratory depression when abused. Ketamine, like phencyclidine (PCP), binds to the NMDA receptor site and blocks the action of excitatory neurotransmission; it affects perceptions, memory, and cognition. More recently, studies suggest it can rapidly reverse treatment-refractory depression.

The treatment for overdoses of all of these drugs is primarily symptomatic.

OPIOIDS

While abuse of all major drug classes increased during the 1990s, the most dramatic increase was seen among new abusers of prescription pain relievers. In 2011, an estimated 4.5 million (1.7%) individuals were active non-medical users of pain relievers.[2] In the US, prescription pain reliever-abuse is considered an epidemic. Many public health problems have been associated with this particular type of drug abuse. The perception of prescription drugs as being less harmful than illicit drugs likely contributed to the problem.[2]

Due to frequency of prescription pain relievers, they are considered an "entry drug" after illicit marijuana. According to the 2012 MFS, 1 out of every 12 high school seniors reported taking prescription pain relievers for non-medical use within the last year.[9] Unfortunately, with the progression of the abuse, many individuals turn to heroin. The latest NSDUH data estimated a significant increase in heroin use in 2007 (373,000) to 2011 (620,000).[2] The major health concerns with increased heroin use are intravenous (IV)-related medical complications.

Nearly one-third (31%) of individuals with acquired immunodeficiency syndrome (AIDS) in the US are related to injection drug use.[10] An estimated 70% to 80% of the new hepatitis C infections occurring in the US each year are among IV drug users. Other public health problems that have emerged over the last decade include increased ED visits and deaths due to overdoses. Specifically, prescription methadone, oxycodone and hydrocodone-related ED visits quadrupled between 2004 and 2008[11] (Figure 27-7).

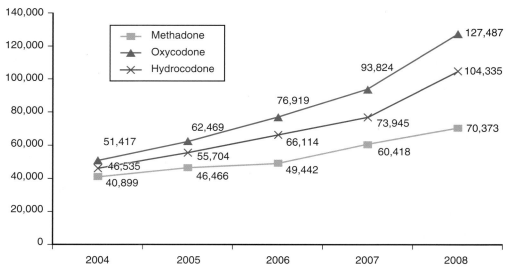

Figure 27-7. Emergency department visits related to methadone, oxycodone and hydrocodone: 2004–2008. DAWN 2008.

Death rates
Deaths per 100,000 population

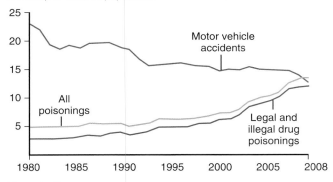

Drug deaths
In thousands

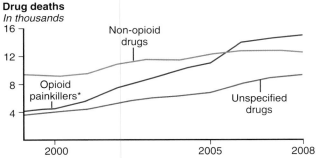

*Note: morphine, hydrocodone, oxycodone, methadone, fentanyl and others

Figure 27-8. Overdose death rates. *(Warner M, Chen LH, Makuc DM, Anderson RN, Miniño AM. Drug poisoning deaths in the United States, 1980–2008. NCHS data brief, no 81. Hyattsville, MD, 2011, National Center for Health Statistics.)*

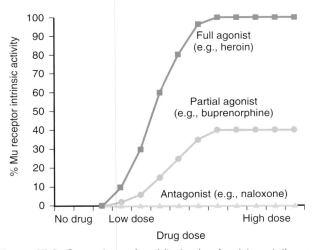

Figure 27-9. Comparison of activity levels of opiates at the mu receptor.

In 2008, there were more poisoning-related deaths than deaths caused by motor vehicle accidents (Figure 27-8). In 2011, pain relievers accounted for 46% of all medical emergencies associated with non-medical use of pharmaceuticals. Since 2007, there were more overdose deaths with prescription pain relievers than there were with heroin and cocaine combined.[12]

Opiates act by binding to the mu opioid receptor (Figure 27-9). Binding to receptors in the ventral tegmental area stimulates the release of dopamine (Figure 27-10), which activates brain reward centers in the nucleus accumbens. Opiates produce a wide range of effects (including analgesia, euphoria,

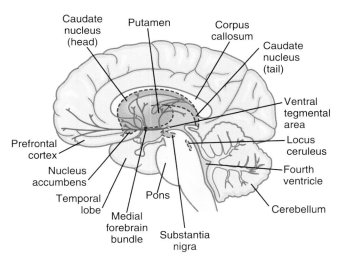

Figure 27-10. Schematic of reward pathways in the brain. *(Redrawn and adapted from Leshner A and the US National Institute on Drug Abuse.* New understandings of drug addiction, Hospital Practice Special Report, *April 1997. New York, 1997, McGraw-Hill.)*

TABLE 27-2 Opioid Agonist Drug Effects

Acute-use effects	Euphoria
	Vomiting
	Constricted pupils
	Depressed respiration
	Drowsiness
	Decreased pain sensation
	Decreased awareness
	Decreased consciousness
Large-dose acute-use effects	Non-responsiveness
	Pin-point pupils
	If severe anoxia, pupils may dilate
	Bradycardia and hypotension
	Skin cyanotic
	Skeletal muscle flaccid
	Pulmonary edema in approximately 50%
	Slow or absent respiration
Chronic-use effects	Physical dependence
	Psychological dependence
	Lethargy and indifference
	Reduction in bowel movement

sedation, decreased secretions, nausea, vomiting, constipation, miosis, urinary hesitation, and hypotension [Table 27-2]). The classic signs of opiate withdrawal are easily recognized and usually begin 8 to 12 hours after the last dose (of a short-lasting agent) (Box 27-1). The patient generally admits the need for drugs and shows sweating, yawning, lacrimation, tremor, rhinorrhea, marked irritability, dilated pupils, piloerection ("gooseflesh"), and an increased respiratory rate. More severe signs of withdrawal occur 24 to 36 hours after the last dose and include tachycardia, hypertension, insomnia, nausea, vomiting, and abdominal cramps. Untreated, the syndrome subsides in 3 to 7 days. Withdrawal symptoms are similar in patients addicted to methadone, but they may not appear until 24 to 36 hours after the last dose (because of methadone's longer half-life) and abate over 2 to 4 weeks. Patients addicted to oxycodone may present with a particularly severe and prolonged withdrawal syndrome and may require high doses of opiates for adequate control.

As the treatment of opioid dependence becomes more commonplace on medical and surgical floors of general hospitals, physicians are challenged to provide proper management, necessitating up-to-date knowledge of FDA regulations

---

BOX 27-1 Signs and Symptoms of Opiate Withdrawal

- Dysphoric mood
- Nausea ± vomiting
- Body aches
- Lacrimation
- Rhinorrhea
- Pupillary dilation
- Sweating
- Piloerection
- Diarrhea
- Yawning
- Mild fever
- Insomnia
- Irritability
- Opioid craving

---

and community treatment resources, as well as competence in the management of detoxification and opiate substitution therapy.

Opiate Substitution Therapy

FDA regulations define opiate substitution therapy (with either methadone, *levo*-alpha-acetylmethadol [LAAM], or buprenorphine) as treatment with an approved opiate that extends beyond 30 days. An addicted individual cannot be placed into a methadone maintenance treatment unless he or she manifests physiological evidence of current addiction (withdrawal signs) and can document a 1-year history of addiction. The only exceptions to this rule are being pregnant and addicted; being addicted and hospitalized for the treatment of a medical, surgical, or obstetric condition; and having been addicted and recently released from incarceration. In the methadone clinic setting, initiation of maintenance treatment begins with an oral dose of 20 to 30 mg per day. Increases are made daily in increments of 10 mg until a dose is achieved that eliminates withdrawal symptoms and blocks craving. More rapid dose escalation runs the risk of excessive sedation and prolongation of the QTc interval. Doses in the range of 80 to 120 mg per day are required to stabilize most addicts and to block the euphoric effect of illicit opiates. Success in methadone maintenance treatment has been associated with higher doses (range 60 to 120 mg daily), long-term treatment, and the provision of comprehensive counseling and rehabilitation services.

In addition to methadone, FDA-approved medications for opiate substitution therapy include LAAM (a synthetic opiate with a duration of action of 48 to 72 hours) and buprenorphine (a long-acting partial opiate agonist). Patients on LAAM must be monitored for evidence of a prolonged QTc interval. Buprenorphine, a partial opioid agonist, produces a milder state of opiate dependence. Because it only partially activates opiate receptors, buprenorphine does not suppress brainstem function and it is relatively safe in overdose (Figure 27-8). Buprenorphine has a high affinity for opiate receptors and is slowly dissociated from the receptor. It will displace most other opiates from the receptor and may precipitate opiate withdrawal in dependent individuals if other opiates are present. To avoid this problem, the initial buprenorphine dose should not be administered until the patient demonstrates mild-to-moderate symptoms of withdrawal.

Buprenorphine can be used in the treatment of patients who meet *Diagnostic and Statistical Manual of Mental Disorders, Fifth Edition* (DSM-5), criteria for opioid dependence.[13] Unlike methadone, treatment with buprenorphine does not require documentation of a 1-year history of addiction. When sublingual (SL) buprenorphine is dispensed in a combination tablet (with naloxone), it has minimal potential for IV abuse and has been effective for maintenance treatment.[14] Buprenorphine has been approved for use in the office-based treatment of opiate dependence and it provides an attractive alternative to methadone treatment for higher-functioning individuals and for those with shorter histories of opiate dependence. To initiate buprenorphine treatment, a patient should be instructed to refrain from the use of heroin, or any other opiate, for at least 24 hours. Once opiate withdrawal is documented (and monitored with an opiate withdrawal scale, such as the Clinical Opiate Withdrawal Scale [COWS]), treatment should begin with 4 mg/1 mg of SL buprenorphine/naloxone. The patient should be observed for 1–4 hours after the initial dose for any signs of precipitated withdrawal. Additional doses of 4 mg/1 mg can be given every 2–4 hours as needed to stabilize the patient. Most clinicians do not prescribe more than 8–12 mg/2–3 mg on the first day. Should precipitated withdrawal occur, more aggressive dosing is recommended to manage the withdrawal symptoms. Most patients can be maintained on SL doses in the range of 12 to 16 mg/day; an adequate stabilizing dose can usually be achieved within 2 to 3 days.

If a patient on methadone maintenance is to be switched to buprenorphine, the methadone dose should be gradually reduced to 30 mg per day. The patient should be maintained on that dose for 1–2 weeks before being transferred to buprenorphine. To avoid precipitated withdrawal, the first buprenorphine dose should not be administered until a mild level of opiate withdrawal is evident (in the range of 5 to 13 on the COWS). Most patients will usually need to wait 24 to 48 hours after their last methadone dose before buprenorphine can be safely administered. The dosing procedure is similar to that described previously for patients using heroin. Long-term methadone patients usually require higher buprenorphine doses (in the range of 16 to 24 mg for stabilization). Because of the ceiling effect seen with partial opiate agonists, there is no pharmacological benefit from doses higher than 32 mg/day. Extensive research has shown that opiate substitution therapy is highly effective. It reduces illicit drug use, the mortality rate, criminal behavior, and transmission of hepatitis and human immunodeficiency virus (HIV) infection, and permits many of those with addictions to attain normal levels of social function.[15] Evaluations conducted under the Drug Addiction Treatment Act of 2000 demonstrated a very positive response to the introduction of buprenorphine treatment for opiate dependence. Of the more than 104,600 individuals that had been treated, approximately 35% had never been in treatment before and 60% were new to treatment with medication[16] (Figure 27-11). Compared to patients on methadone, patients attracted to buprenorphine treatment are more likely to be white, female, better educated, and employed (Figure 27-12).

Opiate Antagonist Therapy

Naltrexone is an opioid receptor antagonist which has been available as an oral agent for many years. It fully occupies the opioid receptor and prevents the euphoric effects of opioid agonists such as heroin, oxycodone etc. Therefore, patients taking naltrexone would not get the reinforcing "high" feeling and that would result in decrease in use pattern. Medication should be given 7–10 days after last opioid use to prevent precipitated withdrawal symptoms. Oral naltrexone has been documented to have better outcomes among motivated heath care professionals and within the criminal justice system population.

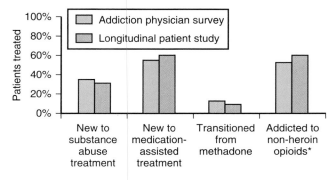

Figure 27-11. Characteristics of patients treated under the buprenorphine waiver program.

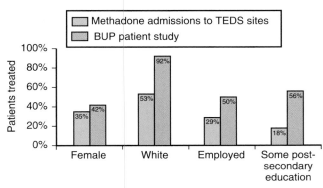

Figure 27-12. Methadone patients and buprenorphine (BUP) patients study sample: demographic differences. (The Treatment Episode Data Set [TEDS] reports primarily on admissions to facilities receiving public funding. Admissions to private facilities are underrepresented.)

In 2010, an injectable form of naltrexone has been approved by FDA. Injectable form of naltrexone (Vivitrol) appears to be a safe and effective alternative in increasing patient compliance and reduce relapse rates.[37]

Managing the Opiate-addicted Hospitalized Patient

If a patient is already receiving opiate substitution treatment before admission to the hospital, the methadone, LAAM, or buprenorphine dose should be confirmed by inpatient staff and should not be changed without consultation with the physician responsible for the patient's outpatient treatment. Under current FDA regulations, hospital-based physicians may prescribe methadone, LAAM, or buprenorphine to any addicted hospitalized person without a specialized treatment waiver or an opioid treatment program registration, as long as the patient was admitted for treatment of a condition other than opiate dependence. The patient should not be withdrawn from opiate substitution therapy unless there is full agreement among the patient, the hospital-based physician, and the outpatient treatment staff on this course of action. Such detoxification is rarely successful, particularly if the patient is under stress from a co-morbid medical or surgical condition. Withdrawal from drugs may complicate the management of the primary illness. The option of detoxification should not be considered until the patient has fully recovered from the condition that required hospitalization. Maintenance treatment should be continued until the individual has fully recovered

from the presenting illness and been referred to an opiate substitution treatment program.

Patients on long-term methadone therapy should continue to receive daily oral methadone treatment while hospitalized. If a switch to parenteral medication is necessary, methadone can be given in IM doses of 5 or 10 mg every 8 hours. This regimen should keep the patient comfortable regardless of the previous oral dose. An alternative method is to give one-third of the daily oral dose intramuscularly every 12 hours. As soon as oral medication can be tolerated, the original oral dose should be re-instated.[17]

Establishing the appropriate dose of methadone for a street addict is a trial-and-error process. Because the quality of street heroin is never certain, the addict's description of the size of the current habit is of minimal value. The safest guide to dosage is to monitor the patient's pulse, respiration, and pupillary size and to use opiate withdrawal scales (such as the COWS). After withdrawal is documented, the patient should receive 10 to 20 mg of methadone orally. Only if the patient is well known as a heavy user should a dose of 30 mg be started. A relatively young patient or a patient who reports a small habit can begin treatment with 10 mg given orally. If vital signs have not stabilized or if withdrawal signs reappear after 2 hours, an additional 5 or 10 mg can be given orally. It is rare for the patient to require more than 40 mg during the first 24 hours. Successful long-term outpatient maintenance treatment generally uses daily doses in the range of 80 to 120 mg, although lower doses may be adequate to control withdrawal symptoms in the inpatient setting. A patient with opioid addiction should be maintained on a single daily oral dose that keeps him or her comfortable and that keeps heart rate and respiratory rate within the normal range. The dose should be reduced by 5 or 10 mg if the patient appears lethargic.

Inpatient Detoxification

If the patient is to be withdrawn from drugs immediately, withdrawal symptoms should first be controlled with methadone. The methadone dose can then be reduced by 10% to 20% each day. If the patient has been maintained on methadone in the hospital for 2 or more weeks or if the patient has been on methadone treatment before admission, detoxification should proceed more slowly. The dose can be reduced by 5 to 10 mg/day until 20 mg/day is reached. Further dosage reduction should occur more gradually, particularly if the patient experiences significant cravings or withdrawal symptoms. Symptoms of chronic pain and anxiety disorders, particularly panic disorder, may also intensify during detoxification. Symptomatic treatment should be provided as needed.

Clonidine, an alpha$_2$-adrenergic agonist, suppresses the noradrenergic symptoms of withdrawal and can be used as an alternative medication for withdrawal. The patient should first be stabilized on methadone. Clonidine should not be substituted for methadone until the methadone dose has been reduced to 20 mg/day. After an initial oral dose of 0.2 mg of clonidine, patients usually require doses in the range of 0.1 to 0.2 mg every 4–6 hours. The total dose should not exceed 1.2 mg/day. Patients on clonidine should be monitored closely for side effects (particularly hypotension and sedation). Clonidine doses should be withheld for a systolic blood pressure below 90 mm Hg, or a diastolic blood pressure below 60 mm Hg. In an inpatient setting, clonidine can be tapered and discontinued over 3–4 days.[18,19] A transdermal clonidine patch is often applied on the third day. Supplemental doses of lorazepam can also be used to moderate withdrawal-related anxiety. Because clonidine does not adequately suppress the subjective symptoms of withdrawal, as does methadone and buprenorphine, and is relatively ineffective for the treatment of muscle aches and insomnia, it is not acceptable for many opioid-dependent patients.

Buprenorphine has also been effective for the short-term inpatient detoxification of opiate addicts. Patients can usually be detoxified over 3 to 5 days. After a patient shows signs of opiate withdrawal, he or she can be dosed up to buprenorphine/naloxone 8 mg/2 mg on day 1, and increased to 12 mg/3 mg on day 2. The dose can be cut to 6 mg/1.5 mg on day 3, with additional 2 mg cuts on each of the following days, if required. Opioid-addicted patients usually report that a buprenorphine detoxification is more comfortable than a detoxification with either methadone or clonidine. Rates for successful completion of opiate detoxification with buprenorphine are almost 65% higher than those reported for clonidine.[20]

Chances for successful treatment of withdrawal are enhanced if the patient is aware of the dose and is able to choose a withdrawal schedule within the limits established by the physician. By involving the patient in the treatment process and by using a flexible withdrawal schedule, the physician can keep withdrawal symptoms to a tolerable level. Rigid adherence to a fixed-dosing schedule is less likely to achieve success, and it may lead to premature termination of treatment.

Other techniques can be used for rapid inpatient detoxification from opiates, but they require more intensive medical management. The patient is first stabilized on clonidine as described previously, and 12.5 mg of naltrexone is added orally. Over the next 3 days, clonidine is gradually reduced, while naltrexone is gradually increased (up to a single dose of 150 mg) by the fourth day. A supplemental benzodiazepine is also given for agitation and insomnia. At the end of 5 days, there are no further withdrawal symptoms and the patient can be discharged directly to an outpatient naltrexone program.[19,21] Serious side effects have been reported with this procedure, including a 25% incidence of delirium that has necessitated termination of treatment.[22] A more rapid experimental protocol using high doses of opiate antagonists given under general anesthesia permits completion of detoxification in 48 hours.[23] This approach has not been adequately evaluated in randomized clinical trials, and it cannot be recommended at this time.

Although techniques that permit a safe, rapid, and medically effective detoxification from opiates seem highly attractive in an era of managed care, clinicians must recognize that detoxification alone is rarely successful as a treatment for any addiction. Unless an opiate addict is directly transferred to a long-term residential treatment program, relapse rates following detoxification are extremely high. The resulting costs to the patient, to society, and to the health care system far outweigh any saving realized from a rapid "cost-effective" detoxification protocol.

Discharge planning should be initiated as quickly as possible after admission. For patients who are not already in treatment, several weeks may be required to arrange admission to a drug-free residential program or to an opiate substitution therapy program. Physicians able to provide office-based buprenorphine treatment can be identified via the "physician locator" at the SAMHSA website (http://www.buprenorphine.samhsa.gov) or at the website maintained by the National Alliance of Advocates for Buprenorphine Treatment (www.naabt.com). Because a serious medical illness usually causes a patient with opioid addiction to re-examine his or her behavior and possibly to choose rehabilitation, the treating physician should always emphasize the need for long-term treatment. No individual should be discharged while still receiving methadone unless he or she is returning to a maintenance program or specifically refuses detoxification. Even

when a physician discharges a patient for disciplinary reasons, medical ethics necessitate that the patient be withdrawn from methadone before discharge.

According to federal regulations, hospital-based physicians can treat patients' withdrawal symptoms for detoxification purposes with methadone or buprenorphine as long as the opioid-dependence diagnosis is incidental for that inpatient admission. Similarly, if a patient who has been maintained on methadone by a methadone program, or buprenorphine by an outpatient provider, gets admitted for medical reasons, the hospital-based physicians can keep patients on methadone or buprenorphine for opioid dependence after the treatment team confirms the dose with the outside provider or the methadone program.[24]

Regardless of the form of opiate substitution therapy employed, all patients require supplemental counseling and rehabilitation services; these should include educational and vocational services as needed. CBT has been shown to be much more effective than drug counseling alone. Contingency management has also helped to reduce illicit drug use in patients on maintenance therapy.

Outpatient Detoxification Treatment

The primary purpose of detoxification treatment is to control withdrawal symptoms while gradually reducing the dose of opiates. According to FDA regulations, maintenance clinics may extend outpatient detoxification treatment from 30 to 180 days if a briefer detoxification program is not successful. The procedures described in the previous section can be easily adapted to the outpatient setting. The primary advantage of outpatient detoxification is that a more gradual procedure greatly reduces the severity of withdrawal symptoms. While the procedures previously described for detoxification with clonidine can be used on an outpatient basis, the risks associated with hypotension and sedation have generally limited the use of clonidine to inpatient settings.

With the approval of SL buprenorphine for the treatment of opiate dependence in office-based settings, clinicians have reported success with this drug for outpatient detoxification. Withdrawal symptoms can be adequately controlled within 48 hours using the dosing-induction procedure described for inpatient detoxification. It is rare for patients to require more than 16 mg/4 mg buprenorphine/naloxone to suppress symptoms. Protocols for dose reduction have ranged from 3 to 28 days, with no general consensus on the optimal duration of treatment. All of these protocols have been reported to produce satisfactory results, either equal to, or superior to, methadone, and consistently superior to clonidine. While those who are addicted almost uniformly prefer buprenorphine detoxification to either methadone or clonidine, it is important to remember that there are few data to support the long-term efficacy of any detoxification treatment. For even the most motivated patients, 12-month relapse rates generally exceed 82%.[15]

Pain Management for Patients Receiving Opiate Substitution

Determining the appropriate dosage of pain medications for a patient receiving opiate substitution therapy is a common clinical problem. The analgesic effect of methadone is minimal in maintenance patients, and, at best, lasts only 6 to 8 hours. If pain control is required, an addicted person should be given standard doses of other narcotics in addition to his or her maintenance dose of methadone. Because of cross-tolerance, a patient on maintenance narcotic therapy metabolizes other narcotics more rapidly and may therefore require more frequent administration of analgesics than might a non-addicted patient. Pentazocine and other partial opiate agonists are contraindicated for such patients. Because of their narcotic antagonist effects, these analgesics produce withdrawal symptoms in opiate addicts. If a patient is maintained on the buprenorphine/naloxone combination tablet and requires additional narcotic analgesia treatment, supplemental 2 mg/0.5 mg SL doses of buprenorphine/naloxone every 4–6 hours can be added to the patient's daily maintenance dose. Similar to methadone, buprenorphine will provide more effective analgesia if the daily maintenance dose is divided and administered on a TID schedule. If the patient requires treatment for severe pain, higher-than-usual narcotic doses may be required to overcome the partial antagonist action of buprenorphine. As long as the supplemental opiate is added following the daily buprenorphine dose, there will be no risk of precipitated withdrawal. Dispensing the other opiate before giving the daily buprenorphine dose must be avoided since buprenorphine will displace the other opiate at the receptor and will precipitate withdrawal. Pain in buprenorphine-maintained patients can also be managed with non-opiate analgesics, regional analgesia, or conscious sedation.[25] Alternatively, such patients can be switched to methadone and can be managed as described previously.

Overdose Prevention and Reversal

Opiate overdoses are medical emergencies and they require immediate attention to the maintenance of airway, breathing, and circulation (i.e., ABCs of resuscitation). Opiate-induced respiratory depression can be treated with 0.4 mg/ml of IV or IM naloxone. This medication can be repeated every 2 minutes, as needed (up to a total dose of 2 mg). If the patient does not respond after 20 minutes, he or she should be treated for a combined drug overdose. Because of the long duration of action of methadone and LAAM, overdoses of these drugs often require an IV naloxone drip.

As a response to the prescription pain-reliever epidemic, many states have implemented intranasal Narcan *overdose-prevention programs*. Practitioners caring for those who abuse, or are addicted to, prescription opioids or heroin are advised to educate their patients, as well as family and friends, about the risk of overdose. Intranasal Narcan can be provided free by state public health agencies or prescribed to such high-risk individuals as well as to household members. Between 2007 and 2011, intranasal Narcan reversed more than 1,000 opiate overdoses in Massachusetts.[26]

BENZODIAZEPINES

In 2011, DAWN estimated 357,836 ED visits for non-medical use of prescription benzodiazepines.[3] Benzodiazepines account for 28.7% of all prescription medication-related ED visits, the second highest following narcotic pain-relievers in this category.

Neurobiology

Benzodiazepines, classified as GABA agonists, bind to a subunit of the GABA receptor; of note, GABA is the major inhibitory neurotransmitter in the CNS. Attachment to the receptor opens chloride ion channels and increases the electric gradient across the cell membrane, thus making the neuron less excitable. Their primary clinical effects are sedation, a reduction in anxiety, and an increase in the seizure threshold. Long-term binding to the GABA receptor can alter the number of receptors or change the affinity of the ligand for the receptor.

BOX 27-2 Sedative-hypnotic Withdrawal Symptoms (DSM-IV Diagnostic Criteria)

- Autonomic hyperactivity (sweating or pulse rate over 100)
- Increased hand tremor
- Insomnia
- Nausea or vomiting
- Transient visual, tactile, or auditory hallucinations or illusions
- Psychomotor agitation
- Anxiety
- Grand mal seizures

BOX 27-3 DSM-5 Diagnostic Criteria: Sedative, Hypnotic, or Anxiolytic Intoxication

A. Recent use of a sedative, hypnotic, or anxiolytic.
B. Clinically significant maladaptive behavioral or psychological changes (e.g., inappropriate sexual or aggressive behavior, mood lability, impaired judgment) that developed during, or shortly after, sedative, hypnotic, or anxiolytic use.
C. One (or more) of the following signs or symptoms developing during, or shortly after, sedative, hypnotic, or anxiolytic use:
   1. Slurred speech
   2. Incoordination
   3. Unsteady gait
   4. Nystagmus
   5. Impairment in cognition (e.g., attention, memory)
   6. Stupor or coma.
D. The signs or symptoms are not attributable to another medical condition and are not better explained by another mental disorder, including intoxication with another substance.

Reprinted with permission from the Diagnostic and statistical manual of mental disorders, *ed 5, (Copyright 2013). American Psychiatric Association.*

Patterns of Chronic Use versus Abuse

Benzodiazepines can produce dependence, especially when used in high doses or for prolonged periods. Up to 45% of patients receiving stable, long-term doses show evidence of physiological withdrawal. Withdrawal symptoms, which are usually the same in both high-dose and low-dose patients, include anxiety, insomnia, irritability, depression, tremor, nausea, vomiting, and anorexia. Seizures and psychotic reactions have also been reported. The more common symptoms are similar to those seen during withdrawal from all of the sedative-hypnotic drugs, and they may be difficult to distinguish from the symptoms for which the benzodiazepine was originally prescribed (Box 27-2 contains DSM-IV diagnostic criteria; refer to Box 27.3 for DSM-5 criteria). In general, withdrawal symptoms abate within 2 weeks.

Benzodiazepines (such as diazepam and alprazolam) with a rapid onset of action seem to be sought out by drug abusers and are generally presumed to have a greater potential for abuse than benzodiazepines with a slower onset of action (e.g., oxazepam). Nonetheless, there is relatively little evidence for the abuse of benzodiazepines when they are prescribed for legitimate medical conditions. Ciraulo and collagues[27] found that the use patterns of benzodiazepines, even among former alcoholics, were similar to those of other psychiatric patients. A study of alcoholics conducted at the Addiction Research Foundation of Ontario found that 40% were recent users of benzodiazepines and that there was a 20% life-time incidence of anxiolytic abuse or dependence.[28] Although these studies suggest that concerns about the abuse of benzodiazepines by alcoholics can be exaggerated, the problem can occur in some patients. Anxiolytics may be prescribed to this population, but they should never be a first-line treatment, and patients must always be carefully monitored for signs of abuse. There is no evidence that anxiolytics are effective as a primary treatment for alcoholism or for drug dependence.

It is important to distinguish between a drug abuser who uses benzodiazepines primarily to get high, often deliberately mixing them with alcohol and other drugs of abuse, and an individual who takes benzodiazepines appropriately under medical supervision. In both cases, the user may develop physiological and psychological dependence. Such dependence, in and of itself, is not evidence of addiction or drug abuse. Unless there is evidence of dose escalation, the deliberate use to produce a high, or dangerous states of intoxication, there is no reason to assume that chronic benzodiazepine users are abusers. Even though clonazepam is the only benzodiazepine with an indication for long-term use, common medical practice supports the merit of the continued use of benzodiazepines in some individuals with chronic medical and psychiatric conditions.

Overdose

Flumazenil, a specific benzodiazepine antagonist, reverses the life-threatening effects of a benzodiazepine overdose. An initial IV dose of 0.2 mg should be given over 30 seconds, followed by a second 0.2 mg IV dose if there is no response after 45 seconds. This procedure can be repeated at 1-minute intervals (up to a cumulative dose of 5 mg). This treatment is contraindicated in individuals dependent on benzodiazepines or those taking tricyclic antidepressants (TCAs), because flumazenil may precipitate seizures in these patients.[29,30] When flumazenil is contraindicated, benzodiazepine overdoses should be handled similarly to other sedative-hypnotic overdoses (see the following section).

Withdrawal

In cases in which there is clear evidence of benzodiazepine abuse or when the patient desires to stop using these medications, it is important that detoxification occurs under medical supervision. During the withdrawal process, patients should be warned about a temporary increase in anxiety symptoms. The simplest approach to detoxification is a gradual reduction in dose that may be extended over several weeks or months; under no circumstances should benzodiazepines be stopped abruptly. When a more rapid detoxification is desired, inpatient dosage reduction can be completed within 2 weeks. For some patients, this rapid withdrawal process produces an unacceptable level of subjective distress. An alternative approach is to switch to a high-potency, long-acting benzodiazepine (such as clonazepam). Most patients seem to tolerate detoxification on clonazepam quite well. Because of the prolonged self-taper after completion of detoxification with clonazepam, patients experience a smoother course of withdrawal with a minimum of rebound anxiety.[31,32] An alternative approach for inpatient detoxification is a 3- to 4-day taper using anticonvulsants. Carbamazepine and valproate are the best-studied medications for this purpose, though topiramate and gabapentin are probably effective.

Withdrawal from the high-potency, short-acting benzodiazepines (such as alprazolam) has been particularly problematic. A rapid tapering of these drugs is often poorly tolerated by patients, and a switch to equivalent doses of a long-acting benzodiazepine often allows acute withdrawal symptoms to emerge. In general, clonazepam is substituted for alprazolam, at a dose ratio of 0.5 mg of clonazepam for each 1 mg of alprazolam. Clonazepam should then be continued for 1 to 3 weeks. A drug taper is not always required, although abrupt discontinuation of even a long-acting agent (such as clonazepam) can be associated with a withdrawal syndrome that includes seizures, but it tends to occur several days after discontinuation. A 2- to 3-week taper is usually adequate.

Supplemental medication is of little use during benzodiazepine withdrawal; beta-adrenergic blockers (e.g., propranolol) and alpha-adrenergic agonists (e.g., clonidine) offer no advantage over detoxification using benzodiazepines alone. Although they tend to moderate the severity of physiological symptoms, they are ineffective in controlling the patient's subjective sense of anxiety, and they do not prevent withdrawal seizures or delirium. Buspirone has no cross-tolerance for the benzodiazepines and does not control withdrawal symptoms from this class of drugs.

SEDATIVE-HYPNOTICS
Abuse

Use of CNS depressants accounts for high rates of ED visits related to suicidal attempts and accidental overdoses (consequent to recreational use and self-medication). Although benzodiazepines have become the most commonly abused sedative-hypnotics in the US, there are still areas where the non-medical use of barbiturates (such as butalbital [Fiorinal and Esgic]), carisoprodol (Soma), and other sedative-hypnotics (such as methaqualone, glutethimide) causes serious clinical problems. More recently, a significant increase with zolpidem-related ED visits has been noted.[33]

Clinical Syndromes

A person intoxicated on a CNS depressant typically has many of the same diagnostic features associated with alcohol intoxication. Slurred speech, unsteady gait, and sustained vertical or horizontal nystagmus that occur in the absence of the odor of alcohol on the breath suggest the diagnosis. Unfortunately, since drug abusers frequently combine alcohol with other sedative-hypnotics, the clinician may be misled by the odor of alcohol. The diagnosis of mixed alcohol–barbiturate intoxication can be missed unless a careful history is taken and blood and urine samples are analyzed for toxic drugs. The behavioral effects of barbiturate intoxication can vary widely, even in the same person, and may change significantly depending on the surroundings and on the expectations of the user. Individuals using barbiturates primarily to control anxiety or stress may appear sleepy or mildly confused as a result of an overdose. In young adults seeking to get high, a similar dose may produce excitement, loud boisterous behavior, and loss of inhibitions. The aggressive and even violent behavior commonly associated with alcohol intoxication may follow. The prescribed regimen for managing an angry alcohol abuser can also be used for the disinhibited abuser of sedative-hypnotics.

As tolerance to barbiturates develops, there is no concomitant increase in the lethal dose, as occurs in opiate dependence. Although the opiate addict may be able to double his or her regular dose and still avoid fatal respiratory depression, as little as a 10%–25% increase over the usual daily dosage may be fatal to the barbiturate addict. Thus, a barbiturate overdose should always be considered potentially life-threatening, especially in a drug abuser.

In overdose, a variety of signs and symptoms may be observed, depending on the drug or the combination of drugs used, the amount of time since ingestion, and the presence of complicating medical conditions (e.g., pneumonia, hepatitis, diabetes, heart disease, renal failure, or head injury). Initially the patient appears lethargic or semi-comatose. The pulse rate is slow, but other vital functions are often normal. As the level of intoxication increases, the patient becomes unresponsive to painful stimuli, reflexes disappear, and there is a gradual depression of the respiratory rate; eventually cardiovascular collapse ensues. Pupillary size is not changed by barbiturate intoxication, but secondary anoxia may cause fixed, dilated pupils. In persons who have adequate respiratory function, pin-point pupils usually indicate an opiate overdose or the combined ingestion of barbiturates and opiates. Such patients should be observed carefully for increased lethargy and for progressive respiratory depression. Appropriate measures for treating overdoses should be instituted as necessary. Patients should not be left unattended until all signs of intoxication have cleared.

Because there is no cross-tolerance between narcotics and barbiturates, special problems are presented by patients receiving methadone or buprenorphine maintenance who continue to abuse sedative-hypnotics. If a barbiturate overdose is suspected, the opiate-dependent patient should be given a narcotic antagonist to counteract any respiratory depression caused by the opiate. Naloxone hydrochloride (Narcan) 0.4 mg is given IM or IV because it is a pure narcotic antagonist and it has no respiratory depressant effect, even in large doses. If respiratory depression does not improve after treatment with naloxone, the patient should be treated for a pure barbiturate overdose. Supportive measures include maintenance of adequate airway, mechanic ventilation, alkalinization of the urine, correction of acid–base disorders, and diuresis with furosemide or mannitol. Severe overdose cases may require dialysis or charcoal resin hemoperfusion.[30]

Withdrawal

Withdrawal from sedative-hypnotics can present with a wide variety of signs and symptoms (including anxiety, insomnia, hyperreflexia, diaphoresis, nausea, and vomiting), or sometimes delirium and convulsions. As a general rule, individuals who ingest 600 to 800 mg/day of secobarbital for more than 45 days develop physiological addiction and show symptoms after taper or discontinuation. Minor withdrawal symptoms usually begin within 24–36 hours after the last dose. Pulse and respiration rates are usually elevated, pupil size is normal, and there may be postural hypotension. Fever may develop, and dangerous hyperpyrexia can occur in severe cases. Major withdrawal symptoms (such as convulsions and delirium) indicate addiction to large doses (more than 900 mg/day of secobarbital).

Because of the danger of convulsions, barbiturate withdrawal should be carried out only on an inpatient basis. Grand mal seizures, if they occur, are usually seen between the third and seventh days, although there have been cases reported of convulsions occurring as late as 14 days after the completion of a medically controlled detoxification. Withdrawal seizures are thought to be related to a rapid drop in the blood barbiturate level. Treatment should therefore be carefully controlled so that barbiturates are withdrawn gradually, with minimal fluctuation in the blood barbiturate level. Theoretically, this should decrease the danger of convulsions. Treatment with phenytoin does not prevent convulsions caused by barbiturate

withdrawal, although it controls convulsions caused by epilepsy.

Withdrawal delirium occurs less frequently than do convulsions, and it rarely appears unless preceded by convulsions. It usually begins between the fourth and sixth days after drug use is stopped and is characterized by both visual and auditory hallucinations, delusions, and fluctuating level of consciousness. The presence of confusion, hyperreflexia, and fever helps distinguish this syndrome from schizophrenia and other nontoxic psychoses.

Treatment for Withdrawal

Several techniques are available for the management of barbiturate withdrawal. The basic principle is to withdraw the addicting agent slowly to avoid convulsions. First, the daily dosage that produces mild toxicity must be established. Because barbiturate addicts tend to underestimate their drug use, it is dangerous to accept the patient's history as completely accurate. Treatment should begin with an oral test dose of 200 mg of pentobarbital, a short-acting barbiturate. If no physical changes occur after 1 hour, the patient's habit probably exceeds 1,200 mg of pentobarbital per day. If the patient shows only nystagmus and no other signs of intoxication, the habit is probably about 800 mg/day. Evidence of slurred speech and intoxication, but not sleep, suggests a habit of 400 to 600 mg/day. The patient can then be given the estimated daily requirement divided into four equal doses administered orally every 6 hours. Should signs of withdrawal appear, the estimated daily dosage can be increased by 25% following an additional dose of 200 mg of pentobarbital given intramuscularly. After a daily dose that produces only mild toxicity has been established, phenobarbital is substituted for pentobarbital (30 mg phenobarbital equals 100 mg pentobarbital) and then withdrawn at a rate of 30 to 60 mg/day[34] (Table 27-3).

The long-acting barbiturate phenobarbital is the drug of choice for managing detoxification for drugs in this class. Cross-tolerance with benzodiazepines is incomplete. A dose of 30 mg of phenobarbital can be substituted for each 100 mg of other barbiturates, or 200 mg of meprobamate or 400 mg of carisoprodol (Soma). An alternative method is to treat emerging withdrawal symptoms orally with 30 to 60 mg of phenobarbital hourly, as needed, for 2–7 days. After the patient has received similar 24-hour doses for 2 consecutive days, the 24-hour stabilizing dose is given in divided doses every 3 to 6 hours. A gradual taper is then instituted as described previously. This latter method is recommended because the use of a long-acting barbiturate produces fewer variations in the blood barbiturate level and should produce a smoother withdrawal.

TABLE 27-3 Equivalent Doses of Common Sedative-Hypnotics

Generic Name	Dose (mg)
BARBITURATES	
Phenobarbital	30
Secobarbital	100
Pentobarbital	100
BENZODIAZEPINES	
Alprazolam	1
Diazepam	10
Chlordiazepoxide	25
Lorazepam	2
Clonazepam	0.5–1
OTHERS	
Meprobamate	400

Inpatient Management and Referral

Those addicted to sedative-hypnotic drugs can present with a variety of psychological management problems. Effective treatment requires a thorough evaluation of the patient's psychiatric problems and the development of long-term treatment plans before discharge. Treatment for withdrawal or overdose presents an opportunity for effective intervention for the addict's self-destructive lifestyle. Drug abuse patients have a reputation for deceit, manipulation, and hostility. They frequently sign out against medical advice. It is rarely acknowledged that these problems are sometimes caused by clinicians who fail to give appropriate attention to the patient's psychological problems. Most of these difficulties can be eliminated by effective medical and psychiatric management. The patient's lack of cooperation and frequent demands for additional drugs are often the result of anxiety and the fear of withdrawal seizures. This anxiety is greatly relieved if the physician thoroughly explains the withdrawal procedure and assures the patient that the staff members know how to handle withdrawal and that convulsions will be avoided if the patient cooperates with a schedule of medically supervised withdrawal.

Physicians sometimes fail to realize that the patient's tough, demanding behavior is a defense against a strong sense of personal inadequacy and a fear of rejection. Addicts have been conditioned to expect rejection and hostility from medical personnel. The trust and cooperation necessary for successful treatment cannot be established unless physicians show by their behavior that they are both genuinely concerned about the patient and medically competent to treat withdrawal. Physicians can expect an initial period of defensive hostility and testing behavior and should not take this behavior personally. Patients need to be reassured that their physician is sincerely concerned about them.

If the patient manifests signs of a character disorder and has a history of severe drug abuse, the setting of firm limits is necessary to ensure successful treatment. Visitors must be limited to those individuals of known reliability. This may mean excluding spouses and other relatives. Urine should be monitored periodically for use of illicit drugs. Family counseling should be started during hospitalization and should focus on the family's role in helping the patient develop a successful long-term treatment program. Hospital passes should not be granted until detoxification is completed; however, passes with staff members as escorts should be used as much as possible. An active program of recreational and physical therapy is necessary to keep young, easily-bored patients occupied. Keys to successful inpatient treatment are summarized in Box 27-4.

BOX 27-4 Inpatient Management and Referral: Keys to Successful Inpatient Treatment

- Perform a psychiatric evaluation
- Develop a long-term treatment plan
- Demonstrate explicit concern and expertise
- Expect testing behavior
- Set appropriate limits
- Limit and monitor visitors
- Supervise passes
- Monitor urine for illicit drug use
- Encourage ward activities and recreation
- Initiate family/network therapy
- Treat with respect

Because treatment for detoxification or for an overdose rarely cures an addict, referrals for long-term outpatient or residential care should be made early in the treatment process. Ideally, the patient should meet the future therapist before discharge. Alcoholics Anonymous and Narcotics Anonymous are useful adjuncts to any outpatient treatment program. If transferring to a halfway house or residential program, the patient should move there directly from the hospital. Addicts are not likely to execute plans for follow-up care without strong encouragement and support.

Bath Salts

Since 2010 there has been a rapid increase in the number of reports of the abuse of various synthetic derivatives of methcathinone, either mephedrone or methylenedioxypyrovalerone (MDPV).[35] These compounds are DEA schedule I substances that are considered illegal only if intended for human consumption. Typically they have been sold legally and labeled "plant food or bath salts, not for human consumption," though it is apparent that they were never intended for use as bath salts. In 2011, the DEA, using its emergency scheduling authority, made sale and possession of these substances illegal in the US. These substances are derived from Khat (or qat; *Catha edulis*), a flowering plant from East Africa. They contain cathione, an amphetamine analogue and they have been chewed in some African cultures for centuries. Recently, cathinone has been isolated from the Khat plant and has been transformed into the more potent methcathinone (ephedrine).[36] It is sold as a white or tan crystalline powder that can be ingested orally, or administered nasally, rectally, IM, or IV. The average dose is 5 to 20 mg; psychoactive effects begin at 3 to 5 mg. The typical package contains 500 mg, thus creating a high risk for overdose. Consumption increases intracellular dopamine and serotonin by their effects on dopamine and serotonin reuptake transporters. Prolonged exposure leads to addictive patterns of use. Subjective effects include euphoria, empathic mood, sexual stimulation, greater mental focus, and enhanced energy (users typically report feelings similar to those produced by MDMA). The peak "rush" occurs at 90 minutes, with effects lasting for 3–4 hours. The total experience lasts for 6–8 hours and it is often followed by a crash. More intense psychic effects can include panic attacks, agitation, paranoia, hallucinations, psychosis, and aggressive, violent, or bizarre self-destructive behavior; use may also lead to anorexia, delirium, and depression. Physical effects included tachycardia, hypertension, mydriasis, arrhythmias, hyperthermia, sweating, rhabdomyolysis, seizures, stroke, cerebral edema, myocardial infarction, cardiovascular collapse, and death. The differential diagnosis includes abuse of cocaine, amphetamines, LSD or PCP, as well as serotonin syndrome, neuroleptic malignant syndrome, or anticholinergic toxicity. Bath salts will not be detected by routine toxic screens. Clinical management usually involves benzodiazepines for acute agitation; antipsychotics should be used with caution because of the risk of rhabdomyolysis, arrhythmias, seizures, and NMS. Cardiac monitoring, and IV fluids are recommended; autonomic instability may require monitoring in an ICU.

MIXED-DRUG ADDICTION

Increasing numbers of patients are addicted to varying combinations of drugs, including benzodiazepines, cocaine, alcohol, and opiates. Accurate diagnosis is difficult because of confusing, inconsistent physical findings and unreliable histories. Blood and urine tests for drugs are required to confirm the diagnosis. A patient who is addicted to both opiates and sedative-hypnotics should be maintained on

TABLE 27-4 Equivalent Doses of Narcotic Pain Medications

Generic Name	Parenteral Dose (mg)
Morphine	10
Oxycodone (Percocet, OxyContin)	5–10
Hydrocodone (Vicodin, Lortab)	10
Meperidine (Demerol)	100
Hydromorphone (Dilaudid)	2.5
Methadone	5
Heroin	10

methadone or buprenorphine while the barbiturate or other sedative-hypnotic is withdrawn. Then the methadone or buprenorphine can be withdrawn in the usual manner. Dose equivalents of narcotics are provided in Table 27-4.

Behavioral problems should be dealt with as previously described. Firm limit-setting is essential to the success of any effective psychological treatment program. Some patients who overdose or have medical problems secondary to drug abuse (such as subacute bacterial endocarditis and hepatitis) are not physiologically addicted to any drug despite a history of multiple-drug abuse. Their drug abuse behavior is usually associated with severe psychopathology. These patients should receive a thorough psychiatric evaluation and may require long-term treatment.

Access a list of MCQs for this chapter at https://expertconsult .inkling.com

REFERENCES

1. O'Brien CP, McLellan AT. Myths about the treatment of addiction. *Lancet* 347:237–240, 1996.
2. Substance Abuse and Mental Health Services Administration. *Results from the 2011 National Survey on Drug Use and Health: Summary of National Findings*, NSDUH Series H-44, HHS Publication No. (SMA) 12-4713, Rockville, MD, 2012, Substance Abuse and Mental Health Services Administration.
3. Substance Abuse and Mental Health Services Administration. *Drug Abuse Warning Network, 2011: National Estimates of Drug-Related Emergency Department Visits*, HHS Publication No. (SMA) 13-4760, DAWN Series D-39, Rockville, MD, 2013, Substance Abuse and Mental Health Services Administration.
4. Boscarino J, Rukstalis M, Hoffman S. Prevalence of prescription opioid-use disorder among chronic pain patients: Comparison of the DSM-5 vs. DSM-4 diagnostic criteria. *J Addict Dis* 30(3):185–194, 2011.
5. Volkow ND, Fowler JS, Wang GJ. The addicted human brain: insights from imaging studies. *J Clin Invest* 111:1444–1451, 2003.
6. Gawin F, Kleber H. Abstinence symptomatology and psychiatric diagnosis in cocaine abusers. *Arch Gen Psychiatry* 43:107–113, 1986.
7. Carroll KM. Relapse prevention as a psychosocial treatment approach: a review of controlled clinical trials. *Exp Clin Psychopharmacol* 4:46–54, 1996.
8. American Psychiatric Association. Practice guidelines: treatment of patients with substance use disorders. *Am J Psychiatry* 163(Suppl.):8, 2006.
9. Johnston LD, O'Malley PM, Bachman JG, et al. *Monitoring the Future national results on drug use: 2012 Overview, Key Findings on Adolescent Drug Use*, Ann Arbor, 2013, Institute for Social Research, The University of Michigan.
10. Centers for Disease Control and Prevention. Reported US AIDS cases by HIV-exposure category—1994. *MMWR* 44:4, 1995.
11. Substance Abuse and Mental Health Services Administration, Center for Behavioral Health Statistics and Quality. *Drug Abuse Warning Network, 2008: National Estimates of Drug-Related Emergency Department Visits*, HHS Publication No. SMA 11-4618, Rockville, MD, 2011, HHS.
12. CDC. Vital Signs: Overdoses of Prescription Opioid Pain Relievers—United States, 1999–2008. *MMWR* 60:1–6, 2011.
13. American Psychiatric Association. *Diagnostic and statistical manual of mental disorders*, ed 5, Washington, DC, 2013, American Psychiatric Association.
14. Ling W, Charuvastra C, Collins JF, et al. Buprenorphine maintenance treatment of opiate dependence: a multicenter, randomized clinical trial. *Addiction* 93:475–486, 1998.
15. Ball JC, Ross A. *The effectiveness of methadone maintenance treatment*, New York, 1991, Springer-Verlag.
16. US Department of Health and Human Services, Substance Abuse and Mental Health Services Administration, Center for Substance Abuse Treatment. *Evaluation of the buprenorphine waiver program*, Presented at American Society of Addiction Medicine. San Diego, May 5, 2006.
17. Fultz JM, Senay EC. Guidelines for the management of hospitalized narcotics addicts. *Ann Intern Med* 82:815–818, 1975.
18. Charney DS, Sternberg DE, Kleber HD, et al. The clinical use of clonidine in abrupt withdrawal from methadone. *Arch Gen Psychiatry* 38:1273–1277, 1981.
19. Jaffe JH, Kleber HD. Opioids: general issues and detoxification. In American Psychiatric Association: *Treatment of psychiatric disorders: a task force report of the American Psychiatric Association*, vol. 2, Washington, DC, 1989, American Psychiatric Association.
20. Fingerhood MI, Thompson MR, Jasinski DR. A comparison of clonidine and buprenorphine in the outpatient treatment of opiate withdrawal. *Subst Abus* 22:193–199, 2001.
21. O'Connor PG, Waugh ME, Carrol KM, et al. Primary care-based ambulatory opioid detoxification. *J Gen Intern Med* 10:255–260, 1995.
22. Golden SA, Sakhrani DL. Unexpected delirium during rapid opioid detoxification (ROD). *Addict Dis* 23(1):65–75, 2004.
23. Legarda JJ, Gossop M. A 24-h inpatient detoxification treatment for heroin addicts: a preliminary investigation. *Drug Alcohol Depend* 35:91–95, 1994.
24. Code of Federal Regulations, Chapter II, Drug Enforcement Administration, Department of Justice (4-1-04 Edition). § 1306.07 Administering or dispensing of narcotic drugs.
25. Alford DP, Compton P, Samet JH. Acute pain management for patients receiving maintenance methadone or buprenorphine therapy. *Ann Intern Med* 144:127–134, 2006.
26. Massachusetts Department of Public Health (MDPH). Overdose Education and Naloxone Distribution (OEND) Program Data, 2011.
27. Ciraulo D, Sands B, Shader R. Critical review of liability for benzodiazepine abuse among alcoholics. *Am J Psychiatry* 145:1501–1506, 1988.
28. Ross HE. Benzodiazepine use and anxiolytic abuse and dependence in treated alcoholics. *Addiction* 88:209–218, 1993.
29. Weinbroum A, Halpern P, Geller E. The use of flumazenil in the management of acute drug poisoning: a review. *Intensive Care Med* 17(Suppl. 1):S32–S38, 1991.
30. Wiviott SD, Wiviott-Tishler L, Hyman SE. Sedative-hypnotics and anxiolytics. In Friedman L, Fleming NF, Roberts DH, et al., editors: *Source book of substance abuse and addiction*, Baltimore, 1996, Williams & Wilkins.
31. Herman JB, Rosenbaum JF, Brotman AN. The alprazolam to clonazepam switch for the treatment of panic disorder. *J Clin Psychopharmacol* 7:175–178, 1987.
32. Patterson JF. Withdrawal from alprazolam dependency using clonazepam: clinical observations. *J Clin Psychiatry* 51:47–49, 1990.
33. SAMHSA, Center For Behavioral Health Statistics and Quality. The Dawn Report. *Emergency department visits for adverse reactions involving the insomnia medication Zolpidem*, Rockville, MD, 2013, SAMHSA.
34. Smith DE, Wesson DR. Phenobarbital technique for treatment of barbiturate dependence. *Arch Gen Psychiatry* 24:56–60, 1971.
35. Ross EA, Watson M, Goldberger B. "Bath salts" intoxication. *N Engl J Med* 365(10):967–968, 2011.
36. Coppola M, Mondola R. Synthetic cathinones: Chemistry, pharmacology and toxicology of a new class of designer drugs of abuse marketed as "bath salts" or "plant food". *Toxicol Lett* 211(2):144–149, 2012.
37. Syed YY, Keating GM. Extended-release intramuscular naltrexone (VIVITROL®): a review of its use in the prevention of relapse to opioid dependence in detoxified patients. *CNS Drugs* 27(10):851–861, 2013.

SUGGESTED READING

Carroll KM. *A cognitive-behavioral approach: treating cocaine addiction. NIDA therapy manuals for drug addiction series (DHHS pub no ADM 98–4308)*, Rockville, MD, 1998, National Institute on Drug Abuse.

Galanter M, Kleber HD, editors: *The American Psychiatric Publishing textbook of substance abuse treatment*, ed 3, Washington, DC, 2004, American Psychiatric Publishing, Inc.

Graham AW, Schultz TK, Mayo-Smith MF, et al., editors: *Principles of addiction medicine*, ed 3, Chevy Chase, MD, 2007, American Society of Addiction Medicine.

Kranzler HR, Ciraulo DA. *Clinical manual of addiction psychopharmacology*, Washington, DC, 2005, American Psychiatric Publishing, Inc.

McNicholas L, Howell EF. *Buprenorphine clinical practice guidelines*, Rockville, MD, 2000, Substance Abuse Mental Health Services Administration, Center for Substance Abuse Treatment. Available at: <http://www.buprenorphine.samhsa.gov>.

Miller WR, Rollnick S. *Motivational interviewing: preparing people for change*, ed 2, New York, 2002, Guilford Press.

Smith DE, Wesson DR. *Diagnosis and treatment of adverse reactions to sedative-hypnotics*, (DHHS pub no ADM 75–144), Rockville, MD, 1974, National Institute on Drug Abuse.

28 Psychosis and Schizophrenia

Oliver Freudenreich, MD, Hannah E. Brown, MD, and Daphne J. Holt, MD, PhD

KEY POINTS

- Schizophrenia is a clinical diagnosis that is based on a combination of characteristic symptoms of sufficient severity (in the absence of other factors that would account for them) that typically begins in adolescence or early adulthood.

- Even if it is successfully treated, function often remains impaired; moreover, there is a high risk of recurrence of psychotic symptoms.

- In addition to psychosis, patients with schizophrenia experience cognitive and negative symptoms, both of which are main contributors to poor psychosocial functioning.

- Schizophrenia is a complex genetic disease; its expression depends on multiple common susceptibility genes with small effects, or rare ones with large effects, that interact with environmental insults. Some of these insults may occur during *in utero* brain development.

- Brain-tissue volumes are on average lower in people with schizophrenia compared to healthy people of a similar age. Studies of pathology have found subtle abnormalities in inter-neurons and pyramidal cells in cortical regions, with loss of neuropil (i.e., atrophy) but no loss of cells.

- Schizophrenia can be viewed as a disorder of brain connectivity where the coordinated coupling of brain activity among regions within large-scale brain networks appears to be disrupted.

- Antipsychotic medications are the mainstay of treatment for schizophrenia; they are most effective in the treatment of acute psychosis and the prevention of relapse.

- Since schizophrenia is a chronic illness, rehabilitation that focuses on optimization of work and social function is as important as symptom control.

- The prognosis of schizophrenia varies from complete recovery (after a period of acute illness) to severe, ongoing symptoms that require institutionalization. For most patients, having schizophrenia means living in the community (and not in an asylum) with some degree of residual symptoms.

- Prevention of suicide and prevention of morbidity and mortality associated with antipsychotic medications, particularly cardiovascular disease, are important goals of management.

OVERVIEW

Psychosis, in a broad sense, signifies impaired reality-testing ability. The most important symptoms of psychosis are delusions and hallucinations, although other signs and symptoms (such as disorganized speech or behavior and catatonia) are also considered psychotic phenomena.

Psychosis is not a specific diagnosis, because it can occur in a wide variety of clinical contexts. Of the psychotic disorders, the prototypical condition is schizophrenia. In schizophrenia, psychotic symptoms occur chronically, without gross organic abnormalities of the brain (hence the term *functional psychosis*) or a severe medical disturbance (as in a delirium). Moreover, psychosis may occur when the mood is normal, thus differentiating it from bipolar disorder or from psychotic depression. While psychosis is a defining (and often the most apparent) clinical feature of schizophrenia, other symptom clusters (e.g., negative symptoms and cognitive symptoms) are largely responsible for the psychosocial disability that usually accompanies this disorder.

Schizophrenia was originally described at the close of the nineteenth century by Emil Kraepelin (who categorized madness into episodic mood disorders and chronic psychotic illnesses; he termed the latter *dementia praecox*, which was later renamed *schizophrenia* by Eugen Bleuler). In the 100 years since the condition was identified, much progress has been made (in large part the result of the discovery of the first antipsychotic, chlorpromazine), turning schizophrenia from an illness treated in asylums (state hospitals) to one treated in community settings (Figure 28-1).[1] The discovery that genetic risk factors are shared between schizophrenia and manic-depressive illness, i.e., bipolar disorder (as well as other psychiatric syndrome),[2] might eventually lead to a new nosology based on genetics and pathophysiology. In the interim, the fundamental Kraepelinian dichotomy between schizophrenia (and related psychotic disorders) and bipolar disorder remains a cornerstone in psychiatric diagnosis.

EPIDEMIOLOGY AND RISK FACTORS

Schizophrenia is a syndrome that occurs in all cultures and in all parts of the world. Epidemiological studies have found incidence rates between 7.7 and 43.0 (median 15.2) new cases per 100,000.[3,4] The point prevalence is approximately 5 per 1,000 and the life-time morbidity risk is approximately 1%. The mortality rate is 2.5 times that of the general population, and this mortality gap continues to grow.[5] Gender differences also exist; men have a 30%–40% higher life-time risk for schizophrenia than women,[6] and the age of onset is roughly 3–4 years later for females.[7]

The old dogma that cited the identical incidence and prevalence rates of schizophrenia around the globe is not quite correct. Clear geographical differences exist, albeit within a fairly narrow range of twofold to threefold differences. The fact that these modest variations in rates exist between cultures, and within subgroups in cultures, likely reflects different risk factors for schizophrenia in different populations (e.g., more infections in one setting, more drug use in another).

The best-established risk factors are not genetic, but environmental (Box 28-1). Immigrant populations have an increased risk,[8] with the highest risks for the children of first-generation immigrants, followed by the immigrants themselves.[9] Urban living increases risk relative to rural living.[10] Etiological insults during brain development include intra-uterine infections, particularly influenza after exposure during the first half of pregnancy,[11] and nutritional deficiencies,

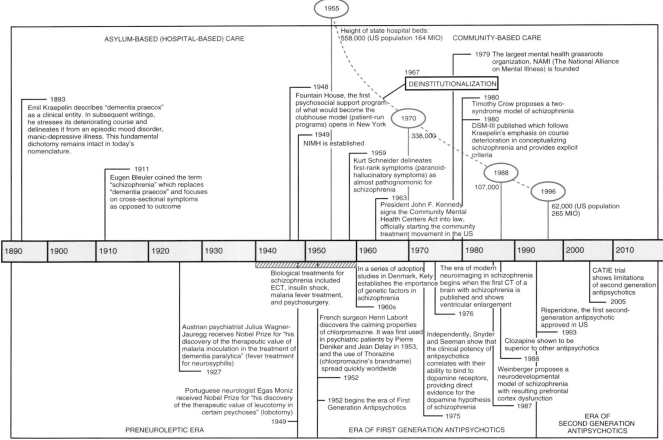

Figure 28-1. Timeline of 100 years of schizophrenia in the United States. *(From Shorter E. A history of psychiatry: from the era of the asylum to the age of Prozac, New York, 1997, John Wiley & Sons; Geller JL. The last half-century of psychiatric services as reflected in psychiatric services,* Psychiatr Serv *51:41–67, 2000.)*

BOX 28-1 Risk Factors for Schizophrenia

NON-GENETIC (ENVIRONMENTAL)
- Prenatal infection (e.g., rubella, influenza, *Toxoplasma gondii*) and starvation
- Obstetric complications (e.g., Rh incompatibility, preeclampsia, hypoxia)
- Season of birth (winter birth)
- Place of birth (urban)
- Immigration
- Head injury
- Drug use (e.g., LSD, cannabis, amphetamines)

GENETIC
- Family history (first- and second-degree relatives)
- Paternal age
- Genetic syndromes (e.g., VCFS, Klinefelter syndrome)
- Specific susceptibility genes (see Table 28-1)

VCFS, Velo-cardio-facial syndrome.

---

including low maternal folate and elevated homocysteine levels.[12,13] Maternal starvation has strong support from two epidemiological studies of famines (the Dutch Hunger winter of 1944–1945[14] and the 1959–1961 Chinese famine[15]). Both studies found a doubling of risk for schizophrenia in offspring of mothers who starved during the first trimester. Other early environmental risk factors include obstetrical complications.[16] Later environmental risk factors are head injury[17] and substance use (particularly cannabis).[18] Frequent pre-morbid cannabis use (i.e., more than 50 uses) increases the risk for the development of schizophrenia by sixfold.[19]

The majority of patients with schizophrenia lack a family history of the disorder. Nevertheless, the fact that genes matter was shown in now-classic twin and adoption studies of the 1960s. For monozygotic twins, the risk of developing schizophrenia approaches 50% for the unaffected twin if the co-twin has schizophrenia. Having siblings or parents (i.e., first-degree relatives) with schizophrenia increases an individual's risk to approximately 10-fold above that seen in the general population. With greater genetic distance, the risk for schizophrenia decreases to a twofold risk over the population risk for second-degree relatives.[20]

Paternal age increases the risk for schizophrenia in a linear fashion. Compared with the children of fathers who are less than 25 years old the relative risk for children increases steadily with paternal age, to about 2.0 for fathers in the 45 to 49 age group, and to almost 3.0 for fathers older than age 50.[21] This increase in risk with paternal age is consistent with the hypothesis that *de novo* mutations contribute to the genetic risk in schizophrenia.[22] New mutations could explain why a disorder associated with lower fertility rates has not disappeared; in men as opposed to women, the germ-line cells, spermatogonia, continue to divide throughout life, allowing replication errors to accumulate and to be transmitted to offspring.

TABLE 28-1 Examples of Susceptibility Genes for Schizophrenia

Gene	Gene Function/Biological Role
NRG1 (Neuregulin 1)	Growth factor with pleomorphic role in brain development and function
Dysbindin or DTNBP1 (dystrobrevin binding protein 1)	Associated with negative symptoms; involved in synaptic function
DISC1 (disrupted in schizophrenia 1)	Interacts with key proteins in signaling pathways and neuronal migration
RGS4 (regulator of G-protein signaling 4)	Modulator of intracellular signaling for G-protein coupled receptor, including the dopamine receptor
GRM3 (metabotropic glutamate receptor type 3 gene)	Involved in glutamatergic neurotransmission and prefrontal function
G72 (G72/G30 gene complex)	Indirectly affects glutamatergic neurotransmission, possibly via interaction with D-amino acid oxidase (DAAO)
CACNA1C (L-type voltage gated alpha 1c subunit)	Calcium channel, mediates influx of calcium ions into cells
ZNF804A (zinc finger transcription factor)	Up-regulates COMT, down-regulates D_2 receptors, affects neuronal connectivity in dorsolateral prefrontal cortex
MIR 137 (microRNA)	Post-trancriptional regulator of messenger RNA
MTHFR	Key enzyme of folate metabolism
HLA-DQB1	Immune system gene

Gene selection based on Zhang J-P, Malhotra AK: Genetics of schizophrenia: what do we know?, Curr Psychiatry 12(3):25–33, 2013.

It is unlikely that a single gene with a significantly large effect will be found that can cause schizophrenia. Most likely, schizophrenia is similar to other non-Mendelian complex disorders where many different common variants of genes each make a small, yet important, contribution to disease vulnerability, or occasionally rarer variants of genes make larger contributions. Such vulnerability gene variants convey susceptibility without directly causing the disease: the disease is only expressed when combined with other genes or certain environmental factors (e.g., infection or drug use). The number of susceptibility genes is unknown; however, many genes can confer risk in a population. Since 2007 when the first genome-wide association studies (GWAS) in schizophrenia was published, GWAS of increasingly larger sample sizes have added susceptibility genes that confer risk for schizophrenia (for a partial list, see Table 28-1).[23] The most promising candidate genes are involved in brain development, frontal lobe function, myelination, synaptic function, and glutamate transmission. Moreover, it appears likely that most gene variants are not specific for schizophrenia; instead, they confer risk for neuropsychiatric disorders that cut across current clinical diagnoses.[2] Several genetic disorders, such as 22q11 deletion syndrome (velo-cardio-facial syndrome [VCFS] or DiGeorge syndrome) or Klinefelter syndrome (XXY syndrome), increase the risk for psychosis in affected individuals.[24,25] In addition, rare structural variants, including microdeletions and microduplications (copy number variants, or CNVs), may also contribute to the illness pathophysiology by disrupting signaling pathways important in neurodevelopment.[26] An interaction between susceptibility genes and environment forms the basis for the neurodevelopmental hypothesis of schizophrenia in which a clinically silent, latent propensity toward schizophrenia (e.g., a genetic vulnerability or insult during brain development, such as intrauterine infections or maternal starvation) gets uncovered when the brain matures (e.g., during the naturally occurring pruning of excessive synapses) or additional insults (e.g., cannabis use) push a vulnerable brain toward psychosis.[27] Since the clinical picture (phenotype) is not solely determined by the gene sequence (genotype), but rather by which genes are expressed (the epigenotype), some gene–environment interactions may occur via epigenetic modifications of the genome. Functionally, a disruption of coordinated activity among regions within (and between) several, distinct networks in the brain has been suggested to account for the emergence of clinical symptoms in this developmental model.

PATHOPHYSIOLOGY

Evidence from neurochemistry, cellular neuropathology, and neuroimaging studies supports the idea that schizophrenia is a brain disease: that is, a disease manifest by abnormalities in brain structure, brain function, or both. The observed abnormalities are, thus far, of limited specificity and sensitivity, and have therefore not yet had clinical relevance for diagnosis and treatment, and are of only limited value in prognostication. Furthermore, there is no single universally accepted theory regarding the brain dysfunction seen in schizophrenia, but rather there are a host of competing and overlapping models.

Neurochemical Changes

The idea that an imbalance in internal chemistry may result in insanity (a notion prevalent since the humoral theories of antiquity) found a modern expression in the "dopamine hypothesis" of schizophrenia.[28] The dopamine hypothesis was built on two pillars of evidence: (1) amphetamines, known dopamine receptor agonists, can produce a schizophrenia-like state in healthy adults; and (2) the discovery that the antipsychotic effect of the phenothiazines was associated with their ability to block the D_2 dopamine receptor. Further work established the tight relationship between the clinical potency of antipsychotic medications and their affinity for D_2 receptors. This confluence of findings suggested that schizophrenia was associated with a hyperdopaminergic state in the mesolimbic system, ameliorated through the use of antipsychotic medication. Modern neuroimaging approaches (such as positron emission tomography [PET] and single-photon emission computed tomography [SPECT]) have directly demonstrated heightened dopamine synthesis and presynaptic release in patients with schizophrenia.[29] Studies have also found alterations in dopamine neurotransmission in people with genetic or clinical risk for schizophrenia—those with a first-degree relative with schizophrenia or with subthreshold psychotic symptoms.[30] Elevated synthesis of dopamine in people who are at risk for schizophrenia may be predictive of the later development of psychosis.[31]

While the dopamine hypothesis remains central to our understanding of the therapeutic action of antipsychotics, hyperdopaminergia seems to explain only the psychotic aspect of schizophrenia.[32] To account for the lack of therapeutic action of antidopaminergic drugs on other symptom clusters of schizophrenia, particularly negative and cognitive symptoms, a hypodopaminergic state was postulated in which there is a lack of stimulation of prefrontal D_1 receptors.[33] In addition, models for schizophrenia involving neurotransmitter systems other than dopamine have been proffered. The impetus for a "glutamate hypothesis" of schizophrenia (with hypofunction of the glutamate system) stems largely from the psychosis-inducing effects of two glutamate antagonists, phencyclidine (PCP) and ketamine.[34] Given the ubiquity of

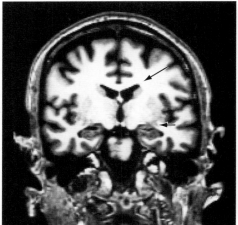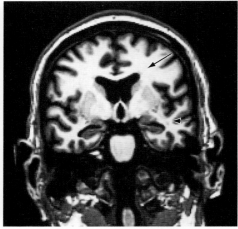

Figure 28-2. MRI of enlarged ventricle in schizophrenia. Example of ventriculomegaly in a patient with schizophrenia. High-resolution magnetic resonance images from a 42-year-old man without mental illness *(left)* and a 46-year-old man diagnosed with schizophrenia *(right)*. Note the expanded volume of both the body *(long arrow)* and temporal horn *(short arrow)* of the lateral ventricle, the latter finding suggestive of hippocampal atrophy.

N-methyl-D-aspartate (NMDA) receptors in the brain and the link between NMDA hyperactivity and excitotoxity, simply enhancing glutamate release to treat schizophrenia is not feasible; increasing activity at the glycine modulatory site on the NMDA receptor, or increasing activity at the glutamatergic alpha-amino-3-hydroxy-5-methylisoxazole-4-propionic acid (AMPA) receptors, has been pursued instead. Acetylcholine, particularly in its actions at intracerebral nicotine receptors, might be a neurotransmitter system target for the amelioration of cognitive deficits and negative symptoms.[35] This relates to the fact that a high percentage of patients with schizophrenia smoke tobacco,[36] consistent with a "self-medication" hypothesis regarding nicotine use. In addition, nicotine appears to have salutatory effects on attention and other cognitive domains know to be affected in these patients. Early work on the development of nicotinic-agonist treatments for schizophrenia is now underway.

Neurocellular Changes

While a unifying neuropathological explanation in the form of a schizophrenia-equivalent of the "plaques and tangles" of Alzheimer's dementia is currently absent (i.e., there is no evidence of neurodegeneration in the form of reactive gliosis), modern stereomorphometric research has uncovered a handful of more subtle abnormalities, primarily within the dorsolateral prefrontal cortex, anterior cingulate gyrus, thalamus, and medial temporal lobe. There is no clear loss of neurons; instead there is subtle disarray in cortical cytoarchitecture and a decreased volume of neuropil (composed of axodendritic processes, glia, and cerebral vasculature).[37,38] Abnormalities in the functioning of several types of cortical gamma amino butyric acid (GABA)-ergic inter-neurons have been described, which might represent compensatory responses to poorly functioning pyramidal cells,[39] or effects of abnormalities in NMDA receptor functioning,[40] and may lead to disrupted communication between emotion and memory centers.[41] Other studies conducted in post-mortem tissue that have measured the expression and downstream molecular effects of genetic variants linked to schizophrenia risk have begun to shed light on the affected neural circuitry and pathophysiological mechanism(s) underlying the risk associated with these genetic variants.[42,43]

Changes in Brain Structure

From the time the first human brain images were obtained, the size of the brain and its ventricular system in schizophrenia has been measured, first using the indirect method of pneumoencephalography, and later with computed tomography (CT) and magnetic resonance imaging (MRI). Soon after the CT became widely available, the landmark study of Johnstone and colleagues[44] revealed that patients with schizophrenia have larger ventricular volumes than demographically matched healthy control subjects. This finding, which has subsequently been replicated many times using MRI, has had a sustained impact on the field and the public perception of the disorder, because it provided the first incontrovertible, visually apparent evidence that schizophrenia is a disease of the brain (Figure 28-2). However, in the decades that followed that initial finding, it became clear that ventricular enlargement is neither specific nor sensitive enough to use as a diagnostic tool; there is a great deal of overlap between the distribution of ventricular sizes of patients with schizophrenia and healthy people (a person with schizophrenia can have ventricular volume well within the normal range). Also, the increase in ventricular volume found in schizophrenia is relatively diffuse (i.e., the entire ventricular system is somewhat affected). Thus, there is no clearly localizable change in brain structure associated with this abnormality.

Subsequent work has attempted to identify specific structural changes within the cerebral cortex and subcortical nuclei in patients with schizophrenia. Structural MRI studies have found abnormal reductions in regional brain volume or cortical thickness in a large number of areas in schizophrenia,[45,46] consistent with post-mortem findings of diminished volumes of cortical and subcortical regions, and increased pyramidal cell packing density.[38,47] For example, meta-analyses of volumetric analyses of imaging data indicate that, on average, hippocampal volumes are 4% smaller in patients with schizophrenia than in matched controls.[48] Other imaging techniques that measure the integrity of the fiber bundles of the brain, such as diffusion tensor imaging (DTI), have found changes in white matter tracts in schizophrenia,[49] suggesting that there may be molecular abnormalities affecting the fiber connections between brain regions in the disorder. Longitudinal imaging studies have found that, although progressive reductions in brain volume normally occur during human brain maturation, the rate of volume change (brain tissue loss) in patients with schizophrenia is more than twice that of healthy subjects.[50] Some of these volume changes might occur during the development of psychosis or during psychotic relapses,[51, 52] and some (including smaller volumes of the anterior cingulate, insular, temporal, parahippocampal cortices) may be present prior to the onset of the illness (during the prodromal state) and predict the later development of full-blown psychosis.[53] However, some of these progressive reductions in brain volume seen in patients with schizophrenia may represent effects of being in poorer physical health, smoking tobacco, or being treated with antipsychotic medication.[54] Distinguishing the changes in the brain that result from the life-style changes and treatments associated with having the illness from those related to the fundamental pathophysiology of schizophrenia remains a challenge for ongoing research.

Changes in Brain Function

Event-related electroencephalography (event-related potentials [ERPs]) and functional magnetic resonance imaging (fMRI) are two technologies used to examine brain function that have distinct advantages: ERPs have excellent temporal resolution, whereas fMRI has superior spatial (anatomical) resolution. Using ERPs, several abnormal physiological effects, sometimes called endophenotypes (if they are also seen in first-degree relatives and appear to be heritable), have been well replicated in patients with schizophrenia.[55] The P_{50}, for example, is an ERP waveform that measures the ability to suppress irrelevant information (sensory gating). The P_{50} is often attenuated in patients with schizophrenia, as well as in their clinically healthy relatives. This endophenotype is linked to genetic polymorphisms of the alpha$_7$ nicotinic receptor, a potential target of treatments for the cognitive deficits of schizophrenia.[56] Another measure of sensory gating, prepulse inhibition (PPI) has been linked to haploinsufficiency of the *Tbx1* gene. This gene is one of the affected genes in the 22q11 deletion syndrome that is associated with increased risk for schizophrenia.[57] Abnormalities in other ERP measurements, such as the P300[58] and "mismatch negativity"[59] have also been found consistently in patients with schizophrenia.

Functional neuroimaging studies have found that frontal cortical regions, including the dorsolateral prefrontal and anterior cingulate cortices, function abnormally in schizophrenia, consistent with the findings of reduced frontal volumes, and impairment in the cognitive domains (executive function, planning, task switching) subserved by these areas, in schizophrenia. However, the direction of findings has been variable; some studies have found reductions in prefrontal responses,[60] whereas other studies have found abnormal increases.[61] These discrepancies appear to depend on the level of difficulty of the cognitive task performed, suggesting that the prefrontal cortex in schizophrenia is in fact "inefficient" in its use of neural resources to execute cognitive tasks.[62] Abnormalities in the function of other regions, such as the hippocampus or lateral temporal or parietal cortex, which receive projections from the prefrontal cortex, has led to the proposal that distributed *networks* of regions (rather than one or two specific brain areas), as well as the connections among these regions, are disrupted in schizophrenia. Thus, whereas cognitive impairment in schizophrenia has been linked to dysfunction of regions known to mediate executive and memory processes, impaired emotional function in schizophrenia (e.g., abnormal assessments of emotional salience or meaning in psychotic states and the impaired motivation seen in patients with negative symptoms) has been linked to changes in networks involved in generating emotional responses and emotional learning and memory.[63-65] In addition, there is evidence for abnormalities in basic sensory processing in schizophrenia.[66,67] Thus, multiple domains of brain functioning are compromised in schizophrenia to varying extents, suggesting that one or more fundamental physiological process is disrupted across several networks.

The theoretical conceptualization of schizophrenia as a "disconnection syndrome"[68] has received recent support from studies of functional connectivity—an fMRI measure of the degree to which regions within a network exhibit coordinated (i.e., correlated) activity. This type of correlated activity or functional coupling within a network is thought to reflect in part the structural integrity of the associated anatomical connections.[69] Patients with schizophrenia exhibit widespread abnormalities (both increases and decreases compared to healthy subjects) in functional connectivity.[70-72] Functional connectivity changes in a frontotemporal circuit have also been found in healthy people and patients with schizophrenia who have a variant of a gene associated with schizophrenia risk.[73,74] Also, several studies have shown that a network that is more active during "resting" states (called the default mode network [see Chapter 72]), which includes the medial prefrontal, posterior cingulate, and lateral temporal-parietal cortices, as well as medial temporal lobe structures, may be disrupted early on in schizophrenia and in people with genetic risk factors for the disorder.[72,75] For example, Figure 28-3 shows that functional connectivity between two central nodes of the default mode network, the medial prefrontal and posterior cingulate cortices, which are each involved in self-referential thinking and other types of social cognition,[76] is markedly diminished in patients with schizophrenia, in comparison to demographically matched healthy control subjects. Future studies will determine the nature of the relationship between changes in functional and structural connectivity measures in schizophrenia and the underlying molecular mechanisms that give rise to these abnormalities.[77]

CLINICAL FEATURES AND DIAGNOSIS

The diagnosis of schizophrenia is made clinically, based on a typical combination of symptoms (present cross-sectionally and longitudinally), in the absence of other psychiatric or medical conditions that would explain the symptoms (see below). The exact number and combination of symptoms, as well as the required duration of symptoms to make a diagnosis of schizophrenia, differ depending on the classification system used (Table 28-2, see Box 28-2 for full DSM-5 diagnostic criteria). Making a diagnosis based on clinical symptomatology and course alone, without the help of genetic markers or biomarkers, can lead to different diagnoses over time (even in the same patient if the clinical picture changes).

Schizophrenia is a disorder with an onset in late adolescence or early adulthood. Most patients (80%) present with schizophrenia between 15 and 45 years of age. Onset during childhood or in late life is possible, but not common. Onset at the extremes of the age range shows continuity with typical-onset schizophrenia, although the onset of psychosis after age 50 should raise suspicion for a secondary psychosis (i.e., secondary to a non-psychiatric medical disorder).

The onset of schizophrenia can be acute (i.e., symptoms develop over a few days) or subacute (i.e., symptoms develop over a month), although a more insidious onset with signs of the illness beginning many months or even years before frank psychosis is usually seen (Figure 28-4). A non-specific prodromal phase can often be ascertained retrospectively. Prodromal symptoms include attenuated psychotic symptoms (e.g., suspiciousness, perceptual distortions, or perplexity), depression and suicidality, obsessive thinking, and sleep problems. Role

Reduced functional connectivity within the default mode network in schizophrenia

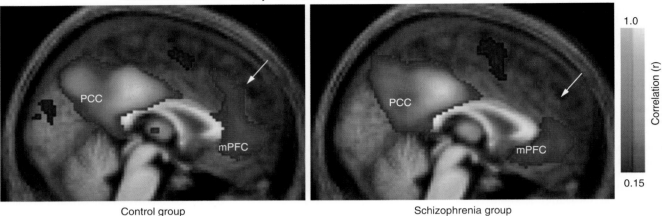

Control group   Schizophrenia group

Figure 28-3. fMRI data demonstrating reduced functional connectivity within the default mode network in schizophrenia. Sagittal views of maps of the average functional connectivity (Pearson's r values) of an area of the posterior cingulate cortex (PCC). In the control group (n = 19, map on the left), the PCC shows robust functional connectivity with the dorsal and ventral medial prefrontal cortex (mPFC). In contrast, in the schizophrenia group (n = 18), there is no connectivity between the PCC and the dorsal mPFC (the white arrows indicate the medial prefrontal area showing the greatest difference in connectivity between the two groups). The PCC and mPFC are two key nodes of the default mode network, which may be particularly affected in schizophrenia (see text). *(Adapted from Figure 2 of Holt DJ, Cassidy BS, Andrews-Hanna JR, et al. An anterior-to-posterior shift in midline cortical activity in schizophrenia during self-reflection, Biol Psychiatry 69(5):415–423, 2011.)*

TABLE 28-2 Key Diagnostic Features in Schizophrenia in DSM-5 and ICD-10

ICD-10	DSM-5
ACTIVE-PHASE SYMPTOMS	
One characteristic symptom from this list:	
Thought echo, insertion, withdrawal, broadcasting*	
Delusions of control, influence, passivity; delusional perception*	
Typical hallucinations (e.g., running commentary, conversing voices)*	
Culturally inappropriate and completely impossible delusions	
OR	
Two symptoms from this list:	*Two symptoms from this list (*one must be a psychotic symptom):*
Other hallucinations with delusions or overvalued ideas	Delusions*
	Hallucinations*
Significant formal thought disorder	Disorganized speech*
Catatonia	Grossly disorganized or catatonic behavior
Negative symptoms	Negative symptoms
DURATION OF SYMPTOMS	
1 month of acute symptoms	6 months of illness (<u>including prodrome</u>); 1 month of acute symptoms
FUNCTIONAL DECLINE	
Not required	Required
EXCLUSION CRITERIA	
Psychosis occurs only in presence of significant mood disorder	Schizoaffective disorder, depression with psychotic features, psychotic bipolar disorder
Alcohol- or drug-related psychosis	Substance use disorders
Organic brain disease	Medical conditions
	Pervasive developmental disorder (unless psychosis is prominent)
SUBTYPES	
Paranoid (mainly delusions and hallucinations)	No subtypes
Hebephrenic (prominent thought disorder)	
Catatonic	
Undifferentiated (syndromal but mixture)	
Residual (no syndromal symptom severity)	
Simple (insidious onset of only negative symptoms)	
Postschizophrenic depression	

(Based on Diagnostic and statistical manual of mental disorders. ed 5. Arlington, VA, 2013, American Psychiatric Association and World Health Organization. The ICD-10 classification of mental and behavioural disorders: diagnostic criteria for research. Geneva, 1993, World Health Organization.)
*These hallucinatory-paranoid symptoms are based on Schneiderian first-rank symptoms.

BOX 28-2 DSM-5 Diagnostic Criteria: Schizophrenia (295.90 (F20.9))

A. Two (or more) of the following, each present for a significant portion of time during a 1-month period (or less if successfully treated). At least one of these must be (1), (2), or (3):
   1. Delusions
   2. Hallucinations
   3. Disorganized speech (e.g., frequent derailment or incoherence)
   4. Grossly disorganized or catatonic behavior
   5. Negative symptoms (i.e., diminished emotional expression or avolition).
B. For a significant portion of the time since the onset of the disturbance, level of functioning in one or more major areas, such as work, interpersonal relations, or self-care, is markedly below the level achieved prior to the onset (or when the onset is in childhood or adolescence, there is failure to achieve expected level of interpersonal, academic or occupational functioning).
C. Continuous signs of the disturbance persist for at least 6 months. This 6-month period must include at least 1 month of symptoms (or less if successfully treated) that meet Criterion A (i.e., active-phase symptoms) and may include periods of prodromal or residual symptoms. During these prodromal or residual periods, the signs of the disturbance may be manifested by only negative symptoms or by two or more symptoms listed in Criterion A present in an attenuated form (e.g., odd beliefs, unusual perceptual experiences).
D. Schizoaffective disorder and depressive or bipolar disorder with psychotic features have been ruled out because either (1) no major depressive or manic episodes have occurred concurrently with the active-phase symptoms, or (2) if mood episodes have occurred during active-phase symptoms, they have been present for a minority of the total duration of the active and residual periods of the illness.
E. The disturbance is not attributable to the physiological effects of a substance (e.g., a drug of abuse, a medication) or another medical condition.

F. If there is a history of autism spectrum disorder or a communication disorder of childhood onset, the additional diagnosis of schizophrenia is made only if prominent delusions or hallucinations, in addition to the other required symptoms of schizophrenia, are also present for at least 1 month (or less if successfully treated).

Specify if:
The following course specifiers are only to be used after a 1-year duration of the disorder and if they are not in contradiction to the diagnostic course criteria:

First episode, currently in acute episode: First manifestation of the disorder meeting the defining diagnostic symptom and time criteria. An *acute episode* is a time period in which the symptom criteria are fulfilled.
First episode, currently in partial remission: *Partial remission* is a period of time during which an improvement after a previous episode is maintained and in which the defining criteria of the disorder are only partially fulfilled.
First episode, currently in remission: Full remission is a period of time after a previous episode during which no disorder-specific symptoms are present.
Multiple episodes, currently in acute episode: Multiple episodes may be determined after a minimum of two episodes (i.e., after a first episode, a remission and a minimum of one relapse).
Multiple episodes, currently in partial remission
Multiple episodes, currently in full remission
Continuous: Symptoms fulfilling the diagnostic symptom criteria of the disorder are remaining for the majority of the illness course, with subthreshold symptom periods being very brief relative to the overall course.
Unspecified.

Specify if:

With catatonia (refer to the criteria for catatonia associated with another mental disorder, pp. 119–120, for definition).

Reprinted with permission from Diagnostic and statistical manual of mental disorders. *ed 5. (Copyright 2013). American Psychiatric Association.*

---

failure and loss of social competence are typical features.[78] However, the progression to the full syndrome of schizophrenia for patients in a putative prodromal state (also referred to as "ultra-high risk state") is not inevitable, with average conversion rates of 18% after 6 months, 22% after 1 year, 29% after 2 years, and 36% after 3 years.[79] Notably, many help-seeking patients who do not convert to psychosis continue to experience mild symptoms and psychosocial difficulties.[80]

Unfortunately, even after the development of clear-cut psychosis, the patient and his or her family and friends often do not recognize it. Even when recognized, the affected individual often resists treatment. This results in untreated psychosis that lasts on average almost 2 years.[81] The duration of untreated illness, which includes the prodromal period and the duration of untreated psychosis (DUP), can last several years, and typically results in disrupted psychological and social development and impaired role function. A shorter DUP is associated with improved symptom-response to antipsychotics and less impairment in overall functioning and better quality of life.[82] The prodromal period is an area of active research, since the functional impairment and cognitive decline seen in schizophrenia occurs before the onset of psychosis and remains stable even after recovery from psychosis.[83] Exactly when the

cognitive decline begins remains uncertain, but early signs of the disturbance (as judged by scholastic records) point toward onset in middle school or even earlier, possibly with further worsening around the time of psychosis and with cumulative damage due to relapse.[52,84]

The hallmarks of acute schizophrenia are hallucinations and delusions, sometimes grouped together as positive symptoms. Hallucinations are perceptions without an external stimulus, and they can occur in any sensory modality (Box 28-3). However, by far the most common type of hallucination is auditory, occurring in at least two-thirds of patients over the course of their illness. Certain types of third-person (Schneiderian) hallucinations are frequently encountered: several voices talking about the patient, often in a derogatory way; a voice giving a running commentary on what the patient is doing; or a voice repeating what the patient is thinking. While hallucinations in other modalities are possible, visual or olfactory hallucinations in particular should raise the suspicion for an organic etiology of the hallucinations.

Delusions are false, non-culturally sanctioned beliefs that are held with great conviction, even in the face of overwhelming evidence to the contrary. Box 28-4 outlines common delusional themes. The delusional idea puts the patient at odds

EARLY COURSE SCHIZOPHRENIA

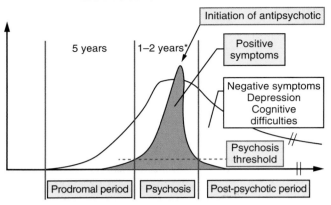

*DUP = duration of untreated psychosis

Figure 28-4. Typical time course of symptoms in a first episode of schizophrenia with a prodromal period and post-psychotic residual symptoms. *(Based on Hafner H, Loffler W, Maurer K, et al. Depression, negative symptoms, social stagnation and social decline in the early course of schizophrenia,* Acta Psychiatr Scandinavica *100(2):105– 118, 1999; Malla AK, Norman RM, Takhar J, et al. Can patients at risk for persistent negative symptoms be identified during their first episode of psychosis?* J Nerv Ment Dis *192(7):455–463, 2004; Malla AK, Takhar JJ, Norman RM, et al. Negative symptoms in first episode non-affective psychosis,* Acta Psychiatr Scandinavica *105(6):431–439, 2002; Green MF, Nuechterlein KH, Gold JM, et al. Approaching a consensus cognitive battery for clinical trials in schizophrenia: the NIMH-MATRICS conference to select cognitive domains and test criteria,* Biol Psychiatry *56(5):301–307, 2004.)*

with his or her culture or subculture. The content of delusions can be non-bizarre (feasible) or bizarre (impossible based on the laws of physics). Bizarre delusions suggest schizophrenia and are less characteristic for delusional disorder.

Patients with schizophrenia usually experience psychotic symptoms at least for part of their illness. Most treated patients, however, do not experience psychotic symptoms every day.

Other symptom domains, although not as dramatic as is florid psychosis, often are more pervasive and account for the difficulties in psychosocial adjustment that characterizes the lives of many patients with schizophrenia (Figure 28-5). These include cognitive deficits and negative symptoms. Negative symptoms are characterized by a loss or diminution of function, typically in the domains of motivation (volition) and emotional expressivity (Figure 28-6). In addition, affective symptoms may occur, including thoughts of suicide. Depression is common early in the course of schizophrenia; patients are particularly vulnerable to depressive symptoms following the resolution of positive symptoms. Motor abnormalities (e.g., catatonic symptoms and dyskinesias) were prominent in the early descriptions of untreated schizophrenia, but are now infrequently observed except in the form of antipsychotic-induced tardive dyskinesia. A formal thought disorder (e.g., with loose associations) can lead to an inability to communicate using language.

Several attempts have been made to reduce heterogeneity in the schizophrenia syndrome and to delineate more homogeneous patient groups that are based on clinical features. For example, the type I and type II distinction described by Crow (1980)[85] distinguished patients with antipsychotic-responsive positive symptoms (type I) from those with largely treatment-unresponsive negative symptoms (type II), the latter correlating with structural brain abnormalities. Later elaborations

BOX 28-3 Types of Hallucinations by Modality in Schizophrenia and Other Conditions

VISUAL HALLUCINATIONS

Visual hallucinations can be simple or elementary (unformed, e.g., a flash of light) or complex (e.g., a face, an animal). While possible in schizophrenia, visual hallucinations (and illusions) are much more typical for, and common in, deliria and dementias. Other non-psychiatric etiologies include migraines and seizures, ocular pathology (including the Charles Bonnet syndrome in visually impaired people), narcolepsy, sleep deprivation, and mid-brain pathology (peduncular hallucinations).

AUDITORY HALLUCINATIONS

Auditory hallucinations can be any sound, such as banging doors, footsteps, music, or voices. Common in schizophrenia are so-called Schneiderian hallucinations, characterized by the voice(s) using the third person when talking about the patient ("He is such a loser."). Depressed patients who hallucinate often experience voices in the self-accusatory second person ("You are such a loser."). Command hallucinations tell a patient to do a certain act and can include homicide, suicide, or self-mutilation.

OLFACTORY HALLUCINATIONS

Olfactory hallucinations are a common symptom in temporal lobe epilepsy. If olfactory hallucinations occur in schizophrenia, the hallucinated smells often have the character of a stench (feces, vomitus), but pleasant smells (e.g., perfume) are also experienced.

TACTILE HALLUCINATIONS

Tactile hallucinations involve the sensation of being touched or of insects crawling on the skin (formication). This is a typical symptom of cocaine or amphetamine use. Tactile hallucinations occur as a fairly isolated symptom in Ekbom's syndrome (delusional parasitosis), where the tactile hallucination is elaborated in a delusional way. It also occurs in alcohol and benzodiazepine withdrawal.

SOMATIC HALLUCINATIONS

Somatic hallucinations involve a sensation arising from within the body; they are fairly common in schizophrenia and are obvious if bizarre (e.g., experiencing movements of the brain). Somatic hallucinations need to be differentiated from symptoms of an as yet undiagnosed disease and from hypochondriacal preoccupation with normal body experiences (e.g., palpitations or bowel peristalsis).

GUSTATORY HALLUCINATIONS

Gustatory hallucinations are very rare in schizophrenia, but they can occur as part of persecutory delusions (e.g., tasting poison in food).

have used a three-symptom cluster model (i.e., reality-distortion, psychomotor poverty, and disorganization) or a further refined five-factor model.[86,87]

Patients with persistent and prominent primary negative symptoms have the deficit syndrome that might represent a biologically distinct group of patients.[88] Negative symptoms are considered primary when they are the result of the presumed schizophrenia disease process and not secondary to another cause such as depression, parkinsonism, or positive symptoms[89] (see Figure 28-6).

Lack of insight into the nature of schizophrenia (i.e., the inability to recognize symptoms, to consider that one is suffering from a disease, or to accept treatment) is a core feature

BOX 28-4 Types of Delusions by Content in Schizophrenia and Other Conditions

PERSECUTORY

Such delusions involve a person or force (e.g., family members, co-workers, government agencies [e.g., the CIA or FBI], or even aliens or the devil) that is interfering with the patient, observing the patient, and wishing to harm the patient (e.g., poisoning him or her). These can be very common themes in delusional disorder or schizophrenia.

REFERENCE

With ideas of reference, random and innocuous events (e.g., a news item in the morning newspaper, an incidental comment or gesture by a stranger) take on personal significance and meaning.

CONTROL

Delusions of control may be manifest by the belief that some agency is taking control of a patient's thoughts, feelings, and behaviors. Patients experience themselves as passive puppets, with their will and thoughts taken away (therefore, the term *delusions of passivity* for delusions of control as well).

SOMATIC

In somatic delusions, part of the body is experienced as being diseased or malfunctioning, or in bizarre cases that the body is physically altered. Often these delusions are accompanied by somatic perceptual abnormalities.

GRANDEUR

In delusions of grandeur there is an unrealistic belief in one's powers and abilities, which can be obvious (a claim of world fame in a common man) or more subtle (a physicist claiming to work at an invention that could change the world). This is the typical mood-congruent delusion of psychotic mania, where patients feel they can move mountains and start believing it.

NIHILISM

Nihilism is an exaggerated belief in the futility of everything. In the extreme, one's own existence is denied and the patient absurdly declares he is literally dead (Cotard syndrome). This type of delusion is usually seen as a mood-congruent delusion in patients with severe depression.

DELUSION OF LOVE

In erotomania (de Clérambault syndrome)—patients feel loved by another person, often of higher status, who is merely an innocent bystander.

JEALOUSY

Jealousy involves suspecting someone of being unfaithful (e.g., alcoholics who suspect their spouse of infidelity).

DELUSIONS OF DOUBLES

In Capgras syndrome, the patient believes that a family member or close friend has been replaced by an identically appearing double. It is associated with neuropsychiatric deficits of facial processing.

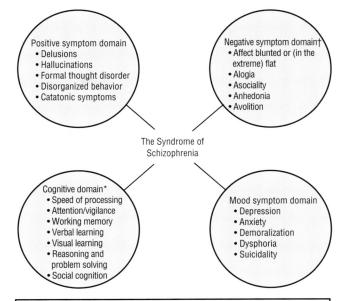

Figure 28-5. Symptom domains and treatment targets for schizophrenia syndrome. *(Figure based on Kirkpatrick B, Fenton WS, Carpenter WT, Jr., et al. The NIMH-MATRICS consensus statement on negative symptoms, Schizophrenia bulletin 32(2):214–219, 2006; and Green MF, Nuechterlein KH, Gold JM, et al. Approaching a consensus cognitive battery for clinical trials in schizophrenia: the NIMH-MATRICS conference to select cognitive domains and test criteria, Biological psychiatry 56(5):301–307, 2004.)*

EVALUATION

The cornerstone of diagnosis is the clinical examination of the patient, with review of symptoms cross-sectionally and historically. The absence of psychotic symptoms at the time of interview, especially if treated, does not argue against a diagnosis of schizophrenia. A family history can be useful if it is positive for schizophrenia or for bipolar disorder, a movement disorder, or another genetic syndrome.

Tests and Laboratory Findings

In the initial evaluation of a psychotic patient, routine laboratory tests to rule out common medical conditions, particularly deliria, are obtained. In the prototypical case, laboratory values will be normal, although minor abnormalities can be seen in agitated patients or in patients who have neglected their health (e.g., as manifest by an increased white blood cell count). A small number of more specific screening tests are often obtained to rule out treatable, reversible conditions (e.g., antibody tests for neurosyphilis), although there is no generally agreed-upon battery of laboratory tests (Box 28-5). A lumbar puncture is indicated in all unclear cases of psychosis if a central nervous system (CNS) infection is a clinical possibility. A good overall rule is to let the clinical presentation guide the appropriate work-up.

A drug-use history supplemented by a urinary drug screen (UDS) is important to exclude unreported drug use. However, a negative UDS cannot prove that drug use is not a relevant factor in a clinical presentation. Many drugs of abuse that can trigger psychosis are not routinely tested for (e.g., ketamine, PCP, LSD), and a positive drug test will depend on timing of

of the illness for many patients with schizophrenia.[90,91] This lack of insight often leads to treatment interruptions or refusal of potentially helpful treatment. Among patients experiencing a first psychotic episode, greater insight is correlated with less schizophrenia psychopathology and increased depressive symptoms, suggesting more self-awareness and self-assessment capabilities.[92]

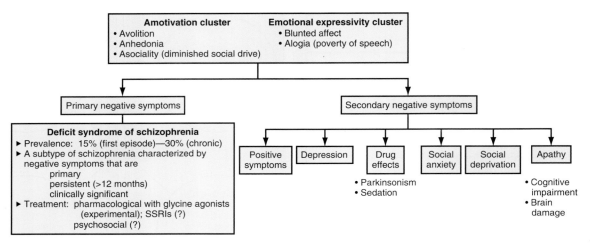

Figure 28-6. Negative symptoms of schizophrenia. *(Based on Kirkpatrick B, Fenton WS, Carpenter WT, Jr., et al. The NIMH-MATRICS consensus statement on negative symptoms,* Schizophr Bull *32(2):214–219, 2006 and Kimhy D, Yale S, Goetz RR, et al. The factorial structure of the schedule for the deficit syndrome in schizophrenia,* Schizophr Bull *32(2):274–278, 2006.)*

BOX 28-5 Initial Medical Work-up for Psychosis

IMAGING STUDIES*
- MRI to rule out demyelinating disease, to rule out brain tumor (e.g., meningioma)

LABORATORY STUDIES
- CBC
- Electrolytes
- BUN/creatinine
- Glucose
- Calcium and phosphorus
- TSH
- Liver function tests
- ESR
- Antinuclear antibodies
- Ceruloplasmin
- HIV screening†
- FTA-Abs for syphilis (RPR not sufficient)
- Vitamin B_{12} and folate
- Urinalysis
- Urine drug screen

This list of tests is not exhaustive but represents merely one possible initial work-up that is recommended in first-episode psychosis.

CLINICAL POINTS REGARDING LABORATORY TESTING IN PSYCHOSIS
- Laboratory testing merely complements the physical examination. Other tests should be considered if the clinical history and the clinical picture suggest that they might be useful (e.g., EEG, chest x-ray, lumbar puncture, neuropsychiatric testing), N-methyl-D-aspartate receptor autoantibodies.
- Broad screening for rare disorders without clinical suspicion risks false-positive results and is generally not recommended.
- Genetic testing is (currently) only indicated if there is clinical suspicion of a genetic syndrome (e.g., VCFS).
- Probably the best safeguard against overlooking important neuropsychiatric or medical disorders causing psychosis is long-term follow-up and vigilance, particularly as new symptoms evolve or the clinical picture changes.

Based on Coleman M, Gillberg C. The schizophrenias. A biological approach to the schizophrenia spectrum disorders. New York, 1996, Springer and Freudenreich O, Schulz SC, Goff DC. Initial medical work-up of first-episode psychosis: a conceptual review, Early Interv Psychiatry 3(1):10–18, 2009.
*Controversial because yield is low. (Sommer IE, de Kort GA, Meijering AL, et al. How frequent are radiological abnormalities in patients with psychosis? A Review of 1379 MRI Scans, Schizophr Bull, 2012.)
†Recommended as part of routine care for all, including psychotic patients.
BUN, Blood urea nitrogen; CBC, complete blood count; EEG, electroencephalogram; ESR, erythrocyte sedimentation rate; FTA-Abs, fluorescent treponemal antibody absorption; MRI, magnetic resonance imaging; RPR, rapid plasma reagin; TSH, thyroid-stimulating hormone; VCFS, velo-cardio-facial syndrome.

---

the test and assay characteristics in relation to the ingestion of the substance. Conversely, a positive UDS does not prove that the substance is responsible for psychosis.

The yield of a routine, standard EEG is low if used as a screening test, particularly given a high base rate of abnormal EEGs in patients diagnosed with schizophrenia (in one first-episode sample, only 43% of patients had a normal EEG).[93] Nevertheless, an EEG should be strongly considered in all cases where delirium cannot be excluded, and in cases with a history of head injury or seizures. Psychosis in the setting of

a seizure disorder can be the direct result of the seizure (e.g., an ictal psychosis) but may also occur in the post-ictal and inter-ictal period. Inter-ictal psychosis only occurs, however, after many years of poorly controlled seizures, and it is unlikely to be the first manifestation of a seizure disorder.[94] While of questionable diagnostic significance, even a subtly abnormal EEG in patients undergoing their first episode of schizophrenia confers a poorer prognosis with regard to positive-symptom remission compared with first-episode patients with a normal EEG after 2 years of follow-up.[93]

Brain Neuroimaging

Whether a brain CT or MRI should be obtained as part of the initial work-up of schizophrenia remains controversial as incidental findings occur at a rate similar to controls.[95] Moreover, only rarely will these tests lead to the discovery of a clinically relevant disorder in the absence of neurological signs (e.g., a frontal lobe tumor that manifests with only psychosis).[96] Nevertheless, given the long-term cost and morbidity of schizophrenia, obtaining a most-likely normal CT or MRI scan in a young person with psychosis serves two functions: it will exclude rare, treatable causes of psychosis, and it will support the diagnosis of schizophrenia, assuring patients that the clinical diagnosis is correct and that treatment needs to proceed. Other imaging modalities, such as PET or SPECT, do not aid in the diagnosis of schizophrenia and should only be ordered if specific conditions are to be ruled out (e.g., epilepsy).

DIFFERENTIAL DIAGNOSIS OF PSYCHOSIS

Schizophrenia is a diagnosis of exclusion. It can only be diagnosed if certain symptoms are present in the absence of other psychiatric or medical etiologies.

Excluding delirium is the most important initial consideration in any patient with psychosis, as hallucinations and delusions are present in about 40% of cases with delirium.[97] Rapid onset of psychosis (over hours or days), particularly if accompanied by a fluctuation in symptoms and a clouded sensorium, in a clinical setting (i.e., a medical unit), and in the wrong age group (i.e., a geriatric patient), strongly argues for a delirium. Medical conditions that can mimic schizophrenia are summarized in Box 28-6. Substance intoxications are next on the list of conditions to be ruled out (Box 28-7). A patient with a known diagnosis of schizophrenia could still be delirious, use drugs, or develop a medical illness. In some cases, serial examinations and longitudinal follow-up are required to establish a diagnosis.

Once medical conditions and intoxications are ruled out, psychiatric illnesses that share characteristic symptoms with schizophrenia must be considered (Box 28-8). Mood episodes, including both mania and depression, can be accompanied by psychotic symptoms at the height of the episode; psychotic depression or bipolar disorder must then be considered. During periods of normal mood, no psychosis is present. While differentiating between schizophrenia, bipolar disorder, or psychotic depression is usually

---

BOX 28-6 Differential Diagnosis of Psychosis: I. Medical Conditions

Epilepsy
Head trauma (history of)
Dementias
- Alzheimer's disease
- Pick's disease
- Lewy body disease
Stroke
Space-occupying lesions and structural brain abnormalities
- Primary brain tumors
- Secondary brain metastases
- Brain abscesses and cysts
- Tuberous sclerosis
- Mid-line abnormalities (e.g., corpus callosum agenesis, cavum septi pellucidi)
- Cerebrovascular malformations (e.g., involving the temporal lobe)
Hydrocephalus
Demyelinating diseases
- MS
- Leukodystrophies (metachromatic leukodystrophy, X-linked adrenoleukodystrophy, Marchiafava-Bignami disease)
- Schilder's disease
Neuropsychiatric disorders
- Huntington's disease
- Wilson's disease
- Parkinson's disease
- Friedreich's ataxia
Autoimmune disorders
- SLE
- Rheumatic fever (history of)
- Paraneoplastic syndromes
- Anti-NMDA receptor encephalitis
- Myasthenia gravis
Infections
- Viral encephalitis (e.g., herpes simplex, measles including SSPE, cytomegalovirus, rubella, Epstein–Barr, varicella)
- Neurosyphilis

- Neuroborreliosis (Lyme disease)
- HIV infection
- CNS-invasive parasitic infections (e.g., cerebral malaria, toxoplasmosis, neurocysticercosis)
- Tuberculosis
- Sarcoidosis
- *Cryptococcus* infection
- Prion diseases (e.g., Creutzfeldt-Jakob disease)
Endocrinopathies
- Hypoglycemia
- Addison's disease
- Cushing's syndrome
- Hyperthyroidism and hypothyroidism
- Hyperparathyroidism and hypoparathyroidism
- Hypopituitarism
- Narcolepsy
- Nutritional deficiencies
- Magnesium deficiency
- Vitamin A deficiency
- Vitamin D deficiency
- Zinc deficiency
- Niacin deficiency (pellagra)
- Vitamin B_{12} deficiency (pernicious anemia)
Metabolic disorders (partial list)
- Amino acid metabolism (Hartnup disease, homocystinuria, phenylketonuria)
- Porphyrias (acute intermittent porphyria, porphyria variegata, hereditary coproporphyria)
- GM-$_2$ gangliosidosis
- Fabry's disease
- Niemann-Pick type C disease
- Gaucher's disease, adult type
Chromosomal abnormalities
- Sex chromosomes (Klinefelter's syndrome, XXY syndrome)
- Fragile X syndrome
- VCFS

CNS, Central nervous system; HIV, human immunodeficiency virus; MS, multiple sclerosis; SLE, systemic lupus erythematosus; SSPE, subacute sclerosing panencephalitis; VCFS, velo-cardio-facial syndrome.

BOX 28-7 Differential Diagnosis of Psychosis: II. Substance Intoxications (Drugs of Abuse, Medications, Toxins)

DRUGS OF ABUSE
Associated with Intoxication
Alcohol
Anabolic steroids
Amphetamine
Cannabis and synthetic cannabinoids
Cocaine
Hallucinogens: LSD, MDMA
Inhalants: glues and solvents
Opioids (meperidine)
Phencyclidine (PCP), ketamine
Sedative-hypnotics: barbiturates and benzodiazepines
New designer drugs: bath salts (methylenedioxypyrovalerone (MDPV))

Associated with Withdrawal
Alcohol
Sedative-hypnotics

MEDICATIONS
Broad Classes with Selected Medications
Anesthetics and analgesics (including NSAIDs)
Anticholinergic agents and antihistamines
Antiepileptics (with high doses)
Antihypertensive and cardiovascular medications (e.g., digoxin)
Anti-infectious medications (antibiotics [e.g., fluoroquinolones, TMP/SMX], antivirals [e.g., nevirapine], tuberculostatics [e.g., INH], antiparasitics [e.g., metronidazole, mefloquine])
Antiparkinsonian medications (e.g., amantadine, levodopa)
Chemotherapeutic agents (e.g., vincristine)
Corticosteroids (e.g., prednisone, ACTH)
Interferon
Muscle relaxants (e.g., cyclobenzaprine)
Over-the-counter medications (e.g., pseudoephedrine, caffeine in excessive doses)

TOXINS
Carbon monoxide
Heavy metals: arsenic, manganese, mercury, thallium
Organophosphates

KEY DIAGNOSTIC QUESTIONS TO DETERMINE CAUSALITY BETWEEN A SUBSTANCE AND PSYCHOSIS
Does the patient have a personal history of psychosis?
Does the patient have a history of illicit drug use?
Did the psychosis start after a medication was started? After the patient came to the hospital?
Is there evidence of delirium?

ACTH, Adrenocorticotropic hormone; INH, isoniazid; LSD, d-lysergic acid diethylamide; MDMA, methylenedioxymethamphetamine; NSAID, non-steroidal antiinflammatory drug; TMP/SMX, trimethoprim-sulfamethoxazole.

BOX 28-8 Differential Diagnosis of Psychosis: III. Psychiatric Syndromes*

CONTINUOUS PSYCHOSIS
Schizophrenia
Schizoaffective disorder, bipolar type (with prominent episodes of mania)
Schizoaffective disorder, depressed type (with prominent depressive episodes)
Paranoia or delusional disorder (prominent delusions as major feature)
Folie à deux or shared psychotic disorder (in which delusions are induced by another person)

EPISODIC PSYCHOSIS
Depression with psychotic features
Bipolar disorder (manic or depressed) with psychotic episodes
Schizophreniform disorder (<6 months' duration)
Brief psychotic disorder (<1 month's duration)

SCHIZOPHRENIA TRAITS
Schizotypal personality disorder
Schizoid personality disorder
Paranoid personality disorder

OTHER
Borderline personality disorder
Attenuated psychosis syndrome (possible prodromal schizophrenia)

*Terminology based on DSM-5 (Association AP. DSM-5. *Diagnostic and statistical manual of mental disorders.* ed 5. (Copyright 2013). American Psychiatric Association.

and such poor reliability that it begs the question why it should be used at all.[100] If the presentation is essentially that of prominent delusions without ancillary symptoms of schizophrenia, delusional disorder is diagnosed. All classification systems specify that schizophrenia can only be diagnosed if symptoms have been present for a sufficient period of time to avoid over-diagnosis. Atypical forms of short-lived psychotic disorders and the absence of a post-psychotic deficit are encountered in clinical practice and known by a variety of names, depending on the locale (e.g., *bouffée délirante*, acute and transient psychotic disorder, and brief psychotic disorder).[101,102] The nosology of such good prognosis cases is unclear, with some cases probably being closer to affective disorders than to schizophrenia. Last, some personality disorders (i.e., schizotypal, schizoid, and paranoid personality disorder) exhibit attenuated symptoms of schizophrenia.

Pharmacological Treatment

The treatment of schizophrenia can be divided into acute phase treatment (i.e., treatment of an acute episode of psychosis) and maintenance phase treatment (Figure 28-7).

Acute Phase

The treatment of the acute episode usually requires the use of antipsychotic medications, followed by maintenance antipsychotic treatment and some degree of psychosocial rehabilitation (for target doses of antipsychotics, see Chapter 42). In the US, second-generation antipsychotics have largely supplanted first-generation antipsychotics, although the issue of relative risk/benefit of one group over the other remains controversial, and the antipsychotic used should be chosen

uncomplicated, enough overlap exists between the disease categories to cause diagnostic uncertainty in some cases. Depressive symptoms are common in the course of schizophrenia, both during episodes of psychotic exacerbation and in the period following resolution of psychosis (post-psychotic depression). Therefore, the presence of depression does not argue against a diagnosis of schizophrenia.[98,99] In clinical practice, however, patients with prominent mood symptoms in the setting of a psychotic disorder are often diagnosed with schizoaffective disorder, a diagnosis of questionable validity

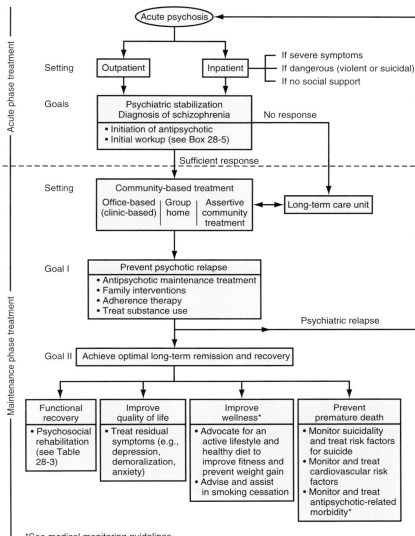

Figure 28-7. Algorithm for comprehensive treatment of schizophrenia.

*See medical monitoring guidelines

based on individual and family risk factors and on clinical tolerability (see Chapter 42).

A psychiatric hospitalization is often necessary during an episode of acute psychosis, particularly if there is diagnostic uncertainty, if the patient is severely ill, if no social support is available, or if there is the risk for suicide or homicide. Regardless of the treatment setting, timely initiation of an antipsychotic treatment is important to induce symptomatic remission. Delay of treatment leads to psychosocial toxicity and possibly to a worse outcome in a first-episode patient.[81,103] All antipsychotics are about equally effective in inducing remission following a first episode of schizophrenia (if defined as a symptomatic [not functional] remission). Depressive symptoms and demoralization are part and parcel of schizophrenia, and they need to be monitored and treated aggressively to prevent suicide.

If antipsychotics are discontinued following treatment of the initial illness episode in narrowly defined schizophrenia (i.e., with signs of the illness for more than 6 months), most patients will relapse within 1 year, and almost all will relapse within the next 2–3 years.[104,105] Therefore, various guidelines have suggested treatment for at least 1–2 years with an antipsychotic following remission of a first episode of psychosis,

and only then gradually discontinuing treatment with close follow-up so that reinstitution of treatment can occur at the earliest sign of relapse. The decision to discontinue an antipsychotic should be made on a case-by-case basis, weighing the risks/benefits.

Maintenance Phase

Multi-episode patients usually require indefinite maintenance treatment with an antipsychotic to prevent a relapse of psychosis.[106] Continuous medication treatment is superior in the prevention of decompensations and hospitalizations when compared with a targeted approach in which treatment is periodically discontinued and re-instituted at signs of relapse.[107] However, even with maintenance treatment, a certain proportion of patients, estimated to be as high as 40%, will relapse each year.[108,109] As in all chronic diseases, poor long-term adherence to antipsychotics is a vexing problem, compounded in schizophrenia by a lack of insight. Poor adherence leads to symptomatic relapse, re-hospitalization, and suicide attempts.[110] An important focus of rehabilitation is improvement of adherence in an attempt to avoid revolving-door admissions to psychiatric hospitals that undermine long-term

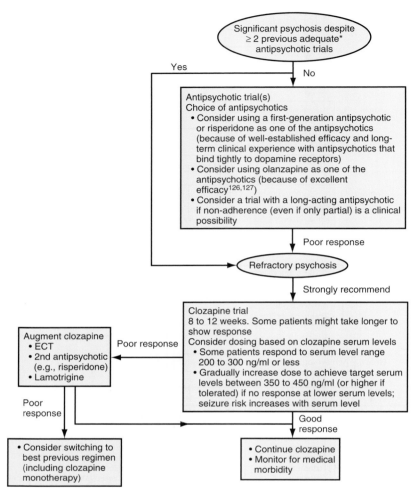

Figure 28-8. Algorithm for treatment-refractory schizophrenia.
Well documented with optimal dose (see Chapter 42 for dose), duration (6 to 8 weeks; some patients have delayed time to response), and adherence; absence of drug use. Diagnoses other than schizophrenia have been excluded. (Based on Kane J, Honigfeld G, Singer J, et al. Clozapine for the treatment-resistant schizophrenic. A double-blind comparison with chlorpromazine, Arch Gen Psychiatry 45(9):789–796, 1988; McEvoy JP, Lieberman JA, Stroup TS, et al. Effectiveness of clozapine versus olanzapine, quetiapine, and risperidone in patients with chronic schizophrenia who did not respond to prior atypical antipsychotic treatment, Am J Psychiatry 163(4):600–610, 2006; Lieberman JA, Stroup TS, McEvoy JP, et al. Effectiveness of antipsychotic drugs in patients with chronic schizophrenia, N Engl J Med 353(12):1209–1223, 2005; Volavka J, Czobor P, Sheitman B, et al. Clozapine, olanzapine, risperidone, and haloperidol in the treatment of patients with chronic schizophrenia and schizoaffective disorder, Am J Psychiatry 159(2):255–262, 2002; VanderZwaag C, McGee M, McEvoy JP, et al. Response of patients with treatment-refractory schizophrenia to clozapine within three serum level ranges, Am J Psychiatry 153(12):1579–1584, 1996; Bell R, McLaren A, Galanos J, et al. The clinical use of plasma clozapine levels, Aust N Z J Psychiatry 32(4):567–574, 1998.)

rehabilitation efforts. Factors that impair adherence (e.g., drug use, side effects of medications, ineffective medication regimen) are an important focus of long-term treatment.[111,112]

Antipsychotics, particularly second-generation antipsychotics, differ sufficiently in their side-effect profile and their efficacy in a given patient to justify sequential medication trials to find the antipsychotic that best balances efficacy with tolerability for a given patient. The choice of the antipsychotic must take into account the compounding effects of antipsychotics on pre-existing medical morbidity. While antipsychotics are generally effective in controlling positive symptoms and in reducing psychotic relapse rates, the National Institute of Mental Health (NIMH)-funded Clinical Antipsychotic Trials of Intervention Effectiveness (CATIE) schizophrenia trial confirmed the limitations of dopamine antagonists for the long-term treatment of schizophrenia.[113] In this large trial, a high antipsychotic discontinuation rate (of greater than 80%) over 18 months of treatment suggested suboptimal overall efficacy or tolerability. This trial also clearly documented high rates of metabolic problems (i.e., weight gain, hyperglycemia, and dyslipidemia) associated with some antipsychotics, which makes long-term adherence challenging.[114]

Approximately 20% of patients with schizophrenia will have an insufficient response to all first- and second-generation antipsychotics, except for clozapine. Clozapine should be offered to refractory patients,[115,116] as well as to suicidal or violent patients, for whom it is also more effective than other antipsychotics (for treatment-refractory schizophrenia, Figure 28-8).[117,118] Clozapine should be offered as soon as

treatment-refractoriness has been detected and not only after years of ineffective treatment with other antipsychotics.[119] In all patients with residual symptoms, it is important to rule out partial adherence, non-adherence, or ongoing drug use in order to avoid mislabeling a patient as refractory.

Only antipsychotics are Food and Drug Administration (FDA)-approved for the treatment of schizophrenia. In clinical practice, many patients receive medications other than antipsychotics (particularly antidepressants for depression and anxiolytics for anxiety) for the symptomatic treatment of residual psychopathology. The role of mood stabilizers for narrowly defined schizophrenia is limited.[120,121] Valproate is useful as an adjunct in acute psychotic exacerbations to hasten response,[122,123] and lamotrigine may augment the therapeutic effects of clozapine.[124-126] Partial and full agonists at the glycine site of the NMDA receptor (e.g., D-cycloserine, glycine, or D-serine) have shown some efficacy for negative symptoms.[127-129] There is some evidence for improvement of negative symptoms and memory consolidation with once-weekly dosing of D-cycloserine.[130] Improving cognition with AMPA modulators or nicotinic agonists is an area of active research, but to date these medications are not available clinically.

REHABILITATION AND LONG-TERM MANAGEMENT

Pharmacotherapy alone does not comprehensively treat schizophrenia. Instead, a broad range of ancillary psychosocial treatments is necessary to address residual symptomatology, skill

TABLE 28-3 Psychosocial Treatments for Schizophrenia

Modality	Goals
Individual supportive therapy	Engage patient in treatment and rehabilitation
Psychoeducation	Improve disease-management skills
Cognitive-behavioral therapy (CBT)	Improve residual symptoms and functioning
Adherence therapy	Improve adherence to medication treatment
Social skills training	Improve social adjustment and independent living skills
Supported vocational rehabilitation	Return to paid employment
Supported employment	Enhance work tenure
Supported housing	Enhance community tenure and prevent homelessness
Family interventions	Improve knowledge and reduce stress for family members through better coping skills; reduce psychiatric hospitalizations
Assertive community treatment	Reduce psychiatric hospitalizations and risk to community
Token economy interventions	Improve adaptive behaviors (personal hygiene, social interactions)
Alcohol/substance use disorders interventions	Motivational enhancement and behavioral strategies for treatment and relapse prevention
Weight management interventions	Weight loss for body mass index > 25

(Based on Royal Australian and New Zealand College of Psychiatrists clinical practice guidelines for the treatment of schizophrenia and related disorders, Aust N Z J Psychiatry 39(1–2):1–30, 2005 and Dixon LB, Dickerson F, Bellack AS, et al. The 2009 schizophrenia PORT psychosocial treatment recommendations and summary statements, Schizophrenia Bulletin 36(1):48–70, 2010.)

deficits, and the functional impairments that accompany schizophrenia (Table 28-3). The scale and scope of these rehabilitation efforts will vary depending on the severity of illness and the residual symptoms. For some patients, meeting basic needs (e.g., housing) is an important goal for initial rehabilitation. Co-morbid substance abuse (dual diagnosis) must be addressed in an integrated treatment setting to reduce non-adherence, psychotic relapse, and violence. In the US, the rate of life-time substance use disorders is approximately 50% for patients with schizophrenia, the most common co-morbidity being alcohol dependence, followed by abuse of cannabis and cocaine.[131]

In a small but important subgroup of patients, violence must be prevented.[132] A past history of violence, drug use, and sociopathic traits are predictors of violence in the patient with schizophrenia. For those patients at highest risk for violence, models of care that include active outreach have been developed (e.g., assertive community treatment [ACT]).[133,134]

The family plays an integral part in the care of patients with schizophrenia, and family interventions are among the most effective interventions when combined with medications. Families can help reduce psychiatric re-hospitalization rates by 50% when an environment with low levels of "expressed emotions," particularly hostile criticism, is created.[135] Most importantly, a recovery orientation (in the way psychiatric services are delivered to patient with schizophrenia), combined with peer-support services, has given many patients alternative views about their illness, counteracting stigma, despair and hopelessness (see Chapter 64).

PROGNOSIS
Morbidity and Mortality Rates

Schizophrenia is a potentially deadly illness. Having schizophrenia reduces the average life expectancy by 15 years,[136] mostly from suicide, but also from premature cardiovascular death.[137] Up to 5% of patients with schizophrenia will die from suicide.[138] Assessment for suicide is therefore an important part of treatment for schizophrenia, particularly during the first few years following diagnosis when patients are at highest risk. Drug use, depressive disorders, and medication non-adherence are important, but treatable, risk factors for suicide in those with schizophrenia.[139] Approximately 40% of patients with schizophrenia suffer from the metabolic syndrome,[114] and patients with schizophrenia have higher rates of the well-established Framingham cardiac risk factors than do matched controls.[140] Paying attention to modifiable cardiac risk factors, particularly smoking, dyslipidemias and diabetes, has therefore become an important part of psychiatric care.[141–143] To this end, chronic disease management (illness self-management) has become an important preventive aspect of care for patients with schizophrenia.[144]

Encouragement of smoking cessation, albeit difficult, is important because as many as two-thirds of patients with schizophrenia smoke, often heavily. In addition, aggressive prevention of weight gain (which can be associated with antipsychotic use) is important (Table 28-4).

Prognosis with Regard to Symptoms and Function

The immediate prognosis for positive-symptom response to antipsychotic medications following a first episode of schizophrenia is good. In one study, three-fourths of patients were considered fully remitted with regard to positive symptoms after 1 year.[145] However, relapse after the initial episode of treatment occurs in approximately 80% of patients within 5 years after antipsychotics are discontinued.[146] Preventing relapse and accrued disability remains an important topic of investigation; unfortunately, it is unclear which patients will not require maintenance treatment. Moreover, less aggressive treatment during the early course of illness (i.e., low-dose approach and attempts to discontinue antipsychotics), while not without risk, might confer long-term benefit with regards to the all-important functioning.[147]

The long-term functional outcome of schizophrenia is less optimistic, although not as inevitably bleak as is sometimes described. A small, yet significant, minority of patients (probably about 10%) will have only one episode from which they recover without sequelae.[148] For most patients, occasional exacerbations of symptoms that require hospitalization are part of the illness. Between hospitalizations, patients struggle

TABLE 28-4 Monitoring Guidelines to Prevent Medical Morbidity in Schizophrenia

	BL	1	2	3	4	5	6	7	8	9	10	11	12
PMHx and FHx	x												x
Smoking status	x	x	x	x	x	x	x	x	x	x	x	x	x
Weight (body mass index [BMI])	x	x	x	x	x	x	x			x			x
Waist circumference	x												x
Fasting glucose*	x			x									x
Fasting lipid profile*	x			x									x
Blood pressure	x			x			x						x
Tardive dyskinesia**	x						x						x
Medical screening⁺	x												x
Lifestyle advice	x						x						x

(From Marder SR, Essock SM, Miller AL, et al. Physical health monitoring of patients with schizophrenia, Am J Psychiatry 161(8):1334–1349, 2004; Goff DC, Cather C, Evins AE, et al. Medical morbidity and mortality in schizophrenia: guidelines for psychiatrists, J Clin Psychiatry 66(2):183–194; quiz 147, 273–184, 2005 and De Hert M, Vancampfort D, Correll CU, et al: Guidelines for screening and monitoring of cardiometabolic risk in schizophrenia: systematic evaluation, Br J Psychiatry 199(2):99–105, 2011.)

*More frequent monitoring may be needed (e.g., patients on clozapine or olanzapine).

**More frequent monitoring in high-risk patients (e.g. elderly patient starting on a first-generation antipsychotic).

⁺Includes review of medical screening needs (e.g., colonoscopy, eye examination), review of vaccination requirements, and review of need for testing for infectious diseases (e.g., human immunodeficiency virus, hepatitis C virus, tuberculosis):
- Recommendations reflect need for increased metabolic monitoring in the initial period after second-generation antipsychotics are instituted.
- More intensive monitoring can be clinically indicated.
- For further guidance, more specific guidelines need to be consulted.

Note: Column heads are the number of months.
BL, Baseline; FHx, family history; PMHx, past medical history.

BOX 28-9 Poor Prognostic Features of Schizophrenia

- Male
- Family history of schizophrenia
- Abnormal brain (e.g., abnormal EEG, abnormal MRI)
- Poor pre-morbid adjustment
- Young age of onset
- Insidious onset
- Lack of insight
- Persistent negative symptoms
- Poor medication response
- Long duration of untreated psychosis
- Living in a developed country

EEG, Electroencephalogram; MRI, magnetic resonance imaging.

BOX 28-10 Current Controversies and Future Considerations

ETIOLOGY AND DIAGNOSIS

Is schizophrenia different from manic-depressive illness (Kraepelinian dichotomy), or are both different clinical expressions of the same genetic vulnerability to psychosis (unitary hypothesis), with some shared genes?

Is there a syndrome of schizophrenia with multiple causes but a final common pathway that links pathophysiology and symptoms?

Are abnormalities of the brain present prior to the onset of the illness in all people who develop schizophrenia, or can the disorder develop in a "normal" brain?

What is the exact genetic architecture of schizophrenia: are there a few major genes, which, if disrupted, contribute to schizophrenia, or are there many genes, each with small contributions?

Does schizophrenia affect the brain globally (e.g., all glutamatergic neurons in every brain region) or are there region-specific abnormalities?

Can schizophrenia be diagnosed in the prodromal state?

TREATMENT

What drugs beyond dopamine blockers are useful for the comprehensive treatment of schizophrenia, particularly for the treatment of non-psychotic symptoms (negative and cognitive symptoms)?

Does treatment with antipsychotics worsen the disease outcome in some patients?

Which psychosocial treatments improve engagement in treatment?

How can high-quality, coordinated, and comprehensive schizophrenia care be delivered?

PREVENTION

Can treatment during the prodrome prevent schizophrenia?

Which approach can reduce the gap in medical morbidity and mortality between patients with schizophrenia and their peers without mental illness?

How can the stigma of schizophrenia be reduced so that patients receive earlier treatment?

---

with varying degrees of residual symptoms.[149] For those patients, living in the community (i.e., not in an asylum), either independently or with some support, is a realistic goal. Very poor outcomes with marginal societal adjustment and with ongoing severe symptoms and the need for continuous hospitalization are possible (i.e., the Kraepelinian subtype of schizophrenia).[150] In the US, a diagnosis of schizophrenia is associated with poor work function. It has been observed that the outcome in rural societies is better.[151] For any individual patient, the eventual outcome is difficult to predict. Poor pre-morbid function, childhood onset, family history of schizophrenia, brain abnormalities (e.g., an abnormal CT or EEG), insidious onset, and drug abuse in a man are poor predictors, whereas a later onset of predominantly positive symptoms in a woman confers a better prognosis (Box 28-9). It should not be ignored that the natural history of any disease, but particularly for psychiatric diseases like schizophrenia, is to a large extent determined by psychosocial factors (e.g., access to care and high-quality treatment; social exclusion due to stigma).[152]

CURRENT CONTROVERSIES AND FUTURE CONSIDERATIONS

Box 28-10 provides a synopsis of current controversies and future considerations.

Access the complete reference list and multiple choice questions (MCQs) online at https://expertconsult.inkling.com

KEY REFERENCES

2. Smoller JW, Craddock N, Kendler K, et al. Identification of risk loci with shared effects on five major psychiatric disorders: a genome-wide analysis. *Lancet* 381(9875):1371–1379, 2013.
11. Brown AS, Derkits EJ. Prenatal infection and schizophrenia: a review of epidemiologic and translational studies. *Am J Psychiatry* 167(3):261–280, 2010.
21. Malaspina D, Harlap S, Fennig S, et al. Advancing paternal age and the risk of schizophrenia. *Arch Gen Psychiatry* 58(4):361–367, 2001.
23. Zhang J-P, Malhotra AK. Genetics of schizophrenia: what do we know? *Curr Psychiatr* 12(3):25–33, 2013.
27. Rapoport JL, Giedd JN, Gogtay N. Neurodevelopmental model of schizophrenia: update 2012. *Mol Psychiatry* 17(12):1228–1238, 2012.
29. Howes OD, Kambeitz J, Kim E, et al. The nature of dopamine dysfunction in schizophrenia and what this means for treatment. *Arch Gen Psychiatry* 69(8):776–786, 2012.
36. Dickerson F, Stallings CR, Origoni AE, et al. Cigarette smoking among persons with schizophrenia or bipolar disorder in routine clinical settings, 1999–2011. *Psychiatr Serv* 64(1):44–50, 2013.
44. Johnstone EC, Crow TJ, Frith CD, et al. Cerebral ventricular size and cognitive impairment in chronic schizophrenia. *Lancet* 2(7992):924–926, 1976.
45. Thompson PM, Vidal C, Giedd JN, et al. Mapping adolescent brain change reveals dynamic wave of accelerated gray matter loss in very early-onset schizophrenia. *Proc Natl Acad Sci U S A* 98(20):11650–11655, 2001.
50. Hulshoff Pol HE, Kahn RS. What happens after the first episode? A review of progressive brain changes in chronically ill patients with schizophrenia. *Schizophr Bull* 34(2):354–366, 2008.
52. Andreasen NC, Liu D, Ziebell S, et al. Relapse duration, treatment intensity, and brain tissue loss in schizophrenia: a prospective longitudinal MRI study. *Am J Psychiatry* 170(6):609–615, 2013.
55. Gottesman II, Gould TD. The endophenotype concept in psychiatry: etymology and strategic intentions. *Am J Psychiatry* 160(4):636–645, 2003.
68. Friston KJ. The disconnection hypothesis. *Schizophr Res* 30(2):115–125, 1998.
70. Garrity AG, Pearlson GD, McKiernan K, et al. Aberrant "default mode" functional connectivity in schizophrenia. *Am J Psychiatry* 164(3):450–457, 2007.

77. Stephan KE, Friston KJ, Frith CD. Dysconnection in schizophrenia: from abnormal synaptic plasticity to failures of self-monitoring. *Schizophr Bull* 35(3):509–527, 2009.
78. Yung AR, McGorry PD. The initial prodrome in psychosis: descriptive and qualitative aspects. *Aust N Z J Psychiatry* 30(5):587–599, 1996.
79. Fusar-Poli P, Bonoldi I, Yung AR, et al. Predicting psychosis: meta-analysis of transition outcomes in individuals at high clinical risk. *Arch Gen Psychiatry* 69(3):220–229, 2012.
82. Hill M, Crumlish N, Clarke M, et al. Prospective relationship of duration of untreated psychosis to psychopathology and functional outcome over 12 years. *Schizophr Res* 141(2–3):215–221, 2012.
83. Hoff AL, Svetina C, Shields G, et al. Ten year longitudinal study of neuropsychological functioning subsequent to a first episode of schizophrenia. *Schizophr Res* 78(1):27–34, 2005.
85. Crow TJ. Molecular pathology of schizophrenia: more than one disease process? *Br Med J* 280(6207):66–68, 1980.
89. Carpenter WT Jr, Heinrichs DW, Wagman AM. Deficit and nondeficit forms of schizophrenia: the concept. *Am J Psychiatry* 145(5):578–583, 1988.
90. David AS. Insight and psychosis. *Br J Psychiatry* 156:798–808, 1990.
95. Sommer IE, de Kort GA, Meijering AL, et al. How frequent are radiological abnormalities in patients with psychosis? A review of 1379 MRI scans. *Schizophr Bull* 39(4):815–819, 2013.
106. Leucht S, Tardy M, Komossa K, et al. Antipsychotic drugs versus placebo for relapse prevention in schizophrenia: a systematic review and meta-analysis. *Lancet* 379(9831):2063–2071, 2012.
113. Lieberman JA, Stroup TS, McEvoy JP, et al. Effectiveness of antipsychotic drugs in patients with chronic schizophrenia. *N Engl J Med* 353(12):1209–1223, 2005.
115. Kane J, Honigfeld G, Singer J, et al. Clozapine for the treatment-resistant schizophrenic. A double-blind comparison with chlorpromazine. *Arch Gen Psychiatry* 45(9):789–796, 1988.
119. Agid O, Arenovich T, Sajeev G, et al. An algorithm-based approach to first-episode schizophrenia: response rates over 3 prospective antipsychotic trials with a retrospective data analysis. *J Clin Psychiatry* 72(11):1439–1444, 2011.
142. Goff DC, Cather C, Evins AE, et al. Medical morbidity and mortality in schizophrenia: guidelines for psychiatrists. *J Clin Psychiatry* 66(2):183–194, 2005.
147. Wunderink L, Nieboer RM, Wiersma D, et al. Recovery in remitted first-episode psychosis at 7 years of follow-up of an early dose reduction/discontinuation or maintenance treatment strategy: Long-term follow-up of a 2-year randomized clinical trial. *JAMA Psychiatry* 2013.

28

29 Mood Disorders: Depressive Disorders (Major Depressive Disorder)

Maurizio Fava, MD, Søren Dinesen Østergaard, MD, PhD, and Paolo Cassano, MD, PhD

KEY POINTS

Incidence

- The annual incidence of major depressive disorder (MDD) is approximately 3%, and the average duration of an episode of MDD is 30 weeks.

Epidemiology

- MDD is a prevalent disorder, with a global point prevalence of approximately 5%. The life-time prevalence rates of MDD in the US and Western European countries are in the range of 10%–20% in the general population.

Pathophysiology

- The pathophysiology of MDD remains largely unknown, but several mechanisms have been proposed, e.g., the monoamine hypothesis, which describes MDD as the consequence of a chemical imbalance in brain serotonin, norepinephrine (noradrenaline), and dopamine.

Clinical Findings

- Typical symptoms of MDD include depressed mood, lack of pleasure/interest/motivation, fatigue, feelings of guilt/worthlessness, anxiety/nervousness, irritability/anger, difficulty concentrating, insomnia/hypersomnia, loss of libido, change in appetite/weight, and recurring thoughts of death/suicide.

Differential Diagnoses

- Common differential diagnoses to MDD are bipolar disorder, psychotic disorders, dementia, substance use disorders, personality disorders, ADHD, anxiety disorders, eating disorders, and various general medical conditions. With the exception of bipolar disorder and psychotic disorders, MDD can also be co-morbid with these conditions.

Treatment Options

- First-line treatment options for MDD include psychotherapy and antidepressant medications (e.g., selective serotonin reuptake inhibitors (SSRIs), serotonin-norepinephrine reuptake inhibitors (SNRIs), tricyclic antidepressants (TCAs), monoamine oxidase inhibitors (MAOIs)). Options for severe and/or treatment-resistant MDD are vagal nerve stimulation (VNS), electroconvulsive therapy (ECT), and deep brain stimulation (DBS).

Complications

- MDD is associated with an increased risk of a number of medical illnesses, such as hypertension, diabetes, and heart disease, and it worsens the course of these illnesses, leading to increased morbidity and mortality. The most severe complication/outcome of MDD is suicide.

Prognosis

- Most episodes of MDD remit. However, the risk of developing further episodes increases progressively with each recurrence, while the recurring episodes tend to become longer and more severe as the number increases.

INTRODUCTION

Depressive disorders, especially major depressive disorder (MDD), are prevalent conditions that are associated with significant suffering, psychosocial impairment, and increased mortality. Despite the availability of numerous effective treatments, these disorders are often under-recognized and under-treated in the community. Several factors contribute to the under-recognition of depressive disorders; these include the stigma of depression itself and the relative lack of systematic ascertainment of depressive symptoms by health care professionals. The public health significance of depression is noteworthy; apart from the direct psychosocial burden, the disorders also heighten the risk of other medical diseases, and increase their associated morbidity and mortality. According to the World Health Organization, MDD ranks among the leading global burdens of disease.[1]

MAJOR DEPRESSIVE DISORDER

Patients who suffer from depressive disorders typically have a constellation of psychological, cognitive, behavioral, and physical symptoms. In the case of MDD, depressed mood and loss of interest/pleasure are considered to be the core features of the condition. Both can be present at the same time, but one of them is sufficient to define MDD, if certain associated symptoms are present. Specifically, the _Diagnostic and Statistical Manual of Mental Disorders_, ed 5 (DSM-5)[2] defines MDD as depressive mood (or irritable mood in children and adolescents) and/or loss of interest/pleasure, accompanied by at least four (only three if both depressed mood and loss of interest/pleasure are present) other depressive symptoms, lasting for at least 2 weeks. The accompanying symptoms (captured in the mnemonic SIG: E CAPS, a prescription for energy capsules) are insomnia/hypersomnia (S), reduced interest/pleasure (I), excessive guilt or feelings of worthlessness (G), reduced energy or fatigue (E), diminished ability to concentrate or make decisions (C), loss or increase of appetite/weight (A), psychomotor agitation/retardation (P), and thoughts of suicide/death or an actual suicide attempt/plan (S). The full DSM-5 diagnostic criteria for MDD are listed in Box 29-1. The degree of functional impairment is essential to distinguish MDD and the other depressive disorders from normal mood variability. That being said, the continuum of depression from mild,

---

BOX 29-1 DSM-5 Diagnostic Criteria: Major Depressive Disorder (296.2-296.3)

A. Five (or more) of the following symptoms have been present during the same 2-week period and represent a change from previous functioning; at least one of the symptoms is either (1) depressed mood or (2) loss of interest or pleasure.
   Note: Do not include symptoms that are clearly attributable to another medical condition.
   1. Depressed mood most of the day, nearly every day, as indicated by either subjective report (e.g. feels sad, empty, hopeless) or observation made by others (e.g. appears tearful). (**Note:** In children and adolescents, can be irritable mood.)
   2. Markedly diminished interest or pleasure in all, or almost all, activities most of the day, nearly every day (as indicated by either subjective account or observation).
   3. Significant weight loss when not dieting or weight gain (e.g. a change of more than 5% of body weight in a month), or decrease or increase in appetite nearly every day. (**Note:** In children consider failure to make expected weight gain.)
   4. Insomnia or hypersomnia nearly every day.
   5. Psychomotor agitation or retardation nearly every day (observable by others, not merely subjective feelings of restlessness or being slowed down).
   6. Fatigue or loss of energy nearly every day.
   7. Feelings of worthlessness or excessive or inappropriate guilt (which may be delusional) nearly every day (either by subjective account or as observed by others).
   8. Diminished ability to think or concentrate, or indecisiveness, nearly every day (either by subjective account or as observed by others).

   9. Recurrent thoughts of death (not just fear of dying), recurrent suicidal ideation without a specific plan, or a suicide attempt or a specific plan for committing suicide.
B. The symptoms cause clinically significant distress or impairment in social, occupational, or other important areas of functioning.
C. The episode is not attributable to the physiological effects of a substance or to another medical condition.
   Note: Criteria A–C represent a major depressive episode.
   Note: Responses to a significant loss (e.g. bereavement, financial ruin, losses from a natural disaster, a serious medical illness or disability) may include the feelings of intense sadness, rumination about the loss, insomnia, poor appetite, and weight loss noted in Criterion A, which may resemble a depressive episode. Although such symptoms may be understandable or considered appropriate to the loss, the presence of a major depressive episode in addition to the normal response to a significant loss should also be carefully considered. This decision inevitable requires the exercise of clinical judgment based on the individual's history and the cultural norms for the expression of distress in the context of loss.[1]
D. The occurrence of the major depressive episode is not better explained by schizoaffective disorder, schizophrenia, schizophreniform disorder, delusional disorder, or other specified and unspecified schizophrenia spectrum and other psychotic disorders.
E. There has never been a manic episode or a hypomanic episode. (**Note:** This exclusion does not apply if all of the manic-like or hypomanic-like episodes are substance-induced or are attributable to the physiological effects of another medical condition.)

[1]In distinguishing grief from a major depressive episode (MDE), it is useful to consider that in grief the predominant affect is feelings of emptiness and loss, while in MDE it is persistent depressed mood and the inability to anticipate happiness or pleasure. The dysphoria in grief is likely to decrease in intensity over days to weeks and occurs in waves, the so-called pangs of grief. These waves tend to be associated with thoughts or reminders of the deceased. The depressed mood of MDE is more persistent and not tied to specific thoughts or preoccupations. The pain of grief may be accompanied by positive emotions and humor that are uncharacteristic of the pervasive unhappiness and misery characteristic of MDE. The thought content associated with grief generally features a preoccupation with thoughts and memories of the deceased, rather than the self-critical or pessimistic ruminations seen in MDE. In grief, self-esteem is generally preserved, whereas in MDE feelings of worthlessness and self-loathing are common. If self-derogatory ideation is present in grief, it typically involves perceived failings vis-à-vis the deceased (e.g., not visiting frequently enough, not telling the deceased how much he or she was loved). If a bereaved individual thinks about death and dying, such thoughts are generally focused on the deceased and possibly about "joining" the deceased, whereas in MDE such thoughts are focused on ending one's own life because of feeling worthless, undeserving of life, or unable to cope with the pain of depression. *Reprinted with permission from the* Diagnostic and statistical manual of mental disorders, *ed 5, (Copyright 2013). American Psychiatric Association.*

---

short-lasting, syndromes toward severe, chronic/recurrent and disabling disorders has been repeatedly stressed.[3,4]

SUBTYPES OF MAJOR DEPRESSIVE DISORDER

MDD is a heterogeneous clinical entity.[5] Therefore, in order to allow clinicians and researchers to differentiate patients with distinct clinical presentations, a number of subtypes have been defined.[2]

Anxious Depression

When patients with depression experience symptoms such as restlessness, tension, excessive worrying or fear of panicking, it is referred to as "anxious depression," which is a relatively common depressive subtype. Among the depressed patients participating in the multi-center Sequenced Treatment Alternatives to Relieve Depression (STAR*D) project, the prevalence of anxious depression was approximately 45%.[6,7] Patients with anxious depression tend to have a slower response to treatment and are less likely to respond to

antidepressant treatment than are those without anxious depression.[8]

Mixed Depression

Patients who, in addition to meeting criteria for depression, also display symptoms of elevated mood, grandiosity, pressured speech, racing thoughts, increased energy, risk-taking, and a decreased need for sleep (without meeting full criteria for hypomania or mania) should be assigned the diagnosis of "mixed depression." These patients are at increased risk of developing bipolar I or bipolar II disorder.

Melancholic Depression

Those with "melancholic depression" are severely depressed patients who are unable to experience pleasure (anhedonia) or who lose normal emotional responsiveness to positive experiences. These patients also exhibit the following characteristics: a distinct quality of depressed mood (despondency, despair, moroseness, or empty mood), a worsening of mood in the morning, excessive/inappropriate guilt, early morning awakening, reduced appetite/weight loss, and psychomotor retardation/agitation.

Atypical Depression

Atypical depression is characterized by mood reactivity (defined as an ability to temporarily respond to positive experiences) accompanied by rejection sensitivity, hypersomnia, hyperphagia, and prominent physical fatigue (leaden paralysis, with feelings of heaviness in the arms and legs).

Psychotic Depression

Patients with psychotic depression suffer from delusions and/or hallucinations in addition to depression. The content of the psychotic symptoms is typically mood-congruent (i.e., consistent with the depressive themes of guilt, nihilism, deserved punishment), but may also be mood-incongruent (e.g. persecutory or self-referential delusions and hallucinations without an affective content). Psychotic depression is typically accompanied by significant cognitive dysfunction and it has shown distinctive responsiveness to treatment with electroconvulsive therapy (ECT) and to the combination of antidepressants and antipsychotics (being superior to either drug alone).[9]

Catatonic Depression

Catatonia is defined by abnormalities of movement and behavior arising as a consequence of a disturbed mental state. Catatonic features include stupor (with a lack of motion/motion-response to environment), posturing (maintenance of a posture held against gravity), negativism (motiveless resistance to all instructions), stereotypy (repetitive purposeless movements), mannerisms (odd/peculiar/circumstantial caricature of normal movements/actions), echolalia (mimicking another person's speech), and echopraxia (mimicking another person's actions).

Peri-partum Depression

Peri-partum depression is characterized by its onset during pregnancy or within 4 weeks of the delivery of a child. The symptomatology does generally not differ from non-peri-partum depressive episodes; however, psychotic features (such as negative delusions involving the newborn infant) are relatively common. Other common symptoms are mood fluctuations, severe anxiety, panic attacks, suicidal thoughts, spontaneous crying, insomnia, and a general disinterest in the infant.

Seasonal Depression

In this subtype of recurrent depression, the onset occurs at a particular time of the year, most often in the fall or winter. Remissions also display a seasonal pattern, i.e., a patient with recurrent depressions during the fall, which will often remit in the spring. Seasonal depression is more prevalent at higher latitudes; a lack of daylight is believed to be an important etiological factor.

EVALUATION OF THE PATIENT WITH POTENTIAL MAJOR DEPRESSIVE DISORDER

When evaluating a patient with potential MDD, clinicians must carefully obtain information regarding the duration and course of all physical and psychological symptoms during the months before the visit, and conduct a thorough physical examination. A routine laboratory test (e.g., with a complete blood count, thyroid function tests, liver enzymes, blood sugar, lipids, C-reactive protein, sodium, potassium, creatinine, calcium, vitamin D, folate, and vitamin B_{12} levels) should also be performed to rule out metabolic disorders, infections, and anemia that may cause symptoms of depression. A full report of any previous/co-morbid psychiatric disorders must also be obtained, including a systematic evaluation of drug or alcohol abuse/dependence (see diagnostic criteria for the significance of substance use). The clinician must then review the medical history and the use of concomitant medications. Finally, a mental status examination must be completed, paying close attention to whether the patient is currently suicidal or has thoughts of hurting others, and whether there are any psychotic symptoms. In their assessment, practitioners should be aware of the societal stigma of depression and, thus, the reluctance of some patients to report psychological distress.

A number of medical conditions must be considered in the differential diagnosis of MDD. The diagnosis of depressive disorders may be complicated by the fact that a patient with certain medical conditions (e.g., cancer, and endocrine, cardiovascular or neurological diseases) may present with physical symptoms that resemble those of depression (e.g., fatigue, weight loss, sleep disturbances). Although MDD is frequently associated with medical illnesses, the DSM-5 specifies that "the depressive episode is not attributable to the physiological effects of a substance or to another medical condition".[2] This hierarchical approach is occasionally ignored by clinicians, who tend to make the diagnosis of MDD even in the presence of medical conditions that may be causally related to the depression itself through pathophysiological mechanisms. In such cases the depression may remit completely with the successful treatment of the underlying medical condition. Therefore, the medical history together with the physical examination and laboratory tests should guide any further diagnostic work-up in order to discover and subsequently treat non-psychiatric medical conditions, which may account for depressive symptoms "mimicking" MDD. However, it is important to stress that many patients will suffer from concomitant non-psychiatric medical conditions and MDD, and should receive treatment for both. Special consideration should be taken into account when evaluating pharmacological treatments that could be responsible for depression, such as use of glucocorticoids.[10] Despite anecdotal reports, beta-blockers do not appear to cause depression.[10]

Other mental disorders may represent differential diagnoses to MDD/other depressive disorders. As specified in the DSM-5 criteria for MDD (Box 29-1): "The occurrence of the major depressive episode is not better explained by schizoaffective disorder, schizophrenia, schizophreniform disorder, delusional disorder, or other specified and unspecified schizophrenia spectrum and other psychotic disorders".[2] Consequently, these disorders represent differential diagnoses for MDD and a patient meeting full diagnostic criteria for a psychotic disorder should be diagnosed as such, despite meeting the symptom criteria for MDD or other depressive disorders. Similarly, a patient with a history of a manic/hypomanic episode should be diagnosed with bipolar disorder, if they meet the symptom criteria for MDD (bipolar depression). These two examples emphasize the need for a thorough assessment of the depressed patient, as the depressive syndrome may be a consequence of a "primary" psychotic disorder or as a depressive episode in the course of bipolar disorder. Distinguishing among psychotic disorders, bipolar disorder, and MDD/other depressive disorders is essential for optimal treatment.

As opposed to the differential diagnoses described above, a number of mental/behavioral disorders may be co-morbid with depression. These include anxiety disorders, obsessive-compulsive disorders, trauma- and stressor-related disorders, eating disorders, substance-related and addictive disorders, personality disorders, and neurodevelopmental disorders (autism, attention-deficit/hyperactivity disorder).[2]

OTHER DEPRESSIVE DISORDERS

Additional categories of depressive disorders listed in DSM-5 are: disruptive mood dysregulation disorder, premenstrual dysphoric disorder, substance/medication-induced depressive disorder, depressive disorder due to another medical condition, other specified depressive disorder, and unspecified depressive disorder. For further information on these disorders, including diagnostic criteria, see the DSM-5.[2]

EPIDEMIOLOGY OF MAJOR DEPRESSIVE DISORDER

A recent systematic review on the epidemiology of depression estimates the global point prevalence of MDD to be approximately 5%[11] and the annual incidence to be 3%.[12] This incidence rate fits very well with the previously reported 30-week average duration of a depressive episode.[13] The life-time prevalence of MDD in the US and most western European countries is in the range of 10%–20%, with rates significantly higher in women than men.[11,14]

MORBIDITY, DISABILITY, AND MORTALITY RATES IN DEPRESSION

MDD is associated with a significant burden of subjective suffering, increased morbidity, and impaired social and work function.[15] Depression is estimated to rival virtually every other known medical illness with regard to its burden of disease morbidity.[1] With respect to physical function, depressed patients score, on average, 77.6% of normal function, with advanced coronary artery disease and angina being 65.8% and 71.6%, respectively, and back problems, arthritis, diabetes, and hypertension ranging from 79% to 88.1%.[16] MDD has also been characterized by increased mortality.[17,18] While in the general population, suicide accounts for about 0.9% of all deaths, depression is the most important risk factor for suicide, with about 21% of patients suffering from recurrent depressive disorders attempting suicide. It has been estimated that about two-thirds of completed suicides occur in depressed patients.[19] Other complications of depressive disorders occasionally encountered in clinical practice include homicidal/aggressive behavior and/or alcohol/substance abuse.[20,21]

Depressive conditions cause substantial disability and cost approximately $86 billion per year (estimate from the year 2000) in the US alone.[22] A study of computerized record systems of a large staff-model health maintenance organization showed that patients diagnosed as depressed had significantly higher annual health care costs ($4,246 versus $2,371, $P < 0.001$) and higher costs for every category of care (e.g., primary care, medical specialty, medical inpatient, pharmacy, and laboratory) than patients who were not depressed.[23] Depressive disorders are likely to cause more disability than many other chronic diseases.[24] Indeed, it has recently been estimated that more than 60 million years of healthy life (number of disability-adjusted life years) are lost every year due to MDD, which ranks the disorder as the 11th largest burden of disease worldwide, above tuberculosis (13th), diabetes (14th), and schizophrenia (43rd).[1] In a large-scale study by the World Health Organization (WHO) concerning patients attending a primary care facility, patients with depressive disorders reported an average of eight days of disability in the

month preceding the referral. The latter was a significantly higher burden of disability compared with the 2 days lost in the non-psychiatric patients.[25] These findings were confirmed among patients with MDD by a study conducted in Western Europe, where the degree of disability was found to be directly related to the severity of depression.[26] While appropriate antidepressant therapy improves daily function and overall health of patients with depressive disorders,[27,28] patients treated for depression still represent a population with significant disability. In fact, the DEPRES-II study found that patients treated for depression by a health care professional were expected to lose on average 30 days of normal activity and 20 days of paid employment during the following 6 months.[29]

IMPACT OF DEPRESSION ON MEDICAL CO-MORBIDITY

Depressed patients often have co-morbid medical illnesses (e.g., arthritis, hypertension, backache, diabetes, and heart problems). The prevalence of these chronic medical conditions in depressed patients is higher regardless of the medical context of recruitment, with an overall rate ranging from 65% to 71% of subjects.[30] Several studies indicate that depression significantly influences the course of concomitant medical diseases. Some degree of depression in patients hospitalized for coronary artery disease is associated with an increased mortality risk, and also with continuing depression over at least the first year following hospitalization.[31] The increased cardiac mortality risk has been confirmed in a large community-dwelling sample with cardiac diseases and either major or minor co-morbid depression. The same study found that, in the community, those without cardiac disease but with depression also had an increased cardiac mortality risk (ranging from 1.5-fold to 3.9-fold).[32] In Type 1 or 2 diabetic patients, depression was associated with a significantly higher risk of diabetes-specific complications (such as diabetic retinopathy, nephropathy, neuropathy, macrovascular complications, and sexual dysfunction).[33] Data from the Hispanic Established Population for the Epidemiologic Study of the Elderly indicated that death rates in this population were substantially higher when a high level of depressive symptoms was co-morbid with diabetes (odds ratio = 3.84).[34] Depression symptom severity is also associated with poor diet/medication adherence, functional impairment, and higher health care costs in primary care diabetic patients.[35]

Under-recognition and under-treatment of depression in the elderly has been associated with increased medical utilization.[36] Among elderly patients (age 65 years or higher), a significant correlation exists between depression and the risk of recurrent falls, with an odds ratio of 3.9 when four or more depressive symptoms co-exist. These data are of particular importance since falls in the elderly are a relevant and well-recognized public health problem.[37]

With respect to the overall mortality risk, the studies that link depression to early death are poorly controlled, but they suggest that depression substantially increases the risk of death, especially death by suicide and other violent causes, but also by non-psychiatric medical illnesses, such as cardiovascular disease.[38] In post–myocardial infarction patients, there is a fourfold increase in mortality rate among those suffering from depression.[39] Patients with cancer and co-morbid depression are also at higher risk of death[40] and at higher risk of longer hospital stays. Unfortunately, despite the impact of depression on overall morbidity, functional impairment, and mortality risk, a significant proportion of sufferers (43%) fail to seek treatment for their depressive symptoms.[26]

IMPACT OF NON-PSYCHIATRIC MEDICAL ILLNESSES ON MAJOR DEPRESSIVE DISORDER

An important aspect of the relationship between depression and non-psychiatric medical illnesses is represented by the potential impact that either the emergence, or changes in the severity of medical illnesses have on the course of depression. This area remains under-studied, as depression is seldom investigated as a secondary outcome in treatment studies of medical illnesses; however, the existing studies stress the importance of this aspect. For example it has been shown that 10 years after the diagnosis, an estimated 48% of a sample of young patients with insulin-dependent diabetes mellitus had developed at least one psychiatric disorder, with MDD being the most prevalent (28%).[41] In addition to diabetes, other non-psychiatric medical illnesses have been associated with an increased risk for MDD. These include other endocrine diseases, cardiovascular disease, musculoskeletal disease, neurological diseases and cancer.[42-44]

DEPRESSION AND PRIMARY CARE

Only 57% of depressed patients actively seek help for their depression, and, interestingly enough, most of them consult a primary care physician (PCP).[26] This finding is of particular importance because it stresses the crucial role of PCPs in the recognition and treatment of depression. Unfortunately, under-recognition of depression is common. It has been estimated through several studies that the rate of missed diagnoses of depression approaches 50%.[26,45] It is crucial to provide clinicians, and especially PCPs, with information concerning risk factors for depression both in the general population and in the health care setting in particular.

RISK FACTORS OF DEPRESSION IN PRIMARY CARE

Four risk factors (female sex, stressful life events, adverse childhood experiences, and certain personality traits) have been consistently associated with MDD, and the level of evidence suggests that at least some of the association is indeed causal. In the National Co-morbidity Study, the life-time prevalence of MDD in the US population was estimated to be 21% in women and 13% in men.[14] A wide range of environmental adversities (such as job loss, marital difficulties, major health problems, and loss of close personal relationships) are associated with a substantial increase in risk for the onset of MDD.[46] A range of difficulties in childhood (including physical and sexual abuse, poor parent–child relationships, and parental discord and divorce) almost certainly increase the risk for development of MDD later in life.[47] Certain personality traits appear to predispose to MDD, with the best evidence available for the trait termed *neuroticism*. Neuroticism is a stable personality trait that reflects the level of emotional stability versus the predisposition to develop emotional upset under stress.[47] A family history of depression is another risk factor, as first-degree relatives of individuals with MDD have a threefold increased risk of being affected by MDD themselves.[47] It is widely accepted that MDD is a heritable disorder, but the genes carrying susceptibility remain to be identified.[48]

ASSOCIATED FEATURES OF DEPRESSION IN PRIMARY CARE

PCPs should also consider associated features of depression, as the presence of such features may increase the sensitivity in detecting MDD. For example, a history of depression may be

significant, as a substantial proportion of patients have their first episode during childhood or adolescence,[47] and the risk of recurrence is greater than 50% after a first episode of MDD.[49] Numerous depressive episodes are an even stronger predictor of recurrence of depression, with 70% and 90% of patients having recurrences of depression after having experienced two and three episodes, respectively.[49] The possibility of depression should certainly be considered in patients with multiple medical problems,[50] unexplained physical symptoms,[51] chronic pain,[52] and among those who use medical services more frequently than expected.[53] Patients affected by chronic and disabling physical illnesses are at higher risk of depressive disorders, with rates being typically over 20%. Among patients with cardiac disease, 20% of have at least some degree of depression.[32] Diabetic patients have a twofold increased prevalence of depression, with 20% and 32% rates in uncontrolled and controlled studies conducted with depression symptom scales, respectively.[54,55] Depression is also more common in obese persons than it is in the general population.[56]

INDICATION FOR REFERRAL TO PSYCHIATRISTS

Physicians should always inquire about suicidal thoughts, since suicide is one of the most serious complications of depressive disorders. Typically, generic questions such as "Have you been thinking lately that life is not worth living?" are appropriate to introduce the subject, and then "Have you also been thinking that you would be better off dead?" and, finally, "Have you considered suicide lately?" and "Have you tried?"[57] Of course, in the event the patient reports suicidal thoughts/intent, referral to a specialist or to a local psychiatric emergency facility (when appropriate) is strongly recommended. History of mania (e.g., with elevated mood, increased energy, and impulsivity), suggested perhaps by a history of uncharacteristic behaviors, buying sprees, and excessive risk-taking behavior, often reported by family members, should lead to referral of depressed patients to a psychiatric specialist for evaluation of potential bipolar disorder. Referral is also indicated in case of treatment-resistant depression, psychotic depression, and whenever there is a danger that the patient will harm someone else.[58]

CONCLUSIONS

The recognition, diagnosis, and treatment of depressive disorders, particularly MDD, has tremendous public health significance. These are highly prevalent conditions that are associated with significant suffering and disability. The main challenges in the recognition and diagnosis of these disorders are that these conditions manifest with a constellation of psychological, behavioral, and physical symptoms and, at the same time, they often co-occur with other psychiatric and non-psychiatric medical disorders.

Access the complete reference list and multiple choice questions (MCQs) online at https://expertconsult.inkling.com

KEY REFERENCES

1. Murray CJ, Vos T, Lozano R, et al. Disability-adjusted life years (DALYs) for 291 diseases and injuries in 21 regions, 1990–2010: a systematic analysis for the Global Burden of Disease Study. *Lancet* 380:2197–2223, 2012.
2. American Psychiatric Association. *Diagnostic and statistical manual of mental disorders*, ed 5, Washington, DC, 2013.
5. Ostergaard SD, Jensen SO, Bech P. The heterogeneity of the depressive syndrome: when numbers get serious. *Acta Psychiatr Scand* 124:495–496, 2011.

7. Fava M, Rush AJ, Alpert JE, et al. What clinical and symptom features and comorbid disorders characterize outpatients with anxious major depressive disorder: a replication and extension. *Can J Psychiatry* 51:823–835, 2006.

11. Kessler RC, Bromet EJ. The epidemiology of depression across cultures. *Annu Rev Public Health* 34:119–138, 2013.

12. Ferrari AJ, Somerville AJ, Baxter AJ, et al. Global variation in the prevalence and incidence of major depressive disorder: a systematic review of the epidemiological literature. *Psychol Med* 43(3):471–481, 2013.

15. Goldney RD, Fisher LJ, Wilson DH, et al. Major depression and its associated morbidity and quality of life in a random, representative Australian community sample. *Aust N Z J Psychiatry* 34:1022–1029, 2000.

16. Wells KB, Stewart A, Hays RD, et al. The functioning and well-being of depressed patients. Results from the Medical Outcomes Study. *JAMA* 262:914–919, 1989.

18. Penninx BW, Geerlings SW, Deeg DJ, et al. Minor and major depression and the risk of death in older persons. *Arch Gen Psychiatry* 56:889–895, 1999.

20. Fishbain DA. The epidemiology of murder-suicide in England and Wales. *Psychol Med* 33:375, 2003.

22. Greenberg PE, Leong SA, Birnbaum HG. Cost of depression: current assessment and future directions. *Exp Rev Pharmacoeconomics Outcomes Res* 1:89–96, 2001.

25. Ormel J, Von Korff M, Ustun TB, et al. Common mental disorders and disability across cultures. Results from the WHO Collaborative Study on Psychological Problems in General Health Care. *JAMA* 272:1741–1748, 1994.

26. Lepine JP, Gastpar M, Mendlewicz J, et al. Depression in the community: the first pan-European study DEPRES [Depression Research in European Society]. *Int Clin Psychopharmacol* 12:19–29, 1997.

28. Katzelnick DJ, Simon GE, Pearson SD, et al. Randomized trial of a depression management program in high utilizers of medical care. *Arch Fam Med* 9:345–351, 2000.

29. Tylee A, Gastpar M, Lepine JP, et al. DEPRES II [Depression Research in European Society II]: a patient survey of the symptoms, disability and current management of depression in the community. DEPRES Steering Committee. *Int Clin Psychopharmacol* 14:139–151, 1999.

31. Frasure-Smith N, Lesperance F. Recent evidence linking coronary heart disease and depression. *Can J Psychiatry* 12:730–737, 2006.

34. Black SA, Markides KS. Depressive symptoms and mortality in older Mexican Americans. *Ann Epidemiol* 9:45–52, 1999.

36. Reynolds CF, Alexopoulos GS, Katz IR, et al. Chronic depression in the elderly: approaches for prevention. *Drugs Aging* 18:507–514, 2001.

38. Wulsin LR, Vaillant GE, Wells VE. A systematic review of the mortality of depression. *Psychosom Med* 61:6–17, 1999.

40. Prieto JM, Atala J, Blanch J, et al. Role of depression as a predictor of mortality among cancer patients after stem-cell transplantation. *J Clin Oncol* 23:6063–6071, 2005.

41. Kovacs M, Goldston D, Obrosky DS, et al. Psychiatric disorders in youths with IDDM: rates and risk factors. *Diabetes Care* 20:36–44, 1997.

42. Fava GA, Sonino N, Morphy MA. Major depression associated with endocrine disease. *Psychiatr Dev* 5:321–348, 1987.

43. Ostergaard SD, Foldager L. The association between physical illness and major depressive episode in general practice. *Acta Psychiatr Scand* 123:290–296, 2011.

47. Fava M, Kendler K. Major depressive disorder. *Neuron* 28:335–341, 2000.

48. Major Depressive Disorder Working Group of the Psychiatric GWAS Consortium. A mega-analysis of genome-wide association studies for major depressive disorder. *Mol Psychiatry* 18(4):497–511, 2013.

49. Kupfer DJ. Long-term treatment of depression. *J Clin Psychiatry* 52(Suppl.):28–34, 1991.

51. Kroenke K, Spitzer RL, Williams JB, et al. Physical symptoms in primary care: predictors of psychiatric disorders and functional impairment. *Arch Fam Med* 3:774–779, 1997.

54. Anderson RJ, Freedland KE, Clouse RE, et al. The prevalence of comorbid depression in adults with diabetes: a meta-analysis. *Diabetes Care* 24:1069–1078, 2001.

56. Wyatt SB, Winters KP, Dubbert PM. Overweight and obesity: prevalence, consequences, and causes of a growing public health problem. *Am J Med Sci* 331:166–174, 2006.

30 Bipolar Disorder

Roy H. Perlis, MD, MSc, and Michael J. Ostacher, MD, MPH, MMSc

KEY POINTS

Incidence

- The lifetime prevalence of bipolar disorders is approximately 2%.

Epidemiology

- Bipolar disorder is associated with significant morbidity, including functional impairment, as well as significant risk for suicide.

Clinical Findings

- Diagnosis of bipolar disorder rests on establishing current or prior manic, hypomanic, mixed, or depressive episodes.

Treatment Options

- Treatments with evidence of efficacy for prevention of recurrence of mood episodes in bipolar disorder include use of lithium, valproate, lamotrigine, and some atypical antipsychotics, as well as psychosocial interventions.

Complications

- Depressive episodes, as well as inter-episode sub-threshold depressive symptoms, contribute substantially to the morbidity of bipolar disorder.

OVERVIEW

Bipolar disorder (BPD) is a group of brain diseases characterized by periods of depressed or elevated/irritable mood that last for weeks to years. Sometimes referred to as manic-depressive illness or manic-depressive disorder, it is traditionally considered a recurrent illness, although a growing body of evidence suggests that symptoms are chronic in many patients. The defining features of BPD are manic or hypomanic episodes; however, depressive symptoms contribute to much of the disability associated with this illness.

EPIDEMIOLOGY AND RISK FACTORS

The National Co-morbidity Survey—Replication (NCS-R) study, in which a random population-based sample of about 9,000 adults was contacted and screened using *Diagnostic and Statistical Manual of Mental Disorders*, ed 4 (DSM-IV)–based questions, estimated a lifetime prevalence of 1% for bipolar I disorder and 1.1% for bipolar II disorder.[1] A previous population-based survey using a validated self-report questionnaire estimated the prevalence of BPD at 3.4% to 3.7%.[2] In the NCS-R, the prevalence of "sub-threshold" BPD—that is, two or more core features of hypomania, without meeting criteria for BPD—was estimated at 2.4%. With this broader definition, the prevalence of all "bipolar spectrum" disorders reaches 4.4%.

The prevalence of BPD is similar for men and women[3] though gender differences may exist in illness features.[4] The risk for BPD also appears to be similar across racial groups and geographical regions. For example, epidemiological studies indicate a lifetime prevalence between 0.3% in Taiwan and 1.5% in New Zealand.[3] Past studies have also suggested that BPD might be under-recognized among non-Caucasians, because of a tendency instead to diagnose these individuals with schizophrenia. However, the NCS-R survey found no differences in the prevalence of BPD by race/ethnicity or by socioeconomic status (defined by family income).[1]

The strongest established risk factor for BPD is a family history of BPD. Individuals with a first-degree relative (a parent or sibling) with BPD have a risk approximately 5 to 10 times that of those in the general population (see the section on genetics, later in this chapter). Importantly, however, their risk for major depressive disorder (MDD) is also increased more than twofold; given the greater prevalence of MDD; this means that family members of bipolar individuals are at greater risk for MDD than BPD, though some authors argue that many of those diagnosed with MDD simply have unrecognized BPD.

A number of putative environmental risks have been described for BPD[5]; these include pregnancy and obstetrical complications, season of birth (winter or spring birth, perhaps indicating maternal exposure to infection), stressful life events, traumatic brain injuries, and multiple sclerosis (MS). In MS, for example, the prevalence of BPD is roughly doubled[6]; this increase does not appear to result from adverse effects of pharmacotherapy. The prevalence may also be increased among individuals with certain neurological disorders, including epilepsy. Another intriguing finding is the association between dietary omega-3 fatty acid consumption and risk of mood disorders. Most such studies focus broadly on depressed mood, although one study reporting on data from 18 countries found greater seafood consumption to be associated with a lower risk for BPD.[7,8]

HISTORICAL CONTEXT

The concept of mood disorders dates back at least to the observations of the ancient Greeks, who recognized melancholia (depression) and mania. Beginning with the Greeks, and continuing through the nineteenth century, multiple authors independently connected the two mood states.[9,10] For example, the French physician Jules Baillarger referred to "la folie a double-forme," the alternation of manic and depressive episodes. Indeed, the concept of a dichotomy between MDD and BPD did not re-emerge until the 1960s, and remains a subject of controversy (see the section on bipolar spectrum illness, later in this chapter).

The modern concept of BPD is attributed to Emil Kraepelin, whose text described the principle of opposing mood states, and more broadly distinguished primary affective disorders from primary psychotic disorders, a distinction that still stands, despite increasing evidence that this distinction is not absolute (see the section on genetics, later in this chapter). Kraepelin's description of phenomenology, based on careful longitudinal evaluation, is instantly recognizable to many modern clinicians. However, some of the nuance of Kraepelin's descriptions has not been transmitted in modern definitions. To cite but one example, the description (by Kraepelin's student Weygandt) of multiple categories of mixed states actually presages modern debates about the overlap between rapid mood cycling, mixed manic and depressive

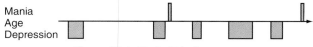

Figure 30-1. Typical bipolar course.

presentations, sub-threshold mood symptoms, and co-morbid anxiety and psychosis.[11]

CLINICAL FEATURES AND PHENOMENOLOGY

BPD is characterized by the presence of mood episodes—that is, periods of change in mood with associated symptoms. These mood episodes are described as depressive, hypomanic, manic, or mixed depending on the predominant mood and the nature of associated symptoms. Criteria for each mood state are included in the DSM-5. Mood episodes are not in and of themselves diagnoses, but rather they form the building blocks for the diagnosis of mood disorders. The key feature for the diagnosis of BPD is the presence of at least one period of mood elevation or significant irritability meeting criteria for a manic, mixed, or hypomanic episode. These episodes typically recur over time; see Figure 30-1 for a graphical illustration of the course of illness in one patient.

A manic episode is identified when a patient experiences an elevated or irritable mood for at least 1 week, along with at least three associated symptoms (described in Box 30-1). An important change in DSM-5 requires the presence of increased activity or energy as a core, or A, criterion, in an effort to improve diagnostic specificity. If the predominant affect is irritable, four rather than three associated symptoms are required. If the symptoms result in hospitalization at any point, the 1-week criterion is not required—for example, a patient hospitalized after 3 days of manic symptoms is still considered to have experienced a manic episode. As with episodes of major depression, DSM-5 criteria also require that symptoms be sufficient to markedly impair occupational or social function, or be associated with psychotic symptoms. The reliability of diagnosis for bipolar I was modest in DSM-5 field trials, with a kappa of 0.56. Hypomanic symptoms are generally similar to, but less severe and impairing than, manic symptoms. DSM-5 criteria require at least 4 days of mood elevation or irritability, along with associated symptoms; as with mania, required core symptoms now include increase in energy or activity. There are three important, but often overlooked, aspects of these criteria that bear highlighting. First, symptoms must be observable by others—that is, a purely subjective report of hypomania is not sufficient for a diagnosis. Second, symptoms represent a change from the individual's baseline; those who are "always" cheerful, impulsive, and talkative are not considered chronically hypomanic (though see the section on hyperthymia, later in this chapter). Third, symptoms by definition do not cause significant functional impairment—hypomanic-like symptoms that lead to loss of a job, for example, could be considered mania. As these criteria may be difficult to operationalize, it is not surprising that inter-rater reliability of hypomania criteria in DSM-5 field trials is somewhat lower.[12]

A major depressive episode is defined exactly as it is in MDD: the presence of depressed mood or loss of interest, most of the day, more days than not, with additional symptoms that include changes in sleep or appetite, poor self-esteem, feelings of guilt, fatigue, poor concentration, psychomotor agitation or slowing, and thoughts of suicide (see Chapter 29 for details). In DSM-IV when criteria were met for both a major depressive and a manic episode nearly every day for at least 1 week, an episode would be characterized as a mixed state. In DSM-5, this mood state is omitted, but a

---

BOX 30-1 DSM-5 Criteria: Manic Episode

A. A distinct period of abnormally and persistently elevated, expansive, or irritable mood and abnormally and persistently increased goal-directed activity or energy, lasting at least 1 week and present most of the day, nearly every day (or any duration if hospitalization is necessary).

B. During the period of mood disturbance and increased energy or activity, three (or more) of the following symptoms (four if the mood is only irritable) are present to a significant degree and represent a noticeable change from usual behaviour:
   1. Inflated self-esteem or grandiosity
   2. Decreased need for sleep (e.g., feels rested after only 3 hours of sleep)
   3. More talkative than usual or pressure to keep talking
   4. Flight of ideas or subjective experience that thoughts are racing
   5. Distractibility (i.e., attention too easily drawn to unimportant or irrelevant external stimuli)
   6. Increase in goal-directed activity (either socially, at work or school, or sexually) or psychomotor agitation
   7. Excessive involvement in pleasurable activities that have a high potential for painful consequences (e.g., engaging in unrestrained buying sprees, sexual indiscretions, or foolish business investments).

C. The mood disturbance is sufficiently severe to cause marked impairment in social or occupational functioning or to necessitate hospitalization to prevent harm to self or others, or there are psychotic features.

D. The episode is not attributable to the physiological effects of a substance (e.g., a drug of abuse, a medication, other treatment) or a general medical condition (e.g., hyperthyroidism).

Note: A full manic episode that emerges during antidepressant treatment (e.g., medication, electroconvulsive therapy) but persists at a fully syndromal level beyond the physiological effect of that treatment is sufficient evidence for a manic episode and, therefore, a bipolar I diagnosis.

Note: Criteria A–D constitute a manic episode. At least one lifetime manic episode is required for the diagnosis of bipolar I disorder.

Reprinted with permission from the Diagnostic and statistical manual of mental disorders, *ed 5, (Copyright 2013). American Psychiatric Association.*

TABLE 30-1 Diagnostic Features of Mood Disorders

	Mania/Mixed	**Depression**
Bipolar I	Yes	Typical but not required
Bipolar II	Hypomania only	Yes
MDD	Never	Yes
Cyclothymia	Never (but periods of elevation)	Symptoms but not full episode within first 2 years

MDD, Major depressive disorder.

---

modifier—"with mixed features"—recognizes the common co-occurrence of manic and depressive features, setting a lower threshold than full syndromal criteria for each episode type.

Having identified the presence and type of current and past mood episodes, the clinician may then categorize the type of mood disorder and make a diagnosis. These diagnostic features are summarized in Table 30-1. Individuals with at least one manic episode are considered to have bipolar I disorder. Those with at least one hypomanic and one depressive episode, but never a manic episode, are considered to have bipolar II disorder. Individuals who have never experienced a period of hypomania, mania, or a mixed state do not have BPD (see the section on bipolar spectrum illness, later in this chapter). Note that individuals with episodes of hypomania but never manic/mixed states must also have had at least one depressive episode to meet criteria for BPD. In practice, the prevalence of hypomania without a single depressive episode is quite rare.

Two additional diagnoses are considered part of the bipolar spectrum in the DSM-5. Individuals with persistent mood instability who never meet full criteria for BPD or MDD are considered to have cyclothymia, a heterogeneous diagnosis whose relationship to other diagnostic categories is poorly understood. Specific criteria include at least 2 years marked by periods of hypomania, as well as periods of depressed mood and no more than 2 months without symptoms. Other specified bipolar and related disorder may be diagnosed in individuals with features of BPD (including mood elevation or depression) who do not meet criteria for another bipolar diagnosis (for example, where too few symptoms of hypomania are present).

ASSOCIATED ILLNESS FEATURES
Bipolar I versus II

The distinction between bipolar I and II disorder formally entered the American diagnostic system in the DSM-IV and continued in DSM-5, though it was initially described in 1976,[13] based on apparent stable differences in course of illness. Indeed, modern studies suggest that transition from bipolar II to bipolar I among adult patients is rare.[14] Some studies suggest that bipolar II patients may experience more frequent episodes and greater risk for rapid cycling,[15] as well as greater burden of depressive symptoms.[16] These differences belie the common misconception that bipolar II is less disabling than bipolar I.

Psychosis

Psychosis is not represented in the diagnostic features for BPD. However, psychotic symptoms are common during both manic/mixed and depressive episodes. A Finnish population-based study found a prevalence of 0.24% for psychotic bipolar I disorder.[17] The lifetime prevalence of psychotic symptoms in a cohort of bipolar patients was approximately 40%.[18] So-called "mood-congruent" psychotic symptoms are often seen—for example, grandiose delusions during mania or delusions of decay and doom during depression. Psychosis typically resolves along with the mood symptoms, though diagnostic criteria acknowledge that psychotic symptoms may linger beyond the end of the mood episode.

Suicide

Suicidal thoughts and attempts are also not required for a diagnosis of BPD, although they are among the criteria for a depressive episode. In one large cohort of bipolar I and II patients, between 25% and 50% reported at least one lifetime suicide attempt.[18] In population-based studies, risk of death from suicide among bipolar patients is estimated at between 10 and 25 times that of the general population,[19,20] similar to that observed in MDD.[20]

Cognitive Symptoms

Increasingly, a subset of patients with BPD has been recognized as experiencing cognitive impairment, both during and outside of mood episodes.[21] Such impairment has been

difficult to characterize because it is likely multi-factorial, but clearly contributes to the profound functional impairments experienced by many bipolar patients.[21] Many commonly used pharmacotherapies (including lithium and anticonvulsants) can affect cognition. Likewise, residual mood symptoms, both depressive and manic, may affect cognition—for example, difficulty with concentrating or distractibility may occur. Attention-deficit/hyperactivity disorder (ADHD) has also been suggested to be prevalent among patients with BPD. This finding may represent "true" ADHD, or simply an overlap in the diagnostic criteria of these diagnoses.

Regardless of potential confounding effects, rigorous studies incorporating neuropsychological testing of relatively euthymic patients suggest a plethora of cognitive complaints.[21] Because these studies often use different cognitive batteries among relatively small numbers of patients, it is difficult to arrive at a single cognitive profile that is typical for BPD. Typical findings on neuropsychological testing include impairment in attention and executive function and, in some studies, deficits in working or verbal memory.

FEATURES OF LONGITUDINAL COURSE
Age at Onset and Prodrome

More recent studies suggest that the age of onset of BPD may be somewhat earlier than previously appreciated. In a large cohort study of adults with BPD, nearly one-third of individuals reported the onset of symptoms before age 13, and another one-third became symptomatic between ages 13 and 18 years.[18] In this study, earlier onset was associated with a more chronic and recurrent course, greater functional impairment, and greater Axis I co-morbidity. Unfortunately, most such studies rely on retrospective reporting, and frequently fail to distinguish between the onset of mood symptoms and the onset of a syndromal mood episode. In the NCS-R survey, the mean age at onset for bipolar I disorder was 18.2 years, and for bipolar II disorder it was 20.3 years.[1]

Mood Episodes and Chronicity

Traditional emphasis on the episodic structure of BPD has been complemented with a recognition that, for many patients, symptoms may be chronic and persist beyond discrete episodes (see Figure 30-1). Indeed, such symptoms likely contribute substantially to the disability associated with BPD, estimated to be one of the 10 greatest medical causes of disability world-wide.[22] In general, while hypomania and mania are considered the defining features of BPD, patients spend a far greater amount of time ill—around two-thirds of the time, in one longitudinal study[23]—with depressive symptoms. In general, persistence of sub-syndromal symptoms appears to be common,[24] which may explain in part persistence of functional impairment as well.[25]

Up to 40% of bipolar I patients experience a mixed state at some point in their disease course.[26] Recently, the concept of sub-threshold mixed states has received increasing attention: patients who do not meet the stringent criteria for a mixed state (who do not meet full criteria for both a manic and a depressive episode simultaneously), but nonetheless have some degree of both types of symptoms. Depressive symptoms are common during manic or hypomanic episodes, underscoring the importance of inquiring about both poles. Conversely, during depressive episodes, patients may experience some degree of hypomanic symptoms, such as racing thoughts. The prognostic implications, if any, of these sub-threshold mixed states has not been well studied. However, the change in DSM-5 to incorporate mixed symptoms as modifiers of a manic or depressive episode rather than distinct states is an effort to better capture such symptoms.

Rapid Cycling

DSM-IV-TR criteria described rapid cycling as a course specifier in BPD—that is, an illness feature that may be present at times but not necessarily throughout the course of the illness. Specifically, individuals with at least four syndromal mood episodes within a single year, separated by full recovery or a switch to the opposite pole, are considered to experience rapid cycling. In one cohort of bipolar patients, prevalence of rapid cycling was 20% assessed retrospectively,[27] and rapid cycling was associated with greater illness burden and chronicity.

Antidepressant-induced Mania/Hypomania

A small number of patients experience the onset of mania or hypomania after initiation of antidepressants, which under DSM-5 is considered to represent BPD. The true prevalence and time course of this phenomenon is difficult to estimate, particularly for a switch to hypomania, because in clinical practice, as well as in randomized controlled trials (RCTs), such symptoms of elevated mood may not be aggressively investigated. A patient who sees his or her clinician, 2 weeks after beginning an antidepressant, feeling "great" and congratulating the clinician on the clinician's excellent skills requires careful questioning about manic/hypomanic symptoms, but more often is congratulated in turn on his or her excellent antidepressant response. In one of the largest prospective antidepressant treatment studies to date in MDD,[28] there was little or no evidence of antidepressant-induced mood elevation. Likewise, most randomized trials in MDD report switch-rates of less than 1%. In a cohort study of BPD, ~20% of subjects transitioned directly from depression to mania/hypomania. Importantly, however, this rate was similar regardless of antidepressant treatment exposure, making the point that such transitions are often not associated with antidepressant treatment and may represent part of the natural history of the disorder.

Such switches are typically described as early (often within 2 weeks) and abrupt, though the time course has not been well established and it is possible that patients "switch" after prolonged antidepressant exposure, and perhaps even after antidepressant discontinuation. Some definitions consider any transition within 8 or 12 weeks of antidepressant initiation to represent a switch. Some patients describe colors being more vivid, or having an abrupt urge to undertake new projects. Importantly, the switch must be discriminated from the immense relief many patients experience with resolution of their depressive symptoms. It does not represent simply the absence of depressive symptoms, but the presence of hypomanic/manic symptoms. Again, close longitudinal follow-up may be required to clarify the diagnosis.

Because of its relative rarity, both the short- and long-term prognosis for patients who only experience hypomania or mania after antidepressant initiation is not known. Even among patients with BPD, induction of a switch with one antidepressant does not necessarily imply induction of a switch with another agent. Still, in general, patients with an antidepressant-induced mood elevation require treatment with mood-stabilizing medications for treatment and prevention of future depressive episodes.

Seasonality and Climate

A relationship between season and course of illness in BPD has been reported, but its precise nature remains unclear.

Multiple studies suggest peaks in admissions for mania, generally occurring in late spring/summer.[29-31] One report suggested that most bipolar patients follow one of two patterns: depression in fall or winter, with elevation in spring/summer, or spring-summer depression, with fall-winter mania.[32] Most recently, a large cohort study found depression peaks in February and July, but only in BPD-II.[33] They found depression to be more prevalent among patients with BPD in more northern regions of the US.

Changes in Episode Frequency

A persistent belief about BPD dating back to Kraepelin's descriptions has been that the interval between episodes decreases over time, at least across the first several episodes. This apparent observation contributed in part to earlier hypotheses that posited a "kindling" effect in which episodes beget subsequent episodes. However, it may actually be the result, at least in part, of a statistical artifact first described more than 70 years ago and referred to as "Slater's fallacy."[34] Indeed, more recent analyses suggest that such worsening with time is not the case for many patients.[35]

NEUROBIOLOGY AND PATHOPHYSIOLOGY
Hypotheses

A number of overlapping hypotheses guide current research into the neurobiology of BPD. One set of observations relates to the mechanism of action of lithium, known to be an effective treatment for BPD (see Chapter 47). While its therapeutic mechanism is not known, it does interact with two key pathways in cell signaling: inositol triphosphate (InsP3)-dependent signaling, and the Wnt signaling pathway, the latter because it inhibits glycogen synthesis kinase 3-beta (GSK3B). The Wnt/GSK3 pathway represents a particular area of interest in BPD because it is a convergent site of action of multiple psychotropics, not just lithium, and because some putative schizophrenia and bipolar liability genes influence this pathway.[36] Other clinically-based hypotheses of current interest include the role of circadian rhythm disruption, because of its prevalence in BPD, and models of stress response.

Animal Models

Research into the pathophysiology of BPD has been hindered by the lack of a convincing animal model.[37] Perhaps the best-studied model is the mouse amphetamine-induced hyperactivity model, which is purported to mimic mania (or sometimes psychosis), at least in terms of inducing psychomotor agitation. Another potential mouse model of mania was created by disrupting a gene important in circadian rhythms, *CLOCK*.[38] Mania-like features in these mice include a marked decrease in sleep and an increase in activity, as well as an increase in the "rewarding" effects of cocaine; most intriguingly, these changes are normalized by the administration of lithium. Circadian rhythm abnormalities have been a focus of investigation because they are so often noted clinically among individuals with BPD.[39] Most recently, additional animal models based on genetic investigation have been reported, with both depressive and manic-like symptoms. In general, results in animal models of BPD highlight the limitations in using rodents to study affective illness.

Post-mortem Studies

Another approach to the study of BPD relies on post-mortem studies of brains from bipolar patients. Neuropathological studies suggest decreased density or morphology of oligodendrocytes.[40] Other studies examine changes in gene expression. Major caveats with this approach include the sensitivity of these studies to post-mortem handling of samples and the mode of death (e.g., duration of agonal period), as well as difficulty in discriminating medication effects from the effects of a primary disease. Still, such studies suggest differences between brains of bipolar patients and normal controls. For example, one small study found down-regulation of genes related to myelination and oligodendrocytes similar to that observed in the brains of patients with schizophrenia.[41] Other recent post-mortem data suggest changes in histone acetylation in some individuals with bipolar disorder.[42]

Neuroimaging Studies

Structural brain imaging has identified regional differences in multiple brain structures among bipolar patients, predominantly cortical and sub-cortical areas implicated in limbic circuitry. While studies of the prefrontal cortex as a whole are inconsistent, a number of reports find decreased volume in individual regions among bipolar patients (reviewed by Strakowski and colleagues[43]). Among sub-cortical structures, perhaps the most consistent findings are of increased volume in the striatum and amygdala. Notably, data from twin and early-onset cohorts suggest that striatal changes may represent "trait" markers of bipolarity, present early in the disease process.

Functional imaging in BPD is complicated by the need to consider variation in mood states, and particularly by practical difficulties in imaging truly manic patients. Region-specific differences by mood state have been noted in regions of prefrontal cortex; for example, one study found decreased perfusion of sub-genual prefrontal cortex during depression and increased perfusion during mania.[44] Similar increases have been noted in basal ganglia perfusion among manic patients.[45] Studying euthymic bipolar patients provides an opportunity to elucidate potential trait markers of bipolarity. In one such study, on a cognitive task, bipolar patients demonstrated greater activation than healthy controls in regions including the ventrolateral prefrontal cortex and amygdala.[46]

Neurochemical studies applied to BPD include positron-emission tomography (PET) and magnetic resonance spectroscopy (MRS). To date, no consistently replicated patterns for binding of serotonergic or dopaminergic ligands have been identified (reviewed by Strakowski and associates[43]). With MRS, multiple studies have reported a decrease in N-acetyl aspartate (NAA) concentration, considered a measure of neuronal health, in the prefrontal cortex.[47] Likewise, in the basal ganglia and anterior cingulate, elevations of choline (considered a marker of integrity of cell membrane) have been identified.[48] Finally, regional changes in other metabolites (i.e., lactate, glutamate/gamma-aminobutyric acid [GABA]) have also been described.[49] Taken together, these results describe an emerging pattern of metabolic abnormalities, though one whose precise nature remains to be elucidated.

Genetic Studies

The familiality of BPD was established by numerous studies indicating that, among first-degree family members of individuals with BPD, the risk for BPD is between 7 and 10 times that found in the general population.[50] Notably, the risk for MDD is also increased roughly twofold. Twin studies indicate that up to 80% of the risk for BPD is inherited. Family and twin studies also indicate an overlap in risk with schizophrenia and schizoaffective disorder (see Chapter 63). Recent studies utilize genome-wide data to estimate the amount of

BPD risk explained by common genetic variation (up to 30%), and provide further support for the genetic overlap of BPD with schizophrenia, MDD, and other psychiatric illness.

To date, at least six areas of the genome have been identified as conferring risk for BPD, including a sub-unit of L-type voltage-gated calcium channels. Studies of rarer chromosomal deletions or duplications have not yet consistently identified areas of risk.

A related area of investigation is the role of epigenetic changes in BPD—in particular, modification of chromatin. Early adversity may increase risk for BPD,[51] and both acute and chronic stress may exert epigenetic effects.[52] Intriguingly, some psychotropics, such as clozapine, appear to influence expression of chromatin-modifying enzymes.[53]

EVALUATION, TESTS, AND LABORATORY WORK-UP
Diagnosis of Bipolar Disorder

The diagnosis of BPD relies on a careful clinical assessment to identify current or past manic, hypomanic, mixed, or major depressive episodes. One study suggested that many patients wait 10 years or more for a "correct" diagnosis of BPD, although that figure may be inflated by the inclusion of patients whose initial episode is depressive.[54] A number of tools have been developed to facilitate diagnosis, but none is a substitute for detailed questioning about the mood and associated symptoms for each episode type.

A crucial and often-overlooked aspect of diagnosis in BPD is the importance of longitudinal assessment. Despite careful history-taking, in the setting of an acute episode it may sometimes be difficult to arrive at a definitive diagnosis. For example, a depressed patient may report "always" being depressed and neglect to recall periods of mood elevation consistent with hypomania.

Differential Diagnosis

A number of Axis I and II disorders may mimic BPD; general medical conditions may also yield symptoms of a mood episode. The following sections review specific diagnoses to be considered in the differential diagnosis, but several principles apply broadly. First, diagnosis requires identification of mood episodes, not simply isolated symptoms of mania or depression. Thus, the substance-abusing patient who reports "mood swings" will not necessarily be diagnosed with BPD. Second, longitudinal follow-up is often the key in clarifying the diagnosis. While difficult to implement in practice, a willingness by the clinician to make a provisional diagnosis, and to re-visit it once additional data have been gathered, eliminates some of the misplaced pressure to make an immediate diagnosis with inadequate data.

Schizophrenia and Schizoaffective Disorder

While psychosis is common among bipolar patients, the key feature that distinguishes schizophrenia and BPD is the presence of psychotic symptoms outside of mood episodes, which is not seen in BPD. In acutely psychotic and agitated patients, it may be difficult to distinguish a schizophrenic psychotic episode from a bipolar mixed state. In such cases longitudinal follow-up is required to clarify the diagnosis: in a bipolar patient, psychotic symptoms should resolve along with mood symptoms.

Schizoaffective patients, like bipolar patients, may experience both depressive and manic episodes. However, once again the presence of psychotic symptoms in the absence of a mood episode defines the diagnosis as a primary psychotic rather than affective one—that is, schizoaffective disorder rather than BPD.

Major Depressive Disorder

To distinguish MDD from BPD requires careful questioning to exclude mixed symptoms and past episodes of mood elevation. For cross-sectional evaluation, such as in a patient having a first episode, there is no single feature (other than identifying a prior episode) that distinguishes bipolar depression from MDD. The first-episode problem is particularly acute given that up to two-thirds of those with BPD recall a depressive episode preceding a manic episode. There are, however, features that may help to stratify risk; these features include current symptoms and sociodemographic/longitudinal factors.

Among current symptoms, those of atypical depression— that is, "reverse" neurovegetative signs (such as increased appetite or carbohydrate craving and hypersomnia) have been associated with bipolar depression. However, atypical depressive features are common among individuals with MDD as well, and the cohesiveness of atypical depression itself has been questioned. Likewise, some authors suggest that irritability during a depressive episode is a marker for bipolarity. Certainly irritability should prompt further questioning for mixed/manic symptoms, but the high prevalence of irritability during depressive episodes again mandates that it not be used to make a diagnosis. Psychotic features may be more commonly seen in BPD than MDD, though here too they are not diagnostic. Last, a comparison of individuals with MDD or BPD participating in RCTs found that overall depression severity was greater among the bipolar subjects, with psychic anxiety more common and somatic symptoms less common in this group.

Among other risk factors, perhaps the best characterized is family history (see the section on risk factors, earlier in this chapter). Another well-investigated risk factor is early age of illness onset. In general, the median age of onset for MDD is later than for BPD. Therefore, those with earlier onset of mood symptoms—particularly onset in childhood or adolescence— must be followed closely for BPD. Greater recurrence of depressive episodes has also been associated with BPD.

Anxiety Disorders

Distinguishing anxiety from BPD is complicated by the high rate of co-morbidity: identifying one disorder does not exclude the other. Between 85% and 90% of individuals in one survey reported at least one co-morbid anxiety disorder;[1] a large cohort study of BPD reported co-morbidity in around 60%.[18] Among the most common co-morbid conditions appear to be social phobia, generalized anxiety, post-traumatic stress disorder (PTSD), and panic disorder. One under-recognized consideration is that patients with severe anxiety may report symptoms suggestive of mania or hypomania. In particular, many anxious patients will report that their thoughts race, or that they experience psychomotor restlessness. These symptoms are often intermittent and worse when patients are most anxious, which may help to distinguish them from those with BPD.

Substance Use Disorders

As with anxiety, rates of co-occurrence between substance use disorders and BPD are quite high; determining that a patient has a substance use disorder does not end the need for screening for BPD, and vice versa. Between 40% and 60% of patients with BPD report a lifetime substance use disorder, with alcohol abuse being the most common.[1,18] What complicates the recognition of BPD is that abused substances may cause symptoms that mimic both depression and mania, as well as mixed states. For example, cocaine binges not only represent injudicious/risk-seeking behavior, but are often associated with a decreased need for sleep, pressured speech, or increased social behavior, and increased impulsivity in other domains. Likewise, the impulsivity experienced during a period of mood elevation may increase the likelihood of substance abuse.

Traditional teaching holds that BPD may be recognized among patients with substance use disorder by identifying mood episodes during periods of sobriety. However, this neglects the common phenomenon of depressive symptoms during early sobriety, as well as the fact that many patients fail to achieve a prolonged period of sobriety during which a mood episode might be detected. More useful may be the principle that mood symptoms among non-bipolar individuals are typically confined to, and change in parallel with, periods of substance intoxication or withdrawal. So, for example, a patient might be impulsive, agitated, and euphoric during a cocaine binge, but these symptoms should parallel the course of intoxication and would be unlikely to persist for days after the last cocaine use. In practice, definitively identifying BPD in a patient with frequent and severe substance use can be difficult.

Borderline Personality Disorder

Many symptoms overlap between DSM-5 definitions of BPD and borderline personality disorder.[55] Notable features in common include irritability, lability, impulsivity, and suicidality. These features may be particularly difficult to distinguish in a patient believed to have current rapid cycling,[56] with rapid fluctuation in mood state. However, several aspects of presentation bear consideration. First, symptoms of personality disorders are typically more pervasive and less episodic; while they may wax and wane over time, they would typically not "remit" in the way a mood episode would. Second, while borderline patients likely satisfy multiple manic or depressive criteria, they would not be expected to meet full criteria at a given time—that is, to have a full-blown hypomanic or manic episode.

Secondary Mania

In 1978, a group of clinicians described a small cohort of patients who developed manic symptoms in the context of medical illness, particularly after exposure to certain medications, such as corticosteroids.[57] Typically, in such cases there are other clues that the culprit is not BPD *per se*: late onset in a patient with no prior mood symptoms, close temporal correlation with a previously implicated medication, or presence of other neurological or systemic symptoms. As noted later, further medical work-up is often warranted when such features are present.

Bipolar Spectrum Illness

Symptoms common in BPD, including irritability, mood lability, and impulsivity, are also seen across many psychiatric disorders. This observation has led some authors to speculate about the concept of a bipolar spectrum: that is, bipolar I and II lie along a continuum with other disorders (such as substance abuse and binge-eating).[58]

The concept of a bipolar spectrum is often invoked in individuals with recurrent MDD, particularly those with features of illness suggestive of BPD: those with irritability or highly recurrent illness, for example.[59] In these cases it is sometimes invoked to justify using bipolar pharmacotherapies by analogy, hypothesizing that recurrent MDD that fails to respond to antidepressants might respond to a drug such as lithium. To date, while the bipolar spectrum is an appealing concept, it is not clear that it is a scientifically useful one. In particular, recent investigations suggest that bipolar spectrum illness as traditionally applied has little or no predictive validity.[60]

CONSEQUENCES OF MISDIAGNOSIS

With the increased attention to recognizing BPD, the consequences of mis-diagnosing BPD also bear a note. Some bipolar pharmacotherapies may be effective in the treatment of other disorders, but in general a patient incorrectly diagnosed with BPD is likely to receive sub-optimal treatment. Moreover, these treatments all carry some degree of potential toxicity, to which these patients may be unnecessarily exposed.

ROLE OF DIAGNOSTIC TESTING (INCLUDING NEUROIMAGING AND OTHER BIOMARKERS)

At present, there is no useful diagnostic test for BPD, nor is there a useful predictor of prognosis. A study of radiographic findings among psychiatric patients underscored the lack of utility for brain imaging in unselected populations. However, such tests may in the proper context be useful for diagnosis by excluding general medical conditions that contribute to so-called secondary mania or other mood symptoms. Medical work-up should be considered in presentations of BPD that appear to be atypical (e.g., with a later onset of illness, with an association with neurological signs, or with evidence of other systemic illnesses). For work-up of depressive symptoms, see Chapter 29. For manic/hypomanic symptoms, structural magnetic resonance imaging (MRI) helps to exclude stroke or tumor; an electroencephalogram (EEG) is rarely useful (because of poor sensitivity) for excluding temporal lobe epilepsy.

TOOLS FOR SCREENING, DIAGNOSIS, AND SYMPTOM MONITORING

Surprisingly, no single screen for BPD has been convincingly validated in clinical populations. One instrument frequently advocated for improving the recognition of BPD is the Mood Disorder Questionnaire (MDQ).[61] This patient-report questionnaire essentially incorporates the DSM criteria for mania and depression. A population-based validation study in which MDQ results were compared to Structured Clinical Interview for Diagnosis (SCID) criteria suggested that its sensitivity is poor (28%) and its specificity is 97%. A similar tool is the Bipolar Spectrum Diagnostic Scale,[62] which also uses self-report for screening. As with any screening measures, their performance depends on the prevalence of the disorder in the population being screened. In general, both measures perform well for excluding BPD when the prior probability is low (approximately 10% prevalence, as might be seen in a cohort of depressed patients), with a negative predictive value of 92% to 97%, but are not useful for confirming a diagnosis, with a positive predictive value as low as 16%—that is, the rate of false positives is extremely high. As such, neither measure can substitute for a clinician's interview, including careful history-taking. They may be most useful in initiating a discussion about BPD, for example, when completed by patients in the office waiting room.

Most research assessment tools for BPD rely on DSM criteria. While cumbersome to use in its entirety in routine practice, the mood and psychosis modules from the SCID require relatively little training to use and are helpful in ensuring comprehensive assessment of mood episodes.

For assessing depressive symptoms, validated self-report measures (the Beck Depression Inventory, the Quick Inventory of Depressive Symptoms) and clinician-rated measures (Hamilton Depression Rating Scale, Montgomery-Asberg Depression Rating Scale) are available. Of note, both the MADRS and the 17-item HAM-D do not capture reverse neurovegetative signs, and the latter weights insomnia relatively strongly, which may limit their application in bipolar depression. Self-report measures are less well-validated in BPD, though there is no reason to imagine they would perform differently in this population. Finally, the 7-point Clinical Global Impression (CGI) scale has been adapted for BPD, with one report suggesting it may capture clinical improvement in randomized trials that is not otherwise measured by other rating scales.[63] Self-report measures of depression can be applied clinically to monitor treatment response or characterize residual symptoms.

Manic symptoms are typically characterized by the Young Mania Rating Scale (YMRS), a clinician-rated scale, or the Mania Rating Scale, derived from the SAD. While a self-report form of the YMRS has been developed, because patient insight into symptoms may be impaired[64] and patients may tend to minimize symptoms during hypomania/mania, its utility could be limited, particularly among more severely ill patients.

In some cases daily mood charting (Figure 30-2) may be applied to quantify the extent of mood elevation or depression. In this approach, patients rate the extent of manic and depressive symptoms each day, along with details, such as medication compliance and sleep schedule. Beyond paper-based charts, a number of electronic mood diaries now make such mood monitoring relatively simple. The value of such charts is primarily in the measurement of changes in symptoms over time in response to different interventions, or in identification of mood cycling.

TREATMENT

Treatment goals in BPD include remission of acute episodes and prevention of recurrence.[65] Less obvious, but also crucial, given the potential chronicity of symptoms and the side-effect burdens with many treatments, treatment is aimed at preventing the consequences of BPD, including functional impairment[21] and suicide.

Determination of Mood State and Symptom Severity

The importance of characterizing mood state before initiation of treatment cannot be over-emphasized. Patients in a mixed state, for example, may complain of depressed mood, and failure to inquire about manic symptoms may result in inappropriate treatment (such as initiation of an antidepressant). More broadly, characterizing symptoms is important in monitoring treatment response, particularly given the prevalence of a partial or an incomplete response to treatment and the consequences (in terms of functional impairment and recurrence risk) of incomplete response.

Treatment strategies are typically divided into two stages: an acute phase (focused on eliminating or managing acute symptoms) and a maintenance phase (focused on prevention of recurrence and maximization of function). To some extent this dichotomy is false: acute treatments are often selected with an eye toward future use in maintenance, while maintenance treatments often require adjustment to manage residual

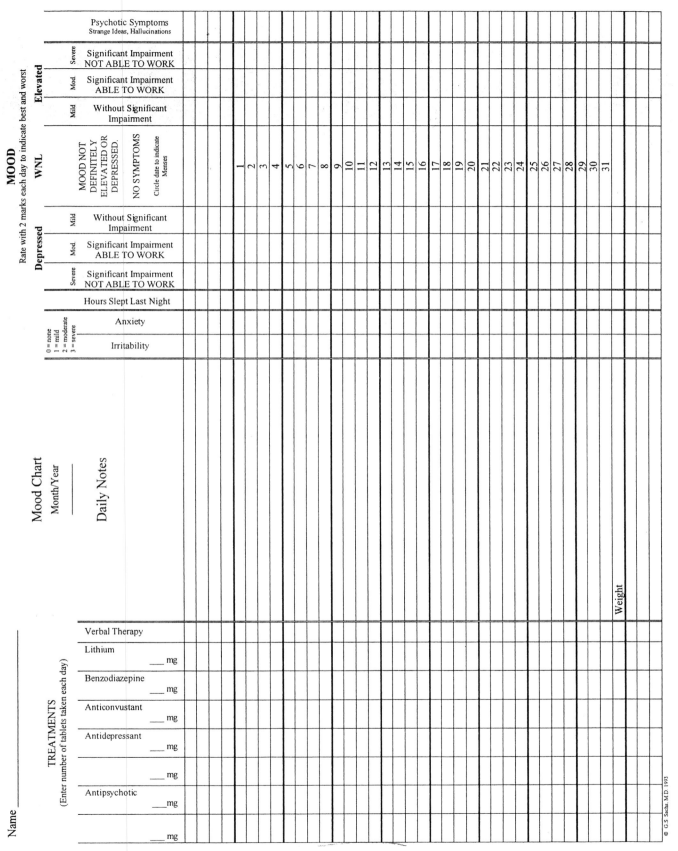

Figure 30-2. Mood chart. *(Source:* www.manicdepressive.org/images/moodchart.pdf. © *G.S. Sachs, MD, 1993.)*

or sub-threshold symptoms. Still, it provides a useful framework for consideration of treatment options.

Treatment Strategies

The number of pharmacological interventions available for the treatment of BPD has grown over the past decade, with increased application of anticonvulsants and antipsychotics. Many of these interventions continue to be actively studied, particularly in the maintenance phase of treatment. Multiple guidelines or algorithms have been developed to aid the clinician in evidence-based treatment of BPD. Internationally, a number of groups have developed their own guidelines, including the Canadian Network for Mood and Anxiety Treatments (CANMAT), the British Association for Psychopharmacology (BAP), and others. In general, these guidelines are remarkably consistent in their approach to treatment. One recent addition is the Clinical Practice Guidelines from the US Department of Veterans Affairs, released in 2010. The following section summarizes evidence-based treatments for each phase of illness. For further details, including information regarding dosing and safety, the interested reader is referred to chapters addressing individual treatment options (see Chapters 42, 43, and 48). Traditional discussions of bipolar pharmacotherapy rely on the concept of a mood stabilizer, most often used as short-hand for lithium, valproate, and in some cases carbamazepine. With the broadening of the bipolar pharmacopoeia in the past decade, however, this term is less useful and more difficult to define.[66] In the following

discussion, interventions are discussed instead in terms of their efficacy in achieving specific treatment goals: acute treatment versus prevention of recurrence, and depression versus mania.

General Treatment Strategies

Most guidelines begin by emphasizing the value of psycho-education and disease management strategies, which are supported by multiple RCTs.[67-69] These approaches focus on educating patients about the illness, and particularly recognizing symptoms, and understanding and adhering to treatment. Recent studies particularly support the utility of group-based cognitive and behavioral interventions.

Approach to Mania

As with any acute episode, the first element of managing mania is to ensure safety for patients and those around them; this may require hospitalization. Medical contributors (including drugs of abuse) to mania should be ruled-out. Antidepressants, which may precipitate or exacerbate mania, should be discontinued.

Multiple first-line agents have been established for mania (Figure 30-3). Those with greatest evidence of efficacy include lithium, valproate, and second-generation antipsychotics (SGAs). Among the SGAs, there appears to be little difference in efficacy.[70] Whether they are used alone or in combination typically depends on the severity of illness—combination therapy may have modestly greater efficacy. If a single

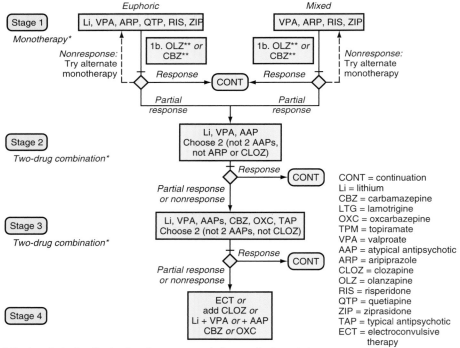

Figure 30-3. Algorithm for treatment of BPD—currently hypomanic/manic. *(Copyright 2005, Texas Department of State Health Services, all rights reserved.)*

pharmacotherapy does not achieve improvement within a short period, a second one may be added, or the patient may be switched to an alternative first-line agent. A number of other pharmacotherapies have been studied in mania; RCTs suggest that gabapentin, topiramate, and lamotrigine are not efficacious in acute treatment (see Chapter 48). Benzodiazepines are sometimes used as adjunctive treatments among manic patients, specifically to reduce agitation and promote sleep; they have shown greater efficacy than placebo in RCTs for agitation.

A question of substantial clinical interest has been whether combining multiple antimanic agents achieves better response than monotherapy. Meta-analyses do suggest modest advantage in efficacy for combination therapy, though this must be weighed against an increase in adverse effects.[70] Generally, monotherapy is preferred for less ill patients, whereas combination therapy is used for those who are more ill (e.g., hospitalized).

Approach to Mixed States

Treatment for mixed states is similar to that for manic states. Most atypical antipsychotics (AAPs) show similar efficacy among mixed and non-mixed manias. While one study suggested that lithium might be less effective in these patients

than in euphoric mania, this is by no means a consistent finding. Valproate and the atypical antipsychotics generally appear to have similar efficacy across forms of mania.[70] Similarly, antimanic agents generally show similar efficacy against psychotic mania, but antipsychotics are typically advised either as monotherapy or combination therapy in these patients.

The approach to mixed states generally follows that of mania. One study suggested that lithium was relatively less effective in mixed mania than in euphoric mania.[71]

Approach to Depression

Multiple strategies have shown efficacy in the treatment of bipolar depression in RCTs (Figure 30-4). Efficacy for lithium, valproate, and carbamazepine has been suggested but not definitively established in RCTs (see Chapters 47 and 48). Multiple SGAs, including quetiapine and olanzapine (the latter in combination with fluoxetine), as well as lurasidone, were more effective than placebo.[25,72] A head-to-head study found slightly greater improvement with the olanzapine–fluoxetine combination than with lamotrigine, despite better tolerability in the lamotrigine arm.[73] The anticonvulsant lamotrigine has also been extensively studied in bipolar depression as well, with suggestive but not consistent evidence

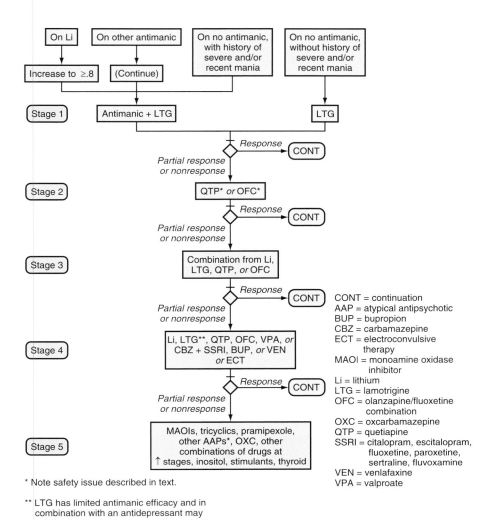

* Note safety issue described in text.

** LTG has limited antimanic efficacy and in combination with an antidepressant may require the addition of an antimanic.

CONT = continuation
AAP = atypical antipsychotic
BUP = bupropion
CBZ = carbamazepine
ECT = electroconvulsive therapy
MAOI = monoamine oxidase inhibitor
Li = lithium
LTG = lamotrigine
OFC = olanzapine/fluoxetine combination
OXC = oxcarbamazepine
QTP = quetiapine
SSRI = citalopram, escitalopram, fluoxetine, paroxetine, sertraline, fluvoxamine
VEN = venlafaxine
VPA = valproate

Figure 30-4. Algorithm for treatment of BPD—currently depressed. *(Copyright 2005, Texas Department of State Health Services, all rights reserved.)* -→ *SUBSTITUTE VA GUIDELINES 2010*

of benefit (see Chapter 48), except in combination with lithium.[74]

The efficacy of antidepressants in patients already treated with an antimanic/prophylactic medication, such as lithium, is not clear. A study of paroxetine or imipramine versus placebo, in addition to lithium, failed to find an advantage for antidepressant treatment, except in a secondary analysis examining individuals with lower (less than 0.8 mEq/L) lithium levels.[75] In the largest study to date, addition of bupropion or paroxetine to a traditional mood stabilizer likewise yielded no benefit compared to placebo.[76]

Furthermore, antidepressants appear to increase the risk of a switch—that is, transitioning directly to manic, hypomanic, or mixed states. While the risk of "switch" into mania is no greater than placebo when these medications are used along with a traditional mood stabilizer,[76,77] in the absence of evidence of efficacy, most guidelines suggest that they are better avoided. However, recent expert consensus statements acknowledge that some individuals with BPD may benefit from antidepressants in conjunction with mood stabilizers.[78] That is, antidepressants may have benefit for some individual patients, even though they fail to benefit bipolar patients as a group; for example, it has not been determined whether they benefit symptoms of co-morbid anxiety in these patients.

Approach to Maintenance Treatment

Most studies of lithium and valproate suggest that they are effective in the prevention of recurrence of mood episodes. The optimum therapeutic dose of each, and their relative benefit for prevention of manic versus depressive recurrence, is debated.[79,80] Two RCTs also found efficacy for lamotrigine in the prevention of depressive recurrence[81] (see Chapter 48). Evidence of benefit in preventing manic recurrence was much more modest. Numerous SGAs have also been shown to prevent recurrence of mood episodes. Despite the efficacy of these interventions, BPD remains highly recurrent for many patients, with residual mood symptoms one of the primary risk factors (Figure 30-5).

As in acute treatment, the role of antidepressants in maintenance is not established. As noted previously, antidepressants may contribute to an increase in mood episode frequency. On the other hand, one study suggested that discontinuing antidepressants among patients who achieved remission was associated with a greater risk of recurrence. In practice, most guidelines suggest avoiding antidepressants in long-term treatment where possible. Long-term benzodiazepine treatment has also been suggested to increase recurrence risk.[82]

Use of Psychosocial Interventions

Psychosocial interventions have received increasing attention in the management of BPD, with some but not all studies showing efficacy. In a large multi-center trial, interventions including cognitive-behavioral therapy (CBT), interpersonal/social rhythm therapy (IPSRT), and family-focused therapy increased rates of recovery from an acute episode.[83] Conversely, IPSRT showed no acute benefit in another randomized trial.[84]

A group psychoeducation approach incorporating elements of CBT also reduced recurrence in one large study.[69] A trial of IPSRT during acute episodes found reduced recurrence regardless of whether IPSRT was continued beyond that episode.[84] On the other hand, a large RCT of CBT found no benefit in preventing recurrence,[85] while another did not reduce recurrence beyond the first year,[86] despite evidence of cost-effectiveness.[87]

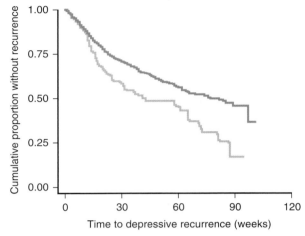

—— With residual manic symptoms			
N = 156	46	16	2
—— Without residual manic symptoms			
N = 702	309	164	19
Total			
N = 858	355	180	21

Figure 30-5. Survival curve (Systematic Treatment Enhancement Program for Bipolar Disorder [STEP-BD]). *(From Perlis RH, Ostacher MJ, Patel JK, et al. Predictors of recurrence in bipolar disorder: primary outcomes from the Systematic Treatment Enhancement Program for Bipolar Disorder (STEP-BD), Am J Psychiatry 163:217–224, 2006.)*

This pattern has persisted with more recent studies: some, but not all, find benefit, not unlike acute pharmacotherapy trials.

SPECIAL CONSIDERATIONS IN TREATMENT
Features of Course

Psychotic symptoms are common during both manic and depressive episodes.[18] Typical management involves the use of an antipsychotic, although at least one study suggested similar efficacy for valproate in psychotic mania.[88] Whether these patients require ongoing treatment with an antipsychotic following the acute episode is not well studied.

There is limited evidence to support the widespread belief that rapid cycling is associated with differential treatment response. Therefore, most treatment guidelines suggest the use of appropriate interventions for the presenting or predominant mood type (e.g., mania, hypomania, depression, and mixed state), with particular effort to avoid the use of standard antidepressants. Clinicians are also encouraged to consider and address other factors that may contribute to cycling, including substance abuse and thyroid disease.

Psychiatric and Medical Co-Morbidity

Alcohol abuse and dependence is extremely prevalent among bipolar patients, and requires concurrent treatment. One RCT suggested efficacy for divalproex among bipolar patients with alcohol abuse.[89] Behavioral strategies have also been shown to be effective. In general, management of co-morbidity in BPD is under-studied, despite its prevalence.

Bipolar II

With a few exceptions, nearly all RCTs in BPD have focused on bipolar I patients, and evidence among bipolar II patients is extremely limited.[90] Therefore, treatment recommendations typically suggest that bipolar II patients be treated "by analogy"—that is, that interventions shown to be effective in bipolar I disorder be used. The two placebo-controlled trials of quetiapine in bipolar depression did include both bipolar I and II patients, with pooled results suggesting less benefit among individuals with bipolar II.

Pregnancy

Most studies find that, on average, recurrence risk neither increases nor decreases during pregnancy. The post-partum period, however, is a period of dramatically increased risk for recurrence, with bipolar patients at particular risk for post-partum psychosis. Whether this is a result of hormonal changes or other factors (such as sleep disruption) during the post-partum period has not been well studied. Treatment of BPD during pregnancy is beyond the scope of this chapter; the interested reader is referred to Viguera and co-workers.[91] In general, all pharmacological treatment strategies carry some risk to the fetus, although this must be balanced against the substantial consequences of recurrence during or after pregnancy.

Childhood, Adolescence, and Geriatric Patients

Regardless of the accuracy with which BPD can be diagnosed in childhood, retrospective studies in adults make it clear that many individuals with BPD were symptomatic before age 18.[18] As such, there remains a need to understand whether adult bipolar interventions are safe and effective in children. In geriatric populations, similar treatment approaches are generally adopted but with more attention paid to potential toxicities. So, for example, lithium may be used but at lower target levels, recognizing that brain levels may correspond poorly to plasma levels in this group. Notably, pharmacovigilance studies suggest that atypical antipsychotics may increase stroke risk among older patients, particularly those with dementia, so use of SGAs requires more caution in this group.

PROGNOSIS

By comparison with other chronic and recurrent medical illnesses, remarkably few data exist to guide clinicians in the estimation of prognosis. The few diagnostic features associated with differential prognosis are rarely replicated, with some exceptions. A greater number of recent episodes, or more days ill in the prior year, do appear to predict earlier recurrence.[92] Also not surprisingly, residual mood symptoms—both manic and depressive—following an acute episode appear to be predictive of earlier recurrence.

Earlier onset of mood symptoms has been associated with a more severe illness course, with greater chronicity, and with recurrence.[18] One study also suggested that individuals with a first depressive rather than manic episode might also be at greater risk for a chronic and depressive course.[93]

An open question is whether interventions targeting those prognostic factors that may be modifiable might improve outcome. For example, more aggressive treatment of residual mood symptoms to target remission, as has been emphasized in MDD, might reduce recurrence risk, though this has not been formally studied.

MEDICAL CO-MORBIDITY AMONG BIPOLAR PATIENTS

A persistent concern is the observation that bipolar patients are at elevated risk of morbidity and mortality from multiple causes, not only suicide.[20,94] In particular, they show elevated incidences of cardiovascular risk factors (including obesity, hyperlipidemia, and diabetes), with risk compounded by greater rates of tobacco use compared to the general population. Several explanations have been suggested for this co-morbidity: it may be another feature of the disorder itself, or a consequence of poorer health maintenance arising from chronic illness. Moreover, many first-line treatments for BPD can precipitate or exacerbate these risk factors. With the discovery that variations in calcium channel genes are associated with BPD risk, it is also possible that systemic effects of such risk genes have previously been overlooked. Indeed, the increased rate of migraine in individuals with BPD may represent one such co-morbidity.

CONTROVERSIES
Child Bipolar

Perhaps no single area of BPD research and clinical practice has prompted as much controversy as the diagnosis and treatment of BPD in children and adolescents. Two key questions for debate are the reliability of the BPD diagnosis, particularly in younger children, and the validity of this diagnosis—that is, to what extent children diagnosed with BPD grow up to be adults with BPD. These issues are often conflated with broader concerns about exposing children to psychotropic medications that are not yet well studied in this population. Cross-sectional/retrospective studies suggest that many bipolar adults are symptomatic as children, while small prospective studies suggest that children diagnosed with BPD often continue to be symptomatic and have a bipolar-like course of illness. To truly understand the continuity between child and adult BPD, long-term prospective cohort studies will be required. Such studies can definitively establish the validity of childhood-onset BPD by examining the proportion of children diagnosed with BPD whose symptoms persist into adulthood.

Access the complete reference list and multiple choice questions (MCQs) online at https://expertconsult.inkling.com

KEY REFERENCES

1. Merikangas KR, Akiskal HS, Angst J, et al. Lifetime and 12–month prevalence of bipolar spectrum disorder in the National Comorbidity Survey Replication. *Arch Gen Psychiatry* 64(5):543–552, 2007.
2. Hirschfeld RM, Calabrese JR, Weissman MM, et al. Screening for bipolar disorder in the community. *J Clin Psychiatry* 64(1):53–59, 2003.
10. Angst J, Marneros A. Bipolarity from ancient to modern times: conception, birth and rebirth. *J Affect Disord* 67(1–3):3–19, 2001.
11. Salvatore P, Baldessarini RJ, Centorrino F, et al. Weygandt's *On the Mixed States of Manic-Depressive Insanity*: a translation and commentary on its significance in the evolution of the concept of bipolar disorder. *Harv Rev Psychiatry* 10(5):255–275, 2002.
16. Judd LL, Akiskal HS, Schettler PJ, et al. A prospective investigation of the natural history of the long-term weekly symptomatic status of bipolar II disorder. *Arch Gen Psychiatry* 60(3):261–269, 2003.
18. Perlis RH, Miyahara S, Marangell LB, et al. Long-term implications of early onset in bipolar disorder: data from the first 1000 participants in the Systematic Treatment Enhancement Program for Bipolar Disorder (STEP-BD). *Biol Psychiatry* 55(9):875–881, 2004.
20. Osby U, Brandt L, Correia N, et al. Excess mortality in bipolar and unipolar disorder in Sweden. *Arch Gen Psychiatry* 58(9):844–850, 2001.
24. Tohen M, Stoll AL, Strakowski SM, et al. The McLean first-episode psychosis project: six month recovery and recurrence outcome. *Schizophr Bull* 18:172–185, 1992.

25. Tohen M, Vieta E, Calabrese J, et al. Efficacy of olanzapine and olanzapine-fluoxetine combination in the treatment of bipolar I depression. *Arch Gen Psychiatry* 60(11):1079–1088, 2003.

29. Lee HC, Tsai SY, Lin HC. Seasonal variations in bipolar disorder admissions and the association with climate: a population-based study. *J Affect Disord* 97(1–3):61–69, 2007.

34. Oepen G, Baldessarini RJ, Salvatore P, et al. On the periodicity of manic-depressive insanity, by Eliot Slater (1938): translated excerpts and commentary. *J Affect Disord* 78(1):1–9, 2004.

38. Roybal K, Theobold D, Graham A, et al. Mania-like behavior induced by disruption of CLOCK. *Proc Natl Acad Sci U S A* 104(15):6406–6411, 2007.

44. Drevets WC, Price JL, Simpson JR Jr, et al. Subgenual prefrontal cortex abnormalities in mood disorders. *Nature* 386(6627):824–827, 1997.

51. Gilman SE, Dupuy JM, Perlis RH. Risks for the transition from major depressive disorder to bipolar disorder in the National Epidemiologic Survey on Alcohol and Related Conditions. *J Clin Psychiatry* 73(6):829–836, 2012. doi:10.4088/JCP.11m06912.

52. Tsankova NM, Berton O, Renthal W, et al. Sustained hippocampal chromatin regulation in a mouse model of depression and antidepressant action. *Nat Neurosci* 9:519–525, 2006. 10.1038/nn1659.

53. Kurita M, Holloway T, Garcia-Bea A, et al. HDAC2 regulates atypical antipsychotic responses through the modulation of mGlu2 promoter activity. *Nat Neurosci* 15:1245–1254, 2012. doi:10.1038/nn.3181.

57. Krauthammer C, Klerman GL. Secondary mania: manic syndromes associated with antecedent physical illness or drugs. *Arch Gen Psychiatry* 35(11):1333–1339, 1978.

60. Perlis RH, Uher R, Ostacher M, et al. Association between bipolar spectrum features and treatment outcomes in outpatients with major depressive disorder. *Arch Gen Psychiatry* 68(4):351–360, 2011. doi:10.1001/archgenpsychiatry.2010.179.

65. Hirschfeld RA, Bowden CL, Gitlin MJ, et al. Practice guideline for the treatment of patients with bipolar disorder (revision). *Am J Psychiatry* 159(Suppl. 4):1–11, 2002.

68. Simon GE, Ludman EJ, Bauer MS, et al. Long-term effectiveness and cost of a systematic care program for bipolar disorder. *Arch Gen Psychiatry* 63(5):500–508, 2006.

70. Perlis RH, Welge JA, Vornik LA, et al. Atypical antipsychotics in the treatment of mania: a meta-analysis of randomized, placebo-controlled trials. *J Clin Psychiatry* 67(4):509–516, 2006.

72. Calabrese JR, Keck PE Jr, Macfadden W, et al. A randomized, double-blind, placebo-controlled trial of quetiapine in the treatment of bipolar I or II depression. *Am J Psychiatry* 162(7):1351–1360, 2005.

73. Brown EB, McElroy SL, Keck PE Jr, et al. A 7-week, randomized, double-blind trial of olanzapine/fluoxetine combination versus lamotrigine in the treatment of bipolar I depression. *J Clin Psychiatry* 67(7):1025–1033, 2006.

74. van der Loos MLM, Mulder PGH, Hartong EG, et al. Efficacy and safety of lamotrigine as add-on treatment to lithium in bipolar depression: a multicenter, double-blind, placebo-controlled trial. *J Clin Psychiatry* 70(2):223–231, 2009. Published online 2008 December 30.

75. Nemeroff CB, Evans DL, Gyulai L, et al. Double-blind, placebo-controlled comparison of imipramine and paroxetine in the treatment of bipolar depression. *Am J Psychiatry* 158(6):906–912, 2001.

79. Perlis RH, Sachs GS, Lafer B, et al. Effect of abrupt change from standard to low serum levels of lithium: a reanalysis of double-blind lithium maintenance data. *Am J Psychiatry* 159(7):1155–1159, 2002.

81. Goodwin GM, Bowden CL, Calabrese JR, et al. A pooled analysis of 2 placebo-controlled 18-month trials of lamotrigine and lithium maintenance in bipolar I disorder. *J Clin Psychiatry* 65(3):432–441, 2004.

82. Perlis RH, Ostacher MJ, Miklowitz DJ, et al. Benzodiazepine use and risk of recurrence in bipolar disorder: a STEP-BD report. *J Clin Psychiatry* 71(2):194–2010, 2010.

83. Miklowitz DJ, Otto MW, Frank E, et al. Psychosocial treatments for bipolar depression: a 1-year randomized trial from the Systematic Treatment Enhancement Program. *Arch Gen Psychiatry* 64(4):419–426, 2007.

87. Lam DH, McCrone P, Wright K, et al. Cost-effectiveness of relapse-prevention cognitive therapy for bipolar disorder: 30-month study. *Br J Psychiatry* 186:500–506, 2005.

92. Perlis RH, Ostacher MJ, Patel JK, et al. Predictors of recurrence in bipolar disorder: primary outcomes from the Systematic Treatment Enhancement Program for Bipolar Disorder (STEP-BD). *Am J Psychiatry* 163(2):217–224, 2006.

31 Psychiatric Illness during Pregnancy and the Post-partum Period

Ruta M. Nonacs, MD, PhD, Betty Wang, MD, Adele C. Viguera, MD, and Lee S. Cohen, MD

KEY POINTS

Epidemiology
- Pregnancy does not protect against psychiatric disorders.

Clinical Findings
- A growing amount of information exists regarding the course of psychiatric illness during pregnancy and the reproductive safety of psychotropic medications.

Complications
- With the exception of one anticonvulsant, sodium valproate, the majority of psychotropics are NOT major teratogens.
- Post-partum depression is the most common complication in modern obstetrics and definitive treatment is essential to minimize maternal morbidity.

OVERVIEW

Psychiatric consultation to obstetric patients typically involves the evaluation and treatment of an array of psychopathology. Once thought to be a time of emotional well-being for women,[1] studies now suggest that pregnancy is not protective with respect to the emergence or persistence of psychiatric disorders.[2-7] Given the prevalence of mood and anxiety disorders in women during the childbearing years,[8,9] and the number of women who receive treatment for these disorders, women frequently present prior to conception for consultation regarding the use of psychotropic medications during pregnancy. In non-puerperal populations, there is increasing evidence of high rates of relapse following discontinuation of psychotropic medications (e.g., antidepressants,[10] mood stabilizers,[11] antipsychotics,[12] and benzodiazepines[13]); thus it is not surprising that many women who attempt to discontinue their medications either prior to or after conception may develop recurrent symptoms. In addition, there are women who experience new-onset psychiatric illness during pregnancy.[2,6,14]

Psychiatric evaluation of women in this setting requires careful assessment of symptoms (such as anxiety or depression), and determination as to whether these symptoms are (1) normative or pathological, (2) manifestations of a new-onset psychiatric disorder, or (3) an exacerbation of a previously diagnosed or undiagnosed psychiatric disorder. Unfortunately, screening for psychiatric disorders during pregnancy and the post-partum period is not consistently performed; however, even when depressed pregnant women are identified, definitive treatment is frequently not delivered.[15] Screening for depression during pregnancy, followed by thoughtful treatment, can minimize maternal morbidity as well as the potential impact of untreated psychiatric disorder on infant development and family functioning.

Pregnancy is an emotionally-laden experience that evokes a spectrum of normal reactions, including heightened anxiety and increased mood reactivity. Normative experiences need to be distinguished from the manifestations of psychiatric disorders. When it is determined that psychiatric illness is present, treatment involves a thoughtful weighing of the risks and benefits of proposed interventions, such as pharmacological treatment, and the documented[16,17] and theoretical risks associated with untreated psychiatric disorders. In contrast to many other clinical conditions, treatment of psychiatric disorders during pregnancy is typically reserved for situations in which the disorder interferes significantly with maternal and fetal well-being; the threshold for the treatment of psychiatric disorders during pregnancy tends to be higher than with other conditions. Moreover, women with similar illness histories often make very different decisions about their care in collaboration with their physicians during pregnancy.

Decisions regarding the initiation or maintenance of treatment during pregnancy must reflect an understanding of the risks associated with fetal exposure to a particular medication but must also take into consideration the risks associated with untreated psychiatric illness in the mother. Psychiatric illness in the mother is not a benign event and may cause significant morbidity for both the mother and her child; thus, discontinuing or withholding medication during pregnancy is not always the safest option.

DIAGNOSIS AND TREATMENT OF MOOD DISORDER DURING PREGNANCY

Although some reports describe pregnancy as a time of affective well-being[1,18-20] that confers "protection" against psychiatric disorders, at least one prospective study describes equal rates of major and minor depression (approximating 10%) in gravid and non-gravid women. Several other recent studies also note clinically-significant depressive symptoms during pregnancy (ante-natal depression).[2,6,21,22] Furthermore, women with histories of major depression appear to be at high risk for recurrent depression during pregnancy, particularly in the setting of antidepressant discontinuation.[5,23]

Diagnosis of depression during pregnancy can be difficult because symptoms frequently experienced during a normal pregnancy, such as changes in sleep and appetite, fatigue, and lower libido, do not necessarily suggest an evolving affective disorder. Clinical features that may support the diagnosis of major depressive disorder (MDD) include anhedonia, feelings of guilt and hopelessness, and thoughts of suicide. Suicidal ideation is not uncommon[24-26]; however, the risk of frank self-injurious or suicidal behaviors appears to be relatively low in women who develop depression during pregnancy.[25,26]

Treatment for depression during pregnancy is determined by the severity of the underlying disorder. Women with mild to moderate depressive symptoms may benefit from non-pharmacological treatments that include supportive psychotherapy, cognitive-behavioral therapy (CBT),[27] or interpersonal psychotherapy (IPT),[28] all of which may ameliorate depressive symptoms. Given the importance of interpersonal relationships in couples who are expecting a child and the significant role transitions that take place during pregnancy and after delivery, IPT is ideally suited for the treatment of depressed pregnant women; preliminary but encouraging data support the efficacy of this intervention.[29] In women who do not respond to non-pharmacological interventions or who have more severe symptoms, pharmacologic treatments must be considered.

Antidepressant Use during Pregnancy

Multiple reviews published over the last decade[23,30-36] have described data regarding the risks associated with fetal exposure to antidepressants. Although data accumulated over the last 30 years suggest that some antidepressants may be used safely during pregnancy, information regarding the full spectrum and relative severity of attendant risks of pre-natal exposure to psychotropic medications is still incomplete.

As is the case with other medications, four types of risk are typically considered with respect to potential use of antidepressants during pregnancy: (1) risk of pregnancy loss or miscarriage, (2) risk of organ malformation or teratogenesis, (3) risk of neonatal toxicity or withdrawal syndromes during the acute neonatal period, and (4) risk of long-term neurobehavioral sequelae. To provide guidance to physicians seeking information on the reproductive safety of various prescription medications, the Food and Drug Administration (FDA) has established a system that classifies medications into five risk categories (A, B, C, D, and X) based on data derived from human and animal studies. Medications in category A are designated as safe for use during pregnancy, whereas category X drugs are contraindicated and are known to pose risks to the fetus that outweigh any benefit to the patient. Most psychotropic medications are classified as category C agents, for which human studies are lacking and for which "risk cannot be ruled out." No psychotropic drugs are classified as safe for use during pregnancy (category A).

Unfortunately, this system of classification is often ambiguous and may lead some to make conclusions that are not warranted. For example, certain tricyclic antidepressants (TCAs) have been labeled as category D agents, indicating "positive evidence of risk," although the pooled available data do not support this assertion and, in fact, suggest that these drugs are safe for use during pregnancy.[35] Therefore, the physician must also consult other sources of information when counseling patients about the potential use of psychotropic medications during pregnancy. Because randomized, placebo-controlled studies examining the effects of medication use on pregnant populations are unethical for obvious reasons, much of the data related to the profile of reproductive safety for a medication are derived from retrospective studies and case reports. More recently, studies evaluating the reproductive safety of antidepressants have used a more rigorous prospective design,[37-43] or have relied on large administrative databases or multi-center birth defect surveillance programs.[44,45]

Several recent reports describing the reproductive safety of selective serotonin re-uptake inhibitors (SSRIs) have recently been published.[34-36] Prospectively-gathered data are available for all of the SSRIs, with the exception of fluvoxamine. The baseline incidence of major congenital malformations in newborns born in the US is estimated to be between 2% and 4%; all studies published have indicated the overall risk of malformations in SSRI-exposed infants does not exceed this baseline level. These reports provide some relative reassurance that as a group of medicines, SSRIs do not constitute major teratogens. However, some[46-49] recent reports have suggested that first trimester exposure to paroxetine is associated with an increased risk of cardiac defects, specifically atrial and ventricular septal defects. While these findings prompted the FDA to change the category label of paroxetine from C to D, even more recently published studies[44,45] do not support an association between paroxetine and increased risk of cardiac defects.

Three prospective and more than 10 retrospective studies have examined the risk of organ malformation in over 400 cases of first-trimester exposure to tricyclic antidepressants (TCAs).[35] When evaluated on an individual basis and when pooled, these studies do not indicate a significant association between fetal exposure to TCAs and risk for any major congenital anomaly. Among the TCAs, desipramine and nortriptyline are often preferred since they are less anticholinergic and the least likely to exacerbate the orthostatic hypotension that may occur during pregnancy.

Bupropion may be an attractive option for women who have not responded well to SSRIs or TCAs. Data thus far have not indicated an increased risk of malformations associated with bupropion use during pregnancy.[50-52] The most recent information from the Bupropion Pregnancy Registry maintained by the manufacturer GlaxoSmithKline includes data from 517 pregnancies involving first-trimester exposure to bupropion. In this sample, there were 20 infants with major malformations. This represents a 3.9% risk of congenital malformation that is consistent with what is observed in women with no known teratogen exposure.

There are limited data available on the use of other antidepressants during pregnancy, including the serotonin-norepinephrine re-uptake inhibitors (SNRIs) venlafaxine (150 exposures)[43] and duloxetine (208 exposures),[31] mirtazapine (n = 104),[37] nefazodone (n = 89),[32] and trazodone (n = 58).[32] These reports did not document any differences in rates of malformation between antidepressant-exposed infants and non-exposed controls. While these initial reports are reassuring, larger samples are required to establish the reproductive safety of these antidepressants. It is estimated that at least 500 to 600 exposures must be collected to demonstrate a two-fold increase in risk for a particular malformation over what is observed in the general population. In general, the SSRIs, specifically fluoxetine, citalopram, and sertraline, are the antidepressants most commonly used during pregnancy.

Scant information is available regarding the reproductive safety of monoamine oxidase inhibitors (MAOIs), and these agents are generally not used in pregnancy as they may produce a hypertensive crisis when combined with tocolytic medications, such as terbutaline.

Despite the growing literature supporting the relative safety of fetal exposure to SSRIs, multiple reports[40,53-55] have described adverse peri-natal outcomes, including decreased gestational age, low birth weight, and poor neonatal adaptation in infants exposed to antidepressants. However, other investigators[38,56,57] have failed to note these same associations. A recent meta-analysis indicates that while in utero exposure to antidepressants may have statistically significant effects on certain pregnancy outcomes, the observed effects were very small: about 3 days shorter gestational age, 75 g lower birth weight, and less than half a point on the 1- and 5-minute Apgar scores.[53] The clinical significance of these findings is likely negligible.

Several recent studies have suggested that exposure to SSRIs near the time of delivery may be associated with poor peri-natal outcomes. Attention has focused on a range of transient neonatal distress syndromes associated with exposure to (or withdrawal from) antidepressants in utero.[58] The most commonly reported symptoms in the newborns include tremor, tachypnea, restlessness, increased muscle tone, and increased crying. Reassuringly, these symptoms appear to be relatively benign and short-lived, resolving within 1 to 4 days after birth without any specific medical intervention.[36]

Another concern has been that maternal SSRI use may be associated with a higher than expected number of cases of persistent pulmonary hypertension of the newborn (PPHN). In the initial report published in 2006, the use of an SSRI antidepressant after the 20th week of gestation was significantly associated with a six-fold greater risk of PPHN, and in that first study it was estimated that PPHN occurs in 1% of infants with late pregnancy exposure to SSRIs.[59] Since the initial report on this topic, three studies have found no association between antidepressant use during pregnancy and PPHN,[60-62] and one study[63] showed a much lower risk than the 1% originally reported. These findings taken together bring into question whether there is an association at all and suggest that, if there is a risk, it is much lower than that reported in the original 2006 report.

Less research has focused on the long-term effects of pre-natal antidepressant exposure. Studies thus far have indicated that there were no differences between the children exposed to fluoxetine or TCAs during pregnancy and children who were not exposed during pregnancy in terms of IQ, language, temperament, behavior, reactivity, mood, distractibility, and activity level.[41,56] In addition, there does not appear to be any difference in levels of internalizing behaviors in children exposed to SSRIs during pregnancy when compared to children of non-depressed mothers not on medication during pregnancy.[64] While the data available are reassuring, further investigation into the long-term neurobehavioral effects of pre-natal exposure to antidepressants is warranted.

A recent study identified an association between antidepressant exposure and increased risk of autism.[65] In a case control study, pre-natal exposure to both SSRIs and non-selective monoamine reuptake inhibitors (MAOIs) was associated with a small but statistically significant increase in the risk of autism spectrum disorders (ASD), particularly milder forms of ASD without intellectual disability. While this initial study raised concerns regarding the long-term effects of SSRI exposure, it must be emphasized that one of the major challenges in doing this type of study is that the results may be confounded by the indication for SSRI use. In other words, if a mother with depression or another psychiatric illness treated with an SSRI is more likely to give birth to a child with an ASD, an erroneous association between SSRI exposure and risk of ASD will be observed.

In a subsequent large population-based study of 626,875 births from Denmark, the use of SSRIs during pregnancy was not associated with a significantly increased risk of ASD.[66] In addition, this report demonstrated that maternal use of SSRIs before but not during pregnancy was associated with an increased risk of ASDs in the offspring. This increased risk associated with SSRI use before pregnancy suggests that any risk associated with SSRI exposure during pregnancy may be related to the indications for its use rather than *in utero* exposure to SSRI.

PHARMACOLOGICAL TREATMENT OF DEPRESSION DURING PREGNANCY: CLINICAL GUIDELINES

The last decade has brought increased attention to the question of how to best manage women who suffer from depression during pregnancy. Clinical lore previously suggested that women enjoyed positive mood during pregnancy, but more recent data suggest that sub-populations of patients may be at risk for recurrence or new onset of depression during pregnancy. There is also a greater appreciation that depression may exert an effect on fetal and neonatal well-being that needs to be taken into account in the risk–benefit decision-making process.[23,30,35,37,67]

The majority of women suffering from depression during pregnancy do not receive adequate treatment, even though this illness is relatively common.[15] Despite the growing number of reviews on the subject, management of ante-natal depression is still largely guided by practical experience, with few definitive data and no controlled treatment studies to inform treatment. In the absence of well-defined guidelines, clinicians must work collaboratively with the patient to arrive at the safest decision based on available information. A patient's psychiatric history, her current symptoms, and her attitude toward the use of psychiatric medications during pregnancy must be carefully assessed and factored into any decision.

In patients with less severe depression, it may be appropriate to consider discontinuation of pharmacological therapy during pregnancy. Though data on the use of IPT or cognitive-behavioral therapy (CBT) to facilitate antidepressant discontinuation prior to conception are not available, it makes clinical sense to pursue such treatment in women on maintenance antidepressant therapy who are planning to become pregnant. These modalities of treatment may reduce the risk of recurrent depressive symptoms during pregnancy, although, as noted previously, this has not been studied systematically. Close monitoring of affective status during pregnancy is essential, even if all medications are discontinued and no need for re-introduction of an antidepressant is apparent. Women with histories of psychiatric illness are at high risk for relapse during pregnancy, and early detection and treatment of recurrent illness may significantly reduce the morbidity associated with recurrent illness during pregnancy.

Many women who discontinue antidepressant treatment during pregnancy experience recurrent depressive symptoms.[68] In one recent study, women who discontinued their medications were five times more likely to relapse as compared to women who maintained their antidepressant treatment across pregnancy.[5] Thus, women with recurrent or refractory depressive illness may decide in collaboration with their clinician that the safest option is to maintain pharmacological treatment during pregnancy in order to minimize the risk for recurrent illness. In this setting, the clinician should attempt to select medications for use during pregnancy that have a well-characterized reproductive safety profile, which may necessitate switching from one psychotropic to another with a better reproductive safety profile. An example would be switching from duloxetine, a medication for which the data on reproductive safety are sparse, to an agent such as fluoxetine or citalopram. In some situations, one may decide to use a medication for which information regarding reproductive safety is lacking. A scenario that highlights this decision is a woman with refractory depressive illness who has responded only to one particular antidepressant for which specific data on reproductive safety are limited (e.g., venlafaxine). She may choose to continue this medication during pregnancy rather than risk potential relapse associated with antidepressant discontinuation or a switch to another antidepressant to which such a patient has no prior history of response.

Women may also experience the new onset of depressive symptoms during pregnancy. For women who present with minor depressive symptoms, non-pharmacological treatment strategies should be explored first. IPT or CBT may be beneficial for reducing the severity of depressive symptoms and may either limit or obviate the need for medications.[27-29] In general, pharmacological treatment is pursued when non-pharmacological strategies have failed or when it is felt that the risks associated with psychiatric illness during pregnancy outweigh the risks of fetal exposure to a particular medication.

In situations in which pharmacological treatment is more clearly indicated, the clinician should attempt to select the safest medication regimen, using, if possible, medications with the safest reproductive profile. Fluoxetine and citalopram, with rather extensive data supporting their reproductive safety, can be considered first-line choices. The TCAs and bupropion have also been relatively well characterized and can be considered reasonable treatment options during pregnancy. Among the TCAs, desipramine and nortriptyline are preferred because they are less anticholinergic and less likely to exacerbate orthostatic hypotension during pregnancy. The amount of literature on the reproductive safety of the newer antidepressants is growing, and these agents may be useful in certain settings.[33,42,66]

When prescribing medications during pregnancy, every attempt should be made to simplify the medication regimen. For instance, one may select a more sedating TCA for a woman who presents with depression and a sleep disturbance instead of using an SSRI in combination with trazodone or a benzodiazepine. In addition, the clinician must use an adequate dosage of medication. Frequently the dosage of a medication is reduced during pregnancy in an attempt to limit risk to the fetus; however, this type of modification in treatment may instead place the woman at greater risk for recurrent illness. During pregnancy, changes in plasma volume and increases in hepatic metabolism and renal clearance may significantly reduce drug levels.[69,70] Several investigators have described a reduction (up to 65%) in serum levels of TCAs during pregnancy.[39,71] As sub-therapeutic levels may be associated with depressive relapse,[39] an increase in daily TCA or SSRI dosage may be required to obtain remission.[72]

With multiple studies supporting the finding of transient jitteriness, tremulousness, and tachypnea associated with peri-partum use of SSRIs,[58,73] some authors (as well as FDA-mandated labeling across the SSRIs) have suggested discontinuation of antidepressants just prior to delivery to minimize the risk of neonatal toxicity. While the recommendation is intuitive, it are not data driven and such a practice may actually carry significant risk as it withdraws treatment from patients precisely as they are about to enter the post-partum period, a time of heightened risk for affective illness.

Severely depressed patients who are acutely suicidal or psychotic require hospitalization, and electroconvulsive therapy (ECT) is frequently selected as the treatment of choice. Two reviews of ECT during pregnancy note the efficacy and safety of this procedure.[74,75] In a review of the 300 case reports of ECT during pregnancy published over the past 50 years, four cases of premature labor and no cases of premature ruptures of membranes were reported. Given its relative safety, ECT may also be considered an alternative to conventional pharmacotherapy for women who wish to avoid extended exposure to psychotropic medications during pregnancy or for women who fail to respond to standard antidepressants.

BIPOLAR DISORDER DURING PREGNANCY

Although the impact of pregnancy on the natural course of bipolar disorder (BPD) is not well described, studies suggest that any "protective" effects of pregnancy on risk for recurrence of mania or depression in women with BPD are limited[76] and the risk for relapse and chronicity following discontinuation of mood stabilizers is high.[77-80] Given these data, clinicians and bipolar women who are either pregnant or who wish to conceive find themselves between a "teratologic rock and a clinical hard place."

Women with BPD have at times been counseled to defer pregnancy (given an apparent need for pharmacological therapy with mood stabilizers) or to terminate pregnancies following pre-natal exposure to drugs such as lithium or valproic acid.

Concerns regarding fetal exposure to lithium, for example, have typically been based on early reports of higher rates of cardiovascular malformations (e.g., Ebstein's anomaly)

following pre-natal exposure to this drug.[81,82] More recent data suggest the risk of cardiovascular malformations following pre-natal exposure to lithium is smaller than previous estimates, and is suggested to be between 1 in 2,000 (0.05%) and 1 in 1,000 (0.1%).[83] Pre-natal screening with a high-resolution ultrasound and fetal echocardiography is recommended at or about 16 to 18 weeks of gestation to screen for cardiac anomalies.

Lamotrigine is another mood stabilizer that is an option for pregnant women with BPD who demonstrate a clear need for prophylaxis with a mood stabilizer. While previous reports did not show an elevated risk of malformations associated with lamotrigine exposure,[84-86] data from the North American Anti-Epileptic Drug registry indicate an increased risk of oral clefts in infants exposed to lamotrigine during the first trimester; the prevalence was approximately 9 per 1,000 births.[87]

Compared with lithium and lamotrigine, pre-natal exposure to some anticonvulsants is associated with a far greater risk for organ malformation. Pre-natal exposure to anticonvulsants, including valproic acid and, to a lesser extent, carbamazepine, has been associated with an increased risk of neural tube defects (3% to 8%) and spina bifida (1%).[88-91] Fetal exposure to anticonvulsants has also been associated with other anomalies, including mid-face hypoplasia, congenital heart disease, cleft lip and/or palate, growth retardation, and microcephaly. Factors that appear to increase the risk for teratogenesis include high maternal anticonvulsant dose (above 1,000 mg of valproic acid per day) and exposure to more than one anticonvulsant (particularly polytherapy with valproic acid).

Information about the reproductive safety of newer anticonvulsants sometimes used to treat BPD, including gabapentin, oxcarbazepine, and topiramate, remains sparse.[92] Preliminary data indicate that there may be a small increase in the risk of oral clefts in children exposed pre-natally to topiramate.[78] Efforts are underway to accumulate data from prospective registries regarding teratogenic risks across a broad range of anticonvulsants.

Pre-natal screening following anticonvulsant exposure for congenital malformations (including cardiac anomalies) with fetal ultrasound at 16 to 18 weeks of gestation is recommended. The possibility of fetal neural tube defects should be evaluated with maternal serum alpha-fetoprotein (MSAFP) levels and ultrasonography. In addition, 4 mg a day of folic acid before conception and in the first trimester for women receiving anticonvulsants is frequently recommended. However, it should be noted that supplemental use of folic acid to attenuate the risk of neural tube defects in the setting of anticonvulsant exposure has not been systematically evaluated.

While there have long been concerns regarding the increased risk of malformations, there is a growing body of literature to indicate that in utero exposure to anticonvulsants, most clearly valproic acid (VPA), may also negatively affect cognitive development.[79,93] In one study, researchers found that the risk of neurodevelopmental disorders was about six times higher in children exposed to valproate monotherapy (12%) than in children with no anticonvulsant exposure (1.87%).[79] This risk was even higher in those exposed to polytherapy with VPA (15%). ASD was the most frequent diagnosis among VPA-exposed children. No significant increase was found among children exposed to carbamazepine or lamotrigine.

Mood stabilizers (including lithium and some anticonvulsants) have become the mainstay of treatment for the management of both acute mania and the maintenance phase of BPD; however, the majority of patients with BPD are not treated with monotherapy. Rather, the use of adjunctive conventional and newer antipsychotics has become common clinical practice for many bipolar patients. Moreover, with growing data supporting the use of atypical antipsychotics as monotherapy in the treatment of BPD, patients and clinicians will seek information regarding the reproductive safety of these newer agents. To date, abundant data exist that supports the reproductive safety of typical antipsychotics; these data will be reviewed elsewhere in this chapter. However, despite their growing use in psychiatry, available reproductive safety data regarding the atypical antipsychotics are limited, but increasing (reviewed in the following section). Some patients who benefit from treatment with atypical antipsychotics may decide with their clinician to discontinue the atypical antipsychotic or switch to a typical antipsychotic with a better-characterized safety profile. Atypical antipsychotics are best avoided if possible, although they are not absolutely contraindicated during pregnancy and should be reserved for use in more challenging clinical situations where treatment with more conventional agents has not been helpful.

The most appropriate treatment algorithm for managing reproductive-age women who wish to conceive or who are pregnant depends on the severity of the individual patient's illness. Patients with histories of a single episode of mania and prompt, full recovery followed by sustained well-being may tolerate discontinuation of mood stabilizer before an attempt to conceive.[76,83] Unfortunately, even among women with histories of prolonged well-being and sustained euthymia, discontinuation of prophylaxis for mania may be associated with subsequent relapse. For women with BPD and a history of multiple and frequent recurrences of mania or bipolar depression, several options may be considered. Some patients may choose to discontinue a mood stabilizer prior to conception as outlined above. An alternative strategy for this high-risk group is to continue treatment until pregnancy is verified and then taper off the mood stabilizer. Because the utero-placental circulation is not established until approximately 2 weeks following conception, the risk of fetal exposure is minimal. Home pregnancy tests are reliable and can document pregnancy as early as 10 days following conception, and with a home ovulation predictor kit, a patient may be able to time her treatment discontinuation accurately. This strategy minimizes fetal exposure to drugs and extends the protective treatment up to the time of conception, which may be particularly prudent for older patients because the time required for them to conceive may be longer than for younger patients.

A potential problem with this strategy is that it may lead to relatively abrupt discontinuation of treatment, thereby potentially placing the patient at increased risk for relapse. With close clinical follow-up, however, patients can be monitored for early signs of relapse, and medications may be re-introduced as needed. Another problem with the strategy of discontinuation of mood stabilizers when the patient is being treated with valproate is that the teratogenic effect of valproate occurs early in gestation between weeks 4 and 5, often before patients even know they are pregnant. In such scenarios, any potential teratogenic insult from valproate may have already occurred by the time the patient actually documents the pregnancy.

For women who tolerate discontinuation of maintenance treatment, the decision of when to resume treatment is a matter for clinical judgment. Some patients and clinicians may prefer to await the initial appearance of symptoms before re-starting medication; others may prefer to limit their risk of a major recurrence by re-starting treatment after the first trimester of pregnancy. Preliminary data suggest that pregnant women with BPD who remain well throughout pregnancy may have a lower risk for post-partum relapse than those who become ill during pregnancy.[76] For women with particularly severe forms of BPD, such as with multiple severe episodes,

and especially with psychosis and prominent thoughts of suicide, maintenance treatment with a mood stabilizer before and during pregnancy may be the safest option. If the patient decides to attempt conception, accepting the relatively small absolute increase in teratogenic risk with first-trimester exposure to lithium or lamotrigine with or without antipsychotic, for example, may be justified because such patients are at highest risk for clinical deterioration if pharmacological treatment is withdrawn. Many patients who are treated with sodium valproate or other newer anticonvulsants, such as gabapentin, for which there are particularly sparse reproductive-safety data, may never have received a trial of lithium prior to pregnancy. For such patients, a lithium trial prior to pregnancy may be a reasonable treatment option.

Even if all psychotropic medications have been safely discontinued, pregnancy in women with BPD should be considered at high risk, because the risk of major psychiatric illness during pregnancy is increased in the absence of treatment with mood-stabilizing medication and is even higher during the post-partum period. Extreme vigilance is required for early detection of an impending relapse of illness, and rapid intervention can significantly reduce morbidity and improve overall prognosis.

PSYCHOTIC DISORDERS DURING PREGNANCY

Although anecdotal reports describe improvement of symptoms in some chronically mentally ill women during pregnancy, as a group these patients are at increased risk for poor pregnancy outcomes.[94,95] First onset of psychosis during pregnancy cannot be presumed to be reactive; it requires a systematic diagnostic evaluation. Psychosis during pregnancy may inhibit a woman's ability to obtain appropriate and necessary pre-natal care or to cooperate with caregivers during delivery.[94-96] Thus, acute psychosis during pregnancy is both an obstetric and psychiatric emergency.

Treatment of psychosis during pregnancy may include use of typical high-potency antipsychotic medications, such as haloperidol or thiothixene, which have not been associated with an increased risk of congenital malformations when used in the first trimester of pregnancy.[97,98] Historically, lower-potency antipsychotics have typically been avoided because of data supporting an increased risk of congenital malformations associated with pre-natal exposure to these compounds.[99,100] However, their use is not absolutely contraindicated.

Less reproductive safety data on the newer "atypical" antipsychotic medications are available as compared to the conventional antipsychotics. Thus far, most of the data on the reproductive safely of atypical agents has been limited to manufacturers' accumulated case series, and some terato-vigilance data reflecting a small number of total drug exposures and spontaneous reports.[101-104] In 2005, one study assessed the outcomes of 151 infants pre-natally exposed to atypical antipsychotics, observing no increase in the risk of congenital malformations.[103] While these preliminary data are reassuring, more research is required to better understand the reproductive safety of these newer antipsychotic agents.

One of the major challenges in assessing the reproductive safety of atypical antipsychotic medications is that they are so commonly used in conjunction with other medications that may influence pregnancy outcomes.[101,102] Studies have observed that exposed neonates were more likely to be born prematurely, were admitted more often to the neonatal intensive care unit, and were more likely to present with poor neonatal adaptation. These adverse neonatal outcomes were found primarily in women receiving polypharmacy.

Decisions regarding the use of these and other psychotropic medications must be made on a case-by-case basis. Given the limited data regarding the reproductive safety of atypical agents, patients taking an antipsychotic drug may choose to discontinue their medication or switch to a better-characterized conventional antipsychotic, such as perphenazine or haloperidol. However, many women do not respond as well to the typical agents or have such severe illness that making any change in their regimen may place them at significant risk. Thus, women and their clinicians may choose to use an atypical agent during pregnancy in order to sustain functioning, while acknowledging information regarding their reproductive safety remains incomplete.

ANXIETY DISORDERS DURING PREGNANCY

Although modest to moderate levels of anxiety during pregnancy are common, some women experience more severe and disabling anxiety disorders, including panic disorder and generalized anxiety disorder (GAD). The course of anxiety disorders in pregnancy is variable. Pregnancy may ameliorate symptoms of panic in some patients and may provide an opportunity to discontinue medication.[105-108] Other studies have noted the persistence or worsening of anxiety symptoms during pregnancy.[4,109,110] Of concern is the finding that anxiety symptoms during pregnancy may be associated with a variety of poor obstetric outcomes, including increased rates of premature labor, lower birth weight, lower Apgar scores, and placental abruption.[111-114]

Consultation requests regarding the appropriate management of anxiety symptoms during pregnancy are common. The use of non-pharmacological treatment, such as CBT and supportive psychotherapy, may be of great value in attenuating symptoms of anxiety in some cases.[115,116] For patients with anxiety disorders who wish to conceive, slow tapering of anti-anxiety medications is recommended. Adjunctive CBT may benefit in helping patients discontinue medications and may increase the time to a relapse.[116] Some patients may conceive inadvertently on anti-anxiety medications and may present for emergent consultation. Abrupt discontinuation of maintenance medications, particularly benzodiazepines, is not recommended given the risk for rebound panic symptoms or a potentially serious withdrawal syndrome. However, gradual taper of benzodiazepine (> 2 weeks) with adjunctive CBT may be pursued in an effort to minimize fetal exposure to medication.

For other patients, especially those with panic disorder or severe generalized anxiety, pharmacological intervention during pregnancy may be necessary. Pharmacotherapy of severe anxiety during pregnancy may include treatment with benzodiazepines, TCAs, SSRIs, or SNRIs. These classes of drugs have all demonstrated efficacy in the management of either GAD[117,118] or panic disorder.[119-121] Pharmacological treatment of severe anxiety during pregnancy may include the use of TCAs or SSRIs. Nonetheless, patients treated with an antidepressant alone for management of anxiety symptoms may not respond optimally. For these patients, benzodiazepines represent a reasonable alternative.

The consequences of pre-natal exposure to benzodiazepines have been debated for over 20 years. Increased risk for oral clefts have been noted in some older studies,[122-124] although other studies do not support this association.[125,126] One meta-analysis that pooled data from multiple samples of patients exposed to different types and doses of benzodiazepines for variable durations of time supported an increased risk of oral clefts following first-trimester exposure to these drugs[127]; this risk for oral clefts was approximately 0.6% following first-trimester exposure.

Although some patients may choose to avoid first-trimester exposure to benzodiazepines given the data on the risk for

cleft lip and palate, benzodiazepines may be used without significant risk during the second and third trimesters and may offer some advantage over antidepressant treatment because they may be used as needed.

With respect to the peri-partum use of benzodiazepines, reports of hypotonia, neonatal apnea, neonatal withdrawal syndromes, and temperature dysregulation[128-134] have prompted recommendations to taper and discontinue benzodiazepines at the time of parturition. The rationale for this course is suspect for several reasons. First, given data suggesting a risk for puerperal worsening of anxiety disorders in women with histories of panic disorder and obsessive-compulsive disorder (OCD),[109,135,136] discontinuation of a drug at or about the time of delivery places women at risk for post-partum worsening of these disorders. Second, data describing the use of clonazepam during labor and delivery at doses of 0.5 to 3.5 mg per day in a group of women with panic disorder did not indicate any adverse events.[137]

ELECTROCONVULSIVE THERAPY DURING PREGNANCY

The use of ECT during pregnancy typically raises considerable anxiety among clinicians and patients. Its safety record has been well documented over the last 50 years.[138-140] Requests for psychiatric consultation on pregnant patients requiring ECT tend to be emergent and dramatic. For example, expeditious treatment is imperative in instances of mania during pregnancy or psychotic depression with suicidal thoughts and disorganized thinking. Such clinical situations are associated with a danger from impulsivity or self-harm. The safety and efficacy of ECT in such settings are well described, particularly when instituted in collaboration with a multi-disciplinary treatment team, including an anesthesiologist, psychiatrist, and obstetrician.[75,140-142] A limited course of treatment may be sufficient, followed by institution of treatment with one or a combination of agents, such as antidepressants, neuroleptics, benzodiazepines, or mood stabilizers.

ECT during pregnancy tends to be under-used because of concerns that treatment will harm the fetus. Despite one report of placental abruption associated with the use of ECT during pregnancy,[143] considerable experience supports its safe use in severely ill gravid women. Thus, it becomes the task of the psychiatric consultant to facilitate the most clinically appropriate intervention in the face of partially informed concerns or objections.

POST-PARTUM MOOD AND ANXIETY DISORDERS: DIAGNOSIS AND TREATMENT

During the post-partum period about 85% of women experience some degree of mood disturbance. For most women the symptoms are mild; however, 10% to 15% of women experience clinically-significant symptoms. Post-partum depressive disorders typically are divided into three categories: (1) post-partum blues, (2) non-psychotic major depression, and (3) puerperal psychosis. Because these three diagnostic sub-types overlap significantly, it is not clear if they actually represent three distinct disorders. It may be more useful to conceptualize these sub-types as existing along a continuum, where post-partum blues is the mildest and post-partum psychosis the most severe form of puerperal psychiatric illness.

Post-partum blues does not indicate psychopathology, but it is common and occurs in approximately 50% to 85% of women following delivery.[144,145] Symptoms of reactivity of mood, tearfulness, and irritability are, by definition, time-limited and typically remit by the tenth post-partum day. As post-partum blues is associated with no significant impairment of function and is time-limited, no specific treatment is indicated. Symptoms that persist beyond 2 weeks require further evaluation and may suggest an evolving depressive disorder. In women with histories of recurrent mood disorder, the blues may herald the onset of post-partum major depression.[21,146]

Several studies describe a prevalence of post-partum major depression of between 10% and 15%.[22,144] The signs and symptoms of post-partum depression usually appear over the first 2 to 3 months following delivery and generally are indistinguishable from characteristics of MDD that occur at other times in a woman's life. The presenting symptoms of post-partum depression include depressed mood, irritability, and loss of interest in usual activities. Insomnia, fatigue, and loss of appetite are frequently described. Post-partum depressive symptoms also co-mingle with anxiety and obsessional symptoms, and women may present with generalized anxiety, panic disorder, or hypochondriasis.[147,148] Although it may sometimes be difficult to diagnose depression in the acute puerperium given the normal occurrence of symptoms suggestive of depression (e.g., sleep and appetite disturbance, low libido), it is an error to dismiss neurovegetative symptoms, such as severe decreased energy, profound anhedonia, and guilty ruminations, as normal features of the puerperium. In its most severe form, post-partum depression may result in profound dysfunction. Risk factors for post-partum depression include pre-natal depression, pre-natal anxiety, and a history of previous depression.

A wealth of literature on this topic indicates that post-partum depression, especially when left untreated, may have a significant impact on the child's well-being and development.[149,150] In addition, the syndrome demands aggressive treatment to avoid the sequelae of an untreated mood disorder, such as chronic depression and recurrent disease. Treatment should be guided by the type and severity of the symptoms and by the degree of functional impairment. However, before initiating psychiatric treatment, medical causes for mood disturbance (e.g., thyroid dysfunction, anemia) must be excluded. Initial evaluation should include a thorough history, physical examination, and routine laboratory tests.

Although post-partum depression is relatively common, few studies have systematically assessed the efficacy of non-pharmacological and pharmacological therapies in the treatment of this disorder. Non-pharmacological therapies are useful in the treatment of post-partum depression, and several preliminary studies have yielded encouraging results. Appleby and associates[151] have demonstrated in a randomized study that short-term CBT was as effective as treatment with fluoxetine in women with post-partum depression. IPT has also been shown to be effective for the treatment of women with mild to moderate post-partum depression.[152]

These non-pharmacological interventions may be particularly attractive to those patients who are reluctant to use psychotropic medications (e.g., women who are breastfeeding) or for patients with milder forms of depressive illness. Further investigation is required to determine the efficacy of these treatments in women who suffer from more severe forms of post-partum mood disturbances. Women with more severe post-partum depression may choose to receive pharmacological treatment, either in addition to, or instead of, non-pharmacological therapies.

To date, only a few studies have systematically assessed the pharmacological treatment of post-partum depression. Conventional antidepressant medications (e.g., fluoxetine, sertraline, venlafaxine) have shown efficacy in the treatment of post-partum depression.[57,151,153-155] In all of these studies,

standard antidepressant doses were effective and well tolerated. The choice of an antidepressant should be guided by the patient's prior response to antidepressant medication and a given medication's side-effect profile. SSRIs are ideal first-line agents because they are anxiolytic, non-sedating, and well tolerated, and bupropion is also another good option. TCAs are used frequently and, because they tend to be more sedating, may be more appropriate for women who have prominent sleep disturbances. Given the prevalence of anxiety in women with post-partum depression, adjunctive use of a benzodiazepine (e.g., clonazepam or lorazepam) may be very helpful.

Some investigators have also explored the role of hormonal manipulation in women who suffer from post-partum depression. The post-partum period is associated with rapid shifts in the reproductive hormonal environment, most notably a dramatic fall in estrogen and progesterone levels, and post-partum mood disturbance has been attributed to a deficiency (or change in the levels) in these gonadal steroids. Although early reports suggested that progesterone may be helpful,[156] no systematically-derived data exist to support its use in this setting. Several studies have described the benefit of exogenous estrogen therapy, either alone or in conjunction with an antidepressant, in women with post-partum depression.[157-159] Although these studies suggest a role for estrogen in the treatment of women with post-partum depression, these treatments remain experimental. Estrogen delivered during the acute post-partum period is not without risk and has been associated with changes in breast-milk production and more significant thromboembolic events. Antidepressants are safe, well tolerated, and highly effective; they remain the first choice for women with post-partum depression.

In cases of severe post-partum depression, inpatient hospitalization may be required, particularly for patients who are at risk for suicide. In Great Britain, innovative treatment programs involving joint hospitalization of the mother and the baby have been successful; however, mother–infant units are much less common in the US. Women with severe post-partum illness should be considered candidates for ECT. The option should be considered early in treatment because it is safe and highly effective. In choosing any treatment strategy, it is important to consider the impact of prolonged hospitalization or treatment of the mother on infant development and attachment.

Although symptoms of post-partum panic attacks and OCD symptoms are frequently included in the description of post-partum mood disturbance, a growing literature supports the likelihood that post-partum anxiety disorders are discrete diagnostic entities.[109,148] Several investigators have described post-partum worsening of panic disorder in women with pre-gravid histories of this anxiety disorder, but with an absence of co-morbid depressive illness.[4] Post-partum OCD has also been described in the absence of co-morbid post-partum major depression. Symptoms often include intrusive obsessional thoughts to harm the newborn in the absence of psychosis. Treatment with anti-obsessional agents, such as fluoxetine or clomipramine, has been effective.[136]

Post-partum psychosis is a psychiatric emergency. The clinical picture is most frequently consistent with mania or a mixed state[19] and may include symptoms of restlessness, agitation, sleep disturbance, paranoia, delusions, disorganized thinking, impulsivity, and behaviors that place mother and infant at risk. The typical onset is within the first 2 weeks after delivery, and symptoms may appear as early as the first 48 to 72 hours post-partum. Although investigators have debated whether post-partum psychosis is a discrete diagnostic entity or a manifestation of BPD, treatment should follow the same algorithm to treat acute manic psychosis, including hospitalization and potential use of mood stabilizers, antipsychotic medications, benzodiazepines, or ECT.

Although it is difficult to reliably predict which women will experience a post-partum mood disturbance, it is possible to identify certain sub-groups of women (i.e., women with a history of mood disorder) who are more vulnerable to post-partum affective illness. At highest risk are women with a history of post-partum psychosis; up to 70% of women who have had one episode of puerperal psychosis will experience another episode following a subsequent pregnancy.[19,160] Similarly, women with histories of post-partum depression are at significant risk, with rates of post-partum recurrence as high as 50%.[161] Women with BPD also appear to be particularly vulnerable during the post-partum period, with rates of post-partum relapse ranging from 30% to 50%.[80,162,163] The extent to which a history of MDD influences risk for post-partum illness is less clear. However, in all women (with or without histories of major depression), the emergence of depressive symptoms during pregnancy significantly increases the likelihood of post-partum depression.[21]

Investigators have explored the potential efficacy of prophylactic interventions in these women at risk.[164-167] Several studies demonstrate that women with histories of BPD or puerperal psychosis benefit from prophylactic treatment with lithium instituted either prior to delivery (at 36 weeks' gestation) or no later than the first 48 hours following delivery.[164-167] Prophylactic lithium appears to significantly reduce relapse rates and diminish the severity and duration of puerperal illness.

For women with histories of post-partum depression, Wisner and colleagues[168] have described a beneficial effect of prophylactic antidepressant (either a TCA or a SSRI) administered after delivery. However, a subsequent randomized, placebo-controlled study from the same group did not demonstrate a positive effect in women treated prophylactically with nortriptyline.[169] The authors have suggested that nortriptyline may be less effective than SSRIs for the treatment of post-partum depression. The efficacy of prophylactic treatment with SSRIs in this population is under investigation.

In summary, post-partum depressive illness may be conceptualized along a continuum, where some women are at lower risk for puerperal illness and others are at higher risk. Although a less aggressive "wait-and-see" approach is appropriate for women with no history of post-partum psychiatric illness, women with BPD or histories of post-partum psychiatric illness deserve not only close monitoring but also specific prophylactic measures.

BREASTFEEDING AND PSYCHOTROPIC DRUG USE

The emotional and medical benefits of breastfeeding to mother and infant are clear. Given the prevalence of psychiatric illness during the post-partum period, a significant number of women may require pharmacological treatment while nursing. Appropriate concern is raised, however, regarding the safety of psychotropic drug use in women who choose to breastfeed while using these medications. Efforts to quantify exposure to psychotropic medications through breastfeeding have been reported.

The data indicate that all psychotropic medications, including antidepressants, antipsychotic agents, lithium carbonate, and benzodiazepines, are secreted into breast milk. However, concentrations of these agents in breast milk vary considerably. The amount of medication to which an infant is exposed depends on several factors[170]: the maternal dosage of medication, frequency of dosing, and rate of maternal drug metabolism. Typically, peak concentrations in the breast milk are attained approximately 6 to 8 hours after the medication is ingested. Thus, the frequency of feedings and the timing of the feedings can influence the amount of drug to which the nursing infant is exposed. By restricting breastfeeding to times during which breast-milk drug concentrations are at their lowest (either shortly before or immediately after dosing medication), exposure may be reduced; however, this approach may not be practical for newborns who typically feed every 2 to 3 hours.

The nursing infant's chances of experiencing toxicity are dependent not only on the amount of medication ingested but also on how well the ingested medication is metabolized. Most psychotropic medications are metabolized by the liver. During the first few weeks of a full-term infant's life, there is a lower capacity for hepatic drug metabolism, which is about one-third to one-fifth that of the adult capacity. Over the next few months, the capacity for hepatic metabolism increases significantly and, by about 2 to 3 months of age, it surpasses that of adults. In premature infants or in infants with signs of compromised hepatic metabolism (e.g., hyperbilirubinemia), breastfeeding typically is deferred because these infants are less able to metabolize drugs and are thus more likely to experience toxicity.

Data have accumulated regarding the use of various psychotropic medications during breastfeeding.[170-173] Much of these data pertain to the use of antidepressants in nursing women. The available data particularly on the TCAs, fluoxetine, paroxetine, and sertraline during breastfeeding have been encouraging and suggest that the amounts of drug to which the nursing infant is exposed is low and that significant complications related to neonatal exposure to psychotropic medications in breast milk appear to be rare.[174-181] Typically very low or non-detectable levels of drug have been detected in the infant serum and one recent report indicates that exposure during nursing does not result in clinically significant blockade of serotonin (5-HT) re-uptake in infants.[181] Although less information is available on other antidepressants, serious adverse events related to exposure to these medications have not been reported.[171,172]

Given the prevalence of anxiety symptoms during the post-partum period, anxiolytic agents often are used in this setting. Data regarding the use of benzodiazepines have been limited; however, the available data suggest that amounts of medication to which the nursing infant is exposed are low.[174] Case reports of sedation, poor feeding, and respiratory distress in nursing infants have been published[63,130]; however, the data, when pooled, suggest a relatively low incidence of adverse events.[171,174]

For women with BPD, breastfeeding may pose more significant challenges. First, on-demand breastfeeding may significantly disrupt the mother's sleep and thus may increase her vulnerability to relapse during the acute post-partum period. Second, there have been reports of toxicity in nursing infants related to exposure to various mood stabilizers, including lithium and carbamazepine, in breast milk. Lithium is excreted at high levels in the mother's milk, and infant serum levels are relatively high, about one-third to one-half of the mother's serum levels,[182-184] thereby increasing the risk of neonatal toxicity. Reported signs of toxicity include cyanosis, hypotonia, and hypothermia.[185] Although breastfeeding typically is avoided in women taking lithium, the lowest possible effective dosage should be used and both maternal and infant serum lithium levels should be followed in mothers who breastfeed. In collaboration with the pediatrician, the child should be monitored closely for signs of lithium toxicity, and lithium levels, thyroid stimulating hormone (TSH), blood urea nitrogen (BUN), and creatinine should be monitored every 6–8 weeks while the child is nursing.

Several recent studies have suggested that lamotrigine reaches infants through breast milk in relatively high doses, ranging from 20% to 50% of the mother's serum concentrations,[186,187] which may be explained by poor neonatal metabolism of lamotrigine. In addition, maternal serum levels of lamotrigine increased significantly after delivery, which may also have contributed to the high levels found in nursing infants. None of these studies have reported any adverse events in breastfeeding newborns. One worry shared by clinicians and new mothers is the risk for Stevens-Johnson syndrome (SJS). This is a severe, potentially life-threatening rash, most commonly resulting from a hypersensitivity reaction to a medication, which occurs in about 0.1% of bipolar patients treated with lamotrigine.[188] Thus far, there have been no reports of SJS in infants associated with exposure to lamotrigine. In fact, it appears that cases of drug-induced SJS are extremely rare in newborns.

Similarly, concerns have arisen regarding the use of carbamazepine and valproic acid. Both of these mood stabilizers have been associated in adults with abnormalities in liver function and fatal hepatotoxicity. Hepatic dysfunction associated with carbamazepine exposure in breast milk has been reported several times.[189,190] Most concerning is that the risk for hepatotoxicity appears to be greatest in children younger than 2 years old; thus, nursing infants exposed to these agents may be particularly vulnerable to serious adverse events. Although the American Academy of Pediatrics has deemed both carbamazepine and valproic acid to be appropriate for use in breastfeeding mothers, few studies have assessed the impact of these agents on fetal well-being, particularly in non-epileptic mothers. In those women who choose to use valproic acid or carbamazepine while nursing, routine monitoring of drug levels and liver function tests is recommended. In this setting, ongoing collaboration with the child's pediatrician is crucial.

Consultation about the safety of breastfeeding among women treated with psychotropic medications should include a discussion of the known benefits of breastfeeding to mother and infant and the possibility that exposure to medications in the breast milk may occur. Although routine assay of infant serum drug levels was recommended in earlier treatment guidelines, this procedure is probably not warranted; in most instances low or non-detectable infant serum drug levels will be evident and, infrequently, serious adverse side effects have been reported. This testing is indicated, however, if neonatal toxicity related to drug exposure is suspected. Infant serum monitoring is also indicated when the mother is nursing while taking lithium, valproic acid, or carbamazepine.

PERINATAL PSYCHIATRY: FROM SCREENING TO TREATMENT

Clinicians who manage the care of female psychiatric patients before, during, and after pregnancy may be called to evaluate women who experience a broad spectrum of difficulties. Symptoms may be mild, although the consultation is typically requested when symptoms become severe. Psychiatric disorders may emerge anew during pregnancy, although more often clinical presentations represent persistence or exacerbation of already existing illness. Physicians, therefore, should screen more aggressively for psychiatric disorders either prior to conception or during pregnancy, integrating questions about psychiatric symptoms and treatment into the obstetric history. Identification of "at-risk" women allows the most thoughtful, acute treatment before, during, and after pregnancy and signals the opportunity to institute prophylactic strategies that prevent psychiatric disturbances in women during the child-bearing years.

One recent report has described the finding that even among women with identified psychiatric illness during pregnancy, definitive treatment is frequently lacking or incomplete.[15] Perhaps one of the reasons for failure to treat women with psychiatric disorders during pregnancy is the concern regarding fetal exposure to psychotropics. Many clinicians can conceptualize the need to weigh relative risks of fetal exposure, on the one hand, with the risk of withholding treatment, on the other. However, given the inability to absolutely quantify these risks, clinicians often defer treatment entirely and consequently put patients at risk for the sequelae of untreated maternal psychiatric illness.

Access the complete reference list and multiple choice questions (MCQs) online at https://expertconsult.inkling.com

KEY REFERENCES

5. Cohen LS, Altshuler LL, Harlow BL, et al. Relapse of major depression during pregnancy in women who maintain or discontinue antidepressant treatment. *JAMA* 295(5):499–507, 2006.

6. O'Hara MW. Social support, life events, and depression during pregnancy and the puerperium. *Arch Gen Psychiatry* 43:569–573, 1986.

7. Frank E, Kupfer DJ, Jacob M, et al. Pregnancy related affective episodes among women with recurrent depression. *Am J Psychiatry* 144:288–293, 1987.

16. Orr S, Miller C. Maternal depressive symptoms and the risk of poor pregnancy outcome. Review of the literature and preliminary findings. *Epidemiol Rev* 17(1):165–171, 1995.

40. Chambers C, Johnson K, Dick L, et al. Birth outcomes in pregnant women taking fluoxetine. *N Engl J Med* 335(14):1010–1015, 1996.

41. Nulman I, Rovet J, Stewart D, et al. Neurodevelopment of children exposed in utero to antidepressant drugs. *N Engl J Med* 336:258–262, 1997.

53. Ross LE, Grigoriadis S, Mamisashvili L, et al. Selected pregnancy and delivery outcomes after exposure to antidepressant medication: A systematic review and meta-analysis. *JAMA Psychiatry* 348:f6932, 2013.

56. Nulman I, Rovet J, Stewart DE, et al. Child development following exposure to tricyclic antidepressants or fluoxetine throughout fetal life: A prospective, controlled study. *Am J Psychiatry* 159(11):1889–1895, 2002.

66. Hviid A, Melbye M, Pasternak B. Use of selective serotonin reuptake inhibitors during pregnancy and risk of autism. *N Engl J Med* 369(25):2406–2415, 2013.

67. Bonari L, Pinto N, Ahn E, et al. Perinatal risks of untreated depression during pregnancy. *Can J Psychiatry* 49(11):726–735, 2004.

73. Moses-Kolko EL, Bogen D, Perel J, et al. Neonatal signs after late in utero exposure to serotonin reuptake inhibitors: Literature review and implications for clinical applications. *JAMA* 293(19):2372–2383, 2005.

75. Leiknes KA, Cooke MJ, Jarosch-von Schweder L, et al. Electroconvulsive therapy during pregnancy: a systematic review of case studies. *Arch Womens Ment Health* 2013.

76. Viguera AC, Baldessarini RJ, Nonacs R. Managing bipolar disorder during pregnancy: Weighing the risks and benefits. *Can J Psychiatry* 47:426–436, 2002.

80. Viguera AC, Nonacs R, Cohen LS, et al. Risk of recurrence of bipolar disorder in pregnant and nonpregnant women after discontinuing lithium maintenance. *Am J Psychiatry* 157(2):179–184, 2000.

83. Cohen LS, Friedman JM, Jefferson JW, et al. A reevaluation of risk of in utero exposure to lithium. *JAMA* 271(2):146–150, 1994.

86. Cunnington M, Tennis P. Lamotrigine and the risk of malformations in pregnancy. *Neurology* 64(6):955–960, 2005.

93. Veiby G, Engelsen BA, Gilhus N. Early child development and exposure to antiepileptic drugs prenatally and through breastfeeding: A prospective cohort study on children of women with epilepsy. *JAMA Neurol* 70(11):1367–1374, 2013.

127. Dolovich L, Antonio A, Vaillancourt JR, et al. Benzodiazepine use in pregnancy and major malformations or oral cleft: Meta-analysis of cohort and case-control studies. *BMJ* 317:839–843, 1998.

149. Murray L. Postpartum depression and child development. *Psychological Med* 27:253–260, 1997.

151. Appleby L, Warner R, Whitton A, et al. A controlled study of fluoxetine and cognitive-behavioral counselling in the treatment of postnatal depression. *BMJ* 314(7085):932–936, 1997.

152. O'Hara MW, Stuart S, Gorman LL, et al. Efficacy of interpersonal psychotherapy for postpartum depression. *Arch Gen Psychiatry* 57(11):1039–1045, 2000.

157. Gregoire AJ, Kumar R, Everitt B, et al. Transdermal estrogen for treatment of severe postnatal depression. *Lancet* 347(9006):930–933, 1996.

164. Austin M-PV. Puerperal affective psychosis: Is there a case for lithium prophylaxis? *Br J Psychiatry* 161:692–694, 1992.

169. Wisner P. Prevention of recurrent postpartum depression: A randomized clinical trial. *J Clin Psychiatry* 62(2):82–86, 2001.

170. Llewellyn A, Stowe Z. Psychotropic medications in lactation. *J Clin Psychiatry* 59(Suppl. 2):41–52, 1998.

171. Burt VK, Suri R, Altshuler L, et al. The use of psychotropic medications during breast-feeding. *Am J Psychiatry* 158(7):1001–1009, 2001.

181. Epperson N, Czarkowski KA, Ward-O'Brien D, et al. Maternal sertraline treatment and serotonin transport in breast-feeding mother-infant pairs. *Am J Psychiatry* 158(10):1631–1637, 2001.

184. Viguera A, Newport DJ, Ritchie J, et al. Lithium in breastmilk and nursing infants: Clinical implications. *Am J Psychiatry* 164(2):342–345, 2007.

32 Anxiety Disorders

Amanda W. Calkins, PhD, Eric Bui, MD, PhD, Charles T. Taylor, PhD, Mark H. Pollack, MD, Richard T. LeBeau, PhD, and Naomi M. Simon, MD, MSc

KEY POINTS

Incidence

- Anxiety disorders are the most prevalent mental health problem in the US, and are associated with marked distress and functional impairments in multiple domains.

Epidemiology/Pathophysiology

- The pathogenesis of anxiety disorders likely resides in the interaction of innate biological vulnerabilities and specific environmental events or stressors.

Clinical Findings/Differential Diagnoses

- Routine screening for anxiety disorders in medical settings is essential; people with anxiety disorders frequently present to primary care and mental health clinics, and anxiety symptoms often mimic common medical conditions.

Treatment Options

- Advances in our understanding of the neurobiological and psychological processes involved in the etiology and persistence of anxiety disorders has contributed to the development of effective pharmacological and psychological interventions for many anxiety disorders.

Complications

- Anxiety disorders commonly co-exist with other psychiatric and medical conditions, which often bodes poorly for the course and prognosis of the disorder.

Prognosis

- Despite current efficacious interventions, many individuals with anxiety disorders fail to respond to first-line treatments or do not achieve high end-state function, highlighting the need for continued efforts directed at elucidating the pathophysiological processes relevant to anxiety.

OVERVIEW

Anxiety disorders are the most common mental health problem in the US, affecting 18.1% of adults in the general population in a given year,[1] and 28.8% of adults at some point during their life-time.[2] Estimates suggest that anxiety disorders cost the US more than $42 billion per year, which amounts to almost one-third of the total direct and indirect mental health "bill".[3] Anxiety itself is a universal human experience; moreover, it is often a normal and beneficial reaction to stressful situations. Determining when anxiety becomes *pathological*, that is, when it deviates from a normal or expected emotional response to an environmental event, can be informed by considering the following criteria: (1) *excessiveness* (i.e., "Would the degree of anxiety experienced be considered disproportionate in relation to the person's current life circumstances or to identifiable environmental stimuli?"); (2) *intensity* (i.e., "How marked is the level of distress experienced by the person?"); (3) *duration* or chronicity (i.e., "Does the anxiety response persist for longer than would be expected under the circumstances?"); (4) *impairment* (i.e., "To what degree is there evidence of significant impairments in social, occupational, educational, health, and/or daily function?"). For the diagnosis of an anxiety disorder to be made, the presence of a specific symptom profile associated with a significant level of distress or impairment is required.

Anxiety is manifest in physical, affective, cognitive, and behavioral domains. Physical expressions of anxiety typically reflect autonomic arousal and include characteristic symptoms (such as palpitations, shortness of breath, muscle tension, dizziness, upset stomach, chest tightness, sweating, and trembling). Emotional manifestations of anxiety range from feelings of uneasiness and edginess to terror and panic. Cognitive manifestations of anxiety include worry, apprehension, and thoughts regarding emotional, bodily, or social threat. Behaviorally, anxiety triggers a multitude of responses concerned with diminishing or preventing the perceived threat and associated distress; these include avoidance, escape, and safety-seeking behaviors. The American Psychiatric Association's (APA's) *Diagnostic and Statistical Manual of Mental Disorders*, Fifth Edition (DSM-5) separates anxiety disorders into discrete categories based on purported similarities in phenomenology, etiology, and pathophysiology. Here, we review four common anxiety disorders, namely (1) panic disorder (PD), and the often co-morbid agoraphobia that has been recently included as an independent disorder, (2) social anxiety disorder (SAD) (or social phobia), and (3) generalized anxiety disorder (GAD). In DSM-5, obsessive compulsive disorder (OCD; Chapter 33) and posttraumatic stress disorder (PTSD; Chapter 34) are no longer listed as anxiety disorders. Common pharmacological and psychological treatments for anxiety-related conditions are reviewed in Chapter 41.

PANIC DISORDER AND AGORAPHOBIA

Introduction

Although officially introduced into the diagnostic nomenclature in 1980 with the publication of the DSM-III, investigations into the phenomenology and treatment of panic-like symptoms appeared decades earlier. Descriptions of PD have remained relatively stable across different versions of the DSM, with the cardinal feature of this condition being the presence of recurrent, unexpected panic attacks accompanied by cognitive (e.g., anxious apprehension) and behavioral sequelae (e.g., interoceptive and situational avoidance) related to perceived consequences of the panic. PD is recognized as a common and often chronic psychiatric condition associated with negative outcomes in emotional and physical health, as well as significant disruptions in several areas of a person's life. Of all the anxiety-related conditions, PD has been most intensively studied over the past several decades, with considerable advancements being made in our understanding of the psychopathology, neurobiology, and treatment of this condition.

Agoraphobia, a condition often co-morbid with PD, was introduced in DSM-III as a distinct disorder, and then linked to the diagnosis of PD in DSM-IV. In DSM-5, agoraphobia is now again a distinct diagnosis. Because of the high co-morbidity between PD and agoraphobia, and because of the lack of research specifically targeting it, agoraphobia is reviewed here together with PD.

Clinical Characteristics and Diagnosis

Panic Disorder

The characteristic feature of PD is the presence of recurrent panic attacks, or paroxysms of extreme anxiety—which are sudden, intense bursts of anxiety or fear accompanied by an array of physical symptoms (e.g., rapid heart rate, dizziness, shortness of breath, sweating, nausea; see Box 32-1 for a complete list of associated symptoms). Panic attacks themselves are relatively common in the general population, with lifetime prevalence rates reported at approximately 28% in a large-scale community sample.[4]

The diagnosis of PD, requires the presence of recurrent unexpected panic attacks, along with at least 1 month of persistent worry about the possibility of future attacks, worry about the implications or consequences of panic attacks, and/or the development of maladaptive behavioral changes related to the attacks (e.g., repeated emergency department [ED] or physician visits due to fears of an undiagnosed medical condition, or efforts to avoid panic attacks, such as avoidance of exercise or unfamiliar situations) (see Box 32-1 for the DSM-5 diagnostic criteria of PD and Box 32-2 for the criteria of agoraphobia). Further, the person must experience marked levels of distress and/or functional impairment that result from their panic symptoms. The difference between people who experience transitory panic episodes and those who go on to develop the full-blown disorder may be explained by differences in pre-existing biological, psychological, or environmental vulnerabilities (see Pathophysiology section below).

Agoraphobia

For a diagnosis of agoraphobia, DSM-5 does not require panic attacks but requires the presence of fear or anxiety about at least 2 of 5 specific types of situations (e.g., public transportation, being in enclosed places or outside the home alone) with associated fear and/or avoidance because of apprehension about having panic-like symptoms or other suddenly incapacitating or embarrassing symptoms (see Box 32-2 for DSM-5 criteria for agoraphobia).

Agoraphobia can therefore occur alone or with PD. Commonly avoided situations include crowded public places (e.g., malls, grocery stores, or movie theatres), enclosed spaces (e.g., elevators or tunnels), driving, traveling far away from home, and standing in line. The presence of agoraphobic avoidance in PD is associated with a variety of poorer outcomes in terms of symptom severity, co-morbidity, and functional impairment.[4] Hence, most treatment-seeking individuals with PD experience some degree of agoraphobia.

Panic Attack Specifier

Clinically, it is important to distinguish episodes of panic that occur in PD from those that occur exclusively in the context of another Axis I condition. Panic attacks are common in other anxiety-related conditions, and are often characterized by the same physical and cognitive symptom constellation as seen in PD (i.e., they are phenomenologically similar). In the latter cases, however, the source of the fearful sensations is clearly identifiable; that is, the panic attacks are cued or triggered. For instance, panic attacks can be provoked when a socially-anxious individual is exposed to situations involving potential observation or evaluation by others, when a person with a specific phobia is exposed to a particular feared stimulus (e.g., heights or spiders), or when a person with PTSD is confronted with reminders of a traumatic event. Conversely, in people with PD, these same types of episodes are experienced, at least initially, as unexpected or as occurring "out of the blue."

BOX 32-1 DSM-5 Diagnostic Criteria: Panic Disorder (300.01 (F41.0))

A. Recurrent unexpected panic attacks. A panic attack is an abrupt surge of intense fear or intense discomfort that reaches a peak within minutes, and during which time four (or more) of the following symptoms occur:
   Note: The abrupt surge can occur from a calm state or an anxious state.
   1. Palpitations, pounding heart, or accelerated heart rate
   2. Sweating
   3. Trembling or shaking
   4. Sensations of shortness of breath or smothering
   5. Feelings of choking
   6. Chest pain or discomfort
   7. Nausea or abdominal distress
   8. Feeling dizzy, unsteady, light-headed, or faint
   9. Chills or heat sensations
   10. Paresthesias (numbness or tingling sensations)
   11. Derealization (feelings of unreality) or depersonalization (being detached from oneself)
   12. Fear of losing control or "going crazy"
   13. Fear of dying.
   Note: Culture-specific symptoms (e.g., tinnitus, neck soreness, headache, uncontrollable screaming or crying) may be seen. Such symptoms should not count as one of the four required symptoms.

B. At least one of the attacks has been followed by 1 month (or more) of one or both of the following:
   1. Persistent concern or worry about additional panic attacks or their consequences (e.g., losing control, having a heart attack, "going crazy").
   2. A significant maladaptive change in behavior related to the attacks (e.g., behaviors designed to avoid having panic attacks, such as avoidance of exercise or unfamiliar situations).
C. The disturbance is not attributable to the physiological effects of a substance (e.g., a drug of abuse, a medication) or another medical condition (e.g., hyperthyroidism, cardiopulmonary disorders).
D. The disturbance is not better explained by another mental disorder (e.g., the panic attacks do not occur only in response to feared social situations, as in social anxiety disorder; in response to circumscribed phobic objects or situations, as in specific phobia; in response to obsessions, as in obsessive-compulsive disorder; in response to reminders of traumatic events, as in posttraumatic stress disorder; or in response to separation from attachment figures, as in separation anxiety disorder).

BOX 32-2 DSM-5 Diagnostic Criteria: Agoraphobia (300.22 (F40.00))

A. Marked fear or anxiety about two (or more) of the following five situations:
   1. Using public transportation (e.g., automobiles, buses, trains, ships, planes)
   2. Being in open spaces (e.g., parking lots, marketplaces, bridges)
   3. Being in enclosed places (e.g., shops, theaters, cinemas)
   4. Standing in line or being in a crowd
   5. Being outside of the home alone.
B. The individual fears or avoids these situations because of thoughts that escape might be difficult or help might not be available in the event of developing panic-like symptoms or other incapacitating or embarrassing symptoms (e.g., fear of falling in the elderly; fear of incontinence).
C. The agoraphobic situations almost always provoke fear or anxiety.
D. The agoraphobic situations are actively avoided, require the presence of a companion, or are endured with intense fear or anxiety.
E. The fear or anxiety is out of proportion to the actual danger posed by the agoraphobic situations and to the sociocultural context.
F. The fear, anxiety, or avoidance is persistent, typically lasting for 6 months or more.
G. The fear, anxiety, or avoidance causes clinically significant distress or impairment in social, occupational, or other important areas of functioning.
H. If another medical condition (e.g., inflammatory bowel disease, Parkinson's disease) is present, the fear, anxiety, or avoidance is clearly excessive.
I. The fear, anxiety, or avoidance is not better explained by the symptoms of another mental disorder—for example, the symptoms are not confined to specific phobia, situational type; do not involve only social situations (as in social anxiety disorder); and are not related exclusively to obsessions (as in obsessive-compulsive disorder), perceived defects or flaws in physical appearance (as in body dysmorphic disorder), reminders of traumatic events (as in posttraumatic stress disorder), or fear of separation (as in separation anxiety disorder).

Note: Agoraphobia is diagnosed irrespective of the presence of panic disorder. If an individual's presentation meets criteria for panic disorder and agoraphobia, both diagnoses should be assigned.

Reprinted with permission from the Diagnostic and statistical manual of mental disorders, ed 5, (Copyright 2013). American Psychiatric Association.

Although many patients who present for treatment may describe their panic as being triggered by a particular situation (e.g., being in crowded public places or enclosed spaces, or on public transportation), or activity (e.g., exercising), a thorough history typically reveals the initial onset of panic as occurring unexpectedly, without clearly identifiable triggers. In those cases, the presence of co-morbid agoraphobia is likely. It is also possible to meet criteria for both PD and another anxiety disorder (with cued panic attacks), as long as some unexpected panic attacks and concern and/or maladaptive behavioral changes about those attacks is present.

Panic attacks have been found to be associated with poorer outcomes across a variety of other psychiatric disorders, including mood disorders, alcohol dependence, psychotic

disorders, somatoform, or eating disorders.[5] As a result, in DSM-5, panic attacks are now a specifier that can be coded across all DSM diagnosis.

Epidemiology

Results from a recent US epidemiological survey reported lifetime and 12-month prevalence rates of panic disorder at 4.7% and 2.4%, respectively.[2,6] Notably, those rates are somewhat higher than findings from the original NCS[7] and the Epidemiological Catchment Area (ECA) study.[8] It is unclear whether these discrepancies represent an increasing prevalence over the past several decades, or are due to differences in diagnostic methods and criteria. Given the salient and distressing physical symptoms experienced by people with PD, it is not surprising that prevalence rates of this condition are even higher in primary medical settings, with reports ranging from 3% to 8%.[9,10]

Despite differences in the reported prevalence of PD over time, the association between PD and several demographic characteristics has remained relatively stable. For instance, PD is consistently diagnosed in about twice as many women as men. PD tends to have an age of onset in late adolescence or early adulthood, although many individuals may exhibit a pre-existing history of anxiety-related symptoms in childhood.[11] Some research suggests a declining prevalence and severity in older adults.[12] For many individuals, the course of the disorder is chronic and unremitting, although symptoms may wax and wane over time with recurrence rates of a remitted PD diagnosis estimated at up to 58% over a 12-year period.[13-15]

Impairment and Quality of Life

PD is associated with significant impairments across domains of functioning. Individuals with PD report disruptions in work, social, and family function, in addition to having more negative life events and an overall diminished quality of life.[16] In terms of academic and vocational outcomes, PD is associated with lower educational achievement, a higher likelihood of unemployment, and diminished work productivity. Socially, patients with PD have impaired interpersonal and marital function, and demonstrate increased financial dependency. Moreover, people with PD report greater health-related problems (both physical and emotional)[17] and PD is often associated with excessive health care utilization, often for presentations of non-psychiatric complaints.[18,19] It is notable that the degree of impairment and reduced quality of life may be similar, if not greater, than that of patients with other serious psychiatric (e.g., depression) and medical problems.[16,20,21]

Co-morbidity

The extant empirical literature suggests that co-morbidity in PD is common, with cases of "pure" PD emerging infrequently in clinical settings. The NCS-R revealed that 83% of the PD-only group and 100% of the PD with agoraphobia group met criteria for one or more life-time co-morbid conditions.[4] Co-occurring anxiety disorders were most common (66% for PD only; 94% for PD with agoraphobia), with specific co-morbidity rates as follows: specific phobias (34% and 75%, respectively), SAD (31% and 67%, respectively), PTSD (22% and 40%, respectively), and GAD (21% and 15%, respectively). PD was also commonly associated with the mood disorders, including major depressive disorder (MDD) (35% and 39%, respectively), bipolar disorders (14% and 33%, respectively), and dysthymia (10% and 15%, respectively).

Substance use disorders were also common, with alcohol abuse or dependence being diagnosed most commonly (25% and 37%, respectively). Interestingly, impulse-control disorders also frequently occurred with PD, with life-time co-morbidity rates of 47% and 60%, respectively.

The presence of co-morbidity in PD bodes poorly for a variety of psychological, functional, and treatment outcomes. For instance, increased rates of suicide and suicide attempts have been associated with PD,[17] with some research suggesting that inflated rates of life-time suicide attempts are the result of co-occurring psychiatric conditions (such as depression or alcohol abuse), although evidence suggests that the presence of PD is associated with increased rates of suicide attempts, even when co-morbidity and a history of childhood abuse is accounted for.[17] Similarly, the life-time risk of suicide attempts in patients with PD and MDD is more than double that of the two disorders independently.[22,23] In the case of co-morbid bipolar disorder, anxiety disorders (including panic) have been associated with an earlier age of onset of bipolar disorder, a worse course of bipolar disorder, a diminished quality of life and function, and heightened levels of suicidal thinking and completion.[24] Further, in a sample of patients with bipolar I disorder, the presence of life-time panic symptoms, in patients with either sub-syndromal or full PD, was associated with poor or delayed response to treatment of bipolar disorder.[25] Finally, not surprisingly, both medical and psychiatric co-morbidities significantly impact quality of life in individuals with PD.[21]

Given that the symptoms characteristic of PD mimic a variety of medical conditions, it is not surprising that afflicted patients commonly present to EDs or primary care clinics; this is reflected in the high degree of health care utilization associated with this disorder.[19,26] Increased utilization of medical services is even greater in panic-disordered patients who present with a co-morbid psychiatric condition.[26] Furthermore, frequent medical visits are associated to a greater extent with panic-disordered patients compared to those with other debilitating psychiatric conditions, including depression and substance use disorders.[27] It is also notable that panic attacks can occur as a symptom of numerous medical conditions (such as hyperthyroidism, and caffeine or stimulant use [e.g., cocaine]). Further, a variety of physical illnesses (such as cardiovascular and respiratory disorders [e.g., mitral valve prolapse, and asthma]) often co-occur with, but are rarely the direct cause of, PD.[28]

The appropriate detection and diagnosis of PD in medical settings can be complicated given the substantial variability that exists in one's ability to accurately describe the experience of anxiety. For instance, anxiety-disordered patients may report a diffuse feeling of uneasiness or describe feeling "not right" in their body, and may generate interpretations that something is physically (not psychologically) wrong with them. An additional complicating factor is that many symptoms of panic attacks (e.g., shortness of breath, chest pain, dizziness) are among the most common complaints of those presenting to medical settings, and research suggests that relatively few patients receive any specific diagnosis for these problems. Thus, professionals working in a variety of health care settings must be particularly vigilant for potential psychiatric underpinnings of the somatic complaints reported by many patients.

Pathophysiology

Consistent with etiological models of other anxiety-related conditions, the pathogenesis and maintenance of PD is likely the result of a complex interaction of biological, psychological, and environmental factors. In support of a genetic transmission of PD, twin studies have demonstrated that monozygotic twins have a significantly greater concordance rate for PD than do dizygotic twins. Further, the risk of PD is increased eight-fold in first-degree relatives of patients with the disorder. A review of twin and family studies suggests that PD has a heritability of approximately 40%, with additional significant contributions from unique environmental effects (greater than 50%), and only a relatively small (less than 10%) contribution from common (familial) environmental factors.[29] Genetic heterogeneity or complex inheritance, with environmental factor interactions and multiple single genes, has been identified as contributing to PD's etiology.[30] Linkage studies have implicated several chromosomal regions; however, recent genome-wide association studies failed to show consistent associations between specific loci and PD.[31,32] Increasing evidence supports the idea that the genes underlying PD overlap significantly and cross diagnostic boundaries (mood and anxiety disorders). Additionally, intermediate phenotypes, such as anxiety-related temperaments, may predispose individuals to PD and the genetics of these phenotypes is the topic of ongoing research.[30]

Stressful life events also appear to be important in the etiology of PD. Previous research has found that approximately 80% of patients with PD report major life stressors within the 12 months preceding the onset of the disorder,[33] suggesting that stressful life events may contribute to the timing of the onset of the disorder.[34] Childhood physical and sexual abuse also appear to increase the risk for the later development of PD.[35] Moreover, symptom severity has been correlated with negative life events (including interpersonal conflicts, physical or health-related problems, and work-related difficulties),[36,37] while the presence of chronic life stressors has been shown to worsen the course of PD.[38] Finally, some work has suggested that teenagers who smoke are at a higher risk of developing PD, although the causal nature of this association remains uncertain.[39] All in all, the extant literature supports a diathesis-stress model of PD, suggesting that exposure to life stressors may trigger a pre-existing vulnerability towards panic. In line with this, recent research has particularly focused on gene × environment interaction.[40]

Neurobiology

Disruptions in the serotonin system have also been implicated in the pathophysiology of PD. One study found that, compared to controls, individuals with PD demonstrated reduced serotonin transport binding in the midbrain, temporal lobe, and thalamus.[41] Additionally, selective serotonin reuptake inhibitors (SSRIs), serotonin-norepinephrine (noradrenaline) reuptake inhibitors (SNRIs), and tricyclic antidepressants (TCAs), all of which have effects on serotonergic neurotransmission, have demonstrated efficacy in the amelioration of panic symptoms.[42]

The widespread use of benzodiazepines in the treatment of PD, has led many to hypothesize that gamma amino butyric acid (GABA), an inhibitory neurotransmitter, is relevant to the underlying pathophysiology of this condition. Benzodiazepines increase GABA-ergic transmission, and have demonstrated efficacy for PD. Consistent with these findings, people with PD display diminished benzodiazepine receptor sensitivity.[43] High densities of benzodiazepine-GABA receptors have been found in brain regions (most notably the amygdala and hippocampus) implicated in anxiety and fear responses.[44] Converging evidence comes from a neuroimaging study that reported reduced GABA levels in the occipital cortex of individuals with PD[45]; interestingly, citalopram, an SSRI effective for a range of depressive and anxiety disorders (including PD), is associated with increases in GABA levels in the occipital cortex of healthy controls.[46]

Advances in neuroimaging techniques over the last 20 years have led to increasing investigation of the neurobiology of anxiety disorders. Research has implicated the limbic system, including most notably the amygdala, as well as the hippocampus, cortical areas (dorsal anterior cingulate cortex [dACC] and ventromedial prefrontal cortex [vmPFC]), the basal ganglia, and the brainstem in the neurobiology of PD (for review, see Dresler et al.[47]). A critical role of the limbic system is to scan the environment for threat-relevant cues, in addition to monitoring interoceptive (bodily) sensations, and to integrate these diverse sources of information to assess the magnitude of threat and the need for action to achieve safety. Neurobiological findings have demonstrated that patients with PD have reduced amygdala volumes,[48-50] as well as reduced cerebral glucose metabolism in the amygdala and hippocampus, along with thalamus and brainstem areas.[51] Hyperactivation of the amygdala and subsequent deficient regulation of the limbic system by cortical regions are supported by the prevailing neurocircuitry models of panic disorder. These findings are bolstered by masked facial affect paradigms as well as fear conditioning and extinction models that have been used to examine the neurobiology underlying fear and anxiety in animals and more recently in humans.[52]

The acquisition and extinction of conditioned fear is also well characterized in animal and human models of fear-based conditions such as panic and agoraphobia, as well as PTSD. Briefly, a conditioned fear response (CR) is acquired when a neutral stimulus (the conditioned stimulus [CS], such as a train, elevator or other situation where escape might be difficult) is repeatedly paired with an intrinsically aversive unconditioned stimulus (UCS), such as physical sensations of panic. With repeated presentation of this pairing, subjects learn that the CS predicts the UCS, causing the CS alone to elicit a fear response, such as heightened skin conductance. The CR can be extinguished by repeatedly presenting the CS without any UCS, leading to a decline in the fear response. Conditioning paradigms are particularly useful in anxiety research as anxiety disorders are characterized by impaired extinction (or extinction learning is not recalled even when specific cues no longer predict threat). This process can be measured in the brain using imaging techniques as valid and sensitive assessments of the associated neural circuitry.[53] Numerous animal and human studies show that this process involves interaction between the prefrontal cortex, basolateral amygdala, and hippocampus (for review, see Quirk et al.[54]). The vmPFC plays a crucial role, with studies suggesting that consolidation of extinction learning leads to potentiation of vmPFC, which inhibits the fear response.[55] The hippocampus encodes the context during both fear acquisition and extinction, and is essential to consolidation of extinction.[56]

Impairments in the fear extinction network have been observed in PD patients using the faces paradigm.[52] In fear conditioning, a recent study showed aberrant responses within the vmPFC, ventral striatum, and the amygdala during the fear acquisition phase in PD patients.[57] Moreover, reduced cortical volume in the dACC as well as the rostral ACC has been reported in PD, indicating structural differences as well as differences in activation in PD.[58] Under conditions of panic provocation, patients show functional differences in insular, cingulate, frontal, and brainstem areas.[47] It has been suggested that PD patients also show deficiencies in prefrontal areas associated with emotion regulation. Ball and colleagues[59] reported reduced dorsomedial PFC (dmPFC) and dorsolateral (PFC) in both PD and GAD patients during an emotion regulation task.

A recent meta-analysis on six studies found gray matter deficits in the right caudate head and the right parahippocampal gyrus.[60] In addition, decreased volume in the temporal, occipital, and frontal lobes has also been consistently reported.[50,61,62] Of interest, a number of recent studies found that successful treatment with an antidepressant was associated with increased brain volumes in some of these areas.[63-66] Similarly, some functional neuroimaging data suggest that cognitive-behavioral therapy (CBT) may have the potential to change brain activity.[67,68] Overall, neurobiology research to date is promising but work remains to be done to understand these conditions and their optimal treatment across patients with panic and/or agoraphobia.

Psychopathological Processes

The psychological construct that has received the most attention in PD research is *anxiety sensitivity* (AS), the belief that anxiety and its related symptoms may lead to deleterious physical, social, and psychological consequences (e.g., fainting, embarrassment, loss of control, going crazy, or death).[69] The empirical evidence demonstrates that AS predicts the onset of panic attacks in a variety of samples (including adolescents, college students, and the general population).[70] The origins of AS are not fully understood, and it is unclear what role genetics and biology play in its development and its specificity to PD. Although the strength of the association may be strongest with PD, AS has also been linked with other anxiety disorders and health related conditions.[71] To date, there are no multi-variate twin studies investigating the genetic and environmental relationships of AS in adults; however, in adolescents AS and anxiety were found to have significant genetic correlations.[72] AS has been also studied in a child twin sample as a broad predictor of anxiety symptoms.[73]

Some experiential contributions to the development of AS likely include repeated exposure to aversive experiences (e.g., a personal history of illness or injury), vicarious observations (e.g., significant illnesses or death among family members), informational learning (e.g., repeated warning messages from parents), parental reinforcement of attention to somatic symptoms, parental modeling of distress in response to bodily sensations, and the occurrence of panic attacks themselves.[74]

AS is posited to maintain panic through two mechanisms. First, it has been argued that panic attacks may become conditioned to themselves, as a conditioned fear of internal cues (i.e., interoceptive conditioning). According to this account, early physical sensations of the anxiety response elicit subsequent intense bursts of anxiety or panic due to previous pairings with the experience of panic.[75] These models offer one psychological explanation for the unexpected nature of panic. Cognitive-behavioral formulations on the other hand suggest that catastrophic misinterpretation of bodily sensations is the core factor responsible for the maintenance of PD.[76] Common misappraisals include the fear that bodily sensations are a sign of imminent death (e.g., heart attack or suffocation), loss of control (e.g., going crazy or fainting), or social catastrophe (e.g., embarrassment or humiliation). In turn, those misinterpretations heighten anxiety (and the associated physical sensations), which triggers further misappraisals. Although many patients can identify particular feared consequences associated with their panic, they may not be aware of specific catastrophic misappraisals in the exact moment of a panic episode, suggesting that misappraisals themselves may also become conditioned stimuli that trigger panic outside of one's conscious awareness. According to both accounts, following an initial exposure to panic, a "fear of fear" develops (i.e., fear of physical sensations associated with a normal fear response), wherein exposure to either physical or cognitive cues associated with prior panic will provoke a state of panic. While AS was initially conceptualized as a trait, it has become clear that AS itself may be reduced both with cognitive-behavioral and pharmacological interventions.[77] Psychometric studies largely support the use of the Anxiety Sensitivity Index (ASI)[78] to measure AS. The ASI is composed of three lower-order factors: physical concerns, cognitive concerns, and social concerns. The physical concerns subscale measures anxiety about the physical health consequences of arousal sensations (e.g., throat tightness leading to choking). The cognitive concerns subscale measures worries that psychological symptoms, such as difficulty concentrating, will lead to mental incapacitation. Finally, the social concerns subscale measures the degree to which publicly observable symptoms of anxiety might lead to embarrassment or rejection. In a recent study, the ASI physical concerns subscale uniquely predicted variance in PD after controlling for other anxiety and depression symptoms.[79] This finding is consistent with the cognitive-behavioral model of AS in PD; the misappraisal of physical symptoms perpetuates panic symptoms.

SOCIAL ANXIETY DISORDER

Although clinical descriptions of social phobia appeared some 40 or more years ago,[80] social phobia did not appear as a unique diagnostic entity until the DSM-III was published in 1980. Originally conceptualized as a "phobic disorder," definitions of social phobia were restricted to specific performance-related situations (e.g., public speaking), while fear of social interaction situations was absent in this early diagnostic nomenclature. The definition of social phobia expanded with the revision of the DSM-III in 1987, and included both performance and social interaction situations. Presently, social anxiety disorder (SAD) is recognized as a prevalent and often incapacitating anxiety disorder characterized by a marked and persistent fear of one or more social or performance situations in which the person is exposed to unfamiliar people or to possible scrutiny by others.[81] Although once referred to as "a neglected anxiety disorder,"[82] the past two decades have witnessed a burgeoning of empirical research dedicated to better understanding the psychology and neurobiology of social fears and anxiety.

Clinical Characteristics and Diagnosis

The fundamental characteristic of SAD is a marked and persistent fear of situations that involve performance, evaluation, or potential scrutiny by others.[81] People with SAD fear that they will act in way or show anxiety symptoms that will be embarrassing or humiliating, or that may result in negative evaluation by others. Consequently, the feared social interaction or performance situations are avoided, or else endured with intense distress and anxiety (see Box 32-3 for DSM-5 diagnostic criteria). Commonly feared and/or avoided situations may include attending parties or social gatherings, meeting new people, initiating or maintaining conversations, participating in group meetings, being the center of attention, interacting with authority figures, being assertive, speaking in public, and eating or drinking in public. Patients often report significant anxiety in anticipation of feared social events, and may report panic attacks upon exposure to such situations.

The DSM-5 recognizes one specifier of SAD, performance-only (similar to the non-generalized subtype in DSM-IV). The performance-only specifier is generally limited to public speaking or to other performance situations and, consequently, is often less disabling, although it may result in impairment at work or school in which regular public presentations may be required.[83] In contrast, SAD with a broader array of fears or anxiety (previously called "generalized") is associated with greater impairment because the anxiety is pervasive and occurs in many social and performance situations. Individuals not meeting criteria for the performance-only

---

BOX 32-3 DSM-5 Diagnostic Criteria: Social Anxiety Disorder (Social Phobia) (300.23 (F40.10))

A. Marked fear or anxiety about one or more social situations in which the individual is exposed to possible scrutiny by others. Examples include social interactions (e.g., having a conversation, meeting unfamiliar people), being observed (e.g., eating or drinking), and performing in front of others (e.g., giving a speech).

Note: In children, the anxiety must occur in peer settings and not just during interactions with adults.

B. The individual fears that he or she will act in a way or show anxiety symptoms that will be negatively evaluated (i.e., will be humiliating or embarrassing; will lead to rejection or offend others).

C. The social situations almost always provoke fear or anxiety.

Note: In children, the fear or anxiety may be expressed by crying, tantrums, freezing, clinging, shrinking, or failing to speak in social situations.

D. The social situations are avoided or endured with intense fear or anxiety.

E. The fear or anxiety is out of proportion to the actual threat posed by the social situation and to the sociocultural context.

F. The fear, anxiety, or avoidance is persistent, typically lasting for 6 months or more.

G. The fear, anxiety, or avoidance causes clinically significant distress or impairment in social, occupational, or other important areas of functioning.

H. The fear, anxiety, or avoidance is not attributable to the physiological effects of a substance (e.g., a drug of abuse, a medication) or another medical condition.

I. The fear, anxiety, or avoidance is not better explained by the symptoms of another mental disorder, such as panic disorder, body dysmorphic disorder, or autism spectrum disorder.

J. If another medical condition (e.g., Parkinson's disease, obesity, disfigurement from burns or injury) is present, the fear, anxiety, or avoidance is clearly unrelated or is excessive.

Specify if:

• **Performance only:** If the fear is restricted to speaking or performing in public.

Reprinted with permission from the Diagnostic and statistical manual of mental disorders, *ed 5, (Copyright 2013). American Psychiatric Association.*

---

specifier often fear and avoid both social interaction situations (e.g., social gatherings and meeting new people), as well as performance situations (e.g., public speaking).

Epidemiology

SAD is a common psychiatric condition, with life-time prevalence rates in Western countries ranging between 7% and 13%.[84] Variations in prevalence rates depend on diagnostic criteria (i.e., DSM-III, DSM-III-R, DSM-IV, or DSM-5), diagnostic threshold (e.g., required level of distress or impairment necessary to meet diagnostic criteria), and method of assessment (e.g., self-report surveys or interviews). Results from the recent National Comorbidity Survey-Replication (NCS-R) indicate that SAD occurs at 12-month prevalence rate of 7.4%, a life-time prevalence of approximately 10.7% in the general population, making it the fourth most prevalent psychiatric disorder, behind MDD, alcohol dependence, and specific phobia.[7,85] Earlier work based on comparable population estimates found that the generalized subtype occurs in about two-thirds of people diagnosed with SAD, with the non-generalized subtype present in one-third.[86]

SAD is more common in women than in men, with a ratio of about 3:2. However, in individuals who present for treatment, men and women are equally represented. Some have argued that this disparity is the result of differential social expectations, gender roles, or differing levels of distress, with symptoms causing more impairment for men than women.[87] Gender, however, does not appear to influence age of onset, duration of illness, or co-morbidity.[88,89] Research conducted within the US has failed to find significant differences in race or ethnicity in SAD within the general population.[90] In some cases, however, prevalence rates have been shown to differ markedly between countries. For example, Asian communities report the lowest life-time prevalence rates (<1%) of SAD.[84]

SAD typically has an early age-of-onset surfacing in either childhood or adolescence, and often persists well into adulthood following a chronic, unremitting course that significantly interferes with the afflicted individual's life.[91] However, evidence from the most recent NCS supported a less chronic course with only 20% of life-time cases of child-adolescent (ages 14–17) SAD meeting criteria for the disorder within the 12 months prior to study participation.[85] This recurrence rate was less than any other anxiety or mood disorder examined and is lower than previously reported recurrence rates of 38%–65%.[15,92] Although the average age of onset of SAD appears to be around 10–16 years of age (with an earlier average age of onset for non-performance-related SAD),[90,93] many patients report being shy or socially anxious since early childhood. Empirical evidence suggests that people with SAD present with a mean duration of illness of around 25 years and low rates of spontaneous recovery.[94] Those striking facts illustrate that, for many, SAD is a life-long illness, and highlight the vast under-utilization of treatment services for this common and debilitating condition. These impairments may be less burdensome for those with the performance-only specifier of SAD. Previous reviews have shown that individuals with the performance-only specifier have a later onset, less behavioral inhibition/shyness, have a stronger physical component of anxiety, and have a better response to beta-blocker treatment.[93]

Impairment and Quality of Life

Functional impairment is common in people with SAD. This condition is associated with educational and occupational under-achievement, impaired social relationships, social isolation, and an overall diminished quality of life.[95] Afflicted individuals tend to be less well educated and of lower socio-economic status compared to people in the general population. Work impairment is also common, with research showing that people with SAD are twice as likely to report at least one disability day in a given 2-week period compared to people without SAD. Evidence also shows that people with SAD report greater physical health-related problems and physical impairment. Individuals with the performance-only specifier tend to have the greatest impairment in their professional (work or school) obligations as opposed to individuals without the performance-only specifier who may have interference in many role domains.[93] The presence of co-morbid psychiatric conditions greatly increases the impairment and disability related to SAD. In terms of social function, socially anxious individuals have been found to have fewer friends, and are less likely to date or to marry compared to people in the general population, as well as relative to patients with

other anxiety disorders.[95,96] Interestingly, even when people with social anxiety do develop friendships and intimate relationships, they often view those relationships as less functional and satisfying than do people without social anxiety.[97,98] Additionally, according to data from the national epidemiologic survey, quality of life improves with anxiety symptom improvement; however, individuals with SAD reported lower quality of life even after symptom reduction than those who were never diagnosed with an anxiety disorder.[99]

Co-morbidity

SAD is highly co-morbid with other psychiatric illnesses. For instance, results from the initial National Comorbidity Survey (NCS) found that 81% of people with SAD met criteria for at least one other life-time DSM-III-R psychiatric diagnosis; 19% reported one other disorder, 14% reported two other disorders, and 48% reported three other disorders.[90] Not surprisingly, individuals with SAD are more likely to suffer from co-morbid mood and anxiety disorders than individuals with the performance subtype.[100] It is particularly notable that the onset of SAD often appears to *precede* the onset of other co-morbid disorders, suggesting that SAD may be a risk factor for the development of other psychopathology.[89,90]

Anxiety disorders are the most commonly reported co-morbid illness, with 57% of people with SAD endorsing criteria for at least one other anxiety-related condition. Data from the NCS revealed the presence of PTSD in 16% of individuals with SAD, in 11% of those with PD, and in 13% of those with GAD.[90] In treatment-seeking populations, the rates of co-morbid anxiety disorders are often higher, with rates of co-morbid SAD reported near 45% in primary PD samples.[101] In primary social phobia, co-morbid GAD has been reported in 24%.[102] Some evidence suggests that in some cases SAD may occur secondarily to trauma or to PTSD.[103]

SAD has also been shown to be highly co-morbid with the spectrum of mood disorders. In the NCS, secondary MDD was present in 37% of those with SAD.[104] Life-time rates of co-morbid MDD in clinical samples have been reported near 60%.[105] Individuals with SAD appear to be at significant risk for the later development of depression, in light of evidence demonstrating that onset of SAD typically occurs many years prior to the onset of depression.[106] In a longitudinal investigation, participants with SAD and depression in adolescence or early adulthood were found to be at greatest risk for subsequent depression, and displayed greater susceptibility to a more difficult course of illness.[107] Research also demonstrates that individuals with SAD are at increased risk of suicidal ideation[89] and have an increased rate of suicide attempts[108] compared to those in the general population. Evidence also suggests that rates of bipolar disorder may also be elevated in people with SAD. In a multi-center study of patients with bipolar I or II disorder, life-time rates of SAD were 22%, which is greater than prevalence rates reported in general community samples.[109]

People with SAD are also at substantially increased risk for the development of substance use disorders. In the NCS, 40% of people with SAD had a co-morbid substance use disorder.[90] It has been argued that alcohol in particular serves as a means to self-medicate anticipatory anxiety and to reduce avoidance of feared social situations.[110] Data from the NCS revealed a 24% life-time prevalence rate for alcohol dependence associated with social anxiety, which translates into a two to three times heightened risk that someone with SAD will develop alcohol abuse or dependence compared to people in the general population.[90] Rates of co-morbid alcohol dependence have been as high as 40% in treatment-seeking populations.

While it is unclear whether early intervention for SAD can prevent co-morbid mood, anxiety, and substance use disorders, all in all, the presence of psychiatric co-morbidity in SAD bodes poorly for affected individuals. Research suggests that people with SAD and co-occurring psychiatric conditions are likely to be more severely affected, with the consequences of the co-morbidity including greater impairment in social and occupational function,[90] increased rates of suicide ideation[89] and suicide attempts, and poorer outcome.[108] Furthermore, some co-morbid conditions, most notably MDD, also appear to adversely impact response to SAD treatment. Those findings highlight the importance of carefully screening for the presence of co-morbid psychiatric conditions, especially alcohol abuse/dependence and depressive disorders, during the initial presentation or detection of SAD.

Pathophysiology

The pathogenesis of SAD has been hypothesized to reside in the interaction between an innately anxious or inhibited disposition and early negative social environments.[111] To fully comprehend the source of dysfunction associated with SAD, one must consider the dynamic interplay between the biological, cognitive, behavioral, and interpersonal aspects of this condition.

The literature provides convincing evidence that heritable, biological processes confer increased risk for the later development of SAD. Evidence from family, twin, and high-risk studies suggests a complex genetic transmission of this disorder. Numerous studies provide evidence for an increased prevalence of SAD in first-degree relatives of probands with the disorder, as well as offspring of individuals diagnosed with SAD.[112,113] Interestingly, evidence from family studies suggests greater familial aggregation for the generalized, compared to the circumscribed, subtype of SAD.[113] Large-scale twin studies provide evidence of higher concordance rates in monozygotic twins (44.4%) compared to dizygotic twins (15.3%), again confirming that SAD is at least partly genetically transmitted.[114] The estimated heritability of SAD is around 51%, consistent with a moderate genetic effect.[115] Finally, studies examining children at high risk for the development of anxiety disorders, including SAD, have shown that those individuals demonstrate heightened physiological responsivity, consistent with the presence of a temperamental predisposition for the development of pathological anxiety.[116] The genetic or familial component of SAD may be less prevalent in individuals with the performance-only specifier of SAD.[93]

A second line of research supporting the presence of an innate vulnerability to SAD comes from Kagan's influential studies on behaviorally inhibited children. For instance, some children, even within the first year of life, display autonomic hypersensitivity to both social and non-social environmental change that operates to inhibit behavior. The presence of behavioral inhibition (BI) early in life has consistently predicted social timidity in childhood and adolescence, and is believed to be the developmental precursor to adult SAD.[117,118] It is notable, however, that not all children identified as behaviorally inhibited early in life continue to be so when they are older. For instance, approximately 25% of children who were extremely timid at 21 months of age were no longer so at age 6, while about the same proportion of children who were not inhibited at 21 months became inhibited by 6 years of age.[117] This suggests that the social environment plays a critical role in shaping the expression of innate dispositions in SAD (excluding performance-only).[93] Ongoing research, however, has begun to identify genetic markers of these anxiety-related temperaments, such as behavioral inhibition, including variation in the gene regulating G protein signaling 2 (RGS2).[119]

The literature highlights three dimensions that have characterized the early social experiences of individuals with SAD: namely, parental over-protection, parental hostility and abuse, and lack of family socializing.[111,120] Developmental studies have revealed that during laboratory-based interactions, mothers of highly anxious-withdrawn children responded to their children's socially-reticent behavior with attempts to direct and control how the child behaved,[121] and were found to display the greatest degree of aversive control compared to mothers of non-anxious and aggressive children.[122] Some patients with SAD also report histories of physical and sexual abuse,[123] and the presence of sexual abuse before the age of 18 was found to increase the risk for developing SAD two- to four-fold.[124] Individuals with SAD also report significantly more emotional abuse and neglect in their childhoods, describing their parents as less affectionate and caring, more rejecting, and more likely to use shame as a form of discipline compared to non-phobic controls.[125,126] Finally, some patients report having limited exposure to social interactions during their development,[125] and in some cases parents have been observed to encourage social avoidance in their anxiety-disordered children.[127,128] Taken together, these findings suggest that there are likely multiple developmental trajectories that contribute to SAD.[111,129]

Developmental models hypothesize a bi-directional relationship between parent and child behavior, suggesting the interplay between innate biological and social developmental factors. For instance, some research has demonstrated that an inhibited temperament can elicit less effective parenting styles.[130,131] In a longitudinal investigation,[130] it was found that parents' perceptions of their child's social wariness predicted their preference for socialization strategies that limited opportunities for the child to develop independence, which in turn, predicted future increases in social reticence. Other research found that physiological indices of behavioral inhibition were moderated by the security of the attachment bond between mother and child.[132] Specifically, children classified as behaviorally inhibited who were also insecurely attached displayed greater autonomic arousal to strangers, compared to similarly inhibited children who were securely attached.

Aside from direct experiences within the family of origin, research provides evidence that social anxiety is associated with a variety of adverse peer social experiences in school situations (including bullying and harassment, rejection, and neglect).[111] Similarly, some adults with social phobia are able to identify a traumatic social event (e.g., being humiliated) in adolescence that marked the onset or an increase in their social anxiety.[133] All in all, the literature implicates a potential role in some cases for the interaction between an innate hypersensitivity to environmental change and negative social developmental experiences throughout childhood in the pathogenesis of SAD. The key question then relates to the underlying neurobiological mechanisms implicated in the etiology and persistence of this condition. Similar to the genetic and behavioral inhibition etiological components of SAD, other childhood factors are less likely to play a causal role in performance-only SAD. For example, the performance-only specifier in DSM-5 is associated with less marital conflict in the parents of the individual with SAD, less physical and sexual abuse, less academic troubles, and a less isolating family environment.[93]

Neurobiology

Although our understanding of the etiological and pathological mechanisms of SAD is in its infancy, exciting advances in psychiatric research have begun to elucidate the neurobiological factors involved in social anxiety and fear. As previously discussed in regards to PD, the neurobiological underpinnings of anxiety have been studied via fear conditioning models. A meta-analysis of emotional processing consistently showed greater activity in the amygdala and insula linked to negative emotional response in socially-anxious patients as compared to matched control subjects.[134] Individuals with SAD also demonstrate decreased activation in prefrontal regions compared with controls. SAD patients show reduced left dlPFC activation in response to emotional and neutral faces compared to scrambled images.[135] Similarly, when undergoing a public speaking challenge task, participants with SAD demonstrated reduced activity in dlPFC and dACC as compared to control subjects.[136] In a study by Goldin and colleagues,[137] SAD patients showed reduced dmPFC and dlPFC activation during a cognitive regulation task, suggesting a reduced ability to utilize an emotion regulation strategy under socially threatening conditions.

Psychophysiology

The psychophysiological response to performance-related social situations in individuals with the performance-only specifier is greater than the psychophysiological response to social situations in individuals without the performance-only specifier. Reviews of the relevant research have shown increased heart rate response and greater anxiety sensitivity in the performance-only specifier.[138,139]

Evidence supporting the role of noradrenaline in autonomic hyperarousal in SAD is mixed. Support for the role of this neurotransmitter in the pathophysiology of SAD comes from research demonstrating that, during anticipation of public speaking, heart rate was elevated in patients with SAD compared to controls. Furthermore, norepinephrine response to the orthostatic challenge test or to the Valsalva maneuver has also been found to be greater in people with SAD compared to controls. Using pharmacological probes, some research demonstrates increased symptomatology in patients with SAD given agents that acutely increase adrenergic activity,[140] while direct infusion of epinephrine failed to cause significant elevations in anxiety.[141] Further, a blunted response of growth hormone to clonidine, an alpha$_2$-adrenergic agonist, despite normal beta-adrenergic receptor number in lymphocytes has been reported. That finding suggests reduced post-synaptic alpha$_2$-adrenergic receptor function related to norepinephrine overactivity in SAD.[142] It is also possible that the blunted growth hormone response to clonidine reflects increased activity of corticotrophin releasing factor (CRF), a critical neuropeptide in the fear response.[143,144]

Research utilizing serotonergic probes has found that patients with SAD display an enhanced sensitivity of specific serotonin receptor subtypes as reflected by increased anxiety and hormonal responses, despite the absence of abnormalities in platelet serotonin transporter density. Specifically, several studies have found elevated cortisol levels, but normal prolactin levels, in response to serotonergic probes in patients with SAD compared to non-anxious controls.[145,146] These findings imply that post-synaptic 5-HT$_2$ receptors may be supersensitized in SAD, while 5-HT$_1$ receptor activity, which regulates prolactin response, may be normal. Moreover, SSRIs have demonstrated effectiveness in the treatment of SAD in numerous controlled trials.[147] Nonetheless, the precise role of serotonin in the regulation of social behavior has yet to be established. Some have speculated that serotonin influences the salience of social reward through the modulation of dopaminergic transmission in mesolimbic reward pathways involving the ventral tegmental area.[148] Interest in the role of dopamine in the pathophysiology of SAD has been piqued by theories that implicate the dopamine system in social

reward.[148] Significantly decreased cerebrospinal fluid (CSF) levels of the dopamine metabolite homovanillic acid (HVA) have been observed in SAD patients relative to controls.[149] Results from neuroimaging studies have found significant reductions in striatal dopamine reuptake binding site density,[150] as well as significantly decreased D$_2$ receptor binding in the striatum[151] of patients with SAD compared to non-anxious controls. Moreover, marginally significant relationships have been found between diminished D$_2$ receptor binding and social anxiety symptom severity,[151] and to trait detachment in healthy participants.[152]

Advances in neuroimaging have implicated several neuroanatomical structures in the pathogenesis of SAD, most notably cortico-limbic pathways, including the amygdala, the prefrontal cortex, and the hippocampus.[153] These brain regions have been reported to play a central role in the cognitive appraisal of environmental stimuli, the integration of social information, and the expression of contextual fear-conditioned behaviors. Adaptive social behavior relies on one's ability to accurately perceive and then flexibly process and react to social cues, which are often complex and ambiguous in nature.

The amygdala is thought to be particularly relevant to understanding the pathophysiology of SAD, given its central role in assigning emotional valence to facial expressions. Patients with SAD exhibit greater amygdala activation in response to human face stimuli compared to non-anxious controls, both when presented with neutral faces[154] and when neutral faces were paired with an aversive stimuli.[155] In the later study, increased regional cerebral blood flow (rCBF) in the hippocampus was also observed. Those findings suggest that people with SAD display biases in assigning threat to human faces, even when depicting neutral expressions. Research examining amygdala response under situations of high social threat (e.g., public-speaking) has found that patients with SAD displayed a greater rCBF response in the right amygdala and peri-amygdaloid cortex, and a decreased rCBF response in cortical regions compared to healthy controls.[156] Taken as a whole, these findings suggest that people with SAD respond to socially relevant stimuli with exaggerated activity within key structures of fear responding (i.e., the amygdala), while displaying a reduction of higher-level cortical processing. Interestingly, one functional neuroimaging (fMRI) study of SAD found that responders to either nine weeks of receiving an SSRI or CBT demonstrated decreases bilaterally in rCBF in the amygdala, while no such changes were observed in the wait-list control group.[157] Another fMRI study of SAD showed exaggerated amygdala activation, positively correlated with SAD symptom severity, which decreased after successful medication treatment.[158] These studies are still in the early stages and the neurobiological literature in SAD is mixed and generally does not distinguish it clearly from other anxiety disorders.[159] Such overlapping findings have led to the notion that there may be core underlying neurobiological features that are present across some of the anxiety disorders, based on symptom clusters (e.g., AS, panic-like symptoms).

Cognitive-behavioral models

Cognitive-behavioral formulations of SAD focus primarily on the information processing and behavioral reactions believed to be responsible for the maintenance of pathological social fear, while acknowledging the importance of biologically based innate sensitivities. Cognitive theorists propose that because of past negative social experiences, socially anxious individuals develop negative beliefs about themselves and their world, which are represented in memory as social threat schemas.[160,161] Current social situations then activate those negative schemas, which lead the anxious individual to anticipate negative social outcomes (e.g., "I will say or do something embarrassing," "The other person will criticize or reject me"). In turn, the activation of the social threat schema is believed to set into motion a constellation of cognitive and behavioral sequelae, most notably heightened processing of threat-relevant cues and the adoption of behaviors intended to protect the individual from perceived social catastrophe (i.e., safety behaviors and avoidance). According to the theory, however, these processes ultimately lead to negative biases in the processing of social information, heighten anxiety, prevent disconfirmation of fear-related beliefs, and may actually create the negative social outcomes the anxious individual is trying to avoid, which serves to maintain the cycle of anxiety.

GENERALIZED ANXIETY DISORDER
Overview

Until recently, GAD had been a relatively poorly understood disorder. Since its introduction in the DSM-III in 1980, GAD has undergone a considerable diagnostic evolution. Once considered by many to be a "wastebasket" or residual category for otherwise unexplained anxiety-related symptomatology, GAD is now recognized as a valid, distinct clinical syndrome with unique phenomenological, etiological, and pathophysiological characteristics. GAD is a common and chronic psychiatric condition, associated with significant distress, functional impairment, and poor health-related outcomes. However, given the significant amount of time required for the diagnosis of GAD to establish validity, research on this condition previously lagged behind other anxiety disorders. Although debate continues regarding the specific diagnostic features that define this disorder and its differentiation from MDD, a renewed focus on GAD has enhanced our understanding of its basic etiological and pathophysiological mechanisms.

Clinical Characteristics and Diagnosis

GAD is characterized by persistent, excessive, and difficult-to-control worry and tension about a variety of events and activities in one's daily life. Common worries concern financial matters, work/school, relationships, minor matters (e.g., punctuality or small household repairs), one's own health or the health/safety of loved ones, and community or world affairs. The worry must be associated with at least three out of six of the following psychological and somatic symptoms: (1) feeling keyed up, restless, or on edge; (2) being easily fatigued; (3) impaired concentration; (4) irritability; (5) muscle tension; and (6) sleep disturbance. Muscle tension has consistently differentiated people with GAD from anxious and non-anxious controls,[162] suggesting that this may represent a particularly important diagnostic feature of GAD. According to the DSM-5, the worry and associated feelings of anxiety and tension must be present for more days than not for at least a *six-month* period to the point where the person experiences significant distress or marked impairment in social, occupational, or day-to-day function (see Box 32-4 for DSM-5 diagnostic criteria).

Broadly defined, worry refers to "a chain of thoughts and images, negatively affect-laden and relatively uncontrollable; it represents an attempt to engage in mental problem-solving on an issue whose outcome is uncertain but contains the possibility of one or more negative outcomes."[163] Given that worry is a universal human experience, current nosologies must be able to distinguish between normal, transient stress reactions and clinically significant generalized anxiety and worry: that is, how does one determine when worry becomes pathological? Although numerous studies have attempted to

---

BOX 32-4 DSM-5 Diagnostic Criteria: Generalized Anxiety Disorder (300.02 (F41.1))

A. Excessive anxiety and worry (apprehensive expectation), occurring more days than not for at least 6 months, about a number of events or activities (such as work or school performance).
B. The individual finds it difficult to control the worry.
C. The anxiety and worry are associated with three (or more) of the following six symptoms (with at least some symptoms having been present for more days than not for the past 6 months):

Note: Only one item is required in children.

1. Restlessness or feeling keyed up or on edge
2. Being easily fatigued
3. Difficulty concentrating or mind going blank
4. Irritability
5. Muscle tension
6. Sleep disturbance (difficulty falling or staying asleep, or restless, unsatisfying sleep).

D. The anxiety, worry, or physical symptoms cause clinically significant distress or impairment in social, occupational, or other important areas of functioning.
E. The disturbance is not attributable to the physiological effects of a substance (e.g., a drug of abuse, a medication) or another medical condition (e.g., hyperthyroidism).
F. The disturbance is not better explained by another mental disorder (e.g., anxiety or worry about having panic attacks in panic disorder, negative evaluation in social anxiety disorder [social phobia], contamination or other obsessions in obsessive-compulsive disorder, separation from attachment figures in separation anxiety disorder, reminders of traumatic events in posttraumatic stress disorder, gaining weight in anorexia nervosa, physical complaints in somatic symptom disorder, perceived appearance flaws in body dysmorphic disorder, having a serious illness in illness anxiety disorder, or the content of delusional beliefs in schizophrenia or delusional disorder).

Reprinted with permission from the Diagnostic and statistical manual of mental disorders, *ed 5, (Copyright 2013). American Psychiatric Association.*

---

delineate differences between the *types* of worries experienced by people with GAD compared to non-anxious controls, results have been largely inconsistent across studies.[164,165] Only worry about minor matters was found to differ between GAD and control participants, with the former group reporting more frequent worries in that domain.[166] Taken as a whole, the literature suggests that people with GAD do not seem to differ from individuals with non-pathological worry in the *content* of their worries.

Other research, however, provides evidence that people who meet diagnostic criteria for GAD differ from non-anxious controls in the severity, pervasiveness, and controllability of their worries. For instance, one study found that a dimensional measure of worry severity had better sensitivity and specificity in identifying people with GAD compared to a measure evaluating the content domains of worry.[167] Further, compared to controls, people with GAD appear to spend more time during the day worrying, describe their worry as uncontrollable, and have greater difficulty identifying the precipitant of the worry.[165]

Despite these differences, questions remain about the validity of certain diagnostic criteria in the *DSM*: for example, the boundaries of the *excessiveness* and *duration* criteria of worry,[2,168] as notable differences continue to exist between DSM-5 and ICD-10 criteria for GAD. First, the ICD-10 does not include *excessive worry* as a requisite for a diagnosis of GAD. Whereas the DSM-5 requires that worry and anxiety be present "more days than not for at least 6 months", the ICD-10 requires that anxiety be present "most days for at least several weeks at a time and usually for several months." There are no specific guidelines regarding the definition of "excessive" worry, and independent assessors most often disagree on the excessiveness criterion, with its elimination leading to a marked increase in inter-rater diagnostic reliability in some research.[169] Although questioned by some, uncontrollability of the worry has continued to be validated as a key feature of GAD[170] and has been retained in DSM-5. Furthermore, the DSM-IV and DSM-5 place greater emphasis on psychological versus somatic or autonomic symptoms compared to the ICD-10 and earlier versions of the DSM (i.e., DSM-III), including just muscle tension amongst key symptoms that might be present but requiring anxiety and difficult to control worry. It is notable, however, that in primary care many anxious patients present with somatic rather than psychological symptoms, suggesting that professionals in health care settings must be aware of the potential underlying psychological contributions to a patient's somatic complaints. Despite these remaining challenges, the increased reliability and validity of the DSM-IV and now DSM-5 diagnoses of GAD compared to earlier versions has fostered an increased awareness of GAD in psychiatric and medical settings.

Epidemiology

Despite considerable changes in the diagnostic criteria for GAD over time, life-time prevalence rates in the general population have remained relatively stable. Recently published data from the National Comorbidity Survey-Replication (NCS-R) found a life-time morbid risk for GAD of 9.0%, with a life-time prevalence of 5.7% (compared to 5.1% found in the original NCS based on DSM-III-R criteria).[85] Slightly higher rates have been reported using ICD-10 criteria (6.5%), which is likely due to the less stringent criteria used in this classification system. GAD is diagnosed more commonly in women than in men (at a ratio of about 2:1), among unmarried individuals, the elderly, racial/ethnic minorities compared to members of majority groups, and among individuals of low socioeconomic status.[171] Data from numerous community surveys and clinical samples suggests that GAD typically begins sometime between the late teens and late twenties,[172] although GAD may begin at any time during the life span. It is notable, however, that in childhood, GAD-like cases were often classified as over-anxious disorder of childhood, which may lead to an elevation in the estimated age of onset. GAD often follows a chronic, unremitting course, with episodes commonly persisting for a decade or longer[173] and 35%-50% of cases exhibiting significant and impairing symptoms of GAD within the last year in one epidemiologic study.[85]

In light of long-standing debates regarding the features that characterize pathological worry and what should be required for a diagnosis of GAD, numerous studies have addressed the consequences of using different definitions of this condition. Interestingly, Kessler and colleagues[2] (in 2005) found that cases of GAD with episodes lasting 1–5 months did not differ substantially from individuals with episodes of six months or longer (as presently defined in the DSM-IV) in terms of onset, persistence, impairment, or co-morbid diagnoses. Further, episode duration was not significantly related to parental history of GAD, as well as most sociodemographic indices (except for age). Importantly, life-time and 12-month prevalence rates increased markedly when moving from a 6-month to one-month duration requirement (6.1% to 12.7%, and 2.9% to 5.5%, respectively),[2] suggesting that many individuals not diagnosed with GAD due to a failure to meet the duration criterion would nonetheless likely meet clinically significant levels of impairment. The six-month requirement has, however, been retained in DSM-5.

Research that evaluated the outcomes of modifying the excessiveness criterion of worry found that "excessive GAD" (as defined by respondents) begins earlier in life, has a more chronic course, and is associated with greater symptom severity and psychiatric co-morbidity than non-excessive GAD.[168] However, even when the excessiveness criterion is removed, individuals who otherwise meet criteria for GAD have considerable persistence and impairment, high rates of treatment-seeking, and significantly elevated co-morbidity compared to individuals without GAD. Strikingly, the life-time prevalence of GAD increased by approximately 40% when the excessiveness criterion was removed. Taken together, recent findings call into question the stringency of the current DSM-5 criteria, and suggest at the very least, that clinicians should not dismiss cases that present with symptoms characteristic of GAD, but that do not meet the excessiveness or six-month duration criteria.[174]

Additionally, the DSM-5 criteria do not include the hierarchical exclusion criteria from DSM-IV (an additional diagnoses of GAD was not assigned in DSM-IV if the symptoms of GAD occurred exclusively within a mood disorder, psychotic disorder, or a pervasive developmental disorder). Given the additional DSM criteria to exclude worry due to another mental or physical health problem (or better explained by another mental disorder), as well as research supporting GAD without the hierarchical criteria as being similar to GAD including the hierarchical exclusion, this change will likely improve the validity of the diagnosis.[174]

Impairment and Quality of Life

GAD is a disabling condition associated with substantial impairments in a number of domains. For instance, one study found that patients with GAD who present to primary care settings reported a significantly higher number of disability days in the past month (4.4) as compared to patients without a psychiatric disorder (1.7).[175] Similarly, GAD is associated with significant reduction in work productivity and activities.[176] Patients with GAD also report greater impairment in social function compared to non-disordered patients.[177] Of note, research has demonstrated that disability and impairment in pure (non-co-morbid) GAD is equivalent to that found in pure mood disorders.[178] Moreover, GAD co-morbid with another mood disorder results in even greater functional impairments and distress relative to either condition alone.[179]

Co-morbidity

Co-morbidity in GAD is high, with "pure" cases of GAD found infrequently in both community and clinical samples. The NCS-R found that 85% of individuals with a diagnosis of GAD in the past 12-months met criteria for another co-occurring psychiatric condition.[177] In mental health settings, 80%-90% of patients with current GAD also have at least one other concurrent psychiatric disorder,[180] with similar rates reported in primary medical settings.[181] High rates of co-morbidity in GAD appear across the life span, including in children and adolescents,[182] and in the elderly.[183]

Considerable attention has been paid to the relationship between GAD and depression.[184] According to data from the original NCS, 39% of people meeting criteria for a current diagnosis of GAD also had current MDD, while 22% met criteria for dysthymia.[185] Similar co-morbidity rates of depressive disorders have been reported in clinical samples. For instance, in the Harvard/Brown Anxiety Disorders Research Program study, 54% of patients with GAD had either current MDD or dysthymia.[186] Other work has demonstrated that between 35% and 50% of patients with current MDD also meet criteria for GAD.[180]

Aside from the commonly reported co-morbidities of GAD and the depressive disorders, GAD also displays high rates of co-morbidity with the other anxiety disorders, most notably SAD and specific phobias. Furthermore, similar to other anxiety-related conditions, GAD frequently co-occurs with substance use disorders, most typically alcohol dependence.[171,187]

GAD is common in patients who present to medical settings with unexplained somatic complaints,[188] and some evidence suggests that GAD may frequently precede the onset of somatic symptoms.[189] These findings are not surprising given previous research that highlights the pervasiveness of somatic symptoms (most notably muscle tension) in people with GAD, and suggest that physicians in primary care must be vigilant to the potential psychological underpinnings of those problems. It is notable that GAD is the least common anxiety disorder reported in mental health settings, but is the most common anxiety disorder in primary care settings[190] and in patients with chronic medical conditions.[191] GAD is commonly associated with numerous physical problems (including chest pain, chronic fatigue syndrome, irritable bowel syndrome, and tension headaches), and chronic medical illnesses (such as hypertension and heart disease). Research also suggests that co-morbidity in GAD increases the burden on health care. For instance, GAD patients with co-morbid psychiatric conditions were shown to have higher medical utilization compared to patients with GAD alone, in that there were higher costs of laboratory tests, hospitalization, and medication; further, they demonstrated greater rates of absenteeism from work.[171]

In general, co-morbid GAD has a poorer prognosis in terms of impairment, course of illness, and treatment response. For example, the NCS demonstrated that people with co-morbid GAD and a mood disorder reported greater interference with life activities, and more interpersonal problems.[192] Similarly, Wittchen and colleagues[176] found that patients with GAD and MDD were slightly more impaired than patients with pure GAD or pure depression. In other work, greater social disability was reported by patients in a primary care setting meeting criteria for both GAD and another psychiatric disorder (46%) compared to patients with GAD alone (25%) and somatic disorders without a psychiatric diagnosis (20%).[190] The remission rate for GAD with a co-morbid disorder appears to be about half the annual remission rate of GAD alone.[173,193] Treatment response is also delayed in patients for whom GAD represents a co-morbid condition. One study found that in patients with MDD, treatment response to either nortriptyline or interpersonal psychotherapy was delayed when GAD was present.[194] Similarly, in GAD patients receiving psychotherapy, the presence of a co-occurring Axis I condition predicted worse outcome.[195] It is promising, however, that in GAD patients with some co-morbid disorders (e.g., SAD) receiving psychotherapy, a significant decrease in co-morbidity was observed,[196] while GAD symptoms were reduced following psychotherapy for PD.[197]

Pathophysiology

Although GAD is one of the most common anxiety disorders, relatively little is known about the biological and psychological mechanisms underlying this condition. Similar to other anxiety-related conditions, research suggests that GAD is at

least partially inherited. A review of twin studies estimates that approximately 32% of the variance in liability to GAD is explained by genetic factors. Data from family studies also suggests a partial genetic transmission of GAD. For instance, one study found that, compared to controls, first-degree relatives of people with GAD had an increased risk for GAD, but not for PD.[198] Interestingly, in a large twin study with females, researchers found that GAD and MDD were largely influenced by the same genetic factors.[199] A recent twin study found GAD genetic risk predicted increases in myo-inositol in the amygdala and, possibly, glutamate/glutamine/GABA alterations in the hippocampus. These data suggest that GAD and its genetic risk factors are likely correlated with volumetric and spectroscopic changes in the amygdala and related limbic structures.[200] Other research has demonstrated overlaps with anxiety, depression, and the personality trait neuroticism, which has been posited to provide one explanation for the high rates of co-morbidity amongst mood and anxiety disorders.[201] Taken as a whole, the literature suggests the existence of a general predisposition toward anxiety rather than specific heritability for GAD, with environmental factors (likely in conjunction with pre-existing biological vulnerabilities) conferring increased risk for specific anxiety disorders, including GAD.

Although the environment has been hypothesized to be important in the pathogenesis of GAD, relatively few studies have directly examined the contribution of environmental factors to the later development of GAD. Rather, most studies have evaluated environmental contributions to anxiety disorders more generally. As with some other anxiety disorders (e.g., SAD), developmental models of GAD highlight the importance of parenting behavior in the etiology of this condition.[202] Specific parenting behaviors may include modeling of anxious or avoidant behavior,[203] encouragement of avoidance,[127] or over-involvement or protection.[204] Existing research does not resolve the issue of whether those outcomes are the result of child effects (i.e., the child's behavior "pulls for" or elicits a certain reaction from parents) or parent effects (e.g., parental anxiety), although contemporary models argue that it is likely due to a dynamic interaction of the two.[202]

A number of studies suggest that stressful life events play a role in the etiology of GAD. For instance, individuals with GAD were more likely than non-anxious controls to report exposure to a potentially traumatic event.[166] GAD has also been associated with an increase in the number of minor stressors, independent of demographic factors. It is notable that early stressful life events can lead to enduring changes in the function of the HPA axis, which may place an individual at a greater risk of developing anxiety-related problems by increasing one's sensitivity to stress.[205] Other researchers propose that perceptions of control mediate the relationship between adverse life events and the development of anxiety.[206] One explanatory model is that early experiences with overly intrusive and controlling parents combined with an innate disposition towards anxiety may lead to diminished perceptions of control over one's environment and future, thereby predisposing a person to frequent worry. It is likely that there are numerous psychological or environmental factors that contribute in part to the development of GAD, likely in individuals with a biological predisposition for anxiety, as has been shown for depression where the severity of environmental stressors interacts with the level of pre-existing neuroticism to predict the development of disorder[207]; this may in part contribute to the heterogeneity of the disorder itself.

Neurobiology

As previously discussed, neuroimaging studies have helped to paint an increasingly clear picture of the neural substrates of the anxiety disorders. Numerous studies indicate the involvement of limbic and paralimbic structures (amygdala, hippocampus, insula) as well as the prefrontal cortex, findings which complement existing knowledge of the neural underpinnings of both fear conditioning[208] and emotion regulation.[209] However, research into the neurobiological mechanisms involved in GAD has been less well studied until recently. Existing evidence supports the general notion that GAD is associated with abnormalities in neurochemical and neurophysiological systems implicated in the pathogenesis of anxiety. Dysregulated neurochemical systems may include: GABA, norepinephrine, serotonin, and CRF. Recent neuroimaging studies have implicated various neural structures involved in anxiety, the amygdala, the insula, the orbitofrontal cortex (OFC), and possibly, the anterior cingulate cortex (ACC) and hippocampus.[210] Several studies have specifically examined GAD, with the majority of findings related to amygdala structure or function,[200] In contrast to the other anxiety disorders discussed in this chapter, there is less data demonstrating an increased amygdala response to emotional stimuli in GAD. In fact, several studies have found evidence of reduced amygdala response in response to threatening faces.[211,212] Comparison of GAD and SAD patients during a facial emotion processing task has led Blair and colleagues to suggest that GAD may be better characterized by alterations in prefrontal regions rather than the amygdala.[211] Several studies support the possibility of hyperactivity in frontal areas in GAD.[211,213,214] These results are in contrast with the previously reported hypoactivity in PFC regions in PD, PTSD, and SAD, which has been conceptualized as contributing to failure to appropriately regulate emotional responding. The opposite pattern may exist in GAD, reflecting an over-engaged cognitive control system.[134]

Conversely, some studies have reported that GAD is characterized by hypoactivity in frontal areas similar to the other anxiety disorders. Ball and colleagues found reduced activation of dmPFC and dlPFC in GAD patients compared to controls during an emotion regulation task.[59] Similarly, Monk and colleagues studied adolescents with GAD, finding increased amygdala responding to masked faces, and noting that the negative coupling of amygdala response and vmPFC activation was weaker in GAD patients than controls.[215]

A few fMRI studies of GAD have supported increased amygdala activation and three studies to date have examined pretreatment neurobiological predictors of treatment response in GAD. Two imaging studies found that greater mPFC (specifically rACC) activation was correlated with better treatment response to venlafaxine,[216,217] while the third study found the greater the amygdala activation pre-CBT treatment, the better the response to treatment in children and adolescents with GAD.[212] While the direction is mixed, and caution should be taken interpreting these results given the age differences across the studies, these studies generally support the amygdala and mPFC as targets for future research in GAD.[159] All in all, an accumulating body of evidence implicates dysregulation in an array of neurobiological systems and disruption of the adaptive response to stress in patients with GAD, with partial overlap with depression and some other anxiety disorders. More work is needed to understand the overlaps and differences in the neurobiology of GAD compared to other disorders such as panic. As increased research utilizes imaging techniques, it is likely a greater understanding of underlying neurobiological and genetic factors and their specificity to GAD will be identified; to date, however, the research is mixed.

Psychopathological processes

Numerous psychopathological models have been developed to account for the development and persistence of GAD. Some theories posit that worry is a mental activity, primarily verbal-linguistic in nature, designed to avoid the occurrence of future catastrophe, distressing thoughts, and emotions.[218] In this way, worry is seen as a form of cognitive and emotional avoidance. Consistent with this notion, people with GAD are more likely to endorse the belief that worry is an effective strategy in distracting oneself from deeply emotional topics.[219] Moreover, research has demonstrated that worry results in the immediate suppression of sympathetic activation to anxiety-provoking material.[220] However, as with other forms of avoidance, worry impedes the processing of emotional material, thereby preventing extinction.

Information-processing biases have also been hypothesized to play a key role in the development and maintenance of GAD. Consistent with these models, research has demonstrated that people with GAD selectively attend to threatening stimuli, and are more likely to interpret ambiguous information in a negative manner.[221,222] Preferential processing of threat-relevant material may well play a role in the etiology of GAD, in that patterns of selective negative processing have been found to precede and predict the development of negative emotional responses to stressful life events.[223] More recently, emerging cognitive-behavioral formulations of GAD propose that intolerance of uncertainty is a central cognitive process involved in worry and GAD but may also be a general factor associated with other anxiety disorders as well.[224,225] Individuals who have difficulties tolerating uncertainty react negatively on an emotional, cognitive, and behavioral level to uncertain situations and events, and may believe that the possibility of a future negative outcome, no matter how small, is unacceptable and should be avoided. Associated features of intolerance of uncertainty include: positive beliefs about the utility of worry (e.g., worrying helps find solutions to problems; worrying protects a person from negative emotions), poor problem orientation (e.g., focusing on uncertain aspects of a problem and appraising them as threats), and cognitive avoidance, all of which have been linked to GAD.[226] Finally, in one other cognitive model, metacognitive appraisals and beliefs are hypothesized to contribute to the development and maintenance of pathological worry seen in GAD.[227] The activation of worry as a means of coping in response to potential future threat is motivated by positive beliefs about worry (described earlier). In turn, a prolonged sequence of worrying activates negative meta-cognitive beliefs about worry, including beliefs about the uncontrollability of worry and about the mental, physical, and/or social consequences of worry (e.g., "Worrying will make me go crazy"). These negative beliefs motivate the use of thought control strategies and safety-seeking behaviors (e.g., reassurance-seeking, distraction, checking), which ultimately disrupts emotional processing and maintains the excessive worry. Although differing in emphasis, contemporary psychopathological models implicate a variety of cognitive and behavioral processes in GAD designed to ward off potential negative future outcomes, as well as distressing thoughts, images, and emotions associated with worry.

CONCLUSION

It is now recognized that anxiety disorders represent serious psychiatric conditions associated with significant distress and morbid sequelae in numerous life domains. While anxiety disorders continue to be the most common mental health problem in the US, significant advances over the past several decades have led to enhanced awareness and understanding of the factors relevant to their etiology and persistence. The pathophysiology of anxiety disorders is complex, and is likely to reside in the dynamic interplay between innate biological vulnerabilities and precipitating life events. Emerging genetic findings promise great hope into elucidating the underlying biological mechanisms associated with pathological anxiety, while developmental and psychopathology research will continue to aid in our understanding of the factors that buffer and protect or, conversely, confer increased risk for the development of an anxiety disorder. Now that efficacious pharmacological and psychological interventions are available, recent efforts have turned to disseminating cost-effective evidence-based pharmacological and psychotherapeutic regimens to the public, improving existing interventions for complicated, treatment-refractory or co-morbid anxiety presentations, and searching for novel approaches with even greater efficacy, tolerability and patient acceptance. Continued advancements in our understanding of the neurobiological and psychological predictors of treatment response and non-response, as well as understanding of their overlap or specificity across the anxiety disorders, will undoubtedly be paramount in fueling future treatment development efforts.

Access the complete reference list and multiple choice questions (MCQs) online at https://expertconsult.inkling.com

KEY REFERENCES

2. Kessler RC, Berglund P, Demler O, et al. Lifetime prevalence and age-of-onset distributions of DSM-IV disorders in the National Comorbidity Survey Replication. *Arch Gen Psychiatry* 62(6):593–602, 2005.

15. Bruce SE, Yonkers KA, Otto MW, et al. Influence of psychiatric comorbidity on recovery and recurrence in generalized anxiety disorder, social phobia, and panic disorder: a 12-year prospective study. *Am J Psychiatry* 162(6):1179–1187, 2005.

17. Goodwin RD, Roy-Byrne P. Panic and suicidal ideation and suicide attempts: results from the National Comorbidity Survey. *Depress Anxiety* 23(3):124–132, 2006.

29. Hettema JM, Neale MC, Kendler KS. A review and meta-analysis of the genetic epidemiology of anxiety disorders. *Am J Psychiatry* 158(10):1568–1578, 2001.

53. Shin LM, Liberzon I. The neurocircuitry of fear, stress, and anxiety disorders. *Neuropsychopharmacology* 35(1):169–191, 2010.

54. Quirk GJ, Garcia R, Gonzalez-Lima F. Prefrontal mechanisms in extinction of conditioned fear. *Biol Psychiatry* 60(4):337–343, 2006.

55. Milad MR, Quirk GJ. Neurons in medial prefrontal cortex signal memory for fear extinction. *Nature* 420(6911):70–74, 2002.

59. Ball TM, Ramsawh HJ, Campbell-Sills L, et al. Prefrontal dysfunction during emotion regulation in generalized anxiety and panic disorders. *Psychol Med* 43(7):1475–1486, 2013.

69. Reiss S. Pavlovian conditioning and human fear: An expectancy model. *Behav Ther* 11(3):380–396, 1980.

71. Olatunji BO, Wolitzky-Taylor KB. Anxiety sensitivity and the anxiety disorders: a meta-analytic review and synthesis. *Psychol Bull* 135(6):974–999, 2009.

85. Kessler RC, Petukhova M, Sampson NA, et al. Twelve-month and lifetime prevalence and lifetime morbid risk of anxiety and mood disorders in the United States. *Int J Methods Psychiatr Res* 21(3):169–184, 2012.

92. Scholten WD, Batelaan NM, van Balkom AJ, et al. Recurrence of anxiety disorders and its predictors. *J Affect Disord* 147(1–3):180–185, 2013.

118. Rosenbaum JF, Biederman J, Bolduc-Murphy EA, et al. Behavioral inhibition in childhood: a risk factor for anxiety disorders. *Harv Rev Psychiatry* 1(1):2–16, 1993.

119. Smoller JW, Paulus MP, Fagerness JA, et al. Influence of RGS2 on anxiety-related temperament, personality, and brain function. *Arch Gen Psychiatry* 65(3):298–308, 2008.

120. Rapee RM, Spence SH. The etiology of social phobia: empirical evidence and an initial model. *Clin Psychol Rev* 24(7):737–767, 2004.

129. Ollendick TH, Hirshfeld-Becker DR. The developmental psychopathology of social anxiety disorder. *Biol Psychiatry* 51(1):44–58, 2002.

139. Hofmann SG, Heinrichs N, Moscovitch DA. The nature and expression of social phobia: toward a new classification. *Clin Psychol Rev* 24(7):769–797, 2004.

153. Kent JM, Rauch SL. Neurocircuitry of anxiety disorders. *Curr Psychiatry Rep* 5(4):266–273, 2003.

174. Andrews G, Hobbs MJ, Borkovec TD, et al. Generalized worry disorder: a review of DSM-IV generalized anxiety disorder and options for DSM-V. *Depress Anxiety* 27(2):134–147, 2010.

179. Romera I, Montejo AL, Caballero F, et al. Functional impairment related to painful physical symptoms in patients with generalized anxiety disorder with or without comorbid major depressive disorder: post hoc analysis of a cross-sectional study. *BMC Psychiatry* 11:69, 2011.

184. Unick GJ, Snowden L, Hastings J. Heterogeneity in comorbidity between major depressive disorder and generalized anxiety disorder and its clinical consequences. *J Nerv Ment Dis* 197(4):215–224, 2009.

200. Hettema JM, Kettenmann B, Ahluwalia V, et al. Pilot multimodal twin imaging study of generalized anxiety disorder. *Depress Anxiety* 29(3):202–209, 2012.

208. Graham BM, Milad MR. The study of fear extinction: implications for anxiety disorders. *Am J Psychiatry* 168(12):1255–1265, 2011.

209. Ochsner KN, Gross JJ. Cognitive Emotion regulation: insights from social cognitive and affective neuroscience. *Curr Dir Psychol Sci* 17(2):153–158, 2008.

211. Blair KS, Geraci M, Smith BW, et al. Reduced dorsal anterior cingulate cortical activity during emotional regulation and top-down attentional control in generalized social phobia, generalized anxiety disorder, and comorbid generalized social phobia/generalized anxiety disorder. *Biol Psychiatry* 72(6):476–482, 2012.

Obsessive-compulsive Disorder and Obsessive-compulsive and Related Disorders

S. Evelyn Stewart, MD, Daniel Lafleur, MD, Darin D. Dougherty, MD, MSc, Sabine Wilhelm, PhD, Nancy J. Keuthen, PhD, and Michael A. Jenike, MD

KEY POINTS

- Obsessive-compulsive disorder (OCD) and obsessive-compulsive-related disorders (OCRDs) now comprise an independent disease category within the DSM-5, as OCD is no longer classified as an anxiety disorder. OCRDs include hoarding disorder (HD), and three body-focused disorders: body dysmorphic disorder (BDD), trichotillomania (hair-pulling disorder) (TTM) and skin-picking (excoriation) disorder (SPD).

Incidence

- OCD and OCRDs are common yet under-recognized, with individual prevalence rates in the range of approximately 1%–2%, except for HD with a reported prevalence of 2%–6%. These rates appear consistent across countries and socioeconomic strata. Moreover, these disorders are highly co-morbid with each other.

Epidemiology

- OCD has peaks of onset in pre-adolescence and early adulthood, whereas the OCRDs typically present in adolescence around puberty. There is no clear gender predominance for either OCD or BDD, although OCD begins earlier in boys than girls. Females are at higher risk for HD, TTM, and SPD, especially in clinical settings.

Pathophysiology

- Research indicates that genetic and environmental factors are fairly equally involved in the etiology of OCD. The orbitofrontal cortex, anterior cingulate cortex, basal ganglia, and thalamic brain structures have been implicated, with dysfunction in corticostriatal pathways including a ventromedial "emotion" circuit and a dorsolateral "cognitive" circuit. Autoimmune processes may play a role in some acute, early-onset, cases. OCRDs have some overlapping and some distinct features with respect to pathophysiology, although studies are preliminary.

Clinical Findings

- Mental status and clinical observation may reveal signs of OCD and OCRDs that differ across individuals and may include red, chapped hands from washing in OCD, cognitive difficulties in HD, dressing in overly concealing clothing in BDD, localized or diffuse areas of baldness in TTM, and extensive scarring and excoriations in SPD.

Differential Diagnoses

- OCD and the OCRDs are characterized by repetitive thoughts and behaviors, and have several overlapping features. Other disorders to consider in the differential diagnosis include eating disorders, autism spectrum disorder, generalized anxiety disorder, impulse control disorders and psychotic disorders.

Treatment Options

- The two main treatment approaches for OCD include cognitive-behavioral therapy (CBT) and serotonin reuptake inhibitors (SRIs), used alone or in combination. OCD exhibits a linear dose-response curve such that higher doses tend to have greater efficacy. CBT is recommended for all OCRDs, although SRIs may be less effective for the management of HD, BDD, TTM, and SPD. There is early evidence for SRI augmentation with atypical antipsychotics and glutamatergic agents for some of these disorders.

Complications

- Delay to diagnosis and treatment is very common, and associated with worse outcomes.
- Access to trained CBT providers for these disorders is frequently challenging. Common prescribing errors include SRI trial attempts with an insufficient duration (<12 weeks) or dosage.

Prognosis

- OCD and OCRDs tend to have chronic courses that wax and wane, although approximately half of OCD cases become subthreshold or remit. Suicide risk is elevated in BDD and HD severity tends to worsen with age.

OVERVIEW

Obsessive-compulsive disorder (OCD) is a common disorder that affects individuals throughout the life span. This disorder has been listed as one of the 10 most disabling illnesses by the World Health Organization.[1] Obsessive-compulsive-related disorders (OCRDs) include hoarding disorder (HD) and body-focused disorders, including body dysmorphic disorder (BDD), trichotillomania (hair-pulling disorder [TTM]) and excoriation (skin-picking) disorder (SPD).

Approximately 1% to 3% of the world's population will be affected by OCD at some point in their lives,[2] and a greater number will suffer from OCRDs. Due to both under-recognition by clinicians and the shame-induced tendency for individuals to hide OCD and OCRD symptoms, the delay in diagnosis and treatment is frequently staggeringly long. The reported mean delay from symptom onset to diagnosis and appropriate treatment is 17 years.[3] Although these disorders tend to have a waxing and waning course, they frequently increase in severity when left untreated, adding to the burden of illness for affected individuals and their family members. The present chapter gives a general description of OCD and OCRDs, followed by characterization of related epidemiology, risk factors, pathophysiology, and clinical features. Practical

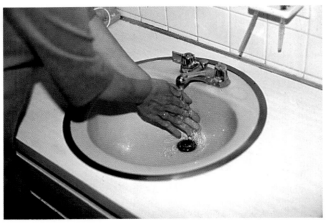

Figure 33-1. Obsessive-compulsive disorder patient demonstrating a typical compulsive behavior of handwashing. Some patients may wash their hands hundreds of times daily, leading to inflamed, erythematous, and cracking skin.

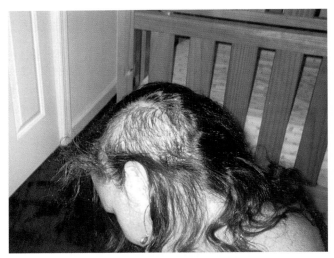

Figure 33-2. Left-side view of a trichotillomania patient's scalp demonstrating areas of alopecia (balding) and hair thinning.

strategies for clinical evaluation and treatment of these illnesses are then discussed.

CLINICAL FEATURES AND DIAGNOSIS

OCD is characterized by recurrent unwanted thoughts, urges, images, and repetitive behaviors or mental acts that are distressing, time-consuming, and affect functioning. The condition is often kept secret because of the shame associated with its particular symptoms. Symptoms experienced by OCD-affected individuals are diverse, with three main groups or "dimensions" that tend to co-occur, including contamination obsessions with cleaning compulsions (Figure 33-1); symmetry obsessions, with ordering and repeating compulsions; and intrusive thoughts related to religious, sexual, aggressive, and somatic themes with checking compulsions.[4] Other common OCD compulsions include reassurance-seeking, counting, praying, mental rituals, and "just right" rituals. OCD-affected individuals frequently experience multiple symptoms at any given time, many of which are driven by the perceived need to achieve certainty, and symptom types tend to change over the course of the illness.

OCRDs are predominantly characterized by the presence of repetitive behaviors, some of which are related to body appearance concerns (BDD), and some of which are associated with repeated attempts to decrease or stop the body-focused behavior (TTM and SPD). What constitutes an OCRD has been a controversial subject.[5] The OCRDs as discussed in this chapter comprise those outlined in the *Diagnostic and Statistical Manual of Mental Disorders*, Fifth Edition (DSM-5)[6] and include hoarding disorder (HD) and the body-focused disorders—body dysmorphic disorder (BDD), trichotillomania (hair-pulling disorder [TTM]) (Figure 33-2) and excoriation (skin-picking) disorder (SPD). Additional OCRDs listed in the DSM-5 (those secondary to a medication, a substance, or a medical condition) will not be discussed here.

HD is a disorder in which individuals have a persistent resistance to, and distress associated with, discarding possessions, regardless of their value. These individuals also experience a strong urge to save items, often resulting in extensive accumulation of items, and clutter in their living areas. Figure 33-3 illustrates the living quarters of a patient with HD.

BDD is a disorder in which individuals suffer from a preoccupation with a slight or imagined defect in appearance that causes significant distress or impairment that is not strictly a manifestation of another disorder.

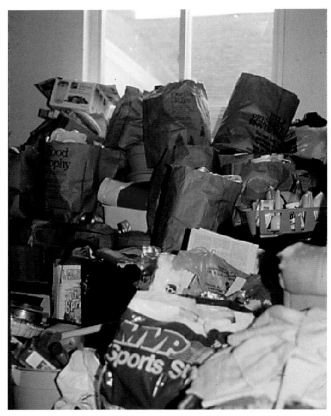

Figure 33-3. Cluttered and overcrowded home of a hoarding disorder patient.

TTM and SPD present with an inability to resist the urge to recurrently pull hair or to pick the skin, respectively, despite recurrent attempts to stop. The differential diagnosis for SPD includes delusional parasitosis. All of these OCRDs are significantly distressing, impairing, and adversely affect quality of life.[7,8] Although many individuals with TTM and SPD report urges to pull or pick prior to, and a sense of relief during, the behavior, these symptoms are not universal.[9]

The publication of the DSM-5 reflects a large shift in the conceptualization of OCD and related disorders, with the emergence of a dedicated chapter and category for these illnesses. Newly defined DSM-5 diagnoses include HD, SPD, substance-/medication-induced OC and related disorder, OC and related disorder due to another medical condition and unspecified OCRDs (such as olfactory reference syndrome and body-focused repetitive behavior disorder). Classification of OCD has been removed from the anxiety disorders; BDD has been moved from the somatoform disorders; and TTM has been moved from the impulse-control disorders. In addition, for OCD, HD and BDD, specifiers related to insight have been expanded to include three options of good or fair insight, poor

insight, and absent insight/delusional beliefs. Moreover, new specifiers include a tic-related specifier for OCD, a "with excessive acquisition" specifier for HD and a muscle dysmorphia specifier for BDD.

A summary of diagnostic criteria changes between DSM-IV and DSM-5 for OCD, BDD, and TTM is provided in Tables 33-1 to 33-3, respectively. DSM-5 diagnostic criteria for OCD appears in Box 33-1, BDD appears in Box 33-2, and TTM appears in Box 33-3. Diagnostic criteria for the new DSM-5 disorders HD and SPD are provided in Box 33-4 and 33-5.

TABLE 33-1 Obsessive-Compulsive Disorder Criteria for DSM-IV and DSM-5

DSM-IV	DSM-5 (300.3(F42))	Summary of Changes
Disease Category		
ANXIETY DISORDERS	OBSESSIVE-COMPULSIVE AND RELATED DISORDERS	NEW CHAPTER CREATED
DIAGNOSTIC CRITERIA FOR OBSESSIVE-COMPULSIVE DISORDER [300.3]		
Either Obsessions or Compulsions		
Obsessions are defined by the following: Recurrent and persistent thoughts, ***impulses***, or images that are experienced, at some time during the disturbance, as intrusive and ***inappropriate*** and that **cause marked anxiety or distress**	Recurrent and persistent thoughts, ***urges***, or images that are experienced, at some time during the disturbance, as intrusive and ***unwanted***, and that ***in most individuals*** cause marked anxiety or distress	• "Impulses" replaced by "urges" • "Inappropriate" changed to "unwanted" • Always cause marked anxiety or distress changed to "in most individuals"
The effort by the affected person to ignore or suppress such thoughts, **impulses**, or images, or to **neutralize** them with some other thought or action	The individual attempts to ignore or suppress such thoughts, **urges**, or images, or to neutralize them with some other thought or action (i.e., **by performing a compulsion**)	• "Impulses" replaced by "urges" • Neutralizing may include performing a compulsion
Thoughts, impulses, or images that are ***not simply excessive worries about real-life problems***		• Criteria removed that would exclude individuals with generalized anxiety disorder moved to exclusion criteria section
Recognition by the affected person that the obsessional thoughts, impulses, or images are ***a product of his or her own mind rather than imposed from without***		• Criteria removed that would exclude individuals with no insight
Compulsions are defined by the following: Repetitive ***activities*** (e.g., handwashing, ordering, checking) or mental acts (e.g., praying, counting, repeating words silently) that the person feels driven to perform in response to an obsession or according to rigid rules that must be applied rigidly	Repetitive ***behaviors*** (e.g., handwashing, ordering, checking) or mental acts (e.g., praying, counting, repeating words silently) that the individual feels driven to perform in response to an obsession or according to rules that must be applied rigidly	• Activities changed to behaviors
Behavior or mental acts aimed at preventing or reducing distress or preventing some dreaded event or situation but either clearly excessive or not connected in a realistic way with what they are designed to neutralize or prevent	The behaviors or mental acts are aimed at preventing or reducing **anxiety** or distress, or preventing some dreaded event or situation; however, these behaviors or mental acts are not connected in a realistic way with what they are designed to neutralize or prevent, or are clearly excessive. **NOTE: Young children may not be able to articulate the aims of these behaviors or mental acts**	• Notation that children can not always explain why they have compulsions
Recognition, by the affected person (unless he or she is a child), at some point during the course of the disorder, that the obsessions or compulsions are **excessive** or unreasonable		• No longer need to recognize as excessive; symptoms
SPECIFIERS Specified as obsessive-compulsive disorder (OCD) with ***poor insight*** if, for most of the time during the current episode, the person does not recognize that the obsessions and compulsions are excessive or unreasonable	**With good or fair insight:** The individual recognizes that obsessive-compulsive disorder beliefs are definitely or probably not true or that they may or may not be true **With poor insight:** The individual thinks obsessive-compulsive disorder beliefs are probably true **With absent insight/delusional beliefs:** The individual is completely convinced that obsessive-compulsive disorder beliefs are true	• Specifiers refined to distinguish between good to fair insight, poor insight and "absent insight/delusional" OCD beliefs • Absent insight now an "option" while retaining OCD diagnosis

Continued on following page

TABLE 33-1 Obsessive-Compulsive Disorder Criteria for DSM-IV and DSM-5 (Continued)

DSM-IV	DSM-5 (300.3(F42))	Summary of Changes
Disease Category		
ANXIETY DISORDERS	OBSESSIVE-COMPULSIVE AND RELATED DISORDERS	NEW CHAPTER CREATED
	Tic-related: The individual has a current or past history of a tic disorder.	• New tic specifier added
FUNCTIONAL IMPACT/EXCLUSION CRITERIA		
Obsessions or compulsions that cause marked distress, are time-consuming (take more than 1 hour per day), or interfere substantially with the person's normal routine, occupational or academic functioning, or usual social activities or relationships	The obsessions or compulsions are time-consuming (e.g., take more than 1 hour per day) or cause clinically significant distress or impairment in social, occupational, or other important areas of functioning	
Content of the obsessions or compulsions not restricted to any other Axis I disorder, such as an obsession with food in the context of an eating disorder that is present	The disturbance is not better explained by the symptoms of another mental disorder (e.g., excessive worries, as in generalized anxiety disorder, preoccupation with appearance, as in body dysmorphic disorder; difficulty discarding or parting with possessions, as in hoarding disorder; hair pulling, as in trichotillomania [hair-pulling disorder]; skin picking, as in excoriation [skin-picking] disorder; stereotypies, as in stereotypic movement disorder; ritualized eating behaviour, as in eating disorders; preoccupation with substances or gambling, as in substance-related and addictive disorders; preoccupation with having an illness, as in illness anxiety disorder; sexual urges or fantasies, as in paraphilic disorders; impulses, as in disruptive, impulse-control, and conduct disorders; guilty ruminations, as in major depressive disorder; thought insertion or delusional preoccupations, as in schizophrenia spectrum and other psychotic disorders; or repetitive patterns of behaviour, as in autism spectrum disorder)	• More examples provided
Disturbance not due to the direct physiological effects of a substance or a general medical condition	The obsessive-compulsive symptoms are not attributable to the physiological effects of a substance *(e.g., a drug of abuse, a medication)* or another medical condition	• Examples of substances added (e.g., a drug of abuse, a medication)

EPIDEMIOLOGY AND RISK FACTORS
Prevalence

Symptoms of OCD are common. Approximately 50% of the general population engage in some ritualized behaviors,[10] and up to 80% experience intrusive, unpleasant, or unwanted thoughts.[11] However, these behaviors do not cause excessive distress, occupy a significant amount of time, or impair function for most individuals, and as such they do not represent OCD. Regarding a clinical diagnosis of OCD in adults, the 1-month prevalence rate is 0.6%,[12] and the reported 12-month prevalence ranges from 0.6% to 1.0% for DSM-IV–defined OCD[13,14] and from 0.8% to 2.3% for DSM-III-R–defined OCD.[15]

Measured life-time prevalence rates for OCD appear to have depended on the version of the DSM used to determine diagnoses. The estimated life-time prevalence is 1.6% using the DSM-IV.[16] Using the DSM-III, the life-time rate was 2.5% in the US Epidemiologic Catchment Area Survey,[15] and the prevalence ranged between 0.7% (in Taiwan) and 2.5% (in Puerto Rico and in seven other countries surveyed).[17] These differences may be due to the fact that the DSM-IV better defined obsessions and compulsions and required significant clinical distress or impairment to confirm a diagnosis.[13]

The prevalence rates of the OCRDs vary. Many of these disorders co-occur with each other and with OCD. HD prevalence

rates have been reported between 2% and 6%, based upon studies in US and Europe.[5] Prevalence of BDD is difficult to accurately estimate given the secrecy of the disorder, although estimates are approximately 2.3% in the general population, and range from 6% to 15% in cosmetic surgery settings.[18] The exact life-time prevalence of TTM is unknown, but rates of DSM-IV-defined TTM range from 1% to 2%.[19] The prevalence is even higher for subclinical hair-pulling, as preceding tension and subsequent gratification are often absent.[19-22] Notably, DSM-5 has removed these criteria. SPD has an estimated prevalence of 1.4%.[6] In patients with OCD, the prevalence of co-morbid broadly-defined OCRDs exceeds that for the general population, with reported rates of over 55%.[23]

Age of Onset

There appears to be a bi-modal age of onset for OCD. Approximately one-third to one-half of adults with OCD develop the disorder in childhood.[17,24] The National Comorbidity Survey Replication reported a median onset at the age of 19 years, with 21% of cases emerging by age 10.[14] Pediatric OCD has a median onset in pre-adolescence.[25] For those who first develop OCD in adulthood, the mean onset age of OCD occurs between 22 and 35 years of age.[26] A few studies report another incidence peak in middle to late adulthood,[27] but it is commonly believed that OCD onset after 50 years old is relatively unusual.[28]

TABLE 33-2 Body Dysmorphic Disorder Criteria for DSM-IV and DSM-5

DSM-IV	DSM-5 (300.7(F45.22))	Summary of Changes
Disease Category		
SOMATOFORM DISORDERS	OBSESSIVE-COMPULSIVE AND RELATED DISORDERS	
BODY DYSMORPHIC DISORDER [300.7] DIAGNOSTIC CRITERIA		
Preoccupation with an imagined defect in appearance. If a slight physical anomaly is present, the person's concern is markedly excessive	Preoccupation with **one or more perceived** defects **or flaws** in physical appearance that are not observable or appear slight to others	• Potential for more than one physical focus of attention clarified
	At some point during the course of the disorder, the individual has performed repetitive behaviors (e.g., comparing his or her appearance with that of others) in response to the appearance concerns	• Addition of repetitive behavior criterion, reflecting inclusion as an obsessive-compulsive-related disorder
FUNCTIONAL IMPACT/EXCLUSION CRITERIA		
The preoccupation causes clinically significant distress or impairment in social, occupational, or other important areas of functioning	The preoccupation causes clinically significant distress or impairment in social, occupational, or other important areas of functioning	• None
The preoccupation is not better accounted for by another mental disorder (e.g., dissatisfaction with body shape and size in anorexia nervosa)	The appearance preoccupation is not better explained by concerns with body fat or weight in an individual whose symptoms meet diagnostic criteria for an eating disorder	• Clarification of eating disorder exclusion
SPECIFIERS		
	With muscle dysmorphia: The individual is preoccupied with the idea that his or her body build is too small or insufficiently muscular. This specifier is used even if the individual is preoccupied with other body areas, which is often the case	• New specifier that predominantly occurs in males
	With good or fair insight: The individual recognizes that the body dysmorphic disorder beliefs are definitely or probably not true or that they may or may not be true **With poor insight:** The individual thinks that the body dysmorphic disorder beliefs are probably true **With absent insight/delusional beliefs:** The individual is completely convinced that the body dysmorphic disorder beliefs are true	• Specifiers refined to distinguish between good to fair insight, poor insight and "absent insight/delusional" body dysmorphic disorder beliefs • Absent insight now an "option" without requiring a concurrent coding of a delusional disorder somatic type diagnosis

TABLE 33-3 Trichotillomania (Hair-Pulling Disorder) Criteria for DSM-IV and DSM-5

DSM-IV	DSM-5 (312.39(F63.2))	Summary of Changes
Disease Category		
IMPULSE-CONTROL DISORDERS NOT ELSEWHERE CLASSIFIED	OBSESSIVE-COMPULSIVE AND RELATED DISORDER	"HAIR-PULLING DISORDER" HAS BEEN ADDED PARENTHETICALLY
TRICHOTILLOMANIA (HAIR-PULLING DISORDER) [312.39] DIAGNOSTIC CRITERIA		
Recurrent pulling out of one's hair resulting in **noticeable** hair loss	Recurrent pulling out of one's hair, resulting in hair loss Repeated attempts to decrease or stop hair pulling	• "Noticeable" removed as descriptor of hair loss • New criterion • Criterion removed
An increasing sense of tension immediately before pulling out the hair or when attempting to resist the behavior		
Pleasure, gratification, or relief when pulling out the hair		• Criterion removed
FUNCTIONAL IMPACT/EXCLUSION CRITERIA		
The disturbance is not better accounted for by another mental disorder and is not due to a general medical condition (e.g., a dermatological condition)	The hair pulling or hair loss is not attributable to another medical condition (e.g., a dermatological condition). The hair pulling is not better explained by the symptoms of another mental disorder (e.g., attempts to improve a perceived defect or flaw in appearance in body dysmorphic disorder)	• Example of mental disorder provided
The disturbance causes clinically significant distress or impairment in social, occupational, or other important areas of functioning	The hair pulling causes clinically significant distress or impairment in social, occupational, or other important areas of functioning	• None

BOX 33-1 DSM-5 Diagnostic Criteria: Obsessive-compulsive Disorder (300.3 (F42))

A. Presence of obsessions, compulsions, or both:
Obsessions are defined by (1) and (2):
1. Recurrent and persistent thoughts, urges, or images that are experienced, at some time during the disturbance, as intrusive and unwanted, and that in most individuals cause marked anxiety or distress.
2. The individual attempts to ignore or suppress such thoughts, urges, or images, or to neutralize them with some other thought or actions (i.e., by performing a compulsion).

Compulsions are defined by (1) and (2):
1. Repetitive behaviors (e.g., hand washing, ordering, checking) or mental acts (e.g., praying, counting, repeating words silently) that the individual feels driven to perform in response to an obsession or according to rules that must be applied rigidly.
2. The behaviors or mental acts are aimed at preventing or reducing anxiety or distress, or at preventing some dreaded event or situation; however, these behaviors or mental acts are not connected in a realistic way with what they are designed to neutralize or prevent, or are clearly excessive.

Note: Young children may not be able to articulate the aims of these behaviors or mental acts.

B. The obsessions or compulsions are time-consuming (e.g., take more than 1 hour per day) or cause clinically significant distress or impairment in social, occupational, or other important areas of functioning.
C. The obsessive-compulsive symptoms are not attributable to the physiological effects of a substance (e.g., a drug of abuse, a medication) or another medical condition.
D. The disturbance is not better explained by the symptoms of another mental disorder (e.g., excessive worries, as in generalized anxiety disorder; preoccupation with appearance, as in body dysmorphic disorder; difficulty discarding or parting with possessions, as in hoarding disorder; hair pulling, as in trichotillomania [hair-pulling disorder]; skin picking as in excoriation [skin-picking] disorder; stereotypies, as in stereotypic movement disorder; ritualized eating behavior, as in eating disorders; preoccupation with substances or gambling, as in substance-related and addictive disorders; preoccupation with having an illness, as in illness anxiety disorder; sexual urges or fantasies, as in paraphilic disorders; impulses, as in disruptive, impulse-control, and conduct disorders; guilty ruminations, as in major depressive disorder; thought insertion or delusional preoccupations, as in schizophrenia spectrum and other psychotic disorders; or repetitive patterns of behavior, as in autism spectrum disorder).

Specify if:

With good or fair insight: The individual recognizes that obsessive-compulsive disorder beliefs are definitely or probably not true or that they may or may not be true.
With poor insight: The individual thinks obsessive-compulsive disorder beliefs are probably ture.
With absent insight/delusional beliefs: The individual is completely convinced that obsessive-compulsive disorder beliefs are true.

Specify if:

Tic-related: The individual has a current or past history of a tic disorder.

Reprinted with permission from the Diagnostic and statistical manual of mental disorders, *ed 5, (Copyright 2013). American Psychiatric Association.*

BOX 33-2 DSM-5 Diagnostic Criteria: Body Dysmorphic Disorder (300.7 (F45.22))

A. Preoccupation with one or more perceived defects or flaws in physical appearance that are not observable or appear slight to others.
B. At some point during the course of the disorder, the individual has performed repetitive behaviors (e.g., mirror checking, excessive grooming, skin picking, reassurance seeking) or mental acts (e.g., comparing his or her appearance with that of others) in response to the appearance concerns.
C. The preoccupation causes clinically significant distress or impairment in social, occupational, or other important areas of functioning.
D. The appearance preoccupation is not better explained by concerns with body fat or weight in an individual whose symptoms meet diagnostic criteria for an eating disorder.

Specify if:

With muscle dysmorphia: The individual is preoccupied with the idea that his or her body build is too small or insufficiently muscular. This specifier is used even if the individual is preoccupied with other body areas, which is often the case.

Specify if:
Indicate degree of insight regarding body dysmorphic disorder beliefs (e.g. "I look ugly" or "I look deformed").

With good or fair insight: The individual recognizes that the body dysmorphic disorder beliefs are definitely or probably not true or that they may or may not be true.
With poor insight: The individual thinks that the body dysmorphic disorder beliefs are probably true.
With absent insight/delusional beliefs: The individual is completely convinced that the body dysmorphic disorder beliefs are true.

Reprinted with permission from the Diagnostic and statistical manual of mental disorders, *ed 5, (Copyright 2013). American Psychiatric Association.*

BOX 33-3 DSM-5 Diagnostic Criteria: Trichotillomania (Hair-Pulling Disorder) (312.39 (F63.2))

A. Recurrent pulling out of one's hair resulting in hair loss.
B. Repeated attempts to decrease or stop hair pulling.
C. The hair pulling causes clinically significant distress or impairment in social, occupational, or other important areas of functioning.
D. The hair pulling or hair loss is not attributable to another medical condition (e.g., a dermatological condition).
E. The hair pulling is not better explained by the symptoms of another mental disorder (e.g., attempts to improve a perceived defect or flaw in appearance in body dysmorphic disorder).

Reprinted with permission from the Diagnostic and statistical manual of mental disorders, *ed 5, (Copyright 2013). American Psychiatric Association.*

BOX 33-4 DSM-5 Diagnostic Criteria: Hoarding Disorder Diagnostic Criteria (300.3 (F42))

A. Persistent difficulty discarding or parting with possessions, regardless of their actual value.

B. This difficulty is due to a perceived need to save items and to the distress associated with discarding them.

C. The difficulty discarding possessions results in the accumulation of possessions that congest and clutter active living areas and substantially compromises their intended use. If living areas are uncluttered, it is only because of the interventions of third parties (e.g., family members, cleaners, authorities).

D. The hoarding causes clinically significant distress or impairment in social, occupational, or other important areas of functioning (including maintaining a safe environment for self and others).

E. The hoarding is not attributable to another medical condition (e.g., brain injury, cerebrovascular disease, Prader-Willi syndrome).

F. The hoarding is not better explained by the symptoms of another mental disorder (e.g., obsessions in obsessive-compulsive disorder, decreased energy in major depressive disorder, delusions in schizophrenia or another psychotic disorder, cognitive deficits in major neurocognitive disorder, restricted interests in autism spectrum disorder).

Specify if:

With excessive acquisition: If difficulty discarding possessions is accompanied by excessive acquisition of items that are not needed or for which there is no available space.

Specify if:

With good or fair insight: The individual recognizes that hoarding-related beliefs and behaviors (pertaining to difficulty discarding items, clutter, or excessive acquisition) are problematic.

With poor insight: The individual recognizes that hoarding-related beliefs and behaviors (pertaining to difficulty discarding items, clutter, or excessive acquisition) are not problematic despite evidence to the contrary.

With absent insight/delusional beliefs: The individual is completely convinced that hoarding-related beliefs and behaviors (pertaining to difficulty discarding items, clutter or excessive acquisition) are not problematic despite evidence to the contrary.

Reprinted with permission from the Diagnostic and statistical manual of mental disorders, *ed 5, (Copyright 2013). American Psychiatric Association.*

BOX 33-5 DSM-5 Diagnostic Criteria: Excoriation (Skin-picking) (698.4 (L98.1))

A. Recurrent skin picking resulting in skin lesions:

B. Repeated attempts to decrease or stop skin picking.

C. The skin picking causes clinically significant distress or impairment in social, occupational, or other important areas of functioning.

D. The skin picking is not attributable to the physiological effects of a substance (e.g., cocaine) or another medical condition (e.g., scabies).

E. The skin picking is not better explained by symptoms of another mental disorder (e.g., delusions or tactile hallucinations in a psychic disorder, attempts to improve a perceived defect or flaw in appearance in body dysmorphic disorder, sterotypes in stereotypic movement disorder, or intention to harm oneself in non-suicidal self-injury).

The age of onset for individuals with OCD appears to be an important clinical variable. Childhood-onset OCD may have a unique etiology and outcome, and it may represent a developmental subtype of the disorder.[29,30] Childhood-onset OCD is also associated with greater severity[29,30] and with higher rates of compulsions without reported obsessions.[29,30] Earlier age of onset within a pediatric sample was associated with higher persistence rates in a meta-analysis of long-term outcomes for childhood-onset OCD.[32] Co-morbid rates of tic disorders,[33] attention-deficit/hyperactivity disorder (ADHD), and anxiety disorders[34] are also higher compared to adult OCD.

HD symptoms tend to begin early in life, between 11 and 15 years of age, increasing in severity with each decade. HD is reportedly three times more common in older adults (between 55 and 94 years) compared to younger adults (between 34 and 44 years old).[6]

BDD tends to present during adolescence. Many individuals with BDD have had life-long sensitivities regarding their appearance. The age of onset for adults with TTM is approximately 13 years.[35] TTM and SPD often begin around the age of puberty.[6]

Gender

The gender profile of OCD differs by age and population type. Clinical samples of individuals with childhood-onset OCD have a male predominance;[30,31,36] however, epidemiological studies of children and adolescents report equal rates of OCD in boys and girls.[37,38] In contrast, a slight female predominance is reported in epidemiological studies of adults with OCD.[17,24,27,39]

There is no clear gender predominance across the OCRDs. While some epidemiological studies indicate a significantly greater prevalence of HD among males, clinical samples are generally female and females tend to display more excessive acquisition.[6] BDD is slightly more common in women,[18] although males are more likely to have genital preoccupation or muscle dysmorphia and females are more likely to have a co-morbid eating disorder.

TTM has a female predominance among adult samples, but a more even gender distribution among younger samples.[40] Overall, TTM has a 10-fold increased rate and SPF has a three-fold increased rate among females.[6]

Race and Cultural Factors

The prevalence of OCD tends to be fairly consistent across countries,[17] suggesting that race and culture are not main causal factors for OCD. However, it is likely that cultural factors influence the content of obsessions and compulsions.[41,42] The disorder is thought to be evenly distributed across socioeconomic strata in most studies, but there tends to be a paucity of minority OCD participants in US epidemiological and clinical studies.[15] Although most research has been conducted on Western, developing countries, HD, BDD, TTM, and SPD appear to be disorders that are universally represented. Nonetheless, the expression of TTM and SPD is thought to be influenced by specific cultural influences related to appearance.[5]

Risk Factors

There are no clearly established environmental risk factors for OCD. However, some patients describe the onset of symptoms after a biologically or emotionally stressful event (such as a pregnancy, divorce, or the death of a loved one), and psychological trauma has been posited as a risk factor for developing OCD.[43] Some preliminary work has found a possible association of OCD with higher recalled rates of perinatal complications[44] and with advanced paternal age.[45] Some studies have associated streptococcal infection with an abrupt, exacerbating–remitting early-onset form of OCD, termed *pediatric autoimmune disorders associated with streptococcus* (PANDAS),[46–48] though the strength of this etiological association persists as a topic of debate.[49,50] More recently, the broader category of *pediatric acute neuropsychiatric syndrome* (PANS) has been proposed to include all cases of acute-onset OCD, independent of *Streptococcus* infection status.[51]

Individuals with HD are more likely to demonstrate characteristics that include indecisiveness, perfectionism, avoidance, procrastination, difficulty planning and organizing tasks, and distractibility, thus making these risk factors.[6] Little is known regarding BDD etiology, although genetic predisposition, serotonin system deficits, perfectionism, an information-processing bias favoring details (versus holistic processing), family biases (e.g., that appearance is highly valued) and specific events (such as teasing) may play a role. A clear understanding of the pathogenesis of TTM remains limited.[52] SPD onset often coincides with a dermatological condition, such as acne.[6]

Genetics

Numerous lines of evidence support a genetic basis for OCD and OCRDs. Twin and family aggregation studies of OCD report higher than expected rates of OCD among relatives.[53–56] This was confirmed in a meta-analysis of five OCD family studies including 1,209 first-degree relatives,[57] reporting a four-fold increased risk of OCD among relatives of probands (8.2%) versus controls (2%). In child and adolescent OCD studies, familial risk appears to be even higher (9.5% to 17%).[58–64] A review of OCD twin studies reinforces these findings, concluding that obsessive-compulsive symptoms are heritable, with genetic influences ranging from 45% to 65% in children with OCD and from 27% to 47% in adults with OCD.[65] Family studies have found that approximately half of the OCD cases do not have a familial pattern.[66–68]

Numerous OCD molecular genetic studies including segregation analyses, linkage studies, candidate gene studies, and genome-wide association studies have been conducted, revealing that this is a complex genetic disorder, for which dozens or hundreds of gene variants are likely to confer vulnerability.[69,70] One gene of ongoing interest is the glutamate transporter gene, *SLC1A1*,[71] although other glutamate genes have also had reported association, such as *GRIK2*.[72]

With respect to genetic studies of OCRDs, significantly higher-than-expected rates of BDD (OR = 5.4) and grooming disorders (OR = 1.8) were reported among the relatives of OCD probands.[73] HD appears to have familial and genetic components, with 50% reporting that they have relatives who do the same, and twin studies reporting a heritability estimate of 50%.[5] It has also been suggested that TTM[52,74,75] and SPD[1] have an underlying genetic basis. A significantly greater concordance rate has been found among monozygotic (31.9%) versus dizygotic (0%) twins for "clinically significant hair-pulling".[76]

PATHOPHYSIOLOGY

The pathophysiology of OCD is incompletely understood, although neurobiological models implicate dysfunction in several corticostriatal pathways,[77,78] including a ventromedial "emotion" circuit and a dorsolateral "cognitive" circuit.[79] OCD is associated with certain neurological conditions, such as multiple sclerosis,[80] Huntington's chorea, and Parkinson's disease.[81,82] The basal ganglia are likely associated with the compulsions of OCD. Damage to this region in human[83] and animal models[84] results in behaviors resembling compulsions. Prefrontal and orbitofrontal regions are responsible for filtering information received by the brain and for suppressing unnecessary responses to external stimuli; these may be more associated with the obsessive symptoms of OCD.

Neuroimaging findings indicate that OCD involves subtle structural and functional abnormalities of the orbitofrontal cortex, the anterior cingulate cortex, the caudate, the amygdala, and the thalamus (Figure 33-4).[77,78,85–87] Nodes of the implicated cortical-basal ganglia-thalamo-cortical circuit are interconnected via two principal white-matter tracts—the cingulum bundle and the anterior limb of the internal capsule. Studies of OCD-affected individuals have inconsistently reported increased gray matter volume, decreased white matter volume, and white matter integrity differences from healthy controls, which suggests a possible developmental etiological process.[88–90]

Neurochemically, serotonergic,[91] dopaminergic,[92] and glutamatergic systems have been implicated in OCD. Other pathophysiological factors may be involved in the etiology of OCD. In rare cases, a brain insult (such as encephalitis, a striatal lesion [congenital or acquired], or head injury) directly precedes the development of OCD.[91,93] As previously noted, some research suggests that autoimmune processes in some childhood-onset cases, associated with beta-hemolytic streptococcal infection, may be associated with childhood-onset cases of OCD.[94–96]

Brain regions implicated in HD include the anterior cingulate cortex, ventromedial prefrontal cortex and insula.[97,98] White matter abnormalities have been reported for SPD[99] and TTM[100] in tracts related to motor generation and suppression, including the anterior cingulate cortex and for BDD in tracts connecting visual with emotion/memory processing regions.[99–101]

EVALUATION, TESTS, AND LABORATORY FINDINGS

To assess an individual with suspected OCD or an OCRD, a systematic approach should be applied. Elements of a standard psychiatric assessment that will assist in management include assessment of the history of present illness, co-morbid psychiatric syndromes, past psychiatric history, family psychiatric history, social and developmental history, review of systems, medical and substance history, medications and drug allergies, and the mental status examination.

Regarding the *history of present illness*, the duration and severity of symptoms and their precipitating, exacerbating, and ameliorating factors should be elucidated. Functional consequences of these symptoms in home, work, and social environments, and the level of insight into, resistance to, and control over symptoms should also be assessed. The Yale-Brown Obsessive Compulsive Scale (Y-BOCS)[102] and checklist may assist in recording the severity and life-time presence of specific symptoms. There is also a children's version of this scale, the Children's Yale-Brown Obsessive Compulsive Scale (CY-BOCS).[103] Family functioning and accommodation of symptoms are important factors to be assessed, which can be accomplished via the OCD Family Functioning (OFF) Scale[104] and the Family Accommodation Scale.[105]

Following initial assessment, co-morbid illnesses or other more responsible disorders should be ruled out. For individuals with OCD, co-morbid OCRDs should be assessed, and vice

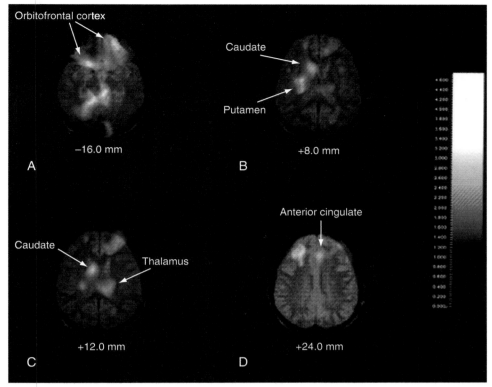

Figure 33-4. Positron-emission tomographic omnibus subtraction images of provoked minus resting conditions for all subjects ($N = 8$; 13 scans per condition) displayed with a "hot iron" scale in units of z score, superimposed over a normal magnetic resonance image transformed to Talairach space, for the purpose of anatomical reference. All images are transverse sections parallel to the anterior commissure–posterior commissure plane, shown in conventional neuroimaging orientation (top = anterior, bottom = posterior, right = left, left = right). Each transverse section is labeled with its z coordinate, denoting its position with respect to the anterior commissure–posterior commissure line (superior > 0). Activation is found within regions of interest corresponding to a prior hypothesis. A, Orbitofrontal cortex bilaterally ($P < 0.008$); B and C, right caudate nucleus ($P < 0.006$); C, left thalamus ($P = 0.07$); and D, anterior cingulate cortex ($P < 0.045$). Other areas of substantial activation include (B) right putamen and (C) left and (D) right middle frontal cortex (not labeled). *(From Rauch SL, Jenike MA, Alpert NM, et al. Regional cerebral blood flow measured during symptom provocation in obsessive-compulsive disorder using oxygen 15–labeled carbon dioxide and positron emission tomography,* Arch Gen Psychiatry, *51:66, 1994.)*

versa. Clinical measures used to record OCRDs include the Saving Inventory-Revised[106] for HD, the BDD Questionnaire for BDD,[107] the Massachusetts General Hospital (MGH) Hair-pulling Scale[108] and the Trichotillomania Scale for Children[109] for TTM and the Skin Picking Scale-Revised[110] and the Skin Picking Impact Scale for SPD.[111] Other co-morbidities occurring at higher than expected rates include depression, anxiety, bipolar disorder, and ADHD.[112-114]

In the assessment of *past psychiatric history*, the duration and maximum dosage of every past medication trial should be recorded. The length and success of past behavioral or cognitive therapies and other psychotherapies are important to establish. Careful attention should be paid to determine whether past CBT included behavioral components (including exposure and response prevention), cognitive interventions, or a combination of the two. It is regrettably all too common for individuals to believe they have had CBT, when they actually received supportive therapy, a modality proven no more effective than placebo for OCD treatment. Other factors that may affect the treatment include a history of substance abuse, which may impede the ability to comply with treatment recommendations. Past mood instability may indicate a risk of developing manic symptoms with administration of serotonergic agents. A history of panic attacks may prompt use of

caution with titrating a serotonergic medication, to best avoid triggering further attacks.

Since OCD and related disorders likely have a genetic component, a thorough *family psychiatric history* should be elicited for the presence of OCD and OCRDs. Furthermore, since medication response may also have an inherited component, information regarding family history of effective treatment trials and negative medication reactions should be gathered.

Medical history is an important component of assessment, with information regarding currently-prescribed, over-the-counter, and birth control medications, as well as drug allergies. Physical and neurological illnesses should be listed, in addition to possible symptoms that may overlap with medication side effects (e.g., insomnia, anergia). A history of thyroid problems, head injuries, or seizures should be noted, and pregnancy should be ruled out especially if a medication trial is anticipated. If the patient is a child with an acute OCD onset that is temporally related to an illness, consideration should be given to obtaining a throat culture and *Streptococcus*-related antibodies, followed by antibiotic management for identified infections.[115,116] In such cases, careful consideration should also be given to other medical conditions that might cause a sudden onset of OCD symptoms, with work-up conducted as indicated.[51,117]

A crucial component is the mental status examination. A general description of the patient and his or her behavior should include any external signs of OCD or OCRDs (e.g., red, chapped hands, repeated behaviors, or bald spots). Abnormal movements (such as tics or choreiform movements) and neurological soft signs should be noted, in addition to abnormalities of speech, the degree of eye contact, and cooperation. Assessments of mood and affect should note levels of expressed anxiety, depression, or anger. Thought form should be assessed with respect to circumstantiality, and thought content with respect to over-valued ideation, delusions, and thoughts of suicide and homicide. The level of insight and degree of judgment exhibited by the patient are also important to note.

Unfortunately, there are no laboratory findings that are diagnostic of OCD or OCRDs. For clinicians who are considering a diagnosis of PANDAS, a positive throat culture for group A beta hemolytic streptococcus or a temporal relationship between *Streptococcus*-related antibodies and OCD symptoms may support that diagnosis, in addition to the fulfilling of other diagnostic criteria. Although characteristic neuroimaging findings have been reported for groups of individuals with OCD, there are no pathognomonic findings to diagnose an individual with the disorder.

TREATMENT

Management of OCD often involves use of medication in combination with other modalities (such as CBT, psychoeducation, and support groups). First-line treatment options for OCD include both CBT and serotonin reuptake inhibitor (SRI) medications. SRIs include selective serotonin reuptake inhibitors (SSRIs), and the tricyclic antidepressant (TCA) clomipramine. Other TCAs with less serotonergic activity are not effective in the treatment of OCD. Effective CBT for OCD includes exposure and response prevention (ERP), which has been well studied in OCD, and also cognitive interventions, which is a promising OCD treatment.[118] ERP works by anxiety habituation following prolonged exposure to a feared OCD stimulus without compulsion performance, whereas cognitive therapy works to directly address distorted OCD beliefs.[119] More recent augmentation approaches that show early promise include Acceptance and Commitment Therapy (ACT)[120] and attention retraining strategies in addition to motivational interviewing.[121]

The decision to initiate an SSRI alone, CBT alone, or a combination depends on individual patient variables. There is evidence to suggest that all three of these approaches, as well as cognitive therapy alone,[122,123] can be effective for OCD. For cases in which potential medication side effects outweigh benefits, an initial trial of CBT alone may be preferable. For those without access to a CBT-trained clinician or with insufficient motivation or insight to engage in effective psychotherapy, an initial trial with an SSRI alone may be optimal. Furthermore, co-morbid depression, psychosis, or other anxiety disorders that may interfere with CBT for OCD may themselves require medication treatment to facilitate overall recovery and treatment focused on specifically on OCD.

A suggested management approach in the treatment of OCD is to initiate SRI treatment with an SSRI rather than clomipramine, given the more problematic side-effect profile associated with clomipramine. If the initial SSRI is not effective, one to two other SSRI trials should be attempted before use of clomipramine. The selection of a specific SSRI is open to clinical judgment, because head-to-head trials and meta-analyses of SSRIs in children and adults with OCD have not found significant differences in efficacy between them. Factors that may be helpful in making this selection include a family

history of a positive response or an adverse reaction to a specific SSRI, potential interactions with other medications, and side-effect profiles.

To determine the effectiveness of a medication, a 10- to 12-week trial, with at least 2–3 weeks at the highest tolerated dose within the advised dose range is required. For treatment of OCD, effective doses are typically higher than are those required for depression due to a linear dose–response curve[124] (Table 33-4). Further, symptom reduction is more common than remission. In clinical trials, "response" is typically defined by either a ≥ 25% or ≥ 35% decrease in Y-BOCS–defined OCD severity. Approximately 40% to 60% of patients respond to SRIs with a reduction of OCD symptoms.[91,125]

Before initiating a medication trial, it is at times necessary to conduct laboratory baseline investigations (such as blood work and an electrocardiogram [ECG]) for clomipramine. It is also necessary to rule-out a previous allergic/negative reaction and to consider potential interactions with other medications in the current regimen. Between each step in the treatment plan, assessment of adherence to, and adverse effects from, the medication regimen should be conducted.

Second-line medication strategies to consider include SRI augmentation with clonazepam, atypical antipsychotics and buspirone. Buspirone and clonazepam are often used before considering atypical antipsychotic agents given the lower risk for weight gain and other side effects, although the level of evidence for atypical agents is much stronger than that for the former. Suggested dosages, common adverse effects, and rare but serious adverse effects of the best-studied second-line agents are found in Table 33-4. It should be noted that distinct adverse effect profiles also exist for certain medications within classes (e.g., citalopram and potential QT prolongation). Moreover, evidence for glutamatergic agents is preliminary and use of these medications would be considered "off label" for OCD. The bottom of the table lists practical suggestions for specific situations, derived from clinical experience of the authors rather than via randomized controlled trials (RCTs).

In situations of treatment resistance and marked severity, additional management approaches to consider include intensive residential treatment[126] or gamma knife surgery.[127] Electroconvulsive therapy (ECT) has not been proven effective for OCD. Repetitive transcranial magnetic stimulation (rTMS) is an effective, non-invasive modality for depression, which requires study in OCD.[128]

Once an effective medication and dose are identified in the treatment of OCD, this should be continued for 6 months to 1 year before considering its discontinuation. A conversation regarding potential risks and benefits is required, and, if a decision is made to stop the medication, this should be conducted very gradually over weeks to months. Unfortunately, the subsequent relapse rate following medication discontinuation is very high, ranging from 24% to 89% at 6-month follow-up.[129-132] For those who have also received CBT, however, relapse risk is diminished (12% with CBT versus 45% without CBT, for clomipramine responders, assessed 12 weeks after discontinuation).[133]

Regarding treatment of OCRDs, large placebo-controlled studies in individuals are lacking and it is difficult to draw firm conclusions on medication use and psychotherapy. However, from available data, CBT strategies offer more promise than pharmacological ones, and while SSRIs appear to have limited value, glutamatergic agents may have some beneficial effect.

Treatment of HD is met by many challenges, including the limited insight and ego-syntonic qualities that characterize this disorder. Whereas family members are typically very distressed about its impacts, those with HD often resist treatment. A team approach is suggested, which may involve CBT components, conceptualizing HD as a consequence of

TABLE 33-4 Obsessive-Compulsive Disorder Medications, Dosages, and Side Effects

Drug (Generic Name)	Drug (Trade Name)	Starting Dose (mg/d)	Target Dose (mg/d)	Adverse Effects (special considerations)
Monotherapy Agents (serotonin reuptake inhibitors)				
SELECTIVE SEROTONIN REUPTAKE INHIBITORS				
Citalopram	Celexa	20	40	Common: insomnia,anxiety, GI upset, decreased sexual function, dizziness, sedation
Escitalopram	Lexapro	10	30	
Fluoxetine	Prozac	20	80	
Fluvoxamine	Luvox	50	300	Rare: rash, headache
Paroxetine	Paxil	20	60	*(monitor weight)*
Sertraline	Zoloft	50	200	
TRICYCLIC ANTIDEPRESSANTS				
Clomipramine	Anafranil	25	250	Common: anti-cholinergic, dizziness, decreased sexual function, weight gain, tremor Rare: ECG changes, seizures *(monitor weight, vital signs, ECG and serum total and metabolite levels)*
AUGMENTING AGENTS (ADD TO SRIS)				
Buspirone	Buspar	10 (divided BID)	10–45 (divided BID)	Common: dizziness, headache, nausea Rare: sedation, rash
BENZODIAZEPINES*				
Clonazepam	Klonopin	0.25–0.5 (PD or divided BID)	0.5–3 (PD or divided BID)	Common: sedation Rare: impaired cognition, disinhibition, ataxia
Lorazepam	Ativan	0.5 (divided BID-TID)	0.5—TID)	*(potential for tolerance—monitor for escalating dose, rebound anxiety)*
ATYPICAL ANTIPSYCHOTICS				
Risperidone	Risperdal	1 (PD or divided BID)	0.5–6	Common: weight gain, dizziness, sedation, constipation, sexual function
Olanzapine	Zyprexa	5	5–20 (PD or divided BID)	Rare: hyperglycemia, elevated prolactin, extrapyramidal symptoms
Quetiapine	Seroquel	50 (divided BID)	500 (divided BID)	*(monitor weight, lipids, cholesterol, and ECG)*
Aripiprazole	Abilify	10	10–30	
Ziprasidone	Geodon	40 (divided BID)	40–160 (divided BID)	
GLUTAMATERGIC AGENTS**				
Memantine	Namenda	10 (divided BID)	20 (divided BID)	Common: dizziness, drowsiness, headache, insomnia, confusion Rare: vomiting, increased libido, cystitis
N-acetylcysteine	Mucomyst	1200 (divided BID)	2400 (divided BID)	Common: dizziness, drowsiness, nausea, vomiting, diarrhea, heartburn Rare: headache, increased ICP
Riluzole	Rilutek		100 (divided BID)	Common: nausea, sedation Rare: liver toxicity *(monitor liver function)*
SSRI AUGMENTATION- PRACTICAL SUGGESTIONS FOR SPECIAL CIRCUMSTANCES***				

	CLASS/SPECIFIC DRUG	PRE/POST-OCD SSRI TRIAL	CONSIDERATIONS	
Co-morbid MDD	Bupropion (Wellbutrin)	post	Seizure risk with comorbid bulimia	
Weight gain	Topiramate (Topamax)	either	Expect 1–2 lb loss weekly	
Mood instability	Lamotrigine (Lamictal)	pre	Reduces SSRI-induced mood switch	
Co-morbid ADHD	Stimulant or atomoxetine	post	Reduces stimulant-induced anxiety	
Impairing tics	Alpha-agonist	pre	Reduces SSRI-induced tic worsening	
Pediatric acute neuropsychiatric syndrome (PANS)	antibiotic + probiotic + NSAID	acute phase only	Probiotic reduces antibiotic-induced *Clostridium difficile*; NSAID reduces inflammation	

BID, Twice a day; ECG, electrocardiogram; GI, gastrointestinal; QD, once daily; TID, three times daily; ICP, intracranial pressure.
* Beneficial while awaiting SRI action. Mixed evidence of efficacy; ** early evidence for efficacy—no RCTs to date; *** based on clinical experience of co-authors.

information-processing deficits, abnormal emotional attachment to objects, and avoidance behaviors.[98] Medication trials have reported variable success, but the presence of hoarding compared to other OCD symptom dimensions has been identified as a predictor of non-remission.[134]

In a meta-analysis of BDD treatment trials, both CBT and medication were effective, although CBT was most useful.[135] Components of CBT for BDD include graded exposure and response prevention, cognitive intervention, perceptual retraining, and a relapse–prevention component.[136] Serotonergic antidepressants (such as SSRIs and clomipramine) appear to be more effective than non-serotonergic antidepressants and antipsychotics,[18] as demonstrated in a crossover trial.[137] Similar to the experience with OCD, high doses of SSRIs are often required for treatment response. There is little evidence for the effectiveness of antipsychotic medications in BDD, although these agents are often used in clinical practice.[138]

Treatment studies of TTM and SPD are limited.[52,139] Behavioral therapy has been demonstrated as superior to placebo and to fluoxetine in several studies.[140,141] Habit reversal appears to be more effective than other CBT approaches in TTM.[52] Serotonergic agent efficacy has not been clearly demonstrated in TTM, with one positive,[142] and one negative[140] RCT of clomipramine and three negative RCTs of fluoxetine.[19,52,141,143] An open study reported that a combination of sertraline and CBT was more efficacious than either approach alone.[144] Other agents studied in TTM include the opioid-blocking agent naltrexone, which was reportedly effective in one study,[145] and the glutamatergic agent, *N*-acetylcysteine, which was positive in an RCT on adults[146] and negative in a similar designed trial in children.[147] Regarding SPD, CBT approaches include habit reversal training (HRT) and acceptance-based behavior therapy. Medication trials have been limited, but have demonstrated preliminary success for SSRIs, *N*-acetylcysteine, and naltrexone.[148]

PROGNOSIS

OCD usually has a gradual onset, although acute onset occurs in some cases (including in PANS). The long-term course of OCD has been studied in both children and adults.

Adult studies of clinical samples report full remission rates ranging between 17% and 27% and partial remission rates between 22% and 28%, whereas child studies report higher full remission rates (40%) and similar partial remission rates of (19%).[32,134,149,150]

In a follow-up study of 144 adult inpatients with OCD after a mean period of 47 years, 20% reported full remission (no symptoms for 5 years), and 28% reported partial remission (5 years of symptoms that were at most subclinical). Forty-six percent of those in remission at the first evaluation remained in remission for at least 30 years.[149] In a study of 213 adult outpatients with OCD after a 5-year follow-up period, 17% reported full remission and 22% reported partial remission. Those who achieved full remission were less likely to relapse (45%) compared to those who only achieved partial remission (70%). Remission predictors included lower OCD severity and shorter duration of illness and relapse predictors included co-morbid obsessive-compulsive personality disorder.[134] Finally, in an Italian 10-year follow-up study, 27% had an episodic course (6 months of full symptom remission), and 73% had a chronic course (with stable or fluctuating symptoms or with deterioration).[112] A long-term outcome study of a community sample of 22 adults with OCD[150] found more optimistic results. At follow-up after a mean of 13 years, 86% were in full remission and 9% were in partial remission.

A meta-analysis[32] conducted on 22 long-term outcome studies for childhood OCD (*N* = 521 subjects) reported that 40% had achieved full remission and 19% achieved partial remission. Remission predictors included older OCD onset, shorter duration of illness, and outpatient status. Hence, in general it appears that childhood OCD can be a chronic illness that exhibits a waxing and waning course, even with treatment. However, most individuals with OCD experience some improvement throughout their illness.

HD tends to increase in severity with each decade,[5] and this tends to have a chronic course. Lower remission rates are reported in HD compared to OCD.[134] BDD is often a lifelong illness when left untreated, although the symptoms may wax and wane over time.[151] For those receiving medication or psychotherapy, 4-year remission rates have been as high as 60%.[152] Of those who remitted, nearly 30% subsequently relapsed, and the risk of remission was associated with initial BDD severity, co-morbid depression, and social phobia. For those who obtained cosmetic interventions in an attempt to alleviate body-related concerns, 83% had either a worsening or no change of their symptoms.[153] People with BDD were found to be more disabled than those with depression, diabetes, or a recent myocardial infarction.[154] Risk of suicide is elevated in both adults and children/adolescents with BDD.[5]

Limited research has been done regarding the prognosis of TTM, although both chronic and remitting forms occur. There is some evidence that self-esteem worsens over the course of the illness.[155] Cases with onset in early childhood have a better prognosis and are more likely to respond to treatment.[151] Both TTM and SPD tend to have chronic courses, with some waxing and waning, although areas of pulling or picking may vary over time.[5]

CURRENT CONTROVERSIES, UNANSWERED QUESTIONS, AND FUTURE CHALLENGES

- Identifying overlapping and common underlying mechanisms for OCD and OCRDs
- Understanding the role of neurochemical factors, such as glutamate modulation, in the pathogenesis of OCD and OCRDs
- Understanding the potential role of autoimmunity in OCD
- Identifying genetic markers that herald OCD or OCRD susceptibility
- Establishing the relative efficacy of somatic treatments for OCD (e.g., transcranial magnetic stimulation, deep brain stimulation, and neurosurgery).

CLINICIAN AND PATIENT RESOURCES

OCD:
  Anxiety Disorders Association of America
    Tel: 301-231-9350
    www.adaa.org
    http://socialanxietysupport.com
  International OCD Foundation
    18 Tremont Street, Suite 903
    Boston, MA 02108
    Tel: 617-973-5801
    Fax: 617-973-5803
    www.ocfoundation.org
  Pediatric Autoimmune Neuropsychiatric Disorders Associated with Streptococcus
    http://pandasnetwork.org
OCDbc:
  http://www.ocdbc.ca
Anxiety BC:
  http://www.anxietybc.com

HD:
  Hoarding website
    http://www.ocfoundation.org/hoarding/
  Clutterers Anonymous
    Tel: (310) 281-6064
    http://www.clutterersanonymous.net
TTM :
  Trichotillomania Learning Center
    Tel: 831-457-1004
    www.trich.org
OTHER:
  National Alliance on Mental Illness
    Tel: 1-800-950-6264; or, 703-524-7600
    http://www.nami.org
  National Institute of Mental Health (NIMH)
    Public Information and Communications Branch
    6001 Executive Boulevard, Room 8184, MSC 9663
    Bethesda, MD 20892-9663
    Tel: 1-866-615-6464
    Fax: 301-443-4279
Peri-partum Medication Use:
  MGH Women's Mental Health Program
    www.womensmentalhealth.com
Children and adolescents:
  American Academy of Child and Adolescent Psychiatry
    3615 Wisconsin Ave., NW
    Washington, DC 20016-3007
    Tel: 202-966-7300
    www.aacap.org/
    www.aacap.org/publications/factsfam/index.htm

Access the complete reference list and multiple choice questions (MCQs) online at https://expertconsult.inkling.com

KEY REFERENCES

9. Lochner C, Grant JE, Odlaug BL, et al. DSM-5 field survey: hair-pulling disorder (trichotillomania). *Depress Anxiety* 29(12):1025–1031, 2012.
18. Castle DJ, Rossell S, Kyrios M. Body dysmorphic disorder. *Psychiatr Clin North Am* 29(2):521–538, 2006.
32. Stewart SE, Geller DA, Jenike M, et al. Long-term outcome of pediatric obsessive-compulsive disorder: a meta-analysis and qualitative review of the literature. *Acta Psychiatr Scand* 110(1):4–13, 2004.
35. Mansueto CS, Stemberger RM, Thomas AM, et al. Trichotillomania: a comprehensive behavioral model. *Clin Psychol Rev* 17(5):567–577, 1997.
51. Swedo SE, Leckman JF, Rose NR. From Research Subgroup to Clinical Syndrome: Modifying the PANDAS Criteria to Describe PANS (Pediatric Acute-onset Neuropsychiatric Syndrome). *Pediatr Ther* 2(2):2012.
63. Chabane N, Delorme R, Millet B, et al. Early-onset obsessive-compulsive disorder: a subgroup with a specific clinical and familial pattern? *J Child Psychol Psychiatry* 46(8):881–887, 2005.
69. Pauls DL. The genetics of obsessive-compulsive disorder: a review. *Dialogues Clin Neurosci* 12(2):149–163, 2010.
70. Stewart SE, Yu D, Scharf JM, et al. Genome-wide association study of obsessive-compulsive disorder. *Mol Psychiatry* 18(7):788–798, 18(7):843 (erratum), 2013.

73. Bienvenu OJ, Samuels JF, Riddle MA, et al. The relationship of obsessive-compulsive disorder to possible spectrum disorders: results from a family study. *Biol Psychiatry* 48(4):287–293, 2000.
92. Pittenger C, Bloch MH, Williams K. Glutamate abnormalities in obsessive compulsive disorder: Neurobiology, pathophysiology, and treatment. *Pharmacol Ther* 132(3):314–332, 2011.
98. Mataix-Cols D, Frost RO, Pertusa A, et al. Hoarding disorder: a new diagnosis for DSM-V? *Depress Anxiety* 27(6):556–572, 2010.
104. Stewart SE, Hu YP, Hezel DM, et al. Development and psychometric properties of the OCD family functioning (OFF) scale. *J Fam Psychol* 2011.
105. Calvocoressi L, Mazure CM, Kasl SV, et al. Family accommodation of obsessive-compulsive symptoms: instrument development and assessment of family behavior. *J Nerv Ment Dis* 187(10):636–642, 1999.
106. Frost RO, Steketee G, Grisham J. Measurement of compulsive hoarding: saving inventory-revised. *Behav Res Ther* 42(10):1163–1182, 2004.
107. Phillips K. Instruments for assessing BDD: the BDDQ: a self-report screening instrument for BDD. *The broken mirror* 321–333, 1996.
108. Keuthen NJ, O'Sullivan RL, Ricciardi JN, et al. The Massachusetts General Hospital (MGH) Hairpulling Scale: 1. development and factor analyses. *Psychother Psychosom* 64(3–4):141–145, 1995.
111. Snorrason I, Olafsson RP, Flessner CA, et al. The Skin Picking Impact Scale: Factor structure, validity and development of a short version. *Scand J Psychol* 54(4):34434–34438, 2013.
121. Merlo LJ, Storch EA, Lehmkuhl HD, et al. Cognitive behavioral therapy plus motivational interviewing improves outcome for pediatric obsessive-compulsive disorder: a preliminary study. *Cogn Behav Ther* 39(1):24–27, 2010.
124. Bloch MH, Landeros-Weisenberger A, Dombrowski P, et al. Systematic review: pharmacological and behavioral treatment for trichotillomania. *Biol Psychiatry* 62(8):839–846, 2007.
126. Greenberg BD, Malone DA, Friehs GM, et al. Three-year outcomes in deep brain stimulation for highly resistant obsessive-compulsive disorder. *Neuropsychopharmacology* 31(11):2384–2393, 2006.
133. Foa EB, Liebowitz MR, Kozak MJ, et al. Randomized, placebo-controlled trial of exposure and ritual prevention, clomipramine, and their combination in the treatment of obsessive-compulsive disorder. *Am J Psychiatry* 162(1):151–161, 2005.
134. Eisen JL, Sibrava NJ, Boisseau CL, et al. Five-year course of obsessive-compulsive disorder: predictors of remission and relapse. *J Clin Psychiatry* 74(3):233–239, 2013.
135. Williams J, Hadjistavropoulos T, Sharpe D. A meta-analysis of psychological and pharmacological treatments for Body Dysmorphic Disorder. *Behav Res Ther* 44(1):99–111, 2006.
136. Wilhelm S, Phillips KA, Steketee G, et al. *Cognitive-behavioral therapy for body dysmorphic disorder a treatment manual*, New York, 2013, Guilford Press. Available from: <http://site.ebrary.com/lib/ubc/Doc?id=10634386>; An electronic book accessible through the World Wide Web.
146. Grant JE, Odlaug BL, Kim SW. N-acetylcysteine, a glutamate modulator, in the treatment of trichotillomania: a double-blind, placebo-controlled study. *Arch Gen Psychiatry* 66(7):756–763, 2009.
148. Grant JE, Odlaug BL, Chamberlain SR, et al. Skin picking disorder. *Am J Psychiatry* 169(11):1143–1149, 2012.
149. Skoog G, Skoog I. A 40-year follow-up of patients with obsessive-compulsive disorder [see comments]. *Arch Gen Psychiatry* 56(2):121–127, 1999.

34 Trauma and Posttraumatic Stress Disorder

Sharon Dekel, PhD, Mark W. Gilbertson, PhD, Scott P. Orr, PhD, Scott L. Rauch, MD, Nellie E. Wood, BA, and Roger K. Pitman, MD

KEY POINTS

Incidence/Epidemiology

- Exposure to events capable of causing posttraumatic stress disorder (PTSD) is the rule rather than the exception. Life-time incidence of exposure to events causing PTSD is greater than 50%. However, development of PTSD following a traumatic event is the exception rather than the rule.

- The overall probability of developing PTSD following a traumatic event is less than 10%. However, assaults and other traumatic events of human design can lead to substantially higher rates. The life-time incidence of DSM-IV PTSD in the general community is approximately 8%.

Pathophysiology

- PTSD is one of the few disorders in DSM-5 for which the cause is considered to be known, viz., exposure to actual or threatened death, serious injury, or sexual violence. Such exposure may set in motion psychological and biological processes including fear conditioning, sensitization, and negative alterations in cognitions and mood that may lead to PTSD symptoms.

- Failure to recover from symptoms over time, e.g., deficient extinction, also plays an important role and likely has a psychological and biological basis.

Clinical Findings

- In adults, PTSD symptomatology is conceptualized within the framework of four symptom clusters: intrusion (DSM-5 criterion B), avoidance (criterion C), negative alterations in cognitions and mood (criterion D), and hyperarousal/hyper(-re)activity (criterion E).

- Duration must be more than 1 month (criterion F).

- Some individuals who fail to meet criteria in all four clusters may nevertheless have clinically significant distress and/or impairment (criterion G).

Differential Diagnoses

- These include adjustment disorder, as well as affective, anxiety, and dissociative disorders precipitated or exacerbated by a traumatic life event. The critical factor in distinguishing PTSD from other disorders (except adjustment disorder) is the presence of trauma-specific intrusion and avoidance symptoms in PTSD.

- In patients who have experienced more than one traumatic event, differential diagnosis of which event(s) caused PTSD may be made by discerning to which event(s) the characteristic intrusion and avoidance symptoms pertain.

Treatment Options

- Despite the presence of helpful psychotherapeutic and pharmacotherapeutic treatments, individuals with PTSD often delay or fail to seek treatment more often than with most other psychiatric disorders.

- Current treatments for PTSD include cognitive-behavioral and other psychotherapeutic modalities, and psychopharmacology. Unfortunately these are typically only partially efficacious. Novel approaches are needed.

Complications

- Complications of PTSD include major depression, substance abuse/dependence, and panic disorder.

- Suicide is a rare outcome of uncomplicated PTSD, but the risk of suicide increases substantially in the presence of complications.

Prognosis

- Recovery from PTSD is most pronounced within the first year following the traumatic event.

- More than 30% of those diagnosed with PTSD fail to show remission and develop a chronic course.

OVERVIEW

The psychopathological impact of exposure to traumatic events has long been recognized, particularly in the context of war. Descriptions of the emotional sequelae of combat date back thousands of years as revealed, for example, in the epic account of Achilles in Homer's *Iliad*. Modern wars have engendered their own unique labels for these sequelae: for example, "nostalgia" or "soldier's heart" (Civil War), "shell shock" (World War I), "battle fatigue" or "combat neurosis" (World War II), and "delayed stress" (Vietnam War). However, stress disorders were largely ignored as a formal psychiatric nosological category and were relegated to "transient" phenomena until the publication of the *Diagnostic and Statistical Manual of Mental Disorders*, Third Edition (DSM-III) in 1980. Consistent with this history, the inclusion of posttraumatic stress disorder (PTSD) in the DSM-III appeared largely in response to the psychiatric difficulties experienced by war veterans, in this case, soldiers returning from Vietnam. As a result, much of the original work underlying the diagnosis of PTSD focused on combat veterans. Since that time, however, the conceptual and empirical basis of PTSD has broadened to include civilian trauma (e.g., assaults, childhood abuse, natural disasters, accidents). Indeed, the most recent editions of the DSM now recognize among the events capable of causing PTSD such things as witnessing the death or injury of others, or learning that the traumatic event occurred in a close family member or close friend. Because the diagnosis of PTSD is frequently associated with trauma that occurs within strong social (e.g., rape or child abuse), political (e.g., war), or legal (e.g., tort civil litigation) contexts, it has frequently engendered controversy; the diagnosis has even been considered by some to reflect a mere "social construction" or a form of "victim advocacy." However, more than two decades of epidemiological, genetic, and biological research has established a firm empirical foundation for PTSD. It is now recognized as a major psychiatric condition with significant social and occupational impact.

DIAGNOSIS
Etiology

The diagnosis of PTSD is nearly unique among psychiatric disorders in that the criteria incorporate a presumptive cause (i.e., a traumatic event) in addition to the typical symptom constellation (see Box 34-1 for the DSM-5 PTSD diagnostic criteria). For this reason, in DSM-5 PTSD has shifted from classification among the anxiety disorders to a new category, "trauma and stressor-related disorders." The stressor criterion in DSM-IV and DSM-5 significantly broadened the concept of a traumatic event from an earlier version of the DSM, which had required that it be "outside the range of usual human experience" (DSM-III-R). This change may have increased the number of stressors that qualify for inclusion by nearly 60%.[1] DSM-5 has also abolished the previously-required subjective element of the stressor criterion, i.e., a response to the

---

BOX 34-1 DSM-5 Diagnostic Criteria: Posttraumatic Stress Disorder (309.81)

Note: The following criteria apply to adults, adolescents, and children older than 6 years. For children 6 years and younger, see corresponding criteria below.

A. Exposure to actual or threatened death, serious injury, or sexual violence in one (or more) of the following ways:
1. Directly experiencing the traumatic event(s)
2. Witnessing, in person, the event(s) as it occurred to others
3. Learning that the traumatic event(s) occurred to a close family member or close friend. In cases of actual or threatened death of a family member or friend, the event(s) must have been violent or accidental
4. Experiencing repeated or extreme exposure to aversive details of the traumatic event(s) (e.g., first responders collecting human remains; police officers repeatedly exposed to details of child abuse).

Note: Criterion A4 does not apply to exposure through electronic media, television, movies, or pictures, unless this exposure is work-related.

B. Presence of one (or more) of the following intrusion symptoms associated with the traumatic event(s), beginning after the traumatic event(s) occurred:
1. Recurrent, involuntary, and intrusive distressing memories of the traumatic event(s).

Note: In children older than 6 years, repetitive play may occur in which themes or aspects of the traumatic event(s) are expressed.

2. Recurrent distressing dreams in which the content and/or effect of the dream are related to the traumatic event(s).

Note: In children, there may be frightening dreams without recognizable content.

3. Dissociative reactions (e.g., flashbacks) in which the individual feels or acts as if the traumatic event(s) were recurring. (Such reactions may occur on a continuum, with the most extreme expression being a complete loss of awareness of present surroundings.)

Note: In children, trauma-specific reenactment may occur in play.

4. Intense or prolonged psychological distress at exposure to internal or external cues that symbolize or resemble an aspect of the traumatic event(s).
5. Marked physiological reactions to internal or external cues that symbolize or resemble an aspect of the traumatic event(s).

C. Persistent avoidance of stimuli associated with the traumatic event(s), beginning after the traumatic event(s) occurred, as evidenced by one or both of the following:
1. Avoidance of, or efforts to avoid, distressing memories, thoughts, or feelings about or closely associated with the traumatic event(s).

2. Avoidance of, or efforts to avoid, external reminders (people, places, conversations, activities, objects, situations) that arouse distressing memories, thoughts, or feelings about or closely associated with the traumatic event(s).

D. Negative alterations in cognitions and mood associated with the traumatic event(s), beginning or worsening after the traumatic event(s) occurred, as evidenced by two (or more) of the following:
1. Inability to remember an important aspect of the traumatic event(s) (typically due to dissociative amnesia and not to other factors such as head injury, alcohol, or drugs).
2. Persistent and exaggerated negative beliefs or expectations about oneself, others, or the world (e.g., "I am bad," "No one can be trusted," "The world is completely dangerous," "My whole nervous system is permanently ruined").
3. Persistent, distorted cognitions about the cause or consequences of the traumatic event(s) that lead the individual to blame himself/herself or others.
4. Persistent negative emotional state (e.g., fear, horror, anger, guilt, or shame).
5. Markedly diminished interest or participation in significant activities.
6. Feelings of detachment or estrangement from others.
7. Persistent inability to experience positive emotions (e.g., inability to experience happiness, satisfaction, or loving feelings).

E. Marked alterations in arousal and reactivity associated with the traumatic event(s), beginning or worsening after the traumatic event(s) occurred, as evidenced by two (or more) of the following:
1. Irritable behavior and angry outbursts (with little or no provocation) typically expressed as verbal or physical aggression toward people or objects.
2. Reckless or self-destructive behavior.
3. Hypervigilance.
4. Exaggerated startle response.
5. Problems with concentration.
6. Sleep disturbance (e.g., difficulty falling or staying asleep or restless sleep).

F. Duration of the disturbance (Criteria B, C, D, and E) is more than 1 month.

G. The disturbance causes clinically significant distress or impairment in social, occupational, or other important areas of functioning.

H. The disturbance is not attributable to the physiological effects of a substance (e.g., medication, alcohol) or another medical condition.

Specify whether:

- **With dissociative symptoms:** The individual's symptoms meet the criteria for posttraumatic stress disorder, and in addition, in

Continued on following page

BOX 34-1 DSM-5 Diagnostic Criteria: Posttraumatic Stress Disorder *(Continued)*

response to the stressor, the individual experiences persistent or recurrent symptoms of either of the following:

- **Depersonalization:** Persistent or recurrent experiences of feeling detached from, and as if one were an outside observer of, one's mental processes or body (e.g., feeling as though one were in a dream; feeling a sense of unreality of self or body or of time moving slowly).
- **Derealization:** Persistent or recurrent experiences of unreality of surroundings (e.g., the world around the individual is experienced as unreal, dreamlike, distant, or distorted).

Note: To use this subtype, the dissociative symptoms must not be attributable to the physiological effects of a substance (e.g., blackouts, behavior during alcohol intoxication) or another medical condition (e.g., complex partial seizures).

   Specify if:

- **With delayed expression:** If the full diagnostic criteria are not met until at least 6 months after the event (although the onset and expression of some symptoms may be immediate).

POSTTRAUMATIC STRESS DISORDER FOR CHILDREN 6 YEARS AND YOUNGER

A. In children 6 years and younger, exposure to actual or threatened death, serious injury, or sexual violence in one (or more) of the following ways:
   1. Directly experiencing the traumatic event(s).
   2. Witnessing, in person, the event(s) as it occurred to others, especially primary caregivers.

Note: Witnessing does not include events that are witnessed only in electronic media, television, movies, or pictures.

   3. Learning that the traumatic event(s) occurred to a parent or caregiving figure.
B. Presence of one (or more) of the following intrusion symptoms associated with the traumatic event(s), beginning after the traumatic event(s) occurred:
   1. Recurrent, involuntary, and intrusive distressing memories of the traumatic event(s).

Note: Spontaneous and intrusive memories may not necessarily appear distressing and may be expressed as play reenactment.

   2. Recurrent distressing dreams in which the content and/or effect of the dream are related to the traumatic event(s).

Note: It may not be possible to ascertain that the frightening content is related to the traumatic event.

   3. Dissociative reactions (e.g., flashbacks) in which the child feels or acts as if the traumatic event(s) were recurring. (Such reactions may occur on a continuum, with the most extreme expression being a complete loss of awareness of present surroundings.) Such trauma-specific reenactment may occur in play.
   4. Intense or prolonged psychological distress at exposure to internal or external cues that symbolize or resemble an aspect of the traumatic event(s).
   5. Marked physiological reactions to reminders of the traumatic event(s).
C. One (or more) of the following symptoms, representing either persistent avoidance of stimuli associated with the traumatic

event(s) or negative alterations in cognitions and mood associated with the traumatic event(s), must be present, beginning after the event(s) or worsening after the event(s):

Persistent Avoidance of Stimuli
   1. Avoidance of or efforts to avoid activities, places, or physical reminders that arouse recollections of the traumatic event(s).
   2. Avoidance of or efforts to avoid people, conversations, or interpersonal situations that arouse recollections of the traumatic event(s).

Negative Alterations in Cognitions
   3. Substantially increased frequency of negative emotional states (e.g., fear, guilt, sadness, shame, confusion).
   4. Markedly diminished interest or participation in significant activities, including constriction of play.
   5. Socially withdrawn behavior.
   6. Persistent reduction in expression of positive emotions.
D. Alterations in arousal and reactivity associated with the traumatic event(s), beginning or worsening after the traumatic event(s) occurred, as evidenced by two (or more) of the following:
   1. Irritable behavior and angry outbursts (with little or no provocation) typically expressed as verbal or physical aggression toward people or objects (including extreme temper tantrums).
   2. Hypervigilance.
   3. Exaggerated startle response.
   4. Problems with concentration.
   5. Sleep disturbance (e.g., difficulty falling or staying asleep or restless sleep).
E. The duration of the disturbance is more than 1 month.
F. The disturbance causes clinically significant distress or impairment in relationships with parents, siblings, peers, or other caregivers or with school behavior.
G. The disturbance is not attributable to the physiological effects of a substance (e.g., medication or alcohol) or another medical condition.

   Specify whether:

- **With dissociative symptoms:** The individual's symptoms meet the criteria for posttraumatic stress disorder, and the individual experiences persistent or recurrent symptoms of either of the following:
  - **Depersonalization:** Persistent or recurrent experiences of feeling detached from, and as if one were an outside observer of, one's mental processes or body (e.g., feeling as though one were in a dream; feeling a sense of unreality of self or body or of time moving slowly).
  - **Derealization:** Persistent or recurrent experiences of unreality of surroundings (e.g., the world around the individual is experienced as unreal, dreamlike, distant, or distorted).

Note: To use this subtype, the dissociative symptoms must not be attributable to the physiological effects of a substance (e.g., blackouts) or another medical condition (e.g., complex partial seizures).

   Specify if:

- **With delayed expression:** If the full diagnostic criteria are not met until at least 6 months after the event (although the onset and expression of some symptoms may be immediate).

traumatic event of intense fear, helplessness, or horror, on the grounds that a substantial minority of persons who don't experience such a subjective response at the traumatic event nevertheless go on to develop the PTSD syndrome.[2]

Clinical Features

In addition to the requisite traumatic event (criterion A) in DSM-5, the symptomatology of PTSD is conceptualized within the framework of four symptom clusters (see Box 34-1): intrusion (criterion B), avoidance (criterion C), negative alterations in cognitions and mood (criterion D), and hyperarousal/hyper(-re)activity (criterion E), with duration of more than 1 month (criterion F). However, some individuals who fail to meet criteria in all four clusters may still have clinically significant distress and/or impairment (criterion G).[3] The requirement that different minimal symptom numbers from different clusters be met in order to qualify for the diagnosis is obviously arbitrary. It may be that this arbitrariness results from the attempt to convert what is in nature a continuum or spectrum of posttraumatic psychopathology into a categorical (present vs. absent) classification (i.e., PTSD). Such taxometric research evidence as exists supports the dimensional model.[4]

In recognition of findings that dissociation, which may operate to minimize the awareness of aversive emotions, is implicated in a substantial minority (perhaps up to 30%) of PTSD cases,[5] DSM-5 has added the optional qualifier, "with dissociative symptoms." In recognition that in a minority of PTSD cases (about 10%), the manifestation may be delayed, DSM-5 has also added the optional qualifier, "with delayed expression." Whereas DSM-IV characterized delayed PTSD as having a symptom *onset* at least 6 months after the trauma, this has been found to be rare. Presently DSM-5 only requires that the diagnostic *threshold* be exceeded more than 6 months after the event. Previous sub-threshold levels of symptomatology may be triggered to threshold levels as a result of new stressful events that re-evoke the original trauma. Delayed onsets that represent exacerbations or re-activations of prior symptoms have been found to account for 38.2% and 15.3%, respectively, of military and civilian cases of PTSD.[6] DSM-5 has also introduced a new diagnostic classification for PTSD in children younger than 6 years. This is the first developmental subtype of an existing disorder in the DSM. It recognizes that young children's expression of their reaction to traumatic events may be more behavioral than verbal, that traumatic re-enactments in play may not necessarily be distressing, and that dreams may be generally fearful rather than trauma-specific. Only a single symptom pertaining to avoidance *or* negative alterations in mood and cognitions is required. Research has suggested that with the new criteria, up to eight times more children would meet the DSM-5 diagnosis compared to DSM-IV.[7] There is still debate as to whether so-called "complex PTSD," which attempts to capture the putative pervasive and negative impact of chronic and repetitive trauma, usually during childhood, should be recognized as a PTSD subtype.

Acute Stress Disorder

DSM-IV introduced a new diagnostic category, acute stress disorder (ASD), to recognize brief stress reactions to traumatic events that are manifest in the first month. Conception was heavily influenced by the theoretical concept of dissociation. To qualify for the ASD diagnosis, both posttraumatic and dissociative symptoms were required (Box 34-2). Because subsequent research has questioned the essential role of dissociation in the short-term psychopathological response to trauma, in DSM-5 symptoms in the dissociative symptom cluster still count towards the diagnosis but are no longer required. Presently any 9 out of the 14 possible intrusion, dissociation, avoidance, and/or arousal symptoms are required, in accordance with the heterogeneity of the condition.[8]

Differential Diagnosis

According to DSM-5, PTSD and ASD need to be differentiated from a number of other disorders. Although adjustment disorder may also result from a traumatic event, it should not be diagnosed if the symptoms that develop following the event qualify for ASD or PTSD. Moreover, adjustment disorder is by definition time-limited, whereas PTSD is not. With regard to anxiety disorders such as panic, generalized anxiety, phobic, and separation anxiety disorders, as well as obsessive-compulsive disorder, although these may share anxiety, unwanted thoughts, and/or avoidance behavior with PTSD, the critical distinction is that in PTSD, the intrusive thoughts and avoidance are specifically related to the causal traumatic event. Thus, it is the DSM-5 B and C criteria (in adults) that are specific to PTSD, whereas the D and E criteria may be shared with other disorders, e.g., depression. PTSD may involve dissociation, but if the full criteria for a dissociative disorder, such as dissociative amnesia or dissociative identity or depersonalization-derealization disorder, are met, this should also be diagnosed. If not, the "with dissociative symptoms" subtype of PTSD should be considered. Differentiating the sensory experiences that may accompany PTSD flashbacks from hallucinations found in psychotic disorders is accomplished by examining whether the sensory experiences are confined to the traumatic event. PTSD is differentiated from ASD by chronology, i.e., time of onset and duration. In patients who have experienced more than one traumatic event, differential diagnosis of which event(s) caused PTSD may be made by discerning to which event(s) the characteristic intrusion and avoidance symptoms pertain.

EPIDEMIOLOGY
Incidence and Prevalence

Because the final DSM-5 criteria for PTSD were only publicized 2 months before this chapter was written, and epidemiological studies take a long time to perform, there have been almost no such studies that have incorporated DSM-5 criteria. For these reasons, it is not possible here to present reliable information regarding the incidence and prevalence of DSM-5-classified PTSD. Instead, this section reviews epidemiological information regarding DSM-IV diagnosis of PTSD, about which more is known. The life-time incidence of DSM-IV PTSD in the general community has been estimated at 8% and its 12-month prevalence at 4%. More than two-thirds of cases manifest moderate to severe functional impairment.[9–11] Women show a higher life-time incidence (10% to 14%) than men (5% to 6%).[12] In mental health treatment–seeking populations, the prevalence of PTSD may be as high as 40% to 50%, including individuals being treated for other conditions not seeking specialized trauma care.[13]

Exposure to *potentially* traumatizing events in the general population is the rule rather than the exception. In the National Comorbidity Survey (NCS), the life-time incidence of exposure to any traumatic event (based on DSM-III-R criteria) was 60% for men and 50% for women.[10] The life-time incidence of exposure to any trauma increases to nearly 90% when the broader DSM-IV exposure criteria are employed.[14] More than half of individuals with trauma exposure report exposure to more than one event.[10] The median number of distinct traumatic events among individuals exposed to any trauma is nearly five.[14]

BOX 34-2 DSM-5 Diagnostic Criteria: Acute Stress Disorder (308.3)

A. Exposure to actual or threatened death, serious injury, or sexual violation in one (or more) of the following ways:
   1. Directly experiencing the traumatic event(s).
   2. Witnessing, in person, the event(s) as it occurred to others.
   3. Learning that the event(s) occurred to a close family member or close friend.

Note: In cases of actual or threatened death of a family member or friend, the event(s) must have been violent or accidental.

   4. Experiencing repeated or extreme exposure to aversive details of the traumatic event(s) (e.g., first responders collecting human remains, police officers repeatedly exposed to details of child abuse).

Note: This does not apply to exposure through electronic media, television, movies, or pictures, unless this exposure is work related.

B. Presence of nine (or more) of the following symptoms from any of the five categories of intrusion, negative mood, dissociation, avoidance, and arousal, beginning or worsening after the traumatic event(s) occurred:

Intrusion Symptoms

   1. Recurrent, involuntary, and intrusive distressing memories of the traumatic event(s).

Note: In children, repetitive play may occur in which themes or aspects of the traumatic event(s) are expressed.

   2. Recurrent distressing dreams in which the content and/or effect of the dream are related to the event(s).

Note: In children, there may be frightening dreams without recognizable content.

   3. Dissociative reactions (e.g., flashbacks) in which the individual feels or acts as if the traumatic event(s) were recurring. (Such reactions may occur on a continuum, with the most extreme expression being a complete loss of awareness of present surroundings.)

Note: In children, trauma-specific reenactment may occur in play.

   4. Intense or prolonged psychological distress or marked physiological reactions in response to internal or external cues that symbolize or resemble an aspect of the traumatic event(s).

Negative Mood

   5. Persistent inability to experience positive emotions (e.g., inability to experience happiness, satisfaction, or loving feelings).
   6. Dissociative symptoms.
   7. An altered sense of the reality of one's surroundings or oneself (e.g., seeing oneself from another's perspective, being in a daze, time slowing).
   8. Inability to remember an important aspect of the traumatic event(s) (typically due to dissociative amnesia and not to other factors such as head injury, alcohol, or drugs).

Avoidance Symptoms

   9. Efforts to avoid distressing memories, thoughts, or feelings about or closely associated with the traumatic event(s).
   10. Efforts to avoid external reminders (people, places, conversations, activities, objects, situations) that arouse distressing memories, thoughts, or feelings about or closely associated with the traumatic event(s).

Arousal Symptoms

   11. Sleep disturbance (e.g., difficulty falling or staying asleep, restless sleep).
   12. Irritable behavior and angry outbursts (with little or no provocation), typically expressed as verbal or physical aggression toward people or objects.
   13. Hypervigilance.
   14. Problems with concentration.
   15. Exaggerated startle response.

C. Duration of the disturbance (symptoms in criterion B) is 3 days to 1 month after trauma exposure.

Note: Symptoms typically begin immediately after the trauma, but persistence for at least 3 days and up to 1 month is needed to meet disorder criteria.

D. The disturbance causes clinically significant distress or impairment in social, occupational, or other important areas of functioning.

E. The disturbance is not attributable to the physiological effects of a substance (e.g., medication or alcohol) or another medical condition (e.g., mild traumatic brain injury) and is not better explained by brief psychotic disorder.

Reprinted with permission from the Diagnostic and statistical manual of mental disorders, *ed 5, (Copyright 2013). American Psychiatric Association.*

Events involving assaultive behavior (e.g., rape, military combat, kidnap/torture, physical assault, molestation) are experienced by roughly 40% of the population, whereas other direct experiences of trauma (e.g., motor vehicle accidents, natural disasters, witnessing others being killed or injured, or being diagnosed with a life-threatening illness) have an estimated life-time prevalence rate of 60%.[14] Events that are only experienced indirectly (e.g., learning that a close friend or relative was assaulted or seriously injured) are reported by over 60% of the population. The nature and type of trauma experienced by men and women differ considerably. NCS data for exposure to trauma are presented in Figure 34-1A. Men more frequently report exposure to physical attacks, combat, being threatened with a weapon, serious accidents, and witnessing others being injured or killed.[10] Men are twice as likely as women to be exposed to assaults, with nearly 35% having been mugged or threatened with a weapon.[14] Women more frequently report having been raped, sexually molested, neglected as children, or physically abused. More than 40% of women have experienced interpersonal violence (including sexual violence and intimate partner violence).[15] Exposure to all classes of trauma in both men and women peaks during late adolescence/early adulthood (ages 16 to 20).[14] This is reflected in the median age of onset (23 years) for PTSD.[16] Exposure to assaultive violence declines precipitously after this period, whereas all other classes of trauma exposure decline only modestly with advancing age or not at all in the case of sudden unexpected death of a close friend or relative (an event that peaks in middle age). In general, the decline in all types of trauma following early adulthood appears to be steeper for women, suggesting that in women the risk of PTSD is especially pronounced during childhood and early adulthood. The demographic variables of race, education, and income level do not appear to affect the risk of exposure to most types of trauma. The clear exception is assaultive violence, in which there is a two-fold increase in exposure prevalence for non-whites vs. whites, for those with less education vs. those with a college education, and for those with low incomes vs. those with high incomes.[14]

NATIONAL CO-MORBIDITY SURVEY

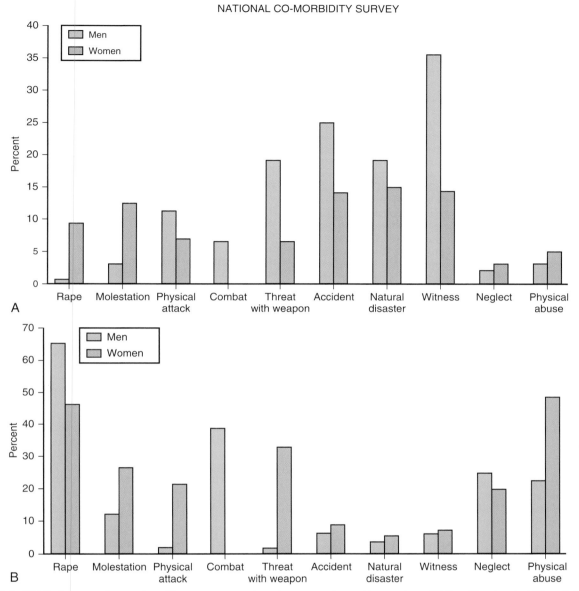

Figure 34-1. (A) Life-time prevalence rates of trauma exposure based upon gender and trauma type. (B) Conditional probabilities of developing PTSD based upon gender and trauma type. *(Data from Kessler RC, Sonnega A, Bromet E, et al. Posttraumatic stress disorder in the National Comorbidity Survey,* Arch Gen Psychiatry *52:1048–1060, 1995.)*

Despite the high prevalence of traumatic exposure, the development of PTSD is the exception rather than the rule. The overall conditional probability of PTSD after a traumatic event is approximately 9%[14]; however, the risk of PTSD varies substantially with the type of trauma experienced. Assaultive violence in general demonstrates the highest probability (over 20%) of leading to PTSD, whereas learning about traumatic events to others carries the lowest probability (2%).[14] Figure 34-1B illustrates the conditional PTSD probabilities associated with specific types of trauma for both men and women based on results from the NCS. Specific traumatic events that carry the highest conditional probability for PTSD include rape (50% or greater), torture/kidnap (50%), combat (nearly 40%), and childhood physical abuse or sexual molestation (25% to 50%).[10,14] Women exposed to trauma are in general more than twice as likely (13% to 20%) to develop PTSD than are men (6% to 8%).[10,14] This general two-fold increase in risk of PTSD

in women is maintained after controlling for the distribution of trauma types. However, women's increased vulnerability to PTSD does not appear to be equally generalizable to all types of trauma. Specifically, the increased risk of a woman developing PTSD occurs predominantly after an assault, in which women demonstrate a PTSD risk with a probability of 35% (vs. 6% in men).[17] A significant portion of this gender difference appears to be attributable to the greater likelihood that women relative to men will meet the avoidance/numbing symptoms (DSM-IV criterion C) required for the diagnosis.

Nearly 40% of all cases of PTSD result from assaultive violence, which reflects the high conditional probability of PTSD associated with this type of trauma.[14] For men, combat exposure alone accounts for a sizeable percentage, approximately 30%, of PTSD.[18] For women, sexual violence accounts for nearly 25% of all PTSD cases, and being "badly beaten up" (including intimate partner violence) constitutes an additional 20% of all cases of PTSD reported by women.[17] Surprisingly, learning of the sudden, unexpected death of a close relative or friend accounts for the second highest proportion of overall PTSD cases (greater than 30%), a finding that reflects the extremely high prevalence for this type of event (60%) despite only a moderate conditional probability for PTSD (14%).[14] Approximately 23% of all PTSD cases result from direct exposure to non-assaultive events (e.g., accidents, natural disasters, witnessing death).

As a final note in considering the rates of DSM-IV PTSD described above, it is important to recognize the "fluid" nature of epidemiological data; that is, reported prevalence rates are estimates that are not written in stone. Epidemiological studies of PTSD have shown that multiple methodological factors can affect the reported prevalence and risk rates of PTSD. Different diagnostic instruments (e.g., the Diagnostic Interview Schedule [DIS] vs. the Structured Clinical Interview for DSM [SCID]) and data-gathering procedures (e.g., telephone vs. in-person interview) can produce widely disparate prevalence estimates in the same population. Methodological variations in the documentation of traumatic events or the validation of symptom status or functional impairment can also have a significant impact on estimates. A recent re-examination of the well-known National Vietnam Veterans Readjustment Study (NVVRS)[19] illustrates this point. The NVVRS is often cited for its estimate of a life-time PTSD prevalence of 30.9% in Vietnam veterans.[20] Employing the same database, the re-examination study provided a more systematic military record documentation of trauma exposure, differentiated war-related from pre-war symptom onset, and factored in distress levels and severity of social/occupational impairment. Based on such refinements, the overall life-time prevalence of PTSD in Vietnam veterans was reduced to approximately 19%, nearly a 40% change from the original estimate. It is unknown to what degree other accepted epidemiological "facts" may be challenged by future refinements. Recognizing the mutable and evolving nature of prevalence and risk estimates for PTSD has important implications regarding the establishment of future public health policy, as well as our understanding of the significance of such constructs as resiliency and "normative" response to trauma.

Empirical studies have suggested that the DSM-IV ASD symptom cluster occurs in 10% to 30% of individuals exposed to trauma. Prospective studies suggest that 72% to 83% of those diagnosed with ASD go on to develop DSM-IV PTSD at 6 months after the trauma, and 63% to 80% have PTSD at 2 years after the trauma.[21] When the dissociation criterion is removed from the DSM-IV ASD diagnosis, comparable rates of subsequent PTSD are observed, i.e., 60% of patients with ASD (minus dissociation) are reported to have PTSD 6 months after the trauma, and 70% report symptoms of PTSD 2 years after the trauma.[22,23] However, the majority of persons who develop PTSD have not had diagnosable ASD.[24] Application of the standard DSM-IV PTSD diagnostic criteria, without the 1-month duration, in the first month following trauma has been as effective as the ASD diagnosis in predicting subsequent and persistent PTSD.[25,26] Some argue that ASD and PTSD represent the same disorder, the latter being merely differentiated by an arbitrary month-long duration criterion. In other words, ASD may simply exemplify "acute PTSD" as defined in the earlier DSM-III.[26] In contrast, others conceptualize ASD as an acute stress response. Regardless, the clinical utility of the ASD diagnosis has been supported by studies that have shown that the employment of specific treatment approaches (e.g., exposure therapy, cognitive therapy, stress management) for such individuals leads to lower rates of later PTSD relative to ASD patients who are either untreated or who receive only general, supportive counseling.[21]

Co-morbidity

Psychiatric co-morbidity is the rule rather than the exception in PTSD. The percentage of a life-time history of other psychiatric disorders in individuals diagnosed with PTSD has been estimated by the NCS at nearly 90% in men and 80% in women. In fact, nearly 60% of men and 45% of women with PTSD report more than three co-morbid psychiatric conditions.[10] Major depressive disorder (MDD) is among the most common of co-morbid conditions for both men and women, affecting nearly 50%. Alcohol abuse (in the majority) and conduct disorder (over 40%) are also highly co-morbid in men. Additionally, there is a three-fold to seven-fold increased risk for both men and women with PTSD of being diagnosed with other anxiety disorders, including generalized anxiety disorder (GAD), panic disorder, and specific phobias. High levels of psychiatric co-morbidity in PTSD may result from the substantial symptom overlap between PTSD and disorders such as MDD (with a loss of interest, social withdrawal, insomnia, and poor concentration) and other anxiety disorders (manifest by hyperarousal and avoidance). NCS results suggest that, more often than not, PTSD is primary with respect to co-morbid affective disorders and substance abuse disorders, but secondary with respect to co-morbid anxiety disorders (and for men, co-morbid conduct disorder).[10] Most studies have failed to find an increased risk of MDD or drug abuse for trauma-exposed individuals who are not diagnosed with PTSD.[12] The same has been found for alcohol abuse or dependence in males, but not females. This suggests that MDD and substance abuse (with the exception of alcohol abuse in women) are not likely to be psychiatric conditions that independently occur outside of PTSD in response to trauma; rather they appear more likely either to be the result of PTSD (i.e., an emotional response to impairment and "self-medication" through substance abuse) and/or of shared antecedent genetic or environmental factors (i.e., a shared liability for both PTSD and depression/substance abuse).

The circumstances of combat in the recent military operations Enduring Freedom and Iraqi Freedom (OEF/OIF) have resulted in a high co-occurrence of PTSD and mild traumatic brain injury (TBI). There is evidence to suggest that persons with mild TBI are at risk for developing PTSD, after adjusting for trauma exposure.[27] This recent research trend contrasts with the notion that TBI prevents PTSD due to impaired consciousness at the time of the traumatic event. The co-occurrence of PTSD and TBI is likely to complicate matters of diagnosis due to symptom overlap. However, there should be no mistake that TBI and PTSD have entirely different causes, i.e., a physical blow to the brain in the former vs. exposure to psychologically distressing information in the latter. The possibility that cognitive impairments seen in TBI could compromise the efficacy of psychological treatments for PTSD that utilize a cognitive approach has yet to be systematically evaluated.

Risk Factors

An understanding of relevant risk factors for the development of PTSD is complicated by the fact that independent risks may exist for an increased exposure to traumatic events as well as for an increased susceptibility for the development of PTSD upon exposure to traumatic events. Research into the heritability of PTSD illustrates this complexity. Combat and civilian twin studies have estimated the heritability of exposure to trauma as between 20% and 50%.[28,29] Furthermore, exposure to different types of trauma may be differentially mediated by genetic factors. The likelihood of exposure to traumatic events involving assaultive violence appears to be highly influenced by genetics, whereas event exposure involving non-assaultive trauma appears to be largely non-genetic.[29] It has been proposed that one pathway underlying genetic predisposition to traumatic exposure may be mediated through heritable personality traits (e.g., neuroticism, antisocial behavior, extroversion, sensation-seeking) that increase the risk of experiencing a traumatic event. It has been reported, for example, that the likelihood of experiencing a violent assault is predicted by antisocial personality traits as well as the more non-pathological personality style of "being open to new ideas and experiences," with genetic factors accounting for upwards of 10% of the relationship between personality and trauma exposure.[30]

Once exposed to a traumatic event, the conditional risk of PTSD also appears to be substantially influenced by genetics. Both combat and civilian trauma twin studies estimate the heritability of PTSD to be approximately 30% to 40% after controlling for trauma exposure.[29,31] Heritability appears to be comparable among the three DSM-IV symptom clusters (i.e., re-experiencing, avoidance/numbing, and arousal). It remains unclear as to whether genetic factors for risk of PTSD are different for men and women or for different trauma types.

Beyond genetics, factors that have been found to be predictive of a vulnerability to PTSD fall into three broad categories: pretraumatic (factors present before trauma exposure), peritraumatic (factors noted at the time of trauma or shortly thereafter), and posttraumatic (factors that may influence not only the development of PTSD but also the capacity to recover from it).[32] Many of the identified pretraumatic factors are not well understood, e.g., whether their impact is attributable to the likelihood of traumatic event exposure or to PTSD liability once exposed; in some cases they are implicated in both. Meta-analytic studies have identified several pretraumatic factors (female gender, previous trauma exposure, a history of MDD or an anxiety disorder, a history of mental disorder in the family, an earlier age of traumatic exposure, and a social/educational/intellectual disadvantage) for an increased risk of PTSD.[32,33]

Previous trauma exposure has been well established as a risk factor for PTSD after subsequent traumas. The impact of previous trauma is particularly significant when prior exposure involves assaultive violence or more than one previous traumatic event (assaultive or non-assaultive). A history of two or more traumatic events of assaultive violence in childhood has been shown to increase the risk of PTSD to an adulthood traumatic event by a factor of five.[34] Combat veterans who develop PTSD are more likely to have histories of childhood abuse (estimated at 25% to 45%).[35,36] The impact of previous assaultive trauma on increasing the rate of PTSD with subsequent trauma appears to persist without a decrement across time. In contrast, the sensitizing impact of previous non-assaultive trauma does appear to weaken over time (estimated at an 8% attenuation rate per year).[34]

Pretraumatic psychiatric symptomatology, especially of MDD, anxiety disorders, neuroticism, and conduct/antisocial personality disorder, is relevant both to the increased risk of traumatic event exposure and to an increased susceptibility to PTSD once exposed. A history of affective disorder may be more prominent as a risk factor in women, whereas a history of anxiety disorder or a parental psychiatric history may be of greater relevance as a risk factor in men.[37] An earlier age of trauma exposure has not been consistently found to be predictive of PTSD; however, an earlier age of onset may constitute a risk for a more chronic course of PTSD. The impact of lower educational and socioeconomic status on heightened PTSD risk has been previously described. In addition, a number of studies (primarily in combat veterans) have identified pre-existing cognitive/intellectual capacity as a risk factor that accounts for 10% to 20% of the variance associated with PTSD

severity.[38,39] Above-average cognitive capacity appears to confer a relative protective effect for those trauma survivors who do not develop PTSD. Such findings are consistent with research that suggests that higher-order cognitive reasoning and verbal encoding of traumatic events may reduce the more persistent negative effects of traumatic exposure.

The most frequently cited peri-traumatic risk factors for PTSD include severity of the trauma, dissociative reactions, excessively heightened arousal, feelings of anger/shame, and reduced social support. Meta-analytic studies of these factors tend to reveal effect sizes in the small to moderate range (0.10 to 0.40 d).[32,33] A significant dose–response relationship is routinely observed between the severity or duration of a traumatic event and the likelihood of developing PTSD. A recent examination of combat veterans employing objective measures of traumatic event severity found the life-time prevalence rates of PTSD to be three-fold to four-fold greater among high-combat-stress veterans vs. low-combat-stress veterans and nearly 30-fold greater when examining the prevalence of PTSD more than 10 years after combat.[19] Findings regarding the significance of traumatic event severity are also reported among most non-combat trauma studies. Likewise, peri-traumatic dissociation (acute feelings of depersonalization, derealization, or amnesia at the time of the traumatic event) has frequently been cited as a significant risk factor for chronic PTSD. A comprehensive meta-analysis has recently reported an average effect size in the moderate range (0.35 d) for studies that examined the risk of PTSD associated with peri-traumatic dissociation.[33] However, some studies have failed to replicate this association and have criticized current estimates on the basis of a failure to control for moderating variables (e.g., dissociation effect is attenuated when controlling for more general personality variables, such as neuroticism) and failure to account for time parameters (e.g., persistent dissociation and emotional disengagement well beyond the traumatic event has been found to be a stronger predictor of PTSD than peri-traumatic dissociation).[40,41] A number of studies have suggested that physiological indices of excessive autonomic arousal following trauma exposure are associated with increased probability of PTSD at 4 months and 2 years.[24,42]

Among posttraumatic risk factors for PTSD, quality of social support and additional life stress have emerged as especially important.[32] Meta-analytic studies have identified effect sizes in the moderate range (0.40 d) regarding the protective effect of social support. Some studies have suggested that the presence of a negative social environment (e.g., blaming, disbelief) has a stronger impact on risk for chronic PTSD than mere absence of perceived positive support. Furthermore, recent research involving victims of violent crime has found that, although men and women were equally likely to report having received positive support, women were significantly more likely to report the presence of negative responses from family and friends.[43] In turn, negative responses were found to be predictive of PTSD at 6 months, with this relationship being stronger among women than men. The presence of anger or guilt has also been found to be predictive of the development and maintenance of PTSD, particularly among crime victims, child abuse survivors, and combat veterans. Those who report persistent feelings of shame are significantly more likely to report a greater presence and severity of all three PTSD symptom clusters both 1 and 6 years following abuse recognition.[44]

PROGNOSIS
Recovery and Course of Illness

Most psychological trauma victims manifest PTSD symptoms shortly following exposure, but fortunately most people recover from these within the first month. It has even been claimed that 94% of victims met PTSD symptom criteria, except for the required 1-month duration, a week following being raped.[45] Following the Oklahoma City bombing, symptoms of PTSD began within 1 day of the bombing in 76% of cases, within the first week in 94%, and within the first month in 98%.[46] For those who go on to meet the full-blown PTSD diagnosis, epidemiological studies suggest a remission rate of approximately 25% at 6 months and 40% at 1 year.[14] The median time to remission has been estimated at 2–3 years.[10,14] Regardless of treatment, more than 30% of individuals diagnosed with PTSD never have their symptoms remit. If PTSD remission has not occurred within six to seven years after the trauma, the chance for significant recovery thereafter appears to be quite small.[10] An estimated 10% to 15% of all Vietnam combat veterans, and nearly 30% of those with high or very high combat exposure, were found to have PTSD 12 years following the cessation of combat.[19,20] Twenty-eight percent of adult survivors of the Buffalo Creek flood failed to show remission from PTSD after 14 years.[47] In a longitudinal study of Israeli veterans from the 1982 Lebanon War, 36% met PTSD criteria 20 years later.[48] Many of the risk factors for the development of PTSD also appear to be relevant to increased risk for a chronic course (e.g., co-morbidity, multiple trauma exposures, negative social support, trauma severity). In addition, the presence and intensity of avoidance and numbing symptoms (DSM-IV criterion C) may specifically predispose toward a chronic, rather than a remitting, course of illness in PTSD.[49]

Suicide Attempts

A number of studies have identified PTSD as a robust risk factor for suicide ideation and attempts irrespective of trauma type. A diagnosis of PTSD has been associated with a threefold to five-fold increase in suicide ideation and a three-fold to six-fold increase in suicide attempts.[50,51] This association has gained increasing recognition in the wake of the wars in Iraq and Afghanistan.[52] In a multivariate prediction model based on NCS suicide data, the diagnosis of PTSD represents one of a limited number of factors identified as most parsimoniously predictive of suicide attempts. At least two additional risk factors (MDD and substance abuse/dependence) have been identified as common co-morbid conditions in PTSD. Based on risk analysis data from the NCS, the probability of a suicide attempt in PTSD patients would be markedly increased by the presence of either MDD or substance abuse (odds ratio = 21) or both (odds ratio = 125).[50] This translates into a life-time conditional probability of making a suicide attempt equal to 17% (per annum probability = 0.1%) for PTSD alone, with a 26% life-time probability (per annum probability = 0.2%) for PTSD plus co-morbid MDD or substance abuse, and a 32% life-time probability (per annum probability = 1%) for PTSD plus both co-morbid MDD and substance abuse. The lethality of suicide attempts or the percentage of successful suicide attempts in individuals diagnosed with PTSD has not been empirically established.

Impairment

Occupational and social impairment secondary to PTSD appears to be substantial.[53,54] Individuals diagnosed with PTSD report an average increase of nearly 1 lost work-day per month, as well as nearly 3 days per month in reduced productivity, due to psychiatric symptomatology.[55] These figures are higher than almost all other psychiatric diagnoses examined (including MDD, dysthymia, and substance abuse disorders), with only GAD and panic disorder demonstrating higher work-day losses. In an examination of the worst 30-day period

in the past year, PTSD patients reported a total work loss of nearly 14 days within that period due to distress about their traumatic experiences.[56] Studies of PTSD in primary care settings report significantly increased numbers of hospitalizations for medical/physical problems, significantly more emergency department visits, and higher utilization of medical care.[57] Significant social impairments in the areas of marital/parenting/family function and general quality of life have frequently been reported for patients with chronic PTSD. During the worst 30-day period (when most upset about traumatic experiences) over the past year, individuals diagnosed with PTSD report nearly 17 of those days in which they spent less time with people and experienced more problems with tension and disagreement. Higher divorce rates, impaired attachment with child, and family violence have been associated with individuals with PTSD more than those without PTSD.[58]

PATHOGENESIS

A critical factor in the path to PTSD is subjective appraisal of the traumatic event. Appraisal helps answer the often-asked question, "How is it that two persons can experience the same traumatic event, and one develops PTSD and the other does not?" The first answer to this question is that two people never experience exactly the same traumatic event. Two soldiers can be in the same foxhole during the same battle but be looking in opposite directions, and their experience will differ. Even if they see the same thing, e.g., enemy soldiers about to over-run their position, one soldier may be thinking that reinforcements will arrive to save them, whereas another may be thinking that everyone is going to be slaughtered. By virtue of different appraisals, the second soldier will be more terrified than the first and hence more likely to develop PTSD. The contributing factors of unpredictability and uncontrollability increase the likelihood of a response manifested by intense fear or helplessness.

Freud characterized traumatic anxiety as the affect that develops when it becomes no longer possible to avoid, or do anything about, a threatening situation, and the ego becomes overwhelmed. A prominent feature of the traumatized response is hyperarousal. A large epidemiological study performed by the Rand Corporation documented that posttraumatic hyperarousal strongly influences, but is not generally influenced by, other PTSD symptom clusters. The investigators concluded that hyperarousal plays a prominent role in the natural course of posttraumatic psychological distress.[59] How hyperarousal contributes to PTSD remains to be elucidated, but it is likely to involve both conditioning and non-conditioning (e.g., sensitization) mechanisms. In support of the latter, results of an identical twin study support the conclusion that increased heart rate response to loud tones, an unconditioned measure of arousal, is acquired as a result of the traumatic event in combat veterans who develop PTSD.[60] It is likely that peripheral sympathetic arousal is secondary to central nervous system changes (e.g., amygdala hyper(re)activity), which are primary in mediating PTSD's pathogenesis (see discussion of neuroimaging findings in PTSD elsewhere in this chapter).

A current translational model of PTSD's pathogenesis posits the following. A traumatic event (unconditioned stimulus) overstimulates endogenous stress hormones, such as epinephrine (unconditioned response); these mediate an over-consolidation of the event's memory traces. Then, recall of the event in response to reminders (conditioned stimulus) releases further stress hormones (conditioned response); these cause further over-consolidation, and the over-consolidated memory generates PTSD symptoms.[61] An important paradox that needs to be clarified in future research is that, although adrenergic mechanisms appear to be critically involved in PTSD's pathogenesis, antidepressant drugs that are thought to act primarily through serotonergic mechanisms represent the pharmacological treatment of choice for this disorder.

The adequacy of the above, static, peri-traumatic model of PTSD's pathogenesis has been challenged by posttraumatic considerations. It has been reported that most persons who are exposed to a traumatic event experience at least some PTSD symptoms in the acute aftermath. However, only a minority qualify for a PTSD diagnosis 1 month later. This observation suggests a role for *failure to recover* from initial posttraumatic symptoms in PTSD's pathogenesis. This ability to recover may be conceptualized from the standpoint of Pavlovian fear extinction. Extinction involves no longer responding with fear to previously-feared stimuli and situations. As with acquisition, this is a learning process. Perhaps even more important is the ability to retain extinction learning, i.e., to remember that a previously-dangerous stimulus or situation is now safe. Recent research has shown that PTSD patients show a psychophysiological extinction retention deficit.[62] The ventromedial prefrontal cortex is critical for extinction retention. PTSD subjects fail to activate this brain area during extinction recall testing[63] (Figure 34-2).

Psychophysiology

For 30 years, findings from psychophysiological research have played an important role in characterizing the psychobiology of PTSD and assessing key features of the disorder as specified in the DSM. The symptom "marked physiological reactions to internal or external cues that symbolize or resemble an aspect of the traumatic event(s)" (DSM-5 criterion B.5) has received considerable attention. A consistent picture has emerged demonstrating greater peripheral (e.g., electrodermal, heart rate, facial electromyogram) reactivity to stimuli that represent or are related to the traumatic events of individuals who develop PTSD.[61,64,65] This heightened reactivity is stable over time[66] and has been observed across individuals with PTSD resulting from a wide range of traumatic events (such as combat, sexual assault, motor vehicle accidents, cancer diagnosis, or witnessing horrific events). When assessed soon after a traumatic event, heightened physiological reactivity to trauma-related cues is predictive of subsequent severity and/or persistence of PTSD symptoms.[67-70] Approximately 60%–70% of individuals who meet diagnostic criteria for PTSD show heightened psychophysiological reactivity when exposed to reminders of their particular traumatic event. The presence or absence of

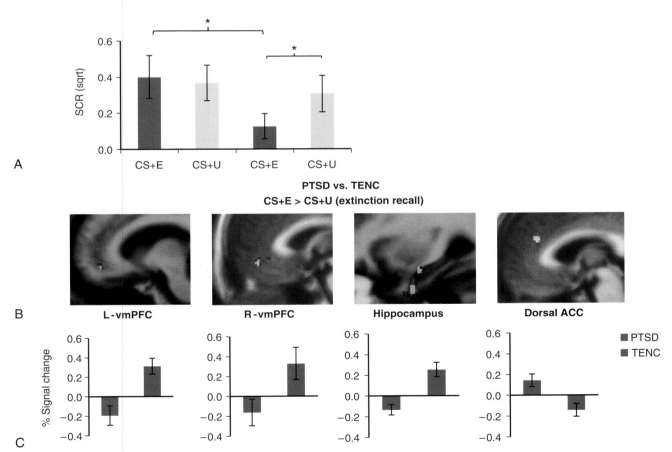

Figure 34-2. Responses of posttraumatic stress disorder (PTSD) and trauma-exposed non-PTSD control (TENC) subjects during extinction recall. (A) Skin conductance responses to the stimulus that was previously extinguished on day 1 (CS+E, dark shading) vs. the CS that was not extinguished on day 1 (CS+U, light shading) in PTSD (red) vs. TENC (blue) subjects. * p < 0.05. (B) Group × Stimulus interactions. Talairach coordinates: left ventromedial prefrontal cortex (L-vmPFC): x = –10, y = 43, z = –11; right vmPFC (R-vmPFC): x = 2, y = 45, z = –12; hippocampus, x = 32, y = –9, z = –27; dorsal anterior cingulate cortex (dACC): x = –2, y = 37, z =18. All images were masked to only show activations/deactivations in hypothesized brain regions. Threshold for displaying the images is set at p = 0.01. (C) Percent signal change extracted from the functional regions of interest shown in B. *(Reproduced from Figure 3 in Milad MR, Pitman RK, Ellis CB, et al. Neurobiological basis of failure to recall extinction memory in posttraumatic stress disorder.* Biol Psychiatry 66(12), 2009.)

heightened psychophysiological reactivity to trauma-related cues could reflect different subtypes of PTSD, e.g., fear-based vs. distress-based PTSD.[66] Few individuals who do not meet diagnostic criteria for PTSD show this heightened reactivity.[71] Psychophysiological reactivity to trauma-related cues has also been found useful as a measure of treatment outcome.[72,73] The fact that some individuals can meet diagnostic criteria for PTSD, yet show little or no psychophysiological reactivity when confronted with trauma-related cues, raises interesting questions regarding whether it is reasonable to assume that self-reported experiences provide an adequate basis on which to establish the PTSD diagnosis.

Another PTSD symptom that has been the focus of considerable psychophysiological investigation is exaggerated startle (DSM-5 criterion E.4). Exaggerated startle has long been recognized as a central feature of post-trauma reactions and may be one of the most reliably reported symptoms of the disorder. However, research support for exaggerated startle, which typically is measured from the eye-blink response to a brief, sudden, loud acoustic stimulus, has been somewhat unreliable.[65,74] Context is an important moderator of the startle response and may help to explain the equivocal findings. Specifically, individuals with PTSD have been found to more reliably show increased startle in the presence of contextual anxiety cues (e.g., anticipation of a threatened shock or needle stick).[74] This suggests that PTSD is associated with a heightened sensitivity to threatening cues or contexts. Findings from prospective studies[75-77] and a study of monozygotic twins discordant for trauma exposure and PTSD[71] suggest that exaggerated eye-blink startle is not a pre-existing marker of risk for PTSD.

Increased heart rate response to repeated presentations of brief loud-tone stimuli has proven to be a reliable feature of PTSD; increased skin conductance and eye-blink electromyogram, less so.[61] Converging data suggest that this increased heart rate response likely reflects reduced parasympathetic activity,[78] whereas the characteristically increased heart rate reactivity to trauma-related reminders observed in individuals with PTSD likely reflects increased sympathetic activity.[60,79] Findings suggest that increased heart rate reactivity to loud tones is not a pretraumatic trait but rather is acquired with the development of PTSD.[71,79,80] A reduction/normalization of increased heart rate reactivity to loud tones has been observed following successful treatment of PTSD symptoms.[81] Whereas eye-blink and heart rate responses to loud-tone/noise stimuli do not appear to be pretraumatic predictors of pretraumatic stress symptoms or PTSD, there is evidence that pretraumatic heightened skin conductance reactivity and/or slower habituation of skin conductance responses to loud-tone/noise stimuli may predict increased risk for post-trauma stress symptoms.[65,75-77]

Over the past decade there has seen a growing focus on the potential relationship between PTSD and conditioned-fear abnormalities. Re-experiencing symptoms, such as psychological distress or physiological reactivity upon exposure to trauma-related cues (DSM-5 criteria B.4 and B.5), are a defining feature of PTSD that can be conceptualized within a fear-conditioning framework. There is some evidence that individuals with, compared to without, PTSD show stronger skin conductance responding to cues paired with an aversive unconditioned stimulus (e.g. a mild electric shock) during acquisition of a conditioned fear response.[82] However, deficits in the ability to extinguish or maintain extinction learning of a conditioned fear response may be more relevant features of PTSD.[83] A study of identical twins discordant for combat exposure and PTSD found that poorer extinction retention of a fear-conditioned skin conductance response is an acquired response of PTSD.[62] On the other hand, pretraumatic poorer

extinction of a conditioned corrugator electromyogram response in police and firefighter recruits predicted greater PTSD-related symptoms following a traumatic event.[76,84]

Biology

Although PTSD is still largely regarded as a psychological phenomenon, over the past three decades the growth of the biological PTSD literature has been explosive, as has recently been reviewed with extensive references.[85] It is tempting to assume that because PTSD by definition is caused by a psychologically-traumatic environmental event, any biological abnormality found to accompany PTSD must also have been traumatically induced. However, it is also possible that an abnormality predated the traumatic event and came to be associated with PTSD because it increased the risk of this disorder's developing upon the traumatic exposure—a psychiatric epitome of gene × environment interaction.

The most replicated structural abnormality found in PTSD is lower volume of the hippocampus.[86] Lower volume of the ventromedial prefrontal cortex (vmPFC) has also been reported.[87] The degree to which these abnormalities represent pre-existing risk factors vs. acquired abnormalities is still being researched. To the extent that diminished volume may underlie diminished function, these findings, whatever their origin, are consistent with a model of PTSD that posits a reduced cortical capacity to inhibit fear and other negative emotional responses. The hippocampus may fail to utilize contextual cues in the environment to signal safety, and the vmPFC may fail to adaptively maintain extinction of conditioned emotional responses once traumatic learning is no longer relevant. Functional neuroimaging studies using positron emission tomography (PET) or functional magnetic resonance imaging (fMRI) have shown hyperactivity in the amygdala (which co-ordinates the fear and other emotional responses), and the dorsal anterior cingulate cortex (dACC), and hypoactivity in the ventromedial prefrontal cortex (vmPFC).[88] Neurocircuitry models of PTSD posit that the vmPFC fails to inhibit the amygdala, leading to attentional bias toward threat, increased fear responses, impaired extinction of traumatic memories and its retention, and deficits in emotion regulation.

Numerous studies have provided compelling evidence for the presence of sympathetic system hyperreactivity in PTSD.[89] It has been suggested that an excessively strong adrenergic response to the traumatic event may mediate the formation of the durable traumatic memories that in part characterize the disorder.[90] In contrast, neuropeptide Y (NPY), which is co-released with norepinephrine (noradrenaline), has protective effects during stress. Lower NPY levels have been associated with more PTSD symptoms. Paradoxically, PTSD is not characterized by elevated tonic cortisol levels, as might be expected in a state of chronic stress. Rather, greater suppression of plasma cortisol after a low dose of dexamethasone is consistent with excessive shutting down of the hypothalamic–pituitary–adrenocortical (HPA) axis due to enhanced sensitivity to negative feedback.[91] A recent study found that high-dose cortisol administration within hours of a traumatic event reduced the subsequent development of PTSD.[92] Levels of the neuroactive steroids allopregnanolone and pregnanolone are negatively associated with PTSD re-experiencing and depressive symptoms.[93]

The genes that increase PTSD risk are not selective in that they typically also confer risk for other mental disorders, such as anxiety disorders and depression. As with other mental disorders, genetic liability to PTSD likely involves the contributions of numerous alleles of small effect, complicating the identification of selected target genes for potential preventive or therapeutic intervention.[85] Further complicating matters, the same gene may confer either risk or resilience depending on such factors as prevalent community crime and unemployment rates,[94] illustrating that genes do not act in isolation, but rather interact with the environment to produce their effects. PTSD itself represents an epitome of this interaction. An exciting frontier of PTSD research is epigenesis, which is the ability of the environment to turn the genome on or off by modifying not the Deoxyribonucleic acid (DNA) sequence itself, but rather its transcription (expression) through the macromolecular mechanisms of DNA methylation and histone deacetylation. Epigenetic effects of traumatic exposure may lie at the heart of PTSD's pathogenesis and may account for trauma's durable effects.[85]

TREATMENT
Utilization

Limited and delayed treatment-seeking significantly contribute to morbidity in PTSD. These factors likely reflect, in part, the avoidance symptoms inherent in the disorder. NCS data suggest that only 7% of individuals make treatment contact within the first year of PTSD onset.[95] This figure compares unfavorably with most other psychiatric disorders, including GAD (33%), panic disorder (34%), MDD (37%), dysthymia (42%), bipolar disorder (39%), and alcohol dependence (21%). The median duration of delay in seeking treatment for PTSD is 12 years. Those who do seek treatment from mental health professionals are seen for an average of 22 visits per year (highest among all psychiatric diagnoses with the exception of non-affective psychosis). The projected life-time proportion of PTSD cases that will make it to treatment is 65% (compared with approximately 90% for MDD and bipolar disorder).[95]

Psychotherapy

A variety of psychological interventions have been advocated for the treatment of PTSD, including prolonged exposure therapy, cognitive therapy, stress management, psychodynamic therapy, and eye movement desensitization and reprocessing (EMDR). The PTSD psychotherapy outcome literature has focused primarily on trauma-focused cognitive-behavioral approaches (prolonged exposure and cognitive processing) and EMDR. These approaches lend themselves readily to randomized-controlled trial (RCT) designs due to their brief duration (generally 6 to 14 sessions) and highly structured nature (easily "manualized" into a standardized treatment package). However, results of studies investigating specific psychodynamic approaches, which have likewise been operationalized into a standardized brief treatment package (e.g., interpersonal therapy which may offer an alternative to individuals who cannot tolerate an exposure treatment component), suggest efficacy that may be comparable to the more empirically, established cognitive-behavioral approaches.[96]

The outcomes of research literature has consistently demonstrated the efficacy of cognitive-behavioral approaches in the treatment of PTSD, which is regarded in many practice guidelines as a first-line treatment. In a meta-analysis, trauma-focused cognitive-behavioral therapy (CBT) was found superior over waiting-list or usual care in improving PTSD symptoms as well as co-morbid symptoms of depression and anxiety.[97] Recent data have suggested that most patients receiving CBT maintained their symptom improvement years after the treatment.[98] Exposure therapy (sometimes known as flooding or implosive therapy) involves confronting traumatic memories by having the patient "re-live" the experience in a safe therapeutic setting, either through mental imagery or when practical by actual exposure to physical reminders, e.g.,

the place where the traumatic event occurred (*in vivo* exposure). Virtual reality may also be employed. Modes of therapeutic action are thought to involve blocking negative reinforcement associated with avoidance, extinction of anxiety/fear responses, incorporation of safety information into the traumatic memory, and differentiation of the traumatic event from the current context. Cognitive processing therapy involves confronting and challenging erroneous or over-generalized beliefs that are developed in the context of trauma and often involve themes of safety, trust, control, and self-esteem (e.g., "The world is unsafe." "I'm incompetent to take care of myself"). Exposure and cognitive therapy approaches often overlap in practice. A meta-analysis of cognitive-behavioral approaches found an average short-term improvement rate of 53% for those completing exposure treatment (42% for individuals who enter treatment, including non-completers, i.e., intent-to-treat sample) and 48% for cognitive therapy completers (38% of intent-to-treat sample).[99]

EMDR involves asking patients to develop a mental image of their traumatic event while tracking an alternating bilateral stimulus (most commonly the therapist's fingers being moved back and forth across the patient's visual field). Unlike the cognitive-behavioral approaches, the development of EMDR was not theory-driven and to date no clear mode of therapeutic action has been established. Questions have been raised regarding the necessity of the visual tracking component and whether EMDR may actually represent a different application of exposure and cognitive-behavioral treatment elements.[100] Nevertheless RCTs have demonstrated the efficacy of EMDR as a treatment modality. The same meta-analysis applied to cognitive-behavioral approaches found a mean improvement rate of 60% in EMDR treatment completers (52% of intent-to-treat sample).[99] These figures are comparable to those reported for cognitive-behavioral approaches.

The majority of meta-analytic and "head-to-head" comparison studies have failed to find differential efficacy among the empirically-studied psychotherapies described previously.[99-102] Nor have combination treatments been found to be more effective than individual approaches alone.[103,104] Furthermore, systematic data are lacking to guide decisions regarding differential effectiveness of various treatments for different types of trauma. Meta-analytic reviews have suggested that some populations may be less responsive to treatment in general (e.g., combat veterans), whereas other populations may be relatively more responsive to treatment (e.g., women). However, specific treatment approaches have not been empirically established as more or less effective for specific trauma populations. Although brief cognitive-behavioral and EMDR approaches have produced substantial post-treatment improvements for individuals diagnosed with PTSD, these approaches have yet to establish long-term effectiveness. Given the chronic nature of PTSD (as described elsewhere), this poses a concern regarding clinical utility.

Outcome studies in PTSD often report percentages of treated patients who no longer "meet criteria for PTSD diagnosis" at the end of treatment. Although these percentages can be impressive, they can also be misleading. Far from suggesting a "cure" or even substantial improvement, a change in a single symptom can move a treatment participant from a diagnosis of PTSD to non-PTSD. Meta-analyses have found average percentages of patients who "lost their PTSD diagnosis" to be higher-than-average percentage of patients who met investigator-defined "improvement" criteria.

As opposed to "efficacy," which has largely been demonstrated in the ivory tower under controlled conditions and in selected populations (i.e., academic research settings), psychotherapies for PTSD have not yet been unequivocally shown to be "effective," that is, helpful for patients encountered in ordinary clinical settings. Dropout rates even in efficacy RCTs of PTSD treatments may in some cases run as high as 40%, with the average dropout rate estimated at nearly 25%.[99,104] In some cases, clinical trials do not account for "dropouts" that occur before treatment randomization, thus underestimating the true rates of treatment implementation failures that would be relevant to a practicing clinician. Furthermore, dropout rates in clinical settings may run even higher. A study of completion rates of cognitive-behavioral treatment for PTSD in a clinical setting (employing few exclusion criteria) found only 28% of patients to complete treatment.[105] Over 40% of those who started exposure therapy did not complete it; 76% of patients who dropped out did so even before starting treatment. Treatment dropout was found to be related to PTSD symptom severity; co-morbid borderline personality disorder; higher depression, avoidance, and arousal levels; and social impairment. Thus, in clinical settings, the potential effectiveness of empirically-supported PTSD therapies must be judged against the backdrop of significant proportions of patients who will fail to engage in or complete such treatments.

Also relevant to effectiveness, it is unclear to what degree the study populations employed in the majority of laboratory-setting RCTs of CBT and EMDR are representative of PTSD cases encountered by clinicians. Nearly one-third of patients referred for treatment for PTSD in RCTs are excluded based on conditions that a typical clinician in practice would not have the option to exclude (e.g., suicidal ideation, substance abuse, co-morbid Axis I or II conditions).[99] Little has been empirically established regarding the differential effectiveness of these treatments with more complex case presentations and the co-morbid presence of serious Axis I or Axis II conditions. For reasons of maintaining internal validity, clinical trials of PTSD treatments are frequently and understandably focused on creating homogeneous populations of relatively "pure" PTSD cases. Given the high rates of co-morbidity in PTSD (as reviewed above), these limitations do not provide clinicians with easy guidelines for applying the empirically-supported therapies to complex, poly-symptomatic patients who may be encountered frequently in ordinary clinical practice.

Few clinicians actually employ the empirically supported therapies described above. In a large-scale survey of psychologists, only 17% used exposure therapy to treat PTSD.[106] Moreover, even among psychologists fully trained in, and familiar with, exposure therapy, one-third did not use exposure therapy at all with their PTSD patients, and a majority of the clinicians used the intervention with less than half of their PTSD patients. Dissemination of empirically-validated therapies remains a challenge.

Recently there have been efforts to implement cognitive-behavioral therapies closer to the occurrence of the traumatic event and more towards secondary prevention as opposed to waiting for patients to enter therapy when PTSD has become chronic. One way to do this is to target patients with ASD in an effort to forestall the development of PTSD. Results obtained so far suggest that this approach is promising.[107] A large RCT of early intervention to prevent PTSD supported the efficacy of prolonged exposure and cognitive therapy, but not of the selective serotonin re-uptake inhibitor (SSRI) escitalopram, in reducing the PTSD outcome compared to a waiting-list control condition.[108]

In the immediate aftermath of exposure to a traumatic event capable of causing PTSD, victims should be advised to make use of available social support systems (e.g., family and friends, clergy, family doctors). Medical assistance should be sought when necessary for physical injury. Interventions involving psychological debriefing whereby the individual is encouraged to talk about their traumatic experience used to be considered helpful, but research data have shown that such debriefing does not appear to produce measurable benefit and may even exacerbate PTSD symptoms.[109] This may be because debriefing may exacerbate arousal in persons who are already over-aroused, enhance the memory of the trauma, and undermine the inhibitory process involved in normal recovery. Trauma victims who wish to ventilate about the traumatic event in the acute aftermath certainly should be allowed to do so, but they should never be forced.

A recent review study reports a growing number of so-called "emerging" treatments.[110] Among them are dialectic behavioral therapy (DBT), mindfulness, yoga, and acceptances approaches. However, these do not have a sufficient evidence base to merit dissemination. Investigators who wish to use these approaches or incorporate them into the more traditional treatments should be aware of this current limitation. The US Army has recently adopted a positive psychology approach that attempts to enhance resilience skills and promote posttraumatic growth[111] in accordance with data documenting posttraumatic growth in various trauma samples.[112] Whether this will work, remains to be seen.

Pharmacotherapy

Because it is so much easier to write out a prescription than to conduct a course of CBT, many patients whose PTSD treatment is started with drugs might do better if it started with psychotherapy. Nevertheless, pharmacotherapy has an important place in the PTSD treatment armamentarium.[113] A related advantage of pharmacotherapy is its ease of administration, given the shorter duration of medication management compared to psychotherapy sessions, and the lesser effort on the part of both the physician and the patient. Another advantage of pharmacotherapy for PTSD is that it has been demonstrated in large-scale studies to be beneficial in settings approaching ordinary clinical settings. In other words, it has been found to be effective.

In contrast, drug side effects, and even adverse effects, constitute a well-known disadvantage of pharmacotherapy. Another important disadvantage in the treatment of PTSD is the need to treat indefinitely. Whereas psychotherapy has been shown to have effects that can last months or years after its completion, long-term follow-up studies have found that discontinuation of drug therapy for PTSD is accompanied by a high risk of relapse. Although current clinical "wisdom" dictates that drug treatment be continued for at least 1 or 2 years after a successful result, there are few data that indicate that treatment for even that long significantly reduces the risk of relapse after discontinuation. Finally, although the two have not been compared head-to-head in sufficient research to draw firm conclusions, comparisons of separate studies of each suggest that pharmacotherapy is somewhat less efficacious than psychotherapy.

Another disadvantage of pharmacotherapy, which it shares with psychotherapy, is partial response. Although data analyses may yield impressive statistical effect sizes, when these are translated into actual improvement on clinical scales by converting standardized into raw scores, the typical improvement in PTSD symptoms turns out to be well less than 50%. The few available studies suggest that a combination of drug therapy and psychotherapy may improve this success rate but not dramatically.

With regard to the types of drugs that have been found to be useful in the treatment of PTSD, 95% of the pharmacotherapeutic history of the disorder may be summed up by one word: antidepressants. The fact that these drugs are called "antidepressants" does not mean that their efficacy is limited to depression. Early studies of monoamine oxidase inhibitors (MAOIs) and tricyclic antidepressants (TCAs) pointed to their efficacy in PTSD, with a possible slight edge for the former. Since the appearance of the SSRIs, however, use of these older-generation antidepressants has become rare. Among the various SSRIs, there is little evidence supporting superior efficacy of any one over the others. The fact that among all of them, only two agents, sertraline and paroxetine, have obtained an indication for PTSD from the US Food and Drug Administration (FDA) reflects strategic marketing decisions on the part of the respective pharmaceutical companies to invest in the costly studies necessary to demonstrate effectiveness to the FDA. Nevertheless, practitioners who reasonably wish to use FDA-approved drugs for FDA-approved indications will necessarily commence treatment with one of these agents. Other considerations in choice of antidepressants include side-effect profile and expense. Dosages and frequency of administration of SSRIs for PTSD are comparable to those for MDD and can readily be obtained from the *Physicians' Desk Reference* or similar sources. Evidence is also emerging that other antidepressants (including serotonin-norepinephrine reuptake inhibitors [SNRIs], bupropion, and mirtazapine) are also efficacious.

It is important to keep in mind that, as routinely practiced, pharmacotherapy for PTSD is plagued by inadequacies that have been found to characterize the treatment of depression, including insufficient dosage, insufficient compliance, insufficient duration of treatment, and insufficient follow-up. Dose should be gradually titrated up toward the maximum recommended limit until either a satisfactory response is achieved or side effects become unacceptable. Three months may be required before concluding that a drug trial is unsuccessful.

Far fewer data are available to guide the use of non-antidepressant drugs in the treatment of PTSD. Given how frequently benzodiazepines are prescribed in common practice, the lack of research data bearing on their efficacy is a serious problem. In view of their abuse potential and deleterious effects on memory, prudence dictates that benzodiazepines only be used for well-defined target symptoms in low-abuse-potential patients, and then only for as long as necessary. Antipsychotics appear to be useful for psychotic symptoms within PTSD and possibly for symptoms beyond that (e.g., agitation, aggression). A variety of antiepileptics, or so-called mood stabilizers (including carbamazepine, valproate, lamotrigine, gabapentin, topiramate, and tiagabine), have been tried for PTSD in small studies and may be useful for such problems as well, or even more generally for PTSD. Prazosin, an alpha$_1$-adrenergic antagonist, was initially reported to reduce PTSD nightmares,[114] but it may also have general PTSD efficacy. A recent approach that is being investigated is secondary pharmacological intervention.[115] This approach involves treating a patient as soon as possible following the traumatic event with agents such as beta-adrenergic blockers or corticosteroids with an eye to forestalling the development of PTSD. Although some progress has been made in this area, no single intervention has yet received sufficient empirical support to merit dissemination.

Current Status of Posttraumatic Stress Disorder Treatment

For a comprehensive overview of current treatment approaches to PTSD and their efficacy, the readers should consult the *Practice Guidelines from the International Society for Traumatic Stress Studies*.[116] A very recent meta-analysis has addressed the efficacy of treatments for PTSD,[117] and its results are sobering. It found the following effect sizes for various psychotherapies: for cognitive therapy g = 1.63, for exposure therapy g = 1.08, for EMDR g = 1.01. With regard to various pharmacotherapies: for paroxetine g = 0.74; for sertraline g = 0.41, for fluoxetine g = 0.43, for risperidone g = 0.41, for topiramate g = 1.20, and

for venlafaxine g = 0.48. At first glance, these effect sizes appear reasonably good. However, the meta-analysis did not go beyond statistical effect sizes, and from a practical clinical standpoint, effect sizes are insufficient and potentially misleading. For example, the state-of-the-art measure of PTSD symptomatology is the Clinician-Administered PTSD Scale (CAPS).[118] Total score on the CAPS ranges from 0 to 136. Based upon data from a large drug study of PTSD,[119] a group of PTSD patients prior to undergoing treatment may be estimated to have a mean CAPS score of 74 with a standard deviation of 16. Therefore, a treatment effect size of 1.00 (about the average in this meta-analysis) translates into a percent symptom reduction of only 21%! Because the meta-analysis did not provide raw symptom improvement data, and means and standard deviations from the studies reviewed may have differed from the above estimates, and there is more than one way to calculate effect size, it is impossible to know the degree to which the pessimistic example presented above actually applies to the results of the meta-analysis, but at least this illustrates the need to move beyond effect sizes in providing useful information to clinicians about the actual improvements they may anticipate when implementing various PTSD treatments. The authors of the meta-analysis discussed above went on to note that because of the tendency to more often report positive than negative results (the so-called "file drawer" problem), the effect sizes it found may actually represent overestimates. Certainly it may be concluded that current PTSD treatments, on average, are far from curative, and that novel approaches to PTSD treatment are needed.

CURRENT CONTROVERSIES AND FUTURE DIRECTIONS

- Is the incidence of PTSD over-estimated? A re-analysis of data from the National Vietnam Veterans Readjustment Survey published in *Science* reduced the original life-time incidence of PTSD from 31% to 19%, a two-fifths reduction. Will downward adjustments of other PTSD incidence rates follow?
- Is PTSD a discrete category, or is it at the far end of a post-traumatic symptom severity spectrum? Preliminary taxometric research supports the latter. Will this call for eventually abandoning the categorical PTSD diagnosis in favor of a dimensional approach?
- In validating biological measures in PTSD research, the gold standard is the interview-based diagnosis. Will it eventually become the other way around, as more is learned about the brain basis of this disorder?
- What novel approaches promise to improve on the limited efficacy of even the best available PTSD treatments?

Access the complete reference list and multiple choice questions (MCQs) online at https://expertconsult.inkling.com

KEY REFERENCES

2. Friedman MJ, Resick PA, Bryant RA, et al. Classification of trauma and stressor-related disorders in DSM-5. *Depress Anxiety* 28(9):737–749, 2011.
4. Forbes D, Haslam N, Williams BJ, et al. Testing the latent structure of posttraumatic stress disorder: a taxometric study of combat veterans. *J Trauma Stress* 18(6):647–656, 2005.
5. Wolf EJ, Miller MW, Reardon AF, et al. A latent class analysis of dissociation and posttraumatic stress disorder: evidence for a dissociative subtype. *Arch Gen Psychiatry* 69(7):698–705, 2012.
6. Andrews B, Brewin CR, Philpott R, et al. Delayed-onset posttraumatic stress disorder: a systematic review of the evidence. *Am J Psychiatry* 164(9):1319–1326, 2007.

8. Bryant RA, Friedman MJ, Spiegel D, et al. A review of acute stress disorder in DSM-5. *Depress Anxiety* 28(9):802–817, 2011.

10. Kessler RC, Sonnega A, Bromet E, et al. Posttraumatic stress disorder in the National Comorbidity Survey. *Arch Gen Psychiatry* 52(12):1048–1060, 1995.

14. Breslau N, Kessler RC, Chilcoat HD, et al. Trauma and posttraumatic stress disorder in the community: the 1996 Detroit Area Survey of Trauma. *Arch Gen Psychiatry* 55(7):626–632, 1998.

16. Kessler RC, Berglund P, Demler O, et al. Lifetime prevalence and age-of-onset distributions of DSM-IV disorders in the National Comorbidity Survey Replication. *Arch Gen Psychiatry* 62(6):593–602, 2005.

19. Dohrenwend BP, Turner JB, Turse NA, et al. The psychological risks of Vietnam for U.S. veterans: a revisit with new data and methods. *Science* 313(5789):979–982, 2006.

20. Kulka RA, Schlenger WE, Fairbank JA, et al. *Trauma and the Vietnam War Generation: Report of Findings from the National Vietnam Veterans Readjustment Study*, New York, 1990, Brunner/Mazel.

21. Harvey AG, Bryant RA. Acute stress disorder: a synthesis and critique. *Psychol Bull* 128(6):886–902, 2002.

29. Stein MB, Jang KL, Taylor S, et al. Genetic and environmental influences on trauma exposure and posttraumatic stress disorder symptoms: a twin study. *Am J Psychiatry* 159(10):1675–1681, 2002.

31. True WR, Rice J, Eisen SA, et al. A twin study of genetic and environmental contributions to liability for posttraumatic stress symptoms. *Arch Gen Psychiatry* 50(4):257–264, 1993.

32. Brewin CR, Andrews B, Valentine JD. Meta-analysis of risk factors for posttraumatic stress disorder in trauma-exposed adults. *J Consult Clin Psychol* 68(5):748–766, 2000.

33. Ozer EJ, Best SR, Lipsey TL, et al. Predictors of posttraumatic stress disorder and symptoms in adults: a meta-analysis. *Psychol Bull* 129(1):52–73, 2003.

53. Holowka DW, Marx BP. Assessing PTSD-related functional impairment and quality of life. In Beck JG, Sloan DM, editors: *Oxford Handbook of Traumatic Stress Disorders*, New York, 2011, Oxford University Press.

54. Rodriguez P, Holowka DW, Marx BP. Assessment of posttraumatic stress disorder-related functional impairment: a review. *J Rehabil Res Dev* 49(5):649–665, 2012.

65. Pole N. The psychophysiology of posttraumatic stress disorder: a meta-analysis. *Psychol Bull* 133(5):725–746, 2007.

74. Orr SP, Metzger LJ, Pitman RK. Psychophysiology of posttraumatic stress disorder. *Psychiatr Clin North Am* 25(2):271–293, 2002.

83. Lissek S, Grillon C. Learning models of PTSD. In Beck JG, Sloan DM, editors: *The Oxford Handbook of Traumatic Stress Disorders*, New York, 2012, Oxford University Press, pp 175–190.

85. Pitman RK, Rasmusson AM, Koenen KC, et al. Biological studies of post-traumatic stress disorder. *Nat Rev Neurosci* 13(11):769–787, 2012.

88. Hughes KC, Shin LM. Functional neuroimaging studies of post-traumatic stress disorder. *Expert Rev Neurother* 11(2):275–285, 2011.

91. Yehuda R. Post-traumatic stress disorder. *N Engl J Med* 346(2):108–114, 2002.

97. Bisson J, Andrew M. Psychological treatment of post-traumatic stress disorder (PTSD). *Cochrane Database Syst Rev* (3):CD003388, 2007.

99. Bradley R, Greene J, Russ E, et al. A multidimensional meta-analysis of psychotherapy for PTSD. *Am J Psychiatry* 162(2):214–227, 2005.

107. Kearns MC, Ressler KJ, Zatzick D, et al. Early interventions for PTSD: a review. *Depress Anxiety* 29(10):833–842, 2012.

108. Shalev AY, Ankri Y, Israeli-Shalev Y, et al. Prevention of post-traumatic stress disorder by early treatment: results from the Jerusalem Trauma Outreach And Prevention study. *Arch Gen Psychiatry* 69(2):166–176, 2012.

113. Ipser JC, Stein DJ. Evidence-based pharmacotherapy of post-traumatic stress disorder (PTSD). *Int J Neuropsychopharmacol* 15(6):825–840, 2012.

115. Searcy CP, Bobadilla L, Gordon WA, et al. Pharmacological prevention of combat-related PTSD: a literature review. *Mil Med* 177(6):649–654, 2012.

116. Effective Treatments for PTSD. *Practice Guidelines from the International Society for Traumatic Stress Studies*, 2nd ed, New York, 2009, Guilford Press.

35 Dissociative Disorders

Steven C. Schlozman, MD, and Ruta M. Nonacs, MD, PhD

KEY POINTS

Epidemiology

- A large segment of the general population will endorse dissociative symptoms in the absence of significant psychopathology, suggesting that these symptoms exist along a spectrum from normal to pathological.
- Dissociative disorders are most often associated with a history of trauma.

Clinical Findings

- Dissociative disorders are a heterogeneous set of psychiatric conditions that are characterized by the lack of a fully integrated consciousness.
- Although dissociative disorders remain controversial, they represent an often unconsidered and therefore missed diagnostic category of diagnoses.

Pathophysiology

- The etiology of dissociation is likely multi-factorial, involving neurobiological responses to significant external stressors.

OVERVIEW

Dissociative disorders are among the most controversial, as well as the most intriguing, psychiatric conditions. Central to the conceptualization of dissociation is the understanding that a person's consciousness may not be fully integrated. Thus, a patient may experience a distinct alteration in personality or experience, in which thoughts, feelings, or actions are not logically integrated with other self-referential experiences.[1] Furthermore, although the concept of dissociation is more than 100 years old, there continues to exist great debate as to the validity of the symptoms of dissociation itself, as to whether the symptoms of dissociative disorders are better accounted for as subsets of different psychiatric conditions (e.g., anxiety disorders, post-traumatic stress disorder [PTSD],[2] brief traumatic reactions, psychotic disorders, and attachment disorders), and as to the extent to which political and even cinematic agendas have contributed to the current conceptualization of dissociative syndromes. Certainly, the most famous of the dissociative conditions, dissociative identity disorder (DID), is featured in more than a half a dozen popular films and is sometimes mentioned in the now somewhat discounted "epidemic" of ritual satanic cults said to spawn new cases of dissociative disorder in the 1980s.

Nevertheless, most clinicians continue to view the concept of dissociation as a rare, albeit possible, response to horrific and traumatic events and experiences. To this extent, dissociative phenomena are often discussed in the setting of trauma studies, and case reports of dissociation detail those who have suffered a single, horrifying event, as well as those who have suffered the repeated neglect and abuse that characterizes early poor attachment. However, it is not the case that trauma is a necessary etiological factor in the development of dissociation. The *Diagnostic and Statistical Manual of Mental Disorders*, Fourth Edition (DSM-IV)[3] was careful to avoid any etiological hypotheses when describing dissociative behavior, and although there have been changes in the terminology and diagnostic entities in DSM-5,[4] there remains a purely descriptive approach to these conditions in the most recent descriptions of these syndromes. Indeed, case reports persist that involve individuals with significant dissociative symptoms that occur in the absence of an identifiable stressor. Given the heterogeneous nature of the syndromes and those who suffer from them, it is no wonder that dissociative disorders are the subject of, at times, intense controversy.

Finally, there are a number of dissociative conditions described in the DSM-5[4] that have undergone re-classifications. These changes include the inclusion of dissociative fugue as a specifier for dissociative amnesia, as well as derealization being added as both a feature of, and part of, the name for the newly coined depersonalization/derealization disorder. Finally, as one might expect given the controversies surrounding dissociative identity disorder, this particular syndrome has undergone the most fundamental changes.[5,6]

This chapter defines the overall concept of dissociation, gives brief summaries of the main dissociative conditions, and discusses etiology and treatment.

History

Dissociative phenomena have been observed and described for hundreds of years. In the late eighteenth century, Franz Mesmer explored the concept of dissociation from the perspective of hypnosis, and, indeed, was likely the first clinician to document the relationship between those who are easily hypnotized and those who are prone to dissociation.[7,8] Nearly a century later, Pierre Janet, building on the work of Sigmund Freud, suggested that the ego fragments in the setting of traumatic events, leading to dissociative states. Importantly, this theory represents a departure from Freud's primary notions regarding trauma and dissociation. While Janet felt that it was primarily a fragile ego that collapsed under the weight of horrifying trauma, thus yielding dissociative symptoms, Freud conceptualized dissociation as the work of a powerful ego defense, in which individuals wall off intense emotional pain as something separate from the self and left to be expressed only in dissociative states.[9] Finally, in the early 1900s, Morton Prince wrote "The Dissociation of a Personality," a lengthy case study that documented his patient, Sally Beauchamp, as "The Saint, the Devil, the Woman." This was the first in-depth analysis of what is today known as DID.[10,11]

As mentioned, dissociative disorders became a much-discussed subject in psychiatry during the 1980s, in which presumed victims of satanic ritual abuse were often diagnosed with DID and discovered their past via hypnosis and the reclamation of lost memories. Much has been written about the increase in recovered memories that is often tied to dissociative states, with some clinicians feeling that these cases represent a barely touched-upon epidemic of dissociation, whereas others feel strongly that these cases were instead the result of suggestible patients being led to express symptoms and memories that had little basis in the suggested etiology of their predicaments. It is clear that controversy still exists regarding these cases.[12]

CAUSES OF DISSOCIATION

Virtually all explorations of dissociation involve trauma. Thus, although the DSM-5[4] specifically avoids etiologic explorations, in research settings the study of trauma and the study of dissociation go hand-in-hand. The majority of academic writing that discusses dissociation occurs in the trauma literature, and scholars have even defined trauma itself as a threat to one's personal integrity. This is in fact one of the main reasons some believe that dissociative behavior is more a subset of PTSD, with the symptoms of disconnection representing the flashbacks, re-experiencing, and numbing that are central to the diagnosis of PTSD.[13,14] There exists as well increased interest in differentiating PTSD from dissociative disorders using newly discovered differences in proposed neurobiological etiologies for each syndrome.[15]

Additionally, those who are more easily hypnotized are also more prone to dissociation. As younger people and especially children are also more easily hypnotized, this finding is perhaps tied to the fact that younger individuals are also more likely to dissociate. Finally, to the extent that deficiencies in early attachment have been tied to dissociation, it may be that children are more prone to dissociation simply because they have more recently experienced the challenges to secure attachment that have been suggested as etiological to dissociation.[16,17]

From a more biological perspective, dissociative-like states have long been observed in patients who are given dissociative anesthetics (such as midazolam), or who use illicit substances such as lysergic acid diethylamide (LSD).[16,18] These findings suggest irregular serotonin activity as playing some role in dissociative phenomena. Additionally, many patients with brain injuries, and especially patients with complex partial seizures, have displayed dissociative behavior.[19-22] These findings suggest that multiple triggers, both biological and psychological in origin, mingle in the formation of dissociation as a pathological state.

However, community samples also document a relatively high degree of dissociation in the general population. Although the reasons for this finding are not clear, dissociation has more recently been characterized as akin to state-dependent learning, in which certain information is more easily retrieved from some individuals in specific states of self. As with many psychiatric phenomena, dissociation may exist along a spectrum, with some expressions of dissociation more closely tied to normal states and other symptoms more obviously representative of significant pathology.[16]

THE EPIDEMIOLOGY OF DISSOCIATION

Estimates as to the prevalence of dissociation vary widely. The overall rate of dissociative disorders is thought to be approximately 10%, based primarily on standardized assessments (such as the Dissociative Experience Scale [DES] and the Structured Clinical Interview for Dissociative Disorders [SCID-D]). Importantly, these assessments have face validity only; therefore, caution must be exercised in interpreting data that stem from these investigations. Additionally, the prevalence of dissociative experiences in the general population is estimated by some to be as high as 75%. It is not clear how to interpret these findings when drawing conclusions regarding the epidemiology of dissociation.[16]

Nevertheless, some important demographic features have emerged from these investigations. First, as already noted, younger people and especially children are more likely to suffer both dissociative events and to meet criteria for dissociative disorders. Second, for symptoms of general dissociation, there appear to be equal male-to-female ratios. However,

---

BOX 35-1	Dissociative Amnesia (DSM-IV Criteria and Exclusions)

A. The predominant disturbance is one or more episodes of inability to recall important personal information, usually of a traumatic or stressful nature, that is too extensive to be explained by ordinary forgetfulness.

B. The disturbance does not occur exclusively during the course of dissociative identity disorder, dissociative fugue, posttraumatic stress disorder, acute stress disorder, or somatization disorder and is not due to the direct physiological effects of a substance (e.g., a drug of abuse, a medication) or a neurological or other general medical condition (e.g., amnestic disorder due to head trauma).

C. The symptoms cause clinically significant distress or impairment in social, occupational, or other important areas of function.

---

specific dissociative syndromes have different gender profiles. While dissociative fugue is more common in men, DID is found more often in women.

DIFFERENT DISSOCIATIVE DISORDERS

The DSM-5[4] lists dissociative amnesia (formerly called psychogenic amnesia), DID (formerly called multiple personality disorder), derealization/depersonalization disorder, and dissociative disorder NOS among the dissociative disorders. Derealization is now part of the symptom structure of depersonalization disorder, and dissociative fugue became a specifier for dissociate amnesia.

Dissociative amnesia has been defined in DSM-IV[3] as "an inability to recall important personal information, usually of a traumatic nature, that is too extensive to be explained by normal forgetfulness." (Box 35-1 lists the DSM-IV[3] criteria of this condition and exclusions to it. See Box 35-2 for updated DSM-5 diagnostic criteria.) Dissociative amnesia may be global, involving a total loss of important personal information, or it may be more localized, in which patients cannot recall specific episodes of behavior or traumatic experiences. These experiences may include self-mutilation, criminal or sexual behaviors, traumatic events, or even marital or financial crises.

The incidence in men and women appears to be equal, and large segments of the general population may suffer brief amnestic periods following a significant large-scale disaster.

The differential diagnosis includes organic syndromes (secondary to brain injuries, lesions, or seizures), as well as factitious disorders and malingering, and the treatment for dissociative amnesia is aimed at the restoration of missing memories, sometimes through psychotherapy and free association, but at times using hypnosis or an amytal interview. Generally speaking, patients with dissociative amnesia recover quickly and completely. However, many patients continue to display a propensity toward amnesia in the setting of trauma.[23]

Dissociative Amnesia

As noted above, dissociative fugue is no longer a distinct diagnosis. DSM-5[4] includes a fugue state as a specifier for dissociative amnesia. This condition remains the rarest of the dissociative disorders. A fugue has been defined as sudden unexpected travel away from one's place of daily activities, with an inability to recall some, or all, of one's past. Often, patients suffering from dissociative fugue will assume entirely

BOX 35-2 DSM-5 Diagnostic Criteria: Dissociative Amnesia (300.12 (F44.0))

A. An inability to recall important autobiographical information, usually of a traumatic or stressful nature, that is inconsistent with ordinary forgetting.

Note: Dissociative amnesia most often consists of localized or selective amnesia for a specific event or events; or generalized amnesia for identity and life history.

B. The symptoms cause clinically significant distress or impairment in social, occupational, or other important areas of functioning.

C. The disturbance is not attributable to the physiological or other medical condition (e.g. alcohol or other drug of abuse, a medication) or a neurological or other medical condition (e.g. partial complex seizures, transient global amnesia, sequelae of a closed head injury/traumatic brain injury, other neurological condition).

D. The disturbance is not better explained by dissociative identity disorder, posttraumatic stress disorder, acute stress disorder, somatic symptom disorder, or major or mild neurocognitive disorder.

• **Coding note:** The code for dissociative amnesia without dissociative fugue is 300.12 (F44.0). The code for dissociative amnesia with dissociative fugue is 300.13 (F44.1).

  Specify if:
  300.13 (F44.1) **With dissociative fugue:** Apparently purposeful travel or bewildered wandering that is associated with amnesia for identity or for other important autobiographical information.

Reprinted with permission from the Diagnostic and statistical manual of mental disorders, ed 5, (Copyright 2013). American Psychiatric Association.

BOX 35-3 Dissociative Fugue (DSM-5 Criteria and Exclusions)

A. The predominant disturbance is sudden, unexpected travel away from home or one's customary place of work, with an inability to recall one's past.

B. There is confusion about personal identity or an assumption of a new identity (partial or complete).

C. The disturbance does not occur exclusively during the course of dissociative identity disorder and is not due to the direct physiological effects of a substance (e.g., a drug of abuse, a medication) or a general medical condition (e.g., temporal lobe epilepsy).

D. The symptoms cause clinically significant distress or impairment in social, occupational, or other important areas of function.

BOX 35-4 Dissociative Identity Disorder (DSM-IV Criteria and Exclusions)

A. There are two or more distinct identities or personality states (each with its own relatively enduring pattern of perceiving, relating to, and thinking about the environment and self).

B. At least two of these identities or personality states recurrently take control of the person's behavior.

C. There is an inability to recall important personal information that is too extensive to be explained by ordinary forgetfulness.

D. The disturbance is not due to the direct physiological effects of a substance (e.g., blackouts or chaotic behavior during alcohol intoxication) or a general medical condition (e.g., complex partial seizures). In children, the symptoms are not attributable to imaginary playmates or other fantasy play.

---

new identities during their fugue episode. (Box 35-3 lists the DSM-IV criteria for this condition and exclusions to it.) Dissociative amnesia appears to be commonly triggered by a traumatic event and thus it appears to be more common during wartime or after natural disasters. Patients may appear normal, though they often become confused and distressed when asked questions about their personal history.

Dissociative amnesia occurs primarily in adults, usually between the second and fourth decades of life. While men appear to be affected as often as women, during war, the incidence of men suffering from dissociative fugue increases, as defined by the DSM-IV.[3] While fugues may last several years,

most episodes last from a few days to a few months. Alternative diagnoses include brain pathology leading to fugue states, drug-induced fugues secondary to alcoholic or drug-related blackouts, and factitious disorders or malingering. In addition, some cultural syndromes (e.g., *amok* and *latah*) may mimic fugue states.

The treatment for dissociative amnesia involves helping the patient to recall the events preceding the fugue, typically with psychotherapy, but sometimes through hypnosis or an amytal interview. The prognosis varies. When fugue states are of short duration, they tend to resolve spontaneously. Longer-lasting episodes, however, may be intractable.[16,24]

Dissociative Identity Disorder

Among the dissociative disorders, DID has received the most attention over the last two decades and has endured considerable controversy. The positive aspects of this controversy involve an ongoing debate regarding the interplay of society on psychiatric nosology, as well as a careful re-examination of all dissociative phenomena and their relationship to consciousness and pathology. As one might expect, DID has also undergone the most revisions with regard to criteria from the DSM-IV[3] to the DSM-5 (Box 35-4,[4] see Box 35-5 for DSM-5 diagnostic criteria). Currently, dissociative identity disorder (DID) retains as its hallmark the presence of two distinct personalities within a single person. These personalities are relatively enduring, and the patient may have limited recollection of the presence of these entities. Furthermore, these entities often "control" behavior and can be seen as responsible for seemingly paradoxical actions of the same patient. The DSM-5[4] has added criteria to the diagnosis of DID to include cases of apparent spiritual or demonic possession, though this aspect of the changed definition remains somewhat controversial.[25] Other, more subtle, changes include the allowance for gaps in memory for everyday events and not just traumatic occurrences, as well as an understanding that the different entities may be observed by others or be self-reported.

An essential aspect of DID is the amnestic quality for alternate personalities displayed by the primary personality. However, in many instances different personality states have varying levels of awareness of other personalities (often called *alters*) and often a dominant personality state exists that is cognizant of all of the various personalities. The term *co-consciousness* has been used to describe the simultaneous experience of multiple entities at one time. Thus, one personality may be aware of another's feelings regarding an ongoing experience.

BOX 35-5 DSM-5 Diagnostic Criteria: Dissociative Identity Disorder (300.14 (F44.81))

A. Disruption of identity characterized by two or more distinct personality states, which may be described in some cultures as an experience of possession. The disruption in identity involves marked discontinuity in sense of self and sense of agency, accompanied by related alterations in affect, behavior, consciousness, memory, perception, cognition, and/or sensory-motor functioning. These signs and symptoms may be observed by others or reported by the individual.

B. Recurrent gaps in the recall of everyday events, important personal information, and/or traumatic events that are inconsistent with ordinary forgetting.

C. The symptoms cause clinically significant distress or impairment in social, occupational, or other important areas of functioning.

D. The disturbance is not a normal part of a broadly accepted cultural or religious practice.

Note: In children, the symptoms are not better explained by imaginary playmates or other fantasy play.

E. The symptoms are not attributable to the physiological effects of a substance (e.g., blackouts or chaotic behavior during alcohol intoxication) or another medical condition (e.g., complex partial seizures).

Reprinted with permission from the Diagnostic and statistical manual of mental disorders, *ed 5, (Copyright 2013). American Psychiatric Association.*

BOX 35-6 Depersonalization Disorder (DSM-IV Criteria and Exclusions)

A. There is a persistent or recurrent experience of feeling detached from, and as if one is an outside observer of, one's mental processes or body (e.g., feeling like one is in a dream).

B. During the depersonalization experience, reality testing remains intact.

C. The depersonalization causes clinically significant distress or impairment in social, occupational, or other important areas of function.

D. The depersonalization experience does not occur exclusively during the course of another mental disorder, such as schizophrenia, panic disorder, acute stress disorder, or another dissociative disorder, and is not due to the direct physiological effects of a substance (e.g., a drug of abuse, a medication) or a general medical condition (e.g., temporal lobe epilepsy).

DID is characterized by high rates of co-morbid depression, and often by affective symptoms that constitute the presenting complaint. In addition, from one-third to one-half of cases of DID experience auditory hallucinations. Some researchers have suggested that these hallucinations are described as "inner voices," helping to differentiate these symptoms from the external voices heard by those suffering from schizophrenia and other psychotic disorders. Also, in contrast to individuals suffering from schizophrenia, patients with DID are unusually hypnotizable and do not display evidence of a formal thought disorder.

DID is reported more commonly in women than in men, and the mean number of distinct personalities is approximately 13. The prevalence rate is estimated at 1%, with co-morbid conditions (such as depression and borderline personality disorder) being relatively common.[26] Additionally, somatic symptoms (including headaches, gastrointestinal distress, and genitourinary disturbances) are also frequent and are associated with increased rates of corresponding conversion symptoms, factitious disorders, and malingering. It is in fact this somewhat messy compilation of diagnoses that contributes to some of the controversy that surrounds DID in general.

DID is usually diagnosed in the third or fourth decade, though those suffering from DID usually report symptoms during childhood and adolescence. Most case series document a chronic, fluctuating course, characterized by relapse and remission. Making the diagnosis of DID in a particular patient is not without controversy. Some clinicians have proposed that the diagnosis must be persistently pursued if a patient's symptoms even subtly hint at the possibility of dissociation. These clinicians describe patients who are either unaware of, or who wish to hide, their disorder, and therefore need to be "educated" about DID. Critics contend that patients with DID are highly suggestible and that clinicians "create" such patients by "suggesting" symptoms. The critics emphasize that clinicians who show interest and enthusiasm in the multiplicity of personalities reinforce the symptoms.

Extended psychotherapy remains the treatment of choice, although approaches vary widely and remain controversial. Some clinicians describe specialized treatment for DID, including delineating and mapping the alters, inviting each to participate in the treatment, and facilitating communication between the various alters. Through careful exploration of all alternate identities, clinicians attempt to understand past episodes of trauma as experienced by each personality. Hypnosis is sometimes employed to reach dissociated states. Other clinicians focus on the function of the dissociative process in the here-and-now of the patient's life and the ongoing treatment. They help patients become aware of using dissociation to manage feelings and thoughts within themselves and to manage the closeness and distance within relationships. All approaches seek to increase affect tolerance and to integrate the dissociated states within the patient.

Psychopharmacological treatments (such as antidepressants and anxiolytics) are often useful in treating the common accompanying complaints of depression and anxiety. However, no pharmacological treatment has been found to reduce dissociation, *per se*. Benzodiazepines reduce anxiety but can also exacerbate dissociation. Although not routinely used for dissociative disorders, neuroleptics are sometimes employed in patients who are grossly disorganized.[16,27,28]

Depersonalization/Derealization Disorder

According to the DSM-IV (Box 35-6[3]; also see Box 35-7 for DSM-5 diagnostic criteria), depersonalization disorder is characterized by "persistent or recurrent episodes. . . . of detachment or estrangement from one's self." Often, patients with symptoms of depersonalization will "feel like an automaton or like he or she is living in a movie." Derealization—the sense that one's surroundings are somehow not real—was added to this nomenclature to account for the fact that depersonalization rarely occurs in the absence of derealization. Additionally, clinicians argue that the inability to separate self from other is a key feature to both derealization and depersonalization. To this end, a more parsimonious diagnostic entity was introduced.

However, reality testing remains intact in those who suffer from depersonalization disorder, representing an important distinction from what would otherwise be seen as primarily a psychotic process.

35

BOX 35-7 DSM-5 Diagnostic Criteria:
Depersonalization/Derealization Disorder
(300.6 (F48.1))

A. The presence of persistent or recurrent experiences of depersonalization, derealization, or both:
   1. **Depersonalization**: Experiences of unreality, detachment, or being an outside observer with respect to one's thoughts, feelings, sensations, body, or actions (e.g., perceptual alterations, distorted sense of time, unreal or absent self, emotional and/or physical numbing).
   2. **Derealization**: Experiences of unreality or detachment with respect to surroundings (e.g., individuals or objects are experienced as unreal, dreamlike, foggy, lifeless, or visually distorted).
B. During the depersonalization or derealization experiences, reality testing remains intact.
C. The symptoms cause clinically significant distress or impairment in social, occupational, or other important areas of functioning.
D. The disturbance is not attributable to the physiological effects of a substance (e.g., a drug of abuse, medication) or another medical condition (e.g., seizures).
E. The disturbance is not better explained by another mental disorder, such as schizophrenia, panic disorder, major depressive disorder, acute stress disorder, posttraumatic stress disorder, or another dissociative disorder.

Reprinted with permission from the Diagnostic and statistical manual of mental disorders, *ed 5, (Copyright 2013). American Psychiatric Association.*

BOX 35-8 Dissociative Disorder NOS (DSM-IV Criteria and Exclusions)

A. Clinical presentations are similar to dissociative identity disorders that fail to meet full criteria for this disorder. Examples include presentations in which (a) there are not two or more distinct personality states, or (b) amnesia for important personal information does not occur.
B. Derealization may be unaccompanied by depersonalization in adults.
C. States of dissociation may occur in individuals who have been subjected to periods of prolonged and intense coercive persuasion (e.g., brainwashing, thought reform, or indoctrination while captive).
D. Dissociative trance disorder: single or episodic disturbances in the state of consciousness, identity, or memory that are indigenous to particular locations and cultures. Dissociative trance involves narrowing of awareness of immediate surroundings or stereotyped behaviors or movements that are experienced as being beyond one's control. Possession trance involves replacement of the customary sense of personal identity by a new identity, attributed to the influence of a spirit, power, deity, or other person, and associated with stereotyped "involuntary" movements or amnesia. Examples include *amok* (Indonesia), *bebainan* (Indonesia), *latah* (Malaysia), *pibloktoq* (Arctic), *ataque de nervios* (Latin America), and possession (India). The dissociative or trance disorder is not a normal part of a broadly accepted collective cultural or religious practice.
E. Loss of consciousness, stupor, or coma is not attributable to a general medical condition.
F. Ganser syndrome involves the giving of approximate answers to questions (e.g., "2 plus 2 equals 5") when not associated with dissociative amnesia or dissociative fugue.

Studies have suggested that as many as 50% of people will at some point endorse transient symptoms of depersonalization based on DSM-IV criteria, and in most cases these symptoms cause little disruption and are not considered pathological. However, frequent depersonalization/derealization can be quite disruptive, interfering with daily function and preventing the integration of new experiences. Also, while transient depersonalization and derealization is roughly equal among men and women, depersonalization disorder is about twice as common in women as it is in men, again as measured by DSM-IV criteria. It is unclear whether these data will change with the addition of derealization as a specifier for depersonalization/derealization.

This syndrome usually begins by late adolescence or early adulthood, with most episodes lasting from hours to weeks at a time. Symptoms of depersonalization and derealization have also been described in those with severe depression or psychosis, among patients taking illicit substances, and as result of specific brain damage, migraines, or seizures.

Treatment is difficult, and patients are often refractory to interventions. Treatment of accompanying psychiatric conditions (such as depression or anxiety) may help. As with other dissociative disorders, exploration of prior traumatic events may prove useful.[16,29,30]

Dissociative Disorder Not Otherwise Specified

This category is reserved for presentations in which the predominant feature is dissociation without meeting criteria for any specific dissociative disorder. (Box 35-8 lists the DSM-IV[4] criteria of this condition and exclusions to it. Box 35-9 lists the DSM-5 update for this disorder Other Specified/Unspecified Dissociative Disorders.) Examples of dissociative disorder NOS vary widely. Additionally, symptoms that result

from torture or brainwashing may be classified in this category. Ganser's syndrome (sometimes called "prison psychosis") is classified as a dissociative disorder NOS. It is characterized by the provision of approximate answers: that is, offering half-correct answers to simple inquiries, such as answering "Five" to the question, "What is two plus two?" The correct set of the response is given, but the answer is inaccurate. Ganser's syndrome is often reported in incarcerated populations.[31-33]

Finally, certain culture-bound syndromes (such as *amok* in Indonesia or *latah* in Malaysia) are often characterized by dissociation and sometimes by violence. These syndromes have often been characterized as dissociative disorder NOS.

FACTITIOUS DISORDERS OR MALINGERING OF DISSOCIATIVE PRESENTATIONS

An additional source of controversy regarding dissociative disorders involves the widely reported imitation of dissociative symptoms among patients seeking secondary gain. These incidences may be more common than previously recognized, with at least one study suggesting that 10% of patients with symptoms of DID were in fact afflicted with factitious disorders, with the assumption of the sick role as their primary motivator. Other patients might feign symptoms for financial gain or to avoid financial responsibility. These cases are very difficult to discern, and certainly the treatment will be radically different from the treatment for those who suffer from true dissociative disorders. Some have noted among patients who feign symptoms that there is often great investment in

BOX 35-9 DSM-5 Diagnostic Criteria: Other Specified Dissociative Disorder (300.15 (F44.89))

This category applies to presentations in which symptoms characteristic of a dissociative disorder that cause clinically significant distress or impairment in social, occupational, or other important areas of functioning predominate but do not meet the full criteria for any of the disorders in the dissociative disorders diagnostic class. The other specified dissociative disorder category is used in situations in which the clinician chooses to communicate the specific reason that the presentation does not meet the criteria for any specific dissociative disorder. This is done by recording "other specified dissociative disorder" followed by the specific reason (e.g., "dissociative trance").

Examples of presentations that can be specified using the "other specified" designation include the following:

A. Chronic and recurrent syndromes of mixed dissociative symptoms: This category includes identity disturbance associated with less-than-marked discontinuities in sense of self and agency, or alterations of identity or episodes of possession in an individual who reports no dissociative amnesia.
B. Identity disturbance due to prolonged and intense coercive persuasion: Individuals who have been subjected to intense coercive persuasion (e.g., brainwashing, thought reform, indoctrination while captive, torture, long-term political imprisonment, recruitment by sects/cults or by terror organizations) may present with prolonged changes in, or conscious questioning of, their identity.
C. Acute dissociative reactions to stressful events: This category is for acute, transient conditions that typically last less than 1

month, and sometimes only a few hours or days. These conditions are characterized by constriction of consciousness; depersonalization; derealization; perceptual disturbances (e.g., time slowing, macropsia); micro-amnesias; transient stupor; and/or alterations in sensory-motor functioning (e.g., analgesia, paralysis).
D. Dissociative trance: This condition is characterized by an acute narrowing or complete loss of awareness of immediate surroundings that manifests as profound unresponsiveness or insensitivity to environmental stimuli. The unresponsiveness may be accompanied by minor stereotyped behaviors (e.g., finger movements) of which the individual is unaware and/or that he or she cannot control, as well as transient paralysis or loss of consciousness. The dissociative trance is not a normal part of a broadly accepted collective cultural or religious practice.

DSM-5 DIAGNOSTIC CRITERIA: UNSPECIFIED DISSOCIATIVE DISORDER (300.15 (F44.9))

This category applies to presentations in which symptoms characteristic of a dissociative disorder that cause clinically significant distress or impairment in social, occupational, or other important areas of functioning predominate but do not meet the full criteria for any of the disorders in the dissociative disorders diagnostic class. The unspecified dissociative disorder category is used in situations in which the clinician chooses not to specify the reason that the criteria are not met for a specific dissociative disorder, and includes presentations for which there is insufficient information to make a more specific diagnosis (e.g., in emergency room settings).

Reprinted with permission from the Diagnostic and statistical manual of mental disorders, *ed 5, (Copyright 2013). American Psychiatric Association.*

the diagnosis and unusual knowledge of the various dissociative syndromes. However, given the ease of access to information that characterizes modern technology, one must guard against false assumptions regarding the well-informed but legitimately dissociating patient. These matters substantially complicate the recognition and treatment of dissociative disorders.[34,35]

CONCLUSION

Dissociative disorders represent a controversial, heterogeneous, and fascinating array of psychiatric syndromes. Though many clinicians might shy away from making the diagnosis of dissociation, and while great caution is required in correctly identifying patients with these relatively rare difficulties, one also runs the risk of missing the diagnosis for patients with legitimate dissociative difficulties. Careful clinical evaluation, judicious use of standardized assessments, and a willingness to remain open-minded regarding these diagnoses will serve the clinician well in recognizing and treating this group of diagnoses.

Access the complete reference list and multiple choice questions (MCQs) online at https://expertconsult.inkling.com

KEY REFERENCES

2. Lanius RA, Brand B, Vermetten E, et al. The dissociative subtype of posttraumatic stress disorder: rationale, clinical and neurobiological evidence, and implications. *Depress Anxiety* 29(8):701–708, 2012.
3. American Psychiatric Association. *Diagnostic and statistical manual of mental disorders*, ed 4, Washington, DC, 1994, American Psychiatric Association Press.

4. American Psychiatric Association. *Diagnostic and statistical manual of mental disorders*, ed 5, Washington, DC, 2013, American Psychiatric Association Press.
5. Brand BL, Lanius R, Vermetten E, et al. Where are we going? An update on assessment, treatment, and neurobiological research in dissociative disorders as we move toward the DSM-5. *J Trauma Dissociation* 13(1):9–31, 2012.
6. Spiegel D, Lewis-Fernández R, Lanius R, et al. Dissociative disorders in DSM-5. *Annu Rev Clin Psychol* 9:299–326, 2013.
8. Bob P. Dissociation and neuroscience: history and new perspectives. *Int J Neuroscience* 113(7):903–914, 2003.
10. Prince M. *The dissociation of a personality*, New York, 1905, Longmans, Green.
12. Mulhern S. Satanism, ritual abuse, and multiple personality disorder: a sociohistorical perspective. *Int J Clin Exp Hypnosis* 42(4):265–288, 1994.
13. van der Hart O, Nijenhuis E, Steele K, et al. Trauma-related dissociation: conceptual clarity lost and found. *Aust N Z J Psychiatry* 38(11–12):906–914, 2004.
14. Candel I, Merckelbach H. Peritraumatic dissociation as a predictor of post-traumatic stress disorder: a critical review. *Compr Psychiatry* 45(1):44–50, 2004.
15. Simeon D, Yehuda R, Knutelska M, et al. Dissociation versus posttraumatic stress: cortisol and physiological correlates in adults highly exposed to the World Trade Center attack on 9/11. *Psychiatry Res* 161(3):325–329, 2008.
16. Coons PM. The dissociative disorders. Rarely considered and underdiagnosed. *Psychiatr Clin North Am* 21(3):637–648, 1998.
17. Kirsch I, Lynn SJ. Dissociation theories of hypnosis [see comment]. *Psychol Bull* 123(1):100–115, 1998.
19. Swinkels WA, van Emde Boas W, Kuyk J, et al. Interictal depression, anxiety, personality traits, and psychological dissociation in patients with temporal lobe epilepsy (TLE) and extra-TLE. *Epilepsia* 47(12):2092–2103, 2006.
20. Mula M, Cavanna A, Collimedaglia L, et al. The role of aura in psychopathology and dissociative experiences in epilepsy. *J Neuropsychiatry Clin Neurosci* 18(4):536–542, 2006.

21. Berthier ML, Posada A, Puentes C. Dissociative flashbacks after right frontal injury in a Vietnam veteran with combat-related posttraumatic stress disorder. *J Neuropsychiatry Clin Neurosci* 13(1):101–105, 2001.

23. Brandt J, Van Gorp WG. Functional ("psychogenic") amnesia. *Semin Neurol* 26(3):331–340, 2006.

25. van Duijl M, Kleijn W, de Jong J. Are symptoms of spirit possessed patients covered by the DSM-IV or DSM-5 criteria for possession trance disorder? A mixed-method explorative study in Uganda. *Soc Psychiatry Psychiatr Epidemiol* 48(9):1417–1430, 2013.

26. Korzekwa MI, Dell PF, Pain C. Dissociation and borderline personality disorder: an update for clinicians. *Curr Psychiatry Rep* 11(1):82–88, 2009.

27. Brand BL, Armstrong JG, Loewenstein RJ. Psychological assessment of patients with dissociative identity disorder. *Psychiatr Clin North Am* 29(1):145–168, 2006.

28. Kluft RP. Dealing with alters: a pragmatic clinical perspective. *Psychiatr Clin North Am* 29(1):281–304, 2006.

29. Bunning S, Blanke O. The out-of-body experience: precipitating factors and neural correlates. *Prog Brain Res* 150:331–350, 2005.

30. Hunter EC, Sierra M, David AS. The epidemiology of depersonalisation and derealisation. A systematic review. *Soc Psychiatry Psychiatr Epidemiol* 39(1):9–18, 2004.

32. Dalfen AK, Anthony F. Head injury, dissociation and the Ganser syndrome. *Brain Inj* 14(12):1101–1105, 2000.

34. LoPiccolo CJ, Goodkin K, Baldewicz TT. Current issues in the diagnosis and management of malingering. *Ann Med* 31(3):166–174, 1999.

36 Sexual Disorders and Sexual Dysfunction

Linda C. Shafer, MD

KEY POINTS

Incidence
- Sexual disorders are common, occurring in 43% of women and 31% of men in the US.

Epidemiology
- Advanced age and co-morbid medical (particularly cardiovascular) and psychiatric conditions are associated with higher rates of sexual dysfunction in both genders. Paraphilic disorders are associated with attention-deficit/hyperactivity disorder (ADHD).

Pathophysiology
- Sexual function depends on a complex interplay of biological, social, cultural, and psychological factors, many of which are poorly understood. The human sexual response cycle is a useful framework for understanding sexual problems.

Clinical Findings
- The new DSM-5 has introduced substantial changes to the classification of sexual disorders. A careful sexual history remains the most important tool for facilitating diagnosis.

Differential Diagnoses
- These include many medical and surgical conditions, adverse effects of medications, and other psychiatric disorders.

Treatment Options
- Phosphodiesterase type 5 (PDE-5) inhibitors have revolutionized the treatment of erectile dysfunction and may benefit some women with SSRI-induced sexual dysfunction. Otherwise, pharmacologic options for sexual disorders remain limited, although many are under study, complemented by therapy.

Complications
- PDE-5 inhibitors are well-tolerated, although adverse effects, such as headache and low blood pressure, may occur. Hormonal agents used in women are linked to potential risks of cardiovascular disease and breast cancer.

Prognosis
- Sexual disorders are often multifaceted and require a multidisclipinary approach to achieve clinically significant improvement.

OVERVIEW

Sexual disorders are extremely common. It has been estimated that 43% of women and 31% of men in the US suffer from sexual dysfunction. Lack of sexual satisfaction is associated with significant emotional distress (e.g., depression, marital conflict) and physical problems (e.g., cardiovascular disease, diabetes mellitus). Individuals with sexual problems are often

reluctant to seek assistance from a physician and may first experiment with any number of self-help methods. However, with the introduction of PDE-5 inhibitors, such as sildenafil (Viagra) for the treatment of erectile dysfunction and the increased interest in pharmacological therapy for female sexual disorders, the frequency of complaints related to sexual dysfunction in primary care practice has risen to nearly 15% to 20% of visits. Nevertheless, the incidence of sexual problems is related to the frequency with which providers take a sexual history.

The new *Diagnostic and Statistical Manual of Mental Disorders*, Fifth Edition (DSM-5), has made several important changes to the classification of sexual disorders. Previously grouped into one chapter, sexual disorders are now separated into three chapters: sexual dysfunctions, paraphilic disorders, and gender dysphoria.

Sexual dysfunction is characterized by a clinically significant disturbance in the ability to respond sexually or to experience sexual pleasure. Previously, it was defined according to the physiological sexual response cycle, a model increasingly felt too simplistic. Criteria are now more precise, requiring 6 months of symptoms and a severity rating. Some disorders are now gender-specific (e.g., male hypoactive sexual desire disorder), and others have been merged (e.g., genito-pelvic pain/penetration disorder instead of vaginismus and dyspareunia), or deleted (e.g., sexual aversion disorder). The sexual dysfunctions are further classified as lifelong or acquired and situational or generalized. The DSM-5 introduces "associated features," such as relationship and medical factors, which support particular diagnoses.

The DSM-5 for the first time distinguishes between paraphilias and paraphilic disorders. Paraphilias are defined as persistent and intense atypical sexual interests and considered normal. Paraphilic disorders are paraphilias that cause distress or impairment to the individual or that result in personal harm or risk of harm to others.

Finally, gender dysphoria replaces gender identity disorder and describes dissatisfaction with one's natal sex. The concepts are similar; however, gender dysphoria abandons the use of "cross-gender," allowing for an "alternative" (undefined) gender. All sexual disorders must cause clinically significant distress or an impairment of social function before a diagnosis can be made.

EPIDEMIOLOGY AND RISK FACTORS

Sexual disorders affect individuals across the epidemiological spectrum. They occur more often in women than in men and are more frequent with advanced age, lower socioeconomic status, obesity, sedentary lifestyle, co-existing medical (e.g., cardiovascular) and psychiatric conditions, and history of sexual trauma. The prototypical paraphilic is young, white, and male and more likely to suffer from ADHD, substance abuse, major depression or dysthymia, and/or a phobic disorder.

PATHOPHYSIOLOGY

Sexual function depends on complex interactions among the brain, hormones, and the vascular system. Neural modulators of sexual desire, arousal, and orgasm include dopamine,

TABLE 36-1 Classification of Sexual Dysfunctions

Impaired Sexual Response Phase	Female	Male
Desire	Female sexual interest/ arousal disorder	Male hypoactive sexual desire disorder
	Other specified sexual dysfunction: sexual aversion	Other specified sexual dysfunction: sexual aversion
Excitement (arousal, vascular)	Female sexual interest/ arousal disorder	Erectile disorder
Orgasm (muscular)	Female orgasmic disorder	Delayed ejaculation Premature ejaculation
Sexual pain	Genito-pelvic pain/ penetration disorder	Other specified or unspecified sexual dysfunction

TABLE 36-2 Medical and Surgical Conditions Causing Sexual Dysfunctions

Organic Disorders	Sexual Impairment
ENDOCRINE	
Hypothyroidism, adrenal dysfunction, hypogonadism, diabetes mellitus	Low libido, impotence, decreased vaginal lubrication, early impotence
VASCULAR	
Hypertension, atherosclerosis, stroke, venous insufficiency, sickle cell disorder	Impotence, but ejaculation and libido intact
NEUROLOGICAL	
Spinal cord damage, diabetic neuropathy, herniated lumbar disk, alcoholic neuropathy, multiple sclerosis, temporal lobe epilepsy	Sexual disorder—early sign, low libido (or high libido), impotence, impaired orgasm
LOCAL GENITAL DISEASE	
Male: Priapism, Peyronie's disease, urethritis, prostatitis, hydrocele	Low libido, impotence
Female: Imperforate hymen, vaginitis, pelvic inflammatory disease, endometriosis	Genito-pelvic pain, low libido, decreased arousal
SYSTEMIC DEBILITATING DISEASE	
Renal, pulmonary, or hepatic diseases, advanced malignancies, infections	Low libido, impotence, decreased arousal
SURGICAL-POSTOPERATIVE STATES	
Male: Prostatectomy (radical perineal), abdominal-perineal bowel resection	Impotence, no loss of libido, ejaculatory impairment
Female: Episiotomy, vaginal repair of prolapse, oophorectomy	Genito-pelvic pain, decreased lubrication
Male and Female: Amputation (leg), colostomy, and ileostomy	Mechanical difficulties in sex, low self-image, fear of odor

melanocortin, estrogen, and testosterone. At the vascular level, nitric oxide (NO) plays a critical role in regulating vaginal smooth muscle tone and intrapenile blood flow. In fact, PDE-5 inhibitors act by prolonging the effects of NO.

The sexual response cycle concept is useful in understanding sexual problems. The stages vary with age and physical status and are affected by medications, diseases, injuries, and psychological conditions (Table 36-1). Three major models have been proposed.

Masters and Johnson developed the first model of the human sexual response, consisting of a linear progression through four distinct phases: (1) excitement (arousal); (2) plateau (maximal arousal before orgasm); (3) orgasm (rhythmic muscular contractions); and (4) resolution (return to baseline). Following resolution, a refractory period exists in men.

Kaplan modified the Masters and Johnson model by introducing a desire stage (neuropsychological input). The Kaplan model consists of three stages: (1) desire; (2) excitement/ arousal; and (3) orgasm (muscular contraction).

Most recently, Basson, recognizing the complexity of the female sexual response, proposed a biopsychosocial model of female sexuality that consists of four overlapping components: (1) biology; (2) psychology; (3) sociocultural factors; and (4) interpersonal relationships. The model acknowledges that many factors may stimulate a woman's receptivity for sex. Indeed, sexual satisfaction may be prompted by such factors as emotional closeness and may still be achieved without direct desire. Additionally, it is known that physical measurements of female arousal (such as increased vaginal secretions) are poorly correlated with sexual satisfaction.

Aging is associated with changes in the normal human sexual response. Men are slower to achieve erections and require more direct genital stimulation. Women have decreased levels of estrogen, leading to decreased vaginal lubrication and narrowing of the vagina. Testosterone levels in both sexes decline with age, which may result in decreased libido.

CLINICAL FEATURES AND DIAGNOSIS

The diagnosis of a sexual problem relies on a thorough medical and sexual history, supplemented by physical examination and laboratory testing. A mixed organic/psychological basis is often present. Physical disorders, surgical conditions (Table 36-2), medications, and use or abuse of drugs (Table 36-3) can affect sexual function directly or cause secondary psychological reactions that lead to a sexual problem. Psychological factors may predispose to, precipitate, or maintain a sexual disorder (Box 36-1).

Approach to Sexual History-taking

The sexual history provides an invaluable opportunity to uncover sexual problems. Patients and physicians alike may be reluctant to discuss sexual problems. Thus, the need to make sexual history-taking a routine part of practice is paramount. Physicians should always attempt to be sensitive and non-judgmental in their interviewing technique, moving from general topics to more specific ones. Questions about sexual function may follow naturally from aspects of the medical history (such as introduction of a new medication, or investigation of a chief complaint that involves a gynecological or urological problem).

Screening questions include: Are you sexually active? With men, women, or both? Is there anything you would like to change about your sex life? Have there been any changes in your sex life? Are you satisfied with your present sex life? To maximize its effectiveness, the sexual history may be tailored to the patient's needs and goals. Physicians should recognize that patients with paraphilic disorders are often secretive about their activities, in part due to legal and societal implications. Patients should be reassured about the confidentiality of their interaction (except in cases where their behavior requires mandatory legal reporting, e.g., as with child abuse).

Clinicians should be aware of the growing numbers of patients with concerns about "hypersexuality" and "sexual addiction," in part spurred by ease of access to Internet pornography and "cybersex" activities. In fact, a "hypersexual disorder," conceptualized as a non-paraphilic sexual desire disorder with an impulsivity component, was proposed for

TABLE 36-3 Drugs and Medicines That Cause Sexual Dysfunction

Drug	Sexual Side Effect
CARDIOVASCULAR	
Methyldopa	Low libido, impotence, anorgasmia
Thiazide diuretics	Low libido, impotence, decreased lubrication
Clonidine	Impotence, anorgasmia
Propranolol	Low libido
Digoxin	Gynecomastia, low libido, impotence
Clofibrate	Low libido, impotence
PSYCHOTROPICS	
Sedatives	
Alcohol	Higher doses cause sexual problems
Barbiturates	Impotence
Anxiolytics	
Alprazolam; diazepam	Low libido, delayed ejaculation
Antipsychotics	
Thioridazine	Retarded or retrograde ejaculation
Haloperidol	Low libido, impotence, anorgasmia
Antidepressants	
MAOIs (phenelzine)	Impotence, retarded ejaculation, anorgasmia
Tricyclics (imipramine)	Low libido, impotence, retarded ejaculation
SSRIs (fluoxetine, sertraline)	Low libido, impotence, retarded ejaculation
Atypical (trazodone)	Priapism, retarded or retrograde ejaculation
Lithium	Low libido, impotence
Hormones	
Estrogen	Low libido in men
Progesterone	Low libido, impotence
GASTROINTESTINAL	
Cimetidine	Low libido, impotence
Methantheline bromide	Impotence
Opiates	Orgasmic dysfunction
Anticonvulsants	Low libido, impotence, priapism

MAOIs, Monoamine oxidase inhibitors; SSRIs, selective serotonin reuptake inhibitors.

BOX 36-1 Psychological Causes of Sexual Dysfunction

PREDISPOSING FACTORS
Lack of information/experience
Unrealistic expectations
Negative family attitudes to sex
Sexual trauma: rape, incest

PRECIPITATING FACTORS
Childbirth
Infidelity
Dysfunction in the partner

MAINTAINING FACTORS
Interpersonal issues
Family stress
Work stress
Financial problems
Depression
Performance anxiety
Gender dysphoria

DSM-5, although ultimately rejected. Nevertheless, the sexual history-taker should actively explore the role of the Internet in the patient's sexual and non-sexual functioning and the potential for excessive and/or compulsive sexual activities.

Physical Examination and Laboratory Investigation

While history-taking is often the most important tool in the diagnosis of sexual disorders, the physical examination and pertinent laboratory testing are useful in excluding an organic cause. There is no "routine" work-up. However, special attention should be paid to the endocrine, neurological, vascular, urological, and gynecological systems.

Tests for systemic illness include: complete blood count (CBC), urinalysis, creatinine, lipid profile, thyroid function studies, and fasting blood sugar (FBS). Endocrine studies (including testosterone, prolactin, luteinizing hormone [LH], and follicle-stimulating hormone [FSH]) can be performed to assess low libido and erectile dysfunction. An estrogen level and microscopic examination of a vaginal smear can be used to assess vaginal dryness. Cervical culture and Papanicolaou (Pap) smear can be performed to investigate a diagnosis of dyspareunia. The nocturnal penile tumescence (NPT) test is

valuable in the assessment of erectile dysfunction (ED). If NPT occurs regularly (as measured by a Rigi-Scan monitor), problems with erection are unlikely to be organic. Penile plethysmography is used to assess paraphilic disorders by measurement of an individual's sexual arousal in response to visual and auditory stimuli.

Diagnostic Features of Specific Sexual Dysfunctions

Male Disorders of Sexual Function

Erectile Disorder. Erectile dysfunction (ED) ("impotence") is characterized by marked difficulty obtaining or maintaining an erection during sexual activity or by a marked decrease in erectile rigidity. Symptoms should be present during 75%–100% of sexual encounters. More than 18 million American men over age 20 suffer from ED, accounting for more than 500,000 ambulatory care visits to health care professionals annually and affecting 40%–50% of men older than 60–70. Between 50% and 85% of cases of ED have an organic basis. Numerous risk factors for ED have been identified (Box 36-2). ED itself may be a symptom of a generalized vascular disease and should prompt further investigation. Depression is a common co-morbidity.

Delayed Ejaculation. Also known as "retarded ejaculation," this uncommon disorder is characterized by a marked delay, infrequency, or absence of ejaculation following normal sexual excitement that is not desired by the individual, occurring in 75%–100% of partnered sexual activity. Patients are usually sexually inexperienced men less than 35 years old. Symptoms are usually restricted to failure to reach orgasm in the vagina during intercourse. Delayed ejaculation must be differentiated from retrograde ejaculation, in which the bladder neck does not close off properly during orgasm, causing semen to spurt backward into the bladder. Delayed ejaculation should also be excluded in couples with infertility of unknown cause; the male may not have admitted his lack of ejaculation to his partner. Men with delayed ejaculation report lower levels of sexual arousal and satisfaction despite strong penile response during psychophysiological testing.

Premature (Early) Ejaculation. This disorder is defined as recurrent ejaculation with minimal sexual stimulation before, on, or shortly after penetration (within approximately 1

> **BOX 36-2** Risk Factors Associated with Erectile Disorder
>
> - Hypertension
> - Diabetes mellitus
> - Smoking
> - Coronary artery disease
> - Peripheral vascular disorders
> - Blood lipid abnormalities
> - Peyronie's disease
> - Priapism
> - Pelvic trauma or surgery
> - Renal failure and dialysis
> - Hypogonadism
> - Alcoholism
> - Depression
> - Lack of sexual knowledge
> - Poor sexual technique
> - Interpersonal problems

minute) and before the person wishes it. Rapid ejaculation is a common complaint reported in 20%–30% of men aged 18–70 internationally. However, only 1%–3% of men would meet the strict DSM-5 criteria for the disorder. Prolonged periods of no sexual activity make premature ejaculation worse. If the problem is chronic and untreated, secondary ED often occurs.

Male Hypoactive Sexual Desire Disorder. This is a new diagnosis in DSM-5 characterized by persistently or recurrently deficient or absent sexual/erotic thoughts or fantasies and desire for sexual activity. (In DSM-IV, there was one diagnosis of "hypoactive sexual desire disorder" applicable to both genders.) The prevalence of problems with sexual desire increases from 6% of men aged 18–24 to 41% of men aged 66–74. However, only 1.8% of men aged 16–44 would meet the strict DSM-5 definition of the disorder requiring symptoms to last at least 6 months.

Female Disorders of Sexual Function

Female Sexual Interest/Arousal Disorder. This disorder replaces the DSM-IV diagnosis "female sexual arousal disorder." It is characterized by absent/reduced interest in sexual activity, erotic thoughts, sexual excitement, arousal, and/or genital sensation and lack of initiation of sexual activity. The prevalence of this disorder as defined by DSM-5 is not known. The lifetime prevalence of its DSM-IV predecessor was estimated at 60%.

Female Orgasmic Disorder. This disorder is defined as a marked delay in, or infrequency or lack of intensity of, orgasm occurring in 75%–100% of occasions of sexual activity. Some women who can have orgasm with direct clitoral stimulation find it impossible to reach orgasm during intercourse. The estimated prevalence of female orgasmic problems ranges from 10% to 42%, but only a fraction of women report associated distress. The ability to reach orgasm increases with sexual experience. Claims that stimulation of the Grafenberg spot, or G spot, in a region in the anterior wall of the vagina will cause orgasm and female ejaculation have never been substantiated. Premature ejaculation in the male may contribute to female orgasmic dysfunction.

Genito-Pelvic Pain/Penetration Disorder. This disorder merges the DSM-IV entities dyspareunia (persistent genital pain associated with sexual intercourse) and vaginismus (recurrent involuntary spasm of the musculature of the outer third of the vagina) into one diagnosis. This change reflects the fact that vaginismus and dyspareunia were difficult to distinguish and tended to occur together. Of note, genito-pelvic pain/penetration disorder is specific to women, whereas dyspareunia could have been diagnosed in men or women. Symptoms of genito-pelvic pain/penetration disorder consist of persistent or recurrent difficulties with vulvovaginal pain or fear of pain during intercourse or penetration. There may be associated marked tensing of the pelvic floor muscles during attempted vaginal penetration. The prevalence is unknown; however, approximately 15% of North American women report recurrent pain during intercourse.

Sexual Dysfunctions Affecting Both Genders

Substance/Medication-Induced Sexual Dysfunction. This disorder (replacing "substance-induced sexual dysfunction" from DSM-IV) is characterized by a clinically significant disturbance in sexual function with objective evidence that the symptoms occurred soon after ingestion of a substance and could have been caused by the substance. It should cause clinically significant distress and not occur during the course of a delirium.

Other Specified and Unspecified Sexual Dysfunction. These diagnoses replace the DSM-IV terminology "sexual dysfunction not otherwise specified" but serve the same purpose. If the clinician wishes to explain why the symptoms do not meet full criteria for another disorder, the "other specified" diagnosis should be used. Otherwise, the "unspecified" diagnosis should be used. The DSM-IV diagnosis "sexual aversion disorder" (persistent extreme aversion to genital sexual contact with a partner) has been eliminated in DSM-5 due to lack of supporting evidence and infrequent use. However, the clinician may elect to use the "other specified" designation followed by "sexual aversion" as the specific reason to indicate this diagnosis.

Diagnostic Features of Specific Paraphilic Disorders

Most paraphilic disorders are thought to have a psychological basis. Individuals with paraphilic disorders have difficulty forming more socialized sexual relationships. Paraphilic disorders may involve a conditioned response in which nonsexual objects become sexually arousing when paired with a pleasurable activity (masturbation). The diagnostic criteria and clinical features of the major paraphilic disorders are summarized in Table 36-4.

Diagnostic Features of Gender Dysphoria

The DSM-5 replaces the older terminology "gender identity disorder" with the newer terminology "gender dysphoria." It also subclassifies gender dysphoria into disorders affecting children and those affecting adolescents and adults.

Gender Dysphoria in Children. Children with this disorder express a strong desire to be of the opposite gender and exhibit behaviors stereotypical of the other sex. They may participate in such activities as cross-dressing and cross-gender roles in fantasy play and prefer toys and sex characteristics of the opposite gender. Children with gender dysphoria may have co-existing separation anxiety, generalized anxiety, and depression and are 2–4.5 times more likely to be natal males.

Gender Dysphoria in Adolescents and Adults. This disorder is similar to the childhood form, but there is emphasis on incongruent sexual identity rather than participation in gender-atypical behaviors. Patients reject their own gender and secondary sex characteristics and desire those of the opposite

TABLE 36-4 Features of Specific Paraphilic Disorders

Disorder	Definition	Features
Exhibitionistic disorder	Exposure of genitals to unsuspecting strangers in public	Primary intent is to evoke shock or fear in victims. Offenders are usually male
Fetishistic disorder	Sexual arousal using non-living objects (e.g., female lingerie) or intense focus on a non-genital body part	Masturbation occurs while holding the fetish object. The sexual partner may wear the object
Frotteuristic disorder	Sexual arousal by touching and rubbing against a non-consenting person	The behavior occurs in a crowded public place from which the offender can escape arrest
Pedophilic disorder	Sexual activity with a prepubescent child. The patient must be at least 16 years of age and be at least 5 years older than the victim	Pedophilia is the most common paraphilic disorder. Most of the victims are girls, often relatives with the perpetrator. Most pedophiles are heterosexual
Sexual masochism disorder	Sexual pleasure comes from physical or mental abuse or humiliation	A dangerous form involves hypoxyphilia, in which oxygen deprivation enhances arousal, and accidental deaths can occur
Sexual sadism disorder	Sexual arousal is derived from causing mental or physical suffering to another person	Sexual sadism is mostly seen in men. It can progress to rape. 50% of those afflicted are alcoholic
Transvestic disorder	Cross-dressing in heterosexual males for sexual arousal	The wife (partner) may be aware of the activity and help in the selection of clothes or insist on treatment
Voyeuristic disorder	Sexual arousal by watching an unsuspecting person who is naked, disrobing, or engaging in sexual activity	Most commonly occurs in men, but it can occur in women. Masturbation commonly occurs
Other specified paraphilic disorder	Paraphilic disorders that do not meet criteria for any of the above categories	Categories include necrophilia (corpses), zoophilia (animals), urophilia (urine), and coprophilia (feces)
Unspecified paraphilic disorder	Paraphilic disorders that do not meet criteria for any of the above categories	Clinician chooses not to specify the reason that criteria are not met. Insufficient diagnostic information

TABLE 36-5 Psychiatric Differential Diagnosis of Sexual Dysfunction

Psychiatric Disorder	Sexual Complaint
Depression (major depression or dysthymic disorder)	Low libido, erectile dysfunction
Bipolar disorder (manic phase)	Increased libido
Generalized anxiety disorder, panic disorder, posttraumatic stress disorder	Low libido, erectile dysfunction, lack of vaginal lubrication, anorgasmia
Obsessive-compulsive disorder	Low libido, erectile dysfunction, lack of vaginal lubrication, anorgasmia, "anti-fantasies" focusing on the negative aspects of a partner
Schizophrenia	Low desire, bizarre sexual desires
Paraphilic disorder	Deviant sexual arousal causing distress and/or harm
Gender dysphoria	Dissatisfaction with one's own sexual preference or phenotype
Personality disorder (passive-aggressive, obsessive-compulsive, histrionic)	Low libido, erectile dysfunction, premature ejaculation, anorgasmia
Marital dysfunction/interpersonal problems	Varied
Fears of intimacy/commitment	Varied, deep intrapsychic issues

(or an alternative) gender. The disorder is equally likely in adolescent natal males and females but is more common in natal males as adults. The overall prevalence in adult natal males and females ranges from 0.005% to 0.014% and 0.002% to 0.003%, respectively. These statistics are based on patients seeking gender reassignment and therefore are likely underestimates. Associations include homosexual or bisexual orientation, anxiety, depression, suicidal ideation or attempts, and paraphilias.

DIFFERENTIAL DIAGNOSIS OF SEXUAL DISORDERS

The differential diagnosis of sexual disorders includes medical and surgical conditions (see Table 36-2), adverse effects of medications (see Table 36-3), and other psychiatric disorders (Table 36-5). Before a primary sexual disorder is diagnosed, it is important to identify potentially treatable conditions (both organic and psychiatric) that manifest as sexual problems. For example, treatment of depression may improve erectile function. While paraphilic disorders often have a psychological basis, an organic cause should be considered if the behavior begins at a late age; there is regression from previously normal sexuality; or there are abnormal physical findings. Box 36-3 lists the psychiatric differential diagnosis of paraphilic disorders. Patients with gender dysphoria generally have normal physical and laboratory findings. The differential diagnosis includes non-conformity to stereotypical sex role behaviors, transvestic fetishism (cross-dressing), and schizophrenia (e.g., with the delusion that one belongs to the other sex).

TREATMENT
Organically-Based Treatment

The essence of treatment for sexual disorders involves treatment of pre-existing illnesses, stoppage of, or substitution for, offending medications, lifestyle modification (e.g., reduction in alcohol and smoking, improvement in diet and exercise), and addition of medications for psychiatric conditions (e.g., depression). Although many medications for the treatment of hypertension inhibit sexual function, the angiotensin II receptor blockers (e.g., losartan) may actually ameliorate sexual problems. Any hormone deficiency should be corrected (e.g., addition of testosterone for hypogonadism, thyroid hormone for hypothyroidism, estrogen/testosterone [Estratest] for post-menopausal females, or bromocriptine for elevated prolactin).

Selective serotonin reuptake inhibitor (SSRI)-induced sexual dysfunction is a frequent complaint that has received significant attention. Treatment strategies include awaiting spontaneous remission, decreasing the dose of the SSRI, taking a drug holiday, switching SSRIs, switching to a non-SSRI, and adding an "antidote" drug, the last two options being the most efficacious. Non-SSRI antidepressants less likely to cause sexual dysfunction include: bupropion (Wellbutrin), mirtazapine (Remeron), possibly duloxetine (Cymbalta), trazodone (Desyrel), vilazodone (Viibryd—limited experience), nefazodone (brand name Serzone withdrawn in US), and transdermal selegiline (EMSAM). Non-approved antidepressants with fewer sexual side effects include: tianeptine (Stablon), reboxetine (Edronax, Vestra), moclobemide (Aurorix, Manerix), agomelatine (Valdoxan, Melitor, Thymanax), and gepirone (Ariza, Variza). PDE-5 inhibitors are the "antidotes" of choice, followed by bupropion and high-dose buspirone (Buspar). Possible antidotes include herbal agents, such as maca root and *gingko biloba*, and a variety of medications including amantadine (Symmetrel), dextroamphetamine (Dexedrine), methylphenidate (Ritalin), granisetron (Kytril), cyproheptadine (Periactin), yohimbine (Yocon), and atomoxetine (Strattera).

Premature Ejaculation

There is no Food and Drug Administration (FDA)–approved treatment for premature ejaculation. However, the SSRIs (e.g., fluoxetine [Prozac], sertraline [Zoloft], and paroxetine [Paxil]), used continuously or intermittently (2 to 12 hours before sex), can cause delayed ejaculation, which can treat premature ejaculation. The tricyclic clomipramine (Anafranil) is also efficacious. Dapoxetine (Priligy), an SSRI with a rapid onset and short half-life, was developed specifically to treat premature ejaculation but is not approved. Tramadol taken on-demand (in re-development for premature ejaculation under the brand name Zertane) appears promising, but as a weak opioid is limited by potential dependency. Topical anesthetic agents under investigation include the lidocaine/prilocaine eutectic mixture (EMLA cream) and topical eutectic-like mixture for premature ejaculation (TEMPE or PSD 502).

However, these can cause skin irritation and penile numbing. Co-existing ED if present should be treated first with PDE-5 inhibitors.

Erectile Disorder

The mainstay of treatment for ED is the use of oral PDE-5 inhibitors, which can help men with a wide range of conditions; they are easy to use and have few adverse effects (Table 36-6). Available agents are sildenafil (Viagra), vardenafil (Levitra; Staxyn orally disintegrating tablet [ODT]), and tadalafil (Cialis). A newer PDE-5 inhibitor, avanafil (Stendra), with faster onset of action, is already FDA-approved but has only been recently marketed in the US (Table 36-6). PDE-5 inhibitors in development include mirodenafil (Mvix), udenafil (Zydena), lodenafil (Helleva), dasantafil, SLx-2101, JNJ-10280205, and JNJ-10287069. Of note, the PDE-5 inhibitors are metabolized by P450 3A4 and 2C9 isoenzyme systems. Patients who take potent inhibitors (including grapefruit juice, cimetidine, ketoconazole, erythromycin, and ritonavir) of these P450 isoenzyme systems should have a lower starting dose of a PDE-5 inhibitor. Statins may also help improve the efficacy of PDE-5 inhibitors.

The only other oral pharmacologic agent FDA-approved for the treatment of ED is yohimbine (Yocon), an α_2-adrenergic inhibitor, although its efficacy is uncertain. Other (non-approved) agents include α-receptor blocker phentolamine (Vasomax), dopamine agonist apomorphine (Uprima), melanocortin agonist bremelanotide (PT-141), amino acid L-arginine (ArginMax), opioid antagonist naltrexone (Depade, Revia) and serotonin/dopamine modulator, clavulanic acid (Zoraxel). 5-HT$_{2C}$ serotonin receptor agonists including trazodone appear to stimulate erections in some studies. Topical agents include alprostadil cream (Topiglan), minoxidil solution, and nitroglycerine ointment. Herbal agents are of uncertain benefit with *P. ginseng*, *B. superba*, and *L. meyenii* (maca root) appearing more promising; some herbals may contain traces of PDE-5 inhibitors. Transdermal testosterone and/or clomiphene citrate (Clomid) may be considered for hypogonadal men with ED.

Second-line treatments for ED include use of intrapenile injection therapy, intraurethral suppository therapy, and vacuum-assisted devices (Table 36-7). Injectable gene therapies for ED, such as hMaxi-K, are promising, but clinical trials are in the early stages. The third-line treatment for ED is surgical implantation of an inflatable or malleable rod or penile prosthesis. Endarterectomy may correct ED in certain patients with underlying vascular disease. Pelvic drug-eluting vascular stents (e.g., zotarolimus) are in investigational stages.

Female Sexual Dysfunction

The only approved medical–surgical intervention for the treatment of female sexual dysfunction is EROS-CTD, a clitoral suction device, which is used to increase vasocongestion and engorge the clitoris for better sexual arousal and orgasm. Additionally, ospemifene (Osphena), an oral selective estrogen receptor modulator, was recently approved for post-menopausal dyspareunia caused by vulvar and vaginal atrophy. Otherwise, most agents used to treat sexual dysfunction in men have been tried in women with limited success. Recent studies did demonstrate a reduction in SSRI-induced adverse sexual effects in women receiving sildenafil. Hormonal agents have been studied extensively, although enthusiasm has been tempered by links with cardiovascular disease and breast cancer. Transdermal/topical preparations include: estrogen/testosterone (Estratest); testosterone (LibiGel—Phase III trials; Intrinsa—rejected by FDA); and prostaglandin E$_1$ (alprostadil). Oral hormonal therapies include estrogen for vasomotor

TABLE 36-6 First-line Treatment for Erectile Dysfunction: Comparison of PDE-5 Inhibitors

Medication	Dose	Onset	Duration	Food Interaction	Advantages	Side Effects	Contraindications
Sildenafil (Viagra)	25–100 mg (maximum)	30–60 min	Up to 12 h	Delayed absorption with high-fat foods	>65% efficacy / Longest track record	Headache, low BP, flushing, dyspepsia, vasodilation, diarrhea, visual changes (blue tinge to vision), hearing loss (rare) / Non-arteritic anterior ischemic optic neuropathy (NAION)—not proven	Active CAD, hypotension / No nitrates for 24 hr after dose / Caution with α-blockers
Vardenafil (Levitra)	2.5–20 mg (maximum)	30–60 min	Up to 10 h	Delayed absorption with high-fat foods	>65% efficacy / Available as ODT preparation (Staxyn)	Headache, low BP, flushing, dyspepsia, vasodilation, diarrhea, visual changes, hearing loss (rare) / NAION—not proven	Active CAD, hypotension / May prolong QTc / May increase LFT / No nitrates for 24 h after dose / Avoid α-blockers Hytrin and Cardura / Cautious use with Flomax or Uroxotra
Tadalafil (Cialis)	2.5–20 mg (maximum) / Only PDE-5 inhibitor approved for daily use (5 mg)	60–120 min	Up to 36 h	None	>65% efficacy / No visual side effects / Can be taken with food	Headache, low BP, flushing, dyspepsia, vasodilation, diarrhea, back pain, myalgias, hearing loss (rare) / NAION—not proven	Active CAD, hypotension / No nitrates for 48 h after dose / Avoid α-blockers Hytrin and Cardura / Cautious use with Flomax or Uroxotra
Avanafil (Stendra)	50–200 mg (maximum)	15–30 min	Up to 6 h	None	Similar efficacy to other PDE-5 inhibitors / Can be taken with food / Shortest onset of action / Shortest duration of action and interaction with nitrates	Headache, low BP, flushing, dyspepsia, nasal congestion, dizziness, hearing loss (rare) / NAION—not proven	No nitrates for 12 hr after dose / Start at lower dose (50 mg instead of 100 mg) if on (stable) α-blocker

BP, Blood pressure; CAD, coronary artery disease; LFT, liver function test. ODT, orally-disintegrating tablet.

TABLE 36-7 Second-line Treatments for Erectile Dysfunction

Treatment	Effects	Advantages	Disadvantages
Intraurethral suppository: alprostadil (MUSE)	Prostaglandin E₁ gel delivered by applicator into meatus of penis Induces vasodilation to cause erection	60% efficacy Less penile fibrosis and priapism than with penile injections Can be used twice daily	Not recommended with pregnant partners Mild penile/urethral pain
Penile self-injection: alprostadil (Caverject and Edex)	Prostaglandin E₁ injected into base of penis Induces vasodilation to cause erection	50%–87% efficacy Few systemic side effects	Can cause penile pain, priapism, fibrosis Not recommended for daily use
Intracavernosal injection: vasoactive intestinal polypeptide (VIP) + phentolamine: aviptadil (Senatek)	VIP causes veno-occlusion while phentolamine increases arterial flow	Associated with less pain than alprostadil and therefore preferred by patients	Less effective than alprostadil
Vacuum constriction device (pump)	Creates vacuum to draw blood into penile cavernosa Elastic band holds blood in penis	67% efficacy No systemic side effects Safe if erection not maintained more than 1 h	May not be acceptable to partner Erection hinged at base; does not allow for external ejaculation

symptoms, novel steroid tibolone (rejected), and dehydroepi-androsterone (DHEA) for women with adrenal insufficiency. The serotonin modulator flibanserin (Girosa) was developed specifically to treat female hypoactive sexual desire disorder (DSM-IV diagnostic criteria) but was withdrawn after a negative FDA report.

Paraphilic Disorders

Pharmacological therapy for paraphilic disorders is aimed at suppression of compulsive sexual behavior. The anti-androgen drugs, cyproterone (CPA—not FDA-approved) and medroxyprogesterone acetate (MPA, Depo-Provera), are used to reduce aberrant sexual tendencies. Treatment with synthetic gonadotropin-releasing hormone analogues (approved for prostate cancer), including leuprorelin (Prostap), triptorelin (Trelstar), and goserelin (Zoladex), is also effective, while oral estrogen (ethinyl estradiol) is less so. The SSRIs and clomipramine (Anafranil) reduce aberrant sexual urges by decreasing the compulsivity/impulsivity of the act. Paraphilic disorders commonly co-exist with ADHD, and the addition of psychostimulants, such as methylphenidate sustained-release (Ritalin-SR), to SSRIs appears beneficial in controlling paraphilic behaviors.

Gender Dysphoria

The major treatment for gender dysphoria disorder is sex-reassignment surgery. Hormone therapy may be necessary to suppress original sex characteristics: that is, with luteinizing hormone-releasing hormone (LH-RH) agonists, CPA, estrogens, or testosterone.

Psychologically-Based Treatments
Sexual Dysfunction

General principles of treatment include improving communication (verbally and physically) between partners, encouraging experimentation, decreasing the pressure of performance by changing the goal of sexual activity away from erection or orgasm to feeling good about oneself, and relieving the pressure of the moment. The PLISSIT model provides a useful framework for approaching treatment of sexual problems and can be tailored to the desired level of intervention. The stages are (1) P: permission; (2) LI: limited information; (3) SS: specific suggestions; and (4) IT: intensive therapy. Permission-giving involves reassuring the patient about sexual

activity, alleviating guilt about activities the patient feels are "bad" or "dirty," and reinforcing the normal range of sexual activities. Limited information includes providing basic knowledge about anatomy and physiology and correcting myths and misconceptions. Specific suggestions include techniques of behavioral sex therapy (Table 36-8). Intensive therapy may be useful for patients with chronic sexual problems or complex psychological issues. While the first three stages (P, LI, SS) may be implemented by any health care provider, the last stage (IT) usual requires an expert with special training in sex therapy.

Paraphilic Disorders

Paraphilic disorders are often refractory to treatment, and recidivism is high, but several non-pharmacological modalities have been used with varying success. Insight-oriented or supportive psychotherapy is relatively ineffective. Cognitive-behavioral therapy can be used to help patients identify aberrant sexual tendencies, alter their behavior, and avoid sexual triggers to prevent relapse. Aversive therapy, via conditioning with ammonia, is used to reduce paraphilic behavior. Orgasmic reconditioning is used to teach the paraphilic patient how to become aroused by more acceptable mental images. Social skills training (individual or group) is used to help the paraphilic form better interpersonal relationships. Surveillance systems (using family members to help monitor patient behavior) may be helpful. Lifelong maintenance is required.

Gender Dysphoria

Individual psychotherapy is useful both in helping patients understand their gender dysphoria and in addressing other psychiatric issues. A thorough psychological evaluation is generally required before sex-reassignment surgery can be performed. Marital and family therapy can help with adjustment to a new gender.

FUTURE OUTLOOK

Sexual disorders remain common and are associated with significant long-term emotional, physical, and psychosocial stress. However, decreasing societal stigma, combined with increasing understanding of the medical basis of sexual disorders, has enabled more patients to feel comfortable seeking treatment. The newly released DSM-5 has made substantial

TABLE 36-8 Specific Behavioral Techniques of Sex Therapy

Sexual Disorder	Suggestions
Male hypoactive sexual desire disorder	Sensate focus exercises (non-demand pleasuring techniques) to enhance enjoyment without pressure Erotic material, masturbation training
Female sexual interest/arousal disorder	Sensate focus exercises Lubrication: saliva, KY Jelly for vaginal dryness
Other specified sexual dysfunction: sexual aversion	Sensate focus exercises For phobic/panic symptoms, use antianxiety/antidepressant medications
Erectile disorder	Sensate focus exercises (non-demand pleasuring techniques) Use female superior position (heterosexual couple) for non-demanding intercourse Female manually stimulates penis, and if erection is obtained, she inserts the penis into the vagina and begins movement Learn ways to satisfy partner without penile/vaginal intercourse
Female orgasmic disorder	Self-stimulation Use of fantasy materials Kegel vaginal exercises (contraction of pubococcygeus muscles) Use of controlled intercourse in female superior position "Bridge technique"—male stimulates female's clitoris manually after insertion of the penis into the vagina
Delayed ejaculation (during intercourse)	Female stimulates male manually until orgasm becomes inevitable Insert penis into vagina and begin thrusting
Premature ejaculation	Increased frequency of sex "Squeeze technique"—female manually stimulates penis until ejaculation is approaching, then squeezes the penis with her thumb on the frenulum; pressure is applied until male no longer feels the urge to ejaculate (15–60 seconds); use the female superior position with gradual thrusting and the "squeeze" technique as excitement intensifies "Stop-start technique"—female stimulates the male to the point of ejaculation, then stops the stimulation; she resumes the stimulation for several stop-start procedures, until ejaculation is allowed to occur
Genito-pelvic pain/penetration disorder	Treat any underlying gynecological problem first Treat insufficient lubrication using, e.g., KY Jelly Female is encouraged to accept larger and larger objects into her vagina (e.g., her fingers, her partner's fingers, Hegar graduated vaginal dilators, syringe containers of different sizes) Recommend use of the female superior position, allowing female to gradually insert erect penis into the vagina Practice Kegel vaginal exercises to develop a sense of control

changes to the classification of sexual disorders. The introduction of stricter criteria for the diagnosis of sexual dysfunctions and "normalization" of certain paraphilias significantly broaden the scope of "acceptable" sexual behavior. While these changes may help to further reassure patients, they could also lead to decreased interest in developing treatment options. The new language also harbors potential legal implications, for example, in regards to equivocally "harmful" paraphilias. Although a "hypersexual disorder" was ultimately not included in the book, clinicians should still recognize such symptoms and proactively inquire about and treat them.

PDE-5 inhibitors remain among the most effective agents for the treatment for sexual dysfunction. Although research continues, to date other pharmacologic options are limited. Further elucidation of the brain mechanisms behind sexual desire and arousal will allow for new therapeutic targets. Genetic research also heralds a new era in drug development aimed at personalized medicine through application of pharmacogenetic principles.

Although sex is increasingly "medicalized," the role of psychological interventions in the treatment of sexual problems should not be overlooked. Evidence-based clinical guidelines for the treatment of sexual disorders may help in optimizing short- and long-term management strategies. Overall, a multidisciplinary approach appears to be advantageous and will continue to evolve with time.

Access a list of MCQs for this chapter at https://expertconsult.inkling.com

SUGGESTED READING

Alwaal A, Al-Mannie R, Carrier S. Future prospects in the treatment of erectile dysfunction: focus on avanafil. *Drug Des Devel Ther* 5:435–443, 2011.

American Psychiatric Association. *Diagnostic and statistical manual of mental disorders*, ed 5, Washington, DC, 2013, American Psychiatric Association, pp 423–459, 685–705.

Basson R. Sexual desire and arousal disorders in women. *N Engl J Med* 354(14):1497–1506, 2006.

Basson R, Schultz WW. Sexual sequelae of general medical disorders. *Lancet* 369(9559):409–424, 2007.

Campbell N, Clark JP, Stecher VJ, et al. Adulteration of purported herbal and natural sexual performance enhancement dietary supplements with synthetic phosphodiesterase type 5 inhibitors. *J Sex Med* 10(7):1842–1849, 2013.

Dean RC, Lue TF. Physiology of penile erection and pathophysiology of erectile dysfunction. *Urol Clin North Am* 32(4):379–395, 2005.

Dording CM, Fisher L, Papakostas G, et al. A double-blind, randomized, pilot dose-finding study of maca root (L. meyenii) for the management of SSRI-induced sexual dysfunction. *CNS Neurosci Ther* 14(3):182–191, 2008.

Dording CM, LaRocca RA, Hails KA, et al. The effect of sildenafil on quality of life. *Ann Clin Psychiatry* 25(1):3–10, 2013.

Feldman HA, Goldstein I, Hatzichristou DG, et al. Impotence and its medical and psychosocial correlates: results of the Massachusetts Male Aging Study. *J Urol* 151(1):54–61, 1994.

Garcia FD, Delavenne HG, Assumpção Ade F, et al. Pharmacologic treatment of sex offenders with paraphilic disorder. *Curr Psychiatry Rep* 15(5):356, 2013.

Goldstein I, Lue TF, Padma-Nathan H, et al. Oral sildenafil in the treatment of sexual dysfunction. *N Engl J Med* 338(20):1397–1404, 1998.

Kafka M. Psychopharmacologic treatments for nonparaphilic compulsive sexual behaviors. *CNS Spectr* 5(1):49–59, 2000.

Kafka MP. Hypersexual disorder: a proposed diagnosis for DSM-V. *Arch Sex Behav* 39(2):377–400, 2010.

Kaplan HS. *The sexual desire disorders: dysfunctional regulation of sexual motivation*, New York, 2013, Brunner/Mazel.

Laumann EO, Paik A, Rosen RC. Sexual dysfunction in the United States. *JAMA* 281:537–544, 1999.

La Torre A, Conca A, Duffy D, et al. Sexual dysfunction related to psychotropic drugs: a critical review—part II: antipsychotics. *Pharmacopsychiatry* 46(6):201–208, 2013.

La Torre A, Giupponi G, Duffy D, et al. Sexual dysfunction related to psychotropic drugs: a critical review part I: antidepressants. *Pharmacopsychiatry* 46(5):191–199, 2013.

McMahon CG. Dapoxetine: a new option in the medical management of premature ejaculation. *Ther Adv Urol* 4(5):233–251, 2012.

Nurnberg HG, Hensley PL, Heiman JR, et al. Sildenafil treatment of women with antidepressant-associated sexual dysfunction: a randomized controlled trial. *JAMA* 300(4):395–404, 2008.

Palacios S. Hypoactive sexual desire disorder and current pharmacotherapeutic options in women. *Womens Health (Lond Engl)* 7(1):95–107, 2011.

Raina R, Pahlajani G, Khan S, et al. Female sexual dysfunction: classification, pathophysiology, and management. *Fertil Steril* 88(5):1273–1284, 2007.

Rosler A, Witztum E. Treatment of men with paraphilia with a long-acting analogue of gonadotropin-releasing hormone. *N Engl J Med* 338(7):416–422, 1998.

Shafer LC. Sexual disorders and sexual dysfunction. In Stern TA, Fricchione GL, Cassem NH, et al., editors: *Massachusetts General Hospital handbook of general hospital psychiatry*, ed 6, Philadelphia, 2010, Elsevier, pp 323–335.

Shafer LC. Sexual disorders and sexual dysfunction. In Stern TA, Herman JB, Gorrindo T, editors: *Massachusetts General Hospital: psychiatry update and board preparation*, ed 3, Boston, 2012, MGH Psychiatry Academy Publishing, pp 171–180.

Shamloul R, Ghanem H. Erectile dysfunction. *Lancet* 381(9861):153–165, 2013.

Shifren JL, Braunstein GD, Simon JA, et al. Transdermal testosterone treatment in women with impaired sexual function after oophorectomy. *N Engl J Med* 343(10):682–688, 2000.

Shifren JL, Monz BU, Russo PA, et al. Sexual problems and distress in United States women: prevalence and correlates. *Obstet Gynecol* 112(5):970–978, 2008.

Thompson IM, Tangen CM, Goodman PJ, et al. Erectile dysfunction and subsequent cardiovascular disease. *JAMA* 294(23):2996–3002, 2005.

Unger CA. Care of the transgender patient: the role of the gynecologist. *Am J Obstet Gynecol* 210(1):16–26, 2014.

Yuan J, Zhang R, Yang Z, et al. Comparative effectiveness and safety of oral phosphodiesterase type 5 inhibitors for erectile dysfunction: a systematic review and network meta-analysis. *Eur Urol* 63(5):902–912, 2013.

37 Eating Disorders: Evaluation and Management

Jennifer J. Thomas, PhD, Diane W. Mickley, MD, FACP, FAED, Jennifer L. Derenne, MD, FACP, FAED, Anne Klibanski, MD, Helen B. Murray, BA, and Kamryn T. Eddy, PhD

KEY POINTS

Incidence

- Eating disorders are prevalent among young women, but they can occur across diverse ages and populations.

Epidemiology

- Eating disorders are associated with serious medical co-morbidity related to nutritional compromise, to low weight, and to chronic bingeing and purging behaviors.

Treatment Options

- The majority of individuals with an eating disorder do not access treatment for this illness.
- Leading evidence-based treatments include cognitive-behavioral therapy for bulimia nervosa and binge-eating disorder; and family-based treatment for adolescent anorexia nervosa.
- Interdisciplinary team management (including primary/specialty medical care, psychotherapy, psychopharmacology, and nutritional counseling) is often necessary for optimal treatment.

Complications

- Although many medical complications of anorexia nervosa resolve with recovery, bone loss may persist and increase the fracture risk life-long.

Prognosis

- Anorexia nervosa has among the highest mortality rates of all mental illnesses (comparable to substance abuse).

OVERVIEW

Eating disorders comprise several phenomenologically-related conditions that are characterized by a disturbance in patterns of eating, often in concert with body image disturbance. Each of the eating disorder diagnoses is associated with substantial distress and psychosocial impairment. Moreover, because the behaviors can result in serious medical complications, these illnesses can have a catastrophic impact on physiological health, as well as on psychological function.

CLASSIFICATION

Current *Diagnostic and Statistical Manual of Mental Disorders, Fifth Edition* (DSM-5) diagnostic categories for eating disorders include anorexia nervosa (AN), bulimia nervosa (BN), binge-eating disorder (BED), and other specified feeding or eating disorder (OSFED).[1] AN is further divided into two subtypes (restricting and binge-eating/purging). DSM-5 specifiers for AN, BN, and BED allow for descriptive indicators of relative severity (mild, moderate, severe, or extreme) and symptomatic improvement (partial vs. full remission). Severity is dictated primarily by body mass index (BMI) for AN,

frequency of binge eating and purging for BN, and frequency of binge-eating for BED. OSFED (previously termed "eating disorder, not otherwise specified" in DSM-IV[2]) allows for specification of sub threshold or atypical symptom presentations. A change from prior versions of DSM, DSM-5 combines both feeding and eating disorders into a single section. Feeding disorders in DSM-5 include pica (persistent ingestion of non-nutritive, non-food substances), rumination disorder (regular regurgitation of previously ingested food), and avoidant/restrictive food intake disorder (limited food intake leading to nutritional deficiency, in the absence of shape and weight concerns). Because research on the etiology, clinical features, and treatment of feeding disorders is ongoing, this chapter will focus specifically on eating disorders (i.e., AN, BN, BED, and OSFED), which are better understood.

EPIDEMIOLOGY

The incidence of eating disorders ascertained by case registries probably underestimates the true incidence for several reasons. Data from the National Comorbidity Survey Replication (NCS-R) indicated that fewer than half of individuals with an eating disorder access any kind of health care service for their illness.[3] Many of those affected are known to avoid or to postpone clinical care for the condition. In addition, both BN and BED may manifest without clinical signs, making them difficult, if not impossible, to recognize in a clinical setting without patient disclosure of symptoms, which may not be forthcoming.[4] Furthermore, whereas AN may manifest with a variety of clinical signs, including emaciation, many patients effectively conceal their symptoms; up to 50% of cases of eating disorders may be missed in clinical settings.[5] The lifetime prevalence of AN has been estimated at 0.9% for adult females, 0.3% for adult males,[3] and 0.3% among adolescent males and females.[6] BN is more common than is AN, with a reported lifetime prevalence in adult women of 1.5% and adult men of 0.5%,[3] and 0.9% in adolescent males and females.[6] BED appears to be the most common eating disorder, with a lifetime prevalence ranging from 2.0% for adult males to 3.5% for adult females[3] and 1.6% in adolescents.[6] In addition, sub threshold presentations (captured by OSFED) are at least twice as common as AN, BN, and BED combined.[7] The prevalence of eating disorders appears to vary by gender, ethnicity, and the type of population studied. Although eating disorders historically have been reported as more common in females than males,[2] males may be under-identified. Eating disorders also occur in culturally, ethnically, and socioeconomically diverse populations. It is thus important for clinicians to remain vigilant for possible eating disorder symptoms regardless of patient demographics.

COURSE, CO-MORBIDITY, AND MORTALITY RATE

AN can onset from childhood to adulthood, but it most commonly begins in post-pubertal adolescence. Likewise, the most common time of onset for BN is in post-pubertal (usually late) adolescence. Both BN and BED can onset in later decades.[3]

Greater than half of those with AN and BN will achieve recovery over long-term follow-up, and more will have symptomatic improvement short of full recovery; approximately 20-33% will have a chronic course.[8,9] Notwithstanding the data and conventional wisdom that AN, in particular, often follows a chronic course, the NCS-R study reported that AN had a significantly shorter course than either BN or BED.[3] These data suggest that there may be more variation in the course of AN than previously thought, possibly due to the fact that some individuals experience remission before seeking care. Outcomes for BED are somewhat more favorable with the majority achieving symptom remission over time but still up to one third remaining more chronically ill.[10] Moreover, there is also considerable diagnostic migration across eating disorder categories, typically reflecting crossover from a primarily restrictive to a bingeing and/or purging presentation over time.[11–13] Eating disorders are associated with high medical co-morbidity (as nutritional derangement and purging behaviors frequently lead to serious medical complications); they are also associated with a high degree of psychiatric co-morbidity. The NCS-R study found that a majority of respondents with each of the full threshold eating disorders (AN, BN, and BED) had a lifetime history of another psychiatric disorder. Of these, 94.5% of respondents with BN had a lifetime history of a co-morbid mental illness.[3] The mortality risk associated with eating disorders is also elevated.[14,15] The risk of mortality may be increased by co-morbid factors, such as substance abuse, and by a longer duration of illness.[16] The high mortality rate is accounted for by both serious medical complications of the behaviors, and by a suicide rate that is 18 times that expected in AN, in particular.[17]

ETIOLOGICAL FACTORS

Although the etiology of eating disorders is likely multifactorial, causal factors are uncertain.[18] Possible sociocultural, biological, and psychological risk factors all have been identified, despite methodological limitations that characterize many studies. In addition to female gender and ethnicity, weight concerns and negative self-evaluation have the strongest empirical support as risk factors for eating disorders.[18] In particular, risk factors for obesity appear to be associated with BED,[19] and risk factors for dieting appear to be associated with BN.[20] Risk for an eating disorder may also be elevated by generic risk factors for mental illness.[18–20]

Sociocultural factors are strongly suggested by population studies that have demonstrated that transnational migration, modernization, and Westernization are associated with an elevated risk for disordered eating among vulnerable subpopulations. Other social environmental factors (such as peer influence, teasing, bullying, and mass media exposure) have been linked with an elevated risk of body image disturbance or disordered eating.[21]

Numerous psychological factors have been identified as either risk factors or retrospective correlates of eating disorders. Among these is exposure to health problems (including digestive problems) in early childhood, exposure to sexual abuse and adverse life events, higher levels of neuroticism, low self-esteem, and anxiety disorders.[18] Furthermore, a cognitive style characterized by weak set-shifting (i.e., difficulty switching between tasks) and poor central coherence (i.e., hyper-focus on minor details to the detriment of grasping the bigger picture) is common in AN and may increase risk for the disorder.[22]

Genetic influences on eating disorders have also been studied. Although family and twin studies support a substantial genetic contribution to the risk for eating disorders and molecular genetic studies hold promise, our understanding of the genetic transmission of risk for eating disorders remains limited. Evolving studies in the area are focusing on the genetic underpinnings of symptoms associated with the eating disorders (rather than diagnoses), as well as gene–environment interactions.[23,24] Emerging evidence from neuroimaging research suggests that, compared to healthy controls, individuals with AN experience an over-activation of neural circuitry in the fear network when presented with food stimuli.[25] In contrast, individuals with BN may binge eat, in part, due to hypoactivation of reward circuitry and impairments in neural networks that contribute to impulse control.[25]

DIAGNOSTIC FEATURES

Considerable phenomenological overlap and diagnostic migration across AN, BN, BED, and OSFED has contributed to a "transdiagnostic" view of eating disorders that highlights similarities in both symptoms and maintaining mechanisms.[26] However, by definition, a diagnosis of one eating disorder is mutually exclusive with another at any particular point in time.

Anorexia Nervosa

AN is characterized and distinguished by a significantly low body weight. A significantly low body weight is assessed in relation to sex, age, and height. Although the clinical context guides whether a particular weight is consistent with AN, a commonly recognized guideline for adults is a BMI less than 18.5 kg/m² (i.e., the lower limit of the normal range). For children and adolescents, the American Academy of Pediatrics and the American Psychiatric Association have set forth practice guidelines that encourage providers to determine an individual adolescent's goal weight range using past growth charts, menstrual history, mid-parental height, and even bone age as guides. The Centers for Disease Control and Prevention (CDC) recommends use of normative growth charts, which plot BMI percentiles for age (2 to 20 years) and sex. Although children who fall below the fifth percentile in BMI for age are generally considered underweight,[1] children who are above the fifth percentile may also be considered underweight particularly in the instance of deviation from growth trajectory. Of note, many physicians note that children and adolescents can be sensitive to the medical consequences of eating disorders even when weight does not appear to be dangerously low.

In addition to a low body weight, AN is often characterized in Western populations by a fear of becoming fat or gaining weight. This may also be manifested in behavior that interferes with gaining weight (e.g., restrictive eating, purging, or compulsive exercising), particularly for those individuals who do not explicitly endorse a fear of fatness.[27] Individuals with AN also often exhibit a disturbance in body experience that can range from a lack of insight or recognition of serious medical consequences to a distorted perception of one's weight and shape and their importance.

Cognitive symptoms can often be assessed by asking about dietary routines, food restrictions, and the patient's desired body weight. Of note, children and adolescents do not always report cognitive symptoms, possibly due to developmental factors.[28] Binge-eating and purging symptoms are common yet often overlooked in AN. The binge-eating/purging subtype of AN is diagnosed in the setting of recurrent binge-eating and purging; otherwise the diagnosis of restricting-type AN is made. Box 37-1 summarizes diagnostic criteria for AN.

Bulimia Nervosa

BN is characterized by recurrent episodes of binge-eating and by behaviors aimed at the prevention of weight gain or purging calories. These behaviors, termed "inappropriate

BOX 37-1 DSM-5 Diagnostic Criteria: Anorexia Nervosa (307.1 (F50.01 restricting type, F50.02 binge-eating/purging type))

A. Restriction of energy intake relative to requirements, leading to a significantly low body weight in the context of age, sex, developmental trajectory, and physical health. *Significantly low weight* is defined as weight that is less than minimally normal or, for children and adolescents, less than that minimally expected.

B. Intense fear of gaining weight or of becoming fat, or persistent behavior that interferes with weight gain, even though at a significantly low weight.

C. Disturbance in the way in which one's body weight or shape is experienced, undue influence of body weight or shape on self-evaluation, or persistent lack of recognition of the seriousness of the current low body weight.

Specify whether:

Restricting type: During the last 3 months, the individual has not engaged in recurrent episodes of binge eating or purging behavior (i.e., self-induced vomiting or the misuse of laxatives, diuretics, or enemas). This subtype describes presentations in which weight loss is accomplished primarily through dieting, fasting, and/or excessive exercise.

Binge-eating/purging type: During the last 3 months, the individual has engaged in recurrent episodes of binge eating or purging behavior (i.e., self-induced vomiting or the misuse of laxatives, diuretics, or enemas).

Specify if:

In partial remission: After full criteria for anorexia nervosa were previously met, Criterion A (low body weight) has not been met for a sustained period, but either Criterion B (intense fear of gaining weight or becoming fat or behavior that interferes with weight gain) or Criterion C (disturbances in self-perception of weight and shape) is still met.

In full remission: After full criteria for anorexia nervosa were previously met, none of the criteria have been met for a sustained period of time.

Specify current severity:

The minimum level of severity is based, for adults, on current body mass index (BMI) (see below) or, for children and adolescents, on BMI percentile. The ranges below are derived from World Health Organization categories for thinness in adults; for children and adolescents, corresponding BMI percentiles should be used. The level of severity may be increased to reflect clinical symptoms, the degree of functional disability, and the need for supervision.

Mild: BMI ≥ 17 kg/m^2
Moderate: BMI 16–16.99 kg/m^2
Severe: BMI 15–15.99 kg/m^2
Extreme: BMI < 15 kg/m^2

Reprinted with permission from the Diagnostic and statistical manual of mental disorders, *ed 5, (Copyright 2013). American Psychiatric Association.*

BOX 37-2 DSM-5 Diagnostic Criteria: Bulimia Nervosa (307.51 (F50.2))

A. Recurrent episodes of binge eating. An episode of binge eating is characterized by both of the following:
   1. Eating, in a discrete period of time (e.g., within any 2-hour period), an amount of food that is definitely larger than what most individuals would eat in a similar period of time under similar circumstances.
   2. A sense of lack of control over eating during the episode (e.g., a feeling that one cannot stop eating or control what or how much one is eating).

B. Recurrent inappropriate compensatory behaviors in order to prevent weight gain, such as self-induced vomiting; misuse of laxatives, diuretics, or other medications; fasting; or excessive exercise.

C. The binge eating and inappropriate compensatory behaviors both occur, on average, at least once a week for 3 months.

D. Self-evaluation is unduly influenced by body shape and weight.

E. The disturbance does not occur exclusively during episodes of anorexia nervosa.

Specify if:

In partial remission: After full criteria for bulimia nervosa were previously met, some, but not all, of the criteria have been met for a sustained period of time.

In full remission: After full criteria for bulimia nervosa were previously met, none of the criteria have been met for a sustained period of time.

Specify current severity:

The minimum level of severity is based on the frequency of inappropriate compensatory behaviors (see below). The level of severity may be increased to reflect other symptoms and the degree of functional disability.

Mild: An average of 1–3 episodes of inappropriate compensatory behaviors per week.
Moderate: An average of 4–7 episodes of inappropriate compensatory behaviors per week.
Severe: An average of 8–13 episodes of inappropriate compensatory behaviors per week.
Extreme: An average of 14 or more episodes of inappropriate compensatory behaviors per week.

Reprinted with permission from the Diagnostic and statistical manual of mental disorders, *ed 5, (Copyright 2013). American Psychiatric Association.*

binge-eating/purging type, although low weight is one helpful feature to draw a distinction between the two. A binge eating episode is considered to take place in a discrete time period, consists of the intake of an unusually large amount of food given the social context, and is subjectively experienced as being out of control. Box 37-2 summarizes the diagnostic criteria for BN.

Binge-eating Disorder

BED is characterized by recurrent episodes of binge-eating. Unlike in individuals with BN, there are no recurrent compensatory behaviors. Binge-eating episodes are accompanied by at least three of five correlates (these include eating rapidly, eating until uncomfortably full, eating when not hungry, or eating alone to avoid embarrassment; and feeling guilty post-binge) and are associated with marked distress. In parallel with the frequency and duration criteria for BN, individuals

compensatory behaviors" in the DSM-5,[1] induced self-induced vomiting; laxative, enema, and diuretic misuse; stimulant abuse; diabetic underdosing of insulin; fasting; and excessive exercise. To meet criteria for the syndrome, patients need to engage in both bingeing and inappropriate compensatory behaviors at least once weekly for at least 3 months. In addition, individuals with BN are excessively concerned with body shape and weight. There can be considerable phenomenological overlap between individuals with BN and AN,

BOX 37-3 DSM-5 Diagnostic Criteria: Binge-Eating Disorder (307.51 (F50.8))

A. Recurrent episodes of binge eating. An episode of binge eating is characterized by both of the following:
   1. Eating, in a discrete period of time (e.g., within any 2-hour period), an amount of food that is definitely larger than what most people would eat in a similar period of time under similar circumstances.
   2. A sense of lack of control over eating during the episode (e.g., a feeling that one cannot stop eating or control what or how much one is eating).
B. The binge-eating episodes are associated with three (or more) of the following:
   1. Eating much more rapidly than normal.
   2. Eating until feeling uncomfortably full.
   3. Eating large amounts of food when not feeling physically hungry.
   4. Eating alone because of feeling embarrassed by how much one is eating.
   5. Feeling disgusted with oneself, depressed, or very guilty afterward.
C. Marked distress regarding binge eating is present.
D. The binge eating occurs, on average, at least once a week for 3 months.

E. The binge eating is not associated with the recurrent use of inappropriate compensatory behavior as in bulimia nervosa and does not occur exclusively during the course of bulimia nervosa or anorexia nervosa.

   Specify if:

In partial remission: After full criteria for binge-eating disorder were previously met, binge eating occurs at an average frequency or less than one episode per week for a sustained period of time.

In full remission: After full criteria for binge-eating disorder were previously met, none of the criteria have been met for a sustained period of time.

   Specify current severity:
   The minimum level of severity is based on the frequency of episodes of binge eating (see below). The level of severity may be increased to reflect other symptoms and the degree of functional disability.

Mild: 1–3 binge-eating episodes per week.
Moderate: 4–7 binge-eating episodes per week.
Severe: 8–13 binge-eating episodes per week.
Extreme: 14 or more binge-eating episodes per week.

Reprinted with permission from the Diagnostic and statistical manual of mental disorders, *ed 5, (Copyright 2013). American Psychiatric Association.*

TABLE 37-1 Differential Diagnosis of Eating Disorders and Their Subtypes by Signs and Symptoms

	Weight Criterion	Body Weight or Shape Concerns	Typical Dietary Pattern	Binge-Eating	Purging or Behaviors to Neutralize Perceived or Real Excessive Caloric Intake
Anorexia nervosa	< Low weight (less than normal or minimally expected)	Yes	Restrictive; recurrent binge-eating	Frequently present; binge-eating/ purging subtype	Frequently present; binge-eating/purging subtype
Bulimia nervosa	No	Yes	Recurrent binge-eating	Yes	Yes
Binge-eating disorder	No, but frequently overweight	No, but frequently present	Recurrent binge-eating	Yes	No
OSFED	No	Frequently present, but not required for diagnosis	Varied	Frequently present, but not required for diagnosis	Frequently present, but not required for diagnosis

OSFED: Other specified feeding or eating disorder.

must experience these episodes (on average) once a week for at least 3 months to meet DSM criteria for BED. Although the diagnostic criteria for BED do not specifically mention the overvaluation of shape and weight that is characteristic of AN and BN, individuals with BED who exhibit this feature have poorer treatment outcomes.[29] Box 37-3 summarizes the diagnostic criteria for BED.

Other Specified Feeding or Eating Disorder

This residual category comprises individuals who experience clinically significant symptoms that do not meet full criteria for AN, BN, or BED. These include sub threshold categories, such as atypical AN (i.e., AN features without low body weight); BN of low frequency and/or limited duration; BED of low frequency and/or limited duration; purging disorder; and night-eating syndrome (NES). Purging disorder resembles BN in terms of purging, but lacks binge-eating episodes. NES involves excessive evening eating that occurs after the evening meal or

in conjunction with night-time awakenings and is associated with distress or functional impairment. Formerly termed eating disorders not otherwise specified (EDNOS), individuals with OSFED often have psychiatric symptoms and physical complications that are just as severe as those associated with full-syndrome disorders.[30] Table 37-1 summarizes distinguishing diagnostic criteria of the eating disorders. Lastly, the diagnosis of unspecified feeding or eating disorder subtypes, for which insufficient information is available to confirm a specific diagnosis (e.g., in an emergency room setting).

EVALUATION AND DIFFERENTIAL DIAGNOSIS

Evaluation of an eating disorder is optimally accomplished with input from mental health, primary care, and dietetic clinicians. Team management is advisable and often essential to clarify diagnosis, to identify psychiatric and medical co-morbidities, and to establish the modalities and level of care best suited safe and effective management. Evaluation is

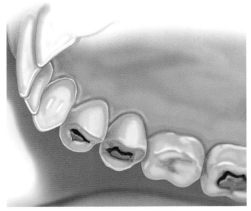

Figure 37-1. Dental erosion resulting from chronic vomiting. *(Adapted and printed with permission from the MGH Department of Psychiatry.)*

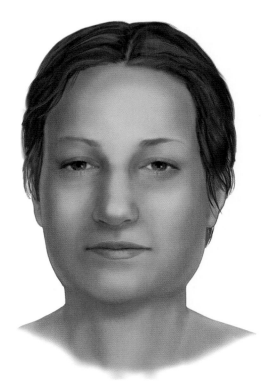

Figure 37-2. Parotid hypertrophy resulting from chronic vomiting. *(Adapted and printed with permission from the MGH Department of Psychiatry.)*

often complicated by a patient's ambivalence about accepting assistance or engaging in treatment. In other situations, it is more appropriate to discuss screening for an eating disorder as a patient may not realize that his or her behaviors are problematic, or may not have decided whether or how to disclose his or her symptoms.

Because BN, BED, and OSFED can present with a normal weight and physical examination, the diagnosis can be missed if a patient is not forthcoming or queried about symptoms. Among individuals who acknowledge eating and weight concerns, only a relatively small percentage report being asked by a doctor about symptoms of an eating disorder.[4] Identification of an occult eating disorder in a primary care or mental health setting can be challenging if a patient is unreceptive to diagnosis or to treatment. Although screening assessments for eating disorders are more frequently used in research than in clinical settings, offering this screening in a primary care setting may provide a practical opportunity for a patient to discuss eating concerns. However, the validity of these assessments rests on a patient's accurate and truthful responses. Certain clinical signs (e.g., a history of extreme weight changes, dental enamel erosion (see Figure 37-1), parotid hypertrophy (see Figure 37-2), or elevated serum amylase) may flag the possibility of an eating disorder, although the disorder can occur in their absence. Occasionally, certain probes in the clinical interview may suggest an eating disorder (Table 37-2). For example, inquiring about maximum, minimum, and desired weights often elicits information about body image concern, weight loss attempts, and overeating. Next, weighing a patient is essential for establishing the weight criterion for AN. The appropriateness of weight for height can be surprisingly difficult to estimate without this objective data. Although clinicians are sometimes reluctant to inquire about purging behaviors, a direct (empathically stated) question has been shown to be useful to elicit a candid response. Data suggest that even patients who have not voluntarily disclosed information to their doctor about an eating disorder are likely to disclose it in response to a direct query.[4]

Evaluation of a patient with a known eating disorder can also be complicated by incomplete disclosure or misrepresentation of the frequency or severity of symptoms. For this reason, it is advisable to obtain additional objective data (such as weight and serum electrolytes). Both the type of symptoms and their severity or frequency will allow classification into one of the eating disorder diagnoses. The latter will be especially helpful in deciding whether a patient is well enough to begin treatment as an outpatient or if he or she would benefit from a more intensive level of care.

The history should elicit the onset of body image and eating disorder disturbances, specific precipitants, if any, and remissions or exacerbations of symptoms. The patient's history of weight fluctuations, as well as minimum and maximum weights and their approximate durations, is useful in gauging how symptomatic the patient has become and where he or she is in relation to his or her illness history. For assessment of body image disturbance, it is useful to probe what the patient's desired weight is in relation to his or her current weight, as well as any behavioral manifestations of shape and weight concerns such as body checking (e.g., seeing if thighs touch, frequent weighing) and experiential avoidance (e.g., hiding one's shape with baggy clothes, avoiding being seen in public). Moreover, probing how preoccupied the patient is with calories or his or her weight can include a straightforward question about it (as well as an inquiry about whether the patient keeps a running tally of calories) or questions about how frequently he or she weighs himself or herself or what effect a weight change has on his or her mood or self-evaluation. Alternatively, how a patient registers and responds to information about medical complications can also signal body image disturbance. Clinicians should ask about current dietary patterns, including a restrictive pattern of eating (e.g., fasting, meal-skipping, calorie restriction, or evidence of restricting intake of specific foods) and overeating (e.g., binge-eating, grazing, or night-eating). Excess water-drinking to produce "fullness" should be asked about and can lead to hyponatremia. Conversely, dehydration from complete avoidance of fluids (due to fear of weight gain) is also commonly observed.[31] In addition to dietary patterns, clinicians should inquire about and inventory attempts to compensate for

TABLE 37-2 Useful Probes for Attitudes and Behaviors Associated with the Eating Disorders

Topic	Suggested Probe Questions
Weight history	• Can you give me a sense of your current height and weight? • Have there been any recent changes in your weight? • What is the least you have weighed at this height? • What is the most you have weighed?
Perception of current shape and size	• Do you see yourself as your friends and family do?
Preoccupations	• How much time do you spend thinking about food/calories/weight/body shape? • Has thinking about these things made it difficult to concentrate on other things?
Dietary patterns	• Do you count calories (in a given day)? • What might you eat for meals (and snacks) on a typical day? • Are there any rules you follow about how much you can eat in a given day? • Are there certain foods that you feel you should not eat or are fearful of? • Are there any rules you follow about how much you can eat during the day? • Are there any rules you follow about certain ways you have to eat?
Binge-pattern eating	• Do you have episodes in which you feel you eat an unusual amount of food and it feels like you cannot control it? • What (amount and kind of food) do you eat during such an episode? • How long does the episode take? • How many times might this happen during 1 day (or over a week)? • How do you feel about it afterward? • Does anything happen before that might be related? What time of day does it normally happen?
Inappropriate compensatory behaviors (ask frequency for each)	• Have you ever made yourself vomit? • Have you ever used laxatives (especially stimulant type), suppositories, enemas, or diuretics to try to control your weight or compensate for calories you have taken in? (To be followed with psychoeducational information; i.e., Do you know that laxatives and diuretics don't remove any calories from your body and may lead to re-weight gain from water retention when you try to stop?) • Have you ever used drugs (prescription or illegal) or caffeine to try to control your appetite or compensate for calories you have taken in? • (Assess adequacy of insulin dosing if diabetic; the nature of the probe used here will depend on the clinical context.) • How often do you exercise? How much exercise do you get on a typical day or in a typical week? • How do you feel if you are unable to exercise on a particular day? • Do you ever skip meals? • Do you ever go a day or more without eating? Without drinking?

binge-eating or to prevent weight gain (see Table 37-2). Some clinicians are reluctant to ask about certain symptoms, out of concern that they may introduce a weight loss strategy that a patient may be tempted to try. Unfortunately, patients have access to information through social media platforms (e.g., Twitter, Tumblr) or "pro-ana" (pro-anorexia) websites about dieting, restrictive pattern eating, purging, and evasion of detection. Patients do not always appreciate how dangerous some behaviors are; therefore, the clinical evaluation provides an invaluable opportunity to intervene in some behaviors that patients use or to suggest that they substitute them for others. Because untreated or poorly treated diabetes can result in weight loss, and because adherence to strict diets and food regimens is part of diabetes management, insulin-dependent diabetic patients present a special challenge in an evaluation. Often patients have been specifically referred for evaluation and management because their blood sugars are poorly controlled and their inappropriate underdosing or withholding of insulin has already come to light. For patients in whom these behaviors have not yet been identified, the most appropriate line of questioning may be more open-ended to determine how they manage their insulin dosing relative to food intake without necessarily suggesting that intentional hyperglycemia would cause weight loss. Excessive exercise is somewhat difficult to assess, as guidelines about the frequency and duration of exercise for health benefits have shifted upward. In this case, it is helpful to determine whether the exercise has a compulsive quality (e.g., does he or she exercise regardless of schedule, weather, injury, or illness) or is greatly in excess of medical or team recommendations.

Other considerations in the evaluation of an eating disorder include the assessment of the supportive or adverse role of family, peers, team members, and other elements of the psychosocial environment. If the patient is participating in an athletic activity (e.g., skating, gymnastics, track, or wrestling) or within an occupation (e.g., dance or modeling) in which low weight is considered highly desirable, it is critical to understand whether there is support for his or her treatment or pressure to remain slim. In addition to the potential benefits of family therapy (especially for adolescents with AN), a family evaluation can play a critical role in psychoeducation for the family. This is particularly useful for patients who live with, or who continue to be dependent on, their family. Parents frequently find themselves in a dilemma, faced with expressing concern about their child's eating (even an adult child) and allowing their child autonomy, and often avoiding a struggle that makes them feel powerless. Some parents benefit from guidance on what constitutes helpful (and unhelpful) input from them, as well as what the signs, symptoms, and health risks of an eating disorder are.

Assessment of motivation for change is often critical for individuals with an eating disorder because it can be predictive of treatment outcome.[32] Although individuals with BN and BED are often distressed by their symptoms, they often are fearful or reluctant about relinquishing them. Individuals with AN are commonly unreceptive to treatment. Cognitive distortions that are typical of the illness make it difficult to motivate a patient to accept treatment that will restore weight. The prescription for recovery—which starts with weight restoration—is exactly what they fear. Moreover, denial of seriousness of medical complications of their low weight is inherent to the illness; therefore, information that might motivate change under other illness scenarios is not always effective for AN. In short, patients with AN are frequently highly invested in their symptoms and unwilling to occupy the conventional sick role, in which patients typically agree to treatment. In addition to sustaining a particular weight that they find acceptable, individuals with an eating disorder often find that their behavioral symptoms (restrictive eating that leads to hunger, binge-eating, or purging) contribute to self-soothing and to self-efficacy, and they are reluctant to relinquish these perceived benefits.

Finally, mental health evaluation must take into account accompanying mood, thought, substance use, personality, and other disorders that are frequently co-morbid with eating disorders. Excessive use of alcohol and cigarettes should be determined as well. Behaviors associated with eating disorders are frequently exacerbated by depression and by anxiety disorders. Conversely, an increase in the frequency or severity of eating disorder symptoms can exacerbate mood symptoms. Moreover, low weight undermines the efficacy of antidepressants. This may be due to nutritional or other unknown factors. Substance abuse sometimes waxes and wanes in relation to disordered eating. A clinician who evaluates a patient with active substance abuse or in early recovery is advised to use particular caution in considering the impact of controlling restrictive eating, bingeing, or purging symptoms if these patterns provide an essential coping mechanism for a patient at risk of relapse for substance abuse or other self-injurious behavior. If the symptoms co-exist, generally the more life-threatening of them will require initial treatment. For BN and BED, the substance abuse disorder generally takes precedence, but the medical and nutritional impact of the eating symptoms requires ongoing surveillance. For severe AN in the setting of substance abuse, it is highly likely that inpatient care is the safest and most effective treatment setting. Finally, assessment of suicidal ideation and behavior is critical in the evaluation of an eating disorder. As noted previously, suicide rates are elevated in eating disorders and the risk and prevention of suicide should always be considered.

MEDICAL COMPLICATIONS

Medical consequences of eating disorders are often occult, yet dangerous. Even subtle laboratory abnormalities, while not intrinsically harmful or worrisome in other settings, may reflect physiological tolls indicative of significant illness.

The devastating physical sequelae of the malnutrition of AN have been well described in the medical literature; children and adolescents are recognized as especially vulnerable. The degree of danger generally parallels the magnitude and speed of the weight loss. Purging augments the risk in all age groups. Major and potentially irreversible effects exist on bones and heart, but no organ system is spared. The physical damage of BN reflects the modalities of purging employed, but frequently affects the gastrointestinal tract, teeth, and electrolytes.

Cardiac consequences of anorexia may be asymptomatic but can turn lethal. Adolescents appear to be particularly at risk.[33] Myocardial hypotrophy occurs, often early, with reduced left ventricular mass and output.[34] The heart of the patient with anorexia has an impaired ability to respond to the increased demands of exercise. Hypotension occurs early and orthostasis follows, possibly enhanced by volume depletion. Bradycardia is common, probably due to increased vagal tone. This should neither be dismissed as innocent, nor be viewed as comparable to that in conditioned athletes. Whereas athletes with bradycardia have increased ventricular mass and myocardial efficiency, in anorexia (even in prior athletes), bradycardia reflects cardiac impairment associated with reduced stroke volume.

Further changes are seen in cardiac anatomy and conduction. Compression of the annulus from reduced cardiac mass may result in mitral valve prolapse, and silent pericardial effusions are common, but generally not of functional significance.[35] Electrophysiologically, the QTc interval and QT dispersion may be increased,[36] and may predispose to ventricular arrhythmias and be harbingers of sudden death.[37] While virtually all aspects of cardiac function normalize with full recovery, some aspects of cardiac function may actually deteriorate during initial treatment.[38]

Although cardiac complications may be the most dangerous for AN patients, low bone mass is among the most permanent. Loss of bone mass can be rapid and remain low despite disease recovery; it represents a life-long risk of increased fractures. The association of low bone mineral density (BMD) is established in adolescent girls as well as boys.[39,40] Of importance, effects on bone mass can be seen with brief disease duration, with very significant reductions in bone mass being reported in girls who have been ill for less than a year. Skeletal impact can be severe.[41] An electron micrograph of an osteoporotic female with multiple vertebral compression fractures is shown in Figure 37-3.

Factors that contribute to low BMD in AN include hormonal and nutritional abnormalities, as well as risks associated with excess exercise, smoking, and alcohol use. Endocrine factors include hypogonadism, low levels of insulin-like growth factor-1 (IGF-1), and hypercortisolemia. In AN, normal puberty is disrupted with prolonged estrogen deficiency, as well as lack of growth hormone (GH) effects mediated by IGF-1. Maximal bone mass is achieved during adolescence and early adult life. Therefore, suppression of bone formation by under-nutrition during adolescence leaves affected girls particularly vulnerable to inadequate peak bone mass formation. Although bone-density measurements in children must be done at a center with access to a normative database, in adults with AN, a screening bone density dual-energy x-ray absorptiometry (DEXA) scan is an important part of the medical evaluation. The results of such a scan in a young woman with AN showing osteoporosis of the spine are shown in Figure 37-4. Using high-resolution CT scans, an important new finding is that bone micro-architecture is also impaired in both girls and boys with AN.[42] Of note, micro-architectural changes may precede a demonstrable change in bone density by traditional DEXA readings. Bone strength, as assessed by finite element analysis techniques, is also decreased compared to healthy-weight girls.[43] A number of neuroendocrine factors, either gut derived, such as ghrelin, PYY, and leptin, may also play a role in low bone mass. Oxytocin, a brain-derived peptide stored in the posterior pituitary, has been shown to be associated with the severity of disordered-eating psychopathology and been shown to relate to low bone mass in AN.[44,45]

The effects of AN on the brain are still being explored but include cortical atrophy with enlarged sulci on computed tomography (CT) scan. Gastrointestinal abnormalities are common and often symptomatic. Gastroparesis is associated with early satiety in AN and can cause significant discomfort during re-feeding. About 50% of patients who vomit regularly have mucosal abnormalities on endoscopy,[46] and many have symptomatic esophagitis. Hematemesis may result from Mallory-Weiss tears, and esophageal or gastric rupture is a rare but fatal complication. Hematological abnormalities reflect bone marrow suppression. They parallel severity of weight loss and may cause anemia, neutropenia, or thrombocytopenia, alone or in combination.[47] In addition, low-weight patients may be unable to mount a febrile response to infection, causing delayed recognition and increased severity.[48] AN is a risk factor

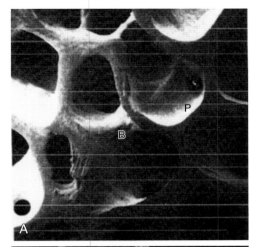

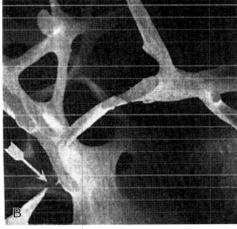

Figure 37-3. (A) Low-power scanning electron micrograph of an autopsy sample of a normal 44-year-old man. (B) Low-power scanning electron micrograph of a 47-year-old osteoporotic woman with multiple vertebral compression fractures. P, Trabecular plate; B, trabecular bar; Field width, 2.6 mm in each. *(From Dempster DW, Shane E, Horbert W, Lindsay R. A simple method of correlative light and scanning electron microscopy of human iliac crest bone biopsies: qualitative observations in normal and osteoporotic subjects, J Bone Miner Res 1:15–21, 1986, with permission from the American Society for Bone and Mineral Research.)*

DXA RESULTS SUMMARY

Region	Area (cm²)	BMC (g)	BMD (g/cm²)	T-score	Z-score
L1	10.41	6.35	0.610	−2.9	−2.7
L2	11.23	8.07	0.718	−2.8	−2.7
L3	13.34	9.72	0.729	−3.2	−3.1
L4	16.32	12.31	0.754	−3.3	−3.1
Total	**51.31**	**36.45**	**0.710**	**−3.1**	**−2.9**

Total BMD CV 1.0%, ACF = 1.008, BCF = 0.990, TH = 5.555 WHO classification: osteoporosis
Fracture risk: high

Figure 37-4. Results of lumbar spine scan of a 22-year-old woman with anorexia nervosa showing marked reduction in bone mass and a Z-score of -2.9 associated with high fracture risk. BMC, bone mineral content; BMD, bone mineral density.

for acute renal injury and nephrolithiasis, and, if chronic, for renal failure.[49] Patients with co-morbid medical illness present an additional challenge. Individuals with type I diabetes have a higher risk of eating disorders and may "purge" by omitting their insulin, resulting in poor glycemic control, rapid development of vascular complications, and episodes of ketoacidosis.

The onset of puberty may be delayed in pre-menarchal girls with AN. Over one-third of pre-pubertal and peri-pubertal girls exhibit delayed menarche. Although the effect of AN on final growth is uncertain, abnormalities in the maximum predicted growth have been reported. Other hormonal abnormalities identified in adults and adolescents with AN include hypercortisolemia, which may have deleterious effects, including suppressed bone formation.

Hypothalamic amenorrhea is a hallmark of AN and precedes the onset of weight loss in a subset of patients. While some individuals have a reliable menstrual weight threshold, others experience a significant delay between weight restoration and the resumption of menses. Normal-weight women with BN may also have irregular, infrequent, or absent menstruation. Of note, some women meeting all the psychiatric criteria of AN may continue to menstruate at very low body weights; low bone mass may still be seen in such women. With full resolution of an eating disorder, frequency of pregnancy has been reported to be comparable to that of the general population. However, a significant number of anovulatory women who seek infertility treatment have sub-syndromal, if not active, eating disorders.

A recent study from Scandinavia documented that more than 10% of women currently bearing children have a past or present eating disorder. This high incidence has stimulated concern about the impact on pregnancy. Although data are limited and at times conflicting, it would appear that women with eating disorders have a significantly increased risk of miscarriage, obstetrical complications, and Cesarean section.[50] Offspring are more likely to show intrauterine growth retardation, low birth weight, and low Apgar scores at delivery.[51] Of additional concern is the high incidence of post-partum depression among women with current or prior eating disorders, raising important questions about pharmacologic management.

The hypothalamic–pituitary–thyroid axis also shows an adaptation to weight loss. Although thyroid-stimulating hormone (TSH) concentrations are typically normal in patients with AN, total T_3 is low (as is leptin), a finding consistent with malnutrition and thought to be part of a complex mechanism to decrease resting energy expenditure.[52] T_3 concentrations increase with weight gain and recovery. It is important not to erroneously diagnose hypothyroidism in the setting of low T_3 levels alone, as administration of thyroid hormone has deleterious metabolic and cardiac effects in a euthyroid patient with AN. Elevations in serum TSH indicate an independent primary cause of hypothyroidism.

The refeeding syndrome is an iatrogenic complication of vigorous initial refeeding of severely emaciated patients, almost always in-hospital. Rapid introduction of calories, particularly carbohydrates, stimulates release of insulin, driving glucose, phosphorus, potassium, and magnesium into the cells. Precipitous drops in phosphorus, in particular, are thought to be responsible for the hemolytic anemia, cardiac arrhythmias, and death that may occur, typically in the first week of re-feeding. Thiamine deficiency can result from the rapid increase in utilization with re-feeding and delirium may occur, especially in the second week.

MEDICAL ASSESSMENT

Taking a medical history provides a crucial opportunity not only to assess but also to educate and engage the patient.

Patients with AN are typically convinced of their well-being despite ominous levels of starvation, and the physician should use every opportunity to affirm the severity of physical compromise, even if it is occult and asymptomatic. BN can generate great shame, and the interviewer can convey acceptance with a sensitive, but open, inquiry that includes the relevant specifics of purging behaviors. In addition to the patient's description of the history of his or her illness (including past and present treatment), it is useful to pose questions that probe for attitudes and behaviors associated with eating disorders (see Table 37-2).

Patients may deny symptoms, but many describe a plaguing preoccupation with food and weight, fatigue or weakness, early satiety, and bloating. Patients with AN may also complain of cold intolerance, impaired concentration, constipation, and hair loss, while patients with BN may note dental problems and the "puffy cheeks" of parotid enlargement. Symptoms of particular medical significance include dizziness, palpitations, orthostasis, or syncope that may herald cardiovascular danger. Gastrointestinal symptoms can be moderated. Hematemesis or rectal bleeding requires emergency intervention. A gynecological history (including age of menarche, duration of amenorrhea, if present, reliable use of contraception, and past or intended pregnancy) is also important.

Physical findings may be minimal despite severe medical compromise. Generally the most crucial medical information comes from the patient's vital signs. Height and weight, percent loss of total body weight, and the current percent of expected body weight are key barometers of health in AN (Box 37-4 and Table 37-3). Patients who have lost a significant percent of total body weight, or are far below expected body weight (EBW), or whose weight loss is rapid, can be in grave medical danger, despite a normal physical examination, laboratory testing, and electrocardiographic findings.

Bradycardia and hypotension are significant indicators of cardiovascular compromise, as are orthostatic changes. Hypothermia is usual with low weight, as is loss of muscle mass and subcutaneous fat. Acrocyanosis is a visible indicator to patients that their smaller, weaker heart is unable to maintain circulation to the periphery. Mitral valve prolapse may occur secondary to constriction of the annulus from reduction in heart size. Parotid enlargement (bilateral and non-tender) occurs in some patients with BN (see Figure 37-2). Submandibular glands may be enlarged as well. Russell's sign—excoriation on the dorsum of a hand—is considered pathognomonic for bulimia. Key potential findings on physical examination are summarized in Table 37-4.

LABORATORY FINDINGS

Laboratory findings are often not useful in establishing the diagnosis or the severity of an eating disorder. The diagnosis may be self-evident with a classic constellation of symptoms, though patients may not always be forthcoming. The clinical history and a directed interview are more useful in establishing the presence of symptoms of an eating disorder; extensive or invasive testing is generally unnecessary and often counterproductive. Laboratory assessment, though sometimes insensitive, is nonetheless essential to exclude other causes of weight loss, or to identify complications of the eating disorder.

Normal laboratory findings do not exclude a serious eating disorder; however, even subtle laboratory abnormalities may signal a major physical toll from the illness. Hypokalemia is diagnostic for purging behavior but is often absent despite significant vomiting, or use of laxatives and/or diuretics. Hyponatremia is sometimes seen with compulsive water-drinking. The tests that may be useful are listed in Table 37-5, and abnormalities associated with eating disorders are shown in Table 37-6.

TREATMENT

Optimal treatment for an eating disorder includes coordinated management of psychological, medical, and nutritional issues. Even if the initial evaluation indicates (and the clinical team believes) that a patient can be safely and effectively managed as an outpatient, early treatment frequently focuses on stabilization of psychological and medical symptoms. It is also beneficial to address contingency plans for intensifying the level of care in the initial phase of treatment. At that time, the clinical team members can establish their respective roles in care (e.g., who will be weighing the patient), their preferred mode of communicating, and parameters for hospitalization. Because it is common for patients to be ambivalent about certain necessary elements of their treatment (such as medical surveillance or hospital admission), these understandings and plans are best arranged before a crisis evolves. A concrete treatment understanding is sometimes very useful, although setting actual parameters can be challenging. Sometimes patients misunderstand these as permission to continue symptomatic behaviors without consequences, until they reach the threshold that has been set. Identifying supportive family members

---

BOX 37-4 Calculation of Body Mass Index (BMI) and Percent Expected Weight in Adults

BMI = Weight (kg)/(Height [m])^2
Expected body weight for adult women =
(100 lb + 5 lb/inch above 5 ft) ± 10%

TABLE 37-3 Relevance of Body Mass Index (BMI) to Health

BMI	Weight Category*
< 14	At risk for re-feeding syndrome
< 18.5	Underweight
18.5–24.9	"Normal weight"
³ 22	Risk of diabetes, HTN, CHD increases
25–29.9	Overweight
> 30	Obese
> 40	Morbidly obese

*Reflects weight categories for adults.
CHD, Coronary heart disease; HTN, hypertension.

TABLE 37-4 Possible Findings Associated with Eating Disorders on Physical Examination

In Low-Weight Patients	In Patients with Induced Vomiting
Bradycardia	Erosion of dental enamel
Hypotension	Russell's sign
Orthostasis	Parotid or salivary gland (or both)
Hypothermia	enlargement
Emaciation	
Flat affect	
Acrocyanosis	
Lanugo	
Click/murmur of mitral	
Valve prolapse	

TABLE 37-5 Useful Laboratory Studies for Evaluating Anorexia Nervosa and Bulimia Nervosa

Patient Population	Suggested Studies
All patients	Electrocardiogram Complete blood count Glucose Blood urea nitrogen, creatinine Electrolytes Calcium, magnesium, phosphorus Liver function
Low-weight patients	Erythrocyte sedimentation rate Serum albumin Thyroid-stimulating hormone Testosterone (for men)
Patients with amenorrhea	Prolactin Estradiol Luteinizing hormone, follicle-stimulating hormone Testosterone Dual-energy x-ray absorptiometry (DEXA)
Patients with additional clinical indications	Urinalysis Amylase Brain magnetic resonance imaging (MRI)

and securing permission to speak with them (to enlist their support) can be useful if the patient is likely to resist a treatment plan.

When treating children and adolescents, clinicians must consider developmental factors. In contrast to adults, children and teenagers with eating disorders rarely seek treatment on their own; worried parents, pediatricians, or teachers most often express concerns. Children and adolescents will often deny there is a problem,[53] and parents may be reluctant to pathologize behavior. Clinicians who treat children and adolescents must be able to coordinate treatment with other health care providers, while also navigating family and school systems. Although it is never appropriate or helpful to blame families for a child's eating problems, it can be helpful to identify stressful situations within a family system that may make recovery difficult. Because parents are the gatekeepers for treatment, it is important that the clinician help them feel comfortable and understood, while also respecting the child's privacy. As such, it can be difficult to engage a child or adolescent in a therapeutic treatment relationship. It is developmentally appropriate for teenagers to rebel against authority and to value the opinions of their peers over those of authority figures. Often, it is helpful to allow for some flexibility in the treatment to strengthen the therapeutic alliance, while also enforcing important limits (such as need for weigh-ins, laboratory studies, and hospitalization if indicated) designed to ensure patient safety.[54]

TABLE 37-6 Possible Laboratory Abnormalities in Patients with Anorexia Nervosa or Bulimia Nervosa

Test	If Abnormal	Details
BLOOD COUNTS		
Hct/Hgb	Low	Normochromic, normocytic
WBC	Low	Reversed neutrophil:lymphocyte ratio
Platelets	Low	Often with anemia and/or leukopenia
ESR	Very low	Helpful in differential
ELECTROLYTES		
Glucose	Low	Especially fasting
	Very high	Type 1 diabetics omitting insulin to purge
BUN	High	Pre-renal
Sodium	High	Dehydration
	Low	Water-loading
Potassium	Low	Only seen with purging
Bicarbonate	High	With vomiting to purge
	Low	With laxatives to purge
CHEMISTRIES		
Magnesium	Low	Perpetuates hypokalemia
Phosphate	Low	May fall rapidly in early re-feeding
	High	In setting of laxative abuse
Transaminases	High	Starvation; early re-feeding
Amylase	Slightly high	Especially salivary if purging
Albumin	Slightly high	Unlike other forms of starvation
Cholesterol	?	May rise or fall
ENDOCRINE		
Total T_3 in the setting of normal TSH	Low	Compensatory and not to be treated
Estradiol (women)	Low	Promotes osteopenia/osteoporosis
Testosterone (men)	Low	Promotes osteopenia/osteoporosis
LH/FSH	Low	Hypothalamic etiology of amenorrhea
Cortisol	High	
ELECTROCARDIOGRAM		
Findings	Low/decreased	Voltage
	Decreased amplitude	P wave
	Increased	QTc interval (may portend sudden death)
	Increased	QTc dispersion
	Low	Heart rate

BUN: Blood urea nitrogen; ESR: erythrocyte sedimentation rate; FSH: follicle-stimulating hormone; Hct: hematocrit; Hgb: hemoglobin; LH: luteinizing hormone; TSH: thyroid-stimulating hormone; WBC: white blood cell.

Medical Management

Effective and safe treatment for an eating disorder requires immediate attention to medical stability. Medical management begins with an assessment of the severity of physical compromise to determine an appropriate level of care. Though there is some variation in the recommendations for hospitalization, suggested parameters are listed in Table 37-7. Patients who require inpatient care should be triaged to an experienced eating disorders treatment program.

Nutritional restoration is the immediate focus in low-weight patients. Meaningful psychological treatment is not possible in an emaciated patient and may engender dangerous delays. Most patients, even those who require hospitalization, can be re-fed orally at experienced programs. Nasogastric tube feeding and total parenteral nutrition (TPN) are very rarely required. Calories should be increased incrementally, but rapidly, to achieve desired weight gains of 1 to 2 pounds weekly in outpatients and 2 to 3 pounds weekly in hospital settings. Patients vary widely in their caloric requirements for weight restoration, but it is not unusual to require up to 4,000 calories a day as re-feeding progresses. Emaciated patients require phosphorus monitoring the first week and often supplementation of phosphorus and magnesium for several weeks, along with cautious caloric increase to avoid a re-feeding syndrome. Orthostasis has been observed to remit after several weeks, at about 80% of expected body weight in adolescents. However, a return to full health requires restoration of normal weight. Relapse rises steeply as the percent of EBW at discharge falls, with 100% minimizing immediate relapse and re-admission rising rapidly as discharge weight falls to 95%, 90%, and 85% of EBW.

Restoration of weight is difficult and uncomfortable for patients. Patients may experience improved energy and affect within several weeks of re-feeding, but generally continue to fear fatness and maintain a tenacious longing for thinness.

Families, however, are often aware of, and gratified by, the returning signs of the patient's health and pre-morbid persona. Dietitians experienced with eating-disordered patients can be a valuable asset in the re-feeding process, providing psycho-educational and cognitive-behavioral treatment, as well as concrete suggestions for incremental increases in the amounts, caloric density, and diversity of intake. Some patients do better with routine foods and others with calorie supplements; many find that they tolerate liquids better than solids. Excess satiety may be lessened by frequent small feedings and by elimination of calorie-free liquids, though some discomfort is generally unavoidable. Prokinetic agents may be used before meals for patients with significant distress.

Exercise should be prohibited at less than 90% of EBW for cardiac safety. This is warranted by extensive data on the inability of the anorexic heart to compensate for exercise. It is not advisable for patients to depart for camp, college, or extended travel below a critical weight, when consistent and intensive monitoring and treatment are still needed. This may engender intense resistance from patients or families, but it should be regarded as a routine and necessary medical recommendation, as would be the case after surgery, a significant orthopedic injury, or a major infectious illness, such as hepatitis. The goal is for the patient to restore physical safety so he or she can return to usual pursuits without danger or damage to health.

Despite the severity of bone loss in those with AN, there is no approved effective therapy for prevention or treatment of low BMD in this population. The single most important factor in improving bone density is weight gain and disease recovery. An improvement in adolescents in bone density is seen after stable weight recovery, but it often remains low despite some gains.

A number of measures can be taken by clinicians to avoid worsening poor bone health. Calcium and vitamin D intake should be normal and supplements given as needed. Some

TABLE 37-7 Criteria for Hospitalization

Domain	General Symptom*	Example†
Weight	Substantially low weight for height and age Rapidly falling weight	<75%–85% expected body weight
Behavioral	Acute food/water refusal Episodes of bingeing and purging of very high or escalating frequency	E.g., bingeing and/or vomiting 10–20 times in a day
Other medical compromise	Abnormal or unstable vital signs Severe medical complications	Bradycardia (e.g., < 40 beats per minute) Orthostatic hypotension (e.g., systolic drop of 30 points, pulse increase of 20 beats per minute) Severe hematemesis Severe neutropenia or thrombocytopenia Severe hypokalemia Uncontrolled type 1 diabetes Syncope
Psychiatric	Substantial risk of self-harm or suicide Co-morbid substance abuse Inability to adhere to treatment plan that will sustain minimal level of safety	
Treatment-related	Lack of substantial progress Necessity of close supervision to maintain symptom control Previously agreed-on criterion for hospitalization based on patient history	E.g., in the setting of chronically low weight and associated medical complications E.g., sustained or persistent inability to eat without supervision or to abstain from intractable purging after food intake E.g., reaching a threshold weight at which the patient repeatedly has rapidly deteriorated

*These criteria may be sufficient but not necessary to indicate inpatient care.
†Weight, vital sign, metabolic, and other parameters for hospitalization are best interpreted within the context of the patient's overall health, medical and psychiatric history, support systems, and engagement in treatment.

exercise in moderation may be clinically indicated as recovery progresses, but excess exercise should be avoided, as should forms of exercise that may predispose to fractures in those with low bone density. Exogenous oral estrogen has not been shown to be effective for prevention or management of osteoporosis in adults and adolescents with AN, despite its well-established role in post-menopausal women.[55,56] However, in a randomized placebo-controlled trial, physiologic estrogen administration, primarily given as a transdermal patch, was shown to improve bone mass accrual in adolescent girls with AN.[57] This is the first intervention shown to increase bone density in this population. Bisphosphonates have been used in many conditions leading to osteoporosis and have been considered for the bone loss of AN. One randomized placebo-controlled trial in adults showed improvement in bone mass using risedronate.[58] However, data in adolescents have not been positive. Because data thus far are few and long-term use of bisphosphonates has been associated with complications (including, very rarely, osteonecrosis of the jaw), and uncertain effects on future pregnancies, their use in treating patients with AN is currently not routinely recommended outside of clinical trials. Several experimental therapies are under investigation.

Patients who induce vomiting may experience symptomatic esophagitis and may benefit from proton pump inhibitors. Although there is no clinical trial data for validation, various recommendations have been made to protect the teeth from erosion in patients who vomit. Most involve neutralizing stomach acid in the mouth after vomiting, using bicarbonate of soda or an alkaline mouthwash. Parotid enlargement, though not painful, can be distressingly obvious. It often remits when vomiting stops, and may be treated with sialagogues, if extreme.

Hypokalemia, from vomiting, laxatives, or diuretics, requires vigorous correction and careful monitoring, in addition to testing for concomitant hypomagnesemia. Patients who are prone to hypokalemia may have their serum potassium levels drop precipitously, in part a reflection of total body potassium deficits and intracellular shifts. Potassium chloride should be used under close medical supervision for replacement, and doses in patients who continue to purge may be quite high. Patients with variable purging may need to titrate doses depending on the frequency of symptoms, taking a baseline amount plus an additional dose the morning after a day with extra purging. Patients generally know when they can hold down potassium or other medication: for example, just before going to sleep at night or just before leaving for work in the morning. Volume depletion will cause continued renal potassium wasting to spare sodium and preserve volume (i.e., secondary hyperaldosteronism), so patients with hypokalemia should be encouraged to have adequate dietary salt. Careful attention to maintenance of normal potassium levels is important to avoid both acute cardiac and respiratory catastrophe and chronically to avoid hypokalemic nephropathy and attendant renal failure. Hyponatremia may be seen with compulsive water-drinking or diuretic abuse and should be carefully monitored because rapidly occurring or very low values can lead to seizures.

Laxatives do not appreciably remove ingested calories. Their futility as a weight loss vehicle notwithstanding, they are the most commonly abused agents used by eating-disordered patients, second only to vomiting as a form of purging. Patients who try to stop their abuse of laxatives may experience both rebound edema and refractory constipation. Protocols are available for abrupt cessation of laxatives and temporary measures to restore normal bowel function. Others find that gradual tapering of laxatives is better tolerated, especially in outpatients.

Fertility may be restored before the first returning menstrual period, and patients should be advised to attend to contraception even while amenorrheic. Patients attempting to conceive, but who experience infertility, should have even subsyndromal eating disorders treated before use of reproductive technology. Pregnancy is a special challenge, with greatest safety for mother and fetus following complete eating disorder recovery. BMI should be no lower than 19 at conception. Women with residual difficulties should be monitored as a high-risk pregnancy, and even women recovered from an eating disorder have a high rate of post-partum depression.

Fortunately, most of the physical tolls of AN and BN, save for bone loss and dental destruction, remit with restoration of normal nutrition and weight and elimination of purging behaviors. After years of illness, physical deficits, as well as the eating disorder itself, become more entrenched with progressive structural damage to various organ systems.

Psychotherapeutic Treatment

In addition to medical monitoring and nutritional support, psychotherapy is a critical component of treatment. Although some patients will also benefit from psychopharmacological management, psychotherapy is the best-supported treatment to address the primary symptoms of an eating disorder. The treatment of choice for adolescent AN is a specialized family-based treatment that empowers the parents to take charge of re-feeding. Interventions for adult AN are less empirically based. In contrast, the gold standard treatment for BN and BED is a specific form of cognitive-behavioral therapy (CBT). In clinical practice, patients with OSFED are typically treated with the modality corresponding to the most similar full syndrome presentation (e.g., CBT for sub threshold BN; family-based treatment for atypical AN).

Anorexia Nervosa

For the treatment of adolescent AN, family-based treatment (FBT) has the strongest evidence base. FBT (sometimes called the "Maudsley method" due to its historical roots at the London-based hospital of the same name) consists of 20 manualized sessions over 12 months.[59] In the first phase, the therapist provides psychoeducation about the medical and psychological consequences of malnutrition. Parents take control of eating and food-related decisions, limit exercise, resist engaging their child in food-related struggles, and work together to persuade their child to eat. During the second phase, as the child engages in treatment and continues to gain weight, the therapist encourages the parents to help their child gradually resume independent eating and developmentally appropriate social activities. When the child is finally able to maintain a stable, healthy weight, the therapist shifts the focus of treatment away from eating and begins to focus on the impact of AN on the child's development, particularly around identity and autonomy.[59] In a large randomized controlled trial (RCT) comparing FBT to individual therapy for adolescent AN, half of those who took part in FBT were remitted at 12-month follow-up, compared to just one-quarter of those who received individual therapy.[60] In a smaller uncontrolled study, 89% of adolescents treated with FBT were weight-restored four years after completing treatment.[61]

In contrast, there is much less empirical support for a particular therapeutic approach in the treatment of adult AN. RCTs attempting to identify a treatment of choice have found low overall recovery rates across diverse modalities including CBT, interpersonal therapy (IPT), and specialist supportive clinical management.[62,63] Given the norm for adolescent onset, adults are more likely to be those whose illness has followed a chronic course. Psychotherapy is, therefore, undermined by the long-term effects of starvation and low body weight on cognition. Low-weight patients often remain perseverative in their preoccupations with food and weight and relatively rigid in their dietary behaviors. Moreover, persuading patients to accept treatment can be challenging due to the ego-syntonic nature of the illness; in a randomized therapy study, 46% of adults with AN dropped out before treatment completion.[64]

In practice with adult AN, clinicians usually select a therapeutic modality based on the history, chronicity, co-morbidity, and underlying factors that brought the patient into treatment. Nonetheless, new interventions are currently being evaluated. A couples-based approach, which enlists a committed partner to gently support the patient in his or her re-feeding efforts has shown preliminary promise.[65] Similarly, an enhanced form of CBT led to weight gain and decreased eating pathology in an uncontrolled trial, though only among the two-thirds of patients who completed treatment.[66] For patients with more than 7 years of illness, a therapeutic approach prioritizing improvements in quality of life (rather than weight gain) may enhance treatment acceptance.[67]

Bulimia Nervosa

Because their symptoms cause significant distress, patients with BN are typically more open to psychosocial interventions, and CBT has greater empirical support than any other therapeutic approach. Originally developed 20 years ago, the most recent or "enhanced" version (CBT-E) comprises four stages.[26] In the first stage, the therapist co-creates a personalized formulation of BN symptoms, highlighting how dieting and negative affect serve to maintain binge/purge behaviors. During this stage, the patient begins self-monitoring daily food intake in order to identify triggers for binge-eating such as under-eating earlier in the day and/or low mood. In the second stage, the therapist and patient collaboratively identify barriers to change, such as perceived benefits of the eating disorder or non-adherence with treatment. In the third stage, maintaining mechanisms—such as basing one's self-worth predominantly on shape and weight—are addressed through behavioral interventions, such as reducing body-checking and avoidance. The fourth stage focuses on relapse prevention. In a recent waitlist-controlled trial, half of BN patients achieved remission (defined as abstinence from bingeing and purging and eating disorder attitudes within one standard deviation of community norms) by the end of the 20-session treatment.[68] Improvements were well maintained over the 1-year follow-up.[68]

To enhance the scalability of this specialized and time-intensive intervention, self-help versions of CBT (typically using Fairburn's book *Overcoming Binge Eating*) have also demonstrated some efficacy in reducing binge/purge frequency in BN.[69] Furthermore, smartphone "apps" make specific components of CBT (e.g., self-monitoring exercises) accessible to a wider cross-section of individuals who may benefit. Guided self-help (i.e., featuring a handful of brief meetings with a therapist to trouble-shoot roadblocks) appears to be more effective than pure self-help, and self-help is contraindicated for AN.[69]

Of course, approximately half of patients do not respond to CBT. Other therapeutic interventions, such as interpersonal psychotherapy, have also been studied, but treatment response is not as rapid as observed in CBT. A new treatment called integrative cognitive-affective therapy (ICAT), which teaches emotional coping skills and aims to reduce the discrepancy between the patient's perceived versus ideal self, may be worthy of further research. In one study, BN patients treated with ICAT had similar abstinence rates after 21 sessions (37.5%) compared to those treated with CBT-E (22.5%).[70]

Binge-Eating Disorder

The psychotherapeutic treatment of BED is very similar to that of BN, and CBT is also the best-established treatment. In a study comparing CBT (with either fluoxetine or placebo) to fluoxetine alone, remission rates (defined as abstinence from binge eating for ≥ 1 month) were 61% for CBT plus placebo, 50% for CBT plus fluoxetine, and 22% for fluoxetine only.[71] Results were maintained at 12-month follow-up for the majority of patients who received CBT, but not those who received fluoxetine alone.[72]

Importantly, most individuals with BED are overweight or obese, and come to treatment hoping to reduce weight in addition to binge-eating. In one study, two-thirds of obese patients seeking treatment for BED had gained a clinically significant amount of weight (i.e., > 5% initial body weight) in the past year.[73] Paradoxically, CBT rarely leads to substantial weight loss, even among obese patients who are able to become abstinent from binge eating.[74] In the study described above, patients in the CBT plus placebo condition lost an average of 5 lb at post-treatment and 10 lb at 12-month follow-up. It is important for clinicians to be empathically aware that these modest losses will feel disheartening to patients, who may be dazzled by the dramatic but unsubstantiated claims of commercially available diet plans. However, in the largest RCT to date comparing behavioral weight loss (BWL) to CBT-guided self-help, CBT was significantly more effective than BWL at eliminating binge-eating, and weight loss was minimal and did not differ significantly between conditions at 2-year follow-up.[74]

PHARMACOLOGICAL TREATMENT

Clinical trials establishing efficacy for pharmacological management of eating disorders include numerous studies on adults with AN, BN, and BED. Notwithstanding these studies, the only agent with Food and Drug Administration (FDA) approval for the treatment of any of the eating disorders is fluoxetine for the treatment of BN. There are few clinical trial data on adolescents with eating disorders and no clinical trials on OSFED. Despite considerable overlap in symptomatology, the respective eating disorders appear to respond differently to medication. Whereas medication has an important adjunctive role in the treatment of BN and in BED, it has a very limited role in the treatment of AN.

Pharmacological Management of Anorexia Nervosa

RCTs of pharmacological agents that address core symptoms of AN suggest few benefits to managing the core features of this illness with psychotropics. Despite the data available, recent estimates suggest that upwards of 50% of patients undergoing treatment for disordered eating are also taking psychotropic medications.[75] Many of them are working with prescribing clinicians to target co-morbid mood and anxiety symptoms, which are likely exacerbated by inadequate nutrition. There is also some speculation that poor nutritional status may impede response to medications.[76] It is noteworthy that a number of RCTs of agents—including chlorpromazine, pimozide, sulpiride, clomipramine, clonidine, and tetrahydrocannabinol[77]—have not demonstrated efficacy in either promoting weight gain or reducing the cognitive symptoms associated with AN. This is unfortunate, but important to emphasize, since patients with AN frequently tolerate medication side effects poorly.

Researchers and clinicians have been quite interested in using the atypical antipsychotics to treat AN, owing to the side effect of significant weight gain in psychiatric patients using these medications for non-eating disorder-related diagnoses.[78] In addition, the core features of AN (including body image distortion and unreasonable fear of weight gain) are frequently compared to psychotic symptoms. Despite this, recruitment for RCTs has been slow, and the data collected so far has been mixed. It is important to note that concerns about weight gain, tardive dyskinesia, and metabolic side effects[79] may prevent patients and families from agreeing to participate in clinical trials. Others are very motivated to try any adjunctive therapies that may improve their course of illness. Initial case reports and trials of olanzapine[80] looked promising, but further investigation and additional studies looking at risperidone, quetiapine, and aripiprazole[81] have not shown any convincing evidence for routine use. Given case reports and anecdotal experience, there may be a role for a trial of olanzapine or, possibly, other atypical or conventional antipsychotics in some patients with AN. However, these agents should be used with caution (start low and titrate slowly) because of potential adverse side-effect profiles (including sedation, prolongation of the QT interval on the electrocardiogram, hyperprolactinemia, and reduction in bone mineral density).[82]

The role of selective serotonin reuptake inhibitors (SSRIs) in the treatment of AN is also quite limited and adjunctive to other treatment. Sertraline[83] and citalopram[84] may improve symptoms of mood and/or anxiety, but do not promote weight restoration. Furthermore, use of citalopram should be closely monitored given risk for prolonged QTc in doses > 40 mg/day. Fluoxetine has not been shown to be beneficial to adult or adolescent low-weight inpatients in treating AN. Fluoxetine has also been studied for stabilization in weight-recovered patients with AN in two RCTs. One of these demonstrated some efficacy (when adjunctive to elective psychotherapy) at a dosage of 20 to 60 mg/day,[76] whereas the other failed to show efficacy compared with placebo when added to CBT (at a target dosage of 60 mg/day).[85]

Pharmacological Management of Bulimia Nervosa

Numerous medications have demonstrated efficacy in treating primary symptoms of BN in at least one RCT (Table 37-8). These include several classes of pharmacological agents, including antidepressants. As a class, antidepressants reduce

TABLE 37-8 Summary of Pharmacological Agents That May Be Useful in Treating Bulimia Nervosa or Binge-eating Disorder Based on Published RCT Data

	Dosage	Comments and Caveats
Bulimia Nervosa		
Fluoxetine	60 mg/day	Best studied; well tolerated; only agent with FDA approval for this indication
Sertraline	100 mg/day	
Fluvoxamine*	Up to 300 mg/day in divided doses	Utility studied for relapse prevention after inpatient care; a second RCT in combination with stepped-care psychotherapy did not show efficacy in remission
Imipramine	Up to 300 mg/day	Potentially undesirable side-effect profile: effects on pulse, blood pressure, and QT interval that potentiate medical complications seen in BN (e.g., QT interval lengthening associated with hypokalemia) High lethality in overdose
Desipramine	Up to 300 mg/day	Potentially undesirable side-effect profile: effects on pulse, blood pressure, and QT interval that potentiate medical complications seen in BN (e.g., QT interval lengthening associated with hypokalemia) High lethality in overdose
Trazodone	Up to 400 mg/day	Potentially undesirable side-effect profile: sedation
Topiramate	Up to 250 mg/day Up to 400 mg/day	Potentially undesirable side-effect profile: Sedation and cognitive changes Weight loss Renal calculi Both studies started at 25 mg/day and titrated upward as tolerated
Naltrexone*	200–300 mg/day	Potentially undesirable side-effect profile: hepatotoxicity
Ondansetron	24 mg/day in 6 divided doses	High cost
Binge-Eating Disorder		
Sertraline	50–200 mg/day	
Citalopram	20–60 mg/day	
Fluoxetine*	20–80 mg/day	
Fluvoxamine*	50–300 mg/day	
Topiramate	50–400 mg/day	Potentially undesirable side-effect profile: sedation and cognitive changes
Orlistat (in combination with CBT)	120 mg TID	
Imipramine (in combination with diet counseling/psychological support)	25 mg TID	Studied in patients meeting criteria similar to BED

*Negative study RCT data also published on this agent for this indication.
BED, Binge-eating disorder; BN, bulimia nervosa; CBT, cognitive-behavioral therapy; FDA, Food and Drug Administration; RCT, randomized clinical trial; TID, three times daily.
From McElroy SL, Hudson JI, Capece KB, et al; for the Topiramate Binge Eating Disorder Research Group: Topiramate for the treatment of binge eating disorder associated with obesity: a placebo-controlled study, Biol Psychiatry 61:1039–1048, 2007.

binge and purge frequency by just over half as compared with an approximately 11% reduction with placebo alone.[86] Despite this, medication is generally not as effective as is psychotherapeutic management of BN, although it has an adjunctive role. For example, augmentation with antidepressants with proven efficacy in BN may further reduce symptoms, and fluoxetine (60 mg/day) appears to be beneficial in reducing symptoms for patients with BN who have not responded well to CBT or IPT.[87] Finally, fluoxetine has some efficacy for treatment of BN in primary care settings, and thus may have a role in management if psychotherapeutic care is unavailable.[88]

Fluoxetine (60 mg/day) is the first-line pharmacological agent in the treatment of BN. It has shown efficacy in the reduction of symptoms of BN compared with placebo in two large RCTs, is generally well tolerated among individuals with BN, shows efficacy in maintenance therapy over the course of a year, and is the only agent with FDA approval for the treatment of BN.[77] Sertraline has also been found to be effective in reducing the number of binge-eating and purging episodes among patients with BN in a small RCT.[89] Finally, fluvoxamine was superior to placebo in a relapse prevention trial for individuals with BN after discharge from inpatient treatment in one controlled trial.[90] The other SSRIs have not been studied in RCTs for this indication.

Although imipramine, desipramine, and trazodone have been found to be effective in reducing symptoms in patients with BN as well, their side-effect profiles limit their utility in this clinical population. Whereas bupropion,[91] phenelzine, and isocarboxazid have each been found to be effective in the reduction of bulimic symptoms, the risk of serious adverse events (i.e., seizures with bupropion and spontaneous hypertensive crises with monoamine oxidase inhibitors [MAOIs]) may be elevated in patients with BN, and these agents are not appropriate for the management of BN.[77] The use of these medications to manage co-morbid depression in the setting of BN is relatively contraindicated as well and warrants careful consideration of risk/benefit ratios in the context of each patient's individualized needs. Other classes of agents also show promise for the reduction of symptoms of BN; these include topiramate—shown to significantly reduce symptoms when compared with placebo in two 10-week RCTs[92]; naltrexone (200 to 300 mg/day)—effective in individuals who did not respond to antidepressant therapy; and ondansetron in patients with severe bulimic symptoms. All are potentially limited by side-effect profile and cost. Topiramate, in particular, is associated with significant cognitive slowing and sedation.[92]

Pharmacological management of BN is a reasonable strategy if psychotherapeutic approaches are ineffective or unavailable. Based on tolerability, efficacy in several large studies, and FDA approval, fluoxetine 60 mg/day is the most appropriate first-line choice for a medication management of BN. If fluoxetine is ineffective, is contraindicated, or cannot be tolerated, consecutive trials of other agents with demonstrated efficacy can be considered. A patient's history of response to a particular agent, co-morbid psychiatric illness, and cost are other important considerations. A dosing schedule that optimizes absorption given a patient's purging habits should be selected for maximum efficacy.

Pharmacological Management of Binge-eating Disorder

Although psychotherapeutic management is considered the first-line treatment of choice for BED, several medications have demonstrated efficacy in reducing symptoms of BED in RCTs, either as a single or as an adjunctive treatment (see Table 37-8). However, none of these medications has FDA approval for this indication, and the majority of the studies have investigated only relatively short-term use of the medication (3 months or less) and little is known about maintenance of symptom reduction after the drug is discontinued. Notably, the majority of these trials also reported a statistically significantly greater weight loss or decrease in BMI in the active drug group compared with placebo, although the weight loss overall was only modest. Only some of these medications have been assessed in BED without co-morbid overweight or obesity.

Pharmacological Considerations in Treating Children and Adolescents

In contrast to the evidence supporting pharmacological management of eating disorders in adults, there are no published RCTs in children and adolescents that support psychotropic medication treatment of eating disorders in this age group. Similar to adult populations, many children and adolescents take psychotropic agents targeting co-morbid conditions. It is important to note that interventions have limited effectiveness when weight is low (re-nourishment is the first priority), and child and adolescent patients may be significantly more susceptible to side effects than are adults. In particular, they may be very sensitive to extrapyramidal symptoms when using antipsychotics (both typical and atypical) aimed at decreasing cognitive distortions. As with adults, there are no studies to support the routine use of antipsychotic medications in children and adolescents with disordered eating.[93] Furthermore, recent data suggest that children and adolescents may be more susceptible to activation and to development of suicidal thinking when taking antidepressants, which has led the FDA to institute a "black box warning" for *all* individuals, particularly those under the age of 24.[94] While not proven effective in the treatment of AN, antidepressants are often used to treat co-morbid anxiety, depression, obsessive-compulsive disorder (OCD), and BN. In an open trial, fluoxetine 60 mg was associated with significant decreases in bingeing and purging, as well as improvement on the Clinical Global Impression-Improvement scale (CGI-I) in adolescents with BN.[83,95] However, when comparing adolescents who have AN (treated with SSRIs relative to those who had not received antidepressants), SSRIs did not appear to have significant effects on BMI, eating disorder core symptom pathology, depression, or OCD symptoms. Because evidence for these medications is limited, clinicians should exercise caution when prescribing antidepressants in this population.

CONCLUSIONS

Eating disorders present challenges to effective management for several key reasons. First, the diagnosis can be difficult to recognize in the clinical setting. The majority of individuals with an eating disorder never access care for this problem. This is both because both BN and BED can occur in the absence of clinical signs and because patients are often reluctant to address symptoms and consequently avoid care. Second, they are associated with serious medical and nutritional complications that must be addressed concomitantly with the psychological aspects of the disorders. Optimal patient care thus almost always requires multi-disciplinary team management. Third, despite some well-supported treatments for the eating disorders, approximately half of patients continue to be symptomatic despite treatment.[8,9] There are some data to suggest that early intervention is beneficial, and when an eating disorder is effectively treated early on, there is a good chance of restored physical well-being. Given the persistence of symptoms in many individuals with an eating disorder and the limited success of preventive interventions, further research on effective therapeutic interventions is urgently needed—especially for AN and the residual category of OSFED.

CURRENT CONTROVERSIES AND FUTURE CONSIDERATIONS

- Etiology of the eating disorders is complex and multifactorial; genetic, psychological, and sociocultural risk factors are being investigated.
- There are few data on effective treatment strategies for adult anorexia nervosa or for OSFED.
- Severity and remission specifiers require investigation regarding their utility and categorization.
- New strategies to address bone loss or failure to achieve peak bone mass during adolescence are critical.
- Treatment strategies are needed for those with BN who do not respond to CBT.
- Novel methods of facilitating weight loss in obese patients with BED also require further research.

Access the complete reference list and multiple choice questions (MCQs) online at https://expertconsult.inkling.com

KEY REFERENCES

1. American Psychiatric Association. *Diagnostic and statistical manual of mental disorders*, ed 5, Arlington, VA, 2013, American Psychiatric Association.
2. American Psychiatric Association. *Diagnostic and statistical manual of mental disorders*, ed 4, text revision, Arlington, VA, 2000, American Psychiatric Association.
3. Hudson JI, Hiripi E, Pope HG, et al. The prevalence and correlates of eating disorders in the National Comorbidity Survey Replication. *Biol Psychiatry* 61(3):348–358, 2007.
4. Becker AE, Thomas JJ, Franko DL, et al. Disclosure patterns of eating and weight concerns to clinicians, educational professionals, family, and peers. *Int J Eat Disord* 38:18–23, 2005.
6. Swanson SA, Crow SJ, LeGrange D, et al. Prevalence and correlates of eating disorders in adolescents: Results from the national comorbidity survey replication adolescent supplement. *Arch Gen Psych* 68:714–723, 2011.
13. Eddy KT, Dorer DJ, Franko DL, et al. Diagnostic crossover in anorexia nervosa and bulimia nervosa: Implications for the DSM-V. *Am J Psychiatry* 165:245–250, 2008.
16. Franko DL, Keshaviah A, Eddy KT, et al. A longitudinal investigation of mortality in anorexia nervosa and bulimia nervosa. *Am J Psychiatr* 170(8):917–925, 2013.

21. Becker AE, Fay K. Socio-cultural issues and eating disorders. In Wonderlich S, de Zwaan M, Steiger H, et al., editors: *Annual review of eating disorders*, Chicago, 2006, Academy for Eating Disorders.
22. Tchanturia K, Hambrook D. Cognitive remediation therapy for anorexia nervosa. In Grilo CM, Mitchell JE, editors: *The treatment of eating disorders*, New York, 2010, Guilford Press, pp 130–149.
24. Trace SE, Baker JH, Peñas-Lledó E, et al. The genetics of eating disorders. *Ann Rev Clin Psychol* 9:589–620, 2013.
25. Friederich H-C, Wu M, Simon JJ, et al. Neurocircuit function in eating disorders. *Int J Eat Disor* 46:425–432, 2013.
30. Thomas JJ, Vartanian LR, Brownell KD. The relationship between eating disorder not otherwise specified (EDNOS) and officially recognized eating disorders: meta-analysis and implications for DSM. *Psychol Bull* 135(3):407, 2009.
32. Clausen L, Lübeck M, Jones A. Motivation to change in the eating disorders: a systematic review. *Int J Eat Disord* 46(8):755–793, 2013.
36. Swenne I, Larsson PT. Heart risk associated with weight loss in anorexia nervosa and eating disorders: factors for QTc interval prolongation and dispersion. *Acta Paediatr* 88:304–309, 1999.
44. Lawson EA, Holsen LM, Santin M, et al. Oxytocin secretion is associated with severity of disordered eating psychopathology and insular cortex hypoactivation in anorexia nervosa. *J Clin Endocrinol Metab* 2012. [Epub ahead of print].
51. Kouba S, Hallstrom T, Lindholm C, et al. Pregnancy and neonatal outcomes in women with eating disorders. *Obstet Gynecol* 105:255–260, 2005.
59. Lock J, Le Grange D, Russell G. *Treatment manual for anorexia nervosa, second edition: a family-based approach*, New York, 2012, Guilford Press.
63. Schmidt U, Oldershaw A, Jichi F, et al. Out-patient psychological therapies for adults with anorexia nervosa: randomised controlled trial. *Br J Psychiatry* 201(5):392–399, 2012.
64. Halmi KA, Agras SW, Crow S, et al. Predictors of treatment acceptance and completion in anorexia nervosa. *Arch Gen Psychiatry* 62:776–781, 2005.
66. Fairburn CG, Cooper Z, Doll HA, et al. Enhanced cognitive behaviour therapy for adults with anorexia nervosa: a UK-Italy study. *Behav Res Ther* 51(1):R2–R8, 2013.
69. Wilson GT, Zandberg LJ. Cognitive-behavioral guided self-help for eating disorders: effectiveness and scalability. *Clin Psychol Rev* 32(4):343–357, 2012.
71. Grilo CM, Masheb RM, Wilson GT. Efficacy of cognitive behavioral therapy and fluoxetine for the treatment of binge eating disorder: a randomized double-blind placebo-controlled comparison. *Biol Psychiatry* 57(3):301–309, 2005.
74. Wilson GT, Wilfley DE, Agras WS, et al. Psychological treatments of binge eating disorder. *Arch Gen Psychiatry* 67(1):94–101, 2010.
81. Kishi T, Kafantaris V, Sunday S, et al. Are antipsychotics effective for the treatment of anorexia nervosa? Results from a systematic review and meta-analysis. *J Clin Psychiatry* 73:6, 2012.
93. Golden NH, Attia E. Psychopharmacology of eating disorders in children and adolescents. *Pediatr Clin N Am* 58:121–138, 2011.

Grief, Bereavement, and Adjustment Disorders

Alicia D. Powell, MD

KEY POINTS

Epidemiology

- Death and loss are part of the human condition; therefore, everyone is at risk for the experience of grief.

Clinical Findings

- Grief may be defined as the physical and emotional pain precipitated by a significant loss.
- Though the course of adjustment disorders is usually brief, the symptoms can be quite severe and may include suicidal ideation; when compared to patients with major depression, individuals with adjustment disorders have a shorter interval between the appearance of their first symptoms and the time of a suicide attempt.

Differential Diagnoses

- The DSM5 has removed the so-called "bereavement exclusion" from the criteria for Major Depressive Disorder, and has added Persistent Complex Bereavement Disorder as a "Condition for Further Study."
- Adjustment disorders comprise a category of emotional or behavioral responses to a stressful event.

Treatment Options

- In a bereaved psychiatric patient, prevention of relapse (of the patient's mental disorder) may be achieved by providing support and optimizing psychotropic medications.
- Psychotherapy can help the patient identify maladaptive responses to stressors, maximize the use of strengths, and provide support.
- Psychopharmacological approaches to adjustment disorders may be necessary, but the use of medications should be brief and be accompanied by psychotherapy.

GRIEF AND BEREAVEMENT
Definition

Grief may be defined as the physical and emotional pain precipitated by a significant loss. The loss may be of a person or pet, but it can also be of a meaningful place, job, or object. A term closely related to grief is *bereavement*, which literally means to be robbed by death. While complicated grief was not defined as a disorder in the *Diagnostic and Statistical Manual of Mental Disorders*, Fourth Edition (DSM-IV), many clinicians observed a need for criteria identifying pathological grief-related conditions.[1] In response, the DSM-5 has removed the so-called "bereavement exclusion" from the criteria for major depressive disorder (MDD) so that even grief of only 2 weeks' duration may be diagnosed as MDD if the patient's symptoms meet criteria. The DSM-5 also defines persistent complex bereavement disorder (PCBD) in its "Conditions for Further Study."[2]

Epidemiology and Risk Factors

Death and loss are part of the human condition; therefore, everyone is at risk for the experience of grief. As death is universally feared, societies and cultures have developed rituals to help deal with the experience of loss and have provided support for survivors. In today's Western society, however, individuals are often distanced from their families or cultures of origin, leaving them to deal with death on their own.

Researchers have found that about 20% of bereaved persons meet criteria for a major depressive episode, with a course and treatment response similar to MDD in non-bereaved individuals.[2,4-6] Those with pre-existing psychiatric disorders appear to be at increased risk for complications secondary to grief.[3,7,8]

The prevalence of PCBD is approximately 2.5%–5%, and is seen in more females than males.[3]

Clinical Findings and Differential Diagnosis

While grief may be universal, each individual's experience of bereavement is unique. When confronted with a grieving person, the physician is often challenged to determine whether the person's grief is proceeding normally, or requires clinical intervention. This determination is often complicated by the fact that grief is shaped by socio-cultural influences, and it does not necessarily develop smoothly from one phase to another.[9-11]

Many investigators have described the stages of adaptive bereavement.[11-13] One useful guideline proposes three overlapping phases: (1) shock, denial, and disbelief; followed by, (2) a stage of mourning that involves physical as well as emotional symptoms and social isolation; eventually arriving at, (3) a reorganization of a life that acknowledges, but is not defined by, the loss of the loved one.

Adaptive bereavement can lead to many symptoms reminiscent of depression: decreased appetite, difficulty with concentration, sleep disturbances, self-reproach, and even hallucinations of the deceased's image or voice (though reality testing remains intact in normal grief). In contrast to depression, however, the sadness of adaptive grief tends to wax and wane, and gradually diminish over time. Qualitatively, the symptoms of normal grief tend to pertain to the deceased, or events surrounding the death.[14] Assessment of various dimensions of the mourner's experience can provide a more complete diagnostic picture[12] (Table 38-1).

The DSM-5 states that in the aftermath of loss, the diagnosis of MDD should not be delayed if the patient's symptoms meet criteria for MDD, are persistent and pervasive, and extend beyond the context of the loss (e.g., feelings of worthlessness not related to the relationship with the deceased). This new designation is supported by research[5] documenting a lack of significant difference between depression related to bereavement and depression associated with other life stressors.

Adding to the difficulty in assessing grief is the lack of consensus regarding a normal duration of bereavement. Manifestations of normal grief (e.g., anniversary reactions) may continue indefinitely, even in otherwise well-functioning individuals. In the acknowledgment of ongoing efforts to better understand ongoing grief, the DSM-5 lists persistent complex bereavement disorder as a "condition for further study." The proposed criteria are listed in Box 38-1.

TABLE 38-1 Dimensions of Grief

Emotional and cognitive responses to the death of a loved one	Reactions may include anger, guilt, regret, anxiety, intrusive images, feelings of being overwhelmed, relieved, or lonely
Coping with emotional pain	Mourners may employ several strategies (e.g., involvement with others, distraction, avoidance, rationalization, the direct expression of feelings, disbelief, or denial, use of faith or religious guidance, or indulgence in "forbidden" activities)
A continuing relationship with the deceased	The mourner's connection with the deceased may be maintained through symbolic representations, adoption of traits of the deceased, cultural rituals, or various means of continued contact (e.g., dreams or attempts at communication)
Changes in daily function	Survivors may experience changes in their mental or physical health or their social, family, or work functions
Changes in relationships	The death of a loved one can profoundly shift the dynamics of a survivor's relationships with family, friends, and co-workers
Changes in self-identity	As the mourning process proceeds, the grieving person may experience himself or herself in new ways that may lead to the development of a new identity (e.g., an orphan, an only child, a widow, or a single parent)

BOX 38-1 Proposed DSM-5 Diagnostic Criteria: Persistent Complex Bereavement Disorder

A. The individual experienced the death of someone with whom he or she had a close relationship.

B. Since the death, at least one of the following symptoms is experienced on more days than not and to a clinically significant degree and has persisted for at least 12 months after the death in the case of bereaved adults and 6 months for bereaved children:
   1. Persistent yearning/longing for the deceased. In young children, yearning may be expressed in play and behavior, including behaviors that reflect being separated from, and also reuniting with, a caregiver or other attachment figure.
   2. Intense sorrow and emotional pain in response to the death.
   3. Preoccupation with the deceased.
   4. Preoccupation with the circumstances of the death. In children, this preoccupation with the deceased may be expressed through the themes of play and behavior and may extend to preoccupation with possible death of others close to them.

C. Since the death, at least six of the following symptoms are experienced on more days than not and to a clinically significant degree, and have persisted for at least 12 months after the death in the case of bereaved adults and 6 months for bereaved children:

REACTIVE DISTRESS TO THE DEATH
   1. Marked difficulty accepting the death. In children, this is dependent on the child's capacity to comprehend the meaning and permanence of death.
   2. Experiencing disbelief or emotional numbness over the loss.
   3. Difficulty with positive reminiscing about the deceased.
   4. Bitterness or anger related to the loss.
   5. Maladaptive appraisals about oneself in relation to the deceased or the death (e.g., self-blame).

   6. Excessive avoidance of reminders of the loss (e.g., avoidance of individuals, places, or situations associated with the deceased; in children, this may include avoidance of thoughts and feelings regarding the deceased).

SOCIAL/IDENTITY DISRUPTION
   1. A desire to die in order to be with the deceased.
   2. Difficulty trusting other individuals since the death.
   3. Feeling alone or detached from other individuals since the death.
   4. Feeling that life is meaningless or empty without the deceased, or the belief that one cannot function without the deceased.
   5. Confusion about one's role in life, or a diminished sense of one's identity (e.g., feeling that a part of oneself died with the deceased).
   6. Difficulty or reluctance to pursue interests since the loss or to plan for the future (e.g., friendships, activities).

D. The disturbance causes clinically significant distress or impairment in social, occupational, or other important areas of functioning.

E. The bereavement reaction is out of proportion to or inconsistent with cultural, religious, or age-appropriate norms.

   Specify if:

With traumatic bereavement: Bereavement due to homicide or suicide with persistent distressing preoccupations regarding the traumatic nature of the death (often in response to loss reminders), including the deceased's last moments, degree of suffering and mutilating injury, or the malicious or intentional nature of the death.

Reprinted with permission from the Diagnostic and statistical manual of mental disorders, *ed 5, (Copyright 2013). American Psychiatric Association.*

An algorithmic presentation of the differential diagnosis of grief and bereavement is provided in Figure 38-1.

Treatment Options

Perhaps the most common treatment of grief involves simply listening to the mourner's experience, and providing support. Most care of mourners is provided by the family, community members, and primary care providers. Two categories of mourners come to the attention of a psychiatrist: those individuals already in treatment for a previously diagnosed psychiatric condition, and those whose concern about grief is the initiating complaint.

Psychiatric patients with any kind of grief reaction may benefit from a review of their psychoactive medications. Besides provision of support during the time of grief, an additional goal of treatment is the prevention of a relapse of the patient's primary mental disorder.

Studies support the use of antidepressant medications if the patient meets criteria for a major depressive episode after the loss of a significant person.[2,6] Psychotherapeutic approaches to bereavement range from psychodynamic to behavioral, and

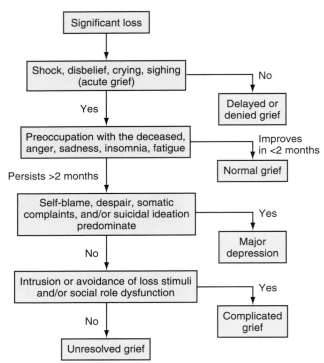

Figure 38-1. Algorithm for differential diagnosis of grief and bereavement.

BOX 38-2 Primary Psychotherapeutic Tasks When Working with a Bereaved Person

- Establish a relationship with the grieving individual, on his or her own terms.
- Explore the loss as fully as possible.
- Review the lost relationship.
- Explore other contributing factors (e.g., financial problems related to the death, and a personal history of responses to death/losses).
- Identify strengths and supports.
- Provide support.
- Look ahead to new roles, relationships, and challenges.

---

from individual to group settings.[15] As the diagnostic criteria and research of treatment for PCBD continue to be investigated, the therapist must rely upon his or her own background, training, and experience to tailor the treatment for each patient. Besides careful attention to the possibility of an emerging Axis I disorder, other key issues in working with a grieving person are summarized in Box 38-2.[15]

Complications

Certain risk factors for poor bereavement outcomes have been identified[16–18] (Table 38-2). Individuals with PCBD frequently report suicidal ideation, and bereavement may increase the risk for completed suicide.[19,20]

Prognosis

The vast majority of bereaved individuals do not experience significant clinical complications due to grief. Those who meet criteria for MDD after a loss have been found to have a

TABLE 38-2 Risk Factors for Poor Bereavement Outcome

| Demographic factors | Advanced age
Lower socioeconomic status |
|---|---|
| Individual factors | Ambivalence or dependency in the relationship with the deceased
Health problems before bereavement |
| Mode of death | Sudden death
Death of a child
Stigmatized (e.g., due to suicide) or traumatic death |
| Circumstances following the loss | Lack of social support
Concurrent crises (e.g., financial problems) |

prognosis not significantly different from those with MDD not associated with bereavement.

ADJUSTMENT DISORDERS
Epidemiology

Estimates of the prevalence of adjustment disorders vary widely depending on the population studied and the methods of assessment used. In outpatient psychiatric settings, the percentage of patients diagnosed with an adjustment disorder ranges from 5% to 20%.[21] Individuals in socio-economically disadvantaged settings often face a high rate of stressors, as do those with chronic medical and psychiatric illness. These individuals may be at higher risk for the development of adjustment disorders than those in the general population. No race, age, or gender differences have been found to be risk factors for adjustment disorder.[22]

Clinical Findings and Differential Diagnosis

DSM-5 diagnostic criteria for Adjustment Disorders are listed in Box 38-3.

Symptoms are described as acute if they last for less than 6 months, and as chronic if they last longer than 6 months. By definition, however, the symptoms cannot persist for more than 6 months after the termination of the stressor. If symptoms persist beyond 6 months without prolonged duration of the stressor, the diagnosis of "Other Specified Trauma- and Stressor-Related Disorder" is given.

Though the course of an adjustment disorder is usually brief, the symptoms can be severe and may include suicidal ideation. Each patient with an adjustment disorder should be evaluated thoroughly for his or her risk of self-injury. Figure 38-2 presents an algorithmic approach to the differential diagnosis of adjustment disorders. Since the prognosis and treatment of mood and other trauma-related conditions differ significantly from adjustment disorder, the clinician is advised to remain alert to the emergence of symptoms meeting criteria for these disorders.

Treatment Options

While no official consensus has been reached on the best treatment for adjustment disorders, psychotherapy is most frequently recommended. Individual therapy can help the patient identify his or her maladaptive responses to the stressor, maximize the use of his or her strengths, and provide support (Box 38-4). Group psychotherapy can be particularly helpful for individuals who share a common stressor (e.g., medical illness, divorce).

Psychopharmacological treatment of adjustment disorders may be necessary if the symptoms are severe, but use of

BOX 38-3 DSM-5 Diagnostic Criteria: Adjustment Disorders

A. The development of emotional or behavioral symptoms in response to an identifiable stressor(s) occurring within 3 months of the onset of the stressor(s).

B. These symptoms or behaviors are clinically significant, as evidenced by one or both of the following:

1. Marked distress that is out of proportion to the severity or intensity of the stressor, taking into account the external context and the cultural factors that might influence symptom severity and presentation.

2. Significant impairment in social, occupational, or other important areas of functioning.

C. The stress-related disturbance does not meet the criteria for another mental disorder and is not merely an exacerbation of a pre-existing mental disorder.

D. The symptoms do not represent normal bereavement.

E. Once the stressor or its consequences have terminated, the symptoms do not persist for more than an additional 6 months.

Specify whether:

309.0 (F43.21) With depressed mood: Low mood, tearfulness, or feelings of hopelessness are predominant.

309.24 (F43.22) With anxiety: Nervousness, worry, jitteriness, or separation anxiety is predominant.

309.28 (F43.23) With mixed anxiety and depressed mood: A combination of depression and anxiety is predominant.

309.3 (F43.24) With disturbance of conduct: Disturbance of conduct is predominant.

309.4 (F43.25) With mixed disturbance of emotions and conduct: Both emotional symptoms (e.g., depression, anxiety) and a disturbance of conduct are predominant.

309.9 (F43.20) Unspecified: For maladaptive reactions that are not classifiable as one of the specific subtypes of adjustment disorder.

Reprinted with permission from the Diagnostic and statistical manual of mental disorders, *ed 5, (Copyright 2013). American Psychiatric Association.*

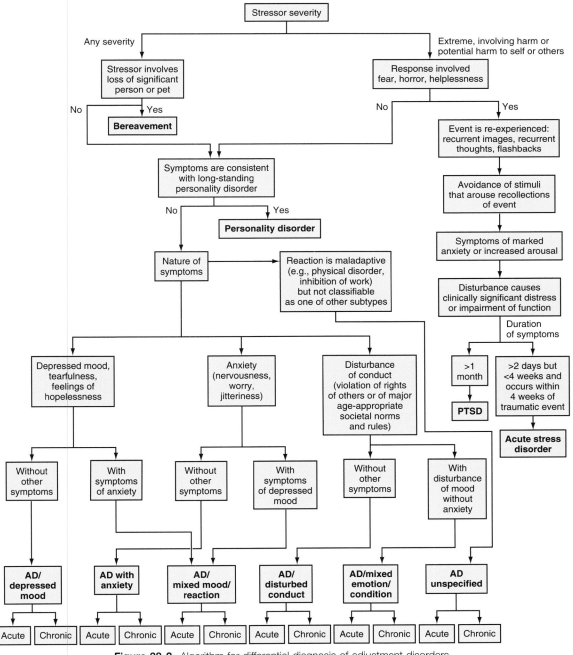

Figure 38-2. Algorithm for differential diagnosis of adjustment disorders.

BOX 38-4 Psychotherapeutic Tasks in Adjustment Disorder

- Examine the stressors in the patient's life.
- Explore ways to reduce or to eliminate the most stressful elements.
- Allow the patient to express concerns and conflicts.
- Search for the meaning of the stressor(s) to the patient and reframe the meaning to allow for an expanded perspective.
- Identify and mobilize the patient's coping strengths.
- Support the patient's use of family and community resources to manage stressors.

---

medications should be brief and be accompanied by psychotherapy. Judicious use of antianxiety or antidepressant agents may be helpful to a patient who suffers from symptoms of anxiety or a mood disorder. Rarely, antipsychotic medications may be indicated for patients who decompensate.

Prognosis

When appropriately treated, most patients with an adjustment disorder will return to their previous level of function within 3 to 6 months. However, the risk of suicide in this population is significant and must be monitored. Studies of suicide have found that when compared to patients with MDD, individuals with an adjustment disorder have a shorter interval between the appearance of their first symptoms and the time of a suicide attempt.[23,24] Limited longitudinal data suggest that adolescents diagnosed with an adjustment disorder are at higher risk of developing a major psychiatric illness.[25]

Access the complete reference list and multiple choice questions (MCQs) online at https://expertconsult.inkling.com

REFERENCES

1. Shear MK, Simon N, Wall M, et al. Complicated grief and related bereavement issues for DSM-5. *Depress Anxiety* 28(2):103–117, 2011.
2. American Psychiatric Association. *Diagnostic and statistical manual of mental disorders*, ed 5, Washington, DC, 2013, APA Press.
3. Piper WE, Ogrodniczuk JS, Azim HF, et al. Prevalence of loss and complicated grief among psychiatric outpatients. *Psychiatr Serv* 52:1069–1074, 2001.
4. Brent D, Melhem N, Donohoe MB, et al. The incidence and course of depression in bereaved youth 21 months after the loss of a parent to suicide, accident, or sudden natural death. *Am J Psychiatry* 166(7):786–794, 2009.
5. Kendler KS, Myers J, Zisook S. Does bereavement-related major depression differ from major depression associated with other stressful life events? *Am J Psychiatry* 165(11):1449–1455, 2008.
6. Zisook S, Shuchter SR, Pedrelli P, et al. Bupropion sustained release for bereavement: results of an open trial. *J Clin Psychiatry* 62(4):227–230, 2001.
7. Ogrodniczuk JS, Piper WE, Joyce AS, et al. Differentiating symptoms of complicated grief and depression among psychiatric outpatients. *Can J Psychiatry* 48(2):87–93, 2003.
8. Zisook S, Lyons L. Bereavement and unresolved grief in psychiatric outpatients. *Omega (Westport)* 20:307–322, 1989–1990.
9. Kleinman A, Good B, editors: *Culture and depression: studies in the anthropology and cross-cultural psychiatry of affect and disorder*, Berkeley, 1985, University of California Press, pp 369–428.
10. Eisenbruch M. Cross-cultural aspects of bereavement: ethnic and cultural variations in the development of bereavement practices. *Cult Med Psychiatry* 8(4):315–347, 1984.
11. Glick IO, Weiss RS, Parkes CM. *The first year of bereavement*, New York, 1974, Wiley.
12. Shuchter SR, Zisook S. The course of normal grief. In Stroebe MS, Stroebe W, Hansson RO, editors: *Handbook of bereavement theory, research, and intervention*, Cambridge, UK, 1993, Cambridge University Press.
13. Brown JT, Stoudemire GA. Normal and pathological grief. *JAMA* 250:378–382, 1983.
14. Lindemann E. Symptomatology and management of acute grief. *Am J Psychiatry* 101:141–148, 1944.
15. Raphael B, Middleton W, Martinek N, et al. Counseling and therapy of the bereaved. In Stroebe MS, Stroebe W, Hansson RO, editors: *Handbook of bereavement theory, research, and intervention*, Cambridge, UK, 1993, Cambridge University Press.
16. Jacobs SC, Kim K. Psychiatric complications of bereavement. *Psychiatr Ann* 20:314–317, 1990.
17. Osterweis M, Solomon F, Green M. *Bereavement: reactions, consequences, and care: a report of the Institute of Medicine, National Academy of Sciences*, Washington, DC, 1984, National Academy Press.
18. Sanders CM. Risk factors in bereavement outcome. *J Soc Issues* 44:97–112, 1988.
19. Ajdacic-Gross V, Ring M, Gadola E, et al. Suicide after bereavement: an overlooked problem. *Psychol Med* 38(5):673–676, 2008.
20. Stroebe M, Stroebe W, Abakoumkin G. The broken heart: suicidal ideation in bereavement. *Am J Psychiatry* 162(11):2178–2180, 2005.
21. Strain JJ. Adjustment disorders. In Gabbard GO, editor: *Treatments of psychiatric disorders*, ed 2, Washington, DC, 1995, APA Press.
22. Billings AG, Moos RH. The role of coping responses and social resources in attenuating the stress of life events. *J Behav Med* 4:139–157, 1981.
23. Polyakova I, Knobler HY, Ambrumova A, et al. Characteristics of suicidal attempts in major depression versus adjustment reactions. *J Affect Disord* 47(1–3):159–167, 1998.
24. Schnyder U, Valach L. Suicide attempters in a psychiatric emergency room population. *Gen Hosp Psychiatry* 19(2):119–129, 1997.
25. Andreasen N, Hoenk P. The predictive value of adjustment disorders: a follow-up study. *Am J Psychiatry* 139:584, 1982.

39 Personality and Personality Disorders

Mark A. Blais, PsyD, Patrick Smallwood, MD, James E. Groves, MD, Rafael A. Rivas-Vazquez, PsyD, ABPP, and Christopher J. Hopwood, PhD

KEY POINTS

Epidemiology

- Personality has evolved to guide both social and interpersonal function.
- Use of dimensional diagnostic systems improves reliability and descriptive breadth.

Clinical Findings

- Normal personality traits and DSM-5 personality disorders share many features.

Treatment Options

- Empirical findings indicate that personality disorders respond positively to a wide range of psychotherapies.
- Targeted pharmacotherapy for personality disorders can be implemented in a rational fashion.

OVERVIEW

The last 30 years have witnessed a remarkable increase in research on, and clinical interest in, personality disorders. Personality disorders are common conditions that affect between 10% and 15% of the general population.[1] Furthermore, between 25% and 50% of individuals who seek outpatient mental health care have either a primary or co-morbid personality disorder. The percentage of psychiatric inpatients with a personality disorder is estimated to be approximately 80%. Personality disorders as a group are among the most frequent disorders treated by psychiatrists.[2]

Personality, as defined, is an enduring pattern of perceiving, relating, and thinking about the environment and oneself that is seen in a wide range of social and personal situations. As such, it is relatively stable and predictable, characterizing an individual in ordinary situations. When non-pathological, it is flexible and adaptable, with less mature coping strategies being held in check. When disordered, it is maladaptive and implacable, with immature and primitive coping strategies rising to the surface and being used in either an inflexible or unpredictable manner as to cause significant distress for the individual and for others. The importance of recognizing, diagnosing, and treating a patient with a personality disorder or disordered traits cannot be emphasized enough. Not only can these disorders affect an individual's ability to function effectively in interpersonal, social, or occupational settings but also they may cause substantial life impairment and suffering. They reduce treatment response for co-morbid Axis I conditions, interfere with educational and occupational achievements, facilitate legal problems, increase suicide rates, lead to substance abuse problems, and lower life satisfaction. Bearing these things in mind, this chapter will provide information that will advance the knowledge and skills of practicing psychiatrists who care for patients with personality disorders.

PERSONALITY THEORY

Gordon Allport,[3] the father of personality psychology, defined *personality* as "the dynamic organization within the individual of those psychophysical systems that determine his characteristic behavior and thought." Understanding what personality is focuses on building comprehensive definitions, such as the following: personality is a stable, organized system composed of perceptual, cognitive, affective, and behavioral subsystems that are hierarchically arranged and that determine how human beings understand and react to others socially. While such a definition has academic merit, it lacks clinical utility. A more useful way of understanding personality is to operationally define it by its functions. One of the chief functions of personality is to guide and regulate our dyadic interpersonal relationships and our small group social interactions. Smooth interpersonal relationships and effective social interactions are crucial to successful life adaptation and to achievement. Evolutionary psychologists believe that personality evolved because improved social and interpersonal function allowed for more effective solutions to the primary problems of human existence (e.g., obtaining food, shelter, protection, and access to reproduction).[4,5] The specific psychological "structures" (functions) and interpersonal skills that allowed our distant ancestors to solve these survival problems evolved into what we now recognize as personality. The evolution of personality, with its emphasis on social effectiveness, may represent one of the more successful survival strategies of our species.[4] Clinically, the advantage of viewing the primary function of personality as the facilitation of effective social and interpersonal interactions is that it allows us to identify when personality becomes disordered: personality is disordered when it interferes with, or complicates, social and interpersonal function.

Guided by the work of Mayer,[6] we can hypothesize that the following three psychological subsystems need to develop for personality to achieve its primary goal of guiding effective social and interpersonal function: a stable and realistic sense of self (the *self-system*); a system for the interpretation of social situations and the understanding of the relational motives and actions of others (the *social system*); and the capacity to observe the self as it relates with others (the *self-in-relation system*).

These components seem to be the irreducible minimum of personality subsystems required for maintenance and regulation of interpersonal function. Figure 39-1 provides a model of personality that uses these three components. The model highlights the fact that personality arises from a combination of complex reciprocal intrapersonal and interpersonal processes that occur simultaneously as we interact with others. Figure 39-1 also shows how these components are organized around, and are influenced, in an ongoing manner by, the maturation and ongoing function of basic cognitive capacities (such as memory, perception, and logical reasoning [association, analysis, and synthesis]).

THE ORIGINS OF PERSONALITY

From birth, infants exhibit differences in activity levels, novelty approach and avoidance, and stimulus threshold. These differences reflect a child's unique temperament. *Temperament* is thought to be the purest expression of the biological basis of personality. Kagan and colleagues[7] have identified two distinct temperaments (*inhibited* or *uninhibited*) in infants. These two temperaments reflect the degree to which infants are fearful of new and unfamiliar situations, and may represent the human

A MODEL OF PERSONALITY ORGANIZATION

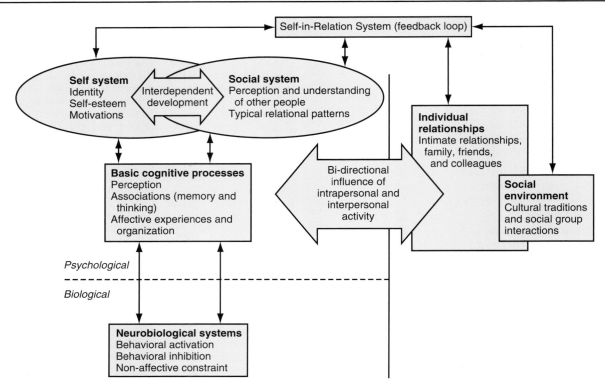

Figure 39-1. A model of the basic personality components, their organization, and their relationship to interpersonal functioning.

version of a universal mammalian tendency for individuals within a species to vary in the degree to which they either approach or avoid unfamiliar situations.

Approximately 15% of infants are *inhibited,* and another 15% are *uninhibited.* Longitudinal research indicates that over 50% of children maintain their initial "inhibited" or "uninhibited" styles well into their teenage years. Inhibited children show less spontaneous speech, less social interaction, and more quiet/vigilant watching of others, whereas uninhibited youngsters are more interactive and talkative. A growing body of knowledge suggests that extremes in these patterns of temperament predispose a child to the development of maladaptive personality traits.

Research with adults has identified three basic temperaments: *positive emotionality, negative emotionality,* and *constraint.*[8-10] *Positive emotionality* and *negative emotionality*[10] are similar to Kagan's inhibited and uninhibited temperaments. Like the inhibited child, the adult who has high negative emotionality tends to perceive and react to the world as if it were a threatening, problematic, and upsetting place,[10] whereas adults who have high positive emotionality are more physically active, happy, and self-confident. Positive emotionality and negative emotionality are primarily associated with the affective tone of an individual's life. *Constraint* refers to how easily an individual acts on an initial emotionally-based evaluation of events and people. In other words, constraint reflects the degree of control an individual exerts over those parts of behavior that are driven by emotion, and can be viewed as the buffering capacity operating in response to emotions. Adults who have a high level of constraint are able to resist their initial impulse to avoid (negative emotionality) or approach

(positive emotionality) a person or situation. This delay allows for the opportunity to evaluate the possible long-term implication of behaviors.[10] Adults who have a low level of constraint, however, act quickly or impulsively on their initial emotional evaluation, and either approach or avoid a person or situation. Constraint may be a precursor to, or foundation of, the adult personality trait of conscientiousness.

The neurobiological network underlying positive emotionality is considered a *behavior activation system* (BAS).[10,11] The BAS is highly sensitive to the effects of positive reinforcement, particularly unconditioned reinforcers (such as food, sex, and safety). With increased cognitive development, the BAS becomes sensitive to the effects of complex secondary (conditioned) reinforcers (e.g., money, social status). The BAS regulates behavior patterns designed to find, identify, and obtain these desired reinforcements. Simply put, the BAS is reward-directed.[11] Depue[12] and Pickering and Gray[11] have suggested that the ascending dopamine (DA) systems found in mesolimbic and mesocortical regions of the brain, long implicated in reward-directed behavior, underlie the BAS.

Negative emotionality, on the other hand, is associated with behavioral inhibition[10,12] and the affective experience of anxiety and fear. The neurobiological network that underlies negative emotionality is a *behavior inhibition system* (BIS). Norepinephrine (noradrenaline) activity in the locus coeruleus appears to underlie the BIS.[11,12]

The neurobiology of constraint is less clear. However, if constraint functions as a response-threshold modifier, neurotransmitters associated with tonic inhibition would likely underlie the trait. Serotonin (5-HT) appears to play a major role in the modulation of a diverse set of functions that includes emotions, motivation, and sensory reactivity.[12] Reduced 5-HT function in animals and humans has been associated with increased irritability, hypersensitivity to sensory stimulation, and impulsivity. From these data, it is plausible that 5-HT networks play a major role in constraint.

Childhood temperament, with its innate, neurobiologically-based behavioral patterns, plays a primary role in the development, expression, and modification of adult personality. Indeed, evidence suggests that there is a moderate degree of stability of childhood temperament through adolescence and into early adulthood.[7] However, the development of adult personality is a complex process that involves more than just biological endowment. In fact, as we mature, the non-biologically based contributions to personality become more influential and more evident in our behavior.

ADULT PERSONALITY TRAITS

Since the mid-1930s, psychologists have devised a number of "dimensional" or "trait" models of adult personality. These models hypothesize that normal personality is composed of between three[13] and sixteen[14] broadly defined traits. Recently, there has been growing agreement that normal adult personality traits can be adequately described using the Five-Factor Model (FFM).[15–17] The FFM is based on the premise that language is the "fossil record" of the personality component of evolutionary psychology. Because language is important for life success in human beings, words had to evolve for all the important observable personality traits. To test this assumption, factor analysis has been used to reduce large lists of descriptive words to their basic psycholinguistic structures. In several such studies, five broad groupings of these trait words have been found. Similar five-factor structures have also been obtained across ethnic groups and languages. The FFM does not argue that all personality traits are represented within the broad domains; however, it provides a reasonably comprehensive coverage of the most important traits that people use to describe themselves and others.[17] The most common names given to these categories are *neuroticism, extroversion, agreeableness, conscientiousness,* and *openness.*

Neuroticism reflects the degree of negative emotion and pessimism a person generally experiences. Individuals who are high in neuroticism tend to be "worriers," and they expect and fear the worst from every experience. Neuroticism is a robust predictor for the development of a psychiatric illness at some point during the life cycle, and it is often associated with low self-esteem, depression, and anxiety. Individuals low in neuroticism are emotionally stable and they deny being bothered by anxiety, irritability, or anger.

Extraversion is associated with positive emotional experiences and an optimistic outlook on life. Individuals who are high in extraversion tend to be outgoing, to like social interactions, to be responsive to intermittent positive reinforcement, and to display high behavioral persistence. High levels of extraversion are thought to be protective against psychiatric illness, and should an illness develop, to respond more consistently to various treatment modalities. The opposite end of the extraversion spectrum is known as *introversion.* Individuals with this trait are often solitary, are socially withdrawn, are less influenced by certain types of positive reinforcement, and have a slower personal pace. Both neuroticism and extraversion have a moderate degree of heritability.[4]

Agreeableness is primarily an interpersonal trait. Individuals who are high in agreeableness are cooperative, are easy going, and tend to have smooth relationships, often at the expense of self-assertion. Individuals who score low on this trait, however, are disagreeable, are oppositional, express their

anger easily, and tend to have relationships that are frequently disrupted by conflict.

Conscientiousness is associated with self-control and a focused and organized approach to life. Individuals high in conscientiousness are achievement-oriented goal-setters who can delay immediate gratification in order to obtain their long-term desired outcome. They are considered responsible, reliable, and dependable. Individuals low in conscientiousness tend to be careless, disorganized, impulsive, and irresponsible. They easily give in to the prospect of immediate or very near-term gratification. Conscientiousness is likely the personality variant of the constraint temperament noted earlier.

Openness describes an individual's interest in, or willingness to engage in, new and varied intellectual and cultural experiences. It is a reflection of curiosity and imagination; it should not to be confused with extraversion. Individuals who are high in openness enjoy a wide range of intellectual and cultural experiences (such as art, theatre, poetry, and philosophy). While openness is moderately correlated with intelligence,[15] individuals who are low on this trait may be no less intelligent but have less interest in esoteric intellectual pursuits. Rather, they concentrate on learning and on experiences that are more practical and applicable to their life. Openness is thought to be associated with the Schizotypal Personality Disorder, but its relationship to the *Diagnostic and Statistical Manual of Mental Disorders* Fifth Edition (DSM-5)[18] personality disorders is less clear than that of the other four Big-5 traits. While the relationship of the DSM-5 personality disorders to temperament and to the FFM personality traits remains unclear, there are persuasive data from many different lines of research that indicate that the FFM dimensions are related to the DSM-5 personality disorders.[19–23] Table 39-1 provides empirically-demonstrated associations among the DSM-5 personality disorders and the domains of the FFM. As Table 39-1 indicates, either alone or in combination, extreme (high or low) forms of these dimensions can explain and deepen our understanding of the DSM-5 personality disorders. For example, the DSM-5 category of *borderline personality disorder* reflects a combination of both high neuroticism and low agreeableness, *histrionic personality disorder* is associated with excessive extraversion, and *antisocial personality disorder* involves low levels of agreeableness and conscientiousness.

Any attempt to integrate the DSM personality disorders with the FFM domains requires some understanding of the conflicts (both historically and conceptually) between the *categorical* and *dimensional* approaches to personality.[24] Medicine has traditionally relied on categorical diagnostic systems for the identification of the presence of a disorder. The categorical approach assumes categories with relatively definite boundaries—"sick" versus "well," pneumonia versus congestive heart failure, schizophrenia versus bipolar disorder, manic episode. It goes back at least to Plato's attempts to "carve nature at the joints." However, categorical models assume that the distribution of the condition is discontinuous (such as pregnancy or death, where there is no gradation). This black-or-white approach contains assumptions that are hard to support (or are even quite misleading) for the personality disorders.

The research is fairly convincing that both normal and abnormal personality traits are continuously distributed throughout the population in a spectrum or on a continuum. The dimensional approach provides a profile or multi-layered picture of personality function that is more realistic than the simple "boxes" that constitute the categories of the categorical approach. And while not mapping directly to the DSM-defined personality disorders or offering treatment guidance, these profiles provide a more individualized and detailed

TABLE 39-1 Relationship of the DSM-5 Personality Disorders (DSM PDs) to the Five-Factor Model Domains

DSM PDs	Neuroticism	Extroversion	Openness	Agreeableness	Conscientiousness
Paranoid	+			−	
Schizoid		−			
Schizotypal	+		+	−	
Antisocial				−	−
Borderline	+			−	
Histrionic		+			
Narcissistic			+	−	
Avoidant	+	−			
Dependent	+			+	
Obsessive		−			+

+, Significant positive associations; −, significant negative associations.
(Based on Widiger TA, Costa PT. Five-factor model personality disorder research. In Widiger TA, Costa PT, editors: Personality disorders and the five-factor model of personality, ed 2, Washington, DC, 2002, American Psychological Association, and the Diagnostic and statistical manual of mental disorders, *ed 5, Washington, DC, 2013, American Psychiatric Association.)*

description of the *person*. Both systems have advantages and disadvantages.

Despite these differences, it seems likely that future versions of the DSM will incorporate some form of a dimensional model for diagnosing or describing personality disorders. In fact, recent findings reveal that a four-factor structure nicely accounts for abnormal personality traits (traits more directly linked to the DSM personality disorders) than to either current systems or the FFM. These factors (emotional dysregulation, dissocial behaviors, inhibition, and compulsivity) closely resemble four of the FFM domains.[25] However, there are other dimensional models of personality. For example, Shedler and Weston[26] have developed a dimensional model for the description and diagnosis of personality disorders that holds considerable clinician utility. Cloninger and Svrakic[8] also have an alternative dimensional model that attempts to account for variations in both normal and abnormal personality. Building on the pioneering ideas of Thomas and Chess, Cloninger and Svrakic's[8] model identifies four basic genetically-determined temperaments (harm-avoidance, novelty-seeking, reward-dependence, and persistence) and three character traits (self-directedness, cooperativeness, and self-transcendent). These seven dimensions interact to form personality. The Temperament and Character Inventory was developed to assess the seven main components and additional subcomponents of the model. This comprehensive model of personality combines findings from the fields of genetics, neurobiology, and trait psychology in a manner that can enhance both the assessment and treatment of personality disorders. Cloninger and Svrakic's[8] ambitious work has generated considerable research activity, but has not been as widely adopted clinically.

DSM-5 PERSONALITY DISORDERS

The DSM-5[18] recognizes 10 personality disorders, which are organized into three clusters (based on shared diagnostic features): (1) cluster A personality disorders, which share the common features of being odd and eccentric (paranoid, schizoid, and schizotypal personality disorders); (2) cluster B personality disorders, which share the common features of being dramatic, emotional, and erratic (antisocial, borderline, histrionic, and narcissistic personality disorders); and (3) cluster C personality disorders, which share the common features of being anxious and fearful (avoidant, dependent, and obsessive-compulsive personality disorders). As a rule, patients often display traits of more than one personality disorder, and if they meet diagnostic criteria for another one, it should be diagnosed along with the primary one.

Cluster A Personality Disorders
Paranoid Personality Disorder

The core feature of *paranoid personality disorder* is a pervasive distrust and suspiciousness of others. Afflicted individuals are reluctant to confide in others; they assume that most people will harm or exploit them in some manner. In new situations, they search for confirmation of these expectations and view even the smallest slight as significant. They unjustifiably question the loyalty of friends and significant others, and, consequently, are often socially isolated and avoid intimacy. They pride themselves on being rational and objective, but they appear to others as unemotional, affectively restricted, and hypervigilant. These individuals bear grudges and collect injustices. When their beliefs are challenged or they are stressed in any significant way, these individuals can show profound anger, hostility, and referential thinking.

The most common differential diagnoses for paranoid personality disorder include delusional disorder (paranoid type), schizophrenia (paranoid type), schizoid personality disorder, and avoidant personality disorder. With delusional disorder and schizophrenia, reality testing is lost; in paranoid personality disorder, formal reality testing is said to remain intact. However, reality testing is a continuum, and it may be difficult to distinguish the degree of reality testing of a person with mild schizophrenia from that of a person with a florid paranoid personality disorder, especially if in the latter certain cultural factors or a potential gain from manipulating the examiner are present. With schizoid and avoidant personality disorder, the amount and degree of paranoia is significantly less, which distinguishes it from paranoid personality disorder.

The prevalence of paranoid personality disorder in the general population is approximately 0.5% to 2.5%. There appears to be an increased incidence in families with schizophrenia and delusional disorder. The diagnosis is far more common in males than it is in females.

Schizoid Personality Disorder

Individuals with a *schizoid personality disorder* are loners who are emotionally detached and indifferent to the world around them. They have little desire for relationships and have few emotional ties, even with family members. They express little or no discomfort over their detachment. With respect to employment, they prefer non-competitive and isolative jobs with non-human themes (such as mathematics, philosophy, or astronomy). They may greatly enjoy solitary pursuits, such as computer games and puzzles. On interview, their thinking is clear and their reality testing is intact. The best caricature of the person with a schizoid personality would be the single, unfashionable, laboratory-oriented, absent-minded professor.

The differential diagnoses for schizoid personality disorder include schizophrenia, as well as paranoid, obsessive-compulsive, and avoidant personality disorders. Intact reality testing, normal abstracting ability, and the absence of a formal thought disorder distinguish schizoid personality disorder from schizophrenia. Patients with a paranoid personality disorder have more socially-oriented ideation than do schizoid patients. Patients with obsessive-compulsive and avoidant personality disorders, while often socially isolated, view loneliness as ego-dystonic or ego-alien and they enjoy a richer interpersonal history than do patients with a schizoid personality disorder.

As currently defined, schizoid personality disorder affects about 7.5% of the population, with men diagnosed twice as often as women. As with paranoid personality disorder, the incidence of psychotic disorders in the relatives of these patients is higher, although this association is less robust. Most affected individuals function reasonably well and have few problems that require intervention.

Schizotypal Personality Disorder

The essential features of the *schizotypal personality disorder* are cognitive, perceptual, and behavioral eccentricities, and a pervasive discomfort with close relationships. Patients with this personality disorder frequently embrace unusual beliefs (such as telepathy, clairvoyance, and magical thinking) to a degree that exceeds cultural and subcultural norms. Socially, they are inept and uncomfortable. The style of their clothing may be inappropriate and strange, further reflecting their eccentric nature. Their speech is often vague, digressive, or inappropriately abstract, and they may talk to themselves in public. The content of that speech may also reflect ideas of reference, bodily illusions, and paranoia, but there is usually an absence of formal thought disorders, and their reality testing is intact. Under periods of stress, however, these patients may decompensate into brief psychotic states.

The differential diagnosis for schizotypal personality disorder includes schizophrenia and several personality disorders. Paranoid and schizoid personality disorders share many of the core features of schizotypal personality disorder, but differ by degree or absence of eccentricity. Borderline personality disorder shares some of the unusual speech and perceptual style, but it demonstrates stronger affect and connection to others. Patients with avoidant personality disorder, while uncomfortable and inept in social settings, are not eccentric and crave contact with others. Schizophrenia differs from schizotypal personality disorder in that the schizotype possesses good reality testing and lacks psychosis.

Schizotypal personality disorder affects about 3% of the population. There is no known sex ratio. While there is no known genetic etiology, there appears to be a higher occurrence of this disorder in the biological relatives of schizophrenic patients, and the disorder is frequently diagnosed in women with fragile X syndrome.

Cluster B Personality Disorders

Personality disorders in this cluster are said to combine abnormalities in both thinking and affect, but not to be predominantly one or the other cluster, such as cluster A (thinking) or cluster C (affect). Disorders in this cluster are very socially interpersonally-focused and to some degree exploitive.

Antisocial Personality Disorder

The key features of *antisocial personality disorder* are repetitive unlawful acts, socially irresponsible behaviors, and a pervasive disregard for the rights of others. Antisocial behaviors develop early in adolescence, before age 15. These individuals are so unconcerned with the feelings and rights of others that they are morally bankrupt and lack a sense of remorse. Such people seem completely unable to project themselves into the feelings of others and they are bereft of empathy. Superficially, they can be charming and engaging, yet beneath the facade lie individuals who live in a world filled with illegal activity, deceit, promiscuity, substance abuse, and assaultive behavior. Because patients with this disorder are so indifferent to how their actions affect others, antisocial personality disorder is the personality disorder most resistant to treatment.

The differential diagnosis for antisocial personality disorder includes antisocial behavior, other cluster B personality disorders, impulse control disorders, mania, psychosis, substance abuse disorders, mental retardation, and personality changes caused by general medical conditions. Patients with borderline personality disorder may perform illegal acts, yet they tend to demonstrate more repetitive suicidal and parasuicidal behaviors, as well as intense affect and self-loathing. When patients with narcissistic personality disorder violate the law, it is typically motivated by a need to maintain their sense of entitlement rather than to meet an instrumental desire (i.e., narcissistic personality disorder is associated with "white collar crime," whereas antisocial personality disorder is associated with "blue collar crime"). Bipolar mania can be difficult to separate from antisocial personality disorder, because patients with antisocial personalities can also have co-morbid bipolar disorders. For the most part, however, patients with bipolar disorder lack a significant degree of childhood conduct problems, and the antisocial behavior is usually limited to manic episodes. Patients with psychotic disorders may also perform criminal acts, but these acts are usually in response to delusions or hallucinations. Substance abuse disorders can be especially difficult to differentiate from antisocial personality disorder, because patients with antisocial personality disorder almost invariably engage in substance use. However, criminal behaviors associated with substance abuse disorders generally center around using and obtaining the drugs.

Antisocial personality disorder affects 3% of men and less than 1% of women. Given the prominence of illegal activity in the diagnostic criteria of this personality disorder, it is not surprising that at least 75% of the prison population carries the diagnosis. Patients with this disorder have an onset of conduct disorder before the age of 15 years, and frequently suffer from co-morbid attention-deficit/hyperactivity disorders, polysubstance disorders, and somatization disorder. The exact etiology is unknown, but this disorder occurs five times more commonly in first-degree relatives of men with the disorder. While the natural history of antisocial personality disorder is variable, some improvement can occur during middle age.

Borderline Personality Disorder

Borderline personality disorder (BPD) has attracted the most research and clinical interest of all the personality disorders. Central to this disorder is an impaired capacity to form stable interpersonal relationships. Other salient features include affective instability (with rapidly shifting mood swings), impulsivity, identity disturbance (described as chronic boredom or emptiness), recurrent manipulative suicidal and parasuicidal behaviors (e.g., self-mutilation), and idealization/

devaluation ("splitting"). When faced with real or perceived separation, these patients often react with intense fear and anger. Under stress, borderline patients may also experience brief reactive psychotic states (also known as "micropsychotic episodes"). Also, they are more likely to have various dissociative phenomena in stressful and affectively intense situations.

It used to be said that this condition was so multifaceted that the diagnosis was non-specific, that it had no "leading edge" or characteristic, and that it was a "wastebasket" diagnosis. This is untrue, however, and the major overarching hallmark of BPD is the presence of dramatic swings in positive or negative affect toward important others in the individual's life, characteristically without any insight into the "switch" in affect—in other words, an "affective amnesia." In 1682 Thomas Sydenham said the following of "hysterics," who are retrospectively recognizable as individuals with BPD: "All is caprice, they love without measure those they will soon hate without reason."[27]

While BPD is a highly co-morbid condition, the differential diagnosis for BPD should focus on other personality disorders, bipolar spectrum disorders, and psychotic disorders. Patients with BPD lack the peculiarity and referential thinking found in those with schizotypal personality disorder and the extreme suspiciousness seen in those with paranoid personality disorder. BPD has extensive overlap with the histrionic, narcissistic, and dependent disorders, but individuals with these conditions tend to have more stable identities and they rarely engage in self-mutilation or chronic suicidal behaviors. Bipolar spectrum disorders can be difficult to distinguish from those with BPD, as the two may co-exist. However, the mood swings displayed by the borderline patient must not meet criteria for manic or hypomanic episodes. Finally, while the borderline patient may experience transient psychotic states, patients with major psychotic disorders generally experience a persistent impairment in reality testing.

Substance abuse disorders, especially alcohol abuse, have a major co-morbidity with BPD. However, well over 10% of patients no longer meet diagnostic criteria for BPD once they are able to maintain a year of sobriety.

BPD is the most prevalent personality disorder in all clinical settings (12% to 15%). It is believed to occur in 2% to 3% of the general population, with a 2:1 female-to-male ratio. There is a high co-occurrence of major depressive disorder in patients with borderline personality, but recent research suggests that this reflects the depressogenic nature of borderline pathology and the consequences of chaotic lifestyles rather than indicating that the two conditions share a common biology. BPD is usually diagnosed before age 40. While the course can be variable, it rarely resolves completely. However, some patients experience a marked decrease in their impulsive and self-injurious behaviors around middle age.

Histrionic Personality Disorder

The most notable features of *histrionic personality disorder* (HPD) are excessive emotionality and an almost insatiable need for attention. These individuals are overly concerned with their physical appearance, they have poor frustration tolerance (with emotional outbursts), and their speech is impressionistic and vague. They view physical attractiveness as the core of their existence, and as such, are often provocative in dress, flamboyant in mannerisms, and inappropriately seductive in behavior. While they appear superficially charming, others tend to view them as vain and lacking in genuineness. Histrionic and narcissistic personality disorders are closely associated.

The differential diagnosis for HPD includes other cluster B personality disorders and somatization disorder. BPD differs from HPD in that the borderline patient displays more despair and suicidal/parasuicidal behaviors. The narcissistic patient is more preoccupied with grandiosity and envy than is the histrionic individual. The person with dependent personality disorder, while sharing the need for acceptance and reassurance, lacks the degree of emotionality seen in histrionic individuals. Somatization disorder can co-exist with HPD, but it is distinguished by the greater emphasis on physical complaints.

This disorder occurs in 2% to 3% of the general population. While women receive the diagnosis more often than do men, many clinicians believe that men are underdiagnosed. This disorder is more common in first-degree relatives of people with this disorder. Like most personality disorders, the course is variable. Some individuals experience an attenuation or softening of the core symptoms during middle age. Others may experience a complicated course, including co-morbid somatization, conversion, pain, and dissociative, sexual, and mood disorders. Two major caveats pertain to this diagnosis. The first is that emotional displays can vary from culture to culture, and what is histrionic in one culture may be identified as normal emotional expression in another. The other concerns the great co-morbidity this disorder has with BPD. Some believe that while not all borderline patents are histrionic, most HPD patients have sufficient borderline traits to merit a diagnosis of BPD.

Narcissistic Personality Disorder

The hallmark of *narcissistic personality disorder* (NPD) is an overwhelming and pathological self-absorption. These individuals possess a grandiose sense of self-importance or uniqueness; they are preoccupied with fantasies of success and feel that the people with whom they associate need also be special and unique. They are blindly ambitious, often breaking conventional rules and exploiting others to meet their self-serving ends. They lack empathy for others (although less so than the antisocial patient), and can react with disappointment and rage when another's needs interfere with their desires. Beneath the facade of self-sufficiency and arrogance lies a fragile individual who is so hypersensitive to issues of self-esteem that if he or she is criticized in even the slightest manner, the reaction is intense emotion and rage. Research suggests that the DSM definition of NPD does not adequately capture the underlying vulnerability seen clinically in many NPD patients.[28]

What makes the differential diagnosis for NPD so difficult is that other cluster B personality disorders often co-exist. Nonetheless, a few distinguishing features are helpful. The borderline patient differs from the narcissistic patient in that the former is more impulsive, has a less cohesive identity, and lives a more chaotic life. The histrionic patient, unlike the narcissistic patient, is more outwardly emotional and deeply involved with others. While the narcissistic patient and the antisocial patient both exploit people, the primary motivation for the narcissistic patient is to maintain his or her grandiose self-image (power and money) rather than short-term material gain.

The exact prevalence of this disorder is unknown. The best estimates are that it occurs in less than 1% of the general population and between 2% and 15% in the clinical population. There are no data concerning familial patterns or sex ratio. However, men are more frequently diagnosed with the condition. Some believe that NPD is actually adaptive in certain specific situations for segments of the life cycle; that is, NPD is actually useful in certain career paths, such as acting, politics, and industry.

The course of this condition is chronic. These patients frequently suffer co-morbid mood disorders, particularly major depression and dysthymia. For some, aging is the ultimate blow to their self-esteem, as many of the qualities that help maintain their identity (e.g., career, health, beauty, youth) must naturally begin to fade. Consequently, the narcissistic patient is prone to severe midlife crises.

Cluster C Personality Disorders

Personality disorders in this cluster are traditionally held to most resemble Axis I disorders characterized by abnormalities of affect, the anxiety disorders, and the depressive disorders.

Avoidant Personality Disorder

The core feature of *avoidant personality disorder* is an excessive discomfort with or fear of intimate and social relationships that results in the pathological avoidance of social interactions (as a means of self-protection). For example, to guard against what they fear might be potentially embarrassing or humiliating situations, these individuals exaggerate the risks of ordinary, but unplanned, tasks so as not to deviate from a safe and predictable daily routine. While genuinely desiring relationships, they are unwilling to enter into them because of real or perceived signs of humiliation, rejection, or negative feedback. If, however, they manage to negotiate a relationship, it is only with the assurance of uncritical acceptance. Because of this pervasive awkwardness and shyness, they suffer from very low self-esteem. Because their chronic avoidant behavior reduces anticipatory anxiety through negative reinforcement (i.e., the removal of a noxious situation), this behavior pattern is powerfully entrenched and difficult to modify.

The differential diagnosis for avoidant personality disorder includes other personality disorders and social phobia. Patients with schizoid personality disorder, unlike avoidant patients, do not desire relationships with others. While dependent personality disorder shares many features with avoidant personality disorder, the former has a greater fear of abandonment, and embraces, rather than avoids relationships. Social phobia can be very difficult to distinguish from avoidant personality disorder, and many clinicians consider them the same. Other clinicians argue, however, that the distinction between the two is that patients with social phobia tend to have more specific fears around social performances.

Avoidant personality disorder is common; it occurs in approximately 1% of the general population and in 10% of clinical samples. Temperament, particularly the inhibited style, and disfiguring physical illnesses may be predisposing factors. There is no information regarding its gender ratio or familial patterns.

Patients with avoidant personality disorder are able to function in relationships, to marry, and to have families, as long as the environment is safe and protective. In the same was as most other personality disorders, they are prone to mood disorders, especially depression and dysthymia. However, they are at especially high risk for anxiety disorders and for social phobia.

Dependent Personality Disorder

Individuals with *dependent personality disorder* display clinging, submissive behavior, and have a strong desire for others to care for them. They are extremely preoccupied with fears of abandonment. They fear being alone and will go to extreme lengths to preserve any relationship, no matter how physically or emotionally abusive it may be. They are submissive and passive toward others, and fear that any direct expression of anger will end in rejection. Consequently, they may volunteer for unpleasant tasks, agree with others who may even be wrong, or look to others for assurance about simple daily decisions, to ensure being liked or cared for.

Dependent personality disorder can be difficult to distinguish from other psychiatric conditions, because many disorders have dependency as an underlying feature. The differential diagnosis for dependent personality disorder includes other personality disorders and agoraphobia. Patients with histrionic personality disorder have issues of dependency, but shorter and more numerous relationships. Borderline patients express more affect and anger around real or perceived abandonment, whereas dependent patients become more placating. When faced with rejection or termination of a relationship, avoidant patients withdraw from further contact, unlike dependent patients, who quickly seek out a new relationship to fill the void. Agoraphobic patients, while displaying dependency, tend to demonstrate a higher level of fear around leaving specific safe environments, especially home.

Dependent personality disorder accounts for about 2.5% of all personality disorders, with women more commonly diagnosed than men. However, this gender difference may reflect a bias in the criteria rather than a true difference in prevalence across the sexes. Patients with a history of childhood separation anxiety or chronic illness may be predisposed to the disorder. There is no known familial pattern of inheritance.

Many patients with this disorder suffer from co-morbid dysthymia, major depression, and alcohol abuse. They may also become victims of physical and emotional abuse due to their dependency and their lack of assertiveness. Because these patients are indecisive, require excessive reassurance, and need so much direction, their careers are unlikely to advance.

Obsessive-compulsive Personality Disorder

The major features of *obsessive-compulsive personality disorder* (OCPD) are perfectionism, inflexibility, and need for interpersonal control. These individuals are so preoccupied with rules, efficiency, trivial details, and procedures that the purpose of the activity is often lost or the job uncompleted. They maintain an inflexible adherence to their own internally strict and excessive standards, and subsequently dislike delegating tasks for fear that others will not meet those standards. When they delegate tasks, they tend to micromanage their subordinates. While mindful of the chain of command, they possess a strong need for control and resist the authority and autonomy of others. To their superiors, they sometimes appear diligent, as they will tolerate protracted work, even at the cost of pleasure and interpersonal relationships. But in certain work situations, their perfectionism creates competition with their managers. To their equals or subordinates, they can be harsh taskmasters with escalating criteria for job perfection, and are stingy with emotions and compliments.

The principal differential diagnosis for OCPD is obsessive-compulsive disorder (OCD). While the two are often confused for each other, they differ significantly: patients with OCD have true obsessions and compulsions that they find ego-dystonic, whereas patients with the personality disorder find that their behaviors are ego-syntonic and rewarded by others. Occasionally, the two disorders co-exist, requiring a diagnosis for each.

This personality disorder is common in the general population, with men receiving the diagnosis more often than women. While the mode of transmission is unknown, it is more common among first-degree relatives of patients with this disorder. There is also an increased concordance in identical twins.

The course for OCPD is variable. However, research suggests that OCPD can be one of the least impairing of the personality disorders, and patients with this condition often achieve substantial success in some life areas.[29]

DSM-5 PERSONALITY DISORDERS

The DSM-IV model of personality disorders has been widely criticized during the last few decades: research has uncovered important flaws, clinicians were reticent to diagnose personality disorders, and insurance companies have not been inclined to reimburse for their treatment. Thus, leading up to the DSM-5, most researchers and clinicians expected that personality disorders would be significantly reformulated. As it turns out, the DSM-IV personality disorders were retained verbatim in Section II (diagnostic criteria and codes) of DSM-5, with the minor exception that there is no longer a not otherwise specified (NOS) category. Instead, a patient with several symptoms who fails to meet criteria for any of the 10 diagnoses would be given a diagnosis of personality disorder, unspecified; whereas a person who met criteria for an unofficial category (e.g., passive-aggressive) would be given the diagnosis of personality disorder, not otherwise specified. The other major change reflects the organization of the DSM-5 in general: namely, that the multi-axial system will no longer be employed. This means that personality disorders will be listed as a primary diagnosis when indicated, rather than separated from other diagnoses on their own "Axis".

Although the DSM-5 personality disorders are essentially the DSM-IV personality disorders, there will also be an alternative formulation of this class of psychopathology in Section III of the DSM (emerging models and measures). This alternative reflects the hybrid model proposed by the personality and personality disorder workgroup that failed to be accepted for full inclusion in the manual. Instead the hybrid model was included in Section III with the goal to continue to research the alternative system so that its evidentiary and clinical basis can be sufficient, with evidence-based modifications, to be offered as the formal diagnostic criteria in the DSM.

DSM-5 Section III: Hybrid Diagnosis

The proposed system divides personality disorder diagnosis into two parts: (a) establishing a diagnosis of personality disorder in general and the severity of personality pathology and, (b) describing the nature of that pathology using a hybrid system involving the use of an evidence-based dimensional system of traits to derive traditional categorical diagnoses.

Criterion A: Level of Personality Functioning

The first step in Section III is to determine whether the patient meets criteria for a personality disorder, in general. This is accomplished with reference to the revised definition of personality pathology, that it involves impairments in self (identity, self-direction) and interpersonal (empathy, intimacy) functioning.[30] These functional difficulties are quantified using the levels of personality functioning scale, which will be available in Section III with specific criteria for each domain. This is in stark contrast to the DSM-IV/DSM-5 Section III model, in which the definition of personality disorder is not quantified, not embedded in formal psychological theories of personality, and contains criteria that are inconsistent with available evidence (e.g., the assumption that personality disorder symptoms are more stable than those of other disorders).[28] In addition to determining the presence of personality and pathology in general, the Section III levels of personality functioning scale provides a quantitative index of the overall severity of personality pathology that can be used for basic triage decisions, such as the level of care most appropriate for a given patient.

Criterion B: Traits and Types

Criterion B involves traits that are embedded in an evidence-based model of individual differences that are organized hierarchically.[31,32] The top level includes five traits: negative affectivity, detachment, antagonism, disinhibition, and psychoticism. Each of these traits has three to seven lower-order traits that describe related behaviors in more specific detail. Interestingly, although this system is very similar to trait models from personality psychology, such as the five-factor model, this was not intentional. The DSM-5 work group assembled a list of 37 traits embedded in the DSM-IV criterion sets. Psychometric analysis in large community and clinical samples winnowed this list to 25, and factor analyses of these 25 revealed the five higher-order traits that are highly similar to the five-factor model.[31] This finding reinforces the strong link between the science of normal personality and the structure of personality disorders.

These traits are used to diagnose one of seven official personality disorders in DSM-5, Section III. Six of these disorders are shared with Section II: antisocial, avoidant, borderline, narcissistic, obsessive-compulsive, and avoidant. The other four were discarded based on insufficient validity evidence and low prevalence.[33] For example, narcissistic personality disorder would be defined by grandiosity and attention-seeking, two of the traits in the antagonism domain. The seventh is personality disorder, trait specified, which is given when a person has a level of functioning consistent with personality disorder but does not have enough of the traits for any of these specific disorders to merit one of those diagnoses. Traits can also be assessed when a person meets criteria for a particular disorder but also has other relevant personality features of concern. Based on substantial evidence that personality functioning is relevant for patients whether or not they have a personality disorder, they can also be assessed in patients who do not meet Criterion A.

DIAGNOSING PERSONALITY DISORDERS

The DSM personality disorders have proven difficult for clinicians to diagnose reliably.[34,35] These difficulties result from a combination of limitations inherent both in the diagnostic system and in standard clinical practice. Problems with the DSM system include high co-morbidity and diagnostic overlap (i.e., arbitrary boundaries) among the personality disorders, low inter-rater agreement for the presence or absence of these disorders, and weak agreement across different diagnostic methods.

Clinicians themselves contribute to the difficulties in diagnosing personality disorders. These difficulties, however, are dynamic and amenable to change, especially if clinicians become more disciplined when following the formal DSM diagnostic process. Research shows that the system becomes more reliable when the clinician ensures that a patient meets the diagnostic criteria for the disorder and does not idiosyncratically or hastily overvalue specific features (e.g., excessive grandiosity indicates narcissistic personality disorders, rage or cutting behavior always indicates borderline personality disorder). Reliability is further increased when clinicians continue to search for co-morbid personality disorders once the more prominent condition has been identified, because patients with one identified personality disorder typically meet criteria for other personality disorders.[34,35]

Clinicians can also increase diagnostic reliability by updating their interviewing styles. Interviewing for signs and symptoms of a personality disorder requires a longitudinal developmental perspective. Such longitudinal interviewing should assess the quality of the patient's social function in the areas of school, career, family, romantic relationships, peer group function, and interactions with authority figures. Across these categories, clinicians should listen for recurring themes of interpersonal conflict, disappointment, exploitation, or emptiness; because these can all indicate a personality disorder.

Some clinicians routinely avoid directly asking about symptoms of a personality disorder, believing that patients are either unwilling or unable to respond accurately. While personality-disordered individuals often use lower-level defense mechanisms, such as projection and denial, and commonly disown responsibility for their actions, they often confirm a public or family consensus about their behavior if couched in sympathetic terms: "Have you ever been unjustly accused of taking things at your various jobs? How often?" "Do people fail to understand and admire your assertiveness and your refusal to get pushed around? Really? Tell me about that."

When making a diagnosis of a personality disorder, clinicians should be cautioned not to rely heavily on behaviors observed while in session. In-session observations, although they provide important information, should be viewed as hypotheses-generating data that need exploration across situations and time. While there is no "gold standard" for clinically diagnosing personality disorders, one approach for improving diagnostic accuracy is the LEAD standard (longitudinal expert evaluation using all data).[36] This approach requires that a clinician obtain and integrate historical/longitudinal data, current life function data, in-session observations, and multiple data sources (e.g., psychological assessment data, informant information) before finalizing a personality disorder diagnosis.

Another way to improve diagnostic accuracy is for the clinician to employ a multi-phase, multi-method approach that combines psychological assessment and clinical interviewing. In the first phase, the patient completes a self-report personality instrument to generate hypotheses about problematic personality styles. Self-report instruments, such as the Millon Clinical Multiaxial Inventory—III (MCMI-III)[37] and the Personality Diagnostic Questionnaire—4 (PDQ-4),[38] provide adequate screening of potential DSM-5 personality disorders. However, as with all self-report measures, these instruments are highly sensitive, but not specific, to the target conditions. In the second phase, after reviewing the assessment findings, the clinician then uses a longitudinally-focused interview to determine the presence, pervasiveness, and impairment of the personality disorders suggested by the self-report test to arrive at a reasonable clinical diagnosis.

TREATMENT OF PERSONALITY DISORDERS
Psychotherapy

Not long ago, skepticism abounded regarding the potential for psychiatric treatment to yield significant improvement in patients who suffer from personality disorders. Such skepticism has now been replaced with growing optimism. The empirical literature on the treatment of personality disorders continues to grow and the number of evidence-based therapies for personality disorders, especially BPD, is expanding. While still limited, the findings in general show that personality-disordered patients can achieve meaningful improvement from individual psychotherapy[39,40] and group psychotherapy.[41] Findings from randomized controlled trials, the "gold standard" for therapeutic evidence, support the efficacy of dialectical behavioral therapy (DBT)[42] and psychodynamic psychotherapy[43] for treating BPD. It appears that cognitive, cognitive-behavioral, and psychodynamic psychotherapies are generally effective treatments for personality disorders, yielding similar degrees of improvement, with no single type of psychotherapy shown to be more effective than any other.[39]

Different personality disorders appear to improve at different rates and to differing degrees. For example, research suggests that patients with cluster C disorders improve more than patients with BPD, while borderline patients improve more than schizotypal and antisocial personality-disordered patients.[40] Schizotypal patients also appear to require a longer duration of treatment to achieve meaningful change. Patients with antisocial personality disorder without co-morbid depression are the least likely to achieve meaningful improvement.

Duration of treatment is also related to overall improvement, with longer treatments generally leading to greater recovery. In their review of psychotherapy studies on personality disorders, Perry and colleagues[40] estimated that it requires 1.3 years (92 sessions) for 50% of personality-disordered patients to achieve recovery (i.e., no longer meeting full criteria for the particular disorder) and 2.2 years (216 sessions) for 75% to recover. This finding is consistent with Howard's phases-of-change model, which also posits that interpersonal function is the last domain to improve with mental health treatment.[44]

Treatment adherence is another determinant of outcome. The literature suggests that personality-disordered patients on average have a dropout rate of between 21% and 31%.[40] However, the dropout rate is quite variable across different personality disorders; patients with a cluster B personality disorder have a dropout rate of 40%, a cluster A disorder of 36%, and a cluster C disorder of 28%. Patients in group therapy have a higher dropout rate than do patients in individual therapy, with up to 51% of personality-disordered patients dropping out of short-term group treatment.[40] Therapeutic alliance is a chief determinant of adherence, and adherence can be significantly enhanced with consistent nonjudgmental attention to the vicissitudes of the therapeutic relationship.[39]

Given that many standard forms of psychotherapy have similar degrees of success in treating personality disorders, a review of their common features may prove informative. The features common to effective psychotherapies include obtaining an adequate pretreatment evaluation, being well structured, having a prominent focus on the therapeutic alliance and treatment adherence, having clear and agreed-on treatment goals, being integrated with other services and caregivers, and being long term.

Pharmacotherapy

While psychotherapy remains the primary treatment modality for personality disorders, many researchers and clinicians assert that pharmacotherapy plays an important role in the comprehensive treatment of personality disorders when applied to well-defined target symptoms.[45] Nevertheless, our knowledge of how psychopharmacology can best be applied to personality disorders is limited. A review of the literature reveals that the majority of pharmacological studies have focused on a few specific disorders, in particular borderline, schizotypal, and antisocial personality disorders.

A consistent neurobiological finding in studies of BPD has been dysregulation in serotonergic neurotransmission, which is hypothesized to subserve impulsive, aggressive, and self-injurious activity, including suicidal behaviors. This has been documented through findings of low levels of serotonin metabolites in cerebrospinal fluid and blunted neuroendocrine responses to serotonergic agonists.[46] Several studies using positron emission tomography (PET) imaging have documented diminished levels of serotonin synthesis and reactivity in the prefrontal cortex and corticostriatal pathways, which appears to correlate with poor regulation of impulsive behavior.[47,48] Reduced glucose metabolism, most notably in subcortical nuclei, prefrontal, and cingulate cortex, has also been identified in a small series of borderline patients without demonstrated co-morbid Axis I disorders.[49] Prossin and colleagues[50] examined the endogenous opioid system, which has been implicated in emotional and stress response regulation, in a small series of patients diagnosed with BPD. They found that, compared to subjects in the normal control group, borderline patients demonstrated greater reactivity in baseline *in vivo* μ-opioid receptor concentrations and decreased opioid system responsiveness to negative emotional challenge. Volumetric analysis of magnetic resonance imaging (MRI) scans has also revealed some structural variability in the frontal lobes and the hippocampi of borderline patients, with the latter being most prominent in borderline patients reporting a history of abuse.[51,52] Studies with schizotypal personality disorder, thought by some to be a schizophrenia spectrum disorder, have consistently revealed abnormal brain morphology and function. Although patients with schizotypal personality disorder seem to share similar processing deficits as schizophrenic patients, most notably sensory gating, working memory, verbal learning, and sustained attention, the pattern of dysfunction appears to be less severe and more focal.[53,54] Results from MRI studies appear to implicate temporal lobe abnormalities, although differences in the corpus callosum and thalamic nuclei have also been identified.[55,56] In contrast to patients with schizophrenia, patients with schizotypal personality disorders do not appear to demonstrate the same degree of diminished frontal lobe volume, which may correlate with the less severe pattern of cognitive and social deterioration demonstrated by patients with schizotypal personality disorder.[57] Moreover, the diminished temporal volume observed in schizotypal patients appears to be a function of cortical gray matter loss with relatively intact subcortical white matter connections, whereas the temporal lobe abnormalities observed in schizophrenia appear to be related to both gray and white matter disruption.[57]

There is less neurobiological data related to antisocial personality disorder, although data continue to implicate subtle frontal dysfunction and reduced autonomic arousal and reactivity in the face of distressing stimuli. Raine and colleagues[58] identified an 11% reduction in prefrontal gray matter volume in patients with antisocial personality disorder who had no history of acquired brain lesions or insults. Studies have also shown that antisocial individuals with increased propensity for violence demonstrate cortical thinning in inferior medial frontal cortices,[59] and decreases in total brain, temporal lobe and putamen volume.[60]

Agents

It should be noted that, to date, no medication has received approval by the Food and Drug Administration for the treatment of a specific personality disorder. In fact, meta-analyses and review of results from placebo-controlled studies have failed to produce either consistent or robust evidence for the use of any specific class or particular agent when applied to personality disorders.[61-67] Methodological issues with these studies, which serve to limit generalizability of results, include short-term trial duration (6 to 12 weeks), small sample size, and variability of outcome measures and inclusion/exclusion criteria.[68] Nonetheless, modest empirical evidence and considerable clinical experience continue to support the use of medications in the overall treatment of personality disorders application of pharmacotherapy, as well as encourage undertaking more rigorous studies.

Antipsychotics. An early study reporting the use of medication for the treatment of personality disorders involved the antipsychotic trifluoperazine.[61] Since then, several conventional antipsychotics have been investigated with variable and modest therapeutic efficacy.[62] Patients in these studies were diagnosed with either borderline or schizotypal personality disorders. Efficacy was obtained not only for cognitive-perceptual distortions but also for impulsive-aggressive symptoms and for affective instability.[63] With the advent of atypical antipsychotics, which have a decreased tendency to produce motor side effects and improved efficacy for negative symptoms, the use of conventional antipsychotics for the treatment of personality disorders has declined. Saunders and Silk[66] examined the results from placebo-controlled trials in which various classes were applied to trait dimensions associated with BPD, and found that the antipsychotic class (including studies using both conventional neuroleptics and the newer atypical agents) had the most evidence across the various trait dimensions. Lieb and colleagues[64] conducted a meta-analysis of 27 trials in which various psychotropics were applied to core symptoms of BPD and found that the atypical antipsychotics were one of the classes demonstrating the most effectiveness.

Several studies provide preliminary data supporting the efficacy of clozapine in the treatment of psychosis, impulsivity, aggression, and the self-mutilation that is seen in BPD.[69-71] Case reports and open-label trials have also suggested that olanzapine and risperidone may have efficacy in borderline patients who display either self-mutilation or depression.[72,73] There has been one report in which risperidone reduced the aggression and impulsivity associated with antisocial personality disorder.[74] In one 12-week RCT assessing the effectiveness of olanzapine versus placebo in treating BPD,[75] the olanzapine group demonstrated improvement, but did not separate from placebo at the study end. A study assessing the efficacy of ziprasidone versus placebo in a 12-week double-blind design failed to demonstrate any difference between treatment conditions.[76] Aripiprazole has been successfully used to treat a broad range of symptoms in patients with BPD, including depression, anxiety, aggression, and thought abnormalities in borderline patients compared to a placebo control group.[77] Resulting from a meta-analysis of antipsychotics on anger and depression occurring with BPD, aripiprazole emerged as having the largest effect size.[65] Based on the meta-analyses conducted by Lieb and colleagues,[64] the most beneficial effects derived for the antipsychotics were found for olanzapine and aripiprazole.

Mood Stabilizers. As a group, mood stabilizers show particular promise for treating personality-disordered patients scoring high on the impulsive-aggressive and affective instability cluster criteria. Lithium was the first mood stabilizer to be studied, with results suggesting some efficacy for aggression and emotional lability displayed by patients with personality disorders.[62] The anticonvulsant carbamazepine has also been studied for personality-disordered patients with behavioral impulsivity, but the results are equivocal.[78] Recent attention has focused on divalproex sodium, with results from several open-label studies indicating efficacy for borderline patients with affective instability, irritability, and impulsive-aggressive behavior.[79,80] These findings have recently been supported by a double-blind, placebo-controlled trial in which divalproex sodium was shown to be more effective than placebo in reducing aggression and depression in patients with BPD.[81] Small placebo-controlled studies of both topiramate[82] and lamotrigine[83] have yielded preliminary data in which these agents have demonstrated efficacy for reducing anger and aggression in patients with BPD for up to 18 months from treatment initiation. Both agents were tolerated well.

Antidepressants. Monoamine oxidase inhibitors (MAOIs) and tricyclic antidepressants (TCAs) have demonstrated variable results in the treatment of personality disorders. These agents have been replaced by newer agents with less cardiotoxicity and other undesirable side effects. The SSRIs have received the most attention, primarily in the treatment of BPD. Fluoxetine has been the most extensively studied, although data are also available for sertraline, with the most dramatic efficacy being noted in the treatment of anger, rage, aggression, depression, irritability, and self-mutilation.[67] These studies have primarily focused on borderline patients, although one study included patients with schizotypal personality disorders.[53] A similar pattern of response should be expected from the other SSRIs, with little reason to suspect that one SSRI will have significantly greater efficacy over another. An open trial using venlafaxine, an antidepressant that has both serotonin and norepinephrine reuptake blocking properties, has demonstrated a global decrease in symptoms and self-injury in a group of borderline patients.[84]

Benzodiazepines. Despite an early finding demonstrating the efficacy of diazepam in patients with personality disorders,[61] benzodiazepines have not been consistently or systematically studied. Case reports and open-label trials of alprazolam and clonazepam suggest some efficacy in decreasing anxiety and fear-related symptoms associated with BPDs.[63] However, there are reports that these agents can lead to behavioral disinhibition and to dyscontrol in patients with personality disorders.[62,85] This, in conjunction with the high potential for abuse and dependence, has served as a strong contraindication for using benzodiazepines in the treatment of patients with personality disorders.[45,86] Use of benzodiazepines in the treatment of patients with personality disorders associated with the anxiety–fear dimension, most notably avoidant personality disorders, dependent personality disorders, and OCPDs, has not been reported.

Opioid Antagonists. Based on findings that self-injurious behavior may be partially produced by dysregulation of endorphins (endogenous opioid-like neuropeptides), the opioid antagonist naltrexone has been used with some success in various patient populations (e.g., children with mental retardation and other developmental disabilities). There is one case report in which naltrexone reduced self-mutilation in a patient with BPD.[87] Results from an open-label trial have also suggested that naltrexone may reduce the duration and intensity of cognitive-perceptual symptoms of dissociation in borderline patients.[88]

Approach to the Pharmacotherapy of Personality Disorders

Based on the neuropsychiatric and pharmacological literature, four clusters of personality disorder symptoms have been proposed as meaningful targets for pharmacotherapy.[84,89] These four clusters reflect difficulties with (1) cognition or perceptual organization, (2) impulsive and aggressive behaviors, (3) mood stability and dysphoria, and (4) anxiety suppression. It has been assumed that the personality disorder symptoms within each cluster share a common neurobiological substrate that can potentially serve as a rationale for treatment selection.[89]

The cognitive–perceptual dimension generally correlates with cluster A disorders, and includes symptoms of psychosis, unusual perceptual experiences, dissociation, suspiciousness, and odd or magical thinking. Behaviors from this dimension may be the result of dysfunction within the dopaminergic neurotransmitter system and can be targeted with antipsychotic medications. Presently there are no definitive data for choosing between a typical and an atypical agent. There is some indication, however, that atypical agents may be best for refractory and self-mutilative patients.[86] Regardless of the agent, lower doses can be effective for these symptoms and benefit may be seen within a few days. Because of potential long-term side effects, discontinuation trials are recommended.

The impulsive-aggressive dimension is a prominent factor in cluster B personality disorders. Anger, aggression, and behavioral disinhibition constitute primary impairments in this dimension, and they are thought to reflect dysfunction in the serotonergic neurotransmitter system. SSRIs should be considered first-line agents for treating impulsivity and aggression in personality-disordered patients. However, if they do not respond well to adequate trials of the SSRIs, augmentation with a mood stabilizer or an anticonvulsant can be considered, because there is some empirical support for the use of divalproex sodium in this patient population.

The mood-instability dimension also appears to be most closely tied to the cluster B disorders, and consists of mood dysregulation, depression, dysphoria, and emotional lability. These behaviors may have broad neurotransmitter underpinnings, possibly related to dysfunction in serotonergic, cholinergic, or noradrenergic systems. Again, SSRIs should be considered first for treatment of these symptoms. If augmentation is needed, buspirone or a long-acting benzodiazepine, such as clonazepam, can be considered. If rage is a prominent component of the mood dysregulation, antipsychotic agents should be considered.

The anxiety-inhibition dimension, predominantly associated with cluster C disorders, consists of anxiety, fear, and manifestations of behavioral inhibition aimed at reducing exposure to anxiety-provoking situations. This dimension may reflect a disturbance in autonomic function, and may be mediated by serotonergic and noradrenergic neurotransmitter systems. While there is very little empirical evidence to draw on, it may be reasonable to start such patients on an SSRI, because these agents have demonstrated efficacy in the treatment of fear and social anxiety. If augmentation is needed, a long-acting anxiolytic, such as clonazepam, can be added under careful supervision to prevent inappropriate dosage escalation.

When using the four-personality symptom clusters as a guide to pharmacotherapy, the clinician should be mindful that the heterogeneity of the DSM personality disorders often results in patients having symptoms from several symptom clusters. For example, patients with BPD tend to demonstrate behaviors from the impulsive-aggressive and mood-instability clusters, but some may also exhibit symptoms within the cognitive-perceptual cluster. This reinforces the concept of selecting pharmacotherapy on the presence of specific target symptoms rather than on a given personality disorder diagnosis. Experienced clinicians tend to use the symptom clusters as medication targets to avoid "chasing" single symptoms to prevent situations in which a patient is prescribed four or more medications without a clear rationale. Clinical experience also suggests following the guidelines for dose and duration for all medications to minimize treatment adjustment. Finally, realistic goals for medication treatment are necessary, and experienced clinicians anticipate only modest benefits in any given situation and consider persistence and patience to be more important than any specific medication.

Access the complete reference list and multiple choice questions (MCQs) online at https://expertconsult.inkling.com

KEY REFERENCES

1. Torgerson S. Epidemiology. In Oldham JM, Skodol AE, Bender DS, editors: *Textbook of personality disorders*, Washington, DC, 2005, American Psychiatric Publishing.
6. Mayer JD. A tale of two visions: can a new view of personality help integrate psychology? *Am Psychol* 60:294–307, 2005.
9. Depue R, Lenzenweger MF. A neurobehavioral dimensional model. In Livesley WJ, editor: *Handbook of personality disorders*, New York, 2001, Guilford Press.
17. Saucier G. Measures of personality factors found recurrently in human lexicons. In Boyle GJ, Matthews G, Saklofske DH, editors: *Handbook of Personality Theory and Assessment*, vol. 2, New York, 2008, SAGE Publications, Inc.
18. American Psychiatric Association. *Diagnostic and statistical manual of mental disorders*, ed 5, Washington, DC, 2013, American Psychiatric Press Inc.
19. Mullins-Sweatt SN, Widiger TA. The five-factor model of personality disorder: a translation across science and practice. In Krueger RF, Tackett JT, editors: *Personality and psychopathology*, New York, 2006, Guilford Press.
20. Blais M. Clinician ratings of the five-factor model of personality and DSM-IV personality disorders. *J Nerv Ment Dis* 185:388–393, 1997.
21. Clark LA, Livesley WJ. Two approaches to identifying the dimensions of personality disorder: convergence on the five-factor model. In Widiger TA, Costa PT, editors: *Personality disorders and the five-factor model of personality*, ed 2, Washington, DC, 2002, American Psychological Association.
26. Shedler J, Weston D. Dimension of personality pathology: an alternative to the five-factor model. *Am J Psychiatry* 161:1743–1754, 2004.
29. Skodol AE, Oldham JM, Bender DS, et al. Dimensional representations of DSM-IV personality disorders: relationship to functional impairment. *Am J Psychiatry* 162:1919–1925, 2005.
30. Bender DS, Morey LC, Skodol AE. Toward a model for assessing level of personality functioning in DSM-5, Part I: A review of theory and methods. *J Pers Assess* 93:332–346, 2011.
31. Krueger RF, Derringer J, Markon KE, et al. Initial construction of a maladaptive personality trait model and inventory for DSM-5. *Psychol Med* 42:1879–1890, 2012.
32. Wright AGC, Thomas KM, Hopwood CJ, et al. The hierarchical structure of DSM-5 pathological personality traits. *J Abnorm Psychol* 121:951–957, 2012.
33. Skodol AE. Personality disorders in the DSM-5. *Annu Rev Clin Psychol* 8:317–344, 2012.
39. Muran JC, Safran JD, Samstag LW, et al. Evaluating an alliance-focused treatment for personality disorders. *Psychother Theory Res Pract Train* 42:532–545, 2005.
40. Perry JC, Bann E, Ianni F. Effectiveness of psychotherapy for personality disorders. *Am J Psychiatry* 156(9):1312–1321, 1999.
42. Linehan MM, Tutek BA, Heard HL, et al. Interpersonal outcome of cognitive behavioral treatment for chronically suicidal borderline patients. *Am J Psychiatry* 151:1771–1776, 1994.
43. Bateman AW, Fonagy P. Randomized control trial of outpatient mentalization-based treatment versus structured clinical management for borderline personality disorder. *Am J Psychiatry* 166:1355–1364, 2009.
45. Cloninger CR, Svrakic DM. Personality disorders. In Sadock BJ, Sadock VA, editors: *Comprehensive textbook of psychiatry*, ed 7, Philadelphia, 2005, Lippincott Williams & Wilkins.
64. Lieb K, Völlm B, Rücker G, et al. Pharmacotherapy for borderline personality disorder: Cochrane systematic review of randomised trials. *Br J Psychiatry* 196:4–12, 2010.
65. Mercer D, Douglass AB, Link PS. Meta-analyses of mood stabilizers, antidepressants and antipsychotics in the treatment of borderline personality disorder: effectiveness for depression and anger symptoms. *J Pers Disord* 23:156–174, 2009.
66. Saunders EF, Silk KR. Personality trait dimensions and the pharmacological treatment of borderline personality disorder. *J Clin Psychopharmacol* 29:461–467, 2009.
67. Stoffers J, Völlm BA, Rücker G, et al. Pharmacological interventions for borderline personality disorder. *Cochrane Database Syst Rev* (6):CD005653, 2010.
68. Biskin RS, Paris J. Management of borderline personality disorder. *CMAJ* 184:1897–1902, 2012.
86. Gunderson JG, Links P. *Borderline personality disorders: a clinical guide*, ed 2, Washington, DC, 2008, American Psychiatric Publishing.

40 Psychiatric Neuroscience: Incorporating Pathophysiology into Clinical Case Formulation

Joan A. Camprodon, MD, MPH, PhD, and Joshua L. Roffman, MD, MMSc

KEY POINTS

- One can approach the study of the brain and its pathophysiology from various perspectives with different levels of resolution: molecular, genetic, cellular, synaptic, systems, and behavioral.

- Pathological processes and therapeutic interventions can target one or more of these levels, leading to a cascade of events that changes each of them.

- Affect, behavior, and cognition are processed in specific brain circuits, and their altered function leads to the signs, symptoms, and syndromes that clinicians identify.

- Neurobiological knowledge often provides mechanistic insight, explanation for behavior, and rationale for treatment, which are important to patients and families, as well as to providers.

- Clinical presentation reflects an interaction of static and dynamic factors, including genetic and environmental ones, often mediated by adaptive or maladaptive plastic changes.

OVERVIEW

People with major mental illness suffer as a result of abnormal brain function. This is the fundamental premise of psychiatric neuroscience, which seeks to identify biological mechanisms underlying mental illness and the effects of psychiatric treatments. An essential goal is to characterize these mechanisms at the different levels of biological resolution that exist in the brain (from ions, to proteins, to DNA, to genes and chromosomes [that encode the structure and function of cells], to synapses, and finally to brain circuits that process affect, behavior, and cognition). This approach does not negate the critical role of psychological, social, and environmental factors; to the contrary, it provides a framework for understanding how these higher levels of resolution affect, and are affected by, neural function. A deeper understanding of brain mechanisms will provide better explanations for patients and families and lead to improvements in diagnosis, treatment, and prognosis.

Psychiatric neuroscience is one of the most interesting and challenging endeavors in all of medicine.[1–5] While a great deal is already known, a wide gap remains between the clinical phenomena of affect, behavior, and cognition and neuroscientific explanations. The brain is extraordinarily complex and less physically accessible than other organ systems, posing

great challenges to researchers. However, recent advances, particularly in neuroimaging and genetics, have provided important tools for tackling these problems. Although progress is difficult, the high prevalence, morbidity, and mortality rates of mental illness make progress essential. Mental health practitioners will need to incorporate the lessons learned from psychiatric neuroscience into everyday practice, and communicate them to patients, families, and members of the general public.

One might ask if the term "psychiatric neuroscience" is still valid. While it has traditionally related to neuroscience research with clinical relevance to disorders embedded within the limits of psychiatry, as opposed to neurology, these boundaries are becoming more porous as knowledge progresses and clinical practice adapts. The unclear limits between the two subspecialties have been defined historically by amorphous criteria, such as differences in clinical attitude (diagnostic vs. therapeutic) or brain function of interest (motor and sensory vs. affective and behavioral, with cognition always occupying an unclear frontier). Neurology once focused mainly on pathologies that resulted in major structural changes that one could observe in an autopsy or under a microscope. Though the label "functional" is at times still casually and inappropriately attached to neurological deficits of presumed "psychological" etiology, a neurobiological re-acquaintance with the original medical meaning of the word emphasizes physiological (functional) over anatomical (structural) pathophysiological mechanisms. This shift led to two very distinct clinical paradigms, one focused on finding the focal lesion and the other on identifying signs and symptoms that present in established syndromal patterns that can then be physiologically investigated.

As new generations of clinician scientists emerge who did not train in psychiatric or neurological neuroscience, but in systems neuroscience, translational efforts are highlighting the common principles of structure, function, pathology, and therapeutics. From this effort, new models are emerging with a clinical focus on brain circuits, as opposed to focal lesions or clinical syndromes. For scientists and clinicians alike it is, and will become increasingly, important to have an understanding of the different levels of biological resolution and how they influence each other in health, in disease, and in therapy.[6] For clinicians treating disorders of affect, behavior, and cognition, it will be particularly important to understand the circuit level, as this is where mental states, including the pathological affective, behavioral, and cognitive states that we treat, are computed.

An important goal of this chapter will therefore be to explain the different levels of biological resolution that determine brain structure and function. A second goal will be to offer a framework with which the biological components of clinical cases may be formulated. This chapter provides an approach to conceptually organizing the biological component of our work with patients, from the dual vantage points of pathophysiology and mechanisms of treatment.

HISTORY OF PSYCHIATRIC NEUROSCIENCE

Psychiatry has a strong neuroscientific tradition. Describing all of the important contributions to brain science made by psychiatric researchers could fill many chapters; here we will cite only a few illustrative examples. Early in the last century, the German psychiatrist and neuropathologist Alois Alzheimer discovered plaques and tangles in the brain of his amnestic patient Mrs. Auguste D. and provided the first description of the clinical syndrome that now bears his name.[7] Together with his colleague and renowned psychiatrist Emil Kraepelin, Alzheimer also described abnormalities in the cortical neurons of patients with dementia praecox, likely representing the first neuropathological studies of schizophrenia.[8] Their discoveries have been extended to the molecular level in modern studies identifying abnormalities in γ-aminobutyric acid (GABA)–ergic neurons of the prefrontal cortex.[9,10] While Alzheimer's passion was neuropathology, he also spent many years caring for patients with mental illness. Reflecting on his life's work, he reportedly said that he "wanted to help psychiatry with the microscope."[11]

Another historical landmark in psychiatric neuroscience was the demonstration of genetic predispositions to major mental illness.[12] Danish adoption studies in the 1960s reported a much greater incidence of schizophrenia in biological as opposed to adoptive relatives of people with schizophrenia, providing key evidence for a significant etiological role of genetics in a psychiatric illness. Other landmark contributions include the work of Julius Axelrod, Ulf von Euler, and Bernard Katz on neurotransmitters and their mechanisms of release, reuptake, and metabolism; their discoveries, recognized with a Nobel Prize in 1970, provide a foundation for much of the content of this chapter.[13] In the 1970s, the discovery that antipsychotic medications targeted brain dopamine receptors led to the influential dopamine hypothesis of schizophrenia.[14,15] Later, converging work characterizing information processing in the brain at a molecular level earned Arvid Carlsson, Paul Greengard, and Eric Kandel the 2000 Nobel Prize at the end of the decade of the brain.[16] These brief highlights emphasize the great progress already attributable to psychiatric neuroscience, and illustrate the great potential for important discoveries in the future.

PSYCHIATRIC DIAGNOSIS: BIOMARKERS AND BIOLOGICAL VALIDITY

In the context of psychiatric neuroscience, the recent diagnostic system (DSM-IV-TR)[17] has both strengths and weaknesses. A major advance of the post-1980s DSM was the development of diagnostic categories of psychiatric illness with good inter-rater reliability, largely based on observation and data collection. This provided a firm starting point for scientific investigation, in contrast to previous diagnostic systems based on unproven etiological theories and associated ill-defined terminology. However, the intentional avoidance of etiological theories in generating DSM diagnoses also makes their biological validity uncertain; the extent to which specific DSM diagnoses correspond to specific pathological neural processes is unknown. Unlike most medical illnesses, the vast majority of psychiatric illnesses have so far not been tightly linked to specific biological markers. The descriptive criteria demarcating current diagnoses are likely several steps removed from core pathological processes.

These diagnostic difficulties can be illustrated by comparing the diagnosis of schizophrenia to that of methicillin-resistant streptococcal pneumonia, a medical diagnosis with obvious biological validity. While pneumonia has a collection of clinical signs and symptoms that may be non-specific and variable (e.g., fever, productive cough, and shortness of breath), it implies a distinct pathophysiology (infection of lung tissue leading to an inflammatory reaction). Subdividing the diagnosis by the infectious agent links it to a specific biological etiology, with tremendous value in guiding prognosis and treatment. In contrast, the diagnosis of schizophrenia, while it has a high level of inter-rater reliability, is not based at present on known biomarkers or pathophysiological mechanisms. It is therefore confined to the syndromic level, comprising a cluster of variable and non-specific clinical features. It can be further divided into more specific clinical subtypes, but these suffer from the same shortcomings. Just as pneumonia may have various specific etiologies, schizophrenia may also have diverse causes; most likely it does not reflect a single "disease." Recent advances in genetics reinforce this conclusion. While schizophrenia is highly heritable, linkage and association studies indicate in the majority of cases that it is a disorder of complex genetics, in which multiple genes of modest effect interact with environmental risk factors to cause the phenotype. In light of these issues, one of the major goals of psychiatric neuroscience is to identify specific biomarkers and pathophysiological mechanisms for each disorder.

METHODS IN PSYCHIATRIC NEUROSCIENCE

Researchers have adopted a variety of methods for studying the neural mechanisms of mental illness and behavior (Box 40-1). Each of these methods has particular strengths and weakness.

Brain Lesions and Behavior

There is a strong tradition within classical neuropsychology and behavioral neurology of understanding neuroanatomical circuitry by studying the emergent or lost behaviors in patients with focal brain lesions.[18] These studies have provided us with a rich view of various brain regions and their relationship to behavior. Perhaps the most famous case is that of Phineas Gage, the Vermont railway worker who suffered a traumatic lesion bilaterally to the medial frontal lobes and developed personality changes.[19] Another famous patient (known by his initials) is H. M., who underwent bilateral medial temporal lobe resection for intractable epilepsy and as a result lost the ability to form new declarative memories.[20] While striking and informative, findings from these rare cases may be difficult to extrapolate to the pathophysiology of common psychiatric illnesses, which generally do not involve focal lesions. Traditionally, biological psychiatry has relied more on biometrics and quantitative methods; these population-based approaches risk losing insights available from rare cases but are more likely to produce broadly generalizable findings.

BOX 40-1 Methods in Psychiatric Neuroscience

Animal models
Brain lesion cases
Brain stimulation and neuromodulation
Genetics and molecular biology
Neuroimaging
Neuropathology
Neurophysiology
Neuropsychology/endophenotypes
Psychopharmacology

Neuropsychology and Endophenotypes

An increasingly important approach in psychiatric neuroscience is to identify and study intermediate phenotypes. These are quantitative phenotypes that are closely associated with the clinical syndrome of interest, but which are less complex and easier to link to the function of specific neural circuits. They can also be used to identify biologically relevant subtypes within a diagnostic category, reducing heterogeneity that may limit the power of scientific investigations. Endophenotypes are intermediate phenotypes that are present both in affected individuals and in their unaffected relatives, therefore reflecting genetic risk independent of actual disease. Neuropsychological tests of cognitive function are commonly used to identify endophenotypes. For example, impairment of working memory, which is closely related to the function of dorsolateral prefrontal cortex, is found within a subgroup of patients with schizophrenia.[21] Endophenotypes thus help bridge the gap between brain circuits, which are amenable to study at the molecular and cellular level, and clinical syndromes, which are less tractable. This approach becomes especially powerful when combined with other methods, such as neuroimaging or genetics.[22]

Neuroimaging

Neuroimaging has provided one of the best modern tools for examining the pathophysiology of mental illness in the living brain. As this topic is covered in greater depth in another chapter, we will only briefly summarize it here. Neuroimaging can provide many different quantitative measures (including morphometry, metabolism, and functional activity). Neuroimaging research using groups of subjects can determine whether mental illness is associated with changes in the size or shape of specific brain regions, the functional activity within these regions, or their concentration of particular neurotransmitters, receptors, or key metabolites.[23] Although neuroimaging methods can be used to measure cellular and molecular phenomena, the currently achievable spatial resolution still represents an important limitation in examining the microscopic pathological changes implicated in psychiatric illness.

Neurophysiology

There is a strong tradition within psychiatric neuroscience of studying the electrical activity of the brain and its relation to function. These methods include electroencephalography (EEG), event-related potentials (ERPs), and, most recently, magnetoencephalography (MEG), and transcranial magnetic stimulation (TMS). Like functional neuroimaging, these modalities provide information about the living, functioning brain. At present, electrophysiological techniques cannot provide anatomical resolution at the level of neurochemistry or synaptic physiology, and are limited to the study of cortical phenomena; however, they can provide excellent temporal and spatial resolution and are invaluable in studying the coordinated function of widely distributed neural circuits. Abnormalities in the timing of oscillations in neural circuit activity have been associated with psychiatric illnesses, and this is an area of intense research activity. For example, the reduction of gamma frequency (30 to 80 Hz) oscillations in schizophrenia has been ascribed to impaired N-methyl-D-aspartate (NMDA) receptor activity on GABA-ergic interneurons.[24] These non-invasive methods are particularly heavily used in studies of brain development and function in children.[25]

Brain Stimulation and Neuromodulation

Brain stimulation and neuromodulation techniques encompass a variety of device-based methodologies able to generate focal electrical currents in pre-selected brain regions. These currents are able to increase or decrease the excitability of the target neurons, and modulate the networks they belong to by acting as a neural pacemaker.[26]

Brain stimulation can be divided among invasive and non-invasive approaches. Invasive techniques require the surgical implantation of stimulating electrodes in the brain, and are therefore exclusively used in therapeutic settings where the risk/benefit analysis is favorable. They include deep brain stimulation (DBS) and vagus nerve stimulation (VNS). Non-invasive methods do not require surgery or anesthesia, are very safe, and alter brain function in ways that are transient and reversible. The better-known and most commonly used methods are transcranial magnetic stimulation (TMS) and transcranial direct current stimulation (tDCS).[27] Chapter 46 describes these methods and their therapeutic applications in detail.

TMS has been used since the mid 1980s as a tool to study brain structure and function. Event-related paradigms using single pulses time-locked to a given stimulus or task have been used to determine the chronometry of the computations in a given brain region with great temporal resolution (in the order of milliseconds).[28] Repetitive TMS (rTMS) can increase or decrease the excitability of a given area beyond the time of stimulation, creating a "virtual lesion" that lasts 15–60 minutes after the stimulation. This virtual lesion approach has been used, following the tradition of classical lesion studies, to understand the functional role of discrete brain regions.[29]

Although neuroimaging and electrophysiological techniques are defined by their spatial and temporal resolution, what sets brain stimulation methods apart is their *causal resolution*. Neuroimaging and electrophysiological methods are observational; they measure patterns of brain activity (the dependent variable) in the context of a given task or disease state (independent variable). Such a design is able to establish correlations among these measures, but can never determine that a given pattern of brain activity is *causing* a mental state (or vice versa). On the other hand, brain stimulation techniques are interventional. They modify the system by changing brain activity (now the independent variable) and measure the behavioral, cognitive or affective changes that follow. This design offers causal explanatory power, which makes it a useful tool to answer a number of questions.[30]

Neuropathology

Many researchers examine post-mortem neural tissue from those who suffered from psychiatric illness during their lifetime. Post-mortem analysis reaches a level of molecular and cellular resolution currently unachievable *in vivo*; however, it is commonly limited by confounds (such as age, effects of chronic medication, and non-specific effects of chronic psychiatric illness).

Neuropathology was clearly in fashion in the late 1800s and early 1900s, when Alzheimer first described plaques in the brain of his patient with dementia,[7] and identified frontal cortex abnormalities in schizophrenia.[8] While some skeptics have described schizophrenia as the "graveyard of neuropathologists,"[31] recent studies have actually provided reproducible descriptions of deficits (such as those in parvalbumin-expressing GABA-ergic interneurons in deep layers 3 and 4, akin to Alzheimer's findings) in the cortex. These neuropathological findings have provided one of the strongest etiological hypotheses for schizophrenia.[9,10]

Psychopharmacology

More than any other methodology in psychiatric neuroscience, pharmacology has been used to understand the neurochemical basis of behavior and to develop hypotheses regarding psycho-pathological mechanisms. Famous examples include the dopamine[32] and glutamate hypotheses of schizophrenia,[33] the catecholamine depletion hypothesis of depression,[34] and the dopaminergic models of attention-deficit/hyperactivity disorder (ADHD) and substance abuse. In relating pharmacological effects to potential disease mechanisms, it is important to note that the effects of drugs on clinical symptoms may reflect mechanisms that are downstream of the core pathophysiology, or even unrelated to core disease mechanisms. By analogy, diuretics can improve the symptoms of congestive heart failure while providing less direct insight into its core pathophysiology. Nonetheless, by clearly connecting cellular and synaptic mechanisms with clinical symptoms, pharmacology provides mechanistic tools and information with enormous clinical and scientific utility.

Animal Experiments

In the authors' opinion, the value of animal experiments has received too little emphasis in psychiatric neuroscience. Clearly, complex psychiatric symptoms (such as delusions) cannot be modeled well in animals, and anthropomorphic interpretations of animal behavior should be taken with due skepticism. Despite these caveats, animal behaviors with known neuroanatomical correlates have been critical in elucidating the neurocircuitry and neurochemistry underlying many psychiatric phenomena. For example, anxiety- and fear-related behaviors have been very productively modeled in animals, leading to a detailed understanding of the role of the amygdala in these behaviors.[35] Of course, animal studies also permit a wider range of experimental perturbations than possible with human investigations. Independent of their value as behavioral models, animal models therefore offer the opportunity to explore cellular and molecular pathophysiology in ways that are ethically or technically impossible in human subjects. For example, the fragile X knock-out mouse is an excellent model for fragile X syndrome, the most common form of inherited cognitive impairment. Studying these mice has led to a deep understanding of relevant defects in dendrite formation and neurophysiology.[36]

Human Genetics and Molecular Biology

Adoption, twin, and familial segregation studies have proven that many psychiatric conditions are highly heritable (i.e., caused in large part by the additive effect of genes).[37] Genetic endeavors in psychiatric neuroscience may be broken up into two broad categories: "forward genetics," or genome-wide attempts to identify genetic loci (genes or their regulatory elements) that underlie susceptibility or contribute to pathophysiology; and "genotype-phenotype" studies, whereby candidate genes are chosen based on *a priori* biological hypotheses and the degree to which a gene plays a role in a given phenotype is assessed. Such phenotypes may be clinical diagnoses, or endophenotypes from neuropsychology or neuroimaging. The promise for human genetics in psychiatry is tremendous,[37] especially for forward genetics, wherein researchers may be led to the core pathophysiology without requiring any *a priori* hypotheses. Yet human genetics research is exceedingly challenging for various reasons that are beyond the scope of the current discussion. In brief, the genetic architecture of neuropsychiatric conditions is heterogeneous and complex. That is, the majority of psychiatric illnesses likely reflect complex interactions of multiple genes, as well as their interaction with environmental factors that are difficult to assess. Despite these difficulties, there have already been a few notable examples of success.

Analysis of rare, large families with early-onset dementia led to the discovery of mutations in amyloid precursor protein (APP) and presenilins in Alzheimer's disease (AD).[38] In these rare families, these mutations are statistically "linked" to disease and considered "highly penetrant." However, the vast majority of AD patients do not have mutations in these genes. Indeed, in psychiatry examples of highly penetrant, simple dominant or recessive gene mutations are rare. That is, examples in neuropsychiatry of a particular gene mutation "causing" a specific condition are exceedingly rare and somewhat controversial, and the generalizability of these findings to the common conditions with more complex inheritance is usually unclear. Nonetheless, the APP pathway has provided an important target for drug development, which may lead to a medicine that stalls the progress of disease.

Genetic association studies through population genetics represent another approach to identifying susceptibility genes in "forward genetics." In this approach, a common variation in the genome, such as single nucleotide polymorphisms (SNPs), is assessed for a statistically significant association with illness. This approach is based on the so-called common disease–common variant hypothesis. That is, psychiatric disorders may be in part due to a disadvantageous combination of a number of common forms of genetic variation as opposed to frank deleterious mutations. Again, a successful example of a gene association in neuropsychiatry comes from the field of AD wherein there is a fairly robust association at the level of population genetics or epidemiology between a common polymorphism in *ApoE4* and susceptibility to AD. However, sometimes even when genetic associations are robust, the amount of the phenotype (i.e., the variance) that is explained by the given gene may be small and therefore the role in causation may be indirect or unclear. In addition, association studies have often used small sample sizes and thereby risked false-positive findings or problems of reproducibility. Now, appropriately-powered association studies (involving thousands of subjects) are underway; many of these use new and more powerful high-density genotype methods, namely "SNP chips" or microarrays. Even still, critical insights into the causative roles of genes in some psychiatric illness may only come from studies of gene–gene or gene–environmental interaction, or by using endophenotypes (such as neuroimaging) that may be closer to the action of the gene.

Methodologies in molecular genetics and molecular neuroscience also promise improved understanding of gene function in the brain. These methods include the following: comparison of gene sequences in human to non-human primate and other animals[39]; a deeper understanding of how non-coding elements within the genome may regulate important brain genes[40] and thereby play a role in psychiatry; the study of gene expression using microarrays[41]; the study of gene function in mice in which specific genes have been modified by recombinant methods (e.g., "knock-out" or "knock-in" studies)[42]; and studies examining how experience and the environment alter gene expression.[43] In summary, genomics and molecular genetics hold great promise for identifying genes and thus biological mechanisms at the core of psychiatric pathophysiology.

BIOLOGICAL CASE FORMULATION: NEUROSCIENTIFIC CONTENT AND PROCESS

Clinical case formulation in psychiatry is structured around the bio-psycho-social model. In this chapter, we offer a framework for formulating the biological aspects of this model. Specifically, neuroscientific explanations may be organized in two broad conceptual areas: process and content. Process refers to dynamic brain mechanisms that lead to illness, while

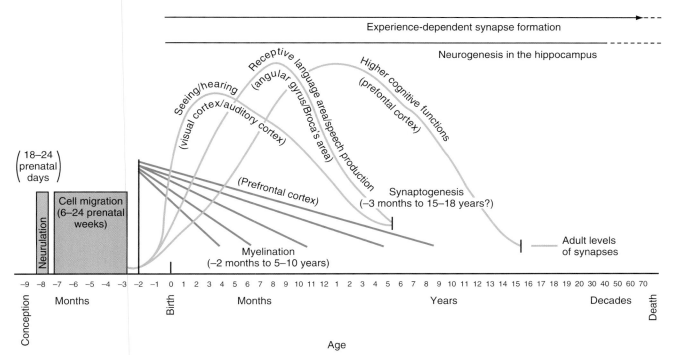

Figure 40-1. A depiction of the processes of brain development, including intrauterine neuronal patterning, neurogenesis, cortical migration, gliogenesis, myelination, and experience-dependent synapse modification. *(From Thompson RA, Nelson CA. Developmental science and the media. Early brain development, Am Psychol 56[1]:5–15, 2001.)*

content refers to the brain properties including neural circuits, brain regions, synapses, cells, and molecules that form the substrate for these changes.

Process

A key concept in basic neuroscience and its clinical specialties is neuroplasticity. Although it is defined in different ways and can be studied at various levels of resolution (e.g., circuits, synapses), this term generally refers to the capacity of the neural system to change in response to external or internal stimuli following predetermined rules. Neuroplasticity provides a great deal of flexibility and adaptive capacity to the brain, permitting variable computational strategies and patterns of connectivity in a changing environment.[44] Despite the significant potential for reactive (and adaptive) change, this happens around an exquisitely regulated homeostatic equilibrium point. Nevertheless, when the plastic changes are restricted, excessive, or occur around an altered equilibrium state, pathology develops. Luckily, the brain remains plastic, and any intervention (e.g., medications, psychotherapy or brain stimulation) that is effective in changing pathological cognition, behavior or affect induces adaptive plasticity. That is, a pathological mental state is sustained by a given pattern of brain activity, and changing this mental state will require changing its associated neural computational algorithm.[45] Therefore, neuroplasticity is a key dynamic property of the brain that allows adaptive change (including learning and memory), but it is also an important source of pathology, and a necessary mechanism of action of effective neuropsychiatric treatments.

Although the specific pathophysiological mechanisms that lead to neuropsychiatric disease are many, we will consider two relevant examples: neurodevelopment, and neurodegeneration. Under neurodevelopment we include related processes that continue into adulthood (such as neurogenesis).

Previously underestimated, adult neurogenesis is now known to continue in select regions of the human brain, most notably the olfactory bulb and the hippocampus. Although the role of adult neurogenesis in humans remains largely unknown, some evidence has connected altered hippocampal neurogenesis to mood disorders.[46]

Neurodevelopmental processes shaping brain circuits have life-long effects on patterns of affect, behavior, and cognition with direct relevance to mental health. The effects of childhood experience have always been central to psychiatric understanding; psychiatric neuroscience has also attempted to provide a biological grounding for this understanding.[43,47] Thus, neurodevelopmental processes include the interacting effects of genes and environment on brain and behavior. Figure 40-1 shows the processes of brain development, including intrauterine neuronal patterning, neurogenesis, cortical migration, gliogenesis, myelination, and experience-dependent synapse modification.[48,49] In the first years and decade of life, the brain undergoes a process of synapse formation and pruning.[50] Initially, neurons form an over-abundance of synapses that are then strengthened and pruned possibly based on experience, learning, or aging (Figure 40-2).

Specific psychiatric disorders may be framed in terms of one or more of these three mechanisms. Autism or attention deficit hyperactivity disorder are examples in which a process of brain development goes awry. At the other end of life, neurodegenerative processes dominate, and can lead to dementias (e.g., Alzheimer's or frontotemporal lobar degeneration) or movement disorders (such as Parkinson's disease). Substance use disorders may reflect a combination of both processes modulated by maladaptive plasticity. Patients with substance dependence may have a susceptibility based on neurodevelopment, including a predisposition to risk-taking behaviors.[51] Substance abuse also causes neuroplastic changes at the level of the synapse.[52] Finally, chronic use of substances can cause neurodegeneration and dementia.[53]

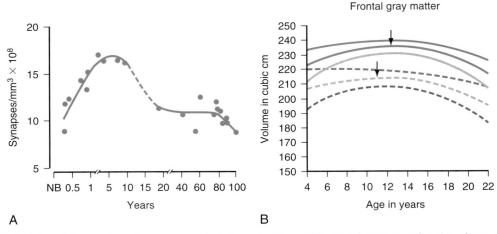

Figure 40-2. (A) A depiction of the number of synapse counts in layer 3 of the middle frontal gyrus as a function of age. (B) A graph of the volume, in cubic centimeters, of frontal gray matter with respect to age in years. Males represented by solid lines and females by dashed lines with 95% confidence intervals, respectively. Arrows indicate peak volume. *(A, Data from Huttenlocher PR. Synaptic density in human frontal cortex: developmental changes and effects of aging,* Brain Res *163[2]:195–205, 1979. B, Data from Lenroot RK, Giedd JN. Brain development in children and adolescents: insights from anatomical magnetic resonance imaging,* Neurosci Biobehav Rev *30[6]:718–729, 2006.)*

Content

The "content" of a psychiatric illness comprises the different structural and functional levels of biological resolution that form the nervous system: ions, proteins, genes, cells, synapses, circuits, behaviors, and mental states. These can all be the target of pathological changes leading to diseases and clinical syndromes. This is the subject of the remaining sections of this chapter. For most conditions, our knowledge of content is incomplete, but this should not lead us to ignore the large amount of information that *is* available for many conditions. Characterizing neuropsychiatric conditions in terms of both biological processes and substrates (content) can provide a framework to facilitate understanding of etiology, loci of intervention, and potential treatments.

OVERVIEW OF THE STRUCTURE OF THE CENTRAL NERVOUS SYSTEM

The structural organization of the central nervous system (CNS) is shown in Figure 40-3A. The human brain is organized into the cerebral cortex, brainstem, subcortical structures (e.g., basal ganglia, brainstem, thalamus, hypothalamus, pituitary), and cerebellum.[3,54,55] These anatomical structures are made of inter-connected elements that create distributed and highly inter-connected circuits. It is in these circuits where cognition, behavior, and affect are processed. This section will provide an overview of neuroanatomy with a structural focus. Chapter 72 describes some of the circuits and systems of clinical relevance in a more detail.

The cerebral cortex is the outermost layer of the cerebrum. The cerebral cortex consists of a foliated structure, encompassing gyri and sulci. Within the most highly evolved cortical regions (isocortex), a six-cell layered structure orchestrates complex brain functions (including perceptual awareness, thought, language, planning, memory, attention, and consciousness). Cortical anatomy can be subdivided in myriad ways, including into anatomical regions (such as the occipital, parietal, temporal, insular, limbic, and frontal lobes) (Figure 40-3B, C, and D). The limbic "lobe" is a ring (limbus) of phylogenetically older cortex surrounding the upper brainstem and includes the hippocampus, amygdala, hypothalamus, parahippocampal gyrus, and cingulate cortex (see Figure 40-3D). Structures within the medial temporal lobe are especially important in psychiatry; the hippocampus plays a critical role in memory, and the amygdala is an important element of fear circuitry and for assigning emotional valence to stimuli.

Functionally, the cortex may be divided into primary sensory or motor (unimodal) regions, and association (multimodal) regions that receive inputs from multiple areas.[54] Association cortex may be subdivided into three areas: frontal (involved in a wide variety of higher functions, such as planning, attention, abstract thought, problem-solving, judgment, initiative, and inhibition of impulses); limbic (involved in emotion and memory); and sensory (e.g., parietal, occipital, temporal), involved in integrating sensory information.

The cortical systems can also be represented in a hierarchical fashion.[54] For example, within sensorimotor sequencing, we see reception of somatosensory, visual, or auditory stimuli in primary sensory cortex; interpretation or representation of the combined sensory modalities in the heteromodal association cortex; integration of this information with the other association cortices (i.e., limbic and frontal); and output via the motor or language system.

In addition to the cerebral cortex, many other brain regions are of critical importance to psychiatry. The cerebellum (see Figure 40-3A and B), traditionally known for its role in motor coordination and learning, has more recently been implicated in cognitive and affective processes as well.[56] The thalamus is a major relay station for incoming sensory information and other critical circuitry, including connections between association cortices (via the mediodorsal nucleus) and outputs regulating motor activity. Interestingly, the mediodorsal nucleus, a critical relay station between association cortices, is a region of the thalamus found to be smaller in some neuropathological studies of patients with schizophrenia.[57,58] Figure 40-3C shows the parts of the basal ganglia, which comprise the striatum (i.e., caudate, putamen, and nucleus accumbens) and globus pallidus rostrally, and the subthalamic nucleus and substantia nigra caudally. The basal ganglia orchestrate multiple functions[59]; the dorsal striatum plays an important role in motor control, and the ventral striatum (in particular, the nucleus accumbens) plays key roles in emotion and learning via connections with the hippocampus, amygdala, and prefrontal cortex. The hypothalamus plays a critical role in neuroendocrine regulation of the internal milieu.[60] Via its effects on pituitary hormone release and connections to other regions

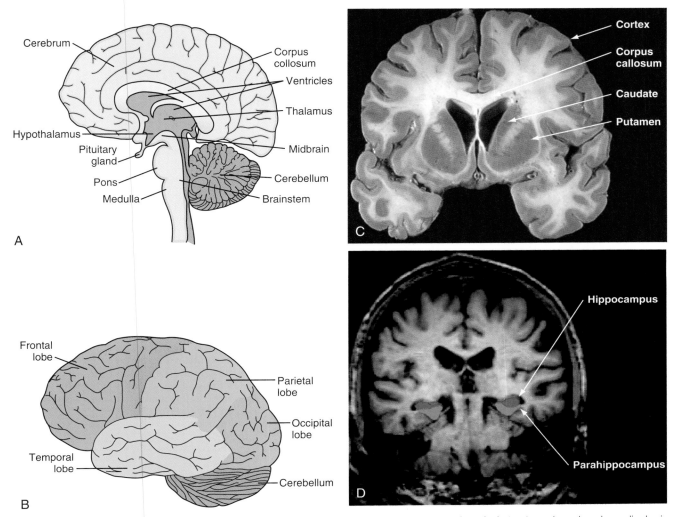

Figure 40-3. (A) Schematic of the human brain organized into the cerebral cortex, brainstem, subcortical structures (e.g., basal ganglia, brain-stem, thalamus, hypothalamus, and pituitary), and cerebellum. (B) Depiction of cortical anatomy divided into anatomical regions (such as the occipital, parietal, temporal, insular, limbic, and frontal lobes). (C) Brain cut demonstrating the limbic "lobe" as a ring (limbus) of phylogenetically older cortex surrounding the upper brainstem. (D) Brain cut highlighting the hippocampus, amygdala, hypothalamus, parahippocampal gyrus, and cingulate cortex. *(C, From* http://library.med.utah.edu/WebPath/HISTHTML/NEURANAT/CNS213A.html. *D, From Dickerson BC, Salat DH, Bates JF, et al. Medial temporal lobe function and structure in mild cognitive impairment,* Ann Neurol *56[1]:27–35, 2004.)*

of the brain, the hypothalamus exerts homeostatic effects on numerous psychiatrically-relevant factors, including mood, motivation, sexual drive, hunger, temperature, and sleep. Finally, a number of discrete nuclei in the brainstem synthe-size key modulatory neurotransmitters, exerting major effects on brain function via their widespread projections to striatal and corticolimbic regions of the brain.[5] These neuromodula-tory nuclei include the dopaminergic ventral tegmental area (VTA) in the midbrain, serotonergic raphe nuclei in the brain-stem, noradrenergic locus coeruleus neurons in the pons, and cholinergic neurons of the basal forebrain and brainstem.

CELLULAR DIVERSITY IN THE BRAIN: NEURONS AND GLIA

The cellular diversity of the primate nervous system is truly fantastic. There are two broad classes of cells in the brain: neurons and glia. The Spanish neuroanatomist Santiago Ramon y Cajal prolifically and painstakingly documented the cellular diversity of the nervous system (Figure 40-4).[61] Images made with modern fluorescent staining techniques also

convey the exquisite beauty of the cells of the CNS (Figure 40-5). Based on his observations, Ramon y Cajal proposed that neurons act as physically discrete functional units within the brain, communicating with each other through specialized junctions. This theory became known as the "neuron doc-trine," and Ramon y Cajal's enormous contributions were rec-ognized with a Nobel Prize in 1906.[62]

Neurons

There are approximately 100 billion neurons in the human brain, and each neuron makes up to 10,000 synaptic connec-tions. At the peak of synapse formation in the third year of life, the total number of brain synapses is estimated at 10,000 trillion, thereafter declining and stabilizing in adulthood to between 1,000 trillion and 5,000 trillion synapses.

Consistent with their functional diversity, neurons come in a wide variety of shapes and sizes. Nonetheless, all neurons share several characteristic features (Figure 40-6), including the cell soma (housing the nucleus with its genomic DNA), the axon, the pre-synaptic axon terminal, and the dendritic field

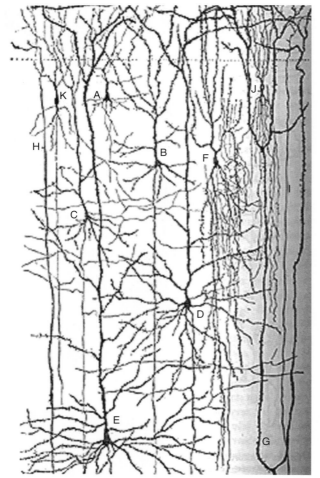

Figure 40-4. Ramon y Cajal's drawing from his classic "Histologie du Système Nerveux de l'Homme et des Vertébrés" showing the cellular diversity of the nervous system. *(From Ramon y Cajal S. Histologie du système nerveux de l'homme et des vertébrés, Paris, 1909, A Maloine.)*

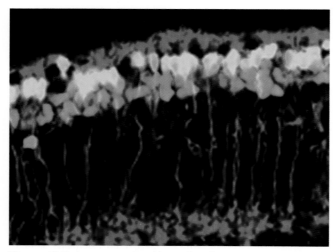

Figure 40-5. Images made with modern fluorescent staining techniques also convey the exquisite beauty of the cells of the CNS. *(From Morrow, et al, unpublished.)*

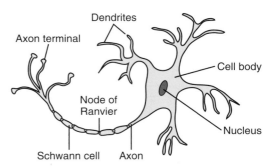

Figure 40-6. Depiction of the neuron with its components.

(the receptive component of the neuron containing post-synaptic dendritic structures). Axon length is highly variable; short axons are found on inhibitory inter-neurons, which make only local connections, while axons many inches long are found on cortical projection neurons, which must reach to the contralateral hemisphere or down to the spinal cord. Motor and sensory neurons have axons that may be several feet long.

There are many ways to classify neurons: by structure (i.e., projection neuron or local inter-neuron); by histology (i.e., bipolar, multipolar, or unipolar); by function (i.e., excitatory, inhibitory, or modulatory); by electrophysiology (i.e., tonic, phasic, or fast-spiking); or by neurotransmitter type.[3] For the purposes of this chapter, classifications using a combination of structural, functional, and neurotransmitter type provide the most useful descriptions. For example, it is useful to appreciate that the major excitatory neurotransmitter is glutamate (commonly used by projection neurons), while the major inhibitory neurotransmitter in the brain is GABA (commonly used by local inter-neurons).

Glia

Although neurons have captured the lion's share of attention since the time of Ramon y Cajal, there are up to 10-fold more glial cells in the brain than neurons. The word "glia" means "glue," aptly summarizing the structural and supportive role traditionally attributed to them. Indeed, glia do support neuronal function in many ways, by supplying nutrition, maintaining homeostasis, stabilizing synapses, and myelinating axons. They also play important roles in synaptic transmission. In the CNS there are two large categories of glia: microglia and macroglia. Microglia are small, phagocytic cells related to peripheral macrophages. Macroglia can be further classified into two types: astrocytes maintain the synaptic milieu, and oligodendrocytes myelinate axons. Astrocytes play an active and critical role in glutamatergic neurotransmission, releasing co-agonists required for glutamate receptor function and transporting glutamate to terminate its synaptic action. New functions of glia continue to be discovered, and belated appreciation of their importance to psychiatric neuroscience continues to grow. Mood disorders are associated with a reduction in the number of glia in select brain regions.[63] In adult-onset metachromatic leukodystrophy, a genetic enzyme deficiency produces diffuse myelin destruction; the illness may manifest in mid-adolescence with neuropsychiatric symptoms resembling schizophrenia.[64] Furthermore, studies looking for genes whose expression is altered in schizophrenia have identified prominent changes in myelin-related genes.[65]

THE STRUCTURE OF THE SYNAPSE

The previous section described how inter-cellular communication serves as an organizing feature of neuroanatomy. Neurons and glia are elegantly situated within the brain to facilitate signaling between adjacent cells, and between cells in distinct brain regions. Depending on the specific neurotransmitters released pre-synaptically, and the specific receptors located post-synaptically, the transmitted signal may have excitatory, inhibitory, or other modulatory effects on the post-synaptic neuron. Detailed knowledge of the neurochemical anatomy of the brain is therefore a prerequisite to the optimal use of psychotropic medicines in psychiatry. Important aspects of neurochemical anatomy include how neurotransmitters are distributed within brain circuits; how these neurotransmitter systems function; and how these systems are altered either by disease or by our treatments.

Neurotransmitters

Neurotransmitters are defined by four essential characteristics (Figure 40-7 and Box 40-2): they are synthesized within the pre-synaptic neuron; they are released with depolarization from the pre-synaptic neuron to exert a discrete action on the post-synaptic neuron; their action on the post-synaptic neuron can be replicated by administering the transmitter exogenously (as a drug); and their action in the synaptic cleft is terminated by a specific mechanism.[3] However, they otherwise differ considerably in structure, distribution, and function. Their chemical make-up (including small molecules [such as amino acids, biogenic amines, and nitrous oxide] as well as larger peptides [such as opioids and substance P]) varies substantially. Certain neurotransmitters are found ubiquitously throughout the cortex, whereas others act in more select locations. Moreover, while certain neurotransmitters are always excitatory (e.g., glutamate) or inhibitory (e.g., GABA in the adult brain), others can exert variable downstream effects based on where they are located and to which receptors they bind.

Nearly 100 neurotransmitters have been identified within the mammalian brain. However, we will focus on several well-characterized neurotransmitter systems with major relevance to neuropsychiatric phenomena (Box 40-3). Each of these neurotransmitters plays an important role in normal brain function; thus, abnormal activity in any of these neurotransmitter systems may contribute to neuropsychiatric dysfunction. We will consider the normal "life cycle" for each neurotransmitter system—including synthesis, synaptic release, receptor binding, neurotransmitter degradation, post-synaptic signaling through ion channels or second messengers, and activity-dependent changes in gene expression and subsequent neuronal activity (see Box 40-2). We will focus particularly on the various points in this cycle that are amenable to pharmacological intervention.

For example, consider the hypothetical synapse in Figure 40-8. Suppose a particular psychiatric symptom was related to abnormally high synaptic concentrations of a specific

---

BOX 40-2 Schema of Neurochemical Systems

Neurotransmitter biosynthesis
Neurotransmitter storage and synaptic vesicle release
Neurotransmitter receptors:
- Post-synaptic
- Pre-synaptic autoreceptors

Post-synaptic ion channels
Post-synaptic second messenger systems
Activity-dependent gene regulation
Neurotransmitter degradation
Neurotransmitter reuptake
Functional neurochemical anatomy

BOX 40-3 Major Neurotransmitter Systems in the Brain

AMINO ACIDS
Glutamate
γ-Aminobutyric acid (GABA)

MONOAMINES
Dopamine
Norepinephrine (noradrenaline)
Epinephrine (adrenaline)
Serotonin
Histamine

SMALL MOLECULE NEUROTRANSMITTER
Acetylcholine

PEPTIDES
Opioids (enkephalins, endorphin, dynorphin)
Hypothalamic factors (CRH, orexins/hypocretins, and others)
Pituitary hormones (ACTH, TSH, oxytocin, vasopressin, and others)
Neuroactive CNS peptides also expressed in the GI system (substance P, VIP, and others)
Others (leptin and others)

ACTH, Adrenocorticotropic hormone; CNS, central nervous system; CRH, corticotropin-releasing hormone; GI, gastrointestinal; TSH, thyroid-stimulating hormone; VIP, vasoactive intestinal polypeptide.

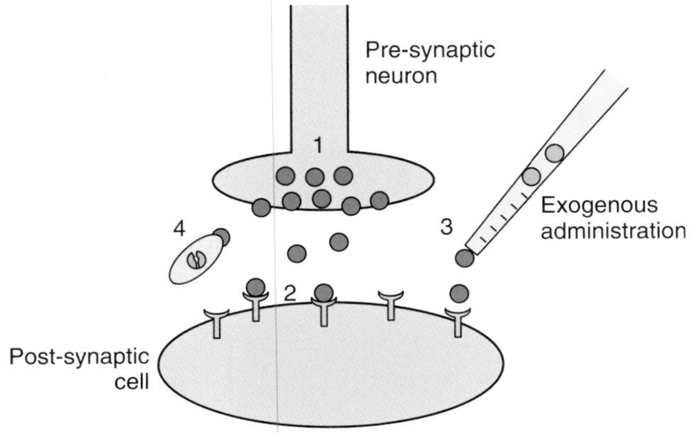

Figure 40-7. Essential characteristics of neurotransmitters.

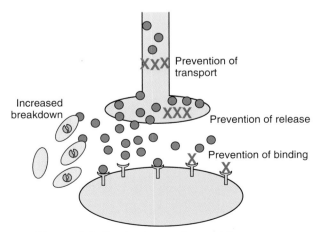

Figure 40-8. Psychopharmacology and the synapse.

neurotransmitter. The diversity of biochemical steps involved in the neurotransmitter cycle provides many targets for pharmacological intervention[5]: one could inhibit neurotransmitter synthesis; interfere with neurotransmitter transport, vesicle formation, or release; block post-synaptic receptor effects; or increase the clearance rate from the synapse by degradation or transport. We will re-visit this model as we consider each of the neurotransmitter systems and their relation to normal and abnormal brain function below.

Synaptic Transmission, Second Messenger Systems, and Activity-Dependent Gene Expression

Neurotransmitter signals alter post-synaptic neuron function via a complex collection of receptors and second messenger systems.[66] These signals ultimately result in changes in neuronal activity, often associated with changes in gene expression. While neurotransmitter receptors are the classic targets of pharmacological intervention, it has become apparent that second messenger systems may also provide important targets for existing and novel therapies.[67,68]

In general, neurotransmitter receptors trigger either rapid or slow effector systems. Rapid-effect neurotransmitter receptors are either themselves ion channels (e.g., NMDA glutamate receptors), or are coupled to ion channels. Ion flux through these transmitter-activated channels rapidly alters membrane potential and neuronal activity. Other neurotransmitter receptors, including the large family of G-protein–coupled receptors (GPCRs), work via slower second messenger systems.[69,70] Such second messenger systems usually involve sequential multi-enzyme cascades. Post-translational modifications, such as protein phosphorylation (introduced by kinase proteins and removed by phosphatase proteins), can act as on–off switches to propagate or terminate the signal at specific branch points. Second messenger systems convert receptor signals into a coordinated set of cellular effects by altering the function of multiple target proteins. These targets include ion channels that control neuronal firing, synaptic proteins that regulate synaptic efficacy, and cytoskeletal elements that determine cellular morphology. While there are over 500 different kinases in the human genome, several that have been heavily studied in psychiatry are worthy of special mention, such as the cyclic AMP (cAMP)–dependent kinase (also known as protein kinase A [PKA]) and calcium/calmodulin-dependent protein kinase (CAMK), which both play critical roles in memory formation.[71] Another second messenger pathway, involving glycogen synthase kinase (GSK), has been proposed to mediate at least some of the therapeutic efficacy of lithium salts in bipolar disorder.[72]

Transcription factors are also critical downstream targets of neurotransmitter signals and second messenger systems. By modifying gene expression in the nucleus, transcription factors can produce persistent changes in neural function. The most widely studied neuronal transcription factors include immediate early genes c-Jun, c-Fos, and cAMP response element binding protein (CREB), whose activity is quickly regulated by neurotransmitter signals.[73] CREB has been shown to be up-regulated and phosphorylated in neurons in response to antipsychotic medication, as well as drugs of abuse,[74–76] and in response to neurotrophic factors, such as brain-derived neurotrophic factor (BDNF).[77] BDNF and related neurotrophic factors are of particular interest to psychiatric neuroscience, as they exert effects both as growth factors during embryonic neurodevelopment and synaptic signaling in adults. BDNF signaling modulates CREB activity and gene expression; both factors play important roles in neural plasticity, and have

been heavily studied in genetic association studies in psychiatric disorders.[78–81]

A REVIEW OF CLINICALLY RELEVANT NEUROTRANSMITTER SYSTEMS

In this section we review the major neurotransmitter systems, all of which have clinical importance in psychiatry. In each subsection, emphasis will be placed on the "content" of neuropsychiatric explanation.

Glutamate

As the major excitatory neurotransmitter in the CNS, glutamate is found ubiquitously throughout the brain. A non-essential amino acid, glutamate does not cross the blood–brain barrier; thus, synthesis of the glutamate neurotransmitter pool relies entirely on conversion from its precursors (glutamine or aspartate) within nerve terminals (Figure 40-9). Aspartate is converted to glutamine via transamination, while glutamine is converted to glutamate within mitochondria via glutaminase. Glutamate is packaged within synaptic vesicles, and, when released into the synapse, binds post-synaptic glutamate receptors. Unable to diffuse across cell membranes, glutamate is cleared from the synapse primarily by sodium (Na^+)–dependent uptake into astrocytic processes that ensheath the glutamatergic synapse ("tripartite synapse"), where it is converted back to glutamine (which is then transported back to the pre-synaptic glutamatergic terminal).

Glutamate receptors are varied in structure and function, capable of imparting either rapid or gradual change in the function of the post-synaptic neuron. The ionotropic family of glutamate receptors, which includes NMDA, α-amino-3-hydroxy-5-methyl-4-isoxazolepropionic acid (AMPA), and kainate (KA) receptors, act rapidly by opening channels for Na^+ and (to a variable degree) calcium (Ca^{2+}) influx. This influx causes post-synaptic depolarization, which, if present in sufficient force, causes the neuron to fire. The metabotropic glutamate receptors (mGluRs) effect gradual change in neuronal function. These seven membrane-spanning G-protein–coupled receptors (GPCRs) are linked to cytoplasmic enzymes via G proteins embedded within the cell membrane. Once activated, these enzymes can induce second messenger cascades that can influence intra-cellular processes, including gene transcription.

The *N*-methyl-D-aspartate Receptor and the Role of Glutamate in Neuropsychiatric Illness

The NMDA receptor deserves special attention due to its role in normal and abnormal cognitive processes. When activated, the NMDA receptor serves as a channel for the influx of Ca^{2+} into the neuron (Figure 40-10). This process relies on both the binding of ligands (such as glutamate and a co-agonist, glycine) to the receptor and on recent depolarization of the post-synaptic cell membrane, which displaces a magnesium (Mg^{2+}) ion that normally blocks the channel. NMDA receptor signaling thus requires near-simultaneous activity of the pre-synaptic and post-synaptic neurons; this provides a molecular mechanism for associating two temporally linked inputs, a key ingredient in basic forms of learning. Indeed, NMDA receptors, along with AMPA receptors, mediate long-term potentiation in the hippocampus, a process critical for hippocampal-dependent memory formation.

When NMDA receptors are activated in sufficient number, however, the resulting large calcium influx can result in cell death, a process known as excitotoxicity (see Figure 40-10). Excitotoxicity is thought to contribute to

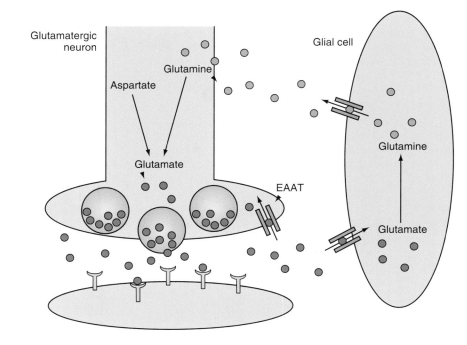

Figure 40-9. The glutamate life cycle.

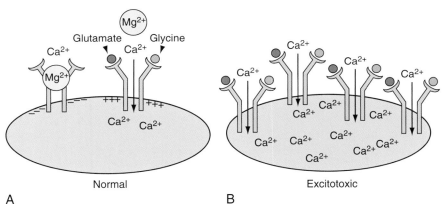

Figure 40-10. *N*-methyl-D-aspartate receptors and excitotoxicity. (A) Normal. (B) Excitotoxic.

neurodegenerative disorders (such as Alzheimer's disease, Huntington's disease, and amyotrophic lateral sclerosis).[82] Memantine, an NMDA antagonist, is used for the treatment of Alzheimer's Dementia Memantine is hypothesized to slow disease progression by dampening excitotoxic injury.[83]

While overactive NMDA receptors may contribute to neurodegeneration and attendant memory loss in dementia, blockade of these receptors can also cause profound cognitive disruption. NMDA antagonists (such as ketamine and phencyclidine [PCP]) produce psychotic symptoms (e.g., disorganization, dissociation, hallucinations, delusions) in healthy people, and exacerbate psychosis in patients with schizophrenia. This pattern, in concert with observed alterations in glutamate-related proteins, has spurred the "glutamate hypothesis" of schizophrenia.[33] The glutamate system thus represents a promising target for the development of new antipsychotic medications. The NMDA receptor, in addition to its binding site for glutamate, also has a co-regulatory site for the amino acids glycine or D-serine, which must be occupied for glutamate to open the channel. Based on the hypothesis of a hypoactive glutamatergic system in schizophrenia, these amino acids, and the related D-cycloserine, are being actively studied as potential augmentation strategies for antipsychotic treatment.

GABA

Another amino acid, γ-aminobutyric acid (GABA), serves as the major inhibitory transmitter in the CNS. When bound to membrane receptors, GABA causes hyperpolarization either directly, by causing chloride channels to open, or indirectly, through second messenger systems. Although found throughout the CNS, GABA is concentrated specifically in both cortical and spinal interneurons, and plays a major role in dampening excitatory signals. As such, GABA receptors have been of considerable interest to researchers concerned about the normal and abnormal function of neural networks.

GABA is synthesized primarily from glucose, which is converted via the Krebs cycle into α-ketoglutarate and then to glutamate (Figure 40-11). Conversion from glutamate to GABA occurs through the action of glutamic acid decarboxylase (GAD). Because GAD is found only in GABA-producing neurons, antibodies to the enzyme have been used to identify GABA-ergic neurons with high specificity. Following depolarization of the pre-synaptic neuron, vesicles containing GABA discharge it into the synapse, where binding to post-synaptic receptors occurs. GABA is then cleared from the synapse and transported into pre-synaptic terminals and surrounding glia. It is then broken down by GABA α-oxoglutarate transaminase

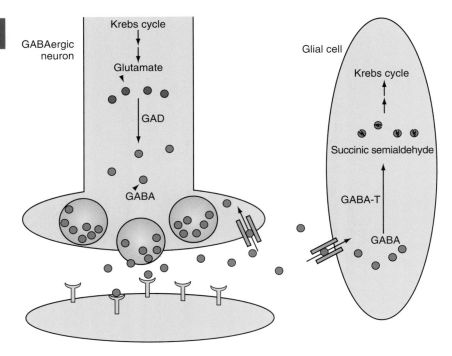

Figure 40-11. The GABA life cycle.

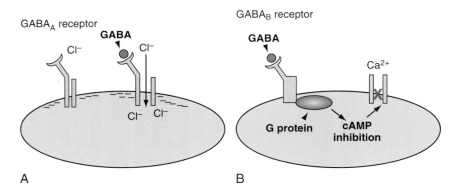

Figure 40-12. GABA receptors. (A) GABA_A receptor. (B) GABA_B receptor.

(GABA-T), and downstream products are returned to the Krebs cycle. GABA synthesis and metabolism are thus referred to as the GABA shunt reaction.

GABA Receptors

There are two major classes of GABA receptors: $GABA_A$ and $GABA_B$ receptors. Binding of GABA to the $GABA_A$ receptor causes a chloride channel to open, which, under most circumstances, renders the post-synaptic membrane potential more negative (Figure 40-12). Of note, several other agents bind allosterically to the $GABA_A$ receptor, including alcohol, barbiturates, and benzodiazepines, and render it more sensitive to GABA. The anticonvulsant activity of benzodiazepines and barbiturates is thought to reflect neural inhibition mediated through the $GABA_A$ receptor.[84]

$GABA_B$ receptors, akin to the metabotropic glutamate receptors, are G-protein–coupled receptors rather than ion channels. Activation of $GABA_B$ causes downstream changes in potassium (K^+) and Ca^{2+} channels, largely via G-protein–mediated inhibition of cAMP. Specific interactions between $GABA_B$ receptors and Ca^{2+} channel activity may be linked to absence seizures.[85]

GABA in Neuropsychiatric Illness

Altered GABA activity may contribute significantly to psychiatric disorders. In schizophrenia, reduced GABA synthesis in a select population of inter-neurons within the dorsolateral prefrontal cortex is thought to affect inhibition of pyramidal neurons in this region. Reduced inter-neuron input may thus disrupt synchronized neuronal activity, which, in turn, may underlie working memory deficits in schizophrenia.[9] Further, although the exact mechanism remains uncertain, the chronic action of alcohol, benzodiazepines, and barbiturates on specific $GABA_A$ receptor subunits is hypothesized to underlie such clinical phenomena as tolerance and withdrawal. GABA-ergic dysfunction has also been posited to contribute to panic disorder.

Dopamine

While glutamate and GABA are found throughout the brain, other neurotransmitter systems are localized to specific neural pathways. The monoamines (e.g., norepinephrine, serotonin, dopamine) and acetylcholine are synthesized in several discrete brainstem nuclei, yet project widely, affecting a majority of brain systems. Dopamine, a catecholamine neurotransmitter, affects many brain regions that are consistently implicated in psychiatric disorders. It is hardly surprising, then, that a host of psychopharmacological interventions target the dopamine system.

Dopamine Pathways and Relevance to Neuropsychiatry

There are four major dopamine projections (Figure 40-13), each with great relevance to neuropsychiatric phenomena. The name of each projection indicates the location of the dopaminergic cell bodies, as well as the region targeted by their axons; for example, the nigrostriatal system consists of dopamine cell bodies in the substantia nigra, with axons projecting to the striatum. Degeneration of the nigrostriatal pathway leads to extrapyramidal motor symptoms (such as tremor, bradykinesia, and rigidity), as seen in Parkinson's disease. An analogous mechanism underlies extrapyramidal symptoms (EPS) associated with antipsychotic medications, which block dopamine receptors in the striatum.

Dopamine neurons in the mesolimbic pathway project from the ventral tegmental area (VTA), also in the mid-brain, to limbic and paralimbic structures, including the nucleus accumbens, amygdala, hippocampus, septum, anterior cingulate cortex, and orbitofrontal cortex. Given the importance of these downstream structures to emotion, sensory perception, and memory, it has been speculated that altered activity in the mesolimbic pathway may underlie the perceptual disturbances common to positive symptoms of schizophrenia, hallucinogen use, and even temporal lobe seizures. The mesolimbic pathway is also implicated in the addictive actions of drugs of abuse, which share the common feature of enhancing dopamine release in the nucleus accumbens. In addition, loss of mid-brain nigrostriatal dopaminergic neurons in Parkinson's disease may spread to VTA neurons, and this may underlie the depressive symptoms commonly seen in Parkinson's disease.

Mesocortical dopamine neurons also have their cell bodies in the VTA, but project to the neocortex, primarily prefrontal cortex. Release of dopamine in the prefrontal cortex is believed to affect the efficiency of information processing, attention, and wakefulness. The relationship between prefrontal dopamine and frontal lobe function does not appear to be linear, but rather reflects an "inverted-U" shape (Figure 40-14).[86] For example, brain activation during working memory tasks, largely mediated by prefrontal activation, is inefficient under conditions of either low or high prefrontal dopamine release. Altered availability of prefrontal dopamine may underlie cognitive impairment in schizophrenia, ADHD, Parkinson's disease, and other neuropsychiatric conditions.

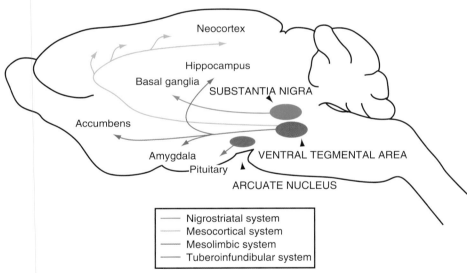

Figure 40-13. Dopaminergic projections. *(Adapted from NIAAA at www.niaaa.nih.gov/Resources/GraphicsGallery/EndocrineReproductiveSystem/ LengthwiseView.htm.)*

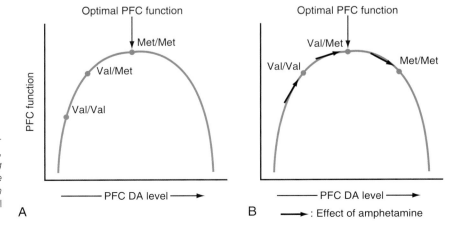

Figure 40-14. (A and B) Dopamine and prefrontal function. PFC, prefrontal cortex; DA, dopamine. *(Adapted from Mattay VS, Goldberg TE, Fera F, et al. Catechol O-methyltransferase val158-met genotype and individual variation in the brain response to amphetamine, Proc Natl Acad Sci U S A 100:6186–6191, 2003.)*

The tuberoinfundibular dopamine system projects from the arcuate nucleus of the hypothalamus to the stalk of the pituitary gland. When released in the pituitary, dopamine inhibits the secretion of prolactin. Individuals who take dopamine-blocking medications (including some antipsychotics) are therefore at risk for hyperprolactinemia, which can in turn cause menstrual cycle abnormalities, galactorrhea, gynecomastia, and sexual dysfunction.

Dopamine Synthesis, Binding, and Inactivation and More Clinical Correlates

The catecholamines (dopamine, norepinephrine, and epinephrine) are synthesized sequentially in the same biosynthetic pathway. First, dopamine is synthesized from tyrosine through the actions of tyrosine hydroxylase (TH, the rate-limiting enzyme for catecholamine synthesis) and 3,4-dihydroxy-L-phenylalanine (Dopa) decarboxylase (Figure 40-15). The dopamine precursor, L-Dopa, crosses the blood–brain barrier and is given systemically to ameliorate symptoms of Parkinson's disease. Dopamine is packaged and stored in synaptic vesicles by the vesicular monoamine transporter (VMAT), and when released binds to post-synaptic dopamine receptors.

Although numerous classes of dopamine receptors have been described, they each affect intra-cellular signaling through second messenger systems. Dopamine receptors fall into one of two families: D_1-like or D_2-like receptors. D_1-like receptors (which include D_1 and D_5) activate adenylyl cyclase, while D_2-like receptors (including D_2, D_3, and D_4) inhibit cAMP production. D_1 and D_2 receptors significantly outnumber other dopamine receptor types. Most typical antipsychotics were developed as D_2 antagonists, while atypical antipsychotics usually have less activity at D_2 receptors (clozapine, for example, has a high affinity for the D_4 receptor).

There are several mechanisms for inactivating dopamine. Within the neuron, extra-vesicular dopamine may be catabolized by the mitochondrial enzymes monoamine oxidase-A or -B (MAO-A or MAO-B). MAO-A metabolizes norepinephrine, serotonin, and dopamine; inhibitors of this enzyme, such as clorgyline and tranylcypromine, are used to treat depression and anxiety. MAO is also present in the liver and gastrointestinal tract, where it degrades dietary amines (such as tyramine and phenylethylamine), thereby preventing their access to the general circulation. Phenylethylamine can cause hypertension when systemically absorbed; thus, patients receiving MAO inhibitors are at risk of hypertensive crisis if they ingest food products containing these amines. MAO-B targets dopamine most specifically, and therefore agents that inhibit this enzyme are used in Parkinson's disease.

Two other molecules, catechol-O-methyltransferase (COMT) and the dopamine transporter (DAT), have the ability to clear dopamine from the synaptic cleft. In the mid-brain and striatum, DAT plays a more substantial role than COMT, while in the prefrontal cortex, COMT predominates. A common, functional polymorphism in the *COMT* gene, Val 108/158 Met, has been identified: individuals with one or more copies of the Met allele have significantly reduced COMT activity. Thus, these individuals presumably have greater concentrations of prefrontal dopamine (see Figure 40-14). In humans, in the setting of a challenging working memory task, healthy individuals homozygous for the Met allele (Met/Met) may exhibit more efficient brain activation than Val/Val or Val/Met subjects. However, if given amphetamine, which blocks dopamine reuptake and increases synaptic dopamine, Val/Val individuals are shifted to a more optimal position in the curve, while those with Met/Met are shifted to the less efficient downward slope of the curve.[87] Among individuals with altered prefrontal dopamine levels, such as patients with schizophrenia and Parkinson's disease, variation in *COMT* genotype may play a significant role in determining prefrontal efficiency, and hence performance on tasks involving planning, sequencing, and working memory. Similarly, patients with velo-cardio-facial syndrome (VCFS) often have psychotic symptoms that may relate to altered COMT function. VCFS is caused by a 3

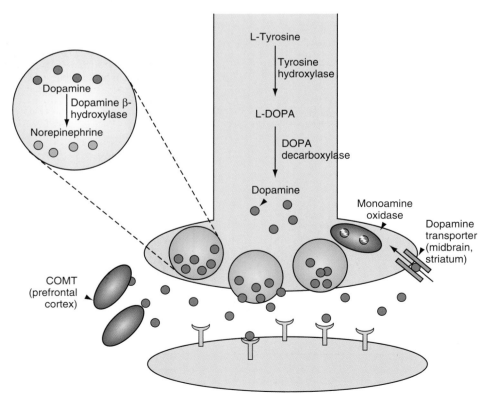

Figure 40-15. The dopamine life cycle.

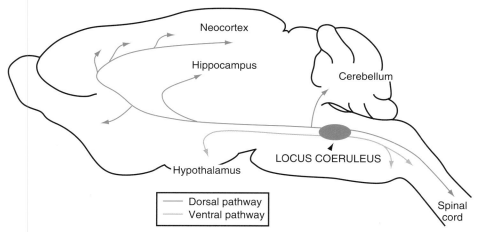

Figure 40-16. Noradrenergic projections. *(Adapted from NIAAA at www.niaaa.nih.gov/Resources/GraphicsGallery/EndocrineReproductiveSystem/ LengthwiseView.htm; and from Siegel GJ, Agranoff BW, Albers RW, et al.* Basic neurochemistry, *ed 6, Philadelphia, 1999, Lippincott-Raven, p. 252.)*

Mb (million base pairs) deletion of the genome on chromosome 22q11.2, which results in the complete loss of one parental copy of approximately 30 genes, one of which is *COMT*. These patients, who exhibit a somewhat variable phenotype (which may also include abnormalities of the heart, thymus, parathyroid, and palate), also have an increased risk for psychotic disorders. Almost 30% of VCFS patients have a psychiatric condition akin to bipolar disorder or schizophrenia.[88]

Norepinephrine

Like dopamine, norepinephrine (noradrenaline [NE]) is a catecholamine neurotransmitter that is present in discrete neural projections. NE cell bodies are concentrated in the locus coeruleus, which is located in the pons near the fourth ventricle (Figure 40-16). This dorsal collection of noradrenergic neurons innervates the cerebral cortex, hippocampus, cerebellum, and spinal cord, while a ventral collection projects to the hypothalamus and other CNS sites.

NE overlaps substantially with dopamine with regard to synthesis and degradation pathways; in fact, dopamine is the immediate precursor to NE, which is produced within synaptic vesicles by dopamine β-hydroxylase (see Figure 40-15). Like dopamine, NE is also degraded by COMT and MAO.

There are three families of noradrenergic receptors: α_1, α_2, and β. Like the dopamine receptors, NE receptors are all coupled to G proteins and thus modify intra-cellular signaling pathways. The α_1 receptors augment protein kinase C activity through the release of inositol 1,4,5-triphosphate and diacylglycerol. While activated α_2 receptors decrease cAMP through inhibition of adenylyl cyclase, β receptors do the opposite, stimulating cAMP production. In this sense, α_2 receptors are somewhat akin to D_2, and β receptors to D_1. In the CNS, α_2 receptors frequently act as "autoreceptors" present pre-synaptically on noradrenergic neurons themselves, providing negative-feedback regulation of noradrenergic output.

Norepinephrine in Opiate Withdrawal

Clonidine, a drug commonly used to treat hypertension, activates CNS α_2 autoreceptors and thereby dampens noradrenergic tone. Use of clonidine in the treatment of opiate withdrawal provides a wonderful example of a case where psychiatric neuroscience has successfully characterized the links between a clinical disorder, therapeutic drug effects, and mechanisms at the molecular, cellular, and neural circuit levels. Acutely,

opiates act through G-protein–coupled receptors to inhibit the cAMP system and reduce the activity of locus coeruleus neurons; this partly mediates their calming and sedating effects. With chronic opiate administration, tolerance develops, in part due to homeostatic up-regulation in the activity of cAMP pathway elements (such as PKA and CREB). In opiate withdrawal, this adaptive up-regulation is no longer balanced by the opiate inhibition. Rebound hyperactivity of the locus coeruleus then occurs, with a great increase in NE release from its widespread projections. This in turn leads to the autonomic and psychological hyperarousal seen during withdrawal; these symptoms are greatly dampened by clonidine.[89]

Serotonin

The serotonin system is involved in many processes in psychiatry, including most prominently mood, sleep, and psychosis.[60,90,91] Serotonin (5-hydroxytryptamine [5-HT]), a monoamine and indolamine, is synthesized from the amino acid tryptophan by tryptophan hydroxylase (TPH) (Figure 40-17). Serotonin is synthesized in mid-line neurons of the brainstem, known as the raphe nuclei.[92] Serotonergic neurons project diffusely to numerous targets (including cerebral cortex, thalamus, basal ganglia, mid-brain dopaminergic nuclei, hippocampus, and amygdala) (Figure 40-18).

Like the catecholamines, serotonin is transported into vesicles by VMAT. Serotonin is subsequently released into the synaptic cleft, and after receptor binding, is inactivated either by pre-synaptic reuptake via the serotonin transporter or degradation via MAO. The serotonin transporter is a critical molecule in neuropsychopharmacology. Drugs that block the serotonin transporter (SERT) prolong serotonin's action; these agents include the selective serotonin reuptake inhibitors (SSRIs) commonly used in treating depression and anxiety disorders. Like the norepinephrine transporter (NET) and dopamine transporter (DAT), SERT is also a common target of drugs of abuse. For example, both cocaine and amphetamine prolong the action of serotonin by inhibiting SERT. Similarly, the club drug ecstasy (MDMA) is a fast-acting SERT inhibitor; MDMA may also be neurotoxic to serotonergic neurons in the dorsal raphe.[93]

The discovery of a common genetic variant in the promoter of the *SERT* gene has had a major impact on psychiatric neuroscience. The "long" form or L-variant (which contains an additional 44-bp sequence) generates more mRNA, and

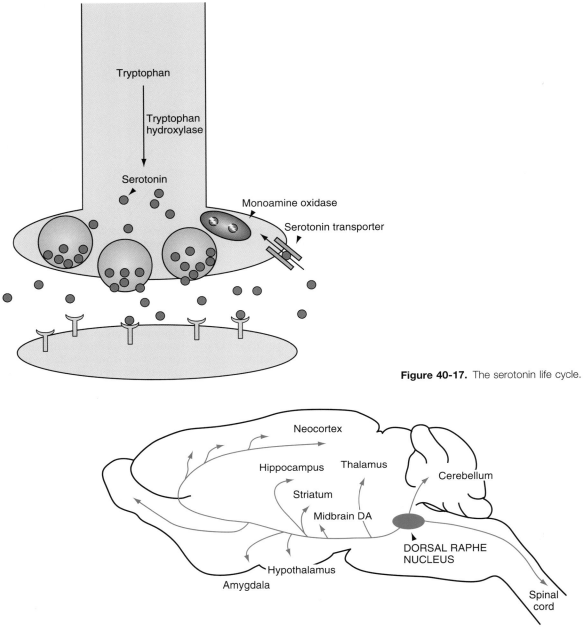

Figure 40-17. The serotonin life cycle.

Figure 40-18. Serotonergic projections. *(Adapted from NIAAA at www.niaaa.nih.gov/Resources/GraphicsGallery/EndocrineReproductiveSystem/ LengthwiseView.htm.)*

thereby protein, than the "short" or S-variant (which lacks this 44-bp sequence). The L-variant thus enhances transporter activity in the synaptic cleft, reducing the duration and intensity of serotonin neurotransmission, while the S-variant leads to lower transporter activity and prolonged serotonin signaling. The S-variant has been implicated in the etiology of depression and anxiety disorders.[94,95]

Seven classes of serotonin receptors exhibit distinct patterns of expression in CNS and peripheral tissues and activate distinct second messenger systems. For example, 5-HT$_{1A}$ receptors are GPCRs that are inhibitory and thereby decrease cAMP; agonists at this receptor (e.g., buspirone) have anxiolytic properties. 5-HT$_2$ receptors (which have three subtypes, A to C) act through a different G protein to activate inositol triphosphate (IP$_3$) and diacylglycerol (DAG) second messenger systems.[96]

5-HT$_2$ signaling is particularly relevant to psychosis: the hallucinogen LSD activates 5-HT$_2$ receptors, while many atypical antipsychotics inhibit them.[91]

Acetylcholine

The first neurotransmitter to be discovered, acetylcholine (ACh) was initially characterized by Otto Loewi as *Vagusstoff*, the mediator of vagal parasympathetic outflow to the heart. As we now know, of course, ACh plays important roles in central as well as peripheral neurophysiology, and cholinergic transmission underlies a host of normal cognitive functions. In recent years, the cholinergic system has become an important target in the psychopharmacology of dementia and movement disorders.

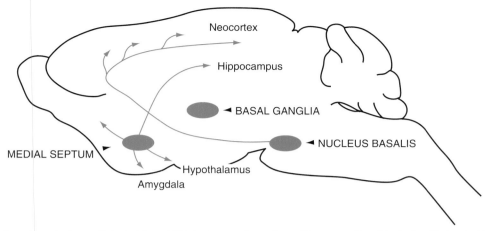

Figure 40-19. Cholinergic projections. *(Adapted from NIAAA at www.niaaa.nih.gov/Resources/GraphicsGallery/EndocrineReproductiveSystem/LengthwiseView.htm.)*

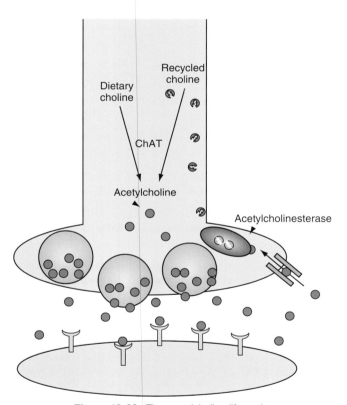

Figure 40-20. The acetylcholine life cycle.

In the periphery, ACh is the neurotransmitter for the neuromuscular junction, for pre-ganglionic neurons in the autonomic nervous system, and for parasympathetic post-ganglionic neurons. In the CNS, cholinergic neurons are concentrated in the nucleus basalis of Meynert in the basal forebrain, and project diffusely to the neocortex (Figure 40-19). There are also cholinergic projections from the septum and diagonal band of Broca to the hippocampus. Cholinergic inter-neurons are found in the basal ganglia.

ACh is formed in nerve terminals through the action of choline acetyltransferase (ChAT; Figure 40-20). Its precursor,

choline, is supplied through both breakdown of dietary phosphatidylcholine, and recycling of synaptic ACh (which is catabolized by acetylcholinesterase to choline and actively transported back into the pre-synaptic terminal).

There are two classes of ACh receptors: muscarinic and nicotinic. While muscarinic receptors are G-protein–coupled, nicotinic receptors are ion channels, which allows for rapid influx of Na^+ and Ca^{2+} into the post-synaptic neuron. Both receptor types are abundant in brain tissue.

Acetylcholine and Cognition

Anticholinergic medications affect the balance of dopamine and ACh in the basal ganglia, which can improve EPS in patients with movement disorders (either primary or secondary to antipsychotic use). However, alterations in cholinergic transmission, due to medications or to underlying disease, can profoundly affect cognition. Anticholinergic medications, such as diphenhydramine, are a common source of delirium in elderly or medically ill patients. Many antipsychotic and tricyclic antidepressant drugs have some anticholinergic activity, which can affect cognition (and also produce significant peripheral side effects, including dry mouth, urinary retention, constipation, and tachycardia). The degeneration of cholinergic neurons in Alzheimer's disease contributes strongly to cognitive decline; acetylcholinesterase inhibitors may slow this effect somewhat, but do not reverse the degeneration process.[97] Nicotine, acting through nicotinic ACh receptors, may produce significant cognitive effects (as well as addictive rewarding effects).

Histamine

Like ACh and NE, histamine serves important functions both in the CNS and peripherally. Histamine is best known for its roles outside the brain in activating immune and inflammatory responses and in stimulating gastric acid secretion. Within the brain, it acts both as a classical neurotransmitter and as a neuromodulator, potentiating the excitability of other neurotransmitter systems.

Histaminergic neurons are concentrated within the hypothalamus, in the tuberomammillary nucleus. They project diffusely to cortical and subcortical targets, as well as to the brainstem and spinal cord. Histamine is derived from its precursor, L-histidine, through the action of L-histidine decarboxylase. Histamine can be broken down either through oxidation (via diamine oxidase) or methylation (via histamine *N*-methyltransferase and, subsequently, MAO).

Three classes of histamine receptors, H_1, H_2, and H_3, have been found both within brain tissue and in the periphery. Each affects second messenger systems through coupling to G proteins. H_3 may also function as an inhibitory autoreceptor. More recently, a fourth class of histamine receptor (H_4) has also been described, but apparently is not expressed in human brain.

Histamine stimulates wakefulness, suppresses appetite, and may enhance cognition through its excitatory effects on brainstem, hypothalamic, and cortical neurons. Drugs with antihistaminic properties can cause significant disruptions of these processes, producing the therapeutic effects of sleep medications, as well as side effects (sedation and weight gain) of some atypical antipsychotics and, in particular, the antidepressant mirtazapine.[98] Animal research shows that histamine depletion adversely affects short-term memory, while H_3 autoreceptor antagonists may have the opposite effect; these findings have fueled the development of H_3 antagonists as a potential treatment for memory disorders.

Other Neurotransmitters, and Interactions among Neurotransmitters

Many additional neurotransmitters mediate important effects in the brain; some with particular relevance to psychiatry include neuropeptides (e.g., endogenous opioids), neurohormones (e.g., corticotropin-releasing hormone), and steroids, cannabinoids, and short-acting gases (such as nitric oxide). And while we have focused on one neurotransmitter at a time, numerous and complex interactions occur among neurotransmitter systems. Although discussion of these other neurotransmitters and neurotransmitter interactions is beyond the scope of this chapter, they are of great importance to psychiatric neuroscience and the subject of intensive research.

GENES, ENVIRONMENT, AND EPIGENETICS

At the outset of this chapter, we stated that major mental illness reflects abnormal brain function, and we have described many genes that could contribute to such dysfunction. However, while neuropsychiatric conditions are frequently highly heritable, the emergence of psychopathology likely requires a complex interaction of a genetic susceptibility and exposure to environmental risk factors. Note that the "environment" must be understood broadly, and includes the prenatal uterine environment as well as peri-natal and post-natal events into childhood, adolescence, and adulthood. Epidemiological studies relating gene–environment interactions to the development of psychiatric conditions have already contributed significantly to psychiatric neuroscience.[99] For example, in a prospective longitudinal study, Caspi and colleagues[100] discovered that genetic variations in the serotonin transporter (*SERT*) promoter interacted with stressful life events to influence depression risk. Individuals with one or two copies of the short S-variant allele (the hypoactive form of the gene) exhibited more depression and suicidality in relation to stressful life events than those carrying two copies of the long L-variant allele. This remarkable study demonstrated that even when genetic susceptibility and environmental exposure do not independently produce a strong increase in risk for psychopathology, in combination they may impressively increase this risk.[100]

Finally, the mechanisms by which experience may interact with genes are various, but one recent study in the field of "epigenetics" merits attention. Epigenetics has various definitions, but includes the idea that a gene function may be changed without a specific alteration in the code, and that this change in gene function also may be heritable.[101] Frequently, this may occur by a change in the structure of the DNA molecule: for example, chromatin, around a gene, which alters gene expression. An important animal model may have shed light on the biological effects of child abuse.[43,102] While it has been widely noted in psychiatry that child abuse or mistreatment can have long-term effects on cognition and behavior, a model system of rodent maternal care has also demonstrated that rodent pups mistreated during development will have long-standing dysfunctional programming of their hypothalamic–pituitary–adrenal axis, and thereby response to stress. Investigators have further demonstrated that these occur due to specific changes in chromatin structure and subsequent gene expression, and have also shown that these changes and downstream effects may be heritable. These effects may be treatable or even reversible with novel medicines that affect chromatic structure,[103] and, indeed, some of our older medicines, most notably valproic acid,[104] may act in part through such mechanisms. This is an important example of how a detailed mechanistic understanding of gene–environment interactions may truly make vast contributions to the understanding and treatment of major mental illness.

CONCLUSION

We are fortunate in psychiatry to have multiple treatment choices for most conditions. However, existing treatments are frequently only partially effective. Side effects may interfere with compliance and produce their own morbidity, and even after successful treatment relapse is common. Despite 50 years of progress in psychopharmacology, we still need better treatments for mental illness. Greater understanding of the biological mechanisms underlying brain function and dysfunction will be essential in the development of new and better remedies. Important insights will also come from clarifying the specific therapeutic mechanisms of existing treatments.

Over the past century psychiatric neuroscience has made great strides in linking neural mechanisms to conditions of abnormal affect, behavior, and cognition. However, because of challenges inherent to the study of psychiatric phenomena and brain function, the gap between mechanistic understanding and clinical practice remains wide for most conditions. Genetics and neuroimaging have dramatically enhanced our ability to bridge these gaps, and the accelerating development of these fields provides great hope.

While our biological knowledge is incomplete, there is already a great deal of information that may be incorporated into our clinical problem-solving. This will be facilitated by applying a systematic framework when evaluating the neuroscientific aspects of clinical cases. Biological formulations should involve consideration of two broad domains: process (the dynamic mechanisms of neurodevelopment, neurotransmission, and neurodegeneration) and content (key regional, cellular, and molecular neural substrates). These biological components of major mental illness, identified through decades of research, are extremely valuable in our explanations to patients and families.

Acknowledgments

The authors would like to thank Stephan Heckers in particular for his rigor and commitment to teaching psychiatric neuroscience at Harvard. This teaching has contributed greatly to the framing of this chapter. We would also like to thank Nicholas Kontos for critical comments of this manuscript.

Access the complete reference list and multiple choice questions (MCQs) online at https://expertconsult.inkling.com

KEY REFERENCES

3. Kandel ER, Schwartz JH, Jessell TM, et al. *Principles of neural science*, ed 5, New York, 2013, McGraw-Hill.

6. Price BH, Adams RD, Coyle JT. Neurology and psychiatry: closing the great divide. *Neurology* 54(1):8–14, 2000.

7. Alzheimer A, Stelzmann RA, Schnitzlein HN, et al. An English translation of Alzheimer's 1907 paper, "Uber eine eigenartige Erkankung der Hirnrinde." *Clin Anat* 8(6):429–431, 1995.

10. Benes FM. Emerging principles of altered neural circuitry in schizophrenia. *Brain Res Brain Res Rev* 31(2–3):251–269, 2000.

13. Snyder SH. Turning off neurotransmitters. *Cell* 125(1):13–15, 2006.

18. Geschwind N. Mechanisms of change after brain lesions. *Ann N Y Acad Sci* 457:1–11, 1985.

19. Fleischman J. *Phineas Gage: a gruesome but true story about brain science*, Boston, 2002, Houghton Mifflin.

20. Corkin S. What's new with the amnesic patient H.M.? *Nat Rev* 3(2):153–160, 2002.

22. Hariri AR, Weinberger DR. Imaging genomics. *Br Med Bull* 65:259–270, 2003.

23. Dougherty DD, Rauch SL, Rosenbaum JF. *Essentials of neuroimaging for clinical practice*, Washington, DC, 2004, American Psychiatric Publishing.

26. Haber SN, Rauch SL. Neurocircuitry: a window into the networks underlying neuropsychiatric disease. *Neuropsychopharmacology* 35(1):1–3, 2010. [Epub 2009/12/17].

29. Pascual-Leone A, Walsh V, Rothwell J. Transcranial magnetic stimulation in cognitive neuroscience—virtual lesion, chronometry, and functional connectivity. *Curr Opin Neurobiol* 10(2):232–237, 2000.

34. Schildkraut JJ. The catecholamine hypothesis of affective disorders. A review of supporting evidence. *Int J Psychiatry* 4(3):203–217, 1967.

35. LeDoux J. The emotional brain, fear, and the amygdala. *Cell Mol Neurobiol* 23(4–5):727–738, 2003.

37. Cowan WM, Kopnisky KL, Hyman SE. The human genome project and its impact on psychiatry. *Annu Rev Neurosci* 25:1–50, 2002.

38. Tanzi RE, Bertram L. Twenty years of the Alzheimer's disease amyloid hypothesis: a genetic perspective. *Cell* 120(4):545–555, 2005.

46. Warner-Schmidt JL, Duman RS. Hippocampal neurogenesis: opposing effects of stress and antidepressant treatment. *Hippocampus* 16(3):239–249, 2006.

47. Rapoport JL, Castellanos FX, Gogate N, et al. Imaging normal and abnormal brain development: new perspectives for child psychiatry. *Aust N Z J Psychiatry* 35(3):272–281, 2001.

52. Hyman SE, Malenka RC, Nestler EJ. Neural mechanisms of addiction: the role of reward-related learning and memory. *Annu Rev Neurosci* 29:565–598, 2006.

54. Mesulam MM. *Principles of behavioral and cognitive neurology*, ed 2, New York, 2000, Oxford University Press.

56. Schmahmann JD. An emerging concept. The cerebellar contribution to higher function. *Arch Neurol* 48(11):1178–1187, 1991.

59. Graybiel AM. The basal ganglia: learning new tricks and loving it. *Curr Opin Neurobiol* 15(6):638–644, 2005.

61. Ramon y Cajal S. *Histology of the nervous system of man and vertebrates*, New York, 1995, Oxford University Press.

63. Ongur D, Drevets WC, Price JL. Glial reduction in the subgenual prefrontal cortex in mood disorders. *Proc Natl Acad Sci U S A* 95(22):13290–13295, 1998.

82. Bossy-Wetzel E, Schwarzenbacher R, Lipton SA. Molecular pathways to neurodegeneration. *Nat Med* 10(Suppl.):S2–S9, 2004.

84. Rowlett JK, Cook JM, Duke AN, et al. Selective antagonism of GABA$_A$ receptor subtypes: an in vivo approach to exploring the therapeutic and side effects of benzodiazepine-type drugs. *CNS Spectr* 10(1):40–48, 2005.

86. Goldman-Rakic PS. The cortical dopamine system: role in memory and cognition. *Adv Pharmacol* 42:707–711, 1998.

90. Arango V, Underwood MD, Mann JJ. Serotonin brain circuits involved in major depression and suicide. *Prog Brain Res* 136:443–453, 2002.

99. Caspi A, Moffitt TE. Gene-environment interactions in psychiatry: joining forces with neuroscience. *Nat Rev* 7(7):583–590, 2006.

101. Petronis A, Gottesman II, Crow TJ, et al. Psychiatric epigenetics: a new focus for the new century. *Mol Psychiatry* 5(4):342–346, 2000.

41 The Pharmacotherapy of Anxiety Disorders

Eric Bui, MD, PhD, Mark H. Pollack, MD, Gustavo Kinrys, MD, Hannah Delong, BA, Débora Vasconcelos e Sá, BA, MSc, and Naomi M. Simon, MD, MSc

KEY POINTS

- A variety of pharmacological agents are effective for the treatment of anxiety disorders.
- The SSRIs and SNRIs are first-line pharmacological agents for the treatment of anxiety disorders.
- Benzodiazepines are effective, rapidly acting and well-tolerated, but are associated with the risk of abuse and dependence, and lack efficacy for co-morbid depression.
- Anticonvulsants, atypical antipsychotics, adrenergic antagonists, and other agents also play role in the treatment of anxiety disorders.
- Many patients remain symptomatic despite standard treatments; this necessitates the creative use of available interventions (alone and in combination), and spurs the development of novel therapeutics.

OVERVIEW

As described elsewhere in this volume (Chapter 32), anxiety disorders are associated with both significant distress and dysfunction. In this chapter we will review the pharmacotherapy of panic disorder with or without co-morbid agoraphobia, generalized anxiety disorder (GAD), and social anxiety disorder (SAD); the treatment of posttraumatic stress disorder (PTSD) is discussed in Chapter 34, and obsessive-compulsive disorder (OCD) is discussed in Chapter 33. Table 41-1 includes dosing information and common side effects associated with the pharmacological agents commonly used for the treatment of anxiety, referred to in the following sections.

PANIC DISORDER AND AGORAPHOBIA

Pharmacotherapy of panic disorder is aimed at preventing panic attacks, diminishing anticipatory and generalized anxiety, reversing phobic avoidance, improving overall function and quality of life, and treating co-morbid conditions (such as depression). As for all anxiety disorders, the goal of pharmacotherapy is to reduce the patient's distress and impairment to the point of remission, and/or to facilitate their participation, if necessary, in other forms of treatment (such as cognitive-behavioral therapy [CBT]).

Antidepressants

The selective reuptake inhibitors (SSRIs) and serotonin-norepinephrine serotonin reuptake inhibitors (SNRIs) have become first-line agents for the treatment of panic disorder as well as other anxiety disorders because of their broad spectrum of efficacy (including benefit for disorders commonly co-morbid with panic disorder, such as major depression), favorable side-effect profile, and lack of cardiotoxicity. Currently, paroxetine, both the immediate ([Paxil] and controlled-release formulations [Paxil-CR]), sertraline (Zoloft), fluoxetine

(Prozac) and extended-release venlafaxine Effexor-XR) are Food and Drug Administration (FDA)-approved for the treatment of panic disorder, though other SSRIs including citalopram (Celexa), and escitalopram (Lexapro),[1] and fluvoxamine (Luvox)[2] have also demonstrated anti-panic efficacy in both open and double-blind trials. A recently introduced SNRI, duloxetine (Cymbalta), has also been reported effective for panic disorder in case reports,[3] and in an open-label trial[4] though no randomized controlled trials (RCTs) are currently reported.

A recent meta-analysis on 50 clinical trials (yielding over 5,000 participants) confirmed that citalopram, paroxetine, fluoxetine, and venlafaxine were superior to placebo in the treatment of panic disorder.[5] Finally, while the majority of data supporting the efficacy of pharmacological agents for panic disorder derive from short-term trials, several long-term studies have also demonstrated sustained efficacy over time.[6]

Because the SSRI/SNRIs have the potential to cause initial restlessness, insomnia, and increased anxiety, and because panic patients are commonly sensitive to somatic sensations, the starting doses should be low, typically half (or less) of the usual starting dose (e.g., fluoxetine 5 to 10 mg/d, sertraline 25 mg/d, paroxetine 10 mg/d [or 12.5 mg/d of the controlled-release formulation], controlled-release venlafaxine 37.5 mg/d), to minimize the early anxiogenic effect. Doses can usually begin to be raised, after about a week of acclimation, to achieve typical therapeutic levels, with further gradual titration based on clinical response and side effects, although even more gradual upward titration is sometimes necessary in particularly sensitive or somatically-focused individuals. Although the nature of the dose–response relationship for the SSRIs in panic is still being assessed, available data support doses for this indication in the typical antidepressant range, and sometimes higher, i.e., fluoxetine 20 to 40 mg/d, paroxetine 20 to 60 mg/d (25 to 72.5 mg/d of the controlled-release formulation), sertraline 100 to 200 mg/d, citalopram 20 to 60 mg/d, escitalopram 10 to 20 mg/d, fluvoxamine 150 to 250 mg/d, and controlled-release venlafaxine 75 to 225 mg/d (although some patients may respond at lower doses). In some cases of refractory panic, even higher doses may be clinically useful, although additional data examining such dosing is needed.

SSRI and SNRI administration may be associated with adverse effects that include sexual dysfunction, sleep disturbance, weight gain, headache, dose-dependent increases in blood pressure (with venlafaxine), gastrointestinal disturbance, potential risk of bleeding (with anticoagulants, aspirin or NSAIDs), and provocation of increased anxiety (particularly at initiation of therapy) that may make their administration problematic for some individuals.[7-9] The SSRIs/SNRIs are usually administered in the morning (though for some individuals, agents such as paroxetine and others may be sedating and better tolerated with bedtime dosing); emergent sleep disruption can usually be managed by the addition of hypnotic agents. The typical 2–3 week lag in onset of therapeutic efficacy for the SSRI/SNRIs can be problematic for acutely distressed individuals. There is also an FDA class warning for risk of emergent suicidal thoughts and behaviors based on short-term studies that suggests close monitoring is advised for individuals age 24 or younger, with use balancing risk and

Other agents

Riluzole

The efficacy of riluzole, an anti-glutamatergic agent, traditionally used in the treatment of amyotrophic lateral sclerosis (ALS) was examined in individuals with GAD, in an 8-week, open-label, fixed-dose study of 100 mg/d.[102] Riluzole appeared to be effective and generally well-tolerated; although its expense makes it unlikely that its use will be widely adopted, the report does suggest a potential role for anti-glutamatergic agents for the treatment of anxiety.

Chamomile

Chamomile as infusion has been commonly used for sleep for decades. Recently, one of its compounds, apigenin, which may have GABA-ergic actions, has been identified as a potential active agent. A small RCT (chamomile 220–1,100 mg, 1.2% apigenin vs. placebo) suggests that chamomile may be useful in the treatment of GAD.[103]

Kava

Similarly, kava roots have been consumed throughout the Pacific Ocean cultures of Polynesia, as a drink with sedative and anesthetic properties. Although earlier reports were inconclusive,[104,105] a recent RCT provides some support for the efficacy of its active agent kavalactones (120–240 mg) in the treatment of GAD.[106]

SOCIAL ANXIETY DISORDER

The pharmacotherapy of social anxiety disorder (SAD) is aimed at reducing the patient's anticipatory anxiety prior to and distress during social interaction and performance situations, reducing avoidance of social and performance situations, and improving associated impairments in quality of life and function.

Selective serotonin Reuptake Inhibitors and Serotonin Norepinephrine Reuptake Inhibitors

Selective serotonin and SNRIs have become first-line pharmacotherapy for the treatment of SAD because of their greater efficacy for this condition, broad-spectrum effects for other anxiety disorders, efficacy for co-morbid depression in contrast to the benzodiazepines, better tolerability than the TCAs, more favorable safety profile than the monoamine oxidase inhibitors (MAOIs), and lack of abuse potential. Currently, the SSRIs paroxetine and sertraline as well as the SNRI venlafaxine (extended-release) have FDA-approved indications for SAD, though available evidence suggests that other agents from these classes, including fluvoxamine,[107–111] citalopram, and escitalopram.[112–114] Regarding fluoxetine, the reported study results have been mixed.[115–117] Finally, some recent data suggest the efficacy of the SNRI duloxetine for the treatment of SAD as well.[118] A meta-analysis of the efficacy of second-generation antidepressants in SAD[119] suggests that escitalopram, paroxetine, sertraline, and venlafaxine produced significantly more responders than placebo and that there were no differences in terms of efficacy among them.

As noted, individuals with SAD are at increased risk for alcohol and other substance abuse, which may in some cases reflect an attempt to "self medicate" anxiety in social situations. A small, randomized placebo-controlled study,[120] in individuals with SAD and active alcohol use disorders, suggested that treatment with the SSRI paroxetine decreased the anxiety and may have reduced the alcohol use as well.

Treatment with the SSRIs and SNRIs for SAD is typically initiated at low doses (e.g., paroxetine 10 mg/d, sertraline 25 mg/d, venlafaxine-extended release 37.5 mg/d) and titrated up against therapeutic response and tolerability (e.g., paroxetine 20–60 mg/d, sertraline 50–200 mg/d, and venlafaxine 75–225 mg/d). There is usually a therapeutic lag in efficacy of 2–3 weeks following initiation of SSRI/SNRI therapy for SAD, although full response can occur over weeks to months, particularly when social anxiety-related avoidance is present, and a return to avoided situations should be encouraged alongside pharmacotherapy to both assess and optimize outcomes. Typical treatment-emergent adverse effects include nausea, headache, dizziness, sedation, increased anxiety, and sexual dysfunction.

Beta-blockers

Beta-blockers, including propranolol (Inderal) and atenolol (Tenormin) are effective for the treatment of non-generalized social anxiety (i.e., "performance anxiety") about public speaking or other performance situations.[121,122] Beta-blockers blunt the symptoms of physiological arousal associated with anxiety or fear, such as tachycardia and tremor, which are often the focus of an individual's apprehension in performance situations and lead to an escalating cycle of arousal, agitation, and further elevations in social anxiety. Beta-blockers are effective for the treatment of performance anxiety, at least in part by blocking these physiological symptoms of arousal, interrupting the escalating fear cycle, and thus mitigating the individual's escalating concern and focus on their anxiety.

Though effective for physiological symptoms of arousal, beta-blockers are not as effective at reducing the emotional and cognitive aspects of social anxiety and thus are not first-line agents for generalized SAD. Results from a double-blind, placebo-controlled study of the beta-blocker atenolol and the MAOI phenelzine found the beta-blocker ineffective for individuals with generalized social anxiety.[123]

Beta-blockers (e.g., propranolol [10–80 mg/d] or atenolol [50–150 mg/d]) are typically administered "as needed" 1–2 hours before a performance situation. The use of beta-blockers may be associated with orthostatic hypotension, lightheadedness, bradycardia, sedation, and nausea. Atenolol is less lipophilic[124] and thus less centrally active than propranolol, and, therefore, may be less sedating. In practice, it is best to administer a "test dose" of the beta-blocker prior to use in an actual performance-related event in order to establish the tolerability of an effective dose and minimize disruptive side effects during a performance that could further increase anxiety.

Monoamine Oxidase Inhibitors

Before they were supplanted by the SSRIs and SNRIs, the MAOIs were the "gold-standard" pharmacological treatment for SAD. Interest in their use in SAD grew in part from initial observations of their efficacy for the atypical subtype of depression characterized in part by marked sensitivity to rejection,[125] and they were subsequently demonstrated effective in RCTs in SAD.[123]

Though clearly effective, the use of MAOIs is associated with troubling side effects including orthostatic hypotension, paresthesias, weight gain, and sexual dysfunction, as well as the need for careful attention to diet and use of concomitant medication because of the risk of potentially fatal hypertensive reactions and serotonin syndrome if the proscriptions are violated. Concerns about the use of MAOIs may have contributed in part to the under-recognition and treatment of SAD[126] that existed until demonstration of the efficacy of the generally safer and easier-to-use SSRIs and SNRIs for this syndrome.

Among the MAOIs, phenelzine has been the best studied for SAD,[123,127,128] although tranylcypromine also appears effective.[129] In a study comparing cognitive-behavioral group therapy (CBGT), phenelzine, an educational-supportive group, and a placebo for the treatment of SAD (n=133),[130] 77% of patients taking phenelzine, were responders at 12 weeks compared to 41% of those in the placebo group (p < 0.005); phenelzine appeared to be more effect than CBGT on some measures during acute treatment, but the psychosocial intervention resulted in better maintenance of benefit after treatment discontinuation.[131]

Phenelzine is typically initiated at 15 mg PO BID, and is less likely than reuptake inhibitors (such as the TCAs, SSRIs, or SNRIs) to exacerbate anxiety during initiation of treatment. The usual therapeutic dose range of phenelzine is 60 to 90 mg/d, with some refractory patients responding to higher doses. Careful attention to adherence to a diet free of tyramine-containing foods and avoidance of sympathomimetic and other serotonergic drugs is important to avoid the risk of hypertensive or serotonergic crisis, and assessment of the ability of an individual patient to maintain these restrictions is a critical component of the risk–benefit analysis of MAOI usage.

Interest in the reversible inhibitors of MAO_A (RIMAs) was stimulated by the significant safety concerns attendant to the administration of the irreversible MAOIs, such as phenelzine. Because they can be displaced from MAO when a substrate (such as tyramine) is presented, the RIMAs do not carry with them the need for strict dietary prohibitions and the risk of hypertensive crisis and serotonin syndrome associated with the irreversible MAOIs. Unfortunately, while some clinical trials have reported positive results with RIMAs (such as moclobemide and brofaromine) for SAD, others have not.[132] Further, while moclobemide is available in some countries, it is generally not perceived as effective as standard MAOIs and is not available in the US. There are no systematic data available to date regarding the efficacy of the selegiline transdermal patch for the treatment of SAD.

Benzodiazepines

Although benzodiazepines are commonly used for many anxiety disorders (including SAD) there are relatively few systematic data addressing their use for this indication. However, the available data do suggest efficacy for these agents with response noted as soon as early as 2 weeks in non-depressed individuals with SAD.[127,133,134] Benzodiazepines may also help enhance response to an antidepressant; results from a randomized, double-blind placebo-controlled study demonstrated that the addition of clonazepam 1–2 mg/d to flexibly, dosed paroxetine (20–40 mg/d) resulted in greater improvement than paroxetine alone in generalized SAD.[135]

As noted, benzodiazepines have the advantage of a relatively rapid onset of effect, a favorable side-effect profile, and efficacy on an as-needed basis for situational anxiety. The use of benzodiazepines, however, may be associated with treatment-emergent adverse effects (including sedation, ataxia, and cognitive and psychomotor impairment), as well as the development of physiological dependence with regular use. Further, they are generally not effective for depression that commonly presents as co-morbid with SAD, and may worsen it. Their potential for abuse in those with a diathesis or a history of alcohol or substance abuse, and their potential negative interaction with concurrent alcohol use, is relevant given the increased rates of alcohol and substance use amongst social phobics. Benzodiazepines are initiated at low dose (e.g., clonazepam 0.25–0.5 mg qHS) to minimize emergent adverse effects (such as sedation) and then titrated up as tolerated to therapeutic doses (e.g., clonazepam 1–4 mg/d or its equivalent).

For maintenance treatment, in order to optimize a continuous anxiolytic effect, longer-acting benzodiazepines (such as clonazepam) are associated with less inter-dose rebound anxiety than shorter-acting agents and are generally preferred, whereas a shorter-acting agent with a more rapid onset of effect (such as alprazolam or lorazepam) may be more appropriate if used on an as-needed basis for performance situations. Monotherapy with as-needed dosing of benzodiazepines alone is not, however, recommended for non-"performance only" social anxiety disorder, and as-needed benzodiazepine use may interfere with the reduction of social anxiety and related avoidance with cognitive behavioral treatments.[136]

Other medications

Although TCAs are useful for a number of anxiety disorders including panic disorder, PTSD, GAD, and, in the case of clomipramine, OCD, results from open[19] and double-blind placebo-controlled trials[137] suggest they are not effective for the treatment of SAD. Small open trials have suggested the efficacy of bupropion in SAD.[138] Although the noradrenergic and serotonergic antidepressant mirtazapine has been reported to be effective for SAD in open-label studies,[139,140] as well as in a RCT conducted specifically in women,[141] a recent randomized placebo-controlled trial failed to replicate these results in a sample (n = 60) including adults of both genders.[142] Available evidence does not support the use of buspirone as a monotherapy for the treatment of SAD, although one report suggests that it may have a role as an adjunct for patients incompletely responsive to SSRI therapy.[79] Small studies and case series suggest the potential efficacy of atypical antipsychotics, including olanzapine,[143] risperidone,[62] and quetiapine[144,145] for the treatment of SAD, but their use is generally reserved for patients remaining symptomatic despite more standard interventions. A number of anticonvulsants have demonstrated potential efficacy for the treatment of SAD. Gabapentin, a GABA (an alpha-$_2$ delta calcium channel antagonist), demonstrated efficacy for SAD in a double-blind, placebo-controlled, parallel-group trial with doses of ranging from 900 to 3,600 mg daily, with most patients receiving greater than 2,100 mg/d.[146] A related compound, pregabalin, currently indicated for the treatment of neuropathic pain and as adjunctive treatment for partial seizures, also demonstrated efficacy for the treatment of SAD at a dose of 600 mg/d, although the side-effect burden at this higher dose was significant.[147] Valproic acid, an anticonvulsant mood-stabilizer, was reported effective for SAD, in an open trial with flexible dosing of 500–2,500 mg/d.[148] Levetiracetam demonstrated promising potential for the treatment of SAD in open trial,[149] but recent RCT data failed to show any efficacy over placebo.[150,151] An open-label trial suggests the potential efficacy of topiramate[152] and tiagabine[153] for the treatment of SAD; however, to date, no RCTs have confirmed these findings.

Though the adjunctive use of pindolol, a beta-blocker with 5-HT$_{1A}$ autoreceptor antagonist properties, has in some, but not all, studies accelerated or augmented response to antidepressants for depression,[154] it was ineffective in one placebo-controlled randomized augmentation trial in social phobics.[155] Other medications, such as the pre-synaptic adrenergic agonist clonidine[156] and the 5-HT$_3$ receptor ondansetron,[157] have been reported helpful for social anxiety in case reports, but there are few systematic data following up on these observations.

CONCLUSIONS AND FUTURE DIRECTIONS

The increased recognition of the prevalence, early-onset, chronicity, and morbid impact of the anxiety disorders has spurred development efforts to find more effective and better-tolerated pharmacotherapies for this condition. Though the SSRIs/SNRIs and benzodiazepines have demonstrated efficacy and favorable tolerability compared to older classes of agents, many patients remain symptomatic despite standard treatment; only a minority remit. In addition to creative uses of available agents alone and in combination, a variety of other pharmacological agents with novel mechanisms of actions, including corticotropin releasing factor (CRF) antagonists, neurokinin (NK)-substance P antagonists, metabotropic glutamate receptor agonists, GABA-ergic agents and receptor modulators, and compounds with a variety of effects on serotonin, noradrenergic, and dopaminergic receptors and their subtypes are in various stages of development. In addition, specific agents targeting ways to enhance outcomes with cognitive-behavioral therapy for anxiety disorders, such as the NMDA receptor antagonist D-cycloserine, remain an active area of translational research.[158,159] These efforts may provide more effective and better-tolerated agents for the treatment of anxiety in the future.

Access a list of MCQs for this chapter at https://expertconsult.inkling.com

REFERENCES

1. Stahl SM, Gergel I, Li D. Escitalopram in the treatment of panic disorder: a randomized, double-blind, placebo-controlled trial. *J Clin Psychiatry* 64(11):1322–1327, 2003.
2. Irons J. Fluvoxamine in the treatment of anxiety disorders. *Neuropsychiatr Dis Treat* 1(4):289–299, 2005.
3. Crippa JA, Zuardi AW. Duloxetine in the treatment of panic disorder. *Int J Neuropsychopharmacol* 9(5):633–634, 2006.
4. Simon NM, Kaufman RE, Hoge EA, et al. Open-label support for duloxetine for the treatment of panic disorder. *CNS Neurosci Ther* 15(1):19–23, 2009.
5. Andrisano C, Chiesa A, Serretti A. Newer antidepressants and panic disorder: a meta-analysis. *Int Clin Psychopharmacol* 28(1):33–45, 2013.
6. Pollack MH, Allgulander C, Bandelow B, et al. WCA recommendations for the long-term treatment of panic disorder. *CNS Spectr* 8(8 Suppl. 1):17–30, 2003.
7. Dannon PN, Iancu I, Cohen A, et al. Three year naturalistic outcome study of panic disorder patients treated with paroxetine. *BMC Psychiatry* 4:16, 2004.
8. Modell JG, Katholi CR, Modell JD, et al. Comparative sexual side effects of bupropion, fluoxetine, paroxetine, and sertraline. *Clin Pharmacol Ther* 61(4):476–487, 1997.
9. Ballenger JC, Wheadon DE, Steiner M, et al. Double-blind, fixed-dose, placebo-controlled study of paroxetine in the treatment of panic disorder. *Am J Psychiatry* 155(1):36–42, 1998.
10. Fava M, Judge R, Hoog SL, et al. Fluoxetine versus sertraline and paroxetine in major depressive disorder: changes in weight with long-term treatment. *J Clin Psychiatry* 61(11):863–867, 2000.
11. Fava M. Prospective studies of adverse events related to antidepressant discontinuation. *J Clin Psychiatry* 67(Suppl. 4):14–21, 2006.
12. Pollack MH, Lepola U, Koponen H, et al. A double-blind study of the efficacy of venlafaxine extended-release, paroxetine, and placebo in the treatment of panic disorder. *Depress Anxiety* 24(1):1–14, 2007.
13. Pollack MH. The pharmacotherapy of panic disorder. *J Clin Psychiatry* 66(Suppl. 4):23–27, 2005.
14. Rosenbaum JF, Pollack MH, Fredman SJ. The pharmacotherapy of panic disorder. In Rosenbaum JF, Pollack MH, editors: *Panic disorder and its treatment*, New York, 1998, Marcel Dekker Inc., pp 153–180.
15. Bakker A, van Dyck R, Spinhoven P, et al. Paroxetine, clomipramine, and cognitive therapy in the treatment of panic disorder. *J Clin Psychiatry* 60(12):831–838, 1999.
16. den Boer JA, Westenberg HG, Kamerbeek WD, et al. Effect of serotonin uptake inhibitors in anxiety disorders; a double-blind comparison of clomipramine and fluvoxamine. *Int Clin Psychopharmacol* 2(1):21–32, 1987.
17. Noyes R Jr, Perry P. Maintenance treatment with antidepressants in panic disorder. *J Clin Psychiatry* 51(Suppl. A):24–30, 1990.
18. Bakish D, Hooper CL, Filteau MJ, et al. A double-blind placebo-controlled trial comparing fluvoxamine and imipramine in the treatment of panic disorder with or without agoraphobia. *Psychopharmacol Bull* 32(1):135–141, 1996.
19. Simpson HB, Schneier FR, Campeas RB, et al. Imipramine in the treatment of social phobia. *J Clin Psychopharmacol* 18(2):132–135, 1998.
20. Sheehan DV, Ballenger J, Jacobsen G. Treatment of endogenous anxiety with phobic, hysterical, and hypochondriacal symptoms. *Arch Gen Psychiatry* 37(1):51–59, 1980.
21. Livingston MG, Livingston HM. Monoamine oxidase inhibitors. An update on drug interactions. *Drug Saf* 14(4):219–227, 1996.
22. Lippman SB, Nash K. Monoamine oxidase inhibitor update. Potential adverse food and drug interactions. *Drug Saf* 5(3):195–204, 1990.
23. van Vliet IM, Westenberg HG, Den Boer JA. MAO inhibitors in panic disorder: clinical effects of treatment with brofaromine. A double blind placebo controlled study. *Psychopharmacology (Berl)* 112(4):483–489, 1993.
24. van Vliet IM, den Boer JA, Westenberg HG. Slaap BR. A double-blind comparative study of brofaromine and fluvoxamine in outpatients with panic disorder. *J Clin Psychopharmacol* 16(4):299–306, 1996.
25. Bakish D, Saxena BM, Bowen R, et al. Reversible monoamine oxidase-A inhibitors in panic disorder. *Clin Neuropharmacol* 16(Suppl. 2):S77–S82, 1993.
26. Loerch B, Graf-Morgenstern M, Hautzinger M, et al. Randomised placebo-controlled trial of moclobemide, cognitive-behavioural therapy and their combination in panic disorder with agoraphobia. *Br J Psychiatry* 174:205–212, 1999.
27. Tiller JW, Bouwer C, Behnke K. Moclobemide and fluoxetine for panic disorder. International Panic Disorder Study Group. *Eur Arch Psychiatry Clin Neurosci* 249(Suppl. 1):S7–S10, 1999.
28. Practice guideline for the treatment of patients with panic disorder. Work Group on Panic Disorder. American Psychiatric Association. *Am J Psychiatry* 155(5 Suppl.):1–34, 1998.
29. Bruce SE, Vasile RG, Goisman RM, et al. Are benzodiazepines still the medication of choice for patients with panic disorder with or without agoraphobia? *Am J Psychiatry* 160(8):1432–1438, 2003.
30. Noyes R Jr, Burrows GD, Reich JH, et al. Diazepam versus alprazolam for the treatment of panic disorder. *J Clin Psychiatry* 57(8):349–355, 1996.
31. Dunner DL, Ishiki D, Avery DH, et al. Effect of alprazolam and diazepam on anxiety and panic attacks in panic disorder: a controlled study. *J Clin Psychiatry* 47(9):458–460, 1986.
32. Charney DS, Woods SW. Benzodiazepine treatment of panic disorder: a comparison of alprazolam and lorazepam. *J Clin Psychiatry* 50(11):418–423, 1989.
33. Schweizer E, Fox I, Case G, et al. Lorazepam vs. alprazolam in the treatment of panic disorder. *Psychopharmacol Bull* 24(2):224–227, 1988.
34. Schweizer E, Pohl R, Balon R, et al. Lorazepam vs. alprazolam in the treatment of panic disorder. *Pharmacopsychiatry* 23(2):90–93, 1990.
35. Stewart SA. The effects of benzodiazepines on cognition. *J Clin Psychiatry* 66(Suppl. 2):9–13, 2005.
36. Nagy LM, Krystal JH, Woods SW, et al. Clinical and medication outcome after short-term alprazolam and behavioral group treatment in panic disorder. 2.5 year naturalistic follow-up study. *Arch Gen Psychiatry* 46(11):993–999, 1989.
37. Pollack MH, Otto MW, Tesar GE, et al. Long-term outcome after acute treatment with alprazolam or clonazepam for panic disorder. *J Clin Psychopharmacol* 13(4):257–263, 1993.
38. Soumerai SB, Simoni-Wastila L, Singer C, et al. Lack of relationship between long-term use of benzodiazepines and escalation to high dosages. *Psychiatr Serv* 54(7):1006–1011, 2003.
39. Nardi AE, Freire RC, Mochcovitch MD, et al. A randomized, naturalistic, parallel-group study for the long-term treatment of panic disorder with clonazepam or paroxetine. *J Clin Psychopharmacol* 32(1):120–126, 2012.
40. Nardi AE, Valenca AM, Freire RC, et al. Randomized, open naturalistic, acute treatment of panic disorder with clonazepam or paroxetine. *J Clin Psychopharmacol* 31(2):259–261, 2011.

41. Pecknold JC, Swinson RP, Kuch K, et al. Alprazolam in panic disorder and agoraphobia: results from a multicenter trial. III. Discontinuation effects. *Arch Gen Psychiatry* 45(5):429–436, 1988.

42. Rickels K, Schweizer E, Weiss S, et al. Maintenance drug treatment for panic disorder. II. Short- and long-term outcome after drug taper. *Arch Gen Psychiatry* 50(1):61–68, 1993.

43. Otto MW, Pollack MH, Sachs GS, et al. Discontinuation of benzodiazepine treatment: efficacy of cognitive-behavioral therapy for patients with panic disorder. *Am J Psychiatry* 150(10):1485–1490, 1993.

44. Kan CC, Hilberink SR, Breteler MH. Determination of the main risk factors for benzodiazepine dependence using a multivariate and multidimensional approach. *Compr Psychiatry* 45(2):88–94, 2004.

45. Gaudreault P, Guay J, Thivierge RL, et al. Benzodiazepine poisoning. Clinical and pharmacological considerations and treatment. *Drug Saf* 6(4):247–265, 1991.

46. Greenblatt DJ, Shader RI, Abernethy DR. Drug therapy. Current status of benzodiazepines. *N Engl J Med* 309(6):354–358, 1983.

47. Mitte K. A meta-analysis of the efficacy of psycho- and pharmacotherapy in panic disorder with and without agoraphobia. *J Affect Disord* 88(1):27–45, 2005.

48. Pollack MH, Simon NM, Worthington JJ, et al. Combined paroxetine and clonazepam treatment strategies compared to paroxetine monotherapy for panic disorder. *J Psychopharmacol* 17(3):276–282, 2003.

49. Goddard AW, Brouette T, Almai A, et al. Early coadministration of clonazepam with sertraline for panic disorder. *Arch Gen Psychiatry* 58(7):681–686, 2001.

50. Simon NM, Otto MW, Worthington JJ, et al. Next-step strategies for panic disorder refractory to initial pharmacotherapy: a 3-phase randomized clinical trial. *J Clin Psychiatry* 70(11):1563–1570, 2009.

51. Sheehan DV, Davidson J, Manschreck T, et al. Lack of efficacy of a new antidepressant (bupropion) in the treatment of panic disorder with phobias. *J Clin Psychopharmacol* 3(1):28–31, 1983.

52. Simon NM, Emmanuel N, Ballenger J, et al. Bupropion sustained release for panic disorder. *Psychopharmacol Bull* 37(4):66–72, 2003.

53. Versiani M, Cassano G, Perugi G, et al. Reboxetine, a selective norepinephrine reuptake inhibitor, is an effective and well-tolerated treatment for panic disorder. *J Clin Psychiatry* 63(1):31–37, 2002.

54. Bertani A, Perna G, Migliarese G, et al. Comparison of the treatment with paroxetine and reboxetine in panic disorder: a randomized, single-blind study. *Pharmacopsychiatry* 37(5):206–210, 2004.

55. Gastfriend DR, Rosenbaum JF. Adjunctive buspirone in benzodiazepine treatment of four patients with panic disorder. *Am J Psychiatry* 146(7):914–916, 1989.

56. Bouvard M, Mollard E, Guerin J, et al. Study and course of the psychological profile in 77 patients expressing panic disorder with agoraphobia after cognitive behaviour therapy with or without buspirone. *Psychother Psychosom* 66(1):27–32, 1997.

57. Sheehan DV, Raj AB, Sheehan KH, et al. Is buspirone effective for panic disorder? *J Clin Psychopharmacol* 10(1):3–11, 1990.

58. Sheehan DV, Raj AB, Harnett-Sheehan K, et al. The relative efficacy of high-dose buspirone and alprazolam in the treatment of panic disorder: a double-blind placebo-controlled study. *Acta Psychiatr Scand* 88(1):1–11, 1993.

59. Munjack DJ, Crocker B, Cabe D, et al. Alprazolam, propranolol, and placebo in the treatment of panic disorder and agoraphobia with panic attacks. *J Clin Psychopharmacol* 9(1):22–27, 1989.

60. Hirschmann S, Dannon PN, Iancu I, et al. Pindolol augmentation in patients with treatment-resistant panic disorder: A double-blind, placebo-controlled trial. *J Clin Psychopharmacol* 20(5):556–559, 2000.

61. Hollifield M, Thompson PM, Ruiz JE, et al. Potential effectiveness and safety of olanzapine in refractory panic disorder. *Depress Anxiety* 21(1):33–40, 2005.

62. Simon NM, Hoge EA, Fischmann D, et al. An open-label trial of risperidone augmentation for refractory anxiety disorders. *J Clin Psychiatry* 67(3):381–385, 2006.

63. Worthington JJ 3rd, Kinrys G, Wygant LE, et al. Aripiprazole as an augmentor of selective serotonin reuptake inhibitors in depression and anxiety disorder patients. *Int Clin Psychopharmacol* 20(1):9–11, 2005.

64. Hoge EA, Worthington JJ 3rd, Kaufman RE, et al. Aripiprazole as augmentation treatment of refractory generalized anxiety disorder and panic disorder. *CNS Spectr* 13(6):522–527, 2008.

65. Prosser JM, Yard S, Steele A, et al. A comparison of low-dose risperidone to paroxetine in the treatment of panic attacks: a randomized, single-blind study. *BMC Psychiatry* 9:25, 2009.

66. Woodman CL, Noyes R Jr. Panic disorder: treatment with valproate. *J Clin Psychiatry* 55(4):134–136, 1994.

67. Lum M, Fontaine R, Elie R. Divalproex sodium's antipanic effect in panic disorder: A placebo-controlled study. *Biol Psychiatry* 27(Suppl. 1):164A–165A, 1990.

68. Uhde TW, Stein MB, Post RM. Lack of efficacy of carbamazepine in the treatment of panic disorder. *Am J Psychiatry* 145(9):1104–1109, 1988.

69. Pande AC, Pollack MH, Crockatt J, et al. Placebo-controlled study of gabapentin treatment of panic disorder. *J Clin Psychopharmacol* 20(4):467–471, 2000.

70. Rickels K, Pollack MH, Feltner DE, et al. Pregabalin for treatment of generalized anxiety disorder: a 4-week, multicenter, double-blind, placebo-controlled trial of pregabalin and alprazolam. *Arch Gen Psychiatry* 62(9):1022–1030, 2005.

71. Bielski RJ, Bose A, Chang CC. A double-blind comparison of escitalopram and paroxetine in the long-term treatment of generalized anxiety disorder. *Ann Clin Psychiatry* 17(2):65–69, 2005.

72. Montgomery SA, Sheehan DV, Meoni P, et al. Characterization of the longitudinal course of improvement in generalized anxiety disorder during long-term treatment with venlafaxine XR. *J Psychiatr Res* 36(4):209–217, 2002.

73. Stocchi F, Nordera G, Jokinen RH, et al. Efficacy and tolerability of paroxetine for the long-term treatment of generalized anxiety disorder. *J Clin Psychiatry* 64(3):250–258, 2003.

74. Rickels K, Downing R, Schweizer E, et al. Antidepressants for the treatment of generalized anxiety disorder. A placebo-controlled comparison of imipramine, trazodone, and diazepam. *Arch Gen Psychiatry* 50(11):884–895, 1993.

75. Rocca P, Fonzo V, Scotta M, et al. Paroxetine efficacy in the treatment of generalized anxiety disorder. *Acta Psychiatr Scand* 95(5):444–450, 1997.

76. Allgulander C, Bandelow B, Hollander E, et al. WCA recommendations for the long-term treatment of generalized anxiety disorder. *CNS Spectr* 8(8 Suppl. 1):53–61, 2003.

77. Ballenger JC. Benzodiazepines. In Schatzberg AF, Nemeroff CB, editors: *Textbook of psychopharmacology*, Washington, DC, 1998, American Psychiatric Press, pp 271–286.

78. Rickels K, Schweizer E. The treatment of generalized anxiety disorder in patients with depressive symptomatology. *J Clin Psychiatry* 54(Suppl.):20–23, 1993.

79. Van Ameringen M, Mancini C, Wilson C. Buspirone augmentation of selective serotonin reuptake inhibitors (SSRIs) in social phobia. *J Affect Disord* 39(2):115–121, 1996.

80. Appelberg BG, Syvalahti EK, Koskinen TE, et al. Patients with severe depression may benefit from buspirone augmentation of selective serotonin reuptake inhibitors: results from a placebo-controlled, randomized, double-blind, placebo wash-in study. *J Clin Psychiatry* 62(6):448–452, 2001.

81. Strand M, Hetta J, Rosen A, et al. A double-blind, controlled trial in primary care patients with generalized anxiety: a comparison between buspirone and oxazepam. *J Clin Psychiatry* 51(Suppl.):40–45, 1990.

82. Chessick CA, Allen MH, Thase M, et al. Azapirones for generalized anxiety disorder. *Cochrane Database Syst Rev* (3):CD006115, 2006.

83. Boschen MJ. A meta-analysis of the efficacy of pregabalin in the treatment of generalized anxiety disorder. *Can J Psychiatry* 56(9):558–566, 2011.

84. Stein DJ, Baldwin DS, Baldinetti F, et al. Efficacy of pregabalin in depressive symptoms associated with generalized anxiety disorder: a pooled analysis of 6 studies. *Eur Neuropsychopharmacol* 18(6):422–430, 2008.

85. Kasper S, Herman B, Nivoli G, et al. Efficacy of pregabalin and venlafaxine-XR in generalized anxiety disorder: results of

a double-blind, placebo-controlled 8-week trial. *Int Clin Psychopharmacol* 24(2):87–96, 2009.
86. Montgomery SA, Tobias K, Zornberg GL, et al. Efficacy and safety of pregabalin in the treatment of generalized anxiety disorder: a 6-week, multicenter, randomized, double-blind, placebo-controlled comparison of pregabalin and venlafaxine. *J Clin Psychiatry* 67(5):771–782, 2006.
87. Feltner DE, Crockatt JG, Dubovsky SJ, et al. A randomized, double-blind, placebo-controlled, fixed-dose, multicenter study of pregabalin in patients with generalized anxiety disorder. *J Clin Psychopharmacol* 23(3):240–249, 2003.
88. Pollack MH, Roy-Byrne PP, Van Ameringen M, et al. The selective GABA reuptake inhibitor tiagabine for the treatment of generalized anxiety disorder: results of a placebo-controlled study. *J Clin Psychiatry* 66(11):1401–1408, 2005.
89. Pollack M, Tiller J, Zie F, et al. *Tiagabine in adult patients with generalized anxiety disorder: results from three randomized, double-blind, placebo-controlled, parallel-group studies.* Submitted for Publication.
90. Pollack MH, Tiller J, Xie F, et al. Tiagabine in adult patients with generalized anxiety disorder: results from 3 randomized, double-blind, placebo-controlled, parallel-group studies. *J Clin Psychopharmacol* 28(3):308–316, 2008.
91. Mendels J, Krajewski TF, Huffer V, et al. Effective short-term treatment of generalized anxiety disorder with trifluoperazine. *J Clin Psychiatry* 47(4):170–174, 1986.
92. Pollack MH, Simon NM, Zalta AK, et al. Olanzapine augmentation of fluoxetine for refractory generalized anxiety disorder: a placebo controlled study. *Biol Psychiatry* 59(3):211–215, 2006.
93. Brawman-Mintzer O, Knapp RG, Nietert PJ. Adjunctive risperidone in generalized anxiety disorder: a double-blind, placebo-controlled study. *J Clin Psychiatry* 66(10):1321–1325, 2005.
94. Snyderman SH, Rynn MA, Rickels K. Open-label pilot study of ziprasidone for refractory generalized anxiety disorder. *J Clin Psychopharmacol* 25(5):497–499, 2005.
95. Bandelow B, Chouinard G, Bobes J, et al. Extended-release quetiapine fumarate (quetiapine XR): a once-daily monotherapy effective in generalized anxiety disorder. Data from a randomized, double-blind, placebo- and active-controlled study. *Int J Neuropsychopharmacol* 13(3):305–320, 2010.
96. Katzman MA, Brawman-Mintzer O, Reyes EB, et al. Extended release quetiapine fumarate (quetiapine XR) monotherapy as maintenance treatment for generalized anxiety disorder: a long-term, randomized, placebo-controlled trial. *Int Clin Psychopharmacol* 26(1):11–24, 2011.
97. Khan A, Joyce M, Atkinson S, et al. A randomized, double-blind study of once-daily extended release quetiapine fumarate (quetiapine XR) monotherapy in patients with generalized anxiety disorder. *J Clin Psychopharmacol* 31(4):418–428, 2011.
98. Merideth C, Cutler AJ, She F, et al. Efficacy and tolerability of extended release quetiapine fumarate monotherapy in the acute treatment of generalized anxiety disorder: a randomized, placebo controlled and active-controlled study. *Int Clin Psychopharmacol* 27(1):40–54, 2012.
99. Mezhebovsky I, Magi K, She F, et al. Double-blind, randomized study of extended release quetiapine fumarate (quetiapine XR) monotherapy in older patients with generalized anxiety disorder. *Int J Geriatr Psychiatry* 28(6):615–625, 2013.
100. Ketter TA, Nasrallah HA, Fagiolini A. Mood stabilizers and atypical antipsychotics: bimodal treatments for bipolar disorder. *Psychopharmacol Bull* 39(1):120–146, 2006.
101. Rapaport MH, Gharabawi GM, Canuso CM, et al. Effects of risperidone augmentation in patients with treatment-resistant depression: Results of open-label treatment followed by double-blind continuation. *Neuropsychopharmacology* 31(11):2505–2513, 2006.
102. Mathew SJ, Amiel JM, Coplan JD, et al. Open-label trial of riluzole in generalized anxiety disorder. *Am J Psychiatry* 162(12):2379–2381, 2005.
103. Amsterdam JD, Li Y, Soeller I, et al. A randomized, double-blind, placebo-controlled trial of oral Matricaria recutita (chamomile) extract therapy for generalized anxiety disorder. *J Clin Psychopharmacol* 29(4):378–382, 2009.
104. Connor KM, Payne V, Davidson JR. Kava in generalized anxiety disorder: three placebo-controlled trials. *Int Clin Psychopharmacol* 21(5):249–253, 2006.
105. Connor KM, Davidson JR. A placebo-controlled study of Kava kava in generalized anxiety disorder. *Int Clin Psychopharmacol* 17(4):185–188, 2002.
106. Sarris J, Stough C, Bousman CA, et al. Kava in the treatment of generalized anxiety disorder: a double-blind, randomized, placebo-controlled study. *J Clin Psychopharmacol* Apr 30 2013.
107. Asakura S, Tajima O, Koyama T. Fluvoxamine treatment of generalized social anxiety disorder in Japan: a randomized double-blind, placebo-controlled study. *Int J Neuropsychopharmacol* 10(2):263–274, 2007.
108. Davidson J, Yaryura-Tobias J, DuPont R, et al. Fluvoxamine-controlled release formulation for the treatment of generalized social anxiety disorder. *J Clin Psychopharmacol* 24(2):118–125, 2004.
109. Owen RT. Controlled-release fluvoxamine in obsessive-compulsive disorder and social phobia. *Drugs Today (Barc)* 44(12):887–893, 2008.
110. Stein MB, Fyer AJ, Davidson JR, et al. Fluvoxamine treatment of social phobia (social anxiety disorder): a double-blind, placebo-controlled study. *Am J Psychiatry* 156(5):756–760, 1999.
111. van Vliet IM, den Boer JA, Westenberg HG. Psychopharmacological treatment of social phobia; a double blind placebo controlled study with fluvoxamine. *Psychopharmacology (Berl)* 115(1–2):128–134, 1994.
112. Furmark T, Appel L, Michelgard A, et al. Cerebral blood flow changes after treatment of social phobia with the neurokinin-1 antagonist GR205171, citalopram, or placebo. *Biol Psychiatry* 58(2):132–142, 2005.
113. Kasper S, Stein DJ, Loft H, et al. Escitalopram in the treatment of social anxiety disorder: randomised, placebo-controlled, flexible-dosage study. *Br J Psychiatry* 186:222–226, 2005.
114. Lader M, Stender K, Burger V, et al. Efficacy and tolerability of escitalopram in 12- and 24-week treatment of social anxiety disorder: randomised, double-blind, placebo-controlled, fixed-dose study. *Depress Anxiety* 19(4):241–248, 2004.
115. Davidson JR, Foa EB, Huppert JD, et al. Fluoxetine, comprehensive cognitive behavioral therapy, and placebo in generalized social phobia. *Arch Gen Psychiatry* 61(10):1005–1013, 2004.
116. Kobak KA, Greist JH, Jefferson JW, et al. Fluoxetine in social phobia: a double-blind, placebo-controlled pilot study. *J Clin Psychopharmacol* 22(3):257–262, 2002.
117. Clark DM, Ehlers A, McManus F, et al. Cognitive therapy versus fluoxetine in generalized social phobia: a randomized placebo-controlled trial. *J Consult Clin Psychol* 71(6):1058–1067, 2003.
118. Simon NM, Worthington JJ, Moshier SJ, et al. Duloxetine for the treatment of generalized social anxiety disorder: a preliminary randomized trial of increased dose to optimize response. *CNS Spectr* 15(7):367–373, 2010.
119. Hansen RA, Gaynes BN, Gartlehner G, et al. Efficacy and tolerability of second-generation antidepressants in social anxiety disorder. *Int Clin Psychopharmacol* 23(3):170–179, 2008.
120. Randall CL, Johnson MR, Thevos AK, et al. Paroxetine for social anxiety and alcohol use in dual-diagnosed patients. *Depress Anxiety* 14(4):255–262, 2001.
121. Brantigan CO, Brantigan TA, Joseph N. Effect of beta blockade and beta stimulation on stage fright. *Am J Med* 72(1):88–94, 1982.
122. Gossard D, Dennis C, DeBusk RF. Use of beta-blocking agents to reduce the stress of presentation at an international cardiology meeting: results of a survey. *Am J Cardiol* 54(1):240–241, 1984.
123. Liebowitz MR, Schneier F, Campeas R, et al. Phenelzine vs atenolol in social phobia. A placebo-controlled comparison. *Arch Gen Psychiatry* 49(4):290–300, 1992.
124. Conant J, Engler R, Janowsky D, et al. Central nervous system side effects of beta-adrenergic blocking agents with high and low lipid solubility. *J Cardiovasc Pharmacol* 13(4):656–661, 1989.
125. Welkowitz LA, Liebowitz MR. Pharmacologic treatment of social phobia and performance anxiety. In Noyes R, Roth M, Burrows GD, editors: *Handbook of anxiety*, vol. 4, London, 1990, Elsevier Science Publishers, pp 233–250.
126. Liebowitz MR, Gorman JM, Fyer AJ, et al. Social phobia. Review of a neglected anxiety disorder. *Arch Gen Psychiatry* 42(7):729–736, 1985.

41

127. Gelernter CS, Uhde TW, Cimbolic P, et al. Cognitive-behavioral and pharmacological treatments of social phobia. A controlled study. *Arch Gen Psychiatry* 48(10):938–945, 1991.

128. Versiani M, Nardi AE, Mundim FD, et al. Pharmacotherapy of social phobia. A controlled study with moclobemide and phenelzine. *Br J Psychiatry* 161:353–360, 1992.

129. Versiani M, Mundim FD, Nardi AE, et al. Tranylcypromine in social phobia. *J Clin Psychopharmacol* 8(4):279–283, 1988.

130. Heimberg RG, Liebowitz MR, Hope DA, et al. Cognitive behavioral group therapy vs phenelzine therapy for social phobia: 12-week outcome. *Arch Gen Psychiatry* 55(12):1133–1141, 1998.

131. Hart TA, Turk CL, Heimberg RG, et al. Relation of marital status to social phobia severity. *Depress Anxiety* 10(1):28–32, 1999.

132. Noyes R Jr, Moroz G, Davidson JR, et al. Moclobemide in social phobia: a controlled dose-response trial. *J Clin Psychopharmacol* 17(4):247–254, 1997.

133. Davidson JR, Potts N, Richichi E, et al. Treatment of social phobia with clonazepam and placebo. *J Clin Psychopharmacol* 13(6):423–428, 1993.

134. Otto MW, Pollack MH, Gould RA, et al. A comparison of the efficacy of clonazepam and cognitive-behavioral group therapy for the treatment of social phobia. *J Anxiety Disord* 14(4):345–358, 2000.

135. Seedat S, Stein MB. Double-blind, placebo-controlled assessment of combined clonazepam with paroxetine compared with paroxetine monotherapy for generalized social anxiety disorder. *J Clin Psychiatry* 65(2):244–248, 2004.

136. Hoge E, Pollack MH. Pharmacotherapy of social anxiety disorder: current practice and future promise. In Pollack M, Simon NM, Otto MW, editors: *Social anxiety disorder: research and practice*, New York, 2003, Professional Publishing Group, Ltd., pp 157–186.

137. Emmanuel N, Johnson M, Villareal G. *Impramine in the treatment of social phobia: a double-blind study.* Presented at American College of Neuropsychopharmacology 36 meeting, 1997, Waikoloa, Hawaii.

138. Emmanuel NP, Brawman-Mintzer O, Morton WA, et al. Bupropion-SR in treatment of social phobia. *Depress Anxiety* 12(2):111–113, 2000.

139. Van Veen JF, Van Vliet IM, Westenberg HG. Mirtazapine in social anxiety disorder: a pilot study. *Int Clin Psychopharmacol* 17(6):315–317, 2002.

140. Mrakotsky C, Masek B, Biederman J, et al. Prospective open-label pilot trial of mirtazapine in children and adolescents with social phobia. *J Anxiety Disord* 22(1):88–97, 2008.

141. Muehlbacher M, Nickel MK, Nickel C, et al. Mirtazapine treatment of social phobia in women: a randomized, double-blind, placebo-controlled study. *J Clin Psychopharmacol* 25(6):580–583, 2005.

142. Schutters SI, Van Megen HJ, Van Veen JF, et al. Mirtazapine in generalized social anxiety disorder: a randomized, double-blind, placebo-controlled study. *Int Clin Psychopharmacol* 25(5):302–304, 2010.

143. Barnett SD, Kramer ML, Casat CD, et al. Efficacy of olanzapine in social anxiety disorder: a pilot study. *J Psychopharmacol* 16(4):365–368, 2002.

144. Schutters SI, van Megen HJ, Westenberg HG. Efficacy of quetiapine in generalized social anxiety disorder: results from an open-label study. *J Clin Psychiatry* 66(4):540–542, 2005.

145. Vaishnavi S, Alamy S, Zhang W, et al. Quetiapine as monotherapy for social anxiety disorder: a placebo-controlled study. *Prog Neuropsychopharmacol Biol Psychiatry* 31(7):1464–1469, 2007.

146. Pande AC, Davidson JR, Jefferson JW, et al. Treatment of social phobia with gabapentin: a placebo-controlled study. *J Clin Psychopharmacol* 19(4):341–348, 1999.

147. Pande AC, Feltner DE, Jefferson JW, et al. Efficacy of the novel anxiolytic pregabalin in social anxiety disorder: a placebo-controlled, multicenter study. *J Clin Psychopharmacol* 24(2):141–149, 2004.

148. Kinrys G, Pollack MH, Simon NM, et al. Valproic acid for the treatment of social anxiety disorder. *Int Clin Psychopharmacol* 18:169–172, 2003.

149. Simon NM, Worthington JJ, Doyle AC, et al. An open-label study of levetiracetam for the treatment of social anxiety disorder. *J Clin Psychiatry* 65(9):1219–1222, 2004.

150. Stein MB, Ravindran LN, Simon NM, et al. Levetiracetam in generalized social anxiety disorder: a double-blind, randomized controlled trial. *J Clin Psychiatry* 71(5):627–631, 2010.

151. Zhang W, Connor KM, Davidson JR. Levetiracetam in social phobia: a placebo controlled pilot study. *J Psychopharmacol* 19(5):551–553, 2005.

152. Van Ameringen M, Mancini C, Pipe B, et al. An open trial of topiramate in the treatment of generalized social phobia. *J Clin Psychiatry* 65(12):1674–1678, 2004.

153. Dunlop BW, Papp L, Garlow SJ, et al. Tiagabine for social anxiety disorder. *Hum Psychopharmacol* 22(4):241–244, 2007.

154. Martinez D, Broft A, Laruelle M. Pindolol augmentation of antidepressant treatment: recent contributions from brain imaging studies. *Biol Psychiatry* 48(8):844–853, 2000.

155. Stein MB, Sareen J, Hami S, et al. Pindolol potentiation of paroxetine for generalized social phobia: a double-blind, placebo-controlled, crossover study. *Am J Psychiatry* 158(10):1725–1727, 2001.

156. Goldstein S. Treatment of social phobia with clonidine. *Biol Psychiatry* 22(3):369–372, 1987.

157. Bell J, De Vaugh-Geiss J. *Multi-center trail of a 5-HT3 antagonist, ondansetron, in social phobia.* Presented at 33rd Annual Meeting of the American College of Neuropsychopharmacology, 1994, San Juan, Puerto Rico.

158. Hofmann SG, Smits JA, Rosenfield D, et al. D-Cycloserine as an augmentation strategy with cognitive-behavioral therapy for social anxiety disorder. *Am J Psychiatry* 170(7):751–758, 2013.

159. Davis M. NMDA receptors and fear extinction: implications for cognitive behavioral therapy. *Dialogues Clin Neurosci* 13(4):463–474, 2011.

42 Antipsychotic Drugs

Oliver Freudenreich, MD, Donald C. Goff, MD, and David C. Henderson, MD

KEY POINTS

- All antipsychotics share dopamine$_2$ blockade as the presumed main mechanism of action.

- Primary symptom targets of antipsychotics are positive symptoms (disorganization, delusions, and hallucinations) and agitation; their efficacy for negative symptoms and cognitive deficits of schizophrenia is questionable. Increasingly, antipsychotics are used for treatment of mood disorders.

- Historically, antipsychotics have been grouped into first-generation antipsychotics (typical or conventional antipsychotics, which are all characterized by their risk of extrapyramidal symptoms [EPS]) and second-generation antipsychotics (with a reduced risk of EPS; hence they are called "atypical" antipsychotics). However, antipsychotics within each class are not necessarily interchangeable.

- The main risks of first-generation antipsychotics are neurological side effects (e.g., dystonias, akathisia, parkinsonism, tardive dyskinesia [TD]); for most second-generation antipsychotics, metabolic problems (e.g., weight gain, dyslipidemia, hyperglycemia) have emerged as major problems.

- First- and second-generation antipsychotics are equally effective for non-refractory patients with schizophrenia. For refractory patients, olanzapine, and in particular clozapine, have been the most efficacious.

- Clozapine has minimal or no risk of inducing EPS and is the most effective antipsychotic. However, its clinical use is limited to refractory patients because of serious side effects (including metabolic problems and agranulocytosis that requires white blood cell count monitoring).

- Currently available antipsychotics have variable efficacy and tolerability and need to be selected on the basis of individualized risk–benefit assessments (i.e., balancing the degree of symptomatic response with day-to-day tolerability and long-term medical morbidity, particularly cardiovascular risk).

INTRODUCTION

In this chapter, we will review the basic pharmacology of antipsychotics, emphasizing the differential efficacy and side-effect profiles between first- and second-generation antipsychotics, including clozapine, based on the schizophrenia literature. While antipsychotics are used more broadly than for the treatment of schizophrenia, antipsychotic agents have received FDA approval for additional indications, particularly for the treatment of mood disorders for which they are used routinely. A recent meta-analysis found that antipsychotics were significantly more effective for mania than were mood stabilizers.[1] The specific treatment considerations with regards to choice of an antipsychotic for the major psychiatric syndromes (e.g. schizophrenia, bipolar disorder, depression, autism) can be found in the chapters on these conditions.

HISTORY
Chlorpromazine and the Early Agents

In 1952, Henri Laborit, a French naval surgeon, was experimenting with combinations of preoperative medications to reduce the autonomic stress of surgical procedures. He tried a newly-synthesized antihistamine, chlorpromazine, and was impressed by its calming effect. He noted that patients seemed indifferent about their impending surgery, yet they were not overly sedated. Convinced that the medication had potential for the care of psychiatric patients, Laborit urged colleagues to test his hypothesis. Eventually a surgical colleague told his brother-in-law, the psychiatrist Pierre Deniker, about Leborit's discovery.

Deniker and Jean Delay, who was the chairman of his department at the Hôpital Sainte-Anne in Paris, experimented with chlorpromazine and found remarkable tranquilizing effects in their most agitated and psychotic patients.[2,3] By 1954, Delay and Deniker had published six papers on their clinical experience with chlorpromazine. They noted in 1955 that both chlorpromazine and the dopamine-depleting agent reserpine shared antipsychotic efficacy and neurological side effects that resembled Parkinson's disease. They coined the term *neuroleptic* to describe these effects. In 1956 Frank Ayd[4,5] described acute dystonia and fatal hyperthermia with chlorpromazine. The first reports of tardive dyskinesia (TD) were published by Sigwald and colleagues in 1959.[6]

Smith Kline purchased chlorpromazine from the French pharmaceutical company Rhône-Poulenc, and in 1954 chlorpromazine received approval from the Food and Drug Administration (FDA) for the treatment of psychosis. Almost immediately the care of psychotic patients was transformed. In the US the traditional practice of life-long "warehousing" of individuals with schizophrenia in large state psychiatric hospitals gave way to the new outpatient community psychiatry movement. An additional 10 antipsychotic compounds were rapidly synthesized and approved for clinical use. This included a series of phenothiazines, the thioxanthenes (that were derived from phenothiazines), and haloperidol, which was synthesized from meperidine by Paul Janssen in 1958. In 1967 haloperidol, the last "neuroleptic," was approved by the FDA and, because of its relative selectivity for dopamine$_2$ (D$_2$) receptors and paucity of non-neurological side effects, became the market leader.

By 1964, several multi-center trials sponsored by the Veterans Administration and the National Institutes of Mental Health (NIMH) were completed, comparing the rapidly growing list of antipsychotic agents. These landmark studies each enrolled several hundred patients and were the first large clinical trials to be conducted in the new field of psychopharmacology. The phenothiazines were found to be highly effective and superior to placebo, barbiturates, and reserpine. With the exception of promazine and mepazine, the phenothiazines were found to be of equivalent efficacy, although they differed in their side-effect profiles. In the NIMH collaborative study of over 400 acutely ill patients, 75% of patients were at least moderately improved with chlorpromazine, thioridazine, or fluphenazine, compared to only 23% with placebo.[7] While reports of efficacy were impressive, the goal of identifying differences in efficacy between drugs that might allow matching of specific drugs with subgroups of patients was not realized.

The discovery by Carlsson and Lindqvist[8] in 1963 that chlorpromazine increased turnover of dopamine in the brain led to the hypothesis that dopamine receptor-blockade was responsible for antipsychotic effects. This was confirmed in 1976 by Creese and colleagues,[9] who demonstrated that the antipsychotic potency of a wide range of agents correlated closely with affinity for the D_2 receptor, which explained the equivalency of efficacy between agents since all were acting via the same mechanism. The dopamine hypothesis led to a reliance on animal models sensitive to D_2 blockade as a screen for discovering potential antipsychotic drugs, with the result that new mechanisms were not intentionally explored.

Clozapine, the First Atypical Antipsychotic

The discovery of the first antidepressant, imipramine, led to the synthesis of related heterotricyclic compounds, among which clozapine, a dibenzodiazepine derivative, was synthesized in 1958 by the Swiss company Wander. Clozapine was initially a disappointment, because it did not produce in animal models the behavioral effects associated with an antidepressant or the neurological side effects associated with an antipsychotic. Clinical trials proceeded in Europe but were halted in 1975 after reports of 17 cases of agranulocytosis in Finland, 8 of which were fatal.[10] However, the impression among researchers that clozapine possessed unique clinical characteristics led the manufacturer, Sandoz, to sponsor a pivotal multicenter trial comparing clozapine with chlorpromazine in neuroleptic-resistant patients prospectively shown to be refractory to haloperidol. The dramatic results reported by Kane and colleagues in 1988[11] demonstrated the superiority of clozapine for essentially all domains of symptoms and a relative absence of neurological side effects, prompting a second revolution in the pharmacotherapy of schizophrenia. To this date, clozapine remains the most effective antipsychotic for treatment-refractory schizophrenia.

Other Atypical Agents

Starting in the mid-1980s, Paul Janssen and colleagues began experimenting with serotonin 5-HT_2 antagonism added to D_2 blockade after demonstrating that this combination reduced neurological side effects of haloperidol in rats.[12] When the 5-HT_2 antagonist ritanserin was added to haloperidol in patients with schizophrenia, EPS were diminished and negative symptoms improved.[13] This led to development of risperidone, a D_2 and 5-HT_{2A} antagonist, the first agent designed to follow clozapine's example as an "atypical antipsychotic" with the goal of reduced EPS and enhanced efficacy. Multicenter trials comparing multiple fixed doses of risperidone with haloperidol at a single, relatively high dose of 20 mg/day demonstrated reduced EPS, improved negative symptoms, and, in a subset of relatively resistant patients, greater antipsychotic efficacy.[14,15] Olanzapine, a chemical derivative of clozapine, similarly demonstrated reduced EPS and superior

TABLE 42-1 Timeline of Antipsychotics in the United States

First-Generation Antipsychotics (11 Agents)*	
Chlorpromazine (Thorazine)	1954
Haloperidol (Haldol)	1967

Second-Generation Antipsychotics (10 Agents)	
Clozapine (Clozaril)	1989
Risperidone (Risperdal)	1993
Olanzapine (Zyprexa)	1997
Quetiapine (Seroquel)	1997
Ziprasidone (Geodon)	2001
Aripiprazole (Abilify)	2002
Paliperidone (Invega)	2006
Iloperidone (Fanapt)	2009
Asenapine (Saphris)	2009
Lurasidone (Latuda)	2010

Note: The year given for each agent denotes the year of FDA approval.
*Only the first and last agents are listed for first-generation antipsychotics.

efficacy compared to haloperidol. Risperidone and olanzapine rapidly replaced the first generation of neuroleptics, particularly after clinicians became convinced that the risk of TD was substantially lower. However, it soon became apparent that risperidone markedly elevated serum prolactin levels and that olanzapine produced weight gain in some patients to a degree previously seen only with clozapine. Quetiapine, ziprasidone, and aripiprazole were subsequently approved in the US, based largely on reduced EPS; these agents did not convincingly demonstrate superior efficacy compared to older neuroleptics. Like risperidone and olanzapine, these last three agents acted via D_2 and 5-HT_{2A} receptors; aripiprazole differed from the other second-generation antipsychotics by possessing partial agonist activity at the D_2 receptor rather than full antagonism. Risperidone became the first atypical agent available as a long-acting injection in the form of "risperidone microspheres". Recently, several additional atypical agents have become available, including a metabolite of risperidone (i.e., paliperidone) and asenapine, iloperidone, and lurasidone (Tables 42-1 and 42-2).

A series of case reports, pharmacoepidemiological studies, and, eventually, direct physiological investigations linked atypical antipsychotics with insulin resistance, a heightened risk for diabetes mellitus (DM), and dyslipidemia (primarily elevation of triglycerides). In response, the FDA issued a class warning for DM, although over time, the evidence most strongly implicated clozapine and olanzapine.

The CATIE Study

In 1999, the NIMH, recognizing that almost all information regarding the new antipsychotics had come from industry-supported efficacy trials of uncertain generalizability, awarded a competitive contract to Dr. Jeffrey Lieberman to conduct a large, multi-center trial to assess the effectiveness and tolerability of these agents under more representative treatment conditions. Results of this seminal Clinical Antipsychotic Trials of Intervention Effectiveness (CATIE) study were first published in 2005 (Figure 42-1).[16] The study was conducted at 57 sites across the US and included 1,493 representative patients with schizophrenia who were randomly assigned to risperidone, olanzapine, quetiapine, ziprasidone, or the conventional comparator, perphenazine, for an 18-month double-blind trial. Dosing was flexible; the range of doses for each

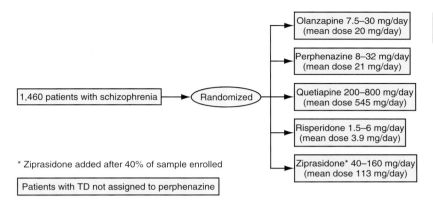

Figure 42-1. CATIE phase 1: double-blind, randomized 18-month trial.

TABLE 42-2 Affinity of Antipsychotic Drugs for Human Neurotransmitter Receptors (Ki, nM)

Receptor	Clozapine	Risperidone	Olanzapine	Quetiapine	Ziprasidone	Aripiprazole	Iloperidone	Haloperidol	Lurasidone
D_1	290	580	52	1,300	130	410	320	120	
D_2	130	2.2	20	180	3.1	0.52	6.3	1.4	1.68
D_3	240	9.6	50	940	7.2	9.1	7.1	2.5	
D_4	47	8.5	50	2,200	32	260	25	3.3	
5-HT_{1A}	140	210	2,100	230	2.5		93	3,600	6.75
5-HT_{1D}	1,700	170	530	>5,100	2			>5,000	
5-HT_{2A}	8.9	0.29	3.3	220	0.39	20	5.6	120	2.03
5-HT_{2C}	17	10	10	1,400	0.72		43	4,700	
5-HT_6	11	2,000	10	4,100	76	160	63	6,000	
5-HT_7	66	3	250	1,800	9.3	15	110	1,100	0.495
α_1	4	1.4	54	15	13	57	1.4	4.7	47.9
α_2	33	5.1	170	1,000	310		160	1,200	40.7
H_1	1.8	19	2.8	8.7	47		470	440	1000
m_1	1.8	2,800	4.7	100	5,100			1,600	1000

(Adapted from Miyamoto S, Duncan GE, Goff DC, et al. Therapeutics in schizophrenia. In Meltzer H, Nemeroff C, editors: Neuropsychopharmacology: the fifth generation of progress, Philadelphia, 2002, Lippincott Williams & Wilkins. The binding affinities for lurasidone were adapted from Ishibashi T, Horisawa T, Tokuda K, et al. Pharmacological profile of lurasidone, a novel antipsychotic agent with potent 5-hydroxytryptamine 7 (5-HT7) and 5-HT1A receptor activity. J Pharmacol Exp Ther 334(1):171–181, 2010.)

drug was selected based on patterns of clinical use (in consultation with the manufacturers). Ziprasidone became available and was added after the study was roughly 40% completed. Patients with TD at study entry were not randomized to perphenazine, and their data were excluded from analyses comparing the atypical agents with perphenazine. Patients who failed treatment with their first assigned agent could be randomized again in subsequent phases; one re-randomization pathway featured open-label clozapine for treatment-resistant patients and one pathway featured ziprasidone for treatment-intolerant patients. The secondary randomization pathway did not include perphenazine.

One striking finding of the CATIE study was that only 26% of subjects completed the 18-month trial still taking their originally-assigned antipsychotic. The primary measure of effectiveness, "all cause discontinuation," significantly favored olanzapine over the other agents. The superior effectiveness of olanzapine was also reflected in significantly fewer hospitalizations and fewer discontinuations due to lack of efficacy. While risperidone-treated patients were numerically less likely to discontinue due to intolerance, this difference was not statistically significant. In addition to greater effectiveness, olanzapine was associated with greater cardiovascular risk; patients treated with olanzapine had more weight gain and elevation

TABLE 42-3 First-Generation Antipsychotic Doses

	Equivalent Dose (mg)*	Typical Dose Acute/maintenance (mg/day)
LOW POTENCY		
Chlorpromazine	100	300–1,000/300–600
Thioridazine	100	300–800/300–600
MEDIUM POTENCY		
Loxapine	10	30–100/30–60
Perphenazine	10	12–64/8–32**
HIGH POTENCY		
Trifluoperazine	5	15–50/15–30
Thiothixene	5	15–50/15–30
Fluphenazine	2	6–20/6–12
Haloperidol	2	6–20/6–12

*Equivalent dose (or "chlorpromazine equivalents") reflects the potency of antipsychotics compared to 100 mg of chlorpromazine as the reference.
**CATIE dose range 8 mg to 32 mg/day.
(Adapted from Buchanan RW, Kreyenbuhl J, Kelly DL, et al. The 2009 schizophrenia PORT psychopharmacological treatment recommendations and summary statements. Schizophrenia Bulletin 36(1):71–93, 2010.)

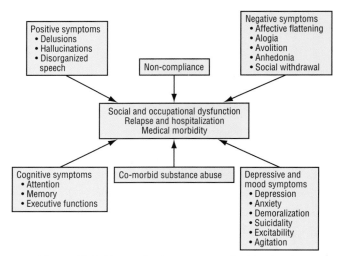

Figure 42-2. Targets for the treatment of schizophrenia.

of hemoglobin A_{1c}, total cholesterol, and triglycerides. The other atypical agents did not significantly differ from perphenazine in either efficacy or tolerability. Overall, the results suggested that no single antipsychotic is likely to be optimal for all, or for most, patients. The duration of the CATIE trial was not long enough to detect differences between agents in the incidence of TD.

CURRENTLY AVAILABLE ANTIPSYCHOTIC AGENTS

All marketed antipsychotic agents share the common property of dopamine (D_2) receptor blockade. The 11 agents approved in the US between 1953 (chlorpromazine) and 1967 (haloperidol) are commonly referred to as *conventional neuroleptics* or *first-generation antipsychotics* (Table 42-3). As a group they possess equivalent efficacy, but differ in their potency and side effects. Reflecting their common property of D_2 blockade, these agents all can produce EPS, TD, and hyperprolactinemia. Clozapine was the first of the *second-generation antipsychotics*, also known as *atypical antipsychotics*. Currently there are 10 atypical antipsychotics approved in the US; these agents generally produce fewer EPS, less elevation of prolactin, and less risk of TD than first-generation antipsychotics. Clozapine has clearly demonstrated greater efficacy than the first-generation agents. Of the other second-generation antipsychotics, only olanzapine was found to be more effective than the first-generation comparator in the CATIE study. Risperidone and its metabolite, paliperidone are unique among the atypical agents in producing marked prolactin elevation. Aripiprazole is the only antipsychotic with partial agonist rather than antagonist activity at the D_2 receptor; this property is believed to limit neurological side effects. Because aripiprazole was not included in the CATIE study, it is unclear if D_2 partial agonism has implications for effectiveness. The most comprehensive meta-analysis, published by Leucht and colleagues in 2013,[17] found substantial differences in side effects and small but statistically significant differences in efficacy between currently available antipsychotics, arguing against a simple categoriza-

tion as first- or second-generation even though this terminology continues to be used (for lack of a better one).

GENERAL CLINICAL CONSIDERATIONS

For schizophrenia, the primary target symptoms for antipsychotic agents fall into three categories: psychotic symptoms (e.g., hallucinations, delusions, disorganization); agitation (e.g., distractibility, affective lability, tension, increased motor activity); and negative symptoms (e.g., apathy, diminished affect, social withdrawal, poverty of speech). Although cognitive deficits are an important contributor to disability in schizophrenia, cognitive deficits usually are not considered a target for antipsychotic agents because they are not very responsive to current agents. Agitation responds to most antipsychotics rapidly and often fully, whereas response of psychotic symptoms is quite variable and negative symptoms rarely exhibit more than modest improvement[18] (Figure 42-2).

The time course of antipsychotic response also can be quite variable. In the 1970s, the treatment of psychosis with relatively large doses of intramuscular (IM) haloperidol, known as "rapid neuroleptization," was advocated, based on the clinical impression that agitation and psychosis responded quickly to this aggressive treatment approach.[19] For the next two decades, the consensus shifted to the view that psychotic symptoms require weeks of antipsychotic treatment before responding. More recently, Kapur and colleagues[20] analyzed data from studies of IM administration of atypical antipsychotics and documented antipsychotic effects within hours of administration, independent of tranquilization. Most likely, tranquilization, or the improvement of agitation and irritability, occurs rapidly with most agents whereas psychotic symptoms may begin to improve quickly in some patients and only after a delay of several weeks in others. Maximal response to antipsychotic treatment can require months. The pharmacological treatment of psychotic symptoms is similar to the treatment of infection with antibiotics—the clinician needs to choose a proper dose and then await therapeutic results while monitoring side effects.

The degree of antipsychotic efficacy ranges from complete resolution of psychosis in a substantial number of patients to minimal or no benefit in others. In between, some patients experience diminished delusional conviction, or may persist in their delusional conviction but no longer interpret new

TABLE 42-4 Antipsychotic Side Effects

	EPS	Tardive Dyskinesia	Prolactin	Anticholinergic Side Effects	Sedation	Weight Gain	Diabetes	Dyslipidemia
Chlorpromazine	++	+++	+++	++++	++++	+++	+++	++
Perphenazine	+++	+++	+++	++	++	++	−	+
Haloperidol	++++	+++	+++	−	+	+− −		
Clozapine	−	−	−	++++	++++	++++	++++	++++
Risperidone	++	+	++++	−	++	++	++	+
Olanzapine	+	+	+	+	+++	++++	++++	++++
Quetiapine	−	?	−	++*	+++	++	+++†	+++†
Ziprasidone	+	?	+	−	+	+	−	−
Aripiprazole	+	?	−	−	+	+	−	−
Asenapine	++	?	+	−	++	+	−?	−?
Iloperidone	−	?	−	−	+	++	++?	?
Lurasidone	+/++	?	+	−	+	+ /−	−	−?

*Elevated urinary hesitancy, dry mouth, constipation in CATIE study, probably not mediated via muscarinic acetylcholine receptors.
†Possibly dose related.(Henderson DC, Copeland PM, Borba CP, et al. Glucose metabolism in patients with schizophrenia treated with olanzapine or quetiapine: a frequently sampled intravenous glucose tolerance test and minimal model analysis. J Clin Psychiatry 67(5):789–797, 2006.)

experiences within the delusional framework. Other patients continue to hear voices, but muted, or less frequently, or with greater insight. Some patients are surprisingly stable and functional despite chronic, attenuated psychotic symptoms. A major benefit from antipsychotics is prevention of relapse by maintenance treatment.[21]

Negative symptoms have been found to respond to both conventional and atypical antipsychotics, although a full resolution of negative symptoms is rare.[18] It remains controversial whether "primary" negative symptoms improve with pharmacotherapy. Examples of "secondary" negative symptoms include social withdrawal resulting from paranoia, and apathy resulting from depression. The most common etiology of secondary negative symptoms is neuroleptic-induced parkinsonism; the improvement of negative symptoms following a switch to an atypical agent sometimes represents resolution of iatrogenic parkinsonian side effects caused by the previous conventional neuroleptic.

DRUG SELECTION

Selection of an antipsychotic agent usually is guided by the side-effect profile and by available formulations (e.g., tablet, rapidly-dissolving or sublingual preparation, liquid, IM immediate-release, or long-acting injectable preparations). The "atypical" antipsychotics have largely supplanted conventional agents because of their reduced burden of neurological side effects, although the good efficacy and tolerability of perphenazine in CATIE has led to a reappraisal of the use of low-dose mid-potency first-generation antipsychotics. TD remains a concern for first-generation antipsychotics (but not limited to them), even if used at low doses. Increasingly, a drug's metabolic side-effect profile is taken into account when selecting an agent. Because of the considerable heterogeneity in response and susceptibility to side effects, it is not possible to predict the optimal agent for an individual patient; sequential trials may be needed. As listed in Table 42-4, side effects likely to influence tolerability and compliance include sedation or activation, weight gain, neurological side effects, and sexual dysfunction. With an increased emphasis on reducing iatrogenic cardiovascular risk factors (i.e., metabolic syndrome), it is becoming more common to switch patients from a high-risk to a low-risk antipsychotic.[22] A switch strategy is often more effective than behavioral interventions.

BOX 42-1 Side Effects Associated with Low-Potency First-Generation Antipsychotics

- Sedation
- Hypotension
- Weight gain
- Anticholinergic symptoms (dry mouth, urinary retention, constipation, blurred vision)
- Impaired heat regulation (hyperthermia or hypothermia)
- Pigmentary retinopathy (thioridazine > 800 mg/day)
- Cardiac conduction effects (chlorpromazine, thioridazine)

The potential therapeutic benefits of clozapine (including greater efficacy for psychosis, negative symptoms, agitation or tension, suicidal ideation, and relapse) are quite broad.[11,23,24] Because of the risk of agranulocytosis, clozapine is reserved for patients who fail to respond to other antipsychotics.

Based on epidemiological studies, all antipsychotics carry a black box warning with regard to an increased risk of death when used for behavioral problems in elderly patients with dementia.[25,26]

FIRST-GENERATION ("TYPICAL") ANTIPSYCHOTICS

Examining representative first-generation antipsychotics, it has been shown that roughly a 65% occupancy of striatal D_2 receptors is necessary for antipsychotic efficacy, whereas neurological side effects emerge when D_2 occupancy levels exceed approximately 80%.[27] Among the conventional antipsychotics, low-potency agents (such as chlorpromazine) have relatively low affinity for the D_2 receptor and hence require higher doses (roughly 50-fold greater than haloperidol). In addition, they are less selective for D_2 receptors and so are associated with a wider range of side effects, including orthostatic hypotension, anticholinergic side effects, sedation, and weight gain (Box 42-1). Perphenazine, which was the conventional antipsychotic selected to represent this class in the CATIE study, is a mid-potency agent that requires doses roughly three-fold greater than are necessary with haloperidol. High-potency conventional agents (such as haloperidol and fluphenazine) are more selective for D_2 receptors and more likely to produce

EPS, such as acute dystonias, parkinsonism, and akathisia. Because affinity for the D_2 receptor is readily measured and is inversely correlated with the typical therapeutic dose for each compound, conversion ratios to calculate equivalent dosing between conventional agents, typically expressed in "chlorpromazine equivalents," can be calculated (see Table 42-3).

Haloperidol is available for parenteral (including intravenous [IV]) administration, and both haloperidol and fluphenazine are available in long-acting injectable depot preparations. Although considerable inter-individual variability exists, daily oral doses of haloperidol between 5 and 15 mg are adequate for the large majority of chronic patients; increasing the dose further may only aggravate side effects without improving antipsychotic efficacy. IM and IV administration require roughly half the dose of oral doses. Great care should be taken with the elderly, in whom 0.5 to 2 mg of haloperidol at bedtime may often be sufficient. If a patient has not previously received antipsychotic medication, it is best to start at a low dose before arriving at a standard therapeutic dose which is between 1 and 4 mg orally. A large number of studies have indicated that an optimal response with haloperidol generally corresponds with trough serum concentrations between 5 and 15 ng/ml,[28] although clinical titration remains the most reliable approach in most situations. In the setting of serious medical illness and delirium, particularly if other medications with anticholinergic or hypotensive side effects are administered, haloperidol is often used. Patients need to be monitored for torsades de pointes if haloperidol is given IV.[29]

The mid-potency antipsychotic loxapine is available as a rapidly-acting aerosolized preparation for inhalation to manage agitation in the setting of psychosis or mania.[30] It shows efficacy within 10 minutes after inhalation and might obviate the need for IM administration of an antipsychotic to patients who need rapid tranquilization.

In the US, fluphenazine and haloperidol are available as long-acting depot preparations (decanoates) that are administered IM. Since 2011, shortages of depot haloperidol and fluphenazine supplies have created disruptions in treatment for some patients and led to uncertainty about the future availability of these medications.

EXTRAPYRAMIDAL SYMPTOMS AND TARDIVE DYSKINESIA

Akathisia is an extremely unpleasant sensation of motor restlessness that is primarily experienced in the lower extremities in patients receiving antipsychotics.[31] Akathisia usually manifests as pacing, although some patients experience akathisia as leg discomfort rather than restlessness, and it can develop after a single dose. Akathisia increases non-adherence and has been associated with self-injurious behaviors, as well as a worsening of psychosis. Untrained staff can mistake akathisia for psychotic agitation, resulting in an unfortunate escalation of the antipsychotic dose. A switch to a different antipsychotic with a low liability for akathisia usually resolves the problem. Because akathisia is dose dependent, lowering the dose may provide relief. Alternatively, propranolol 10 to 20 mg two to four times daily is often helpful.[32] The antidepressant mirtazepine which has antagonism at serotonin$_{2A}$ receptors that are implicated in the pathophysiology of akathisia has been shown in double-blind trials to reduce akathisia.[33]

Dystonias are sustained spasms that can affect any muscle group. Neuroleptic-induced dystonias usually occur within the first 4 days of initiating neuroleptic treatment, or after a dose increase, and often affect the neck, tongue, or back. Dystonia may also manifest as lateral deviation of the eyes (opisthotonus) or stridor (laryngeal spasm). Younger patients started on high-potency first-generation antipsychotic

medication are at high risk for developing acute dystonic reactions during the first week of exposure to antipsychotic medication.[34] The incidence of dystonia decreases by about 4% per year of age until it is almost negligible after age 40. Dystonia is a frightening and uncomfortable experience. The occurrence of dystonia early in treatment seriously jeopardizes future compliance with antipsychotic medication, so it is important to anticipate and treat this side effect aggressively. The best method of prevention comes from use of a second-generation atypical antipsychotic. When high-potency neuroleptics are started, prophylaxis with anticholinergic agents (such as benztropine 1 to 2 mg twice daily) substantially reduces the likelihood of dystonic reactions in high-risk patients.[35] Prophylaxis with anticholinergics is risky in the elderly because of their sensitivity to adverse effects, but is usually unnecessary since the elderly are at very low risk for dystonia. Dystonia is uncommon with atypical agents and occurs very rarely with quetiapine and clozapine.

Antipsychotic-induced parkinsonism mimics the tremor, stiffness, gait disturbance, and diminished facial expression characteristic of idiopathic Parkinson's disease. It easily can be mistaken for depression or for negative symptoms of schizophrenia,[36] although the presence of tremor and rigidity usually distinguishes this side effect. Parkinsonian side effects are most common with high-potency first-generation antipsychotics and occur in a bi-modal age distribution with maximal risk in the young and in the elderly. Symptoms frequently improve with a reduction in the dose of the antipsychotic or with addition of an antiparkinsonian agent (such as benztropine 1 to 2 mg twice daily or amantadine 100 mg twice or three times daily).[37] Because anticholinergic agents can produce an array of troublesome side effects (including constipation, dry mouth, dental caries, blurred vision, urinary retention, and memory impairment), particularly in the elderly, long-term use of these agents should be avoided. In addition, anticholinergics might impede cognitive gains hoped for when using cognitive-behavioral therapy or cognitive remediation.[38,39] The atypical agents as a class produce substantially fewer parkinsonian side effects, and both clozapine and quetiapine are essentially free of EPS, making them the drugs of choice for patients with idiopathic Parkinson's disease complicated by psychosis.[40] Box 42-2 describes EPS.

TD rarely appears after less than 6 months of treatment with an antipsychotic agent, but once present it may be

---

BOX 42-2 Extrapyramidal Symptoms

AKATHISIA

Restlessness in lower extremities; often results in pacing
Can occur after the first dose
Risk factors: use of high-potency first-generation agents in high doses

DYSTONIA

Acute muscle spasm: can be very distressing
Usually occurs within the first 4 days after starting the drug
Risk factors: youth and use of high-potency first-generation antipsychotics

PARKINSONISM

Tremor, bradykinesia, rigidity—often confused with negative symptoms
Usually does not become evident until after several weeks of treatment
Risk factors: use of high-potency first-generation antipsychotics, high doses, youth, and old age

irreversible.[39] TD usually takes the form of involuntary, choreiform (quick, non-rhythmic) movements of the mouth, tongue, or upper extremities, although a dystonic form has also been described.[41] The risk for developing TD with first-generation agents is about 5% per year of exposure, with a life-time risk possibly as high as 50% to 60%.[42] The incidence of TD is much higher in the elderly, although a substantial proportion of these cases may represent spontaneously occurring dyskinesias.[43] Patients who develop parkinsonian side effects early in the course of treatment also appear to be at heightened risk for TD. The best treatment of TD is prevention since options are limited once TD is established. Clozapine has not been linked to TD, and switching a patient who develops TD to clozapine increases the likelihood of spontaneous improvement of TD.[44] Lowering the dose of a first-generation antipsychotic or switching to a second-generation agent can occasionally produce "withdrawal dyskinesias," which typically resolve within 6 weeks, or may unmask an underlying dyskinesia that was previously suppressed by the antipsychotic medication.[45] In severe cases, tetrabenazine or deep brain stimulation can been tried.[46,47] Box 42-3 describes TD.

NEUROLEPTIC MALIGNANT SYNDROME

Neuroleptic malignant syndrome (NMS) is a rare, potentially lethal complication of neuroleptic treatment characterized by hyperthermia, rigidity, confusion, diaphoresis, autonomic instability, elevated creatine phosphokinase (CPK), and leukocytosis (Box 42-4).[48] The symptoms of NMS may evolve gradually over time, usually starting with mental status changes and culminating in fever and elevated CPK. NMS probably occurs in fewer than 1% of patients receiving conventional antipsychotic agents, although subsyndromal cases may be much more common.[49,50] Parallels have been drawn between NMS and malignant hyperthermia (resulting from general anesthesia), largely on the basis of common clinical characteristics. Patients with a history of either NMS or malignant hyperthermia, however, appear to be at no increased risk for developing the other syndrome, and analysis of muscle biopsy specimens has not consistently demonstrated a physiological link between the two conditions.[49] Lethal catatonia is a spontaneously occurring syndrome that may be indistinguishable from NMS and has been described in the absence of neuroleptic treatment.[51] In addition, antipsychotic agents may impair temperature regulation and so may produce low-grade fever in the absence of other symptoms of NMS.[52] The clinician's immediate response to NMS should be to discontinue medication and hospitalize the patient to provide IV fluids and cooling. Whether bromocriptine or dantrolene facilitates recovery remains the subject of debate.[53] It is important that re-institution of antipsychotic medication be delayed at least 2 weeks until after the episode of NMS has resolved.[54] NMS has been described with all antipsychotics including clozapine.[55] It has been suggested that a variant of NMS without rigidity may result from use of second-generation antipsychotics, although if such a syndrome occurs, it is probably quite rare: perhaps with the exception of clozapine where NMS can display few EPS, second-generation antipsychotics produce the typical clinical picture of NMS with rigidity.[56]

SECOND-GENERATION ("ATYPICAL") ANTIPSYCHOTICS

The second-generation agents (Table 42-5) are generally better tolerated with regards to EPS, producing fewer neurological side effects (dystonia, akathisia, and parkinsonism) than the first-generation agents and possibly less TD (see Table 42-4). While relatively free of EPS in most patients at doses of less than 6 mg daily, risperidone (and its metabolite paliperidone) requires careful titration to avoid EPS at higher doses and is unique among the atypical agents in producing sustained hyperprolactinemia.[57] However, attention over the past decade has focused on effects of second-generation antipsychotics on glucose metabolism and lipids[58] and the associated metabolic syndrome (Table 42-6). A large number of cases of treatment-emergent DM have been reported, which in some cases resolved after discontinuation of the antipsychotic.[59,60] In the CATIE study, olanzapine produced significantly greater weight gain, impairment of glucose metabolism, and dyslipidemia than the other agents[16]; this has since been confirmed in a meta-analysis that found clozapine and olanzapine to be the drugs with the highest metabolic liability.[61] Nonetheless, intermediate risk drugs, such as quetiapine, may carry similar risks when used in doses necessary to treat psychotic symptoms.[62] Possible differences between second-generation antipsychotics in risk for causing DM may be obscured in part by the considerable variability between individual patients for weight gain, the potential delay between initiation of treatment and elevation of glucose levels, and a possible propensity for abnormal glucose metabolism associated with schizophrenia independent of drug treatment.[63] All patients treated with an antipsychotic should therefore be monitored regularly for weight gain, DM, and hyperlipidemia, with particular attention paid to more frequent monitoring for patients who receive high-risk drugs (i.e., olanzapine and clozapine) (Table 42-7). Olanzapine and aripiprazole have few or no cardiac effects and can be initiated at a full therapeutic dose. Clozapine, risperidone, quetiapine, ziprasidone, and iloperidone have α-adrenergic effects that necessitate dose titration to avoid orthostatic hypotension. Clozapine produces more

---

BOX 42-3 Tardive Dyskinesia

Late-developing, chronic choreiform (non-rhythmic, quick) movements, most commonly oral-buccal muscles and tongue

RISK FACTORS
Old age
More than 6 months of first-generation neuroleptic exposure
History of parkinsonian side effects
Diabetes
Risk is reduced with second-generation agents

BOX 42-4 Neuroleptic Malignant Syndrome

TRIAD
1. Rigidity
2. Fever
3. Altered mental status

PRESENTATION (MAY GRADUALLY EVOLVE, USUALLY IN THE FOLLOWING ORDER):
- Confusion and fluctuating levels of consciousness
- Rigidity (can be less pronounced with clozapine)
- Diaphoresis
- Mutism
- Autonomic instability
- Hyperthermia
- Elevated creatine phosphokinase

(Based on Gurrera RJ, Caroff SN, Cohen A, et al. An international consensus study of neuroleptic malignant syndrome diagnostic criteria using the Delphi method. J Clin Psychiatry 72(9):1222–1228, 2011.)

TABLE 42-5 Second-Generation Antipsychotic Doses

	Typical Dose (mg/day)	High Dose* (mg/day)	Potential Dose-Limiting Side Effects
Risperidone	3–6	6–12	EPS
Olanzapine	10–20	30–40	Sedation
Quetiapine	300–600	600–1,200**	Sedation
Ziprasidone	80–160	160–320***	Akathisia
Aripiprazole	10–20	20–40	
Clozapine	100–400	400–900****	Sedation, orthostatic hypotension, seizures
Iloperidone	12–24	24	Orthostatic hypotension
Asenapine	10–20	20	Sedation; EPS
Lurasidone	40–80	160	EPS

*Evidence for benefit of higher dose available for olanzapine only.
**Two controlled trials have <u>not</u> found benefit from high-dose quetiapine.[111,112]
***One controlled trial has not found benefit from high-dose ziprasidone.[114]
****Dose should be guided by clozapine serum levels. An optimal highest dose has not been established. (Remmington G, Agid O, Foussias G, et al. Clozapine and therapeutic drug monitoring: is there sufficient evidence for an upper threshold? *Psychopharmacology* 225(3):505–518, 2013.)
EPS, Extrapyramidal symptom.

TABLE 42-6 Identification of the Metabolic Syndrome

Risk Factor (three or more required for diagnosis)	Defining Level
Abdominal obesity	Waist circumference
Men	>40 in (> 102 cm)
Women	>35 in (> 88 cm)
Triglycerides	≥150 mg/dl
HDL cholesterol	
Men	<40 mg/dl
Women	<50 mg/dl
Blood pressure	≥130/85 mmHg
Fasting blood glucose	≥100 mg/dl

HDL, High-density lipoprotein.
(Adapted from Expert panel on detection, evaluation, and treatment of high blood cholesterol in adults. JAMA 285:2486–2497, 2001.)

BOX 42-5 Clozapine

CLINICAL EFFICACY

Effective in 30% of treatment-resistant patients at 6 weeks
Prevents relapse
Stabilizes mood
Improves polydipsia and hyponatremia
Reduces hostility and aggression
Reduces suicidality
Possibly reduces cigarette smoking and substance abuse

ADVERSE EFFECTS

Common Side Effects

Sedation
Tachycardia
Sialorrhea (impairs esophageal motility)
Dizziness
Constipation (can lead to bowel impaction)
Hypotension
Fever (usually within first 3 weeks, lasting a few days)
Weight gain

Serious Side Effects

Agranulocytosis*
Seizures*
Myocarditis*
Orthostatic hypotension with syncope or cardiorespiratory arrest*
Pulmonary embolus
Diabetes mellitus

*Clozapine-specific black box warnings

hypotension and tachycardia than other atypical agents; both are generally easily managed. Ziprasidone's approval was delayed when it became clear that it prolongs the QT interval more than other second-generation antipsychotics (but less than thioridazine).[64]

Clozapine

Clozapine (Box 42-5) is a tricyclic dibenzodiazepine derivative approved for the treatment of treatment-resistant schizophrenia and for the reduction of suicidal behavior in patients with schizophrenia or schizoaffective disorder. Clozapine binds to a wide array of central nervous system (CNS) receptors (including dopaminergic [all five subtypes], muscarinic cholinergic receptors, histaminergic, noradrenergic, and serotonergic). In addition, it appears to modulate glutamatergic NMDA-receptor sensitivity and the release of brain-derived neurotropic factor (BDNF). The absence of neurological side effects has been attributed to serotonin $5\text{-}HT_{2A}$ antagonism, a high D_2 dissociation constant (loose binding) that results in relatively low levels of D_2 receptor occupancy at therapeutic doses, strong anticholinergic activity, and preferential binding to limbic over striatal dopamine receptors. However, the exact mechanism by which clozapine achieves greater efficacy than other agents remains a mystery, despite almost 20 years of research.

Peak plasma levels of clozapine are attained approximately 2 hours after oral administration. It is metabolized primarily by hepatic microsomal enzymes CYP 1A2 and, to a lesser extent, 3A4 and 2D6, with a mean half-life of 8 hours following a single dose and 12 hours after repeated dosing. Only the desmethyl metabolite is active. Clozapine blood levels are significantly lowered by cigarette smoking and by other hepatic enzyme-inducers (including phenytoin and rifampin) and elevated by CYP 1A2 and 3A4 inhibitors (such as fluvoxamine and erythromycin). Fluvoxamine has been shown to increase clozapine plasma concentrations by as much as four-fold.[65] Some patients may experience a doubling of clozapine blood levels after smoking cessation, with attendant sedation and worsening of other side effects. Several studies have indicated that clozapine is most likely to be effective at trough serum concentrations of 350 ng/ml or greater.[66] In a prospective, double-blind trial, patients randomly assigned to treatment with a clozapine dose adjusted to produce a serum concentration between 200 and 300 ng/ml responded more fully than

TABLE 42-7 Recommendations for Monitoring Patients Starting Antipsychotics*

	Baseline	4 Weeks	8 Weeks	12 Weeks	Quarterly	Annually
Personal/family history	X					X
Weight (body mass index [BMI])	X	X	X	X	X	
Waist circumference	X			X	X	
Blood pressure	X			X	X	
Fasting plasma glucose†	X			X		X**
Fasting lipid profile	X			X		X**

Consider an intervention (weight reduction program or switch antipsychotic) if:
- 5% or greater increase in weight
- 1 point increase in BMI
- 1 inch or greater increase in waist circumference
- Criteria met for metabolic syndrome

*The monitoring recommendations are derived from the literature about second-generation antipsychotics. However, first-generation antipsychotics (particularly low-potency antipsychotics) are not devoid of metabolic problems.
**More frequent monitoring (e.g., every 3 months until stable, then every 6 months) is indicated for patients on high-risk drugs (clozapine, olanzapine)
†Hemoglobin A1c can be used insteadHemoglobin A1c can be used instead.
(Adapted in part from American Diabetes Association, American Psychiatric Association, American Association of Clinical Endocrinologists, North American Association for the Study of Obesity. Consensus development conference on antipsychotic drugs and diabetes and obesity. Diabetes Care 27:596–601, 2004 and Goff DC, Cather C, Evins AE, et al. Medical morbidity and mortality in schizophrenia: guidelines for psychiatrists. J Clin Psychiatry 66(2):183–194; quiz 147, 273–184, 2005.)

did patients assigned to lower concentrations; moreover, their response was comparable to patients assigned to higher concentrations.[67]

In the pivotal study comparing clozapine to chlorpromazine in patients prospectively defined as treatment resistant, clozapine produced significantly greater improvement in measures of psychosis, negative symptoms, depression, and anxiety.[11] Thirty percent of the clozapine-treatment group responded compared to 4% treated with chlorpromazine; a subsequent study indicated that the response rate may increase to as high as 60% with trials lasting 6 months or longer.[68] Clozapine has also been found to improve aggression and hostility,[69] reduce relapse,[70] and decrease suicidality.[24,70] Open-label studies have found impressive mood-stabilizing effects of clozapine in patients with refractory bipolar or schizoaffective disorder.[71] Clozapine may also improve polydipsia with hyponatremia,[72] reduce arrest rates,[73] and facilitate a decrease in cigarette smoking.[74]

Potentially serious side effects (such as agranulocytosis, seizures, DM, and myocarditis) have limited clozapine treatment to the most refractory patients; the more common side effects of weight gain, sialorrhea, orthostatic hypotension, constipation, and sedation further complicate its use (see Box 42-5).[75] Because of the risk of agranulocytosis, patients must meet a minimum threshold for their neutrophil count before starting the drug and must continue to meet safety criteria with weekly blood tests during the first 6 months of treatment, biweekly tests for the second 6 months, and then monthly bloods tests for as long as the patient takes the drug (Box 42-6 and Box 42-7). Results of all white blood cell (WBC) counts are monitored and stored in national databases; an analysis of these records from the period 1990 to 1991 indicated that 0.8% of patients who were started on clozapine developed agranulocytosis, and 0.01% of patients died of agranulocytosis.[76] The risk of developing agranulocytosis peaked in the 3rd month. While most cases of agranulocytosis occur during the first 6 to 12 months of treatment, 10% of patients developed agranulocytosis after 2 years of treatment, even after a decade.[77] Patients usually recover from clozapine-induced agranulocytosis within 14 to 24 days of stopping the drug, but re-challenge with clozapine is not allowed because of the very high rate of recurrence.[78,79]

Some patients with habitually low WBC counts due to ethnicity (benign ethnic neutropenia [BEN]) can safely be treated with clozapine if they are pre-treated with lithium,

---

BOX 42-6 Clozapine-Induced Agranulocytosis

- Granulocytes < 500/mm³
- Risk factors: Ashkenazi Jews (HLA-B38, DR4, DQw3) and Finns
- Preservation of other cell lines (platelets and RBCs)
- Maximum risk: 4–18 weeks (77% of cases)
- Recovery usually within 14 days if drug stopped
- No cross-reactivity with other drugs, but avoid carbamazepine, captopril, sulfonamides, propylthiouracil, and other drugs that might affect bone marrow or WBCs
- Because of sensitization: Do not rechallenge!

RBCs, Red blood cells; WBCs, white blood cells.

BOX 42-7 Monitoring for Agranulocytosis

WBC count must be ≥ 3,500 and ANC ≥ 2,000 to initiate clozapine
Weekly CBC for 6 months, if all WBC counts ≥ 3,500 and ANCs ≥ 2,000; then biweekly for 6 months, then monthly
Repeat CBC if:
- ANC = 1,500–2,000 or WBC count = 3,000–3,500, or
- WBC count drops by 3,000 or ANC drops by 1,500 from previous test, or
- Three consecutive weekly drops

If ANC = 1,500–2,000 or WBC count = 3,000–3,500, proceed with twice-weekly CBCs
Hold drug if ANC < 1,500 or WBC count < 3,000
Discontinue if ANC < 1,000 or WBC count < 2,000: *do not re-challenge*

ANC, Absolute neutrophil count; CBC, complete blood count; WBC, white blood cell.

---

which stimulates the bone marrow to boost WBC counts to levels acceptable for prescribing clozapine.[80]

Of additional concern are the recent findings of myocarditis and cardiomyopathy occurring in 0.01% to 0.2% of patients treated with clozapine, of which approximately 20% were fatal.[81] These cases commonly manifested within the first month of treatment with fever, dyspnea, a "flu-like illness," and chest pain; abnormal laboratory findings included a reduced ventricular ejection fraction on echocardiogram, T-wave changes on the electrocardiogram (ECG), eosinophilia, and an elevated CPK.[82,83]

Seizures have been reported in 5% to 10% of patients treated with clozapine.[84] Seizure risk appears to be related to both rapid dose escalation and to high plasma concentrations. High rates of obesity, DM, and dyslipidemia have also been associated with clozapine. In one 5-year naturalistic study, weight gain with clozapine reached a mean plateau of 31 lb after approximately 4 years and almost 37% of patients developed DM.[58] Whereas the striking abdominal adiposity associated with clozapine treatment might explain the elevated rate of DM, markedly decreased insulin sensitivity has been documented in non-obese patients treated with clozapine compared to risperidone-treated patients matched for age and weight.[85]

Given the rare but serious risks of agranulocytosis and myocarditis and the more common risks of seizures and metabolic complications, clozapine should be reserved for patients who fail at least two other trials of antipsychotics. However, the potential therapeutic benefits of clozapine often outweigh the risks of medical morbidity. One study using the Clozapine National Registry found a higher mortality rate in patients after they stopped clozapine than while they were taking it, due to an almost 90% reduction in suicide associated with clozapine treatment.[86] A second epidemiological study (FIN11 study) found a lower all-cause mortality rate and no increased deaths from cardiovascular causes over an 11-year period for clozapine-treated patients compared to other antipsychotics.[87]

Risperidone and Paliperidone

Risperidone is a benzisoxazole derivative that received FDA approval for the treatment of schizophrenia in 1994 and later for bipolar mania. It is characterized by a very high affinity for the 5-HT$_{2A}$ receptor and by moderate affinity for D$_2$, H$_1$, and α_1- and α_2-adrenergic receptors. Risperidone has essentially no activity at muscarinic acetylcholine receptors. Risperidone has a high affinity and low dissociation constant for the D$_2$ receptor, making it "tightly bound" and thereby more likely to produce EPS at high doses than some more "loosely bound" agents. At typical clinical doses, risperidone was found to occupy 65% to 69% of D$_2$ receptors 12 to 14 hours after the last dose; a mean occupancy of 79% was found in patients treated with a risperidone dose of 6 mg/day.[88]

Risperidone is rapidly absorbed after oral administration with peak plasma levels achieved within 1 hour. It is metabolized by hepatic microsomal enzyme CYP 2D6 to form the active metabolite 9-hydroxyrisperidone, which exhibits a pattern of receptor binding similar to that of the parent compound. 9-Hydroxyrisperidone is in turn metabolized by N-dealkylation. The half-life of the "active moiety" (risperidone plus 9-hydroxyrisperidone) is approximately 20 hours. CYP 2D6 activity, which varies dramatically between "rapid" and "poor" metabolizers, determines the ratio of risperidone to 9-hydroxyrisperidone serum concentrations and influences the half-life of the active moiety. Drugs that inhibit CYP 2D6, such as paroxetine and fluoxetine, may increase risperidone levels with the risk of neurological side effects.[89]

In the North American registration trials, risperidone doses of 6, 10, and 16 mg/day (but not 2 mg/day) produced significantly greater reductions compared to high-dose haloperidol (20 mg/day) in all five domains of the Positive and Negative Syndromes Scale (PANSS),[90] whereas risperidone was similar in efficacy to the first-generation antipsychotic perphenazine in the CATIE trial and in an earlier study.[16] In a flexibly-dosed, double-blind, randomized study, Csernansky and colleagues[91]

found almost twice the relapse rate with haloperidol compared to risperidone. Increasing the risperidone dose above 8 mg/day has not improved response in patients who did not fully respond to a treatment with a typical dose.[92]

Risperidone is well tolerated at doses low enough to avoid EPS (generally below 6 mg/day). In the CATIE trial, risperidone at a mean dose of 3.9 mg/day was the best-tolerated agent, although differences between agents were not statistically significant. Weight gain with risperidone is intermediate compared to other atypical agents and is quite variable. Woerner and colleagues[93] found a cumulative TD rate of 7.2% over 2 years of treatment in elderly, antipsychotic-naive patients who were prospectively followed. Risperidone causes a small increase in the QTc interval (a mean prolongation of 10 ms at a dose of 16 mg/day).[94]

Risperidone differs from other second-generation antipsychotics in causing persistent hyperprolactinemia. In one large study, galactorrhea or amenorrhea occurred in 8% to 12% of women treated with risperidone (4 to 6 mg/day), and sexual dysfunction or gynecomastia was reported in 15% of men.[95] Side effects tend not to correlate with serum prolactin concentrations. Hyperprolactinemia in patients with pituitary tumors has been shown to lower estrogen and testosterone levels, which may secondarily result in osteopenia. Similarly, risperidone-induced hyperprolactinemia might increase the risk for osteoporosis.[96]

The active metabolite of risperidone, 9-hydroxyrisperidone, was re-named paliperidone and approved for the treatment of schizophrenia in 2006. It is equipotent to risperidone with which it shares its receptor and side-effect profile including significant prolactin elevation. Its typical dose range is 3 to 6 mg/day but doses up to 12 mg/day can be given. As the end-product of oxidative metabolism, paliperidone is primarily renally excreted and does not rely on P450 metabolism (59% excreted unchanged in urine).

Both risperidone and paliperidone are available as long-acting injectable formulations. The long-acting risperidone formulation (Consta) consists of polymer microspheres containing risperidone, which, immediately before injection, are suspended in a water-based diluent. Following injection, the microspheres begin to release risperidone after a delay of 3 to 4 weeks, after which levels persist for about 4 weeks. Microspheres are administered by gluteal injection every 2 weeks (dose range 12.5 and 50 mg); oral dosing of risperidone should continue until the third injection (4 weeks after the first). If an increase in the dose is necessary, oral supplementation should be provided for 3 to 4 weeks after increasing the dose of risperidone microspheres. Paliperidone is also available as a long-acting injectable formulation (paliperidone palmitate) for monthly IM injections at a dose between 39 and 234 mg. A loading strategy (i.e., 234 mg once, followed by 117 mg 1 week later) produces therapeutic steady-state drug levels rapidly and can be started in inpatient settings. After treatment initiation it is given as a monthly IM injection at a dose between 39 mg and 234 mg. Before administering a long-acting injectable antipsychotic, tolerability of the oral preparation should first be established.

Olanzapine

Olanzapine, a thienobenzodiazepine derivative chemically related to clozapine, was approved by the FDA in 1997 for the treatment of schizophrenia and subsequently approved for bipolar mania. Olanzapine binds to dopamine D$_1$, D$_2$, D$_4$, and D$_5$; serotonin 5-HT$_{2A}$ and 5-HT$_{2C}$; muscarinic M$_{1-5}$; histaminergic H$_1$; and α_1-adrenergic receptors.

Following oral administration, olanzapine is well absorbed, producing peak concentrations in 4 to 6 hours. Olanzapine is metabolized via glucuronidation and oxidation by CYP 450 1A2 with a mean half-life of 24 to 36 hours. Like clozapine, olanzapine's metabolism is induced by cigarette smoking and slowed by CYP 1A2 inhibitors, although to a lesser degree because of alternative metabolic pathways.

In an early fixed-dose registration trial, olanzapine (at doses ranging from 5 to 15 mg/day) displayed a near-linear dose–response relationship; antipsychotic effects were comparable to haloperidol at 15 mg/day, but olanzapine (15 mg/day) demonstrated significantly greater improvement of negative symptoms, fewer EPS, and less prolactin elevation compared to haloperidol at 15 mg/day.[97] A larger flexible-dose trial found higher completion rates, response rates, and greater improvement over a broad range of symptom domains with a mean olanzapine dose of 13 mg/day compared to a mean haloperidol dose of 12 mg/day.[98] Additional analyses of data from these studies found a significant reduction in rates of TD with olanzapine,[99] and a path analysis suggested that olanzapine's superior efficacy for negative symptoms was a primary effect and not due to effects on EPS or depression.[100] In contrast, Rosenheck and colleagues[101] found in a study conducted at Veterans Affairs Medical Centers that outcomes were quite similar between patients randomized to olanzapine and to haloperidol plus prophylactic benztropine except for reduced rates of akathisia and TD. In the CATIE study, olanzapine at a mean dose of 20 mg/day was the antipsychotic with the best efficacy.[16] Since the original designation of 10 mg/day as the recommended dose at the time of olanzapine's introduction, typical clinical doses have steadily climbed to the 15 to 20 mg/day range. One study indicated that escalation of the mean dose to 30 mg/day may improve efficacy in some treatment-resistant patients.[92]

Olanzapine may cause sedation, which some patients experience as a welcome treatment for insomnia whereas others are distressed by difficulty awakening in the morning. Even at high doses, olanzapine is relatively free of EPS[92] and prolactin elevation. However, weight gain and dyslipidemia and metabolic dysregulation are common and a major long-term concern. In the CATIE study, patients randomized to olanzapine gained an average of 2 lb per month and 30% gained more than 7% of their body weight.[16] Olanzapine was also associated with significant elevation of glycosylated hemoglobin, triglycerides, and total cholesterol. Weight gain or metabolic side effects caused 9% of olanzapine-treated patients to discontinue their medication. Both olanzapine and clozapine have been linked to insulin resistance and to DM—an effect that may occur in the absence of obesity.[85] Patients should be carefully screened for metabolic risk factors before initiating olanzapine and should be monitored according to established guidelines (see Table 42-7).[102,103]

A long-acting injectable olanzapine formulation (olanzapine pamoate) can be given every 2 to 4 weeks. Very rarely (approximately 1 event per 1,700 injections), the injection can cause confusion, severe drowsiness or coma due to excessive olanzapine plasma concentrations, resembling alcohol intoxication.[104,105] Termed post-injection delirium/sedation syndrome (PDSS), it requires patients to be observed for 3 hours after receiving the injection which can only be given by certified prescribers and facilities who are able to manage PDSS.

Quetiapine

Quetiapine was approved in 1997 for the treatment of schizophrenia and later for the treatment of acute bipolar mania. Quetiapine has a high affinity for serotonin 5-HT$_{2A}$, α_1- and α_2-adrenergic, and histaminergic H$_1$ receptors and a relatively low affinity for D$_2$ receptors. Whereas maximal D$_2$ occupancy levels of approximately 60% are achieved 2 to 3 hours after a single dose, because of quetiapine's high dissociation constant and short half-life, D$_2$ occupancy drops to less than 30% after 12 hours.[106]

Quetiapine is rapidly absorbed following oral administration, with peak plasma concentrations achieved in 1 to 2 hours. It is primarily metabolized via CYP P450 3A4, producing two active metabolites. Quetiapine metabolism is significantly influenced by drugs that inhibit 3A4 (such as ketoconazole) or induce 3A4 (such as carbamazepine). The half-life of quetiapine is approximately 6 hours; despite this short half-life, quetiapine is frequently prescribed as a once-daily dose, at bedtime, with good results.[107] No significant association has been identified between quetiapine blood levels and clinical response.[108]

In controlled clinical trials, quetiapine demonstrated efficacy for global psychopathology, psychotic symptoms, and negative symptoms greater than placebo and it was comparable to haloperidol or chlorpromazine. Whereas one large multiple fixed-dose trial found no dose–response relationship within a range of doses from 150 to 750 mg/day,[109] another study found superior efficacy when patients were randomly assigned to a higher range of doses (approximately 750 mg/day) compared to low (approximately 250 mg/day).[110] In the CATIE study, quetiapine at a mean dose of 543 mg/day was less effective than olanzapine but it did not differ statistically from the other antipsychotics in tolerability or effectiveness.[16] Doses above 800 mg/day have not been found to have added therapeutic benefit.[111,112]

Common side effects reported with quetiapine include somnolence and dizziness. Quetiapine is very sedating; however, because of its short half-life, bedtime dosing may minimize daytime sedation. Mild orthostatic hypotension was observed in trials that followed a conservative schedule of dose titration, starting with quetiapine 25 mg twice daily. Initiation at higher doses may cause significant orthostatic hypotension, particularly in the elderly, due to quetiapine's adrenergic effects. Reports of dry mouth are probably attributable to its adrenergic mechanisms, since quetiapine is essentially free of muscarinic activity. Quetiapine has consistently demonstrated extremely low levels of EPS and prolactin elevation, comparable to placebo. Quetiapine is intermediate among the second-generation antipsychotics in producing weight gain and in estimates for risk for producing dyslipidemia and DM. In the CATIE study, quetiapine was similar to risperidone in producing a mean 0.5 lb weight gain per month, compared to a 2 lb per month weight gain with olanzapine and weight loss with perphenazine and ziprasidone.[18] Early concerns about a possible link with cataracts have not been supported in post-marketing surveillance, nor was a link detected in the CATIE study. While QTc prolongation is not clinically significant at typical doses, quetiapine overdoses have been associated with cardiac arrhythmias.[113]

Ziprasidone

Ziprasidone was approved in 2001 for the treatment of schizophrenia. Like other second-generation agents, it has a favorable ratio of serotonin 5-HT$_2$ to dopamine D$_2$ affinities. In addition, it is an antagonist with high affinity for serotonin 5-HT$_{1D}$ and 5-HT$_{2C}$ receptors and an agonist at the 5-HT$_{1A}$ receptor. Ziprasidone differs from other agents in its moderate reuptake blockade of serotonin and norepinephrine (noradrenaline).

After oral administration, absorption of ziprasidone is significantly more rapid when administered within 1 hour of a meal compared to fasting. In one study, a fatty meal increased total absorption compared to fasting by 68% and decreased the serum half-life from 6.6 hours to 4.7 hours.[104] Ziprasidone is metabolized by several pathways. Approximately two-thirds of ziprasidone's metabolism is via aldehyde oxidase and the remainder is by CYP450 3A4 and 1A2 hepatic microsomal enzymes. Clinically significant drug–drug interactions have not been reported.

In early trials, ziprasidone exhibited efficacy comparable to haloperidol at doses above 120 mg/day,[105] but with fewer EPS and without sustained elevation of prolactin. Ziprasidone did not become available for inclusion in the CATIE trial until after approximately 40% of subjects had entered and been randomized. At a mean dose of 113 mg/day ziprasidone was less effective than olanzapine and did not differ from the other antipsychotics. Notably, ziprasidone was associated with a mean weight loss of 0.3 lb per month, normalization of lipids, and a lowering of prolactin levels. In a recent study of patients with schizophrenia who remained symptomatic after at least 3 weeks of treatment with ziprasidone at a dose of 160 mg/day, increasing the dose to a maximum of 320 mg/day did not improve outcomes.[114]

Side effects commonly associated with ziprasidone include insomnia or somnolence, nausea, anxiety, and headache. The finding of a mean QTc prolongation of 15.9 ms raised concerns about the risk of torsades de pointes, particularly when administered to patients with underlying cardiac conduction defects or other cardiac risk factors. However, QTc intervals greater than 500 ms have been extremely rare, and a large post-marketing surveillance study of over 18,000 patients (Ziprasidone Observational Study of Cardiac Outcomes [ZODIAC]) did not find an increased rate of non-suicide deaths compared to olanzapine-treated patients.[115] Despite the reassuring safety data, cardiac risk factors should be assessed before initiating this agent.

Aripiprazole

Aripiprazole is a dihydroquinolinone, structurally unrelated to the other antipsychotics. It was approved for the treatment of schizophrenia in 2002 and subsequently for bipolar or mixed mania. It exhibits a novel mechanism of action as a partial agonist at the D_2 receptor with approximately 30% activity compared to dopamine. In addition, aripiprazole has high affinity as a partial agonist at serotonin 5-HT_{1A} and as a full antagonist at 5-HT_{2A}. Aripiprazole has moderate affinity for α_1-adrenergic and histamine H_1 receptors, as well as the serotonin reuptake site. At typical clinical doses of 15 to 30 mg/day, aripiprazole exhibited D_2 receptor occupancy greater than 80%[116] and was not associated with EPS at occupancy levels greater than 90%, presumably the result of partial agonism.

Aripiprazole is well absorbed and reaches peak plasma levels within 3 to 5 hours of an oral dose. It is metabolized primarily by CYP 450 2D6 and 3A4 to dehydroaripiprazole, an active metabolite with a pharmacological profile similar to aripiprazole. The half-lives of aripiprazole and dehydroaripiprazole are 75 and 94 hours, respectively. Because of this unusually long half-life, a period of approximately 2 weeks is required to achieve steady-state drug levels following a change in dosing. Aripiprazole's metabolism may be altered by inhibitors and inducers of CYP 450 3A4 and 2D6.

In registration studies, aripiprazole at doses ranging from 15 to 30 mg/day exhibited efficacy comparable to haloperidol (10 mg/day) and risperidone (6 mg/day). Compared to haloperidol, patients treated with aripiprazole had significantly less prolactin elevation, had less akathisia, and required less anticholinergic treatment for EPS. No differences in efficacy or tolerability were identified between aripiprazole doses of 15, 20, and 30 mg/day. In a 26-week placebo-controlled

trial, aripiprazole was found to prevent relapse.[117] Because aripiprazole was not included in the CATIE trial, its relative effectiveness compared to other agents remains unclear.

Aripiprazole has generally been found to be well tolerated, with side effects largely restricted to insomnia, somnolence, headache, agitation, nausea, and anxiety. It has not differed from placebo in prolactin elevation, EPS, or QTc prolongation. Aripiprazole can lower prolactin (to below the lower normal of prolactin levels in some cases), and it can be used adjunctively to reverse antipsychotic-induced hyperprolactinemia.[118] In a prospective study of first-time users of antipsychotics, aripiprazole caused weight gain, but does not seem to have major effects on glucose or lipid metabolism.[119]

A long-acting injectable aripiprazole formulation (extended-release suspension for monthly IM injections) was approved in 2013 for the maintenance treatment of schizophrenia. This preparation has been shown to reduce relapse rate in a 1-year trial.[120]

Iloperidone

Iloperidone was approved for the treatment of schizophrenia in 2009. Like risperidone, it belongs to the class of benzisoxazole antipsychotics. It has high affinity for D_2/5-HT_{2A} receptors, consistent with other atypicals, and the D_3 and norepinephrine α_1-receptor. In addition, it has moderate affinities for D_4, 5-HT_6 and 5-HT_7 receptors. It is not anticholinergic.

Iloperidone is well absorbed in 2 to 4 hours. While food slows its absorption, it does not alter overall bioavailability and can be given without regards to meals. It is extensively metabolized by 3A4 and 2D6, leading to two active metabolites, P88 and P95.

The effective dose range for iloperidone is 12 to 24 mg/day, given as twice daily dosing (half-life 18 hours). Iloperidone needs to be titrated slowly over the course of at least 1 week or more (e.g., starting with 1 mg twice daily, and daily increases by a maximum of 2 mg twice daily [4 mg/day]; to 2 mg, 4 mg, 6 mg, 8 mg, 10 mg, and 12 mg twice daily) to minimize orthostatic hypotension.[121] In registration trials, orthostatic hypotension was observed in 5% of patients given 20 to 24 mg/day of drug versus 1% given placebo. Consistent with iloperidone's prominent α-blocking properties, retrograde ejaculation and priapism have been observed. Other side effects reported in clinical trials include tachycardia, dizziness, dry mouth, nasal congestion, somnolence, and dyspepsia. Headache, insomnia, and anxiety were reported as well. Iloperidone can cause modest prolactin elevation but little EPS, which might be a relative advantage. It has been associated with dose-dependent weight gain but its overall propensity for metabolic problems remains to be defined. Iloperidone can increase the QTc interval in a dose-dependent fashion.[122] Its use needs thus to be preceded by an assessment of cardiac safety, including possible drug interactions that could alter iloperidone drug levels. In known poor metabolizers of 2D6, half the dose should be used.

Asenapine

Asenapine was approved in 2009 for the treatment of schizophrenia and the acute treatment of manic or mixed mood episodes of bipolar disorder, either as monotherapy or in conjunction with lithium or valproate. Its chemical structure is unique among antipsychotics (a dibenzo-oxepino pyrrole). It has high affinity for a host of receptors, including dopamine$_{1-4}$, 5-HT_{1A} (partial agonist)/$_B$, 5-$HT_{2A,B,C}$, 5-$HT_{5/6/7}$; and $\alpha_{1/2}$-receptors; it has negligible muscarinic receptor affinity but moderate $H_{1/2}$ receptor affinity.

Due to poor gastrointestinal absorption, asenapine is formulated as a sublingual tablet that gets rapidly absorbed. For 10 minutes after the dose, there should be no eating or drinking; if asenapine is swallowed as an oral tablet, the bioavailability is less than 2%.[123] For schizophrenia and adjunctive treatment of mood episodes, the starting dose is 5 mg twice daily that can be adjusted to 10 mg twice daily; for mania monotherapy, the recommended starting dose is 10 mg twice daily. Asenapine is cleared via glucuronidation by UGT1A4 and oxidative metabolism, mostly via CYP1A2.

The most prominent side effects in asenapine registration trials were somnolence and EPS, dose-related akathisia and oral hypoesthesia as well as dizziness and dysgeusia. Asenapine is not weight-neutral but its propensity for weight gain and metabolic disturbances remains to be elucidated. In a 52-week extension trial, 15% of patients gained 7% of body weight or more.[124] Allergic reactions and syncope have been reported as rare but dangerous side effects. Prolactin levels can be increased with asenapine. The registration trials found modest QTc prolongation ranging from 2 to 5 ms for doses up to 40 mg/day, which should be taken into account before prescribing asenapine.

Lurasidone

In 2010, the benzisothiazole antipsychotic lurasidone was approved by the FDA for schizophrenia. It has high affinity binding for dopamine$_2$ receptors, 5-HT$_{2A}$ receptors, and 5-HT$_7$ receptors.[125] Moderate binding exists for α_{2C}; partial antagonism 5-HT$_{1A}$; antagonism for α_{2A}. It does not appreciably bind histamine$_1$ and muscarinic M$_1$ receptors. Lurasidone has a half-life of 18 hours. Its total absorption is increased by two-fold with food, and it should be taken with a meal of at least 350 calories (no effect of fat composition). It is mostly metabolized via 3A4 and blood levels of lurasidone may be significantly affected by CYP3A4 inducers or inhibitors. The recommended starting dose, which is also an effective dose, is 40 mg/day given once daily but doses up to 160 mg/day have been studied.[126] Lurasidone can increase prolactin levels, and it can cause insomnia and EPS including akathisia, particularly at higher doses.[127] In contrast, its propensity for weight gain and metabolic disturbances seems to be low.[128] It effects on the QTc interval are minimal.

DRUG INTERACTIONS WITH ANTIPSYCHOTIC AGENTS

Antipsychotic drugs are most likely to interact with other medications as a result of alterations of hepatic metabolism or when combined with drugs that produce additive side effects (such as anticholinergic effects) or when combined with drugs that impair cardiac conduction. Most conventional antipsychotic agents are extensively metabolized by the 2D6 isoenzyme of the hepatic P450 enzyme system, whereas atypical agents generally have more variable hepatic metabolism, typically involving isoenzymes 3A4, 1A2, and 2D6.[129] Fortunately, because the therapeutic index (risk ratio) of antipsychotic drugs is quite large, interactions with agents that inhibit hepatic metabolism are unlikely to be life-threatening but may increase side effects. Among the atypical antipsychotics, clozapine can produce the most serious adverse effects when blood levels are dramatically elevated; obtundation and cardiovascular effects have been associated with inhibition of clozapine metabolism by fluvoxamine or erythromycin.[65,130] Addition of 2D6 inhibitors (e.g., some SSRIs) to conventional antipsychotics would be expected to increase EPS, but in one placebo-controlled trial this was not clinically significant despite

substantial increases in blood levels of haloperidol and fluphenazine.[131] Drugs that induce hepatic metabolism (such as certain anticonvulsants [e.g., carbamazepine, phenobarbital, phenytoin]) may lower antipsychotic blood concentrations substantially and cause loss of therapeutic efficacy.[132]

Great care must be taken if low-potency agents (such as chlorpromazine, thioridazine, and clozapine) are combined with other highly anticholinergic drugs because the additive anticholinergic activity may produce confusion, urinary retention, or constipation. In addition, low-potency antipsychotic agents can depress cardiac function and can significantly impair cardiac conduction when added to class I antiarrhythmic agents (such as quinidine or procainamide). Ziprasidone and iloperidone also significantly affect cardiac conduction and should not be combined with low-potency phenothiazines or the antiarrhythmic agents.[64]

ONGOING CHALLENGES

Two major challenges remain: antipsychotics are not effective for all patients with psychosis, and they pose significant long-term medical risks to patients who need maintenance treatment. Very little guidance is available from controlled trials for additional interventions if a schizophrenia patient remains symptomatic despite treatment with an adequate dose of clozapine. Early reports described improvement of positive and negative symptoms with the addition of risperidone to clozapine, consistent with the hypothesis that achieving a higher degree of D$_2$ blockade might enhance clozapine's effectiveness for some patients.[133] Subsequent placebo-controlled trials produced inconsistent results, and therefore the role of clozapine augmentation in refractory cases remains controversial and poorly substantiated.[134] As a result, polypharmacy for refractory disease remains a widely used, expensive practice with little support from clinical trials, particularly for patients with serious mental illness. Some forms of secondary psychosis (e.g., psychosis in setting of dementia) show little if any benefit from a treatment which in addition might increase mortality.

For those patients who benefit sufficiently from treatment, prevention of antipsychotic-induced metabolic problems has become a major clinical focus, and creating integrated treatment settings that allow for appropriate medical management of psychiatric patients who receive antipsychotics is a major health care systems goal. Currently, even simple preventive measures (i.e., guideline-concordant metabolic monitoring) remain a major hurdle in many settings,[135] hindering progress in preventing premature death from iatrogenic contributions.[136] The use of metformin to blunt antipsychotic-induced weight gain and metabolic problems has been shown to be an effective prevention strategy in both early course[137] and chronic schizophrenia patients.[138] Patients can benefit from a switch to antipsychotics with less metabolic liability,[22] and some patients can safely reduce polypharmacy.[139] Such proactive management strategies are necessary to reduce the multi-morbidity that characterizes many patients who are treated with antipsychotics.[140] In addition to metabolic problems, there remain concerns about neurotoxicity from antipsychotics over and above disease-related changes as suggested by brain volume loss in treatment studies of patients with schizophrenia.[141,142] Recently, a long-term follow-up of a randomized first episode clinical trial comparing early antipsychotic drug discontinuation with maintenance treatment in symptomatically remitted first-episode patients found that the less aggressive approach with early drug discontinuation led to better long-term functional outcomes compared to those patients assigned to maintenance treatment.[143]

Despite the short-comings of antipsychotics, not treating patients with schizophrenia with an antipsychotic has been shown to have an increased overall mortality rate that needs to be taken into account when considering the risk–benefit equation.[87,144-147]

⊗ Access the complete reference list and multiple choice questions (MCQs) online at https://expertconsult.inkling.com

KEY REFERENCES

9. Creese I, Burt DR, Snyder SH. Dopamine receptor binding predicts clinical and pharmacological potencies of antischizophrenic drugs. *Science* 192(4238):481–483, 1976.

11. Kane J, Honigfeld G, Singer J, et al. Clozapine for the treatment-resistant schizophrenic. A double-blind comparison with chlorpromazine. *Arch Gen Psychiatry* 45(9):789–796, 1988.

16. Lieberman JA, Stroup TS, McEvoy JP, et al. Effectiveness of antipsychotic drugs in patients with chronic schizophrenia. *N Engl J Med* 353(12):1209–1223, 2005.

17. Leucht S, Cipriani A, Spinelli L, et al. Comparative efficacy and tolerability of 15 antipsychotic drugs in schizophrenia: a multiple-treatments meta-analysis. *Lancet* 328(9896):951–962, 2013.

20. Kapur S, Arenovich T, Agid O, et al. Evidence for onset of antipsychotic effects within the first 24 hours of treatment. *Am J Psychiatry* 162(5):939–946, 2005.

21. Leucht S, Tardy M, Komossa K, et al. Antipsychotic drugs versus placebo for relapse prevention in schizophrenia: a systematic review and meta-analysis. *Lancet* 379(9831):2063–2071, 2012.

22. Stroup TS, Byerly MJ, Nasrallah HA, et al. Effects of switching from olanzapine, quetiapine, and risperidone to aripiprazole on 10-year coronary heart disease risk and metabolic syndrome status: results from a randomized controlled trial. *Schizophr Research* 146(1–3):190–195, 2013.

24. Meltzer HY, Alphs L, Green AI, et al. Clozapine treatment for suicidality in schizophrenia: International Suicide Prevention Trial (InterSePT). *Arch Gen Psychiatry* 60(1):82–91, 2003.

27. Farde L, Wiesel FA, Halldin C, et al. Central D2-dopamine receptor occupancy in schizophrenic patients treated with antipsychotic drugs. *Arch Gen Psychiatry* 45(1):71–76, 1988.

42. Kane JM, Woerner M, Weinhold P, et al. Incidence of tardive dyskinesia: five-year data from a prospective study. *Psychopharmacol Bull* 20(3):387–389, 1984.

48. Gurrera RJ, Caroff SN, Cohen A, et al. An international consensus study of neuroleptic malignant syndrome diagnostic criteria using the Delphi method. *J Clin Psychiatry* 72(9):1222–1228, 2011.

58. Henderson DC, Cagliero E, Gray C, et al. Clozapine, diabetes mellitus, weight gain, and lipid abnormalities: A five-year naturalistic study. *Am J Psychiatry* 157(6):975–981, 2000.

76. Alvir JM, Lieberman JA, Safferman AZ, et al. Clozapine-induced agranulocytosis. Incidence and risk factors in the United States. *N Engl J Med* 329(3):162–167, 1993.

83. Ronaldson KJ, Fitzgerald PB, Taylor AJ, et al. A new monitoring protocol for clozapine-induced myocarditis based on an analysis of 75 cases and 94 controls. *Aust N Z J Psychiatry* 45(6):458–465, 2011.

85. Henderson DC, Cagliero E, Copeland PM, et al. Glucose metabolism in patients with schizophrenia treated with atypical antipsychotic agents: a frequently sampled intravenous glucose tolerance test and minimal model analysis. *Arch Gen Psychiatry* 62(1):19–28, 2005.

87. Tiihonen J, Lonnqvist J, Wahlbeck K, et al. 11-year follow-up of mortality in patients with schizophrenia: a population-based cohort study (FIN11 study). *Lancet* 374(9690):620–627, 2009.

93. Woerner MG, Correll CU, Alvir JM, et al. Incidence of tardive dyskinesia with risperidone or olanzapine in the elderly: results from a 2-year, prospective study in antipsychotic-naive patients. *Neuropsychopharmacology* 36(8):1738–1746, 2011.

102. Goff DC, Cather C, Evins AE, et al. Medical morbidity and mortality in schizophrenia: guidelines for psychiatrists. *J Clin Psychiatry* 66(2):183–194, 2005.

115. Strom BL, Eng SM, Faich G, et al. Comparative mortality associated with ziprasidone and olanzapine in real-world use among 18,154 patients with schizophrenia: The Ziprasidone Observational Study of Cardiac Outcomes (ZODIAC). *Am J Psychiatry* 168(2):193–201, 2011.

134. Sommer IE, Begemann MJ, Temmerman A, et al. Pharmacological augmentation strategies for schizophrenia patients with insufficient response to clozapine: a quantitative literature review. *Schizophr Bull* 38(5):1003–1011, 2012.

137. Wu RR, Zhao JP, Jin H, et al. Lifestyle intervention and metformin for treatment of antipsychotic-induced weight gain: a randomized controlled trial. *JAMA* 299(2):185–193, 2008.

138. Jarskog LF, Hamer RM, Catellier DJ, et al. Metformin for weight loss and metabolic control in overweight outpatients with schizophrenia and schizoaffective disorder. *Am J Psychiatry* 170(9):1032–1040, 2013.

139. Essock SM, Schooler NR, Stroup TS, et al. Effectiveness of switching from antipsychotic polypharmacy to monotherapy. *Am J Psychiatry* 168(7):702–708, 2011.

141. Andreasen NC, Liu D, Ziebell S, et al. Relapse duration, treatment intensity, and brain tissue loss in schizophrenia: a prospective longitudinal MRI study. *Am J Psychiatry* 170(6):609–615, 2013.

143. Wunderink L, Nieboer RM, Wiersma D, et al. Recovery in remitted first-episode psychosis at 7 years of follow-up of an early dose reduction/discontinuation or maintenance treatment strategy: Long-term follow-up of a 2-year randomized clinical trial. *JAMA Psychiatry* 70(9):913–920, 2013.

144. Buchanan RW, Kreyenbuhl J, Kelly DL, et al. The 2009 schizophrenia PORT psychopharmacological treatment recommendations and summary statements. *Schizophr Bull* 36(1):71–93, 2010.

43 Antidepressants

Maurizio Fava, MD, and George I. Papakostas, MD

KEY POINTS

- The immediate mechanism of action of modern antidepressants ("immediate effects") involves influencing the function of one or more monoamine neurotransmitter systems (serotonin, norepinephrine [noradrenaline], or dopamine).

- Influencing monoaminergic function has been shown to result in several changes in second-messenger systems and gene expression/regulation ("downstream effects").

- "Downstream effects" may explain the delayed onset of antidepressant response seen with all contemporary agents (most patients improve following at least 3 weeks of treatment).

- For the most part, all contemporary antidepressants are equally effective when treating major depressive disorder.

- There are significant differences in the relative tolerability and safety of contemporary antidepressants.

OVERVIEW

A large number of compounds have been developed to treat depression. Traditionally, these compounds have been called "antidepressants," even though most of these drugs are also effective in the treatment of a number of anxiety disorders (such as panic and obsessive-compulsive disorder [OCD]) and a variety of other conditions (Box 43-1). The precursors of two of the major contemporary antidepressant families, the monoamine oxidase inhibitors (MAOIs) and the tricyclic antidepressants (TCAs), were discovered by serendipity in the 1950s.

Specifically, the administration of iproniazid, an antimycobacterial agent, was first noted to possess antidepressant effects in depressed patients suffering from tuberculosis.[1] Shortly thereafter, iproniazid was found to inhibit MAO, which is involved in the catabolism of serotonin, norepinephrine (noradrenaline), and dopamine.

In parallel, imipramine was initially developed as an antihistamine, but Kuhn[2] discovered that of some 500 imipramine-treated patients with various psychiatric disorders, only those with endogenous depression with mental and motor retardation showed a remarkable improvement during 1 to 6 weeks of daily imipramine therapy. The same compound was also found to inhibit the re-uptake of serotonin and norepinephrine.[3,4] Thus, it was the discovery of the antidepressant effects of iproniazid and imipramine that led to the development of the MAOIs and TCAs, and this discovery was instrumental in the formulation of the monoamine theory of depression. In turn, guided by this theory, the subsequent development of compounds selective for the re-uptake of either serotonin or norepinephrine or both was designed, rather than accidental. As a result, over the last few decades, chemical alterations of these first antidepressants have resulted in the creation of a wide variety of monoamine-based antidepressants with a variety of mechanisms of action. The antidepressant drugs are a heterogeneous group of compounds that have been traditionally subdivided into major groups according to their chemical structure or, more commonly, according to their effects on monoamine neurotransmitter systems: selective serotonin re-uptake inhibitors (SSRIs); TCAs and the related cyclic antidepressants (i.e., amoxapine and maprotiline); MAOIs; serotonin norepinephrine re-uptake inhibitors (SNRIs); norepinephrine re-uptake inhibitors (NRIs); norepinephrine/dopamine re-uptake inhibitors (NDRIs); serotonin receptor antagonists/agonists; and alpha$_2$-adrenergic receptor antagonists. Because they overlap, the mechanisms of action and the indications for use for the antidepressants are discussed together, but separate sections are provided for their method of administration and their side effects.

MECHANISM OF ACTION

The precise mechanisms by which the antidepressant drugs exert their therapeutic effects remain unknown, although much is known about their immediate actions within the nervous system. All of the currently marketed antidepressants interact with the monoamine neurotransmitter systems in the brain, particularly the norepinephrine and serotonin systems, and to a lesser extent the dopamine system. Essentially all currently marketed antidepressants have as their molecular targets components of monoamine synapses, including the re-uptake transporters (that terminate the action of norepinephrine, serotonin, or dopamine in synapses), monoamine receptors, or enzymes that serve to metabolize monoamines. What remains unknown is how these initial interactions produce a therapeutic response.[5] The search for the molecular events that convert altered monoamine neurotransmitter function into the lifting of depressive symptoms remains a matter of very active research.

Since TCAs and MAOIs were the first antidepressants to be discovered and introduced, this was initially interpreted as suggesting that antidepressants work by increasing noradrenergic or serotonergic neurotransmission, thus compensating for a postulated state of relative monoamine "deficiency." However, this simple theory could not fully explain the action of antidepressant drugs for a number of reasons. The most important of these include the lack of convincing evidence that depression is characterized by a state of inadequate or "deficient" monoamine neurotransmission. In fact, the results of studies testing the monoamine depletion hypothesis in depression have yielded inconsistent results.[5] Moreover, blockade of monoamine re-uptake or inhibition of monoamine degradation occurs rapidly (within hours) following monoamine re-uptake inhibitor or MAOI administration, respectively. However, treatment with antidepressants for less than 2 weeks is unlikely to result in a significant lifting of depression; it has been consistently observed and reported that remission of depression often requires 4 weeks of treatment or more. These considerations have led to the idea that inhibition of monoamine re-uptake or inhibition of MAO by antidepressants represents an initiating event. The actual therapeutic actions of antidepressants, however, result from slower adaptive responses within neurons to these initial biochemical perturbations ("downstream events").[6] Although research geared toward understanding the therapeutic actions of antidepressants has been challenging, receptor studies have been useful in

- Major depressive disorder and other unipolar depressive disorders
- Bipolar depression
- Panic disorder
- Social anxiety disorder
- Generalized anxiety disorder
- Post-traumatic stress disorder
- Obsessive-compulsive disorder (e.g., clomipramine and SSRIs)
- Depression with psychotic features (in combination with an antipsychotic drug)
- Bulimia nervosa
- Neuropathic pain (tricyclic drugs and SNRIs)
- Insomnia (e.g., trazodone, amitriptyline)
- Enuresis (imipramine best studied)
- Atypical depression (e.g., monoamine oxidase inhibitors)
- Attention-deficit/hyperactivity disorder (e.g., desipramine, bupropion)

SNRIs, Serotonin norepinephrine re-uptake inhibitors; SSRIs, selective serotonin re-uptake inhibitors.

understanding and predicting some of the side effects of contemporary antidepressants. For example, the binding affinity of antidepressants at muscarinic cholinergic receptors generally parallels the prevalence of certain side effects during treatment (e.g., dry mouth, constipation, urinary hesitancy, poor concentration). Similarly, treatment with agents that have high affinities for histamine H_1 receptors (e.g., doxepin and amitriptyline) appears to be more likely to result in sedation, and increased appetite. Such information is very useful to clinicians and patients when making treatment decisions or to researchers when attempting to develop new antidepressants.

The architecture of the monoamine neurotransmitter systems in the central nervous system (CNS) is based on the synthesis of the neurotransmitter within a restricted number of nuclei within the brainstem, with neurons projecting widely throughout the brain and, for norepinephrine and serotonin, the spinal cord as well.[5] Norepinephrine is synthesized within a series of nuclei in the medulla and pons, of which the largest is the nucleus locus coeruleus. Serotonin is synthesized in the brainstem raphe nuclei. Dopamine is synthesized in the substantia nigra and the ventral tegmental area of the midbrain. Through extensive projection networks, these neurotransmitters influence a large number of target neurons in the cerebral cortex, basal forebrain, striatum, limbic system, and brainstem, where they interact with multiple receptor types to regulate arousal, vigilance, attention, sensory processing, emotion, and cognition (including memory).[7]

Norepinephrine, serotonin, and dopamine are removed from synapses after release by re-uptake, mostly into presynaptic neurons.[5] This mechanism of terminating neurotransmitter action is mediated by specific norepinephrine, serotonin, and dopamine re-uptake transporter proteins. After re-uptake, norepinephrine, serotonin, and dopamine are either re-loaded into vesicles for subsequent release or broken down by MAO. MAO is present in two forms (MAO_A and MAO_B), which differ in their substrate preferences, inhibitor specificities, tissue expression, and cell distribution. MAO_A preferentially oxidizes serotonin and is irreversibly inactivated by low concentrations of the acetylenic inhibitor clorgyline. MAO_B preferentially oxidizes phenylethylamine (PEA) and benzylamine and is irreversibly inactivated by low concentrations of pargyline and deprenyl.[5] Dopamine, tyramine, and tryptamine are substrates for both forms of MAO. Catecholamines are also broken down

by catechol O-methyltransferase (COMT), an enzyme that acts extracellularly.

The classification of antidepressant drugs has perhaps focused too narrowly on synaptic pharmacology (i.e., "immediate effects"), and has certainly failed to take into account molecular and cellular changes in neural function that are brought about by the chronic administration of these agents.[5] For example, it has been postulated that changes in post-receptor signal transduction may account for the aforementioned characteristic lag-time between the time a drug is administered and the drug-induced resolution of a depressive episode. In fact, studies have shown that hippocampal neurogenesis occurs following chronic antidepressant treatment in animal models.[8] In parallel, rapid activation of the TrkB neurotrophin receptor and PLC gamma-1 signaling has been described with almost all antidepressant drugs, a possible mechanism by which the process of neuronal neurogenesis observed following chronic administration of antidepressants may occur.[9] Alternatively, one could postulate that this lag phase in antidepressant action may be related to a re-organization of neuronal networks, postulated as a potential "final common pathway" for antidepressant effects to occur.[5] Nevertheless, further research is urgently needed in order to help us understand the specific effects of the antidepressants and what constitutes illness and recovery in depression.

Mechanism of Action of Selective Serotonin Re-uptake Inhibitors

At therapeutically relevant doses, the SSRIs exhibit significant effects primarily on serotonin re-uptake in the human brain.[10] Some SSRIs also appear to have effects on other monoamine transporters, with sertraline demonstrating modest dopamine re-uptake inhibition, and paroxetine and fluoxetine demonstrating modest norepinephrine re-uptake inhibition.[10] In addition, fluoxetine, particularly the R-isomer, has mild 5-HT_{2A} and 5-HT_{2C} antagonist activity. Non-monoaminergic effects have also been described for some of the SSRIs, including moderate and selective effects on glutamate receptor expression and editing.[11] The SSRIs have minimal or no affinity for muscarinic cholinergic, histaminergic, and adrenergic receptors, with the exception of paroxetine (which is a weak cholinergic receptor antagonist), citalopram (which is a weak antagonist of the histamine H_1 receptor), and sertraline (which has weak affinity for the alpha$_1$ receptors).[10] Overall, the affinity of these agents for these specific receptors is lower than those of the TCAs, resulting in a milder side-effect profile. Similarly, the lack of significant action for the remaining SSRIs on these receptors is also thought to contribute to the milder side-effect profile of these agents compared with the TCAs.

Mechanism of Action of Serotonin Norepinephrine Re-uptake Inhibitors

Unlike the TCAs, SNRIs inhibit the re-uptake of serotonin more potently than the re-uptake of norepinephrine.[10] Similar to most SSRIs, the SNRIs have minimal or no affinity for muscarinic cholinergic, histaminergic, and adrenergic receptors.[10] Interestingly enough, administration of these drugs has been shown to prevent a decrease in cell proliferation and BDNF expression in rat hippocampus observed with chronic stress, in a study that offers further insights into the "downstream effects" of these agents.[12] In parallel, studies suggest that chronic treatment with the SNRI duloxetine not only produces a marked up-regulation of BDNF mRNA and protein but may also affect the sub-cellular re-distribution of neurotrophin, potentially improving synaptic plasticity.[13]

Mechanism of Action of Norepinephrine Re-uptake Inhibitors

At therapeutically relevant doses, the NRIs have significant effects primarily on norepinephrine re-uptake, although the NRI atomoxetine is also a weak inhibitor of serotonin uptake.[14] NRIs also appear to have several non-monoaminergic properties. Specifically, the NRI reboxetine also appears to functionally inhibit nicotinic acetylcholine receptors.[15] In addition, in rats, atomoxetine has been shown to increase in vivo extracellular levels of acetylcholine (ACh) in cortical but not subcortical brain regions, with a mechanism dependent on norepinephrine alpha$_1$ and/or dopamine D$_1$ receptor activation.[16] Furthermore, the major human metabolite of atomoxetine (4-hydroxyatomoxetine) is a partial agonist of the kappa-opioid receptor.[17] Finally, reboxetine has also been found to be the antidepressant that affects glutamate receptors (GluR) most, with a decrease of GluR3 expression.[11]

Mechanism of Action of Serotonin Receptor Agonist/Antagonists

Both trazodone and nefazodone are relatively weak inhibitors of serotonin and norepinephrine uptake, and they primarily block serotonin 5-HT$_{2A}$ receptors (in some cases, demonstrating partial agonist properties as well).[18–21] They also share a metabolite, m-chlorophenylpiperazine (mCPP), which acts as a serotonin 5-HT$_{2C}$ agonist and appears to be able to release serotonin pre-synaptically.[22] Trazodone also appears to stimulate the mu$_1$- and mu$_2$-opioid receptors[23] and is a potent agonist of the serotonin 5-HT$_{2C}$ receptors, which, when activated,[24,25] may inhibit NMDA-induced cyclic GMP elevation. Since trazodone is also a weak inhibitor of serotonin re-uptake as well, the overall effect of trazodone appears to be an increase in extracellular levels of serotonin in the brain.[26] This effect explains the fact that trazodone treatment has been associated with the occurrence of a serotonin syndrome.[27] Both trazodone and (although to a lesser degree) nefazodone are potent blockers of the alpha$_1$-adrenergic receptor.

Agomelatine, available in Europe as an antidepressant, is a selective 5-HT$_{2C}$ antagonist and acts as a melatonin MT$_1$ and MT$_2$ receptor agonist. The 5-HT$_{2C}$ antagonism properties of agomelatine have been thought to be responsible for increases in frontocortical dopaminergic and adrenergic activity in animals during administration of agomelatine.[28]

Buspirone and gepirone act as full agonists at serotonin 5-HT$_{1A}$ autoreceptors and are generally, but not exclusively, partial agonists at post-synaptic serotonin 5-HT$_{1A}$ receptors.[29] Neither buspirone or gepirone are approved for depression, but buspirone is FDA-approved for the treatment of anxiety. Buspirone and gepirone show weak alpha$_1$-adrenoceptor affinity, but significant and selective alpha$_1$-adrenoceptor intrinsic efficacy, which was expressed in a tissue- and species-dependent manner.[30] Buspirone also shows binding with high affinity to recombinant human D$_3$ and D$_4$ receptors (~98 and ~29 nm respectively).[31] Buspirone and gepirone are thought to lead to excitation of noradrenergic cell firing,[32] antagonizing primarily pre-synaptic inhibitory dopamine D$_2$ autoreceptors at dopaminergic neurons.[33] Buspirone also has potent alpha$_2$-adrenoceptor antagonist properties via its principal metabolite, 1-(2-pyrimidinyl)-piperazine.[34,35] Vilazodone is a serotonin 5-HT$_{1A}$ receptor partial agonist and a selective serotonin re-uptake inhibitor that induces maximal serotonin levels that are similar in the medial and the lateral cortex and are up to six-fold higher than those induced by SSRIs tested in parallel, when serotonin levels are measured in two sub-regions of the rat prefrontal cortex by microdialysis.[36] It appears that the net effect of vilazodone at release-regulating 5-HT$_{1A}$ autoreceptors is inhibitory, leading to markedly increased serotonin output.

Vortioxetine is a recently-approved antidepressant with multi-modal activity that functions as a serotonin 5-HT$_3$, 5-HT$_7$ and 5-HT$_{1D}$ receptor antagonist, serotonin 5-HT$_{1B}$ receptor partial agonist, serotonin 5-HT$_{1A}$ receptor agonist and inhibitor of the serotonin transporter in vitro.[37] Vortioxetine has shown to be able to increase extracellular serotonin, dopamine, and norepinephrine in the medial prefrontal cortex and ventral hippocampus,[38] and to significantly increase cell proliferation and cell survival and stimulate maturation of immature granule cells in the sub-granular zone of the dentate gyrus of the hippocampus after 21 days of treatment.[37]

Mechanism of Action of Norepinephrine/ Dopamine Re-uptake Inhibitors

The NDRIs primarily block the re-uptake of dopamine and norepinephrine and have minimal or no affinity for pre-synaptic or post-synaptic monoamine receptors. The mechanism of action of bupropion has not been fully elucidated, although it appears to primarily block the re-uptake of both dopamine and norepinephrine.[39] Bupropion and its metabolites have been shown to be able to inhibit striatal uptake of the selective dopamine transporter (DAT)-binding radioligand (11)C-betaCIT-FE in vivo,[40] and to have mild affinity for the norepinephrine transporter,[41] although some researchers have argued that the effect of bupropion on norepinephrine is primarily through an increase in pre-synaptic norepinephrine release.[42] Whatever the exact mechanism may be, it appears that the overall effect of bupropion is a dose-dependent increase in brain extracellular dopamine and norepinephrine concentrations.[43] It also appears that bupropion acts as an antagonist at alpha$_3$beta$_2$ and alpha$_3$beta$_4$ nAChRs in rat striatum and hippocampus, respectively, across the same concentration range that inhibits DAT and norepinephrine transporter (NET) function.[44]

Mechanism of Action of Alpha$_2$-Adrenergic Receptor Antagonists

The alpha$_2$-adrenergic receptor antagonists (e.g., mirtazapine and mianserin) appear to enhance the release of both serotonin and norepinephrine by blocking auto- and hetero-alpha$_2$ receptors.[45] Since mirtazapine appears to be a blocker of serotonin 5-HT$_2$ and 5-HT$_3$ receptors as well, it is thought to enhance the release of norepinephrine and also enhance 5-HT$_{1A}$–mediated serotonergic transmission.[46] Mirtazapine was the first alpha$_2$-adrenergic receptor antagonist to be approved by the Food and Drug Administration (FDA) for depression. Mirtazapine is also a potent histaminergic H$_1$-receptor antagonist.[10] Mianserin, also an alpha$_2$-noradrenergic receptor antagonist and a serotonin 5-HT$_2$ antagonist, is available in Europe and is not FDA-approved.

Mechanism of Action of Tricyclic Antidepressants

TCAs, referred to as such because they share a chemical structure with two joined benzene rings, have been in use for almost half a century for the treatment of depression. With the exception of clomipramine, and in contrast with the SNRIs, the TCAs inhibit the re-uptake of norepinephrine more potently than the re-uptake of serotonin. Recent studies have also shown that five of the TCAs bind to the S1S2 domain of the GluR2 subunit of the AMPA receptor, suggesting an effect of TCAs on the glutamergic system.[47] In addition, doxepin, amitriptyline, and nortriptyline also inhibit glycine uptake by blocking the glycine transporter 1b ($GLYT_{1b}$) and glycine transporter 2a ($GLYT_{2a}$) to a similar extent.[48] Amoxapine displays a selective inhibition of $GLYT_{2a}$ behaving as a 10-fold more efficient inhibitor of this isoform than of $GLYT_{1b}$[48] and is also a dopamine D_2 receptor antagonist.[49] Interestingly, *in vitro* data suggest that trimipramine and clomipramine have comparable affinity for the dopamine D_2 receptor.[50] The TCAs, to varying degrees, are also fairly potent blockers of histamine H_1 receptors, serotonin 5-HT_2 receptors, muscarinic acetylcholine receptors, and alpha$_1$-adrenergic receptors.[10,50]

Mechanism of Action of Monoamine Oxidase Inhibitors

MAOIs act by inhibiting MAO, an enzyme found on the outer membrane of mitochondria, where it catabolizes (degrades) a number of monoamines including dopamine, norepinephrine, and serotonin. Specifically, following their re-uptake from the synapse into the pre-synaptic neuron, norepinephrine, serotonin, and dopamine are either loaded into vesicles for subsequent re-release or broken down by MAO. MAO is present in two forms (MAO_A and MAO_B), which differ in their substrate preferences, inhibitor specificities, tissue expression, and cell distribution. MAO_A preferentially oxidizes serotonin and is irreversibly inactivated by low concentrations of the acetylenic inhibitor clorgyline. MAO_B preferentially oxidizes phenylethylamine (PEA) and benzylamine and is irreversibly inactivated by low concentrations of pargyline and deprenyl. Dopamine and the dietary (exogenous) amines, tyramine and tryptamine, are substrates for *both* forms of MAO.[51] In the gastrointestinal (GI) tract and the liver, MAO catabolizes a number of dietary pressor amines (such as dopamine, tyramine, tryptamine, and phenylethylamine).[52] For this reason, consumption of certain foods (that contain high levels of dietary amines) while on an MAOI may precipitate a hypertensive crisis, characterized by hypertension, hyperpyrexia, tachycardia, tremulousness, and cardiac arrhythmias.[53] The same reaction may also occur during co-administration of dopaminergic agents and MAOIs, while the co-administration of MAOIs with other antidepressants that potentiate serotonin could result in serotonin syndromes due to toxic CNS serotonin levels. The serotonin syndrome is characterized by alterations in cognition (e.g., disorientation and confusion), behavior (e.g., agitation and restlessness), autonomic nervous system function (e.g., fever, shivering, diaphoresis, and diarrhea), and neuromuscular activity (e.g., ataxia, hyperreflexia, and myoclonus).[54-56] Since MAO enzymatic activity requires approximately 14 days to be fully restored, such food or medications should be avoided for 2 weeks following the discontinuation of an irreversible MAOI ("MAOI washout period"). Serotonergic and dopaminergic antidepressants are typically discontinued 2 weeks before the initiation of an MAOI, with the exception of fluoxetine, which needs to be discontinued 5 weeks in advance because of its much longer half-life.

Older MAOIs, including phenelzine, tranylcypromine, and isocarboxazid, irreversibly inhibit the enzymatic activity of both MAO_A and MAO_B, while newer ones are relatively selective (brofaromine and moclobemide preferentially inhibit MAO_A; oral selegiline selectively inhibits MAO_B). Reversible MAO_A-selective inhibitors are designed to minimize the risk of hypertensive crises, and patients on conventional doses of moclobemide do not need to strictly adhere to the low-tyramine diet, although, at very high doses (e.g., 900 mg/day of moclobemide), inhibition of MAO_B also occurs.[57] All MAOIs available in the US are irreversible inhibitors of MAO_A and MAO_B activity.

More recently, additional pharmacological properties for the MAOIs have been revealed. MAOIs, for instance, also appear to inhibit the binding of [3H] quinpirole, a dopamine agonist with high affinity for D_2 and D_3 dopamine receptors.[58,59] To complicate the pharmacology of MAOIs further, two of the MAOIs, selegiline and tranylcypromine, have methamphetamine and amphetamine as metabolites.[60,61] In addition, phenelzine also elevates brain gamma-aminobutyric acid (GABA) levels, and as yet unidentified metabolites of phenelzine may be responsible for this effect.[61] R($-$)- but not S($+$)- selegiline also appears to induce dopamine release by directly modulating ATP-sensitive potassium channels.[62] Finally, ($+$)-tranylcypromine (TCP) has been shown to be more potent than ($-$)-TCP as an inhibitor of 5-HT uptake, whereas ($-$)-TCP has been shown to be more potent than ($+$)-TCP as an inhibitor of dopamine and norepinephrine uptake.[63]

Although the risk for serotonin syndromes may be lower than with the older MAOIs, and a number of studies suggested the safety of combining moclobemide with SSRIs,[64-66] there have been a number of non-fatal[67,68] and fatal serotonin syndromes involving the co-administration of moclobemide and SSRIs.[69-74] For these reasons, the concomitant use of moclobemide and serotonergic agents should be avoided. In addition, the co-ingestion of moclobemide and SSRIs in overdose may result in death, which needs to be taken into account for patients at risk for suicide.[70]

CLINICAL USES OF ANTIDEPRESSANTS

Since the introduction of fluoxetine, the SSRIs and the SNRIs have become the most often prescribed initial pharmacological treatment for major depressive disorder (MDD). The success of these newer agents in displacing TCAs as first-choice agents is not based on established differences in efficacy, but rather on a generally more favorable side-effect profile (such as a lack of anticholinergic and cardiac side effects, and a high therapeutic index, i.e., the ratio of lethal dose to therapeutic dose), combined with ease of administration. Furthermore, with certain co-morbidities of depression (such as OCD), SSRIs offer advantages in efficacy over the TCAs. Nonetheless, the TCAs remain useful alternatives for the treatment of some patients with depression. In contrast, because of their inferior safety profile, the traditional MAOIs are a class of drugs reserved for patients in whom other treatments have failed. Clearly, the newer antidepressants (SSRIs, SNRIs, NRIs, NDRIs, and serotonin receptor antagonists) all have major safety or tolerability advantages over the TCAs and MAOIs. The recently-approved serotonin receptor antagonist vortioxetine may have the additional advantage of distinctive pro-cognitive effects.

Continuation and Maintenance of Antidepressant Treatment

Originally, based on studies with TCAs, patients with unipolar depressive disorders were observed to be at high risk for relapse when treatment was discontinued within the first 16 weeks of therapy. Therefore, in treatment-responders, most experts favor a continuation of antidepressant therapy for a minimum of 6 months following the achievement of remission. The value of continuation therapy for several months to prevent relapse into the original episode has also been established for virtually all of the newer agents.[75] Risk of recurrence after this 6- to 8-month continuation period (i.e., the development of a new episode after recovery from the index episode) is particularly elevated in patients with a chronic course before recovery, residual symptoms, and multiple prior episodes (three or more).[76] For these individuals, the optimal duration of maintenance treatment is unknown, but is assumed to be much longer (measured in years). In fact, based on research to date, prophylactic efficacy of an antidepressant has been observed for as long as 5 years with clear benefit.[77] In contrast to the initial expectation that maintenance therapy would be effective at dosages lower than that required for acute treatment, the current consensus is that full-dose therapy is required for effective prophylaxis.[78] About 20% to 30% of patients who are treated with each of the classes of antidepressants will experience a return of depressive symptoms despite continued treatment. In such patients, a dose increase of the antidepressant is typically the first-line approach.[79]

Suicide Risk

Unlike the SSRIs and other newer agents, the MAOIs, TCAs, and related cyclic antidepressants (maprotiline and amoxapine) are potentially lethal in overdose. Thus, a careful evaluation of impulsiveness and suicide risk influences not only the decision as to the need for hospitalizing a person with depression but also the choice of an antidepressant. For potentially suicidal or highly impulsive patients, the SSRIs and the other newer agents would be a better initial choice than a cyclic compound or an MAOI. Patients at elevated suicide risk who cannot tolerate these safer compounds or who do not respond to them should not receive large quantities or refillable prescriptions for TCAs or MAOIs. Generally, patients who are new to treatment or those at more than minimal risk for suicide or whose therapeutic relationship is unstable should receive a limited supply of any medication. Evaluation for suicide risk must continue even after the initiation of treatment. Although suicidal thoughts are often among the first symptoms to improve with antidepressant treatment, they may also be slow to respond to treatment, and patients may become demoralized before therapeutic efficacy is evident. Side effects (such as agitation and restlessness) and, most important, inter-current life events may exacerbate suicidal thoughts before a full therapeutic response. Thus, rarely, for a variety of reasons, patients may temporarily become more suicidal following the initiation of treatment. Should such worsening occur, appropriate interventions may include management of side effects, more frequent monitoring, discontinuation of the initial treatment, or hospitalization. In 2004, the FDA asked manufacturers of almost all the newer antidepressant drugs to include in their labeling a warning statement that recommends close observation of adult and pediatric patients treated with these drugs for worsening depression or the emergence of suicidality. This warning was based on the analyses of clinical trials data that compared the relative risk of emergence of suicidal ideation on these drugs compared to placebo following initiation of treatment. The difference was small, but statistically significant. This finding underscores the need for good practice, which includes education of patients (and families if the patient is a child) about side effects of drugs (including the possible emergence of suicidal thoughts and behaviors), close monitoring (especially early in treatment), and the availability of a clinician in case suicidality emerges or worsens. A general consensus remains, however, that the risks associated with withholding antidepressant treatment from patients, including pediatric patients, with serious depression vastly outweighs the risks associated with the drugs by many orders of magnitude.

CHOICE OF AN ANTIDEPRESSANT

A large number of antidepressants are available (Table 43-1), including SSRIs, SNRIs, NRIs, NDRIs, serotonin receptor antagonists/agonists, the alpha$_2$-adrenergic receptor antagonists, TCAs and related compounds, and MAOIs. The available formulations and their typical dosages are listed in Table 43-1, and aspects of their successful use are listed in Box 43-2.

Selective Serotonin Re-uptake Inhibitors

The overall efficacy of the SSRIs in the treatment of depression is equivalent to that of older agents, including the TCAs and the MAOIs moclobemide[80] and phenelzine,[81] while all SSRIs appear to be equally effective in the treatment of depression.[82] However, there is some evidence suggesting that that the SSRI escitalopram may be more effective than the remaining five SSRIs in the treatment of MDD,[83] although this evidence remains controversial.

Because of their favorable side-effect profile, the SSRIs are used as first-line treatment in the overwhelming majority of cases, with more than 90% of clinicians in one survey indicating that SSRIs were their first-line treatment.[84] Despite the tolerability and the widespread efficacy of the SSRIs, there is mounting evidence to suggest that depressed patients with certain characteristics (including co-morbid anxiety disorders[85] and a greater number of somatic symptoms [such as pain, headaches, and fatigue][86]) respond less well to SSRIs than those without such characteristics.

TABLE 43-1A Available Preparations of Antidepressants: Selective Serotonin Re-uptake Inhibitors (SSRIs)

Drug	Therapeutic Dosage Forms	Usual Daily Dose (mg/day)	Extreme Dosage (mg/day)	Plasma Levels (ng/ml)
Fluoxetine (Prozac and generics)	C: 10, 20, 40 mg LC: 20 mg/5 ml Weekly: 90 mg	20–40	5–80	
Fluvoxamine (Luvox and generics)*	T: 50, 100 mg	50–150	50–300	
Paroxetine (Paxil and generics)	T: 10, 20, 30, 40 mg LC: 10 mg/5 ml CR: 12.5, 25, 37.5 mg	20–40 25–50	10–50 12.5–50	
Sertraline (Zoloft and generics)	T: 25, 50, 100 mg LC: 20 mg/ml	50–150	25–300	
Citalopram (Celexa and generics)	T: 10, 20, 40 mg LC: 10 mg/5 ml	20–40	10–60	
Escitalopram (Lexapro and generics)	T: 10, 20 mg	10–20	10–30	

*Not marketed for depression in the US.
C, Capsules; CR, controlled release; LC, liquid concentrate or solution; T, tablets.

TABLE 43-1B Available Preparations of Antidepressants: Serotonin Norepinephrine Re-uptake Inhibitors (SNRIs)

Drug	Therapeutic Dosage Forms	Usual Daily Dose (mg/day)	Extreme Dosage (mg/day)	Plasma Levels (ng/ml)
Venlafaxine (Effexor and generics)	T: 25, 37.5, 50, 75, 100 mg XR: 37.5, 75, 150 mg	75–300	75–450	
Duloxetine (Cymbalta and generics)	C: 20, 30, 60 mg	60–120	30–180	
Desvenlafaxine (Pristiq)	T: 50, 100 mg	50–100	25–200	
Levomilnacipran ER (Fetzima)	C: 20, 40, 80, 120 mg	40–120	20–240	

C, Capsules; T, tablets; XR, extended-release.

TABLE 43-1C Available Preparations of Antidepressants: Norepinephrine Re-uptake Inhibitors (NRIs)

Drug	Therapeutic Dosage Forms	Usual Daily Dose (mg/day)	Extreme Dosage (mg/day)	Plasma Levels (ng/ml)
Reboxetine*	T: 4 mg	4–10	4–12	
Atomoxetine (Strattera)	T: 10, 18, 25, 40, 60 mg	40–80	40–120	

*Not marketed for depression in the US.
T, tablets.

TABLE 43-1D Available Preparations of Antidepressants: Serotonin Receptor Antagonists/Agonists

Drug	Therapeutic Dosage Forms	Usual Daily Dose (mg/day)	Extreme Dosage (mg/day)	Plasma Levels (ng/ml)
Trazodone (Desyrel and generics)	T: 50, 100, 150, 300 mg	200–400	100–600	
Trazodone Extended Release (Oleptro)	T: 150, 300 mg	150–300	75–600	
Nefazodone (Serzone and generics)	T: 50, 100, 150, 200, 250 mg	200–400	100–600	
Vilazodone (Viibryd)	T: 10, 20, 40 mg	40–80	20–160	
Vortioxetine (Brintellix)	T: 5, 10, 20 mg	10–20	5–40	

T, tablets.

TABLE 43-1E Available Preparations of Antidepressants: Norepinephrine Dopamine Re-uptake Inhibitors (NDRIs)

Drug	Therapeutic Dosage Forms	Usual Daily Dose (mg/day)	Extreme Dosage (mg/day)	Plasma Levels (ng/ml)
Bupropion (Wellbutrin and generics)	T: 75, 100 mg XR: 100, 150, 200 mg XL: 150, 300 mg Soltabs: 15, 30, 45 mg	200–300	100–450	

Soltabs, orally disintegrating tablet; T, tablets; XL, extended-release; XR, extended-release.

TABLE 43-1F Available Preparations of Antidepressants: Alpha$_2$-receptor Antagonists

Drug	Therapeutic Dosage Forms	Usual Daily Dose (mg/day)	Extreme Dosage (mg/day)	Plasma Levels (ng/ml)
Mirtazapine (Remeron and generics)	T: 15, 30, 45 mg Soltabs: 15, 30, 45 mg	15–45	7.5–90	

Soltabs, orally disintegrating tablet; T, tablets.

Dosage

Because of their relatively low side-effect burden, the starting dose of SSRIs is often the minimally effective daily dose: 10 mg for escitalopram (Lexapro); 20 mg for fluoxetine (Prozac), paroxetine (Paxil), and citalopram (Celexa); 50 mg for sertraline (Zoloft); 25 mg for paroxetine CR (Paxil CR); and 100 mg for fluvoxamine (Luvox). Starting at lower doses and increasing the dose shortly thereafter (i.e., after 1 to 2 weeks) may further improve tolerability. Maximum therapeutic doses for SSRIs are typically one-fold to four-fold greater than the starting dose. The dosages and formulations of the SSRIs marketed in the US are listed in Table 43-1. Only one of the SSRIs, fluvoxamine, is not approved for the treatment

TABLE 43-1G Available Preparations of Antidepressants: Tricyclic Antidepressants (TCAs) and Other Cyclic Compounds

Drug	Therapeutic Dosage Forms	Usual Daily Dose (mg/day)	Extreme Dosage (mg/day)	Plasma Levels (ng/ml)
Imipramine (Tofranil and generics)	T: 10, 25, 50 mg C: 75, 100, 125, 150 mg INJ: 25 mg/2 ml	150–200	50–300	>225*
Desipramine (Norpramin and generics)	T: 10, 25, 50, 75, 100, 150 mg C: 25, 50 mg	150–200	50–300	>125
Amitriptyline (Elavil and generics)	T: 10, 25, 50, 75, 100, 150 mg INJ: 10 mg/ml	150–200	50–300	>120†
Nortriptyline (Pamelor and generics)	C: 10, 25, 50, 75 mg LC: 10 mg/5 ml	75–100	25–150	50–150
Doxepin (Adapin, Sinequan, and generics)	C: 10, 25, 50, 75, 100, 150 mg LC: 10 mg/ml	150–200	25–300	100–250
Trimipramine (Surmontil and generics)	C: 25, 50, 100 mg	150–200	50–300	
Protriptyline (Vivactil and generics)	T: 5, 10 mg	10–40	10–60	
Maprotiline (Ludiomil and generics)	T: 25, 50, 75 mg	100–150	50–200	
Amoxapine (Asendin and generics)	T: 25, 50, 100, 150 mg	150–200	50–300	
Clomipramine (Anafranil and generics)	C: 25, 50, 75 mg	150–200	50–250	

*Sum of imipramine plus desipramine.
†Sum of amitriptyline plus nortriptyline.
C, Capsules; INJ, injectable form; LC, liquid concentrate or solution; T, tablets.

TABLE 43-1H Available Preparations of Antidepressants: Monoamine Oxidase Inhibitors (MAOIs)

Drug	Therapeutic Dosage Forms	Usual Daily Dose (mg/day)	Extreme Dosage (mg/day)	Plasma Levels (ng/ml)
Phenelzine (Nardil and generics)	T: 15 mg	45–60	15–90	
Tranylcypromine (Parnate and generics)	T: 10 mg	30–50	10–90	
Isocarboxazid (Marplan and generics)	T: 10 mg	30–50	30–90	
Selegiline Transdermal System (patch) (Emsam)	P: 6, 9, 12/day	6–12	6–18	

T, tablets.

BOX 43-2 Requirements for Successful Use of Antidepressants

1. Good patient selection as determined by a thorough and comprehensive diagnostic evaluation. In particular, attention should be paid to co-morbid psychiatric and medical disorders.
2. Choice of a drug with an acceptable side-effect profile for the given patient.
3. Adequate dosage. In the absence of side effects and response, dose escalations within the recommended range should be pursued aggressively.
4. Use of the antidepressant for at least 6–12 weeks to determine whether it is helping or not.
5. Consideration of drug side effects. Although there are some differences in efficacy across the class of antidepressants for sutypes of depression, the major clinically significant differences among the antidepressants are in their side effects.
6. Use of a drug that was clearly effective in the past if it was well tolerated by the patient.
7. Selection of an appropriate agent for patients with initial insomnia, for example, a sedating secondary amine TCA (e.g., nortriptyline) given at bedtime (a strategy used by some clinicians), avoidance of agents with anticholinergic and cardiovascular side effects (therefore, the sleep-enhancing, alpha₂-adrenergic receptor antagonist mirtazapine would be preferred, with the expectation that daytime sedation will abate over time with these medications). An alternative to prescribing a sedating antidepressant is the temporary use of a short-acting benzodiazepine or other hypnotic combined with an SSRI or another non-sedating newer antidepressant, with the expectation of tapering and discontinuing the hypnotic when the depression has improved. Trazodone at lower doses (50–300 mg at bedtime) has been used in place of benzodiazepines or other hypnotics to treat insomnia, particularly middle to late insomnia, in patients treated for depression with an SSRI.
8. Consideration of effects on sexual function. In particular, decreased libido, delayed orgasm or anorgasmia, arousal difficulties, and erectile dysfunction have been reported with almost all of the classes of antidepressants.
9. Awareness of co-morbid conditions. The co-morbid disorder should influence initial treatment selection in choosing an agent thought to be efficacious for the co-morbid condition, as well as the depression, as with SSRIs and OCD or the NDRI bupropion and attention-deficit disorder.
10. Consideration of metabolic effects on drug levels and elimination half-life. The elderly may have alterations in hepatic metabolic pathways, especially so-called phase I reactions, which include demethylation and hydroxylation, which are involved in the metabolism of both SSRIs and cyclic antidepressants. In addition, renal function may be decreased, and there may be increased end-organ sensitivity to the effects of antidepressant compounds. Because the elimination half-life of antidepressants can be expected to be significantly greater than what it is in younger patients, accumulation of active drug will be greater and occur more slowly. Clinically this means that the elderly should be started on lower doses, that dosage increases should be slower, and that the ultimate therapeutic dose may be lower than in younger patients.

NDRI, Norepinephrine/dopamine re-uptake inhibitor; OCD, obsessive-compulsive disorder; SSRI, selective serotonin re-uptake inhibitor.

of depression in the US, as it is approved only for the treatment of OCD, although several placebo-controlled trials have demonstrated the efficacy of fluvoxamine in MDD.[87,88]

Side-effect Profile

The most common side effects of the SSRIs are nausea, tremor, excessive sweating, flushing, headache, insomnia, activation or sedation, jitteriness, dizziness, rash, and dry mouth.[89] Sedation does not appear to occur more often with any particular SSRI, while the SSRIs appear to be equally well tolerated and effective in the treatment of depressed patients, regardless of whether they cause insomnia, activation, or sedation.[82] The use of SSRIs is also associated with the emergence of sexual dysfunction (including decreased libido, delayed ejaculation, impotence, and anorgasmia), or the worsening of pre-existing sexual dysfunction in depression.[90] These side effects tend to improve rapidly after temporary ("drug holiday") discontinuation of the SSRIs, particularly those SSRIs with a shorter half-life,[91] although prolonging such drug holidays carries a risk of withdrawal effects and of depressive relapse. Some patients treated with SSRIs may also experience cognitive symptoms (such as mental slowing and worsened attention), psychological symptoms (such as apathy and emotional blunting),[92] and motor symptoms (such as bruxism and akathisia).[93,94] Other, less common, adverse events associated with SSRI treatment include diarrhea, tremor, bruxism, rash, hyponatremia, hair loss, and the syndrome of inappropriate antidiuretic hormone (SIADH) secretion. There are also case reports of the SSRIs worsening motor symptoms in patients with Parkinson's disease,[95–97] as well as creating increased requirements for levodopa in Parkinson's patients following initiation of an SSRI for depression.[98] SSRIs have been associated with abnormal bleeding (e.g., bruising and epistaxis) in children and adults who have unremarkable routine hematological laboratory results, except for abnormal bleeding time or platelet counts.[99] A systematic study of this issue has failed to reveal abnormalities in platelet aggregation, hematopoiesis, or coagulation profile in SSRI-treated patients.[100] Although many patients may also experience reduced appetite and weight loss during the acute phase of treatment with SSRIs,[101,102] any beneficial effects of the SSRIs with respect to weight loss do not seem to be sustained during the continuation and maintenance phases of treatment,[101,102] while one study reveals a greater risk for significant weight gain during long-term treatment with paroxetine, but not fluoxetine or sertraline.[103] Although SSRI-induced side effects appear to be well tolerated by most patients,[104] for depressed patients who are unable to tolerate one SSRI, switching to another SSRI has been effective and well tolerated in most cases.[105–108] For patients complaining of GI side effects with paroxetine, the continued-release formulation (Paxil CR), reported to have a lower incidence of nausea, may be used in place of the standard formulation.[109] As with other antidepressants, the potential adverse neuroendocrine and skeletal effects of the SSRIs have yet to be systematically explored.[110] However, a study from our group has shown that 4.5% of men and 22.2% of women with MDD developed new-onset hyperprolactinemia following SSRI treatment,[111] and daily SSRI use in adults 50 years and older was associated with a two-fold increased risk of fractures after adjustment for potential co-variates.[112] The SSRIs also appear to possess extremely low toxicity in overdose.[113] Finally, of all antidepressants, fluoxetine has the most extensive literature supporting its reproductive safety.[114]

Selective Serotonin Re-uptake Inhibitors Discontinuation Syndrome

A number of reports also describe discontinuation-emergent adverse events after abrupt cessation of SSRIs, including dizziness, insomnia, nervousness, irritability, nausea, and agitation.[115,116] The risk of such adverse events occurring seems to be inversely related to the half-life of the SSRI, with fluoxetine reported as having a significantly lower risk than paroxetine in two studies.[115,117] For more severe discontinuation-related adverse events, re-institution of the SSRI and slow taper may be necessary to alleviate these symptoms.[118]

Drug Interactions

With the exception perhaps of citalopram, and its stereoisomer escitalopram,[119] SSRIs may inhibit cytochrome P (CYP) 450 isoenzymes to varying degrees, potentially causing substrate levels to rise, or reducing conversion of a substrate into its active form. Concern about drug interactions, however, is pertinent to patients who take medications with narrow therapeutic margins that are metabolized by isoenzymes inhibited by an SSRI and if the prescriber is unfamiliar with or unable to determine the appropriate dose adjustment. Given their vast availability, reports of clinically significant interactions with the SSRIs are remarkably rare. Among the SSRIs, fluvoxamine is a potent CYP 1A2 and CYP 2C19 inhibitor, and a moderate CYP 2C9, CYP 2D6, and CYP 3A4 inhibitor, while fluoxetine and paroxetine are potent CYP 2D6 inhibitors, and fluoxetine's main metabolite, norfluoxetine, has a moderate inhibitory effect on CYP 3A4.[119] Sertraline is a moderate CYP 2D6 inhibitor, while citalopram and escitalopram appear to have little effect on the major CYP isoforms.[119] However, for all of the SSRIs, some vigilance is reasonable concerning the possibility of increased therapeutic or toxic effects of other co-prescribed drugs metabolized by P450 2D6. In particular, if combining a TCA with an SSRI, the TCA should be initiated with low doses, and plasma levels should be monitored. Given the high capacity of the CYP 450 3A3/3A4 system, inhibition of this isoenzyme is not a major concern for the SSRIs, although fluvoxamine, and less so fluoxetine, can inhibit it to some extent. Of little importance to drug interactions is the high rate of protein-binding of the SSRIs because, if other drugs are displaced from carrier proteins, the result is simply an increase in the rate and amount of free drug being metabolized. The augmentation and combination of SSRIs with other serotonergic agents, tryptophan, 5-HT, or MAOIs may also result in the serotonin syndrome; SSRIs should never be used concomitantly with MAOIs, because there have been a number of reports of fatal cases of serotonin syndrome due to the simultaneous use of these classes of drugs or to the inadequate washout period between the two.[54–56]

Use of Selective Serotonin Re-uptake Inhibitors in Pregnancy and the Post-partum Period

There is accumulating information about the use of SSRIs in pregnancy, although the bulk of the available data are on fluoxetine. One prospective study of 128 pregnant women who took fluoxetine,[120] 10 to 80 mg/day (mean 25.8 mg), during their first trimester did not find elevated rates of major malformations compared with matched groups of women taking TCAs or drugs thought not to be teratogenic. There was a higher, albeit not statistically significant, rate of miscarriages in the fluoxetine (13.5%) and TCA (12.2%) groups compared with the women exposed to known non-teratogenic drugs (6.8%). Whether this increased rate of miscarriages is biologically significant and, if so, whether it relates to the drugs or to the depressive disorder could not be determined from this study. Decisions on continuing antidepressant drugs during pregnancy must be individualized, but it must be recalled that the effects of severe untreated depression on maternal and fetal health may be far worse than the unknown risks of fluoxetine or tricyclic drugs. A large registry of fluoxetine exposure during pregnancy is consistent with generally reassuring data from the TCA era that antidepressant agents are not evidently teratogens.

On the other hand, infants exposed to SSRIs during late pregnancy may be at increased risk for serotonergic CNS adverse effects, although the incidence of these events has not been well established. Recently, the FDA has issued a warning for all SSRIs, reporting an increased risk for neonatal toxicity and recommending cessation of treatment before delivery. However, in clinical practice, the risk of post-partum depression often warrants continued treatment and close monitoring of the newborn.

Whenever possible, unnecessary exposure to any drug should be minimized, and thoughtful pre-pregnancy treatment planning and consideration of alternative interventions, such as psychotherapies (e.g., cognitive-behavioral therapy [CBT]), are to be recommended.

SSRIs are secreted in breast milk. Because their effects on normal growth and development are unknown, breast-feeding should be discouraged for mothers who are on SSRIs.

Serotonin Norepinephrine Re-uptake Inhibitors

Venlafaxine, duloxetine, desvenlafaxine, and levomilnacipran share the property of being relatively potent re-uptake inhibitors of serotonin and norepinephrine and are therefore considered SNRIs. They are all approved for the treatment of depression in the US.

Venlafaxine and Desvenlafaxine

Venlafaxine (Effexor) was the first SNRI to gain FDA approval for the treatment of depression. At daily doses greater than 150 mg,[121] venlafaxine inhibits the re-uptake of both serotonin and norepinephrine, while mostly inhibiting the re-uptake of serotonin at lower doses.[122,123] The augmentation and combination of venlafaxine with other serotonergic agents, tryptophan, 5-HT, or MAOIs may also result in the serotonin syndrome. Venlafaxine lacks significant cholinergic, antihistaminergic, and alpha$_1$-adrenergic–blocking effects. Venlafaxine is metabolized by CYP 450 2D6, of which it is also a very weak inhibitor. The half-lives of venlafaxine and its active metabolite O-desmethylvenlafaxine are about 5 and 11 hours, respectively. The drug and this metabolite reach steady state in plasma within 3 days in healthy adults. Venlafaxine is generally effective at daily doses at or above 150 mg, and is often started at 75 mg or even 37.5 mg, typically in its extended-release (XR) formulation.[124] Several meta-analyses suggest venlafaxine to be more effective than the SSRIs in the treatment of MDD,[125–127] with the exception of escitalopram, whose relative efficacy appears to be comparable.[83]

Venlafaxine, along with the SSRIs and bupropion, is also commonly chosen as a first-line treatment for depression.[84] Venlafaxine is also used in treatment-refractory depression as a "next-step" strategy,[128–135] reported as the most popular switch strategy for refractory depression in one large survey of clinicians.[136]

Common side effects of venlafaxine include nausea, insomnia, sedation, sexual dysfunction, headache, tremor, palpitations, and dizziness,[137] as well as excessive sweating, tachycardia, and palpitations. There are also reports of bruxism.[138,139] Venlafaxine's potential for sexual dysfunction appears to be comparable to that of the SSRIs.[140,141] The incidence of GI side effects and dizziness appears to be lower with the use of the XR formulation than the immediate-release formulation.[142] Between 2% and 6% of patients also experience an increase in diastolic blood pressure,[143] which appears to be dose-related.[144] The abrupt discontinuation of venlafaxine, given its short half-life, also carries a risk of

discontinuation-related adverse events similar to those described for the SSRIs.[145] Finally, in one uncontrolled study, 4 of 13 patients treated with venlafaxine during electroconvulsive therapy (ECT) experienced asystole.[146] Although the authors noted that this serious adverse event only occurred in patients on daily doses of venlafaxine greater than 300 mg and in patients anesthetized with propofol, in the absence of further data the use of venlafaxine in patients requiring ECT and perhaps even general anesthesia should be avoided.

Desvenlafaxine (Pristiq) is a major active metabolite of venlafaxine and an SNRI with little affinity for muscarinic, histaminic, or adrenergic receptors. Desvenlafaxine is metabolized by CYP 450 3A4 and it is a very weak inhibitor of 2D6. The half-life of desvenlafaxine is about 10 hours. The augmentation and combination of desvenlafaxine with other serotonergic agents, tryptophan, 5-HT, or MAOIs may also result in the serotonin syndrome. Desvenlafaxine was found to be more effective than placebo in the treatment of MDD in two separate randomized, double-blind clinical trials. Side effects reported in those studies included nausea, dry mouth, sweating, somnolence, anorexia, constipation, asthenia, vomiting, tremor, nervousness, abnormal vision, and sexual dysfunction. There have been reports of increases in diastolic blood pressure, and the abrupt discontinuation of desvenlafaxine carries a risk of discontinuation-related adverse events similar to those described for the SSRIs. There are also reports of an increase in liver enzymes among patients treated with desvenlafaxine. Desvenlafaxine is commonly used at doses between 50 and 100 mg daily in a single administration.

Duloxetine

Duloxetine (Cymbalta) also inhibits the re-uptake of both serotonin and norepinephrine.[147] Duloxetine appears to be as effective as the SSRIs in the treatment of MDD, although in more severe depression there may be some advantages.[148]

Duloxetine lacks significant cholinergic, antihistaminergic, and alpha$_1$-adrenergic blocking effects. Duloxetine is extensively metabolized to numerous metabolites that are primarily excreted into the urine in the conjugated form. The major metabolites in plasma are glucuronide conjugates of 4-hydroxy duloxetine (M6), 6-hydroxy-5-methoxy duloxetine (M10), 4,6-dihydroxy duloxetine (M9), and a sulfate conjugate of 5-hydroxy-6-methoxy duloxetine (M7). Duloxetine is metabolized by CYP 450 2D6, of which it is also a moderate inhibitor, intermediate between paroxetine and sertraline. Drugs that inhibit this enzyme may increase duloxetine concentrations. The half-life of duloxetine is about 12.5 hours. Abrupt discontinuation of duloxetine is associated with a discontinuation-emergent adverse event profile similar to that seen with SSRIs and SNRI antidepressants.[149] Therefore, duloxetine's discontinuation should be accomplished with a gradual taper (over at least 2 weeks) to reduce the risk of discontinuation-emergent adverse events. Duloxetine is commonly used at daily doses of 60 to 120 mg, often started at 30 mg. Duloxetine also appears to be effective in the treatment of somatic symptoms of depression, such as pain.[150,151] Common side effects associated with duloxetine include dry mouth, headache, nausea, somnolence, sweating, insomnia, and fatigue.[152] Duloxetine does not appear to cause hypertension.[152]

Levomilnacipran and Milnacipran

Levomilnacipran (Fetzima) is an SNRI and is the 1S-2R enantiomer of milnacipram, an SRNI approved for depression in Europe (brand names: Dalcipran, Ixel). Levomilnacipran is metabolized by CYP 450 3A4 and it is not an inhibitor of CYP 450 systems. Its half-life is about 12 hours. The augmentation and combination of milnacipran or levomilnacipran with other serotonergic agents, tryptophan, 5-HT, or MAOIs may also result in the serotonin syndrome. A number of studies had demonstrated that the SNRI milnacipran[153] is equivalent to the SSRIs[154–157] and the TCAs[158–162] and superior to placebo in the treatment of depression.[163,164] Similarly, several studies have shown that the norepinephrine and serotonin re-uptake inhibitor levomilnacipran is superior to placebo in the treatment of depression.[165–167] Because of the potent norepinephrine re-uptake inhibition, levomilnacipran appears to be particularly effective in treating fatigue in depression. Common side effects reported during treatment with milnacipran include headaches, dry mouth, dysuria, tremor, tachycardia, weight gain, and sedation, although the incidence of weight gain and sedation with milnacipran is lower than with the TCAs.[162] Levomilnacipran's frequently reported adverse events (≥ 5% in levomilnacipran ER and twice the rate of placebo) are nausea, dizziness, constipation, tachycardia, urinary hesitation, hyperhidrosis, insomnia, vomiting, and elevated blood pressure. Daily doses of milnacipran range from 50 to 200 mg, often divided in twice-daily dosing, whereas the usual dose of levomilnacipran ER is 40–120 mg once/daily

Norepinephrine Re-uptake Inhibitors

Reboxetine

Reboxetine[168] acts by selectively inhibiting the norepinephrine transporter, thereby increasing synaptic norepinephrine levels. Reboxetine, a morpholine compound, is chemically unrelated to the other antidepressants. It is highly protein-bound and has a plasma half-life of about 13 hours. The drug does not appear to be a meaningful inhibitor of the CYP 450 system and is metabolized itself by CYP 450 3A4 isozyme with two inactive metabolites. Increased blood pressure has been reported to be a problem for some patients, particularly those with a genetic variant of the norepinephrine transporter (SCL6A2). Reboxetine has not received FDA approval for the treatment of depression, but is available in Europe for the treatment of depression (brand name: Edronax). Double-blind, placebo-controlled trials suggest reboxetine to be more effective than placebo[169–172] and as effective as fluoxetine[170] in the treatment of MDD. The starting daily dose is usually 8 mg but can be as low as 4 mg, with effective daily doses ranging from 8 to 10 mg given in divided doses (twice a day). Common side effects include insomnia, headache, dry mouth, diaphoresis, and constipation,[170] as well as urinary hesitancy. The incidence of nausea, headache, fatigue,[170] and sexual dysfunction[173] appears to be more common during treatment with the SSRIs than with reboxetine. The urinary hesitancy and constipation do not appear to reflect anticholinergic, but rather noradrenergic, effects.

Atomoxetine

Atomoxetine also selectively inhibits the re-uptake of norepinephrine.[174] In vitro, ex vivo, and in vivo studies have shown that atomoxetine is a highly selective antagonist of the pre-synaptic norepinephrine transporter, with little or no affinity for other noradrenergic receptors or other neurotransmitter transporters or receptors, with the exception of a weak affinity for the serotonin transporter. Atomoxetine is rapidly absorbed, with peak plasma concentrations occurring 1 to 2 hours after dosing, and its half-life hovers around 3 to 4 hours. While atomoxetine is an FDA-approved treatment for attention-deficit/hyperactivity disorder (ADHD) (brand name: Strattera), there is a single open trial of atomoxetine in depression involving 10 patients, with daily doses ranging from 40 to 70 mg.[175] Common side effects reported so far include decreased appetite, insomnia, and increased blood pressure.[176]

Atomoxetine has also been associated with mild increases in blood pressure and pulse that plateau during treatment and resolve after discontinuation. There have been no effects seen on the QT interval. It is a substrate of CYP 2D6 and its biotransformation involves aromatic ring hydroxylation, benzylic oxidation, and N-demethylation. At high therapeutic doses, atomoxetine inhibits CYP 2D6 and CYP 3A activity, although in vivo studies clearly indicate that atomoxetine administration with substrates of CYP 2D6 and CYP 3A does not result in clinically significant drug interactions.

Norepinephrine/Dopamine Re-uptake Inhibitors

Bupropion

The NDRI bupropion appears to be as effective as the SSRIs in the treatment of depressive[177,178] and anxiety symptoms in depression,[179] and more effective than the SSRIs in the treatment of sleepiness and fatigue in depression.[180] Interestingly, bupropion has been shown to be as effective as the SNRI venlafaxine in the treatment of MDD.[181]

Bupropion is a phenethylamine compound that is effective for the treatment of MDD. Bupropion is structurally related to amphetamine and the sympathomimetic diethylpropion, and it primarily blocks the re-uptake of dopamine and norepinephrine and has minimal or no affinity for post-synaptic receptors. Although some researchers have argued that the NDRI bupropion's effect on norepinephrine is primarily through an increase in pre-synaptic release, there is still convincing evidence for binding of both norepinephrine and dopamine transporters. Bupropion is rapidly absorbed after oral administration and demonstrates biphasic elimination, with an elimination half-life of 11 to 14 hours. It is converted to three active metabolites, hydroxybupropion, threohydrobupropion, and erythrohydrobupropion, all of which have been demonstrated to have antidepressant activity in animal models. Bupropion lacks anticholinergic properties and does not cause postural hypotension or alter cardiac conduction in a clinically significant manner. It is a substrate of CYP 450 2B6 and appears to have CYP 450 2D6 inhibition potential, which suggests that, when it is combined with fluoxetine or paroxetine, both 2D6 substrates, levels of the SSRI may increase. One advantage of treatment with bupropion compared to the SSRIs is the lower risk of sexual dysfunction.[140,141,182–187] Treatment with bupropion is also associated with a lower incidence of GI side effects (e.g., nausea and diarrhea)[185,186] and sedation[177,179,185] than the SSRIs. Although a difference in terms of weight changes in bupropion and SSRI-treated depressed patients is not immediately apparent during the acute phase of treatment in randomized trials,[183,185,186,188–190] there is evidence to suggest that any beneficial effects of SSRIs in terms of weight reduction during the acute phase are not sustained during the continuation and maintenance phases.[101,102] In fact, long-term treatment with some SSRIs may also result in long-term weight gain.[103] In contrast, long-term (44 weeks) bupropion treatment appears to result in weight changes no different than those of placebo in MDD.[191] Thus, long-term treatment with bupropion may carry a lower risk of weight gain than long-term treatment with the SSRIs.

The dose range for the sustained-release (SR) formulation of bupropion (Wellbutrin SR) is 150 to 450 mg in twice a day or three times a day dosing, with 100 or 150 mg being a common starting dose. A once-daily dose formulation (Wellbutrin XL), available in 150 and 300 mg doses, was subsequently introduced. Common side effects include agitation, insomnia, weight loss, dry mouth, headache, constipation, and tremor.[189] The major medically important adverse event associated with bupropion is seizure. With the immediate-release formulation the rate is 0.4% (4 per 1,000) at doses up to 450 mg/day, whereas with bupropion SR the rate is of 0.1% (1 per 1,000) at doses up to the target antidepressant dose of 300 mg/day (Wellbutrin SR Prescribing Information).[192] SSRI antidepressants are also associated with seizures at a similar rate of approximately 0.1% (Wellbutrin SR Prescribing Information). Patients should only be administered bupropion with extreme caution if a predisposition to seizure is present. For this reason, the maximum daily dose for bupropion SR and bupropion XL is 450 mg, with no single dose above 200 mg for the SR formulation. In addition, bupropion may be more likely to induce seizures in patients with bulimia nervosa and histories of head trauma and it should not be used in these patients. Since the risk of seizure appears to be dose-related and related to the peak plasma concentrations, the SR and XL formulations are thought to be associated with a somewhat lower seizure risk, estimated at 0.1% for daily doses lower than 450 mg.[192]

Serotonin Receptor Antagonists/Agonists

Trazodone

Although the serotonin receptor antagonists trazodone (Desyrel) and nefazodone (Serzone) have been shown to be as effective as the SSRIs in the treatment of depression,[193] they are used extremely infrequently as monotherapy for depression.[84] Trazodone is rapidly absorbed following oral administration, achieving peak levels in 1 to 2 hours. It has a relatively short elimination half-life of 3 to 9 hours and is excreted mainly in urine (75%); its metabolite mCPP has a similar pharmacokinetic profile. Despite the short half-life, once-daily dosing at bedtime is the usual route of administration because of its sedating properties. When used as monotherapy for the treatment of depression, a patient is typically started on 100 to 150 mg daily either in divided doses or in a single bedtime dose and gradually increased to 200 to 300 mg/day. An extended-release formulation of trazodone (Oleptro) is available. The dose range for the extended-release is between 150 and 300 mg qHS. For optimal benefit, doses in the range of 400 to 600 mg may be needed for either formulation. Low-dose trazodone (25 to 150 mg at bedtime) is commonly used in the treatment of insomnia secondary to antidepressant use,[194] a strategy that may also result in an improvement in depressive symptoms.[195] The most common side effects of trazodone are sedation, orthostatic hypotension, and headaches. Trazodone lacks the quinidine-like properties of the cyclic antidepressants but has been associated in rare cases with cardiac arrhythmias, which may be related to trazodone's ability to inhibit potassium channels. Thus, trazodone should be used with caution in patients with known cardiac disease. A rare but serious side effect of trazodone is priapism of both the penis and clitoris,[196,197] which requires immediate medical attention. Priapism has been attributed to the alpha-adrenoceptor blocking properties of trazodone by interference with the sympathetic control of penile detumescence.[198] Rare cases of hepatotoxicity have been associated with the use of trazodone,[199] and fatal cases of trazodone overdose have also been reported.[200] In one review, trazodone was reported to carry one of the lowest risks for seizure of all antidepressants examined.[201] The minimal effective dose for trazodone is usually 300 mg daily.

Nefazodone

Nefazodone has less affinity for the alpha$_1$-adrenergic receptor and is therefore less sedating. The half-life of nefazodone is approximately 5 hours. The usual starting dosage is 50 mg/day given at bedtime or twice a day, titrated up in the absence of daytime sedation as rapidly as tolerated to achieve a usually effective antidepressant dosage in the 450 to 600 mg/day range in divided doses. Slower dose titration is recommended in the elderly. Nefazodone has been found to inhibit CYP 3A4 and to result in serotonin syndrome when combined with SSRIs. Common side effects include somnolence, dizziness, dry mouth, nausea, constipation, headache, amblyopia, and blurred vision.[202] An unusual but occasional adverse effect is irritability (possibly related to its mCPP metabolite, which may occur in higher levels in the presence of a CYP 450 2D6 inhibitor). Treatment with nefazodone has the advantage of a lower risk of long-term weight gain than the SSRIs or TCAs,[97] perhaps because of the appetite-reducing effects of mCPP.[203] Nefazodone also has the advantage of a lower risk of sexual side effects than the SSRIs.[140,141,204] A rare but serious side effect of nefazodone is priapism of both the penis and clitoris,[205,206] which requires immediate medical attention. In addition, an increasing number of reports suggest that treatment with nefazodone is associated with an increase risk of hepatotoxicity (approximately 29 cases per 100,000 patient years),[207] often severe (more than 80% of cases), and often appearing during the first 6 months of treatment.[208] To date, there has even been one reported death due to such hepatotoxicity.[209] Therefore, this agent should be avoided in patients with current or a history of liver abnormalities; liver enzymes should be checked periodically in patients on nefazodone. The minimal effective doses for nefazodone are usually 300 mg daily, with 600 mg daily being the optimal dose.

Vilazodone

Vilazodone (Vibryd) is a serotonin 5-HT$_{1A}$ receptor partial agonist and a selective serotonin re-uptake inhibitor. Studies have shown its superiority over placebo in the treatment of depression.[210] The augmentation and combination of vilazodone with other serotonergic agents, tryptophan, 5-HT, or MAOIs may also result in the serotonin syndrome. Vilazodone lacks significant cholinergic, antihistaminergic, and alpha$_1$-adrenergic–blocking effects. Vilazodone is metabolized primarily by CYP 450 3A4 and is a moderate inhibitor of 2C19 and 2D6. The terminal half-life of vilazodone is about 25 hours. Vilazodone therapy is typically initiated at a dosage of 10 mg once daily and incrementally adjusted over 14 days to the recommended target daily dose of 40 mg; for optimal bioavailability and effectiveness, it should be taken after a light or high-fat meal. The adverse effects most commonly reported in clinical trials of vilazodone were diarrhea, nausea, vomiting, dizziness, insomnia and dry mouth. Treatment-related sexual side effects may be less likely than with SSRIs: in three placebo-controlled studies, 8.0% of vilazodone-treated patients and 0.9% of placebo-treated patients reported ≥ 1 sexual-function-related treatment-emergent adverse event (P< 0.001)).[211] Vilazodone was not associated with clinically-relevant weight change in the short-term trials. In an open-label 1-year study of vilazodone, mean weight increased by 1.7 kg among the observed cases.[212]

Vortioxetine

Vortioxetine (Brintellix) is a recently-approved antidepressant with multi-modal activity that functions as a serotonin 5-HT$_3$, 5-HT$_7$ and 5-HT$_{1D}$ receptor antagonist, serotonin 5-HT$_{1B}$ receptor partial agonist, serotonin 5-HT$_{1A}$ receptor agonist and inhibitor of the serotonin transporter *in vitro*. Vortioxetine has shown to be able to increase extracellular serotonin, dopamine, and norepinephrine levels in the medial prefrontal cortex and ventral hippocampus. The augmentation and combination of vortioxetine with other serotonergic agents, tryptophan, 5-HT, or MAOIs may result in the serotonin syndrome. Vortioxetine lacks significant cholinergic, anti-histaminergic, and alpha$_1$-adrenergic–blocking effects. Vortioxetine is metabolized primarily by CYP 450 2D6. The terminal half-life of vortioxetine is about 66 hours. Vortioxetine therapy is typically initiated at a dosage of 10 mg once daily and incrementally adjusted 20 mg once daily, if necessary; the dose can be lowered to 5 mg daily, if necessary based on tolerability issues. Nausea, dry mouth, diarrhea, nasopharyngitis, headache, dizziness, somnolence, vomiting, dyspepsia, constipation and fatigue were reported in ≥ 5% of patients receiving vortioxetine.[213] Rates of treatment-emergent sexual dysfunction (TESD) in the vortioxetine dosing groups were similar to placebo.[213] In a 52-week open-label extension study, vortioxetine was associated with minimal weight gain.[214] Recently presented data suggest that vortioxetine may have the additional advantage of distinctive pro-cognitive effects.

Ritanserin

Ritanserin, a serotonin 5-HT$_{2A}$ and 5-HT$_{2C}$ antagonist, is not FDA-approved, but is available in Europe. One placebo-controlled study revealed ritanserin to be effective in the treatment of dysthymic disorder,[215] while a separate study found ritanserin to be as effective as amitriptyline in patients with depression and chronic headaches.[216] Ritanserin appears to be effective for depression at doses above 5 mg.

Agomelatine

Agomelatine, a newer agent, is a selective 5-HT$_{2C}$ antagonist and acts as a melatonin MT$_1$ and MT$_2$ receptor agonist. To date, at least two placebo-controlled trials have found agomelatine (25 mg) to be more effective than placebo and as effective as the SSRIs in the treatment of MDD,[217-219] and as effective as the SSRI paroxetine in MDD.[217] Agomelatine is approved for the treatment of depression in Europe, but not in the US.

Buspirone and Gepirone

Buspirone (BuSpar) and gepirone (Ariza) act as full agonists at serotonin 5-HT$_{1A}$ autoreceptors and are generally, but not exclusively, partial agonists at post-synaptic serotonin 5-HT$_{1A}$ receptors.[29] Buspirone is FDA-approved as a treatment for anxiety and not for depression, while gepirone has not been FDA-approved. Nevertheless, a number of double-blind trials report buspirone[220-223] and gepirone[224-228] to be more effective than placebo in the treatment of MDD. One advantage of gepirone and perhaps buspirone is that their use does not appear to be related to a greater incidence of weight gain or sexual side effects than placebo, at least during the acute phase of treatment of depression.[228] Effective doses for buspirone and gepirone for depression range between 30 and 90 mg and 20 and 80 mg, respectively. Side effects are similar for these two agents and include headache, dizziness, light-headedness, nausea, and insomnia.[222,229]

Alpha$_2$-Adrenergic Receptor Antagonists
Mirtazapine

Mirtazapine is as effective as the SSRIs[230] and venlafaxine[231,232] in the treatment of MDD. Mirtazapine shows linear pharmacokinetics over a dose range of 15 to 80 mg and its elimination half-life ranges from 20 to 40 hours, consistent with its time to reach steady state (4 to 6 days). Biotransformation is mainly mediated by the CYP 2D6 and CYP 3A4 isoenzymes. Inhibitors of these isoenzymes, such as paroxetine and fluoxetine, cause modestly increased mirtazapine plasma concentrations, while mirtazapine has little inhibitory effects on CYP isoenzymes; therefore, the pharmacokinetics of co-administered drugs are hardly affected by mirtazapine. Mirtazapine is associated with more sedation and weight gain than the SSRIs.[233-236] The widespread use of mirtazapine as a first-line agent in depression has been primarily limited by its sedative effects and weight gain.[237] In addition to sedation and weight gain, common side effects associated with mirtazapine include dizziness, dry mouth, constipation, and orthostatic hypotension. Due to blockade of 5-HT$_2$ and 5-HT$_3$ receptors, mirtazapine is associated with a lower risk of headaches[233] and nausea[233-235,238,239] than the SSRIs. Treatment with mirtazapine is also associated with a lower incidence of sexual dysfunction than the SSRIs.[141,234] In addition, switching to mirtazapine may alleviate SSRI induced sexual dysfunction in SSRI-remitters.[240] Severe neutropenia has been rarely reported (1 in 1,000) with an uncertain relationship to the drug, but as with other psychotropics, the onset of infection and fever should prompt the patient to contact his or her physician. The drug is most efficacious at doses of 30 to 45 mg (although 60 mg/day has been used in refractory cases) usually given in a single bedtime dose. Available in 15, 30, and 45 mg scored tablets and in an orally soluble tablet formulation (Soltab) at 15, 30, and 45 mg, the lower dose may be sub-optimal, and compared with 15 mg, the 30 mg dose also may be less or at least not more sedating, possibly as a consequence of the noradrenergic effects being recruited at that dose. The starting daily dose can be as low as 7.5 mg in the elderly.

Mianserin

Mianserin is approved for depression in Europe (brand name: Lantanon) and is not FDA-approved. Double-blind studies report the efficacy of mianserin in the treatment of MDD to be equivalent to the TCAs.[241-243] The most common side effects include somnolence, weight gain, dry mouth, sleep problems, tremor, and headaches.[244] Effective daily doses for mianserin range from 30 to 60 mg, usually given at bedtime.

Tricyclic and Related Cyclic Antidepressants

Oral preparations of TCAs and related drugs are rapidly and completely absorbed from the GI tract; a high percentage of an oral dose is metabolized by the liver as it passes through the portal circulation (first-pass effect). The TCAs are metabolized by the microsomal enzymes of the liver; the tertiary amines are first monodemethylated to yield compounds that are still active. Indeed, the desmethyl metabolites of amitriptyline and imipramine are nortriptyline and desipramine, respectively, and are marketed as antidepressants. Other major metabolic pathways include hydroxylation (which may yield partially active compounds) and conjugation with glucuronic acid to produce inactive compounds. TCAs are highly lipophilic, meaning the free fraction passes easily into the brain and other tissues. They are also largely bound to plasma proteins. Given their lipophilicity and protein-binding, they are not removed effectively by hemodialysis in cases of overdose. The time course of metabolism and elimination is biphasic, with approximately half of a dose removed over 48 to 72 hours and the remainder, strongly bound to tissues and plasma proteins, slowly excreted over several weeks. There is considerable variation among individuals in their metabolic rate for cyclic antidepressants based on genetic factors, age, and concomitantly taken drugs. In fact, when metabolic differences are combined with variation in the degree of protein-binding, as much as a 300-fold difference in effective drug levels may be found among individuals.

Although TCAs' overall efficacy in treating depression is equivalent to that of the SSRIs,[245] they tend to have considerably more side effects and, due to their ability to block the aforementioned receptors, as well as the sodium channel,[246] TCAs are often arrythmogenic[247] and epileptogenic[248] when taken in very large (supra-therapeutic) quantities. As a result, they are rarely chosen as first-line agents in the treatment of depression.[84] Furthermore, several studies also suggest that TCAs may be more effective than the SSRIs in the treatment of melancholic depression, or in the treatment of depressed patients with certain co-morbid medical conditions.[249-253] In addition, perhaps due to their ability to inhibit the re-uptake of both serotonin and norepinephrine, as well as their ability to block sodium channels, TCAs appear to be more effective in treating neuropathic pain than the SSRIs.[254] In fact, the results of a separate meta-analysis reveal that the TCAs are superior to the SSRIs in the treatment of a number of somatic/pain disorders (including headaches, fibromyalgia, irritable bowel disorder, idiopathic pain, tinnitus, and chronic fatigue) often diagnosed in patients with chronic depression.[255] The TCAs may be sub-divided into tertiary amines and secondary amines (their demethylated secondary amine derivatives). In addition, maprotiline (Ludiomil), which is classified as a tetracyclic antidepressant, is commonly grouped with the TCAs, due to similarities in dosing, mechanism of action, and side effects. Tertiary amine TCAs include amitriptyline (Elavil, Adepril), imipramine (Tofranil, Antidepril), trimipramine (Surmontil, Herphonal), clomipramine (Anafranil, Clopress), and doxepin (Sinequan, Deptran). Secondary amine TCAs are nortriptyline (Pamelor, Aventyl), desipramine (Norpramin, Metylyl), protriptyline (Vivactil, Concordin), and amoxapine (Ascendin, Defanyl).

Side-effect Profile

In general, the side effects of the TCAs and related cyclic antidepressants are more difficult for patients to tolerate than are the side effects of the newer drugs (Table 43-2) and they probably account for higher drop-out rates than are associated with the SSRIs.[256] Thus, treatment is typically initiated at lower doses (e.g., 10 mg/day for imipramine) in order to minimize the risk of adverse events and premature treatment discontinuation. The side-effect profile of the TCAs can be sub-categorized in terms of their relative affinity for a number of monoamine receptors and transporters. Overall, secondary amine TCAs tend to cause fewer anticholinergic, antihistaminergic, and anti-alpha$_1$–related side effects than tertiary amine TCAs.

Amoxapine is the only TCA with documented, significant dopamine D$_2$ receptor antagonism.[49] Therefore, there have been case reports of tardive dystonia and dyskinesia associated with amoxapine treatment,[257,258] and amoxapine should be avoided in patients with co-morbid depression and Parkinson's disease.[259]

Anticholinergic-related side effects result from the affinity of TCAs for muscarinic cholinergic receptors and typically include dry mouth, blurred vision, constipation, urinary hesitancy, tachycardia, memory difficulties, and ejaculatory difficulties. Finally, due to their anticholinergic effects, TCAs should be avoided in patients with narrow-angle glaucoma and prostatic hypertrophy, as symptoms related to these conditions may worsen because of such anticholinergic effects.

Antihistaminergic-related side effects result from histaminergic H$_1$-receptor blockade and typically include increased appetite, weight gain, sedation, and fatigue. Weight gain with TCAs can be substantial, averaging 1 to 3 lb per month of treatment.[260] As a result, TCAs may complicate the management of diabetes and worsen glycemic control, and should be avoided whenever possible in diabetics.[261] TCAs may also have hyperlipidemic effects, thus complicating their long-term use in patients with hyperlipidemia.[262] Xerostomia secondary to anticholinergic and antihistaminergic effects may also increase the risk of oral pathology, particularly dental caries.[263]

Orthostatic hypotension and reflex tachycardia may result from alpha$_1$-adrenergic receptor antagonism. Nortriptyline is generally thought to be less likely to cause orthostatic hypotension than tertiary amine TCAs, such as imipramine[264,265]; however, nortriptyline's affinity for the alpha$_1$-adrenergic receptor, although less than the affinity of most TCAs, is actually much greater (e.g., by a factor of two) than the affinity of desipramine and protriptyline.[50] In addition, homozygosity for 3435T alleles of *ABCB1*, the multi-drug resistance gene that encodes a P-glycoprotein (P-gp) regulating the passage of many substances across the blood–brain barrier, appears to be a risk factor for occurrence of nortriptyline-induced postural hypotension.[266] Antidepressant-induced postural hypotension in the elderly may, in turn, increase the risk of falls and fractures (e.g., hip fractures).[267] Although less likely to suffer a fall or fracture, the sedative potential of various TCA antidepressants is also a serious consideration in younger depressed patients as well, as this effect may increase the mortality risk from

TABLE 43-2 Tricyclic Antidepressants and Monoamine Oxidase Inhibitors Side-effect Profile

Category and Drug	Sedative Potency	Anticholinergic Potency	Orthostatic Hypotensive Potency	Usual Adult Daily Dose (mg/day)	Dosage (mg/day)
Tricyclic and Related Cyclic Compounds*					
Amitriptyline	High	Very high	High	150–200	75–300
Amoxapine	Low	Moderate	Moderate	150–200	75–300
Clomipramine	High	High	High	150–200	75–250
Desipramine	Low	Moderate (lowest of the tricyclics)	Moderate	150–200	75–300
Doxepin	High	High	Moderate	150–200	75–300
Imipramine	Moderate	High	High	150–200	75–300
Maprotiline	Moderate	Low	Moderate	150–200	75–225
Nortriptyline	Moderate	Moderate	Lowest of the tricyclics	75–100	40–150
Protriptyline	Low	High	Low	30	10–60
Trimipramine	High	Moderate	Moderate	150–200	75–300
Monoamine Oxidase Inhibitors					
Isocarboxazid	—	Very low	High	30	20–60
Phenelzine	Low	Very low	High	60–75	30–90
Tranylcypromine	—	Very low	High	30	20–90

*All of the tricyclic and related cyclic compounds have well-established cardiac arrhythmogenic potential.
(From Rosenbaum JF, Arana GW, Hyman SE, et al., editors: Handbook of psychiatric drug therapy, ed 5, Philadelphia, 2005, Lippincott Williams & Wilkins.)

automobile accidents. In fact, in a recent review,[268] sedating antidepressants (dothiepin, amitriptyline, imipramine, doxepin, and mianserin) were found to result in driving impairments on a standardized road test comparable to impairments found in drivers with a blood alcohol level of 0.8 mg/ml, whereas non-sedating antidepressants (moclobemide, fluoxetine, paroxetine, venlafaxine, and nefazodone) were not found to adversely affect driving performance. TCAs may also cause sexual dysfunction and excessive sweating.

The ability of TCAs to inhibit the sodium channel may also result in electrocardiographic changes in susceptible individuals (e.g., in post–myocardial infarction patients, as well as in patients with bifascicular heart block, left bundle branch block, or a prolonged QT interval), even at therapeutic doses,[269] and, given that contemporary psychopharmacologists have access to a multitude of alternative treatment options, TCAs should be avoided in these patients. Due to the inhibition of sodium channels and cholinergic receptors, the TCAs also carry a risk of seizure. Maprotiline and clomipramine are considered the TCAs with the greatest risk of seizures.[270] This combined risk of seizure and arrhythmia renders the TCAs as the least safe during overdose.[271]

Prescribing Tricyclic and Related Cyclic Antidepressants

Aside from the electrocardiogram (ECG), no other tests are generally indicated in healthy adults before starting a TCA. TCAs are started at a low dose followed by gradual increases until the therapeutic range is achieved. Finding the right TCA dose for a patient often involves a process of trial and error. The most common error leading to treatment failure is inadequate dosage. In healthy adults, the typical starting dose is 25 to 50 mg of imipramine or its TCA equivalent. Nortriptyline is about twice as potent; thus, its starting dose is 10 to 25 mg. In some clinical situations, especially in the elderly and patients with panic disorder, it may be necessary to start with lower doses (as low as 10 mg of imipramine or the equivalent) because of intolerance to side effects. Generally, TCAs are administered once a day at bedtime to help with compliance and, when the sedating compounds are used, to help with sleep. Divided doses are used if patients have side effects due to high peak levels. The dosage can be increased by 50 mg every 3 to 4 days, as side effects allow, up to a dose of 150 to 200 mg of imipramine or its equivalent at bedtime (see Table 43-1). If there is no therapeutic response in 3 to 4 weeks, the dosage should be slowly increased, again as side effects allow. The maximum dosage of most TCAs is the equivalent of 300 mg/day of imipramine, although uncommonly, patients who metabolize the drug rapidly may do well on higher dosages. Of the currently available cyclic antidepressants, only four drugs (imipramine, desipramine, amitriptyline, and nortriptyline) have been studied well enough to make generalizations about the value of their blood levels in treatment of depression. Serum levels of the other cyclic antidepressants have not been investigated well enough to be clinically meaningful, although they can confirm presence of the drug or document extremely high serum levels. There is a wide range of effective doses for TCAs. Typical antidepressant doses are 100 to 300 mg/day for imipramine. There is evidence to suggest a relationship between serum levels of TCAs and clinical response. Perry and colleagues[272] pooled and analyzed all available studies examining the relationship between TCA blood levels and clinical response with the use of receiver operating-characteristics curves. The relationship between clinical response and blood levels for desipramine was linear, with the threshold concentration in plasma for therapeutic response being greater than or equal to 116 ng/ml (response rates: 51% versus 15% for patients with levels above or below that threshold, respectively). The

remaining TCAs exhibited a curvilinear (inverse "U"–shaped curve) relationship between blood level and clinical response. The optimal ranges for nortriptyline, "total" imipramine (imipramine plus desipramine), and "total" amitriptyline (amitriptyline plus nortriptyline) (with their corresponding response rates within versus outside the level range) were 58 to 148 ng/ml (66% versus 26%), 175 to 350 ng/ml (67% versus 39%), and 93 to 140 ng/ml (50% versus 30%), respectively.

Nortriptyline levels have been the best studied of the antidepressants. Some researchers believe that such studies reveal a more complex pattern than with imipramine or desipramine—an inverted U-shape correlation with clinical improvement, which is sometimes referred to as a therapeutic window. Clinical improvement correlates with levels of 50 to 150 ng/ml. The reason for the poorer response with doses above 150 ng/ml is not known, but it does not appear to relate to any measurable toxicity. On the other hand, the number of subjects in well-designed studies that indicate a window is small, so not all researchers believe there is adequate evidence in favor of a therapeutic window. Studies of amitriptyline levels have resulted in disagreement about the utility of levels, with linear, curvilinear, and lack of relationship reported by different investigators. When used, blood levels should be drawn when the drug has achieved steady-state levels (at least 5 days after a dosage change in healthy adults; longer in the elderly) and 10 to 14 hours after the last oral dose. Abrupt discontinuation symptoms may emerge with TCAs and in part represent cholinergic rebound, and include GI distress, malaise, chills, coryza, and muscle aches.

Use of Tricyclic and Related Cyclic Antidepressants during Pregnancy and the Post-partum Period

There are limited data on the use of TCAs during pregnancy. There have been reports of congenital malformations in association with TCA use, but there is no convincing causal association. Overall, the TCAs may be safe, but given the lack of proven safety, the drugs should be avoided during pregnancy, unless the indications are compelling. Pregnant women who are at risk for serious depression might be maintained on TCA therapy. This decision should always be made very carefully and with extensive discussion of the risk–benefit factors. Due to more clinical experience, older agents, such as imipramine, may be preferred to newer drugs during pregnancy. TCAs appear to be secreted in breast milk. Because their effects on normal growth and development are unknown, breast-feeding should be discouraged for mothers who are on tricyclics.

Overdoses with Tricyclic and Related Cyclic Antidepressants

Acute doses of more than 1 g of TCAs are often toxic and may be fatal. Death may result from cardiac arrhythmias, hypotension, or uncontrollable seizures. Serum levels should be obtained when overdose is suspected, both because of distorted information that may be given by patients or families and because oral bioavailability with very large doses of these compounds is poorly understood. Nonetheless, serum levels of the parent compound and its active metabolites provide less specific information about the severity of the overdose than one might hope. Serum levels of greater than 1,000 ng/ml are associated with serious overdose, as are increases in the QRS duration of the ECG to 0.10 second or greater. However, serious consequences of a TCA overdose may occur with serum levels under 1,000 ng/ml and with a QRS duration of less than 0.10 second. In acute overdose, almost all symptoms develop within 12 hours.

BOX 43-3 Drug Interactions with Cyclic Antidepressants

WORSEN SEDATION

Alcohol
Antihistamines
Antipsychotics
Barbiturates, chloral hydrate, and other sedatives

WORSEN HYPOTENSION

α-Methyldopa (Aldomet)
β-Adrenergic blockers (e.g., propranolol)
Clonidine
Diuretics
Low-potency antipsychotics

ADDITIVE CARDIOTOXICITY

Quinidine and other type 1 antiarrhythmics
Thioridazine, mesoridazine, pimozide, ziprasidone

ADDITIVE ANTICHOLINERGIC TOXICITY

Anti-histamines (diphenhydramine and others)
Anti-parkinsonians (benztropine and others)
Low-potency antipsychotics, especially thioridazine
Over-the-counter sleeping medications
Gastrointestinal antispasmodics and anti-diarrheals (Lomotil and others)

OTHER

Tricyclics may increase the effects of warfarin
Tricyclics may block the effects of guanethidine

(From Rosenbaum JF, Arana GW, Hyman SE, et al., editors: Handbook of psychiatric drug therapy, ed 5, Philadelphia, 2005, Lippincott Williams & Wilkins.)

Anti-muscarinic effects are prominent, including dry mucous membranes, warm dry skin, mydriasis, blurred vision, decreased bowel motility, and, often, urinary retention. Either CNS depression (ranging from drowsiness to coma) or an agitated delirium may occur. The CNS depressant effects of cyclic antidepressants are potentiated by concomitantly ingested alcohol, benzodiazepines, and other sedative-hypnotics. Seizures may occur, and in severe overdoses, respiratory arrest may occur. Cardiovascular toxicity presents a particular danger (Box 43-3). Hypotension often occurs, even with the patient supine.

A variety of arrhythmias may develop, including supraventricular tachycardia, ventricular tachycardia, or fibrillation, and varying degrees of heart block, including complete heart block.

Drug Interactions

The cyclic antidepressants have a variety of important pharmacodynamic and pharmacokinetic drug–drug interactions that may worsen the toxicity of other drugs (see Box 43-3).

Monoamine Oxidase Inhibitors

The MAOIs are well absorbed after oral administration. A transdermal form of selegiline (Emsam) is also available and approved by the FDA for the treatment of depression. Since MAOIs irreversibly inhibit the enzymes, return of enzyme function after discontinuation may require 2 weeks (the time it takes for *de novo* synthesis of the enzyme). The metabolism of MAOIs is not well understood. Selegiline and tranylcypromine have meta-amphetamine and amphetamine as

metabolites. There is controversy as to whether phenelzine is cleaved and acetylated in the liver. It is known that a sizable number of people are slow acetylators (a high percentage of Asians and about 50% of whites and blacks), but there is little evidence that the rate of acetylation is clinically significant for this class of drugs. Of clinical importance is the observation that metabolism of MAOIs does not seem to be affected by use of anticonvulsants.

Although the overall efficacy of MAOIs does not differ from that of other commonly used antidepressants in the treatment of MDD, their use is considerably limited by the risk of potentially lethal adverse events, such as hypertensive crises and serotonin syndromes, and by the strict dietary restrictions required to minimize such risks. As a result, they are rarely chosen as first-line agents in the treatment of depression[84]; their use is mainly limited to the treatment of treatment-refractory depression, either as a "next-step" strategy in TCA-resistant depression,[273-279] or even depression resistant to a number of antidepressants.[280-284] High doses of the MAOI tranylcypromine (90 to 170 mg daily) may also be effective in depressed patients who do not experience sufficient improvement during treatment with lower doses.[285] In addition, perhaps due to their ability to inhibit the re-uptake of dopamine in addition to serotonin and norepinephrine, MAOIs appear to be more effective than TCAs[286] in the treatment of atypical depression (characterized by mood reactivity in addition to symptoms such as hypersomnia, hyperphagia, extreme fatigue, and rejection sensitivity). In parallel, while the MAOIs also seem to be effective in the treatment of fatigue in fibromyalgia or chronic fatigue syndrome,[287-291] four of five studies do not show any effect of the SSRIs on fatigue.[292-296] Although, to date, there are no double-blind studies that compare the relative efficacy of MAOIs versus the SSRIs or TCAs in the treatment of fatigue in depression, these studies suggest a potential advantage for MAOIs over SSRIs.

In the GI tract and the liver, MAO catabolizes a number of dietary pressor amines (such as dopamine, tyramine, tryptamine, and phenylethylamine).[52] For this reason, consumption of foods containing high levels of dietary amines while on an MAOI may precipitate a hypertensive crisis, characterized by hypertension, hyperpyrexia, tachycardia, tremulousness, and cardiac arrhythmias.[53] The same reaction may also occur during co-administration of dopaminergic agents and MAOIs, while the co-administration of MAOIs with other antidepressants that potentiate serotonin could result in serotonin syndromes due to toxic CNS serotonin levels. The serotonin syndrome is characterized by alterations in cognition (disorientation, confusion), behavior (agitation, restlessness), autonomic nervous system function (fever, shivering, diaphoresis, diarrhea), and neuromuscular activity (ataxia, hyperreflexia, and myoclonus).[54-56] Since MAO enzymatic activity requires approximately 14 days to be restored, such food or medications should be avoided for 2 weeks after the discontinuation of an irreversible MAOI ("MAOI washout period"). Serotonergic and dopaminergic antidepressants are typically discontinued 2 weeks before the initiation of an MAOI, with the exception of fluoxetine, which needs to be discontinued 5 weeks in advance due to its relatively longer half-life. In addition to its oral formulation, selegiline is also available in a transdermal form (patch), designed to minimize the inhibition of the MAO enzymes found in the lining of the GI tract. Treating MDD with transdermal selegiline appears to be effective[297,298] and also safe, even in the absence of a tyramine-restricted diet.[298] Although rare, serotonin syndrome may occur when oral selegiline is combined with serotonergic agents, particularly the SSRIs.[299] The risk of such drug interactions with the transdermal formulation of selegiline has not been studied.

Side-effect Profile

The most common side effects of MAOIs include postural hypotension, insomnia, agitation, sedation, and sexual dysfunction, although the incidence of sexual dysfunction is lower than with the SSRIs.[300] Other side effects include weight change, dry mouth, constipation, and urinary hesitancy.[51] Peripheral neuropathies have been reported, and may be prevented by concomitant therapy with pyridoxine.[301] A list of side effects with MAOIs is reported in Table 43-2. Elderly patients may develop constipation or urinary retention. Alternatively, nausea and diarrhea have been reported by some patients. Sweating, flushing, or chills may occur. Rarely, hepatotoxicity (which may be serious) may occur with phenelzine. Peripheral edema likely reflecting effects of the drug on small vessels may prove difficult to manage. Finally, some patients complain of muscle twitching or electric shock–like sensations.

Dietary Restrictions and Drug Interactions

As discussed previously, treatment with MAOIs carries a risk of hypertensive crisis. To minimize this risk, patients on MAOIs need to adhere to a strict dietary regimen that excludes foods and beverages that have a high content of dietary amines, including all aged cheeses; sour cream; yogurt; fermented or dried meats (sausages, basderma, pastrami, pepperoni, louza, lingiça, chorizo); offal (liver, sweetbread, kidney, tripe, brains); fava and broad bean pods (lima, lentils, snow-peas); marmite yeast extract; sauerkraut; soy sauce and other soy products; over-ripe bananas and avocado; eggplant; spinach; pickled, dried, or salted fish; caviar; fish roe (tarama); and foods containing monosodium glutamate (MSG). Patients should also avoid consumption of caffeinated drinks, and most alcoholic beverages, especially tap beer and red wine, but also certain white wines, including those that are resinated (retsina), botrytized (sauternes, cadillac, loupiac, monbazillac, coteaux du layon, Alsace vendage tardive, tokaji aszú, trockenbeerenausle), aged (sherry), and others (Riesling, vermouth). Sympathomimetics, both prescribed and over-the-counter (pseudoephedrine, ephedrine, oxymetazoline, dextroamphetamine, and methylphenidate), potent noradrenergic and dopaminergic antidepressants, dextromethorphan, and meperidine (Demerol) may also precipitate a hypertensive crisis. In addition, as mentioned previously, combining MAOIs with potent serotonergic agents (such as the TCAs, SSRIs, and others) carries a risk of serotonergic syndrome. MAOIs must be used with caution in patients with diabetes (due to possible potentiation of oral hypoglycemics and worsened hypoglycemia).

Dosage

The optimal dosages for MAOIs vary from agent to agent. Initially, MAOIs are administered at low doses, with gradual increases as side effects allow. Some tolerance may develop to side effects, including postural hypotension. Phenelzine is usually started at 15 mg twice daily (7.5 to 15 mg/day in the elderly), isocarboxazid at 10 mg twice daily, and tranylcypromine at 10 mg twice daily (5 to 10 mg/day in the elderly). Dosages can be increased by 15 mg weekly for phenelzine and 10 mg weekly for isocarboxazid and tranylcypromine (as side effects allow) to 45 to 60 mg/day for phenelzine (30 to 60 mg/day in the elderly) and 30 to 40 mg/day for the others. Dosages as high as 90 mg/day of these drugs may be required, although these exceed the manufacturer's recommendations. Once depressive symptoms remit, full therapeutic doses are protective against relapse, although in managing patients on MAOIs, dose adjustments over time to manage side effects or clinical response are common. For transdermal selegiline, the minimal effective dose reported is 6 mg/day. It is prudent to taper MAOIs over 2 weeks or more when discontinuing them because discontinuation reactions have been reported with abrupt discontinuation. There is little experience with the use of MAOIs in pregnancy. For this reason, their use should be avoided.

Patients have reported weight gain on all MAOIs and occasionally weight loss (more commonly on tranylcypromine). Anticholinergic-like side effects occur, although they are not due to muscarinic antagonism. These side effects are less severe than those seen with TCAs, although patients on phenelzine may experience dry mouth. Elderly patients may develop constipation or urinary retention. Nausea and diarrhea have been reported by some patients. Sweating, flushing, or chills also may occur. Rarely, hepatotoxicity may occur with phenelzine, which may be serious. Peripheral edema likely reflecting effects of the drug on small vessels may prove difficult to manage. Finally, some patients complain of muscle twitching or electric shock–like sensations. The latter may respond to clonazepam, although the emergence of neurological or neuropathic symptoms may reflect interference with absorption of vitamin B_6 that should improve with dietary supplementation of pyridoxine (vitamin B_6) 50 to 100 mg/day.

TABLE 43-3 Interactions of Monoamine Oxidase Inhibitors with Other Drugs*

Drug	Effect
Sympathomimetics (e.g., amphetamines, dopamine, ephedrine, epinephrine [adrenaline], isoproterenol [Isuprel], metaraminol, methylphenidate, oxymetazoline [Afrin], norepinephrine, phenylephrine [Neo-Synephrine], phenylpropanolamine, pseudoephedrine [Sudafed])	Hypertensive crisis
Meperidine (Demerol and others)	Fever, delirium, hypertension, hypotension, neuromuscular excitability, death
Oral hypoglycemics	Further lowering of serum glucose
L-dopa	Hypertensive crisis
Tricyclic antidepressants,† duloxetine, venlafaxine, SSRIs, clomipramine, tryptophan	Fever, seizures, delirium Nausea, confusion, anxiety, shivering, hyperthermia, rigidity, diaphoresis, hyperreflexia, tachycardia, hypotension, coma, death
Bupropion	Hypertensive crisis

*This may include selegiline even at low doses.
†Tricyclics and MAOIs are occasionally used together.
SSRIs, Selective serotonin re-uptake inhibitors.
(From Rosenbaum JF, Arana GW, Hyman SE, et al., editors: Handbook of psychiatric drug therapy, *ed 5, Philadelphia, 2005, Lippincott Williams & Wilkins.)*

Overdose

MAOIs are extremely dangerous in overdose. Because they circulate at very low concentrations in serum and are difficult to assay, there are no good data on therapeutic or toxic serum levels. Manifestations of toxicity may appear slowly, often taking up to 12 hours to appear and 24 hours to reach their peak; thus, even if patients appear clinically well in the emergency department, they should be admitted for observation after any significant overdose. After an asymptomatic period, a serotonin syndrome may occur, including hyperpyrexia and autonomic excitation. Neuromuscular excitability may be severe enough to produce rhabdomyolysis, which may cause renal failure. This phase of excitation may be followed by CNS depression and cardiovascular collapse. Death may occur early due to seizures or arrhythmias, or later due to asystole, arrhythmias, hypotension, or renal failure. Hemolysis and a coagulopathy also may occur and contribute to morbidity and mortality risk.

Drug Interactions

Important drug interactions with MAOIs are listed in Table 43-3.

Access the complete reference list and multiple choice questions (MCQs) online at https://expertconsult.inkling.com

KEY REFERENCES

5. Fava M, Kendler KS. Major depressive disorder. *Neuron* 28(2):335–341, 2000.
51. Fava M, Rosenbaum JF. Pharmacotherapy and somatic therapies. In Beckham EE, Leber WR, editors: *Handbook of depression,* New York, 1995, Guilford.
76. Thase ME. Preventing relapse and recurrence of depression: a brief review of therapeutic options. *CNS Spectr* 11(12 Suppl. 15):12–21, 2006.
78. Papakostas GI, Perlis RH, Seifert C, et al. Antidepressant dose-reduction and the risk of relapse in major depressive disorder. *Psychother Psychosom* 76(5):266–270, 2007.
79. Fava M, Detke MJ, Balestrieri M. Management of depression relapse: re-initiation of duloxetine treatment or dose increase. *J Psychiatr Res* 40(4):328–336, 2006.
80. Papakostas GI, Fava M. A meta-analysis of clinical trials comparing moclobemide with selective serotonin reuptake inhibitors for the treatment of major depressive disorder. *Can J Psychiatry* 51(12):783–790, 2006.
82. Fava M, Hoog SL, Judge RA, et al. Acute efficacy of fluoxetine versus sertraline and paroxetine in major depressive disorder including effects of baseline insomnia. *J Clin Psychopharmacol* 22(2):137–147, 2002.
85. Fava M, Uebelacker LA, Alpert JE, et al. Major depressive subtypes and treatment response. *Biol Psychiatry* 42(7):568–576, 1997.
90. Fava M, Rankin M. Sexual functioning and SSRIs. *J Clin Psychiatry* 63(Suppl. 5):13–16, discussion 23–25, 2002.
92. Fava M, Graves LM, Benazzi F, et al. A cross-sectional study of the prevalence of cognitive and physical symptoms during long-term antidepressant treatment. *J Clin Psychiatry* 67(11):1754–1759, 2006.
103. Fava M, Judge R, Hoog SL, et al. Fluoxetine versus sertraline and paroxetine in major depressive disorder: changes in weight with long-term treatment. *J Clin Psychiatry* 61(11):863–867, 2000.
106. Thase ME, Ferguson JM, Lydiard RB, et al. Citalopram treatment of paroxetine-intolerant depressed patients. *Depress Anxiety* 16(3):128–133, 2002.
107. Thase ME, Blomgren SL, Birkett MA, et al. Fluoxetine treatment of patients with major depressive disorder who failed initial treatment with sertraline. *J Clin Psychiatry* 58(1):16–21, 1997.
116. Fava M. Prospective studies of adverse events related to antidepressant discontinuation. *J Clin Psychiatry* 67(Suppl. 4):14–21, 2006.
125. Thase ME, Entsuah AR, Rudolph RL. Remission rates during treatment with venlafaxine or selective serotonin reuptake inhibitors. *Br J Psychiatry* 178:234, 2001.
140. Clayton AH, Pradko JF, Croft HA, et al. Prevalence of sexual dysfunction among newer antidepressants. *J Clin Psychiatry* 63(4):357–366, 2002.
144. Thase ME. Effects of venlafaxine on blood pressure: a meta-analysis of original data from 3744 depressed patients. *J Clin Psychiatry* 59(10):502–508, 1998.
145. Fava M, Mulroy R, Alpert J, et al. Emergence of adverse events following discontinuation of treatment with extended-release venlafaxine. *Am J Psychiatry* 154(12):1760–1762, 1997.
157. Papakostas GI, Fava M. A meta-analysis of clinical trials comparing milnacipran, a serotonin-norepinephrine reuptake inhibitor, with a selective serotonin reuptake inhibitor for the treatment of major depressive disorder. *Eur Neuropsychopharmacol* 17(1):32–36, 2007.
178. Papakostas GI. Dopaminergic-based pharmacotherapies for depression. *Eur Neuropsychopharmacol* 16(6):391–402, 2006.
179. Trivedi MH, Rush AJ, Carmody TJ, et al. Do bupropion SR and sertraline differ in their effects on anxiety in depressed patients? *J Clin Psychiatry* 62(10):776–781, 2001.
180. Papakostas GI, Nutt DJ, Hallett LA, et al. Resolution of sleepiness and fatigue in major depressive disorder: a comparison of bupropion and the selective serotonin reuptake inhibitors. *Biol Psychiatry* 60(12):1350–1355, 2006.
193. Papakostas GI, Fava M. A meta-analysis of clinical trials comparing the serotonin (5HT)-2 receptor antagonists trazodone and nefazodone with a selective serotonin reuptake inhibitor for the treatment of major depressive disorder. *Eur Psychiatry* 22(7):444–447, 2007.
230. Papakostas GI, Homberger CH, Fava M. A meta-analysis of clinical trials comparing mirtazapine with a selective serotonin reuptake inhibitor for the treatment of major depressive disorder. *J Psychopharmacol* 22(8):843–848, 2008.
237. Schatzberg AF, Kremer C, Rodrigues HE, et al. Mirtazapine vs. Paroxetine Study Group: Double-blind, randomized comparison of mirtazapine and paroxetine in elderly depressed patients. *Am J Geriatr Psychiatry* 10(5):541–550, 2002.
260. Fava M. Weight gain and antidepressants. *J Clin Psychiatry* 61(Suppl. 11):37–41, 2000.
274. McGrath PJ, Stewart JW, Nunes EV, et al. A double-blind cross-over trial of imipramine and phenelzine for outpatients with treatment-refractory depression. *Am J Psychiatry* 150(1):118–123, 1993.
279. McGrath PJ, Stewart JW, Harrison W, et al. Treatment of tricyclic refractory depression with a monoamine oxidase inhibitor antidepressant. *Psychopharmacol Bull* 23(1):169–172, 1987.
286. Thase ME, Trivedi MH, Rush AJ. MAOIs in the contemporary treatment of depression. *Neuropsychopharmacology* 12(3):185–219, 1995.

44 Pharmacological Approaches to Treatment-Resistant Depression

Ji Hyun Baek, MD, Andrew A. Nierenberg, MD, and Maurizio Fava, MD

KEY POINTS

Background

- Treatment-resistant depression (TRD) refers to an inadequate response to at least one antidepressant given in sufficient doses and for an appropriate duration.

History

- Despite the recent advances in treatment of depression, only 30%–40% of patients achieve remission following initial treatment.

Clinical and Research Challenges

- Inadequate response usually means failure to achieve remission. However, the, importance of functional recovery in treatment has also been emphasized.

- Staging methods to include the types and numbers of failed antidepressant trials might help clinicians and researchers to plan treatment strategies.

- Various strategies including switching antidepressant, combining two different antidepressants, augmentation, and non-pharmacological approaches, can be applied to TRD. However, the standard approach for TRD has not been established mainly due to lack of comprehensive investigations.

- Biomarkers to identify the predicting factors of TRD can help clinicians determine an appropriate treatment plan.

Practical Pointers

- Many patients with TRD are either inadequately treated or misdiagnosed. Clinicians need to systematically re-evaluate the primary diagnosis of depression as well as search for medical and psychiatric co-morbidities.

- Switching antidepressants, combining two antidepressants and applying augmentation strategies are the most commonly used approaches.

- More rigorous studies on definition, clinical trials, and biomarkers of TRD are necessary.

OVERVIEW

Treatment-resistant depression (TRD) refers to an inadequate response to adequate antidepressant treatment. TRD is common in clinical settings. In the Sequenced Treatment Alternatives to Relieve Depression (STAR*D), only 36.8% of patients with major depressive disorder (MDD) who were initially treated with citalopram achieved remission.[1] A recent meta-analytic study reviewed 91 antidepressant monotherapy randomized controlled trials and showed an average remission rate of 44%.[2]

TRD leads to poorer psychosocial functioning[3,4] and raises the risk of suicide,[5] which increases the disease burden of MDD. Cases of TRD tend to be highly recurrent, with up to 80% of patients requiring multiple treatments. The clinical outcomes of patients who fail to remit are usually worse than those of first-episode patients.[6]

DEFINITION OF TREATMENT-RESISTANT DEPRESSION

Although it appears simple, defining "inadequate response" and "adequate antidepressant treatment" remains controversial.

Inadequate response typically means failure to achieve remission; patients who improve but who fail to remit with initial treatment are more likely to have a recurrence. In clinical trials, remission is usually defined by scores on depression symptom severity scales (e.g., a Hamilton Depression Rating Scale-17 $\leq$ 7). Several researchers have suggested that functional recovery also needs to be taken into consideration when defining adequate response.[7]

At least one trial with an antidepressant with established efficacy in MDD (with sufficient duration and doses) is considered to be "adequate antidepressant treatment." However, defining sufficient duration and dose is difficult. Sufficient dose is either the minimum dosage that will produce the expected effect or the maximum dosage that the patient can tolerate until the expected effect is achieved. Typically, sufficient duration of an antidepressant is considered to be long enough to produce a robust therapeutic effect.[8] In clinical trials 4–6 weeks has been used as the threshold for sufficient duration, but some researchers suggest using a longer period, up to 8–12 weeks.[9] In STAR*D, many patients who initially failed to achieve remission or response, eventually achieved remission or a response by 14 weeks.[10]

STAGING MODELS OF TREATMENT-RESISTANT DEPRESSION

Another important characteristic of TRD is the number of failed trials. As previously mentioned, most clinical studies use a definition of TRD as failure to remit to at least one antidepressant. In other words, those with TRD can fail a number of antidepressant trials. Although there is no clear method of defining the severity of TRD, it is generally thought that as the number of failed trials increases, the chance of remission will diminish. In STAR*D, 30.6% of patients achieved remission at Level 2 and about 13% of subjects achieved remission at Level 3.[1]

Several staging models have been suggested involving the number of non-response to adequate treatment strategies and the types of antidepressants used.[8,11] However, several factors have not been fully studied. In the staging models, non-response to two agents of different classes has been thought to be more difficult to treat than non-response to two agents of the same class. In addition, there is an implicit hierarchy of antidepressant treatments, with monoamine oxidase inhibitors (MAOIs) being considered as superior to tricyclic antidepressants (TCAs) and SSRIs, and TCAs being considered as more effective than SSRIs in some populations. These two concepts have never been fully investigated.[8] A recent study showed no significant difference in remission rates between venlafaxine-treated and sertraline-treated patients who had not responded to other SSRIs.[12] Similarly, a meta-analysis of antidepressants and a cross-over trial of imipramine[13] and setraline[14] did not prove superior to TCAs.

CLINICAL FEATURES ASSOCIATED WITH TREATMENT-RESISTANT DEPRESSION

Several clinical conditions (e.g., substance abuse and co-morbid anxiety disorder) have been associated with TRD.[10,15] Co-morbid personality disorders, subtypes of depression (including atypical depression, melancholic depression, and chronic depression) have also been associated with worse response to antidepressants; however, the studies have had mixed results.[15] Co-morbid personality disorders also have been associated with poorer outcome, but not all studies support these findings.[8] Medical co-morbidities also contribute to a poorer response to antidepressants.

CLINICAL APPROACH TO TREATMENT-RESISTANT DEPRESSION

Pseudo-resistance refers to non-response associated with inadequate treatment.[16] When patients with MDD show an inadequate response (i.e., not achieving remission) with adequate antidepressant treatment, clinicians should consider the possibility of pseudo-resistance.

Misdiagnosis of mood disorders is a relatively common problem in clinical practice. This may involve recall bias associated with retrospective evaluations. When remission does not occur, we recommend that clinicians re-do the diagnostic evaluation using a structured clinical interview. Psychiatric co-morbid conditions also need to be examined thoroughly.

It is also important to assess whether a patient actually receives an "adequate antidepressant treatment." Clinicians need to evaluate whether an antidepressant was used in an adequate dose for a sufficient amount of time and whether the patient actually took medication as prescribed. Medical co-morbidities (including hypothyroidism, fibromyalgia, and neurologic conditions) can also confound the treatment response. Conducting routine blood work and a physical examination can provide additional clues. Also, co-administered medication can affect antidepressant metabolism (via inducing cytochrome P450 enzymes). In some cases, a patient might be a rapid metabolizer of a drug and result in a lower blood level.

COMMON TREATMENT STRATEGIES FOR TREATMENT-RESISTANT DEPRESSION

Once TRD is confirmed, more rigorous treatment is necessary. Various strategies have been investigated, although the best sequence of treatment has not been established. In general, switching antidepressants, combining two antidepressants, and using augmenting strategies are the most reasonable for TRD. However, the optimal method has not been determined. A retrospective analysis from STAR*D showed no significant differences (in terms of remission rate, response rate, time to remission, and time to response) between switching and augmentation strategies.[17]

Switching an Antidepressant

One of the most common strategies is switching antidepressants; however, the superiority of switching to a different class (e.g., from a SSRI to a SNRI) or switching within the same class has not been proven. In STAR*D, switching treatments in Level 2 (i.e., those who had unsatisfactory results or intoler-

ance of citalopram) involved use of sertraline, venlafaxine, or bupropion sustained-release (SR). No significant difference was observed in terms of remission rates (24.8% for venlafaxine XR, 21.3% for bupropion SR, and 18.1% for sertraline).[1] In addition, the ARGOS study did not find significant differences (in terms of remission rates) between venlafaxine XR and other second-generation-antidepressants (mostly SSRIs) (59.3% for venlafaxine XR, 51.5% for another antidepressant).[18] On the contrary, two of four randomized controlled trials (RCTs) demonstrated that switching from a SSRI to venlafaxine was superior to the switching to a second SSRI.[19] One RCT compared the efficacy of mirtazapine, venlafaxine, and paroxetine after failure of two antidepressant trials did not find statistically significant differences in remission rates.[20] A meta-analysis of four clinical trials found only modest, but statistically significant increases after switching to a non-SSRI in patients with SSRI-resistant depression.[21]

Combining Two Antidepressants with Different Mechanisms of Action

Combining two antidepressants with different mechanisms of action is an attractive approach for managing TRD. Combination of an SSRI or an SNRI with a norepinephrine-dopamine re-uptake inhibitor (bupropion) or a serotonin-norepinephrine antagonist (mirtazapine or mianserin) is a commonly used combination, with expected synergistic effects of their pharmacodynamic properties.

A double blind placebo-controlled study found significant benefit using mirtazapine for augmentation after failing to respond to an antidepressant. Blier et al.[22] conducted a RCT of mirtazapine in combination with fluoxetine, venlafaxine, or bupropion compared with fluoxetine monotherapy and found that combination therapies were associated with approximately twice the remission rate of fluoxetine monotherapy. In contrast, in single-blind studies, no significant differences in remission rates were found with escitalopram plus placebo, bupropion SR plus escitalopram, or venlafaxine ER plus mirtazapine.[19]

When using combination treatments, clinicians should be mindful of pharmacokinetic and phamacodynamic interactions. Serotonin syndrome or the effects associated with increased drug levels (due to cytochrome P450 enzyme inhibition, e.g., CYP2D6 inhibition by fluoxetine or paroxetine) might develop.

Augmentation

Lithium

Lithium is one of the most common augmenting agents in TRD. A minimum daily dose of 900 mg is generally recommended. The efficacy of lithium augmentation (with either a TCA or an SSRI) has been supported by randomized, placebo-controlled double-blind studies. In a meta-analysis, lithium augmentation was found to be significantly more effective than placebo (OR = 3.1; 95% confidence interval [CI] 1.8–5.4).[23]

Triiodothyronine (T_3)

A meta-analysis of T_3 augmentation of TCA (8 clinical trials, n = 292),[24] showed that T_3 augmentation almost doubled the response rate. Limited data on the effect of T_3 augmentation of SSRIs is available. A recent double-blind, RCT[25] compared the effects of T_3 plus sertraline and sertraline plus placebo in MDD at treatment initiation. No significant difference was noted in remission rates, response rates, or time-to-response between two groups. In the STAR*D study, T_3 and lithium augmentation was used in patients who failed to achieve remission after two trials. Although no statistical significant difference was observed (remission rate of T_3 was 24.7% and that of lithium was 15.9%), use of T_3 had superior tolerability and adherence. While T_3 augmentation appears safe, there is a limited evidence to guide its long-term adjunctive use. More controlled trials are needed to determine the efficacy of T_3 as an adjunctive medication.[26]

Atypical Antipsychotics

Recently, use of atypical antipsychotics as adjunctive agents has been increasing. A meta-analysis by Nelson and Papakostas[27] of the adjunctive use of olanzapine, quetiapine, aripiprazole, and risperidone (16 trials, n = 3480) demonstrated that use of adjunctive atypical antipsychotics was significantly more effective than use of placebo (remission: odds ratio = 2.00 95% CI = 2.68–5.72). Aripiprazole, quetiapine, and olanzapine-fluoxetine combinations are appropriate for use in TRD in the US. Newer atypical antipsychotics, i.e., ziprasidone, paliperidone, asenapine, and iloperidone, have not been examined for their efficacy in controlled trials.

Atypical antipsychotics are apt to induce adverse effects, including extrapyramidal symptoms, tardive dyskinesia, and metabolic syndrome. Discontinuation rates due to such adverse effects are also high. Use of newer atypical antipsychotics with fewer metabolic concerns might be reasonable, although limited evidence is available.

Buspirone

Buspirone is a serotonin$_{1A}$ receptor partial agonist. In the STAR*D study, adjunctive use of buspirone showed a similar remission rate to that of adjunctive bupropion SR in citalopram non-responders (30.1% vs. 29.7%). While there have been positive data from open-label studies, two randomized placebo-controlled trials have failed to find a significant benefit from buspirone.[28]

L-Methylfolate

Folate is an essential co-factor involved in methylation reactions, which are crucial for monoamine synthesis and homocysteine regulation. Abnormal folate metabolism has long been associated with mood disorders. L-Methylfolate is a biologically-active form of dietary folate. In a recent study Papakostas et al.[29] examined use of L-Methylfolate as an augmentation strategy for poor responder to SSRIs. The response rate was 32.3% compared to 14.6% for placebo over the course of two trials. Since L-Methylfolate is a neutraceutical, it is safe and has few (minor) side effects. Considering its safety and tolerabililty, it may be a promising candidate as an augmentation agent for TRD.

S-adenosyl-L-methionine

S-adenosyl-L-methionine (SAMe) is the major donor for methyl group in synthesis of neurotransmitters. Along with folic acid, SAMe also has received attention as a promising complementary alternative medicine for the treatment of depression. In a 6-week, double-blind, randomized trial of adjunctive SAMe with SSRI non-responders, remission rates were significantly higher for patients treated with SAMe than with placebo (25.8% vs. 11.7%).[30] It is also safe and has few adverse effects.

Novel Therapeutic Agents

New drugs with mechanisms that fall outside of those associated with the classical monoamine receptor hypothesis of depression offer great promise for the treatment of TRD.[19]

Ketamine, an NMDA receptor antagonist, has shown rapid antidepressant effects. Recently, several open-label studies[31,32] with repeated intravenous ketamine infusions have shown promising results. Inflammation is thought to be associated with treatment response in depression. In this context, anti-inflammatory agents may be effective. Aspirin, celecoxib, infliximab, N-acetylcysteine have all been studied; however, no definite answer has been reached about their benefits.[19]

Non-pharmacological Interventions

Adjunctive psychotherapy can be helpful in TRD. In the STAR*D study, cognitive therapy was included in Level 2. No significant difference was observed in remission rates between the cognitive therapy group and the medication-only group. A randomized trial investigating the effects of cognitive-behavioral therapy (CBT) in women with TRD (n = 469), adding CBT to usual care, significantly increased treatment response compared with usual care at 6 months (46% vs. 22%). However, the efficacy of other types of psychotherapy has not been investigated in TRD.

Brain stimulation focuses on the direct or indirect alteration of brain function by electrical or magnetic methods. Electroconvulsive therapy (ECT), the oldest brain stimulation methods, has long been viewed as an effective treatment for severe depression.[33] Cognitive impairment is its most common side effect. Vagus nerve stimulation (VNS) therapy stimulates the left vagus nerve repetitively using small electrical pulse from an neurostimulator implanted on patients' neck. In an open study with patients afflicted with chronic MDD who had failed to respond to more than four adequate antidepressant treatments, the response rate to VNS was approximately 30%. Recently, it has been approved as an adjunctive treatment for TRD in the US. Side effects (such as voice alteration, dyspnea, and neck pain) of VNS are generally mild. However, it requires an invasive procedure, and most of the studies done so far had relatively small sample sizes. Deep brain stimulation (DBS) was initially developed for the treatment of Parkinson's disease. DBS therapy stimulates targeted brain region via electrodes which are permanently implanted. Subcallosal cingulate white matter, the ventral caudate, the ventral striatum, and the subcallosal cingulate white matter are commonly targeted. Several small open studies have shown promise.[34]

In severe TRD, psychosurgery also has been tried. Subcaudate tractomy, anterior cingulatomy, limbic leucotomy, and anterior capsulotomy are the most common methods. Its efficacy has been established, but its use is still limited.

RESEARCH CHALLENGES

As previously mentioned, a precise definition of TRD is necessary. Staging models to identify the degree of TRD also need to be conducted.

Several antidepressant combination strategies have not been confirmed through placebo-controlled RCTs. Newer antidepressants with novel mechanisms of action may be promising. Innovative treatment strategies need to be evaluated through more collaborative, multi-center, controlled trials.

Predictive factors to identify which patients are likely to respond well to treatment remain elusive. Biomarkers can help to predict responses to certain treatments. Several studies have suggested that BDNF, inflammatory markers, and abnormalities in default mode network may be potential biomarkers for antidepressant response, but definitive answers are lacking.

CONCLUSIONS

TRD is common, although its definition is not exactly clear. Since some cases of TRD could actually be pseudo-resistance, or non-response due to suboptimal treatment, clinicians should re-do diagnostic evaluations and check patients' drug compliance when remission does not develop. Optimal treatment strategies for TRD are not well established. In order to develop efficacious treatment guidelines for TRD, more rigorous studies with collaborative, multi-center, controlled trials need to be done with a variety of promising agents. Identifying mechanisms and predicting factors of poor response to antidepressants will be important. Further studies on biomarkers for TRD are warranted.

Access a list of MCQs for this chapter at https://expertconsult.inkling.com

REFERENCES

1. Rush AJ, Trivedi MH, Wisniewski SR, et al. Acute and longer-term outcomes in depressed outpatients requiring one or several treatment steps: a STAR*D report. *Am J Psychiatry* 163:1905–1917, 2006.
2. Sinyor M, Schaffer A, Smart KA, et al. Sponsorship, antidepressant dose, and outcome in major depressive disorder: meta-analysis of randomized controlled trials. *J Clin Psychiatry* 73:e277–e287, 2012.
3. Ansseau M, Demyttenaere K, Heyrman J, et al. Objective: remission of depression in primary care The Oreon Study. *Eur Neuropsychopharmacol* 19:169–176, 2009.
4. Fekadu A, Wooderson SC, Markopoulou K, et al. What happens to patients with treatment-resistant depression? A systematic review of medium to long term outcome studies. *J Affect Disord* 116:4–11, 2009.
5. Kiloh LG, Andrews G, Neilson M. The long-term outcome of depressive illness. *Br J Psychiatry* 153:752–757, 1988.
6. Demyttenaere K, Adelin A, Patrick M, et al. Six-month compliance with antidepressant medication in the treatment of major depressive disorder. *Int Clin Psychopharmacol* 23:36–42, 2008.
7. Zimmerman M, McGlinchey JB, Posternak MA, et al. How should remission from depression be defined? The depressed patient's perspective. *Am J Psychiatry* 163:148–150, 2006.
8. Fava M. Diagnosis and definition of treatment-resistant depression. *Biol Psychiatry* 53:649–659, 2003.
9. Donovan SJ, Quitkin FM, Stewart JW, et al. Duration of antidepressant trials: clinical and research implications. *J Clin Psychopharmacol* 14:64–66, 1994.
10. Trivedi MH, Rush AJ, Wisniewski SR, et al. Evaluation of outcomes with citalopram for depression using measurement-based care in STAR*D: implications for clinical practice. *Am J Psychiatry* 163:28–40, 2006.
11. Thase ME, Rush AJ. When at first you don't succeed: sequential strategies for antidepressant nonresponders. *J Clin Psychiatry* 58(Suppl. 13):23–29, 1997.
12. Lenox-Smith AJ, Jiang Q. Venlafaxine extended release versus citalopram in patients with depression unresponsive to a selective serotonin reuptake inhibitor. *Int Clin Psychopharmacol* 23:113–119, 2008.
13. Mace S, Taylor D. Selective serotonin reuptake inhibitors: a review of efficacy and tolerability in depression. *Expert Opin Pharmacother* 1:917–933, 2000.
14. Thase ME, Rush AJ, Howland RH, et al. Double-blind switch study of imipramine or sertraline treatment of antidepressant-resistant chronic depression. *Arch Gen Psychiatry* 59:233–239, 2002.
15. Souery D, Oswald P, Massat I, et al. Clinical factors associated with treatment resistance in major depressive disorder: results from a European multicenter study. *J Clin Psychiatry* 68:1062–1070, 2007.
16. Nierenberg AA, Amsterdam JD. Treatment-resistant depression: definition and treatment approaches. *J Clin Psychiatry* 51(Suppl.): 39–47, discussion 48–50, 1990.
17. Gaynes BN, Dusetzina SB, Ellis AR, et al. Treating depression after initial treatment failure: directly comparing switch and augmenting strategies in STAR*D. *J Clin Psychopharmacol* 32:114–119, 2012.
18. Baldomero EB, Ubago JG, Cercos CL, et al. Venlafaxine extended release versus conventional antidepressants in the remission of depressive disorders after previous antidepressant failure: ARGOS study. *Depress Anxiety* 22:68–76, 2005.
19. Carvalho AF, Berk M, Hyphantis TN, et al. The integrative management of treatment-resistant depression: a comprehensive review and perspectives. *Psychother Psychosom* 83:70–88, 2014.
20. Fang Y, Yuan C, Xu Y, et al. Comparisons of the efficacy and tolerability of extended-release venlafaxine, mirtazapine, and paroxetine in treatment-resistant depression: a double-blind, randomized pilot study in a Chinese population. *J Clin Psychopharmacol* 30:357–364, 2010.
21. Papakostas GI, Fava M, Thase ME. Treatment of SSRI-resistant depression: a meta-analysis comparing within- versus across-class switches. *Biol Psychiatry* 63:699–704, 2008.
22. Blier P, Ward HE, Tremblay P, et al. Combination of antidepressant medications from treatment initiation for major depressive disorder: a double-blind randomized study. *Am J Psychiatry* 167:281–288, 2010.
23. Crossley NA, Bauer M. Acceleration and augmentation of antidepressants with lithium for depressive disorders: two meta-analyses of randomized, placebo-controlled trials. *J Clin Psychiatry* 68:935–940, 2007.
24. Aronson R, Offman HJ, Joffe RT, et al. Triiodothyronine augmentation in the treatment of refractory depression. A meta-analysis. *Arch Gen Psychiatry* 53:842–848, 1996.
25. Garlow SJ, Dunlop BW, Ninan PT, et al. The combination of triiodothyronine (T3) and sertraline is not superior to sertraline monotherapy in the treatment of major depressive disorder. *J Psychiatr Res* 46:1406–1413, 2012.
26. Rosenthal LJ, Goldner WS, O'Reardon JP. T3 augmentation in major depressive disorder: safety considerations. *Am J Psychiatry* 168:1035–1040, 2011.
27. Nelson JC, Papakostas GI. Atypical antipsychotic augmentation in major depressive disorder: a meta-analysis of placebo-controlled randomized trials. *Am J Psychiatry* 166:980–991, 2009.
28. Connolly KR, Thase ME. If at first you don't succeed: a review of the evidence for antidepressant augmentation, combination and switching strategies. *Drugs* 71:43–64, 2011.
29. Papakostas GI, Shelton RC, Zajecka JM, et al. L-methylfolate as adjunctive therapy for SSRI-resistant major depression: results of two randomized, double-blind, parallel-sequential trials. *Am J Psychiatry* 169:1267–1274, 2012.
30. Papakostas GI, Mischoulon D, Shyu I, et al. S-adenosyl methionine (SAMe) augmentation of serotonin reuptake inhibitors for antidepressant nonresponders with major depressive disorder: a double-blind, randomized clinical trial. *Am J Psychiatry* 167:942–948, 2010.
31. Haile CN, Murrough JW, Iosifescu DV, et al. Plasma brain derived neurotrophic factor (BDNF) and response to ketamine in treatment-resistant depression. *Int J Neuropsychopharmacol* 17:331–336, 2014.
32. Shiroma PR, Johns B, Kuskowski M, et al. Augmentation of response and remission to serial intravenous subanesthetic ketamine in treatment resistant depression. *J Affect Disord* 155:123–129, 2014.
33. Kellner CH, Greenberg RM, Murrough JW, et al. ECT in treatment-resistant depression. *Am J Psychiatry* 169:1238–1244, 2012.
34. Gaynes BN, Lux LJ, Lloyd SW, et al. Nonpharmacologic interventions for treatment-resistant depression in adults. Rockville MD 2011.

45 Electroconvulsive Therapy

Charles A. Welch, MD

KEY POINTS

- Remission rates of 70%–90% have been reported in clinical trials of electroconvulsive therapy (ECT) and ECT is currently the most promising prospect for addressing the unmet worldwide need for effective treatment of individuals suffering from depression.

- The symptoms that predict a good response to ECT are those of major depression (e.g., anorexia, weight loss, early morning awakening, impaired concentration, pessimistic mood, motor restlessness, increased speech latency, constipation, and somatic or self-deprecatory delusions).

- Psychotic illness is the second most common indication for ECT; ECT is effective in up to 75% of patients with catatonia, regardless of the underlying cause, and is the treatment of choice as a primary treatment for most patients with catatonia.

- The greatest challenge facing ECT patients is the high rate of relapse after a successful index course of ECT. There is an urgent need to improve on current strategies of continuation ECT and continuation pharmacotherapy.

- The use of ultra-brief pulse waveform (0.3 ms) is becoming the standard of practice worldwide because of its extremely low side-effect profile. Nevertheless, some patients still require standard waveform (1.0 ms) to achieve full remission of symptoms.

OVERVIEW

Electroconvulsive therapy (ECT) remains an indispensable treatment because of the large number of depressed patients who are unresponsive to drugs or who are intolerant to their side effects. In the largest clinical trial of antidepressant medication, only 50% of depressed patients achieved a full remission, while an equal percentage were non-responders or achieved only partial remission.[1] On the other hand, remission rates of 70%–90% have been reported in clinical trials of ECT with response rates as high as 95% in delusional depression.[2,3] Depression requires effective treatment because it is associated with increased mortality (mainly due to cardiovascular events or suicide).[4] Furthermore, among all diseases, depression currently ranks fourth in global disease burden, and is projected to rank second by the year 2020.[5] ECT is currently the most promising prospect for addressing the unmet worldwide need for effective treatment of individuals suffering from medication-resistant depression.

INDICATIONS FOR ELECTROCONVULSIVE THERAPY

Major depression is the most common indication for ECT. The symptoms that predict a good response to ECT are those of major depression (e.g., anorexia, weight loss, early morning awakening, impaired concentration, pessimistic mood, motor restlessness, increased speech latency, constipation, and delusions).[6,7] The cardinal symptom is the acute loss of interest in activities that formerly gave pleasure. These are exactly the same symptoms that constitute the indication for antidepressant drugs, and at the present time there is no way to predict which patients will ultimately be drug-resistant. There is currently little consensus on the definition of drug-resistant depression,[8] and the designation of drug failure varies with the adequacy of prior treatment.[9] Medical co-morbidities are also important to this definition. Young, healthy patients can safely receive four or more different drug regimens before moving to ECT, whereas older depressed patients may be unable to tolerate more than one drug trial without developing serious medical complications.

Other factors also affect the threshold for moving from drug therapy to ECT. Suicidal ideation and intent respond to ECT 80% of the time,[10] and are an indication for an early transition from drug therapy.[11] Lower response rates to ECT have been reported in depressed patients with a co-morbid personality disorder,[12] and a longer duration of depression,[13] but there is conflicting evidence in the literature as to whether a history of medication-resistance is associated with a lower response rate to ECT. However, none of these factors constitute a reason to avoid ECT if neurovegetative signs are present.

Psychotic illness is the second most common indication for ECT. Although it is not a routine treatment for schizophrenia, ECT, in combination with a neuroleptic, may result in sustained improvement in up to 80% of drug-resistant patients with chronic schizophrenia.[14,15] Young patients with psychosis conforming to the schizophreniform profile (i.e., with acute onset, positive psychotic symptoms, affective intactness, and medication-resistance) are more responsive to ECT than are those with chronic schizophrenia, and they may have a full and enduring remission of their illness with treatment.[16–18]

Bipolar depression has over a 50% remission rate with ECT. Mania also responds well to ECT,[19,20] but drug treatment remains the first-line therapy. Nevertheless, in controlled trials, ECT is as effective as lithium (or more so), and in drug-refractory mania, more than 50% of cases have remitted with ECT.[21] ECT is highly effective in the treatment of medication-resistant mixed affective states[22] and refractory bipolar disorder in adolescents.[23]

Although most patients initially receive a trial of medication regardless of their diagnosis, several groups of patients (see below) are appropriate for ECT as a primary treatment. These include: patients who are severely malnourished, dehydrated, and exhausted due to protracted depressive illness (they should be treated promptly after careful re-hydration); patients with complicating medical illness (such as cardiac arrhythmia or coronary artery disease) because these individuals are often more safely treated with ECT than with antidepressants; patients with delusional depression (as they are often resistant to antidepressant therapy,[24] but respond to ECT 80%–90% of the time)[25–27]; patients who have been unresponsive to medications during previous episodes (because they are often better served by proceeding directly to ECT); and, the majority of patients with catatonia (as they respond promptly to ECT).[28–30] Although the catatonic syndrome is most often associated with an affective disorder, catatonia may also be a manifestation of schizophrenia, metabolic disorders, structural brain lesions, anti-NMDA receptor encephalitis, or systemic lupus erythematosus. Prompt treatment is essential because the mortality of untreated catatonia is as high as 50%, and even its non-fatal complications (including pneumonia, venous embolus, limb contracture, and decubitus ulcer) are serious. ECT is effective in up to 75% of patients with catatonia, regardless of the underlying cause, and is the treatment of choice as a primary treatment for most patients with catatonia.[31] Lorazepam has also been effective for short-term treatment of catatonia,[32] but its long-term efficacy has not been confirmed. While neuroleptic malignant syndrome (NMS) may be clinically indistinguishable from catatonia,[33] high fever, opisthotonos, and rigidity are more common in the former. ECT has been reported effective in NMS,[34] but intensive supportive medical treatment, discontinuation of neuroleptic therapy, use of dantrolene, and use of bromocriptine are still the essential steps of management.

RISK FACTORS ASSOCIATED WITH ELECTROCONVULSIVE THERAPY

As the technical conduct of ECT has improved, factors that were formerly considered absolute contraindications to ECT have become relative risk factors. The patient is best served by weighing the risk of treatment against the morbidity or lethality of remaining depressed. The prevailing view is that there are no longer any absolute contraindications to ECT, but the following conditions warrant careful work-up and management.

The heart is physiologically stressed during ECT.[35] Cardiac work increases abruptly at the onset of the seizure initially because of sympathetic outflow from the diencephalon, through the spinal sympathetic tract, to the heart (Figure 45-1). This outflow persists for the duration of the seizure and is augmented by a rise in circulating catecholamine levels that peak about 3 minutes after the onset of seizure activity (Figure 45-2A).[36,37] After the seizure ends, parasympathetic tone remains strong, often causing transient bradycardia and hypotension, with a return to baseline function in 5–10 minutes (see Figure 45-2B).

The cardiac conditions that most often worsen under this autonomic stimulus are ischemic heart disease, hypertension, congestive heart failure (CHF), and cardiac arrhythmias. These conditions, if properly managed, have proved to be surprisingly tolerant to ECT. The idea that general anesthesia is contraindicated within 6 months of a myocardial infarction (MI) has acquired a certain sanctity, which is surprising considering the ambiguity of the original data.[38] A more rational approach involves careful assessment of the cardiac reserve, a reserve that is needed as cardiac work increases during ECT.[39] Vascular aneurysms should be repaired before ECT if possible, but in practice, they have proved surprisingly durable during treatment.[40,41] Critical aortic stenosis should be surgically corrected before ECT to avoid ventricular overload during the seizure. Patients with cardiac pacemakers generally tolerate ECT uneventfully, although proper pacer function should be ascertained before treatment. Implantable cardioverter defibrillators should be converted from demand mode to fixed mode by placing a magnet over the device during ECT.[42] Patients with compensated CHF generally tolerate ECT well, although a transient decompensation into pulmonary edema for 5–10 minutes may occur in patients with a baseline ejection fraction below 20%. It is unclear whether the underlying cause is a neurogenic stimulus to the lung parenchyma or a reduction in cardiac output because of increased heart rate and blood pressure.

The brain is also physiologically stressed during ECT. Cerebral oxygen consumption approximately doubles, and cerebral blood flow increases several-fold. Increases in intracranial pressure and the permeability of the blood–brain barrier also develop. These acute changes may increase the risk of ECT in patients with a variety of neurological conditions.[43]

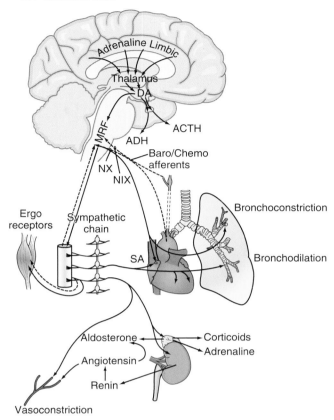

DA - Defense area in hypothalamus
MRF - Medullary reticular formation
SA - Sinoatrial node

Figure 45-1. Schematic of sympathetic outflow from the diencephalon to the heart and other organs.

Space-occupying brain lesions were previously considered an absolute contraindication to ECT, and earlier case reports described clinical deterioration when ECT was given to patients with brain tumors.[44] However, more recent reports indicate that with careful management patients with brain tumor or chronic subdural hematomas may be safely treated.[45–48] Recent cerebral infarction probably represents the most common intracranial risk factor. Case reports of ECT after recent cerebral infarction indicate that the complication rate is low,[43] and consequently ECT is often the treatment of choice for post-stroke depression.[49] The interval between infarction and time of ECT should be determined by the urgency of treatment for depression.

ECT has been safe and efficacious in patients with hydrocephalus, arteriovenous malformations, cerebral hemorrhage, multiple sclerosis, systemic lupus erythematosus, Huntington's disease, and mental retardation. Patients with depression and Parkinson's disease experience improvement of both disorders with ECT, and Parkinson's disease alone may constitute an indication for ECT.[50] Depressed patients with pre-existing dementia are likely to develop especially severe cognitive deficits secondary to ECT, but most return to their baseline after treatment, and many actually improve.[51,52]

The pregnant mother who is severely depressed may require ECT to prevent malnutrition or suicide. Although reports of ECT during pregnancy are reassuring,[53] fetal monitoring is recommended during treatment. The fetus may be protected from the physiological stress of ECT by nature of its lack of

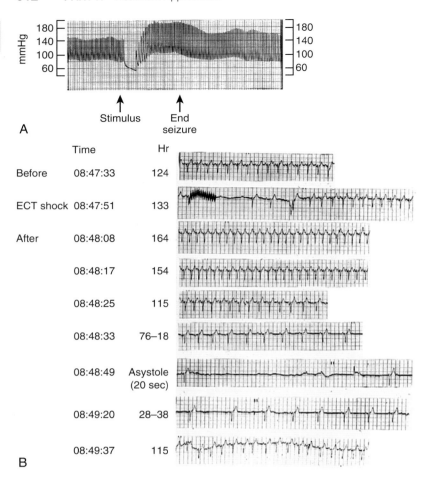

Figure 45-2. (A) Graphic of the impact of electroconvulsive therapy (ECT) on catecholamine levels and blood pressure following a seizure. (B) Graphic of the effects of ECT on cardiac rhythm.

direct neuronal connection to the maternal diencephalon, which spares it the intense autonomic stimulus experienced by maternal end organs during the ictus.

TECHNIQUE FOR CONDUCTING ELECTROCONVULSIVE THERAPY

The routine pre-ECT work-up usually includes a thorough medical history and physical examination, along with: a chest film; an electrocardiogram (EKG); a urinalysis; a complete blood count; and determination of blood glucose, blood urea nitrogen, and electrolytes. Additional studies may be necessary, at the clinician's discretion. In a patient with cognitive deficits, it is sometimes difficult to decide whether a CNS work-up is indicated because depression itself is usually the cause of this deficit. A metabolic screen, computed tomography (CT) scan, and magnetic resonance imaging (MRI) are often useful to rule out causes of impaired cognition unrelated to depression. Whenever a question of primary dementia arises, neurological consultation should be requested. Neuropsychological testing may be diagnostically helpful in making the distinction between primary dementia and depressive pseudomentia.[54,55]

It is essential that the patient's medical condition be optimized before starting treatment. Elderly patients often arrive at the hospital severely malnourished and dehydrated, and ECT should be delayed until they have had several days of re-hydration, with alimentation via feeding tube, if necessary. Antihypertensive regimens should be optimized before treatment to reduce the chance of a severe hypertensive reaction during treatment. Most diabetic patients are more stable if the

morning dose of insulin is held until after their treatment. The insulin requirement usually decreases as a diabetic patient recovers from depression, and blood glucose levels must be monitored frequently during the course of ECT.

Antidepressant medications do not necessarily have to be discontinued prior to ECT, since there is little evidence of a harmful interaction. Indeed, there is preliminary evidence that neuroleptics, tricyclic antidepressants (TCAs), selective serotonin re-uptake inhibitors (SSRIs), and mirtazapine are not only safe to prescribe during a course of ECT, but also may enhance the therapeutic effectiveness of the treatment.[56] Monoamine oxidase inhibitors (MAOIs) may be safely given during a course of ECT, as long as sympathomimetic drugs are not administered.[57] Early case reports described excessive cognitive disturbance and prolonged apnea in a small percentage of patients receiving lithium during ECT, but more recent data indicate that this is a rare complication, and that concurrent administration of lithium is usually safe.[58] Benzodiazepines are antagonistic to the ictal process and should be discontinued.[59] Even short-acting benzodiazepines may have a long half-life in a sick, elderly person and make effective treatment less likely. For sedation, patients receiving ECT usually do well with a sedating atypical antipsychotic, such as quetiapine, or a non-benzodiazepine hypnotic, such as hydroxyzine. Anticonvulsants, prescribed as mood stabilizers, are usually discontinued prior to ECT, but in a recent series of bipolar patients the concurrent administration of lamotrigine did not interfere with treatment, and facilitated transition to maintenance pharmacotherapy.[60] In the patient with a pre-existing seizure disorder, the anticonvulsant regimen should be continued for patient safety. The elevated seizure threshold can almost always be over-ridden with an ECT stimulus, and patients managed in this manner usually have the same clinical response as patients not taking anticonvulsants.[61]

Because of the profound systemic physiological responses unique to this treatment, anesthesia for ECT should be performed by an anesthesiologist familiar with it. ECT presents special challenges in anesthetic management, and a careful reading of the pertinent literature is essential preparation for the anesthesiologist.[62] The use of cardiac monitoring and pulse oximetry on all patients undergoing general anesthesia has been endorsed by the American Society of Anesthesiologists. Most existing ECT machines record the EKG only during the treatment itself, but recording of baseline and post-ictal rhythms is essential, and a separate operating room monitor with paper recording capability is therefore necessary to monitor the EKG adequately.

Prior to induction, atropine or glycopyrrolate may be administered routinely to all patients, but in many treatment centers their use is reserved for patients who are prone to bradycardia. Atropine does not reduce oral secretions in ECT.[63]

The four most commonly used induction agents are methohexital, propofol, etomidate, and ketamine, and each has its pros and cons.[64] Methohexital does not affect the seizure threshold, and has been extensively studied. Propofol increases seizure threshold, and is associated with shorter seizures, a higher intensity of the stimulus, and a higher number of treatments.[65] Nevertheless, overall therapeutic response rates with propofol are no worse than with the other agents, and it has a uniquely smooth emergence syndrome. Etomidate lowers seizure threshold and is associated with longer seizures,[66] but has the disadvantage of causing adrenal suppression, even in single doses. Ketamine also lowers the seizure threshold, and is associated with less memory disturbance than etomidate.[67] Both methohexital and propofol cause a significant drop in blood pressure on induction, while etomidate and ketamine do not. In most treatment centers, either methohexital or propofol is used as the routine induction agent, while etomidate or ketamine is reserved for patients with high seizure thresholds or a fragile cardiovascular status.

Sevoflurane, an inhaled anesthetic, is a proven ECT-induction agent for patients with severe needle phobia, agitation, or poor tolerance of intravenous (IV) induction agents.[68] For children it is often the least traumatic induction method. It can be used as the only induction agent, or it can be augmented with IV agents once the patient is unconscious.

Paralytic drugs are essential to the safe conduct of ECT. Prior to the use of paralytic agents, over 30% of ECT patients suffered compression fractures of the spine. The standard agent is succinylcholine, which is a depolarizing muscle relaxant. Depolarizing drugs cause a rise in serum potassium, which is usually well tolerated, but may be exaggerated in patients who are inactive or bed-ridden, paretic secondary to stroke or injury, or who have the suffered recent major burns. In these patients, a non-depolarizing muscle relaxant offers important advantages, since it does not cause a rise in serum potassium.[69] Cisatrocurium and rocuronium are the two shortest acting non-depolarizing agents currently available, but both have a duration of action of 10–20 minutes, which is several-fold longer than succinylcholine.

Short-acting IV β-blockers effectively reduce stress on the heart. These agents attenuate hypertension, tachycardia, ectopy, and cardiac ischemia, and with proper use they rarely result in hypotension or bradycardia. Esmolol (2–4 mg/kg) or labetalol (0.2–0.4 kg/mg) given IV immediately before the anesthetic induction is usually sufficient, but higher doses may be necessary in individual patients.[70] Esmolol has the advantage of being much shorter-acting than labetalol. Although theoretically these drugs may result in decompensa-

tion of CHF, this has not been reported in practice. Nitroglycerine (infused at 0.5 to 3.0 mg/kg/minute) may be used to blunt the hypertensive response of patients who are already receiving β-blockers or calcium channel blockers and who require additional antihypertensives. For patients refractory to these approaches, nitroprusside delivered by slow IV infusion is highly effective, but requires blood pressure monitoring with an intra-arterial line to avoid overshooting the blood pressure target.

Treating hypertension adequately before a course of ECT usually reduces the hypertensive response during the treatment itself. Maintenance β-blockers (such as atenolol 25–50 mg orally every day) may render the use of a short-acting antihypertensive during treatment unnecessary.

Conduction system abnormalities during treatment have been reported in 20% to 80% of ECT patients,[71] but such abnormalities are usually transient. Persistent or severe arrhythmias occasionally require treatment, and the approach depends on the type of arrhythmia. Supraventricular tachycardias generally are best treated with calcium channel blockers, whereas ventricular ectopy is most rapidly stabilized with IV lidocaine. Many arrhythmias can be prevented by pre-treatment with a short-acting IV β-blocker before subsequent treatments.

Decompensation of CHF is usually treatable with oxygen and with elevation of the head. Occasionally, IV furosemide and morphine become necessary, but this is extremely rare. Most patients re-compensate within 10 to 15 minutes of the treatment without aggressive intervention.

Cardiac arrest is a rare complication of ECT. The majority of patients have some degree of sinus pause after the ECT stimulus that may last up to eight seconds, and this may be mistaken for a true arrest.[35] Patients who receive non-convulsive stimuli may be especially at risk for extended sinus pauses. Because the intense parasympathetic outflow caused by the stimulus is not counteracted by the sympathetic outflow of the seizure itself, severe bradycardia or arrest may ensue. Immediately following the cessation of ictal activity, parasympathetic tone is predominant and bradycardia is common. However, a full cardiac arrest may also occur during the immediate post-ictal interval.

The relative efficacy of unilateral and bilateral electrode placement remains unclear, but for most patients, a unilateral stimulus, when performed under optimal conditions, is as effective as a bilateral stimulus.[72,73] Ineffective unilateral ECT is associated with use of threshold stimulus intensity.[74] Consequently, a unilateral stimulus should be well over threshold with the electrodes placed in the d'Elia position (Figure 45-3A and 45-3B). Recent studies report equal efficacy as long as unilateral ECT is performed with a stimulus intensity well above seizure threshold.[75] Bifrontal electrode placement has not been extensively studied, but evidence thus far indicates that it has equal effectiveness when compared to bitemporal and right unilateral electrode placement.[76,77]

Use of brief pulse waveform has become standard practice in the US (Figure 45-4). Brief pulse waveform is efficient at inducing seizure activity and is associated with little post-treatment confusion and amnesia.[78] Recently, modification of brief pulse waveform, by reducing pulse width and extending the stimulus duration, has resulted in a stimulus referred to as ultra-brief pulse.[79-81]

Generalization of the seizure to the entire brain is essential for efficacy.[82] The standard way to monitor seizure generalization is to inflate a blood pressure cuff on an arm or ankle above systolic pressure, just before injection of succinylcholine. The convulsion can then be observed in the unparalyzed extremity. In unilateral ECT, the cuff is placed on the limb ipsilateral to the stimulus. Most ECT instruments have a built-in single-channel electroencephalographic monitor, but this is not always a reliable indicator of full seizure generalization because partial seizures may also generate a typical seizure tracing.

Following ECT, patients should not be left in the supine position but should be turned on their side to allow better drainage of secretions. Patients should be monitored carefully by a recovery nurse; vital signs should be taken regularly and pulse oximetry employed. Some patients, typically young, healthy individuals, may develop an agitated delirium with a vacant stare, disorientation, and automatisms immediately

following treatment. This clinical picture is usually due to tardive seizures; it clears promptly with midazolam (2–5 mg IV), diazepam (5–10 mg IV) or propofol (20–40 mg IV). Post-treatment agitation may be preemptively treated with propofol 30–50 mg intravenously immediately after cessation of the seizure. Post-treatment nausea may be effectively treated with droperidol (1.25–2.5 mg IV), and prevented in subsequent treatments with pre-medication using ondansetron (4 mg IV).

The average number of ECT procedures necessary to treat major depression is consistently reported to be between 6 and 12 treatments, but occasional patients may require up to 30. The customary timing is three sessions per week with one full seizure per session. The use of more than one seizure per session (multiple monitored ECT) has no proven advantages. The most objective comparison of single and multiple ECT was performed by Fink,[83] who concluded, "Multiple ECT carried more risks and fewer benefits than conventional ECT for our patients."

ADVERSE EFFECTS OF ELECTROCONVULSIVE THERAPY

Survey data indicate a mortality rate of 0.03% in patients who undergo ECT.[84] Although there is no evidence for structural brain damage as a result of ECT,[85] there are important effects on cognition. Memory impairment varies greatly in severity and is associated with bilateral electrode placement, high stimulus intensity, inadequate oxygenation, prolonged seizure activity, advanced age, alcohol abuse, and lower premorbid cognitive function.[86] Difficulty recalling new information (anterograde amnesia) is usually experienced during the ECT series, but it normally resolves within a month after the last treatment. Difficulty remembering events before ECT (retrograde amnesia) is usually more severe for events closer to the time of treatment. Bilateral ECT causes more memory disturbance than does unilateral, and this is true for both retrograde and anterograde memory function and for both verbal and non-verbal recall.[87]

A meta-analysis of cognitive function testing in 2,981 patients in 84 studies[88] found significant decreases in cognitive performance scores 0 to 3 days after completion of a series of ECT. However, within 15 days of the last ECT treatment, almost all mean test scores were at or above pre-ECT levels. After 15 days, improvements compared to baseline were observed in processing speed, working memory, anterograde memory, and aspects of executive function.

Severe encephalopathy associated with ECT may require discontinuation of treatment. Usually, substantial improvement occurs within 48 hours after the last treatment. If symptoms become more severe with time after cessation of treatment, a full neurological work-up is indicated to assess whether there is an underlying cause other than ECT.

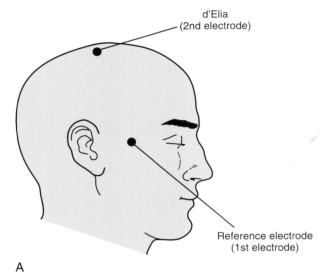
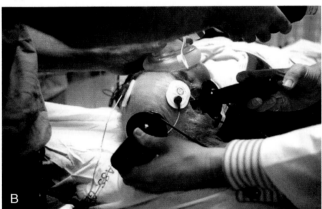

Figure 45-3. (A) Schematic of electrode placements during electroconvulsive therapy (ECT). (B) Photograph of electrodes being placed during ECT.

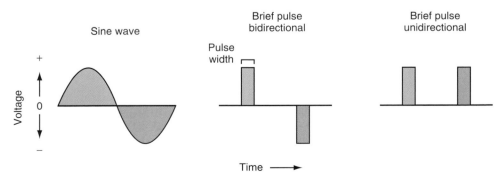

Figure 45-4. Schematic of sine wave and brief pulse stimuli for electroconvulsive therapy.

MAINTENANCE ELECTROCONVULSIVE THERAPY TREATMENT

Following successful treatment with ECT, without any continuation therapy the risk of depressive relapse is greater than 80% at 6 months.[89] Continuation therapy with nortriptyline plus lithium is associated with a relapse rate of about 50% at 6 months.[89-91] Continuation therapy with venlafaxine plus lithium is associated with a relapse rate of approximately 40% at 6 months.[91] In a recent comparison of pharmacotherapy alone versus ECT plus pharmacotherapy, relapse rates at 1 year were 61% with pharmacotherapy alone and 32% with pharmacotherapy plus maintenance ECT.[92] Continuation ECT alone (weekly for 4 weeks, biweekly for 8 weeks, and monthly for 3 months) lowers the relapse rate at 6 months to below 40%.[90] Large controlled trials of other antidepressant drugs after ECT have not yet been conducted. Although questions remain about the relative effectiveness of continuation ECT and continuation pharmacotherapy, the cumulative evidence over the last decade indicates that continuation ECT is a valuable and effective strategy for most patients.

ELECTROCONVULSIVE THERAPY IN CHILDREN

The first meta-analysis of published reports of ECT in children, published in 1997, reported response rates of 63% in depression, 80% in mania, 42% in schizophrenia, and 80% in catatonia.[93] In 2004, the American Academy of Child and Adolescent Psychiatry published its *Practice Parameter for Use of Electroconvulsive Therapy with Adolescents*,[94] in which it recognized the high effectiveness of ECT in children, set forth guidelines for safe administration of ECT in adolescents, and addressed the ethical and legal issues involved with ECT in this age group. Recent published reviews have addressed ECT for children with catatonia,[95] autism,[96] schizophrenia,[97] and maintenance ECT.[98] There is a rapidly growing body of evidence that ECT in children and adolescents is safe, effective, well tolerated, and long lasting.[99,100]

CONCLUSION

ECT continues to undergo reduction in side effects, improved effectiveness, more exact indications, and enhanced safety. Although the mechanism of action remains unknown, current research into these issues will ultimately produce important insights into the pathophysiology of mood disorders. In view of its unique effectiveness in patients unresponsive to other therapies, it is likely that the technique of ECT will continue to be refined, and its indications expanded. It is likely that ECT will not only be a cornerstone of psychiatric treatment for the foreseeable future but also an important window on the pathophysiology of mood disorders and psychosis.

Access a list of MCQs for this chapter at https://expertconsult.inkling.com

REFERENCES

1. Rush A. STAR*D: what have we learned? *Am J Psychiatry* 164:201–204, 2007.
2. Petrides G, Fink M, Husain MM, et al. ECT remission rates in psychotic versus non-psychotic depressed patients: a report from CORE. *J ECT* 17:244–253, 2001.
3. Koh KH, van Vreeswijk MA, Simpson S, et al. A meta-analysis of electroconvulsive therapy efficacy in depression. *J ECT* 19:139–147, 2003.
4. Angst F, Stassen HH, Clayton PJ, et al. Mortality of patients with mood disorders: follow-up over 34–38 years. *J Affect Disorders* 68:167–181, 2002.
5. Murray CJL, Lopez AD. Alternative projections of mortality and disability by cause 1990–2020: Global Burden of Disease Study. *Lancet* 349:1498–1504, 1997.
6. Carney MWP, Roth M, Garside RF. The diagnosis of depressive syndromes and the prediction of ECT response. *Br J Psychiatry* 3:659–674, 1965.
7. Swartz CM, editor: *Electroconvulsive and neuromodulation therapies*, Cambridge, 2009, Cambridge University Press.
8. Souery D, Papakostas GI, Trivedi MH. Treatment-resistant depression. *J Clin Psychiatry* 67(Suppl. 6):16–26, 2006.
9. Sackeim HA. The definition and meaning of treatment-resistant depression. *J Clin Psychiatry* 62(Suppl. 16):10–17, 2001.
10. Kellner CH, Fink M, Knapp R, et al. Relief of expressed suicidal intent by ECT: a consortium for research in ECT study. *Am J Psychiatry* 162:977–982, 2005.
11. Patel M, Patel S, Hardy DW, et al. Should electroconvulsive therapy be an early consideration for suicidal patients? *J ECT* 22:113–115, 2006.
12. Feske U, Mulsant BH, Pilkonis PA, et al. Clinical outcome of ECT inpatients with major depression and comorbid borderline personality disorder. *Am J Psychiatry* 161:2073–2080, 2004.
13. Dombrovski AY, Mulsant BH, Haskett RF, et al. Predictors of remission after electroconvulsive therapy in unipolar major depression. *J Clin Psychiatry* 66:1043–1049, 2005.
14. Braga RJ, Petrides G. The combined use of electroconvulsive therapy and antipsychotics in patients with schizophrenia. *J ECT* 21:75–83, 2005.
15. Painuly N, Chakrabarti S. Combined use of electroconvulsive therapy and antipsychotics in schizophrenia: the Indian evidence. A review and meta analysis. *J ECT* 22:59–66, 2006.
16. Fink M, Sackeim HA. Convulsive therapy in schizophrenia? *Schizophr Bull* 22:27–39, 1996.
17. Ucok A, Cakir S. Electroconvulsive therapy in the first-episode schizophrenia. *J ECT* 22:22–38, 2006.
18. Suzuki K, Atawa S, Takano T, et al. Improvement of psychiatric symptoms after electroconvulsive therapy in young adults with intractable first episode schizophrenia and schizophreniform disorder. *Tohoku J Exp Med* 210:213–220, 2006.
19. Dierckx B, Heijnen WT, van den Broek WW, et al. Efficacy of electroconvulsive therapy in bipolar versus unipolar major depression: a meta-analysis. *Bipolar Disord* 14:146–150, 2012.
20. Mukherjee S, Sackeim HA, Schnur DB. Electroconvulsive therapy of acute manic episodes: a review of 50 years experience. *Am J Psychiatry* 151:169–176, 1994.
21. Mukherjee S, Sackeim HA, Lee C. Unilateral ECT in the treatment of manic episodes. *Convuls Ther* 4:74–80, 1988.
22. Devanand DP, Polanco P, Cruz R, et al. The efficacy of ECT in mixed affective states. *J ECT* 16:32–37, 2000.
23. Kutcher S, Robertson HA. Electroconvulsive therapy in treatment-resistant bipolar youth. *J Child Adolesc Psychopharmacol* 5:167–175, 1995.
24. Wheeler Vega JA, Mortimer AM, Tyson PJ. Somatic treatment of psychotic depression: review and recommendations for practice. *J Clin Psychopharmacol* 20:504–519, 2000.
25. Kroessler D. Relative efficacy rates for therapies of delusional depression. *Convuls Ther* 1:173–182, 1985.
26. Janicak PG, Easton M, Comaty JE, et al. Efficacy of ECT in psychotic and nonpsychotic depression. *Convuls Ther* 5:314–320, 1989.
27. Spiker DG, Stein J, Rich CL. Delusional depression and electroconvulsive therapy: one year later. *Convuls Ther* 1:167–172, 1985.
28. Mann SC, Caroff SN, Bleier HR, et al. Lethal catatonia. *Am J Psychiatry* 143:1374–1381, 1986.
29. Mann SC, Caroff SN, Bleier HR, et al. Electroconvulsive therapy of the lethal catatonia syndrome. *Convuls Ther* 6:239–247, 1990.
30. Rohland BM, Carroll BT, Jacoby RG. ECT in the treatment of the catatonic syndrome. *J Affect Disord* 29:255–261, 1993.
31. Fink M. Is catatonia a primary indication for ECT? *Convuls Ther* 6:1–4, 1990.
32. Rosebush PI, Hildebrand AM, Furlong BG, et al. Catatonic syndrome in a general psychiatric inpatient population: frequency, clinical presentation, and response to lorazepam. *J Clin Psychiatry* 51:357–362, 1990.
33. Fink M. Neuroleptic malignant syndrome and catatonia: one entity or two? *Biol Psychiatry* 39:1–4, 1996.

34. Davis JM, Janicak PG, Sakkas P, et al. Electroconvulsive therapy in the treatment of the neuroleptic malignant syndrome. *Convuls Ther* 7:111–120, 1991.

35. Welch CA, Drop LJ. Cardiovascular effects of ECT. *Convuls Ther* 5:35–43, 1989.

36. Khan A, Nies A, Johnson G, et al. Plasma catecholamines and ECT. *Biol Psychiatry* 20:799–804, 1985.

37. Liston EH, Salk JD. Hemodynamic responses to ECT after bilateral adrenalectomy. *Convuls Ther* 6:160–164, 1990.

38. Goldman L. Multifactorial index of cardiac risk of non-cardiac surgical procedures. *N Engl J Med* 297:845–850, 1977.

39. Drop JD, Welch CA. Anesthesia for electroconvulsive therapy in patients with major cardiovascular risk factors. *Convuls Ther* 5:88–101, 1989.

40. Drop LJ, Bouckoms AJ, Welch CA. Arterial hypertension and multiple cerebral aneurysms in a patient treated with electroconvulsive therapy. *J Clin Psychiatry* 49:280–282, 1988.

41. Viguera A, Rordorf G, Schouten R, et al. Intracranial hemodynamics during attenuated responses to electroconvulsive therapy in the presence of an intracerebral aneurysm. *J Neurol Neurosurg Psychiatry* 64:802–805, 1998.

42. Dolenc TJ, Barnes RD, Hayes DL. Electroconvulsive therapy in patients with cardiac pacemakers and implantable cardioverter defibrillators. *Pace* 27:1257–1263, 2004.

43. Hsiao JK, Messenheimer JA, Evans DL. ECT and neurological disorders. *Convuls Ther* 3:121–136, 1987.

44. Maltbie AA, Wingfield MS, Volow MR, et al. Electroconvulsive therapy in the presence of brain tumor: case reports and an evaluation of risk. *J Nerv Ment Dis* 168:400–405, 1980.

45. Fried D, Mann JJ. Electroconvulsive treatment of a patient with known intracranial tumor. *Biol Psychiatry* 23:176–180, 1988.

46. Malek-Ahmadi P, Beceiro JR, McNeil BW, et al. Electroconvulsive therapy and chronic subdural hematoma. *Convuls Ther* 6:38–41, 1990.

47. Zwil AS, Bowring MA, Price TRP, et al. Prospective electroconvulsive therapy in the presence of intracranial tumor. *Convuls Ther* 6:299–307, 1990.

48. Patkar AA, Hill KP, Weinstein SP, et al. ECT in the presence of brain tumor and increased intracranial pressure: evaluation and reduction of risk. *J ECT* 16:187–189, 2000.

49. Currier MB, Murray GB, Welch CA. Electroconvulsive therapy for post-stroke depressed geriatric patients. *J Neuropsychiatry Clin Neurosci* 4:140–144, 1992.

50. Fink M. ECT for Parkinson's disease? *Convuls Ther* 4:189–191, 1988.

51. Steif BL, Sackeim HA, Portnoy S, et al. Effects of depression and ECT on anterograde memory. *Biol Psychiatry* 21:921–930, 1986.

52. Nelson JP, Rosenberg DR. ECT treatment of demented elderly patients with major depression: a retrospective study of efficacy and safety. *Convuls Ther* 7:157–165, 1991.

53. Ferrill MJ, Kehoe WA, Jacisin JJ. ECT during pregnancy: physiologic and pharmacologic considerations. *Convuls Ther* 8:186–200, 1992.

54. Austin MP, Mitchell K, Wilhelm G, et al. Cognitive function in depression: a distinct pattern of frontal impairment in melancholia? *Psychol Med* 29:73–85, 1999.

55. Austin MP, Mitchell P, Goodwin GM. Cognitive deficits in depression: possible implications for functional neuropathology. *Br J Psychiatry* 178:200–206, 2001.

56. Baghi TC, Marcuse A, Brosch M, et al. The influence of concomitant antidepressant medication on safety, tolerability, and clinical effectiveness of electroconvulsive therapy. *World J Biol Psychiatry* 7:82–90, 2006.

57. Dolenc TJ, Habl SS, Barnes RD, et al. Electroconvulsive therapy in patients taking monoamine oxidase inhibitors. *J ECT* 20:258–261, 2004.

58. Dolenc TJ, Rasmussen KG. The safety of electroconvulsive therapy and lithium in combination. A case series and review of the literature. *J ECT* 21:165–170, 2005.

59. Greenberg RM, Pettinati HM. Benzodiazepines and electroconvulsive therapy. *Convuls Ther* 9:262–273, 1993.

60. Penland HR, Ostroff RB. Combined use of lamotrigine and electroconvulsive therapy in bipolar depression: a case series. *J ECT* 22:142–147, 2006.

61. Lunde ME, Lee EK, Rasmussen KG. Electroconvulsive therapy in patients with epilepsy. *Epilepsy & Behavior* 9:355–359, 2006.

62. Ding Z, White PF. Anesthesia for electroconvulsive therapy. *Anesth Analg* 94:1351–1364, 2002.

63. Bouckoms AJ, Welch CA, Drop LJ, et al. Atropine in electroconvulsive therapy. *Convuls Ther* 5:48–55, 1989.

64. Avramov MN, Husain MM, White PF. The comparative effects of methohexital, propofol, and etomidate for electroconvulsive therapy. *Anesth Analg* 81:596–602, 1995.

65. Vaidya P, Anderson E, Bobb A, et al. A within-subject comparison of propofol and methohexital anesthesia for electroconvulsive therapy. *J ECT* 28(1):14–19, 2010.

66. Khalid N, Atkins M, Kirov G. The effects of etomidate on seizure duration and electrical stimulus dose in seizure-resistant patients during electroconvulsive therapy. *J ECT* 22:184–188, 2006.

67. McDaniel WW, Sahota AK, Vyas BV, et al. Ketamine appears associated with better word recall than etomidate after a course of 6 electroconvulsive therapies. *J ECT* 22:103–106, 2006.

68. Rasmussen KG, Spackman TN, Hooten MW. The clinical utility of inhalational anesthesia with sevoflurane in electroconvulsive therapy. *J ECT* 21:239–242, 2005.

69. Mirzakhani H, Welch C, Eikermann M, et al. Neuromuscular blocking agents for electroconvulsive therapy: a systematic review. *Acta Anaesthesiol Scand* 56(1):3–16, 2012.

70. Castelli I, Steiner A, Kaufmann MA, et al. Comparative effects of esmolol and labetolol to attenuate hyperdynamic states after electroconvulsive therapy. *Anesth Analg* 80:557–561, 1995.

71. Gerring JP, Shields HM. The identification and management of patients with a high risk for cardiac arrhythmias during modified ECT. *J Clin Psychiatry* 43:140–143, 1982.

72. Ottoson JO. Is unilateral nondominant ECT as efficient as bilateral ECT? A new look at the evidence. *Convuls Ther* 7:190–200, 1991.

73. Sackeim HA, Prudic J, Devanand DP, et al. A prospective, randomized, double-blind comparison of bilateral and right unilateral electroconvulsive therapy at different stimulus intensities. *Arch Gen Psychiatry* 57:425–434, 2000.

74. Sackeim H, Decina P, Prohovnik I, et al. Seizure threshold in electroconvulsive therapy: effects of sex, age, electrode placement, and number of treatments. *Arch Gen Psychiatry* 44:355–360, 1987.

75. McCall WV, Dunn BA, Rosenquist PB, et al. Markedly suprathreshold right unilateral ECT versus minimally suprathreshold bilateral ECT: antidepressant and memory affects. *J ECT* 18:126–129, 2002.

76. Delva NJ, Brunet D, Hawken ER, et al. Electrical dose and seizure threshold: relations to clinical outcome and cognitive effects in bifrontal, bitemporal, and right unilateral ECT. *J ECT* 16:361–369, 2000.

77. Rankesh F, Barekatian M, Kuchakian S. Bifrontal versus right unilateral and bitemporal electroconvulsive therapy in major depressive disorder. *J ECT* 21:207–210, 2005.

78. Squire LR, Zouzounis JA. ECT and memory: brief pulse versus sine wave. *Am J Psychiatry* 143:596, 1986.

79. Sackeim H, Prudic J, Nobler M, et al. Effects of pulse width and electrode placement on the efficacy and cognitive effects of electroconvulsive therapy. *Brain Stimul* 1:71–83, 2008.

80. Sienaert P, Vansteelandt K, Demyttenaere K, et al. Absence of cognitive side effects after ultrabrief electroconvulsive therapy. *J ECT* 24:44–49, 2008.

81. Loo C, Sheehan P, Pigot M, et al. A comparison of right unilateral ultra-brief pulse (0.3ms) ECT and standard right unilateral ECT. *J ECT* 24:51–55, 2008.

82. Ottoson JO. Experimental studies on the mode of action of electroconvulsive therapy. *Acta Psychiatr Neural Scand* 35(Suppl. 145):1–141, 1960.

83. Fink M. *Convulsive therapy: theory and practice*, New York, 1979, Raven Press.

84. Kramer B. Use of ECT in California, 1977–1983. *Am J Psychiatry* 142:1190–1192, 1985.

85. Devanand DP, Dwork AJ, Hutchinson ER, et al. Does ECT alter brain structure? *Am J Psychiatry* 151:957–970, 1994.

86. Sackeim HA, Prudic J, Fuller R. The cognitive effects of electroconvulsive therapy in community settings. *Neuropsychopharmacology* 32:244–254, 2007.

87. Daniel WF, Crovitz HP. Acute memory impairment following electroconvulsive therapy: 2. effects of electrode placement. *Acta Psychiatr Scand* 67:57–68, 1983.

statistically significant efficacy on the primary outcome measure, the Hamilton Depression Rating Scale (a clinician-administered scale). However, the VNS group did demonstrate statistically significant greater improvement on a secondary outcome measure, the Inventory of Depressive Symptomatology—Self-Report (a self-report scale). After the acute 8-week trial, patients in both groups (with a total of 205 patients) went on to receive open active adjunctive treatment (continuing treatment-as-usual) with VNS therapy for 1 year in the second clinical trial.[46] At the 1-year follow-up, 27.2% of patients receiving adjunctive VNS responded and 15.8% met criteria for remission. In addition, the rates of response and remission doubled from 3 months to 12 months, suggesting that longer-term treatment may be required with VNS. The third clinical trial compared the patients receiving adjunctive VNS therapy during the 1-year follow-up study to a matched group of 124 treatment-refractory MDD patients who received only treatment-as-usual.[47] Response rates between VNS plus treatment-as-usual (19.6%) versus treatment-as-usual only (12.1%) were not statistically significant. However, there was a statistically significant difference between remission rates with VNS therapy plus treatment-as-usual (13.2%) and treatment-as-usual alone (3.2%). Last, this study found that one-half of VNS plus treatment-as-usual responders at 3 months remained responders at 12 months, while only one treatment-as-usual only responder at 3 months remained a responder at 12 months.

Adjustment of the stimulation parameters is performed by using a device that communicates transcutaneously with the IPG. The dose parameters used by the clinician for VNS therapy include the magnitude of the electrical charge delivered to the left vagus nerve, the stimulation frequency, the stimulation pulse width, and the duration of stimulation. Settings used in the clinical trials submitted to the FDA for approval of the device for TRD included a median output of 0.75 mA (range 0 to 1.5 mA), a median signal frequency of 20 Hz, a median pulse width of 500 μS, a median on-time of 30 seconds, and a median off-time of 5 minutes.[45] In practice, many clinicians use higher-output currents; it should be noted that higher-output currents of 3 mA are routinely used in patients with treatment-resistant epilepsy. In patients who are not responding to VNS, many clinicians will increase the charge duty cycle. As described above, a 10% duty cycle (30 seconds on, 5 minutes off) was used in the clinical trials submitted for FDA approval. However, decreasing the off-time to 2 or 3 minutes or increasing the on-time to 60 seconds (or both) can increase the duty cycle to as high as 50%. Duty cycles higher than 50% should not be used, as animal studies suggest potential vagus nerve damage at duty cycles higher than 50%. Finally, decreasing the stimulation pulse width or stimulation frequency is often helpful for addressing potential side effects associated with VNS therapy.

Potential risks associated with VNS include standard risks associated with the surgical procedure itself. Most common side effects associated with active VNS therapy are likely due to the fact that the electrodes are attached to the left vagus nerve near the laryngeal and pharyngeal branches of the left vagus nerve. The most common side effect is voice alteration (seen in 54% to 60% of patients). Other side effects include cough, neck pain, paresthesias and dyspnea.[46] These side effects typically decrease or dissipate over time. Strategies such as decreasing the stimulation frequency or pulse width are often helpful for reducing these side effects as well. Despite these side effects, the device is well tolerated, with only seven patients withdrawing from the clinical trial due to adverse events. Patients also have the ability to turn off the device at any time by placing a magnet provided by the manufacturer over the IPG. The IPG will remain off (i.e., no stimulation will occur) as long as the magnet is in place. When the magnet is removed, the IPG returns to its previously set stimulation parameters.

In summary, the clinical trial data suggest that VNS plus treatment-as-usual is more efficacious than treatment-as-usual alone. In addition, the side effects are typically tolerable as demonstrated by the fact that only 7 of 205 patients in the 1-year clinical trial discontinued the trial due to adverse events. It is important to note that the FDA-approval language states that VNS is an adjunctive treatment for TRD and that it should be used in patients with severe, chronic, recurrent TRD who have failed at least four adequate antidepressant trials.

ELECTROCONVULSIVE THERAPY

Electroconvulsive therapy (ECT) is discussed in detail elsewhere in this volume (see Chapter 45). ECT has been used to treat depression since the 1930s, and many consider it the "gold standard" of antidepressant treatment. ECT involves delivery of an electrical current to the brain through the scalp and skull in order to induce a generalized seizure. While the mechanism by which generalized seizures alleviate depressive symptoms is not fully understood, the efficacy of ECT for depression has been demonstrated in a large number of clinical trials. A recent meta-analysis that included most of these clinical trials found that active ECT was significantly more effective than sham ECT and more effective than pharmacotherapy.[48] However, many patients relapse unless they receive periodic maintenance treatments; there are common side effects, such as memory loss, that are associated with ECT.[49]

TRANSCRANIAL MAGNETIC STIMULATION

Transcranial magnetic stimulation (TMS) is a non-invasive neuromodulation modality that uses powerful and rapidly changing magnetic fields applied over the surface of the skull to generate targeted electrical currents in the brain, painlessly and without the need for surgery, anesthesia, or the induction of seizures. Since its development in the mid-1980s; it has become a widely used tool for neuroscience research and clinical applications (diagnostic and therapeutic). In 2008, the FDA approved the use of high-frequency repetitive TMS (rTMS) over the left dorsolateral prefrontal cortex (DLPFC) for the treatment of MDD, and in 2013 the use of deep TMS H-coils for the treatment of MDD was also approved.

One of the primary advantages of TMS is its non-invasive nature, which is made possible by the application of Faraday's principle of electromagnetic induction. Briefly (and overly simplified), this principle states that a changing electrical current flowing through a circular coil will generate a magnetic field tangential to the plane of the coil. If this magnetic field comes in contact with another conductive material (e.g., a pick-up coil) it will generate a secondary electrical current (Figure 46-3A). TMS systems use an electrical capacitor to generate a brief powerful current that flows through the TMS coil, which is a circular loop of wire (usually copper) connected to the capacitor and embedded in a protective plastic case. According to Faraday's principle, when the electrical current flows through the circular coil, a rapidly changing magnetic field is generated. If the TMS coil is placed on the surface of the skull, this magnetic field will travel towards the intra-cranial space unaltered by the different structures it will cross (e.g., soft tissue, bone, CSF), until it reaches the electrically conductive neurons of the cortex. These neurons will act as an organic pick-up coil, and a secondary electrical current will be generated able to trigger action potentials and force brain cells to fire (Figure 46-3B). It is important to note that the stimulation of neurons is actually electrical, not magnetic,

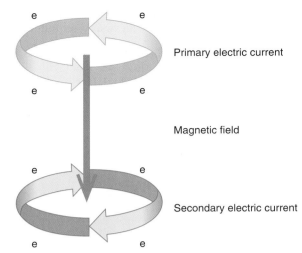

Primary electric current

Magnetic field

Secondary electric current

Figure 46-3. (A) This schematic illustrates the principle of electromagnetic induction, by which a primary electrical current generates a perpendicular magnetic field that, when in contact with a conductive material, leads to a secondary electrical current in the same plane, but opposite sense than the primary. (B) This drawing shows how this principle of physics is applied in TMS, placing a coil on the scalp surface leading to electrical stimulation of the cortex. *(Redrawn from Jalinous R. A guide to magnetic stimulation, Whitland, Carmarthenshire, Wales, UK, 1998, Magstim Company Ltd.)*

and the term "magnetic stimulation" is a misnomer. Magnetic pulses are used only as a vehicle to non-invasively transfer the electrical currents from the coil to the cortex. This avoids the need for surgical access to the intra-cranial space or the painful application of strong electrical currents on the skull.

Another important technical fact to take into account relates to the depth of TMS modulation. Although the magnetic field is practically unaltered by the various structures it finds on its path to the cortex, the strength of the field weakens as it moves away from its source in the TMS coil. As a result, the 1 to 2 Tesla magnetic pulse originated in the coil becomes too weak to generate neuronal action potentials 2–4 cm away from its origin on the surface of the skull. This sets a practical limitation to this technique, as only superficial cortical structures can be directly stimulated by TMS. Nevertheless, the effects of TMS are not only local but circuit-wide; once an action potential is generated in a cortical neuron, the volley of activation will travel through its axon and stimulate the post-synaptic neuron, leading to a cascade of events through the entire neural circuit (including deep cortical, sub-cortical and contralateral regions). This cascade of electrical events is specific to the brain circuit our target region is connected to, and not generalized like the effects of ECT. Therefore, although it is true that TMS can only directly modulate superficial cortical nodes, these nodes act as windows that provide modulatory access to an entire functional network of cortical and sub-cortical neurons.[50]

The effects of TMS are not only specific to the target of stimulation but also to the parameters used. This is important as we consider statements such as "TMS is (or is not) effective for a given condition", which lack meaning and are not informative. Alternatively, "TMS applied over a determined anatomical target at a specific frequency and dose for a particular condition" would be more clinically and neuroscientifically meaningful. Since the effects of TMS are specific to the stimulated region and the parameters used, we could certainly expect that stimulating prefrontal cortical areas that process

---

BOX 46-1 Transcranial Magnetic Stimulation Parameters

ANATOMICAL
1. Location (can be optimized with neuroimaging and neuronavigation).
2. Focality (depends primarily on coil architecture, also on intensity).
3. Depth (also depends primarily on coil architecture and partially on intensity).

PHYSIOLOGICAL
1. Frequency (can facilitate or inhibit a target region).
2. Intensity of stimulation (usually expressed as a percentage of the motor threshold).
3. Number of pulses per session (will also determine the duration of the session).
4. Number of sessions (treatment protocols require multiple sessions over weeks).

---

working memory or spatial attention would have little effect on mood, anhedonia, or neurovegetative symptoms of depression. Similarly, inhibiting a pathologically hypoactive region will most likely worsen a patient's condition, though its activation may prove therapeutic. Last, applying 2 weeks of stimulation when 6 or more weeks are needed should have minimal or no therapeutic impact. This highlights the need to have a basic understanding of the TMS parameters that clinicians and scientists are able to manipulate: the location or target of stimulation, the focality and depth, the frequency, and the dose of stimulation (which is a composite measure of stimulation intensity and duration) (Box 46-1). As mentioned above, the choice of the anatomical site of stimulation is crucial, as this will grant us access to modulate a specific functional network of interest. Recent developments in image-guided TMS using neuro-navigation have proved to increase the anatomical specificity and clinical efficacy of TMS,[51,52] but although this approach is common in cognitive neuroscience research it is still rare in clinical practice. Similarly, the focality of stimulation will be of relevance as the clinical impact and specificity won't be the same if one modulates a cortical area of 0.25 or 1 cm². Although the intensity of stimulation has an influence on the focality of its effects (the stronger the magnetic field, the deeper and less focal its effects),[53] focality is primarily controlled by the choice of TMS coil. Various types of coils are manufactured with differences in their internal architecture that allow varying degrees of focality and depth.[54] The most common types remain the circular coil (less focal) and the figure-of-eight or butterfly coil (more focal).[54,55] A new generation of deep TMS coils, such as the H-coil, have been developed in recent years and received FDA approval for the treatment of MDD in 2013.[56] Once these anatomical parameters are determined (location, focality, and depth), it is important to focus on physiological variables. Notably, TMS is able to either inhibit (down-regulate) or activate (up-regulate) populations of neurons, and these selective effects are primarily determined by the frequency of stimulation. With parameters similar to the ones leading to long-term depression (LTD) or long-term potentiation (LTP), low frequencies of 1 Hz are known to be inhibitory[57] while high frequencies of > 5 Hz (typically 10 or 20 Hz) are activating.[58] Newer TMS protocols with more complex patterns of stimulation (such as theta burst stimulation or TBS) have been developed in recent years.[59] Although the use of TBS in therapeutic settings has not been thoroughly tested, it is likely to have significant impact given its longer-lasting behavioral effects despite a significantly shorter stimulation time (a traditional therapeutic protocol for MDD lasts 37.5 minutes, while TBS can performed in 40 seconds). Once the target of stimulation and direction of modulation are set, the dose will be determined by deciding the strength of the magnetic field (pulse intensity) and the total number of pulses (duration). Duration also relates to the total number of sessions; typically, daily sessions over the course of weeks. Other more complex variables, such as the waveform of the electromagnetic current, are also relevant to define the dose.[60] As we improve our understanding of the mechanism of action of TMS, the parameter space available becomes more complex and rich, granting greater control and specificity to clinicians and scientists.[61]

The safety profile of TMS is notoriously benign, given its non-invasive nature. Nevertheless, it is an intervention and attention to safety and iatrogenic effects are important. The only contraindication considered to be absolute is the presence of metallic hardware in the area of stimulation, such as cochlear implants, brain stimulators, or medication pumps.[61] Still, the use of TMS on patients with DBS has been tested and considered relatively safe when the DBS system is off, although data are still very limited and extreme caution (in addition to an accurate risk/benefit analysis) should be used in these cases.[62] The primary safety concern with TMS remains the induction of seizures with repetitive trains, even if this is a very rare phenomenon; approximately 20 seizures have been reported out of the estimated 300,000 sessions (clinical or research) since its development in the early 1980s.[61] Since the 2008 FDA approval of the NeuroStar TMS Therapy® system (Neuronetics, Inc.), seven seizures have been reported in the USA from 250,000 treatment sessions in 8,000 patients.[63] This represents 1 case in 35,000 patients, which is similar or fewer than the seizure risk of most antidepressant medications. It should be noted that TMS may trigger a seizure but not cause epilepsy; seizures are always during (not after) rTMS, and do not lead to spontaneous events afterwards. Nevertheless, one should screen patients for a personal history of epilepsy and possible risk factors that increase their seizure risk (such as brain lesions or medications that lower the seizure threshold). Other less severe but more common side effects include headaches, local discomfort in the area of stimulation, facial twitching, tinnitus, anxiety, and vasovagal syncope.[61]

TMS is routinely used for diagnostic applications, primarily in clinical neurophysiology.[64] Therapeutic applications for various neurological and psychiatric conditions have been investigated since the development of repetitive TMS. In this chapter we will focus on therapeutic studies for MDD, since it is the most widely used indication and the only one with FDA approval in the US (although in other countries TMS is approved for other neuropsychiatric indications as well). The evidence for the use of high-frequency rTMS to the left DLPFC or low-frequency rTMS to the right DLPFC is supported by multiple clinical studies including over 2,000 patients and summarized in more than 10 meta-analyses and critical reviews.[65–78] Although conclusions from these analyses confirm the clinical efficacy of TMS, early trials used highly heterogeneous study designs and stimulation parameters, which in retrospect were often sub-therapeutic (e.g., only 2 weeks of stimulation or less than 1,000 pulses per session). This is to be expected in the early phases of any treatment development because the limits of safety are not well defined, but it was particular in TMS as most seizures occurred in the initial years, increasing the caution of researchers in the field. As a result, meta-analyses that included early studies were often burdened with excessive variability that compromised the capacity to extract clinically meaningful conclusions. Indeed, Gross and colleagues compared the efficacy of clinical trials published in 2007 against all previously published studies, and demonstrated the therapeutic superiority of recent studies.[69] Naturally, as the field developed, the use of more effective protocols became more consistent, and larger studies with more appropriate parameters were conducted.

In 2007, O'Reardon and colleagues published the first large multi-center, randomized clinical trial (RCT).[79] This trial was industry-sponsored and its data led to the FDA approval of the Neurostar TMS Therapy ® system (Neuronetics Inc.). Similarly, large RCTs, initiated by academic researchers and sponsored by the National Institutes of Health, have subsequently been conducted with similar results.[80] The Neurostar TMS trial conducted by O'Reardon and colleagues,[79] enrolled 325 patients with moderate to severe MDD who had failed at least one, but no more than four antidepressant treatments in the current episode. Patients started with a 1-week washout period in which medications were discontinued, as the study aimed to determine the effects of TMS monotherapy. Sessions occurred Monday to Friday over the course of 6 weeks, and were followed by a 3-week taper period. The parameters of stimulation were 10 Hz rTMS over the left DLPFC at 120% of the motor threshold, using 3,000 pulses per session. The left DLPFC was identified as the point 5 cm anterior to the primary motor cortex (where the motor threshold was calculated). Using this TMS regimen, which was much more aggressive than previously tested parameters, they proved this intervention to be very safe, not causing any seizures and only minimum-risk side effects, such as discomfort under the site of stimulation or headaches. Most importantly, TMS proved to be an effective antidepressant with response rates of 23.9%–24.5% (compared to 12.3%–15.1% for placebo) and remission rates of 14.2%–17.4% (compared to 5.5%–8.2% for placebo) after 6 weeks of treatment. It is significant to note that remission rates doubled from week 4 to week 6, with outcomes continued to improve during the taper phase, with response rates increasing from 23.9% to 27.7% and remission rates from 14.2% to 20.6% using the primary outcome (Montgomery-Asberg Depression Rating Scale or MADRS).

From a safety perspective, these data demonstrated how conservative TMS protocols in previous studies had been, as the upper limit of tolerable risks seems to be far even from this more aggressive regimen. In terms of efficacy, these results provided robust evidence for the dose-dependent antidepressant effects of TMS, as stimulation over weeks 4, 6, and the taper period continued to improve response and remission rates, and further separated active from placebo arms.

While RCTs are imperative to prove the efficacy of any treatment compared to placebo in a very controlled manner, the generalizability of these studies is usually limited by their strict inclusion and exclusion criteria that do not reflect the prototypical patient in standard clinical settings (e.g., suffering from multiple medical and psychiatric co-morbidities, undergoing concomitant treatments). This is why naturalistic effectiveness studies are needed to complement RCTs. Carpenter and colleagues[81] conducted a multi-site open label naturalistic trial in which they enrolled 339 patients who, on average, were more refractory, had a longer duration for the current episode and presented with more complex co-morbidities than the cohort in the Neurostar TMS trial[79]; i.e., they were sicker and more representative of the average patient. All participants were naïve to TMS but were allowed to continue with their ongoing pharmacological and psychotherapeutic treatments in addition to TMS. They received the same TMS protocol as reported by O'Reardon, consisting of 6 weeks of daily left prefrontal 10Hz TMS.[79] After 6 weeks of treatment, response rate for the primary outcome (Clinical Global Impressions—Severity or CGI-S) was 58% and remission rate 37.1%. Secondary outcome measures showed a range of response and remission rates of 41.5%–58% and 26.5%–37.1%, respectively. Age and severity of the current episode were negative predictors of response, but unlike patient in the Neurostar TMS trial, the number of previously failed medication trials did not negatively predict therapeutic response, as both mild and severely refractory patients presented with very similar outcomes. Other naturalistic studies have reported similar results.[82] These studies present effectiveness data in less controlled but more realistic settings, which better describe the outcomes expected for patients treated in clinics and hospitals with current standard protocols.

As TMS has entered clinical practice with more homogeneous protocols leading to greater effects sizes and decreased variability, researchers have explored what variables may predict the antidepressant response of TMS. Fregni and colleagues analyzed the pooled data for 195 patients from six independent studies.[83] They reported that age and the number of previously failed medication trials were negative predictors of response, i.e., younger and less refractory patients had better outcomes. Lisanby and colleagues analyzed the data from the Neurostar TMS trial and also identified the number of previously failed trials as a predictor of poor response, in addition to the duration of the current episode and the presence of co-morbid anxiety.[84] Interestingly, these clinical variables are not specific to TMS, but they seem to predict antidepressant response across treatment modalities including pharmacological and psychotherapeutic interventions. As the field moves towards identifying not only clinical or demographic variables but also biological markers that predict response to treatment, the hope is that the biomarkers linked to the therapeutics targets specifically modulated by the different treatment modalities will help stratify patients and individually select the most effective treatments.[85]

In summary, TMS is a powerful research and clinical tool with FDA approval for diagnostic applications in clinical neurophysiology and antidepressant therapy in the USA, although therapeutic indications are wider in other countries. Its non-invasive nature and benign safety profile, added to its proven antidepressant efficacy, have contributed to its introduction in community and academic clinics as standard of care. Future developments should advance our understanding of the efficacy of different parameters and present new stimulation protocols that expand the indications to other disorders and increase the cost-effectiveness of this consolidated treatment.

CONCLUSION

In this chapter, we have provided an overview of neurotherapeutic interventions for psychiatric disorders that are currently available or are being studied in clinical trials. Some of these treatments have been available for many years (e.g., ECT and ablative limbic system surgery), some (such as VNS, DBS or TMS) have only recently been approved by the FDA for psychiatric indications. Systems neuroscience and translational neuropsychiatry research are in the path to expand our therapeutic armamentarium even further with new indications and protocols for these treatments and novel technologies. These innovations will change how we practice, maximizing safety and efficacy and allowing us to individualize treatment decisions in the near future.

Access the complete reference list and multiple choice questions (MCQs) online at https://expertconsult.inkling.com

KEY REFERENCES

5. Dalgleish T, Yiend J, Bramham J, et al. Neuropsychological processing associated with recovery from depression after stereotactic subcaudate tetractomy. *Am J Psychiatry* 161:1913–1916, 2004.
6. Dougherty DD, Baer L, Cosgrove GR, et al. Prospective long-term follow-up of 44 patients who received cingulotomy for treatment-refractory obsessive-compulsive disorder. *Am J Psychiatry* 159:269–275, 2002.
11. Hardesty DE, Sackeim HA. Deep brain stimulation in movement and psychiatric disorders. *Biol Psychiatry* 61(7):831–835, 2007.
14. Corse D, Chou T, Arulpragasam AR, et al. Deep brain stimulation for obsessive-compulsive disorder. *Psychiatr Ann* 43(8):351–357, 2013.
26. Malone DA Jr, Dougherty DD, Rezai AR, et al. Deep brain stimulation of the ventral capsule/ventral striatum for treatment-resistant depression. *Biol Psychiatry* 65(4):267–275, 2009.
28. Mayberg HS, Lozano AM, Voon V, et al. Deep brain stimulation for treatment-resistant depression. *Neuron* 45(5):651–660, 2005.
29. Lozano AM, Mayberg HS, Giacobbe P, et al. Subcallosal cingulate gyrus deep brain stimulation for treatment-resistant depression. *Biol Psychiatry* 64(6):461–467, 2008.
31. Holtzheimer PE, Kelley ME, Gross RE, et al. Subcallosal cingulate deep brain stimulation for treatment-resistant unipolar and bipolar depression. *Arch Gen Psychiatry* 69(2):150–158, 2012.
32. Schlaepfer TE, Cohen MX, Frick C, et al. Deep brain stimulation to reward circuitry alleviates anhedonia in refractory major depression. *Neuropsychopharmacology* 33(2):368–377, 2008.
34. Kaur N, Chou T, Corse AK, et al. Deep brain stimulation for treatment-resistant depression. *Psychiatr Ann* 43(8):358–365, 2013.
39. Arulpragasam AR, Chou T, Kaur N, et al. Future directions of deep brain stimulation: current disorders, new technologies. *Psychiatr Ann* 43(8):366–373, 2013.
42. Nemeroff CB, Mayberg HS, Krahl SE, et al. VNS therapy in treatment-resistant depression: clinical evidence and putative neurobiological mechanisms. *Neuropsychopharmacology* 31:1345–1355, 2006.
47. George MS, Rush AJ, Marangell LB, et al. A one-year comparison of vagus nerve stimulation with treatment as usual for treatment-resistant depression. *Biol Psychiatry* 58:364–373, 2005.
48. The UK ECT Review Group. Efficacy and safety of electroconvulsive therapy in depressive disorders: a systematic review and meta-analysis. *Lancet* 361:799–808, 2003.
78. Slotema CW, Blom JD, Hoek HW, et al. Should we expand the toolbox of psychiatric treatment methods to include repetitive transcranial magnetic stimulation (rTMS)? A meta-analysis of the efficacy of rTMS in psychiatric disorders. *J Clin Psychiatry* 71(7):873–884, 2010.

47 Lithium and Its Role in Psychiatry

Roy H. Perlis, MD, MSc, and Michael J. Ostacher, MD, MPH, MMSc

KEY POINTS

- Lithium remains a first-line treatment for all phases of bipolar disorder, including mania, depression, and prevention of recurrence.
- While not examined in a controlled trial, abundant evidence supports a role for lithium in decreasing the risk of suicide.
- Lithium has a narrow therapeutic window, necessitating careful titration and close monitoring of plasma levels.
- Lithium toxicity may cause confusion and ataxia.
- Drugs that affect lithium levels include non-steroidal anti-inflammatory drugs (NSAIDs) and diuretics.

HISTORICAL CONTEXT

The history of lithium's use in psychiatry parallels the development of modern psychopharmacology. The first specific description of the application of lithium to treat mania occurred in 1949, by an Australian named John Cade, who observed that lithium had calming effects on animals and then treated a series of 10 agitated manic patients. In fact, however, descriptions of lithium treatment date back to at least the United States Civil War. An 1883 textbook by Union Army Surgeon General William Hammond recommended the use of lithium bromide to treat manic or agitated patients, though he later downplayed the importance of lithium. In the early 1900s, a Danish physician, Lange, published a case series reporting the treatment of manic patients with lithium carbonate. There is little evidence that lithium was studied further, however, until Garrod proposed that lithium urate could be used to treat gout, opening the door to its broader therapeutic application.

Unfortunately, despite early studies by Mogen Schou and others, lithium's wider adoption in the US was hindered by concerns about lithium toxicity. Lithium chloride had been used as a sodium substitute in the 1940s, until several deaths were reported from lithium toxicity among hyponatremic patients. Thus, lithium was initially perceived as too dangerous for clinical application, and it was only in 1970 that lithium was approved by the United States Food and Drug Administration (FDA) for the treatment of mania.[1]

LITHIUM'S MECHANISM OF ACTION

The mechanisms by which lithium exerts its therapeutic effects are not entirely clear, but the signaling pathways with which it interacts are becoming better understood. Two major pathways are influenced by lithium. In the first, re-cycling of inositol is inhibited by lithium, which influences inositol 1,4,5-triphosphate (InsP$_3$)-dependent signaling.[2-4] InsP$_3$ signaling acts in part by regulating intra-cellular calcium release and protein kinase activation, with broad effects. At a neuronal level, lithium, like valproate, has been shown to increase the spread of growth cones, which are necessary for synapse formation. This effect is reversed by addition of myoinositol, providing some support for the importance of InsP$_3$ in lithium's effect.

In the second, lithium inhibits glycogen synthesis kinase 3-beta (GSK3B),[4-7] an important enzyme in pathways including the Wnt signaling cascade.[8] Notably, mice expressing lower levels of GSK3B exhibit behaviors similar to mice treated chronically with lithium.[9] Signaling through the GSK3B pathway may also be central to the observed neuroprotective effects of lithium.[10] Of course, both InsP$_3$ and GSK3B pathways have convergent effects—both influence the serine/threonine kinase Akt-1,4 for example. Expression of other genes (typically in lymphocytes) has been shown in single studies to be influenced by lithium administration, though the relevance of these effects to lithium's effects on mood or other phenotypes is unknown.

PHARMACOKINETICS AND PHARMACODYNAMICS

Lithium is absorbed through the gut and distributes rapidly through body water, achieving peak plasma concentrations 1 to 2 hours after a single dose. (Slower-release forms may require 4 to 5 hours to reach peak concentration, because of transit time through the gut.) As a monovalent cation like sodium, lithium's clearance relies entirely on renal function. It is not metabolized by the liver, nor is it significantly protein bound while circulating. In general, the half-life for renal excretion is approximately 24 hours, so steady-state serum levels are typically reached after 5 days. For this reason, lithium levels are typically checked about 5 days after initiation or dose change. Because lithium distributes throughout the body, it is influenced by lean body mass—for example, among geriatric patients, lithium levels for a given dose tend to be greater than among younger patients with greater lean body (including muscle) mass. Magnetic resonance spectroscopy studies suggest that brain lithium levels are highly correlated with plasma levels, though less so in patients at the extremes of age—that is, it is possible to have supra-therapeutic levels in the central nervous system (CNS) while maintaining a normal plasma lithium level.

Drugs that affect renal function, particularly re-absorption, can have profound effects on lithium clearance. Perhaps most notably from a clinical perspective, non-steroidal anti-inflammatory drugs (NSAIDs) or other COX-2 inhibitors may decrease renal blood flow and thereby increase lithium levels by up to 25%. Diuretics likewise affect lithium levels, though the nature of their effect depends on their site of action. In the kidney, lithium is primarily re-absorbed in the proximal renal tubules, with some subsequent absorption in the loop of Henle. Importantly, in contrast to sodium, no significant absorption occurs in the distal tubules. Therefore, thiazide diuretics, which act distally, will tend to increase lithium levels by up to 50%, while those that act more proximally generally have less of an effect on lithium levels.

More broadly, hydration status can affect lithium levels: individuals who become salt-avid (e.g., because of hypovolemia or hyponatremia, perhaps in the context of vomiting and diarrhea or self-induced injury, such as long-distance-running) will cause their lithium levels to increase.

EVIDENCE FOR LITHIUM'S EFFICACY
Lithium in Acute Mania

Beginning with Schou's study of lithium versus placebo for acute mania, lithium has repeatedly shown efficacy for the treatment of mania,[11] with the first large randomized study of lithium treatment of acute mania finding lithium comparably effective to the antipsychotic chlorpromazine.[12] Since then, multiple studies have found lithium to be superior to placebo and comparable or superior to other agents in the acute management of bipolar mania; few studies have found superiority for other drugs over lithium. A systematic review found 12 acute mania trials comparing lithium to placebo or another agent that met their criteria for data-pooling. This review of studies of lithium for acute mania found superiority for lithium over placebo and chlorpromazine, with equivalence to valproate and carbamazepine.[13]

As pointed out by Grunze,[14] however, few studies of lithium in acute mania were undertaken with the methodological rigor required today for regulatory approval of a drug's use. By coincidence, the first rigorously designed study to demonstrate the efficacy of lithium for acute mania was Bowden's seminal study of divalproex sodium for the treatment of acute mania in 1994, which was designed to study that drug for FDA approval; by including lithium as an active comparator, the study also demonstrated lithium's efficacy.[15] This study was adequately powered (i.e., it included a large enough sample of patients to find a high probability of finding a statistically significant difference between treatments with a low probability of error), compared a drug to an agent known to be effective (lithium), and it included a placebo arm. Additionally, it was not biased by inclusion based on prior response to lithium. In this 3-week study, lithium was superior to placebo and equivalent in efficacy to divalproex sodium with a 50% response rate (defined as a 50% drop in mania scale scores) for lithium compared to 26% for placebo.[15] Since that study, pooled data from trials of topiramate for mania failed to demonstrate a benefit for that drug, but it did re-confirm the efficacy of lithium for acutely manic patients.[16] The percentage of patients with a 50% or greater reduction in the Young Mania Rating Scale (YMRS) at day 21 was 28% with placebo (n = 427), 27% with topiramate (n = 433), and 46% with lithium (n = 227). Lithium was statistically better than placebo and topiramate on all psychometric measures other than the Montgomery-Asberg Depression Rating Scale (MADRS).

Monotherapy treatment in any phase of bipolar disorder, however, is increasingly rare, and is especially so in the treatment of acute mania.[17] It appears that mania outcomes, in terms of time to response and proportion of patients who remit, may be improved with the addition of antipsychotics to lithium.[18] The adjunctive use of typical (including haloperidol) and atypical (e.g., aripiprazole, asenapine, olanzapine, quetiapine, and risperidone) antipsychotics with lithium carbonate has been found to improve outcomes compared to lithium alone. The atypical antipsychotic ziprasidone, however, did not improve outcomes significantly compared to placebo when added to lithium.

Lithium in Acute Bipolar Depression

The options for the pharmacological treatment of major depressive episodes in bipolar disorder, unlike those for mania, remain few. In spite of being recommended as first-line treatment in recent bipolar treatment guidelines, there are few data to support the use of lithium as an acute antidepressant in bipolar disorder. A comprehensive review by Bauer and Mitchner[19] identified only three placebo-controlled trials of lithium for bipolar depression (with a total of 62 subjects).

While these trials showed a positive benefit for lithium, none was a randomized, parallel-group study; instead, they used a within-subject design in which each subject was started on lithium or placebo and then switched to the other. It is unlikely, unfortunately, that there will be any large, well-designed trials of lithium to answer this question, most prominently because there is no pharmaceutical manufacturer producing lithium that has any financial incentive to undertake such a study.

Lithium, used as monotherapy, appears to be as effective for the treatment of bipolar depression as the combination of lithium and an antidepressant. In a study comparing imipramine, paroxetine, and placebo added to lithium carbonate for the treatment of a major depressive episode in bipolar disorder, neither antidepressant added benefit beyond lithium alone.[20] Response rates (defined as a Hamilton Depression Rating Scale [HAM-D] score of 7 or lower) were 35% for lithium alone, compared to 39% for imipramine, and 46% for paroxetine. In a secondary analysis, subjects with lower lithium levels (less than 0.8 mEq/L) had a lower response rate compared to the adjunctive antidepressant group, suggesting, perhaps, that higher lithium levels are as effective as lithium plus an antidepressant in the treatment of bipolar depression.

Lithium for Maintenance Treatment and Relapse Prevention of Bipolar Disorder

Lithium is the archetypal maintenance treatment for bipolar disorder. From Prien's first maintenance study of lithium (comparing it to chlorpromazine), to more recent studies using lithium as a comparator for maintenance studies of other drugs, lithium has clear benefit for maintaining response and preventing relapse in bipolar disorder.[12,21] Lithium's clearest benefit in long-term use is in the prevention of relapse to mania, although relapse to depression is more common in patients with bipolar disorder. As is the case with lithium in acute mania, lithium's efficacy compared to placebo was only confirmed in later studies designed to establish regulatory approval for newer drugs, including divalproex sodium and lamotrigine. Earlier studies were beset with methodological problems, including on–off rather than parallel group designs, lack of diagnostic clarity (e.g., the inclusion of unipolar patients), and rapid or abrupt lithium discontinuation in stable patients. Concerns about sudden discontinuation of lithium are genuine, as there is a high rate of manic relapse in these patients; inclusion of patients from these studies might artificially inflate the difference between lithium and placebo in maintenance treatment.[22,23]

Geddes and colleagues[24] have completed the definitive systematic review of lithium for maintenance treatment in bipolar disorder. Having reviewed 300 studies, they included only five in their meta-analysis, limiting inclusion to randomized, double-blind, placebo-controlled trials. They found that lithium was more effective than placebo in preventing relapses to any mood episode (random effects relative risk = 0.65, 95% confidence interval [CI] = 0.50 to 0.84) and to mania (relative risk = 0.62, 95% CI = 0.40 to 0.95), with a non-significant effect on relapse to depression (relative risk = 0.72, 95% CI = 0.49 to 1.07).[24] The average risk of relapse of any kind in 1 to 2 years of follow-up was 60% for placebo, compared to 40% for lithium; this can be understood as lithium preventing one relapse for every five patients treated compared to placebo. Relapse rates to mania were 14% for lithium compared to 24% for placebo, while relapse rates to depression were 25% for placebo compared to 32% for lithium. There are some limitations and criticisms of this study, however. The outcomes were not defined uniformly across the included studies; one study included in the analysis had exclusively bipolar II subjects, and the follow-up period of 1 to 2 years is too short to adequately evaluate the benefit of lithium (as some have argued that the maintenance benefit of lithium is only apparent after 2 years of treatment).[23,25]

Lithium was compared to olanzapine for the prevention of relapse of bipolar I disorder in a randomized, controlled, double-blind trial.[26] Bipolar I patients were stabilized on a combination of lithium and olanzapine, randomized to one or the other drug, and followed for 12 months. There was no difference between drugs on the primary outcome measure or time to symptomatic relapse (YMRS or HAM-D scores of 15 or greater), although there were fewer relapses to mania/mixed (but not depressive) episodes in the olanzapine-treated group.

A number of studies have examined outcomes for subjects stabilized on an antipsychotic added to lithium or valproate and then randomized to remain on lithium or valproate and the antipsychotic or lithium or valproate plus placebo. Notably, these studies include aripiprazole, quetiapine, and ziprasidone; they are enriched designs intended to study the impact of the antipsychotic primarily, but do suggest that those patients who are stabilized on lithium or valproate plus one of those antipsychotics remain on both drugs.

A study was completed specifically to examine whether combination treatment with lithium and valproate together is more effective than either of those two drugs as monotherapy to prevent recurrence in bipolar I disorder. BALANCE is a randomized, open-label trial of lithium, divalproex sodium, or the combination for maintenance treatment in bipolar disorder. Participants were stabilized on both drugs during a 4 to 8-week open-label run-in phase (to screen for tolerability), then randomized to continue on lithium (titrated to at 0.4–1.0 mmol/L), divalproex sodium (750 mg, 1,250 mg, or valproic acid serum concentration at least 50 µg/ml), or the combination, with the primary outcome measure being time to intervention for a mood episode. While combination treatment was superior to divalproex sodium (hazard ratio 0.59, 95% CI 0.42–0.83) and lithium was also superior to divalproex (HR 0.71, 95% CI 0.71–1.00), combination therapy was not superior to lithium (HR 0.82, 95% CI 0.58–1.17). This suggests that the role for valproate monotherapy (i.e., not in combination with lithium) is limited, and that lithium alone or in combination with valproate is the preferred treatment.

There remains some controversy about what adequate maintenance lithium levels should be. In order to minimize adverse effects and to increase patient acceptance of lithium treatment, lowest effective doses should be the goal. A randomized, double-blind study by Gelenberg and co-workers[27] stabilized patients on a standard serum level of lithium (0.8 to 1 mmol/L), then assigned them to either remain at that level or to be maintained with a lower serum lithium level (0.4 to 0.6 mmol/L). Patients in the higher lithium level group had fewer relapses than those randomly assigned to lower lithium levels.[27] A re-analysis of the data, however, controlling for the rate at which the lithium dose was lowered, found no difference between groups, suggesting that lower maintenance lithium levels may be adequate for some patients.[28]

Lithium in Rapid-cycling Bipolar Disorder

Rapid cycling is no longer included as a course specifier in DSM-5, but continues to be used conceptually by clinicians. Rapid-cycling is defined in DSM-IV-TR as four or more distinct mood episodes (either of opposite poles, or of the same pole after at least 8 weeks of partial or full recovery) within a 12-month period; patients with this course are notoriously difficult to treat and to stabilize. Some have concluded that lithium is less effective than other drugs (e.g., divalproex

sodium) for this specific course of bipolar disorder, but an ambitious clinical trial and a large body of naturalistic data suggest that lithium is no less ineffective than other compounds for rapid-cycling.[29–32] Calabrese and colleagues[31] compared lithium to divalproex sodium in rapid-cycling patients stabilized on both drugs and found no difference between drugs on time-to-episode-recurrence. As testament to the difficulty of treating rapid-cycling, only 60 of the original 254 subjects, who were randomized to the two study conditions, achieved stabilization. In a cohort of 360 patients treated for bipolar disorder in Sardinia, time to recurrence was no different for the patients with or without a rapid-cycling course.[32]

Lithium in Suicide Prevention

Lithium may have anti-suicide effects in patients with mood disorders. While there are no prospective, randomized studies designed to examine lithium's potential to reduce suicide and suicide attempts, a number of meta-analyses, smaller independent studies, and a study from two large health insurance databases generally substantiate lithium's value as a prophylactic agent against suicidal behavior in bipolar disorder.

The strongest evidence for decreased suicide in patients treated with lithium comes from a meta-analysis by Cipriani and co-workers[33] of all randomized studies of lithium (either versus placebo or another drug) in mood disorders (including bipolar disorder and major depressive disorder [MDD]).[33]

They found that lithium-treated patients had significantly fewer suicides and deaths from all causes. In an examination of 32 trials, 1,389 patients were randomly assigned to lithium treatment and 2,069 to other compounds. Seven trials reported any deaths by suicide; subjects treated with lithium were less likely to commit suicide (2 versus 11 suicides; odds ratio = 0.26; 95% CI = 0.09 to 0.77). When suicides plus suicidal behavior (i.e., deliberate self-harm) were examined, the results also favored the lithium-treated group (odds ratio = 0.21; 95% CI = 0.08 to 0.50). In the 11 trials reporting any deaths, all-cause mortality was lower in the lithium group (data from 11 trials; 9 versus 22 deaths; odds ratio = 0.42, 95% CI = 0.21 to 0.87).

In an analysis of databases from two large health maintenance organizations in the US, Goodwin and Goldstein[34] found a strong effect favoring lithium compared to divalproex sodium or other anticonvulsants. The incidence of emergency department admissions for suicide attempts (31.3 versus 10.8 per 1,000 person-years; P < 0.001), suicide attempts resulting in hospitalization (10.5 versus 4.2 per 1,000 person-years; P < 0.001), and death by suicide (1.7 versus 0.7 per 1,000 person-years; P = 0.04) was lower in the group receiving at least one prescription for lithium. When adjusted for a number of demographic factors (including age and psychiatric and medical co-morbidity), they found that the risk of death by suicide was 2.7 times that for patients prescribed divalproex for a diagnosis of bipolar disorder compared to those prescribed lithium (95% CI = 1.1 to 6.3; P = 0.04).[34] The non-randomized nature of the sample, however, leaves open the concern that the groups were clinically different, and the results confounded by indication.[35] For instance, it is not known how many of the patients in the divalproex group had previously failed to respond to lithium and were thus a treatment-resistant group, and whether there were co-morbidities (such as anxiety disorders, personality disorders, or substance use disorders) that were present to a greater degree in the non–lithium-treated subjects. In any case, the results are strongly in favor of lithium and are consistent with other examinations of the effect of lithium on suicide.

Another meta-analysis of 33 studies investigating long-term lithium treatment between the years 1970 and 2000 yields a result that favors lithium as a potential means of suicide prevention.[36] Of the 19 studies comparing groups with and without lithium treatment, 18 found a lower risk of suicide in the treatment group and one had no suicides in either group.[36] Overall, the meta-analysis demonstrated a 13-fold reduction in suicidality for patients with an affective illness, leading to a largely reduced suicide risk (which nevertheless remained larger than that estimated for the general population). The rates of suicide associated with lithium treatment (0.109% to 0.224% annually) are 10 times greater than the international base rate (0.017%).[36]

Lithium discontinuation itself may increase suicide risk. Rapid or accelerated lithium discontinuation (as may be practiced by non-compliant individuals who decide to simply stop taking their medications) may increase risk for suicidal behavior. In a sample of 165 patients who decided to discontinue lithium for a variety of reasons (whether electively or for some medical reason), there was a 14-fold increase in all suicidal acts following discontinuation of lithium.[37] It is unclear whether the risk of suicide following lithium discontinuation exceeds that found in untreated affective illness. Lithium discontinuation may increase suicidal behavior due to higher relapse rates, higher than would be expected even if subjects had been treated with placebo or had been on no medication at all.[23] Ultimately, although the effects of lithium are promising in the realm of suicide prevention, they have not yet been definitively determined (and are likely never to be).

Lithium in Children and Adolescents
Pediatric Bipolar Disorder

There are no randomized, controlled, parallel group trials of lithium treatment of acute mania in children or adolescents. This is unfortunate, as the use of lithium in children without clear benefit may be inappropriate due to its known side effects. Open-label data are suggestive of an anti-manic effect, but without randomization or a control group, these data are difficult to interpret.[38] Kafantaris and co-workers[39] published a discontinuation study of adolescents with acute mania who were stabilized for 4 weeks on lithium, then randomly assigned to double-blind discontinuation over 2 weeks. They found no differences in rate of symptom-worsening between the group continued on lithium (10 of 19, 52.6%) versus the group switched to placebo (13 of 21, 61.9%), but their follow-up period may have been too short to detect a meaningful difference.[39]

A small, randomized, placebo-controlled, 6-week study of lithium in adolescents (n = 25, average age 16.3 years) with bipolar disorder and substance dependence disorder (including alcohol, cannabis, stimulants, and sedative/hypnotics) showed that lithium (average serum level 0.9 mEq/L) appears to improve both disorders.[40] Urine screens and measures of psychopathology improved in this group, although the results were preliminary and have yet to be replicated in a larger sample using more rigorous methodology.

Conduct Disorder

Lithium has been of some interest for use in treating symptoms of aggression associated with conduct disorder in children. In the largest study of this, 40 children (33 boys, 7 girls, with an average age of 12.5 years) were randomly assigned to lithium or placebo for 4 weeks.[41] Sixteen of 20 subjects in the lithium-treated group were considered responders on consensus ratings compared to 6 of 20 in the placebo group (P = 0.04), while Overt Aggression Scale scores decreased significantly for the lithium group compared to the placebo group (P = 0.04). There were significant side effects, however,

potentially limiting the utility of the treatment, and the follow-up period was short.

Other Uses of Lithium

While well validated for use in the treatment of bipolar disorder, lithium has been studied with greater or lesser success through randomized trials in the treatment of other psychiatric illnesses, including unipolar MDD, schizophrenia, and alcohol dependence.

Augmentation of Antidepressants in Treatment-refractory Major Depressive Disorder

The use of lithium as an agent to prevent relapse in MDD has been somewhat controversial, although the accumulation of evidence suggests that it may be effective in a small number of difficult-to-treat, refractory patients. While some of the earlier placebo-controlled trials found lithium augmentation to be of no benefit, a few larger studies with improved methodology suggested a benefit for lithium over placebo; a meta-analysis that included nine double-blind, placebo-controlled trials found a statistically significant difference in response rates to lithium augmentation compared to placebo in trials that used a minimum lithium carbonate dose of 800 mg/day or a serum level of 0.5 mEq/L or greater.[42] More recently, however, a small, double-blind, placebo-controlled trial of lithium augmentation found no benefit for lithium, and a recent large head-to-head comparison between lithium carbonate and triiodothyronine (T_3) found that only a small proportion of patients improved with lithium.[43,44]

Nierenberg and associates[43] found no benefit for lithium in a placebo-controlled trial. Thirty-five non-responders to 6 weeks of treatment with nortriptyline were treated with lithium carbonate or placebo; only 12.5% of the lithium-treated subjects improved, compared to 20% on placebo. As part of the Sequential Treatment Alternatives to Relieve Depression (STAR*D) study, lithium carbonate was compared to T_3 as an augmentation strategy in a 14-week randomized, open-label trial for 142 patients who had failed to improve on citalopram followed by a second treatment (either a switch to another antidepressant or augmentation with another agent), and found similarly low response rates for lithium.[44]

Remission rates were 15.9% with lithium augmentation (mean dose = 859.8 mg, SD = 373.1) and 24.7% with T_3 augmentation (mean dose = 45.2 µg, SD = 11.4) after a mean of 9.6 weeks of treatment, although the difference between treatments was not statistically significant. Lithium, however, was more frequently associated with side effects than was T_3 (P = 0.045), and more participants in the lithium group left treatment because of side effects (23.2% versus 9.6%; P = 0.027).

Relapse Prevention in Major Depressive Disorder

Several efforts have been made to examine the potential benefit of lithium in preventing relapse in MDD. In an early study, Prien and colleagues[45] found no additional benefit of the combination of lithium and imipramine over imipramine monotherapy. Lithium monotherapy was less successful than imipramine or combination treatment in this study.

In a small cohort (n = 29) of patients who responded to lithium augmentation in a 6-week open-label treatment phase and remained well over a 2- to 4-week stabilization period, those randomized to continue lithium had lower relapse rates in 4 months of follow-up (0 of 14) compared to those on placebo (7 of 15, including one suicide).[42] Serum lithium levels were moderate, averaging between 0.65 and

study was not designed to compare valproate and lithium monotherapies directly, although it appeared that lithium monotherapy was more effective than valproate alone. Thus valproate monotherapy is not recommended for maintenance therapy of BPD. For patients on valproate alone, the study indicates there is a potential benefit of adding lithium for maintenance, although the question remains whether patients should simply be on lithium alone in the first place. It is intriguing that the same investigators who demonstrated a role for divalproex sodium in acute mania treatment conducted a second, randomized double-blind study of the same drug in the same setting, but subsequently found no difference between divalproex sodium and placebo in acute mania.[15] The investigators attributed this discrepancy to methodological differences in study design (lower drug dose, allowance of early study termination, more liberal use of adjunctive medications, and 2:1 randomization in favor of study drug); however, in the context of other well-established options for acute mania treatment and BPD maintenance therapy, one wonders whether overall use of valproate for any phase of BPD should be limited.

Anticonvulsants, including valproate, are often viewed as more effective in rapid cycling than is lithium. However, it appears that this may not be the case. In a rigorous and ambitious double-blind study, rapid-cycling patients were stabilized on open-label lithium and divalproex sodium and then randomized in a double-blind fashion to either lithium or divalproex and followed prospectively.[16] There were no significant differences between the lithium-treated or the valproate-treated groups in time to drop-out or time to additional psychopharmacology.

Lastly, there is inadequate data to support a role for valproate in acute bipolar depression. Two independent meta-analyses of four randomized placebo-controlled trials suggested possible efficacy in acute depressive symptoms of BPD; however, the study sizes were very small (n = 9–28).[17,18] These findings will need to be replicated before valproate can be recommended for this indication.

Lamotrigine

Lamotrigine represents a significant advance in the long-term management of bipolar depression, especially given the prominent burden of depression and depressive relapses in BPD.[19–23] Lamotrigine is approved for the maintenance treatment of BPD, and is efficacious when compared to placebo in maintenance studies.[24] Long-term studies found an overall reduction in bipolar depressive relapse compared with placebo. In a key study in which patients who were most recently depressed were first stabilized on lamotrigine and randomly assigned to maintenance treatment with lamotrigine, lithium, or placebo, the overall sustained response rate was 57% with lamotrigine, compared with 46% for lithium, and 45% for placebo; this indicates that lamotrigine is effective in the prevention of relapse to depression when compared with placebo.[21] It is important to note, however, that a substantial proportion (43%) of bipolar patients remained unprotected against a depression relapse by continuation lamotrigine.

The evidence for efficacy of lamotrigine in the treatment of acute bipolar depression, on the other hand, remains limited. No single trial of the drug for acute bipolar depression found the drug better than placebo on the primary outcome measure of the study.[25] One widely referenced study found that while lamotrigine was not statistically different from placebo for total Hamilton Depression Rating Scale (HDRS) scores, it was superior on several other measures, including the Montgomery-Asberg Depression Rating Scale (MADRS) and the Clinical Global Impression Improvement (CGI-I) scale.[19]

This effect has never been replicated in individual trials, but a meta-analysis and meta-regression of pooled individual data from all five lamotrigine trials in acute bipolar depression (both bipolar I and II disorders) found that response (defined as a ≥ 50% decrease in scores) on both the HDRS and the MADRS was significantly greater than for placebo.[26] The effect size was small, however, and the number-needed-to-treat was about 11; a finding the authors note is at the "margins" of clinical utility. Remission was greater than placebo on the MADRS, but not the HDRS. The antidepressant effect of lamotrigine was greatest in the most severely depressed subjects in a subgroup analysis. These data suggest that any potential benefit of lamotrigine in acute depression is likely to be small, except perhaps in severely depressed patients. It is notable that the study of lamotrigine in maintenance of bipolar depression was designed to follow patients after they were first stabilized on lamotrigine for an acute depressive episode[21]; taken together, these studies suggest that lamotrigine should be continued for maintenance therapy in patients who responded to lamotrigine during acute bipolar depression, and that the patients most likely to respond are those who are most severely depressed.

A small randomized, double-blind study was performed comparing lamotrigine versus placebo as add-on medications to lithium in acutely depressed bipolar patients, and showed that lamotrigine plus lithium significantly improved MADRS scores at the end of week 8 versus lithium alone.[27] In order to be eligible for the study, however, patients had to be depressed despite taking a therapeutic dose of lithium for at least 2 weeks (most had been taking for at least 3 months), suggesting that this study population was likely enriched for non-responders to lithium monotherapy. The study also consisted of only 124 patients, and needs to be replicated. Subsequent follow-up of these patients showed that lamotrigine plus lithium was approximately as effective as lithium alone for preventing mood relapse or recurrence up to 68 weeks; however, the small sample size and the study design precluded formal statistical analyses.[28] At this point, evidence for any additional benefit of lamotrigine–lithium combination therapy in treating BPD, versus either of these medications alone, remains limited.

Lamotrigine has not demonstrated efficacy for the acute treatment of mania. Multiple treatments meta-analysis of antimanic drugs also indicated that lamotrigine is not more effective than placebo in treating acute mania.[11] No single trial found benefit for lamotrigine in the prevention of manic episodes; however, pooled analysis revealed a small but significant effect size for the prevention of mania.[21,24,29] While lamotrigine is more effective than lithium in the prevention of depressive episodes, lithium appears to be more effective than lamotrigine in preventing manic episodes.

No validated treatments for treatment-refractory bipolar depression exist, but a small, randomized, open-label trial of adjunctive lamotrigine, risperidone, or inositol in subjects who had depression in spite of trials of two consecutive standard antidepressants of adequate dose and duration was conducted as part of the Systematic Treatment Enhancement Program for Bipolar Disorder (STEP-BD).[30] An equipoise randomization process allowed subjects to choose to be randomized to any pair of the study treatments. While no differences were found in primary pair-wise comparisons in randomized patients (n = 66), a secondary, post-hoc analysis found that 8 weeks of sustained recovery were seen in 23.8% of the lamotrigine-treated patients, 17.4% of inositol-treated patients, and 4.6% of risperidone-treated patients. These data must be viewed cautiously, as they are from a secondary analysis, but they represent one of few studies for the treatment of refractory bipolar depression.

Carbamazepine

Carbamazepine was the first anticonvulsant studied as a treatment of mania. More than 19 studies (most of which were small case series or open trials) evaluated carbamazepine for the treatment of mania, and until recently it was used in BPD despite little scientific support for its use. More recently, carbamazepine (in extended-release form) was found to be effective for acute mania in two large placebo-controlled trials.[31,32] Multiple treatments meta-analysis of anti-manic drugs showed that carbamazepine was similar to valproate in terms of efficacy and acceptability in treating acute mania; however, all anticonvulsants as a class were outperformed by atypical antipsychotics.[11] There are no data directly establishing carbamazepine as an effective maintenance treatment in BPD. A meta-analysis of four small studies comparing efficacy of carbamazepine versus lithium in BPD maintenance suggested a possible similarity in relapse rates; however, this was tempered by the finding that carbamazepine use was associated with significantly more study withdrawals due to adverse effects.[33] At present, there are insufficient data to suggest that carbamazepine is more effective in these patients than any other treatment.

PHARMACOKINETICS, PHARMACODYNAMICS, ADVERSE EFFECTS, AND MONITORING

Valproic Acid

Valproic acid (di-n-propylacetic acid) is an anticonvulsant drug chemically unrelated to other psychiatric medications. One of the more commonly used preparations is divalproex sodium (Depakote), a compound of sodium valproate and valproic acid in a 1:1 molar ratio. Valproate is available as tablets (both delayed- and extended-release), capsules, enteric-coated capsules, sprinkles, and syrup. Absorption is different across the different preparations and it is delayed by ingestion of food. This may be of some importance when one switches from one preparation to another. Peak plasma levels are achieved between 2 and 4 hours after ingestion of the direct-release preparation, and the half-life ranges from 6 to 16 hours. More than 90% of plasma valproic acid is protein-bound. The time of dosing is determined by possible side effects, and, if tolerated, a once-a-day dosing could be employed. The therapeutic plasma levels generally used for the treatment of mania are the same as those used for anticonvulsant therapy (50–100 μg/ml), and the total daily dosage required to achieve these levels ranges from 500 mg to greater than 1,500 mg, although one study suggests a direct relationship between plasma valproate levels and response in acute mania, suggesting optimal levels in acute treatment of greater than 90 μg/ml.[12]

Valproic acid is metabolized by the hepatic CYP 2D6 system but, unlike carbamazepine, does not auto-induce its own metabolism. Concomitant administration of carbamazepine will decrease plasma levels of valproic acid, and drugs that inhibit the CYP system (e.g., selective serotonin reuptake inhibitors [SSRIs]) can cause an increase in valproic acid levels. Valproate is known to increase the plasma levels of lamotrigine, so it is recommended that the lamotrigine dose be lowered in patients taking valproate. Dose-related and common initial side effects include nausea, tremor, and lethargy. Gastric irritation and nausea can be reduced by dividing the dose or by using enteric-coated preparations. Valproic acid has been associated with potentially fatal hepatic failure, usually occurring within the first 6 months of treatment and most frequently occurring in children under age 2 years and in persons with pre-existing liver disease. Transient, dose-related elevations in liver enzymes can occur in up to 44% of patients. Any change in hepatic function should be followed closely, and patients should be warned to report symptoms of hepatic failure (such as malaise, weakness, lethargy, edema, anorexia, or vomiting). Multiple cases of valproate-associated pancreatitis have also been reported, as has multi-organ failure. These can occur at any point during treatment.

Valproic acid may produce teratogenic effects, including spina bifida (1%) and other neural tube defects. Other potential side effects include weight gain, inhibition of platelet aggregation, hair loss, and severe dermatological reactions (such as Stevens-Johnson syndrome).

There is additional worry that valproate may cause endocrine abnormalities in women. Two hundred and thirty women were evaluated for polycystic ovarian syndrome (PCOS) as part of an ancillary study during the Systematic Treatment Enhancement Program for Bipolar Disorder (STEP-BD). Criteria for PCOS are met when oligomenorrhea (defined as ≤ 9 cycles in the past year) coincides with at least one feature of hyperandrogenism (including hirsutism, acne, male-pattern alopecia, or elevated serum androgen levels); it can ultimately result in an increased risk of type 2 diabetes mellitus, cardiovascular disease, and some types of cancer.[34] Joffe and associates[34] compared the rate of new-onset PCOS in women with BPD taking valproate compared to the rate in those taking other anticonvulsants and lithium. Nine (10.5%) of the 86 valproate users developed treatment-emergent oligomenorrhea with hyperandrogenism, compared to 2 (1.4%) of the 144 valproate non-users. The relative risk for developing PCOS on valproate versus on non-valproate mood stabilizers was 7.5 (95% confidence interval, 1.7 to 34.1, p = 0.02).[34] The onset of oligomenorrhea usually began within 12 months of the beginning of valproate treatment.[34] A later analysis found that discontinuation of valproate in women with valproate-associated PCOS may result in an improvement of the PCOS reproductive features, as these symptoms resolved in three of the four women who discontinued valproate, but persisted in all three women who continued on valproate.[35]

Because of the risk of PCOS in women of child-bearing age who are exposed to valproate-containing products, the use of valproate as a first-line treatment for BPD is not recommended in these patients.

Lamotrigine

Lamotrigine was originally developed and approved for use as an anticonvulsant. The mechanism of action of lamotrigine in BPD is not precisely known, although lamotrigine appears to block voltage-gated sodium channels *in vitro*, and decrease pre-synaptic release of glutamate.[36] Lamotrigine is a weak dihydrofolate reductase inhibitor *in vitro* and in animal studies, but no effect on folate concentrations has been noted in human studies.[36] It is absorbed within 1–3 hours and has a half-life of 25 hours. Non-serious rash can arise in approximately 8% of adults, but serious rash that requires hospitalization is seen in up to 0.5% of lamotrigine-treated individuals.[36] Because of the possibility of Stevens-Johnson syndrome, toxic epidermal necrolysis, or angioedema, all rashes should be regarded as potentially serious and monitored closely, and to minimize serious rashes the dose should be increased at the rate suggested in the package insert. One randomized, open-label trial of rash precautions during the use of lamotrigine found no benefit from taking additional dermatological precautions (e.g., avoiding use of any other new drugs during dosage titration), but found an overall rash rate of approximately 8% while also finding that only 5.3% of subjects discontinued lamotrigine due to this adverse effect.[37] Dosing is adjusted upward for patients who are simultaneously taking antiepileptics, such as carbamazepine, that induce the metabolism of lamotrigine, and downward for those patients who are simultaneously taking antiepileptics, such as valproate, that may inhibit the clearance of the drug. There is no known relationship between lamotrigine drug levels and response in BPD.

Post-marketing surveillance has revealed an increased risk of fetal anomalies in children born to women exposed to lamotrigine during early pregnancy, specifically oral cleft deformities.[36] One study in the US found five cases of oral clefts in infants in a study of 684 pregnancies (i.e., 7.3 in 1,000 cases) where the mother was taking lamotrigine and no other antiepileptic drugs.[38] This is 10.4-times higher (95% confidence interval 4.3 to 24.9) than a comparison group of unexposed infants (where the prevalence was 0.7 in 1,000).[38] Other large-scale studies have not found such an elevated rate, however, and it remains controversial whether the rate elevation is due to reporting bias.[39]

Carbamazepine

Carbamazepine, an anticonvulsant drug structurally related to the tricyclic antidepressants (TCAs), has variable absorption and metabolism. Carbamazepine is rapidly absorbed (peak plasma levels within 4–6 hours). Eighty percent of plasma carbamazepine is protein-bound. Half-life ranges from 13 to 17 hours. Carbamazepine is metabolized by the hepatic CYP 2D6 system.

Carbamazepine induces the CYP enzymes, causing an increase in the rate of its own metabolism over time (as well as that of other drugs metabolized by the CYP system). Because of this, the dose of the drug should be monitored by serum levels every 2 to 3 months and raised if necessary. Concomitant administration of carbamazepine with oral contraceptives, warfarin, theophylline, doxycycline, haloperidol, TCAs, or valproic acid leads to decreased plasma levels of these other drugs. Concomitant administration of drugs that inhibit the CYP system will increase plasma levels of carbamazepine. These drugs include fluoxetine, cimetidine, erythromycin, isoniazid, calcium channel blockers, and propoxyphene. Concomitant administration of phenobarbital, phenytoin, and primidone causes a decrease in carbamazepine levels through induction of the CYP enzymes.

Based on its use as an anticonvulsant, dosages of carbamazepine typically range from 400 mg to 1,200 mg/day, and therapeutic plasma levels range from 4 to 12 µg/ml. The relationship between blood levels and response in mania is unknown.

Carbamazepine frequently causes lethargy, sedation, nausea, tremor, ataxia, and visual disturbances during the acute-treatment phase. Some patients can develop mild leukopenia or thrombocytopenia during this phase, although it typically does not progress. Carbamazepine causes a rare but severe form of aplastic anemia or agranulocytosis—estimated to occur with an incidence of about 2 to 5 per 100,000, which is 11 times the incidence in the general population. Although the vast majority of these reactions occur during the first 3 months of therapy, some cases have been reported as late as 5 years after the start of therapy treatment. If the white blood cell count drops below 3,000 cells/mm³, the medication should be discontinued.

Carbamazepine has also been associated with fetal anomalies, including a risk of spina bifida (1%), low birth weight, and small head circumference. It has also been shown to have effects on cardiac conduction, slowing atrioventricular conduction. Other reported side effects include inappropriate secretion of antidiuretic hormone with concomitant hyponatremia, decreased thyroid hormone levels without changes in levels of thyroid-stimulating hormone, severe dermatological reactions (such as Stevens-Johnson syndrome), and hepatitis.

Because of the cardiac, hematological, endocrine, and renal side effects associated with carbamazepine, patients should have the drug initiated with care. A recent physical examination, complete blood count (CBC) with platelet count, liver function tests, thyroid function tests, and renal function tests are necessary before the start of the drug. The CBC (with platelets) and liver function tests should be monitored every 2–3 weeks during the initial 3–4 months of treatment, and yearly after stabilization of the dose. Any abnormalities in the tests listed above should be evaluated, especially decreases in neutrophils and sodium. As with TCAs, carbamazepine shares the risk of hypertensive crisis when co-administered with monoamine oxidase inhibitors, and so this combination should be avoided.

OTHER ANTICONVULSANTS
Oxcarbazepine

Oxcarbazepine, a keto-analog of carbamazepine, is purported to have fewer side effects and drug–drug interactions than carbamazepine, but evidence of its efficacy in mania is absent. There are no published placebo-controlled studies of oxcarbazepine in adults with BPD, and the single published double-blind, placebo-controlled trial of oxcarbazepine in children and adolescents with BPD found no difference between drug and placebo.[40] There are a few small studies comparing oxcarbazepine with other anti-manic agents that have not found any difference in efficacy.[41] Because it is now available as a generic drug, it is unlikely that any definitive trials of this drug for BPD will ever be completed.

Gabapentin

Gabapentin was for a time a popular treatment for mania, likely because of perceptions of good tolerability and ease of use and because of aggressive marketing by the drug's manufacturer, Warner-Lambert. Two double-blind studies failed to detect anti-manic or antidepressant effect of gabapentin (one found an antidepressant effect for lamotrigine, however).[42] One double-blind, placebo-controlled study of adjunctive gabapentin in acute mania actually found that the anti-manic response to placebo was statistically significantly greater than for the drug.[43] Current evidence does not support the use of gabapentin in any phase of BPD.

Levetiracetam

Levetiracetam is an adjunctive treatment for complex partial seizures, and its mechanism of antiepileptic action remains unknown. It has had mixed results in several open-label trials as monotherapy or adjunctive therapy in bipolar mania. In one open-label trial, a proportion of the subjects had marked mood worsening.[44] Recently, a randomized, double-blind trial of adjunctive levetiracetam versus placebo in the treatment of acute bipolar depression showed no difference between the two groups in mean change of HDRS ratings at week 6.[45] At this time, more evidence is needed to determine the safety and efficacy of the compound before it can be used in BPD.

Pregabalin

Pregabalin binds voltage-gated calcium channels, and is used in the treatment of fibromyalgia and neuropathic pain. It has also been approved in Europe, but not the US, for the treatment of anxiety. A recent meta-analysis of randomized controlled trials in generalized anxiety disorder showed a small, but statistically significant, effect of pregabalin on the Hamilton Anxiety Rating Scale (HARS), compared to placebo.[46] For BPD, one open-label trial found that the use of adjunctive pregabalin in treatment-refractory bipolar patients improved mood in 41% of patients, as measured by CGI-BP; however, these data are preliminary.[47] The authors of the study also cited an unpublished double-blind, placebo-controlled trial by Pfizer, Inc., that showed no difference between pregabalin and placebo in the treatment of acute mania. Thus, further data are needed to support the use of pregabalin in the treatment of BPD, although there is substantial evidence supporting its use in generalized anxiety disorder.

Tiagabine

Tiagabine is a potent selective inhibitor of the principal neuronal gamma-aminobutyric acid (GABA) transporter (GAT-1) in the cortex and hippocampus, and it is marketed as an anti-epileptic compound. There are no published parallel-group trials of tiagabine in BPD. While there has been hope for this drug as a monotherapy or adjunctive treatment for mania, there have been serious concerns about adverse effects in patients treated with it, including syncope and seizures. A recent Cochrane review found little rigorous data for tiagabine in BPD to recommend its use.[48]

Topiramate

Topiramate is an anticonvulsant that inhibits voltage-gated sodium channels, antagonizes kainate and alpha-amino-3-hydroxy-5-methyl-4-isoxazole propionic acid (AMPA) glutamate receptors, and potentiates the $GABA_A$ receptor, although its mechanism of action in the treatment of seizures remains unknown. Although case reports and uncontrolled trials suggested efficacy for topiramate in the treatment of acute bipolar mania, controlled trials have not demonstrated this effect.[49] These do not appear to be failed trials (i.e., ones in which the study was not able to demonstrate an effect that was actually there), as the active comparator in some of the trials, lithium, was effective in reducing manic symptoms in those studies.

Zonisamide

The antiepileptic mechanism of zonisamide is unknown. Recently, a randomized, double-blind trial of adjunctive zonisamide in the treatment of acute bipolar mania/hypomania showed no difference in efficacy between zonisamide and placebo adjunctive groups.[50] In a large, open-label, 56-week trial of zonisamide for acute and continuation treatment in BPD, McElroy and associates[51] found that while some patients may have had improvements in mood, a high proportion of subjects dropped out of the study due to adverse effects or worsening of mood. Any beneficial effects of zonisamide on weight loss may be mitigated by concerns about the safety of the drug in BPD.

CONCLUSION

In spite of great promise, anticonvulsants, as a class of medications, have limited usefulness in the treatment of BPD (Table 48-1). Three anticonvulsants have proven effective in different phases of BPD (valproate, lamotrigine, and carbamazepine), but each has specific (and not broad) efficacy in the disorder. Other anticonvulsants have proved ineffective in rigorous trials or have not been adequately studied.

It is difficult to argue that unproven anticonvulsants have a place in the treatment of any phase of BPD—even if they have

TABLE 48-1 Anticonvulsants for Bipolar Disorder

	Acute Mania	Acute Depression	Maintenance
Valproate	+	−	−
Carbamazepine	+	−	−
Lamotrigine	−	+/−	+

a theoretically favorable side-effect profile—as there are now multiple evidence-based treatments for acute mania, acute depression, and relapse prevention in BPD. There is ongoing concern in the epilepsy literature that anticonvulsants, such as zonisamide and topiramate, may induce mood syndromes in patients with seizure disorders.[52] While BPD is often a life-threatening and disabling illness, anticonvulsants without proven efficacy in BPD must be used with caution in this illness, and it is prudent to wait until firm evidence allows clinicians and patients to make informed decisions regarding defined benefits and known harm before initiating these agents.

Access a list of MCQs for this chapter at https://expertconsult.inkling.com

REFERENCES

1. Post RM, Uhde TW, Putnam F, et al. Kindling and carbamazepine in affective illness. *J Nerv Ment Dis* 170(12):717–731, 1982.
2. Post RM. Cocaine psychoses: a continuum model. *Am J Psychiatry* 132(3):225–231, 1975.
3. Lenzer J. Pfizer pleads guilty, but drug sales continue to soar. *BMJ* 328(7450):1217, 2004.
4. Bender RE, Alloy LB. Life stress and kindling in bipolar disorders: review of the evidence and integration with emerging biopsychosocial theories. *Clin Psychol Rev* 31(3):383–398, 2011.
5. Turvey CL, Coryell WH, Solomon DA, et al. Long-term prognosis of bipolar I disorder. *Acta Psychiatr Scand* 99(2):110–119, 1999.
6. Bialer M. Why are antiepileptic drugs used for nonepileptic conditions? *Epilepsia* 53(Suppl. 7):26–33, 2012.
7. Rogawski MA, Loscher W. The neurobiology of antiepileptic drugs for the treatment of nonepileptic conditions. *Nature Med* 10(7):685–692, 2004.
8. Bowden CL, Swann AC, Calabrese JR, et al. A randomized, placebo-controlled, multicenter study of divalproex sodium extended release in the treamtent of acute mania. *J Clin Psychiatry* 67(10):1501–1510, 2006.
9. Pope HG, McElroy SL, Keck PE, et al. Valproate in the treament of acute mania. A placebo-controlled study. *Arch Gen Psychiatry* 48(1):62–68, 1991.
10. Bowden C, Gogus A, Grunze H, et al. A 12-week, open, randomized trial comparing sodium valproate to lithium in patients with bipolar I disorder suffering from a manic episode. *Int Clin Psychopharm* 23(5):254–262, 2008.
11. Cipriani A, Barbui C, Salanti G, et al. Comparative efficacy and acceptability of antimanic drugs in acute mania: a multiple-treatments meta-analysis. *Lancet* 378(9799):1306–1315, 2011.
12. Allen MH, Hirschfeld RM, Wozniak PJ, et al. Linear relationship of valproate serum concentration to response and optimal serum levels for acute mania. *Am J Psychiatry* 163(2):272–275, 2006.
13. Bowden CL, Calabrese JR, McElroy SL, et al. A randomized, placebo-controlled 12-month trial of divalproex and lithium in treatment of outpatients with bipolar I disorder. Divalproex Maintenance Study Group. *Arch Gen Psychiatry* 57:481–489, 2000.
14. BALANCE investigators and collaborators, Geddes J, Goodwin GM, et al. Lithium plus valproate combination therapy versus monotherapy for relapse prevention in bipolar I disorder (BALANCE): a randomised open-label trial. *Lancet* 375(9712):385–395, 2010.
15. Hirschfeld RMA, Bowden CL, Vigna NV, et al. A randomized, placebo-controlled, multicenter study of divalproex sodium extended-release in the acute treatment of mania. *J Clin Psychiatry* 71(4):426–432, 2010.

16. Calabrese JR, Shelton MD, Rapport DJ, et al. A 20-month, double-blind, maintenance trial of lithium versus divalproex in rapid cycling bipolar disorder. *Am J Psychiatry* 162:2152–2161, 2005.

17. Bond DJ, Lam RW, Yatham LN. Divalproex sodium versus placebo in the treatment of acute bipolar depression: a systematic review and meta-analysis. *J Affect Disord* 124(3):228–234, 2010.

18. Smith LA, Cornelius VR, Azorin JM, et al. Valproate for the treatment of acute bipolar depression: systematic review and meta-analysis. *J Affect Disord* 124(3):228–234, 2010.

19. Calabrese JR, Bowden CL, Sachs GS, et al. A double-blind placebo-controlled study of lamotrigine monotherapy in outpatients with bipolar I depression. Lamictal 602 Study Group. *J Clin Psychiatry* 60:79–88, 1999.

20. Calabrese JR, Suppes T, Bowden CL, et al. A double-blind, placebo-controlled, prophylaxis study of lamotrigine in rapid-cycling bipolar disorder. Lamictal 614 Study Group. *J Clin Psychiatry* 61:841–850, 2000.

21. Calabrese JR, Bowden CL, Sachs G, et al. A placebo-controlled 18-month trial of lamotrigine and lithium maintenance treatment in recently depressed patients with bipolar I disorder. *J Clin Psychiatry* 64:1013–1024, 2003.

22. Judd LL, Akiskal HS, Schettler PJ, et al. The long-term natural history of the weekly symptomatic status of bipolar I disorder. *Arch Gen Psychiatry* 59:530–537, 2002.

23. Judd LL, Akiskal HS, Schettler PJ, et al. A prospective investigation of the natural history of the long-term weekly symptomatic status of bipolar II disorder. *Arch Gen Psychiatry* 60:261–269, 2003.

24. Goodwin GM, Bowden CL, Calabrese JR, et al. A pooled analysis of 2 placebo-controlled 18-month trials of lamotrigine and lithium maintenance in bipolar I disorder. *J Clin Psychiatry* 65:432–441, 2004.

25. Calabrese JR, Huffman RF, White RL, et al. Lamotrigine in the acute treatment of bipolar depression: results of five double-blind, placebo-controlled clinical trials. *Bipolar Disord* 10(2):323–333, 2008.

26. Geddes JR, Calabrese JR, Goodwin GM. Lamotrigine for treatment of bipolar depression: independent meta-analysis and meta-regression of individual patient data from five randomised trials. *Br J Psychiatry* 194(1):4–9, 2009.

27. van der Loos MDM, Mulder PGH, Hartong EGThM, LamLit Study Group. Efficacy and safety of lamotrigine as add-on treatment to lithium in bipolar depression: a multicenter, double-blind, placebo-controlled trial. *J Clin Psychiatry* 70(2):223–231, 2009.

28. van der Loos MDM, Mulder P, Hartong EGThM, LamLit Study Group. Long-term outcome of bipolar depressed patients receiving lamotrigine as add-on to lithium with the possibility of the addition of paroxetine in nonresponders: a randomized, placebo-controlled trial with a novel design. *Bipolar Disord* 13(1):111–117, 2011.

29. Bowden CL, Calabrese JR, Sachs G, et al. A placebo-controlled 18-month trial of lamotrigine and lithium maintenance treatment in recently manic or hypomanic patients with bipolar I disorder. *Arch Gen Psychiatry* 60:392–400, 2003.

30. Nierenberg AA, Ostacher MJ, Calabrese JR, et al. Treatment-resistant bipolar depression: a STEP-BD equipoise randomized effectiveness trial of antidepressant augmentation with lamotrigine, inositol, or risperidone. *Am J Psychiatry* 163:210–216, 2006.

31. Weisler RH, Kalali AH, Ketter TA, SPD417 Study Group. A multicenter, randomized, double-blind, placebo-controlled trial of extended-release carbamazepine capsules as monotherapy for bipolar disorder patients with manic or mixed episodes. *J Clin Psychiatry* 65(4):478–484, 2004.

32. Weisler RH, Keck PE Jr, Swann AC, SPD417 Study Group. Extended-release carbamazepine capsules as monotherapy for acute mania in bipolar disorder: a multicenter, randomized, double-blind, placebo-controlled trial. *J Clin Psychiatry* 66(3):323–330, 2005.

33. Ceron-Litvoc D, Soares BG, Geddes J, et al. Comparison of carbamazepine and lithium in treatment of bipolar disorder: a systematic review of randomized controlled trials. *Hum Psychopharmacol Clin Exp* 24:19–28, 2009.

34. Joffe H, Cohen LS, Suppes T, et al. Valproate is associated with new-onset oligoamenorrhea with hyperandrogenism in women with bipolar disorder. *Biol Psychiatry* 59(11):1078–1086, 2006.

35. Joffe H, Cohen LS, Suppes T, et al. Longitudinal follow-up of reproductive and metabolic features of valproate-associated polycystic ovarian syndrome features: a preliminary report. *Biol Psychiatry* 60(12):1378–1381, 2006.

36. Lamictal (lamotrigine) package insert, 2006, GlaxoSmithKline.

37. Ketter TA, Greist JH, Graham JA, et al. The effect of dermatologic precautions on the incidence of rash with addition of lamotrigine in the treatment of bipolar I disorder: a randomized trial. *J Clin Psychiatry* 67(3):400–406, 2006.

38. Holmes LB, Baldwin EJ, Smith CR, et al. Increased frequency of isolated cleft palate in infants exposed to lamotrigine during pregnancy. *Neurology* 70(22):2152–2158, 2008.

39. Hunt SJ, Craig JJ, Morrow JI. Comment on: Increased frequency of isolated cleft palate in infants exposed to lamotrigine during pregnancy. *Neurology* 72(12):1108, 2009.

40. Wagner KD, Kowatch RA, Emslie GJ, et al. A double-blind, randomized, placebo-controlled trial of oxcarbazepine in the treatment of bipolar disorder in children and adolescents. *Am J Psychiatry* 163(7):1179–1186, 2006.

41. Vasudev A, Macritchie K, Vasudev K, et al. Oxcarbazepine for acute affective episodes in bipolar disorder. *Cochrane Database Syst Rev* 7(12):CD004857, 2011.

42. Frye MA, Ketter TA, Kimbrell TA, et al. A placebo-controlled study of lamotrigine and gabapentin in refractory mood disorders. *J Clin Psychopharmacol* 20:607–614, 2000.

43. Pande AC, Crockatt JG, Janney CA, et al. Gabapentin in bipolar disorder: a placebo-controlled trial of adjunctive therapy. Gabapentin Bipolar Disorder Study Group. *Bipolar Disord* 2:249–255, 2000.

44. Post RM, Altshuler LL, Frye MA, et al. Preliminary observations on the effectiveness of levetiracetam in the open adjunctive treatment of refractory bipolar disorder. *J Clin Psychiatry* 66(3):370–374, 2005.

45. Saricicek A, Maloney K, Muralidharan A, et al. Levetiracetam in the management of bipolar depression: a randomized, double-blind, placebo-controlled trial. *J Clin Psychiatry* 72(6):744–750, 2011.

46. Boschen MJ. A meta-analysis of the efficacy of pregabalin in the treatment of generalized anxiety disorder. *Can J Psychiatry* 56(9):558–566, 2011.

47. Schaffer LC, Schaffer CB, Miller AR, et al. An open trial of pregabalin as an acute and maintenance adjunctive treatment for outpatients with treatment resistant bipolar disorder. *J Affect Disord* 147(1–3):407–410, 2013.

48. Vasudev A, Macritchie K, Rao SNK, et al. Tiagabine in the maintenance treatment of bipolar disorder. *Cochrane Database Syst Rev* 7(12):CD005173, 2012.

49. Kushner SF, Khan A, Lane R, et al. Topiramate monotherapy in the management of acute mania: results of four double-blind placebo-controlled trials. *Bipolar Disord* 8(1):15–27, 2006.

50. Dauphinais D, Knable M, Rosenthal J, et al. Zonisamide for bipolar disorder, mania, or mixed states: a randomized, double blind, placebo-controlled adjunctive trial. *Psychopharmacol Bull* 44(1):5–17, 2011.

51. McElroy SL, Suppes T, Keck PE Jr, et al. Open-label adjunctive zonisamide in the treatment of bipolar disorders: a prospective trial. *J Clin Psychiatry* 66(5):617–624, 2005.

52. Mula M, Sander JW. Negative effects of antiepileptic drugs on mood in patients with epilepsy. *Drug Saf* 30(7):555–567, 2007.

49 Pharmacotherapy of Attention-Deficit/Hyperactivity Disorder across the Life Span

Jefferson B. Prince, MD, Timothy E. Wilens, MD, Thomas J. Spencer, MD, and Joseph Biederman, MD

KEY POINTS

- Attention-deficit/hyperactivity disorder (ADHD) is a common disorder in children, adolescents, and adults.
- While the phenotype of ADHD changes across the life span, ADHD persists in many children, adolescents, and adults.
- Formulations of stimulant and non-stimulant medications are Food and Drug Administration-approved as pharmacological treatments for ADHD in children, adolescents, and adults.
- Co-morbid psychiatric and learning disorders are common in patients with ADHD across the life span.
- When treating ADHD and co-morbid disorders, clinicians must prioritize and treat the most severe condition first, and regularly re-assess the symptoms of ADHD and the co-morbid disorder.

OVERVIEW

Attention-deficit/hyperactivity disorder (ADHD) is a common psychiatric condition shown to occur in 3% to 10% of school-age children worldwide, up to 8% of adolescents and up to 4% of adults.[1-5] The classic triad of impaired attention, impulsivity, and excessive motor activity characterizes ADHD, although many patients may manifest only inattentive symptoms.[6,7] ADHD usually persists, to a significant degree, from childhood through adolescence and into adulthood.[8,9] Most children, adolescents, and adults with ADHD suffer significant functional impairment(s) in multiple domains,[10] as well as co-morbid psychiatric or learning disorders.[5,11-18]

Studies demonstrate that ADHD is frequently co-morbid with oppositional defiant disorder (ODD), conduct disorder (CD), multiple anxiety disorders (panic disorder, obsessive-compulsive disorder [OCD], tic disorders), mood disorders (e.g., depression, dysthymia, and bipolar disorder [BPD]), learning disorders (e.g., auditory processing problems and dyslexia), and substance use disorders (SUDs) and often complicates the development of patients with autism spectrum disorders (ASDs). Co-morbid psychiatric, learning, and developmental disorders need to be assessed in all patients with ADHD and the relationship of these symptoms with ADHD delineated.[1,19,20]

Before using medications, clinicians should complete a through clinical evaluation that includes a complete history of symptoms, a differential diagnosis, a review of prior assessments/treatments, a medical history, and a description of current physical symptoms (including questions about the physical history, including either a personal or family history of cardiovascular symptoms or problems). Before treatment with medications, it is usually important to measure baseline levels of height, weight, blood pressure, and pulse and to monitor them over the course of treatment (see http://

www.fda.gov/Drugs/DrugSafety/PostmarketDrugSafety InformationforPatientsandProviders/DrugSafetyInformation forHeathcareProfessionals/ucm165858.htm for the most recent recommendations by the Food and Drug Administration [FDA] about monitoring for children and http://www.fda .gov/drugs/drugsafety/ucm279858.htm for the most recent recommendations about monitoring for adults). Clinicians and patients/families should select an initial treatment, either a stimulant or a non-stimulant; decide on a target dose (either absolute or weight-based) titration schedule; and decide how to monitor tolerability and response to treatment (using rating scales, anchor points, or both). Patients should be educated about the importance of adherence, safely maintaining medications (e.g., as in college students), and additional types of treatment (e.g., coaching and organizational help) that may be helpful.

STIMULANTS

For over 60 years stimulants have been used safely and effectively in the treatment of ADHD[21] and they are among the most well-established treatments in psychiatry.[22,23] The stimulants most commonly used include methylphenidate (MPH), a mixture of amphetamine salts (MAS) and dextroamphetamine (DEX). The recent development of various novel delivery systems has significantly advanced the pharmacotherapy of ADHD (see Table 49-1 for a list of these medications).

Pharmacodynamic Properties of Stimulants

Stimulants increase intra-synaptic concentrations of dopamine (DA) and norepinephrine (NE).[24-27] MPH primarily binds to the DA transporter protein (DAT), blocking the re-uptake of DA, increasing intra-synaptic DA.[25,27] While amphetamines diminish pre-synaptic re-uptake of DA by binding to DAT, these compounds also travel into the DA neuron, promoting release of DA from reserpine-sensitive vesicles in the pre-synaptic neuron.[25,26] In addition, stimulants (amphetamine > MPH) increase levels of NE and serotonin (5-HT) in the inter-neuronal space.[24] Although group studies comparing MPH and amphetamines generally demonstrate similar efficacy,[19,20] their pharmacodynamic differences may explain why a particular patient may respond to, or tolerate, one stimulant preferentially over another. It is necessary to appreciate that while the efficacy of amphetamine and MPH is similar, their potency differs, such that 5 mg of amphetamine is approximately equally potent to 10 mg of MPH.

Methylphenidate

As originally formulated, MPH was produced as an equal mixture of d,l-threo-MPH and d,l-erythro-MPH. The erythro isomers of MPH appear to produce side effects, and thus MPH is now manufactured as an equal racemic mixture of d,l-threo-MPH.[28] Behavioral effects of immediate-release MPH peak 1 to 2 hours after administration, and tend to dissipate within 3 to 5 hours. After oral administration immediate-release MPH is readily absorbed, reaching peak plasma concentration in 1.5 to 2.5 hours, and has an elimination half-life of

TABLE 49-1 Available FDA-approved Treatments for Attention-Deficit/Hyperactivity Disorder

Generic Name (Brand Name)	Formulation and Mechanism	Duration of Activity	How Supplied	Usual Absolute and (Weight-based) Dosing Range	FDA-approved Maximum Dose for ADHD
MPH (Ritalin)*	Tablet of 50:50 racemic mixture d,l-threo-MPH	3–4 hours	5, 10, and 20 mg tablets	(0.3–2 mg/kg/day)	60 mg/day
Dex-MPH (Focalin)*	Tablet of d-threo-MPH	3–5 hours	2.5, 5, and 10 mg tablets (2.5 mg Focalin equivalent to 5 mg Ritalin)	(0.15–1 mg/kg/day)	20 mg/day
MPH (Methylin)*	Tablet of 50:50 racemic mixture d,l-threo-MPH	3–4 hours	5, 10, and 20 mg tablets	(0.3–2 mg/kg/day)	60 mg/day
MPH-SR (Ritalin-SR)*	Wax-based matrix tablet of 50:50 racemic mixture d,l-threo-MPH	3–8 hours Variable	20 mg tablets (amount absorbed appears to vary)	(0.3–2 mg/kg/day)	60 mg/day
MPH (Metadate ER)*	Wax-based matrix tablet of 50:50 racemic mixture d,l-threo-MPH	3–8 hours Variable	10 and 20 mg tablets (amount absorbed appears to vary)	(0.3–2 mg/kg/day)	60 mg/day
MPH (Methylin ER)*	Hydroxypropyl methylcellulose base tablet of 50:50 racemic mixture d,l-threo-MPH; no preservatives	8 hours	10 and 20 mg tablets 2.5, 5, and 10 mg chewable tablets 5 mg/5 ml and 10 mg/5 ml oral solution	(0.3–2 mg/kg/day)	60 mg/day
MPH (Ritalin LA)*	Two types of beads give bimodal delivery (50% immediate-release and 50% delayed-release) of 50:50 racemic mixture d,l-threo-MPH	8 hours	20, 30, and 40 mg capsules; can be sprinkled	(0.3–2 mg/kg/day)	60 mg/day
D-MPH (Focalin XR)	Two types of beads give bimodal delivery (50% immediate-release and 50% delayed-release) of d-threo-MPH	12 hours	5, 10, 15, 20, 25, 30, 35, and 40 mg capsules	0.15–1 mg/kg/day	30 mg/day in youth; 40 mg/day in adults
MPH (Metadate CD)*	Two types of beads give bimodal delivery (30% immediate-release and 70% delayed-release) of 50:50 racemic mixture d,l-threo-MPH	8 hours	20 mg capsule; can be sprinkled	(0.3–2 mg/kg/day)	60 mg/day
MPH (Daytrana)*	MPH transdermal system	12 hours (patch worn for 9 hours)	10, 15, 20, and 30 mg patches	0.3–2 mg/kg/day	30 mg/day
MPH (Concerta)*	Osmotic pressure system delivers 50:50 racemic mixture d,l-threo-MPH	12 hours	18, 27, 36, and 54 mg caplets	(0.3–2 mg/kg/day)	72 mg/day
MPH (Quillivant XR)	Extended-release liquid	12 hours	25 mg/5 ml	(0.3–2 mg/kg/day)	60 mg/day
AMPH† (Dexedrine Tablets)	d-AMPH tablet	4–5 hours	5 mg tablets	(0.15–1 mg/kg/day)	40 mg/day
AMPH† (Dextrostat)	d-AMPH tablet	4–5 hours	5 and 10 mg tablets	(0.15–1 mg/kg/day)	40 mg/day
AMPH† (Dexedrine Spansules)	Two types of beads in a 50:50 mixture short and delayed-absorption of d-AMPH	8 hours	5, 10, and 15 mg capsules	(0.15–1 mg/kg/day)	40 mg/day
Mixed salts of AMPH† (Adderall)	Tablet of d,l-AMPH isomers (75% d-AMPH and 25% l-AMPH)	4–6 hours	5, 7.5, 10, 12.5, 15, 20, and 30 mg tablets	(0.15–1 mg/kg/day)	40 mg/day
Mixed salts of AMPH*‡ (Adderall-XR)	Two types of beads give bimodal delivery (50% immediate-release and 50% delayed-release) of 75:25 racemic mixture d,l-AMPH	At least 8 hours (but appears to last much longer in certain patients)	5, 10, 15, 20, 25, and 30 mg capsules; can be sprinkled	(0.15–1 mg/kg/day)	30 mg/day in children Recommended dose is 20 mg/day in adults

Continued on following page

TABLE 49-1 Available FDA-approved Treatments for Attention-Deficit/Hyperactivity Disorder *(Continued)*

Generic Name (Brand Name)	Formulation and Mechanism	Duration of Activity	How Supplied	Usual Absolute and (Weight-based) Dosing Range	FDA-approved Maximum Dose for ADHD
Lisdexamfetamine (Vyvanase)*	Tablets of dextroamphetamine and L-lysine	12 hours	30, 50, and 70 mg tablets		70 mg/day
Atomoxetine*‡ (Strattera)	Capsule of atomoxetine	5 hour plasma half-life but CNS effects appear to last much longer	10, 18, 25, 40, 60, and 80 mg capsules	1.2 mg/kg/day	1.4 mg/kg/day or 100 mg
Guanfacine ER** (Intuniv)	Extended-release tablet of guanfacine	Labeled for once-daily dosing	1,2,3 & 4 mg tablets	Up to 4 mg per day	Up to 4 mg per day
Clonidine ER**(Kapvay)	Extended-release tablet of clonidine	Labeled for twice-daily dosing	0.1 mg tablet	0.1–0.2 mg twice daily	Up to 0.4 mg daily

*Approved to treat ADHD age 6 years and older.
†Approved to treat ADHD age 3 years and older.
‡Specifically approved for treatment of ADHD in adults.
**Approved to treat ADHD in youth 6–17 years old as monotherapy or as adjunctive treatment with stimulant.

2.5–3.5 hours. After oral administration, but prior to reaching the plasma, the enzyme carboxylesterase (CES-1), which is located in the walls of the stomach and liver, extensively metabolizes MPH via hydrolysis and de-esterification, with little oxidation.[29,30] Individual differences in CES-1's hydrolyzing activity may result in variable metabolism and serum MPH levels.[31] While generic MPH has a similar pharmacokinetic profile to Ritalin, it is more rapidly absorbed and peaks sooner.[32] Due to its wax-matrix preparation, the absorption of the sustained-release MPH preparation (Ritalin-SR) is variable,[33] with peak MPH plasma levels in 1 to 4 hours, a half-life of 2 to 6 hours, and behavioral effects that may last up to 8 hours.[34] The availability of the various new extended-delivery stimulant formulations has greatly curtailed use of MPH-SR.

Concerta (OROS-MPH) uses the Osmotic Releasing Oral System (OROS) technology to deliver a 50:50 racemic mixture of d,l-threo-MPH.[35] OROS-MPH, indicated for the treatment of ADHD in children and adolescents, is available in 18, 27, 36, and 54 mg doses and is indicated in doses up to 72 mg daily. The 18 mg caplet of OROS-MPH provides an initial bolus of 4 mg of MPH, delivering the remaining MPH in an ascending pattern, such that peak concentrations are generally reached around 8 hours after dosing; it is labeled for 12 hours of coverage.[28,36] A single morning dose of 18, 27, 36, 54,or 72 mg of OROS-MPH is approximately bioequivalent to 5, 7.5, 10,15,or 20 mg of immediate-release MPH administered three times daily, respectively. The effectiveness and tolerability of OROS-MPH have been demonstrated in children,[37–39] adolescents,[40] and adults[41] with ADHD. Data support OROS-MPH's continued efficacy in many of those with ADHD over the course of 24 months of treatment.[42]

Metadate CD (MPH MR), the first available extended-delivery stimulant preparation to employ beaded technology, is available in capsules of 10, 20, 30, 40, 50, and 60 mg, which may be sprinkled. Using Eurand's Diffucaps technology, MPH MR contains two types of coated beads, IR-MPH and extended-release-MPH (ER-MPH). Metadate delivers 30% of d,l-threo-MPH initially, and 70% of d,l-threo-MPH several hours later. MPH MR is designed to simulate twice-daily (BID) dosing of IR MPH providing approximately 8 hours of coverage. The efficacy of MPH MR capsules has been demonstrated,[43] and it is approved for treatment in youth with ADHD in doses of up to 60 mg/day.[28] An extended-delivery tablet form of Metadate (Metadate ER) is also available in doses of 10 and 20 mg.

Ritalin-LA (MPH-ERC), another beaded-stimulant preparation, which may be sprinkled,[28] is available in capsules of 10, 20, 30, and 40 mg, essentially equivalent to 5, 10, 15 and 20 mg of IR-MPH delivered BID. MPH-ERC uses the beaded Spheroidal Oral Drug Absorption System (SODAS) technology to achieve a bi-modal release profile that delivers 50% of its d,l-threo-MPH initially and another bolus approximately 3 to 4 hours later, providing around 8 hours of coverage. The efficacy of MPH-ERC has been demonstrated in youth with ADHD.[44]

The primarily active form of MPH appears to be the d-threo isomer,[45–47] which is available in both immediate-release tablets (Focalin 2.5, 5, and 10 mg) and, employing the SODAS technology, extended-delivery capsules (Focalin XR 5, 10, 15, and 20 mg). The efficacy of D-MPH is well established in children, adolescents, and adults under open- and double-blind conditions.[48–51] D-MPH is approved to treat ADHD in children, adolescents, and adults in doses of up to 20 mg per day and has been labeled to provide a 12-hour duration of coverage.[28] Although not definitive, 10 mg of MPH appears to be approximately equivalent to 5 mg of d-MPH, and clinicians can reasonably use this estimate in clinical practice.[52]

The MPH transdermal system (MTS; Daytrana) delivers MPH through the skin via the DOT Matrix transdermal system. The patches are applied once daily and intended to be worn for 9 hours, although in clinical practice they can be worn for shorter and longer periods of time. The MTS usually takes effect within 2 hours and provides coverage for 3 hours after removal. MTS is available in 10, 15, 20, and 30 mg patches.[53–55] Since the MPH is absorbed through the skin, it does not undergo first-pass metabolism by CES-1 in the liver, resulting in higher plasma MPH levels.[56] Therefore, patients may require lower doses with MTS compared to oral preparations (10 mg of MTS = 15 mg of extended-release oral MPH). MTS may be a particularly useful treatment option for patients who have difficulty swallowing or tolerating oral stimulant formulations or for patients who need flexibility in the duration of medication effect.

Recently an extended-delivery MPH oral suspension formulation became available (MEROS or Quillivant XR 25 mg/5 ml). Although head-to-head trials haven't been published and clinical experience to date is limited, this formulation appears to provide similar efficacy and duration of effect as other extended-delivery MPH preparations.[57,58] This preparation may be particularly helpful for youth who prefer a liquid preparation or who experience skin reactions to the transdermal patch. Prior to dosing, the manufacturer recommends shaking the contents in the bottle to ensure an even distribution of medication.

Amphetamines

Amphetamine is available in three forms, dextroamphetamine (DEX; Dexedrine), mixed amphetamine salts (MAS; Adderall), and lisdexamfetaminedimesylate (LDX, Vyvanase). DEX tablets achieve peak plasma levels 2 to 3 hours after oral administration, and have a half-life of 4 to 6 hours. Behavioral effects of DEX tablets peak 1 to 2 hours after administration, and last 4 to 5 hours. For DEX spansules, these values are somewhat longer. MAS consist of equal portions of d-amphetamine saccharate, d,l-amphetamine asparate, d-amphetamine sulfate, and d,l-amphetamine sulfate, and a single dose results in a ratio of approximately 3:1 d- to l-amphetamine.[28] The two isomers have different pharmacodynamic properties, and some patients with ADHD preferentially respond to one isomer over another. The efficacy of MAS tablets is well established in ADHD youth[59] and adults.[60] An extended-delivery preparation of MAS is available as a capsule containing two types of Micotrol beads (MAS XR; Adderall XR). The beads are present in a 50:50 ratio, with immediate-release beads designed to release MAS in a fashion similar to MAS tablets, and delayed-release beads designed to release MAS 4 hours after dosing. The efficacy of MAS XR is well established in children,[61,62] adolescents,[63] and adults.[64,65] Furthermore, open treatment with MAS XR appears to be effective in the treatment of many ADHD youths over a 24-month period.[66]

LDX is FDA-approved for treatment of ADHD in children, adolescents, and adults. LDX[28] is an amphetamine pro-drug in which L-lysine, a naturally occurring amino acid, is covalently linked to d-amphetamine. After oral administration, the pro-drug is metabolically hydrolyzed in the body to release d-amphetamine. LDX appears to reduce abuse liability (e.g., misuse, abuse, and overdose) as intravenously and intranasally administered LDX results in similar effects as oral administration.[67,68] It is available in capsules of 20, 30, 40, 50, 60, and 70 mg that appear to be comparable to MAS XR doses of 10, 15, 20, 25, 30, and 35 mg, respectively.

Clinical Use of Stimulants

Guidelines and recent excellent clinical reviews regarding the use of stimulant medications in children, adolescents, and adults in clinical practice have been published.[1,7,19,20,69–72] Treatment with immediate-release preparations generally starts at 5 mg of MPH or amphetamine once daily and is titrated upward every 3 to 5 days until an effect is noted or adverse effects emerge. Typically, the half-life of the short-acting stimulants necessitates at least twice-daily dosing, with the addition of similar or reduced afternoon doses dependent on breakthrough symptoms. In a typical adult, dosing of immediate-release MPH is generally up to 30 mg three to four times daily or amphetamine 15 to 20 mg three to four times a day. Currently, most adults with ADHD will be treated with a stimulant that has an extended delivery. Since there is no way to determine which stimulant will be best tolerated and most effective, it is wise to consider including trials with extended-delivery preparations of both MPH and amphetamine.[73]

Side Effects of Stimulants

Although generally well tolerated, stimulants can cause clinically significant side effects (including anorexia, nausea,

difficulty falling asleep, obsessiveness, headaches, dry mouth, rebound phenomena, anxiety, nightmares, dizziness, irritability, dysphoria, and weight loss).[1,20,74–77] Rates and types of stimulant side effects appear to be similar in ADHD patients, regardless of age. In patients with a current co-morbid mood/anxiety disorder, clinicians should consider whether an adverse effect reflects the co-morbid disorder, a side effect of the treatment, or an exacerbation of the co-morbidity. Moreover, while stimulants can cause these side effects, many ADHD patients experience these problems before treatment; therefore, it is important for clinicians to document these symptoms at baseline.[76] Recommendations about management of some common side effects are listed in Table 49-2.

Growth

The impact of stimulant treatment on growth remains a concern, and the data are conflicting. For instance, in the MTA study, ADHD youth, treated with a stimulant medication continuously over a 24-month period, experienced a deceleration of about 1 cm per year. Despite this slowing, except for those subjects in the lowest percentile for height, these children remained within the normal curves.[78] Recently, Biederman and colleagues reported on growth trajectories in two case-control samples of boys and girls with ADHD compared to controls.[79] Over 10–11 years of follow-up these authors found no significant impact of ADHD or its treatment on growth parameters except in subjects with ADHD and depression, where girls were larger and boys smaller. Despite reassuring data clinicians, parents and patients healthy physical development and these difficulties do not usually pose significant clinical problems for most patients. To effectively address these concerns the AACAP practice parameters for ADHD recommend routine monitoring of height and weight, including serial plotting of growth parameters.[1,20] Crossing two percentile lines of height and/or weight may indicate a clinically significant change in growth that should be addressed clinically. A variety of options may be considered, including a medication holiday, dose adjustment, a change in medication, and/or consultation. Ultimately impact on growth should be balanced with the overall benefits of treatment.

Sleep

Parents often report sleep disturbances in their children with ADHD before[80–83] and during treatment.[84–87] Various strategies (including improving sleep hygiene, making behavioral modifications, adjusting timing or type of stimulant, and switching to an alternative ADHD treatment) have been suggested to help make it easier for patients with ADHD to fall asleep.[88,89] Complementary pharmacological treatments to consider include the following: melatonin (1 to 3 mg), clonidine (0.1 to 0.3 mg),[90] diphenhydramine (25 to 50 mg), trazodone (25 to 50 mg), and mirtazapine (3.75 to 15 mg). Recently, interest in the use of melatonin, a hormone secreted by the pineal gland that helps regulate circadian rhythms,[91] to address sleep problems in children has been growing.[92] Melatonin used alone[93] and in conjunction with sleep hygiene techniques[94] appears to improve sleep in youths with ADHD. In these two well-designed but small studies, the most concerning adverse events included migraine (n = 1), nightmares (n = 1), and aggression (n = 1). Although not yet studied, another consideration is ramelteon, a synthetic melatonin receptor agonist.[95]

Appetite Suppression

Patients treated with stimulants often experience a dose-related reduction in appetite, and in some cases weight loss.[74] Although appetite suppression often decreases over time,[42] clinicians

TABLE 49-2 Pharmacological Strategies in Challenging Cases of Attention-Deficit/Hyperactivity Disorder

Symptoms	Interventions
Worsening or unchanged ADHD symptoms (inattention, impulsivity, hyperactivity)	Change medication dose (increase or decrease) Change timing of dose Change preparation, substitute stimulant Evaluate for possible tolerance Consider adjunctive treatment (antidepressant, alpha-adrenergic agent, cognitive enhancer) Consider adjusting non-pharmacological treatment (cognitive-behavioral therapies or coaching or re-evaluating neuropsychological profile for executive function capacities)
Intolerable side effects	Evaluate if side effect is drug-induced Assess medication response versus tolerability of side effect Aggressive management of side effect (change timing of dose; change preparation of stimulant; adjunctive or alternative treatment)
Symptoms of rebound	Change timing of dose Supplement with small dose of short-acting stimulant or alpha-adrenergic agent 1 hour before symptom onset Change preparation Increase frequency of dosage
Development of tics or Tourette's syndrome (TS) or use with co-morbid tics or TS	Assess persistence of tics or TS If tics abate, re-challenge If tics are clearly worsened with stimulant treatment, discontinue Consider stimulant use with adjunctive anti-tic treatment (haloperidol, pimozide) or use of alternative treatment (antidepressants, alpha-adrenergic agents)
Emergence of dysphoria, irritability, acceleration, agitation	Assess for toxicity or rebound Evaluate development or exacerbation of co-morbidity (mood, anxiety, and substance use [including nicotine and caffeine]) Reduce dose Change stimulant preparation Assess sleep and mood Consider alternative treatment
Emergence of major depression, mood lability, or marked anxiety symptoms	Assess for toxicity or rebound Evaluate development or exacerbation of co-morbidity Reduce or discontinue stimulant Consider use of antidepressant or anti-manic agent Assess substance use Consider non-pharmacological interventions
Emergence of psychosis or mania	Discontinue stimulant Assess co-morbidity Assess substance use Treat psychosis or mania

should give guidance on improving the patient's nutritional options with higher caloric intake to balance the consequences of decreased food intake.[19] While appetite suppression is a common side effect of stimulants, little research has been done studying remedies. Cyproheptadine, in doses of 4 to 8 mg, has recently been reported to improve appetite in ADHD patients with stimulant-associated appetite suppression.[96]

Medication Interactions with Stimulants

The interactions of stimulants with other prescription and non-prescription medications are generally mild and not a major source of concern.[97,98] Concomitant use of sympatho-mimetic agents (e.g., pseudoephedrine) may potentiate the effects of both medications. Likewise, excessive intake of caffeine may potentially compromise the effectiveness of the stimulants and exacerbate sleep difficulties. Although data on the co-administration of stimulants with tricyclic antidepressants (TCAs) suggest little interaction between these compounds,[99] careful monitoring is warranted when prescribing stimulants with either TCAs or anticonvulsants. Although administering stimulants with ATMX is common in clinical practice, and appears to be safe, well tolerated, and effective based on clinical experience, to date only small samples have been studied; therefore, patients taking this combination

should be monitored closely.[100] In fact, co-administration of stimulants with MAOIs is the only true contraindication.

Despite the increasing use of stimulants for patients with ADHD, many of them may not respond, experience untoward side effects, or manifest co-morbidity, which stimulants may exacerbate or be ineffective in treating.[17,101] Over the last 10 years ATMX has been systematically evaluated and is FDA-approved for the treatment of ADHD in children, adolescents, and adults.[28]

ATOMOXETINE

Unlike the stimulants, atomoxetine (ATMX; Strattera) is unscheduled; therefore, clinicians can prescribe refills. ATMX acts by blocking the NE re-uptake pump on the pre-synaptic membrane, thus increasing the availability of intra-synaptic NE, with little affinity for other monoamine transporters or neurotransmitter receptors.[102] In addition to prominent effects of ATMX on NE re-uptake inhibition, pre-clinical data also show that the noradrenergic pre-synaptic re-uptake protein regulates DA in the frontal lobes and that by blocking this protein ATMX increases DA in the frontal lobes.[103] ATMX is rapidly absorbed following oral administration; food does not appear to affect absorption, and C_{max} occurs 1 to 2 hours after dosing.[104] While the plasma half-life appears to be around 5 hours, the central nervous system (CNS) effects appear to last over 24 hours.[105] ATMX is metabolized primarily in the liver to 4-hydroxyatomoxetine by the cytochrome (CYP) P450 2D6 enzyme.[106,107] Although patients identified as "poor metabolizers" (i.e., with low 2D6 activity) appear to generally tolerate ATMX, these patients seem to have more side effects, and a reduction in dose may be necessary.[108,109] Therefore, in patients who are taking medications that are strong 2D6 inhibitors (e.g., fluoxetine, paroxetine, quinidine), it may be necessary to reduce the dose of ATMX. Clinically, ATMX is often prescribed in conjunction with stimulants. Although the safety, tolerability, and efficacy of this combination have not been fully studied, reports suggest that this combination is well tolerated and effective.[100,110,111] Therefore, although the full safety of administering stimulants and ATMX together has not been fully established, there are good data from which to extrapolate, and clinicians must balance the risks and benefits in each patient.

Clinical Use of Atomoxetine

ATMX should be initiated at 0.5 mg/kg/day and after a few days increased to a target dose of 1.2 mg/kg/day. Although ATMX has been studied in doses of up to 2 mg/kg/day, current dosing guidelines recommend a maximum dosage of 1.4 mg/kg/day. Although some patients have an early response, it may take up to 10 weeks to see the full benefits of ATMX treatment.[112–114] In the initial trials, ATMX was dosed BID (typically after breakfast and after dinner); however, recent studies have demonstrated its efficacy and tolerability in many patients dosed once a day.[115–117] Although the effects of ATMX dosed once daily in the morning or at bedtime appear to be similar (with a mean dose of 1.25 mg/kg/morning or 1.26 mg/kg/night), once-daily ATMX appears to be best tolerated when dosed in the evening. To date, plasma levels of ATMX have not been used to guide dosing. However, Dunn and colleagues[118] found that patients with a plasma level of ATMX greater than 800 ng/ml had more robust responses, although patients treated with higher doses also experienced more side effects.

ATMX may be particularly useful when anxiety, mood symptoms, or tics co-occur with ADHD. For example, a large, 14-week multi-site study of ATMX in adults with ADHD and social anxiety disorder reported clinically significant effects on both ADHD and on anxiety.[119] Although untested, because of its lack of abuse liability,[120] ATMX may be particularly of use in adults with current substance use issues. For instance, Wilens and associates[121] demonstrated in a 12-week controlled trial that treatment with ATMX in recently abstinent alcoholics was associated with improved ADHD and reduced drinking, although absolute abstinent rates were unaffected. Moreover, ATMX has not been reported to have significant or serious drug interactions with alcohol or marijuana.[122]

Side Effects of Atomoxetine

Although generally well tolerated, the most common side effects in children and adolescents taking ATMX include reduced appetite, dyspepsia, and dizziness,[28] although height and weight in long-term use appear to be on target.[113] In adults, ATMX treatment may be associated with dry mouth, insomnia, nausea, decreased appetite, constipation, decreased libido, dizziness, and sweating.[123] Furthermore, some men taking ATMX may have difficulty attaining or maintaining erections. Several easy strategies can be used to manage ATMX's side effects. When patients experience nausea, the dose of ATMX should be divided and administered with food. Sedation is often transient, but may be helped by either administering the dose at night or by dividing the dose. If mood swings occur, patients should be evaluated and their diagnosis reassessed.

Although ATMX treatment is associated with mean increases in heart rate of 6 beats per minute, and increases in systolic and diastolic blood pressure of 1.5 mm Hg, the impact of ATMX on the cardiovascular system appears to be minimal.[124–126] Extensive electrocardiogram (ECG) monitoring indicates that ATMX has no apparent effect on QTc intervals, and ECG monitoring outside of routine medical care does not appear to be necessary. Adults should have their vital signs checked prior to initiating treatment with ATMX and periodically thereafter.

Concerns have been raised that treatment with ATMX may increase the risk of hepatitis. During post-marketing surveillance, two patients (out of 3 million exposures) developed hepatitis during treatment with ATMX.[127] Patients and families should contact their doctors if they develop pruritus, jaundice, dark urine, right upper quadrant tenderness, or unexplained "flu-like" symptoms.[28]

The FDA issued a public health advisory, and the manufacturer later added a black box warning regarding the development of suicidal ideation in patients treated with ATMX.[28] Similar to the selective serotonin re-uptake inhibitors (SSRIs), there was a slight increase in suicidal thinking in controlled trials. Parents and caregivers should be made aware of any such occurrences and should monitor unexpected changes in mood or behavior.

Alpha-adrenergic Agonists

Clonidine, an imidazoline derivative with alpha-adrenergic agonist properties, has been primarily used in the treatment of hypertension.[128] At low doses, it appears to stimulate inhibitory, pre-synaptic autoreceptors in the CNS.[129] In 2010 the FDA approved an extended delivery oral formulation of clonidine, clonidine ER (Kapvay) as a treatment for ADHD in youth aged 6–17 years.[28] This formulation is approved both as monotherapy and as adjunctive treatment with stimulants. Although clonidine reduces symptoms of ADHD,[130] its overall effect is less than the stimulants,[131] and likely smaller than ATMX, TCAs, and bupropion. Clonidine appears to be particularly helpful in patients with ADHD and co-morbid CD or ODD,[132–134] tic disorders,[135,136] ADHD-associated sleep disturbances,[90,137] and may reduce anxiety and hypervigilance in traumatized children.[138]

Clonidine is a relatively short-acting compound with a plasma half-life ranging from approximately 5.5 hours (in children) to 8.5 hours (in adults). Clonidine ER is usually initiated a dose of 0.1 mg HS for several days and titrated up to a maximum recommended dose of 0.2 mg BID. Immediate release clonidine usually initiated at the lowest manufactured dose of a half or quarter tablet of 0.1 mg. Usual daily doses ranges from 3 to 10 μg/kg given generally in divided doses, BID, three times daily (TID), or four times daily (QID), and there is a transdermal preparation. The most common short-term adverse effect of clonidine is sedation, which tends to subside with continued treatment. It can also produce, in some cases, hypotension, dry mouth, vivid dreams, depression, and confusion. A recent summary of the safety of Kapvay is available at http://www.fda.gov/downloads/Advisory Committees/CommitteesMeetingMaterials/PediatricAdvisory Committee/UCM319363.pdf. Overdoses of clonidine in children under 5 years of age may have life-threatening consequences.[139] Since abrupt withdrawal of clonidine has been associated with rebound hypertension, slow tapering is advised.[140,141] In addition, extreme caution should be exercised with the co-administration of clonidine with beta-blockers or calcium channel blockers.[142] Although concerns about the safety of co-administration of clonidine with stimulants have been debated,[143] recent data supports the tolerability, safety, and efficacy of this combination.[144] Current guidelines are to monitor blood pressure when initiating and tapering clonidine, but ECG monitoring is not usually necessary.[145]

Guanfacine, the most selective alpha$_{2A}$-adrenergic agonist currently available, appears to act by mimicking NE binding in the pre-frontal cortex.[146] In 2009, an extended delivery formulation guanfacine ER (Intuniv) was FDA-approved for the treatment of ADHD as monotherapy or as adjunctive treatment with stimulants.[28] Guanfacine ER is usually started at 1 mg daily at bedtime and titrated to a maximum dose of 4 mg. Possible advantages of guanfacine over clonidine include less sedation, a longer duration of action, and since it has little affinity for the brainstem imidazoline I1 receptors, may have a milder cardiovascular profile.[146] Recent information from the FDA about post-marketing experience with Intuniv is available at http://www.fda.gov/downloads/AdvisoryCommittees/CommitteesMeetingMaterials/PediatricAdvisoryCommittee/UCM255105.pdf. Anecdotal information suggests that guanfacine may be more useful in improving the cognitive deficits of ADHD. School-aged children with ADHD and co-morbid tic disorder, treated with immediate release guanfacine in doses ranging from 0.5 mg BID to 1 mg TID, showed reduction in both tics and ADHD.[147,148] Guanfacine treatment is associated with minor, clinically insignificant decreases in blood pressure and pulse rate. The adverse effects of guanfacine include sedation, irritability, and depression. Several cases of apparent guanfacine-induced mania have been described, but the impact of guanfacine on mood disorders remains unclear.[149] Alpha-adrenergic medications may be particularly useful in youth with primarily a hyperactive/impulsive and/or aggressive component.[150] However, there is a dearth of data on using the alpha agonists in adults with ADHD.

SUGGESTED MANAGEMENT STRATEGIES ACROSS THE LIFE SPAN

Having made the diagnosis of ADHD, the adult needs to be familiarized with the risks and benefits of pharmacotherapy, the availability of alternative treatments, and the likely adverse effects. Patient expectations need to be explored and realistic goals of treatment need to be clearly delineated.[151] Likewise, the clinician should review with the patient the various pharmacological options available and that each will require systematic trials of the anti-ADHD medications for reasonable durations of time and at clinically meaningful doses. Patients with ADHD who have psychiatric co-morbidity, residual symptomatology despite treatment, or report psychological distress related to their ADHD (e.g., self-esteem issues, self-sabotaging patterns, interpersonal disturbances) should be directed to appropriate psychotherapeutic intervention with clinicians knowledgeable in ADHD treatment.

Recognizing the morbidity associated with ADHD, its effect on psychological, social, and emotional development, as well as co-morbid/residual psychiatric and ADHD symptoms, it is necessary to tailor a comprehensive treatment plan. The foundations of such planning involve education, pharmacotherapy, and psychosocial treatments. Support with educational planning, social interactions, and the work environment is often helpful and complimentary to pharmacotherapy.

The stimulant medications, ATMX, guanfacine ER, and clonidine ER are FDA-approved and are considered the first-line therapy for ADHD across the life span. Although there are no evidence-based guidelines in selecting a first choice of medication for patients with ADHD, it is important to consider issues of co-morbidity, tolerability, efficacy, and duration of action.[1,19,20,70,72] The European Network Adult ADHD published a consensus outlining guidelines regarding ADHD treatment with stimulants. The guidelines recommended that the severity of ADHD and co-morbid disorders should be the first guide to select treatments, with stimulants being the medication of choice. Long-lasting, extended-release formulations are preferred for reasons of adherence to treatment, for protection against abuse, to avoid rebound symptoms, and to provide symptomatic relief throughout the day without the need for multiple doses. Every few days the dose may be increased to optimize response. Frequently, patients benefit from adding immediate-release amphetamine or MPH in combination with longer-acting preparations in order to sculpt the dose to the patient's individual needs,[152] although the efficacy of this practice is not well studied. Additionally, psychotherapy is recommended in combination with stimulant treatment in order to relieve additional impairments.[70]

Consideration of another stimulant or ATMX is recommended when symptoms aren't unresponsive or the patient experiences clinically significant side effects to the initial medication. Given their pharmacodynamic differences,[26] if a MPH product was initially selected, then moving to an amphetamine-based medication is appropriate. Although some patients are able to take ATMX once daily, many benefit from BID dosing.[123] Patients must also be made aware that the full benefits of ATMX may not occur for several weeks and they may not "feel" anything like they may have with the stimulants. Monitoring routine side effects, vital signs, and the misuse of the medication is warranted.

SAFETY OF MEDICATIONS USED TO TREAT ATTENTION-DEFICIT/HYPERACTIVITY DISORDER

The FDA's Pediatric Drugs Advisory Committee (PDAC) reviewed data concerning the cardiovascular (CV) effects of medications used to treat ADHD, as well as concerns regarding psychosis, mania, and suicidal thinking.

Cardiovascular Safety of Attention-Deficit/Hyperactivity Disorder Treatments

Treatment with stimulants is associated with small increases in heart rate and blood pressure that are weakly correlated with dose. There has been concern about CV safety/risk in patients receiving stimulants.[153] However, recent work has shed light on the CV risk of stimulants in adults. Habel and colleagues retrospectively investigated serious CV events in a large group of medication users and non-users (n = 443,198 adults aged 25–64). The authors reported on 806,182 person-years of follow-up (median, 1.3 years per person), and found no relationship between past or current ADHD medication use and serious CV or stroke outcomes. As highlighted by these authors[125] among young and middle-aged adults, current or new use of ADHD medications, compared with non-use or remote use, was not associated with an increased risk of serious cardiovascular events. These results mirror the findings of a similarly-designed study in youth with ADHD[126] and a recent review of the cardiovascular literature related to stimulant exposure in ADHD[154] and seems to suggest that the vital sign changes seen acutely and chronically are usually not clinically significant. Please see Table 49-3 for one way to screen for CV symptoms prior to the initiation of pharmacotherapy and while monitoring treatment.

The PDAC cited the baseline rate of sudden unexplained death in the pediatric population to range from 0.6 to 6 occurrences per 100,000 patient-years.[155] From the FDA's research, the PDAC presented data indicating that the rates of sudden unexplained death in the pediatric population between 1992 and February 2005, treated with MPH, amphetamine, or ATMX, were 0.2, 0.3, and 0.5 cases per 100,000 patient-years,

TABLE 49-3 A Strategy to Screen for Cardiovascular Symptoms

Cardiovascular History	Yes	No	Comment
PERSONAL HISTORY			
Congenital or acquired cardiac disease?			
Coronary artery disease?			
Chest pain?			
Palpitations?			
Shortness of breath?			
Dizziness?			
Syncope?			
Change in exercise tolerance or tolerance to usual physical activities?			
FAMILY HISTORY (<30 YEARS OF AGE)			
Early myocardial infarction?			
Cardiac death?			
Significant arrhythmia(s)?			
Long QT syndrome?			
OBJECTIVE			
Baseline (off medication) blood pressure and heart rate within normal limits			

This tool may be useful for screening at initial assessment and prior to initiation of medication(s) used to treat ADHD. As a part of follow-up visits this tool may be used as one way to monitor ongoing treatment as well as prior to changing medication dose(s). During ongoing treatment we encourage clinicians to inquire about current cardiovascular symptoms, measure pulse and blood pressure as well as changes to family history
[a]Copyright Timothy E. Wilens, MD Published with permission.
[b]If positive on an item, recommend referral to primary care physician or cardiology for further assessment prior to initiating medications
(Adapted from Massachusetts General Hospital Cardiovascular Screen[a,b])

respectively. Based on these data, the PDAC *rejected* adding a black box warning, but recommended that current labeling language for amphetamine drugs on CV risks in patients with structural cardiac abnormalities should be extended to all medications approved for the treatment of ADHD. Details regarding these issues are provided in two recent reviews.[156,157]

The American Heart Association has previously commented on CV monitoring of youths taking psychotropic medications.[145] Despite the generally benign CV effects of these medications, caution is warranted in the presence of a compromised CV system (e.g., untreated hypertension, arrhythmias, and known structural heart defects). It remains prudent to monitor symptoms referable to the CV system (e.g., syncope, palpitations, and chest pain) and vital signs at baseline and with treatment in all patients with ADHD. For most pediatric patients it is not necessary to check an ECG at baseline or with treatment. In patients at risk for CV symptoms, it is important to collaborate with the patient's primary care physician and to ensure that hypertension is not an issue. Recent data from an open-label study of ADHD treatment in adults suggest that if hypertension is well controlled, stimulants may be safely used in the short term.[158] Safety remains the paramount concern; thus, in each case the physician and patient must weigh the risks and benefits of treatment.

Aggression during Treatment with Attention-Deficit/Hyperactivity Disorder Medications

From the FDA's research, the PDAC presented data reporting episodes of aggression with all ADHD medications during clinical trials and in post-marketing surveillance. However, aggression in patients with ADHD usually responds to stimulant treatment.[159] During clinical trials, rates of aggression were observed to be similar with active and placebo treatment. The PDAC recommended that the decision about whether to continue therapy following an aggression event is complex and that the physician and parent should evaluate whether the

risks outweigh the benefits that the child obtains from the treatment.

Psychotic or Manic Symptoms during Treatment with Attention-Deficit/Hyperactivity Disorder Medications

The FDA has received hundreds of reports of psychotic or manic symptoms, particularly hallucinations, associated with ADHD medication use in children and adolescents. FDA drug-safety analysts recommended adding warnings to ADHD medication-labeling advising that ADHD medications should be stopped if a patient experiences signs and symptoms of psychosis or mania. A recent review of stimulant trials revealed that psychotic-like or manic-like symptoms might occur in approximately 0.25% of children (or 1 in 400) treated with stimulant medications.[160]

In conclusion, the PDAC recommended that a medication guide be issued for all ADHD medications describing the potential psychiatric, aggression, and CV risks and that these risks be clearly elucidated in the product labeling of all ADHD medications. However, the PDAC concluded that potential episodes of psychosis, aggression, suicidality, and cardiac events during treatment with ADHD medications in children do not warrant a black box warning.

Currently the only black box warning for stimulants warns about the potential for substance abuse.

ALTERNATIVE (NOT FDA-APPROVED) TREATMENTS FOR ATTENTION-DEFICIT/HYPERACTIVITY DISORDER
Bupropion

Bupropion hydrochloride (Wellbutrin), a unicyclic aminoketone, approved for treatment of depression and as an aid for smoking cessation in adults,[28] has been reported to be moderately helpful in reducing ADHD symptoms in children, adolescents,[161–163] and adults.[164–167] Although helpful, the magnitude of effect of bupropion is less than that seen with either stimulants or ATMX. Bupropion is often used in patients with ADHD and co-morbidities and has been studied in small groups of adolescents with ADHD and nicotine dependence,[168] substance use and mood disorders,[169] substance abuse and conduct disorder,[170] and depression.[171] In light of the high rates of marijuana use in patients with ADHD,[172] it is important for clinicians to note that adolescents treated with bupropion may experience increased irritability during marijuana withdrawal.[173] In addition, bupropion has been helpful in ADHD adults with BPD,[174] substance use[175,176] or with co-existing cardiac abnormalities.[177]

Bupropion modulates both NE and DA. It appears to be more stimulating than other antidepressants, may cause irritability, has been reported to exacerbate tics,[178] and is associated with higher rates of drug-induced seizures than other antidepressants.[28] These seizures appear to be dose-related (>450 mg/day) and more likely to occur in patients with bulimia or a seizure disorder, and thus should be avoided in patients with these problems. In ADHD adults, bupropion IR and SR should be given in divided doses, with no single dose of the IR exceeding 150 mg, or SR 200 mg. Dosing for ADHD appears to be similar to that for depression. The once-daily preparation of bupropion is usually initiated at 150 mg XL once in AM and titrated every 7–14 days to maximum dose of 450 mg XL daily. Common side effects include insomnia, edginess, tremor, and a risk for seizures, primarily with immediate-release preparations.

Tricyclic Antidepressants

Although controlled trials in ADHD youths[179] and adults[180] demonstrate TCAs' efficacy, the effects are less robust than with stimulants. Compared to the stimulants, TCAs have negligible abuse liability, have once-daily dosing, and may be useful in patients with co-morbid anxiety, ODD,[181] tics,[182] and, theoretically, depression (adults). However, given concerns about potential cardiotoxicity and the available of ATMX, guanfacine ER and clonidine ER, use of the TCAs has been significantly curtailed.

Before treatment with a TCA, a baseline ECG should be obtained (as well as inquiry into any family history of early-onset or sudden cardiac arrhythmias).[183] Dosing for ADHD appears to be similar to that for depression. ECGs should be obtained as the dose is increased. Monitoring serum levels of TCAs is more helpful in avoiding toxicity than it is in determining optimal levels for response.

Common short-term adverse consequences of the TCAs include dry mouth, blurred vision, orthostasis, and constipation. Since the anticholinergic effects of TCAs limit salivary flow, they may cause dental problems. Following the sudden death of a number of children receiving desipramine (DMI), concerns were raised regarding the possible cardiac toxicity of TCAs in children.[184] However, epidemiological evaluation of the association between DMI and sudden death in children has not supported a causal relationship.[185] TCAs predictably increase heart rate and are associated with conduction delays, usually affecting the right bundle, thus requiring ECG monitoring.[186] However, these effects, when small, rarely seem to be pathophysiologically significant in non-cardiac patients with normal baseline ECGs. In patients with documented congenital or acquired cardiac disease, pathological rhythm disturbances (e.g., atrioventricular block, supraventricular tachycardia, ventricular tachycardia, and Wolff-Parkinson-White syndrome), family history of sudden cardiac death or cardiomyopathy, diastolic hypertension (>90 mm Hg), or when in doubt about the CV state of the patient, a complete (non-invasive) cardiac evaluation is indicated before initiation

of treatment with a TCA to help determine the risk–benefit ratio of such an intervention. A serious adverse event associated with use of TCAs is overdose. Hence, close supervision of the administration and storage of TCAs is necessary.

Modafinil

Modafinil, a novel stimulant that is distinct from amphetamine, is approved for the treatment of narcolepsy.[28] Unlike the broad activation observed with amphetamine, modafinil appears to activate specific hypothalamic regions.[187,188] Although one controlled trial in ADHD adults was positive,[189] a recent large (n = 330) multi-center (18 locations) randomized, double-blind treatment study in adults with ADHD did not find significant reductions in subjects treated with modafinil compared to those treated with placebo.[190] However, these investigators noted that certain subjects experienced significant benefit and suggest that this agent may warrant further investigation. Although controlled trials of modafinil in children with ADHD demonstrated efficacy,[191-193] the FDA PDAC voted that modafinil is "not approvable" for pediatric ADHD due to possible Stevens-Johnson syndrome (SJS) and toxic epidermal necrolysis (TEN). Clinically, it may be reasonable to consider combining modafinil with stimulants,[194,195] and clinicians should be aware of the potential to exacerbate mania.[196]

NOVEL TREATMENTS FOR ATTENTION-DEFICIT/HYPERACTIVITY DISORDER
Nicotinic Agents

Given the cognitive enhancing properties of nicotine,[197] nicotinic agents have been studied in the treatment of ADHD. Whereas smaller cross-over studies of nicotinic analogs with either full or partial agonist properties demonstrated efficacy in adults with ADHD,[198-200] follow-up larger multi-site parallel design studies failed to show a significant effect of this compound on reducing ADHD symptomatology[201] and the role of nicotinic agents remains investigational.

Medications Used in the Treatment of Alzheimer's Disease

Although compelling based on efficacy in Alzheimer's disease and some positive initial experience in ADHD patients[202] trials in ADHD adults with donepezil[203] and galantamine[204] were negative. At this time there are no data to support the use of these cholinergic agents in the treatment of ADHD. Recently, Surman and colleagues[205] openly treated 34 ADHD adults with the N-methyl-D-aspartate (NMDA) receptor antagonist memantine. In this pilot study, memantine, titrated to a maximum dose of 10 mg BID, was generally well tolerated and resulted in improvements in measures of ADHD symptoms and neuropsychological measures. These encouraging but preliminary results warrant controlled study.

Metadoxine

Recently, MG01CI, an extended-release formulation of metadoxine has been studied in adults with ADHD. Metadoxine is an ion-pair salt of pyridoxine (vitamin B$_6$) and 2-pyrrolidone-5-carboxylate used in Europe for over 30 years in the treatment of acute alcohol intoxication and withdrawal. In a short-term controlled trial with MG01CI, subjects experienced improvements in ADHD symptoms as well as neuropsychological measures and overall functioning.[206]

Selegiline

Selegiline (l-deprenyl), an irreversible type B monoamine oxidase inhibitor (MAOI) that is metabolized into amphetamine and methamphetamine, has been compared to MPH in two trials of ADHD youths[207,208] and alone in adults.[209] Previous work with selegiline in children with ADHD and Tourette's syndrome suggests that it may reduce symptoms of ADHD.[210,211] Although to date its role in the treatment of ADHD has been limited by both the availability of alternative treatments and potential for the "cheese reaction," its formulation as a patch,[212] which may diminish this reaction, may increase interest in its use.

PHARMACOTHERAPY OF ATTENTION-DEFICIT/ HYPERACTIVITY DISORDER AND COMMON CO-MORBID PSYCHIATRIC DISORDERS

Attention-Deficit/Hyperactivity Disorder and Aggression

The importance of aggression should not be underestimated, as these patients often suffer severe psychopathology, adversely affect their families/communities, and have high rates of service utilization.[213] Although medications are usually effective in reducing symptoms of ADHD and impulsive aggression,[22,23] these patients usually benefit from multi-modal treatment.[214–216] Medications should initially treat the most severe underlying disorder, after which targeting specific symptoms (e.g., irritability, hostility, hypervigilance, impulsivity, fear, or emotional dysregulation) is appropriate.[217,218] These patients often display aggression before, and during, the course of treatment, making it imperative to document their aggressive behaviors before the introduction of medications and to make these behaviors an explicit target of treatment. The PDAC of the FDA suggests that if and when a patient displays worsening of aggressive behaviors during medication treatment for ADHD, the clinician should make a judgment regarding the tolerability and efficacy of the treatment (see www.fda.gov for the most recent recommendations).

In patients with co-morbid ADHD and ODD/CD, the clinician should first attempt to optimize the pharmacotherapy of ADHD[219] followed by augmentation with behavioral treatments. Supporting this strategy, a meta-analysis of studies from 1975 to 2001 found that stimulants significantly reduced both overt and covert aggression as rated by parents, teachers, and clinicians.[159] During the MTA trial, ADHD youths with and without ODD or CD responded robustly and equally well to stimulant medication.[220] Furthermore, in the MTA study, behavioral therapy without concomitant medication was less effective in subjects with ADHD and ODD/CD. Similarly, in ADHD youth treatment with ATMX, MAS XR, and OROS-MPH reduced ODD symptoms.[42,221–223] While these interventions are often sufficient, a significant number of these patients have severe symptoms that necessitate treatment with additional or alternative medications. Neuroleptic use should be limited to those ADHD patients with severe aggression or disruptive or mood disorders.[224,225]

In recent years the use of atypical antipsychotics in pediatric populations has increased considerably.[226] The American Academy of Child and Adolescent Psychiatry has published treatment recommendations for the use of antipsychotic medications in aggressive youth.[215,216] Clinicians are encouraged to optimize psychosocial/educational interventions, followed by appropriate pharmacotherapy of the primary psychiatric disorder, followed by use of an atypical antipsychotic medication. Treatment with atypical antipsychotics warrants careful monitoring as various side effects may be anticipated. These include sedation or extrapyramidal symptoms (EPS), which usually occur during initiation of therapy, while others, such as akathisia or dyskinesia/dystonias, may develop after several months of therapy. Clinicians are encouraged to monitor these side effects and to document abnormal movements using the Abnormal Involuntary Movement Scale (AIMS) on a periodic basis. Patients treated with atypical antipsychotics should also be monitored for sedation, hyperprolactinemia, CV symptoms, weight gain, and development of a metabolic syndrome. Although not specifically written for children, the American Diabetes Association recommends that while treating patients with atypical antipsychotics clinicians should inquire about a family history of diabetes, as well as regularly monitor patients' body mass index, waist circumference, blood pressure, fasting blood glucose, and fasting lipid profile.[227,228] Safety remains the paramount consideration, and after a period of remission of the aggressive symptoms, consideration should be given to tapering off of the atypical antipsychotic. Tapering atypical antipsychotics should proceed slowly in order to prevent withdrawal dyskinesias and to allow adequate time to adjust to the reduced dose. If there is evidence of severe mood instability, other mood stabilizers should be considered (see below).

Attention-Deficit/Hyperactivity Disorder Plus Anxiety Disorders

Anxiety disorders, including agoraphobia, panic, over-anxious disorder, simple phobia, separation anxiety disorder, and OCD, frequently occur in children, adolescents, and adults with ADHD.[5,11,23,229] The effect of stimulant treatment in youths with ADHD and anxiety has been variable. Earlier studies found increased placebo response, increased side effects, and a reduced response to stimulants in patients with both conditions,[230–232] whereas others observed stimulant treatment to be well tolerated and effective.[23,220,233] Many youths with ADHD and anxiety experience robust improvements with stimulant treatment and may not experience exacerbations of anxiety.[234,235] Of interest, ATMX is reported to reduce anxiety in ADHD youths[236] and adults.[119] The Texas Medication Algorithm Project (TMAP) Consensus Panel recommends beginning pharmacotherapy for patients with ADHD and a co-morbid anxiety disorder with either ATMX aimed at both the ADHD and anxiety or prescribing a stimulant first to address the ADHD, then adding an SSRI to address the anxiety if necessary.[219]

Attention-Deficit/Hyperactivity Disorder Plus Obsessive-compulsive Disorder

Considerable overlap exists between pediatric ADHD and OCD,[237] including rates of ADHD in up to 51% of children and 36% of adolescents with OCD.[238,239] In general, patients with OCD and ADHD require treatment for both conditions. The SSRIs, especially in combination with cognitive-behavioral therapy (CBT), are well-established treatments for pediatric and adult OCD.[240] Although stimulants may exacerbate tics, obsessions, or compulsions, they are frequently used in patients with these conditions, often in combination with SSRIs.[19,241,242] Therefore, clinicians should identify and prioritize treatment of the most severe condition first, then address secondary concerns, while monitoring for signs of worsening symptoms while recognizing that patients successfully treated have much residual morbidity and that CBT is an essential component of long-term management.

Attention-Deficit/Hyperactivity Disorder Plus Tic Disorders

Tics and tic disorders commonly occur in patients with ADHD,[241] as well as in students receiving special education services.[243] A community-based study of 3,006 children (6 to 12 years of age) found that 27% with ADHD also had tics, and 56% with tics had ADHD.[244] Tics occurred more commonly in males (2:1 to 6:1) and in youths with combined-type ADHD. Children, adolescents, and adults may suffer the triad of tics, ADHD, and OCD.[245] Pharmacotherapy of youths with ADHD and tic disorders is challenging. First-line treatment about tics is education. In most patients, tics are mild to moderate in severity, have a fluctuating course, even when taking a tic-suppressing medication and generally decline by early adulthood. Although stimulants may exacerbate tics and are listed as a contraindication to the use of MPH,[28] stimulants have been well tolerated and effective in these patients.[241,242,246,247] Randomized treatment with MPH (26.1 mg/day), clonidine (0.25 mg/day), or MPH plus clonidine (26.1 mg/day plus 0.28 mg/day) was studied in 136 children with ADHD and chronic tic disorders.[241] While MPH treatment improved ADHD and clonidine reduced tics, the greatest effect was observed with the combination treatment. Tic severity reduced with all active treatments and in the following order: clonidine plus MPH, clonidine alone, and MPH alone. No clinically significant CV adverse events were noted. The frequency of tic worsening was similar, and not significantly different, in subjects treated with MPH (20%), clonidine (26%), and placebo (22%). Follow-up of children with ADHD and tics treated with MPH over a 2-year period observed improvements in ADHD symptoms without worsening of tics.[242] Given the data on clonidine, interest in guanfacine treatment has grown, and it appears to be effective in reducing symptoms of both ADHD and tics.[147,148]

Palumbo and colleagues[248] observed similar rates of tics during short-term blinded treatment with placebo (3.7%), IR-MPH (2.3%), or OROS-MPH (4.0%). During 24-month open-label treatment with OROS-MPH, the rate of tics remained steady. However, clinicians must still discuss these issues and obtain informed consent from patients and families before using stimulants in patients with tic disorders. Investigations have demonstrated utility of noradrenergic agents, including DMI[182] and ATMX.[249] Although treatment with ATMX was not associated with significant reductions in tics compared to placebo (with reductions of Yale Global Tic Severity Scale −5.5 ± 6.9 versus −3.3 ± 8.9; P = 0.063), tic severity did not worsen and symptoms of ADHD were significantly improved. In patients who do not tolerate or respond to treatment with stimulants, noradrenergic agents, or alpha-adrenergic agents, or their combination, consideration should be given to treatment with a neuroleptic.[219]

Attention-Deficit/Hyperactivity Disorder Plus Depression

Depression and dysthymia are commonly co-morbid with ADHD.[5,11,17,250,251] In ADHD patients, depression is not an artifact,[252] and it must be distinguished from demoralization.[253] Although there are no formal evidence-based guidelines, clinicians should, in general, assess the severity of ADHD and depression and direct their initial treatment toward the most impairing condition. In treating pediatric depression, clinicians must keep in mind recent black box warnings about antidepressants and the risk of suicide. Excellent information for professionals, parents, and patients can be found at www.parentsmedguide.org. Clinicians are also directed to a review of the treatment of pediatric depression.[254] In adults

with ADHD and depression, TCAs remain a reasonable choice and may be helpful for both conditions. As discussed previously, the use of TCAs requires close monitoring.

Attention-Deficit/Hyperactivity Disorder Plus Bipolar Disorder

Although BPD is recognized in ADHD patients, ADHD may complicate the presentation, diagnosis, and treatment of BPD.[255-257] Differentiating BPD from ADHD can be challenging as these disorders share many features (including symptoms of distractibility, hyperactivity, impulsivity, talkativeness, and sleep disturbance).[258-263] Clinicians are faced with the challenging and important task of differentiating BPD, ADHD, ADHD with emotional dysregulation and the new DSM-5 diagnosis of Disruptive Mood Dysregulation Disorder.[264] Data to guide clinicians in this area are emerging, but often conflicting and may be confusing.[265-268] Previous data show that BPD appears to occur at increased rates in ADHD children and adolescents of both genders at baseline (11%) and during longitudinal 4-year follow-up (23%) compared to matched non-ADHD controls (P < 0.01).[269] A large study of BPD in adults funded by the National Institute of Mental Health (NIMH), the Systematic Treatment Enhancement Program for Bipolar Disorder (STEP-BD), observed that 9.5% of adults who present for treatment of BPD had lifetime co-morbid ADHD, with 6% meeting current criteria.[270,271] An array of information about and rating scales to evaluate BPD can be found at www.manicdepressive.org, www.bpkids.org, and www.schoolpsychiatry.org.

Given the severe morbidity of pediatric BPD, families and patients usually benefit from an integrated and coordinated treatment plan that includes medications (often more than one is necessary and appropriate), psychotherapies (individual, group, and family), educational/occupational interventions (accommodations or modifications in school or work), and psychoeducation and parent/family support (available through national organizations such as the National Alliance for the Mentally Ill and the Child and Adolescent Bipolar Foundation).

Medications are usually a fundamental part of the treatment plan of all patients with BPD. The reader is referred to practice guidelines for both pediatric patients[272] and adults.[273] The adult guidelines do not specifically address pharmacotherapy of BPD in the context of co-morbid ADHD; clinicians should first ensure mood stability before the initiation of treatment for ADHD. Patients with BPD type I without symptoms of psychosis should receive monotherapy with either a mood stabilizer (e.g., lithium, valproic acid, or carbamazepine) or an atypical antipsychotic (e.g., risperidone, olanzapine, or quetiapine).[272,274] In patients with only a partial response, the initial medication should be augmented with either an additional mood stabilizer or an atypical antipsychotic. The combination of lithium and valproic acid has been shown to substantially reduce symptoms of mania and depression in children, and in patients with BPD type I with psychosis, both a mood stabilizer and an atypical antipsychotic should be started concurrently (following the same augmentation strategy).

In patients with ADHD plus BPD, for example, the risk of mania or hypomania needs to be addressed and monitored during treatment of ADHD. Once the mood is euthymic, conservative introduction of anti-ADHD medications along with mood-stabilizing agents should be considered.[275] Scheffer and colleagues[276] recently demonstrated the tolerability and efficacy of MAS XR in reducing ADHD symptoms over the short-term in pediatric bipolar patients after successful mood stabilization with VPA. Similarly, in a small short-term trial in bipolar adults, bupropion successfully reduced symptoms of

ADHD without exacerbating mania.[174] McIntyre and colleagues treated 40 mood-stabilized bipolar I/II adults with LDX for their co-morbid ADHD.[277] Short-term (9-week) treatment with a mean dose of 60 ± 10 mg daily subjects reported significant improvements in self-ratings of ADHD and clinicians observed significant improvements in ADHD symptoms and functioning without exacerbations on mania. Case reports also describe successful treatment of ADHD symptoms in bipolar patients with ATMX[278] alone and in combination with OROS-MPH.[279] However, clinicians should advise patients (and perhaps their families) to monitor any induction or exacerbation/worsening of mania or cycling during treatment with ADHD medications.[280–286] In such situations it is necessary to prioritize the mood stabilization, which may also necessitate the discontinuation of the ADHD treatment until euthymia has been achieved.[272,287]

Attention-Deficit/Hyperactivity Disorder Plus Substance Use Disorders

Many adolescents and young adults with ADHD have either a past or current alcohol or drug use disorder, and co-morbidity within ADHD increases the risk.[17,172,288,289] Patients with ADHD frequently misuse a variety of substances (including alcohol, marijuana, cocaine, stimulants, opiates, and nicotine). In fact, children with ADHD start smoking nicotine an average of 2 years earlier than their non-ADHD peers[290] and have increased rates of smoking as adults, more difficulty quitting smoking,[291,292] and nicotine dependence (achieved more rapidly and lasting longer compared to controls).[293,294] Since the rates of substance abuse in patients with ADHD are increased,[295] concerns persist that stimulant treatment contributes to subsequent substance abuse. Wilens and colleagues[296] performed a pooled analysis of six studies that examined the relationship between stimulant treatment and substance abuse. Their meta-analysis revealed that stimulant treatment resulted in a 1.9-fold reduction in risk for later substance abuse among youths treated with a stimulant for ADHD, as compared to those youths receiving no pharmacotherapy for their ADHD.[296] The protective effect was greater through adolescence and less into adulthood. Longitudinal follow-ups also suggest that stimulant pharmacotherapy of ADHD does not increase risk of developing SUD.[297–299]

A careful history of substance use/misuse/abuse should be completed as part of the ADHD evaluation in adolescents and adults.[300] When substance misuse/abuse/dependence is a clinical concern, the clinician should assess the relative severity of the ADHD and the SUD. Furthermore, addictions often affect cognition, behavior, sleep, and mood/anxiety, which make it challenging to assess ADHD symptoms. Stabilizing the addiction and addressing co-morbid disorder(s) are generally the priority when treating ADHD patients with SUD. Treatment for patients with ADHD and SUD usually includes a combination of addiction treatment/psychotherapy and pharmacotherapy.[301] Patients with ongoing substance abuse or dependence should generally not be treated for their ADHD until appropriate addiction treatments have been undertaken and the patient has maintained a drug- and alcohol-free period. The clinician should begin pharmacotherapy with medications that have little likelihood of diversion or low liability, such as bupropion[175] and ATMX,[121] and, if necessary, progress to the stimulants. When using stimulants in this patient population, it is wise to prescribe an extended-delivery formulation with minimal risk of misuse (e.g., MTS or LDX), as well as to agree on a method for monitoring the SUD and adherence to the treatment plan. Moreover, since stimulants are Schedule II medications, concerns remain regarding their addictive potential. Concerns about possible diversion and

misuse of stimulant medications remain, making careful monitoring necessary.[302–304] In these populations use of extended-delivery stimulant preparations, which are more difficult to misuse, or non-stimulants should be considered.[301] When administered orally in their intended dosages, stimulants do not appear to cause euphoria, nor do they appear to be addictive.[305,306]

Attention-Deficit/Hyperactivity Disorder Plus Autism Spectrum Disorders

Children, adolescents and adults with ASD may display a persistent and impairing pattern of hyperactivity, impulsivity, and inattention[307–311]; and when these symptoms can be distinguished from core features of ASD, DSM-5 allows clinicians to diagnose ADHD.[264] In treating this group of patients, clinicians, in collaboration with parents, balance the risks and benefits of treatments. In general, the philosophy is to identify target symptoms and to prioritize impairments.

Interest in the pharmacotherapy of ADHD and ASDs is growing. Although earlier work in small samples supported the use of MPH in doses of 0.3 to 0.6 mg/kg/day, these patients often experienced side effects (such as irritability) that limited stimulant use.[312,313] One of the Research Units in Pediatric Psychopharmacology (RUPP) compared placebo to low, medium, and high doses of MPH in 72 children with pervasive developmental disorder and ADHD.[314] In these subjects, although MPH treatment significantly improved attention and reduced distractibility, hyperactivity, and impulsivity, the effect sizes, according to parent and teacher ratings, were smaller than those usually observed in ADHD children. Furthermore, adverse effects, primarily irritability, led to MPH discontinuation in 18%, and occurred most often during treatment with either the medium or high MPH doses. A recent trial in 24 youth with ASD and ADHD found that MPH was generally well tolerated and efficacious in reducing symptoms of hyperactivity and impulsivity.[315] Similarly, data suggest that ATMX may be useful in ASD patients with ADHD symptoms.[316,317] For a full review of pharmacological treatments in ASDs, the interested reader is referred to excellent recent reviews.[318–320]

Attention-Deficit/Hyperactivity Disorder Plus Epilepsy

Children with epilepsy often display difficulties with behavior and cognition, and anticonvulsants may have cognitive side effects. On the other hand, treatment with anticonvulsants may lead to improved seizure control and result in improved cognition and behavior. Although there is ongoing concern that treatment with stimulants may lower the seizure threshold,[28] recent reviews and data challenge the traditional warning and provide evidence for the safe and effective use of stimulants in patients with epilepsy when appropriate antiepileptic treatment is used.[321–324] Current recommendations for evaluation, diagnosis, and treatment of ADHD acknowledge inconsistent findings in the literature on the overlap of ADHD and epilepsy, but do not recommend the use of routine electroencephalograms (EEGs) in the assessment of ADHD.[1,20,70]

MANAGING SUB-OPTIMAL RESPONSES

Despite the availability of various agents for adults with ADHD, there appear to be a number of individuals who either do not respond to, or are intolerant of adverse effects of, medications used to treat their ADHD. In managing difficult cases, several therapeutic strategies are available (see Table 49-2). If psychiatric adverse effects develop concurrent with a poor medication response, alternative treatments should be pursued. Severe psychiatric symptoms that emerge during the acute phase can be problematic, irrespective of the efficacy of the medications for ADHD. These symptoms may require re-consideration of the diagnosis of ADHD and careful re-assessment of the presence of co-morbid disorders. For example, it is common to observe depressive symptoms in an adult with ADHD when symptoms are independent of the ADHD or treatment. If reduction of dose or change in preparation (i.e., regular versus slow-release stimulants) does not resolve the problem, consideration should be given to alternative treatments. Neuroleptic medications should be considered as part of the overall treatment plan in the face of co-morbid BPD or extreme agitation. Concurrent non-pharmacological interventions (such as behavioral or cognitive therapy) may assist with symptom reduction and functional improvements.

CONCLUSION

In conclusion, the aggregate literature supports that pharmacotherapy provides an effective treatment for children, adolescents, and adults with ADHD and co-morbid disorders. Effective pharmacological treatments for ADHD include stimulants and non-stimulants. Structured psychotherapy may be effective when used adjunctly with medications. Groups focused on coping skills, support, and interpersonal psychotherapy may also be very useful for these patients. For adults who are considering advanced schooling, educational planning and alterations in the school environment may be necessary. Further controlled investigations assessing the efficacy of single and combination agents for patients with ADHD are necessary, with careful attention paid to diagnostics, symptom and neuropsychological outcome, long-term tolerability, and efficacy, as well as their use in specific ADHD sub-groups.

Access the complete reference list and multiple choice questions (MCQs) online at https://expertconsult.inkling.com

KEY REFERENCES

1. Wolraich M, Brown L, Brown RT, et al. ADHD: Clinical practice guideline for the diagnosis, evaluation, and treatment of attention-deficit/hyperactivity disorder in children and adolescents. *Pediatrics* 128(5):1007–1022, 2011.
4. Merikangas KR, He JP, Burstein M, et al. Service utilization for lifetime mental disorders in U.S. adolescents: results of the National Comorbidity Survey-Adolescent Supplement (NCS-A). *J Am Acad Child Adolesc Psychiatry* 50(1):32–45, 2011.
5. Kessler RC, Adler L, Barkley R, et al. The prevalence and correlates of adult ADHD in the United States: results from the National Comorbidity Survey Replication. *Am J Psychiatry* 163(4):716–723, 2006.
7. Volkow ND, Swanson JM. Clinical practice: Adult attention deficit-hyperactivity disorder. *N Engl J Med* 369(20):1935–1944, 2013.
11. Biederman J, Monuteaux MC, Mick E, et al. Young adult outcome of attention deficit hyperactivity disorder: a controlled 10-year follow-up study. *Psychol Med* 36(2):167–179, 2006.
17. Biederman J, Faraone SV, Spencer T, et al. Patterns of psychiatric comorbidity, cognition, and psychosocial functioning in adults with attention deficit hyperactivity disorder. *Am J Psychiatry* 150:1792–1798, 1993.
18. Biederman J, Newcorn J, Sprich S. Comorbidity of attention deficit hyperactivity disorder with conduct, depressive, anxiety, and other disorders. *Am J Psychiatry* 148:564–577, 1991.
19. Greenhill LL, Pliszka S, Dulcan MK, et al. Practice parameter for the use of stimulant medications in the treatment of children, adolescents, and adults. *J Am Acad Child Adolesc Psychiatry* 41(2 Suppl.):26S–49S, 2002.

20. Pliszka S. Practice parameter for the assessment and treatment of children and adolescents with attention-deficit/hyperactivity disorder. *J Am Acad Child Adolesc Psychiatry* 46(7):894–921, 2007. [Epub 2007/06/22].
21. Bradley C. The behavior of children receiving benzedrine. *Am J Psychiatry* 94:577–585, 1937.
23. Moderators and mediators of treatment response for children with attention-deficit/hyperactivity disorder: the Multimodal Treatment Study of children with attention-deficit/hyperactivity disorder. *Arch Gen Psychiatry* 56(12):1088–1096, 1999.
36. Spencer TJ, Biederman J, Ciccone PE, et al. PET study examining pharmacokinetics, detection and likeability, and dopamine transporter receptor occupancy of short- and long-acting oral methylphenidate. *Am J Psychiatry* 163(3):387–395, 2006.
70. Kooij SJ, Bejerot S, Blackwell A, et al. European consensus statement on diagnosis and treatment of adult ADHD: The European Network Adult ADHD. *BMC Psychiatry* 10:67, 2010.
71. Wilens TE, Morrison NR, Prince J. An update on the pharmacotherapy of attention-deficit/hyperactivity disorder in adults. *Expert Rev Neurother* 11(10):1443–1465, 2011.
72. Weiss MD, Weiss JR. A guide to the treatment of adults with ADHD. *J Clin Psychiatry* 65(Suppl. 3):27–37, 2004.
73. Ramtvedt BE, Roinas E, Aabech HS, et al. Clinical gains from including both dextroamphetamine and methylphenidate in stimulant trials. *J Child Adolesc Psychopharmacol* 23(9):597–604, 2013.
75. Graham J, Banaschewski T, Buitelaar J, et al. European guidelines on managing adverse effects of medication for ADHD. *Eur Child Adolesc Psychiatry* 20(1):17–37, 2011.
79. Biederman J, Spencer TJ, Monuteaux MC, et al. A naturalistic 10-year prospective study of height and weight in children with attention-deficit hyperactivity disorder grown up: sex and treatment effects. *J Pediatr* 157(4):635–640, 40 e1, 2010.
86. Barrett JR, Tracy DK, Giaroli G. To sleep or not to sleep: a systematic review of the literature of pharmacological treatments of insomnia in children and adolescents with attention-deficit/hyperactivity disorder. *J Child Adolesc Psychopharmacol* 23(10): 640–647, 2013.
89. Cortese S, Brown TE, Corkum P, et al. Assessment and management of sleep problems in youths with attention-deficit/hyperactivity disorder. *J Am Acad Child Adolesc Psychiatry* 52(8):784–796, 2013.
102. Arnsten AF, Pliszka SR. Catecholamine influences on prefrontal cortical function: relevance to treatment of attention deficit/hyperactivity disorder and related disorders. *Pharmacol Biochem Behav* 99(2):211–216, 2011.
125. Habel LA, Cooper WO, Sox CM, et al. ADHD medications and risk of serious cardiovascular events in young and middle-aged adults. *JAMA* 306(24):2673–2683, 2011.
126. Cooper WO, Habel LA, Sox CM, et al. ADHD drugs and serious cardiovascular events in children and young adults. *N Engl J Med* 365(20):1896–1904, 2011.
145. Gutgesell H, Atkins D, Barst R, et al. *Cardiovascular monitoring of children and adolescents receiving psychotropic drugs*, Dallas, 1999, American Heart Association, pp 979–982.
146. Arnsten AF. The use of alpha-2A adrenergic agonists for the treatment of attention-deficit/hyperactivity disorder. *Expert Rev Neurother* 10(10):1595–1605, 2010.
151. Haavik J, Halmoy A, Lundervold AJ, et al. Clinical assessment and diagnosis of adults with attention-deficit/hyperactivity disorder. *Expert Rev Neurother* 10(10):1569–1580, 2010.
154. Hammerness PG, Perrin JM, Shelley-Abrahamson R, et al. Cardiovascular risk of stimulant treatment in pediatric attention-deficit/hyperactivity disorder: update and clinical recommendations. *J Am Acad Child Adolesc Psychiatry* 50(10):978–990, 2011.
157. Wilens TE, Prince JB, Spencer TJ, et al. Stimulants and sudden death: what is a physician to do? *Pediatrics* 118(3):1215–1219, 2006.
160. Ross RG. Psychotic and manic-like symptoms during stimulant treatment of attention deficit hyperactivity disorder. *Am J Psychiatry* 163(7):1149–1152, 2006.
183. Gutgesell H, Atkins D, Barst R, et al. AHA scientific statement: Cardiovascular monitoring of children and adolescents receiving psychotropic drugs. *J Am Acad Child Adolesc Psychiatry* 38(8):979–982, 1999.

219. Pliszka SR, Crismon ML, Hughes CW, et al. The Texas Children's Medication Algorithm Project: revision of the algorithm for pharmacotherapy of attention-deficit/hyperactivity disorder. *J Am Acad Child Adolesc Psychiatry* 45(6):642–657, 2006.

220. Jensen PS, Hinshaw SP, Kraemer HC, et al. ADHD comorbidity findings from the MTA study: comparing comorbid subgroups. *J Am Acad Child Adolesc Psychiatry* 40(2):147–158, 2001.

224. Loy JH, Merry SN, Hetrick SE, et al. Atypical antipsychotics for disruptive behaviour disorders in children and youths. *Cochrane Database Syst Rev* (9):CD008559, 2012.

225. Linton D, Barr AM, Honer WG, et al. Antipsychotic and psychostimulant drug combination therapy in attention deficit/hyperactivity and disruptive behavior disorders: a systematic review of efficacy and tolerability. *Curr Psychiatry Rep* 15(5):355, 2013.

235. Abikoff H, McGough J, Vitiello B, et al. Sequential pharmacotherapy for children with comorbid attention-deficit/hyperactivity and anxiety disorders. *J Am Acad Child Adolesc Psychiatry* 44(5):418–427, 2005.

241. Group TTsSS. Treatment of ADHD in children with tics: A randomized controlled trial. *Neurology* 58(4):527–536, 2002.

251. McIntyre RS, Kennedy SH, Soczynska JK, et al. Attention-deficit/hyperactivity disorder in adults with bipolar disorder or major depressive disorder: results from the international mood disorders collaborative project. *Prim Care Companion J Clin Psychiatry* 12(3):2010.

252. Milberger S, Biederman J, Faraone S, et al. Attention deficit hyperactivity disorder and comorbid disorders: Issues of overlapping symptoms. *Am J Psychiatry* 152(12):1793–1799, 1995.

258. Biederman J, Faraone SV, Wozniak J, et al. Clinical correlates of bipolar disorder in a large, referred sample of children and adolescents. *J Psychiatr Res* 39(6):611–622, 2005.

262. Birmaher B, Axelson D, Goldstein B, et al. Four-year longitudinal course of children and adolescents with bipolar spectrum disorders: the Course and Outcome of Bipolar Youth (COBY) study. *Am J Psychiatry* 166(7):795–804, 2009.

263. Mick E, Spencer T, Wozniak J, et al. Heterogeneity of irritability in attention-deficit/hyperactivity disorder subjects with and without mood disorders. *Biol Psychiatry* 58(7):576–582, 2005.

266. Axelson D, Findling RL, Fristad MA, et al. Examining the proposed disruptive mood dysregulation disorder diagnosis in children in the Longitudinal Assessment of Manic Symptoms study. *J Clin Psychiatry* 73(10):1342–1350, 2012.

268. Barkley RA. Differential diagnosis of adults with ADHD: the role of executive function and self-regulation. *J Clin Psychiatry* 71(7):e17, 2010.

274. Kowatch RA, Youngstrom EA, Horwitz S, et al. Prescription of psychiatric medications and polypharmacy in the LAMS cohort. *Psychiatr Serv* 64(10):1026–1034, 2013.

289. Wilens TE, Martelon M, Joshi G, et al. Does ADHD predict substance-use disorders? A 10-year follow-up study of young adults with ADHD. *J Am Acad Child Adolesc Psychiatry* 50(6):543–553, 2011.

296. Wilens T, Faraone S, Biederman J, et al. Does stimulant therapy of attention-deficit/hyperactivity disorder beget later substance abuse? A meta-analytic review of the literature. *Pediatrics* 111(1):179–185, 2003.

297. Biederman J, Monuteaux MC, Spencer T, et al. Stimulant therapy and risk for subsequent substance use disorders in male adults with ADHD: a naturalistic controlled 10-year follow-up study. *Am J Psychiatry* 165(5):597–603, 2008.

302. McCabe SE, Knight JR, Teter CJ, et al. Non-medical use of prescription stimulants among US college students: prevalence and correlates from a national survey. *Addiction* 100(1):96–106, 2005.

306. Swanson JM, Volkow ND. Serum and brain concentrations of methylphenidate: implications for use and abuse. *Neurosci Biobehav Rev* 27(7):615–621, 2003.

310. Johnston K, Dittner A, Bramham J, et al. Attention deficit hyperactivity disorder symptoms in adults with autism spectrum disorders. *Autism* 6(4):225–236, 2013.

315. Pearson DA, Santos CW, Aman MG, et al. Effects of extended release methylphenidate treatment on ratings of attention-deficit/hyperactivity disorder (ADHD) and associated behavior in children with autism spectrum disorders and ADHD symptoms. *J Child Adolesc Psychopharmacol* 23(5):337–351, 2013.

324. Santos K, Palmini A, Radziuk AL, et al. The impact of methylphenidate on seizure frequency and severity in children with attention-deficit-hyperactivity disorder and difficult-to-treat epilepsies. *Dev Med Child Neurol* 655(7):654–660, 2013.

50 Drug–Drug Interactions in Psychopharmacology

Jonathan E. Alpert, MD, PhD

KEY POINTS

- Drug–drug interactions refer to alterations in drug levels or drug effects (or both) related to the administration of two or more prescribed, recreational, or over-the-counter agents in close temporal proximity.

- Although some drug–drug interactions involving psychotropic medications are life-threatening, most interactions manifest in more subtle ways through increased side-effect burden, aberrant drug levels, or diminished efficacy.

- Pharmacokinetic drug–drug interactions involve a change in the plasma level or tissue concentration of one drug following co-administration of one or more other drugs due to an action of the co-administered agents on one of four key pharmacokinetic processes: absorption, distribution, metabolism, or excretion.

- Pharmacodynamic drug–drug interactions involve an effect of one or more drugs on another drug at biological receptor sites of action and do not involve a change in plasma level or tissue concentration.

- The potential for drug–drug interactions should be carefully considered whenever prescribing medications associated with interactions that are uncommon but catastrophic (e.g., hypertensive crises, Stevens-Johnson syndrome, or cardiac arrhythmias) and medications with low therapeutic indices (e.g., warfarin) or narrow therapeutic windows (e.g., cyclosporine), and when prescribing for frail or clinically brittle patients for whom small variations in side effects or efficacy may be particularly troublesome.

OVERVIEW

An understanding of drug–drug interactions is essential to the practice of psychopharmacology.[1,2] As in other areas of medicine, polypharmacy has become an increasingly accepted approach in psychiatry for addressing difficult-to-treat disorders.[3] Moreover, general medical co-morbidity is common among patients with psychiatric disorders, elevating the likelihood of complex medication regimens.[4,5] Similarly, the widespread use of over-the-counter (OTC) supplements by patients receiving treatment for psychiatric disorders may invite additional risk of drug–drug interactions.[6] When they occur, drug–drug interactions may manifest in myriad ways, from perplexing laboratory tests to symptoms that are difficult to distinguish from the underlying psychiatric and physical conditions under treatment. The comprehensive evaluation of patients with psychiatric disorders therefore requires a careful assessment of potential drug–drug interactions.

Drug–drug interactions refer to alterations in drug levels or drug effects (or both) attributed to the administration of two or more prescribed, illicit, or OTC agents in close temporal proximity. Although many drug–drug interactions involve drugs administered within minutes to hours of each other,

some drugs may participate in interactions days or even weeks after their discontinuation because of prolonged elimination half-lives (e.g., fluoxetine) or due to their long-term impact on metabolic enzymes (e.g., carbamazepine). Some drug–drug interactions involving psychotropic medications are life-threatening, such as those involving the co-administration of monoamine oxidase inhibitors (MAOIs) and drugs with potent serotonergic (e.g., meperidine) or sympathomimetic (e.g., phenylpropanolamine) effects.[7-9] These combinations are therefore absolutely contraindicated. However, most drug–drug interactions in psychopharmacology manifest in somewhat more subtle ways, often leading to poor medication tolerability and compliance due to adverse events (e.g., orthostatic hypotension, sedation, or irritability), diminished medication efficacy, or puzzling manifestations (such as altered mental status or unexpectedly high or low drug levels). Drug combinations that can produce these often less than catastrophic drug–drug interactions are usually not absolutely contraindicated. Some of these combinations may, indeed, be valuable in the treatment of some patients while wreaking havoc for other patients. The capacity to anticipate and to recognize both the major, but rare, and the more subtle, but common, potential drug–drug interactions allows the practitioner to minimize the impact of these interactions as an obstacle to patient safety and to therapeutic success. This is both an important goal and a considerable challenge in psychopharmacology.

While drug–drug interactions are ubiquitous, few studies have systematically assessed *in vivo* drug–drug interactions of most interest to psychiatrists. Fortunately, well-designed studies of drug–drug interactions are an increasingly integral part of drug development. Beyond these studies, however, the literature on drug–drug interactions remains a patchwork of case reports, post-marketing analyses, extrapolation from animal and *in vitro* studies, and extrapolation from what is known about other drugs with similar properties. While these studies often shed some light on the simplest case of a single drug (drug B) exerting an effect on another (drug A), they rarely consider the common clinical scenario in which multiple drugs with numerous potential interactions among them are co-administered. Under these circumstances, the range of possible, if not well-delineated, drug–drug interactions often seems overwhelming.

Fortunately, an increasing range of resources are available (including prescribing software packages and regularly updated websites, such as www.drug-interactions.com) that allow for the prevention and detection of potential interactions. In addition, it is important to recall that numerous factors contribute to inter-individual variability in drug response.[10,11] These factors include treatment adherence, age, gender, nutritional status, disease states, and genetic polymorphisms that may influence risk of adverse events and treatment resistance (Figure 50-1). Drug–drug interactions are an additional factor that influence how patients react to drugs. The importance of these interactions depends heavily on the clinical context. In many cases, the practical impact of drug–drug interactions is likely to be very small compared with other factors that affect treatment response, drug levels, and toxicity. It is reasonable, therefore, to focus special attention on the contexts in which drug–drug interactions are most likely to be clinically problematic.

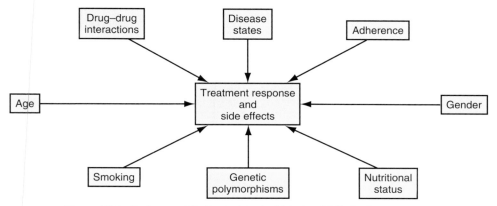

Figure 50-1. Factors contributing to inter-individual variability in drug response.

First, it is crucial to be familiar with the small number of drug–drug interactions in psychopharmacology that, though uncommon, are associated with potentially catastrophic consequences. These include drugs associated with ventricular arrhythmias, hypertensive crisis, serotonin syndrome, Stevens-Johnson syndrome, seizures, and severe bone marrow suppression. In addition, drug–drug interactions are important to consider when a patient's drugs include those with a low therapeutic index (e.g., lithium, digoxin, or warfarin) or a narrow therapeutic window (e.g., indinavir, nortriptyline, or cyclosporine) such that relatively small alterations in pharmacokinetic or pharmacodynamic behavior may jeopardize a patient's well-being. In addition, it is worthwhile to consider potential drug–drug interactions whenever evaluating a patient whose drug levels are unexpectedly variable or extreme, or a patient with a confusing clinical picture (such as clinical deterioration), or with unexpected side effects. Finally, drug–drug interactions are likely to be clinically salient for a patient who is medically frail or elderly, owing to altered pharmacokinetics and vulnerability to side effects, as well as for a patient heavily using alcohol, cigarettes, or illicit drugs, or being treated for a drug overdose.

CLASSIFICATION

Drug–drug interactions may be described as pharmacokinetic, pharmacodynamic, idiosyncratic, or mixed, depending on the presumed mechanism underlying the interaction (Box 50-1). Pharmacokinetic interactions are those that involve a change in the plasma level or tissue distribution (or both) of one drug by virtue of co-administration of another drug. These interactions occur due to effects at one or more of the four pharmacokinetic processes by which drugs are acted on by the body: absorption, distribution, metabolism, and excretion. Because of the importance of these factors, particularly metabolism, in drug–drug interactions, a more detailed description of pharmacokinetic processes follows. An example of a pharmacokinetic drug–drug interaction is the inhibition of the metabolism of lamotrigine by valproic acid,[12] thereby raising lamotrigine levels and increasing the risk of potentially serious adverse events, including hypersensitivity reactions (such as Stevens-Johnson syndrome). In contrast, pharmacodynamic interactions are those that involve a known pharmacological effect at biologically-active (receptor) sites. These interactions occur due to effects on the mechanisms through which the body is acted on by drugs and do not involve a change in drug levels. An example of a pharmacodynamic drug–drug interaction is the interference of the antiparkinsonian effects of a dopamine receptor agonist (such as pramipexole) by a dopamine receptor antagonist (such as risperidone). Mixed interactions are

BOX 50-1 Classification of Drug–Drug Interactions

PHARMACOKINETIC
Alteration in blood level or tissue concentration (or both) resulting from interactions involving drug absorption, distribution, metabolism, or excretion
PHARMACODYNAMIC
Alteration in pharmacological effect resulting from interactions at the same or inter-related biologically-active (receptor) sites
MIXED
Alterations in blood levels and pharmacological effects due to pharmacokinetic and pharmacodynamic interactions
IDIOSYNCRACTIC
Sporadic interactions among drugs not accounted for by their currently known pharmacokinetic or pharmacodynamic properties

those that are believed to involve both pharmacological and pharmacodynamic effects. Symptoms of serotonin toxicity, such as agitation and confusion that have been observed in some individuals on the combination of paroxetine and dextromethorphan, for example, may reflect the shared pharmacodynamic effect of the two agents at serotonin receptor sites as well as the elevation of dextromethorphan levels due to inhibition of its cytochrome P450 metabolism by paroxetine. Finally, idiosyncratic interactions are those that occur sporadically in a small number of patients in ways that are not yet predicted by the known pharmacokinetic and pharmacodynamic properties of the drugs involved.

PHARMACOKINETICS

As described earlier, pharmacokinetic processes refer to absorption, distribution, metabolism, and excretion, factors that determine plasma levels and tissue concentrations of a drug.[2,11,13] Pharmacokinetics refers to the mathematical analysis of these processes. Advances in analytic chemistry and computer methods of pharmacokinetic modeling and a growing understanding of the molecular pharmacology of the liver enzymes responsible for metabolism of most psychotropic medications have furnished increasingly sophisticated insights into the disposition and interaction of administered drugs. Although pharmacokinetics refers to only one of the two broad mechanisms by which drugs interact, pharmacokinetic interactions involve all classes of psychotropic and nonpsychotropic medications. An overview of pharmacokinetic processes is a helpful prelude to a discussion of drug–drug interactions by psychotropic drug class.

Absorption

Factors that influence drug absorption are generally of less importance to drug–drug interactions involving psychiatric medications than are factors that influence subsequent drug disposition, particularly drug metabolism. Factors relevant to absorption generally pertain to orally rather than parenterally administered drugs, for which alterations in gastrointestinal drug absorption may affect the rate (time to reach maximum concentration) or the extent of absorption or both. The extent or completeness of absorption, also known as the fractional absorption, is measured as the area under the curve (AUC) when plasma concentration is plotted against time. The bioavailability of an oral dose of drug refers, in turn, to the fractional absorption for orally compared with intravenously (IV) administered drug. If an agent is reported to have a 90% bioavailability (e.g., lorazepam), this would indicate that the extent of absorption of an orally administered dose is nearly that of an IV-administered dose, although the rate of absorption may well be slower for the oral dose.

Because the upper part of the small intestine is the primary site of drug absorption through passive membrane diffusion and filtration and both passive and active transport processes, factors that speed gastric emptying (e.g., metoclopramide) or diminish intestinal motility (e.g., opiates or marijuana) may facilitate greater contact with, and absorption from, the mucosal surface into the systemic circulation, potentially increasing plasma drug concentrations. Conversely, antacids, charcoal, kaolin-pectin, and cholestyramine may bind to drugs, forming complexes that pass unabsorbed through the gastrointestinal lumen. Changes in gastric pH associated with food or other drugs alter the non-polar, un-ionized fraction of drug available for absorption. In the case of drugs that are very weak acids or bases, however, the extent of ionization is relatively invariant under physiological conditions. Properties of the preparation administered (e.g., tablet, capsule, or liquid) may also influence the rate or extent of absorption, and, for an increasing number of medications (e.g., lithium, bupropion, valproate, and methylphenidate), preparations intended for slow release are available. Finally, the local action of enzymes in the gastrointestinal tract (e.g., monoamine oxidase [MAO] and cytochrome P450 3A4) may be responsible for metabolism of drug before absorption. As described later, this is of critical relevance to the emergence of hypertensive crises that occur when excessive quantities of the dietary pressor tyramine are systemically absorbed in the setting of irreversible inhibition of the MAO isoenzymes for which tyramine is a substrate.

Distribution

Drugs distribute to tissues through the systemic circulation. The amount of drug ultimately reaching receptor sites in tissues is determined by a variety of factors, including the concentration of free (unbound) drug in plasma, regional blood flow, and physiochemical properties of drug (e.g., lipophilicity or structural characteristics). For entrance into the central nervous system (CNS), penetration across the blood–brain barrier is required. Fat-soluble drugs (such as benzodiazepines, neuroleptics, and cyclic antidepressants) distribute more widely in the body than water-soluble drugs (such as lithium), which distribute through a smaller volume of distribution. Changes with age, typically including an increase in the ratio of body fat to lean body mass, therefore result in a net greater volume of lipophilic drug distribution

and potentially greater accumulation of drug in adipose tissue in older than in younger patients.

In general, psychotropic drugs have relatively high affinities for plasma proteins (some to albumin but others, such as antidepressants, to α_1-acid glycoproteins and lipoproteins). Most psychotropic drugs are more than 80% protein-bound. A drug is considered highly protein-bound if more than 90% exists in bound form in plasma. Fluoxetine, aripiprazole, and diazepam are examples of the many psychotropic drugs that are highly protein-bound. In contrast, venlafaxine, lithium, topiramate, zonisamide, gabapentin, pregabalin, milnacipran, and memantine are examples of drugs with minimal protein-binding and therefore minimal risk of participating in drug–drug interactions related to protein-binding. A reversible equilibrium exists between bound and unbound drug. Only the unbound fraction exerts pharmacological effects. Competition by two or more drugs for protein-binding sites often results in displacement of a previously bound drug, which in the free state becomes pharmacologically active. Similarly, reduced concentrations of plasma proteins in a severely malnourished patient or a patient with a disease that is associated with severely lowered serum proteins (such as liver disease or nephrotic syndrome) may be associated with an increase in the fraction of unbound drug potentially available for activity at relevant receptor sites. Under most circumstances, the net changes in plasma concentration of active drug are, in fact, quite small because the unbound drug is available for redistribution to other tissues and for metabolism and excretion, thereby off-setting the initial rise in plasma levels. Nevertheless, clinically significant consequences can develop when protein-binding-interactions alter the unbound fraction of previously highly protein-bound drugs that have a low therapeutic index (e.g., warfarin). For these drugs, relatively small variations in plasma level may be associated with serious untoward effects.

An emerging understanding of the drug transport proteins, of which P-glycoproteins are the best characterized, indicates a crucial role in regulating permeability of intestinal epithelia, lymphocytes, renal tubules, the biliary tract, and the blood–brain barrier. These transport proteins are thought to account for the development of certain forms of drug resistance and tolerance, but are increasingly seen as likely also to mediate clinically-important drug interactions.[2] Little is known yet about their relevance to drug interactions involving psychiatric medications; the capacity of St. John's wort to lower blood levels of several critical medications (including cyclosporine and indinavir) is hypothesized to be related, at least in part, to an effect of the botanical agent on this transport system.[14]

Metabolism

Metabolism is the best-characterized mechanism of all of the pharmacokinetic processes implicated in known drug–drug interactions. Metabolism refers to the biotransformation of a drug to another form, a process that is usually enzyme-mediated and that results in a metabolite that may or may not be pharmacologically active and may or may not be subject to further biotransformations before eventual excretion. Most drugs undergo several types of biotransformation, and many psychotropic drug interactions of clinical significance are based on interference with this process. A growing understanding of hepatic enzymes, and especially the rapidly emerging characterization of the cytochrome P450 isoenzymes and other enzyme systems including the uridine-diphosphate glucuronosyltransferases (UGTs), flavin-containing monooxygenases (FMOs), methyltransferases, and sulfotransferases, has significantly advanced a rational understanding and prediction of drug interactions and individual variation in drug responses.[2,15]

Phase I reactions include oxidation, reduction, and hydrolysis, metabolic reactions that typically result in intermediate metabolites, which are then subject to phase II reactions (including conjugation [e.g., glucuronidation and sulfation] and acetylation). Phase II reactions typically yield highly polar, water-soluble metabolites suitable for renal excretion. Most psychotropic drugs undergo both phase I and phase II metabolic reactions. Notable exceptions include valproic acid and a subset of benzodiazepines (i.e., lorazepam, oxazepam, and temazepam), which skip phase I metabolism and undergo phase II reactions only. In addition, certain medications, including lithium and gabapentin, do not undergo any hepatic biotransformation before excretion by the kidneys.

The synthesis or activity of hepatic microsomal enzymes is affected by metabolic inhibitors and inducers, as well as by distinct genetic polymorphisms (stably inherited traits). Table 50-1 lists enzyme inducers and inhibitors common in clinical settings. These should serve as red flags that beckon further scrutiny for potential drug–drug interactions when they are found on a patient's medication list. Imagine two drugs, drug A and drug B, which are both associated with a metabolic enzyme. Drug B may be an inhibitor or an inducer of that enzyme. Drug A may be normally metabolized by that enzyme and would therefore be called a substrate. If drug B is an inhibitor with respect to the metabolic enzyme, it will impede the metabolism of a concurrently administered substrate (drug A), thereby producing a rise in the plasma levels of that substrate. If drug B is an inducer of that enzyme, it will enhance the metabolism of the substrate (drug A), resulting in a decline in the plasma levels of that substrate (Figure 50-2). In some circumstances an inhibitor (such as grapefruit juice) or inducer (e.g., a cruciferous vegetable, such as brussels sprouts) may not be a drug but rather another ingested substance. Moreover, in some circumstances a drug is not only a substrate of an enzyme but it can also inhibit the metabolism of other substrates relying on that enzyme, in which case it is considered an inhibitor as well as a substrate. Although inhibition is usually immediate, occurring by one or more of a variety of mechanisms (including competitive inhibition or inactivation of the enzyme), induction, which requires enhanced synthesis of the metabolic enzyme, is typically a more gradual process. A fall in plasma levels of a substrate may not be apparent for days to weeks following introduction of the inducer. This is particularly important when a patient's care is being transferred to another setting where clinical deterioration may be the first sign that drug levels have declined. Reciprocally, an elevation in plasma drug concentrations could reflect the previous discontinuation of an inducing factor (e.g., cigarette smoking or carbamazepine) just as it could reflect the more recent introduction of an inhibitor (e.g., fluoxetine or valproic acid).

Although the cytochrome P450 isoenzymes represent only one of the numerous enzyme systems responsible for drug

TABLE 50-1 Commonly Used Drugs and Substances That Inhibit or Induce Hepatic Metabolism of Other Medications

Inhibitors	Inducers
Antifungals (ketoconazole, miconazole, itraconazole)	Barbiturates (e.g., phenobarbital, secobarbital)
Macrolide antibiotics (erythromycin, clarithromycin, triacetyloleandomycin)	Carbamazepine
Fluoroquinolones (e.g., ciprofloxacin)	Oxcarbazepine
Isoniazid	Phenytoin
Antiretrovirals	Rifampin
Antimalarials (chloroquine)	Primidone
Selective serotonin reuptake inhibitors (fluoxetine, fluvoxamine, paroxetine, sertraline)	Cigarettes
Duloxetine	Ethanol (chronic)
Bupropion	Cruciferous vegetables
Nefazodone	Charbroiled meats
β-Blockers (lipophilic) (e.g., propranolol, metoprolol, pindolol)	St. John's wort
Quinidine	Oral contraceptives
Valproate	Prednisone
Cimetidine	
Calcium channel blockers (e.g., diltiazem)	
Grapefruit juice	
Ethanol (acute)	

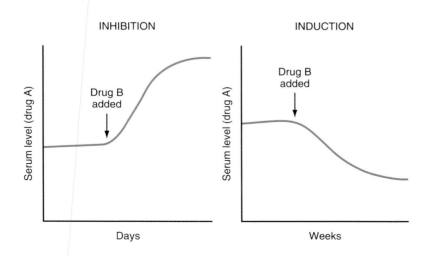

Figure 50-2. Metabolic inhibition and induction. Serum concentrations of drug A rise abruptly if co-administered drug B is an inhibitor of its metabolism, but serum concentrations fall gradually if co-administered drug B is an inducer of its metabolism.

metabolism, they are responsible for metabolizing, at least in part, over 80% of all prescribed drugs. In addition, growing awareness in the 1990s about the capacity of many of the newer antidepressants to inhibit cytochrome P450 isoenzymes fueled great interest in the pattern of interaction of psychotropic and other drugs with these enzymes in the understanding and prediction of drug–drug interactions. The cytochrome P450 isoenzymes represent a family of more than 30 related heme-containing enzymes, largely located in the endoplasmic reticulum of hepatocytes (but also present elsewhere, including the gut and brain), which mediate oxidative metabolism of a wide variety of drugs, as well as endogenous substances (including prostaglandins, fatty acids, and steroids). The majority of antidepressant and antipsychotic drugs are metabolized by, or inhibit, one or more of these isoenzymes. Table 50-2 summarizes the interactions of psychiatric and non-psychiatric drugs with a subset of isoenzymes that have been increasingly well characterized (1A2, 2C subfamily, 2D6, and 3A4). Further information about the relevance of these and other interactions is highlighted in a later section of this chapter in which clinically important drug–drug interactions are reviewed.

In addition to being influenced by pharmacological inducers or inhibitors, a patient's metabolic status is also under genetic control. Knowledge continues to evolve concerning genetic polymorphisms that affect drug metabolism. Within the group of cytochrome P450 isoenzymes, there appears to be a polymodal distribution of metabolic activity in the population with respect to certain isoenzymes (including 2C19 and 2D6). Most individuals are normal ("extensive") metabolizers with respect to the activity of these isoenzymes. A smaller number are "poor metabolizers" with deficient activity of the isoenzyme. Probably very much smaller numbers are ultra-rapid metabolizers (who have more than normal activity of the enzyme) and intermediate metabolizers (who fall between extensive and poor metabolizers). Individuals who are poor metabolizers with respect to a particular cytochrome P450 isoenzyme are expected to have higher plasma concentrations of a drug that is metabolized by that isoenzyme, thereby potentially being more sensitive to, or requiring lower doses of that drug than, a patient with normal activity of that enzyme. They may also have higher-than-usual plasma levels of metabolites of the drug that are produced through other metabolic pathways that are not altered by the polymorphism, thereby potentially incurring pharmacological activity or adverse effects related to these alternative metabolites. Poor metabolizers are relatively impervious to drug interactions involving inhibition of the particular isoenzyme system for which they are already deficient. When the polymorphism is related to an isoenzyme required for conversion of a pro-drug (e.g., tamoxifen, codeine, or tramadol) to its active form, poor metabolizers are also likely to demonstrate a diminished response to those treatments. Studies on genetic polymorphisms affecting the cytochrome P450 system suggest ethnic differences.[16] Approximately 15% to 20% of Asian Americans and African Americans appear to be poor metabolizers with respect to P450 2C19 compared with 3% to 5% of Caucasians. Conversely, the proportion of frankly poor metabolizers with respect to P450 2D6 appears to be higher among Caucasians (approximately 5% to 10%) than among Asian Americans and African Americans (approximately 1% to 3%). Current understanding of the clinical relevance of genetic polymorphisms in drug therapy in psychiatry remains rudimentary. Commercial genotyping tests for polymorphisms of potential relevance to drug–drug metabolism are increasingly available. Further systematic study of their relevance to the understanding and prediction of drug response is needed before such testing can be meaningfully incorporated into routine psychopharmacological practice.

TABLE 50-2 Selected Cytochrome P450 Isoenzyme Substrates, Inhibitors, and Inducers

1A2	Substrates	Acetaminophen, aminophylline, asenapine, caffeine, clozapine, cyclobenzaprine, estradiol, fluvoxamine, haloperidol, mirtazapine, ondansetron, olanzapine, phenacetin, procarcinogens, propranolol, ramelteon, riluzole, ropinirole, tacrine, tertiary amine tricyclic antidepressants (TCAs), theophylline, verapamil, warfarin, zileuton, zolmitriptan
	Inhibitors	Amiodarone, cimetidine, fluoroquinolones, fluvoxamine, grapefruit juice, methoxsalen, ticlopidine
	Inducers	Charbroiled meats, tobacco (cigarette smoking), cruciferous vegetables, modafinil, omeprazole
2C	Substrates	Barbiturates, diazepam, fluvastatin, glipizide, glyburide, irbesartan, losartan, mephenytoin, NSAIDs, nelfinavir, phenytoin, primidone, propranolol, proguanil, proton pump inhibitors, rosiglitazone, tamoxifen, tertiary TCAs, THC, tolbutamide, R-warfarin, S-warfarin
	Inhibitors	Armodafinil, fluoxetine, fluvoxamine, ketoconazole, modafinil, omeprazole, oxcarbazepine, sertraline
	Inducers	Carbamazepine, norethindrone, prednisone, rifampin, secobarbital
2D6	Substrates	Amphetamines, aripiprazole, atomoxetine, β-blockers (lipophilic), codeine, debrisoquine, dextromethorphan, diltiazem, donepezil, duloxetine, encainide, flecainide, galantamine, haloperidol, hydroxycodone, iloperidone, lidocaine, mCPP, metoclopramide, mexiletine, nifedipine, ondansetron, phenothiazines (e.g., thioridazine, perphenazine), promethazine, propafenone, risperidone, SSRIs, tamoxifen, TCAs, tramadol, trazodone, venlafaxine
	Inhibitors	Amiodarone, antimalarials, bupropion, cimetidine, citalopram, duloxetine, escitalopram, fluoxetine, methadone, metoclopramide, moclobemide, paroxetine, phenothiazines, protease inhibitors (ritonavir), quinidine, sertraline, terbinafine, TCAs, yohimbine
	Inducers	Dexamethasone, rifampin
3A3/4	Substrates	Alfentanil, alprazolam, amiodarone, amprenavir, aripiprazole, armodafinil, bromocriptine, buspirone, cafergot, calcium channel blockers, caffeine, carbamazepine, cisapride, clozapine, cyclosporine, dapsone, diazepam, disopyramide, efavirenz, estradiol, fentanyl, HMG-CoA reductase inhibitors (lovastatin, simvastatin), indinavir, lidocaine, loratadine, lurasidone, methadone, midazolam, modafinil, nimodipine, pimozide, prednisone, progesterone, propafenone, quetiapine, quinidine, ritonavir, sildenafil, tacrolimus, testosterone, tertiary amine TCAs, triazolam, vinblastine, warfarin, zolpidem, zaleplon, ziprasidone
	Inhibitors	Antifungals, calcium channel blockers, cimetidine, efavirenz, indinavir, fluvoxamine, fluoxetine (norfluoxetine), grapefruit juice, macrolide antibiotics, mibefradil, nefazodone, ritonavir, verapamil, voriconazole
	Inducers	Armodafinil, carbamazepine, glucocorticoids, modafinil, oxcarbazepine, phenobarbital, phenytoin, pioglitazone, rifabutin, rifampin, ritonavir, St. John's wort, troglitazone

HMG-CoA, Hydroxymethylglutaryl coenzyme A; mCPP, m-chlorophenylpiperazine; NSAIDs, non-steroidal anti-inflammatory drugs; SSRIs, selective serotonin reuptake inhibitors; THC, tetrahydrocannabinol.

Excretion

Because most antidepressant, anxiolytic, and antipsychotic medications are largely eliminated by hepatic metabolism, factors that affect renal excretion (glomerular filtration, tubular reabsorption, and active tubular secretion) are generally far less important to the pharmacokinetics of these drugs than to lithium, for which such factors may have clinically-significant consequences. Conditions resulting in sodium deficiency (e.g., dehydration, sodium restriction, use of thiazide diuretics) are likely to result in increased proximal tubular reabsorption of lithium, resulting in increased lithium levels and potential toxicity. Lithium levels and clinical status must be monitored especially closely in the setting of vomiting, diarrhea, excessive evaporative losses, or polyuria. Factors, such as aging, that are associated with reduced renal blood flow and glomerular filtration rate (GFR) also reduce lithium excretion. For this reason, as well as for their reduced volume of distribution for lithium because of relative loss of total body water with aging, elderly patients typically require lower lithium doses than younger patients, and a low starting dose (i.e., 150 to 300 mg/day) is often prudent. Apparently separate from pharmacokinetic effects, however, elderly patients may also be more sensitive to the neurotoxic effects of lithium even at low therapeutic levels. Factors associated with an increased GFR, particularly pregnancy, may produce an increase in lithium clearance and a fall in lithium levels.

For other medications, renal excretion may sometimes be exploited in the treatment of a drug overdose. Acidification of the urine by ascorbic acid, ammonium chloride, or methenamine mandelate increases the rate of excretion of weak bases (such as the amphetamines and phencyclidine [PCP]). Therefore, such measures may be important in the emergency management of a patient with severe PCP or amphetamine intoxication. Conversely, alkalinization of the urine by administration of sodium bicarbonate or acetazolamide may hasten the excretion of weak acids (including long-acting barbiturates, such as phenobarbital).

ANTIPSYCHOTICS

Antipsychotic or neuroleptic drugs include the phenothiazines (e.g., chlorpromazine, fluphenazine, perphenazine, thioridazine, and trifluoperazine), butyrophenones (haloperidol), thioxanthenes (thiothixene), indolones (molindone), diphenylbutylpiperidines (pimozide), dibenzodiazepines (loxapine), and the newer atypical agents (clozapine, olanzapine, risperidone, quetiapine, ziprasidone, aripiprazole, iloperidone, paliperidone, asenapine, and lurasidone).[17] As a class, they are generally rapidly, if erratically, absorbed from the gastrointestinal tract after oral administration (peak plasma concentrations ranging from 30 minutes to 6 hours). They are highly lipophilic and distribute rapidly to body tissues with a large apparent volume of distribution. Protein-binding in the circulation ranges from approximately 90% to 98% except for molindone, paliperidone, and quetiapine, which are only moderately protein-bound. The antipsychotics generally undergo substantial first-pass hepatic metabolism (primarily oxidation and conjugation reactions), reducing their systemic bioavailability when given orally compared with intramuscular (IM) administration, the fractional absorption of which nearly approximates that of IV administration. Most of the individual antipsychotics have several pharmacologically active and inactive metabolites. Because of their propensity to sequester in body compartments, the elimination half-life of antipsychotics is quite variable, generally ranging from approximately 20 to 40 hours. For butyrophenones, however, elimination pharmacokinetics appear to be especially complex, and

the disappearance of drug from the systemic circulation, and even more so from brain, may take much longer, as it does for the newer agent, aripiprazole (and its active metabolite, dehydro-aripirazole), whose half-life may exceed 90 hours.

The lower-potency antipsychotics (including chlorpromazine, mesoridazine, thioridazine, and clozapine) are generally the most sedating and have the greatest anticholinergic, antihistaminic, and α_1-adrenergic antagonistic effects, whereas the higher-potency antipsychotics (including haloperidol, loxapine, molindone, and the piperazine phenothiazines, such as trifluoperazine), are more likely to be associated with an increased incidence of extrapyramidal symptoms (EPS), including akathisia, dystonia, and parkinsonism. The atypical antipsychotics generally have multiple receptor affinities, including antagonism at dopamine D_{1-4} receptors, serotonin 5-HT_1, 5-HT_5, and 5-HT_2 receptors, α_1- and α_2-adrenergic receptors, histamine-H_1 receptors, and cholinergic muscarinic receptors, with variations across agents; thus, for example, clozaril and olanzapine have notably greater affinity at the muscarinic receptors than the other agents and aripiprazole is a partial agonist at the D_2 receptor. Although the more complex pharmacological profile of these newer atypical agents, as well as the older low-potency antipsychotics, has generally been associated with a lower risk of EPS, the same broad range of receptor activity also poses greater risk of pharmacodynamic interactions.

Lower-potency drugs, as well as some atypical antipsychotics, can produce significant hypotension when combined with vasodilator or antihypertensive drugs related to α_1-adrenergic blockade (Table 50-3).[18,19] Hypotension can also occur when low-potency antipsychotics and atypical antidepressants are combined with tricyclic antidepressant (TCA) and MAOI antidepressants. Severe hypotension has been reported when chlorpromazine has been administered with the angiotensin-converting enzyme (ACE) inhibitor captopril. Paradoxical hypotension can develop when epinephrine is administered with low-potency antipsychotics. In this setting, the β-adrenergic stimulant effect of epinephrine, resulting in vasodilation, is thought to be unopposed by its usual pressor effect because α_1-adrenergic receptors are occupied by the antipsychotic. A similar effect may result if a low-potency neuroleptic is administered to a patient with a pheochromocytoma. Finally, hypotension may develop when low-potency antipsychotics are used in combination with a variety of anesthetics (such as halothane, enflurane, and isoflurane).

In addition, the low-potency antipsychotics have quinidine-like effects on cardiac conduction (and may prolong Q-T and P-R intervals).[20] Ziprasidone may also cause Q-T prolongation, although clinically-significant prolongation (QTc > 500 ms) appears to be infrequent when administered to otherwise healthy subjects. Significant depression of cardiac conduction, heart block, and life-threatening ventricular dysrhythmias may result from the co-administration of low-potency antipsychotics or ziprasidone with class I antiarrhythmics (e.g., quinidine, procainamide, disopyramide), as well as when administered with high doses of the TCAs, which have quinidine-like activity on cardiac conduction, and when administered in the context of other aggravating factors (including hypokalemia, hypomagnesemia, bradycardia, or congenital prolongation of the QTc). Pimozide also can depress cardiac conduction as a result of its calcium channel blocking action, and the combination of pimozide with other calcium channel blockers (e.g., nifedipine, diltiazem, verapamil) is contraindicated.

Another clinically-significant pharmacodynamic interaction arises when low-potency antipsychotics, as well as atypical antipsychotics, particularly clozapine or olanzapine, are administered with other drugs that have anticholinergic effects (including TCAs, benztropine, and diphenhydramine). When

TABLE 50-3 Selected Drug Interactions with Antipsychotic Medications

Drug	Potential Interaction
Antacids (aluminum-magnesium containing), fruit juice	Interference with absorption of antipsychotic agents
Carbamazepine	Decreased antipsychotic drug plasma levels; additive risk of myelosuppression with clozapine
Cigarettes	Decreased antipsychotic drug plasma levels; reduced extrapyramidal symptoms
Rifampin	Decreased antipsychotic drug plasma levels
TCAs	Increased TCA and antipsychotic drug plasma levels; hypotension, depression of cardiac conduction (with low-potency antipsychotics)
SSRIs	Increased SSRI and antipsychotic drug plasma levels; arrhythmia risk with thioridine and pimozide
Bupropion, duloxetine	Increased antipsychotic drug plasma levels; arrhythmia risk with thioridazine
Fluvoxamine, nefazodone	Increased antipsychotic drug plasma levels; arrhythmia risk with pimozide; seizure risk with clozapine
β-Blockers (lipophilic)	Increased antipsychotic drug plasma levels; improved akathisia
Anticholinergic drugs	Additive anticholinergic toxicity; reduced extrapyramidal symptoms
Antihypertensive, vasodilator drugs	Hypotension (with low-potency antipsychotics and risperidone)
Guanethidine, clonidine	Blockade of antihypertensive effect
Epinephrine	Hypotension (with low-potency antipsychotics)
Class I antiarrhythmics	Depression of cardiac conduction; ventricular arrhythmias (with low-potency antipsychotics, ziprasidone)
Calcium channel blockers	Depression of cardiac conduction; ventricular arrhythmias (with pimozide)
Lithium	Idiosyncratic neurotoxicity

SSRIs, Selective serotonin reuptake inhibitors; TCAs, tricyclic antidepressants.

these drugs are combined, there is greater risk of urinary retention, constipation, blurred vision, impaired memory and concentration, and increased intraocular pressure in the setting of narrow-angle glaucoma. With overdose, a severe anticholinergic syndrome can develop, including delirium, paralytic ileus, tachycardia, and dysrhythmias. Elderly patients are likely to be at increased risk for toxicity due to anticholinergic effects. The high-potency agents and non-anticholinergic atypical agents (e.g., risperidone) are indicated when anticholinergic effects need to be minimized.

The sedative effects of low-potency agents and atypical antidepressants are also often additive to those of the sedative-hypnotic medications and alcohol. In patients for whom sedative effects may be especially dangerous, including the elderly, the cautious selection and dosing of antipsychotics should always take into account the overall burden of sedation from their concurrent medications. For these patients, starting with a low, divided dose is often an appropriate first step.

Because dopamine receptor blockade is a property common to all antipsychotics, they are all likely to interfere, although to varying degrees, with the efficacy of levodopa and direct dopamine receptor agonists in the treatment of Parkinson's disease. When antipsychotic treatment is necessary in this setting, clozapine and the newer atypical agents, or the lower-potency conventional agents, have been preferred. Reciprocally, antipsychotics are likely to be less effective in the treatment of psychosis in the setting of levodopa, stimulants (e.g., dextroamphetamine), and direct agonists (e.g., ropinirole) that facilitate dopamine transmission. Nevertheless, these agents have been combined with antipsychotics in cautious, modestly successful efforts to treat the negative symptoms of schizophrenia (including blunted affect, paucity of thought and speech, and social withdrawal). In addition, elevated prolactin is common on antipsychotics, particularly higher-potency conventional agents and risperidone; it manifests with irregular menses, galactorrhea, diminished libido, or hirsutism. If these agents are necessary and other causes of hyperprolactinemia have been excluded, there is an

appropriate role for concurrent, cautious use of dopamine agonists, particularly bromocriptine, to lower prolactin.

The risk of agranulocytosis, which occurs rarely with the low-potency antipsychotics, is much higher with clozapine, with an incidence as high as 1% to 3%. For this reason, the combination of clozapine with other medications associated with a risk of myelosuppression (e.g., carbamazepine) should be avoided. Similarly, as clozapine lowers the seizure threshold to a greater extent than other antipsychotics, co-administration with other medications that significantly lower the seizure threshold (e.g., maprotiline) should be avoided or combined use with an anticonvulsant should be considered.

The co-administration of lithium with antipsychotic agents (most notably haloperidol) has been associated, very rarely, with potentially irreversible neurotoxicity, characterized by mental status changes, EPS, and, perhaps in some cases, cerebellar signs and hyperthermia.[21] Related to this concern is the unconfirmed suggestion that lithium co-administration with an antipsychotic may increase the risk of neuroleptic malignant syndrome (NMS). Other clinical variables, including dehydration and poor nutrition, are likely to be of greater significance as putative risk factors for NMS. At present, the evidence is not sufficient to warrant avoidance of the widely used combination of lithium and neuroleptics. Such a possibility, however, should be considered when a patient receiving these medications has neuropsychiatric toxicity of unclear origin.

Pharmacokinetic drug interactions are common among the antipsychotic drugs.[18,19] Plasma levels of the neuroleptics, however, may vary as much as 10-fold to 20-fold between individuals even on monotherapy, and, as a class, antipsychotics fortunately have a relatively wide therapeutic index. Therefore, factors that alter antipsychotic drug metabolism may not have deleterious clinical consequences in many instances. Exceptions include those antipsychotic drugs linked to risk of arrhythmia, most notably thioridazine and pimozide. Related to cytochrome P450 isoenzyme inhibition, agents that interfere with P450 2D6 (such as fluoxetine, paroxetine, duloxetine, or bupropion) can greatly increase levels of low-potency agents, including thioridazine, and thus increase the risk of arrhythmia. Similarly, agents that interfere with P450 3A4 (such as erythromycin, fluvoxamine, or nefazodone) entail similar risk when combined with pimozide. These combinations are contraindicated. The concurrent administration of potent P450 3A4 inhibitors with ziprasidone may increase levels and theoretically increase QTc and risk of arrhythmias. Another exception has to do with patients who are maintained on antipsychotics carefully tapered to the lowest effective dose. In these patients, a small decrease in antipsychotic levels, as may occur with the introduction of a metabolic inducer or an agent that interferes with absorption, may bring them below the threshold for efficacy.

Antipsychotic drug levels may be lowered by aluminum-containing or magnesium-containing antacids, which reduce their absorption and are best given separately. Mixing liquid preparations of phenothiazines with beverages, such as fruit juices, presents the risk of causing insoluble precipitates and inefficient gastrointestinal absorption. Carbamazepine, known to be a potent inducer of hepatic enzymes, including P450 3A4 and others, has been associated with reduction of steady-state antipsychotic drug plasma levels by as much as 50%. This effect is especially important to bear in mind as a potential explanation when a neuroleptic-treated patient appears to deteriorate in the weeks following the introduction of carbamazepine. Oxcarbazepine may also induce antipsychotic drug metabolism, as can a variety of other anticonvulsants, including phenobarbital and phenytoin. Cigarette smoking may also be associated with a reduction in antipsychotic drug levels through enzyme metabolism. As inpatient units and community residential programs have widely become "smoke-free," there are often substantial differences in smoking frequency between inpatient and outpatient settings. Among patients who smoke heavily, consideration should be given to the impact of these changes in smoking habits on antipsychotic dose requirements.

When an antipsychotic drug is given together with a TCA, the plasma level of each agent may rise, presumably because of mutual inhibition of microsomal enzymes. Reciprocally, when a patient with psychotic depression is tapered off an antipsychotic, it is important to remember that the plasma level of TCAs may also decline. Selective serotonin reuptake inhibitors (SSRIs) and other antidepressants with inhibitory effects on cytochrome P450 isoenzymes may also produce an increase in the plasma levels of a concurrently administered antipsychotic agent (see Table 50-1). Thus, increases in clozapine, olanzapine, asenapine, and haloperidol plasma levels may occur when co-administered with fluvoxamine. Increases in risperidone, aripiprazole, iloperidone, and typical antipsychotic levels may follow initiation of fluoxetine, paroxetine, bupropion, duloxetine, or sertraline. Quetiapine, lurasidone, and ziprasidone levels may rise following addition of nefazodone, fluvoxamine, or fluoxetine. Phenothiazine drug levels may be increased when co-administered with propranolol, another inhibitor of hepatic microenzymes. Because propranolol is often an effective symptomatic treatment for neuroleptic-associated akathisia, the combined use of the β-blocker with an antipsychotic drug is common. When interactions present a problem, the use of a water-soluble β-blocker, such as atenolol, which is not likely to interfere with hepatic metabolism, provides a reasonable alternative.

MOOD STABILIZERS
Lithium

Lithium is absorbed completely from the gastrointestinal tract.[17] It distributes throughout total body water and, in contrast to most psychotropic drugs, does not bind to plasma

TABLE 50-4 Selected Drug Interactions with Lithium

Drug	Potential Interaction
Aminophylline, theophylline, acetazolamide, mannitol, sodium bicarbonate, sodium chloride load	Decreased lithium levels
Thiazide diuretics	Increased lithium levels; reduction of lithium-associated polyuria
Non-steroidal anti-inflammatory drugs, COX-2 inhibitors, tetracycline, spectinomycin, metronidazole, angiotensin II receptor antagonists, angiotensin-converting enzyme inhibitors	Increased lithium levels
Neuromuscular blocking drugs (succinylcholine, pancuronium, decamethonium)	Prolonged muscle paralysis
Antithyroid drugs (propylthiouracil, thioamide, methimazole)	Enhanced antithyroid efficacy
Calcium channel blockers (verapamil, diltiazem)	Idiosyncratic neurotoxicity
Antipsychotic drugs	Idiosyncratic neurotoxicity

proteins and is not metabolized in the liver. It is filtered and reabsorbed by the kidneys, and 95% of it is excreted in the urine. Lithium elimination is highly dependent on total body sodium and fluid balance; it competes with sodium for reabsorption in the proximal tubules. To a lesser extent, lithium is also reabsorbed in the loop of Henle but, in contrast to sodium, is not reabsorbed in the distal tubules. Its elimination half-life is approximately 24 hours; clearance is generally 20% of creatinine clearance but is diminished in elderly patients and in patients with renal disease. The risk of toxicity is increased in these patients, as well as in patients with cardiovascular disease, dehydration, or hypokalemia. The most common drug–drug interactions involving lithium are pharmacokinetic. Because lithium has a low therapeutic index, such interactions are likely to be clinically significant and potentially serious (Table 50-4).[22]

A number of medications are associated with decreased lithium excretion and therefore increased risk of lithium toxicity. Among the best studied of these interactions involve thiazide diuretics. These agents decrease lithium clearance and thereby steeply increase the risk of toxicity. Thiazide diuretics block sodium reabsorption at the distal tubule, producing sodium depletion, which, in turn, results in increased lithium reabsorption in the proximal tubule. Loop diuretics (e.g., furosemide, bumetanide) appear to interact to a lesser degree with lithium excretion, presumably because they block lithium reabsorption in the loop of Henle, potentially off-setting possible compensatory increases in reabsorption more proximally.[23,24] The potassium-sparing diuretics (e.g., amiloride, spironolactone, ethacrynic acid, triamterene) also appear to be somewhat less likely to cause an increase in lithium levels, but close monitoring is indicated when introduced. The potential impact of thiazide diuretics on lithium levels does not contraindicate their combined use, which has been particularly valuable in the treatment of lithium-associated polyuria. Potassium-sparing diuretics have also been used for this purpose. When a thiazide diuretic is used, a lithium dose reduction and frequent monitoring of lithium levels are required. Monitoring of serum electrolytes, particularly potassium, is also important when thiazides are introduced, because hypokalemia enhances the toxicity of lithium. Although not contraindicated with lithium, ACE inhibitors (e.g., captopril) and angiotensin II receptor antagonists (e.g., losartan) can elevate lithium levels, and close monitoring of levels is also required when these agents are introduced. Many of the non-steroidal anti-inflammatory drugs (NSAIDs) (including ibuprofen, indomethacin, naproxen, ketorolac, meloxicam, and piroxicam) have also been reported to increase serum lithium levels, potentially by as much as 50% to 60% when used at full prescription strength. This may occur by inhibition of renal clearance of lithium by interference with a prostaglandin-dependent mechanism in the renal tubule. The COX-2 inhibitors may also raise lithium levels. Limited available data suggest that aspirin is less likely to affect lithium levels.[25,26]

Finally, a number of antimicrobials are associated with increased lithium levels, including tetracycline, metronidazole, and parenteral spectinomycin. In the event that these agents are required, close monitoring of lithium levels and potential dose adjustment are recommended.

Conversely, a variety of agents can produce decreases in lithium levels, thereby increasing risk of psychiatric symptom breakthrough and relapse. The methylxanthines (e.g., aminophylline, theophylline) can cause a significant decrease in lithium levels by increasing renal clearance; close blood level monitoring is necessary when co-administration occurs. A reduction in lithium levels can also result from alkalinization of urine (e.g., with acetazolamide or sodium bicarbonate), osmotic diuretics (e.g., urea or mannitol), or from ingestion of a sodium chloride load, which also increases lithium excretion.

A probable pharmacodynamic interaction exists between lithium and agents (e.g., succinylcholine, pancuronium, decamethonium) used to produce neuromuscular blockade during anesthesia. Significant prolongation of muscle paralysis can occur when these agents are administered to the lithium-treated patient. Although the mechanism is unknown, the possible inhibition by lithium of acetylcholine synthesis and release at the neuromuscular junction is a potential basis for synergism.

Lithium interferes with the production of thyroid hormones through several mechanisms, including interference with iodine uptake, tyrosine iodination, and release of triiodothyronine (T_3) and thyroxine (T_4). Lithium may therefore enhance the efficacy of antithyroid medications (e.g., propylthiouracil, thioamide, methimazole) and has also been used preoperatively to help prevent thyroid storm in the surgical treatment of Graves' disease.

There are isolated reports of various forms of neurotoxicity, usually but not always reversible, when lithium has been combined with SSRIs, serotonin norepinephrine reuptake inhibitors (SNRIs), and other serotonergic agents, calcium channel blockers, antipsychotics, and anticonvulsants (such as carbamazepine). In some cases, features of the serotonin syndrome or NMS have been present. While it is worthwhile to bear this in mind when evaluating unexplained mental status changes in a lithium-treated patient, the combination of lithium with these classes of medication is neither contraindicated nor unusual.

Valproic Acid

Valproic acid is a simple branched-chain carboxylic acid that, like several other anticonvulsants, has mood-stabilizing properties. Valproic acid is 80% to 95% protein-bound and is rapidly metabolized primarily by hepatic microsomal glucuronidation and oxidation. It has a short elimination half-life of about 8 hours. Clearance is essentially unchanged in the elderly and in patients with renal disease, whereas it is significantly reduced in patients with primary liver disease.

In contrast to some other major anticonvulsants (such as carbamazepine and phenobarbital), valproate does not induce hepatic microsomes. Rather, it tends to act as an inhibitor of oxidation and glucuronidation reactions, thereby potentially

TABLE 50-5 Selected Drug Interactions with Valproate and Carbamazepine

Drug	Interaction with Valproate
Carbamazepine	Decreased valproate plasma levels; increased plasma levels of the epoxide metabolite of carbamazepine; variable effects on plasma levels of carbamazepine
Phenytoin	Decreased valproate plasma levels; variable effects on phenytoin plasma levels
Phenobarbital	Decreased valproate plasma levels; increased phenobarbital plasma levels
Oral contraceptives	Decreased valproate plasma levels
Carbapenem antibiotics	Decreased valproate plasma levels
Lamotrigine	Increased lamotrigine levels; hypersensitivity reaction
Aspirin	Increased unbound (active) fraction of valproate
Cimetidine Fluoxetine	Increased valproate plasma levels
Clonazepam	Rare absence seizures

Drug	Interaction with Carbamazepine
Phenytoin Phenobarbital Primidone	Decreased carbamazepine plasma levels
Macrolide antibiotics Isoniazid Fluoxetine Verapamil Diltiazem Danazol Propoxyphene	Increased carbamazepine plasma levels
Oral contraceptives Corticosteroids Thyroid hormones Warfarin Cyclosporine Phenytoin Ethosuximide Carbamazepine Valproate Lamotrigine Tetracycline Doxycycline Theophylline Methadone Benzodiazepines TCAs Antipsychotics Methylphenidate Modafinil	Induction of metabolism by carbamazepine
Thiazide diuretics Furosemide	Hyponatremia

TCAs, Tricyclic antidepressants.

increasing levels of co-administered hepatically-metabolized drugs, notably including lamotrigene as well as some TCAs, such as clomipramine, amitriptyline, and nortriptyline (Table 50-5).[27-29] A complex pharmacokinetic interaction occurs when valproic acid and carbamazepine are administered concurrently. Valproic acid not only inhibits the metabolism of carbamazepine and its active metabolite, carbamazepine-10,11-epoxide (CBZ-E), but also displaces both entities from protein-binding sites. Although the effect on plasma carbamazepine levels is variable, the levels of the unbound (active) epoxide metabolite are increased with a concomitant increased risk of carbamazepine neurotoxicity. Conversely, co-administration with carbamazepine results in a decrease in plasma valproic acid levels. Nevertheless, the combination of valproate and carbamazepine has been used successfully in the treatment of patients with bipolar disorder who were only partially responsive to either drug alone. Oral contraceptives as well as carbapanem antibiotics have also been associated with decreases in plasma valproic acid levels; enhanced monitoring of levels and valproate dose adjustments are recommended when these agents are used.

Cimetidine, a potent inhibitor of hepatic microsomal enzymes, is associated with decreased clearance of valproic acid resulting in increased levels. Dose reductions of valproic acid may be necessary in the patient starting cimetidine but not for other H_2-receptor antagonists. Elevated levels of valproic acid have also been reported sporadically with fluoxetine and other SSRIs. Aspirin and other salicylates may displace protein-binding of valproic acid, thereby increasing the unbound (free) fraction, which may increase risk of toxicity from valproate even though total serum levels are unchanged.

Absence seizures have been reported with the combination of clonazepam and valproate, although this is likely to be rare and limited to individuals with neurological disorders.

Lamotrigine

Lamotrigine is a phenyltriazine anticonvulsant that is moderately (50% to 60%) protein-bound and metabolized primarily by glucuronidation. Its most serious adverse effect is a life-threatening hypersensitivity reaction with rash, typically, but not always, occurring within the first 2 months of use. The incidence among individuals with bipolar disorder is estimated at 0.8 per 1,000 among patients on lamotrigine monotherapy and 1.3 per 1,000 among patients on lamotrigine in combination with other agents.

The risk of adverse effects including hypersensitivity reactions and tremor is increased when lamotrigine is combined with valproic acid. As much as a two-fold to three-fold increase in lamotrigine levels occurs when valproic acid is added, related to inhibition of glucuronidation of lamotrigine.[12,28] Accordingly, the *Physicians' Desk Reference* (PDR) provides guidelines for more gradual dose titration of lamotrigine and lower target doses when introduced in a patient already taking valproate. When valproate is added to lamotrigine, the dose of the latter should typically be reduced by one-half to two-thirds.

Conversely, lamotrigine levels can be decreased by as much as 50% when administered with metabolic inducers, particularly other anticonvulsants (including carbamazepine and phenobarbital). Guidelines have therefore been developed for the dosing of lamotrigine in the presence of these metabolic-inducing anticonvulsants. Of particular note, similar magnitude reductions in lamotrigine levels have been reported in patients on oral contraceptives, requiring an increase in the dose of lamotrigine.[30] Lamotrigine levels and symptom status should be monitored closely when oral contraceptives or metabolic-inducing anticonvulsants are started.

Carbamazepine

Carbamazepine is an iminostilbene anticonvulsant structurally related to the TCA imipramine. It is only moderately (60% to 85%) protein-bound. It is poorly soluble in gastrointestinal fluids, and as much as 15% to 25% of an oral dose is excreted unchanged in the feces. Its carbamazepine-10,11-epoxide (CBZ-E) metabolite is neuroactive. Carbamazepine, a potent inducer of hepatic metabolism, can also induce its own metabolism such that elimination half-life may fall from 18 to 55 hours to 5 to 20 hours over a matter of several weeks, generally reaching a plateau after 3 to 5 weeks.[17]

Most drug–drug interactions with carbamazepine occur by pharmacokinetic mechanisms.[29,31,32] The metabolism of a wide variety of drugs (e.g., valproic acid, phenytoin, ethosuximide, lamotrigine, alprazolam, clonazepam, TCAs, antipsychotics, methylphenidate, doxycycline, tetracycline, thyroid hormone, corticosteroids, oral contraceptives, methadone, theophylline, warfarin, oral hypoglycemics, cyclosporine) is induced by carbamazepine, thereby lowering drug levels and potentially leading to therapeutic failure or symptom relapse (see Table 50-5). Patients of childbearing potential on oral contraceptives must be advised to use an additional method of birth control.

Several drugs inhibit the metabolism of carbamazepine, including the macrolide antibiotics (e.g., erythromycin, clarithromycin, triacetyloleandomycin), isoniazid, fluoxetine, valproic acid, danazol, propoxyphene, and the calcium channel blockers verapamil and diltiazem. Because of its low therapeutic index, the risk of developing carbamazepine toxicity is significantly increased when these drugs are administered concurrently. Conversely, co-administration of phenytoin or phenobarbital, both microsomal enzyme inducers, can increase the metabolism of carbamazepine, potentially resulting in subtherapeutic plasma levels.

Carbamazepine has been associated with hyponatremia. The combination of carbamazepine with thiazide diuretics or furosemide has been associated with severe, symptomatic hyponatremia, suggesting the need for close monitoring of electrolytes when these medications are used concurrently. Carbamazepine has also been associated with bone marrow suppression, and its combination with other agents that interfere with blood cell production (including clozapine) should generally be avoided.

Oxcarbazepine appears to be a less potent metabolic inducer than carbamazepine, although it still may render certain important agents, particularly P450 3A4 substrates, less effective due to similar pharmacokinetic interactions. Women of childbearing potential should therefore receive guidance about supplementing oral contraceptives with a second non-hormonal form of birth control, as with carbamazepine. Similarly, like carbamazepine, oxcarbazepine is also associated with risk of hyponatremia.

ANTIDEPRESSANTS

The antidepressant drugs include the TCAs, the MAOIs, the SSRIs, the atypical agents (bupropion, trazodone, nefazodone, and mirtazapine), and the SNRIs (duloxetine, venlafaxine, and desvenlafaxine). Although the TCAs and MAOIs are used infrequently, they continue to serve a valuable role in the treatment of more severe, treatment-resistant depressive and anxiety disorders despite the wide range of drug–drug interactions they entail.

Selective Serotonin Reuptake Inhibitors and Other Newer Antidepressants

The SSRIs (fluoxetine, sertraline, paroxetine, fluvoxamine, citalopram, escitalopram, and vilazodone) share similar pharmacological actions, including minimal anticholinergic, antihistaminic, and α_1-adrenergic blocking effects, and potent pre-synaptic inhibition of serotonin reuptake. Vilazodone is also a partial agonist at the 5-HT$_{1A}$ receptor while vortioxetine is an antagonist, agonist or partial agonist at multiple serotonin receptor subtypes. There are important pharmacokinetic differences, which account for distinctions among them with respect to potential drug interactions (Table 50-6).[2,3,33] Nefazodone, similar to trazodone, is distinguished from classic SSRIs by its antagonism of the 5-HT$_2$ receptor (and differs from trazodone in its lesser antagonism of the α_1-adrenergic receptor). Mirtazapine also blocks the 5-HT$_2$ receptor, though it also blocks the 5-HT$_3$ receptor and α_2-adrenergic receptors. Venlafaxine,

TABLE 50-6 Potential Drug Interactions with the Selective Serotonin Reuptake Inhibitors and Other Newer Antidepressants

Drug	Potential Interaction
MAOIs	Serotonin syndrome
Secondary amine TCAs	Increased TCA levels when co-administered with fluoxetine, paroxetine, sertraline, bupropion, duloxetine
Tertiary amine TCAs	Increased TCA levels with fluvoxamine, paroxetine, sertraline, bupropion, duloxetine
Antipsychotics (typical) and risperidone, aripiprazole	Increased antipsychotic levels with fluoxetine, sertraline, paroxetine, bupropion, duloxetine
Thioridazine	Arrhythmia risk with P450 2D6 inhibitory antidepressants
Pimozide	Arrhythmia risk with P450 3A4 inhibitory antidepressants (nefazodone, fluvoxamine)
Clozapine and olanzapine	Increased antipsychotic levels with fluvoxamine
Diazepam	Increased benzodiazepine levels with fluoxetine, fluvoxamine, sertraline
Triazolobenzodiazepines (midazolam, alprazolam, triazolam)	Increased levels with fluvoxamine, nefazodone, sertraline
Carbamazepine	Increased carbamazepine levels with fluoxetine, fluvoxamine, nefazodone
Theophylline	Increased theophylline levels with fluvoxamine
Type 1C antiarrhythmics (encainide, flecainide, propafenone)	Increased antiarrhythmic levels with fluoxetine, paroxetine, sertraline, bupropion, duloxetine
β-Blockers (lipophilic)	Increased β-blocker levels with fluoxetine, paroxetine, sertraline, bupropion, duloxetine
Calcium channel blockers	Increased levels with fluoxetine, fluvoxamine, nefazodone

MAOIs, Monoamine oxidase inhibitors; TCAs, tricyclic antidepressants.

desvenlafaxine, levomilnacipran, and duloxetine, similar to TCAs, inhibit serotonin and norepinephrine reuptake but, in contrast to TCAs, are relatively devoid of post-synaptic anticholinergic, antihistaminic, and α_1-adrenergic activity. Milnacipran is also an SNRI, though FDA-approved only for fibromyalgia. While venlafaxine is predominantly serotonergic at low to moderate doses, duloxetine is a potent inhibitor of both the norepinephrine and serotonin transporters across its clinical dose range. Although not an approved antidepressant, the norepinephrine reuptake inhibitor atomoxetine, indicated for the treatment of attention-deficit/hyperactivity disorder (ADHD), may have a role in depression pharmacotherapy as single agent or as adjunctive treatment. It is neither a significant inhibitor nor an inducer of the P450 cytochrome system, but owing to its adrenergic effects, the risk of palpitations or pressor effects is likely to be greater than with serotonergic agents when combined with prescribed and OTC sympathomimetics, and its use with MAOIs is contraindicated.

All of the SSRIs, as well as nefazodone, are highly protein-bound (95% to 99%), with the exception of fluvoxamine (77%), citalopram (80%), and escitalopram (56%). Mirtazapine and bupropion are moderately protein-bound (85%). The SNRI duloxetine is highly protein-bound (90%), though venlafaxine, desvenlafaxine, and levomilnacipran are minimally protein-bound (15% to 30%). All of the antidepressants are hepatically metabolized, and all of them (except paroxetine and duloxetine) have active metabolites. The major metabolites of sertraline and citalopram, however, appear to be minimally active. Elimination half-lives range from 5 hours for venlafaxine and 11 hours for its metabolite, O-desmethylvenlafaxine, to 2 to 3 days for fluoxetine and 7 to 14 days for its metabolite, norfluoxetine. Nefazodone, similar to venlafaxine, has a short half-life (2 to 5 hours), with fluvoxamine, sertraline, paroxetine, citalopram, escitalopram, bupropion, mirtazapine, and duloxetine having half-lives in the intermediate range of 12 to 36 hours. Food may have variable effects on antidepressant bioavailability, including an increase for sertraline and vilazodone but a decrease for nefazodone, and no change for escitalopram.

The growing knowledge about the interaction of the newer antidepressants with the cytochrome P450 isoenzymes has revealed differences among them in their pattern of enzyme inhibition that are likely to be critical to the understanding and prediction of drug–drug interactions.

P450 2D6

Fluoxetine, norfluoxetine, paroxetine, bupropion, duloxetine, sertraline (to a moderate degree), and citalopram and escitalopram (to a minimal extent) inhibit P450 2D6, which accounts for their potential inhibitory effect on TCA clearance and the metabolism of other P450 2D6 substrates. Other drugs metabolized by P450 2D6 whose levels may rise in the setting of P450 2D6 inhibition include the type 1C antiarrhythmics (e.g., encainide, flecainide, propafenone), as well as lipophilic β-blockers (e.g., propranolol, timolol, metoprolol), antipsychotics (e.g., risperidone, haloperidol, aripiprazole, iloperidone, thioridazine, perphenazine), TCAs, and trazodone. P450 2D6 converts codeine and tramadol into their active form; hence the efficacy of these analgesics may be diminished when concurrently administered with a P450 2D6 inhibitor. So too, as P450 2D6 converts tamoxifen into its active N-desmethyl tamoxifen form for treatment of neoplasms, the use of inhibitors of 2D6 should be carefully re-evaluated during tamoxifen treatment. These observations underscore the need to exercise care and to closely monitor when prescribing these SSRIs, bupropion, or duloxetine in the setting of complex medical regimens. Plasma TCA levels do not routinely include levels of active or potentially toxic metabolites, which may be altered by virtue of shunting to other metabolic routes when P450 2D6 is inhibited. Therefore, particularly in the case of patients at risk for conduction delay, electrocardiography, as well as blood level monitoring, is recommended when combining TCAs with SSRIs, duloxetine, or bupropion.

P450 3A4

Fluoxetine's major metabolite (norfluoxetine), fluvoxamine, nefazodone, and, to a lesser extent, sertraline, desmethylsertraline, citalopram, and escitalopram inhibit P450 3A4. All of these agents have some potential therefore for elevating levels of pimozide and cisapride (arrhythmia risks), methadone, oxycodone, fentanyl (respiratory depression risks), calcium channel blockers, the "statins," carbamazepine, midazolam, and many other important and commonly prescribed substrates of this widely recruited P450 isoenzyme.

P450 2C

Serum concentrations of drugs metabolized by this subfamily may be increased by fluoxetine, sertraline, and fluvoxamine. Reported interactions include decreased clearance of diazepam on all three SSRIs, a small reduction in tolbutamide clearance on sertraline, and increased plasma phenytoin concentrations reflecting decreased clearance on fluoxetine. Warfarin is also metabolized by this subfamily, and levels may be increased by the inhibition of these enzymes. SSRIs may interact with warfarin and potentially increase bleeding diathesis by still other, probably pharmacodynamic, mechanisms (such as depletion of platelet serotonin). Although the combination is common, increased monitoring is recommended when SSRIs are prescribed with warfarin.

P450 1A

Among the SSRIs, only fluvoxamine appears to be a potent inhibitor of P450 1A2. Accordingly, increased serum concentrations of theophylline, haloperidol, clozapine, olanzapine, asenapine, and the tertiary amine TCAs (including clomipramine, amitriptyline, and imipramine) may occur when co-administered with this SSRI. Because theophylline and TCAs have a relatively narrow therapeutic index and because the degree of elevation of antipsychotic blood levels appears to be substantial (e.g., up to four-fold increases in haloperidol concentrations), additional monitoring and consideration of dose reductions of these substrates are necessary when fluvoxamine is co-administered.

Mirtazapine, although neither a potent inhibitor nor inducer of the P450 cytochrome isoenzymes, has numerous pharmacodynamic effects, including antagonism of the histamine-H_1, α_2-adrenergic, 5-HT_2 and 5-HT_3, and muscarinic receptors, creating the possibility of myriad pharmacodynamic interactions (including blockade of clonidine's antihypertensive activity) but also the possible benefit of attenuated nausea and sexual dysfunction that may occur with SSRIs.

The serotonin syndrome is a potentially life-threatening condition characterized by confusion, diaphoresis, hyperthermia, hyperreflexia, muscle rigidity, tachycardia, hypotension, and coma.[9,34] Although the serotonin syndrome may develop whenever an SSRI is combined with a serotonergic drug (e.g., L-tryptophan, clomipramine, venlafaxine, triptans) and drugs with serotonergic properties (e.g., lithium, mirtazapine, dextromethorphan, tramadol, meperidine, pentazocine), the greatest known risk is associated with the co-administration of an SSRI or SNRI with an MAOI, which constitutes an absolute contraindication. In view of the long elimination half-life of fluoxetine and norfluoxetine, at least 5 weeks must elapse after fluoxetine discontinuation before an MAOI can be safely introduced. With the other SSRIs and SNRIs, an interval of 2 weeks appears to be adequate. Because of the time required for the MAO enzymes to regenerate, at least 2 weeks must elapse after discontinuation of an MAOI before an SSRI or other potent serotonergic drug is introduced. The weak, reversible MAOI antimicrobial linezolid, used for treatment of multi-drug-resistant Gram-positive infections, has been implicated in a small number of post-marketing cases of serotonin syndrome in patients on serotonergic antidepressants, typically patients on SSRIs, as well as other medications (including narcotics). Patients on serotonergic antidepressants receiving linezolid should be monitored for the occurrence of symptoms suggesting serotonin syndrome. The co-administration of SSRIs with other serotonergic agents is not contraindicated but should prompt immediate discontinuation in any patient on this combination of drugs who has mental status changes, fever, or hyperreflexia of unknown origin.

Tricyclic Antidepressants

TCAs are thought to exert their pharmacological action by inhibiting the pre-synaptic neuronal reuptake of norepinephrine and serotonin in the CNS with subsequent modulation of both pre-synaptic and post-synaptic β-adrenergic receptors. TCAs also have significant anticholinergic, antihistaminic, and α-adrenergic activity, as well as quinidine-like effects on cardiac condition, in these respects resembling the low-potency antipsychotic drugs that are structurally similar.

TCAs are well absorbed from the gastrointestinal tract and subject to significant first-pass liver metabolism before entry into the systemic circulation, where they are largely protein-bound, ranging from 85% (trimipramine) to 95% (amitriptyline). They are highly lipophilic with a large volume of distribution. TCAs are extensively metabolized by hepatic microsomal enzymes, and most have pharmacologically-active metabolites.

With two methyl groups on the terminal nitrogen of the TCA side-chain, imipramine, amitriptyline, trimipramine, doxepin, and clomipramine are called *tertiary amines*. The demethylation of imipramine, amitriptyline, and trimipramine yields the secondary amine TCAs, desipramine, nortriptyline, and protriptyline, which are generally less sedating and have less affinity for anticholinergic receptors. The demethylation of imipramine relies on cytochrome P450 isoenzymes 1A2 and 3A3/4, whereas that of amitriptyline appears to rely primarily on 1A2. These tertiary amines, as well as their secondary amine offspring, are then hydroxylated via cytochrome P450 2D6, a step sensitive to inhibition by a wide variety of other drugs. The hydroxymetabolites of the most commonly prescribed TCAs can be active. Furthermore, the hydroxymetabolite of nortriptyline may block the antidepressant effect of the parent drug, and some hydroxymetabolites of the TCAs may be cardiotoxic.

Additive anticholinergic effects can occur when the TCAs are co-administered with other drugs possessing anticholinergic properties (e.g., low-potency antipsychotics, antiparkinsonian drugs), potentially resulting in an anticholinergic syndrome. SSRIs, SNRIs, atypical antidepressants, and MAOIs are relatively devoid of anticholinergic activity, although the MAOIs may indirectly potentiate the anticholinergic properties of atropine and scopolamine. Additive sedative effects are not uncommon when TCAs are combined with sedative-hypnotics, anxiolytics, narcotics, or alcohol (Table 50-7).

TCAs possess class 1A antiarrhythmic activity and can lead to depression of cardiac conduction, potentially resulting in heart block or ventricular arrhythmias when combined with quinidine-like agents (including quinidine, procainamide, and disopyramide, as well as the low-potency antipsychotics).[35,36] The antiarrhythmics quinidine and propafenone, inhibitors of cytochrome P450 2D6, may additionally result in clinically significant elevations of the TCAs, thus increasing the risk of cardiotoxicity through both pharmacodynamic and pharmacokinetic mechanisms.

The arrhythmogenic risks of a TCA are enhanced in an individual with underlying coronary or valvular heart disease, recent myocardial infarction, or hypokalemia, and in a patient receiving sympathomimetic amines, such as dextroamphetamine.

TABLE 50-7 Selected Drug Interactions with Tricyclic Antidepressants

Drug	Potential Interaction
Carbamazepine	Decreased TCA plasma levels
Phenobarbital	
Rifampin	
Isoniazid	
Antipsychotics	Increased TCA plasma levels
Methylphenidate	
SSRIs	
Quinidine	
Propafenone	
Antifungals	
Macrolide antibiotics	
Verapamil	
Diltiazem	
Cimetidine	
Class I antiarrhythmics	Depression of cardiac conduction; arrhythmias
Low-Potency Antipsychotics	
Guanethidine	Interference with antihypertensive effect
Clonidine	
Sympathomimetic amines (e.g., isoproterenol, epinephrine)	Arrhythmias, hypertension
Antihypertensives, vasodilator drugs	Hypotension
Anticholinergic drugs	Additive anticholinergic toxicity
MAOIs	Delirium, fever, convulsions
Sulfonylurea hypoglycemics	Hypoglycemia

MAOIs, Monoamine oxidase inhibitors; SSRIs, selective serotonin reuptake inhibitors; TCA, tricyclic antidepressant.

TCAs also interact with several antihypertensive drugs. TCAs can antagonize the antihypertensive effects of guanethidine, bethanidine, debrisoquine, or clonidine via interference with neuronal reuptake by noradrenergic neurons. Conversely, TCAs can cause or aggravate postural hypotension when co-administered with vasodilator drugs, antihypertensives, and low-potency neuroleptics.

Hypoglycemia has been observed on both secondary and tertiary TCAs, particularly in the presence of sulfonylurea hypoglycemic agents, suggesting the need for close monitoring.

Pharmacokinetic interactions involving the TCAs are often clinically important. The antipsychotic drugs (including haloperidol, chlorpromazine, thioridazine, and perphenazine) are known to increase TCA levels by 30% to 100%. Cimetidine can also raise tertiary TCA levels as predicted by microsomal enzyme inhibition, as can methylphenidate. The antifungals (e.g., ketoconazole), macrolide antibiotics (e.g., erythromycin), and calcium channel blockers (e.g., verapamil and diltiazem) as inhibitors of cytochrome P450 3A4 may also impair the clearance of tertiary amine TCAs, thereby requiring a TCA dose reduction. SSRIs, particularly fluoxetine, paroxetine, and, to a lesser extent, sertraline, have been associated with clinically-significant increases in TCA plasma levels, believed to be the result of inhibition primarily but not exclusively of cytochrome P450 2D6. Similar elevations in TCA levels would be expected with other potent P450 2D6 inhibitor antidepressants (including duloxetine and bupropion).

Inducers of P450 enzymes can increase the metabolism of TCAs. Thus, plasma levels of TCAs may be significantly reduced when carbamazepine, phenobarbital, rifampin, or isoniazid are co-administered or in the setting of chronic alcohol or cigarette use.

Monoamine Oxidase Inhibitors

Monoamine oxidase (MAO) is an enzyme located primarily on the outer mitochondrial membrane and is responsible for intracellular catabolism of the monoamines. It is found in high concentrations in brain, liver, intestines, and lung. In pre-synaptic nerve terminals, MAO metabolizes cytoplasmic monoamines. In liver and gut, MAO catabolizes ingested bioactive amines, thus protecting against absorption into the systemic circulation of potentially vasoactive substances, particularly tyramine. Two subtypes of MAO have been distinguished: intestinal MAO is predominantly MAO_A, whereas brain MAO is predominantly MAO_B. MAO_A preferentially metabolizes norepinephrine and serotonin. Both MAO subtypes metabolize dopamine and tyramine. The traditional MAOIs that have been used for treatment of depression—phenelzine, tranylcypromine, and isocarboxazid—are nonspecific inhibitors of both MAO_A and MAO_B. More recently, selegiline, available in transdermal form, has been approved for treatment of depression. At low doses, selegiline is primarily an inhibitor of MAO_B, though it is a mixed MAO_A and MAO_B inhibitor at higher doses. When patients are using MAOIs, dietary[37,38] and medication restrictions must be closely followed to avoid serious interactions. The MAOIs are therefore generally reserved for use in responsible or supervised patients when adequate trials of other classes of antidepressants have failed.

The two major types of MAOI drug–drug interaction are the serotonin syndrome and the hypertensive (also called hyperadrenergic) crisis.[7,8,33] Hypertensive crisis is an emergency characterized by an abrupt elevation of blood pressure, severe headache, nausea, vomiting, and diaphoresis; intracranial hemorrhage or myocardial infarction can occur. Prompt intervention to reduce blood pressure with the α_1-adrenergic antagonist phentolamine or the calcium channel blocker nifedipine may be life-saving. Potentially catastrophic hypertension appears to be due to release of bound intraneuronal stores of norepinephrine and dopamine by indirect vasopressor substances. The reaction can therefore be precipitated by the concurrent administration of vasopressor amines, stimulants, anorexiants, and many OTC cough and cold preparations; these include L-dopa, dopamine, amphetamine, methylphenidate, phenylpropanolamine, phentermine, mephentermine, metaraminol, ephedrine, and pseudoephedrine. By contrast, direct sympathomimetic amines (e.g., norepinephrine, isoproterenol, epinephrine), which rely for their cardiovascular effects on direct stimulation of post-synaptic receptors, rather than on pre-synaptic release of stored catecholamines, may be somewhat safer when administered to individuals on MAOIs, although they are also contraindicated.

Hypertensive crises may also be triggered by ingestion of naturally-occurring sympathomimetic amines (particularly tyramine), which are present in various food products, including aged cheeses (e.g., stilton, cheddar, blue cheese, or camembert, rather than cream cheese, ricotta cheese, or cottage cheese), yeast extracts (e.g., marmite and brewer's yeast tablets), fava (broad) beans, over-ripened fruits (e.g., avocado), pickled herring, aged meats (e.g., salami, bologna, and many kinds of sausage), chicken liver, fermented bean curd, sauerkraut, many types of red wine and beer (particularly imported beer), and some white wines. Although gin, vodka, and whiskey appear to be free of tyramine, their use should be minimized during the course of MAOI treatment, as with other antidepressants, because of the risk of exaggerated side effects and reduced antidepressant efficacy. Other less stringent requirements include moderated intake of caffeine, chocolate, yogurt, and soy sauce. Because MAO activity may remain diminished for nearly 2 to 3 weeks following the discontinuation of MAOIs, a tyramine-free diet and appropriate medication restrictions should be continued for at least 14 days after an MAOI has been discontinued. The lowest dose available of transdermal selegiline has been shown to have minimal risks of hypertensive crisis on a normal diet and therefore does not require the same level of restriction; however, doses of 9 mg/24 hours and above carry the same dietary recommendations as oral MAOIs.

The serotonin syndrome, the other major drug–drug interaction involving the MAOIs, occurs when MAOIs and serotonergic agents are co-administered. Potentially fatal reactions most closely resembling the serotonin syndrome can also occur with other drugs with less selective serotonergic activity, most notably meperidine, as well as dextromethorphan, a widely available cough suppressant. Both of these medications, similar to the SSRIs, SNRIs, and clomipramine, are absolutely contraindicated when MAOIs are used. The 5-HT$_1$ agonist triptans, used in the treatment of migraine, have been implicated in serotonin syndrome when administered to patients on MAOIs. This may be a particular problem on the triptans that are metabolized in part through the MAO enzymes, including sumatriptan, rizatriptan, and zolmitriptan. Other serotonergic medications (e.g., buspirone and trazodone), although not absolutely contraindicated, should be used with care. Other narcotic analgesics (e.g., propoxyphene, codeine, oxycodone, morphine, alfentanil, or morphine) appear to be somewhat safer alternatives to meperidine, but, in conjunction with MAOIs, their analgesic and CNS depressant effects may be potentiated and rare serotonin syndrome–like presentations have been reported.[33,39] If opioid agents are necessary, they should be started at one-fifth to one-half of the standard doses and gradually titrated upward, with monitoring for untoward hemodynamic or mental status changes.

Extremely adverse, although reversible, symptoms of fever, delirium, convulsions, hypotension, and dyspnea were reported on the combination of imipramine and MAOIs. This has contributed to a general avoidance of the once popular TCA–MAOI combinations. Nevertheless, although incompletely studied, the regimen has been observed in some instances to be successful for exceptionally treatment-refractory patients. When combined, simultaneous initiation of a TCA–MAOI or initiation of the TCA before, but never after the MAOI has been recommended, although avoidance of the more serotonergic TCAs (including clomipramine, imipramine, and amitriptyline) is prudent.

The sedative effects of CNS depressants (including the benzodiazepines, barbiturates, and chloral hydrate) may be potentiated by MAOIs. MAOIs often cause postural hypotension, and severe additive effects have occurred when co-administered with vasodilator or antihypertensive medications or low-potency antipsychotics.

The MAOIs, similar to the TCAs, have also been observed to potentiate hypoglycemic agents, including insulin and sulfonylurea drugs, suggesting the need for more frequent glucose monitoring when MAOIs are co-administered with hypoglycemic medications.

Phenelzine has been associated with lowered serum pseudocholinesterase levels and prolonged neuromuscular blockade. The concurrent use of MAOIs is not a contraindication to surgery or electroconvulsive therapy (ECT), although it requires a detailed pre-procedure consultation with the anesthesiologist.

St. John's Wort

Although the efficacy of St. John's wort for depression has not been well established, it has emerged as one of the most carefully studied herbal preparation when it comes to drug–drug interactions. Initial concerns about the generally weak, though potentially variable, MAOI activity of this botanical and the associated risk of serotonin syndrome when combined with serotonergic agents have only been weakly borne out, with few cases of serotonin syndrome reported despite widespread concurrent use of St. John's wort with serotonergic

antidepressants. However, both case reports and clinical trials indicate that some critical medications may be rendered less effective in some patients concurrently taking St. John's wort.[14,40] These medications include immunosuppressants (such as cyclosporine and tacrolimus), coumarin anticoagulants, antiretrovirals, theophylline, digoxin, amitriptyline, and oral contraceptives. Although the precise mechanisms and herbal constituents responsible for these effects remain to be elucidated, the primary focus has been on P450 3A4 and P-glycoprotein. A paucity of systematic information exists concerning potential drug interactions and adverse effects of other natural products, including a possible risk of increased bleeding in patients on *gingko biloba* and warfarin and of hepatotoxicity in patients on certain kava preparations.[6]

BENZODIAZEPINES

The benzodiazepines are a class of widely-prescribed psychotropic drugs that have anxiolytic, sedative, muscle-relaxant, and anticonvulsant properties. Their rate of onset of action, duration of action, presence of active metabolites, and tendency to accumulate in the body vary considerably and can influence both side effects and the success of treatment.[17] Most benzodiazepines are well absorbed on an empty stomach, with peak plasma levels achieved generally between 1 and 3 hours, although with more rapid onset on some (e.g., diazepam, clorazepate) than others (e.g., oxazepam). Duration of action of a single dose of benzodiazepine generally depends more on distribution from systemic circulation to tissue than on subsequent elimination (e.g., more rapid for diazepam than lorazepam). With repeated doses, however, the volume of distribution is saturated, and elimination half-life becomes the more important parameter in determining duration of action (e.g., more rapid for lorazepam than diazepam). A benzodiazepine that is comparatively short-acting on acute administration may, therefore, become relatively long-acting on long-term dosing. Benzodiazepines are highly lipophilic and distribute readily to the CNS and to tissues. Plasma protein-binding ranges from approximately 70% (alprazolam) to 99% (diazepam).

Of the benzodiazepines, only lorazepam, oxazepam, and temazepam are not subject to phase I metabolism. Because phase II metabolism (glucuronide conjugation) does not produce active metabolites and is less affected than phase I metabolism by primary liver disease, aging, and concurrently used inducers or inhibitors of hepatic microsomal enzymes, the 3-hydroxy-substituted benzodiazepines are often preferred in older patients and patients with liver disease.

Perhaps the most common and clinically significant interactions involving benzodiazepines are the additive CNS-depressant effects, which can occur when a benzodiazepine is administered concurrently with barbiturates, narcotics, or ethanol. These interactions can be serious because of their potential to cause excessive sedation, cognitive and psychomotor impairment, and, at higher doses, potentially fatal respiratory depression. An interesting pharmacodynamic interaction exists between benzodiazepines and physostigmine, which can act as a competitive inhibitor at the benzodiazepine receptor, antagonizing benzodiazepine effects. The specific benzodiazepine antagonist flumazenil, however, is now more commonly the treatment of choice in managing a severe benzodiazepine overdose.

Pharmacokinetic interactions include a decreased rate, but not extent, of absorption of benzodiazepines in the presence of antacids or food. This is more likely to be a factor in determining the subjective effects accompanying the onset of benzodiazepine action for single-dose rather than the overall efficacy of repeated-dose administration. Carbamazepine, phenobarbital, and rifampin may induce metabolism, lowering levels of benzodiazepines that are oxidatively metabolized. In contrast, potential inhibitors of cytochrome P450 3A4 (including macrolide antibiotics, antifungals [e.g., ketoconazole, itraconazole], nefazodone, fluvoxamine, and cimetidine) may be associated with decreased clearance and therefore increased levels of the triazolobenzodiazepines, as well as the non-benzodiazepine sedative-hypnotics (zolpidem, zaleplon, and eszopiclone), which are metabolized through this pathway.[2] The metabolism of diazepam depends in part on cytochrome P450 2C19. Decreased diazepam clearance has been reported with concurrent administration of a variety of agents (including fluoxetine, sertraline, propranolol, metoprolol, omeprazole, disulfiram, low-dose estrogen containing oral contraceptives, and isoniazid).

PSYCHOSTIMULANTS AND MODAFINIL

A variety of miscellaneous drug–drug interactions involving the psychostimulants have been reported.[41] These include increased plasma levels of TCAs (and possibly other antidepressants); increased plasma levels of phenobarbital, primidone, and phenytoin; increased prothrombin time on coumarin anticoagulants; attenuation or reversal of the guanethidine antihypertensive effect; and increased pressor responses to vasopressor drugs. The risk of arrhythmias or hypertension should be considered when combining psychostimulants with TCAs. Although methylphenidate has been implicated in putative drug interactions more often than dextroamphetamine or mixed amphetamine salts, drug interactions involving psychostimulants have been insufficiently studied to draw firm conclusions about their comparative suitability for use among patients on complex medical regimens. Although contraindicated because of the risk of hypertensive crisis, the combination of psychostimulants and MAOIs has been cautiously used in patients with exceptionally treatment-refractory depression or in patients with limiting hypotension on MAOIs that proved resistant to other measures.[42,43] Urinary alkalinization (e.g., with sodium bicarbonate) may result in amphetamine toxicity, most likely because of increased tubular reabsorption of un-ionized amphetamine.

Modafinil and armodafinil interact with the P450 cytochrome isoenzymes as a minimal to moderate inducer of 1A2 and 3A4 and yet as an inhibitor of the 2C isoforms.[2] Modafinil and armodafinil may thereby engage in drug–drug interactions with common substrates, including oral contraceptives (whose levels may decrease) and lipophilic β-blockers, TCAs, clozapine, and warfarin (whose levels may increase), therefore requiring monitoring and patient education. It is important to advise use of a second non-hormonal form of contraception in modafinil and armodafinil-treated patients on oral contraceptives. Like St. John's wort, modafinil has also been implicated as a factor in lowered cyclosporine levels, presumably through P450 3A4 induction, and should be used with extreme care in patients on immunosuppressants that rely on this enzyme for metabolism. Although modafinil and armodafinil have been widely combined with SSRIs and other first-line antidepressants, its safety in combination with MAOIs is unknown.

Access the complete reference list and multiple choice questions (MCQs) online at https://expertconsult.inkling.com

KEY REFERENCES

1. Ciraulo DA, Shader RI, Greenblatt DJ, et al., editors: *Drug interactions in psychiatry*, ed 3, Baltimore, 2005, Williams & Wilkins.
2. Wynn GH, Cozza KL, Armstrong SC, et al. *Clinical manual of drug interaction principles for medical practice*, Washington, DC, 2008, American Psychiatric Publishing Inc.
3. Preskorn SH, Flockhart D. 2010 guide to psychiatric drug interactions. *Prim Psychiatry* 16(12):45–74, 2009.
4. Owen JA. Psychopharmacology. In Levenson JL, editor: *The American Psychiatric Publishing textbook of psychosomatic medicine: psychiatric care of the medically ill*, ed 2, Washington DC, 2011, American Psychiatric Publishing Inc.
5. Alpert JE. Drug-drug interactions in psychopharmacology. In Stern TA, Herman JB, Gorrindo T, editors: *Massachusetts General Hospital psychiatry update and board preparation*, ed 3, New York, 2012, McGraw-Hill, pp 401–409.
6. Mills E, Wu P, Johnston B, et al. Natural health product-drug interactions: a systematic review of clinical trials. *Ther Drug Monit* 27(5):549–557, 2005.
7. Livingston MG, Livingston HM. Monoamine oxidase inhibitors: an update on drug interactions. *Drug Saf* 14:219–227, 1997.
8. Flockhart DA. Dietary restrictions and drug interactions with monoamine oxidase inhibitors: an update. *J Clin Psychiatry* 73(Suppl. 1):17–24, 2012.
9. Boyer EW, Shannon M. Current concepts: the serotonin syndrome. *N Engl J Med* 352(11):1112–1120, 2005.
10. Wilkinson GR. Drug metabolism and variability among patients in drug response. *N Engl J Med* 352:2211–2221, 2005.
11. Buxton ILO, Benet LZ. Pharmacokinetics: the dynamics of drug absorption, distribution, and elimination. In Chabner BA, Knollman BC, editors: *Goodman and Gilman's the pharmacological basis of therapeutics*, ed 12, New York, 2011, McGraw-Hill.
12. Patsalos PN, Froscher W, Pisani F, et al. The importance of drug interactions in epilepsy therapy. *Epilepsia* 43(4):365–385, 2002.
13. Kahn AY, Preskorn SH. Pharmacokinetic principles and drug interactions. In Soares JC, Gershon S, editors: *Handbook of medical psychiatry*, New York, 2003, Marcel Dekker.
14. Zhou S, Chan E, Pan SQ, et al. Pharmacokinetic interactions of drugs with St. John's wort. *J Psychopharmacol* 18:262–276, 2004.
17. Rosenbaum JF, Arana GW, Hyman SE, et al. *Handbook of psychiatric drug therapy*, ed 5, Boston, 2005, Lippincott Williams & Wilkins.
18. Freudenreich O, Goff DC. Antipsychotics. In Ciraulo DA, Shader RI, Greenblatt DJ, et al., editors: *Drug interactions in psychiatry*, ed 3, Baltimore, 2005, Williams & Wilkins.
19. Spina E, de Leon J. Metabolic drug interactions with newer antipsychotics: a comparative review. *Basic Clin Pharmacol Toxicol* 100:4–22, 2007.
22. Sarid-Segal O, Creelman WL, Ciraulo DA, et al. Lithium. In Ciraulo DA, Shader RI, Greenblatt DJ, et al., editors: *Drug interactions in psychiatry*, ed 3, Baltimore, 2005, Williams & Wilkins.
27. DeVane CL. Pharmacokinetics, drug interactions, and tolerability of valproate. *Psychopharmacol Bull* 37(Suppl. 2):25–42, 2003.
28. Fleming J, Chetty M. Psychotropic drug interactions with valproate. *Clin Neuropharmacol* 28(2):96–101, 2005.
29. Circaulo DA, Pacheco MN, Slattery M. Anticonvulsants. In Ciraulo DA, Shader RI, Greenblatt DJ, et al., editors: *Drug interactions in psychiatry*, ed 3, Baltimore, 2005, Williams & Wilkins.
33. Ciraulo DA, Creelman WL, Shader RI, et al. Antidepressants. In Ciraulo DA, Shader RI, Greenblatt DJ, et al., editors: *Drug interactions in psychiatry*, ed 3, Baltimore, 2005, Williams & Wilkins.
34. Keck PE, Arnold LM. The serotonin syndrome. *Psychiatr Ann* 30:333–343, 2000.
36. Witchel HJ, Hancok JC, Nutt DJ. Psychotropic drugs, cardiac arrhythmia and sudden death. *J Clin Psychopharmacol* 23:58–77, 2003.
41. Markowitz JS, Morrison SD, DeVane CL. Drug interactions with psychostimulants. *Int Clin Psychopharmacol* 14:1–18, 1999.

51 Side Effects of Psychotropic Medications

Jeff C. Huffman, MD, Scott R. Beach, MD, and Theodore A. Stern, MD

KEY POINTS

Background

- A systematic approach to side effects of medications should include consideration of the nature, severity, and timing of symptoms to facilitate optimal management of such side effects.

History

- Many medications (e.g., nefazodone) previously used in psychiatric disorders, but shown to have serious adverse side effects, have been removed from the market over the years.

Clinical and Research Challenges

- Rates of medication side effects may be difficult to quantify.
- Though some side effects may be class effects, others are specific to individual agents.
- It is difficult to predict who will suffer side effects; some side effects are idiosyncratic.

Practical Pointers

- Tricyclic antidepressants are associated with cardiac effects and can be dangerous in overdose.
- Use of monoamine oxidase inhibitors requires education about dietary limitations and drug–drug interactions.
- Selective serotonin reuptake inhibitors and other newer antidepressants are generally well tolerated and safer in overdose than older agents, but still may cause clinically significant side effects.
- Some selective norepinephrine (noradrenaline)-serotonin reuptake inhibitors have been associated with increased blood pressure (e.g., venlafaxine) and liver dysfunction (e.g., duloxetine).

- Bupropion is known to lower the seizure threshold and has also been associated with an increase in panic symptoms.
- Mirtazapine is associated most commonly with sedation and weight gain.
- Lithium and anticonvulsant mood stabilizers are associated with a variety of side effects, including cognitive slowing, weight gain, and neurological symptoms.
- Lamotrigine is the mood stabilizer most associated with the development of Stevens-Johnson syndrome, a rare but life-threatening skin disease.
- Typical antipsychotics are associated with tardive dyskinesia and, of them, the high-potency typical antipsychotics commonly cause extrapyramidal symptoms.
- Several atypical antipsychotics are linked to weight gain and metabolic side effects.
- Most antipsychotics can cause prolongation of the QTc interval, which may increase the risk for lethal ventricular arrhythmias.
- Stimulants have a propensity to cause increased heart rate and blood pressure, and their use is not recommended for patients with underlying ventricular arrhythmias.
- Benzodiazepines are associated with a variety of side effects (including falls, dizziness, and ataxia).
- Short-acting sedative-hypnotic agents, such as zolpidem, have been associated with various sleep-related behaviors, including eating and driving.

OVERVIEW

Side effects of psychotropics, which can range from minor nuisances to life-threatening conditions, can seriously affect the quality of a patient's life and his or her ability to comply with psychopharmacological treatments. For these reasons, it is important for clinicians who prescribe psychotropic medications to know their potential side effects and how such side effects can be managed.

Determining which medication is causing a specific side effect, and whether *any* medication is to blame for a given adverse effect, can be difficult. For example, more than half of all patients with untreated melancholic depression report headache, constipation, and sedation; these same symptoms are frequently attributed to side effects of antidepressant medications.[1] A stepwise approach to the assessment of a potential side effect can help to ensure that true side effects are quickly addressed, while knee-jerk reactions that result in the discontinuation of well-tolerated treatments can be avoided. This approach (Box 51-1) involves an assessment of the nature and severity of the effect, a thoughtful investigation into the

causality of the effect, and the appropriate management of the symptom.

In this chapter, the most common and most dangerous side effects of psychotropics will be discussed in an effort to guide clinicians to treatment decisions and management of adverse effects. For each agent or class of agents, we will review common initial side effects, frequent long-term side effects, severe but rare adverse events, consequences of overdose, and (where applicable) withdrawal symptoms.

ANTIDEPRESSANTS

Tricyclic Antidepressants

Tricyclic antidepressants (TCAs) have a number of common side effects that require careful management. Anticholinergic effects (including dry mouth, blurry vision, urinary hesitancy, constipation, tachycardia, and delirium) that result from the blockade of muscarinic cholinergic receptors can occur with use of TCAs. In addition, anticholinergic effects can also be dangerous to patients with pre-existing glaucoma (leading to

---

BOX 51-1 A Systematic Approach to Medication Side Effects

NATURE OF THE SIDE EFFECT

What exactly are the signs and symptoms? In some cases (e.g., drug rash) this can be easily ascertained, while in others (e.g., a severely demented patient with worsening agitation, possibly consistent with akathisia, restlessness, constipation) it may be difficult.

When did the symptom start?

Has this ever happened before?

Are there associated symptoms?

SEVERITY OF THE SIDE EFFECT

What subjective distress does the symptom cause?

What impact is it having on function and quality of life?

What medical dangers are associated with the side effect?

CAUSALITY OF THE SIDE EFFECT

Did the side effect start in the context of a new medication or a dosage change?

What other medications/remedies are being taken?

Have there been other changes in medication, medical issues, diet, environment, or psychiatric symptoms?

Are the current signs and symptoms consistent with known side effects of a given medication?

MANAGEMENT OF THE SIDE EFFECT

If it appears that a specific medication is causing the side effect, options for management include:

Discontinue the medication

Decrease the dose

Change the dosing schedule (e.g., splitting up dose, taking medication during meals)

Change the preparation (e.g., to longer-lasting formulation)

Add a new medication to treat the side effect (e.g., propranolol for akathisia)

BOX 51-2 Management of Antidepressant Side Effects

GENERAL PRINCIPLES

- Carefully consider whether the side effect is from the antidepressant.
- Consider the timing, dosing, and the nature of effect, as well as the impact of concomitant medications, environmental changes, and medical conditions.
- Consider drug–drug interactions as the cause of the adverse effects, rather than the effects of the antidepressant acting in isolation.
- If an antidepressant appears to be causing non-dangerous side effects, consider lowering the dose (temporarily or permanently), dividing the dose, or changing medications.

MANAGEMENT OF SPECIFIC SIDE EFFECTS

- Anticholinergic effects (e.g., dry mouth, urinary hesitancy, constipation): Symptomatic treatment (use hard candies for dry mouth, use laxatives for constipation); use bethanechol (25–50 mg/day) for refractory symptoms.
- Sedation: Move the dose to bedtime, divide the dose, or add a psychostimulant (e.g., methylphenidate, 5–15 mg each morning) or modafinil (100–200 mg each morning).
- Orthostatic hypotension: Increase fluid intake, divide the dose or move it to bedtime, or add a stimulant/mineralocorticoid.
- Gastrointestinal side effects: Divide the dose, take it with meals, give it at bedtime, or use an H_2 blocker (e.g., ranitidine 150 mg twice daily).
- Insomnia: Move the dose to the morning or add trazodone (25–100 mg), a sedative-hypnotic (e.g., zolpidem 5–10 mg), or another sedating agent.
- Weight gain: Use diet and exercise, and consider addition of an H_2 blocker, topiramate, or sibutramine.
- Sexual dysfunction: Options include switching to another agent (to bupropion, mirtazapine, or another agent not associated with sexual dysfunction), employing a drug holiday (often ineffective), or augmenting with a variety of agents (e.g., sildenafil, methylphenidate, bupropion, amantadine, buspirone, or yohimbine).

---

acute angle-closure glaucoma), benign prostatic hypertrophy (leading to acute urinary retention), and dementia (leading to acute confusional states). TCAs can also cause sedation that results from blockade of H_1 histamine receptors, and orthostatic hypotension, due to blockade of alpha$_1$ receptors on blood vessels. All three of these side-effect clusters are more common with tertiary amine TCAs (e.g., amitriptyline, doxepin, clomipramine, imipramine) than with secondary amine TCAs (e.g., nortriptyline, desipramine, protriptyline). TCAs may also cause increased sweating. Longer-term side effects of TCAs include weight gain (related to histamine receptor blockade) and sexual dysfunction. Box 51-2 describes the management of common side effects of TCAs and other antidepressants.

In addition to these common initial and long-term side effects, TCAs may have more serious but uncommon side effects; many of them are cardiac in nature. These agents are structurally similar to class I antiarrhythmics that are actually pro-arrhythmic in roughly 10% of the population; approximately 20% of patients with pre-existing conduction disturbances have cardiac complications while taking TCAs.[2] TCAs are associated with cardiac conduction disturbances and their use can lead to prolongation of the PR, QRS, and QT intervals on the electrocardiogram (ECG) and have been associated with all manner of heart block. Some have suggested that effects on cardiac conduction are most severe with desipramine, while other studies have found amitriptyline and maprotiline to be most associated with torsades de pointes.[3] Furthermore, these agents have been associated with an increased risk of

myocardial infarction (MI) when compared to selective serotonin reuptake inhibitors (SSRIs).[4] In addition to cardiac effects, other serious adverse events include the serotonin syndrome that occurs most often when TCAs are combined with other serotonergic agents, especially monoamine oxidase inhibitors (MAOIs). This syndrome can include confusion, agitation, and neuromuscular excitability (including seizures), and is more comprehensively discussed in Chapter 55.

Adverse effects associated with TCA overdose include the exacerbation of standard side effects (e.g., severe sedation, hypotension, anticholinergic delirium). Ventricular arrhythmias and seizures can also result from TCA overdose. TCA overdose is frequently lethal, with death most often occurring via cardiovascular effects. Figure 51-1 shows an ECG (with characteristic QRS interval widening) of a patient following TCA overdose.[5] A withdrawal syndrome (manifested by malaise, nausea, muscle aches, chills, diaphoresis, and anxiety) can occur following abrupt discontinuation of TCAs; the syndrome is thought to result from cholinergic rebound.

Selective Serotonin Reuptake Inhibitors

Selective serotonin reuptake inhibitors (SSRIs) are generally well tolerated. The most common side effects of SSRIs include gastrointestinal side effects (e.g., nausea, diarrhea, heartburn) that likely result from interactions with serotonin receptors

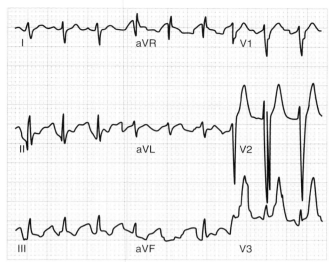

Figure 51-1. ECG showing findings consistent with tricyclic antidepressant poisoning, including sinus tachycardia with widened QRS complex (110 ms) and marked deviation of the terminal portion of the QRS complex in lead I (deep S wave) and aVR (large R wave). *(Re-drawn from Van Mieghem C, Sabbe M, Knockaert D, et al. The clinical value of the ECG in noncardiac conditions, Chest 125:1561– 1576, 2004.)*

(primarily 5-HT$_3$ that line the gut), central nervous system (CNS) activation (e.g., anxiety, restlessness, tremor, insomnia), and sedation that appear within the first few days of treatment. Gastrointestinal side effects may be most common with sertraline and fluvoxamine, CNS activation with fluoxetine, and sedation with paroxetine. Headache and dizziness can also occur early in treatment. These symptoms often improve or resolve within the first few weeks of treatment. Rarely, akathisia or other extrapyramidal symptoms (EPS) may occur (sertraline appears to be the most frequent offender due to its dopamine-blocking properties). Nausea, insomnia, and somnolence are adverse effects that most often lead to discontinuation of SSRIs. It is notable that the rate of discontinuation due to side effects is higher with fluvoxamine than with other SSRIs.

Longer-term side effects associated with SSRIs include sexual dysfunction, which occurs in 30% or more of SSRI-treated patients; SSRI-induced sexual dysfunction occurs in both men and women, affecting both libido and orgasms. Weight gain, fatigue, and apathy are infrequent long-term side effects; weight gain may occur more frequently with paroxetine. The syndrome of inappropriate antidiuretic hormone secretion (SIADH) can occur with all SSRIs, though it may be more frequent with fluoxetine.[6] Finally, SSRIs may increase the risk of bleeding, primarily due to the effects of these agents on serotonin receptors of platelets, resulting in decreased platelet activation and aggregation; it appears that the bleeding risk associated with use of SSRIs is similar to that of low-dose non-steroidal anti-inflammatory agents.[7] SSRIs are relatively safe in overdose. The serotonin syndrome can occur when these agents are combined with other serotonergic compounds, or, very rarely, when used alone.

SSRIs are generally considered safe in terms of cardiovascular side effects. Recently, concern has arisen regarding the possibility of SSRIs leading to prolongation of the QTc interval and increasing the risk for torsades de pointes, a potentially lethal ventricular arrhythmia. In fact, all SSRIs have been associated in case reports with QTc prolongation at therapeutic doses and in overdose.[8] In particular, citalopram has been

shown to have a modest QT-prolonging effect, which resulted in a recommendation from the Food and Drug Administration (FDA) in August 2011 to limit the maximum daily dose of citalopram to 40 mg (20 mg in patients with hepatic impairment or those older than 60 years) because of the increased risk of QTc prolongation at higher doses, and to declare its use contraindicated in patients with congenital long-QT syndrome. Less stringent recommendations were issued in March 2012, but citalopram remains not recommended for use at doses greater than 40 mg per day. No QTc-related recommendations have been issued for other SSRIs, though escitalopram appears to have a more modest, dose-dependent effect on prolongation of the QTc interval.[9]

Finally, abrupt withdrawal from SSRIs can lead to a withdrawal syndrome characterized by several somatic symptoms. The syndrome includes disequilibrium (dizziness, vertigo, and ataxia), flu-like symptoms (headache, lethargy, myalgias, rhinorrhea, and chills), gastrointestinal symptoms (nausea, vomiting, and diarrhea), sensory disturbances (paresthesias and sensations of electrical shock), and sleep disturbances (insomnia, fragmented sleep, and vivid, often frightening, dreams). In addition, a number of psychological symptoms (e.g., agitation, irritability, anxiety, crying spells) are associated with SSRI discontinuation.

Symptoms of the discontinuation syndrome typically begin 1 to 3 days after withdrawal of an SSRI, though when associated with a longer–half-life agent (fluoxetine in particular), symptoms may begin as long as 7 to 10 days after its discontinuation. Symptoms usually resolve within 2 weeks. If the original antidepressant is restarted, or another SSRI is substituted, the symptoms resolve, usually within 24 hours of re-initiation. This syndrome is most common with SSRIs with shorter half-lives (paroxetine and fluvoxamine); it rarely occurs with fluoxetine, whose metabolite has a half-life of more than 1 week. The syndrome is thought to result from diminished synaptic serotonin levels at serotonin receptors that have been desensitized in the context of serotonin reuptake inhibition.

Serotonin-Norepinephrine Reuptake Inhibitors
Venlafaxine

Venlafaxine's initial side effects are similar to those of the SSRIs. Nausea and CNS activation appear to occur somewhat more commonly than with the SSRIs; in addition, dry mouth and constipation may be associated with venlafaxine use despite lack of effects on muscarinic cholinergic receptors. Increased blood pressure, presumably related to effects on norepinephrine (noradrenaline), can occur with immediate-release venlafaxine, with 7% of patients taking 300 mg per day or less and 13% taking doses greater than 300 mg having elevation of blood pressure; this resolves spontaneously in approximately one-half of cases.[10] The extended-release (XR) formulation appears to be associated with lower rates of hypertension. Sexual dysfunction occurs at approximately the same rate as occurs with SSRIs. Venlafaxine does not appear to have substantial adverse effects on the cardiovascular system, though at least one study has suggested the possibility of QTc prolongation.[11] Among more serious side effects, SIADH and serotonin syndrome have been reported with venlafaxine.

Overdose of venlafaxine generally causes symptoms similar to those of SSRI overdose. However, venlafaxine, according to one large epidemiological study in the United Kingdom,[12] has been associated with a high rate of death in overdose (possibly via seizure and cardiovascular effects); other (smaller) studies have not found an increased lethality with overdose. Finally, due to the short half-life of venlafaxine, the discontinuation syndrome reported with SSRIs is common in patients who abruptly stop taking this antidepressant.[13]

Duloxetine

In general, duloxetine's common side effects are similar to those of SSRIs. Nausea, dizziness, headache, and insomnia may be somewhat more frequent than with SSRIs, but overall this agent is well tolerated.[14] Duloxetine does not appear to have significant effects on blood pressure or other cardiovascular parameters, including the QTc interval. Sexual dysfunction appears in concert with duloxetine use, but may be less common than with SSRIs such as paroxetine.[15] Duloxetine has not shown significant affinity for histaminic or cholinergic receptors, and thus sedation, weight gain, and anticholinergic effects are uncommon.

With respect to more severe adverse effects, SIADH has been reported with duloxetine use, and serotonin syndrome may develop with this agent because of its significant serotonin reuptake inhibition. Increased levels of hepatic transaminases develop in a small percentage of patients taking duloxetine; this is usually asymptomatic, but patients with chronic liver disease or cirrhosis have experienced elevated levels of bilirubin, alkaline phosphatase, and transaminases, and currently it is recommended that duloxetine should not be given to patients who consume substantial amounts of alcohol or who exhibit evidence of chronic liver disease.[16] Duloxetine does not appear to have increased rates of death in cases of overdose. A discontinuation syndrome similar to that seen with SSRIs and venlafaxine can occur with abrupt withdrawal of duloxetine,[17] though it is probably less likely than with venlafaxine or paroxetine due to its longer half-life.

Monoamine Oxidase Inhibitors

Tranylcypromine and phenelzine are the most commonly used oral MAOIs and are both irreversible inhibitors. Tranylcypromine is associated with anxiety, restlessness, insomnia, and tremor, while phenelzine is more associated with sedation, mild anticholinergic effects, and orthostatic hypotension (though this last effect can occur with both agents). Both agents are associated with headache, dry mouth, and gastrointestinal side effects. With regard to long-term side effects, weight gain and sexual dysfunction can occur with all MAOIs, though perhaps more commonly with phenelzine. MAOIs can result in symptoms of pyridoxine deficiency, including paresthesias and weakness. Finally, MAOIs have been associated with elevated liver transaminases, though true hepatotoxicity is exceedingly rare.

Hyperadrenergic crises, characterized by occipital headache, nausea, vomiting, diaphoresis, tachycardia, and severe hypertension, can occur in patients taking MAOIs. These most commonly occur when tyramine-containing foods are consumed or when adrenergic agonists (such as sympathomimetics) are taken in combination with MAOIs. Box 51-3 lists tyramine-containing foods that should be avoided by patients on MAOIs.[18] Serotonin syndrome can also occur with MAOIs when these agents are taken with SSRIs, TCAs, or other serotonergic agents (Box 51-4 lists medications that should be avoided by patients taking MAOIs). MAOI overdose is quite dangerous, with rates of death higher than those for SSRIs and other newer antidepressants[12]; with serotonin syndrome, neuromuscular excitability, seizures, arrhythmias, and cardiovascular collapse are all possible.

The transdermal MAOI (selegiline) patch does not require dietary modification at its lowest dose. At this lowest dose (6 mg/24 hours) transdermal selegiline appears to have an

---

BOX 51-3 Foods to Be Avoided by Patients Taking Monoamine Oxidase Inhibitors

- All matured or aged cheeses (fresh cottage, cream, ricotta, and processed cheese are tolerated)
- Pizza, lasagne, and other foods made with cheese
- Fermented/dried meat (e.g., pepperoni, salami, or summer sausage)
- Improperly stored meat and fish
- Fava or broad bean pods
- Banana peel (banana and other fruit are tolerated, but do not use more than 1/4 pound of raspberries)
- All tap beer (two or less cans/bottles of beer or 4 oz glasses of wine per day)
- Sauerkraut
- Soy sauce and other soybean products (soy milk is acceptable)
- Marmite yeast extract (other yeast extract are acceptable)

Data from Gardner DM, Shulman KI, Walker SE, et al. The making of a user friendly MAOI diet, J Clin Psychiatry 57:99–104, 1996.

BOX 51-4 Medications to Be Avoided by Patients Taking Monoamine Oxidase Inhibitors

INCREASED RISK OF SEROTONIN SYNDROME
- SSRIs
- TCAs
- Mirtazapine
- Nefazodone
- Vilazodone
- Trazodone
- Buspirone
- Lithium
- Dextromethorphan
- Tramadol
- Methadone
- Carbamazepine
- Sumatriptan and related compounds
- Cocaine
- MDMA
- St. John's wort
- SAMe
- Linezolid

INCREASED RISK OF HYPERADRENERGIC CRISIS
- Dopamine
- L-dopa
- Psychostimulants
- Bupropion
- Amphetamine
- Cold remedies or weight loss products containing pseudoephedrine, phenylpropanolamine, phenylephrine, or ephedrine
- Other
- Meperidine (may cause seizures and delirium)

MDMA, 3,4-methylenedioxy-N-methylamphetamine; SAMe, S-adenosyl-methionine; SSRIs, selective serotonin reuptake inhibitors; TCAs, tricyclic antidepressants.

---

incidence of orthostatic hypotension, gastrointestinal side effects, weight gain, and sexual dysfunction that is greater than placebo, but lower than with orally-ingested MAOIs; skin irritation at the patch sites has been the most common adverse effect. At doses above 6 mg/24 hours, dietary modification is required, and at all doses concomitant medications that increase catecholamines or serotonin should be avoided as with the oral MAOIs.

Other Antidepressants
Bupropion

Bupropion, an agent that does not directly affect serotonin neurotransmission, has initial side effects that differ from those of SSRIs and dual-action agents. Its most common and important initial side effects include headache, dizziness, dry mouth, anxiety, restlessness, anorexia, nausea, and insomnia. Long-term side effects are rare; rates of sexual dysfunction and weight gain are equal to placebo (weight loss can occur in some patients), and this agent has minimal cardiovascular effects, even in overdose. The most serious side effect associated with bupropion use is seizure. The risk of seizure with the immediate-release preparation is 0.1% at doses less than 300 mg/day, and 0.4% at doses from 300 to 400 mg/day; the risk of seizure may be lower with longer-acting preparations, but guidelines to keep the total daily dose at or below 450 mg/day remain. In addition, maximum single doses should not exceed 150 mg for the immediate-release form and 200 mg for the sustained-release form. The longest-acting preparation, Wellbutrin XL, can be given as a single dose of up to 450 mg. Because of its increased risk of seizure, bupropion should not be used in those patients with a history of seizures, or in those at increased risk of seizures (e.g., those with eating disorders, head trauma, or alcohol abuse). Overdose is infrequently life-threatening, though seizures, arrhythmias, and death have occurred in overdose. There is no withdrawal syndrome associated with abrupt discontinuation of bupropion.

Mirtazapine

The most common initial side effects associated with mirtazapine include sedation and increased appetite due to histamine receptor blockade; sedation may be less prevalent at higher doses (i.e., 30 mg/day or greater) than at lower doses due to recruitment of noradrenergic effects at higher doses. Less frequently, dry mouth, constipation, and dizziness have been associated with mirtazapine use; orthostatic hypotension can occur occasionally. Gastrointestinal side effects, anxiety, insomnia, and headache are all less common than with use of most other antidepressants. Weight gain is the most common long-term side effect, and elevated lipids occur in approximately 15% of patients who use mirtazapine. Rare, but more serious, side effects have included an increase in liver transaminases (in approximately 2% of patients), and neutropenia (in 0.1%). Mirtazapine appears to be associated with less sexual dysfunction than the SSRIs and it has minimal cardiovascular effects; it has no withdrawal syndrome. There is also a low mortality rate in overdose.

Trazodone

Trazodone is associated with significant sedation. Other common initial side effects can include dry mouth, nausea, and dizziness; orthostasis is much more common than with nefazodone, with reports of syncope.[19] Weight gain and sexual dysfunction are rare, and trazodone is not associated with hepatotoxicity. Trazodone has, very infrequently, been associated with cardiac arrhythmias and QTc prolongation,[20] possibly due to effects on potassium channels, and it should be used with caution in patients with a propensity for, or a history of, arrhythmias. Priapism occurs in approximately 1 in 6,000 male patients who take trazodone; this effect usually occurs within the first month of treatment.[21] In overdose, sedation and hypotension are the most common adverse effects; isolated trazodone overdose is rarely fatal. There is no discontinuation syndrome.

Vilazodone

Vilazodone, a newer antidepressant, has diarrhea, nausea, and headache as its most common side effects, all of which are typically transient. The dose is typically titrated incrementally to avoid gastrointestinal side effects. Dry mouth, dizziness, insomnia, and abnormal dreams have also been reported. Vilazodone has not been shown to have adverse cardiac effects and appears to have minimal effects on weight gain. Though purported to cause less sexual dysfunction than other antidepressants, the FDA reports that vilazodone does not meet the minimal criteria to make this claim.[22]

MOOD STABILIZERS
Lithium

Lithium has many associated adverse effects, summarized in Box 51-5. Gastrointestinal and neurological side effects (e.g., sedation, tremor), along with increased thirst, often occur early in therapy, while effects on thyroid and renal function occur more chronically. Box 51-6 summarizes potential treatments for lithium-induced side effects; change in dosing and formulation can reduce gastrointestinal side effects, while other side effects require additional therapies. Lithium has some effects on sino-atrial node transmission and (less commonly) an atrio-ventricular conduction. However, it has not been commonly associated with other effects on the cardiovascular system, and cardiac disease (aside from sick sinus syndrome) is not an absolute contraindication for lithium use. Lithium has a low therapeutic index and lithium toxicity (whether intentional or unintentional) can lead to a variety of symptoms, including neurological (e.g., severe sedation,

---

BOX 51-5 Common Adverse Effects of Lithium

NEUROLOGICAL
- Sedation
- Tremor (fine action tremor)
- Ataxia/incoordination
- Cognitive slowing

GASTROINTESTINAL
- Nausea and vomiting
- Diarrhea
- Abdominal pain
- Weight gain
- Renal
- Polydipsia/polyuria
- Nephrogenic diabetes insipidus
- Interstitial nephritis

DERMATOLOGICAL
- Acne
- Psoriasis
- Edema

CARDIOVASCULAR
- T-wave inversion on electrocardiogram
- Sinoatrial node slowing
- Atrioventricular blockade
- Other
- Hypothyroidism
- Leukocytosis
- Hypercalcemia

BOX 51-6 Management of Selected Lithium
Side Effects

TREMOR
- Propranolol (10–30 mg twice or three times daily); primidone is a second-line option (25–100 mg per day)
- Gastrointestinal
- Change the formulation to a longer-lasting oral preparation or lithium citrate syrup

POLYDIPSIA/POLYURIA
- Amiloride (5–20 mg/day); hydrochlorothiazide (50 mg/day) is a second-line option (halve the lithium dose and follow lithium levels closely)

EDEMA
- Spironolactone (25 mg/day); follow lithium levels closely

HYPOTHYROIDISM
- Treat with thyroid hormone and continue lithium therapy

---

tremor, dysarthria, delirium, anterograde amnesia, myoclonus, seizure), gastrointestinal (e.g., nausea, vomiting), and cardiovascular (e.g., arrhythmia) effects; renal function often is impaired, and dialysis may be required to treat lithium toxicity if supportive measures and intravenous (IV) normal saline to aid lithium excretion are ineffective. Lithium does not have a characteristic discontinuation syndrome, but rapid withdrawal of lithium therapy is associated with substantially higher rates of relapse than when lithium is tapered.[23]

Valproic Acid

Common initial side effects of valproate therapy include gastrointestinal side effects (nausea, vomiting, diarrhea, and abdominal cramps), sedation, tremor, and alopecia; gastrointestinal side effects are less frequent with divalproex sodium (Depakote) than with other preparations, and tremor can be treated with propranolol, as can lithium-induced tremor. Alopecia is sometimes transient and may be reduced by using a multivitamin with zinc and selenium. Longer-term side effects include weight gain and perhaps cognitive slowing. More serious adverse effects associated with valproic acid therapy include pancreatitis (occurring in approximately 1 in 3,000 patients), elevated transaminases (leading very rarely to liver failure), hyperammonemia (at times leading to confusion), thrombocytopenia, platelet dysfunction, and leukopenia. These effects are all quite rare, with the exception of elevated hepatic transaminase levels. There is some controversy regarding whether valproic acid is associated with polycystic ovarian syndrome (PCOS) in women[24]; some studies have suggested that this agent is associated with the development of PCOS, whereas other studies have indicated that bipolar disorder itself may be associated with menstrual irregularities. Practitioners are advised to watch for hirsutism, acne, menstrual irregularities, and weight gain in their female patients who take valproic acid and to initiate evaluation for PCOS if such symptoms arise. Valproate overdose can lead to CNS depression, but it is rarely fatal; dialysis has been used on occasion to aid removal of valproate. Abrupt withdrawal can theoretically increase the risk of seizure, especially in those patients on long-term therapy or with a seizure disorder, but there is no withdrawal syndrome.

Carbamazepine

Initial side effects of carbamazepine include gastrointestinal side effects (nausea, vomiting), neurological side effects (sedation, ataxia, vertigo, diplopia, and blurry vision), and rash. The rash is often benign (occurring in approximately 5% to 10% of patients), but the drug should be stopped if the rash is widespread, or if the rash is associated with systemic signs of illness, facial lesions, or mucous membrane involvement, as Stevens-Johnson syndrome has been reported with this agent. With respect to longer-term side effects, there is usually less weight gain than with use of either valproic acid or lithium. More serious side effects, in addition to Stevens-Johnson syndrome, can include hyponatremia (from SIADH), elevated liver transaminases (though less frequently than with valproic acid), and aplastic anemia and other blood dyscrasias (which occur in approximately 1 in 10,000 to 150,000 of treated patients). Carbamazepine also slows cardiac conduction and should be avoided in patients with high-grade atrioventricular block and sick sinus syndrome. Low free T_3 and T_4 values can occur with carbamazepine use; these levels are usually not of clinical significance, but hypothyroidism should be considered if refractory depression or clinical signs of hypothyroidism exist. Overdose of carbamazepine results in exacerbation of neurological side effects, the potential for high-grade atrio-ventricular (AV) block, and stupor/CNS depression; supportive care is required, and hemodialysis is ineffective. When possible, carbamazepine should be tapered rather than discontinued abruptly to minimize lowering of the seizure threshold.

Oxcarbazepine

Initial side effects from the related compound, oxcarbazepine, are very similar to those of carbamazepine, with gastrointestinal and neurological side effects being the most common. Rash is much less common with oxcarbazepine, but it does occur more frequently than with placebo. The neurological side effects (including cognitive difficulties, incoordination, visual changes, and sedation) associated with oxcarbazepine are reported to be less frequent than with carbamazepine but occur substantially more frequently than in patients who take placebo. Like carbamazepine, it appears to be associated with less weight gain than with lithium or valproic acid. With regard to more serious effects, oxcarbazepine can lead to elevation of transaminases, and it is thought to be associated with higher rates of hyponatremia than carbamazepine. Patients taking oxcarbazepine are at elevated risk of Stevens-Johnson syndrome and other serious dermatological syndromes; low T_4 values can also occur in isolation. However, oxcarbazepine has not been associated with blood dyscrasias. Overdose with oxcarbazepine has been managed supportively and symptomatically.

Lamotrigine

Initial side effects of lamotrigine include neurological side effects (such as dizziness, ataxia, visual changes [diplopia and blurred vision], sedation, and headache); nausea, vomiting, and uncomplicated rash may also occur. All of these initial effects, however, are uncommon, at least in part because of the slow dose escalation required to reduce the risk of dangerous dermatological conditions. Lamotrigine does not have significant long-term side effects; weight gain is rare, and neither hepatoxicity nor cardiovascular effects have been described at usual doses. However, the best-known and most important adverse effects associated with lamotrigine are dermatological conditions related to serious rash. Both Stevens-Johnson syndrome (Figure 51-2) and toxic epidermal necrolysis have occurred in association with lamotrigine use; the risk appears to be greater in pediatric patients, with rapid escalation of the dose, and with concomitant use of valproic acid (which inhibits lamotrigine metabolism). The risk of life-threatening rash appears to be between 0.1% and 0.3% (as opposed to an approximately 10% prevalence of benign rash), and it has been on the lower end of this continuum in trials of lamotrigine for psychiatric illness. Any patient who develops rash on lamotrigine should be promptly evaluated by a medical professional; furthermore, rash with significant facial involvement, mucous membrane involvement (e.g., dysuria, tongue/mouth lesions), or systemic symptoms (such as fever or lymphadenopathy) prompt great concern for life-threatening rash and require immediate emergency evaluation. Lamotrigine overdose can be fatal; the most common symptoms include stupor, convulsions, and intraventricular conduction delay, and treatment is largely supportive.

ANTIPSYCHOTICS
Typical Antipsychotics

Table 51-1 shows the relative frequencies of the common adverse effects of antipsychotics; chlorpromazine

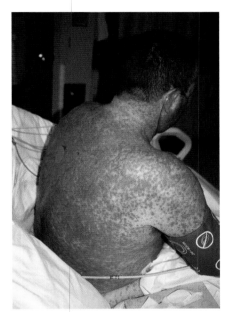

Figure 51-2. Stevens-Johnson syndrome. *(From The Stevens Johnson Syndrome Foundation, SJSmaleback1. Available at www.sjsupport.org.)*

(low-potency), perphenazine (mid-potency), and haloperidol (high-potency) are listed as the prototype agents in the classes of typical antipsychotics. Initial side effects of the low-potency typical agents are similar to those of the TCAs: sedation (due to H_1 receptor blockade), anticholinergic effects (dry mouth, urinary hesitancy, constipation, blurred vision, tachycardia, and risk of confusion, due to the blockade of muscarinic receptors), and orthostatic hypotension (due to $alpha_1$-receptor blockade); these effects can occur to a lesser degree with mid-potency agents and are relatively uncommon with high-potency agents. In contrast, EPS are common in patients taking high-potency typical antipsychotics, but their incidence decreases with decreasing potency (Box 51-7; see also Table 51-1). Common long-term side effects of typical antipsychotics include weight gain (greatest with low-potency agents), photosensitivity (perhaps greatest with chlorpromazine), sexual dysfunction (due to effects on $alpha_2$-receptors), and hyperprolactinemia (which can lead to amenorrhea, galactorrhea, infertility, and osteoporosis). Tardive dyskinesia (TD) (see Box 51-7) is another long-term potential side effect associated with use of all typical antipsychotics, occurring at a rate of approximately 5% per year.[25]

Rarer, but serious, side effects of low-potency antipsychotics include neuroleptic malignant syndrome (NMS; see Box 51-7), QTc prolongation, and torsades de pointes ventricular arrhythmias (especially with use of thioridazine, the antipsychotic most commonly associated with torsades de pointes, and IV haloperidol; Figure 51-3).[26] In addition, chlorpromazine has been associated with cholestatic jaundice (at a rate of approximately 0.1%) and thioridazine has been associated with irreversible pigmentary retinopathy (at doses > 800 mg/day) that can lead to blindness. Overdose of typical antipsychotics has been associated with lethargy, delirium, cardiac arrhythmias, hypotension, EPS, seizure, and death; symptomatic treatment is required and dialysis is not of benefit.

Atypical Antipsychotics

In general, most atypical antipsychotics have significantly lower rates of TD and EPS than do the typical antipsychotics, and (aside from clozapine) have relatively negligible anticholinergic effects; they are generally quite well tolerated. However, several of the atypical antipsychotics have been associated with significant weight gain and with metabolic side effects; these effects appear to be greatest with clozapine and olanzapine, moderate with iloperidone, risperidone,

TABLE 51-1 Selected Side Effects of Antipsychotic Medications

Agent	Sedation	Orthostasis	Ach	EPS	TD	Weight Gain	DM Risk	HyperPRL	QTc Prolongation
Chlorpromazine	Sev	Sev	Sev	Mod/Sev	Mod	Mod/Sev	Mild	Mild	Mod
Perphenazine	Mod	Mod	Mod	Mod	Mod	Mild	Mild	Mild	Mod
Haloperidol	Mild	0	0	Sev	Mod	Mild	0	Mod	Mod (PO form); Sev (IV form)
Risperidone	Mild	Mod/Sev	0	Mod/Sev	Mild	Mod	Mod	Sev	Mod
Ziprasidone	0	Mild	0	Mild[a]	Mild	Mild	Mild	Mild	Sev
Olanzapine	Mod	0	Mild	Mild	Mild	Sev	Sev	Mild	Mod
Aripiprazole	Mild	0	0	Mild[a]	Mild	Mild	Mild	0	0
Quetiapine	Mod	Mod	Mild	0/Mild	0	Mod	Mod	0	Mod
Clozapine	Sev	Mod/Sev	Sev	0	0	Sev	Sev	?	?
Iloperidone*	Mild	Sev	Mild	Mod	?	Mod/Sev	Mod/Sev	Mild	Mod/Sev
Paliperidone	Mild	Mod/Sev	0	Mod	Mild	Mod	Mod	Sev	Mild
Asenapine*	Mod	Mod/Sev	Mild	Mild[a]	?	Mild	Mild	Mild	Mod
Lurasidone*	Mild	Mild	0	Mod	?	Mild	Mild	Mod	0

Ach, Anticholinergic effects; DM, diabetes mellitus; EPS, extrapyramidal symptoms; HyperPRL, hyperprolactinemia; TD, tardive dyskinesia; 0, no effect; Mild, mild effect; Mod, moderate effect; Sev, severe effect; ?, insufficient data.
[a]Moderate frequency and intensity of akathisia.
*Newer agent; somewhat limited clinical experience available.

BOX 51-7 Extrapyramidal Symptoms

ACUTE DYSTONIA

Signs and Symptoms

Localized muscular contraction leading to jaw protrusion, torticollis, tongue protrusion, opisthotonos, extremity contraction, or a fixed upward gaze of the eyes (oculogyric crisis) with associated pain

Risk Factors

Age < 30, male gender, high-potency typical antipsychotics, intramuscular (IM) administration, increased dose, rapid titration of dose

Time Course

Usually occurs within the first several days of initiation or a dose increase

Treatment

Moderate-to-severe reaction: IM diphenhydramine (25–50 mg, repeat as needed) or benztropine (1–2 mg, repeat as needed)
Mild-to-moderate reaction: decrease of antipsychotic dose, addition of oral anticholinergic (e.g., benztropine 0.5–1 mg BID-TID, diphenhydramine 25 mg BID)

ANTIPSYCHOTIC-INDUCED PARKINSONISM

Signs and Symptoms

Muscular rigidity, bradykinesia, shuffling gait, masked facies, and resting (usually non–pill-rolling) tremor

Risk Factors

Female gender, advanced age, high-potency typical antipsychotics, and possibly increased dose

Time Course

Usually gradual in onset, occurs during first 3 months of treatment

Treatment

Decrease the dose or switch the agent; if this is ineffective or not feasible, the addition of an anticholinergic (diphenhydramine or benztropine) or amantadine can reduce symptoms; benzodiazepines or beta-blockers may be helpful in refractory cases

AKATHISIA

Signs and Symptoms

Internal, uncomfortable feeling of restlessness; frequent pacing, inability to remain seated

Risk Factors

High-potency typical antipsychotics (mid-potency typicals, risperidone, and aripiprazole to a lesser degree), higher dosage, rapid titration of dose; possibly advanced age, and diabetes mellitus

Time Course

Usually occurs within the first several days of initiation or a dose increase

Treatment

Reduction of dose (or change of agent); addition of propranolol (e.g., 10–20 mg BID-TID); benzodiazepines may be effective in refractory cases or when beta-blockers are contraindicated; anticholinergics are occasionally helpful, especially when other EPS also present

TARDIVE DYSKINESIA

Signs and Symptoms

Repetitive, involuntary, non-rhythmic movements, most frequently of the tongue and mouth, but potentially including facial (e.g., grimacing), extremity (e.g., repetitive hand gestures), truncal (e.g., opisthotonos), and ocular (e.g., oculogyric crisis) movements

Risk Factors

Typical antipsychotics (risperidone to a lesser degree), time of exposure, advanced age; possibly mood disorders, organic brain disease, and female gender

Time Course

Approximate incidence of 4% per year for first 5 years of treatment with typical antipsychotics; incidence may somewhat slow thereafter, but the prevalence continues to grow with increased time of exposure

Treatment

Few clear treatment options; change of agent, especially to clozapine, may lead to reduction of symptoms; other treatments (e.g., vitamin E, benzodiazepines, botulinum toxin, or reserpine) do not appear to be broadly effective

NEUROLEPTIC MALIGNANT SYNDROME (NMS; SEE ALSO CHAPTER 55)

Signs and Symptoms

Confusion, lethargy, rigidity, fever, autonomic instability (with abnormal laboratory values, including significantly increased creatine phosphokinase, elevated hepatic transaminases, and mild leukocytosis)

Risk Factors

Include dehydration, agitation, use of physical restraint, increased or titration of dose, high-potency typical antipsychotics (though NMS can appear with any antipsychotic), IM administration, and history of catatonia or NMS

Time Course

Usually occurs within the first several days of treatment

Treatment

Discontinuation of the offending agent and supportive care to prevent aspiration pneumonia, deep venous thrombosis, renal failure, and other complications in all cases of NMS; dopamine agonists (e.g., bromocriptine), muscle relaxants (e.g., dantrolene), benzodiazepines, and electroconvulsive therapy are all options in refractory or severe cases

---

paliperidone, and quetiapine, and low with aripiprazole, ziprasidone, asenapine and lurasidone (see Table 51-2 regarding weight gain and Table 51-3 regarding monitoring guidelines for metabolic side effects).[27–29] In addition, increased rates of cardiovascular events and death have been associated with the use of atypical antipsychotics among patients with dementia, with a 1.6- to 1.7-fold mortality rate increase in a pooled analysis of over 5,000 patients in 17 clinical trials.[30] These findings have led to a "black box warning" in the package inserts of these agents; of note, a larger analysis found

that the rate of stroke with atypical antipsychotics was not significantly greater than with typical antipsychotics among patients with dementia.[31] More information is needed to determine whether there is a differential risk between agents.

Risperidone

Common initial side effects of risperidone include dizziness and orthostatic hypotension (due to alpha$_1$ blockade), headache, and sedation, though sedation is less frequent with this

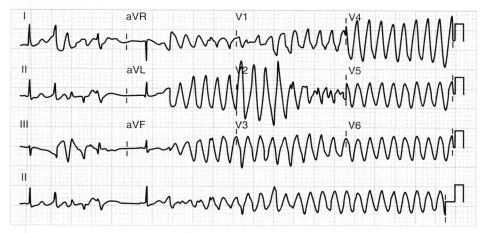

Figure 51-3. Torsades de pointes ventricular arrhythmia. *(Re-drawn from Khan IA. Twelve-lead electrocardiogram of torsades de pointes,* Tex Heart Inst J *28:69, 2001.)*

TABLE 51-2 Weight Gain Associated with 10 Weeks of Antipsychotic Treatment

Agent	Gain at 10 Weeks (kg) Estimated Weight	Estimated Weight Gain at 10 Weeks (lb)
Clozapine	4.45	9.8
Olanzapine*	4.15	9.1
Chlorpromazine	2.58	5.7
Risperidone*	2.10	4.6
Perphenazine	1.33	2.9
Haloperidol†	1.08	2.4
Ziprasidone†	0.04	0.1

*Weight gain associated with quetiapine appears to be intermediate between olanzapine and risperidone.
†Weight gain associated with aripiprazole appears to be intermediate between haloperidol and ziprasidone.
(Adapted from Allison DB et al. Antipsychotic-induced weight gain, Am J Psychiatry *156: 1686–1696, 1999.)*

TABLE 51-3 American Diabetes Association Guidelines for Monitoring Patients Taking Antipsychotics

Monitor	Baseline	4 Weeks	8 Weeks	12 Weeks	1 Year	5 Years
Weight	X	X	X	X*	X	X
Blood pressure	X				X	X†
Lipid panel	X			X	X	X
Fasting glucose	X			X	X†	

*Weight should be monitored quarterly after 12 weeks.
†Blood pressure and glucose should be monitored yearly after 1 year.
(Adapted from ADA guidelines. American Diabetes Association, American Psychiatric Association, American Association of Clinical Endocrinologists, North American Association for the Study of Obesity: Consensus development conference on antipsychotic drugs and obesity and diabetes, Diabetes Care *27(2):596–601, 2004.)*

agent than with low- and mid-potency typical antipsychotics and many of the other atypicals. With respect to longer-term side effects, hyperprolactinemia is greatest with risperidone among all antipsychotics, and weight gain and risk of diabetes are intermediate between high-potency typical antipsychotics (low rates) and olanzapine and clozapine (very high rates). Risperidone also has one of the highest rates of EPS among atypicals. TD has been described with risperidone, at lower rates than with typical antipsychotics (0.6% per year versus 4.1% per year with haloperidol in one study),[32] but generally at higher rates than other atypicals when high doses of risperidone are used. NMS has also been reported in over 20 patients taking risperidone.[33] Risk of QTc prolongation appears to be intermediate compared with other atypicals.[29] Overdose with risperidone most commonly results in hypotension and sedation.

Paliperidone

Paliperidone is a metabolite of risperidone, and side effects are therefore similar. It is excreted primarily by the kidney and does not undergo processing by the liver. The most commonly reported side effects with paliperidone are headache, nausea, dizziness, insomnia, and dyspepsia. Sedation has been reported, though paliperidone appears to be less associated with sedation than many other atypicals.[29] Despite early claims that paliperidone was not as highly associated with EPS as risperidone, several studies have suggested rates of EPS of up to 20%.[34] Paliperidone has very high rates of hyperprolactinemia.[29] Paliperidone is thought to have effects on weight gain and metabolic parameters that are comparable to that of risperidone. Paliperidone has been associated with prolongation of the QTc interval, though less so than most other atypicals.

Iloperidone

Patients taking iloperidone have high rates of orthostasis, and the dose typically must be titrated very slowly to avoid this. Common side effects include dizziness, headache, dry mouth and insomnia. Weight gain with iloperidone is greater than with risperidone, and in a recent meta-analysis it appears that such weight gain may even approach rates seen with clozapine in the short-term, though longer-term studies are lacking.[29] EPS and hyperprolactinemia are less common than with risperidone. Iloperidone has been associated with QTc prolongation of 9.1 msec, which is similar in scope to that of ziprasidone and greater than is associated with oral haloperidol.[35]

Asenapine

Common side effects of asenapine include somnolence, dizziness and headache. These are likely due to prominent actions at histaminergic and alpha$_1$ receptors. Rates of somnolence are comparable to those seen with olanzapine. Oral hypoesthesia is a side effect seen in up to 7% of patients that appears to be unique to this agent.[36] Weight gain appears to be less common with asenapine than with risperidone, though long-term metabolic effects are unclear at this time. Up to 12% of patients report EPS, with akathisia being the most common manifestation. Hyperprolactinemia has also been reported, though appears to be uncommon. The effects of asenapine on the QTc interval appear comparable to those of risperidone, with a mean increase of 4.4 msec in one study.[36] Finally, serious hypersensitivity reactions have occurred following a single dose of asenapine.

Lurasidone

Sedation is the side effect most commonly reported with lurasidone. Alpha$_1$-antagonist properties also contribute to a risk of orthostatic hypotension and tachycardia. Other common side effects include headache, dry mouth and constipation. Lurasidone has been suggested to have higher rates of hyperprolactinemia and EPS, particularly akathisia and parkinsonism, than other atypical antipsychotics. As many as 13% of patients in a 6-week study experienced EPS, with 7% exhibiting parkinsonism and 8% exhibiting akathisia.[37] Weight gain and metabolic effects appear to be lower than with many other atypical antipsychotics. Lurasidone appears to be least associated with QTc prolongation.[29]

Ziprasidone

Neurological (dizziness, sedation, and headache) and gastrointestinal (nausea and dyspepsia) side effects are common with ziprasidone administration, but they are usually mild. Sedation with ziprasidone is equivalent to that seen with quetiapine. Akathisia is frequently reported, though some apparent akathisia may be a result of activating properties at lower doses. TD appears at much lower rates with ziprasidone than with typical antipsychotics, but can occur[38]; more long-term data are needed. Orthostasis can also uncommonly occur because of alpha$_1$ blockade. With respect to longer-term side effects, weight gain, risk of diabetes, and hyperprolactinemia appear to be lower with this agent. Risk for prolactin increase is moderate. Ziprasidone has been associated with QTc prolongation—greater than with other atypicals and oral haloperidol[39]—but in the clinical setting, this has not been a major issue (there has been a single report of torsades de pointes associated with ziprasidone monotherapy). Overdose with ziprasidone alone has appeared to be relatively safe; cardiotoxicity has not occurred, and the major symptoms have been sedation and dysarthria.

Aripiprazole

The most common initial side effects of aripiprazole include headache, anxiety, insomnia, akathisia, and gastrointestinal side effects (nausea, vomiting, and constipation). Sedation may also occur at higher doses, but is less common than with other atypicals. Akathisia is a common side effect of aripiprazole, and indeed aripiprazole may cause the most akathisia across all atypicals; other EPS are rare. As with ziprasidone, significant weight gain and glucose intolerance are less common with aripiprazole; furthermore, this agent appears to have no significant cardiovascular effects, including no prolongation of the QTc interval. Additionally, it is considered the only antipsychotic that does not cause hyperprolactinemia and may actually lower prolactin levels.[29] The risk of TD appears to be quite low. Aripiprazole overdose appears to be relatively safe, with the most common effects being sedation, vomiting, tremor, and orthostatic hypotension; however, more clinical experience is needed.

Olanzapine

Patients using olanzapine can initially experience sedation, dry mouth, constipation, increased appetite, dizziness (occasionally with orthostatic hypotension), and tremor. EPS occur more frequently than with placebo, but they are less frequent than with use of risperidone or high-potency typical antipsychotics. The major long-term side effects of olanzapine are metabolic. Weight gain occurs frequently with olanzapine; patients on average gain approximately 10 lb in the first 10 weeks of treatment (see Table 51-2) and they can continue to gain weight during ongoing treatment, with one-third to one-half of patients gaining significant weight (as defined by greater than 7% increase in body weight).[40] In addition, olanzapine has been associated with the development of diabetes mellitus; in one study the risk of developing diabetes was approximately six times greater than the risk of diabetes with placebo, and approximately four times the risk for patients on typical antipsychotics.[41] It appears that both insulin resistance and weight gain contribute to this increase in diabetes risk. Diabetic ketoacidosis (DKA) is rare but has been reported in patients taking olanzapine, often occurring within the first month of treatment. Hyperlipidemia, likely in the context of increased food intake and weight gain, is also common with long-term olanzapine therapy. The risks of these metabolic side effects are approximately equivalent to those associated with clozapine; greater than those for quetiapine, low-potency typical antipsychotics, and risperidone; and much greater than for use of the high-potency typicals. Given the risk of these side effects, the American Diabetes Association has developed guidelines for the monitoring of metabolic and cardiovascular parameters for patients taking antipsychotics (see Table 51-3).[27] Hyperprolactinemia is uncommon, but it can occur with olanzapine, especially at higher doses. TD and NMS can occur, but again are rare and less common than with use of typical antipsychotics; rates of TD are generally between 0.5% and 1% per year of treatment.[42] NMS with olanzapine manifests with fewer motor symptoms than with use of typical antipsychotics. Elevation of hepatic transaminases, without progression to liver failure, occurs in approximately 2% of patients; olanzapine has little effect on cardiac conduction. In overdose, olanzapine is relatively safe, with lethargy seen as the most common effect.

Clozapine

Clozapine has many initial side effects. Anticholinergic side effects, sedation, and orthostatic hypotension are common. Sialorrhea occurs frequently, especially at night, and it can be

TABLE 51-4 Monitoring Guidelines for Clozapine

Blood Count	Clozapine Administration	Monitoring
WBC > 3.5K	Continue	Obtain CBC weekly for first 6 months of treatment, then every other week throughout clozapine treatment
WBC between 3–3.5K, or drop of greater than 3K within 3 weeks	Continue	Repeat the value; if unchanged, obtain a CBC twice weekly until the WBC is > 3.5K; monitor for fever, sore throat, and other signs of infection
WBC between 2–3K or absolute neutrophil count (ANC) between 1–2K	Discontinue temporarily	Obtain a CBC daily until WBC is >3K and the ANC is > 2K; then check the WBC twice weekly until the WBC is > 3.5K; monitor for signs of infection
WBC < 2K or ANC less than 1K	Discontinue permanently	Daily CBC until the WBC is > 3.5K and the ANC is > 2K; monitor for infection

ANC, Absolute neutrophil count; CBC, complete blood count; WBC, white blood cell count.
(Adapted from Clozapine (Clozaril) package insert, *East Hanover, NJ, January 2003, Novartis.)*

quite upsetting to patients; clonidine, glycopyrrolate, or atropine drops administered on the tongue may reduce this symptom. Patients who take clozapine can also have drug-induced fever and tachycardia during the initial days of treatment. Long-term side effects are similar to those of olanzapine, with weight gain, development of diabetes, and hyperlipidemia all significantly prevalent; for both clozapine and olanzapine, weight gain is especially common among adolescents. Fortunately, TD does not seem to be associated with clozapine (with reports of TD improvement on switching to clozapine)[43]; this agent also appears to be prolactin-sparing.

There are several rare but serious adverse effects associated with clozapine. Agranulocytosis is the best-known adverse effect of clozapine; it was initially thought to occur in 1% to 2% of clozapine patients, but subsequent rates have been approximately 0.4% to 0.8%,[44,45] with the institution of mandatory weekly blood count monitoring for the first 6 months and twice-monthly monitoring for the remainder of treatment. Agranulocytosis occurs most frequently within the first 6 months of treatment, and appears to be more likely in women and in those of Ashkenazi Jewish descent; advanced age may also be a minor risk factor.[44] Specific guidelines (Table 51-4) serve to guide the clinician regarding when to stop treatment and when to check complete blood counts more frequently when leukocyte levels drop.[46] Seizures are another risk of clozapine treatment, and risk increases with increasing dose; 4% to 6% of patients treated with doses of 600 mg or more per day will have seizures. If clozapine is necessary, patients having seizures on clozapine can be re-started on the agent once adequate anticonvulsant treatment has been initiated. Uncommonly, cardiac complications occur and include myocarditis (characterized by chest pain, dyspnea, fatigue, and tachycardia, and occurring in approximately 0.2%) and cardiomyopathy (0.1% with long-term treatment). There have been more than 20 reports of NMS with clozapine, with classic symptoms aside from lack of rigidity. Hepatotoxicity can occur, though it is exceedingly rare.[47] Clozapine overdose can result in delirium, lethargy, tachycardia, hypotension, and respiratory failure. Cardiac arrhythmias and seizures have occurred in a minority of cases, and overdose can be fatal. Hemodialysis does not remove clozapine, and management is generally supportive and symptomatic.

ANTIANXIETY AND SLEEP AGENTS
Benzodiazepines

The most common initial side effects of benzodiazepines are sedation and associated daytime fatigue; these effects are frequently transitory and can be managed by lowering the dose or moving the dose to bedtime. Other potential side effects include dizziness, nausea, incoordination, ataxia, anterograde amnesia, and muscle weakness. Uncommon, but possible, psychological effects include increased irritability/hostility and paradoxical disinhibition. Cognitive effects appear to be greatest in the elderly, in those with dementia, and in delirious patients. Long-term side effects are uncommon; a minority of patients report increased depressive symptoms while taking benzodiazepines, and memory impairment and motor incoordination may persist. Furthermore, initial side effects can persist and occasionally worsen, especially with longer-acting agents (such as diazepam), or in patients with liver failure or otherwise impaired hepatic metabolism. Such effects may be less serious when using short-acting benzodiazepines and those agents (lorazepam, oxazepam, temazepam) that do not undergo hepatic oxidative metabolism.

Serious adverse events associated with benzodiazepine use include an increased risk of falls in the elderly, with one study finding an increased risk of hip fractures in the elderly, especially with use of higher doses of benzodiazepines.[48] Furthermore, patients who take benzodiazepines appear to be at higher risk for motor vehicle accidents and for accidental injuries, the risk of the latter being greatest during the initial period (2 weeks to 1 month) of therapy. Finally, respiratory depression can occur in the context of benzodiazepine use, especially in patients with pre-existing respiratory illness. Benzodiazepine overdose in isolation is usually non-fatal, with sedation, dysarthria, confusion, ataxia, and incoordination being common; however, respiratory depression, hypotension, and coma can occur, and deaths have resulted.

Benzodiazepines cause physiological dependence and have a characteristic and potentially dangerous withdrawal syndrome. The withdrawal syndrome usually appears within the first 12 to 48 hours of discontinuation of short-lasting benzodiazepines (such as lorazepam); it may not appear until 2 to 5 days after discontinuation in those patients taking longer-lasting agents (such as clonazepam or diazepam). Given this risk, benzodiazepines should be slowly tapered in all patients; short-lasting agents should be carefully tapered, and at times a switch to a longer-lasting agent (followed by taper of the longer-acting agent) may be required when taper of the shorter-acting agent proves problematic.[49] The withdrawal syndrome from benzodiazepines includes anxiety, tremor, diaphoresis, nausea, insomnia, and irritability; vital signs—especially blood pressure and heart rate—are often elevated in untreated benzodiazepine withdrawal. Generalized tonic-clonic seizures may result, usually early in the course of the syndrome. As withdrawal continues, delirium may result, characterized by more intense withdrawal symptoms, significant autonomic instability, and, frequently, psychotic symptoms. Delirium from benzodiazepine withdrawal is associated with significant risk of fall, congestive heart failure, aspiration, deep venous thrombosis, and other serious medical complications. For the vast majority of patients, development of benzodiazepine abuse is rare and significant dose escalation is uncommon; in fact, many patients who take benzodiazepines have residual symptoms that could benefit from additional therapy.[50] However, patients with ongoing substance use disorders have relatively high rates of benzodiazepine abuse,[51,52] and patients with prior substance use disorders appear to be at increased risk of abuse of prescribed benzodiazepines.

Short-acting Sedative-Hypnotic Sleep Agents (Zolpidem, Zaleplon, and Eszopiclone)

The initial side effects of these agents are similar to those of the benzodiazepines, though they appear to be less frequent. Sedation—their desired effect—is common and occasionally may result in daytime somnolence or fatigue. Dry mouth and headache are other common initial effects. Incoordination, memory disturbance, nausea, and dizziness are uncommon when these agents are used at standard doses in patients without impaired metabolism. An unpleasant taste has been reported by a minority of patients taking eszopiclone. Long-term side effects appear to be uncommon, though these agents have, for the most part, only been studied in short-term use. Tolerance and dose escalation are uncommon. Physiological dependence is also generally uncommon when used as prescribed, but withdrawal syndromes, similar to those seen with benzodiazepines, can occur occasionally when these agents are abruptly discontinued after long-term use; rates of withdrawal are much lower than with the short-lasting benzodiazepines.[53]

The one serious adverse effect that has been reported with zolpidem use involves sleep-associated behavior disorders, including somnambulism and night-eating disorder. These agents are relatively safe in isolated overdose, though respiratory and cardiovascular adverse effects can occur rarely. Treatment of overdose is generally supportive and symptomatic.

Ramelteon

Initial side effects associated with this melatonin receptor agonist are uncommon, but can include dizziness, sedation, nausea, and fatigue. Long-term and serious side effects appear to be rare. Overdose has not been reported, but ramelteon was administered in single doses up to 160 mg in an abuse liability trial, and no safety or tolerability concerns were seen. There is no characteristic withdrawal syndrome with discontinuation of ramelteon.

Buspirone

Buspirone is generally well tolerated. Headache, dizziness, and nausea are the most common side effects, and restlessness, insomnia, and increased anxiety may also occur. Sedation, incoordination, and cognitive effects do not appear to be associated with buspirone use. There are no known common long-term side effects, and there is no physiological dependence or withdrawal syndrome. There have been single case reports of the induction[54] and disappearance[55] of psychosis in the setting of buspirone initiation. Overdose with buspirone appears to be relatively safe, with dizziness, vomiting, and sedation among the most common effects; seizures occurred in the context of one buspirone overdose.[56]

Gabapentin

Gabapentin is frequently used to treat anxiety. Common initial side effects are similar to those of other anticonvulsants: sedation, dizziness, nausea, ataxia, headache, tremor, and visual changes. In general, these side effects are relatively mild and are often transient. Weight gain can occur as a long-term side effect, but it appears to be less common than with valproic acid. Gabapentin undergoes minimal hepatic metabolism and thus is not associated with hepatotoxicity; cardiovascular effects are few as well. In overdose, gabapentin is relatively safe, in part because of dose-limited absorption from the gut, but it is associated with sedation, ataxia, and diplopia; hemodialysis can be used if necessary.

OTHER AGENTS USED IN THE TREATMENT OF PSYCHIATRIC CONDITIONS

Beta-blockers

Initial side effects of the beta-blockers can include bradycardia, dizziness/orthostasis, fatigue, nausea, diarrhea, and insomnia. The effects of beta-blockers can affect a number of medical conditions (Table 51-5), including exacerbation or causation of bronchospasm in vulnerable individuals; in such patients a more β_1-selective agent (such as atenolol or metoprolol) may be required instead of less-selective agents (such as propranolol and pindolol) that act equally at β_1 and β_2 receptors. Patients who take beta-blockers for extended periods may develop sexual dysfunction or depressive symptoms. However, a large meta-analysis examining beta-blockers' link with fatigue, sexual dysfunction, and depression found that such associations were quite weak, with no significant associations between depression and the use of beta-blockers; furthermore, rates of fatigue (one additional report per 57 patient-years) and sexual dysfunction (one report per 1,999 patient-years) were very similar to placebo,[57] though idiosyncratic reactions can occur. Overdose of beta-blockers is serious and can cause bradycardia, hypotension, and more serious cardiac adverse events, up to and including cardiac arrest. Somnolence and lethargy are common in overdose, and propranolol has been associated with seizures in overdose. Abrupt withdrawal after pronged use of beta-blockers has, on occasion, led to angina, myocardial infarction, and, rarely, death in patients with (diagnosed or undiagnosed) coronary artery disease (CAD), and therefore these medications should be tapered after long-term use, especially in patients with CAD or with cardiac risk factors.

Clonidine

Dry mouth, sedation, fatigue, and dizziness are the most common side effects of clonidine. Hypotension (and

TABLE 51-5 Medical Conditions Adversely Affected by Use of Beta-blockers

Medical Condition	Beta-blockers' Effects Related to the Condition
Diabetes	May impair the adrenergic response (tachycardia, diaphoresis, and tremor) to hypoglycemia May inhibit glucose mobilization after hypoglycemia, preventing rapid recovery
Reactive airway disease (e.g., asthma)	Beta-blockers with β_2 activity produce bronchospasm and can lead to hypoxia and respiratory distress
Raynaud's syndrome	Increase the risk of peripheral vasoconstriction
Hypertension	May combine with patients' antihypertensive regimen to have additive effects on cardiac conduction and hypotension (especially true for calcium channel blockers)

orthostasis) can occur, especially among those patients taking other antihypertensive agents. Somewhat less common side effects include nausea, headache, restlessness, and irritability. Vivid dreams, nightmares and sexual dysfunction are infrequent, but have been reported among patients taking clonidine. In overdose, a variety of significant adverse events (including bradycardia, hypotension, respiratory depression, and lethargy) may occur, and in large overdoses, cardiac conduction defects, seizures, and coma can result. Abrupt withdrawal from clonidine has resulted in restlessness, agitation, tremor, and rebound hypertension, and has led rarely to hypertensive encephalopathy or cerebrovascular accidents.

Stimulants

Frequent side effects of the most commonly used psychostimulants (e.g., methylphenidate, dextroamphetamine, mixed amphetamine salts) include anxiety, insomnia, restlessness, and decreased appetite. Increased blood pressure and heart rate can occur in both children and adults, and these effects are generally dose-dependent. Stimulants have been associated with the development of tics; however, controlled studies, even those in children with co-morbid tic disorders, have not found elevated rates of tics among children who are taking psychostimulants.[58,59] In addition, there have been reports of growth retardation among children who receive psychostimulants; however, as with tics, controlled studies have not found a consistent association with growth retardation.[60] More serious adverse effects can include psychosis and disorientation, which are rare except in overdose. Overdose can also be characterized by hyperpyrexia, arrhythmias, seizures, and rhabdomyolysis. There is no characteristic withdrawal syndrome, though abrupt cessation of stimulants after long-term use can be associated with lethargy, dysphoria, irritability, and psychomotor slowing similar to that seen during withdrawal from illicit amphetamine use.

Modafinil

The most common side effects of modafinil include headache, nausea, anxiety, and insomnia. Hypertension and tachycardia occur infrequently (in less than 5% of patients), but have occurred more often than with placebo. This agent has not been extensively studied in patients with significant cardiac disease (such as patients with a history of MI). Modafinil has been associated with Stevens-Johnson syndrome, angioedema, and multi-organ hypersensitivity. Symptoms most commonly associated with modafinil overdose include restlessness, gastrointestinal symptoms, disorientation/confusion, and cardiovascular symptoms (tachycardia, hypertension, and chest pain); death has not occurred with modafinil overdose taken in isolation. There is no known withdrawal syndrome.

Atomoxetine

Initial side effects of atomoxetine include gastrointestinal side effects (decreased appetite, nausea, and vomiting), anticholinergic effects (e.g., urinary hesitancy/retention, dry mouth, constipation), dizziness, palpitations, and insomnia. Heart rate and blood pressure are elevated in a small percentage of patients; in pre-marketing trials, approximately 4% of pediatric patients had mean increases of heart rate of 25 or greater beats to a heart rate of 110 beats per minute. With regard to long-term effects, atomoxetine is associated with sexual dysfunction in both men and women. In addition, growth appears to initially slow in the first 9 months of treatment in pediatric patients, then appears to normalize over the course of 36 months of treatment. Rare, but more serious, side effects of atomoxetine include liver dysfunction, which has occurred in

at least three patients since its release, all of whom have recovered after discontinuation of atomoxetine; systematic monitoring of liver function tests has not been recommended.[61] In addition, suicidal ideation emerged in a small percentage (approximately 4 in 1,000) of patients in pre-marketing trials; no suicide attempts were made. In overdose, fatalities have not been reported, and sedation/agitation, gastrointestinal symptoms, and tachycardia appear commonly. There appear to be no withdrawal symptoms associated with discontinuation of atomoxetine.

Anticholinergics

The most common side effects of anticholinergic medications (such as benztropine and diphenhydramine) include dry mouth, constipation, urinary hesitancy, tachycardia, thickening of secretions, and dry skin (related to effects on muscarinic cholinergic receptors). In addition, sedation is common, especially with diphenhydramine and related compounds, because of their effects on histaminic receptors. Dizziness, tremor, incoordination, dyspepsia, and hypotension can also occur, and these agents should not be used in patients with narrow-angle glaucoma or benign prostatic hypertrophy because of their potential to worsen the effects of these conditions. Long-term effects are generally extensions of the usual initial side effects. Anticholinergic medications can lead to daytime fatigue, slowed thinking, and frank delirium, especially in those with risk factors for the development of delirium (e.g., the elderly and those with dementia or another organic brain syndrome). Overdose of anticholinergic medications can lead to a variety of effects (including ataxia, disorientation/confusion, psychosis/hallucinations, agitation, tachycardia, a prolonged QTc interval, hypotension, cardiovascular collapse, seizure, and coma). In most cases, treatment is supportive; vasopressors can be used for hypotension. In patients with refractory symptoms, physostigmine can be used; this agent is often effective, but it can cause bradyarrhythmias, asystole, seizures, and significant gastrointestinal effects, and it is contraindicated in patients with prolonged PR or QRS intervals. However, it is effective, and one study found physostigmine to be safer and more effective than benzodiazepines in the treatment of delirious patients with anticholinergic toxicity.[62]

Topiramate

The anticonvulsant topiramate is not an established mood stabilizer, but it has been used in the treatment of alcohol and cocaine use disorders. The most prominent initial side effects of topiramate are neurological side effects (including paresthesias, impaired memory and attention, dizziness, sedation, fatigue, anxiety, and impaired taste); insomnia and visual impairment are less common. Cognitive impairment occurs in up to one-third of patients. Gastrointestinal side effects (e.g., nausea, anorexia, dyspepsia, diarrhea) are also somewhat common with topiramate. Most of these effects—aside from decreased appetite, paresthesias, and cognitive slowing—tend to improve over time. Longer-term side effects include weight loss (in approximately 7% of patients who receive 200 to 400 mg/day).[63] Nephrolithiasis, resulting from inhibition of carbonic anhydrase, can also occur in about 1% of patients. One rare, but serious, adverse effect associated with topiramate is acute myopia with secondary angle-closure glaucoma; this syndrome causes bilateral ocular pain and blurred vision, and is a result of increased intraocular pressure. It usually occurs in the first month of treatment and resolves with discontinuation of topiramate. Metabolic acidosis can also occur, and it has been recommended that serum bicarbonate levels be checked intermittently during topiramate treatment. Topiramate does not have significant cardiac effects, and it has not been associated with liver failure when used alone. Overdose can lead to severe lethargy, confusion, impaired vision, and significant metabolic acidosis, though it is usually not fatal; hemodialysis can be used as needed.

Acamprosate

Acamprosate is used in the treatment of alcohol use disorder to reduce the risk of relapse. Diarrhea and GI upset are the most common side effects reported with acamprosate, causing discontinuation rates of up to 2%. Pruritus has also been reported with some frequency. Erythema multiforme has been noted as a complication in case reports, though it appears to be an extremely rare event. Acamprosate is contraindicated in patients with severe renal impairment, and dose adjustment must be made for patients with moderate renal impairment. Diarrhea is the most common manifestation of overdose; treatment is generally symptomatic and supportive.

Naltrexone

Naltrexone is used in the treatment of substance use disorders to reduce craving and improve abstinence rates. The most frequent side effects reported with naltrexone include nausea, dizziness, asthenia, and headache. Naltrexone is contraindicated in individuals with acute hepatitis or liver failure. Naltrexone has been associated with elevation of liver enzymes in some patients, and some clinicians may elect to monitor liver function tests prior to (and periodically after) initiation. Given its opioid receptor antagonism, it may precipitate acute withdrawal if given to patients who have used opioids in the past 7–10 days, and should be avoided in such patients. Overdose is generally managed supportively.

Buprenorphine

The partial opioid receptor agonist buprenorphine is used in patients with opioid use disorder both for management of acute withdrawal and as a maintenance treatment for relapse prevention. Naloxone is commonly added to buprenorphine in the sublingual formulation used to treat opioid use disorder to prevent IV injection of this agent. Side effects of buprenorphine parallel those of other opioids—sedation, nausea, dizziness, constipation, cognitive effects, and urinary retention—and respiratory depression, likewise, is possible with this agent, especially at high doses. However, respiratory depression is less likely than with full opioid agonists due to a ceiling effect.

Access the complete reference list and multiple choice questions (MCQs) online at https://expertconsult.inkling.com

KEY REFERENCES

2. Roose SP, Laghrissi-Thode F, Kennedy JS, et al. Comparison of paroxetine and nortriptyline in depressed patients with ischemic heart disease. *JAMA* 279(4):287–291, 1998.
3. Vieweg WV, Wood MA. Tricyclic antidepressants, QT interval prolongation, and torsade de pointes. *Psychosomatics* 45(5):371–377, 2004.
7. Weinrieb RM, Auriacombe M, Lynch KG, et al. Selective serotonin re-uptake inhibitors and the risk of bleeding. *Expert Opin Drug Saf* 4(2):337–344, 2005.
8. Beach SR, Celano CM, Noseworthy PA, et al. QTc prolongation, torsades de pointes, and psychotropic medications. *Psychosomatics* 54(1):1–13, 2013.
9. Castro VM, Clements CC, Murphy SN, et al. QT interval and antidepressant use: a cross sectional study of electronic health records. *BMJ* 346:f288, 2013.
10. Thase ME. Effects of venlafaxine on blood pressure: a meta-analysis of original data from 3744 depressed patients. *J Clin Psychiatry* 59(10):502–508, 1998.
11. Waring WS, Graham A, Gray J, et al. Evaluation of a QT nomogram for risk assessment after antidepressant overdose. *Br J Clin Pharmacol* 70(6):881–885, 2010.
13. Haddad PM. Antidepressant discontinuation syndromes. *Drug Saf* 24(3):183–197, 2001.
15. Delgado PL, Brannan SK, Mallinckrodt CH, et al. Sexual functioning assessed in 4 double-blind placebo- and paroxetine-controlled trials of duloxetine for major depressive disorder. *J Clin Psychiatry* 66(6):686–692, 2005.
18. Gardner DM, Shulman KI, Walker SE, et al. The making of a user friendly MAOI diet. *J Clin Psychiatry* 57(3):99–104, 1996.
22. Laughren TP, Gobburu J, Temple RJ, et al. Vilazodone: clinical basis for the US Food and Drug Administration's approval of a new antidepressant. *J Clin Psychiatry* 72(9):1166–1173, 2011.
25. Latimer PR. Tardive dyskinesia: a review. *Can J Psychiatry* 40(7 Suppl. 2):S49–S54, 1995.
27. Allison DB, Mentore JL, Heo M, et al. Antipsychotic-induced weight gain: a comprehensive research synthesis. *Am J Psychiatry* 156(11):1686–1696, 1999.
28. American Diabetes Association, American Psychiatric Association, American Association of Clinical Endocrinologists, North American Association for the Study of Obesity. Consensus development conference on antipsychotic drugs and obesity and diabetes. *Diabetes Care* 27(2):596–601, 2004.
29. Leucht S, Cipriani A, Spineli L, et al. Comparative efficacy and tolerability of 15 antipsychotic drugs in schizophrenia: a multiple-treatments meta-analysis. *Lancet* 2013.
30. Schneider LS, Dagerman KS, Insel P. Risk of death with atypical antipsychotic drug treatment for dementia: meta-analysis of randomized placebo-controlled trials. *JAMA* 294(15):1934–1943, 2005.
31. Wang PS, Schneeweiss S, Avorn J, et al. Risk of death in elderly users of conventional vs. atypical antipsychotic medications. *N Engl J Med* 353(22):2335–2341, 2005.
34. Wang SM, Han C, Lee SJ, et al. Paliperidone: a review of clinical trial data and clinical implications. *Clin Drug Investig* 32(8):497–512, 2012.
35. Citrome L. Iloperidone: a clinical overview. *J Clin Psychiatry* 72(Suppl. 1):19–23, 2011.
36. Citrome L. Asenapine for schizophrenia and bipolar disorder: a review of the efficacy and safety profile for this newly approved sublingually absorbed second-generation antipsychotic. *Int J Clin Pract* 63(12):1762–1784, 2009.
37. Loebel A, Cucchiaro J, Sarma K, et al. Efficacy and safety of lurasidone 80 mg/day and 160 mg/day in the treatment of schizophrenia: a randomized, double-blind, placebo- and active-controlled trial. *Schizophr Res* 145(1–3):101–109, 2013.
41. Koro CE, Fedder DO, L'Italien GJ, et al. Assessment of independent effect of olanzapine and risperidone on risk of diabetes among patients with schizophrenia: population based nested case-control study. *BMJ* 325(7358):243, 2002.
44. Alvir JM, Lieberman JA, Safferman AZ, et al. Clozapine-induced agranulocytosis. Incidence and risk factors in the United States. *N Engl J Med* 329(3):162–167, 1993.
45. Honigfeld G. Effects of the clozapine national registry system on incidence of deaths related to agranulocytosis. *Psychiatr Serv* 47(1):52–56, 1996.
48. Wang PS, Bohn RL, Glynn RJ, et al. Hazardous benzodiazepine regimens in the elderly: effects of half-life, dosage, and duration on risk of hip fracture. *Am J Psychiatry* 158(6):892–898, 2001.
57. Ko DT, Hebert PR, Coffey CS, et al. Beta-blocker therapy and symptoms of depression, fatigue, and sexual dysfunction. *JAMA* 288(3):351–357, 2002.
58. Law SF, Schachar RJ. Do typical clinical doses of methylphenidate cause tics in children treated for attention-deficit hyperactivity disorder? *J Am Acad Child Adolesc Psychiatry* 38(8):944–951, 1999.
59. Tourette's Syndrome Study G. Treatment of ADHD in children with tics: a randomized controlled trial. *Neurology* 58(4):527–536, 2002.
61. Lim JR, Faught PR, Chalasani NP, et al. Severe liver injury after initiating therapy with atomoxetine in two children. *J Pediatrics* 148(6):831–834, 2006.
62. Burns MJ, Linden CH, Graudins A, et al. A comparison of physostigmine and benzodiazepines for the treatment of anticholinergic poisoning. *Ann Emerg Med* 35(4):374–381, 2000.

52 Natural Medications in Psychiatry

Felicia A. Smith, MD, and David Mischoulon, MD, PhD

KEY POINTS

- Complementary and alternative medical therapies are made up of a diverse spectrum of practices (including natural medications) that often overlap with more traditional medical practice.

- The use of natural medications is growing considerably in the US and around the world, and patients often do not report use of natural medications to their physicians.

- Historical lack of scientific research in this area has contributed to deficiencies in knowledge with respect to safety and efficacy of many of the natural remedies on the market today.

- Natural medications are used for the psychiatric indications of mood disorders, anxiety, insomnia, menstrual and menopausal symptoms, and dementia (among others).

OVERVIEW

Complementary and alternative medical therapies are made up of a diverse spectrum of practices and beliefs that often overlap with current medical practice. The National Institutes of Health (NIH) defines *complementary and alternative medicine* (CAM) as "healthcare practices outside the realm of conventional medicine, which are yet to be validated using scientific methods."[1] The National Center for Complementary and Alternative Medicine (NCCAM) is one of the NIH institutes and is the federal government's lead agency responsible for scientific research on complementary and alternative medicine. NCCAM distinguishes four domains within complementary medicine: mind–body medicine, energy medicine, manipulative and body-based practices, and biologically-based practices.[2] This chapter will focus on the biologically-based practices including natural medications. *Natural medications* are medications that are derived from natural products, and are not approved by the Food and Drug Administration (FDA) for their proposed indication.[3] Natural medications may include a wide variety of types of products such as hormones, vitamins, plants, herbs, fatty acids, amino acid derivatives, and homeopathic preparations. Natural medications have been used in Asia for thousands of years. Their use in the US has, however, been much more recent, with a dramatic increase over the past decade and a half. In fact, the National Health Interview Survey conducted in 2002 revealed that 62% of a randomly-sampled US population used some form of CAM, including prayer, for health reasons within the past year. When prayer was excluded, 36% of those sampled admitted to using some form of CAM.[4-6] Moreover, between 1990 and 1997 the prevalence of herbal remedy use increased by 380%, while high-dose vitamin use increased by 130%.[7] Between 1998 and 2002 CAM use doubled in the over-65 population.[6] Ethnic considerations also appear to be important, with African Americans being the group least likely in the US to try natural remedies and Hispanics being the most prone to their use.[8] Given the considerable portion of the US population trying natural remedies, it is clearly becoming increasingly important to be informed about these medications in order to provide comprehensive patient care. This chapter provides an overview of the use of natural medications in psychiatry. General safety and efficacy are discussed first. This is followed by an examination of some of the primary remedies used for psychiatric indications including mood disorders, anxiety and sleep disorders, menstrual disorders, and dementia.

EFFICACY AND SAFETY

Although both governmental agencies (including the NIH and NCCAM) and the pharmaceutical industry are sponsoring more clinical research involving natural medications, data regarding effectiveness still lag behind. The actual benefits of natural remedies are often unclear in a setting where relatively few systematic studies have adequately addressed the question of effectiveness.[9] The FDA does not routinely regulate natural medications, leaving questions of safety at the forefront. Consumers often believe that because a remedy is "natural," it is therefore safe. Moreover, since these remedies are most often purchased over the counter (OTC), there is no clear mechanism for reports of toxicity to reach those who use them. Another significant problem lies in the limited information regarding the safety and efficacy of combining natural medications with more conventional ones.[9] In cases where interactions are known, the psychiatrist faces the reality that patients frequently do not disclose their use of CAM therapies to their physicians. In one study, fewer than 40% of CAM therapies used were disclosed to a physician.[7] Asking very specific questions about a patient's use of both prescribed and OTC medications may improve disclosures in this regard. Finally, since natural medications are not regulated as more conventional ones are, significant variability exists among different preparations. Preparations often vary in purity, quality, potency, and efficacy while side effects may vary. The increase in government- and industry-sponsored studies may further clarify the potential uses, safety, and efficacy of these medications; until such results are available, caution should still be used in recommending those that are less well understood. The remainder of this chapter outlines the current understanding of some of the primary natural medications with potential psychiatric indications.

MOOD DISORDERS

Numerous natural medications have been used to treat mood disorders, including omega-3 fatty acids, St. John's wort (SJW), *S*-adenosylmethionine (SAMe), folic acid, vitamin B_{12}, and inositol (Table 52-1). Dehydroepiandrosterone (DHEA) may also have a role in the treatment of depression; however, further description of this adrenal steroid is reserved for the cognition and dementia section later in this chapter. The efficacy, possible mechanisms of action, dosing, adverse effects, and drug interactions of each of these medications are discussed in the following section.

TABLE 52-1 Natural Medications for Mood Disorders

Medication	Active Components	Possible Indications	Possible Mechanisms of Action	Suggested Doses	Adverse Events
Omega-3 fatty acids	Essential fatty acids (primarily EPA and DHA)	Depression, bipolar disorder, schizophrenia, ADHD	Effects on neurotransmitter signaling receptors; inhibition of inflammatory cytokines; lowering plasma norepinephrine (noradrenaline)	1,000–2,000 mg/day	Fishy taste and odor, GI upset, theoretical risk of bleeding
Folic acid	Vitamin	Depression, dementia	Neurotransmitter synthesis	400–800 mcg/day; 15 mg/day 5-MTHF (Deplin)	Masking of B_{12} deficiency, lowers seizure threshold in high doses, and adverse interactions with other drugs
Inositol	Six-carbon ring natural isomer of glucose	Depression, panic, OCD, and possibly bipolar disorder	Second messenger synthesis	12–18 g/day	Mild GI upset, headache, dizziness, sedation, and insomnia
SAMe	Biological compound involved in methylation reactions	Depression	Neurotransmitter synthesis	300–1,600 mg/day	Mild anxiety, agitation, insomnia, dry mouth, GI disturbance; also possible switch to mania and serotonin syndrome
St. John's wort *(Hypericum perforatum L.)*	Hypericin, hyperforin, polycyclic phenols, pseudohypericin	Depression	Inhibition of cytokines, decreased serotonin receptor density, decreased neurotransmitter reuptake, MAOI activity	900–1,800 mg/day	Dry mouth, dizziness, GI disturbance, and phototoxicity; also possible serotonin syndrome when taken with SSRIs and adverse interactions with other drugs
Vitamin B_{12}	Vitamin	Depression	Neurotransmitter synthesis	500–1,000 mcg/day	None

ADHD, Attention-deficit/hyperactivity disorder; DHA, docosahexaenoic acid; EPA, eicosapentaenoic acid; GI, gastrointestinal; MAOI, monoamine oxidase inhibitor; OCD, obsessive-compulsive disorder; SAMe, *S*-adenosylmethionine; SSRI, selective serotonin reuptake inhibitor.
(Adapted from Mischoulon D, Nierenberg AA. Natural medications in psychiatry. In Stern TA, Herman JB, editors: Psychiatry update and board preparation, ed 2, New York, 2004, McGraw-Hill.)

Omega-3 Fatty Acids

Omega-3 fatty acids are polyunsaturated lipids derived from fish oil and certain land-based plants (e.g., flax). Omega-3 fatty acids have been shown to have benefits in numerous medical conditions, including rheumatoid arthritis, Crohn's disease, ulcerative colitis, psoriasis, immunoglobulin A (IgA) nephropathy, systemic lupus erythematosus, multiple sclerosis, and migraine headache, among others.[10] Cardioprotective benefits have also been demonstrated,[11] although recent systematic reviews have been less supportive of their role as preventive agents for cardiovascular disease.[12-14] From a psychiatric standpoint, omega-3 fatty acids may have a role in the treatment of unipolar depression, post-partum depression, bipolar disorder, schizophrenia, and attention-deficit/hyperactivity disorder (ADHD).[15-19] The most promising data, however, are in the treatment of both bipolar disorder and unipolar depression; positive studies have been reported in each of these domains,[15,20-22] yet recent meta-analyses have also cast doubt on the degree of antidepressant efficacy of the omega-3s.[20-26] In countries with higher fish consumption, lower rates of depression and bipolar disorder provide a clue that omega-3 fatty acids may play a protective role in these disorders.[20] Although there are several types of omega-3 fatty acids, eicosapentaenoic acid (EPA) and docosahexaenoic acid (DHA) are thought to be psychotropically active.[3] While their mechanism of action is not completely clear, several have been proposed. These run the gamut from effects on membrane-bound receptors and enzymes that regulate neurotransmitter signaling, to the regulation of calcium ion influx through calcium channels, to the lowering of plasma norepinephrine (noradrenaline)

levels, or possibly to the inhibition of secretion of inflammatory cytokines that result in decreased corticosteroid release from the adrenal gland.[27-30] Omega-3 fatty acids may be consumed naturally from a variety of sources, including fatty fish (e.g., salmon), flax seeds, chia seeds, hemp seeds, and enriched eggs. Commercially available preparations of omega-3 fatty acids in pill form vary in composition, and the suggested ratio of EPA:DHA is at least 3:2 in favor of EPA.[25] Psychotropically-active doses are generally thought to be in the range of 1 to 2 g per day, with dose-related gastrointestinal (GI) distress being the major side effect. There is also a theoretical risk of increased bleeding, so concomitant use with high-dose non-steroidal anti-inflammatory drugs (NSAIDs) or anticoagulants is not recommended. There are thus far no known interactions with other mood stabilizers or antidepressants.

In sum, the use of omega-3 fatty acids remains promising, particularly given the range of potential benefits and the relatively low toxicity seen thus far. However, larger and more definitive studies are still needed.

St. John's Wort

St. John's wort (SJW) *(Hypericum perforatum)* is one of the biggest-selling natural medications on the market. It has been shown to be more effective than placebo in the treatment of mild-to-moderate depression.[31-34] Studies have further suggested that SJW is as effective as low-dose tricyclic antidepressants (TCAs) (e.g., imipramine 75 mg, maprotiline 75 mg, or amitriptyline 75 mg).[27,31] When compared with selective serotonin reuptake inhibitors (SSRIs), the efficacy of SJW has been comparable and better than placebo in some studies of mild depression. For example, SJW was shown to be as effective as sertraline and fluoxetine in the treatment of mild-to-moderate depression in at least two cases.[35,36] However, in other studies, SJW has not shown an advantage over placebo.[37,38] These mixed results may be explained by more severely depressed study populations in studies with negative outcomes.[27] *Hypericum* is thought to be the main antidepressant ingredient in SJW, while polycyclic phenols, pseudohypericin, and hyperforin are also thought to be active ingredients. As far as the mechanism of action of SJW is concerned, there are several proposed theories. These include the inhibition of cytokines, a decrease in serotonin (5-HT) receptor density, a decrease in reuptake of neurotransmitters, and monoamine oxidase inhibitor (MAOI) activity.[9,27] Since SJW has MAOI activity, it should not be combined with SSRIs because of the possible development of serotonin syndrome. Suggested doses range from 900 to 1,800 mg per day depending on the preparation, and adverse effects include dry mouth, dizziness, constipation, and phototoxicity. Care should be taken in patients with bipolar disorder due to the possibility of a switch to mania.[39] Finally, there are a number of important drug–drug interactions with SJW that are of particular note. Hyperforin is metabolized through the liver and induces cytochrome P-3A4 expression, which may reduce the therapeutic activity of a number of common medications, including warfarin, cyclosporine, oral contraceptives, theophylline, digoxin, and indinavir.[40,41] Transplant recipients should not use SJW since transplant rejections have been reported as a result of interactions between SJW and cyclosporine.[42] Individuals with human immunodeficiency virus (HIV) infection on protease inhibitors also should avoid SJW because of drug interactions.

In sum, SJW appears to be better than placebo and equivalent to low-dose TCAs for the treatment of mild depression. Emerging data also suggest that SJW may also compare favorably to SSRIs for mild depression. Data also seem to suggest that SJW may not be effective for more severe forms of depression. There are important drug–drug interactions that should be considered as outlined previously.

S-Adenosylmethionine

S-Adenosylmethionine (SAMe) is a compound found in all living cells that is involved in essential methyl group transfers. It is the principal methyl donor in the one-carbon cycle with SAMe levels depending on levels of the vitamins folate and B_{12} (Figure 52-1). SAMe is involved in the methylation of neurotransmitters, nucleic acids, proteins, hormones, and phospholipids—its role in the production of norepinephrine, serotonin, and dopamine may explain SAMe's antidepressant properties.[3,9,43,44] SAMe has been shown to elevate mood in depressed patients in doses of between 300 and 1,600 mg per day. Studies support antidepressant efficacy of SAMe when compared with placebo and TCAs.[44–46] Recent studies have demonstrated efficacy as augmentation for SSRI and SNRI partial responders.[47,48] Oral preparations of SAMe are somewhat unstable, making high doses required for adequate bioavailability. Since the medication is relatively expensive (and not covered by conventional medical insurance plans), the high cost may be prohibitive for many patients. Potential adverse effects are relatively minor and include anxiety, agitation, insomnia, dry mouth, bowel changes, and anorexia. Sweating, dizziness, palpitations, and headaches have also been reported. Psychiatrists should also watch for a potential switch to mania. Furthermore, suspected serotonin syndrome was reported when SAMe was combined with clomipramine in an elderly woman.[49] Finally, there have not yet been reports of significant drug–drug interactions or hepatoxicity with SAMe.

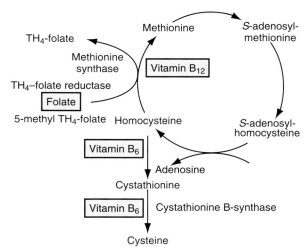

Figure 52-1. One-carbon cycle with SAMe, folate, and vitamin B_{12}. *(Redrawn from Dinavahi R, Bonita Falkner B. Relationship of homocysteine with cardiovascular disease and blood pressure,* J Clin Hypertens 6:495, 2004. © 2004 Le Jacq Communications, Inc.)

SAMe therefore is a natural medication that appears to be relatively safe and shows promise as an antidepressant. Further study will help clarify its efficacy and safety.

Folate and Vitamin B_{12}

Folate and vitamin B_{12} are dietary vitamins that play a key role in one-carbon metabolism in which SAMe is formed[50] (see Figure 52-1). SAMe then donates methyl groups that are crucial for neurological function and play important roles in the synthesis of central nervous system (CNS) neurotransmitters (e.g., serotonin, dopamine, norepinephrine), as discussed previously. Folate and vitamin B_{12} deficiency states may cause or contribute to a variety of neuropsychiatric and general medical conditions (e.g., macrocytic anemia, neuropathy, cognitive dysfunction/dementia, depression). Folate deficiency, to start, has a number of potential etiologies. These include inadequate dietary intake, malabsorption, inborn errors of metabolism, or an increased demand (e.g., as seen with pregnancy, infancy, bacterial overgrowth, rapid cellular turnover). Drugs (such as anticonvulsants, oral contraceptives, sulfasalazine, methotrexate, triamterene, trimethoprim, pyrimethamine, and alcohol, among others) may also contribute to folate defiency.[51] Like folate, vitamin B_{12} deficiency may also be a result of inadequate dietary intake, malabsorption, impaired utilization, and interactions with certain drugs. Colchicine, H_2 blockers, metformin, nicotine, oral contraceptive pills, cholestyramine, K-Dur, and zidovudine are some examples of these.[40] From a psychiatric standpoint, deficiency of both folate and vitamin B_{12} has been linked with depression, though the association with folate seems to be greater.[50,52–54] Moreover, low folate levels have been associated with delayed onset of clinical improvement of depression in at least one study.[55] Studies suggest that folate deficiency may lessen antidepressant response,[52] and that folate supplementation may be a beneficial adjunct to SSRI-refractory depression.[56] A recent study on a prescription form of 5-methyl tetrahydrofolate (5-MTHF; Deplin) supports its efficacy as an augmenter of antidepressants at doses of 15 mg/day.[57] This form crosses the blood–brain barrier directly, without requiring enzymatic inter-conversion, and may theoretically deliver more active product to the brain. Metabolically significant vitamin B_{12} deficiency, in turn, has been shown to be associated with a two-fold risk of severe (not mild) depression in a population of geriatric women.[58] Low vitamin B_{12} levels have also been associated with poor cognitive status and psychotic depression in the geriatric population.[59,60] Although the data are somewhat mixed, folic acid and vitamin B_{12} supplementation in daily doses of 800 mcg and 1 mg, respectively, has been suggested to improve outcomes in depressed patients.[50] Adequate levels of each of these is thought to provide optimal neurotransmitter synthesis that may aid in reversing depression. One caveat is that supplementation with folate alone may "mask" vitamin B_{12} deficiency by correcting macrocytic anemia while neuropathy continues, so vitamin B_{12} levels should be routinely measured when high doses of folate are given. Folate may also reduce the effectiveness of other medications (e.g., phenytoin, methotrexate, and pheno-barbital) and has been reported to lower the seizure threshold since high doses disrupt the blood–brain barrier.[61,62]

In summary, correction of folate deficiency (and perhaps vitamin B_{12} deficiency) may improve depression or at least augment therapy with other medications. Folate (and maybe B_{12}) supplementation may also shorten the latency of response and enhance response in the treatment of depressed patients even with normal levels. While overall data are not conclusive, psychiatrists should at minimum be on the lookout for potential deficiency states as outlined here by checking serum levels in patients at risk of deficiencies or who have not responded to antidepressant treatment.

Inositol

Inositol is a natural isomer of glucose that is present in common foods. Inositols are cyclic carbohydrates with a six-carbon ring, with the isomer myo-inositol being the most common in the CNS of mammals (Figure 52-2). Myo-inositol is thought to modulate interactions between neurotransmitters, receptors, cell-signaling proteins, and drugs through its activity in the cell-signaling pathway, and is the putative target of the mood-stabilizing drug lithium.[63] There is also emerging evidence for a role of inositol in the mechanism of valproate and car-bamazepine.[64] Inositol has been found in various small studies to be effective in the treatment of depression, panic disorder, obsessive-compulsive disorder (OCD), and possibly bipolar depression.[65–69] While there are some promising findings, negative monotherapy trials with inositol have also been seen in a variety of psychiatric illnesses, including schizophrenia, dementia, ADHD, premenstrual dysphoric disorder, autism, and electroconvulsive-therapy (ECT)-induced cognitive impairment.[9,68] Effective doses are thought to be in the range of 12 to 18 g/day. Adverse effects are generally mild and include GI upset, headache, dizziness, sedation, and insomnia. There is no apparent toxicity or known drug interactions at this time.[3,9]

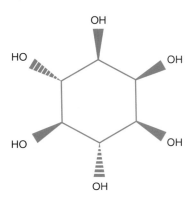

Figure 52-2. Myo-inositol (MI) cyclic carbohydrate with six-carbon ring.

In summary, treatment with inositol in the spectrum of illness treated with SSRIs and mood stabilizers as discussed previously appears to be safe and remains promising.

ANXIETY AND INSOMNIA
Valerian

Valerian *(Valeriana officinalis)* is a flowering plant extract that has been used to promote sleep and to reduce anxiety for over 2,000 years. Common names also include *all heal* and *garden heliotrope.* Typical preparations include capsules, liquid extracts, and teas made from roots and underground stems. A national survey of US adults in 2002 revealed that 1.1% of those surveyed had used valerian in the past week.[4] Since the data regarding valerian and sleep are much more substantial than that of valerian and anxiety,[70–73] sleep will be the focus of the rest of this section. Valerian is thought to promote natural sleep after several weeks of use by decreasing sleep latency and by improving overall sleep quality; however, methodological problems in the majority of studies conducted limit firm conclusions in this area.[71] A proposed mechanism involves decreasing γ-aminobutyric acid (GABA) breakdown.[72,73] Sedative effects are dose-related with usual dosages in the range of 450 to 600 mg about 2 hours before bedtime. Dependence and daytime drowsiness have not been problems. Adverse effects, including blurry vision, GI symptoms, and headache, seem to be uncommon. Although data are limited, valerian should probably be avoided in patients with liver dysfunction (due to potential hepatic toxicity). Major drug interactions have not been reported.

In summary, valerian has been used as a hypnotic for many years with relatively few reported adverse effects.

Melatonin

Melatonin is a hormone made in the pineal gland that has been shown to help travelers avoid jet lag and to decrease sleep latency for those suffering with insomnia. It may be particularly beneficial for night-shift workers as well. Melatonin is derived from serotonin (Figure 52-3) and is thought to play a role in the organization of circadian rhythms via interaction with the suprachiasmatic nucleus.[74,75] Low-dose melatonin treatment has been shown to increase circulating melatonin levels to those normally observed at night and thus to facilitate sleep onset and sleep maintenance without changing sleep architecture.[76] Melatonin generally facilitates falling asleep within 1 hour, independent of when it is taken. Optimal doses are not completely known, although they are thought to be in the range of 0.25 to 0.30 mg per day. Some preparations, however, contain as much as 5 mg of melatonin.[3,9] Higher doses have been noted to cause daytime sleepiness and confusion; other potential adverse effects include decreased sex drive, retinal damage, hypothermia, and fertility problems. Melatonin is contraindicated in pregnancy and in those who are immunocompromised.[3,9] There are few reports of drug–drug interactions.

Melatonin seems to be a relatively safe hypnotic and an organizer of circadian rhythms when taken in appropriate doses. Caution should be taken in at-risk populations and with use of higher doses (as discussed previously).

Kava

Kava *(Piper methysticum)* is derived from a root originating in the Polynesian Islands, where it is used as a social and ceremonial herb. Though it is thought to have mild anxiolytic and hypnotic effects, study results have been mixed. The mechanism of action is attributed to kavapyrones, which are central muscle relaxants that are thought to be involved in blockade of voltage-gated sodium ion channels, enhanced binding to GABA$_A$ receptors, diminished excitatory neurotransmitter release, reduced reuptake of norepinephrine, and reversible inhibition of MAO$_B$.[77] The suggested dose is 60 to 120 mg per day. Major side effects include GI upset, headaches, and dizziness.[3,9] Toxic reactions, including ataxia, hair loss, respiratory problems, yellowing of the skin, and vision problems, have been seen at high doses or with prolonged use. There have also been more than 70 published reports of severe hepatotoxicity worldwide,[78] including some that have required liver transplantation.[79] For this reason, several countries have pulled kava off the market. In the US, the FDA has issued a

warning regarding the use of kava and NCCAM has suspended investigations involving kava since that warning.[80]

While kava appears to be somewhat efficacious in the treatment of mild anxiety, current concerns about safety make its use risky. Table 52-2 summarizes the natural medications discussed here for the treatment of insomnia and anxiety.

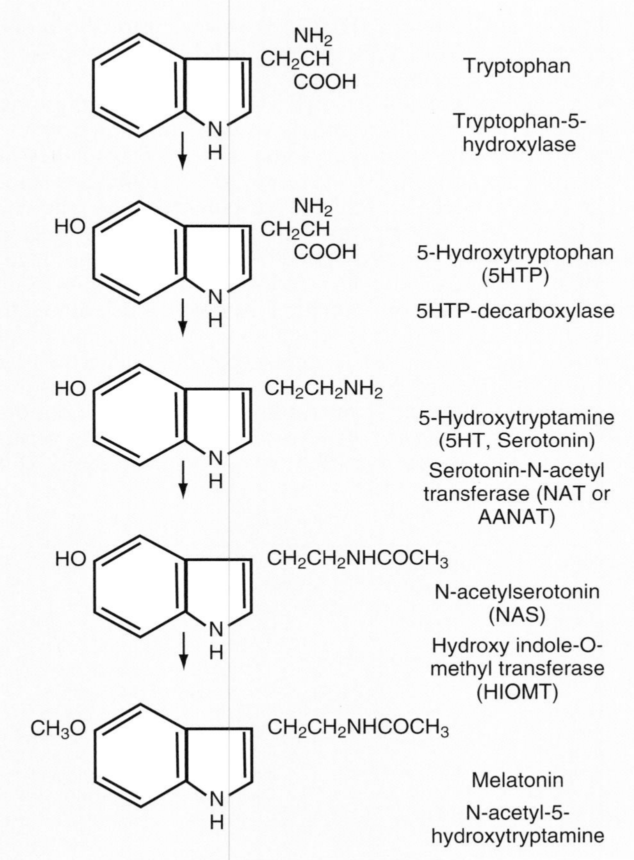

PREMENSTRUAL AND MENOPAUSAL SYMPTOMS
Black Cohosh

Black cohosh (Cimicifuga racemosa) is a member of the buttercup family native to the northeastern US. The available natural supplement, derived from the root of the plant, at a dose of 40 mg per day has been shown to reduce physical and psychological menopausal symptoms, as well as dysmenorrhea.[81,82] Active ingredients are thought to be triterpenoids, isoflavones, and aglycones, which may participate in suppression of luteinizing hormone in the pituitary gland,[3,9] though studies in humans have shown mixed results.[82] Effects on breast cancer proliferation are also inconsistent.[82] Headache, dizziness, GI upset, and weight gain are among the generally mild side effects reported. Limited data have not revealed specific toxicity or drug interactions. Black cohosh is not recommended for individuals who are pregnant or breast-feeding or who have heart disease or hypertension. Those with adverse reactions to aspirin should also avoid black cohosh since it contains salicylates. Beneficial effects and safety profiles will be further elucidated as more data are obtained.

Chaste Tree Berry

Chaste tree berry (Vitex agnus castus) is derived from the dried fruit of the chaste tree; it has been used since ancient Greece to help alleviate female reproductive complaints.[82] Its name comes from its earlier use to help monks keep their vow of chastity through decreasing the sex drive. The mechanism in both instances is thought to be via prolactin inhibition by binding dopamine receptors in the anterior pituitary,[82] though this remains under investigation. It is most commonly used to alleviate premenstrual syndrome (PMS) in suggested doses of 200 to 400 mg per day.[3,9] Side effects such as increased acne, increased menstrual flow, and GI disturbance seem to be minor. While there are no clear drug–drug interactions, there is a theoretical risk of decreased efficacy of birth control due to its effects on prolactin. Since it is thought to be a dopamine agonist, there may also be interactions with other dopamine agonists or antagonists.[82] A summary of the natural medica-

Figure 52-3. Melatonin synthesis.

TABLE 52-2 Natural Medications for Anxiety and Insomnia

Medication	Active Components	Possible Indications	Possible Mechanisms of Action	Suggested Doses	Adverse Events
Kava (Piper methysticum)	Kavapyrones	Anxiety	Central muscle relaxant, enhanced GABA$_A$ receptor binding, reversible inhibition of MAO$_B$	60–120 mg/day	Gastrointestinal disturbance, headaches, dizziness, ataxia, hair loss, visual problems, respiratory problems, rash, severe liver toxicity
Melatonin	Hormone made in pineal gland	Insomnia	Regulates circadian rhythm in suprachiasmatic nucleus	0.25–0.3 mg/day (may increase up to 5 mg/day if needed)	Sedation, confusion, hypothermia, retinal damage, decreased sex drive, infertility
Valerian (Valeriana officinalis)	Valepotriates (from roots and underground stems)	Insomnia	Decrease GABA breakdown	450–600 mg/day	Blurry vision, headache, and possible hepatotoxicity

GABA, γ-aminobutyric acid; MAO, monoamine oxidase.
Adapted from Mischoulon D, Nierenberg AA. Natural medications in psychiatry. In Stern TA, Herman JB, editors: Psychiatry update and board preparation, ed 2, New York, 2004, McGraw-Hill.

tions discussed here for premenstrual and menopausal symptoms is found in Table 52-3.

COGNITION AND DEMENTIA
Ginkgo biloba

Ginkgo biloba has been used in Chinese medicine for thousands of years. This natural medication comes from the seed of the gingko tree, and has generally been used for the treatment of impaired cognition and affective symptoms in dementing illnesses; however, a possible new role has also emerged in the management of antidepressant-induced sexual dysfunction.[83] As far as its role in cognition is concerned, target symptoms in patients with dementia include memory and abstract thinking. Studies have shown modest but significant improvements in both cognitive performance and social function with doses of 120 mg per day.[84-88] Evidence suggests that progression of disease may be delayed by 6 to 12 months, while those with mild dementia show greatest improvement and those with more severe disease may at most stabilize.[85] Recent studies have suggested that ginkgo may be effective in combination with registered nootropic agents, the cholinesterase inhibitors.[86] Furthermore, one study of healthy young volunteers taking *Ginkgo biloba* made significant improvements in speed of information processing, executive function, and working-memory, suggesting that gingko may also enhance learning capacity.[87] Flavonoids and terpene lactones are thought to be the active components, which may work by stimulating still functional nerve cells.[3,9] They may also play a role in protecting cells from pathological effects (such as hypoxia and ischemia). Since ginkgo has been shown to inhibit platelet-activating factor and has been associated with increased bleeding risk (though results are mixed), it should probably be avoided in those at high risk of bleeding until further data are available.[88] Other noted side effects include headache, GI distress, seizures in epileptics, and dizziness. The suggested dose of *Ginkgo biloba* is 120 to 240 mg per day, with a minimum 8-week course of treatment; however, it may take up to a year to appreciate the full benefit.

Ginkgo biloba appears to be a safe and efficacious cognition-enhancing medication. It may have an additional role in reducing antidepressant-induced sexual dysfunction. Further studies are needed to fully understand its complete and long-term effects.

Dehydroepiandrosterone

Dehydroepiandrosterone (DHEA) is an androgenic hormone synthesized primarily in the adrenal glands, and converted to testosterone and estrogen.[89] DHEA is thought to play a role in enhancing memory and in improving depressive symptoms, though studies in this regard have had mixed results.[89-91] Possible mechanisms of action may include modulation of *N*-methyl-D-aspartate (NMDA) receptors and GABA$_A$ receptor antagonism.[89] DHEA is available for purchase in a synthetic oral formulation and an intra-oral spray with doses ranging from 5 to 100 mg per day. Strength and purity are not regulated, as is the case with most other natural remedies. Side effects are principally hormonally driven with a risk of weight gain, hirsutism, menstrual irregularity, voice changes, and headache in women. Men may experience gynecomastia and prostatic hypertrophy. The effects on hormone-sensitive tumors are not known.[89] Larger studies will help flesh out the promising early data for DHEA use, and clarify risks versus benefits before it may be safely recommended. Table 52-4

TABLE 52-3 Natural Medications for Premenstrual and Menopausal Symptoms

Medication	Active Components	Possible Indications	Possible Mechanisms of Action	Suggested Doses	Adverse Events
Black cohosh (*Cimicifuga racemosa*)	Triterpenoids, isoflavones, aglycones	Menopausal and premenstrual symptoms	Suppression of luteinizing hormone (LH) in the pituitary gland	40 mg/day	Gastrointestinal upset, headache, weight gain, and dizziness, unclear effects on breast cancer proliferation
Chaste tree berry (*Vitex agnus castus*)	Unknown	Premenstrual symptoms	Prolactin inhibition by binding to dopaminergic receptors in the anterior pituitary	200–400 mg/day	Minor GI disturbance, increased acne, increased menstrual flow, possible decreased efficacy of birth control

GI, Gastrointestinal.
Adapted from Mischoulon D, Nierenberg AA. Natural medications in psychiatry. In Stern TA, Herman JB, editors: Psychiatry update and board preparation, *ed 2, New York, 2004, McGraw-Hill.*

TABLE 52-4 Natural Medications for Cognition and Dementia

Medication	Active Components	Possible Indications	Possible Mechanisms of Action	Suggested Doses	Adverse Events
Dehydroepiandrosterone (DHEA)	Androgenic hormone synthesized in adrenal glands	Depression and dementia	Modulation of NMDA receptors and GABA$_A$ receptor antagonism	5–100 mg/day	Weight gain, hirsutism, menstrual irregularity, voice changes in women, gynecomastia and prostatic hypertrophy in men
Ginkgo biloba	Flavonoids, terpene lactones	Dementia and sexual dysfunction	Nerve cell stimulation and protection and free radical scavenging	120–240 mg/day	Mild GI disturbance, headache, irritability, dizziness, seizures in epileptics

GABA, γ-aminobutyric acid; GI, gastrointestinal; NMDA, *N*-methyl-D-aspartate.
Adapted from Mischoulon D, Nierenberg AA. Natural medications in psychiatry. In Stern TA, Herman JB, editors: Psychiatry update and board preparation, *ed 2, New York, 2004, McGraw-Hill.*

outlines the natural medications described here for cognitive dysfunction and dementia.

CONCLUSION

Complementary and alternative medical therapies are becoming increasingly popular in the US and around the world. The spectrum of CAM therapies is quite diverse and may have significant overlap with more traditional medical practice. Lack of scientific research in this area historically has contributed to deficiencies in knowledge with respect to safety and efficacy of many of the natural remedies on the market today. This should be improved by a recent surge in funding by governmental and industry sources. Current knowledge about a few such therapies in the psychiatric realm has been outlined in this chapter; these include proposed treatments for mood disorders, anxiety and sleep disorders, menstrual disorders, and dementia. Many of these therapies may prove to be a valuable addition to the armamentarium of treatments available to psychiatrists in the future. There are also important drug–drug interactions and potential side effects as outlined in the prior sections. A general knowledge of these therapies and routine questioning about their use is an essential part of comprehensive care by the current psychiatrist.

Access the complete reference list and multiple choice questions (MCQs) online at https://expertconsult.inkling.com

KEY REFERENCES

3. Mischoulon D, Nierenberg AA. Natural medications in psychiatry. In Stern TA, Herman JB, Gorrindo T, editors: *Psychiatry update and board preparation*, ed 3, Boston, 2012, MGH Psychiatry Academy.
15. Freeman MP, Hibbeln JR, Wisner KL, et al. Omega-3 fatty acids: evidence basis for treatment and future research in psychiatry. *J Clin Psychiatry* 67(12):1954–1967, 2006.
23. Lin PY, Su KP. A meta-analytic review of double-blind, placebo-controlled trials of antidepressant efficacy of omega-3 fatty acids. *J Clin Psychiatry* 68(7):1056–1061, 2007.
24. Appleton KM, Rogers PJ, Ness AR. Updated systematic review and meta-analysis of the effects of n-3 long-chain polyunsaturated fatty acids on depressed mood. *Am J Clin Nutr* 91(3):757–770, 2010.
25. Sublette ME, Ellis SP, Geant AL, et al. Meta-analysis of the effects of eicosapentaenoic acid (EPA) in clinical trials in depression. *J Clin Psychiatry* 72(12):1577–1584, 2011.
26. Bloch MH, Hannestad J. Omega-3 fatty acids for the treatment of depression: systematic review and meta-analysis. *Mol Psychiatry* 17(12):1272–1282, 2012.
27. Mischoulon D. Update and critique of natural remedies as antidepressant treatments. *Psychiatr Clin North Am* 30(1):51–68, 2007.
33. Sarris J. St. John's wort for treatment of psychiatric disorders. *Psychiatry Clin North Am* 36(1):65–72, 2013.
38. Hypericum Depression Trial Study Group. Effect of *Hypericum perforatum* (St John's wort) in major depressive disorder: a randomized controlled trial. *JAMA* 287(14):1807–1814, 2002.
43. Mischoulon D, Fava M. Role of S-adenosyl-L-methionine in the treatment of depression: a review of the evidence. *Am J Clin Nutr* 76(5):1158S–1161S, 2002.
45. Papakostas GI, Alpert JE, Fava M. S-Adenosyl methionine in depression: a comprehensive review of the literature. *Curr Psychiatry Rep* 5:460–466, 2003.
46. Alpert JE, Papakostas G, Mischoulon D, et al. S-Adenosyl-L-methionine (SAMe) as an adjunct for resistant major depressive disorder: an open trial following partial or nonresponse to selective serotonin reuptake inhibitors or venlafaxine. *J Clin Psychopharmacol* 24(6):661–664, 2004.
47. Papakostas GI, Mischoulon D, Shyu I, et al. S-adenosyl methionine (SAMe) augmentation of serotonin reuptake inhibitors (SRIs) for SRI- non-responders with major depressive disorder: A double-blind, randomized clinical trial. *Am J Psychiatry* 167:942–948, 2010.
49. Coppen A, Bolander-Gouaille C. Treatment of depression: time to consider folic acid and vitamin B$_{12}$. *J Psychopharmacol* 9(1):59–65, 2005.
56. Papakostas GI, Shelton RC, Zajecka JM, et al. L-methylfolate as adjunctive therapy for SSRI-resistant major depression: Results of two randomized, double-blind, parallel-sequential trials. *Am J Psychiatry* 169:1267–1274, 2012.
65. Benjamin J, Agam G, Levine J, et al. Inositol treatment in psychiatry. *Psychopharmacol Bull* 31(1):167–175, 1995.
69. Mischoulon D. Herbal remedies for anxiety and insomnia: kava and valerian. In Mischoulon D, Rosenbaum J, editors: *Natural medications for psychiatric disorders: considering the alternatives*, ed 2, Philadelphia, 2008, Lippincott Williams & Wilkins.
72. Miyasaka LS, Atallah AN, Soares BG. Valerian for anxiety disorders. *Cochrane Database Syst Rev* 4:CD004515, 2006.
73. Zhdanova V, Friedman L. Melatonin for treatment of sleep and mood disorders. I: Mischoulon D, Rosenbaum J, editors: *Natural medications for psychiatric disorders: considering the alternatives*, ed 2, Philadelphia, 2008, Lippincott Williams & Wilkins.
81. Tesch BJ. Herbs commonly used by women: an evidence-based review. *Am J Obstet Gynecol* 188(5 Suppl.):S44–S55, 2002.
83. Le Bars PL, Katz MM, Berman N, et al. A placebo-controlled, double-blind, randomized trial of an extract of *Ginkgo biloba* for dementia: North American EGb Study Group. *JAMA* 278(16):1327–1332, 1997.
84. Le Bars PL, Velasco FM, Ferguson JM, et al. Influence of the severity of cognitive impairment on the effect of the *Ginkgo biloba* extract EGb 761 in Alzheimer's disease. *Neuropsychobiology* 45(1):19–26, 2002.
89. Wolkowitz OM, Reus VI, Roberts E, et al. Dehydroepiandrosterone (DHEA) treatment of depression. *Biol Psychiatry* 41(3):311–318, 1997.
90. Wolkowitz OM, Reus VI, Keebler A, et al. Double-blind treatment of major depression with dehydroepiandrosterone. *Am J Psychiatry* 156(4):646–649, 1999.

53 The Suicidal Patient

Rebecca Weintraub Brendel, MD, JD, Christina A. Brezing, MD, Isabel T. Lagomasino, MD, MSHS, Roy H. Perlis, MD, MSc, and Theodore A. Stern, MD

KEY POINTS

- Suicide, or intentional self-harm with the intent of causing death, is one of the most common causes of death in the US.

- For every completed suicide, between 8 and 25 attempts are made.

- Psychiatric illness is the most powerful risk factor for both completed and attempted suicide; mood disorders are responsible for a majority of suicides.

- Medical illness, especially of a severe or chronic nature, is associated with an increased risk of suicide; familial, genetic, and social factors also have an impact on suicide risk.

- The approach to the patient at risk for suicide should be non-judgmental, supportive, and empathic; specific questions concerning potential suicide plans and preparation must follow any admission of suicidal ideation or intent.

- A clinician may experience personal feelings and attitudes toward a patient at risk for suicide, which must be recognized and which must not be allowed to interfere with the delivery of appropriate patient care.

OVERVIEW

Suicide, or intentional self-harm with the intent of causing death, is the 10th leading cause of death in the US, accounting for between 30,000 and 40,000 deaths each year.[1] Non-lethal self-inflicted injuries are even more prevalent, accounting for more than 500,000 emergency department (ED) visits per year[1] and reflecting the high ratio of suicide attempts to completed suicides. Psychiatric disorders are associated with more than 90% of completed suicides[2,3] and with the majority of attempted suicides.[4-6] Therefore, psychiatrists must be familiar with the evaluation and treatment of patients who contemplate, threaten, or attempt suicide. Although guided by knowledge of epidemiological risk factors for suicide (Box 53-1), the clinician must rely on a detailed examination and on clinical judgment in the evaluation of current suicide risk.

EPIDEMIOLOGY AND RISK FACTORS

Epidemiology

Suicide accounts for 1.3% of the total number of deaths in the US each year.[1,7] For every person who completes suicide, approximately 8 to 10 people attempt suicide.[8,9] Although no nation-wide data on annual attempted suicides are available, research indicates that for every completed suicide, approximately 8 to 25 attempts are made[10-12]; that is, some individuals make more than one unsuccessful attempt. Each year, EDs treat over 500,000 suicide attempters.[1,13,14] These visits represent approximately 0.5% of all annual emergency department visits.[1,2,15]

Use of firearms is the most common method of committing suicide for both men and women in the US, accounting for between 50% and 60% of annual suicides.[11,12] Suffocation, including hanging, is the second most common cause of suicide overall in the US, and the second most common cause in men, accounting for over 9,000 suicide deaths in 2010.[1] Poisoning, including drug ingestion, is the third most common cause of completed suicide in the US and the second most common cause in women, accounting for approximately 5,500–6,500 deaths per year.[1,14,15] Historically, drug ingestion has accounted for the majority of unsuccessful suicide attempts.[16,17]

Suicide rates differ by age, gender, and race. Rates generally increase with age; people older than age 65 are 1.5 times more likely to commit suicide than are younger individuals, while white men over the age of 85 have an even higher rate of suicide.[13,18,19] The number of suicides in the elderly is disproportionately high; the elderly appear to make more serious attempts on their lives and are less apt to survive when medical complications from an attempt ensue—one out of four attempts in this group results in a completed suicide.[18-20] Although the elderly have the highest suicide rates, suicide in young adults (between ages 15 and 24) rose three-fold between 1950 and 1990, becoming the third leading cause of death following unintentional injuries and homicide.[11,21,22] Since that time, the suicide rate has declined in adolescents.[22] Men are more likely to complete suicide than are women, although women are more likely to attempt suicide than are men. Four times more men than women complete suicide,[7,23] although women are three to four times more likely than men to attempt suicide.[23,24] The reasons for these disparities have not been established clearly.

Whites and Native Americans attempt and commit suicide more than non-whites.[4,11,23] African Americans and Hispanics have approximately half the suicide rate of whites.[23,25,26]

Psychiatric Risk Factors

Psychiatric illness is the most powerful risk factor for both completed and attempted suicide. Psychiatric disorders are associated with more than 90% of completed suicides[2,3,23,27] and with the vast majority of attempted suicides.[4-6] Mood disorders, including major depressive disorder (MDD) and

---

BOX 53-1 Risk Factors for Suicide

Psychiatric illness
- Major depression
- Bipolar disorder
- Alcoholism and drug dependence
- Schizophrenia
- Character disorders
- Organic brain syndrome
- Panic disorder

Race
Marital status (widowed, divorced, or separated)
Living alone
Recent personal loss
Unemployment
Financial/legal difficulties
Co-morbid medical illness (having chronic illness, pain, or terminal illness)
History of suicide attempts or threats
Male gender
Advancing age
Family history of suicide
Recent hospital discharge
Firearms in the household
Hopelessness

TABLE 53-1 Percentage of Suicides with a Given Psychiatric Disorder

Condition	Percentage of Suicides
Affective illness	50
Drug or alcohol abuse	25
Schizophrenia	10
Character disorders	5
Secondary depression	5
Organic brain syndromes	2
None apparent	2

bipolar disorder, are responsible for approximately 50% of completed suicides, alcohol and drug abuse for 25%, psychosis for 10%, and personality disorders for 5%[28,29] (Table 53-1).

Up to 15% of patients with MDD or bipolar disorder complete suicide, almost always during depressive episodes[30]; this represents a suicide risk 30 times greater than that of the general population.[31,32] True life-time risk may be somewhat lower, because these estimates (and those for the other diagnoses discussed later) typically derive from hospitalized patient samples.[28] The risk appears to be greater early in the course of a life-time disorder, early on in a depressive episode,[10,33] in the first week following psychiatric hospitalization,[34] in the first month following hospital discharge,[34] and in the early stages of recovery.[34] The risk may[35] or may not[36] be elevated by co-morbid psychosis. A 10-year follow-up study of almost 1,000 patients found that those who committed suicide within the first year of follow-up were more likely to be suffering from global insomnia, severe anhedonia, impaired concentration, psychomotor agitation, alcohol abuse, anxiety, and panic attacks, whereas those who committed suicide after the first year of follow-up were more likely to be suffering from suicidal ideation, severe hopelessness, and a history of suicide attempts.[35]

Approximately 15% to 25% of patients with alcohol or drug dependence complete suicide,[33,37] of which up to 84% suffer from both alcohol and drug dependence.[37] The suicide risk appears to be greatest approximately 9 years after the commencement of alcohol and drug addiction.[2,38] The majority of patients with alcohol dependence who commit suicide suffer from co-morbid depressive disorders,[33,39,40] and as many as one-third have experienced the recent loss of a close relationship through separation or death.[41]

Nearly 20% of people who complete suicide are legally intoxicated at the time of their death.[42] Alcohol and drug abuse are associated with more pervasive suicidal ideation, more serious suicidal intent, more lethal suicide attempts, and a greater number of suicide attempts.[43] Use of alcohol and drugs may impair judgment and foster impulsivity.[34,44]

Approximately 10% of patients with schizophrenia complete suicide, mostly during periods of improvement after relapse or during periods of depression.[40,45,46] The risk for suicide appears to be greater among young men who are newly diagnosed,[46–48] who have a chronic course and numerous exacerbations, who are discharged from hospitals with significant psychopathology and functional impairment, and who have a realistic awareness and fear of further mental decline.[46,48] The risk may also be increased with akathisia and with abrupt discontinuation of neuroleptics.[33] Patients who experience hallucinations (that instruct them to harm themselves) in association with schizophrenia, mania, or depression with psychotic features are probably at greater risk for self-harm and they should be protected.[49]

Between 4% and 10% of patients with borderline personality disorder and 5% of patients with antisocial personality disorder commit suicide.[50] The risk appears to be greater for those with co-morbid unipolar depression or alcohol abuse.[51,52] Patients with personality disorders often make impulsive suicidal gestures or attempts; these attempts may become progressively more lethal if they are not taken seriously. Even manipulative gestures can turn fatal.[49]

As many as 15% to 20% of patients with anxiety disorders complete suicide,[53] and up to 20% of patients with panic disorder attempt suicide.[54] Although the risk of suicide in patients with anxiety and panic disorders may be elevated secondary to co-morbid conditions (e.g., MDD and alcohol or drug abuse), the suicide risk remains almost as high as that of major depression, even after co-existing conditions are taken into account.[55] The risk for suicide attempts may be elevated for women with an early onset and with co-morbid alcohol or drug abuse.[54]

Medical Risk Factors

Medical illness, especially of a severe or chronic nature, is generally associated with an increased risk of suicide and is thus considered a risk factor for completed suicide even though there is a most likely a multi-factorial relationship between medical illness and suicide.[15,56,57] Medical disorders are associated with as many as 35% to 40% of suicides[58] and with as many as 70% of suicides in those older than age 60.[59] Acquired immunodeficiency syndrome (AIDS), cancer, head trauma, epilepsy, multiple sclerosis, Huntington's chorea, organic brain syndromes, spinal cord injuries, hypertension, cardiopulmonary disease, peptic ulcer disease, chronic renal failure, Cushing's disease, rheumatoid arthritis, and porphyria have each been reported to increase the risk of suicide. Notably, however, few investigations concerning the increased risk for suicide in these populations have controlled for the effects of age, gender, race, psychiatric disorders, other medical disorders, or use of medications.

Patients with AIDS appear to have a suicide risk that is greater than that of the general population, and estimates of the increased risk range from 7 to 66 times that of the general population.[28,60,61] It is generally accepted that the risk of suicide in human immunodeficiency virus (HIV) infection is increased approximately seven-fold.[15,60] Testing for antibodies to HIV has resulted in an immediate and substantial decrease in suicidal ideation in those who turned out to be sero-negative; no increase in suicidal ideation was detected in those who were seropositive.[62] A study in 2012, found that individuals with HIV/AIDS who had a recent diagnosis, psychiatric co-morbidity, and frequent, more intensive hospital care for medical problems were at an even greater risk.[63] Sexual orientation among men, in and of itself, has not been identified as an independent risk factor for completed suicide.[11,64]

Cancer patients have a suicide rate that is almost twice as great as that of the general population and seem to be at higher risk in the first 2 years after they are diagnosed.[59,65] Head and neck malignancies are associated with an 11 times greater risk of suicide compared with those in the general population, possibly due to increased rates of tobacco and alcohol use in this population and the resultant facial disfigurement and loss of voice.[59] In men, gastrointestinal cancers are associated with a greater risk of suicide, and in both genders lung and upper airway malignancies are also associated with greater suicide risk.[59] Other factors, including poor prognosis, poor pain control, fatigue, depression, hopelessness, delirium, disinhibition, prior suicide attempts, recent losses, and a paucity of social supports, may place cancer patients at greater risk.[66,67]

Like cancer patients, individuals with head trauma, multiple sclerosis, and peptic ulcer disease have approximately twice the risk of suicide as those in the general population.[59,68,69] In patients with head injuries, the risk appears to be greater in those who suffer severe injuries and in those who develop dementia, psychosis, character changes, or epilepsy.[67-70] In patients with multiple sclerosis, the risk may be higher for those diagnosed before age 40 and within the first 5 years after diagnosis.[71] In patients with peptic ulcer disease, the increased risk is hypothesized to be due to co-morbid psychiatric and substance use (especially alcohol) disorders.[59,72]

Between the increased risk of suicide of approximately two-fold for cancer, head trauma, multiple sclerosis, and peptic ulcer disease, and the increased risk in HIV-infected/AIDS patients estimated to be at least nearly seven-fold, there are a number of medical illnesses with intermediate increases in suicide risk. These illnesses include epilepsy, systemic lupus erythematosus, spinal cord injuries, Huntington's disease, organic brain syndromes, and chronic renal disease. Patients with end-stage renal disease on hemodialysis may have the highest relative risk of all subgroups.[59,72] As many as 5% of patients with chronic renal failure who receive hemodialysis die from suicide; those who travel to medical centers for dialysis have a higher suicide rate than those who are dialyzed at home.[8] The risk for suicide among these patients may be as high as 400 times that of the general population.[73]

Patients with epilepsy are five times more likely than those in the general population to complete or to attempt suicide.[59,74-76] Sufferers of temporal lobe epilepsy, with concomitant psychosis or personality changes, may be at greater risk.[59,74,75,77]

Delirious and confused patients may suffer from agitation and destructive impulses and be unable to protect themselves from harm.[66] In victims of spinal cord injury, the risk is actually greater for those with less severe injuries.[78,79]

Hypertensive patients[70] and those with cardiopulmonary disease[49] may also have a higher risk for suicide than those in the general population. Although previous reports suggested that beta-blockers could contribute to increased risk by promoting depression,[70] recent studies suggest that beta-blockers do not increase the risk of developing depression.[80] Finally, an association between suicide and very low cholesterol levels has been reported, but the connection is still under investigation.[15,28]

Familial and Genetic Risk Factors

A family history of suicide, a family history of psychiatric illness, and a tumultuous early family environment have each been found to have an important impact on the risk for suicide.[11,58] As many as 7% to 14% of persons who attempt suicide have a family history of suicide.[81] A family history of suicide confers approximately a two-fold increase in risk for suicide after family psychiatric history is controlled for.[82] This increased suicide risk may be mediated through a shared genetic predisposition for suicide, psychiatric disorders, or impulsive behavior,[33,47,83] or through a shared family environment in which modeling and imitation are prominent.[84]

Genetic factors are supported by evidence that monozygotic twins have a higher concordance rate for suicide and suicide attempts than dizygotic twins and by evidence that biological parents of adoptees who commit suicide have a higher rate of suicide than do biological parents of non-suicidal adoptees.[28,83,85] However, little is known about the specific genetic factors that confer this risk.[28] Study has largely focused on serotonin neurotransmission, including genetic mutations in the rate-limiting enzyme in serotonin synthesis, L-tryptophan hydroxylase, serotonin receptors, and the serotonin transporter, but this investigation is still preliminary.[82,86-88] While there is partial overlap with vulnerability to depression, predisposition to suicide is separate.[89] Overall, it is estimated that one-third to one-half the risk of suicide is genetically mediated.[82]

Recent evidence suggests that epigenetics, particularly alterations in promoter DNA methylation patterns, play an important role in the neurobiology of suicide.[90-96] Numerous familial environmental factors, that may be mediated through epigenetic changes, contribute to suicide risk.[94-96] A tumultuous early family environment (including factors of early parental death, parental separation, frequent moves, and emotional, physical, or sexual abuse) increases the risk for suicide.[97] Children's risk of future suicidal behavior may also be increased by suicidal behavior in important family members through modeling.[28]

Social Risk Factors

Widowed, divorced, or separated adults are at greater risk for suicide than are single adults, who are at greater risk than married adults.[98,99] Married adults with young children appear to carry the lowest risk.[34,49,58] Living alone substantially increases the risk for suicide, especially among adults who are widowed, divorced, or separated.[34] Social isolation from family, relatives, friends, neighbors, and co-workers also increases the chance of suicide.[47,58] Conversely, the presence of social supports is protective against suicide.[82]

Significant personal losses (including diminution of self-esteem or status[58,59]) and conflicts also place individuals, particularly young adults and adolescents, at greater risk for suicide.[2,100] Bereavement following the death of a loved one increases the risk for suicide over the next 4 or 5 years, particularly for people with a psychiatric history (including suicide attempts) and for people who receive little family support.[33] Unemployment, which may produce or exacerbate psychiatric illness or may result from psychiatric illness,[33] increases the likelihood of suicide and accounts for as many as one-third to one-half of completed suicides.[42,58] This risk may be particularly elevated among men.[34] Financial and legal difficulties also increase the risk for suicide.[11,34,101]

The presence of one or more firearms in the home appears to increase the risk of suicide independently for both genders and all age groups, even when other risk factors, such as depression and alcohol abuse, are taken into account.[6,100,102] For example, adolescents with a gun in the household have suicide rates between 4 and 10 times higher than other adolescents.[23,103]

Recently, rates of suicide in US military personnel are increasing. Studies regarding rates of suicide in this population have historically drawn conflicting conclusions. Compared to the US population, Vietnam War and Gulf War veterans have similar rates of suicide.[104–109] However, Vietnam War veterans with trauma as reflected by a diagnosis of post-traumatic stress disorder (PTSD), hospitalization for combat wounds, or multiple wounds had significantly increased rates of suicide compared to those in the general population.[110,111] Before the wars in Afghanistan and Iraq, rates of suicide in military personnel, when adjusted for age and gender, were consistently lower as compared to national rates from 1980 to 1992.[112,113] However, suicide in the US Army increased 80% in 2004–2008 compared to previous decades[114] and in 2008, the age and gender-adjusted suicide rate in the Army was greater than the average suicide rate in the general population for the first time.[115,116] This trend continued and the US military reported that deaths from suicide surpassed deaths from combat from January to June 2012.[115] Veterans of Operations Enduring Freedom or Iraqi Freedom (OEF/OIF) as a whole trended towards having higher rates of suicide following deployment compared to those in the US general population.[117] OEF/OIF veterans who were in active duty units and therefore more likely exposed to combat trauma or those diagnosed with a mental disorder had statistically significant higher rates of suicide than in the general population.[117] The impact of combat exposure, deployment, and their relationships on psychiatric illness in OEF/OIF veterans appear to be risk factors for suicide; however, a study looking at data of current and former US military personnel from 2001 to 2008 found that the risk of suicide was independently associated with male gender and psychiatric co-morbidity and found no association to risk of suicide with military-specific variables (i.e., unique stressors, such as combat deployment).[118] Clinicians treating this population should also screen for evidence of sleep disturbances as warning signs for suicide, be aware of the parallel between increased prescribing and overuse of opioid analgesics in patients with PTSD, and restrict access to firearms.[115]

Past and Present Suicidality

A history of suicide attempts is one of the most powerful risk factors for completed and attempted suicide.[11,119] As many as 10% to 20% of people with prior suicide attempts complete suicide.[9,16,120] The risk for completed suicide following an attempted suicide is almost 100 times that of the general population in the year following the attempt; it then declines but remains elevated throughout the next 8 years.[33] People with prior suicide attempts are also at greater risk for subsequent attempts and have been found to account for approximately 50% of serious overdoses.[121] The clinical use of past suicide attempts as a predictive risk factor may be limited in the elderly because the elderly make fewer attempts for each completed suicide.[18–20,58]

The lethality of past suicide attempts slightly increases the risk for completed suicide,[33] especially among women with psychiatric illness.[39] The dangerousness of an attempt, however, may be more predictive of the risk for suicide in those individuals with significant intent to suicide and a realization of the potential lethality of their actions.[122]

The communication of present suicidal ideation and intent must be carefully evaluated as a risk factor for completed and attempted suicide. As many as 80% of people who complete suicide communicate their intent either directly or indirectly.[58] Death or suicide may be discussed, new wills or life insurance policies may be written, valued possessions may be given away, or uncharacteristic and destructive behaviors may arise.[58]

People who intend to commit suicide may, however, be less likely to communicate their intent to their health care providers than they are to close family and friends.[45] Although 50% of people who commit suicide have consulted a physician in the month before their death, only 60% of this group communicated some degree of suicidal ideation or intent to their physician.[2,45] In a study of 571 cases of completed suicide who had met with their health care professional within 4 weeks of their suicide,[123] only 22% discussed their suicidal intent. Many investigators believe that ideation and intent may be more readily discussed with psychiatrists than with other physicians.[123,124]

Hopelessness, or negative expectations about the future, is a stronger predictor of suicide risk than is depression or suicidal ideation,[125,126] and may be both a short-term and long-term predictor of completed suicide in patients with major depression.[45]

Contact with Physicians

Nearly half of the people who commit suicide have had contact with their primary care provider (PCP) within 1 month of committing suicide.[35,46,127] Approximately three-quarters of people who commit suicide saw a PCP in the year before the suicide.[127] Many of these individuals seek treatment from their PCP for somatic rather than psychiatric complaints.[128] Rates of psychiatric encounters in the period before completed suicides are lower than those for primary care contacts.[128] In the month before a completed suicide, approximately one-fifth of suicide completers obtained mental health services, and in the year before a completed suicide, approximately one in three suicide completers had contact with a mental health professional.[128]

PATHOPHYSIOLOGY

Suicide is a behavioral outcome with a large number of contributing factors, rather than a disease entity in itself. Therefore, in order to understand the pathophysiology of suicidality, it is necessary to examine the differences between individuals with a given set of predisposing factors who do not attempt or complete suicide and those who do. Research has focused on a wide array of neurobiological and psychological topics in an attempt to better understand the pathophysiology of suicide. Neurobiological inquiries have included neurotransmitter analyses, genetic studies, neuroendocrine studies, biological markers, and imaging studies.[15] Psychological aspects of suicide typically focus on psychodynamic and cognitive perspectives.

Neurobiology

Of all the neurotransmitters, the relationship of serotonin to suicidality has been most widely studied.[15] An association between decreased cerebrospinal fluid (CSF) levels of the serotonin metabolite 5-hydroxyindoleacetic acid (HIAA) and serious suicide attempts was first described in the 1970s.[129] Since then, evidence of an association between the serotonergic system and suicidality has continued to grow, with most subsequent studies finding decreased CSF 5-HIAA levels in individuals who attempt suicide.[130,131] There have also been reports of a blunted prolactin response to fenfluramine challenge, a marker for serotonergic dysfunction.[82,131,132] This finding is independent of underlying psychiatric diagnosis: that is, it is consistent for suicide attempters with major depression, schizophrenia, and personality disorders compared to diagnosis-matched controls without a history of attempting suicide.[130,131] Low levels of 5-HIAA are associated with more serious attempts, and are negatively correlated with the degree of injury in the most recent suicide attempt or most serious past attempt[130-132]: that is, higher-lethality past attempts are associated with lower CSF 5-HIAA levels. Finally, low CSF 5-HIAA has also been shown to predict future attempted and completed suicide.[133]

Similarly, post-mortem brainstem analysis has shown a reduction in serotonin and its metabolite 5-HIAA in suicide completers.[28,130,134,135] This reduction in serotonin and 5-HIAA was similar for depressed, schizophrenic, personality-disordered, and alcoholic patients, showing that decreased brainstem serotonin activity correlates with completed suicide irrespective of diagnosis.[130,136] Other brainstem abnormalities associated with suicide victims are the presence of an increased number of serotonin neurons compared to controls.[15,28,137]

Serotonin receptors, in particular the serotonin transporter (SERT), have also been implicated in the neurophysiology of suicide. There is evidence for both pre-synaptic and post-synaptic changes in the prefrontal cortex of suicide completers, although not all studies have demonstrated these findings.[28,130] Specific findings in the prefrontal cortex of suicide victims include a decrease in pre-synaptic serotonin transporter binding on nerve terminals and increases in post-synaptic serotonin$_{1A}$ and serotonin$_{2A}$ receptors.[15,28,130,137] Changes in receptor expression and binding are also accompanied by changes in intra-cellular signaling.[131,138,139] Abnormalities include low protein kinase C activity in the prefrontal cortex, low cyclic adenosine monophosphate-(cAMP)-mediated activity in the hippocampus and prefrontal cortex, and a decreased number of G-protein alpha subunits.[131,138-140]

Changes in norepinephrine (noradrenaline) transmission in suicide have also been investigated, but to a lesser degree than have serotonergic changes. As a result, the implications of studies on the noradrenergic system remain comparatively preliminary. Post-mortem brainstem analysis of the locus coeruleus of suicide victims with major depression has revealed a decreased number of noradrenergic neurons.[130,132,140,141] However, this finding may be the result of illness, a stress-related phenomenon, or other factors.[130,131,140,141] Specifically, because of stress-related changes in the noradrenergic system during stress, the stress preceding suicide may be the cause of other observed changes in the brainstems of suicide victims, which include alterations in adrenergic receptor populations and tyrosine hydroxylase activity, the rate-limiting step in norepinephrine synthesis.[28,82,140] Overall, CSF studies have shown no significant difference in norepinephrine metabolites in suicidal behavior.[82,142]

Although some investigation into the role of dopamine in suicidal behavior and suicide has been done, overall, the data are relatively inconclusive. Post-mortem studies are too few to determine whether there are changes in levels of dopamine and its metabolites in the brains of suicide victims.[140] CSF levels of dopamine metabolites have, in general, not been shown to differ in individuals with suicidal behavior compared to others.[82,142,143] Low levels of the dopamine metabolite homovanillic acid (HVA) have been shown in individuals with major depression who attempted suicide.[140] However, it is unclear whether a relationship between dopamine and suicide exists independent of the known association of major depression and dopamine down-regulation.[140]

The hypothalamic–pituitary–adrenal (HPA) axis has been implicated in the pathophysiology of suicide, although not all studies of the relationship between the HPA axis abnormalities and suicidal behavior have reached the same conclusions.[15,28,82,140] In general, heightened HPA axis activity, as evidenced by abnormal dexamethasone suppression test (DST) results, has been shown in major depression and thought to be associated with suicidality.[15,28,82,131,140] However, while some studies of the relationship between HPA axis activity and suicidality have shown a relationship between dexamethasone non-suppression and suicidality, other recent investigations have not found a correlation.[82] Urinary cortisol production has been shown to be elevated in suicidal behavior, and this finding has been replicated in CSF studies and post-mortem brain analysis.[16] Elevated urinary cortisol and dexamethasone non-suppression have also been shown to correlate with future suicidality.[28,82,131,140]

Psychological, Psychodynamic, and Neuropsychological Perspectives

The psychodynamic and psychological understanding of suicide encompasses a vast literature; nonetheless, according to one expert, "The psychological operation of this extraordinary phenomenon, whatever its neurochemical matrix may be, is far from obvious."[144] In conceptualizing the notion of murder turned against the self, Freud described confusion between the self and another person who is both loved and hated as central to suicide.[144,145] Suicide can, then, be conceptualized as anger turned on one's self or anger toward others directed at the self.[144-146] Suicide has also been seen as motivated by three driving forces: the wish to die, the wish to kill, and the wish to be killed.[146] Deficits in ego functioning have also been postulated to predispose to suicide,[144] as have poor object relations.[146] Maltsberger has identified a core set of principles that are generally true in suicide; these include a central connection to object loss, mental anguish, confusion of parts of the self with others, the presence of fantasies of resurgence into a new life, and difficulty in self-regulation.[144]

Hopelessness is a central psychological correlate of suicide. Extensive study on hopelessness has shown a stronger correlation among hopelessness, suicidal ideation, and suicide than hopelessness and depression, and depression and suicide.[82] Hopelessness may be the best overall predictor of suicide.[82] Shame, worthlessness, and poor self-esteem are also key concepts in the understanding of suicide; individuals with early traumatic relationships may be particularly vulnerable to narcissistic wounds.[146] Shneidman,[147] in setting forth his psychological approach to suicide, has argued that the psychology of suicide involves intense psychological pain, which he has termed *psychache*. This psychache occurs due to unmet psychological needs (specifically the vital needs individuals require when under duress).[147] He has identified five clusters of psychological pain that predispose to suicide: these center on thwarted love; acceptance and belonging, fractured control, assaulted self-image and avoidance of shame; ruptured key relationships; and excessive rage; anger, and hostility.[147] Poor coping skills, antisocial traits, hostility, hopelessness, dependency, and self-consciousness have also been associated with suicide.[146]

One recent report found that depressed patients with either thoughts of death or suicidal ideation had lower self-confidence, over-dependency on others, and high intropunitiveness compared with depressed patients without thoughts of death or suicide.[148] Other research has postulated correlations between observed neuroanatomic, neurotransmitter, and neuroendocrine findings in suicide and attendant cognitive traits of loser status, no escape, and no rescue as central to understanding suicidal behavior.[131]

CLINICAL FEATURES AND DIAGNOSIS

The patient at risk for suicide varies along a continuum (from an individual with private thoughts of wanting to be dead or to commit suicide, to a gravely ill individual who requires emergent medical attention as the result of a self-inflicted injury aimed to end his or her life). Therefore, there is no characteristic presentation of the suicidal patient. As a result, the evaluation of suicide risk depends on clinical assessment of suicide risk in all patients and, in particular, on a detailed clinical examination of the patient who has contemplated, threatened, or attempted suicide. The thoughts and feelings of the individual must be elicited and placed in the context of known risk factors for suicide.

Although useful as a guide to patient populations who may be more likely to commit or to attempt suicide, risk factors alone are neither sensitive nor specific in the prediction of suicide. Their pervasive prevalence in comparison with the relatively low incidence of suicide in the general population may also lead to high false-positive rates. A multiple logistic regression model that used risk factors (such as age, gender, psychiatric diagnoses, medical diagnoses, marital status, family psychiatric history, prior suicide attempts, and suicidal ideation) failed to identify any of the 46 patients who committed suicide over a 14-year period from a group of 1,906 people with affective disorders.[149] Similarly, a multiple regression analysis aimed at predicting risk classification by treatment disposition of individuals after suicide attempts had only slightly more than a two-thirds concordance with the decisions made by the treating clinician.[150]

An evaluation for suicide risk is indicated for all patients who have made a suicide attempt, who have voiced suicidal ideation or intent, who have admitted suicidal ideation or intent on questioning, or whose actions have suggested suicidal intent despite their protests to the contrary. All suicide attempts and thoughts of suicide should be taken seriously, regardless of whether the actions or thoughts appear manipulative in nature. The work group on suicidal behaviors of the American Psychiatric Association has outlined the four critical features of a comprehensive assessment of patients with suicidal behaviors in its 2006 practice guideline: a thorough psychiatric evaluation, specific inquiry about suicidality, establishment of a multi-axial diagnosis, and estimation of suicide risk.[146] The key facets of each of these components are detailed in Box 53-2.

The approach to the patient at potential risk for suicide should be non-judgmental, supportive, and empathic. The initial establishment of rapport may include an introduction, an effort to create some degree of privacy in the interview setting, and an attempt to maximize the physical comfort of the patient for the interview.[49] The patient who senses interest, concern, and compassion is more likely to trust the examiner and to provide a detailed and accurate history. Often ambivalent about their thoughts and plans, suicidal patients may derive significant relief and benefit from a thoughtful and caring evaluation.[47,49]

The patient should be questioned about suicidal ideation and intent in an open and direct manner. Patients with suicidal thoughts and plans are often relieved and not offended when they find someone with whom they can speak about the unspeakable. Patients without suicidal ideation do not have the thoughts planted in their mind and do not develop a greater risk for suicide.[47,49,151] General questions concerning suicidal thoughts can be introduced in a gradual manner while obtaining the history of present illness. Questions such as "Has it ever seemed like things just aren't worth it?"[49] or "Have you had thoughts that life is not worth living?"[47] may lead to a further discussion of depression and hopelessness.

BOX 53-2 Components of the Suicide Evaluation

Conduct a thorough psychiatric examination
- Establish initial rapport
- Combine open-ended and direct questions
- Gather data from family, friends, and co-workers
- Conduct a mental status examination

Suicide assessment
- Ask specifically about thoughts of suicide and plans to commit suicide
- Examine the details of the suicide plan
- Determine the risk:rescue ratio
- Assess the level of planning and preparation
- Evaluate the degree of hopelessness
- Identify precipitants

Establish a multi-axial diagnosis
- Obtain history
- Use data from a psychiatric examination
- Incorporate data from prior or current treaters

Estimate suicide risk
- Evaluate risk factors
- Evaluate available social supports

"Have you gotten so depressed that you've considered killing yourself?"[49] or "Have you had thoughts of killing yourself?"[46] may open the door to a further evaluation of suicidal thoughts and plans.

Specific questions concerning potential suicide plans and preparations must follow any admission of suicidal ideation or intent. The patient should be asked when, where, and how an attempt would be made, and any potential means should be evaluated for feasibility and lethality. An organized and detailed plan involving an accessible and lethal method may place the patient at higher risk for suicide.[42] The seriousness of the wish or the intent to die must also be assessed. The patient who has begun to carry out the initial steps of a suicide plan, who wishes to be dead, and who has no hopes or plans for the future may be at greater risk. The last-mentioned domain (plans for the future) may be assessed by asking questions such as "What do you see yourself doing five years from now?" or "What things are you still looking forward to doing or seeing?"[49]

Many clinicians have addressed the issues of lethality and intent by means of the risk:rescue ratio.[146,152] The greater the relative risk or lethality and the lesser the likelihood of rescue of a planned attempt, the more serious is the potential for a completed suicide. Although often useful, the risk:rescue ratio cannot be merely applied as a simple formula; instead, one must examine and interpret the particular beliefs of a given patient. For example, a patient may plan an attempt with a low risk of potential harm but may sincerely wish to die and believe that the plan will be fatal; the patient may thus have a higher risk for suicide. Conversely a patient may plan an attempt that carries a high probability of death, such as an acetaminophen overdose, but may have little desire to die and little understanding of the severity of the attempt; the patient may thus have a lower risk.[42,146]

The clinician must attempt to identify any possible precipitants for the present crisis in an effort to understand why the patient is suicidal. The patient who must face the same problems and stressors following the evaluation or who cannot or will not discuss potential precipitants may be at greater risk for suicide.[42] The clinician must also assess the social support in place for a given patient. A lack of outpatient care providers, family, or friends may elevate potential risk.[47,58]

The examiner who interviews a patient after a suicide attempt needs to evaluate the details, seriousness, risk:rescue ratio, and precipitants of the attempt. The patient who carries out a detailed plan, who perceives the attempt as lethal, who thinks that death will be certain, who is disappointed to be alive, and who must face unchanged stressors will be at a continued high risk for suicide. The patient who makes a calculated, premeditated attempt may also be at a higher risk for a repeat attempt than the patient who makes a hasty, impulsive attempt (out of anger, a desire for revenge, or a desire for attention), or the patient who is intoxicated.[49]

A thorough psychiatric, medical, social, and family history of the patient who may be at risk for suicide should be completed to evaluate the presence and significance of potential risk factors. Particular attention should be paid to the presence of MDD, alcohol or drug abuse, psychotic disorders, personality disorders, and anxiety disorders. The presence of multiple significant risk factors may confer an additive risk.

A careful mental status examination allows the clinician to detect psychiatric difficulties and to assess cognitive capacities. Important aspects to evaluate in the examination include level of consciousness, appearance, behavior, attention, mood, affect, language, orientation, memory, thought form, thought content, perception, insight, and judgment.[152,153] A psychiatric review of systems aids in the detection of psychiatric disease.

The clinician should interview the family and friends of the patient at risk to corroborate gathered information and to obtain new and pertinent data. The family may provide information that a patient is hesitant to provide and that may be essential to his or her care.[42,47,49] A patient who refuses to discuss an attempt or insists that the entire event was a mistake may speak in an open and honest manner only when confronted with reports from his or her family. The evaluation of suicidal risk and the protection of the patient at risk are emergent procedures, which may take precedence over the desire of the patient for privacy and the maintenance of confidentiality in the physician–patient relationship. Concern over a life-or-death situation may obviate obtaining formal consent from the patient before speaking to family and friends.[49]

TREATMENT OF SUICIDE RISK

The treatment of suicide risk begins with stabilization of medical sequelae of suicidal behaviors. Attention to current or potential medical conditions must be prompt, and medical evaluations must be complete. The severity of the psychiatric presentation should not distract a clinician from his or her obligation to provide good medical care.[42] Once the patient is medically stable, or if the patient is suicidal but has not acted on suicidal impulses, the focus of treatment can shift to initiation of treatment for the underlying causes of the desire for death. Components of the treatment of suicide risk include providing a safe environment for the patient, determining an appropriate treatment setting, developing a treatment plan involving appropriate somatic and psychotherapeutic interventions, and reassessing safety, suicide risk, psychiatric status, and treatment response in an ongoing fashion[146] (Box 53-3).

Throughout the evaluation and treatment of the suicidal patient, safety must be ensured until the patient is no longer at imminent risk for suicide. Appropriate intervention and the passage of time may aid in the resolution of suicidal ideation and intent.[42,49] A patient who is at potential risk for suicide and who threatens to leave before an adequate evaluation is completed must be detained, in accordance with statutes in most states that permit the detention of individuals deemed dangerous to themselves or others.[154] Patients who attempt to leave nonetheless should be contained by locked environments or restraints.[42]

BOX 53-3 Treatment of Suicide Risk

Stabilize the medical situation
Create a safe environment
- Remove potential means for self-harm
- Provide frequent supervision
- Use restraints as needed
- Detain involuntarily if necessary

Identify and treat underlying mental illness
Identify and modify other contributing factors

Potential means for self-harm should be removed from the reach of a patient at risk. Sharp objects (such as scissors, sutures, needles, glass bottles, and eating utensils) should be removed from the immediate area. Open windows, stairwells, and structures to which a noose could be attached must be blocked. Medications or other dangerous substances that patients may have in their possession must be secured by staff in a location out of the patient's access.[42] Appropriate supervision and restraint must be provided at all times for a patient at risk for suicide. Frequent supervision, constant one-to-one supervision, physical restraints, and medications may be used alone or in combination in an effort to protect a patient at risk. The least restrictive means that ensures the safety of the patient should be used.

A decision about the appropriate level of care and treatment setting for the suicidal patient is critical. The patient's safety is paramount, and decisions about level of care—from discharge home with outpatient follow-up to involuntary hospitalization—should be based on risk determinations and methods most likely to protect the patient from self-harm, even when the patient disagrees. Those who are at high risk for suicide, or who cannot control their suicidal urges, should be admitted to a locked psychiatric facility. A patient who is at high risk but who refuses hospitalization should be committed involuntarily.

A patient who requires hospitalization should be informed of the disposition decision in a clear, direct manner. Possible transfers should proceed as quickly and efficiently as possible because a patient may become quite tense and ambivalent about the decision to hospitalize. Those who agree to voluntary hospitalization and who cooperate with caregivers may have the highest likelihood of successful treatment.[49] A 3-year study of patients at a university emergency room in Zurich found that older patients were more likely to be hospitalized after a suicide attempt and that nearly half of patients admitted for psychiatric treatment were voluntary.[150] In a regression analysis of the same sample, more aggressive methods of suicide attempt (defined as not overdose or cutting), a history of previous inpatient treatment, and a current diagnosis of psychosis or schizophrenia were associated with inpatient admission.[150]

The clinician should always take a conservative approach to the treatment of suicidal risk and the maintenance of patient safety and err, if necessary, on the side of excess restraint or hospitalization. From a forensic standpoint, the clinician sued for battery secondary to the use of restraints or to involuntary commitment would be easier to defend than the clinician sued for negligence secondary to a completed suicide. Acting in accordance with good clinical judgment in the best interest of the patient brings little danger of liability.[49] Adequate documentation should include the thought processes behind decisions to supervise, restrain, discharge, or hospitalize.[49]

Although managed care may place pressure on a clinician to avoid hospitalization through the use of less costly alternatives, there is no substitute for sound clinical judgment.[146] In particular, safety contracts or suicide prevention contracts, while intended to manage risk, are generally overvalued and of limited utility.[146,155] Specifically, suicide contracts depend on the subjective beliefs of the psychiatrist and the patient and not on objective data; they have never been shown to be clinically efficacious.[146,155] In addition, many suicide attempters and completers had suicide contracts in place at the time of the suicidal act.[146,156,157] Finally, a suicide contract is not a legal contract and it has limited utility, if any, if litigation should ensue from a completed suicide.[146,158,159]

Somatic therapies to target underlying psychiatric illness are a mainstay of the management of the suicidal patient. However, while psychiatric illness is a significant risk factor for suicide and treatment of underlying psychopathology is associated with decreased suicide risk, with few exceptions psychiatric medications have not independently been associated with a decrease in suicide. The two notable exceptions are long-term treatment with lithium (in affective illness)[160,161] and clozapine (in schizophrenia).[162,163]

Because depression is the psychiatric diagnosis most associated with suicide, psychopharmacological treatment of depression is a central facet of management of suicide risk. However, antidepressants have not been shown to decrease suicide risk.[146,164] Although one recent study found a higher rate of suicide after discontinuation of antidepressants compared with during antidepressant treatment, the study was small and further investigation is required.[165]

Controversy regarding the relationship of selective serotonin reuptake inhibitor (SSRI) antidepressant medications and suicide has now spanned two decades. In the early 1990s, reports of a possible increase in suicidal ideation and suicidal behavior in both adults and children on SSRIs emerged.[166,167] In 2004, the Food and Drug Administration (FDA) issued a "black box warning" for all antidepressant drugs related to the risk of suicide in pediatric patients[168] and in more recent years extended this warning for individuals up to age 24.[169] Nonetheless, controversy about SSRIs and suicide persists, in both adults and children. For example, in 2004, before the FDA advisory opinion, the American College of Neuropsychopharmacology's Task Force on SSRIs and Suicidal Behavior in Youth failed to find an association between SSRIs and increased suicidality in children.[170] Another study also showed an improvement in depression and a reduction in suicidal thinking with fluoxetine and with fluoxetine combined with cognitive-behavioral therapy (CBT), when compared with placebo and CBT alone.[171] Additionally, prescription fills for SSRIs decreased by 58% in the years following the 2004 FDA black box warning with significant spillover effect into the adult population with decreases in diagnosis and treatment of depression.[172] These decreases were associated with increases in rates of suicidality in pediatric patients.[173]

In adults, there has been similar controversy about a possible relationship between SSRIs and increased suicidality and self-harm. Multiple large studies that assessed the risk of suicide and self-harm have been conducted; they largely determined that SSRIs were not associated with a greater risk of suicide or violence.[146,174-176] However, debate has continued.[177] Most recently (2005), three papers published in the *British Medical Journal* reached varying conclusions and raised some questions about the data used in a previous analysis. One analysis of 477 randomized control trials with more than 40,000 patients found no evidence that SSRIs increased the risk of suicide, but found weak evidence of an increased risk of self-harm.[178] A second review of randomized controlled trials with a total of 87,650 patients reached the opposite conclusion, finding an association between suicide attempts and the use of SSRIs.[179] A case-control study of 146,095

individuals with a first prescription for depression found no greater risk of suicide or non-fatal self-harm in adults prescribed SSRIs as opposed to those prescribed tricyclic antidepressants (TCAs), although there was some weak evidence for increased non-fatal self-harm with use of SSRIs in patients under age 18 years.[180] What is clear from review of the data on SSRIs is that more study is needed. Because SSRIs are prescribed for treatment of an underlying illness characterized by anxiety, agitation, and suicidality, it is difficult to separate out drug effect from illness effect.[146] Despite there being an association between SSRIs and emergent suicidal ideation and behavior, treatment with antidepressants has not been demonstrated to increase completed suicide,[181] and rates of suicide mortality have decreased as SSRI usage has increased.[182,183] Notwithstanding the continuing controversy, SSRIs do have the obvious advantage over TCAs and monoamine oxidase inhibitor (MAOI) antidepressants of being relatively safe in overdose. FDA warnings regarding the possible induction of suicidality have also been issued for antiepileptic drugs, varenicline, and tetrabenazine, but the clinical implications at this time are unclear.[169] In general, physicians should be aware of the potential for SSRIs and other medications to have suicide-inducing effects in a vulnerable subset of patients and therefore careful assessments, psychoeducation to patients and families, close monitoring, and follow-up care is indicated when initiating antidepressant treatment. However, the well-known beneficial effects of SSRIs need to be weighed against the risks.

Finally, because pharmacotherapy for depression typically requires several weeks for onset of efficacy, electroconvulsive therapy (ECT) may be indicated in cases in which suicide risk remains high or antidepressants are contraindicated.[146,184] ECT is associated with a decrease in short-term suicidal ideation.[146] Its use is best established for depression, and it may also be recommended for pregnant patients and for patients who have not responded to pharmacological interventions.[146]

Psychotherapeutic interventions are widely used to manage suicide risk, although few studies have addressed psychotherapy outcomes regarding the reduction of suicidality. Nonetheless, clinical practice and consensus supports the use of psychotherapy and other psychosocial interventions, notwithstanding the need for further study.[146] There is emerging evidence of the efficacy of multiple psychotherapeutic modalities in the treatment of depression, borderline personality disorder, and suicide risk *per se*, including psychodynamic psychotherapy, CBT, dialectical behavioral therapy, and interpersonal psychotherapy.[146]

DIFFICULTIES IN THE ASSESSMENT OF SUICIDE RISK

Clinicians may encounter obstacles with certain patients, or within themselves, during the evaluation of suicide risk. They must be adept in the examination of patients who are intoxicated, who threaten, or who are uncooperative, and they must be aware of personal feelings and attitudes (e.g., anxiety, anger, denial, intellectualization, or over-identification) to allow for better assessment and management of the patient at risk (Box 53-4).

A patient who is intoxicated may voice suicidal ideation or intent that is (frequently) retracted when sober. A brief initial evaluation while the patient is intoxicated and his or her psychological defenses are impaired may reveal the depth of suicidal ideation or the reasons behind a suicide attempt.[49] A more thorough examination when he or she is sober must also be completed and documented.[42,49]

A patient who threatens should be evaluated in the presence of security officers and should be placed in restraints as necessary to protect both the individual and the staff.[49] Those

BOX 53-4 Common Reactions of Clinicians to Suicide	
Anger	Indifference
Anxiety	Intellectualization
Depression	Over-identification
Denial	Rejection
Helplessness	

who are uncooperative may refuse to answer questions despite all attempts to establish rapport and to create a supportive and empathic connection. Stating "I'd like to figure out how to be of help, but I can't do that without some information from you" in a calm but firm manner might be helpful. Patients should be informed that safety precautions will not be discontinued until the evaluation can be completed and that they will not be able to sign out against medical advice. Their capacity to refuse medical treatments should be carefully questioned.[49] A patient who refuses to cooperate until restraints are removed should be reminded of the importance of the evaluation and should be enlisted to cooperate with the goal of removing the restraints in mind. Statements such as "We both agree that the restraints should come off if you don't need them. I am very concerned about your safety, and I need you to answer some questions before I can decide if it's safe to remove the restraints" might be helpful.[49]

A clinician may experience personal feelings and attitudes toward a patient at risk for suicide, which must be recognized and which must not be allowed to interfere with appropriate patient care.[144] Clinicians may feel anxious because of the awareness that an error in judgment might have fatal consequences. They may feel angry at a patient with a history of multiple gestures or at a patient who has used trivial methods, often resulting in poor evaluations and punitive interventions. Angry examiners may inappropriately transfer a patient with a low risk for suicide to a psychiatric facility or may discharge a patient with a high risk to home.[49]

Some clinicians are prone to experience denial as they evaluate and treat patients at risk for suicide. They may conspire with the patient or family in the stance that voiced suicidal ideation was "just talk" or that an attempt was "just an accident." Others may practice intellectualization and choose to believe that suicide is "an act of free will" and that patients should have the personal and legal right to kill themselves.[42]

Clinicians commonly over-identify with patients with whom they share personal characteristics. The thought "I would never commit suicide" may become translated into the thought "This patient would never commit suicide," and serious risk may be missed.[49] The examiner may try to assure patients that they will be fine or may try to convince them that they do not feel suicidal. Patients may thus be unable to express themselves fully and may not receive proper evaluation and treatment.

A clinician who performs evaluations for patients who have made suicide attempts and who have been admitted to general hospital floors has to be aware of his or her own reactions to the patient, as well as to those of the staff. In addition, medical and surgical staff often develop strong feelings toward patients who have attempted suicide and at times they wish that these patients were dead. The clinician must diffuse such charged situations, perhaps by holding group meetings for those involved to make them more aware of their negative feelings so that they are not acted out.[185] Such intervention may prevent mismanagement and premature discharge.

Access the complete reference list and multiple choice questions (MCQs) online at https://expertconsult.inkling.com

KEY REFERENCES

1. National Center for Injury Prevention and Control, Centers for Disease Control and Prevention. FastStats: suicide and self-inflicted injury, <http://www.cdc.gov/nchs/fastats/suicide.htm>; [Accessed on August 3, 2013].
10. Malone KM, Haas GL, Sweeney JA, et al. Major depression and the risk of attempted suicide. *J Affect Dis* 34:173–185, 1995.
11. Moscicki EK. Epidemiology of suicidal behavior. *Suicide Life Threat Behav* 25:22–35, 1995.
13. Gaynes BN, West SL, Ford CA, et al. Screening for suicide risk in adults: a summary of the evidence for the U.S. Preventive Services Task Force. *Ann Intern Med* 140:822–835, 2004.
19. O'Connell H, Chin A, Cunningham C, et al. Recent developments: suicide in older people. *BMJ* 329:895–899, 2004.
26. Earls F, Escobar JI, Manson SM. Suicide in minority groups: epidemiologic and cultural perspectives. In Blumenthal SJ, Kupfer DJ, editors: *Suicide over the life cycle: risk factors, assessment, and treatment of suicidal patients*, Washington, DC, 1990, American Psychiatric Press.
28. Mann JJ. A current perspective of suicide and attempted suicide. *Ann Intern Med* 136:302–311, 2002.
37. Miller NS, Giannini AJ, Gold MS. Suicide risk associated with drug and alcohol addiction. *Cleve Clin J Med* 59:535–538, 1992.
39. Appleby L. Suicide in psychiatric patients: risk and prevention. *Br J Psychiatry* 161:749–758, 1992.
42. Buzan RD, Weissberg MP. Suicide: risk factors and therapeutic considerations in the emergency department. *J Emerg Med* 10:335–343, 1992.
44. Weiss R, Hufford MR. Substance abuse and suicide. In Jacobs DG, editor: *The Harvard Medical School guide to suicide assessment and intervention*, San Francisco, 1999, Jossey-Bass.
49. Shuster JL, Lagomasino IT, Okereke OI, et al. Suicide. In Irwin RS, Rippe JM, editors: *Intensive care medicine*, ed 5, Philadelphia, 2003, Lippincott-Raven.
56. Silverman MM, Goldblatt MJ. Physical illness and suicide. In Maris RW, Berman AL, Silverman MM, editors: *Comprehensive textbook of suicidology*, New York, 2000, Guilford Press.
57. Hughes K. Kleepies P. Suicide in the medically ill. *Suicide Life Threat Behav* (Suppl.):48–60, 2001.
59. Conwell Y, Duberstein PR. Suicide among older people: a problem for primary care. *Prim Psychiatry* 3:41–44, 1996.
60. Kelly MJ, Mufson MJ, Rogers MP. Medical settings and suicide. In Jacobs DG, editor: *The Harvard Medical School guide to suicide assessment and intervention*, San Francisco, 1999, Jossey-Bass.
63. Jia CX, Mehlum L, Qin P. AIDS/HIV infection, comorbid psychiatric illness, and risk for subsequent suicide: a nationwide register linkage study. *J Clin Psychiatry* 73(10):1315–1321, 2012.
65. Massie MJ, Gagnon P, Holland JC. Depression and suicide in patients with cancer. *J Pain Symptom Manage* 9:325–340, 1994.
72. Kurella M, Kimmel PL, Yang BS, et al. Suicide in the United States End-Stage Renal Disease Program. *J Am Soc Nephrol* 16(3):774–781, 2005.
82. Joiner TE Jr, Brown JS, Wingate LR. The psychology and neurobiology of suicidal behavior. *Annu Rev Psychol* 56:287–314, 2005.
85. Roy A, Segal NL, Sarchiapone M. Attempted suicide among living co-twins of twin suicide victims. *Am J Psychiatry* 152:1075–1076, 1995.
86. Baldessarini RJ, Hennen J. Genetics of suicide: an overview. *Harv Rev Psychiatry* 12:1–13, 2004.
88. Hranilovic D, Stefulj J, Furac E, et al. Serotonin transporter gene promoter (5-HTTLPR) and Intron 2 (VNTR) polymorphisms in Croatian suicide victims. *Biol Psychiatry* 54:884–889, 2003.
93. McGown PO, Sasaki A, D'Alessio AC, et al. Epigenetic regulation of the glucocorticoid receptor in human brain associates with childhood abuse. *Nat Neuroscience* 12:342–348, 2009.
97. Lagomasino IT, Stern TA. The suicidal patient. In *MGH guide to primary care psychiatry*, New York, 2004, McGraw-Hill.
111. Eaton KM, Messer SC, Garvey Wilson AL, et al. Strengthening the validity of population-based suicide rate comparisons: an illustration using US military and civilian data. *Suicide Life Threat Behav* 36(2):182–191, 2006.
114. Lineberry TW, O'Connor SS. Suicide in the US Army. *Mayo Clinic Proc* 87(9):871–878, 2012.
115. Rozanov V, Carli V. Suicide among war veterans. *Int J Environ Res Public Health* 9:2504–2519, 2012.

117. LeardMann CA, Powell MS, Smith TC, et al. Risk factors associated with suicide in current and former US military personnel. *JAMA* 310(5):496–506, 2013.

127. Luoma JB, Martin CE, Pearson JL. Contact with mental health and primary care providers before suicide: a review of the evidence. *Am J Psychiatry* 159:909–916, 2002.

130. Mann JJ, Arango V. The neurobiology of suicidal behavior. In Jacobs DG, editor: *The Harvard Medical School guide to suicide assessment and intervention*, San Francisco, 1999, Jossey-Bass.

131. Van Heeringen K. The neurobiology of suicide and suicidality. *Can J Psychiatry* 48:292–300, 2003.

134. Nordstrom P, Samuelsson M, Asberg M, et al. CSF 5-HIAA predicts suicide risk after attempted suicide. *Suicide Life Threat Behav* 24:1–9, 2004.

142. Placidi GPA, Oquendo MA, Malone KM, et al. Aggressivity, suicide attempts, and depression: relationship to cerebrospinal fluid monoamine metabolite levels. *Biol Psychiatry* 50:783–791, 2001.

144. Maltsberger JT. The psychodynamic understanding of suicide. In Jacobs DG, editor: *The Harvard Medical School guide to suicide assessment and intervention*, San Francisco, 1999, Jossey-Bass.

146. American Psychiatric Association. Practice guideline for the assessment and treatment of patients with suicidal behaviors. *Am J Psychiatry* 160(11 Suppl.):1–60, 2003.

148. Fountoulakis K, Iacovides A, Fotiou F, et al. Neurobiological and psychological correlates of suicide attempts and thoughts of death in patients with major depression. *Neuropsychobiology* 49:42–62, 2004.

150. Hepp U, Moergeli H, Trier S, et al. Attempted suicide: factors leading to hospitalization. *Can J Psychiatry* 49:736–742, 2004.

154. Amchin J, Wettstein RM, Roth RH. Suicide, ethics, and the law. In Blumenthal SJ, Kupfer DJ, editors: *Suicide over the life cycle: risk factors, assessment, and treatment of suicidal patients*, Washington, DC, 1990, American Psychiatric Press.

156. Hall RC, Platt DE, Hall RC. Suicide risk assessment: a review of risk factors for suicide in 100 patients who made severe suicide attempts: evaluation of suicide risk in a time of managed care. *Psychosomatics* 40:18–27, 1999.

159. Miller MC, Jacobs DG, Gutheil TG. Talisman or taboo: the controversy of the suicide-prevention contract. *Harv Rev Psychiatry* 6:78–87, 1998.

161. Baldessarini RJ, Tondo L, Hennen J. Lithium treatment and suicide risk in major affective disorders: update and new findings. *J Clin Psychiatry* 64(Suppl. 5):44–52, 2003.

164. Gibbons RD, Hur K, Bhaumik DK, et al. The relationship between antidepressant medication use and rate of suicide. *Arch Gen Psychiatry* 62:165–172, 2005.

168. Gillmore JM, Chan CH. Suicide: a focus on primary care. *Wisc Medical J* 103(6):88–92, 2004.

169. Reeves RR, Ladner ME. Antidepressant-induced suicidality: Implications for clinical practice. *Southern Med J* 102(7):713–718, 2009.

170. American College of Neuropsychopharmacology, Executive Summary. Preliminary report of the Task Force on SSRIs and Suicidal Behavior in Youth, 2004.

171. Treatment for Adolescents with Depression Study Team. Fluoxetine, cognitive-behavioral therapy, and their combination for adolescents with depression. *JAMA* 292:807–820, 2004.

172. Sussman N. FDA warnings and suicide rates: unintended consequences. *Prim Psychiatry* 15:22–232, 2008.

180. Fergusson D, Doucette S, Glass KC, et al. Association between suicide attempts and selective serotonin reuptake inhibitors: systematic review of randomized controlled trials. *BMJ* 330:396–402, 2005.

181. Reith DM, Edmonds L. Assessing the role of drugs in suicidal ideation and suicidality. *CNS Drugs* 21:463–472, 2007.

54   Psychiatric Consultation to Medical and Surgical Patients

Nicholas Kontos, MD, and John Querques, MD

KEY POINTS

- Consultation psychiatry encompasses the evaluation and management of affective, behavioral, and cognitive symptoms in medical and surgical patients in general hospitals.

- Effective psychiatric consultation requires clear communication with the referring physician to hone the consultation question, to provide a useful response, and to facilitate optimal patient care.

- A temporal orientation to history-taking and a hierarchical approach to neuropsychological screening are keys to effective patient assessment.

- Some special clinical situations in the consultation arena include working with consultees, negotiating medically-unexplained symptoms, and dealing with difficult and hateful patients.

OVERVIEW

The heart of consultation psychiatry is the provision of psychiatric consultation to hospitalized medical and surgical patients who are thought by their primary caretakers to have a psychiatric problem. Implied in this task is the education of the consultee, nurses, and medical students about common affective, behavioral, and cognitive disorders in the general hospital. Some consultation psychiatrists formalize this implicit educative role in undertaking *liaison* work, which can include rounding with teams; provision of psychological support to medical and nursing staff; and application of general psychological principles to the health care delivery system.

This chapter reviews the epidemiology, diagnostic features, differential diagnosis, principles of evaluation, treatment, and special situations of psychopathology in the general hospital population.

EPIDEMIOLOGY AND DIFFERENTIAL DIAGNOSIS

Despite the high prevalence of psychiatric disorders among patients in general hospitals, rates of psychiatric consultation in this population are quite low and vary due to patient population, nature and severity of illness, length of stay, and idiosyncratic styles of referring physicians and consulting psychiatrists.[1] At the Massachusetts General Hospital, the rate of psychiatric consultation is 11–13%.[1] The most common stated reasons for psychiatric consultation are listed in

Box 54-1, while the diagnoses the consulting psychiatrist usually makes fall into the five categories listed in Box 54-2.

PRINCIPLES OF PSYCHIATRIC EVALUATION OF MEDICAL AND SURGICAL PATIENTS

The key steps in the process of psychiatric consultation are listed in Box 54-3. Each is explained in detail below.

Speak with the Consultee

Rarely does the referring physician's stated request for consultation tell the entire story of why the primary caretakers want or need assistance from a psychiatrist. More often, the stated request is effectively a "calling card" to get the psychiatrist to come, a label signifying the team recognizes that something is psychologically amiss with the patient but about which they cannot be more specific. Only in speaking directly with the consultee will the consultant figure this out and determine what the "real" problem is.

Review the Record

Busy consultants should resist the temptation to allow the referring physician's synopsis of the patient's medical history and hospital course to substitute for a thorough review of the hospital record. Often the written and electronic records contain important data the referring physician may not even be aware of or pay attention to. For example, notes from nurses, nutritionists, and physical, occupational, and speech therapists frequently prove invaluable in assessing a patient's affective, behavioral, and cognitive states. Of all the patient's physicians, the psychiatric consultant may be the only physician to study these important entries. Ambulance "run" sheets and emergency department notes are also helpful. For example, knowing whether the patient initiated or cooperated with the process of getting to the hospital can be hugely useful in capacity evaluations and in assessments after suicide attempts. Anesthesia flow sheets may reveal periods of hypotension or hypoxia during an operative procedure, suggesting the occurrence of clinically-significant cerebral hypoperfusion. In most instances, previous records do not have to be reviewed quite as exhaustively, but electronic medical records (EMRs) have enhanced the ease of doing so; the consultant wishing to avoid reinventing the wheel is well advised to take advantage of them.

Review Medications

The most definitive way to determine the medications the patient is actually receiving is a thorough review of the

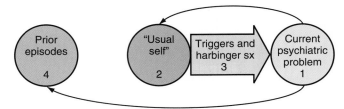

Figure 54-1. Organizing the interview.

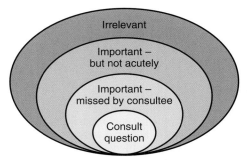

Figure 54-2. Areas of inquiry.

("they *won't*"). In these cases, information from collateral sources (e.g., family, friends, primary care physician, previous treaters, and old records) is invaluable. However, information from these collateral sources is not necessarily more reliable or more valid than data gleaned from the patient. Therefore, no one source of information should be prized over any other.

Interview the Patient

The psychiatric interview of a patient in the general hospital is identical in principle to that performed in most other venues. Areas of inquiry are identified; a diagnosis is pursued; and contributing factors from other aspects of the patient's background, current circumstances, and personal characteristics are elicited. A longitudinal conceptualization of the problem is useful (Figure 54-1). Thorough description of the presenting problem should be followed by an appraisal of the patient's psychological baseline. The patient should be asked when she last felt like her "usual self" rather than when she last felt "normal" or "good," since some patients do not view themselves in these terms. Descriptions of that time should be provided and detailed questions should be asked (e.g., "How did you spend your time then?" and "Would I notice a difference about you if I met you then?"). The patient should be invited to speculate on how her "usual self" might cope differently with her medical situation. If the answer is "the same," this provides an opportunity to explore characterological vulnerabilities. If not, this becomes an opportunity to look at intervening psychopathology or at demoralization. Next, triggers or harbinger symptoms of the presenting problem are identified. Lastly, a history of similar problems in the past is elicited. While many patients cannot be interviewed in such an orderly fashion, the history can still be organized this way in the note.

A schema for understanding the scope of the consulting psychiatrist's interview is presented in Figure 54-2. Although the consultee's question must be kept in mind throughout the interview, consultees often misidentify psychopathology and thus the consultation question should be taken only as a *suggestion*.[2–4] At the same time, the psychiatrist should not function as the local "biopsychosocial expert," for whom just

medication administration record (MAR). Computerized and handwritten order entries convey only the medications the patient is ordered to receive, not the agents he or she actually received. In reviewing the MAR, standing, as-needed, and one-time orders should be examined in order to capture a complete appraisal of the patient's treatment. This scrutiny is particularly useful in tracking alcohol detoxification, levels of sedation and agitation in delirium, and suspected "medication seeking." Attention should also be paid to medications the patient has recently stopped taking or has had erroneously continued. While "medication reconciliation" has never been easier or more emphasized than it currently is, clinical laxity should be resisted. For certain classes of medications, such oversight can cause mental status aberrations of relevance to the consulting psychiatrist. For example, a benzodiazepine a patient has received for several weeks while in the intensive care unit may be mistakenly discontinued when the patient is transferred to a regular nursing unit, thereby precipitating acute benzodiazepine withdrawal.

Gather Information from Family and Others

Patients in the general hospital are frequently poor historians. Because of delirium, dementia, substance intoxication or withdrawal, and sundry other causes of altered mental status, patients evaluated by psychiatric consultants may be *unable* to report the details of their medical and psychiatric histories ("they *can't*"). For various other reasons (e.g., personality disorder, factitious disorder, malingering, shame, or misguided modesty), patients may be *unwilling* to divulge personal data

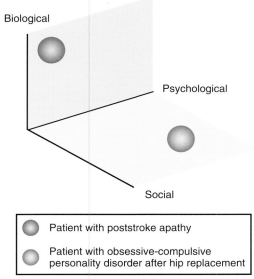

Figure 54-3. Prioritizing biopsychosocial inquiries.

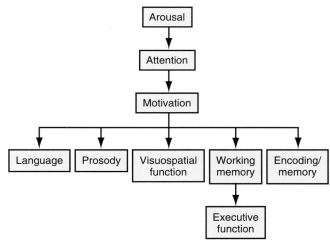

Figure 54-4. Basic hierarchy of neuropsychological functions.

TABLE 54-1 Examples of Screening Tasks for Selected Cognitive Domains

Cognitive Domain	Screening Task
Arousal	• Note the intensity of the stimulus needed to rouse the patient and to maintain arousal • Describe the quality of alertness
Attention	• Test digit span • Use backward recitation of over-learned information (e.g., days of week)
Motivation	• Compare spontaneous versus elicited cognitive performance • Ask explicit questions
Language	• Monitor fluency • Make absurd statements to assess comprehension • Test repetition • Test naming
Memory	• Obtain spontaneous recall of recent events • Review 5-minute recall • Place objects in the room for subsequent location and identification
Executive function	• Use a clock-drawing test • Test Luria hand maneuvers • Draw alternating figures • Generate word lists • Test go/no-go tasks

about anything in the patient's life is worthy of attention.[5] Rather, the consultant generally situates himself or herself just outside the border of the "MISSED BY CONSULTEE" circle and just inside the "IMPORTANT—BUT NOT ACUTELY" circle. Keeping the interview in this area requires clinical judgment beyond simply "being biopsychosocial." For example, a patient with acute apathy after a stroke has very different needs from the patient with obsessive-compulsive tendencies who is driving his family and the hospital staff to distraction after a hip replacement (Figure 54-3).

Conduct a Mental Status Examination

There are no unexaminable patients in consultation psychiatry. Even a profoundly delirious patient who cannot maintain alertness can have his level of arousal assessed. Non-cognitive aspects of the mental status examination (MSE) are the same as in routine psychiatric practice and are discussed in Chapter 2. This section focuses on principles of neuropsychological assessment and screening. We use the term *screening* to distinguish what the physician does at the patient's bedside from *testing*, a more rigorous and quantitative task usually performed by a neuropsychologist.

Neuropsychological assessment of the hospitalized patient begins not with specific screens, but with the interview itself.[6] Acutely ill patients may be unmotivated to engage in a cognitive screening battery. Since motivation plays a key role in task performance, the consultation psychiatrist closely observes the patient's spontaneous processes, and subtly evokes them during the interview. For example, the patient who can discuss the up-to-the-minute details of her hospital course yet recalls none of the three items on the Folstein Mini-Mental State Examination (MMSE)[7] does not have severe anterograde amnesia.

A fundamental principle of neuropsychological assessment is that mental functions are hierarchical: that is, some functions cannot be assessed validly if the faculties "above" them are disrupted. The broadest distinction in this ranking is that of state-dependent versus channel-dependent functions.[8] State-dependent functions include arousal, attention, and motivation. Subordinate to these are channel-dependent functions, comprising language, prosody, visuospatial function,

executive function, praxis, comportment, and the various forms of memory (Figure 54-4). We now briefly review the state-dependent functions and those channel-dependent functions that are of particular value to the consulting psychiatrist.[9,10] Table 54-1 gives a summary.

Arousal

Unless the patient is clearly alert, the examination begins with an assessment of arousal. The Glasgow Coma Scale may be used for profoundly impaired patients.[11] The terms *lethargic*, *somnolent*, and *obtunded* should be avoided since most physicians use them imprecisely. A three-parameter description of the patient's level of arousal is more useful:

• What type and intensity of stimulus wakens the patient (e.g., saying the patient's name with normal volume or vigorously shaking the patient's shoulder)?
• What quality of alertness is produced (e.g., coherent or incoherent verbalization)?
• What stimulus is required to maintain alertness?

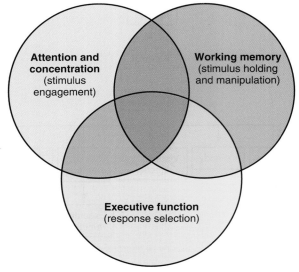

Figure 54-5. Overlapping domains of "focus."

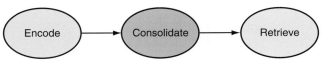

Figure 54-6. Aspects of memory.

Attention

Attention and *concentration* refer to the abilities to engage appropriate stimuli without distraction by irrelevant inputs. *Working memory* refers to the ability to hold and manipulate selected information.[12] *Executive function* involves response selection and guides the "work" of working memory. These three cognitive functions share dorsolateral-prefrontal-subcortical circuitry. The complex overlap among them is simplified in Figure 54-5. Assessment of attention begins with simple observation of the patient during the interview while watching for distraction by extraneous internal or external stimuli. Forward digit span is the gold standard for screening attention at the bedside. Backward digit span or backward recitation of over-learned information (e.g., months of the year) uses information that is less influenced by education or culture than is a spelling or a mathematical task. The cognitive "work" required is simple, and, though it invokes working memory, we see it as occupying the overlap area in Figure 54-5.

Motivation

There are no specific bedside tests to assess motivation. The astute clinician can usually gain some sense of the patient's motivation from observation and interaction. Simply asking the patient about level of interest in the examiner's tests may be sufficient. Many patients with acute somatic illness will quite justifiably indicate that psychiatric consultation, let alone cognitive screening, is not high on their list of priorities. Comparing spontaneous and elicited cognitive performances, as noted previously, may provide a clue to the patient's engagement and effort, but is by no means conclusive.

Language

Fluency, comprehension, repetition, and naming are the basic components of language testing.[13] The intactness of the first two is usually apparent from the interview alone. Fluency should not be mistaken for comprehensibility (e.g., patients with Wernicke's aphasia speak fluently but non-sensically). The comprehension of the non-communicative or minimally-communicative patient can sometimes be discerned by asking absurd questions (e.g., "Do helicopters in Panama eat their young?" [Cassem NH, personal communication, 2000]). Naming should include components of objects (e.g., the face

of a watch or the cap of a pen), as well as whole objects (e.g., a watch or a pen).

Memory

When assessing memory, one needs to keep in mind the type, timing, and component of it that is being scrutinized. *Declarative* or *explicit memory*, which includes both *episodic* (experiential) and *semantic* (factual) memory, is the type usually screened at the bedside.[14] *Recent* memory operates on a scale of minutes to days, *remote* memory on a scale of days to years.[15] Note that problems of *encoding, consolidation,* and *retrieval* (Figure 54-6) all produce errors of *recall*.[13] Before resorting to prompts, it is sometimes helpful to ask the patient who "can't remember any" items to "just try to think of one" rather than all three. Many patients surprise themselves. Storage and retrieval errors can be distinguished by giving the patient categorical, then multiple-choice, prompts. Consistent accuracy aided by prompts suggests a retrieval rather than an encoding or a consolidation problem, and perhaps a frontal-subcortical circuit perturbation rather than a hippocampal one. Errors of recall might trigger other bedside tests, such as hiding objects (e.g., bills or coins of various denominations, which enhance the patient's affective engagement with the task) around the room and asking the patient to identify and locate them after several minutes.

Executive Function

Executive functions, construed most broadly as response selection,[16] are manifested in strategic pursuit of goals, set-shifting, independence from environmental cues, and using language to guide action.[17] Executive dysfunction is often subtle, yet it is pervasive in consultation psychiatry; it is found in neuropsychiatric syndromes, idiopathic psychopathologies, and general medical illnesses.[18] During the interview, one watches for signs of frontal-subcortical dysfunction, such as environmental dependency (e.g., imitating the examiner's movements or manipulating objects left within arm's reach)[19] and perseverative thought process. The latter—an inability to shift cognitive set—should be distinguished from voluntary persistence with a topic foremost on the patient's mind. Useful bedside screens include clock-drawing,[20] cognitive estimations,[21] Luria hand maneuvers, alternating figures,[6] word-list generation, and the go/no-go task.[9] Errors on these tasks are multiply determined but often suggest disruption of the brain's frontal-subcortical circuitry, particularly the dorsolateral prefrontal circuit. Such disruptions can occur through functional or anatomical lesions that affect the cortex, basal ganglia, thalamus, or intervening white matter[17]; or indirectly via lateral cerebellar lesions[22] or depletion of brainstem monoamine (especially dopamine) nuclei.

Structured Instruments

When guided by clinical acumen, brief structured instruments can bring added rigor and breadth to one's exam. The Folstein MMSE[7] and the Montreal Cognitive Assessment[23] are the most commonly used tools; recently the latter has gained traction for its relatively greater emphasis on frontal-subcortical functions. The CLOX is an informative systematization of the commonly used clock-drawing task.[20] Cutoff scores are of some utility, but one should also "dissect" these examinations to see where a patient's greatest difficulties lie.[24] Confinement of errors to a particular domain might lead to deceptively low scores and should trigger scrutiny of that function and others that could confound it.

Conduct Physical and Neurological Examinations

Arguably categorically obsolete,[25,26] the taboo against psychiatrists' touching their patients certainly has no place in consultation psychiatry. The consulting psychiatrist should be able to perform a competent neurological examination and at least a serviceable and targeted physical examination. Many psychiatric presentations are associated with demonstrably organic causes. In addition, psychiatric patients are at greater risk for somatic illnesses, yet often get medical short shrift, particularly when they have atypical complaints. The consulting psychiatrist may need to advocate for these patients[27] and will lack both information and credibility if concerns are not backed up by action.

Write a Note

The consultation note should be a model of succinct, concise writing, free of psychiatric jargon and irrelevant data. A lengthy recapitulation of the patient's medical history and current hospital course is unnecessary; the consultee already knows this information. A brief summary is sufficient to indicate that the consultant has reviewed and considered the record in forming his or her opinion. Here again, EMRs can be both blessing and curse.[28] Items should not be "cut and pasted" into one's note unless they were actually reviewed and judged relevant. The diagnostic impression and treatment recommendation sections should be especially clear because this is "where the rubber hits the road" in the entire consultative process. These sections address what the referring physician really wants to know: What's wrong with the patient and how do I fix it?

Speak with the Consultee

The consultative process ends as it begins: with a conversation with the consultee. Obviously it is important in urgent situations, and even in less urgent ones, and it is courteous and effective practice, to communicate one's findings in person or on the phone rather than just to leave a written note.

TREATMENT

The consulting psychiatrist's therapeutic recommendations fall into various combinations of three domains: biological, psychological, and social. As noted earlier, the consultant uses clinical judgment to gauge the situation-weighted relevance of each domain for each patient.

Biological

Biological management often involves recommendations about psychoactive agents. It is best to proceed in an orderly fashion. Attention should first be turned to those medications the patient is already prescribed. Does the patient need them? If so, is the dose correct? If not, can they simply be stopped or is tapering required? Are they causing problems? Just because a patient is on various psychiatric medications as an outpatient does not mean that he or she necessarily needs them in the hospital. For example, a patient who is floridly agitated because of delirium after cardiac surgery probably does not need the stimulant medication he or she takes at home for attention-deficit disorder and most likely will do

better without it. The psychiatric consultant can be particularly helpful to medical and surgical teams unfamiliar with psychiatric medications and thus leery of stopping agents the patient is prescribed at home for fear of precipitating an acute crisis. Likewise, the consultant often needs to advise the consultee when the latter is unaware of adverse psychiatric effects of medications with which he or she is comfortable (e.g., delirium-inducing effects of diphenhydramine or akathisia-inducing effects of prochlorperazine).

The consultant can then focus attention on psychotropic agents the patient may need while in the hospital. Returning to the patient who is delirious after cardiac surgery, this patient may benefit from haloperidol. In recommending various medications, the consultant needs to appreciate the patient's medical and psychiatric histories, current medical situation and laboratory values, and current medication regimen in order to assess pharmacokinetics, drug–drug interactions, and adverse effects. In our experience, patients seen as "psychiatric" tend to be scrutinized closely for any possible signs of "behavior problems" or "anxiety." Thus, doses and frequencies of any recommended as-needed medications should be clearly spelled out.

Beyond medications, biological "management" often involves advice for further general medical work-up. Such is the case when the etiology of delirium is unknown, when "secondary" psychopathology is suspected, and when staff, patients, and families require education about the biological underpinnings of known neuropsychiatric conditions. In addition, the psychiatrist should feel obliged to be on the lookout for general medical issues that the consultee might have overlooked even if they do not have direct bearing on the reason for the consultation. This issue receives further attention under Special Situations later in this chapter.

Psychological

While a hospital unit may not be a suitable venue for exploratory, insight-oriented psychotherapy, it may be an appropriate place for brief, supportive psychotherapy. A patient in the midst of a protracted hospitalization for a complicated illness may benefit greatly from acknowledgment of his or her suffering; support in bearing it; bolstering of adaptive coping mechanisms; and opportunities for ventilation and catharsis. Even when family, friends, and other supportive associates are plentiful, the psychiatrist may be the only resource available to the patient for such emotional release and relief. For some patients, it can be appropriate to offer limited interpretations of their illness experiences against the backdrop of their biographical themes and events. Viederman's "life narrative" is one such technique and sees certain aspects of the hospitalized patient's vulnerability (e.g., regression, self-examination) as opportunities for empathic intervention.[29]

Knowledge of different personality profiles is key to working with patients in the general hospital. The psychiatric consultant can make an accurate and practically articulated assessment of the patient's personality style and help the primary team tailor its interactions with the patient accordingly. For example, a patient who needs to be in control may be allowed to decide when he receives his morning medications or undergoes physical therapy. The patient's feeling that he has at least some control over what otherwise feels like an out-of-control illness probably is more important than the exact time of various ministrations. This topic is explored in greater depth in Chapter 9.

Social

Recommendations in the social realm frequently involve the issues enumerated in Box 54-4.[30] Psychiatric consultants also

---

BOX 54-4 Common Social Issues

Decisions about end-of-life care
- Do-not-resuscitate orders
- Do-not-intubate orders

Discharge planning
- Rehabilitation hospital
- Home with services
- Assisted living facility
- Skilled nursing facility
- Nursing home

Short-term disability

Probate guardianship

Involuntary psychiatric commitment

TABLE 54-2 Potential Symptom–Diagnosis Mismatches

Patient Reports/ Displays	Consultee Concludes	Consultant Concludes*
"Depression"	Major depressive disorder	• Delirium • Adjustment disorder • Demoralization
"Mood swings"	Bipolar disorder	• Delirium • Personality disorder • Emotional incontinence • Mixed messages from staff
"Panic"	Panic disorder	• Delirium • Fear • Hypoxia • Angina
"Hallucinations" "Paranoia"	Schizophrenia or psychosis	• Delirium • Fear • Dementia • Intoxication • Affective psychosis
"Anxiety"	Anxiety disorder	• Delirium • Fear • Adjustment disorder • Misinformation • Pain

*Illustrative, not exhaustive, differential diagnoses.

---

make recommendations about various types of restraints (e.g., soft restraints, leather restraints, Posey vests, mitts) and continuous 1:1 patient observation for patients who present a risk of harm to themselves or to others.

SPECIAL SITUATIONS

Some of the most challenging aspects of consultation psychiatry are products of the consultation arena itself. Here we briefly review some areas of particular challenge and potential reward in working with providers who are not psychiatrists and their sometimes "psychiatry-averse" patients.

Diagnosis, Treatment, and Patient Advocacy

In "The Devil's Dictionary," Ambrose Bierce defined "physician" as "one upon whom we set our hopes when ill and our dogs when well."[31] Such can be the plight of the consultation psychiatrist, who may feel regarded as quack or disposition planner one day, behavior-altering potentate the next. This admittedly caricatured portrayal captures the clinical reality that conflicts sometimes occur on consultation services; when they occur between psychiatric consultant and consultee, matters of diagnosis, treatment, or patient advocacy are usually at issue.

Disagreements over patients' diagnoses often stem from confusion over the difference between experiences and symptoms on the one hand and diagnoses on the other. Experiences and symptoms may or may not be part of a psychopathological entity. Unfortunately, many common psychiatric diagnoses share names with psychological experiences and lay terms.[32] This terminology can lead to confusion in consultees who will then disagree with a consultant's assessment that does not confirm their own diagnosis.[33] Table 54-2 provides examples of potential symptom–diagnosis mismatches. When these mismatches arise, the communication and the educational aspects of the consultant role become quite important. Often the consultee has accurately detected that psychopathology is present; this can be pointed out and clarification offered. At other times, there is no psychopathology present, and the consultant must be able to defend this position because the consultee is presumably worried about the patient and will therefore have a hard time accepting that "nothing is wrong." Both situations offer an opportunity for the consultation psychiatrist to demonstrate commonalities in practice patterns with the rest of medicine. The lack of availability of concrete data and, therefore, of certainty must be acknowledged. However, one must be clear in communicating how elicitation of symptom clusters and examination signs, plus longitudinal organization of information, lead to psychiatric diagnoses.

Most consultees are no strangers to uncertainty in their practices and should appreciate the consultant's description of a medical approach to patient assessment.

Treatment recommendations will flow from the consultant's diagnostic assessment. Often a consultee has already initiated treatment before asking for assistance. The consulting psychiatrist should be prepared to recommend discontinuation of any unnecessary medications. These may be psychiatric, in the case of incorrect preconsultation diagnosis and treatment, or non-psychiatric, in the case of unrecognized, iatrogenically-exacerbated delirium (see Chapter 18). For patients and families struggling with pain, fear, or other *normal* psychological fallout of serious illness, psychiatric input can be of great value. In these cases, however, no one is being done any favors when the psychiatrist is seen as taking on a "psychotherapy" role. The patient is inherently "pathologized" by being thrust into the psychiatrist's domain; the treating physician is inappropriately absolved of involvement in important aspects of the doctor–patient relationship; and the psychiatrist risks conflation of his or her role with that of the "unit holistic humanist."[5] A psychiatrist may have considerable skill in identifying and addressing some patients' psychological needs. However, there is much more positive potential in helping patients and their physicians address non-psychopathological issues on their own.

Consulting psychiatrists may also need to advocate for optimal general medical care for psychiatric patients, particularly the chronically mentally ill. Severe mental illness provides a convenient, but dangerous, substrate for the application of Occam's razor to complex medical presentations. Thus, atypical presentations, odd (or absent) self-expression, and biases about mental illness may jeopardize the health of the severely mentally ill.[34] The consulting psychiatrist must be attentive to the patient's manner of expressing distress, to incongruities between objective information and patient care, and to his or her own role as a physician. Certainly, a psychiatrist is not expected to have comprehensive knowledge of every medical specialty, but general medical vigilance is part of the consulting psychiatrist's mandate. Any concerns should be backed up by specific findings on mental status and physical examinations, plus available laboratory and radiological

BOX 54-5 Reasons for Psychiatric Referral of Patients with Medically-Unexplained Symptoms

- To rule out a somatoform disorder
- To rule out malingering
- To rule out co-morbid psychopathology
- To assess "stressors"
- To persuade the patient that the problem is psychiatric
- To take the patient off the consultee's hands

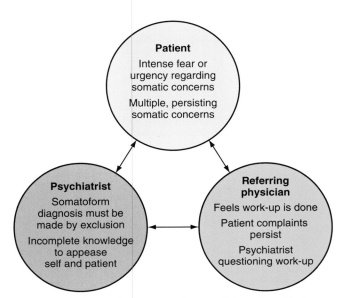

Figure 54-7. Competing concerns in consultations to patients with medically unexplained symptoms.

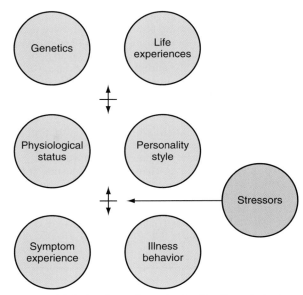

Figure 54-8. A scheme for understanding illness behavior.

studies. Simply saying, "I think this patient is sick," is not acceptable and will cause frustration on all sides.[35]

Somatic Symptom Disorders

Patients with medically-unexplained symptoms (MUS) usually come to the psychiatrist by way of consultation rather than on their own initiative. They are often befuddled or irritated by the referral, mirroring the consultee's befuddlement or irritation by these patients, who, left to their own devices, are high utilizers of most medical services except, interestingly, psychiatric services.[36] Common reasons for psychiatric consultation for these patients are listed in Box 54-5. Diagnosis and treatment of patients with MUS are as challenging for the psychiatrist as they are for the non-psychiatrist. Different ideas of what constitutes exclusion of primary somatic causes can lead to mutually interacting and anxiety-generating concerns from the patient, the referring physician, and the psychiatrist (Figure 54-7). General medical awareness—plus frequent, collegial, and assertive, yet humble, communication with the consultee—are the best ways to align these competing priorities. When it comes to assessing patients with MUS, it is most important for the consulting psychiatrist to do the following:

- Be satisfied with the medical evaluation carried out to date
- Determine whether the patient is significantly impaired by, or pursuing inordinate medical attention to, MUS
- Diagnose a DSM-5[32] somatic symptom disorder, if it is present

- If it is not, conceptualize the problem in another way that will be helpful to the consultee[37]

Treatment options for the patient with somatic symptom disorders and other problematic presentations of MUS are covered in Chapter 24. There are, however, some specific targeted interventions that the consulting psychiatrist might recommend for patients with MUS. In doing so, the psychiatrist must respect the often fierce opposition these patients may mount to any challenge to their ardent "physical" etiological convictions. At the same time, the psychiatrist must also be aware that these convictions can be associated with worse outcomes.[38] Patient acceptability of diagnoses has no place in the codification of diagnostic schemes,[39] but in the clinical interaction with somatizing patients a stance of etiological neutrality can be useful. The psychiatrist may help the patient and the consultee with:

- diagnosing and treating co-morbid mood and anxiety disorders
- referring the patient, when appropriate, to cognitive-behavioral therapy for the purpose of symptom control[40,41]
- assisting the patient and consultee with "meaning-making" of the patient's experience[42,43]

"Meaning-making" in particular can be delicate but profitable. Helping the patient to understand how genetics, life events, and personality style come together to produce normal and abnormal physiological states, as well as individualized experiences of those states (Figure 54-8), can place symptoms into a larger context with more possible points for intervention.

The Reticent Patient

In consultation psychiatry, patients usually do not ask to see the psychiatrist. Further, there are rarely any coercive legal measures that force the interaction, as there may be in psychiatric emergency departments and inpatient settings. As a result, many patients muster a sort of "pseudoengagement," in which they speak with the psychiatrist in a polite but superficial or guarded way. These patients might be dismissed as "difficult historians" if one is not attentive to the signs and potential causes of pseudoengagement (Box 54-6).

Obstacles to genuine engagement of patients with normal levels of arousal and attention almost always involve unstated (or indirectly stated) wishes or fears on the part of the patient. In general, the quality of the interview will be greatly improved if the psychiatrist directly addresses these issues with the patient. It is not terribly important that the psychiatrist's hunch be correct. Most patients appreciate the effort, which may in itself either diffuse their reticence or lead them to discuss their actual concerns.

An exception is the patient with an agenda that relies on deception (e.g., malingering). In these cases, the psychiatrist should complete the interview, however compromised, before airing his or her suspicions. This tactic allows time for self-examination of personal motives in "exposing" the patient, which may then lead to a decision not to confront the patient at all. If it is decided to confront the patient, one has already obtained clinical information before the engagement is further sabotaged or the patient is left able to hold the psychiatrist hostage with newly-voiced suicidal ideation or other subjective urgent complaints.

Difficult and Hateful Patients

Sometimes, in the hospital, it can seem that Jean-Paul Sartre was correct that "hell is other people."[44] As the scope, legitimacy, and appreciation of mental illness increase, psychiatric consultation is sought, with hope or desperation, as a remedy for various forms of interpersonal unpleasantness. The language used to describe the patients involved in this unpleasantness has changed significantly over the years, with the more intellectualized adjective "difficult" now favored over the more limbic (and probably honest) one, "hateful." Notably, the two terms seem to describe essentially the same group of patients, and Table 54-3 compares Groves' original conceptualization with that arrived at in a more recent review.[45,46]

Psychiatric consultants are often called to see patients who create problems in their own care, disrupt the care of other patients, or simply irk their doctors. The latter can be important to get out in the open, but by itself is not grounds for clinical action, and is seldom the sole reason behind these consultations. Instead, our umbrella formulation for a hateful and difficult patient is one under which a given patient's stated goals and expectations regarding his own health and providers' duties are unaccompanied by that patient's actual demonstrations of investment in health and respect for providers' privileges (Figure 54-9).[47]

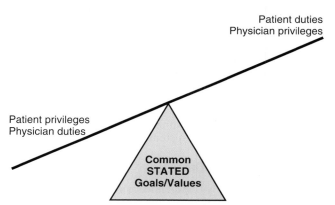

Figure 54-9. Privileges and duties at play with hateful and difficult patients.

BOX 54-6 Signs and Causes of "Pseudoengagement"

SIGNS
- Minimalist responses
- Categorically-positive (or negative) self-presentation
- Improbable or incongruous positivity (or negativity)
- Inconsistent history to different providers
- Inconsistent information from collateral sources
- Irritability without overt hostility
- Continuous returning to a particular psychosocial topic

WISHES
- Attention to an area of personal importance
- Information/education/reassurance about medical situation
- Peace and quiet (from psychiatrist, family, and/or providers)
- Controlled substances
- Financial gain
- Relief from societal obligations

FEARS
- Being "analyzed"
- Being psychiatrically labeled
- Being psychiatrically medicated
- Not being taken seriously by one's primary physician
- Use of coercive measures (e.g., psychiatric commitment or guardianship)
- Being exposed to oneself or others as "weak"

TABLE 54-3 Hateful and Difficult Patients

Groves' Category—"Hateful"	Koekkoek's Category—"Difficult"	Approach
Entitled demander	Demanding care claimer	Avoid confronting entitlement Identify obstacles to "best care"
Dependent clinger	Demanding-ambivalent claimer-seeker	Avoid power/rescue fantasies Set clear, non-threatening limits
Manipulative help-rejecter	Ambivalent care seeker	Share pessimism Affirm engagement
Self-destructive denier	Unwilling care avoider	*Based on character*: • Recognize own aversion • Recognize limitations • *Based on psychosis, depression, dementia, etc.*: • Treat underlying pathology • Assess capacity

Adapted from Groves JE. Taking care of the hateful patient. N Engl J Med 298:883–887, 1978 and Koekkoek B, van Meijel B, Hutschemaekers G. "Difficult patients" in mental health care: a review. Psychiatric Serv 57:795–802, 2006.

TABLE 54-4 Ethical Dilemmas in Hateful and Difficult Patients

	Principle	Concern	Physician Feels	Resolution
Autonomy "Versus"	Beneficence	Incongruent patient–physician values	Paternalisic	Gain understanding of patient's values
	Nonmaleficence	Patient elicits aversion	Guilty	Act based on reasonable limits
	Justice	Unreasonable patient demands (system level)	Conflicted about obligations	Have frank discussion with patient
	Autonomy (others')	Unreasonable patient demands (family level)	Detached	Discuss with patient and family

Adapted from Kontos N, Freudenreich O, Querques J. Beyond capacity: identifying ethical dilemmas underlying capacity evaluation requests,. Psychosomatics. 2013;54: 103–110, 2013.

Interventions in these situations, viewed medically, depend on diagnosis (Table 54-3). Thus the consultant must first determine what, if any, psychopathology is driving the patient's behavior. The manic patient's irritability and inappropriateness are dealt with very differently from those of a psychiatrically unafflicted patient. The latter scenario is important to keep in mind, since undesirable conduct is not *ipso facto* evidence of psychopathology. In the gray zone of personality disorders, what reasonable "limit setting" looks like is a matter of clinical judgment. Again, some basic advice is found in Table 54-3. Confrontation is reserved for patients who are assessed as accountable for their behavior; is conducted as an interaction between respectful, honest adults; and, in order to be handled responsibly, is focused purely on the imbalance between privileges and duties described above.[47]

Finally, psychiatric consultation for help with a difficult or hateful patient might occur under the guise of a capacity evaluation request, which itself is reflexive shorthand for any ethical dilemma. Prototypes for these situations include ones where a patient's values are not in sync with his/her physician's, where hatred of the patient leads to paradoxical indulgence of his/her misbehavior, or where a patient's decisions/desires exert unfair demands on the "system" or put his/her family in an unreasonable position. Sometimes, once everyone's cards are on the table, it turns out that the patient is not difficult at all and agreements can be reached. At other times, the consultant can be helpful in identifying the actual problem and participating in, but not necessarily effecting, its resolution. These situations can involve challenging medical presumptions about value neutrality, allowing anger-avoidant equanimity, or considering the wider impact of decisions made by and for individual patients.[48] A sample schematic for these types of problems is shown in Table 54-4.

CONCLUSIONS

- Psychiatric conditions are highly prevalent among medical and surgical patients in general hospitals.
- Effective psychiatric consultants must consider a vast array of information sources and domains for each patient assessment.
- The general hospital presents special challenges and opportunities in the provision of effective, medically-minded patient care.

Access the complete reference list and multiple choice questions (MCQs) online at https://expertconsult.inkling.com

KEY REFERENCES

3. Boland RJ, Dias S, Lamdan RM, et al. Overdiagnosis of depression in the general hospital. *Gen Hosp Psychiatry* 18:28–35, 1996.
5. Murray GB. The liaison psychiatrist as busybody. *Ann Clin Psychiatry* 1:265–268, 1989.
6. Malloy PF, Richardson ED. Assessment of frontal lobe functions. *J Neuropsychiatry Clin Neurosci* 6:399–410, 1994.
10. Freedman M, Stuss DT, Gordon M. Assessment of competency: the role of neurobehavioral deficits. *Ann Intern Med* 115:203–208, 1991.
13. Devinsky O. *Behavioral neurology 100 maxims*, Boston, 1992, Mosby–Year Book.
15. Cummings JL, Mega MS. *Neuropsychiatry and behavioral neuroscience*, New York, 2003, Oxford University Press.
17. Mega MS, Cummings JL. Frontal-subcortical circuits and neuropsychiatric disorders. *J Neuropsychiatry Clin Neurosci* 6:358–370, 1994.
20. Royall DR, Cordes JA, Polk M. CLOX: an executive clock drawing task. *J Neurol Neurosurg Psychiatry* 64:588–594, 1998.
22. Schmahmann JD. The role of the cerebellum in cognition and emotion: personal reflections since 1982 on the dysmetria of thought hypothesis, and its historical evolution from theory to therapy. *Neuropsychol Rev* 20:236–260, 2010.
23. Nasreddine ZS, Phillips NA, Bedirian V, et al. The Montreal cognitive assessment, MoCA: a brief screening tool for mild cognitive impairment. *J Am Geriatr Soc* 53:695–699, 2005.
28. Hartzband P, Groopman J. Off the record—avoiding the pitfalls of going electronic. *N Engl J Med* 358:1656–1658, 2008.
33. Kontos N, Freudenreich O, Querques J, et al. The consultation psychiatrist as effective physician. *Gen Hosp Psychiatry* 25:20–23, 2003.
34. Freudenreich O, Stern TA. Clinical experience with the management of schizophrenia in the general hospital. *Psychosomatics* 44:12–23, 2003.
35. Kontos N, Freudenreich O, Querques J. Ownership, responsibility and hospital care: lessons for the consultation psychiatrist. *Gen Hosp Psychiatry* 30:257–262, 2008.
37. Meador CK. *Symptoms of unknown origin*, Nashville, 2005, Vanderbilt University Press.
39. Starcevic V. Somatoform disorders and DSM-V: conceptual and political issues in the debate. *Psychosomatics* 47:277–281, 2006.
43. Barsky AJ. Patients who amplify bodily sensations. *Ann Intern Med* 91:63–70, 1979.
45. Groves JE. Taking care of the hateful patient. *N Engl J Med* 298:883–887, 1978.
47. Kontos N, Querques J, Freudenreich O. Fighting the good fight: responsibility and rationale in the confrontation of patients. *Mayo Clin Proc* 87:63–66, 2012.
48. Kontos N, Freudenreich O, Querques J. Beyond capacity: identifying ethical dilemmas underlying capacity evaluation requests. *Psychosomatics* 54:103–110, 2013.

55

Life-threatening Conditions in Psychiatry: Catatonia, Neuroleptic Malignant Syndrome, and Serotonin Syndrome

Gregory L. Fricchione, MD, Scott R. Beach, MD, Jeff C. Huffman, MD, George Bush, MD, MMSc, and Theodore A. Stern, MD

KEY POINTS

Background

- Catatonia, neuroleptic malignant syndrome (NMS), and serotonin syndrome are neuropsychiatric conditions with prominent motor, behavioral, and systemic manifestations.
- Catatonia is a syndrome with multiple medical, neurological, and psychiatric etiologies that requires a systematic approach for diagnosis.
- NMS is a form of malignant catatonia.
- Serotonin syndrome (SS), caused by an excess of serotonin, shares many features in common with catatonia and NMS.

History

- Catatonia was first described in 1847 by Karl Kahlbaum.

Clinical and Research Challenges

- There is no universal agreement on the number of signs required to make the diagnosis of catatonia, as the Bush-Francis Catatonia Rating Scale requires only two features, whereas the DSM-5 requires three.
- Patients with catatonia may present with highly variable signs and symptoms, and many clinicians have a very narrow concept of how the syndrome may appear.
- Very few neuroimaging studies involving patients with catatonia have been completed, and the underlying pathophysiology of the disorder remains unclear.

Practical Pointers

- Examination of patients who present with a mood disorder should always include assessment of catatonic features.

- Patients with encephalitis may be particularly susceptible to developing catatonia.
- Though stuporous catatonia is the most common subtype, many patients display an excited catatonia that may include excessive motor activity and increased speech production.
- Delirious mania is a syndrome involving manic features, disorientation, and catatonia that often requires emergency treatment.
- Catatonia likely reflects disruption in the basal ganglia-thalamocortical loop system.
- Lorazepam and electroconvulsive therapy (ECT) are important therapies for catatonic states.
- Neuroleptics may worsen catatonia or predispose patients to the development of a malignant catatonia called NMS and should be used with extreme caution.
- Risk factors for NMS include exposure to high-potency neuroleptics, a history of catatonia or NMS, agitation, dehydration, exhaustion, a low serum iron, basal ganglia disorders, and withdrawal from alcohol or sedatives.
- NMS is typically self-limited once neuroleptics are stopped and supportive measures instituted, though the mortality rate is approximately 10%.
- Lorazepam can be effective for NMS but ECT is the definitive treatment; re-challenging a patient who has NMS with neuroleptics remains controversial.
- Serotonin syndrome is usually self-limiting once the offending serotonergic agents are discontinued and supportive measures are initiated.

OVERVIEW

The syndromes described in this chapter each involve a complex mixture of motor, behavioral, and systemic manifestations that are derived from unclear mechanisms. What *is* clear is that neurotransmitters, such as dopamine (DA), gamma-aminobutyric acid (GABA), and glutamate (GLU), are of major importance in catatonia and neuroleptic malignant syndrome (NMS), and serotonin (5-hydroxytryptamine [5-HT]) is crucial to the development of serotonin syndrome (SS).

As medications with potent effects on the modulation of monoamines have proliferated, the diagnosis and management of these complex disorders has become even more important; without question, these syndromes have signs, symptoms, and treatments that overlap.

CATATONIA
Definition

The catatonic syndrome comprises a constellation of motor and behavioral signs and symptoms that often occur in relation to neuromedical insults. Structural brain disease, intrinsic brain disorders (e.g., epilepsy, toxic-metabolic derangements, infectious diseases), systemic disorders that affect the brain, and idiopathic psychiatric disorders (such as affective and schizophrenic psychoses) have all been associated with catatonia. Catatonia was first named and defined in 1847 by Karl Kahlbaum, who published a monograph that described 21 patients with a severe psychiatric disorder.[1]

Kahlbaum believed that patients with catatonia passed through several phases of illness: a short stage of immobility (with waxy flexibility and posturing), a second stage of stupor or melancholy, a third stage of mania (with pressured speech, hyperactivity, and hyperthymic behavior), and finally, after repeated cycles of stupor and excitement, a stage of dementia.[1]

Kraepelin[2] included catatonia in the group of deteriorating psychotic disorders named "dementia praecox." Bleuler[3] adopted Kraepelin's view that catatonia was subsumed under the heading of severe idiopathic deteriorating psychoses, which he renamed "the schizophrenias." It is curious that while Kraepelin and Bleuler both seemed to understand that catatonic symptoms could emerge as part of a mood disorder or could result from neurologic, toxic-metabolic, and infectious etiologies, they persisted in categorizing it exclusively with the severe dilapidating psychoses.

As a result of their influence, catatonia was strongly linked with schizophrenia until the 1990s, and until fairly recently catatonia could only be diagnosed in the setting of schizophrenia. Thanks in large part to the work of Fink and Taylor,[4] the *Diagnostic and Statistical Manual of Mental Disorders*, ed 4 (DSM-IV) was the first to include criteria for mood disorders with catatonic features and for catatonic disorder secondary to a general medical condition, as well as for the catatonic type of schizophrenia.[5] In some measure due to lobbying from catatonia researchers, in DSM-5, catatonia is now subdivided into Catatonia Associated with Another Mental Disorder, Catatonic Disorder due to Another Medical Condition, and Unspecified Catatonia.[6,7] The catatonic subtype of schizophrenia has been removed.

Under DSM-5, catatonia, whether a consequence of medical illness or a mental disorder, is diagnosed when the clinical picture includes at least three of the following 12 features: catalepsy, waxy flexibility, stupor, agitation, mutism, negativism (characterized by an apparently motiveless resistance to all instructions or by the maintenance of a rigid posture against attempts to be moved), posturing, mannerism, stereotypy, grimacing, and echolalia or echopraxia.

Epidemiology and Risk Factors

Catatonia is a non-specific syndrome associated with a variety of etiologies.[8] The rate of catatonia in the general psychiatric population varies according to the study design and diagnostic criteria. Prospective studies on patients hospitalized with acute psychotic episodes place the incidence of catatonia in the 7% to 17% range.[9] In patients who suffer from mood disorders, rates have ranged from 13% to 31%. Catatonia appears commonly in those with bipolar disorder, with some suggesting that 20% of manic patients display at least one sign of catatonia.[9] Some have contended that the incidence of catatonia has diminished in schizophrenia, but diagnostic and study design variations make this interpretation problematic. Patients with autism-spectrum disorders and developmental disorders appear to be at higher risk for developing catatonia.[10] Personality disorders or conversion disorder have been cited as etiologic in a minority of catatonia cases.

Risk factors include: a history of catatonia; extrapyramidal symptoms (EPS); a mood disorder with psychomotor retardation or excitement (manic delirium); perinatal infectious disease; epilepsy or migraine; frontal, basal gangliar, brainstem, or cerebellar disease; dehydration; hyponatremia; weight loss; medications that lower seizure threshold, block dopamine, reduce $GABA_A$, or increase serotonin; long-term benzodiazepine or antiparkinsonian use with recent withdrawal or a decrease in dose; and low levels of serum iron.[8,11-14]

Neuromedical "organic" etiologies account for 4% to 46% of cases in various series, underscoring the need for a thorough neuromedical work-up when catatonic signs are present. Though the current nosology does not allow for the diagnosis of catatonia in the setting of delirium, clinical experience suggests that delirium is often present in patients with catatonia. In a recent retrospective cohort analysis, encephalitis was the diagnosis most commonly associated with catatonia due to a medical condition.[15] Absence of psychiatric history and a history of seizures predicted a primary medical, as opposed to primary psychiatric, etiology. Catatonia is idiopathic in 4% to 46% of cases in various case series.[8]

Recently, attention has been drawn to cases of limbic encephalitis that are classically responsible for catatonic presentations. These can be secondary to paraneoplastic or immune causes.[16,17] Acute or subacute onset (usually of less than 12 weeks), history of a tumor, infection, autoimmune disease along with lack of psychiatric history, and evidence of central nervous system (CNS) inflammation/infection (CSF pleocytosis, protein increase, positive culture; MRI and PET findings) are helpful in considering the many paraneoplastic, autoimmune, and infectious etiologies. Serum autoantibody titers are also available and can be helpful in determining etiology. Management is directed at the causative condition and includes surgical removal of an ovarian or testicular teratoma or other offending tumors and anti-inflammatory treatments (such as medications, intravenous IgG, and plasmaphoresis). However, use of lorazepam and electroconvulsive therapy (ECT) should not be neglected as potential treatments in cases with catatonia.

Subtypes

Several subtypes of catatonia have been described. Catatonic withdrawal, or stuporous catatonia, is characterized by psychomotor slowing, whereas catatonic excitement is characterized by hyperactivity. These presentations may alternate during the course of a catatonic episode. Catatonia that is associated with fever and autonomic instability is classified as lethal or malignant catatonia. Untreated malignant catatonia is now estimated to be fatal in 10%–20% of cases.[11,18]

Kraepelin identified a "periodic" catatonia (with an onset in adolescence) characterized by intermittent excitement, followed by catatonic stupor and a remitting and relapsing course.[19] In the 1930s this disorder was further described and distinguished by the rapid onset of a manic delirium, high temperatures, catatonic stupor, and a mortality rate in excess of 50%. Cases from the pre-neuroleptic era classically began with 8 days of intense, uninterrupted motor excitement; three out of four cases were fatal.[18] In later cases, 60% of patients who received neuroleptics died. Afflicted patients were often bizarre and violent, refused to eat, and manifested intermittent mutism, posturing, catalepsy, and rigidity that alternated with excitement. When hyperactive, they were febrile, diaphoretic, and tachycardic. This stage would be followed by exhaustion, characterized by stupor and by high temperatures. Once stupor and rigidity emerged, patients were clinically indistinguishable from those with NMS.[20] Periodic catatonia has been associated with various neuromedical and psychiatric etiologies.

The excited phase of the syndrome that Kraepelin referred to as periodic catatonia appears similar in many ways to the phenomenon currently termed "delirious mania." Delirious mania has been described as a nightmarish overactive state with acute onset of disorientation, sleeplessness, amnesia, confabulation, frightening perceptual changes, bizarre behavior, agitation, echophenomena, rambling and often incoherent speech with flight of ideas sometimes alternating with short periods of mutism, negativism, and automaticity.[21]

TABLE 55-1 Modified Bush-Francis Catatonia Rating Scale

Catatonia can be diagnosed by the presence of two or more of the first 14 signs listed below.

1. Excitement	Extreme hyperactivity, and constant motor unrest, which is apparently non-purposeful. Not to be attributed to akathisia or goal-directed agitation.	
2. Immobility/stupor	Extreme hypoactivity, immobility, and minimal response to stimuli.	
3. Mutism	Verbal unresponsiveness or minimal responsiveness.	
4. Staring	Fixed gaze, little or no visual scanning of environment, and decreased blinking.	
5. Posturing/catalepsy	Spontaneous maintenance of posture(s), including mundane (e.g., sitting/standing for long periods without reacting).	
6. Grimacing	Maintenance of odd facial expressions.	
7. Echopraxia/echolalia	Mimicking of an examiner's movements/speech.	
8. Stereotypy	Repetitive, non–goal-directed motor activity (e.g., finger-play, or repeatedly touching, patting, or rubbing oneself); the act is not inherently abnormal but is repeated frequently.	
9. Mannerisms	Odd, purposeful movements (e.g., hopping or walking on tiptoe, saluting those passing by, or exaggerating caricatures of mundane movements); the act itself is inherently abnormal.	
10. Verbigeration	Repetition of phrases (like a scratched record).	
11. Rigidity	Maintenance of a rigid position despite efforts to be moved; exclude if cogwheeling or tremor is present.	
12. Negativism	Apparently motiveless resistance to instructions or attempts to move/examine the patient. Contrary behavior; one does the exact opposite of the instruction.	
13. Waxy flexibility	During reposturing of the patient, the patient offers initial resistance before allowing repositioning, similar to that of a bending candle.	
14. Withdrawal	Refusal to eat, drink, or make eye contact.	
15. Impulsivity	Sudden inappropriate behaviors (e.g., running down a hallway, screaming, or taking off clothes) without provocation. Afterward, gives no or only facile explanations.	
16. Automatic obedience	Exaggerated cooperation with the examiner's request or spontaneous continuation of the movement requested.	
17. *Mitgehen*	"Anglepoise lamp" arm raising in response to light pressure of finger, despite instructions to the contrary.	
18. *Gegenhalten*	Resistance to passive movement that is proportional to strength of the stimulus; appears automatic rather than willful.	
19. Ambitendency	The appearance of being "stuck" in indecisive, hesitant movement.	
20. Grasp reflex	Per neurologic examination.	
21. Perseveration	Repeatedly returns to the same topic or persistence with movement.	
22. Combativeness	Usually aggressive in an undirected manner, with no or only facile explanation afterward.	
23. Autonomic abnormality	Abnormal temperature, blood pressure, pulse, or respiratory rate, and diaphoresis.	

The full 23-item Bush-Francis Catatonia Rating Scale (BFCRS) measures the severity of 23 signs on a 0–3 continuum for each sign. The first 14 signs combine to form the Bush-Francis Catatonia Screening Instrument (BFCSI). The BFCSI measures only the presence or absence of the first 14 signs, and it is used for case detection. Item definitions on the two scales are the same.
From Bush G, Fink M, Petrides G, et al. Catatonia I. Rating scale and standardized examination, Acta Psychiatr Scand *93:129–136, 1996.*

Clinical Features and Diagnosis

Signs and symptoms of catatonia are outlined in Table 55-1 (the Bush-Francis Catatonia Rating Scale). Catatonia may be caused by a host of syndromes (Boxes 55-1, 55-2, 55-3, and 55-4).[22] Efforts should of course be made to identify the etiology of catatonia and treat it, if possible.

Fortunately, while no one test can confirm the diagnosis of catatonia, some studies (e.g., the electroencephalogram [EEG], neuroimaging of the brain, optokinetic and caloric testing) may help identify the etiology. A personal and family history of psychiatric illness is important, although not diagnostic.

The specific number and nature of the signs and symptoms required to make a diagnosis of catatonia remains controversial. Some authors[23] have contended that even one cardinal characteristic conveys as much clinical confidence as the presence of seven or eight characteristics and they have noted that evidence does not support a relationship among the number of catatonic features, the diagnosis, and the response to treatment. Fink and Taylor[4] considered that a minimum of two classic symptoms was sufficient to diagnose the syndrome, and, more recently, Bush and colleagues[24] developed a rating

---

BOX 55-1 Primary Psychiatric Etiologies of the Catatonic Syndrome

- Acute psychoses
- Conversion disorder
- Dissociative disorders
- Mood disorders
- Obsessive-compulsive disorder
- Personality disorders
- Schizophrenia

Most common medical conditions associated with catatonic disorder from literature review done by Carroll BT, Anfinson TJ, Kennedy JC, et al. Catatonic disorder due to general medical conditions, *J Neuropsychiatry Clin Neurosci* 6:122–133, 1994.
From Philbrick KL, Rummans TA: Malignant catatonia, J Neuropsychiatry Clin Neurosci 6:1–13, 1994.

---

scale and guidelines for the diagnosis of catatonia. They found that two or more signs identified all of their patients with catatonia (Table 55-1, Box 55-5). DSM-5 now requires the presence of three or more catatonic signs.

BOX 55-2 Neurological Etiologies of the Catatonic Syndrome

CEREBROVASCULAR
- Arterial aneurysms
- Arteriovenous malformations
- Arterial and venous thrombosis
- Bilateral parietal infarcts
- Temporal lobe infarct
- Subarachnoid hemorrhage
- Subdural hematoma
- Third ventricle hemorrhage
- Hemorrhagic infarcts

OTHER CENTRAL NERVOUS SYSTEM CAUSES
- Akinetic mutism
- Alcoholic degeneration and Wernicke's encephalopathy
- Cerebellar degeneration
- Cerebral anoxia
- Cerebromacular degeneration
- Closed head trauma

- Frontal lobe atrophy
- Hydrocephalus
- Lesions of thalamus and globus pallidus
- Narcolepsy
- Parkinsonism
- Limbic encephalitides and post-encephalitic states
- Seizure disorders
- Surgical interventions
- Tuberous sclerosis

NEOPLASM
- Angioma
- Frontal lobe tumors
- Gliomas
- Langerhans' carcinoma
- Paraneoplastic limbic encephalitis
- Periventricular diffuse pinealoma

Most common medical conditions associated with catatonic disorder from literature review done by Carroll BT, Anfinson TJ, Kennedy JC, et al. Catatonic disorder due to general medical conditions, *J Neuropsychiatry Clin Neurosci* 6:122–133, 1994.

BOX 55-3 Medical Etiologies of the Catatonic Syndrome

POISONING
- Coal gas
- Organic fluorides
- Tetraethyl lead poisoning

INFECTIONS
- Acquired immunodeficiency syndrome
- Bacterial meningoencephalitis
- Bacterial sepsis
- General paresis
- Malaria
- Mononucleosis
- Subacute sclerosing panencephalitis
- Tertiary syphilis
- Tuberculosis
- Typhoid fever
- Viral encephalitides (especially herpes)
- Viral hepatitis

METABOLIC AND OTHER MEDICAL CAUSES
- Acute intermittent porphyria
- Addison's disease

- Cushing's disease
- Diabetic ketoacidosis
- Glomerulonephritis
- Hepatic dysfunction
- Hereditary coproporphyria
- Homocystinuria
- Hyperparathyroidism

IDIOPATHIC HYPERADRENERGIC STATE
- Multiple sclerosis
- Pellagra
- Idiopathic
- Peripuerperal
- Systemic lupus erythematosus
- Thrombocytopenic purpura
- Uremia

Most common medical conditions associated with catatonic disorder from literature review done by Carroll BT, Anfinson TJ, Kennedy JC, et al. Catatonic disorder due to general medical conditions, *J Neuropsychiatry Clin Neurosci* 6:122–133, 1994.
From Philbrick KL, Rummans TA. Malignant catatonia, *J Neuropsychiatry Clin Neurosci 6:1–13, 1994.*

BOX 55-4 Drug-Related Etiologies of the Catatonic Syndrome

- Neuroleptics
- Non–neuroleptics
  - Alcohol
  - Antidepressants (tricyclics, monoamine oxidase inhibitors, and others)
  - Anticonvulsants (e.g., carbamazepine, primidone)
  - Aspirin
  - Disulfiram
  - Metoclopramide
  - Dopamine depleters (e.g., tetrabenzine)

- Dopamine withdrawal (e.g., levodopa)
- Hallucinogens (e.g., mescaline, phencyclidine, and lysergic acid diethylamide)
- Lithium carbonate
- Morphine
- Sedative-hypnotic withdrawal
- Steroids
- Stimulants
  - Amphetamines, methylphenidate, and possibly cocaine

Most common medical conditions associated with catatonic disorder from literature review done by Carroll BT, Anfinson TJ, Kennedy JC, et al. Catatonic disorder due to general medical conditions, *J Neuropsychiatry Clin Neurosci* 6:122–133, 1994.
From Philbrick KL, Rummans TA. Malignant catatonia, *J Neuropsychiatry Clin Neurosci 6:1–13, 1994.*

BOX 55-5 Standardized Examination for Catatonia

The method described here is used to complete the 23-item Bush-Francis Catatonia Rating Scale (BFCRS) and the 14-item Bush-Francis Catatonia Screening Instrument (BFCSI). Item definitions on the two scales are the same. The BFCSI measures only the presence or absence of the first 14 signs.

Ratings are based solely on observed behaviors during the examination, with the exception of completing the items for "withdrawal" and "autonomic abnormality," which may be based on directly observed behavior or chart documentation.

As a general rule, only items that are clearly present should be rated. If the examiner is uncertain as to the presence of an item, rate the item as "0."

PROCEDURE

1. Observe the patient while trying to engage in a conversation.
2. The examiner should scratch his or her head in an exaggerated manner.
3. The arm should be examined for cogwheeling. Attempt to reposture and instruct the patient to "keep your arm loose." Move the arm with alternating lighter and heavier force.

4. Ask the patient to extend his or her arm. Place one finger beneath his or her hand and try to raise it slowly after stating, "Do not let me raise your arm."
5. Extend the hand stating, "Do not shake my hand."
6. Reach into your pocket and state, "Stick out your tongue. I want to stick a pin in it."
7. Check for grasp reflex.
8. Check the chart for reports from the previous 24-hour period. Check for oral intake, vital signs, and any incidents.
9. Observe the patient indirectly, at least for a brief period each day, regarding the following:

Activity level	Waxy flexibility
Abnormal movements	*Gegenhalten*
Abnormal speech	*Mitgehen*
Echopraxia	Ambitendency
Rigidity	Automatic obedience
Negativism	Grasp reflex

From Bush G, Fink M, Petrides G, et al. Catatonia. I. Rating scale and standardized examination. Acta Psychiatr Scand 93(2):129–136, 1996.

Pathophysiology

Catatonia is thought to reflect a disruption in basal ganglia thalamocortical tracts (including the motor circuit [rigidity], the anterior cingulate/medial orbitofrontal circuit [akinetic mutism and perhaps through lateral hypothalamic connections hyperthermia and dysautonomia], and the lateral orbitofrontal circuit [imitative and repetitive behaviors]) (Figure 55-1).[25-27] Such disruption may lead to a relative state of hypodopaminergia in these circuits through reduced flow in the medial forebrain bundle, the nigrostriatal tract, and the tuberoinfundibular tract. Dopamine (DA) activity in the dorsal striatum and in the ventral striatum and paralimbic cortex is reduced, perhaps secondary to reduced $GABA_A$ inhibition of $GABA_B$ substantia nigra (SN) and ventral tegmentum (VTA) interneurons. This would explain improvement with the use of benzodiazepines, as activation at $GABA_A$ would indirectly disinhibit DA cell activity.[28,29] Support for alterations in $GABA_A$ function also comes from the observation that patients with catatonia tolerate high doses of benzodiazepines without sedation. Another possible site of pathophysiology involves reduced $GABA_A$ inhibition of frontal corticostriatal tracts leading to NMDA changes in the dorsal striatum and indirectly in the SN and VTA.[29] $GABA_A$ receptors have been shown to be decreased in the left sensorimotor cortex of patients with catatonia. Any disease process affecting the basal ganglia, thalamus, or paralimbic or frontal cortices will thus have the potential to disrupt basal ganglia-thalamocortical circuits, leading to the phenomenology of catatonia.[25]

Fink and Taylor[11] have proposed an epilepsy model of catatonia, noting the overlap of symptoms between catatonia and certain types of seizures. They suggest that electrical discharges may occur in the frontal lobes and anterior limbic system. EEG findings in catatonia sometimes include diffuse background slowing and a dysrhythmic pattern similar to that seen in nonconvulsive status epilepticus. This theory could also explain why benzodiazepines, anticonvulsants, and ECT are effective treatments, as all are also used to treat seizures.

Research on regional cerebral blood flow has shown basal ganglia asymmetry (with left-sided hyperperfusion), hypoperfusion in the left medial temporal area, and decreased perfusion in the right parietal cortex. During working memory tasks and with emotional-motor activation, the orbitofrontal cortex appears to be altered in several cases studied with functional magnetic resonance imaging (fMRI).[30]

Management and Treatment

Catatonia is accompanied by significant morbidity and mortality from systemic complications (Box 55-6). In addition, many of the physical illnesses responsible for catatonia can be dangerous. Thus, timely diagnosis and treatment are essential. If a neurological or medical condition is found, treatment for that specific illness is indicated. Box 55-7 reviews the management principles of catatonia.

Lorazepam has been found to be effective in certain cases of catatonia secondary to medical illness, and it has become the first-line treatment for catatonia regardless of etiology. In 1983, both Lew and Tollefson[31] (reporting on the usefulness of IV diazepam) and Fricchione and colleagues[32] (reporting on the benefit of IV lorazepam given to patients in neuroleptic-induced catatonic states [including NMS]) suggested the use of IV benzodiazepines in primary psychiatric catatonia. Lorazepam administered intravenously appears to provide clinical actions not shared by other benzodiazepines. Despite having a shorter elimination half-life than some other benzodiazepines, the effective clinical activity may be longer because tissue distribution is less rapid and extensive.[33] Lorazepam also demonstrates a higher binding affinity for the $GABA_A$ receptor. For these reasons, IV lorazepam also remains the treatment of choice for status epilepticus, a possibly related condition.[34]

A typical algorithm for the use of lorazepam in catatonia is outlined in Box 55-8. IV lorazepam is typically initiated with a test dose of 2 mg (with reduced dosing in the elderly or in those with respiratory compromise), and is continued at a frequency of every 8 hours around the clock, with doses held for respiratory compromise, but not for sedation. A switch to regular doses of lorazepam or diazepam may maintain the therapeutic effect following initial IV administration, though many would advocate for continued use of the IV form over at least the first 24–48 hours. If IV access is not present, intramuscular lorazepam administered in the deltoid is more reliably absorbed than with other benzodiazepines. If the

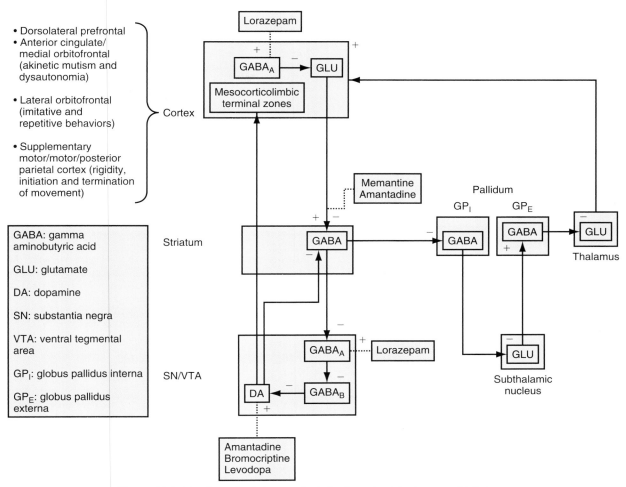

Figure 55-1. Basal ganglia thalamocortical circuits and catatonia: a candidate loop.

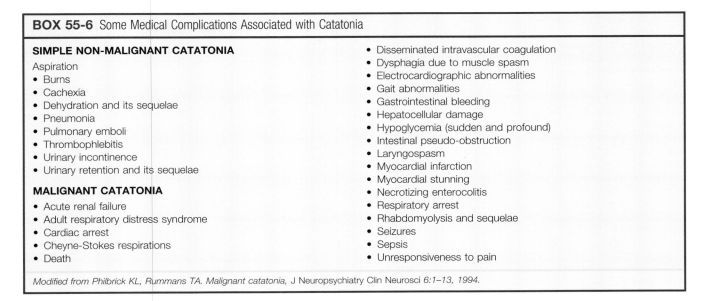

BOX 55-6 Some Medical Complications Associated with Catatonia

SIMPLE NON-MALIGNANT CATATONIA

Aspiration
- Burns
- Cachexia
- Dehydration and its sequelae
- Pneumonia
- Pulmonary emboli
- Thrombophlebitis
- Urinary incontinence
- Urinary retention and its sequelae

MALIGNANT CATATONIA
- Acute renal failure
- Adult respiratory distress syndrome
- Cardiac arrest
- Cheyne-Stokes respirations
- Death

- Disseminated intravascular coagulation
- Dysphagia due to muscle spasm
- Electrocardiographic abnormalities
- Gait abnormalities
- Gastrointestinal bleeding
- Hepatocellular damage
- Hypoglycemia (sudden and profound)
- Intestinal pseudo-obstruction
- Laryngospasm
- Myocardial infarction
- Myocardial stunning
- Necrotizing enterocolitis
- Respiratory arrest
- Rhabdomyolysis and sequelae
- Seizures
- Sepsis
- Unresponsiveness to pain

Modified from Philbrick KL, Rummans TA. Malignant catatonia, J Neuropsychiatry Clin Neurosci 6:1–13, 1994.

parenteral form is unavailable or not feasible, sublingual lorazepam is preferred. Diazepam (10 to 50 mg/day) and clonazepam (1 to 5 mg/day) also have been used successfully, as has midazolam.[35]

With clinical improvement, the dose should be gradually tapered over a matter of days, rather than abruptly stopped,

in order to prevent re-emergence of catatonia. On occasion, lorazepam must be continued for longer periods to maintain a catatonia-free state. A switch in the patient's clinical course to lorazepam-induced sedation may signal the time to taper.

Catatonia secondary to schizophrenia may be less responsive to lorazepam. In these patients, IV amantadine (available in Europe) and more recently memantine has shown some anecdotal effectiveness in isolated cases, suggesting NMDA antagonists are therapeutic in this condition.[36,37] IV amobarbital also leads to rapid resolution in some patients with catatonic stupor.[38] However, these effects tend to be short-lived. Muscle relaxants, calcium channel blockers, carbamazepine, topiramate, zonisamide, anticholinergics, lithium, thyroid medication, stimulants, and corticosteroids have each been anecdotally associated with resolution of catatonia.[22] Valproic acid and zolpidem have also been successfully used.[39,40] Oral bromocriptine has been used successfully for catatonia that preceded neuroleptic exposure.[41]

Historically, neuroleptics have been used frequently to treat catatonia, as well as the psychosis and agitation that may accompany it. However, beyond the variable response of catatonia to these drugs, neuroleptics may complicate matters, as their use has precipitated malignant catatonia and NMS.[42] Moreover, among the 292 patients with malignant catatonia reviewed by Mann and colleagues,[43] 78% of those solely treated with a neuroleptic died, compared with an overall mortality rate of 60%. While avoidance of neuroleptic medications is recommended and preferred, if antipsychotic treatment is

required, maintenance of lorazepam to buffer against catatonia re-emergence is prudent. If the catatonia has been malignant but a neuroleptic is still felt to be necessary, a waiting period of at least 2 weeks is justified, although there are no systematic studies confirming this. Before starting a neuroleptic in such a situation, use of ECT should be strongly considered.

ECT has been used to treat lupus patients with catatonia[44] and other secondary catatonias and remains the most effective treatment for catatonia.[45] ECT should be considered for patients who fail to respond fully to benzodiazepines and has been shown to be effective in cases refractory to lorazepam.[24,46] Two or three ECT treatments are usually sufficient to lyse the catatonic state in routine cases, though a course of four to six treatments is usually given to prevent relapse, and 10 to 20 treatments are sometimes needed in difficult cases, often when catatonia has lasted for more than a month. For severe forms, bilateral ECT is recommended,[24] and daily treatments are sometimes required.[11] Some 85% of catatonia cases respond to ECT.[47] Continuation of pharmacotherapy is recommended during treatment. Fatality rates of 50% or more were the rule before the introduction of ECT.[48] Because of the life-saving benefits of ECT, especially in patients with malignant catatonia, we recommend initiating consent procedures prior to a lorazepam treatment trial and commencing ECT treatment within 5 days of malignant catatonia's onset.[22]

Prognosis and Complications

In patients with catatonia, the long-term prognosis is fairly good in almost half the cases.[49] Those with an acute onset, depression, or a family history of depression have a better prognosis.[50] Periodic catatonias have good short- and long-term prognoses. Neuromedically-induced catatonias vary in prognosis in relation to their particular etiologies. Treatment with ECT offers a good short-term prognosis for most catatonias, and maintenance ECT may often improve long-term prognosis.

NEUROLEPTIC MALIGNANT SYNDROME
Epidemiology and Risk Factors

Estimates of the risk for NMS have varied widely (from 0.02% to more than 3%). Different diagnostic criteria, survey techniques, population susceptibilities, prescribing habits, and treatment settings all contribute to the variance. In one center with a large number of patients treated with antipsychotics, 1 out of every 500 to 1,000 patients was thought to develop NMS.[51] Schizophrenia, mood disorders, neuromedical "organic" brain disorders, and substance use disorders have each been associated with NMS. While NMS can occur in association with any disorder treated with a neuroleptic, presence of certain conditions may elevate the risk.

The fact that NMS is now considered by most a form of malignant catatonia suggests that many risk factors are shared with those for catatonia.[11,26] Age and gender do not appear to be reliable risk factors, though young adult males may be more prone to EPS. The fact that NMS occurs around the world suggests that environmental factors are not significant predictors. A history of catatonia is a major risk factor, as is a history of NMS, with up to one-third of patients with NMS having a subsequent episode when re-challenged. The period of withdrawal from alcohol or sedative-hypnotics may increase the risk of NMS due to aberrant thermoregulation and autonomic dysfunction. Agitation, dehydration, and exhaustion may also increase the risk for NMS. Basal ganglia disorders (e.g., Parkinson's disease, Wilson's disease, Huntington's disease, tardive dystonia) are thought to place patients

---

BOX 55-9 Diagnostic Criteria for Neuroleptic Malignant Syndrome

Treatment with neuroleptics within 7 days of onset (2–4 weeks for depot neuroleptics)
Hyperthermia (≥38°C)
Muscle rigidity
Five of the following:
1. Change in mental status
2. Tachycardia
3. Hypertension or hypotension
4. Tachypnea or hypoxia
5. Diaphoresis or sialorrhea
6. Tremor
7. Incontinence
8. Creatine phosphokinase elevation or myoglobinuria
9. Leukocytosis
10. Metabolic acidosis
Exclusion of other drug-induced, systemic, or neuropsychiatric illness

Adapted from Caroff SN, Mann SC, Lazarus A, et al. Neuroleptic malignant syndrome: diagnostic issues, Psychiatr Ann 21:130–147, 1991.

TABLE 55-2 Catatonia and Neuroleptic Malignant Syndrome: Associated Features

	NMS	Catatonia
CLINICAL SIGNS		
Hyperthermia	Yes	Often
Motor rigidity	Yes	Yes
Mutism	Often	Often
Negativism	Often	Yes
Altered consciousness	Yes	Yes
• Stupor or coma	Yes	Yes
Autonomic dysfunction	Yes	Often
• Tachypnea	Yes	Often
• Tachycardia	Yes	Often
• Abnormal BP	Yes	Yes
• Diaphoresis	Yes	Yes
LABORATORY RESULTS		
CPK elevated	Yes	Often
Serum iron reduced	Yes	Probable
Leukocytosis	Yes	Often

BP, Blood pressure; CPK, creatine phosphokinase; NMS, neuroleptic malignant syndrome.

---

at increased risk. Low serum iron levels appears to be a state-specific finding in NMS, and patients with low serum iron in the context of catatonia may be at greater risk for NMS if placed on neuroleptic medications. NMS may be caused by typical or atypical antipsychotic agents, with high-potency neuroleptics producing an elevated risk and more intense cases of NMS. It should be noted that withdrawal from antiparkinsonian agents or benzodiazepines has been reported to cause NMS-like states. Studies have not supported any particular genetic predisposition, although case reports have implicated an association with CYP 2D6.[51]

Clinical Features and Diagnosis

Philbrick and Rummans[22] suggested using the term *malignant catatonia* rather than lethal catatonia (since not all cases are lethal) to describe critically ill cases marked by autonomic instability or hyperthermia. The causes of malignant catatonia are the same as those of simple catatonia. *Pernicious catatonia* has also been used to describe this catatonic variant.[52]

NMS is characterized by autonomic dysfunction (with tachycardia and elevated blood pressure), rigidity, mutism, stupor, and hyperthermia (associated with diaphoresis), sometimes in excess of 42°C. Hyperthermia is reported in 98% of cases.[51] The rigidity can become "lead-pipe" in nature. Parkinsonian features, including cogwheel rigidity, may be present. Mental status changes occur in 97% of cases.[51] Most often patients will be in a catatonic state; such patients may be alert, delirious, stuporous, or comatose. Diagnostic criteria for NMS are found in Box 55-9,[53] and their overlap with features of catatonia are displayed in Table 55-2.

A variant of NMS, known as "atypical NMS," has been described in association with the use of atypical antipsychotics. Atypical NMS may occur without rigidity or other EPS or creatine phosphokinase (CPK) elevation.

EEGs are abnormal in roughly half of cases of NMS, most often with generalized slowing that is consistent with encephalopathy.[51] In contrast, computed tomography (CT) of the brain and cerebrospinal fluid (CSF) studies are normal in 95% of NMS cases.[51]

Most commonly, NMS develops over a few days. The course is usually self-limited, lasting from 2 days to 1 month (once

neuroleptics are stopped and supportive measures are begun).[51] Although the mortality rate has been reduced through better recognition and management, there is still an approximately 10% risk of death.[51] Myoglobinuric renal failure may have long-term consequences.

Management and Treatment

Approaches to treating malignant catatonia and NMS are similar to those used to treat catatonia. In a study of lorazepam treatment for NMS, rigidity and fever abated in 24 to 48 hours, whereas secondary features of NMS dissipated within 64 hours (without adverse effects).[54]

Philbrick and Rummans[22] reviewed 18 cases of malignant catatonia; 11 out of 13 patients treated with ECT survived, whereas only 1 out of 5 not treated with ECT survived. In terms of NMS, 39 cases of ECT treatment have been reported; 34 of them improved. The message is clear—when a patient has malignant catatonia of any type, ECT should be used expeditiously.

Adrenocorticotropic hormone and corticosteroids also have been reported to work in cases of malignant catatonia.[43] Dopaminergic agents, such as bromocriptine and amantadine, have been used successfully in NMS, though efficacy continues to be debated.[44,55]

Re-challenging a patient who has had NMS with an antipsychotic is controversial. Most investigators suggest that antipsychotics should not be given until at least 2 weeks after an episode of NMS has resolved and that re-challenge should be with an atypical antipsychotic.

SEROTONIN SYNDROME
Definition

Serotonin is involved in many psychiatric disorders. As serotonin levels become excessive, adverse CNS effects and toxicity may arise. Heightened clinical awareness is necessary to prevent and to intervene when a toxic syndrome secondary to serotonin excess emerges. Serotonin syndrome (SS) may occur in the setting of overdose on serotonergic agents or the use of multiple serotonergic agents concomitantly. Signs of SS include mental status changes (e.g., confusion, anxiety, irritability, euphoria, dysphoria), gastrointestinal symptoms (e.g., nausea, vomiting, diarrhea, incontinence), behavioral manifestations (e.g., restlessness, agitation), neurological findings (e.g., ataxia or incoordination, tremor, myoclonus, hyperreflexia, ankle clonus, muscle rigidity), and autonomic nervous system abnormalities (e.g., hypertension, hypotension, tachycardia, diaphoresis, shivering, sialorrhea, mydriasis, tachypnea, hyperthermia).[56,57]

Epidemiology

The incidence of SS is unknown. There are no data to suggest that gender differences confer any particular vulnerability to the syndrome. Given the overlap of symptoms with NMS, SS is often mistaken for it and thus may be underreported. The existence of the syndrome in varying degrees also may confound its recognition, as can unawareness on the part of the majority of physicians.[57] SS occurs most often in individuals being treated with psychotropics. It occurs in about 14% to 16% of selective serotonin reuptake inhibitor (SSRI) overdose patients.[58]

Clinical Features and Diagnosis

As with NMS, taking a detailed history is crucial. Use of two or more serotonergic agents confers a greater risk of developing SS. Obtaining a history of neuroleptic use is especially important because NMS shares many clinical features with SS.

Based on his review of 38 cases, Sternbach[59] proposed the first operational definition of the syndrome in humans. According to this schema (in addition to at least three of the following features: mental status changes, agitation, myoclonus, hyperreflexia, diaphoresis, shivering, tremor, diarrhea, and incoordination), diagnosis requires: an increase in, or addition of, a serotonergic agent to an established medication regimen; other etiologies to be ruled out; and that a neuroleptic must not have been started or increased in dosage before the onset of the signs and symptoms previously listed.

Keck and Arnold[56] modified Sternbach's criteria to include restlessness, autonomic nervous system dysfunction, hyperthermia, and muscle rigidity. Hunter Serotonin Toxicity Criteria have also been proposed.[60] Under these criteria, SS can be diagnosed in the setting of recent serotonergic drug exposure with any of the following symptom combinations: spontaneous clonus alone; either inducible or ocular clonus and either agitation or diaphoresis; either inducible or ocular clonus and hypertonicity and temperature greater than 38°C; tremor and hyperreflexia. This approach to SS diagnosis may be more sensitive to serotonin toxicity and less prone to produce false-positive cases.

A temporal relationship between the start of pharmacotherapy and the development of the syndrome exists. The syndrome ranges from mild to severe, with a mildly affected patient showing restlessness, tremor, tachycardia, shivering, diaphoresis, and the start of hyperreflexia. Moderate cases will show tachycardia, hypertension, fever (sometimes as high as 40°C), mydriasis, strong bowel sounds, hyperreflexia, and clonus (greater in the lower extremities than in the upper ones). Horizontal ocular clonus will also be seen in moderate cases, and there will be mental status changes of agitation, pressured speech, and autonomic hyperactivity. Head rotation movement with neck extension has also been reported. In severe cases, there will be severe autonomic hyperactivity and severe hyperthermia with temperatures sometimes over 41.1°C. There is an agitated delirium accompanied by severe muscular rigidity. This severe hypertonicity may obscure the appearance of clonus and hyperreflexia and thereby confound the diagnosis.

Laboratory abnormalities are mostly non-specific or are secondary to the medical complications of the syndrome. A complete laboratory evaluation is nevertheless essential to rule out other etiologies. Leukocytosis, rhabdomyolysis, and liver function test abnormalities have all been reported in SS, along with hyponatremia, hypomagnesemia, and hypocalcemia. It is thought that these latter disturbances are related to fluid and electrolyte abnormalities.

It is interesting to note that certain secreting tumors (e.g., carcinoid, small cell carcinoma) have been associated with SS. Therefore, X-ray examinations and imaging of the abdomen and lungs may sometimes be helpful in working up SS. An EEG and neuroimaging of the brain are often useful in uncovering a seizure disorder or another neurological condition. Drugs associated with SS are included in Box 55-10. MAOI–SSRI combinations are most commonly implicated. Because of the potential problems of using an MAOI and any medicine with serotonergic properties, caution on the part of the prescribing physician is required. With this in mind, a 2-week washout interval is required following discontinuation of an MAOI before starting any serotonergic medication. In the case of fluoxetine discontinuation, there should be a minimum 5-week washout period before an MAOI is initiated.

Pathophysiology

From both animal and human studies, the role of 5-HT has been implicated in the pathogenesis of SS. Nucleus raphe serotonin nuclei (located in the midbrain and arrayed in the midline down to the medulla) are involved in mediating thermoregulation, appetite, nausea, vomiting, wakefulness, migraine, sexual activity, and affective behavior. Ascending serotonergic projections are likely to play a role in the presentation of SS, particularly in the development of hyperthermia, mental status, and autonomic changes. The 5-HT_{2A}[58] and 5-HT_{1A} receptors appear to be overactive in this condition. There also appears to be CNS norepinephrine (noradrenaline) overactivity, and clinical outcomes may be associated with hypersympathetic tone.[57] The roles of catecholamines and 5-HT_2 and 5-HT_3 receptor interactions are unclear, as are the contributions of glutamate, GABA, and DA.

Management and Treatment

No prospective studies have looked at treatment of SS and recommendations remain anecdotal. SS is often self-limited, and removal of the offending agents will frequently result in resolution of symptoms within 24 hours. The next step is to provide supportive measures to prevent potential medical complications. These supportive measures include the use of antipyretics and cooling blankets (to reduce hyperthermia), monitoring and support of the respiratory and cardiovascular systems, IV hydration (to prevent renal failure), use of benzodiazepines (for myoclonic jerking), use of anticonvulsants (if seizures arise), and use of antihypertensive agents (for significantly elevated blood pressures). In severe cases with very high temperatures, patients should be intubated, sedated, and paralyzed. The syndrome rarely leads to respiratory failure. When it does, it usually is because of aspiration, and artificial ventilation may then be required.

Management (with benzodiazepines) of agitation, even when mild, is essential in the SS. Benzodiazepines, such as diazepam and lorazepam, can reduce autonomic tone and temperature and thus may have positive effects on survival.[57] Physical restraints should be avoided if at all possible because muscular stress can lead to lactic acidosis and to elevated temperature.

Specific 5-HT receptor antagonism has occasionally been advocated for the treatment or prevention of the symptoms associated with SS. Cyproheptadine, a 5-HT_{2A} antagonist, has been recommended.[57] Mirtazapine, a 5-HT_3 and 5-HT_2

BOX 55-10 Central Nervous System Serotonergic Agents

ENHANCED SEROTONIN SYNTHESIS
- L-Tryptophan

INCREASED SEROTONIN RELEASE
- Amphetamines
- Cocaine
- Dextromethorphan
- Fenfluramine
- Meperidine
- 3,4-Methylenedioxymethamphetamine (MDMA, "ecstasy")
- Sibutramine

SEROTONIN AGONISTS
- Buspirone
- Dihydroergotamine (DHE)
- Lithium
- Meta-chlorophenylpiperazine (mCPP)
- Sumatriptan
- Trazodone
- Vilazodone

INHIBITED SEROTONIN CATABOLISM
- Isocarboxazid
- Linezolid
- Moclobemide
- Phenelzine
- Selegiline
- Tranylcypromine

INHIBITED SEROTONIN REUPTAKE
- Amitriptyline
- Bromocriptine
- Citalopram
- Clomipramine
- Desipramine
- Dextromethorphan
- Escitalopram
- Fenfluramine
- Fluoxetine
- Fluvoxamine
- Imipramine
- Meperidine
- Methadone
- Mirtazapine
- Nefazodone
- Nortriptyline
- Olanzapine
- Paroxetine
- Pethidine
- Quetiapine
- Sertraline
- Tramadol
- Trazodone
- Venlafaxine
- Vilazodone

Modified from Keck PE, Arnold LM. The serotonin syndrome, Psychiatr Ann 30:336, 2000.

antagonist, has also been used in a small number of cases. For hypertension, nitroprusside and nifedipine, and for tachycardia, esmolol, have been advocated.[57] Since the rise in temperature is muscular in origin, antipyretics are of no use in SS, and paralytics are required when fever is high.

Prognosis and Complications

Typically, SS starts usually within hours of medication initiation, a dose increase, or overdose. SS will continue as long as the serotonergic agents remain in the system. Severe SS can lead to death from medical complications.

In SS, rhabdomyolysis is the most common and serious complication; it occurs in roughly one-fourth of cases.[51] Generalized seizures occur in approximately 10%, with 39% of these patients dying. Myoglobinuric renal failure accounts for roughly 5% of medical complications, as does diffuse intravascular coagulation (DIC). Unfortunately, nearly two-thirds of patients with DIC die.

Access the complete reference list and multiple choice questions (MCQs) online at https://expertconsult.inkling.com

KEY REFERENCES
4. Fink M. Catatonia: a separate category in DSM-IV? *Integr Psychiatry* 7(25):1991.
6. Francis A, Fink M, Appiani F, et al. Catatonia in diagnostic and statistical manual of mental disorders, fifth edition. *J ECT* 26(4):246–247, 2010.
8. Caroff SNMS, Campbell EC, Sullivan KA. *Epidemiology*, Washington, DC, 2004, American Psychiatric Publishing.
9. Braunig P, Kruger S, Shugar G. Prevalence and clinical significance of catatonic symptoms in mania. *Compr Psychiatry* 39(1):35–46, 1998.
11. Fink M. *Catatonia: a clinician's guide to diagnosis and treatment*, Cambridge, UK, 2003, Cambridge University Press.
18. Mann SC, Caroff SN, Bleier HR, et al. Lethal catatonia. *Am J Psychiatry* 143(11):1374–1381, 1986.
20. Caroff SN. The neuroleptic malignant syndrome. *J Clin Psychiatry* 41(3):79–83, 1980.
22. Philbrick KL, Rummans TA. Malignant catatonia. *J Neuropsychiatry Clin Neurosc* 6(1):1–13, 1994.
23. Taylor MA. Catatonia: a review of a behavioral neurologic syndrome. *Neuropsychiatry Neuropsychol Behav Neurol* 3:48–72, 1990.
24. Bush G, Fink M, Petrides G, et al. Catatonia. I. Rating scale and standardized examination. *Acta Psychiatr Scand* 93(2):129–136, 1996.
26. Mann SC, Fricchione GL, Campbell EC, et al. *Malignant catatonia*, Washington, DC, 2004, American Psychiatric Publishing.
29. Fricchione GL, Bush G, Fozdar M, et al. Recognition and treatment of the catatonic syndrome. *J Intensive Care Med* 12:135–147, 1997.
30. Northoff G. *Neuroimaging and neurophysiology*, Washington, DC, 2004, American Psychiatric Publishing.
47. Hawkins JM, Archer KJ, Strakowski SM, et al. Somatic treatment of catatonia. *Int J Psychiatry Med* 25(4):345–369, 1995.
49. Levenson JL. *Prognosis and complications*, Washington, DC, 2004, American Psychiatric Publishing.
53. Caroff SN, Mann SC, Lazarus A, et al. Neuroleptic malignant syndrome: diagnostic issues. *Psychiatr Ann* 21:130–147, 1991.
55. Caroff SN, Mann SC. Neuroleptic malignant syndrome. *Med Clin North Am* 77(1):185–202, 1993.
56. Keck PE. The serotonin syndrome. *Psychiatr Ann* 30:333–343, 2000.
57. Boyer EW, Shannon M. The serotonin syndrome. *N Engl J Med* 352(11):1112–1120, 2005.

56 Psycho-oncology: Psychiatric Co-morbidities and Complications of Cancer and Cancer Treatment

Carlos Fernandez-Robles, MD, Donna B. Greenberg, MD, and William F. Pirl, MD, MPH

KEY POINTS

- By exploring the patient's capacity to consider choices, psychiatrists convey respect and enhance the patient's conviction of influence on the world. The sense of purpose adds value to life regardless of time frame. Additional psychosocial interventions combine education, relaxation skills, and social support.

- So that treatable psychiatric syndromes do not interfere with quality cancer care, psychiatrists diagnose and plan specific treatment. They also may use stimulants for fatigue, tranquilizers for nausea, and antidepressants for hot flushes.

- In patients with cancer, major depressive disorder is associated with poor quality of life, worse adherence to treatment, longer hospital stays, greater desire for death, and an increased suicide and mortality rate.

- Delirium in patients with cancer results from infection, opiates, recent surgery, hyponatremia, hypercalcemia, brain tumors, and leptomeningeal disease. Specific causes of delirium may be associated with specific cancers, hyperviscosity syndrome, Cushing's syndrome, paraneoplastic encephalomyelitis, and limbic encephalitis.

- Neuropsychiatric cancer-drug-induced side effects are most associated with biologicals, steroids, and interferon. White matter injury from chemotherapy and central nervous system radiation can cause learning difficulties and behavioral syndromes in survivors.

THE ROLE OF PSYCHIATRY IN THE CARE OF CANCER PATIENTS

The seriousness of the diagnosis of cancer challenges the capacity to survive, to set a course in life, and to fulfill hopes and dreams. Over the twentieth century, even as cancer treatments improved and some patients were cured, psychiatrists in the tradition of humane psychiatry used their skills to stand by patients who were overwhelmed, to help them to speak in their own voices, to make complex treatment choices, and to shape the rest of their life or the end of life. Psychiatrists have offered expert diagnosis and management of co-morbid psychiatric syndromes and collaborated with oncologists so that treatable psychiatric illness does not stand in the way of technical oncological care. Specific cancer-related or cancer-treatment-related neuropsychiatric syndromes (Boxes 56-1 to 56-4)[1-5] can be recognized and treated. Psychiatrists can help patients to cope with physical symptoms, developmental losses, changes in relationships, and the effects of cancer on families.

Since Weisman and co-workers explored how to help patients cope with cancer when they are demoralized,[6-8] psychiatrists have tried to understand who the patient was before

the diagnosis and the nature of the existential predicament. The psychiatric interview can assess the personal past, present plight, anticipated future, regrets, salient concerns, physical symptoms, disabilities, coping strategies, and psychiatric vulnerability (Table 56-1).[7]

Denial and "Middle Knowledge"

Patients often seem to know and want to know about the gravity of their illness, yet they often talk as if they do not know and do not want to be reminded about their cancer.[9] Weisman used the expression "middle knowledge" for the space between open acknowledgment of death and its utter repudiation. Patients may deny facets, implications, or mortal threat of an illness.[9] Middle knowledge is most apparent at transition points (such as a recurrence of cancer). However, denial is an unstable state, almost impossible to maintain against even the reluctant patient's inner perceptions. To preserve a relationship, patients often deny their knowledge of impending death to different people at different times.[10] Tactful discussion of mortality allows patients to be responsive to those most close as long as possible.[9]

Hope and the Doctor–Patient Relationship

Physicians convey respect by exploring the patient's capacity to cope. That respect allows the patient to nurture courage and resiliency.[11] Trust between the patient and the physician is borne out of mutual respect. Patients regain a sense of control as they appraise and re-appraise what choices to make. Presenting the facts about an illness does not break trust between a patient and a doctor. Furthermore, hope is not merely related to prognosis. The patient's capacity to hope is also related to an ego ideal and to the conviction of one's influence on the world. As the physician sustains the patient's self-esteem, a sense of purpose adds value to life regardless of the time frame. The psychiatrist's capacity to listen to a patient in a non-judgmental way allows patients to express doubts and weaknesses, to accept who they are and why they see things as they do. The physician's presence there protects patients from abandonment and offers a place where they can explore what is meaningful.[11,12]

Medical Choices

The psychiatrist also clarifies with the patient the medical understanding of what choices are feasible. Unfazed by personal shock, anxiety, and denial, and armed with a medical education, the psychiatrist is in an excellent position to understand (better than the patient) the individualized medical plan. Diagnosis, treatment, and prognostic decisions are complex as set forth by medical experts. As the psychiatrist learns how the patient thinks, and if necessary, adds appropriate psychopharmacological treatment for symptoms or Axis I diagnoses, the psychiatrist can maintain a focus on necessary anticancer treatments that are most likely to give the best outcome. Focusing on problems, setting priorities, making clear what the patient is doing and not doing about

---

BOX 56-1 Neuropsychiatric Side Effects of Cancer Drugs

HORMONES[1]

Anti-estrogens

Tamoxifen, toremifene: hot flushes, insomnia, mood disturbance; at high doses tamoxifen can cause confusion

Anastrazole (Arimidex), letrozole (Femara), exemestane (Aromacin): hot flushes, fatigue, mood swings, and irritability; cognitive effects are not known

Raloxifene (Evista): no cognitive side effects noted

Leuprolide (Lupron), goserelin (Zoladex): hot flushes, fatigue, and mood disturbance

Androgen Blockade

Leuprolide (Lupron), goserelin (Zoladex): hot flushes, fatigue, and mood disturbance

Flutamide (Eulexin), bicalutamide (Casodex), nilutamide (Nilandron): as above

Glucocorticoids

Dose-related, variable psychiatric side effects including insomnia, hyperactivity, hyperphagia, depression, hypomania, irritability, and psychosis

Treated by *ad hoc* antipsychotics easily with cancer patients

Other drugs with benefit: lithium, valproate, lamotrigine, and mifepristone

Dexamethasone (Decadron) 9 mg equals 60 mg of prednisone; psychiatric side effects are associated with this dose level

Steroids used as part of an antiemetic treatment with chemotherapy infusion, with lymphoma protocols as high as prednisone 100 mg for 5 days, with nervous system radiation treatment to reduce swelling, with taxanes to reduce side effects

---

BOX 56-2 Biologicals

INTERFERON-ALPHA[2,3]

Depression, cognitive impairment, hypomania, psychosis, fatigue, and malaise

Responsive to antidepressants, hypnotics, antipsychotics, stimulants, and antianxiety agents

Associated with autoimmune thyroiditis that may increase or decrease thyroxine; check thyroid function

May inhibit metabolism of some antidepressants by P450 enzymes CYP1A2, CYP2C19, CYP2D6

Interferon-beta has less neurotoxicity

INTERLEUKIN-2

Delirium, flu-like syndrome, dose-dependent neurotoxicity, and hypothyroidism

---

BOX 56-3 Chemotherapy

VINCRISTINE (ONCOVIN), VINBLASTINE (VELBAN), VINORELBINE (NAVELBINE)

Neurotoxicity is dose-related and usually reversible. Fatigue and malaise are noted. Seizure and SIADH are uncommon. Postural hypotension may be an aspect of autonomic neuropathy.

Less toxicity is noted with vinblastine and vinorelbine.

PROCARBAZINE (MATULANE)

Mild reversible delirium, depression, and encephalopathy

A weak MAO inhibitor

Antidepressant use must consider the timing of procarbazine or risk serious interactions

Disulfiram-like effect; avoid alcohol

ASPARAGINASE (ELSPAR)

Depression, lethargy, and delirium with treatment

CYTARABINE (ARA-CELL, ALEXIN)

High-dose IV treatment (over 18 g/m^2/course) can cause confusion, obtundation, seizures and coma, cerebellar dysfunction, and leukoencephalopathy. Older patients with multiple treatments are more susceptible. Delirium and somnolence can be seen 2–5 days into treatment. Those with renal impairment are more vulnerable.

FLUDARABINE (FLUDARA)

Rare somnolence, delirium, and rare progressive leukoencephalopathy

5-FLUOROURACIL (5-FU)

The primary neurotoxicity is cerebellar, but encephalopathy with headache, confusion, disorientation, lethargy, and seizures has also been seen.

Rare deficiency of enzyme that metabolizes dihydropyrimidine dehydrogenase (DPD) is associated with greater exposure and more toxicity.

Fatigue is the most common side effect.

Cerebellar syndrome and rarely seizure or confusion or parkinsonism may be noted.

High-dose IV thymidine may be an antidote for toxicity.

CAPECITABINE (XELODA)

Related to 5-FU, but with less neurotoxicity

METHOTREXATE

Causes neurotoxicity particularly when the route is intrathecal or high-dose IV (usually over 1 g/m^2). The toxicity, which is usually reversible, is related to peak level and duration of exposure. Leptomeningeal disease or other conditions that break the blood–brain barrier may impair drug clearance. Prolonged exposure allows the drug to pass through the ependyma of the ventricles to cause leukoencephalopathy. The risk is greater in patients also exposed to cranial radiation. Intrathecal methotrexate may also cause seizures, motor dysfunction, chemical arachnoiditis, and coma. Serum levels are followed closely; folinic acid (leucovorin) rescue is an antidote. Alkalinization may lower the serum level.

There is a dose- and route-related risk of delirium.

BOX 56-3 Chemotherapy (continued)

PEMETREXED (ALIMTA)

An antifolate given with supplements of folate, intramuscular vitamin B_{12}, and dexamethasone. It is associated with a 10% rate of depression and fatigue.

GEMCITABINE (GEMSAR)

Fatigue, flu-like syndrome, and a rare autonomic neuropathy

ETOPOSIDE (EPOSIN)

Postural hypotension and rare disorientation

CARMUSTINE (BCNU)

Delirium, only at high dose, rare leukoencephalopathy
Thiotepa
Rare leukoencephalopathy

IFOSFAMIDE (IFEX)

Transient delirium, lethargy, seizures, drunkenness, parkinsonism, and cerebellar signs that improve within days of treatment
Risk factors: liver and kidney impairment
Hyponatremia
Leukoencephalopathy
Thiamine or methylene blue may be antidotes

CISPLATIN

Rare reversible posterior leukoencephalopathy, parietal, occipital, frontal with cortical blindness.
Peripheral neuropathy, poor proprioception, and rarely autonomic
Hypomagnesemia secondary to renal wasting
Vitamin E (300 mg), amifostine may limit peripheral toxicity
Hearing is decreased due to dose-related sensorineural hearing loss

CARBOPLATIN

Neurotoxicity only at high doses

OXALIPLATIN (ELOXATIN)

Acute dysesthesias of hands, feet, perioral region, jaw tightness, and pharyngo-laryngodysesthesias

PACLITAXEL (TAXOL)

Sensory peripheral neuropathy not worse with continued treatment
Rarely seizures and transient encephalopathy, and motor neuropathy
Given with steroids

DOCETAXEL (TAXOTERE)

Like paclitaxel but less neurotoxicity

IV, Intravenous; MAO, monoamine oxidase; SIADH, syndrome of inappropriate antidiuretic hormone.

BOX 56-4 Inhibitors of Kinase Signaling Enzymes[4,5]

The newest class of medications, specific inhibitors of kinase signaling enzymes, do not typically cause major behavioral side effects. However, their toxicity related to overlapping effects on several kinase pathways has not been fully defined. Hypertension has been an important side effect related to inhibition of the vascular endothelial growth factor (VEGF). Asthenia or feelings of weakness are commonly reported.

IMATINIB (GLEEVEC)

Can cause fluid retention and fatigue, rarely low phosphate; confusion and papilledema

SUNITINIB (SUTENT)

Hypothyroidism, TSH should be checked every 3 months

SORAFENIB (NEXAVAR)

Fatigue and asthenia and rarely hypophosphatemia

BEVACIZUMAB (AVASTIN)

A monoclonal antibody that blocks VEGF-binding, causes fatigue, and rarely causes reversible posterior leukoencephalopathy

THALIDOMIDE

Drowsiness and somnolence improve over 2–3 weeks, dose-related, associated with dizziness, orthostatic hypotension, tremor, loss of libido, hypothyroidism, and rarely confusion

BORTEZOMIB (VELCADE)

Postural hypotension and asthenia; confusion, psychosis, and suicidal thoughts have been reported

RITUXIMAB (RITUXAN)

Headache and dizziness

TRASTUZUMAB (HERCEPTIN)

Headache, insomnia, and dizziness

TSH, Thyroid-stimulating hormone.

---

a problem, and exploring strategies are key elements of care. This technique allows patients to make the decisions that are most critical to them. Meanwhile, the psychiatrist, in collaboration with oncology staff, sorts through differential diagnoses as new psychological symptoms develop and the medical condition and treatment progress. The psychiatric assessment includes evaluation of physical symptoms, psychiatric diagnosis, and the differential diagnosis. The work includes education about how to support significant others and how to allow help or to relinquish control to those who have shown themselves trustworthy. The goal of honest communication is to support acceptance, to reduce bitterness, and to replace denial with the courage to confront what cannot be changed.[10]

Distress

Emotional distress is common following cancer diagnosis and its treatment; it is estimated that 25% of outpatient cancer patients experience significant psychological distress, and it occurs in up to 60% of those receiving specialist palliative care.[13] The National Comprehensive Cancer Network (NCCN) Distress Management Guidelines Panel defines distress as "a multifactorial unpleasant emotional experience of a psychological (cognitive, behavioral, emotional), social, and/or spiritual nature that may interfere with the ability to cope effectively with cancer, its physical symptoms and its treatment. Distress extends along a continuum, ranging from common and normal feelings of vulnerability, sadness, and

TABLE 56-1 Concerns of Patients with Specific Cancer Types

Cancer Type	Likely Concerns
Prostate cancer	Significance of serum prostate-specific antigen (PSA) test results: anxiety Once diagnosed, the initial choices are watchful waiting, surgery, or radiation treatment Side effects of surgery or radiation: incontinence or erectile dysfunction Sexual function and dysfunction Androgen blockade and its effects on fatigue and loss of sexual interest
Breast cancer	Body image related to mastectomy or to reconstruction Adjuvant chemotherapy and its side effects: alopecia, weight gain, fatigue, and impaired concentration Menopausal symptoms: insomnia, sexual dysfunction, and hot flushes related to adjuvant treatment, antiestrogens, or aromatase inhibitors The question of prophylactic mastectomy Sexuality and fertility (or infertility)
Colon cancer	Adjustment to surgery or an ostomy Body image and sexual function Bowel dysfunction
Lung cancer	Physical limitations of reduced lung capacity Post-thoracotomy neuralgia Cough Guilt about nicotine addiction (past and present)
Ovarian cancer	Anxiety about the tumor marker CA125 Sexual dysfunction and infertility Pain and recurrent bowel obstruction
Pancreatic cancer	Maintenance of adequate nutrition Poor appetite Bowel function (and the need for pancreatic enzymes and laxatives) Pain Diabetes Depressed mood
Head and neck cancer	Facial deformity Dry mouth Poor nutrition A weak voice and difficulty with communication Post-treatment hypothyroidism Alcohol and nicotine dependency
Lymphoma	Corticosteroid-induced mood changes The need for recurrent chemotherapy and its effects
Hodgkin's disease	Post-treatment hypothyroidism Fatigue
Osteosarcoma	Amputation/prosthesis vs. bone graft Impaired mobility Post-thoracotomy neuralgia

fears to problems that can become disabling, such as depression, anxiety, panic, social isolation, and existential and spiritual crisis."[14] Underlying psychopathology, limited financial and social support, substance abuse, troubled relationships, and burden from illness have been associated with higher levels of distress.[15] Weisman and associates found that vulnerable patients were unable to generate alternative coping strategies, and tend to overuse strategies that are ineffective for finding relief and resolution.[7] They defined a treatment to reduce distress, to correct deficits in coping, to reclaim personal control, and to improve morale and self-esteem. Patients were asked to examine their plight in relation to cancer (their current concerns); to articulate their understanding of what might interfere with good coping; and by looking beyond, to use options that were feasible for finding satisfactory solutions. Staff took the view that change was possible and that patients could be helped to take steps on their own behalf, as problems were broken down into manageable proportions. They focused on coping and adaptation rather than on psychopathology; they conveyed an expectation of positive change, a sense that options and alternatives are seldom completely exhausted, and an awareness that flexibility in perceiving problems helps to attain additional information and support. They compared a brief psychodynamic and behavioral technique; both were effective in reducing distress and denial.[7]

Screening

Starting in 2015, cancer programs seeking accreditation from the American College of Surgeons Commission on Cancer will be required to offer cancer patients screening for distress a minimum of one time per patient at a pivotal medical visit and link patients in distress with psychosocial services offered on-site or by referral.[16] The widely used distress thermometer, a simple visual nomogram developed by the NCCD, serves as a rough initial single-item question screen, which identifies distress arising from any source, even if unrelated to cancer.[17] Tools such as the Weisman and Worden's Omega instrument help identify patients at risk for psychosocial vulnerability and ineffective coping.[7] More efficient tools such as the Brief Symptom Inventory (BSI) and the General Health Questionnaire (GHQ) can help identify those with more somatic symptoms.[18,19]

Psychosocial Interventions

In addition to trying to extend survival, the oncology community increasingly recognizes the value of considering how well people live.[20] A principal goal of psychosocial care is to recognize and address the effects that cancer and its treatment have on mental status and emotional well-being of patients.[21] Analyses of clinical trials implementing psychosocial interventions, such as educational programs, cognitive-behavioral therapy, supportive-expressive group therapy, relaxation training and mindfulness, have been shown to reduce distress, positively impact medical outcome, alleviate symptoms, such as pain and fatigue, and overall improve patients' quality of life.[22-25] A Cochrane Database review on psychosocial interventions for women with metastatic breast cancer found it was not only effective in reducing distress symptoms but could also improve 12-month survival rates.[26] As a strategy to improve the quality of psychosocial care provided, large cancer centers (e.g., Memorial Sloan-Kettering Cancer Center and Massachusetts General Hospital) have created integrative care programs that facilitate on-site access to complementary alternative services.[27,28]

ANXIETY SYNDROMES

Anxiety is part of the emotional reaction that accompanies a diagnosis of cancer. The roller coaster ride of life-threatening experiences and uncertainty associated with cancer treatment parallels the unpredictable aversive stimuli that provoke conditioned helplessness and depression.[29] A common mistake among patients and providers is to consider anxiety as normal even when it is both excessive and significantly impairing. Clinically-significant anxiety is present in up to 34% of cancer patients.[30] A history of anxiety predisposes individuals to reactivating premorbid anxiety following a diagnosis of cancer.[31,32]

Anxiety as a symptom can arise from a wide variety of causes. In oncology patients it can be classified in four separate categories: situational anxiety, organic anxiety, psychiatric anxiety, and existential anxiety.[33] Patients anticipate the results of cancer markers and scans; their mood rises and falls with the results or news of progressive disease.[34] Most patients are alert to physical symptoms after treatment and worry that such symptoms signify recurrent disease. A visit to the doctor can be reassuring for most; but for some, the alarm of danger does not turn off. They remain preoccupied with fear, as every symptom signals cancer recurrence. Metabolic derangements, such as hypercalcemia and hypoglycemia,[35] hypoxia related to parenchymal or mediastinal disease, pulmonary embolism, pleural effusions or pulmonary edema,[36] structural brain lesions leading to complex partial seizures,[37] and side effects of medications, such as steroids and antiemetics, can be all misdiagnosed as anxiety.[38] Pre-existing psychiatric disorders can be activated by cancer and its care. Claustrophobia becomes clinically important when magnetic resonance imaging (MRI) is required for careful physical evaluation or when patients are trapped in bed by orthopedic care (e.g., a repair of a leg with osteogenic sarcoma). Needle phobias, which can be problematic, may be treated with rapid desensitization.[39]

Post-traumatic stress disorder (PTSD) is uncommon (occurring in 3% to 10%) in patients treated for cancer[40]; however, Pitman and colleagues[41] have shown that women with breast cancer have a physiological response 2 years after hearing a narrative of the two most stressful experiences during their cancer. Leukemia survivors who developed anticipatory nausea with treatment are also more apt to become nauseated in response to reminders of their treatment.[42] Specific cancer-related symptoms (e.g., embarrassment related to unexpected diarrhea) can contribute to anticipatory anxiety and agoraphobia. Disability and poor quality of life have also been associated with co-morbid anxiety disorders and physical conditions.[43]

The management of anxiety symptoms should include both pharmacologic and non-pharmacologic interventions. Antidepressant medications suppress the chronic state of alarm and reduce chronic anxiety. Benzodiazepines are best used for specific anxiety-provoking procedures. Cognitive-behavioral therapy and stress management offer patients the opportunity to learn adaptive skills for coping with stressors.[44]

Nausea and Vomiting

Approximately one half of cancer patients will experience nausea or vomiting during the course of their disease either because of the cancer itself or because of their treatment.[45] Delayed nausea, which comes after the first days of chemotherapy, significantly compromises quality of life even more than vomiting does.[46] As a result of vomiting during chemotherapy, patients can develop conditioned nausea and anxiety associated with the smells and sights linked with treatment. They may have nausea and vomit even before arriving at the hospital for treatment.[47] Anticipatory nausea and vomiting are more likely to occur in younger patients, in those who have had more emetic treatments, and in those who have trait anxiety.[47] Conditioned nausea morphs into anticipatory anxiety, insomnia, and aversion to treatment. The best treatment for anticipatory nausea is the control of chemotherapy-induced nausea and vomit (CINV).[48] Addition of neurokinin 1 receptor antagonists to 5-hydroxytryptamine-$_3$ [5-HT$_3$] receptor antagonists and/or steroids significantly reduce the occurrence of CINV.[49] Hypnosis, cognitive-behavioral techniques, and antianxiety agents (e.g., alprazolam or lorazepam) can reduce phobic responses, as well as anticipatory nausea and vomiting (both during and after chemotherapy).[50]

DEPRESSION

In people with cancer, MDD is associated with poor quality of life, worse adherence to treatment, longer hospital stays, greater desire for death, and an increased suicide and mortality rate.[51-54] Reports of its prevalence (10% to 25%) in people with cancer have varied widely.[55] People with histories of MDD are more likely to develop MDD after the diagnosis of cancer, but about half of the cases occur in people without a history of MDD.[56]

As in people without cancer, the diagnosis of MDD is made with DSM-5 criteria. However, the diagnosis can be complicated by symptoms that overlap with cancer and cancer treatments. To address this issue, alternative criteria have been proposed, such as the Endicott criteria, that suggest somatic symptoms (e.g., anorexia, insomnia, fatigue) be replaced by non-somatic symptoms (e.g., tearfulness, social withdrawal, self-pity).[57] The Hospital Anxiety and Depression Scale (HADS) is a valid instrument in the assessment of emotional distress in cancer patients and follows a similar approach.[58]

Similar to the evaluation of other medically ill patients who appear depressed, it is critical to consider possible medical contributions in the differential diagnosis. Untreated pain, hypothyroidism, and medications, such as corticosteroids and chemotherapies (e.g., alpha interferon, pemetrexed, and taxane drugs) may contribute to MDD. Delirium, especially the hypoactive subtype, can be mistaken for depression. Although mood symptoms occur as part of delirium, key features include a generalized impairment of attention and cognition, a waxing and waning severity of symptoms, and a sleep–wake disturbance. Fatigue is a common cancer-related symptom that is prevalent and that can be difficult to tease apart from MDD. Anhedonia may be the best distinguishing factor for MDD.[58] Apathy (e.g., that results from a lesion in the frontal lobes) can also be reminiscent of MDD. With apathy there are delayed responses, cognitive impairment, and a loss of spontaneous action or speech.

The treatment (primarily consisting of antidepressant medications and/or psychotherapy) of MDD in people with cancer is based on the treatment of MDD in people without medical co-morbidity. Severe cases of MDD, especially those with wasting because of MDD, may be treated with electroconvulsive therapy (ECT). Although complementary treatments (such as herbal preparations, acupuncture, and massage) are available, there are currently few data on their efficacy for treating MDD in cancer patients.[59]

While antidepressants are commonly used to treat MDD that is co-morbid with cancer, placebo-controlled trials of their efficacy in cancer are scarce. A recent meta-analysis focusing exclusively on pharmacological interventions, reported that treatment with antidepressants was found to improve depressive symptoms more than placebo.[60] Furthermore, it found that subsyndromal depressive symptoms may improve with antidepressants as well.[60] When using antidepressants, close attention should be paid to side effects, such as gastrointestinal and anticholinergic effects, as they can worsen pre-existing conditions. Often antidepressant medications are chosen for their side-effect profile (such as sedation or increased appetite), which may be desirable in some cases. Some of the selective serotonin reuptake inhibitors (SSRIs) (e.g., fluoxetine, fluvoxamine, and paroxetine) and bupropion can interfere because of their effects on cytochrome P450 2D6 system with the metabolism of commonly used medications in oncology.[61] Stimulant medications (such as methylphenidate and dextroamphetamine) may also be beneficial (i.e., may lift mood, increase appetite, and improve fatigue), but there is limited evidence to support this practice.[62] When response to stimulants develops, it is usually seen within 1 week.

Although little research has been conducted on medications for MDD in people with cancer, there are a bevy of studies that confirm the efficacy of psychosocial interventions.[55] The severity of cancer-related symptoms (such as fatigue and nausea) and the demanding schedules for anticancer treatments may limit a patient's ability to participate in the traditional weekly 50-minute psychotherapy visit. Therefore, psychotherapy visits need to be flexible and include shorter visits, meet during chemotherapy treatments, and involve more phone contact.

FATIGUE

Fatigue (the most commonly reported symptom in people with cancer and the symptom that causes the most functional impairment)[63] in people with cancer can often be confused with MDD.[64] Although fatigue is not a psychiatric disorder, psychiatric contributions can cause fatigue; therefore, fatigue could be considered a psychosomatic illness.

Prevalence

The prevalence (estimated at 60% to 90% of patients)[65,66] of fatigue in people affected by cancer varies widely because of differing measures of fatigue and heterogeneous populations studied.

Diagnosis

Fatigue can arise before the diagnosis of cancer, during active cancer treatment, and into the survivorship years. The diagnosis is made primarily by asking questions about the presence and severity of the symptoms. While there are validated instruments for the measurement of fatigue[64] (e.g., the Functional Assessment of Chronic Illness Therapy—Fatigue scale [FACIT-F]), administration of these questionnaires may not be feasible in busy clinical settings. The National Comprehensive Cancer

Network (NCCN) recommends screening for fatigue at visits with a one-item, 0-to-10 scale, similar to that used for screening of pain, with 0 being "no fatigue" and 10 being "the most severe fatigue." Scores of 4 or greater should prompt further evaluation. (The full set of guidelines that also includes a review of the literature can be viewed at www.nccn.org.)[65]

The NCCN recommends that primary evaluation include exploration of modifiable causes of fatigue (such as anemia, pain, sleep disturbance [insomnia, difficulty staying asleep, and sleep apnea], emotional distress [MDD and anxiety], poor nutrition, inactivity/deconditioning, medications, and chemotherapies that cause fatigue [e.g., gemcitabine, corticosteroids, narcotics, antiemetics, and beta-blockers], and other medical conditions [e.g., hypothyroidism, hypogonadism, adrenal insufficiency, hypercalcemia, hepatic failure, and cardiovascular or pulmonary compromise]). Fatigue can also be a side effect of radiation therapy.

Treatment

The primary treatment for fatigue is modification of the contributing factors; for fatigue this should be done in conjunction with the patient's oncologist or primary care provider. Mental health clinicians can provide treatment for any underlying psychiatric disorder, as well as offer interventions that are fatigue-specific (including stimulants, exercise, and behavioral interventions).

Stimulants

A Cochrane Review of drug treatment of cancer-related fatigue, after combining five randomized controlled studies, concluded that current evidence supports the use of psychostimulants for this condition.[67] NCCN guidelines recommend the use of methylphenidate after other non-pharmacological approaches have failed.[65] However, stimulants can raise blood pressure and heart rate and should be used with caution in patients with cardiac disease. Common side effects include constipation, sleep disturbance, anxiety, and (at higher doses) anorexia.

Exercise

Abundant evidence exists for exercise as a treatment of fatigue, with several studies demonstrating the benefit of exercise for fatigue in people with cancer.[68] Mental health clinicians can encourage exercise through motivational interviewing and through behavioral changes. Because patients can have serious physical morbidities, such as large bone metastases that could lead to fracture, consultation with the oncologist is recommended before initiating exercise. A physical therapist can assist in designing an exercise program that contains both strength and aerobic training, and that is appropriate for a person with physical limitations from cancer or cancer treatments. For more medically-complicated patients, exercise might best be done in a cardiovascular or pulmonary rehabilitation center.

Behavioral Interventions

Behavioral interventions (such as cognitive-behavioral therapy [CBT] and energy conservation) may be beneficial as both primary and adjunctive treatments for fatigue in cancer patients. CBT emphasizes management of fatigue, rather than a cure for it.[69] Energy conservation is similar to that with CBT in some respects; it focuses on prioritizing activities and delegating, problem-solving around difficulties caused by the fatigue, and improving organizational skills.[70]

CONFUSION AND COGNITIVE IMPAIRMENT

In cancer, delirium is highly prevalent; its incidence ranges between 10% and 27% in early stages,[71] but can increase to up to 44% in patients admitted to a hospital,[72] and over 85% in patients with terminal illness.[73] Common causes include infection, hypoxia, metabolic abnormalities, pain, substance withdrawal, and side effects of medications (e.g., anticholinergic agents, opioids). In the majority of cancer patients, delirium is multifactorial, with a median number of three precipitating factors per delirious episode.[74] Older patients, as well as patients with structural brain disease, vascular disease, or lung, kidney, or liver impairment, are predisposed to delirium.[75] Specific cancer-related syndromes of cognitive impairment that may cause psychiatric symptoms in oncology patients are listed below.

Hypercalcemia

Hypercalcemia (in patients with metastatic lesions to the bone or with tumor-related ectopic production of parathyroid-hormone-related protein) secondary to cancer can cause nausea, vomiting, constipation, progressive mental impairment, and if not corrected can progress to coma and renal failure. A serum protein-bound calcium may initially appear normal, when the free calcium is elevated or when serum albumin is low and not taken into consideration. Hypercalcemia can be treated by use of diphosphonates, hydration, and diuresis.

Hyponatremia

Hyponatremia can result from the syndrome of inappropriate antidiuretic hormone (SIADH) that occurs as a paraneoplastic syndrome (especially from small cell carcinoma, but also from non-small-cell lung cancer, mesothelioma, pancreatic cancer, duodenal cancer, lymphoma, endometrial cancer, and leukemia), lung infections, cerebral tumors, brain injury, and complications of many psychotropic medications (e.g., phenothiazines, SSRIs, carbamazepine, and tricyclic antidepressants [TCAs]). Lethargy and confusion are attributable to cerebral edema caused by the movement of water across the osmotic gradient created by a reduction in the serum sodium[76]; chronic hyponatremia is associated with falls and inattention in the elderly.[77]

Brain Tumors

The incidence of primary brain tumors is 6.6 per 1,000,000, but the rate of metastatic brain tumors is higher (ranging from 8 to 11 per 100,000). Virtually any tumor can metastasize to the brain, the most common being non-small and small cell lung cancers, breast cancer, melanoma, and gastrointestinal cancers.[78] In patients with small cell lung cancer, brain metastases are anticipated, and prophylactic whole brain radiation is often recommended.[79] Isolated brain metastases from non-small cell lung cancer may be treated surgically, and modern radiation techniques target small areas of the brain.

Consciousness deterioration can occur in 33% to 85% of patients with space-occupying lesions, and full agitation and delirium in 15% to 19%.[80,81] Tumors (particularly of the frontal, temporal, and limbic lobes) that affect the hardwiring of motivation, attention, mood stability, and memory come to psychiatric attention. Temporal lobe epilepsy can be associated with psychological symptoms (e.g., memory dysfunction, anxiety, hypergraphia, and viscosity). For these patients, neuropsychiatric consultation, testing, and cognitive rehabilitation may be critically important to define and to treat the specific loss. Multimodal interventions for attention, memory, word-retrieval, and problem-solving abilities may be appropriate.[82] Loved ones can understand more clearly the basis of some limitations, and the patient can acknowledge his or her deficits and take whatever control is possible. Psychotropic medications, used appropriately, are adjuncts to anticonvulsants and to anticancer treatment.

Leptomeningeal Disease

Leptomeningeal disease or carcinomatous meningitis, seen most often in breast cancer, lung cancer, melanoma and non-Hodgkin's lymphomas, can lead to diffuse encephalopathy due to changes in brain metabolism or reductions in regional cerebral blood flow. If there are no focal signs or findings on neuroimaging, the associated malaise may be thought of as psychiatric. In addition to mental changes, headache, difficulty with walking, limb weakness, and seizures are common. Dizziness and sensorineural deafness have also been noted. Malignant cells in CSF confirm the diagnosis, but a large enough fluid sample improves the chance for a positive diagnosis; half to 70% may be falsely negative. A brain MRI may be unremarkable in 20%, but more likely will show hydrocephalus, brain metastases, or contrast enhancement of the sulci or cisterns.[83,84]

Delirium in Hematopoietic Stem Cell Transplantation

The incidence of delirium among patients undergoing hematopoietic stem cell transplantation (HSCT) is high, 43–50%, with most cases developing within the first 2 weeks post-transplantation.[85,86] An engraftment syndrome may cause delirium with fever, headache, and rash. Usually this syndrome occurs when the neutrophil count is greater than 500/mm^3 and with a cytokine effect of the hematopoietic colony-stimulating factors.[87]

In the transplant setting, immunosuppressive drugs (e.g., cyclosporine, tacrolimus, or the antifungal drug amphotericin B) can cause delirium. Hypertension, use of steroids, uremia, and previous radiation to the brain are risk factors.[88] Drug serum levels may facilitate diagnosis; tremor occurs in 40%, and paresthesias in 11%. Hypomagnesemia increases the risk of seizures. Immunosuppressants are rarely associated with a syndrome of reversible posterior leukoencephalopathy that causes headache, visual loss or blurring, visual hallucinations, and confusion.[89] Parkinsonism, ataxia, or dystonia can also occur. White matter edema is documented in the parieto-occipital area on fluid-attenuated inversion recovery (FLAIR) sequences. If this syndrome has occurred with one immunosuppressant, either tacrolimus or cyclosporine, the other may be used.[90]

Hyperviscosity Syndrome

Hyperviscosity syndromes, seen in multiple myeloma and lymphomas, present with the triad of confusion, vision abnormalities, and bleeding. A serum viscosity level above 4.0 centipoise (1.56 to 1.68 cp) has been associated with symptoms.[91]

Cushing's Syndrome

Cushing's syndrome may cause delirium, psychosis, and muscle weakness in adrenocortical carcinoma or tumors with paraneoplastic production of adrenocorticotropic hormone (ACTH). Psychiatric disorders are a feature of the syndrome of ectopic ACTH production in 53% of patients. Specific treatments for this syndrome include steroidogenesis inhibitors or glucocorticoid receptor antagonists (e.g., ketoconazole, metyrapone, aminoglutethimide, opDDD, etomidate, or mifepristone).[92]

Paraneoplastic Neurological Disorders

Paraneoplastic neurological disorders include a myasthenic syndrome, cerebellar degeneration, or diffuse encephalomyelitis.[93] These syndromes may manifest before the cancer is diagnosed. An afflicted patient may develop an immune reaction against neural tissue when exposed to a tumor antigen that reacts against normal nervous system in the setting of dying tumor cells. The exact mechanism of the immune reaction has not been established. Typically there are more T and B cells and plasma cells in these tumors. Small cell lung cancer is the tumor most commonly associated with this syndrome, and anti-Hu antibody syndromes are often noted.[94]

Paraneoplastic Limbic Encephalitis

Paraneoplastic limbic encephalitis (PLE) is a specific autoimmune encephalopathy that causes memory difficulties, anxiety, depression, agitation, confusion, hallucinations, and complex partial seizures. This syndrome been most commonly associated with small cell carcinoma of the lung, but it also occurs with Hodgkin's lymphoma, thymoma, and cancers of the testes, breasts, ovaries, stomach, uterus, kidney, thyroid, and colon.[95] Typical presentations consist of progressive confusion and deficits in short-term memory. Less commonly, patients experience visual and auditory hallucinations, delusions, or frank paranoia.[95] Detection of antibodies directed against onconeural antigens in the serum or the CSF may assist in diagnosis. MRI findings, if present, include abnormal hyperintensity on the T_2-weighted image, sometimes with contrast. Removal is key to the treatment of the syndrome; first-line immunotherapy (steroids, intravenous immunoglobulin, plasmapheresis) minimize autoimmune response and neural inflammation and can resulting in improvement in up to half of the cases.[96] Second-line immunotherapy (rituximab, cyclophosphamide), is usually effective when first-line treatments fail.[96] Anticonvulsants and neuroleptics have been used in the symptomatic treatment of psychiatric manifestations.[95]

Toxic Leukoencephalopathy

White matter injury can be an early, a temporary, or a late consequence of cancer treatment. Whole brain radiation and certain anticancer drugs can injure the projection fibers, association fibers, and commissural tracts that affect cognition and emotion. These drugs include methotrexate, carmustine, cisplatin, levamisole, fludarabine, thiotepa, ifosfamide, cytarabine, and fluorouracil. Acutely, confusion is related to patchy, reversible edema and later to widespread edema and demyelination. More severe delayed consequences result from loss of myelin and axons related to vascular necrosis and thrombosis. Risk of leukoencephalopathy is related to patient age, total dose of radiation, fraction size, and timing of chemotherapy. In most cancer protocols, the doses and timing have been adjusted to minimize these adverse effects. However, sometimes patients with vulnerable brains or delayed metabolism of the drug may be unexpectedly affected. Neurobehavioral sequelae occur in 28% of patients acutely and are a consideration in cancer survivors.[97]

The frontal lobes, the lobes with the most white matter tracts, are the ones most likely to be injured. Patients with mild leukoencephalopathy may complain of difficulty with concentration and vigilance and problems with attention. Apathy, anxiety, irritability, depression, or changes in personality may be seen with memory loss, slowed thinking, and failure of executive oversight. In more severe cases, dementia, abulia, stupor, and coma occur with necrotic areas and diffuse hyperintensity of white matter on MRI. This injury, unlike that seen in Alzheimer's disease, spares language, praxis, perceptions, and procedural memory. The key bedside tests on mental status examination are the elements that test attention (e.g., digit span, serial sevens, three-word delayed recall, and clock-drawing for visuospatial skills and alternating motor sequences for frontal function). The contribution of white matter injury should be documented on T_2-weighted MRI.[98]

This toxicity is seen in patients who have had high-dose methotrexate and radiation treatment for childhood acute lymphoblastic leukemia (ALL) or primary CNS lymphoma. In the latter, a rapidly progressive subcortical dementia with psychomotor slowing, executive and memory dysfunction, behavioral changes, ataxia, and incontinence can be seen. Diffuse white matter disease and cortical-subcortical atrophy are also noted.[99]

Toxic effects of drugs or radiation may add to white matter damage of hydrocephalus, trauma, alcoholism, and hypertension. Patients with a history of psychosis or affective disorder also tend to have more evidence of abnormal white matter on imaging.

Chemotherapy-related Cognitive Impairment

Chemotherapy-related cognitive impairment (CRCI) is commonly reported following treatment in patients with cancer. A recent meta-analysis examining the effects of chemotherapy in seven cognitive domains established evidence for memory and executive function impairments.[100] One study looking at the impact of CRCI found that the deficits had a significant negative impact on self-esteem, self-confidence, work performance, and social relationships.[101] The symptoms of CRCI are transient and reversible, but take at least several years to disappear.[102] Interventions to help alleviate the symptoms of CRCI include non-pharmacologic treatment, such as cognitive-behavioral therapy and pharmacologic treatment, such as recombinant human erythropoietin and psychostimulant drugs, such as modafinil.[103,104]

Effects of Hormonal Therapy in Cancer Patients

Treatment of hormonal-sensitive tumors involves the use of medications aimed at reducing the availability of sex hormones. Patients who receive adjuvant treatment for breast cancer often develop menopausal symptoms because of a direct effect on the ovary that decreases hormone levels and hastens menopause. Menopause is a goal of treatment for those with estrogen-receptor-positive tumors.[105]

Tamoxifen is a mixed agonist/antagonist of estrogen that is associated with hot flushes and insomnia. Aromatase inhibitors reduce estradiol to barely detectable concentrations. There seem to be no distinctions in quality-of-life measures in women taking tamoxifen or an aromatase inhibitor (e.g., anastrozole). Vasomotor symptoms are frequent with both drugs, and about 10% of patients report mood swings and irritability.[106] Men receiving androgen ablation for prostate cancer experience hot flushes that are more frequent, severe, and longer lasting.[107] Venlafaxine and all SSRIs reduce the frequency and severity of hot flushes and improve mood, sleep, anxiety, and quality of life in patients undergoing hormonal deprivation therapy for hormone-sensitive tumors.[107] Gabapentin and pregabalin have also been beneficial decreasing hot flushes in cancer patients.[108,109]

Finally, gonadotropin releasing hormone (GnRH) agonists (i.e., leuprolide and goserelin), have been associated with depression in non-cancer populations; however, in prostate cancer patients, clinical trials have showed diverse results, and well-controlled prospective studies have suggested that even though depression occurs, fatigue is more prevalent and may be mistaken for depression.[110]

Survivors of Childhood Cancer

The most common diagnoses for children with cancer are leukemia, lymphoma, brain tumors, osteogenic sarcoma, Ewing's sarcoma, and Wilms' tumor. Childhood cancer is now more commonly considered a serious chronic illness rather than a uniformly terminal illness. A child psychiatrist works side-by-side in the outpatient setting with the pediatric hematology-oncology team to treat the emotional needs of the child in age-appropriate ways during active treatment and thereafter. With consideration of the child's stage of development, the psychiatrist can judge what the child will understand and what the child will want and need to know.

The most common consultation questions include evaluation of the child with anticipatory anxiety, sleep disturbances, behavioral problems, or mood changes. Anticipatory anxiety still affects many children despite advances in antiemetic medication. The child may feel nauseated or vomit on approaching the hospital, clinic, or phlebotomist. Behavioral modification, visualization and relaxation, and medication are helpful. Sleep disturbances may be related to children's worries about the illness or to medications, such as steroids. Child psychiatrists are also consulted for behavioral problems in younger children who become more aggressive or difficult to manage. The emphasis in treatment of depression or withdrawn states is on the child's ability to enjoy life. Overall, children tend to be quite resilient. Although children and parents are very distressed at the time of diagnosis, the prevalence of psychological problems among survivors of childhood cancer is similar to that in the community.[111]

Children treated for ALL or for a brain tumor with cranial irradiation are at risk for cognitive decline.[112] Cognitive decline is progressive over at least 10 years. A radiation-induced progressive microvasculopathy may account for this progression. Babies are particularly prone to radiotoxicity in the first 2 years of life because of the rapid growth of the brain and white matter development in those years. Cognitive defects have been seen in verbal comprehension, perceptual organization, distractibility, and memory in survivors of ALL. Visuomotor integration, sequential memory, fine motor coordination, processing speed, and math abilities may also be affected. Risk factors include young age, female gender, and time since radiation. The volume and dose of radiation are also thought to be factors. The combination of radiation treatment and intrathecal methotrexate increases the risk of cognitive impairment. Children exposed to cranial irradiation may also suffer hypothyroidism and growth hormone deficiency. Children who have been treated for leukemia or brain tumors should be monitored for cognitive and endocrine dysfunction.

Access the complete reference list and multiple choice questions (MCQs) online at https://expertconsult.inkling.com

KEY REFERENCES
11. Weisman AD. *The vulnerable self: conquering the ultimate questions*, New York, 1993, Plenum Press.
14. Network NCC. NCCN Clinical Practice Guidelines in oncology: Version 2.2013 Distress Management. <http://www.nccn.org/professionals/physician_gls/PDF/distress.pdf>; [Accessed July 1, 2013].
23. Faller H, Schuler M, Richard M, et al. Effects of psycho-oncologic interventions on emotional distress and quality of life in adult patients with cancer: systematic review and meta-analysis. *J Clin Oncol* 31:782–793, 2013.
26. Mustafa M, Carson-Stevens A, Gillespie D, et al. Psychological interventions for women with metastatic breast cancer. *Cochrane Database Syst Rev* (6):CD004253, 2013.
44. Traeger L, Greer JA, Fernandez-Robles C, et al. Evidence-based treatment of anxiety in patients with cancer. *J Clin Oncol* 30:1197–1205, 2012.
46. Bloechl-Daum B, Beuson RR, Mavros P, et al. Delayed nausea and vomiting continue to reduce patients' quality of life after highly and moderately emetogenic chemotherapy despite antiemetic treatment. *J Clin Oncol* 24:4472–4478, 2006.
50. Andrykowski MA. The role of anxiety in the development of anticipatory nausea in cancer chemotherapy: a review and synthesis. *Psychosom Med* 54:458–475, 1990.
54. Breitbart W, Rosenfeld B, Pessin H, et al. Depression, hopelessness, and desire for hastened death in terminally ill patients with cancer. *JAMA* 284:2907–2911, 2000.
55. Pirl WF. Evidence report on the occurrence, assessment, and treatment of depression in cancer patients. *JNCI Monograph* 32:32–39, 2004.
60. Laoutidis ZG, Mathiak K. Antidepressants in the treatment of depression/depressive symptoms in cancer patients: a systematic review and meta-analysis. *BMC Psychiatry* 13:140, 2013.
64. Pirl W. Fatigue. In Holland JC, Greenberg DB, Hughes MK, editors: *Quick reference for oncology clinicians: the psychiatric and psychological dimensions of cancer symptom management*, Charlottesville, VA, 2006, American Psychosocial Oncology Society.
65. Network NCC. NCCN Clinical Practice Guidelines in Oncology: Version 1.2013 Cancer related fatigue. <http://www.nccn.org/professionals/physician_gls/pdf/fatigue.pdf>; [Accessed July 1, 2013].
67. Minton O, Richardson A, Sharpe M, et al. Drug therapy for the management of cancer-related fatigue. *Cochrane Database Syst Rev* (7):CD006704, 2010.
71. Morrison C. Identification and management of delirium in the critically ill patient with cancer. *AACN Clin Issues* 14:92–111, 2003.
80. Pace A, Di Lorenzo C, Guariglia L, et al. End of life issues in brain tumor patients. *J Neurooncol* 91:39–43, 2009.
84. DeAngelis LM. Current diagnosis and treatment of leptomeningeal metastasis. *J Neurooncol* 38:245–252, 1998.
86. Fann JR, Roth-Roemer S, Burington BE, et al. Delirium in patients undergoing hematopoietic stem cell transplantation. *Cancer* 95:1971–1981, 2002.
91. Stern TA, Purcell JJ, Murray GB. Complex partial seizures associated with Waldenström's macroglobulinemia. *Psychosomatics* 26:890–892, 1985.
92. Ilias I, Torpy DJ, Pacak K, et al. Cushing's syndrome due to ectopic corticotrophin secretion: twenty years' experience at the National Institutes of Health. *J Clin Endocrinol Metab* 90:4955–4962, 2005.
95. Foster AR, Caplan JP. Paraneoplastic limbic encephalitis. *Psychosomatics* 50:108–113, 2009.
96. Titulaer MJ, McCracken L, Gabilondo I, et al. Treatment and prognostic factors for long-term outcome in patients with anti-NMDA receptor encephalitis: an observational cohort study. *Lancet Neurol* 12:157–165, 2013.
97. Filley CM. Neurobehavioral aspects of cerebral white matter disorders. *Psychiatr Clin North Am* 28:685–700, 2005.
100. Hodgson KD, Hutchinson AD, Wilson CJ, et al. A meta-analysis of the effects of chemotherapy on cognition in patients with cancer. *Cancer Treat Rev* 39:297–304, 2013.
104. Joly F, Rigal O, Noal S, et al. Cognitive dysfunction and cancer: which consequences in terms of disease management? *Psychooncology* 20:1251–1258, 2011.
106. Fallowfield L, Cella D, Cuzick J, et al. Quality of life of postmenopausal women in the Arimidex, Tamoxifen, Alone or in Combination (ATAC) adjuvant breast cancer trial. *J Clin Oncol* 22:4261–4271, 2004.
107. Adelson KB, Loprinzi CL, Hershman DL. Treatment of hot flushes in breast and prostate cancer. *Expert Opin Pharmacother* 6:1095–1106, 2005.
111. Sawyer M, Antoniou G, Toogood I, et al. Childhood cancer: a two-year prospective study of the psychological adjustment of children and parents. *J Am Acad Adolesc Psychiatry* 36:1736–1743, 1997.
112. Duffner PK. Long-term effects of radiation therapy on cognitive and endocrine function in children with leukemia and brain tumors. *Neurologist* 6:293–310, 2004.

57 Psychiatric Aspects of HIV Infection and AIDS

John Querques, MD, and Oliver Freudenreich, MD

KEY POINTS

- Highly active antiretroviral therapy (HAART) has transformed infection with the human immunodeficiency virus (HIV) from a terminal illness to a chronic, treatable condition.

- Psychiatric and substance use disorders are frequent concomitants of HIV infection and complicate its diagnosis and treatment.

- Evaluation of affective, behavioral, and cognitive symptoms must be broad and include primary psychiatric disorders and secondary conditions related to HIV infection, opportunistic infections, and neoplasms.

- Because both psychotropic and antiretroviral agents are metabolized by the cytochrome P-450 enzyme system, pharmacokinetic interactions between these two classes of medication must be considered when treating psychiatric disorders in HIV-infected patients.

- Successful psychiatric treatment can be lifesaving if poor adherence to HAART is due to untreated psychiatric illness.

OVERVIEW

Once a dread illness that portended certain death after years— or even just months—of inexorable decline, infection with HIV has become a chronic, treatable illness. The advent of HAART in 1995 marked a critical turning point in the pandemic. Various combinations of potent medications, each targeting a different step in the virus's hijacking of its human host, reduced the incidence of the acquired immunodeficiency syndrome (AIDS) and improved life expectancy for many patients with HIV infection.[1] Well into the fourth decade of the epidemic, now nearly 30 medications in five classes are available, at least in developed nations and increasingly in developing areas.

The successes of the past 30 years notwithstanding, diagnosis with HIV infection still foreshadows an arduous course of frequent examinations, serial monitoring of cell count and viral load, and difficult treatments with potentially disabling and disfiguring adverse effects (e.g., neuropathy, lipodystrophy). Effective treatment is not obtainable in all parts of the world, and, even in countries where medications are available, not all patients have access to them. At each step of what has been termed the *HIV care cascade*, significant attrition curtails the number of patients who receive the evaluation and care required to achieve the most critical outcome—full viral suppression.[2,3] For example, in the US in 2009, 81.9% of HIV-infected people knew their status, 65.8% received care, 36.7% stayed in treatment, 32.7% received HAART, and only 25.3% achieved viral suppression.[2] Blacks and Hispanics/Latinos were significantly less likely to be aware of their HIV status; young people were significantly more adversely affected at each level of the cascade. Closing these gaps in care will require overcoming several barriers, including health beliefs,

mental illness, and stigma around HIV, sexual orientation, and substance use.[3]

For the reasons listed in Box 57-1, the general psychiatrist— regardless of venue and type of practice—will be called on to evaluate and to treat a fair share of patients with HIV infection. This chapter reviews the epidemiology, basic biology, classification, and diagnosis of HIV infection; a general approach to psychiatric care of HIV-infected patients; psychiatric and neurological disorders common in this population and their treatments; and special clinical problems encountered in HIV psychiatry.

EPIDEMIOLOGY

At the end of 2011, 34 million people were living with HIV infection worldwide.[4] Sub-Saharan Africa remains the epicenter of the pandemic, followed by the Caribbean. In the US, at the end of 2011, 1.3 million people were living with HIV infection.[4] Since 2001, approximately 50,000 new infections have occurred yearly.[4] Of these, the largest proportion continue to occur in men who have sex with men (MSM).[5]

BASIC BIOLOGY

The HIV (Figure 57-1) is a retrovirus—a virus containing ribonucleic acid and the enzyme reverse transcriptase for replication—that affects the immune system and the central nervous system (CNS), gaining entry to cells (e.g., T lymphocytes, monocytes, macrophages) that express the CD4 receptor on their membranes. The life cycle of the virus once inside an infected cell is depicted in Figure 57-2. All of the currently available antiretroviral medications target one of five key steps and enzymes in this process: fusion of the virus with the host cell membrane; entry into the cell; reverse transcriptase; integrase; and protease.

During the first weeks after infection, the population of CD4+ T lymphocytes (i.e., the CD4 count) decreases as the amount of virus in the blood (i.e., the viral load) increases (Figure 57-3). Following a weak and short-lived rebound, the CD4 count steadily declines. At the same time, the viral load oscillates around a "set-point" until ultimately viral replication intensifies and peripheral viremia surges. Administration of HAART, when effective, halts this process. Opportunistic infections (OIs), neoplasms, and neuropsychiatric conditions occur with increasing frequency as the immune deficiency worsens; prophylaxis for certain OIs (e.g., *Pneumocystis jirovecii* [formerly *Pneumocystis carinii*] pneumonia and toxoplasmosis) is instituted during the course of infection according to the CD4 count.

CLASSIFICATION AND DIAGNOSIS

According to the Centers for Disease Control and Prevention (CDC),[6] AIDS is defined by a CD4 count below 200 cells/μl (or less than 14% of total lymphocytes) or the presence of an AIDS-defining condition (Box 57-2).

Infection with HIV is usually diagnosed in two steps. The initial test is an enzyme-linked immunosorbent assay (ELISA). A positive result on this test is then confirmed by a Western blot test. Because one-fifth of HIV-infected people in the US are unaware of their serostatus, the CDC and the United States

BOX 57-1 Why are the Principles of HIV
Psychiatry Important?

- Many patients with HIV infection have psychiatric problems,
  both antecedent and consequent to contracting the virus.
- Many patients with psychiatric problems have HIV infection, in
  part related to poor judgment.
- Patients with HIV infection develop medical problems that can
  manifest as psychiatric illness.
- Patients with HIV infection take medications with affective,
  behavioral, and cognitive effects and that interact with
  psychotropic agents.

HIV, Human immunodeficiency virus.

HIV-1 VIRION

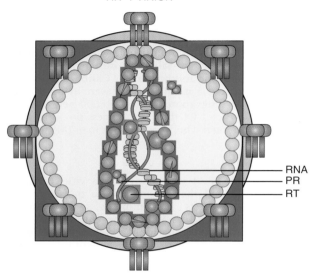

Figure 57-1. Human immunodeficiency virus. PR, Protease; RNA,
ribonucleic acid; RT, reverse transcriptase. *(Modified from Cohen J,
Powderly WG, editors. Infectious diseases, ed 2. Philadelphia, 2004,
Elsevier, p. 1252.)*

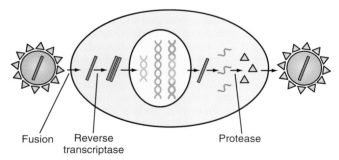

Fusion Reverse Protease
transcriptase

Figure 57-2. Life cycle of HIV. *(Adapted from Cohen J, Powderly WG,
editors. Infectious diseases, ed 2. Philadelphia, 2004, Elsevier, p. 1254.)*

Preventive Services Task Force (USPSTF) recommend that HIV
testing be done as part of routine clinical care for *all* patients,
regardless of risk factors.[7,8]

GENERAL APPROACH TO PSYCHIATRIC CARE

The approach to the psychiatric care of the patient with HIV
infection focuses on accurate diagnosis; an appreciation of the

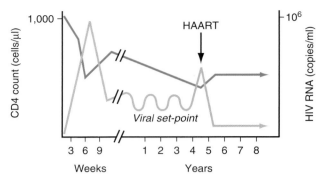

Figure 57-3. History of HIV infection with HAART. *(Adapted from
Bartlett JG, Gallant JE. 2001–2002 medical management of HIV infection. Available at www.hopkins-aids.edu.)*

BOX 57-2 AIDS-defining Conditions

- Candidiasis
- Cervical cancer, invasive
- Coccidioidomycosis
- Cryptococcosis
- Cryptosporidiosis
- Cytomegalovirus disease or retinitis
- Herpes simplex virus infection
- Histoplasmosis
- HIV-related encephalopathy
- HIV-related wasting syndrome
- Isosporiasis
- Kaposi's sarcoma
- Lymphoma (Burkitt's, immunoblastic, or primary CNS)
- Mycobacterial infection (*M. avium* complex, *M. kansasii, M.
  tuberculosis,* or other species)
- *Pneumocystis jirovecii* pneumonia
- Pneumonia, recurrent
- Progressive multifocal leukoencephalopathy
- *Salmonella* septicemia, recurrent
- Toxoplasmosis, cerebral

AIDS, Acquired immunodeficiency syndrome; CNS, central nervous
system; HIV, human immunodeficiency virus.
*Adapted from Centers for Disease Control and Prevention. 1993 revised
classification system for HIV infection and expanded surveillance case
definition for AIDS among adolescents and adults. MMWR 41(RR-
17):1–23, 1992.*

differences in response to, and tolerability of, psychotropic
medications; and the prognostic importance of optimal adherence to effective antiretroviral treatment, which psychiatric
illness often compromises.

Psychiatric symptoms in a patient with HIV infection may
be primary or secondary (Box 57-3); the CD4 count provides
useful initial guidance in making this differential diagnosis. A
CD4 count greater than 500 cells/μl suggests a primary psychiatric cause, whereas a CD4 count less than 200 cells/μl, and
a fortiori less than 50 cells/μl, suggests the psychiatric problem
is secondary to the effects of immune compromise. For
example, a patient who has just been told that he is HIV-
positive but whose CD4 count is still normal and whose viral
load is low may become depressed as part of an adjustment
disorder (a primary psychiatric problem). However, 10 years
later, when he again has depressed mood and his CD4 count
is 100 cells/μl, he may very likely have an OI or a neoplasm
affecting his CNS and causing depression (a secondary psychiatric problem).

BOX 57-3 Differential Diagnosis of Psychiatric Symptoms in the HIV-Infected Patient

Delirium
Substance intoxication or withdrawal
Primary HIV syndromes
    Seroconversion illness
    Acute HIV meningoencephalitis
    HIV-associated neurocognitive disorder
Opportunistic infections
    Fungi
      • *Aspergillus fumigatus*
      • *Candida albicans*
      • *Coccidioides immitis*
      • *Cryptococcus neoformans*
      • *Histoplasma capsulatum*
      • Mucormycosis
    Protozoa/parasites
      • Amebas
      • *Toxoplasma gondii*
    Viruses
      • Adenovirus type 2
      • Cytomegalovirus (CMV)
      • Herpes simplex virus
      • JC virus
      • Varicella-zoster virus
    Bacteria
      • Gram-negative organisms
      • *Listeria monocytogenes*
      • *Mycobacterium avium-intracellulare*
      • *Mycobacterium tuberculosis*
      • *Nocardia asteroides*
      • *Treponema pallidum*
Neoplasms
    Primary CNS lymphoma
    Non-Hodgkin's lymphoma
    Metastatic Kaposi's sarcoma (rare)
Medication side effects
Endocrinopathies and nutrient deficiencies
    Addison's disease (CMV, *Cryptococcus*, HIV, ketoconazole)
    Hypothyroidism
    Hypogonadism
    Vitamins A, B_6, B_{12}, and E deficiencies
Non–HIV-related conditions

HIV, Human immunodeficiency virus.
Adapted from Querques J, Freudenreich O, Gandhi R. HIV infection and AIDS. In: Stern TA, Herman JB, Gorrindo T, editors. Massachusetts General Hospital psychiatry update and board preparation. *ed 3. Boston, 2012, MGH Psychiatry Academy Publishing, pp. 226.*

BOX 57-4 Adverse Effects of Substance Use in the Context of HIV Infection

• Impaired judgment
• Disinhibition
• Risky sexual practices
• Viral transmission
• Interactions with psychotropic medications
• Poor adherence to antiretroviral therapy
• Possible immune suppression

HIV, Human immunodeficiency virus.

PSYCHIATRIC DISORDERS
Substance Use Disorders

Substance use disorders are well represented among HIV-infected patients. The 12-month prevalence of drug dependence in the HIV Cost and Services Utilization Study (HCSUS)—a study of a nationally representative sample of nearly 3,000 HIV-infected adults in the US—was 12.5%.[9] Substance use disorders affect the transmission, course, and treatment of HIV infection in numerous ways (Box 57-4).

So-called "club drugs"—methylenedioxymethamphetamine (MDMA, "ecstasy"), gamma-hydroxybutyrate (GHB, "liquid ecstasy"), and ketamine ("special K")—and other related compounds (e.g., methamphetamine [speed, crystal meth]) have become increasingly popular drugs of abuse, in part because of their effects on social disinhibition and sexual enhancement. As a result, they can pave the way to HIV transmission. By virtue of pharmacokinetic interactions with the cytochrome P-450 system, the co-administration of "club drugs" with antiretroviral medications can have harmful consequences. Adverse effects of MDMA and GHB, thought to be due to interactions with protease inhibitors, have been reported.[10,11] Protease inhibitors, especially ritonavir, may inhibit the metabolism of amphetamines and ketamine.[10]

Many stressors during the course of HIV infection threaten both the establishment and the maintenance of sobriety in patients with substance use disorders (Box 57-5).

Interactions between methadone and various antiretroviral agents are presented in Box 57-6. While these interactions may produce measurable changes in methadone plasma levels, such alterations do not consistently result in clinical manifestations.[12] Withdrawal phenomena have been observed with efavirenz, nevirapine, and nelfinavir.[13]

Less is known about buprenorphine, which, like methadone, is metabolized by cytochrome P-450 3A4.[14] The co-administration of buprenorphine/naloxone and efavirenz to 10 volunteers did not precipitate opioid withdrawal, despite decreased buprenorphine exposure; efavirenz plasma levels remained therapeutic.[15] The combination of ritonavir and atazanavir caused symptoms consistent with opioid excess when given to three patients also taking buprenorphine; pharmacokinetic measures of buprenorphine and the two protease inhibitors were not reported.[16] Buprenorphine's *partial* agonism at opioid receptors limits its utility in patients who require narcotic analgesics, as many HIV-infected patients do.[17]

The oral solution (but not the capsules) of amprenavir contains propylene glycol, which is metabolized by aldehyde dehydrogenase. Disulfiram inhibits this enzyme and can thus lead to propylene glycol toxicity; therefore, the combination of disulfiram and amprenavir oral solution is contraindicated.

Distinguishing between primary and secondary causes has therapeutic implications because results of standard psychiatric treatment for secondary problems may be inferior to those achieved if the problem were primary. As in a patient with traumatic brain injury, stroke, dementia, or advanced age, the brain of a patient with HIV infection can be considered to be more sensitive to psychotropics and to have less reserve capacity. Thus a standard dose of a psychotropic medication may have a more (or less) profound effect in an HIV-infected patient or may cause adverse effects that usually occur only at higher dosages.

Optimum treatment of HIV infection and related conditions is essential for effective psychiatric care. Close collaboration between the psychiatrist and the physician providing the HIV care (usually a specialist in infectious diseases) is crucial.

BOX 57-5 Stressors during HIV Infection

Diagnosis and Treatment
- Testing seropositive
- Serial determinations of CD4 count and viral load
- Initiation of highly active antiretroviral therapy
- Initiation of prophylaxis for opportunistic infections
- First hospitalization
- Transfer to hospice care

Experience of Symptoms
- Wasting
- Diarrheal illness
- Treatment-resistant pain and insomnia
- Vision-impairing disease (e.g., cytomegalovirus retinitis)
- Cognitive and motor dysfunction
- Side effects of medications (e.g., fat redistribution syndrome)

Psychosocial Consequences
- Disclosure of HIV serostatus
- Disclosure of sexual orientation (e.g., leading to loss of family support)
- Loss of employment and health insurance
- Application for welfare and disability insurance
- Financial and social impoverishment (e.g., loss of friends to AIDS)

AIDS, Acquired immunodeficiency syndrome; HIV, human immunodeficiency virus.
Data from Querques J, Worth JL. HIV infection and AIDS. In Stern TA, Herman JB, editors. Massachusetts General Hospital psychiatry update and board preparation. ed 2. New York, 2004, McGraw-Hill, p. 208.

BOX 57-6 Interactions between Methadone and Antiretroviral Agents

Antiretrovirals that decrease methadone concentrations
- Amprenavir
- Efavirenz
- Fosamprenavir
- Lopinavir/ritonavir
- Nelfinavir
- Nevirapine
- Ritonavir

Methadone decreases the concentration of:
- Didanosine
- Stavudine

Methadone increases the concentration of:
- Zidovudine

Depressive and Anxiety Disorders

Mood and anxiety disorders are two of the most frequent major psychiatric concomitants of HIV infection. In the HCSUS, 36% screened positive for major depression, 26.5% for dysthymia, 15.8% for generalized anxiety disorder, and 10.5% for panic attack.[9] While individual studies have failed to document a greater risk for depressive disorders in HIV-positive patients compared to HIV-negative controls, a meta-analysis found the frequency of major depressive disorder to be nearly twice as high in the HIV-positive group.[18] This finding may suggest that the various consequences of HIV infection (e.g., effects of the virus within the CNS, immune dysfunction, and systemic viral burden) exert a depressogenic effect.

BOX 57-7 Differential Diagnosis of Depression and Anxiety in the HIV-infected Patient

- Normal depressed or anxious mood
- Grief
- Primary depressive disorder (first or recurrent episode)
- Primary anxiety disorder
- HIV-associated neurocognitive disorder
- Hypoactive delirium
- Secondary causes (see Box 57-3)

HIV, Human immunodeficiency virus.

The differential diagnosis of depression and anxiety is broad (Box 57-7). The patient's complaint of "depression" or "anxiety" should be taken solely as a description of his subjective feeling state rather than as a proclamation of his diagnosis. The patient may simply have a depressed mood or feel anxious, isolated from other symptoms and signs of psychiatric illness. Such a state, for example, would not be unusual in a patient who was recently told that he is HIV-positive or in a patient who is starting an antiretroviral regimen. Dysphoria or apprehension in this situation may be more consistent with grief over loss of health. Moreover, because of their drug use or sexual orientation, many HIV patients have friends who also are HIV-positive. When these friends die of the disease, bereavement can overwhelm the surviving members of their social circles. Many patients, particularly women, will have experienced psychological trauma due to childhood abuse and partner violence and may have post-traumatic stress disorder, which can be easily missed without specific inquiry.[19]

At later stages of illness, OIs and neoplasms affecting the CNS, other complications of advanced disease, cognitive disorders, and adverse effects of HAART can cause secondary depressive disorders. Delirium and HIV-associated neurocognitive disorder (HAND), including HIV-associated dementia (HAD), are characterized by apathy and psychomotor slowing that can easily be mistaken for a depressive disorder.

Treatment of depression and anxiety includes the usual modalities: psychopharmacology, psychotherapy, and electroconvulsive therapy (ECT).

Choice of psychotropic medication is not usually limited by the presence of HIV infection *per se*. However, owing to the sensitivity of the brain in HIV-infected patients, especially at later stages, initiation of treatment with half the usual starting dose and titration at half the usual speed is recommended; most patients will ultimately tolerate (and need) standard doses. Tricyclic antidepressants (TCAs) may have an advantage in this regard because their serum levels can be measured to gauge any pharmacokinetic effects of interactions between them and HAART. If apathy or psychomotor slowing is prominent—due to depression, dementia, or both (or in unclear cases)—psychostimulants, bupropion, or desipramine can be particularly effective. Bupropion is metabolized by cytochrome P-450 isoform 2B6, which is inhibited by ritonavir, nelfinavir, and efavirenz[20] and induced by nevirapine. The triazolobenzodiazepines—alprazolam, midazolam, and triazolam—are metabolized by cytochrome P-450 3A4, an isoform inhibited by protease inhibitors (PIs), which can thus enhance the effects of these anxiolytics. Use of those benzodiazepines in patients on HAART is relatively contraindicated; other benzodiazepines should be considered.

ECT can be lifesaving when a more rapid response is required and when catatonia is present.

Psychotic Disorders

HIV-associated Psychosis

Psychosis can occur at any time during the course of HIV disease and complicate its treatment. The differential diagnosis for new-onset psychosis in a patient with HIV infection is very broad; it includes delirium, HAD, OIs, other illnesses (e.g., neurosyphilis), side effects of medications, and drug use. Special weight should be given to past stimulant and sedative use disorders, because these increase the risk for the later development of psychosis.[21] In cases of secondary psychosis, cognitive impairment is typically seen.[22] In the US, new-onset psychosis without other signs of AIDS is only rarely the presenting sign of HIV infection. In one study of 246 patients with new-onset psychosis referred to a military hospital, none was positive for HIV.[23] In some HIV-infected patients, psychosis will mark the onset of schizophrenia and will be unrelated to the infection.

The treatment of psychosis in the setting of HIV infection involves treating both any underlying disorder and psychosis symptomatically with antipsychotics. Second-generation antipsychotics are often preferred over first-generation agents because of the latter's higher risk for inducing extrapyramidal symptoms (EPS) in patients with HIV disease. However, the similar metabolic side-effect profiles of second-generation antipsychotics and HAART (i.e., glucose intolerance and dyslipidemias) complicate the risk–benefit equation with regard to long-term cardiovascular mortality. While clozapine can be used in patients with HIV disease, the additive bone marrow toxicities from clozapine and many medications used in HIV care should be seen as a relative contraindication.

Antipsychotics do not significantly inhibit or induce P-450 enzymes and can safely be added to HAART regimens without fear of causing HAART failure or toxicity. HAART regimens may accelerate the metabolism of antipsychotics (leading to antipsychotic failure) or inhibit the metabolism of antipsychotics (leading to a higher risk of dose-related antipsychotic side effects), depending on the combination used. Potentially cardiotoxic antipsychotics—particularly pimozide, droperidol, and thioridazine—should not be combined with HAART.

To avoid further brain compromise, anticholinergic medications to manage antipsychotic-induced EPS should not be used over the long term. Instead, antipsychotics that do not require the concomitant use of anticholinergics are preferred.

"AIDS Mania"

A clinical entity of mania with cognitive impairment but without a personal or family history of bipolar disorder has been termed *AIDS mania*, a form of secondary mania that tends to occur in late-stage HIV disease.[24] In one study from Uganda, a country with high HIV prevalence, 61 (43%) of 141 hospital admissions for acute mania were for HIV-related secondary mania.[25] Clinically, the full manic syndrome is present, often more severe than primary mania and accompanied by significant psychosis. The mood is typically irritable and paranoid and rarely euphoric. Profound sleep disturbance causes patients to be confused and up all night; delirium must be excluded. Treatment includes initiating or optimizing HAART, but it is otherwise identical to standard management of bipolar disorder. In more severely ill HIV-infected patients, antipsychotics are preferred over anti-manic mood stabilizers because of relatively poor clinical tolerability for lithium and carbamazepine and because of increased risk for liver toxicity for valproate. Valproate can enhance the risk for bone marrow toxicity when combined with zidovudine because of increased zidovudine blood levels.

COGNITIVE DISORDERS
Delirium

Delirium must be considered in a patient with HIV infection who has any alteration in mental status, including new-onset psychosis. Delirium is often mistaken for depression or anxiety, which can overshadow the cognitive impairments. Causes of delirium in this population are myriad and some are listed in Box 57-3; often, several causative factors are present simultaneously. Evaluation of delirium in HIV-infected patients must include rare causes. In immunocompromised patients, delirium might be the sole sign of an infection. Delirium is discussed at greater length in Chapter 18.

HIV-associated Neurocognitive Disorder

Perhaps because HIV invades the brain shortly after infection, cognitive complaints and problems at some point during the life course are common in HIV-infected patients.[26] Before HAART, the majority of patients developed cognitive problems, including a late-stage subcortical dementia, currently termed HAD (previously referred to as AIDS dementia or AIDS dementia complex), part of a wider spectrum of neurocognitive impairments collectively called HIV-associated neurocognitive disorder (HAND).[27] While the incidence of HAD has declined since the introduction of HAART, that even HAART-treated patients can manifest the less severe forms of HAND—asymptomatic neurocognitive impairment and mild neurocognitive disorder—is increasingly recognized.[28] It is likely that phenotypic differences exist among HAD patients[29]; some patients have irreversible deficits (accrued in the absence of HAART during times of prolonged and high viremia and poor immune function), whereas newly diagnosed patients might recover substantially if treated with HAART, even if they have HAD.[30,31] Some cohorts might have other pathophysiological processes adding insult to injury. For example, the hepatitis C virus (HCV) has been shown to be neurotropic,[32] and significant past or active drug use can further impair brain function.

As a subcortical dementia, HAD is characterized by disturbances of mood, memory, and motor function (Box 57-8).

BOX 57-8 Clinical Features of Cognitive Disorders in the HIV-infected Patient*

Mood
- Apathy
- Depression
- Anxiety
- Hypomania
- Disinhibition
- Poor judgment
- Personality change

Memory
- Impaired attention
- Impaired concentration
- Impaired memory

Motor Function
- Mental and psychomotor slowing
- Incoordination
- Gait problems

*If mild with no functional disruption, asymptomatic neurocognitive impairment; if moderate with some functional disruption, mild neurocognitive disorder; if severe with functional impairment, HIV-associated dementia.

HIV, Human immunodeficiency virus.

Impairments in attention, new learning, processing speed, and executive function cause significant disability. Depression and anxiety are often present and can eclipse the cognitive problems. Motor and cognitive slowness can be pronounced. Behavioral problems ranging from apathy to hypomania and disinhibition can greatly complicate management, particularly if judgment is impaired.

Any HIV-infected patient should be carefully assessed for cognitive problems, particularly if periods of high viremia and low CD4 counts occurred in the past. It is useful to screen for cognitive problems with the HIV Dementia Scale (HDS)[33] or its modified form (Table 57-1), supplemented by other bedside tests (e.g., Luria hand maneuvers and verbal forms of the Trail-making Tests A and B). The Folstein Mini-Mental State Examination (MMSE) is not sensitive for subcortical dementias, particularly if mild. Because it does not include timed tasks, it is relatively poor at detecting the psychomotor slowing that is the hallmark of HAD.

Comprehensive neuropsychological testing should be ordered to clarify the diagnosis, for longitudinal assessments, and to delineate further the nature and severity of detected or suspected deficits. However, there can be a discrepancy between test scores and functional capability, and a patient's complaint about cognitive difficulties should not be dismissed. In addition, depression should be considered and a time-limited antidepressant trial be offered when the diagnosis is unclear.

Recognition of cognitive impairment is important since patients with executive dysfunction and poor memory, left to their own devices, may be unable to participate in their HIV treatment and to adhere optimally to HAART, thus setting up a vicious cycle of exacerbated brain dysfunction. Any treatment recommendations must take these limitations into account, and sufficient support must be provided to compensate for these deficits.

The optimal HAART regimen for patients with CNS disease (or to prevent CNS disease) remains to be established. While it is unclear if regimens with antiretrovirals that penetrate the CNS (i.e., zidovudine, stavudine, abacavir, and nevirapine) are superior to other regimens,[34,35] there is consensus that optimal peripheral viral suppression is necessary. Treatments for the dementia itself are experimental (e.g., selegiline or memantine). Sometimes, stimulants are beneficial, particularly if apathy and slowness are prominent. Medications that adversely affect brain function (e.g., anticholinergics) should be minimized or avoided and substance use disorders treated. Any patient who is suspected to have a primary depressive or anxiety disorder must also be assessed for HAD. Often, the issue cannot be resolved on clinical grounds, and an antidepressant trial is initiated in conjunction with HAART

TABLE 57-1 HIV Dementia Scale*

Maximum Score	Score	
		MEMORY—REGISTRATION
		Give four words to recall (dog, hat, green, peach), 1 second to say each. Then ask the patient to say all four after you have said them.
4	___	**ATTENTION**
		Anti-saccadic eye movements: 20 commands.
		≤ 3 errors = 4 6 errors = 1
		4 errors = 3 > 6 errors = 0
		5 errors = 2
6	___	**PSYCHOMOTOR SPEED**
		Ask the patient to write the alphabet in uppercase letters horizontally across a page and record time: ___ seconds.
		≤ 21 seconds = 6 30.1–33 seconds = 2
		21.1–24 seconds = 5 33.1–36 seconds = 1
		24.1–27 seconds = 4 > 36 seconds = 0
		27.1–30 seconds = 3
4	___	**MEMORY—RECALL**
		Ask for the four words from Registration above. Give 1 point for each correct. For words not recalled, prompt with a "semantic" cue, as follows: animal (dog); piece of clothing (hat); color (green); fruit (peach). Give ½ point for each correct after prompting.
2	___	**CONSTRUCTION**
		Copy the cube below; record time: ___ seconds.
		< 25 seconds = 2
		25–35 seconds = 1
		> 35 seconds = 0
Total Score	___ /16	

*The modified version excludes the attention task.
HIV, Human immunodeficiency virus.
Adapted from Power C, Selnes OA, Grim JA, McArthur JC. HIV dementia scale: a rapid screening test. J Acquir Immune Defic Syndr Hum Retrovirol 8:273–278, 1995.

optimization. A dementing illness coupled with impulsivity increases suicide risk.

NEUROLOGICAL DISORDERS

Several central neurological conditions are AIDS-defining conditions (Box 57-2): cytomegalovirus (CMV) encephalitis, cryptococcal meningitis, HAD, primary CNS lymphoma, progressive multifocal leukoencephalopathy (PML; Figure 57-4), and cerebral toxoplasmosis (Figure 57-5). Boxes 57-9 and 57-10 provide a more extensive list of neurological conditions associated with HIV infection. Patients with these disorders are usually acutely ill, and they are treated by neurologists and internists in hospital settings. Psychiatrists get involved when behavioral manifestations (e.g., depression or psychosis) are prominent and when, following the acute treatment phase, patients have to adjust to a new diagnosis (which might include AIDS) and new disabilities (e.g., loss of brain function after treatment of CNS lymphoma or visual impairment from CMV).

One peripheral neurological complication—distal sensory polyneuropathy (DSP)—has emerged as a significant clinical problem. It is the most common neurological complication of HIV disease, affecting approximately one-third of all patients.[36] The etiology of DSP is often a mixture of macrophage-driven nerve damage and mitochondrial dysfunction caused by nerve-toxic nucleoside reverse transcriptase inhibitors (NRTIs) (the dideoxynucleosides or "d drugs": ddI, d4T, and ddC) resulting in an axonal neuropathy. Many patients bear the burden of additional toxins (e.g., alcoholism, OI prophylaxis, or past treatment with vincristine for HIV-related cancers). A lower CD4 count is one recognized risk factor; others include older age, lower hemoglobin, and higher viral set-point. Thus DSP encompasses two phenotypically-identical neuropathies: HIV-associated DSP and antiretroviral toxic neuropathy (ATN).

As the most common neurological condition, DSP is important for psychiatrists for two reasons: (1) many long-term patients suffer from it, resulting in a chronic pain syndrome that can be excruciating, resulting in disability, depressive overlay, and reduced quality of life; and (2) CNS-active

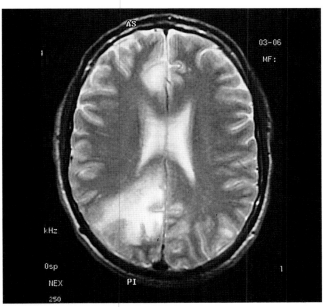

Figure 57-4. Progressive multifocal leukoencephalopathy. *(Courtesy of Dr. Jane Anderson.)*

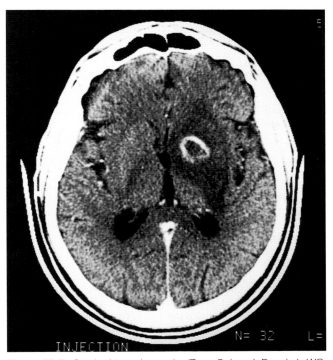

Figure 57-5. Cerebral toxoplasmosis. *(From Cohen J, Powderly WG, editors.* Infectious diseases, *ed 2, Philadelphia, 2004, Elsevier, p 1293.)*

BOX 57-9 Neurological Complications of HIV Infection

HIV-associated neurocognitive disorder (HAND)
Myelopathy (spinal cord disease)
- Vacuolar
- Pure sensory

Focal central nervous system (CNS) lesions
- Toxoplasmosis
- Primary CNS lymphoma
- Progressive multifocal leukoencephalopathy

Meningitis
- Aseptic
- Cryptococcosis
- Tuberculosis

Neurosyphilis

Kaposi's sarcoma
Chagas reactivation
Encephalitis
- Cytomegalovirus (CMV)
- Herpes simplex virus

Neuropathies (see also Box 57-10)
- HIV-associated distal sensory polyneuropathy
- Antiretroviral toxic neuropathy (due to the "d drugs": ddI, ddC, d4T)
- Inflammatory polyneuropathies
- CMV polyradiculopathy
- Mononeuritis multiplex

Myopathy

HIV, Human immunodeficiency virus.

BOX 57-10 Important Causes of Peripheral Neuropathy in the HIV-infected Patient

HIV-associated distal sensory polyneuropathy
Antiretroviral toxic neuropathy (due to the "d drugs")
- ddC (zalcitabine)
- ddI (didanosine)
- d4T (stavudine)

Diabetes mellitus
Alcoholism
Disulfiram
Vitamin B$_{12}$ deficiency
Diffuse infiltrative lymphocytosis syndrome
Antibiotics
- Dapsone (used to treat *Pneumocystis jirovecii* pneumonia and toxoplasmosis)
- Isoniazid (used to treat tuberculosis)
- Metronidazole (used to treat amebic dysentery)

Cancer drugs
- Paclitaxel
- Thalidomide (used to treat aphthous ulcers and wasting)
- Vincristine (used to treat Kaposi's sarcoma)

HIV, Human immunodeficiency virus.

---

medications are often required to treat the pain, adding iatrogenic morbidity (e.g., fatigue).

DSP is a rather pure sensory neuropathy with symptoms typical of sensory neuropathies (i.e., tingling, pain, and burning on the soles of the feet). In addition, ankle reflexes are often absent.

The diagnosis can be suspected on clinical grounds in the right setting and with typical symptoms. Nerve conduction studies demonstrate an axonal neuropathy. In unclear situations, particularly when severe symptoms are not supported by signs, an outpatient punch skin biopsy can clarify the situation. In patients with DSP, the intra-epidermal nerve fiber density is reduced.

Treatment involves removal of toxic agents; if the offending agents can be discontinued, the neuropathy might resolve. Since many HAART medications do not cause neuropathy, regimens that do not contain high-risk drugs (i.e., the "d drugs") can usually be found. Treatment of confounding conditions (e.g., alcoholism, diabetes) must be optimized. In many cases, symptomatic treatment will be necessary. Treatments include pain medications, anti-epileptic drugs, and TCAs. In one well-controlled trial, lamotrigine was effective.[37] Carbamazepine is difficult to use in this population because of a higher rate of rashes and leukopenia.

TREATMENT

The key therapeutic modalities for HIV-infected patients are psychopharmacology and psychotherapy, often combined with providing social support and crisis intervention.

In general, patients with HIV infection—particularly those at advanced stages of illness—have less lean body mass, metabolize drugs more slowly, and are sensitive to drug side effects. Because of blood–brain barrier compromise, the HIV-infected brain may "see" higher levels of drug. Therefore, when starting a psychotropic, start at half the usual starting dose, titrate half as fast as usual, and aim for low therapeutic levels. These clinical rules of thumb should not be taken as excuses for prescribing subtherapeutic doses over prolonged periods of time, because most patients will tolerate and need standard regimens.

TABLE 57-2 Antiretroviral Medications

Generic Name	Brand Name	Abbreviation
NUCLEOSIDE REVERSE TRANSCRIPTASE INHIBITORS (NRTIs)		
Abacavir	Ziagen	ABC
Didanosine	Videx	ddI
Emtricitabine	Emtriva, Coviracil	FTC
Lamivudine	Epivir	3TC
Stavudine	Zerit	d4T
Tenofovir*	Viread	TDF
Zalcitabine	Hivid	ddC
Zidovudine	Retrovir	AZT, ZDV
NON-NUCLEOSIDE REVERSE TRANSCRIPTASE INHIBITORS (NNRTIs)		
Delavirdine	Rescriptor	
Efavirenz	Sustiva	
Etravirine	Intelence	
Nevirapine	Viramune	
Rilpivirine	Edurant	
PROTEASE INHIBITORS (PIs)		
Amprenavir	Agenerase	
Atazanavir	Reyataz	
Darunavir	Prezista	
Fosamprenavir	Lexiva	
Indinavir	Crixivan	
Lopinavir/ritonavir	Kaletra	
Nelfinavir	Viracept	
Ritonavir	Norvir	
Saquinavir	Invirase, Fortovase	
Tipranavir	Aptivus	
FUSION INHIBITOR		
Enfuvirtide	Fuzeon, T-20	
ENTRY INHIBITOR		
Maraviroc	Selzentry	
INTEGRASE INHIBITORS**		
Elvitegravir		
Raltegravir	Isentress	
COMBINATION FORMULATIONS		
Efavirenz/emtricitabine/ tenofovir	Atripla	
Lamivudine/zidovudine	Combivir	
Emtricitabine/rilpivirine/ tenofovir	Complera	
Abacavir/lamivudine	Epzicom	
Elvitegravir/cobicistat/ emtricitabine/tenofovir	Stribild	
Abacavir/lamivudine/ zidovudine	Trizivir	
Emtricitabine/tenofovir	Truvada	

*Nucleotide reverse transcriptase inhibitor.
**Integrase strand transfer inhibitors.

Several classes of antiretroviral agents are currently available to combat HIV infection (Table 57-2), and some have neuropsychiatric side effects. The NNRTI efavirenz carries the highest liability for a broad range of neuropsychiatric symptoms (e.g., vivid dreams, dizziness, insomnia, depressive symptoms), affecting up to half of patients. However, these side effects (mostly mild in nature and possibly related to plasma levels) are usually limited to the period of initiation of efavirenz.[38,39] High-dose AZT has been linked to mania.[40]

Potential interactions between antiretroviral and psychotropic medications are numerous. The University of Liverpool maintains a comprehensive online database of these and other interactions at www.hiv-druginteractions.org, to which the interested reader is referred for the latest information on this topic.

All of the NNRTIs and PIs are metabolized by the cytochrome P-450 system—especially the 3A4 isoform—and many

BOX 57-11 Features of the "Marathon Model" in Psychotherapy

Training
- How have you coped with adversity in the past?
- Personal team
- Who comprises your personal support system?

Pit stops
- Can you take a break from being sick by scheduling a week without doctors' appointments?

Corporate support
- Do you have a primary care physician, HIV specialist, psychiatrist, hospital, health insurance, and employer?

HIV, Human immunodeficiency virus.

BOX 57-12 Factors Affecting Adherence to Highly Active Antiretroviral Therapy

- Depression*
- *Active* substance use (particularly cocaine use and alcohol use)
- Cognitive impairment
- Psychosis
- Personality factors that lead to chaotic lives with no routines
- "Medication fatigue"
- Demoralization
- Age < 35 years
- Non-disclosed status
- Health illiteracy

*Strongest remediable risk factor.

BOX 57-13 Differential Diagnosis of Fatigue in the HIV-infected Patient

Stress
Sleep deprivation
- Insomnia
- Pain

Dysphoric mental states
- Anxiety
- Depression

Obesity
Deconditioning
Drug and alcohol use
Medication-induced sedation
- Highly active antiretroviral therapy
- Psychotropics

HIV/AIDS-related conditions
- Wasting
- Diarrhea
- Infections
- Anemia
- Hypogonadism
- Cardiac disease
- Adrenal disease

AIDS, Acquired immunodeficiency syndrome; HIV, human immunodeficiency virus.

also induce or inhibit it (as well as other, non-P-450-enzyme systems). Ritonavir is the most potent 3A4 inhibitor if given at full dose (low-dose ritonavir is often added to other PIs to "boost" their levels), saquinavir the least. Some antiretroviral agents (e.g., efavirenz) have complex interactions with the P-450 system, both inhibiting and inducing it, thus complicating prediction of psychotropic drug levels, especially with multiple-drug regimens. In all cases, a high index of suspicion and close clinical follow-up are the best safeguards against drug interactions. The most dangerous drug interactions are those that block the metabolism of psychotropics with dose-related toxicity (e.g., pimozide, clozapine, triazolobenzodiazepines, TCAs). The NRTIs and the fusion inhibitor enfuvirtide have no P-450-mediated drug interactions with psychotropics. The entry inhibitor maraviroc and the integrase inhibitor raltegravir have limited potential for interactions with psychotropics. A combination pill, Stribild (brand name), contains cobicistat, a potent 3A inhibitor, that could potentially increase plasma levels of co-administered psychotropics.

Psychotherapy with the HIV-infected patient is more often supportive and crisis-centered than exploratory and insight-oriented. Frequently, one or more of the stressors listed in Box 57-5 brings the patient to therapy. The four key questions of the "marathon model" (Box 57-11) identify the strengths the patient brings to bear on the stressful situation and the weaknesses that will render its resolution difficult.[41] Through education, guidance, and advice, psychosocial assets are enhanced and deficits remedied.

SPECIAL CLINICAL PROBLEMS
Adherence

A high degree of adherence to HAART is necessary to minimize the risk of medication failure and the development of resistant HIV strains. For non-boosted PI-based HAART regimens, adherence approaching 100% is required to suppress viral replication,[42] although adherence requirements for other regimens (e.g., those containing the more potent NNRTIs) might be more "forgiving."[43] Maintaining adherence over an entire lifetime often proves challenging, even for the most industrious patient.

Psychiatrists can contribute their part to optimizing adherence to HAART by identifying and treating those psychiatric factors that can lead to poor adherence (Box 57-12). Psychiatrists should routinely assess HAART adherence and educate patients about the importance of optimally controlled HIV disease for their mental health. In many instances of poor adherence (e.g., if there is cognitive impairment), merely focusing on simpler HAART (or psychotropic) regimens is insufficient and more active approaches are required, including enlisting the help of other people to ensure proper taking of medications (e.g., providing directly observed therapy [DOT]). Treating depression with fluoxetine in homeless patients using DOT has been shown to be an effective intervention in achieving control of HIV.[44]

Fatigue

Clinically-impairing fatigue affects at least one-third of patients with HIV/AIDS.[45] That the etiology can be multi-factorial (Box 57-13) should not dissuade a vigorous pursuit for remediable causes (Box 57-14). Poor sleep quality and insomnia are often present in HIV disease and can be targeted symptomatically. Psychological factors are an important consideration, particularly in patients with well-controlled HIV disease who complain about fatigue. While not all fatigue signifies depression, fatigue is a core symptom of depressed patients in primary

---

BOX 57-14 Evaluation of Fatigue in the HIV-infected Patient

History
Medication review
Focused laboratory work-up
- Complete blood cell count
- Chemistries
- Thyroid-stimulating hormone
- Folate
- Vitamin B_{12}
- Testosterone (in males)
- Pregnancy test
- Erythrocyte sedimentation rate
Substance use screening
Rating scales
- Anxiety
- Depression
- Sleep quality
Polysomnography (if indicated)
Work-up for cardiac disease and adrenal insufficiency (if indicated)

HIV, Human immunodeficiency virus.

BOX 57-15 Risk Factors for Suicide in the HIV-infected Patient

- Male gender
- Depression
- Substance use
- Cognitive impairment
- Same-gender sexual orientation
- Stressors associated with living with a complex disorder
- Recent diagnosis of HIV disease
- Terminal stage of illness

HIV, Human immunodeficiency virus.

---

care settings. Accordingly, all HIV-infected patients should be screened for depression, anxiety, and substance use as main contributors to insomnia and fatigue.[46] Management of fatigue involves specific treatment of identified causes of fatigue (e.g., replacement of testosterone for hypogonadism, analgesics for pain at night, or antidepressants for depression). If no specific cause is identified or remedied, stimulants and modafinil can be used symptomatically. Fatigue can easily be rated (e.g., with a simple visual analogue scale) before, and following, treatment to judge the efficacy of the intervention.

Suicide

After HAART was introduced, the suicide rate in the HIV population decreased.[47] However, all elements of suicidal burden (i.e., thoughts, deliberate self-injury, and completed suicides) are elevated among HIV-positive patients.[48] In many instances, a diagnosis of HIV infection is simply one additional stressor in a life already complicated by substance use and psychiatric morbidity (Box 57-15). If HIV infection *per se* confers any additional risk beyond generally known suicide risk factors, particularly substance use and depression, is unknown. More specific associations between HIV infection and suicide might exist (e.g., HAD with mood lability, impulsivity, and poor judgment may increase the risk for suicide). Even when

depression and substance use are controlled for, an association between homosexuality and suicide persists.

Serious Mental Illness

A small minority of patients with schizophrenia and other serious mental illnesses (SMIs) are infected with HIV, with estimates ranging from 3.1% to 8%. This population is often overlooked as being at risk, despite a high rate of lifetime substance use and other risk factors, including trading sex for money.[49] In one survey, patients with schizophrenia were rather misinformed about the transmission of HIV. Screening for HIV risk factors and provision of modified education about HIV infection that takes into account cognitive limitations have become important roles of providers who treat patients with SMI. Importantly, substance use more than SMI *per se* is the driving force behind newly acquired HIV infection.[50]

Complex treatment regimens are best avoided, and second-generation antipsychotics are preferred over first-generation agents to avoid EPS and the need for anticholinergics. Drug interactions between antipsychotics and HAART should be anticipated, and antipsychotic drug levels should be measured to ensure adequate concentrations and avoid psychotic relapse. Because of the severity and chronicity of their mental illness, many patients with SMI are well connected to psychiatric and medical services and live in supervised settings, so adding HIV treatment poses fewer difficulties than usually feared. However, a group of so-called "triply diagnosed" patients—HIV infection, SMI, and substance use—poses particular challenges in treatment engagement and adherence. If a psychotic exacerbation occurs in a patient with SMI and HIV disease, causes related to HIV, its complications, or its treatment must be ruled out before attributing the exacerbation to the psychiatric illness.

Co-infection with HIV and Hepatitis C

Approximately 15% to 30% of patients with HIV disease are also infected with HCV. This "co-infected cohort" is rather different from HIV "mono-infected" patients with regard to risk factors and psychiatric illnesses. Most patients have acquired HCV from injection drug use, the main mode of transmission for HCV; the group is marginalized with high rates of homelessness; and there might be a higher rate of antisocial tendencies or personality disorder.[51] Accordingly, psychiatric treatment focuses on cessation of substance use and prevention of relapse.

Alcoholism is often present and can lead to additional liver damage. However, recent outbreaks of acute hepatitis C infections have confirmed a role for sexual transmission of HCV as well, particularly among MSM. As treatment of, and survival with, HIV disease have improved, liver failure from hepatitis C infection has become a major concern in this cohort, and patients are increasingly treated as the newly available directly acting antivirals telaprevir and boceprevir when combined with interferon, have improved the outlook for clearing hepatitis C infection.[52] Neuropsychiatric side effects of interferon are common and can lead to depression, suicide, and relapse to substance use.

Cigarette Smoking

As mortality due to HIV-related causes has steadily decreased, intervention has focused on other causes of premature death, including cardiovascular disease. A major contributor to cardiac risk as well as cancer and pneumonia in HIV-infected patients is smoking. An estimated 40% to 80% of persons with HIV are current smokers.[53] With expertise in addictions,

BOX 57-16 Useful Internet Resources

AEGIS (AIDS Education Global Information System)
- www.aegis.org

AIDSinfo (U.S. Department of Health and Human Services)
- www.aidsinfo.nih.gov

American Psychiatric Association AIDS Resource Center
- www.psych.org/aids

Centers for Disease Control and Prevention
- www.cdc.gov

Joint United Nations Programme on HIV/AIDS
- www.unaids.org

Project Inform (HIV information for the lay public)
- www.projectinform.org

The Body Pro (HIV/AIDS resource for health care professionals)
- www.thebodypro.com

University of Liverpool's drug interaction website
- www.hiv-druginteractions.org

psychiatrists can be critically involved in motivational interviewing and assisting motivated smokers to quit smoking, using standard approaches including nicotine replacement therapy. Varenicline appears to be as efficacious and tolerable in HIV-infected patients as in the general population.[54]

INTERNET RESOURCES

Numerous websites that contain useful information about HIV infection, AIDS, and the psychiatric aspects of the medical care of patients with HIV/AIDS are available. Some of them are listed in Box 57-16.

Access the complete reference list and multiple choice questions (MCQs) online at https://expertconsult.inkling.com

KEY REFERENCES

1. Huang L, Quartin A, Jones D, et al. Intensive care of patients with HIV infection. *N Engl J Med* 355:173–181, 2006.
2. Hall HI, Frazier EL, Rhodes P, et al. Differences in human immunodeficiency virus care and treatment among subpopulations in the United States. *JAMA Intern Med* 173(14):1337–1344, 2013.
3. Christopoulos KA, Havlir DV. Overcoming the human immunodeficiency virus obstacle course. *JAMA Intern Med* 173(14):1344–1345, 2013.
8. Moyer VA. Screening for HIV: U.S. Preventive Services Task Force recommendation statement. *Ann Intern Med* 159(1):51–60, 2013.

17. Sullivan LE, Fiellin DA. Buprenorphine: its role in preventing HIV transmission and improving the care of HIV-infected patients with opioid dependence. *Clin Infect Dis* 41:891–896, 2005.
18. Ciesla JA, Roberts JE. Meta-analysis of the relationship between HIV infection and risk for depressive disorders. *Am J Psychiatry* 158:725–730, 2001.
19. Machtinger EL, Wilson TC, Haberer JE, et al. Psychological trauma and PTSD in HIV-positive women: a meta-analysis. *AIDS Behav* 16:2091–2100, 2012.
21. Sewell DD, Jeste DV, Atkinson JH, et al. HIV-associated psychosis: a study of 20 cases. *Am J Psychiatry* 151:237–242, 1994.
24. Lyketsos CG, Schwartz J, Fishman M, et al. AIDS mania. *J Neuropsychiatry Clin Neurosci* 9:277–279, 1997.
25. Nakimuli-Mpungu E, Musisi S, Kiwuwa Mpungu S, et al. Primary mania versus HIV-related secondary mania in Uganda. *Am J Psychiatry* 163:1349–1354, 2006.
26. Clifford DB. Human immunodeficiency virus–associated dementia. *Arch Neurol* 57:321–324, 2000.
27. Antinori A, Arendt G, Becker JT, et al. Updated research nosology for HIV-associated neurocognitive disorders. *Neurology* 69:1789–1799, 2007.
28. Heaton RK, Clifford DB, Franklin DR Jr, et al. HIV-associated neurocognitive disorders persist in the era of potent antiretroviral therapy: CHARTER Study. *Neurology* 75:2087–2096, 2010.
29. McArthur JC. HIV dementia: an evolving disease. *J Neuroimmunol* 157:3–10, 2004.
31. Ghafouri M, Amini S, Khalili K, et al. HIV-1 associated dementia: symptoms and causes. *Retrovirology* 19:28, 2006.
35. Nath A, Sacktor N. Influence of highly active antiretroviral therapy on persistence of HIV in the central nervous system. *Curr Opin Neurol* 19:358–361, 2006.
38. Kenedi CA, Goforth HW. A systematic review of the psychiatric side-effects of efavirenz. *AIDS Behav* 15:1803–1818, 2011.
42. Paterson DL, Swindells S, Mohr J, et al. Adherence to protease inhibitor therapy and outcomes in patients with HIV infection. *Ann Intern Med* 133:21–30, 2000.
44. Tsai AC, Karasic DH, Hammer GP, et al. Directly observed antidepressant medication treatment and HIV outcomes among homeless and marginally housed HIV-positive adults: a randomized controlled trial. *Am J Public Health* 103:308–315, 2013.
47. Keiser O, Spoerri A, Brinkhof MW, et al. Suicide in HIV-infected individuals and the general population in Switzerland, 1988–2008. *Am J Psychiatry* 167:143–150, 2010.
48. Catalan J, Harding R, Sibley E, et al. HIV infection and mental health: suicidal behaviour—systematic review. *Psychol Health Med* 16:588–611, 2011.
50. Prince JD, Walkup J, Akincigil A, et al. Serious mental illness and risk of new HIV/AIDS diagnoses: an analysis of Medicaid beneficiaries in eight states. *Psychiatric Serv* 63:1032–1038, 2012.
52. Liang TJ, Ghany MG. Current and future therapies for hepatitis C virus infection. *N Engl J Med* 368:1907–1917, 2013.
53. Lifson AR, Lando HA. Smoking and HIV: prevalence, health risks, and cessation strategies. *Curr HIV/AIDS Rep* 9:223–230, 2012.

58

Organ Transplantation: Pre-transplant Assessment and Post-transplant Management

Laura M. Prager, MD

KEY POINTS

- Solid organ transplantation is a viable treatment option for patients with end-organ failure.
- Psychiatrists are integral members of multi-disciplinary transplant teams, involved in both pre-operative and post-operative assessment and care.
- The emotional well-being of the transplant patient can influence outcome.
- Neuropsychiatric sequelae attend both the complications of end-organ failure and the medications used to treat the rejection and infection that follows transplantation.
- Ethical issues in transplantation include determination of selection criteria for recipients and degree of risk acceptable for informed, voluntary living organ donors.

OVERVIEW

Solid organ transplantation is an accepted, successful, and commonly employed treatment option for patients with end-organ failure. Transplant recipients who have received a heart, kidney, liver, pancreas, lung, or small intestine now live longer with an overall improved quality of life. Progress in the development of immunosuppressive therapies and in methods of organ procurement and distribution has also facilitated the transplant process. Even patients with infectious diseases, such as HIV infection, or a history of certain cancers are now potentially eligible for transplant.

In the US, the United Network for Organ Sharing (UNOS), a non-profit organization endowed by Congress but reporting to the Department of Health and Human Services, regulates the allocation and distribution of donor organs. UNOS has two branches: the Organ Procurement and Transplant Network (OPTN) and the Scientific Registry of Transplant Recipients (SRTR). The OPTN divides the country into 11 distinct geographical regions or donation service areas (DSA); each region has its own waiting list. Allocation of organs generally follows a local, regional, and national progression, where local refers to the boundaries of the DSA. The length of time spent on the waiting list can differ greatly among regions.

Determination of priority is organ specific. For kidneys, the length of time on the waiting list is the primary determining factor, although patients listed simultaneously for transplant of a kidney and another solid organ have greater priority. In addition, full human leukocyte antigen (HLA) compatibility (zero antigen mismatch) confers priority. Pediatric recipients (those patients age 18 and under) of kidneys and livers take priority over adults. Within the last few years, OPTN/UNOS Kidney Transplantation Committee has reviewed this allocation procedure and drafted new guidelines taking into account a candidate's ability to survive on the waiting list and creating a measure of kidney quality that would allow for optimizing the match between donors and recipients.[1] The Lung Allocation Score (LAS) is a calculated score for patients over 12 years of age that identifies, among other things, the severity of illness and the likelihood of a successful transplant outcome. The score undergoes frequent modifications based on, among other things, shifts in the characteristics of the candidate cohort, with the consistent goal of reducing time spent on the waiting list. That score, in addition to other factors, includes age, blood type, and geographical location, and determines waiting-list placement for potential lung transplantation recipients. OPTN limits the allocation of lungs to patient's less than 12 years of age to donors within the same age range. This policy has come under scrutiny due to a highly publicized case in which the parents of a 10-year-old girl appealed to a federal judge to allow the patient access to lungs from the adult donor pool.[2] Increasingly, patients with acute respiratory failure have been placed on a mechanical circulatory support (MCS) device, an extracorporeal membrane oxygenator (ECMO), as a bridge to transplant.[3] The Model for End-Stage Liver Disease (MELD) is also a calculated score that predicts how urgently a patient over 12 years of age will need a transplant within the next 3 months. The only exception to the MELD system is a special category known as "Status 1." Status 1A patients have suffered acute hepatic failure and might die within hours or days without a transplant. Boxes 58-1 and 58-2 list the LAS and MELD criteria. Since 1999, heart transplant recipients, likewise, receive organs based on medical urgency. Guidelines from 2006 dictate local and regional allocation and allow critically ill patients within a 500 nautical mile radius of the donor's hospital to take priority over less sick patients within the local zone.[4]

Several factors limit the success of organ transplantation. First, there is the ever-present potential for allograft rejection. In addition, immunocompromised hosts are vulnerable to bacteria, viruses, and fungi that are not considered pathogenic in the normal population. Finally, the side effects of immunosuppressive medications that are used to manage rejection can be debilitating, disfiguring, or life-threatening, and increase the risk for neoplasm, problems with bone metabolism, a cushingnoid body habitus, nephrotoxicity, posterior-reversible encephalopathic syndrome (PRES), and the development of diabetes mellitus.

Societal mores also impose limitations. The scarcity of cadaveric organs creates a mismatch between the number of patients who need transplantation and the number who can undergo transplantation. Currently, there are 118,725 active waiting-list candidates for a solid organ transplantation, but only 14,105 transplants were done between January and July of 2013.[5] In recent years, transplant centers have attempted to expand the donor pool by harvesting organs from donors after circulatory death (DCD) and expanded criteria donors (ECD) in addition to harvesting organs from persons who have been declared dead by neurological criteria (i.e., brain death).[6] In response to this problem, the Institute of Medicine (IOM) created a committee to study ways in which the supply of transplantable organs can be increased. The committee's report, released in May 2006, recommended the following: vigorous public education about organ donation; provision of

---

BOX 58-1 Criteria for Lung Allocation Score (LAS)*
(Age 12 and Older)

- Diagnosis
- Age
- Body mass index (BMI)
- Presence of diabetes
- New York Heart Association Functional Classification
- Distance walked in 6 minutes
- Forced vital capacity (FVC)
- Pulmonary artery pressure (PAP)
- Pulmonary capillary wedge pressure (PCWP)
- Creatinine
- Continuous oxygen requirement
- Requirement for ventilatory support
- Current, highest, and lowest pCO_2

*Adapted from United Network for Organ Sharing (UNOS): www.unos.org.

BOX 58-2 Model for End-Stage Liver Disease (MELD)*
(Age 12 and Older)

- Bilirubin (BR)
- Prothrombin time (international normalized ratio [INR])
- Serum creatinine
- Score ranges from 6 to 40
- Represents urgency for need of transplant within 3 months of calculation

*Adapted from United Network for Organ Sharing (UNOS): www.unos.org.

---

more opportunities for registration as an organ donor; easier access to state donor registries; and renewed attention to improvement of organ procurement systems.[7] A more recent effort includes the establishment of the Transplant Growth and Management Collaborative in 2007,[6] and, in 2008, legislation that gave the Department of Health and Human Services a mandate to issue a National Medal honoring organ donors.[8] Some European countries follow the doctrine of "presumed consent" for post-mortem donation, but the US has not embraced this idea. In fact, New York State Assemblyman Richard Brodsky was unable to attract support for his bill that would assume presumed consent for New York residents.

Organ donation by living donors is an increasingly important potential source of transplantable kidneys, livers, and lungs. This is especially true in Japan where there are no defined criteria for determination of brain death and therefore few cadaveric organs are available for harvest.[9] In the US, living donors may be: related to the recipient; unrelated but emotionally connected; or anonymous, altruistic strangers. According to data from OPTN (from 2013) 11,216 transplanted organs came from deceased donors and 2,889 organ transplants (kidney, liver, lung) came from live donors.[5] Parent-to-child liver transplantation (of the left lateral lobe) is an option, as is adult-to-adult transplantation of the right hepatic lobe. Living-lung donation is also an option for carefully selected candidates, but it requires a lower lobe from two different donors for each single potential recipient. The source of the donated organ (i.e., from a deceased donor or living donor) does not affect recipient outcome.

Living organ donation raises several ethical questions: What is true informed consent regarding both short- and long-term risks for the donor? Is the donor's offer (be it from an emotionally connected or unrelated person) truly voluntary?

It is difficult to determine what level of risk is acceptable for a healthy, altruistic donor.[10,11]

Several retrospective studies of the long-term medical and psychological sequelae in living organ donors have been conducted. Short-term risks for live kidney donors include the morbidity secondary to surgery and anesthesia (e.g., bleeding, infection) and salary loss during the weeks of recovery. For kidney donors, long-term health risks include the development of microalbuminuria and the potential for renal failure in the remaining kidney.[12] The mortality rates for kidney donors is 0.05%[13]; with adult-to-adult liver donation there is a significant degree of morbidity, and mortality rate estimates approach 0.1% for left lateral donation and 0.5% for right lateral donation.[14] To date, no deaths have resulted from living lobar lung donation. One study found that donors lose 15% to 20% of their total lung volume and often experience a decrease in exercise capacity.[15] Another study demonstrated that both the forced vital capacity (FVC) and forced expiratory volume at 1 minute (FEV1) returned to 90% of baseline at 1 year post-lobectomy.[16]

PSYCHIATRIC EVALUATION OF THE TRANSPLANT PATIENT

Psychiatrists and other mental health professionals are involved in many different aspects of the transplantation process. In some centers, a designated psychiatrist works with a specific team: for example, the kidney transplant team. Other transplant centers rely on general hospital psychiatric consultation services, psychologists, or social workers to provide case-by-case consultation. The "involvement" of mental health professionals ranges from the pre-operative evaluation of candidates and living donors, to the short- and long-term post-operative management of solid organ recipients.

The psychiatrist or other mental health professional plays an important role in the evaluation of the patient who is approaching a transplant. Initially, the psychiatrist conducts a thorough psychiatric evaluation of the potential recipient to determine suitability for transplant. The psychiatrist must be familiar with medical and surgical problems facing the patient (both before and after transplantation), in order to educate both the patient and the family members about the risks and benefits of transplantation.

The psychiatrist may also act as a liaison between the patient (and family members) and the transplant team. The patient will need support, direction, and clarification of the transplant team's expectations and concerns. The transplant team may require help interpreting a patient's behavior. The psychiatrist can direct the team's attention on ethical dilemmas that may arise, particularly in the area of directed living donation by a related or unrelated donor.

After transplantation, the psychiatrist will be instrumental in guiding the family through the patient's often difficult and unpredictable post-operative course, as well as in managing the neuropsychiatric sequelae secondary to graft rejection, infection, and immunosuppression.

Pre-transplant Psychiatric Evaluation

There are no universally-accepted guidelines for the psychiatric evaluation of potential candidates for organ transplantation and little reliable or predictive data regarding "suitability for transplantation." Some centers routinely offer a face-to-face clinical interview with a mental health provider, whereas other centers administer formal psychological testing or offer a structured or semi-structured interview. Transplant centers differ in their determination of who is an "acceptable" candidate and what degree of risk they are willing to assume.

BOX 58-3 Psychosocial Exclusion Criteria for Lung Transplantation

ABSOLUTE
- Active substance abuse
- Active psychotic symptoms that interfere with function
- Suicidal ideation with intent or plan
- Dementia

RELATIVE
- Poor social supports
- Personality disorders that cause interpersonal difficulties with members of the transplant team
- Non-adherence to medication regimen or to recommendations for procedures

---

Common psychosocial and behavioral exclusion criteria include active substance abuse, active psychotic symptoms, suicidal ideation (with intent or plan), dementia, or a felony conviction. Relative contraindications include poor social supports with inability to arrange for pre-transplant or post-transplant care, personality disorders that interfere with a working relationship with a transplant team, non-adherence to a medication regimen, and neurocognitive limitations[17] (Box 58-3).

The pre-transplantation psychiatric evaluation should be primarily diagnostic, but it can also be both educational and therapeutic. General objectives of the psychiatric evaluation include screening of potential recipients for the presence of significant Axis I and II diagnoses that might complicate management or interfere with the patient's ability to comply with the treatment team's recommendations after transplantation. The diagnosis of a major Axis I disorder (such as major depressive disorder, schizophrenia, or bipolar disorder) should not be a contraindication to transplant if the patient has been stable for an extended period on appropriate medications and has adequate outpatient care and support. Transplantation is possible even in pre-morbidly cognitively impaired (e.g., mentally retarded) individuals with end-organ failure. Such patients may have family members who will assume legal responsibility for medical decision-making and oversee adherence to post-transplant protocols. The relationship between cognitive dysfunction secondary to end-organ failure and post-transplant function has not been well studied. Personality disorders (listed on Axis II) are more difficult to diagnose in a cross-sectional interview, but, when present, can complicate the patient's interactions with members of the treatment team. Patients with borderline personality disorder and anti-social personality disorder are particularly problematic given their affective dysregulation, unstable personal relationships, and potential for lack of impulse control. Transplant psychiatrists must carefully assess the individual patient's history of interpersonal relationships, substance abuse, potential for self-injurious behavior, adherence to treatment recommendations, and interactions with caregivers before making a decision as to whether such a patient can work successfully with the team.

Psychiatrists are often asked to predict a patient's motivation for transplantation and risk for non-compliance with medication regimens. Life following transplant requires consistent attention to, and compliance with, medical protocols. Post-transplant patients often take as many as 20 medications daily, attend regular clinic appointments, self-monitor blood pressure and blood sugar, maintain good nutrition, and frequently endure uncomfortable procedures and tests.

Evaluators may also wish to assess the patient's resilience and ability to persevere despite setbacks, as well as the availability of social supports that will allow for continued care in the community and easy transportation to and from the hospital. There is controversy as to whether or not the transplant team should explore social media sites in order to verify the patient's report of his/her lifestyle choices. Most mental health professionals who work with this population do not engage in what some have referred to as "patient-targeted googling,"[18] but others feel strongly that they must use whatever means they have in order to make a decision about a candidate's ability to comply with the demands of transplantation. (Personal communication, TransplantPsychiatry@googlegroups.com, 2013.)

Frequently the question arises as to whether or not there is a conflict of interest if, as is often the case, the psychiatrist who conducts the initial screening for transplant candidacy is the same psychiatrist who works with the multi-disciplinary transplant team to decide who is listed. Again, there are no national guidelines and individual transplant teams must address and resolve this ethical issue. The psychiatrist may choose to handle this situation by informing the patient and the family at the beginning of the evaluation that the information presented will be shared with other members of the team.

The issue of substance abuse in the pre-transplant population is particularly challenging because of the risk for relapse with possible non-adherence post-transplant. Most transplant programs require 6 months to 1 year of sustained sobriety before initiation of the transplant evaluation, although this policy has not been shown to affect outcome.[19] Some programs require patients to participate in a substance abuse counseling program in addition to Alcoholics Anonymous (AA) or Narcotics Anonymous (NA) as a prerequisite for listing if they appear to be at high risk for relapse. Cigarette smoking or any form of tobacco use is an absolute contraindication to lung transplantation. Patients must demonstrate sustained abstinence from cigarettes and undergo random measurements of urinary cotinine and/or serum carboxyhemoglobin as part of the evaluation process. In the end, individual transplant centers determine what degree of risk they are willing to tolerate.

Pre-transplant Psychiatric Disorders

Many psychiatric disorders (such as depression, anxiety, adjustment disorders, and substance abuse) are common in the pre-transplant candidate population, regardless of the type of end-stage organ failure. Other disorders are unique to patients who suffer from a particular type of end-organ failure.

Usually, there is a significant wait between the time of listing for transplant and the transplant itself. Many patients with heart failure must wait in a hospital's intensive care unit (ICU) attached to a cardiac monitor or an intra-aortic balloon pump (IABP). Years can go by while the patient with lung disease waits at home, sometimes far from a transplant center, becoming gradually sicker and more sedentary. The wait is stressful. A call from a member of the transplant team saying that an organ is available can come at any time or not at all. Sometimes a patient arrives at the hospital only to learn that the quality of the harvested organs is not good enough—the so-called "false start" or "dry run." Loss of physical strength and productivity (with accompanying role change within the family or community) can lead to an adjustment disorder and to depression.

As many as 25% of dialysis-dependent patients with end-stage renal disease (ESRD) manifest symptoms of clinical depression.[20] Disorders in endocrine function (e.g., hyperparathyroidism), and chronic anemia can also contribute to depression. The dialysis-dysequilibrium syndrome with resultant cerebral edema, as well as uremia, can precipitate a change in mental status or even a frank encephalopathy.

Patients with renal failure are prone to delirium from the accumulation of toxins (e.g., aluminum) or prescribed medications that are normally cleared through the kidney.

Patients with cardiac failure are also at risk for depression and delirium. These patients can spend long periods in the ICU awaiting transplantation with little contact with the outside world. Delirium can be caused by decreased cerebral blood flow, by multiple small ischemic events, or by IABP treatment.[21] The development of the ventricular assist device (VAD) as a bridge to heart transplantation offers a chance for improved quality of life and functional status in this population.

Hepatic failure (e.g., from cirrhosis) is also associated with a high degree of depression and subclinical or frank encephalopathy. Treatment of the mood disorder can result in a more positive outlook and in better self-care. Suicide attempt by toxic ingestion (e.g., of acetaminophen) can result in sudden, drastic hepatic failure and in an immediate need for transplantation. These patients are more difficult to assess because they are often on ventilators. The psychiatric consultant must therefore rely on collateral sources of information about the patient's pre-morbid function.

Patients with end-stage lung disease are likely to suffer from anxiety disorders, particularly panic disorder, in addition to adjustment disorders, depression, and delirium. Most patients who are not anxious pre-morbidly become anxious in the setting of increasing shortness of breath. They often describe anticipatory anxiety (in the setting of planned exertion), panic attacks, and agoraphobia, despite adequate oxygen supplementation. A decreasing radius of activity leads to both adjustment disorder and, sometimes, major depression, as patients struggle to cope with their relentless and progressive inability to perform even simple activities of daily living (ADLs). Extremely compromised patients with pulmonary failure may become delirious from hypoxia or hypercapnia or from medications (such as intravenous benzodiazepines and narcotics) used to treat their anxiety and pain. Patients on ECMO as a bridge to transplant pose a new challenge. These patients are awake and alert, but aware of their tenuous condition and their total dependence on the machine and the staff. In this setting, they often become demanding and angry and deplete the energy and patience of the ICU team.

TREATMENT OF THE PRE-TRANSPLANT PATIENT

Psychiatric care of the pre-transplant patient is based on the bio-psycho-social approach. Psychotropic medications are often a mainstay of treatment. Psychotherapeutic intervention can be helpful as well. Enhancement of a network of social support from family members, neighbors, and friends is crucial. Substance abuse counseling may be required for at-risk patients. Transplant centers may offer support groups run by mental health professionals or clinical nurse specialists that welcome both pre-transplant and post-transplant patients.

Psychopharmacological management of the pre-transplant patient follows the adage, "start low and go slow." Choice of medication and dosage depends on the patient's diagnosis, as well as on the type and degree of organ failure.

The selective serotonin reuptake inhibitors (SSRIs) are usually the first-line treatment of depressive disorders, given their benign side-effect profile and anxiolytic effects. For patients who also struggle to refrain from cigarette smoking, bupropion may be a good choice. Antidepressants are metabolized in the liver, and it is wise to use lower doses for patients with hepatic disease. In addition, there is some evidence to suggest that SSRIs can put patients at increased risk for upper gastrointestinal bleeding and therefore should be used with caution in patients with portal vein hypertension and with

cirrhosis.[22] SSRIs must also be used with caution in patients with resistant bacterial infections who require the antibiotic linezolid (a weak monoamine oxidase inhibitor [MAOI]) because of the risk of serotonin syndrome.[23] With the exception of paroxetine, the SSRIs are well tolerated in patients with ESRD. Likewise, clearance of venlafaxine is reduced in renal failure and the metabolites of bupropion hydrochloride (which are excreted by the kidney) may accumulate and cause seizures in these vulnerable patients.[24]

Benzodiazepines are the mainstay of anxiety management; nonetheless, some transplant teams are unwilling to use them because of their addictive potential. Shorter-lasting agents (such as lorazepam) are preferable because longer-lasting agents (such as chlordiazepoxide) have active metabolites that can accumulate (particularly in patients with hepatic failure) and cause toxicity. Low-dose atypical antipsychotics (such as risperidone or olanzapine) can also be helpful in the treatment of anxiety in those patients who cannot tolerate benzodiazepines because of the risk of respiratory depression or abuse. Risperidone and olanzapine can worsen diabetes mellitus, which often occurs in patients with ESRD, and these agents should be used with caution.

Patients who require mood stabilizers (such as lithium, valproic acid, or carbamazepine) and neuroleptics can continue to take them before transplantation. Because the mood-stabilizing medications have a high level of plasma protein-binding, much lower doses are required in patients with ESRD. Lithium is completely eliminated by dialysis; therefore, serum levels should be obtained just before dialysis and a dose should be given just after dialysis. For patients with hepatic failure, one should adjust the dose of valproic acid or carbamazepine, both of which are metabolized in the liver.

Psychotherapy can also be an extremely important therapeutic intervention for patients approaching a transplant. Even the relatively brief psychiatric pre-transplant evaluation can serve as a good opportunity for patients to share their hopes and dreams for the future, as well as their fears of ongoing illness and of death either before or after transplant. Some psychiatrists will refer pre-transplant patients to other mental health providers for therapy because they feel that they cannot maintain the patients' confidentiality and continue to report to other members of the transplant team (personal communication, TransplantPsychiatry@googlegroups.com, 2006). Common issues raised in psychotherapy include grief over loss of productivity, guilt over dependent status, adaptation to a changing role within the family and community, sexual dysfunction, cognitive slowing secondary to use of medications, and conflict between the reluctance to wish anyone ill and the desire for a deceased donor's organ.

CARE OF THE POST-TRANSPLANT PATIENT

The post-operative period is unpredictable. Some patients recover rapidly and are able to leave the hospital within several weeks. Others can be less fortunate and spend many weeks or even months in the ICU, endure lengthy stays on the transplant unit, and face discharge to a rehabilitation facility. Common sequelae in the immediate post-operative period include delirium, anxiety, and depression. Over the long term, patients can manifest continued anxiety and depression, develop problems with body image, fail to adhere to post-transplant medication regimens, and even revert to active substance abuse.

Short-term Care

The hallmark of the early post-operative period for almost all transplant patients is delirium. The etiology can be

TABLE 58-1 Potential Psychiatric Side Effects of Immunosuppressant Agents

Immunosuppressant Agent	Description	Psychiatric Side Effects	Laboratory Findings
Cyclosporine (Neoral; Sandimmune)	Polypeptide fungal product	Tremor, restlessness, delirium, psychotic symptoms; periventricular leukoencephalopathy	Side effects more prominent with intravenous administration, high dosages, and high serum values, which resolve as serum levels decrease; avoid simultaneous administration of psychotropics that inhibit cytochrome P-450 3A4
Tacrolimus (Prograf, FK 506)	Macrolide antibiotic	Headache, restlessness, insomnia, anxiety; delirium can be seen with high serum levels	Side effects more prominent at high serum values
Mycophenolate (Cellcept)	Suppresses T- and B-cell proliferation cyclosporine or tacrolimus	Anxiety, depression	
Muromonab-CD3 (OKT3)	Monoclonal antibody that suppresses CD3 T-cell function; given immediately post-operatively to prevent rejection	Aseptic meningitis; hallucinations during administration	
Corticosteroids	Very high doses used initially then tapered over weeks to months; most patients remain on small doses indefinitely	Increased appetite, anxiety, depression, mood lability, mania, paranoia	Side effects more prominent at high doses

multi-factorial but it usually represents a combination of medication effects or withdrawal states, metabolic changes, or infectious processes. Heart transplantation patients are at risk for intra-operative cerebral ischemia that may predispose them to delirium in the very early post-operative period. Lung transplantation patients may become hypoxic. All of the immunosuppressive medications can cause psychotic symptoms (such as paranoid delusions and auditory and visual hallucinations [with or without accompanying delirium]). Cyclosporine and tacrolimus can also cause PRES. High-dose steroids can precipitate hypomanic or manic behaviors with psychotic symptoms (Table 58-1).

Management of delirium demands a search for the etiology and treatment of the underlying disorder. Cautious use of neuroleptics (such as haloperidol) can offer relief from disabling and frightening symptoms. Haloperidol is usually the first choice because it can be given intravenously and it is primarily metabolized by the process of glucuronidation rather than by the cytochrome P-450 isoenzymes. Gabapentin can be helpful in the management of steroid-induced psychosis (if the patient can take oral medication), with dosage adjustment made for renal insufficiency. When patients are unable to tolerate haloperidol, dexmedetomidine, an alpha agonist, can be a good choice for management of refractory delirium.

Early symptoms of depression (e.g., mood changes, sleep disturbance, irritability, poor concentration) may be secondary to medications (such as beta-blockers or steroids) or may represent a recurrence of a pre-morbid mood disorder. Sometimes, new symptoms of depression herald the development of infectious processes (such as cytomegalovirus [CMV] or *Mycobacterium avium* complex [MAC]). Treatment with the SSRIs can be helpful both for their antidepressant and anxiolytic effects.

Anxiety symptoms in the early post-operative period can result from rapid adjustments in benzodiazepines or narcotics, from early immunosuppressive toxicity, or from sepsis. In lung transplant patients, anxiety can accompany acute rejection, pneumonia, or pleural effusion. Treatment strategies include a gradual tapering of high-dose intravenous or oral benzodiazepines and/or narcotics followed by maintenance with a low-dose, short-lasting benzodiazepine (such as lorazepam). Patients who have a pre-morbid generalized

anxiety or panic disorder that recurs may be managed with a combination of an SSRI and a benzodiazepine.

Long-term Care

Patients undergoing solid organ transplantation are effectively exchanging one set of problems, those related to end-organ failure, for another set: rejection of the allograft; side effects of immunosuppressive medications; and possible progression of an underlying systemic disease. Although transplant teams certainly inform potential recipients of the risks and benefits of the procedure, many of those recipients (and their families) have unrealistic expectations of their rate of recovery and their overall quality of life following transplantation.

Disappointment and dashed hopes can precipitate mood changes. Frequent medical setbacks, understood by the treatment team as part of the normal course of events, discourage patients and family members. Family members can aggravate the situation by expecting too much, too soon from the transplant recipient. Alternatively, family members or friends who have served as caretakers for many years may be unable to relinquish control, even when the recipient is clearly stronger and better able to care for himself or herself.

Transplant recipients have spent many years in and around hospitals. After a transplant, they gradually move back into their community. Initially, clinic visits can be bi-weekly. As time goes by, patients come into the hospital less and less often. Many transplant patients get anxious as they transition from the close monitoring provided by the medical and surgical teams to a more independent status. Phone contact with a member of the team can be helpful in such circumstances. These patients also benefit from regular attendance at a transplantation support group where, under the guidance of a knowledgeable team leader, they can share their experiences with other transplant recipients.

Almost all transplant recipients take steroids, and most have some visible changes in body habitus. Patients exhibit a cushingoid distribution of body fat and can suffer, among other things, hirsutism and easy bruising. Young women patients in particular struggle with these bodily changes and may be more likely than other transplant recipients to refuse to take the steroids as prescribed. This level of non-compliance is extremely worrisome because it can result in potentially life-threatening acute or chronic rejection. Prompt psychiatric evaluation of the non-compliant transplant recipient for the presence of an underlying mood or adjustment disorder is essential to prevent rejection of the allograft. Ideally, use of supportive psychotherapy might help such patients understand the potentially self-destructive nature of their actions and devise strategies that could ensure better adherence.

Substance abuse can also re-emerge in the post-transplant period, even though the patient may have had years of sobriety before transplantation. Members of transplant teams often have difficulty managing the liver transplant recipient who begins drinking again or the lung transplant recipient who picks up a cigarette not only because of their concern regarding risk to the allograft but also because of their tremendous disappointment in the patient's behavior.

PEDIATRIC TRANSPLANTATION

In 2013, pediatric patients accounted for approximately 6% (865) of all organ transplants done in the US (14,105). Forty percent of those transplants were for children between the ages of 11 and 17 years.[5]

Pediatric transplant patients differ from adult transplant patients in a number of ways. A parent or appointed legal guardian makes the medico-legal decisions for the child; the children (infants, toddlers, and school-age children) are not responsible for the decision to proceed with transplant or for pre-transplant and post-transplant care. Most young patients require a transplant because of a congenital disorder (such as biliary atresia, cardiac malformations, or pulmonary atresia) and are not held responsible for their disease. A child's ability to understand the serious nature of his or her illness and the risks and benefits of transplant depends on the child's age and developmental stage. Many transplant patients have never had the chance to enjoy age-appropriate activities. The severity of their illness might have imposed limitations on school attendance and social interactions and bred a profound dependence on parents and other caregivers.

The primary goal of the psychiatrist who cares for a pediatric transplant patient is to help the child maintain a normal developmental trajectory in the face of life-threatening illness. The psychiatrist must also attempt to balance the needs of the child with the needs of parents, siblings, and involved members of the extended family. No one wants to deny a child the chance for a longer life. However, children, like adults, may not be appropriate candidates for transplantation. Sometimes a child is disqualified for transplantation because of the inability of adult caregivers to provide adequate monitoring or to follow the instructions of the treatment team. The psychiatrist who works with young patients with end-organ failure must also be able to understand and to withstand the anger and disappointment of members of the treatment team when faced with such a situation.

Pre-transplant Evaluation

Unlike with adults, however, the order and style of the pre-transplant psychiatric interview depend on the child's age and developmental stage. With a pre-pubertal child, it is appropriate to meet first with the parents or guardians to obtain a coherent, chronological history and to assess the parents' understanding of the risks and benefits, as well as their history of compliance in obtaining care for their child. With an adolescent, it is helpful to interview the child alone, before speaking with the parents, in order to support his or her independence and wish for autonomy. Again, the psychiatric evaluation should address the following issues: presence of significant

Axis I disorders (such as mood disorders, anxiety disorders, and learning disabilities) in the patient or in a caregiver; history of past or current substance abuse; relationship with caregivers; patient's and family's motivation for transplant; ability of the caregivers to comply with treatment recommendations (medication regimen and appointments); adequacy of social supports; and assessment of stressors within the family, such as marital discord or financial problems.

Although parents or guardians must be the ones to give "consent" for the surgery and post-operative care, a verbal child must be able to "assent" to the surgery and be willing to participate in treatment. Both parents and children must be fully engaged in preparation for transplant, as well as be able and willing to work together toward a common goal.

The dilemma of the adolescent transplant candidate who abuses substances is particularly important. Adolescents are less likely than adults to have long-standing struggles with substance abuse, but they are often recreational users of alcohol or street drugs, particularly in social situations. The normal adolescent's need for autonomy and independence often leads to substance use, despite an intellectual appreciation of the grave risks. Some teens with liver disease drink alcohol, and some teens with lung disease smoke cigarettes or marijuana. This behavior usually stops as the illness progresses and the patient becomes more medically compromised. It is difficult to know, however, whether this change reflects a true understanding of the risks, or whether it is simply a short-term response to the fear of jeopardizing their transplant candidacy.

Adolescents often struggle to comply with medication regimens and treatment recommendations before transplantation. They are seeking to forge their own identity and to separate themselves from their parents. At the same time, they desperately want to be part of their peer group and to look just like everyone else. Often this translates into, for example, a teenager with cystic fibrosis who refuses to take enzymes at lunch in the cafeteria, or go to the nurse for an insulin injection in the middle of the day. Because non-adherence is a major cause of graft rejection in adolescents, a history of this kind of behavior pattern in a pre-transplant candidate is worrisome—even though it is consistent with the patient's age and developmental stage.

In some instances, the evaluator may use the 17-item Pediatric Transplant Rating Instrument (P-TRI) to assess an adolescent's understanding of the transplant process, history of adherence to medication regimens and the recommendations of his/her treatment team, presence or absence of psychiatric problems and/or substance use, and degree of family engagement.[25] Although this screening tool can be helpful, it is important to remember that the P-TRI is not intended to determine eligibility for transplantation because the data linking patients' scores to transplant outcome are lacking.[26]

Post-transplant Care

The post-operative care of the pediatric transplant patient is similar to that of the adult. Delirium is a common occurrence. The immunosuppressive medications can cause neuropsychiatric symptoms, and high-dose steroids can precipitate psychosis. Cautious use of intravenous haloperidol remains the mainstay of treatment.

Evidence suggests that the extent to which pediatric patients with life-threatening illnesses feel traumatized both by the procedure and by its sequelae correlates with the parents' sense of stress.[27] In fact, although parents (and primary caregivers) have a relatively high rate of post-traumatic stress disorder (PTSD) in the first few years following their child's transplant,[28] the transplant recipients themselves experience symptoms of PTSD at rates comparable to those of children with other life-threatening conditions. Interestingly, the likelihood of experiencing such symptoms (e.g., re-experiencing, having flashbacks, or manifesting avoidance) does not seem to be related to the type of organ transplant and is more common in those adolescents with relatively mild complications, or in those whose organ failure occurred abruptly.[29] In one more recent study, the authors found that children and parents differed in their assessment of psychological health following transplant. Children generally under-reported their psychological distress and parents reported that their children were more distressed than a normal cohort.[30]

In general, however, pediatric transplant patients do well. They feel better, return to school, and resume many of their activities. They do not demonstrate significant new psychopathology, although pre-morbid psychiatric illness may recur. Pediatric liver transplantation patients demonstrate significant neuropsychological deficits and developmental delays in intellectual and academic functioning, both before and after transplantation, thought to be related to the effect of elevated levels of bilirubin pre-transplant and total number of days in the hospital in the first year following transplant.[31] Other studies have shown persistent cognitive deficits in pediatric heart transplant recipients,[28] but a recent study found that 89% of children who underwent heart transplantation following VAD bridging demonstrated normal cognitive function.[32]

CONCLUSION

The patient with end-organ failure, adult or child, who is approaching transplantation has few real options. These patients are profoundly physically disabled and emotionally drained. They are often depressed and anxious, even sometimes quite desperate. Recognition and treatment of psychiatric disorders, both before and after transplant, can improve their quality of life.

The role of the transplant psychiatrist is challenging but also immensely rewarding. It requires a sophisticated appreciation of the medical and surgical issues facing patients with end-organ failure, an understanding of the mechanism of action and side-effect profiles of their medications, and the ways in which those medications interact with psychotropic medications. As a member of a multi-disciplinary team, the psychiatrist must act as a liaison to the patient, the family, and other medical providers and serve as a resource for other team members. The transplant psychiatrist plays a central role in the selection of transplant candidates and potential living donors, necessitating an understanding of the ethical issues inherent in a system where resources are limited.

Access a list of MCQs for this chapter at https://expertconsult.inkling.com

REFERENCES

1. Smith JM, Biggins SW, Hasselby DG, et al. Kidney, pancreas and liver allocation and distribution in the United States. *Am J Transplant* 12:3191–3212, 2012.
2. Ladin K, Hanto DW. Rationing lung transplants—procedural fairness in allocation and appeals. *N Engl J Med* 369:599–601, 2013.
3. Lang G, Taghavi S, Aigner C, et al. Primary lung transplantation after bridge with extracorporeal membrane oxygenation: a plea for a shift in our paradigms for indications. *Transplantation* 93(7):729–736, 2012.
4. Colvin-Adams M, Valapour M, Hertz M, et al. Lung and heart allocation in the United States. *Am J Transplant* 12:3213–3234, 2012.
5. <http://optn.transplant.hrsa.gov/data/>; [Accessed September 14, 2013].
6. Wynn JJ, Alexander DE. Increasing organ donation and transplantation: the U.S. experience over the past decade. *Transpl Int* 24:324–332, 2011.
7. <http://www.iom.edu/Reports/2006/Organ-Donation-Opportunities-for-Action.aspx>; [Accessed September 14, 2013].
8. <http://organdonor.gov/legislation/timeline.html>; [Accessed September 14, 2013].
9. Nudeshima J. Obstacles to brain death and organ transplantation in Japan. *Lancet* 338:1063–1066, 1991.
10. Childress JF. How can we ethically increase the supply of transplantable organs? *Ann Intern Med* 145(3):224–225, 2006.
11. Surman OS. The ethics of partial-liver donation. *N Engl J Med* 346:1038, 2002.
12. Ingelfinger JR. Risks and benefits to the living donor. *N Engl J Med* 353:447–449, 2005.
13. Trotter JF, Everhart JE. Outcomes among living liver donors. *Gastroenterology* 142(2):207–210, 2012.
14. Wakade VA, Mathur SK. Donor safety in live-related liver transplantation. *Indian J Surg* 74(1):118–126, 2011.
15. Prager LM, Wain JC, Roberts DH, et al. Medical and psychological outcome of living lobar lung transplant donors. *ISHLT* 25(10):1206–1212, 2006.
16. Chen F, Fujinaga T, Shoji T, et al. Outcomes and pulmonary function in living lobar lung transplant donors. *Transpl Int* 35:153–157, 2012.
17. Dobbels F, Verleden G, Dupont L, et al. To transplant or not? The importance of psychosocial and behavioral factors before lung transplantation. *Chron Respir Dis* 3:39–47, 2006.
18. Clinton BK, Silverman BS, Brendel DH. Patient-targeted googling: the ethics of searching on line for patient information. *Harv Rev Psychiatry* 18(2):103–112, 2009.
19. Parker R, Armstrong MJ, Corbett C, et al. Alcohol and substance abuse in solid-organ transplant recipients, <wwwtransplantjournal.com>; 2013.
20. Zalai D, Szeifert L, Novak M. Psychological distress and depression in patients with chronic kidney disease. *Semin Dial* 25(4):428–438, 2012.
21. Sanders KM, Stern TA, O'Gara PT, et al. Delirium during IABP therapy: incidence and management. *Psychosomatics* 33:35–44, 1992.
22. Weinrieb R, Auriacombe M, Lynch KG, et al. A critical review of selective serotonin reuptake inhibitor–associated bleeding: balancing the risk of treating hepatitis C–infected patients. *J Clin Psych* 64:1502–1510, 2003.
23. Taylor JJ, Wilson JW, Estes LL. Linezolid and serotonergic drug interactions: a retrospective survey. *Clin Infect Dis* 43(2):180–187, 2006.
24. Cohen LM, Tessier EG, Germaine MJ, et al. Update on psychotropic medication use in renal disease. *Psychosomatics* 45:34–48, 2004.
25. Fung E, Shaw RJ. Pediatric Transplant Rating Instrument—a scale for the pretransplant psychiatric evaluation of pediatric organ transplant recipients. *Pediatr Transplant* 12:57–68, 2008.
26. Fisher M, Storfer-Isser A, Shaw RJ, et al. Inter-rater reliability of the pediatric transplant rating instrument (P-TRI): challenges to reliably identifying adherence risk factors during pediatric pretransplant evaluations. *Pediatr Transplant* 15:142–147, 2011.
27. Stuber ML, Kazak AE, Meeske K, et al. Predictors of posttraumatic stress symptoms in childhood cancer survivors. *Pediatrics* 100:958–964, 1997.
28. Stuber ML. Psychiatric issues in pediatric organ transplantation. *Child Adolesc Psychiatr Clin N Am* 19(2):285–300, 2010.
29. Mintzer LL, Stuber ML, Seacord D, et al. Traumatic stress symptoms in adolescent organ transplant recipients. *Pediatrics* 115:1640–1644, 2003.
30. Wu YP, Aylward BS, Steele RG, et al. Psychosocial functioning of pediatric renal and liver transplant recipients. *Pediatr Transplant* 12:582, 2008.
31. Krull K, Fuchs C, Yurk H, et al. Neurocognitive outcome in pediatric liver transplant recipients. *Pediatr Transplant* 7:111–118, 2003.
32. Stein ML, Bruno JL, Konopack KL, et al. Cognitive outcomes in pediatric heart transplant recipients bridged to transplantation with ventricular assist devices. *J Heath Lung Transplant* 32(2):212–220, 2013.

59 Approaches to Collaborative Care and Primary Care Psychiatry

BJ Beck, MSN, MD

KEY POINTS

Background

- Changes in psychiatry and the US health care system mandate the development of innovative models to provide high-quality, cost-effective, and efficient psychiatric care in the general medical setting.

History

- Patients generally prefer to receive treatment for their psychiatric problems in the general medical setting, but patient, provider, and system factors interfere with appropriate recognition and treatment.

Clinical and Research Challenges

- Psychiatric symptoms are common in primary care populations, though many patients do not meet criteria for a diagnosable disorder.

- Primary care patients are different from those who seek specialty care; they may seek treatment earlier in the course of their illness; they frequently present with somatic complaints, rather than psychiatric symptoms; they often improve with relatively short courses of what psychiatrists would consider sub-therapeutic doses of medication.

- The real-time, documentation and productivity demands on primary care providers may limit their ability or interest to diagnose, treat, or research psychiatric problems in their practices.

Practical Pointers

- Collaboration begins with education.

- The four major goals of collaboration are to improve access, treatment, outcomes, and communication.

- Careful attention to documentation and dissemination of clinical outcomes and cost-offset or cost-effectiveness is necessary to inform future systemic and reimbursement policies.

OVERVIEW

Historical trends in the research, education, and clinical practice of psychiatry[1] over the last century mirrored concerns and developments in the more general US health care system[2] that called for system redesign to provide safe, personal, cost-effective, high-quality health care. This included innovative approaches to the psychiatric care of patients in the general medical setting, where most patients still prefer to receive care, and the only available resource for many. Advances in psychopharmacology greatly facilitated the development of such models, which were designed to address quality, cost-containment, and allocation of limited resources. Psychiatric consultation and care provided to medically ill patients was primarily hospital-based, but ever-shorter inpatient stays pre-dominantly relocated these services to outpatient settings. This paralleled the trend for shorter inpatient psychiatric

hospitalizations (without increased community mental health resources),[3] which left primary care providers (PCPs) to treat more acute psychiatric illness in their outpatient practices. Innovative psychiatrists heeded the mandate to collaborate with their medical colleagues to develop and implement pragmatic, cost-effective, outpatient models of high-quality psychiatric care that could be delivered in the primary care setting.

The realization of limited health care resources and rapid escalation of health care expense also forced a change in focus from patient- to population-based care.[4] Although inherently painful in our individualistic society, this transition exposed the tremendous fiscal burden of psychiatric morbidity. The psychiatrically-disordered population experiences increased *physical* health care utilization, work absenteeism, unemployment, subjective disability,[5-7] and mortality rates. Though more difficult to demonstrate, there is also a cost-offset of appropriate and timely psychiatric treatment.[8-10]

Changes in health care reimbursement resulted in conflicted PCP incentives.[11] On the one hand, pre-paid, provider-risk plans (i.e., capitated programs), such as health maintenance organizations (HMOs), exposed the expensive use of general medical services by patients with untreated or poorly managed psychiatric illness. There was an incentive for the PCP to initiate treatment for the more common psychiatric problems seen in primary care. On the other hand, the PCP gate-keeper system, which evolved to manage the expense of specialty care, created a disincentive to recognize more serious mental illness (or any mental condition the PCP was not comfortable treating). Limited formularies, varying by plan, with onerous, time-consuming prior authorization requirements, further complicated and deterred treatment initiation. Managed care organizations (MCOs) often carved-out substance use and mental health (collectively called behavioral health [BH]) benefits management to managed BH organizations (MBHOs),[12] some with limited referral networks not inclusive of the PCP's psychiatric colleagues. This was not only a major referral disincentive but also complicated future communication and collaboration between BH and physical health providers. While many MBHOs have spearheaded initiatives to promote primary care treatment of common psychiatric problems, most do not credential or contract with non-psychiatric physicians, so this essentially cost-shifts expense from the MBHO to the [medical] MCO.

Passage of the 2010 health care reform legislation (Patient Protection and Affordable Care Act [PPACA]) has pushed the envelope to create more inclusive, accessible, coordinated, and integrated care systems,[13] and to achieve the "triple aim" (i.e., improved quality, improved outcomes, reduced total health care cost).[14] These initiatives include the patient-centered medical home, the health home, accountable care organizations, and integrated programs for the "dual eligible" populations (i.e., those eligible for both Medicare and Medicaid, either the elderly and indigent, or the disabled and poor).[15] To be successful, there is an important and recognized role for consultant psychiatrists in each of these initiatives.[16] Medical and health homes share some features, but have notable differences, which are summarized in Table 59-1.[13] Health homes specifically focus on care for patients with certain chronic conditions, recognizing that care for patients with multiple

TABLE 59-1 How are Health Homes Different from Patient-Centered Medical Homes?[13]

Category	Health Homes	Medical Homes
Population served	Individuals with approved chronic conditions	All populations served
Staffing	May include primary care practices, community mental health centers, federally qualified health centers, health home agencies, ACT teams, etc.	Are typically defined as physician-led care practices, but also mid-level practitioners
Payers	Currently are a Medicaid-only construct	In existence for multiple payers: Medicaid, commercial insurance, etc.
Care focus	Strong focus on behavioral health (including substance abuse treatment), social support, and other services (including nutrition, home health, coordinating activities, etc.)	Focused on the delivery of traditional care: referral and lab tracking, guideline adherence, electronic prescribing, provider–patient communication, etc.
Technology	Use of IT for coordination across continuum of care, including in-home solutions such as remote monitoring in patient homes	Use of IT for traditional care delivery

(From Morgan L. Health homes vs. medical homes: big similarities and important differences. OPEN MINDS Management Newsletter, *April 2012. http://www.openminds.com/market-intelligence/premium/2012/040112/040112f.htm? Accessed on 8/9/2013.)*

BOX 59-1 Core Services of Health Homes[13]

1. Comprehensive care management
2. Care coordination and health promotion
3. Comprehensive transitional care from inpatient to other settings, including appropriate follow-up
4. Individual and family support
5. Referral to community and social support services
6. Use of health information technology to link services

---

chronic illnesses is seven times as costly as the care of patients with only one such condition. Serious mental illness is one of the identified chronic conditions because 68% of affected adults have other medical conditions, and they die, on average, 25 years earlier than the general population primarily from preventable medical issues. Collaborative care for this population has been shown to improve outcomes for both physical and psychiatric conditions.[17] Health homes are required to offer six core services, listed in Box 59-1, designed to integrate physical health care, BH care, and social services.[13]

EPIDEMIOLOGY

The Epidemiologic Catchment Area (ECA) Study, conducted in the early 1980s, attempted to quantify the prevalence of psychiatric problems in community residents of the US. Within a 6-month span, roughly 7% sought help for a BH problem. More than 60% never saw a BH professional, but sought care in a medical setting (e.g., emergency department [ED], PCP's office).[18] Even among those who met full criteria for a diagnosable psychiatric disorder, 75% were seen only in the general medical (rather than BH) setting.[19] Psychiatric distress therefore was exceedingly common among primary care populations. About half of general medical outpatients had some psychiatric symptoms. The use of structured diagnostic interviews detected a prevalence of 25% to 35% for diagnosable psychiatric conditions in this patient population. However, roughly 10% of primary care patients had significant psychiatric distress without meeting diagnostic criteria for a psychiatric disorder.[20] The majority of diagnosable disorders were mood disorders (80%), depression being the most prevalent (60%) and anxiety was a distant second (20%). The more severe disorders (e.g., psychotic disorders) were more likely to be treated by BH professionals.[19]

The National Comorbidity Survey (NCS), conducted between 1990 and 1992), demonstrated a 50% life-time prevalence of one or more psychiatric disorders in US adults, with a 30% 1-year prevalence of at least one disorder.[21] Alcohol dependence and major depression were the most common disorders.

A rigorous replication of the NCS (NCS-R), in 2001–2002, also measured severity, clinical significance, overall disability, and role impairment.[22] The NCS-R found the risk of major depression was relatively low until early adolescence, when it begins to rise in a linear fashion. The slope of that line has increased (i.e., becoming steeper) for each successive birth cohort since World War II. The life-time prevalence of significant depression was 16.2%; the 12-month prevalence was 6.6%. Two findings, however, were of particular interest. First, 55.1% of depressed community respondents seeking care received that care in the BH sector. The other significant finding, attributable to advances in pharmacotherapy and educational efforts, was that 90% of respondents treated for depression in any medical setting received psychotropic medication. While this suggested improved community depression treatment, that was tempered by the finding that only 21.6% of patients received what recent, evidence-based guidelines (American Psychiatric Association [APA], Agency for Healthcare Research and Quality [AHRQ]) considered minimally adequate treatment (64.3% treated by BH providers, and 41.3% of those treated by general medical providers), and almost half (42.7%) of patients with depression still received no treatment.[22]

Older studies documented PCPs' failure to diagnose over half of the full criteria mental disorders of their patients,[23,24] but later studies demonstrated that PCPs recognized their more seriously depressed[25] or anxious[26] patients. These studies also demonstrate that higher-functioning, less severely symptomatic primary care patients have relatively good outcomes, even with short courses of relatively low doses of medications. This highlights the diagnostic difficulty for PCPs. Primary care patients are different from those who seek specialty care (i.e., the population in whom most psychiatric research is done). Primary care patients may seek treatment earlier in the course of their illness, since they have an established relationship with their PCP that is not dependent on their having a psychiatric disorder. They frequently present with somatic complaints, rather than psychiatric symptoms. Since the soma is the rightful domain of the PCP, this further obscures the diagnosis. Primary care patients often present with acute psychiatric symptoms that clear quickly (i.e., before therapeutic medication levels are reached), suggesting they might benefit as much from watchful waiting and the empathic support of their PCP. There is a high noise-to-signal ratio in psychiatrically-distressed primary care patients: that is, as many as one-third of these significantly distressed patients have sub-syndromal disorders not meeting criteria for diagnosable mental disorders. This diagnostic ambiguity, coupled with relatively good outcomes after brief trials of sub-therapeutic medication doses,[23,27] is cause to reconsider the significance of the PCP's "failure" to diagnose. Much primary care patient angst resolves spontaneously, either with resolution of an initiating event, expressed caregiver concern, or the placebo effect of a few days of medication. It may be attributable to an adjustment disorder.

Barriers to Treatment

Symptom recognition is necessary but not sufficient to ensure primary care treatment of psychiatric problems.[28] Even when PCPs are informed of standardized screening results, they may not initiate treatment. PCP, patient, and system factors collude to inhibit the discussion necessary to promote treatment ("don't ask/don't tell").[29]

Physician factors ("don't ask") include the failure to take a social history or to perform a mental status examination (MSE).[30] This may be attributed to deficits in training of medical students and residents,[31] to time and productivity pressures, and to personal defenses (e.g., identification, denial,[32] isolation of affect). PCPs are more experienced and comfortable addressing physical complaints. Some PCPs fear their patients will leave the practice if asked about BH issues. Like many patients, the PCP may not believe treatment will help. Not having a ready response or approach is a major deterrent to identification of a new problem within the context of a 15-minute primary care visit. Denial or avoidance may prevail when the time-pressured PCP feels unsure of how, or whether, to treat or to refer.

Stigma, prevalent among patients and providers, is a major patient deterrent to bringing up psychiatric symptoms. Often patients "don't tell" because of shame or embarrassment. Patients may not know they have a diagnosable or treatable BH disorder.[33] They may equate psychiatric problems with personal weakness, and assume their PCP shares that view. For these and other reasons, primary care patients frequently present with physical complaints, increasing diagnostic complexity[34] since medical disorders may simulate psychiatric disorders, psychiatric disorders may lead to physical symptoms, and psychiatric and medical disorders may co-exist.

System factors include the ever-changing health care finance and reimbursement climate (e.g., managed care, "carve-outs," provider risk, capitation, fee-for-service, coding nuances, differential formularies, prior authorization) that promotes financial imperatives to contain cost and to increase efficiency. This systemic instability, confusion, and administrative time-creep easily dwarfs the impulse to pursue the treatment of a possibly self-limited condition. BH carve-outs have complicated the possibility of reimbursing PCP treatment of BH disorders, while pre-paid plans (e.g., HMOs) decrease incentives to offer anything "extra."[35] The necessity to increase productivity has excessively shortened the "routine visit," now often less than 15 minutes, while the excessive burden of required documentation further erodes clinically-available time. Although the electronic medical record [EMR] has standardized and improved screening, documentation, and follow-up,[36] it is also a source of clinical time depletion. The care-promoting advent of new, safer, more tolerable psychotropic medications has been offset by soaring pharmacy costs and by restrictive (and possibly short-sighted[37]) formularies. The practice of primary care has reached a crisis point: the pressures are so overwhelming that few PCPs can sustain full-time clinical practice.

THE GOALS OF COLLABORATION

Now that effective, evidence-based treatments exist, access and quality of care remain significant issues, best addressed through the collaboration of psychiatry and primary care. The four major goals of collaboration are to improve access, treatment, outcomes, and communication.

Access

Collaborative care in the primary care setting addresses both physician and patient factors that limit the patient's access to appropriate assessment and treatment. Most patients are familiar with the general medical setting and feel more comfortable and less stigmatized there. Conversely, they may believe the mental health clinic is for "crazy people," not a (perceived) clientele with whom they identify. Even a defined BH unit in the primary care setting may be stigmatizing and thus a barrier to treatment access. Most patients do not know of a psychiatrist or how to access care from one and may not feel certain that they need one. The unaided decision to foray into the BH arena may be fraught with shame and anxiety, powerful deterrents to making that first call. Calling the PCP's office and making an appointment for fatigue, sleep problems, weight loss, or palpitations is infinitely less threatening.

An established relationship between the PCP and a trusted, accessible psychiatric consultant eases the burden of recognizing, treating, or referring patients with mental disorders. PCPs more readily identify psychiatric distress and initiate treatment when they have expert clinical back-up available.

Treatment

Historically, PCPs often prescribed insufficient doses of medications (e.g., amitriptyline 25 mg) for major depression.[38] Since the advent of safer, well-tolerated medications (e.g., selective serotonin reuptake inhibitors [SSRIs]), PCPs' prescriptive choices have improved,[39,40] although the doses used often remain suboptimal. Benzodiazepines have been prescribed by PCPs more frequently than any other class of psychotropic medication, even for major depression,[41] but they now are appropriately surpassed by antidepressant prescriptions.[40] Collaboration with the consultation psychiatrist can improve the choice, dose, and management of psychotropic medications. Collaboration is also helpful when the PCP's preferred medication is off-formulary for a given patient. Such a treatment deterrent may instead become an opportunity for brief, pragmatic education.

Outcomes

Several studies have demonstrated better outcomes for seriously depressed primary care patients treated collaboratively by their PCP and a psychiatrist.[42–44] Cost-offset, however, is difficult to demonstrate because of the hidden costs of psychiatric disability.[6,45,46] Nonetheless, there is evidence for decreased total health care spending when BH problems are adequately addressed.[10] Even if this were not so, the case for cost-effectiveness could be made.[8,47–49] That is, care for the patient's psychiatric problem is more cost-effective than spending the same amount of money addressing the often non-responsive, somatic complaints of high-utilizing medical patients.

Communication

Collaboration ends the PCP's justifiable complaint of the "black box" of psychiatry because communication is implicit in these care models. Information must flow in both directions to assist the psychiatrist and the PCP in the provision of quality care. Referrals by PCPs provide pertinent information and state the clinical question. In addition to the target psychiatric symptoms, the PCP has, and provides, important information about the medical history, allergies, treatments, and medications. The collaborating psychiatrist shares findings, diagnostic impressions, and treatment recommendations. Information about referrals and consultations should be written, and, whenever possible, provided verbally to ensure an understanding between collaborating care providers. Secure e-mail, EMR staff messaging, or other IT solutions may also provide nearly instantaneous feedback, and focus on pertinent details for the busy PCP.

Patients, of course, must be aware of the collaborative relationship between the PCP and the psychiatrist, as well as their shared communication.

ROLES, RELATIONSHIPS, AND EXPECTATIONS

Successful collaboration requires a clear understanding and definition of roles. All parties, including the patient, should recognize the PCP's responsibility for the patient's overall care. The PCP is the broker and overseer of all specialty services. The psychiatrist is a consultant to the PCP, and sometimes a co-treater, depending on the model. Collaboration does not breach patient confidentiality because the PCP and the psychiatrist are now within the circle of care, and the patient is informed of this relationship.

This free flow of communication and documentation has reasonable limitations. If a patient asks that particular details not be placed in his or her general medical record and these details do not directly affect the patient's medical care (e.g., a history of childhood incest), it is reasonable to respect this wish. The pertinent information (e.g., the experience of childhood trauma) can be expressed in more general terms. If, however, information could affect medical treatment (e.g., current or past drug addiction) or safety (e.g., suicidal or homicidal intent, or previous suicide attempt), such information cannot be withheld from the PCP, and the patient should be so informed.

When the PCP refers the patient to the psychiatrist, the patient should understand what to expect from the visit. It is also the psychiatrist's responsibility to clearly describe the parameters of the contact (e.g., whether it will be a one-time consultation, with or without the possibility of medication follow-up, or possible referral for therapy). If the psychiatrist

sees the patient more than once, the relationships (i.e., between the PCP and the psychiatrist, as well as between the patient and the psychiatrist) may need to be reiterated. The clarity of the providers' roles and relationship serves to spare the patient a sense of abandonment, either by the PCP when the patient is referred to the psychiatrist, or by the psychiatrist when the patient is returned to the PCP for ongoing psychiatric management.

In collaborative models of care, it is common for the psychiatric notes to be placed in the general medical record, which may raise issues of confidentiality and privacy. Most states require a specific release for mental health or substance use treatment records. BH notes in the general medical record should be color-coded or otherwise flagged, so they can be removed when records are copied for general medical release of information. With an EMR, there may be software coding solutions to avoid the inadvertent release of this information. (As BH issues are increasingly treated by PCPs, the question of how to document and protect such information is a growing concern, preferably to be addressed in a way that does not further complicate and deter such treatment.)

MODELS OF COLLABORATION

Collaborative models differ in terms of where the patient is seen, whether there is a single medical record, how providers communicate, whether the psychiatrist recommends or initiates treatment, and whether the psychiatrist sees the patient (at all, once, more than once) or is an ongoing treater. Another important variable is whether both providers belong to the same medical staff and how available (physically, electronically, or telephonically) the psychiatrist is to the PCP. Table 59-2 summarizes these differences.

Outpatient Consultation Models

Consultation implies collaboration in that the PCP refers or presents the patient to the psychiatrist to obtain expert advice or recommendations. Depending on the setting or the system, one medical record may be shared, or providers may maintain separate records and share pertinent information. Patients may be seen in either the psychiatric or the primary care setting.

TABLE 59-2 Models of Collaboration

Model	Records	See Pt[1]	Tx/Rec[2]	Communication[3]	Locus[4]	Staff[5]	Availability (Patient/PCP)[6]
CONSULTATION							
Specialty psychiatry clinic	Separate	1+ or cont	T	W (V, E)	Psy	N	App/Arr
Consult psychiatrist	Variable	1+	R	W (P,V, or E)	PC or Psy	N	App/Arr
Teleconsultation	n/a	0	R	W & V	n/a	N	0/RT, V
Three-component model (TCM)	Shared	0, 1+	R	CM (P, V, E)	PC	N	0, App/Sch (RT)
Staff consultant	Shared	1+	R, T	W & (P,V, or E)	PC	Y	App/Arr
Parallel care	Variable	Cont	T	W or P or V or E	PC(Psy)	Y	App/Arr
Collaborative management	Shared	2	T & R	W & (P,V, or E)	PC	Y	App/Sch (RT)
Primary care–driven	Shared	1, 2	T & R	W & (P,V, or E)	PC	Y	0, App, RT/RT (P,V,E)

Key:
[1]0 = patient is not seen by psychiatrist; 1 = seen once; 1+ = seen once or more; 2 = may be seen several times, but not for ongoing care; Cont = patient is seen continuously (ongoing care).
[2]T = initiate treatment; R = make recommendations; R,T = depending on prior agreement, may recommend and/or treat; T & R = initiate treatment and follow up with recommendations for primary care physician (PCP).
[3]W = written, hard copy note or evaluation; P = in person; V = phone or voice mail; E = secure e-mail or electronic medical record (EMR); CM = liaison with care manager, standardized log, etc.; ( ) = modes that may be available.
[4]Psy = psychiatrist's office or clinic; PC = primary care setting; PC(Psy) = primary care or psychiatric or mental health unit within the primary care setting.
[5]N = psychiatrist is not necessarily on the same medical staff with the PCP; Y = PCP and psychiatrist are staff colleagues.
[6]App = by appointment; Arr = as arranged between PCP and consultant; 0 = patient is not seen by psychiatrist; RT = real time; Sch = regularly scheduled times on a repeating basis; P = in person; V = phone or voice mail; E = secure e-mail or EMR.

This differs from the practice of private psychiatrists with established referral sources in the primary care sector in that these providers generally do not develop a truly collaborative relationship, with ongoing communication or shared records. They treat in parallel, rarely in collaboration.

Specialty Psychiatric Clinics

Specialty psychiatric clinics (e.g., eating disorders clinic), usually in teaching hospitals or tertiary care centers, generally maintain separate records, require the patient to be seen in the psychiatric clinic, and develop some means of ongoing, clinically relevant PCP communication. Patients typically need to have well-defined problems to get referred. Although stigma may interfere with patient adherence to such a referral, one major advantage of such clinics is the expert, multidisciplinary approach they provide for patients with complex psychiatric and medical problems.

Consultation Psychiatrists

Consultation psychiatrists[50,51] may render a one-visit opinion in the primary care clinic (or in the consultant's office, similar to other specialty consultations). Like inpatient consultation, the consultation request and report should be in the primary care record. Immediate verbal communication, in person, whenever possible, or by phone, e-mail, or voice mail, greatly enhances the utility of such consultations. The consultant generally does not initiate treatment but makes practical recommendations. The role of the PCP and occurrence in the primary care setting enhances patient participation and decreases stigma. This model also promotes opportunities for ongoing informal education between the PCP and the consultant.

Three-component Model

Supported by the MacArthur Initiative on Depression in Primary Care, the three-component model (TCM)[52] is a formalized system of consultative care that promotes the primary care treatment of depression as a chronic disease, with regular measures of adherence and outcome to guide the evidence-based protocol of medication and other treatment adjustments. Educational modules exist for PCPs, consultant psychiatrists, phone-based care managers, and patients. The Patient Health Questionnaire—9 (PHQ-9), a 10-item, 1-page, self-administered tool that quantifies the patient's neurovegetative symptoms of depression,[53] is repeatedly used to track the patient's progress. Multiple measures of symptoms and treatment adherence are recorded on a standard form that facilitates consultation, communication, and organized treatment review, planning, and adjustment.

Dissemination of the TCM and its standardized materials, manuals, and educational modules addresses the need to improve care for this large population (i.e., patients receiving depression treatment in primary care) while also providing data to inform policy (and payment) decisions. Similar evidence-based endeavors include the Health Disparities Collaboratives (the combined effort of the Department of Health and Human Services, the Health Resources and Services Administration, and the Bureau of Primary Health Care) and the IMPACT model[54] (initially funded by the John A. Hartford, California HealthCare, Hogg, and Robert Wood Johnson Foundations).

Psychiatrist on the Primary Care Clinic Medical Staff

When the psychiatrist is a medical staff colleague of the PCP, there are enhanced possibilities for collaboration and shared care. This PCP–consultant proximity facilitates communication, formal and informal education, immediate access to curbside consultation, and heightened PCP awareness of psychiatric problems in their patients. This arrangement can also provide an excellent opportunity for training of both psychiatric and primary care residents. Patients appreciate being seen in the more familiar primary care setting, and they feel less stigmatized.

Several models of care have evolved or been developed to utilize the services of an in-house psychiatrist. The psychiatrist may (1) consult as a member of the medical team, (2) evaluate and treat patients in parallel with the PCP, (3) alternate visits with the PCP while treatment is initiated,[9,44,54] or (4) evaluate, stabilize, and return the patient to the PCP with recommendations for continued care, or facilitate referrals to outside mental health providers.[55]

Staff Consultant

Consultations, as above, are written in the regular medical record. The permanency of the psychiatrist allows for a more finely-tuned consultant–PCP relationship. For instance, with a previously established agreement, the consultant may initiate the recommended treatment. The consultation psychiatrist may offer clinically, relevant suggestions during case conferences or discussions of more complex patients. The psychiatrist may also see the patient with the PCP during the primary care visit, capitalizing on the PCP's extensive knowledge of, and long-term relationship with, the patient to provide more timely treatment recommendations. In one such consultation model, a consultant and several clinicians travel to several primary care clinics within the larger health care system, and provide a variety of consultative, educational, and treatment services.[51]

Parallel Care

If the psychiatrist assumes the ongoing psychiatric care of patients in parallel with the PCP, some clinics have separate mental health charts. This option requires some overt means of communication to keep all providers informed. In clinics with an EMR, a single up-to-date medication list will at least keep both providers aware of current medications and medication changes.

Some primary care clinics incorporate a mental health unit or clinic. If this is an identifiable, geographical locus within the clinic, it is fraught with the same stigma that occurs when the clinics are truly separate. Although still within the circle of care, the larger the clinic and more separate the clinical services, the greater the diligence required on the part of each provider to meet the challenge of continued communication.

The psychiatric capacity of primary care clinics that offer these services is often inadequate to meet the needs of the total clinic patient population. This situation can be problematic and delay access because most patients would like to be treated in this setting. Uniform criteria facilitate the triage of patients for in-house treatment or outside referral. These criteria include such justifiable considerations as diagnosis, available community resources, language requirements, or payment source. Certain unstable or less common psychiatric problems may be better served in the BH sector, either in community clinics with "wrap-around" services or in specific subspecialty clinics. In most communities, English-speaking patients have more options for treatment. Depending on the location and availability of appropriate, non-English-speaking services, patients may be preferentially kept in-house, or referred out. When otherwise appropriate, capitation will favor treating the patient in-house. Patients with insurance will generally have more options outside the primary care setting than those who are uninsured, and some insurance plans with BH carve-outs may not cover psychiatric care in the same setting in which they cover medical services.

Collaborative Management

In collaborative management,[44,56] the patient alternates visits between the psychiatrist and the PCP in the primary care setting during initiation of treatment (i.e., the first 4 to 6 weeks). The PCP then assumes responsibility for the patient's continued psychopharmacological treatment. This model was developed as a research protocol for the treatment of depressed, primary care patients (and has been extended to the treatment of panic disorder[8] and patients with persistent depressive symptoms[56]). Patients are referred by the PCP, usually after an initial ineffective trial of medication. This intensive program of care has been cost-effective for more severely depressed primary care patients.

Implicit in this model are certain underlying assumptions. Collaborative management assumes that PCPs can initiate appropriate treatment for depression, manage the care of patients stabilized on antidepressant medications, and better care for more seriously depressed patients with the collaboration of an in-house psychiatric consultant.[57] This model also assumes that such collaboration begins with PCP education and training. In addition, PCPs participate in regular teaching conferences. A psychoeducational module for patients is also an integral part of the treatment.

Primary-care-driven Model

The primary-care-driven model[55] evolved from the practical necessity to assist PCPs in the provision of quality psychiatric care for their own primary care patients with limited psychiatric resources. This model incorporates elements of consultation and collaborative management, with the goal of maximizing the treatment of appropriate primary care patients, in the primary care setting. Established criteria are used for triage, with the appropriateness of PCP management being the first consideration. Copies (either photocopies or electronic copies) of all psychiatric notes and evaluations are sent to the PCP, as well as being placed in the regular medical record (or EMR). The clinic provides psychiatric training for both psychiatric and primary care residents. Underlying assumptions of this model include those of the collaborative management model, but are more extensive, reflective of the broader diagnostic scope. These assumptions are listed in Box 59-2.

BOX 59-2 Underlying Assumptions of the Primary-care-driven Model

1. Collaboration begins with education of primary care providers (PCPs) *and* psychiatrists.
2. Patients' psychiatric needs should be met in the primary care setting when consistent with good care.
3. PCPs can manage the care of patients stabilized on psychiatric medications.
4. PCPs can initiate appropriate treatment for some psychiatric disorders.
5. PCPs can better care for the psychiatric needs of more patients with the collaboration of in-house psychiatric consultation.
6. Some patients and some disorders are unlikely to be stable enough for PCP management.
7. Responsibility for total care requires communication between the PCP and any other involved care provider or consultant.

In this model, the written request for consultation or referral comes from the PCP. The referral includes the clinical issue to be addressed and any PCP-initiated medication trials. PCPs are also encouraged to call or to stop by the psychiatrist's office, located within the primary care clinical area, for more general information about diagnoses, medications, or behavioral management.

An array of psychiatric services are available, including formal evaluation with stabilization over several visits and return of the patient to the PCP's care (with recommendations on how to take, and how long to continue, medications and when to re-refer). The psychiatrist also provides informal "curbside" consultation to the PCP, brief consultation with the patient and the PCP during the patient's primary care visit, and behavioral treatment planning for the difficult-to-manage patient. Re-evaluation of patients previously seen occurs when there is a change, such as *roughening* (the recurrence of symptoms during apparent adherence to previously effective treatment), the development of new psychiatric symptoms, medication side effects, or a change in medical condition or medications that affect psychiatric symptoms or medications. When a patient does not meet criteria for in-house treatment, the psychiatrist facilitates the referral to appropriate outside services (e.g., community mental health center, private psychiatrist, therapist).

A premise of the primary-care-driven model is that not all patients are appropriate for PCP management. The psychiatrist should help the PCP recognize which patients are better served by ongoing specialty care and assist with appropriate referral. Patients not recommended for PCP management include those with suicidal ideation (or high risk factors), severe personality disorders, primary addiction disorders, inherently unstable conditions (e.g., psychotic disorders, bipolar disorder), or complicated medication regimens that require close monitoring.

Other available in-house BH services include focused, short-term, goal-oriented individual or group therapy (with master's-level clinicians located within the primary care clinical area), and collaborative care management, a service that helps broker and coordinate the care of patients with complicated medical, mental health, or addiction problems who use services in multiple (otherwise discontinuous) settings. It bridges the communication needs when patients access services outside the primary care setting. After a comprehensive diagnostic and functional assessment, necessary releases are signed to allow the care manager to serve as a liaison between the PCP and all other care providers. The care manager involves the patient and all treaters in the development of a comprehensive treatment plan within a network of services, and tracks the patient from site to site throughout this plan. As a member of the discharge planning team, the care manager ensures that the patient returns to the appropriate network of services after care in a hospital, a detoxification program, or another residential/institutional setting. The lack of sustainable reimbursement sources severely limited this useful program (which may now be reinvented to meet the new mandates of health and medical homes).

CHOOSING THE RIGHT MODEL

The choice of model depends on a variety of practice factors, such as patient population, payer mix, range of available community resources, and the location, type, and size of the practice. Patients with higher educational or socioeconomic status may feel less stigmatized and be more able and willing to seek and to pay for outside psychiatric services.[58] Some patients feel more comfortable in private practice settings that allow the greatest possible privacy. BH problems are less acceptable or even shameful in some cultures. These patient populations will favor a more integrated and "invisible" system within the primary care setting. Capitation would most clearly demonstrate the cost-offset and cost-effectiveness of in-house, collaborative models. The primary-care-driven model requires adequate community resources to refer patients not considered appropriate for primary care management. Suburban or rural areas that lack these resources are better served by parallel, or shared, care models. Small groups or solo practitioners may favor consultation models, either with a part-time but regularly scheduled consultant or through access to an outside consultant, as needed. Large practices, and especially training facilities, will benefit most from the full range of in-house consultative and collaborative services that include formal education, case conferences, curbside consultation, and collaborative care management. The current Affordable Care Act promotion of integrated care will likely employ or enhance some of these same features, and hopefully provide the necessary and sustainable funding for their continued success.

CONCLUSION

PCPs have held (and will continue to hold) an important front-line position in total health care, population-based care, and all levels of prevention.[59] Though mandated by changes in the health care system, collaborative models serve to increase access and improve treatment for patients who would be unable or unlikely to receive psychiatric care outside of the primary care setting. A number of considerations determine the best model for a given practice setting. Such factors include size, patient population, available community resources, payer mix, and other reimbursement sources. To remain viable, high-quality and cost-effective models will need to adapt and to evolve with the changing health care system. Psychiatrists and PCPs will need to be flexible and innovative in their approaches to patient care and to be diligent in the documentation of cost-offset to encourage payers to reimburse their services.[60,61] Medical,[62] psychiatric, and patient education will need to reflect these changes in caregiver roles and expectations.

Access the complete reference list and multiple choice questions (MCQs) online at https://expertconsult.inkling.com

KEY REFERENCES

2. Committee on Quality Health Care in America, Institute of Medicine. *Crossing the quality chasm: a new health system for the 21st century*, Washington, DC, 2001, National Academy Press.
3. Leslie DL, Rosenheck R. Shifting to outpatient care? Mental health care use and cost under private insurance. *Am J Psychiatry* 156:1250–1257, 1999.
4. Katon W, Von Korff M, Lin E, et al. Population-based care of depression: effective disease management strategies to decrease prevalence. *Gen Hosp Psychiatry* 19:169–178, 1997.
8. Katon WJ, Roy-Byrne P, Russo J, et al. Cost-effectiveness and cost offset of a collaborative care intervention for primary care patients with panic disorder. *Arch Gen Psychiatry* 59:1098–1104, 2002.
9. Katon WJ, Russo JE, Von Korff M, et al. Long-term effects on medical costs of improving depression outcomes in patients with depression and diabetes. *Diabetes Care* 31:1155–1159, 2008.
10. Simon GE, Khandker RK, Ichikawa L, et al. Recovery from depression predicts lower health service costs. *J Clin Psychiatry* 67:1226–1231, 2006.
11. Pincus HA. Assessing the effects of physician payment on treatment of mental disorders in primary care. *Gen Hosp Psychiatry* 12:23–29, 1990.
13. Morgan L. Health homes vs. medical homes: big similarities and important differences. *OPEN MINDS Management Newsletter*. <http://www.openminds.com/market-intelligence/premium/2012/040112/040112f.htm?>; April, 2012 [Accessed on 8/9/2013].
14. Berwick DM, Nolan TW, Whittington J. The triple aim: care, health and cost. *Health Aff* 27:759–769, 2008.
15. Neuman P, Lyons B, Rentas J, et al. Dx for a careful approach to moving dual-eligible beneficiaries into managed care plans. *Health Aff* 31:1186–1194, 2012.
16. Katon W, Unützer J. Consultation psychiatry in the medical home and accountable care organizations: achieving the triple aim. *Gen Hosp Psychiatry* 33:305–310, 2011.
17. Katon WJ, Lin EHB, Von Korff M, et al. Collaborative care for patients with depression and chronic illness. *N Engl J Med* 363:2611–2620, 2010.
22. Kessler RC, Berglund P, Demler O, et al. The epidemiology of major depressive disorder: results from the National Comorbidity Survey Replication (NCS-R). *JAMA* 289:3095–3105, 2003.
25. Coyne JC, Schwenk TL, Fechner-Bates S. Nondetection of depression by primary care physicians reconsidered. *Gen Hosp Psychiatry* 17:3–12, 1995.
39. Olfson M, Marcus SC, Druss B, et al. National trends in the outpatient treatment of depression. *JAMA* 287:203–209, 2002.
42. Druss BG, Rohrbaugh RM, Levinson CM, et al. Integrated medical care for patients with serious psychiatric illness. *Arch Gen Psychiatry* 58:861–868, 2001.
46. Stewart WF, Ricci JA, Chee E, et al. Cost of lost productive work time among US workers with depression. *JAMA* 289:3135–3144, 2003.
49. Katon WJ, Schoenbaum M, Fan MY, et al. Cost-effectiveness of improving primary care treatment of late-life depression. *Arch Gen Psychiatry* 62:1313–1320, 2005.
52. Oxman T, Dietrich AJ, Williams JW, et al. A three-component model for reengineering systems for the treatment of depression in primary care. *Psychosomatics* 43:441–450, 2002.
59. Druss BG, Mays RA, Edwards VJ, et al. Primary care, public health, and mental health. *Prev Chronic Dis* 7:A04, 2010. <http://www.cdc.gov/pcd/issues/2010/jan/09_0131.htm>; [Accessed on 8/9/2013].

60 Psychiatric and Ethical Aspects of Care at the End of Life

Guy Maytal, MD, Lucy A. Epstein Hutner, MD, Ned H. Cassem, MA, PhL, MD, SJ, BD, and Rebecca Weintraub Brendel, MD JD

KEY POINTS

- Psychiatrists face multiple challenges when caring for a dying patient, encompassing issues of diagnosis and treatment, as well as larger ethical and legal considerations.
- Psychiatrists may be uniquely effective in helping a dying patient by ensuring optimization of palliative care and by assisting the patient and his or her family in the dying process.
- Psychiatric issues (such as depression, anxiety, delirium, substance dependence, and problematic coping) are commonly seen in patients at the end of life.
- Suicidal thoughts should not be considered solely as "understandable" and should be addressed actively by the psychiatrist.
- Psychiatrists play an important role in the mediation of important ethical and legal considerations that occur at the end of life.

OVERVIEW

With nearly 2.5 million deaths each year in the US,[1] providing both competent and compassionate care for patients at the end of life is a crucial task for physicians. Caring for patients at the end of life occurs amidst an often complex background of medical, psychiatric, ethical, and legal concerns. This chapter provides an overview of the central principles of care, diagnosis, and treatment of the dying patient from the psychiatric perspective. It also examines current concepts in ethics, as well as legal precedents that surround this evolving area of medicine—where advances in medical technology and practice have extended the human life span and led to the emergence of novel ethical conflicts. In particular, end-of-life care may create tension between two essential medical principles: to do no harm (*primum non nocere*) and to relieve suffering. For example, prescribing an opioid medication for pain relief may unintentionally (but predictably) hasten a patient's death via respiratory suppression.

Caring for patients at the end of life is further complicated when the medically ill also suffer from psychiatric co-morbidities, such as major depression and anxiety, as well as cognitive disorders or delirium. Finally, end-of-life decisions occur in a dynamic societal and legal context. For example, recent attention regarding end-of-life issues has focused on physician-assisted suicide and on legal cases that surround withdrawal of life-sustaining treatments.

GOALS OF TREATMENT

An important first step in the treatment of the dying patient is for the psychiatrist and the patient to define treatment goals.

According to Saunders,[2] the primary aim of care is to help patients "feel like themselves" for as long as possible. Care at the end of life also offers an important opportunity, according to Kübler-Ross, to address and to complete "unfinished business."[3] Common themes in this category include reconciliation with estranged friends or family, resolution of conflicts with loved ones, and the pursuit of goals and hopes. With the rise of multi-disciplinary team-based care at the end of life, the psychiatrist should be in close communication with the patient's other medical caregivers regarding overall treatment goals.

Additionally, according to Kübler-Ross,[3] patients who are dying can go through a transformational process (that includes, but is not limited to, the stages of denial, anger, bargaining, guilt/depression, and eventual acceptance). Kübler-Ross wrote that these stages may occur in a unique order, may occur simultaneously, and may last for variable amounts of time. More recently, Maciejewski and colleagues[4] reported on an empirical analysis of the stage theory of grief. Studying 233 bereaved individuals over 3 years, these researchers found that the five grief indicators each peaked in the sequence predicted by the stage theory of grief: disbelief, yearning, anger, depression, and acceptance. Given that all of them peak about 6 months post-loss, anyone who continues to suffer from negative grief indicators may benefit from evaluation and treatment. Psychiatrists and other physicians may assist the dying patient in the transition through these often difficult stages toward acceptance—especially if the negative factors persist.

Hackett and Weisman[5] also developed five goals for "appropriate death" that help to focus therapeutic efforts for the treatment of a dying patient. These goals include freedom from pain, optimal function within the constraints of disability, satisfaction of remaining wishes, recognition and resolution of residual conflict, and yielding of control to trusted individuals.

It is perhaps more important than any other principle in the treatment of the dying patient that the patient's treatment be tailored to his or her individual circumstances. Within all the general goals and guidelines, each patient's unique characteristics will necessitate careful tailoring of clinical interventions. This case-by-case approach can be accomplished only by getting to know the patient and his or her family, by responding to his or her needs and interests, by proceeding at his or her pace, and by allowing him or her to shape the manner in which those in attendance behave. Psychiatrists and other medical caregivers should resist the urge to try to force the patient to fit into any particular model of the dying process. In other words, there is no one "best" way to die.

Hospice care often serves an important function for the dying patient by incorporating spiritual and family support, pain management, respite services, and a multi-disciplinary approach to medical and nursing care. When St. Christopher's Hospice opened in 1967 with Dame Cicely Mary Saunders as medical director, it was dedicated to enabling a patient, "to live to the limit of his or her potential in physical strength, mental and emotional capacity, and social relationships."[2]

Since then, hospice care has become a widely accepted means of providing care for the terminally ill outside of a

652

hospital setting. Hospices can provide a spectrum of services for patients (including home nursing, family support, spiritual counseling, pain treatment, medication, medical care, and some inpatient care). In 1994,[6] about 340,000 terminally ill patients received hospice care in the US. In 2011, that figure rose to 1.1 million, associated with 45% of the deaths in the US.

Since the US Congress enacted the Medicare hospice benefit in 1982, the vast majority of hospice services have been paid for by Medicare. In 2011, nearly 85% of hospice patients received services through their Medicare benefits.[6] To qualify for hospice benefits, potential recipients of hospice care must be terminally ill and their physician and the hospice medical director must certify that the patient will live for 6 or fewer months if their illness runs its normal course.[7]

Just as hospice care has grown outside of hospital settings, palliative medicine has developed as a discipline in general hospitals to address the "care and management of the physical, psychological, emotional and spiritual needs of patients (of all ages) and their families with chronic, debilitating, or life threatening illness."[8] This includes establishing goals of care, addressing symptoms (such as pain and respiratory distress), working with patients' families, and educating medical teams about the unique needs of dying patients. The number of palliative care programs has grown rapidly. From 2000 to 2010, the number of palliative care teams in hospital settings increased from 658 (accounting for 25% of US hospitals) to 1635 (accounting for 66% of US hospitals).[9]

THE ROLE OF THE PSYCHIATRIST

Psychiatric expertise is crucial to the care of patients at the end of life. Psychiatrists, by virtue of their training and experience, appreciate the impact of disease process on behavior, cognition, and affect. In addition, they understand the highly subjective and individual factors that contribute to the personal significance of illness, personality styles and traits, and maladaptive responses to illness.[10,11] Consequently, the psychiatrist may serve many functions—including facilitating medical treatment, enhancing communication among the patient and his or her caregivers, and modeling those qualities that may be helpful for the patient.

Above all, the psychiatrist's primary role is the diagnosis and management of psychiatric symptoms and conditions. As with all other patients, a consideration of the factors that contribute to psychiatric suffering—including biological illnesses, psychological style, psychosocial factors, and functional capacity—is essential. The most common issues that lead to psychiatric interventions for the dying patient include major depression, anxiety, personality disorders, delirium and other organic brain syndromes, refractory pain, substance abuse, cognitive impairment (including dementia), and difficulties surrounding bereavement.[12,13]

Depression

The more seriously ill a person becomes, the more likely the person is to develop major depression.[14] Contrary to the popular misconception, depression is not a "normal" part of the dying process. Rather, it is a syndrome that occurs with predictable prevalence (10%–25% depending on the specific cancer), and one that can be treated.[15,16] Risk factors associated with depression in cancer patients include a high disease burden, lower functionality, insecure attachments, low self-esteem, and younger age.[17] Careful vigilance for depression is necessary, as symptoms of depression and the impact of depression on other aspects of the patient's life and medical care are problematic. For example, Ganzini and colleagues[18]

documented that severely depressed patients made more restricted advance directives when depressed, and then changed them after their depression remitted.

Thus, aggressive treatment of depression is a cornerstone of care, as it dramatically decreases suffering and improves the quality of life. In terms of specific treatments, data supports pharmacologic and psychotherapeutic treatments (especially cognitive-behavioral therapy) for the treatment of depression in cancer patients.[19] Psychiatrists may consider the use of both antidepressants (such as the selective serotonin reuptake inhibitors [SSRIs]) as well as more rapidly-acting treatments (including psychostimulants) that target specific symptoms (e.g., decreased energy and appetite). Psychostimulants have several advantages over traditional antidepressants, including the rapid onset of improved mood, and potentiation of co-administered narcotics (with less accompanying sedation).

Thoughts of suicide should not be thought of solely as an "understandable" response to terminal illness, but rather as a condition that warrants immediate investigation and treatment.[13] It is also important to differentiate suicidal ideation from a stated desire to hasten death. The desire to hasten death has been identified consistently among a minority of terminally ill patients.[18–20] While the desire to hasten death is frequently associated with depression, other factors (such as pain, existential concerns, loss of function, and social circumstances) also play critical roles.[17,20–28] It is important to note that patients expressing a desire for hastened death are likely communicating distress, and are not necessarily planning to harm themselves. Therefore, the psychiatric consultant needs to listen carefully to the patient who desires hastened death, to treat any underlying psychiatric or physical problem, and to take steps to lessen distress.[29]

Anxiety

Anxiety frequently occurs as the end of life and requires psychiatric attention.[12,13] Impending death can generate severe anxiety in those who face death themselves, as well as their family members, friends, and caregivers. The patient who experiences anxiety surrounding death may not necessarily be able to articulate his or her fears, which may be expressed as anger, isolative behavior, or worry. Common fears associated with death include helplessness or loss of control, feelings of guilt and punishment, physical pain or injury, or abandonment.[12–14,28–30] The psychiatrist can be helpful by addressing these fears and by exploring issues related to isolation, abandonment, and suffering. Mindfulness-based techniques to reduce stress and anxiety can be effective.[31] Appropriate attention should also be directed toward psychopharmacological management of anxiety.

Personality Considerations

The terminally ill patient who has a personality disorder (such as narcissistic or borderline personality disorder) or problematic coping (e.g., associated with a history of trauma or posttraumatic stress disorder) can present a particular challenge for care providers. Such patients can find it difficult, if not impossible, to accept help and to trust their caregivers. This can interfere with a patient's ability to accept comfort from others.[10,12,13] For such a patient, much of the situation is out of his or her immediate control; this elicits regression and the use of more primitive defenses (such as splitting). This may manifest as poor communication with treaters, inadequate pain control, and difficulty in the resolution of interpersonal conflicts.[13] Psychiatrists may find it useful to call on psychodynamic diagnostic and treatment skills to assist such a person in accepting palliative care.[12] In particular, symptom-focused psychotherapeutic management can limit patient aggression and self-destructiveness, as well as enhance staff empathy for the patient.[32] Working closely with family and friends of the patient, as well as the medical team, is important in these situations.[12,13]

Delirium and Cognitive Changes

As terminal illness progresses, medical complications (such as delirium and other cognitive changes) can occur. These complications can manifest as confusion, psychosis, agitation, or a multitude of other symptoms and can be caused by the medical illness, by its treatment, by a reaction to the illness, or by a combination of causes. Effective management of changes in affect, behavior, and cognition due to delirium is of clinical importance, as it can indicate worsening of medical illness and can greatly affect the quality of time spent with friends, family, and caretakers.[12,13]

Pain

Pain management offers complex challenges that require extensive expertise. Freedom from pain is basic to every care plan, and it should be achievable in most cases.[12] However, for a multitude of reasons, pain is often under-treated by medical staff.[33-37] Several studies have revealed that as many as one out of every two cancer patients has pain that is under-treated.[35] Pain management may be particularly challenging for those with a history of substance dependence; such individuals are more likely to obtain inadequate pain treatment than those without a history of substance abuse or dependence.[11,38,39] This may be due to concerns about higher-than-expected (and escalating) doses of opiates, potential misuse or diversion of drugs, and fears of legal consequences of prescribing narcotics to a patient with substance dependence.[38,40,41] Evidence of abuse may include unexpectedly positive toxicology screening, frequent requests for higher doses, recurrent reports of lost prescriptions, and multiple visits to various providers or emergency departments for prescription refills.[42]

Caring for terminally ill patients with a history of an addiction raises several issues. Overuse and opioid-induced toxicity, with its associated delirium, myoclonus, and seizures, diminishes the quality of life for the patient.[43] However, restrictive prescribing practices for patients with addiction histories may lead individuals with pain to develop 'pseudoaddiction', a syndrome of abnormal behavior caused by inadequate pain management.[44] Optimal relief of suffering mandates acknowledgment and treatment of active substance abuse issues.[45] The goal of care requires the physician to separate the management of the patient's pain from the management of addiction and to treat both.[11,46]

Having a uniform set of clinical practices for the care of such patients is essential for avoidance of patient and staff distress.[47] Specifically, careful monitoring of a patient's narcotic use, use of a multi-disciplinary team, encouragement of substance abuse treatment, limitation of prescribing power to a single provider, and utilization of screening tests (e.g., urine toxicology) may all be useful in the management of the terminally ill person with substance dependence.[48]

Psychosocial Considerations

Optimal end-of-life care involves an understanding of the major areas of psychosocial concern (such as family, work, religion, faith, ethnicity, and culture). The presence of the family is crucial to help a patient resolve long-standing conflicts (if possible) and to provide a context for honoring and remembering the patient.[12] Psychiatrists and other mental health professionals can aid the family in a variety of ways, including exploring the story of illness and families' ways of coping, assessing and supporting family communication and cohesiveness, and exploring how family members relate to one another.[13,49] At the same time, an understanding of the complexities of family interactions (both positive and negative) helps prevent harm to a potentially fragile family system. For example, a recent randomized clinical trial of family-focused grief therapy found that it could help prevent pathological grief in family members; however, it had the potential to increase conflict in families where the level of hostility was high.[50] As with family relationships, a sense of vocational identity can help create meaning for a patient at the end of life.[12] Work is important to self-esteem and the self-concept of a large proportion of the population. As one patient stated, "What you do is what you are."[51] As a patient can begin to feel less valued when work ceases or retirement arrives, the presence of former and current colleagues can be quite supportive. Similarly, thoughtful discussion about a patient's beliefs and faith can provide an opportunity for a patient to further his or her sense of meaning and thoughts about an after-life.[13]

Many patients are grateful for the chance to express thoughts about their faith. The patient's own religious leader, if available, can provide valuable information and insights about the patient and family and help smooth the course before death. For most Americans, religious belief plays an essential part of their understanding of the world and their role in it. For example, 86% of Americans believe in a personal God who answers prayers, 79% believe in miracles, 70%–85% pray regularly for good or better health, and 72% believe God can cure people given no chance of survival by medical science.[52] Psychiatrists should attend to patients' religious attitudes and beliefs regarding illness and death, and seek consultation with local clergy or hospital chaplaincy, as appropriate.

Writers, such as Feifel,[53] have contrasted an extrinsic religious orientation (in which religion is mainly a means to social status, security, or relief from guilt) with an intrinsic religious orientation (in which the values appear to be internalized and subscribed to as ends in themselves). Experimental work[54] and clinical experience[12] indicate that an extrinsic value system, without internalization, appears to offer less assistance in coping with a fatal illness than intrinsic religious commitment (which can offer considerable stability and strength).

Patients from under-served communities or minority populations within the US may have needs that may not be served by the current health care system. Unfortunately, the same institutional, cultural, and individual factors that generate disparities in care for minority populations also affect care at the end of life.[55,56] These factors include lack of access to care, under-treatment of pain, and mistrust of the health care system.[55-58] Furthermore, important differences among ethnic groups and cultures can be found at all segments of end-of-life care. For example, several studies have shown that African American patients, as well as older individuals from other ethnic backgrounds (such as Latino, Asian, or Native American), are somewhat less likely to have arranged for an advance directive as compared to Caucasian patients.[59] There are also important differences in terms of preferences for life-sustaining treatment. For example, in a study involving multiple ethnic groups, African Americans had the highest rate of preferring life-sustaining treatment, and European Americans had the lowest rates.[60]

Multiple other studies have demonstrated a preference by African Americans to choose more life-sustaining treatment and cardiopulmonary resuscitation in the face of terminal illness.[61-64] Additionally, culture may also influence the decision-making process. For example, family-centered (rather than individual-centered) decision-making is common in certain ethnic groups within the US, which challenges the traditional Western model of the importance of individual autonomy.[55] Studies have found that family-centered decision-making (which is more common among Latino and Asian groups in the US) may include the decision to disclose (or not to disclose) the diagnosis of a terminal illness to an individual patient.[59] Thus, cultural sensitivity and respectful curiosity on the part of psychiatrists plays a significant role in mediating end-of-life care for patients from all ethnicities and cultures.

CHALLENGES FOR CARE PROVIDERS

The emotional intensity associated with providing empathy and support for the dying patient may challenge and exhaust caregivers (both family and professional staff). Caregivers may feel helpless and despondent in the face of their powerlessness over a patient's imminent death. If left unaddressed, these feelings may lead the caregiver to retreat, to avoid the patient, or even to lash out (e.g., expressing that the patient is a burden to care for). This could be devastating to the helpless patient who looks to his or her caregiver for hope and compassionate care.

Hence, among the greatest psychological burdens for caregivers is learning to live with negative feelings (rather than enact them) and being mindful of urges to avoid the patient. For caregivers with certain ways of relating to others, these empathic requirements can be daunting. For example, a caregiver with a dependent style may expect the patient to appreciate, to thank, to love, and to nurture them. These caregivers are at risk of exhausting themselves because they "can't do too much." This may be sustainable for a patient with the capacity to routinely acknowledge and appreciate the caregiver, but it could lead to a disastrous outcome if the patient is depleted or hostile. In the latter case, the harder the caregiver strives, the less rewarding the work becomes. Exhaustion and demoralization follow.

ETHICS AND END-OF-LIFE CARE
Principles

End-of-life care, by its nature, is linked to a host of ethical questions that the psychiatrist is likely to encounter. A brief discussion of principles is not intended to supplant the need for concrete individualized judgments for every patient. Principles provide anchor points from which clinical reasoning can proceed—specifically, when limitation of life-supporting treatment is proposed.

The primary obligation of the physician to the patient in traditional medical ethics has been expressed in both positive and negative terms. The negative goal, always referred to first, is not to harm the patient (*primum non nocere*). The positive obligation is to restore health, to relieve suffering, or both. Our contemporary dilemma, as Slater[65] has pointed out, arose because we now have many situations in which these two aims come into conflict (i.e., the more aggressive the efforts to reverse an incurable illness, the more suffering is inflicted on the patient). Medicine routinely tolerates this conflict when the prognosis is one of recovery (e.g., the months of difficult surgeries and rehabilitation for a young victim of a car crash). However, the dilemma regarding these two values is more striking when intervention cannot lead to meaningful recovery or quality of life. For example, if a 70-year-old man with large cell cancer of the lung is found to have metastatic disease, any treatment of the cancer is likely to make him feel worse and would be unlikely to prolong his survival.

Second, modern medicine respects the patient's right to autonomy. This principle guarantees any competent patient the right to refuse any treatment, even a life-saving one. This was the emphasis of the field of medical ethics in the 1970s and 1980s, when it focused on the right of a patient to refuse life-prolonging treatment, such as mechanical ventilation; and, more recently, the right to refuse nutrition and hydration. Honoring such refusals presupposes that the patient is competent. It is important to remember that competent patients may make decisions that providers may view as irrational.[66] However, a patient cannot insist that the physician provide treatment that the physician considers ineffective or counter to good clinical care.[67-70] Defining "futility" continues to be controversial in medical ethics. Some continue to insist that an objective definition of futility is attainable, and it simply needs to balance patient autonomy to opt for aggressive treatment and the physician's duty not to offer or provide treatments that are ineffective or even harmful.[71] However, others argue that the notion of an objective definition of futility is unattainable and impractical. They point out that the notion of futility simply masks a conflict of values between two views of the same situation. For example, relatives of a dying patient may think that keeping their loved one alive at all costs even for a few hours is worthwhile, while the clinical team may not and instead call those efforts "futile." These ethicists argue for a process-oriented approach around conflicts at the end of life that enhances communication among clinicians, relatives, and patients.[72]

Limitation of Life-sustaining Treatment

One salient concept for psychiatrists to understand is the limitation of life-sustaining treatment. Whenever the risks or burdens of a treatment appear to outweigh the benefits, use of that treatment should be questioned by both the physician and the patient. Limitation of life-prolonging treatment is generally reserved for three categories of patients. First, patients whose illness is judged to be irreversible, who are moribund, and who need to be protected from needlessly burdensome treatments may refuse life-sustaining treatment. This is widely accepted for patients who will die with or without treatment (such as the patient with advanced metastatic cancer). Second, because of the right to refuse treatment, competent patients who are not moribund but who have an irreversible illness often choose to have life-sustaining treatments stopped. Last, competent patients with a reversible illness have the right to refuse any treatment, including life-saving treatments.

However, complications emerge when a patient is unable to make or to voice a decision regarding his or her wishes. In the absence of this information, it is often up to surrogate decision-makers to decide what the patient would have wanted in these circumstances. If no surrogate decision-maker is available, then the medical team (often in consultation with the hospital's legal counsel) will resort to the "reasonable person standard:" asking what would a "reasonable person" opt to do in these situations.

From a legal perspective, the state has a recognized legal interest in preserving life, and it may be difficult to ascertain whether the patient had a countervailing autonomy interest. One historical example is the case of Karen Ann Quinlan, a 21-year-old woman who in 1976 fell into an irreversible coma while at a party. This case became a legal battle between the right of Quinlan's mother (who as her guardian wished to withdraw life-sustaining treatment from her daughter and allow her daughter to die) and the state's interest in preserving life. In the end, the Supreme Court of New Jersey decided that, if it was believed, to a reasonable degree, that the coma was irreversible, life-sustaining treatment (e.g., with a respirator) could be removed.[73] Now, more than 30 years later, the standard medical recommendation in the case of irreversible coma is to stop all treatment (including nutrition and hydration). This judgment is made on the principle of the inevitability of death and the futility of any treatments to prevent this.

For patients in a persistent vegetative state (PVS) (a state in which patients have a functioning brainstem but total loss of cortical function) a complicated scenario emerges.[74-77] The diagnosis of a PVS is made when a patient is unaware of himself or herself and his or her environment and there is no prospect of any change in this state by any means. The clinical characteristics and diagnosis of the condition are established, but given the spectrum from PVS to full awareness, the clinical reality is that the diagnosis of PVS cannot be absolutely certain. Furthermore, there is no standard test of awareness and data on prognosis are limited.[77] In the absence of clinical clarity, values conflict has emerged.

There have been several notable legal cases of patients in PVS where there was conflict around whether or not they could be allowed to die (most notably the Nancy Cruzan case in 1990).[78,79] The complicated scenario of the PVS was recently encountered in the Theresa Schiavo case from 1998 to 2005.[80] In this highly public and controversial case, Theresa Schiavo was determined to be in a PVS in 1990. In 1998, her husband, who was her legal guardian, wished to withdraw life-sustaining nutrition and hydration from her, in accordance with what he believed her wishes would have been. However, her parents opposed removal of the life-sustaining measures because they believed Mrs. Schiavo to be conscious.[80] This case highlights the confusion and controversy that surrounds the withdrawal of medical care for patients with a PVS.[81] The case revived public debate about withdrawal of care at the end of life. And many states began debating the level of proof required to establish that an incompetent patient, when competent, would have opted to have his or her life-sustaining care withdrawn.

As a whole, the legal cases regarding end-of-life decision-making explicitly give patients the right to exercise their autonomy regarding what care they receive at the end of life. Competent patients can make these wishes known through the use of advance directives, which take effect in the event of future incapacity to make or to express decisions about their care. These directives may be instructional, may appoint a substitute decision-maker, or both. Instructional directives placing limits on life-sustaining treatment, however, may be difficult to interpret on clinical grounds. Advance directives that appoint a substitute decision-maker with whom the patient has discussed his or her wishes may be a more flexible way to enact a patient's wishes. Specifically, a substitute decision-maker can use his or her knowledge of the patient's prior expressed wishes in combination with the actual clinical scenario in order to effect (more reliably) the outcome that the patient would have wanted, if they were competent.

Physician-assisted Suicide

Although patients have broad rights of autonomy in expressing their wishes for end-of-life care, there are limits on a patient's ability to control his or her death. Specifically, a patient may express the wish to have a physician end his or her life (euthanasia). However, euthanasia, even when requested by the patient, is illegal in all 50 states and all US districts and territories. Unlike euthanasia, physician-assisted suicide has become legal in the states of Oregon, Washington, Montana, and most recently in Vermont. For patients who meet specific criteria (including having a prognosis of less than 6 months and being evaluated by at least two physicians regarding their request to die), physician-assisted suicide allows physicians to help patients acquire the means to end their lives (by prescribing a lethal dose of medications) but

does not permit the physician to actually administer those means. Although Oregon has legalized the practice, organized medicine (including organized psychiatry) opposes the practice. The debate over physician-assisted suicide will no doubt continue as other states consider passing laws that authorize physician-assisted suicide.

CONCLUSION

In conclusion, the aim of end-of-life care is to maximize the quality of life and to minimize the suffering of patients who are terminally ill. For many patients, the end of life marks an important opportunity to reflect, reconcile, and pursue remaining hopes. The psychiatrist can play an important role both in the diagnosis and treatment of psychiatric illness in this setting, as well as facilitating treatment, enhancing communication, and modeling caregiver qualities for families. From a psychiatric perspective, major depression and anxiety are commonly seen; and suicidality should not be considered "understandable" or "normal" in this setting. Delirium, pain, and difficulties with coping are also common reasons for consultation requests. As in all other forms of psychiatric evaluation and treatment, it is crucial to consider any medical contribution to psychiatric symptoms. Aggressive treatment of depression, anxiety, and other psychiatric symptoms is a crucial part of holistic management. Additionally, psychosocial factors may also play an important (and, at times, complicating) role in the care of these patients. Psychiatrists also should be aware of, and prepared to manage, many of the complex ethical and legal issues that arise in the care of these patients.

Physicians have clear obligations in caring for their patients, and patients have rights to autonomy in their decision-making. Sound clinical and ethical practice requires that the physician assist the terminally ill patient in the complex and often simultaneous processes of grieving and celebrating, reconciling conflicts and completing unfinished business, achieving last hopes and accepting unrealized goals, while alleviating suffering and maximizing autonomy and personhood until death.

Access the complete reference list and multiple choice questions (MCQs) online at https://expertconsult.inkling.com

KEY REFERENCES

1. Centers for Disease Control and Prevention Faststats website. <www.cdc.gov/nchs/fastats/deaths.htm>; [accessed August 15, 2013].
3. Kübler-Ross E. *On death and dying*, New York, 1969, MacMillan.
4. Maciejewski PK, Zhang B, Block SD, et al. An empirical examination of the stage theory of grief. *JAMA* 297(7):716–723, 2007.
5. Hackett TP, Weisman AD. The treatment of the dying. *Curr Psychiatr Ther* 2:121–126, 1962.
6. National Hospice and Palliative Care Organization. NHPCO's facts and figures—2012 findings. Available at http://www.nhpco.org/sites/default/files/public/Statistics_Research/2012_Facts_Figures.pdf>; [accessed September 1, 2013].
10. Kim HF, Greenberg DB. Coping with medical illness. In Stern TA, Herman JB, editors: *Massachusetts General Hospital psychiatry update and board preparation*, ed 2, New York, 2004, McGraw-Hill.
12. Brendel RW, Wei M, Epstein LA, et al. Care at the end of life. In Stern TA, Fricchione GL, Cassem NH, et al, editors: *Massachusetts General Hospital handbook of general hospital psychiatry*, ed 6, Philadelphia, 2010, Saunders.
16. Pirl WF. Evidence report on the occurrence, assessment, and treatment of depression in cancer patients. *J Natl Cancer Inst Monogr* 32P:32–39, 2004.
20. Breitbart W, Rosenfeld B, Pessin H, et al. Depression, hopelessness, and desire for hastened death in terminally ill patients with cancer. *JAMA* 284(22):2907–2911, 2000.

25. Maytal G, Stern TA. The desire for death in the setting of terminal illness: a case discussion. *Prim Care Companion J Clin Psychiatry* 8(5):299–305, 2006.

29. Chochinov HM, Hack T, Hassard T, et al. Dignity in the terminally ill: a cross-sectional, cohort study. *Lancet* 360(9350):2026–2030, 2002.

31. Smith JE, Richardson J, Hoffman C, et al. Mindfulness-based stress reduction as supportive therapy in cancer care: systematic review. *J Adv Nurs* 52(3):315–327, 2005.

42. Ballantyne JC, Mao J. Opioid therapy for chronic pain. *N Engl J Med* 349(20):1943–1953, 2003.

45. Passik SD, Theobald DE. Managing addiction in advanced cancer patients: why bother? *J Pain Symptom Manage* 19(3):229–234, 2000.

48. Kirsh KL, Passik SD. Palliative care of the terminally ill drug addict. *Cancer Invest* 24(4):425–431, 2006.

50. Kissane DW, McKenzie M, Bloch S, et al. Family focused grief therapy: a randomized, controlled trial in palliative care and bereavement. *Am J Psychiatry* 163:1208–1218, 2006.

53. Feifel H. Religious conviction and fear of death among the healthy and the terminally ill. *J Sci Study Relig* 13:353–360, 1974.

56. Siriwardena AN, Clark DH. End-of-life care for ethnic minority groups. *Clin Cornerstone* 6(1):43–48, discussion 49, 2006.

57. Hazin R, Giles CA. Is there a color line in death? An examination of end-of-life care in the African American community. *J Natl Med Assoc* 103(7):609–613, 2011.

62. Garrett JM, Harris RP, Norburn JK, et al. Life-sustaining treatments during terminal illness: who wants what? *J Gen Intern Med* 8(7):361–368, 1993.

66. Brock DW, Wartman SA. When competent patients make irrational choices. *N Engl J Med* 322:1595–1599, 1990.

67. Consensus report on the ethics of forgoing life-sustaining treatments in the critically ill. Task Force on Ethics of the Society of Critical Care Medicine. *Crit Care Med* 18:1435–1439, 1990.

72. Truog RD, Brett AS, Frader J. The problem with futility. *N Engl J Med* 326(23):1560–1564, 1992.

77. Wade DT. Ethical issues in diagnosis and management of patients in the permanent vegetative state. *BMJ* 322(7282):352–354, 2001.

81. Mueller PS. The Terri Schiavo saga: ethical and legal aspects and implications for clinicians. *Pol Arch Med Wewn* 119(9):574–581, 2009.

61 Psychiatric Epidemiology

Albert S. Yeung, MD, ScD, and Trina E. Chang, MD, MPH

KEY POINTS

- Epidemiology is the study of the distribution and determinants of disease frequency in humans to inform the natural history, service needs, and etiology of illness.

- The frequency of disease can be expressed in different concepts, including cumulative incidence, incidence density, point prevalence, lifetime prevalence, and so on.

- Epidemiological studies frequently rely on assessment instruments to evaluate psychiatric disorders. It is important to first establish the reliability (or consistency) and validity (or truthfulness) of these assessment instruments.

- Based on the recent National Comorbidity Survey (NCS) in the US, the most common psychiatric disorders were major depression and alcohol dependence, followed by social and simple phobias. Approximately one in four respondents met criteria for a substance use disorder, one in four for an anxiety disorder, and one in five for an affective disorder in their lifetime.

- Epidemiological studies in the US and in European countries showed that, in general, individuals with a psychiatric disorder underutilize mental health services. Among those who sought treatment, there was significant delay in seeking help.

OVERVIEW

Epidemiology is the study of the distribution and determinants of disease frequency in man. Epidemiological studies typically examine large groups of individuals, and by providing data on the distribution and frequency of diseases, they help describe the natural history of illness, assess service needs in the community or in special institutions, and shed light on the etiology of illness.

Epidemiology is based on two fundamental assumptions: first, that human disease does not occur at random, and second, that human disease has causal and preventive factors that can be identified through systematic investigation of different populations in different places or at different times. By measuring disease frequency, and by examining who gets a disease within a population, as well as where and when the disease occurs, it is possible to formulate hypotheses concerning possible causal and preventive factors.[1]

EPIDEMIOLOGICAL MEASURES OF DISEASE FREQUENCY

The frequency of disease or some other outcome within a population group is described using different concepts: the rate at which new cases are observed, or the proportion of a given population that exhibits the outcome of interest.

Incidence refers to the number of new events that develop in a population over a specified period of time (t_0 to t_1). If this incidence rate is described as the number of events (outcomes) in proportion to the population at risk for the event, it is called the *cumulative incidence* (CI), and is calculated by the following equation:

$$CI = \frac{\text{Number of new cases, } t_0 \text{ to } t_1}{\text{Population at risk at } t_0}$$

The denominator equals the total number of persons at risk for the event at the start of the time period (t_0) without adjustment for any subsequent reduction in the cohort size for any reason, for example, loss to follow-up, death, or reclassification to "case" status. Therefore, CI is best used to describe stable populations where there is little reduction in cohort size during the time period of interest. An example would be a study of the incidence of major depressive disorder (MDD) in a residential program. If, at the beginning of the study, 8 of the 100 residents have MDD, and of the 92 remaining patients, 8 develop MDD over the next 12 months, the CI for MDD would be $(8/92 \times 100) = 8.7\%$ for this period (i.e., 1 year). Note that the denominator does not include those in the population with the condition at t_0, since they are not at risk for newly experiencing the outcome.

When patients are followed for varying lengths of time (e.g., due to loss to follow-up, death, or reclassification to "case" status) and the denominator value representing the population-at-risk changes significantly, incidence density provides a more precise measure of the rate at which new events occur. *Incidence density* (ID) is defined as the number of events occurring per unit population per unit time:

$$\text{Incidence density} = \frac{\text{Number of new cases, } t_0 \text{ to } t_1}{\text{Total person-time of observation}}$$

The denominator is the population that is actively at risk for the event, and is adjusted as people no longer belong in that pool. In a study of psychosis, for instance, if a person develops hallucinations and delusions, he or she becomes "a case" and no longer contributes to the denominator. Similarly, a person lost to follow-up would also contribute to the denominator only so long as he or she is being tracked by the study. To illustrate, suppose in a 100-person study of human immunodeficiency virus (HIV) infection, 6 people are lost to follow-up at the end of 6 months, and 4 develop HIV infection at the end of the third month, the person-years of observation would be calculated as follows: $(90 \times 1 \text{ year}) + (6 \times 0.5 \text{ year}) + (4 \times 0.25 \text{ year}) = 94$ person-years, and incidence density = $(4 \text{ cases})/(94 \text{ person-years}) = 4.26$ cases/100 person-years of observation.

Prevalence is the proportion of individuals who have a particular disease or outcome at a point or period in time. In most psychiatric studies, "prevalence" refers to the proportion of the population that has the outcome at a particular point in time, and is called the *point prevalence*:

$$\text{Point prevalence} = \frac{\text{Number of existing cases at } t_0}{\text{Population at } t_0}$$

In stable populations, prevalence (P) can be related to incidence density (ID) by the equation $P = ID \times D$, where D is the average duration of the disease before termination (by death or remission, for example). At times, the numerator is expanded to include the number of all cases, existing and new, in a specified time period; this is known as a *period prevalence*. When the period of interest is a lifetime, it is a type of period prevalence called *lifetime prevalence*, which is the proportion of people who have ever had the specified disease or attribute in their lifetime.

Lifetime prevalence is often used to convey the overall risk for someone who develops an illness, particularly psychiatric ones that have episodic courses, or require a certain duration of symptoms to qualify for a diagnosis (e.g., depression, anxiety, or post-traumatic stress disorder). In practice, however, an accurate lifetime prevalence rate is difficult to determine since it often relies on subject recall and on sampling populations of different ages (not necessarily at the end of their respective "lifetimes"). It is also an overall rate that does not account for changes in incidence rates over time, nor for possible differences in mortality rates in those with or without the condition.

CRITERIA FOR ASSESSMENT INSTRUMENTS

There are a number of concepts that are helpful in the evaluation of assessment instruments. These involve the consistency of the results that the instrument provides, and its fidelity to the concept being measured.

Reliability is the degree to which an assessment instrument produces consistent or reproducible results when used by different examiners at different times. Lack of reliability may be the result of divergence between observers, imprecision in the measurement tool, or instability in the attribute being measured. *Inter-rater reliability* (Figure 61-1) is the extent to which different examiners obtain equivalent results in the same subject when using the same instrument; *test-retest reliability* is the extent to which the same instrument obtains equivalent results in the same subject on different occasions.

		Rater A		
		Disorder present	Disorder absent	Total
Rater B	Disorder present	a	b	a+b
	Disorder absent	c	d	c+d
	Total	a+c	b+d	n

Figure 61-1. Inter-rater reliability.

Reliability is not sufficient for a measurement instrument—it could, for example, consistently and reliably give results that are neither meaningful nor accurate. However, it is a necessary attribute, since inconsistency would impair the accuracy of any tool. The demonstration of the reliability of an assessment tool is thus required before its use in epidemiological studies. The use of explicit diagnostic criteria, trained examiners to interpret data uniformly, and a structured assessment that obtains the same types of information from all subjects can enhance the reliability of assessment instruments.

There are several commonly used measures to indicate the degree of consistency between sets of data, which in psychiatry is often used to quantify the degree of agreement between raters. The kappa statistic (κ) is used for categorical or binary data, and the intra-class correlation coefficient (ICC, usually represented as r) for continuous data. Both measures have the same range of values (-1 to $+1$), from perfect negative correlation (-1), to no correlation (0), to perfect positive correlation ($+1$). For acceptable reliability, the kappa statistic value of 0.7 or greater is generally required; for the ICC, a value of 0.8 or greater is generally required.

Calculation of the kappa statistic (κ) requires only arithmetic computation, and accounts for the degree of consistency between raters with an adjustment for the probability of agreement due to chance. When the frequency of the disorder is very low, however, the kappa statistic will be low despite having a high degree of consistency between raters; it is not appropriate for the measurement of reliability of infrequent disorders.

$$\kappa = \frac{P_o - P_c}{1 - P_c}$$

where P_o is the observed agreement and P_c is an agreement due to chance. $P_o = (a + d)/n$ and $P_c = [(a + c)(a + b) + (b + d)(c + d)]/n^2$. Calculation of the ICC is more involved and is beyond the scope of this text.

Validity is a term that expresses the degree to which a measurement instrument actually measures what it purports to measure. When translating a theoretical concept into an operational instrument that purports to assess or measure it, several aspects of validity need to be accounted for.

For any abstract concept, there are an infinite number of criteria that one might use to assess it. For example, if one wants to develop a questionnaire to diagnose bipolar disorder, one should ask about mood, thought process, and energy level, but probably not whether the subject owns a bicycle. *Content validity* is the extent to which the instrument adequately incorporates the domain of items that would accurately measure the concept of interest.

Criterion validity is the extent to which the measurement can predict or agree with constructs external to the construct being measured. There are two types of criterion validity generally distinguished, predictive validity and concurrent validity. *Predictive validity* is the extent to which the instrument's measurements can predict an external criterion. For instance, if we devise an instrument to measure math ability, we might postulate that math ability should be correlated to better grades in college math courses. A high correlation between the measure's assessment of math ability and college math course grades would indicate that the instrument can correctly predict as it theoretically should, and has predictive validity. *Concurrent validity* refers to the extent to which the measurement correlates to another criterion at the same point in time. For example, if we devise a measure relying on visual inspection of a wound to determine infection, we can correlate it to a bacteriological examination of a specimen taken at the same time. A high correlation would indicate concurrent validity, and suggest that our new measure gives valid results for determining infection.

Construct validity refers to the extent to which the measure assesses the underlying theoretical construct that it intends to measure. This concept is the most complex, and both content and criterion validity point to it. An example of a measure lacking construct validity would be a test for assessing algebra skills using word problems that inadvertently assesses reading skills rather than factual knowledge of algebra. Construct validity also refers to the extent that the construct exists as theorized and can be quantified by the instrument. In psychiatry, this is especially difficult since there are no "gold standard" laboratory (e.g., chemical, anatomical, physiological) tests, and the criteria if not the existence of many diagnoses are disputed. To establish the validity for any diagnosis, certain requirements have been proposed, and include an adequate clinical description of the disorder that distinguishes it from other similar disorders and the ability to correlate the diagnosis to external criteria, such as laboratory tests, familial transmission patterns, and consistent outcomes, including response to treatment.

Because there are no "gold standard" diagnostic tests in psychiatry, efforts to validate diagnoses have focused around such efforts as increasing the reliability of diagnostic instruments—by defining explicit and observationally-based diagnostic criteria (DSM-III and subsequent versions), or employing structured interviews, such as the Diagnostic Interview Schedule (DIS)—and conducting genetic and outcome studies for diagnostic categories. The selection of a "gold standard" criterion instrument in psychiatry, however, remains problematic.

Assessment of New Instruments

If we assume that a reliable criterion instrument that provides valid results exists, the assessment of a new measurement instrument would involve comparing the results of the new instrument to those of the criterion instrument. The criterion instrument's results are considered "true," and a judgment of the validity of the new instrument's results are based on how well they match the criterion instrument's (Figure 61-2).

Sensitivity is the proportion of true cases, as identified by the criterion instrument, who are identified as cases by the new instrument (also known as the *true positive rate*).

Specificity is the proportion of non-cases, as identified by the criterion instrument, who are identified as non-cases by the new instrument (also known as the *true negative rate*).

For any given instrument, there are tradeoffs between sensitivity and specificity, depending on where the threshold

limits are set to distinguish "case" from "non-case." For example, in the Hamilton-Depression Scale (HAM-D) instrument, the cutoff value for the diagnosis of MDD (often set at 15) would determine whether an individual would be identified as "case" or "non-case." If the value were instead set at 5, which most clinicians would consider "normal" or not depressed, the HAM-D would be an unusually sensitive instrument (e.g., using a structured clinical interview as the criterion instrument) since most anyone evaluated with even a modicum of depressive thinking would be considered a "case" as would anybody typically considered to have major depression. However, the test would not be especially specific, since it would be poor at identifying those without depression. Conversely, if the cutoff value were set at 25, sensitivity would be low but the specificity high.

In practice, the threshold values in any given evaluation instrument, whether creatine kinase (CK) levels for determining myocardial infarction, the number of colonies on a Petri dish to determine infection, or criteria to determine attention-deficit/hyperactivity disorder (ADHD) (e.g., 6 of 9 from group one, 6 of 9 from group two), are chosen to balance the need for both sensitivity and specificity. To improve both these measures without a tradeoff, either the instrument itself or its administration must be improved, or efforts made to ensure maximum stability of the attribute being measured (e.g., administering them concurrently, or in similar circumstances, such as at the same time of day, or a similar clinical setting).

Two other useful measures are the *positive predictive value* (PPV), the proportion of those with a positive test that are true cases as determined by the criterion instrument. *Negative predictive value* (NPV) is the proportion of those with a negative test that are true non-cases as determined by the criterion instrument.

Study Designs

There are six basic study types, presented here in the order of their respective ability to infer causality.

Descriptive Studies

The weakest of all study designs, these studies simply describe the health status of a population or of a number of subjects. Case series are an example of descriptive studies, and are simply descriptions of cases, without a comparison group. They can be useful for monitoring unusual patients, and in generating hypotheses for future study. One example is Teicher and colleagues' 1990 case series of six patients who developed suicidal ideation on fluoxetine, which informed future studies that ultimately led to black box warnings for all antidepressants.[2] Case series can also be misleading, though, as in the early 1980s when physicians began describing male homosexuals with depressed immune systems. The use of amyl nitrate-based sexual stimulants was a suspected cause, and studies on the effects of amyl nitrates on the immune system were under way when HIV was discovered.

Ecological Studies

In these types of studies, groups of individuals are studied as a whole, and the overall occurrence of disease (outcome) is correlated with the aggregate level of exposure to a risk factor. The groups being studied can be differentiated by geographical region or by other criteria, such as school, workplace, or clinic. Data are usually collected at different times for different reasons, and do not include data on individuals. Ecological studies are helpful for generating hypotheses, and are generally inexpensive and not time-consuming (since they are often based on data that are routinely published, such as death and

| | | Criterion instrument | | |
		Disorder present	Disorder absent	Total
New instrument	Disorder present	a	b	a+b
	Disorder absent	c	d	c+d
	Total	a+c	b+d	n

Sensitivity = a/(a+c)
Specificity = d/(b+d)
Positive predictive value = a/(a+b)
Negative predictive value = d/(c+d)

Figure 61-2. Validity of a new instrument.

disease rates, per capita income, religious affiliation, or food consumption). However, these studies are limited in showing causality because of the lack of individual data, the temporal ambiguity of the data (it is not known if a given risk factor precedes the outcome, for example), and problems with using data in an aggregate form to generalize about individuals. One such study that helped generate a helpful hypothesis included an intercountry comparison of prevalence rates for coronary artery disease (CAD); it showed that CAD was highest in those countries with the highest mean serum cholesterol values. This eventually led to more rigorous studies that confirmed a causal link between cholesterol levels and CAD.

Cross-sectional Studies

Cross-sectional studies examine individuals and determine their case status and risk factor exposures at the same time. Outcome rates between those with exposure can then be compared to those without. Data are collected by surveys, laboratory tests, physical measurements, or other procedures, and there is no follow-up or other longitudinal component. Cross-sectional studies are also called prevalence studies (more precisely, they are *point prevalence* studies), and, as with ecological studies, are relatively inexpensive and are useful for informing future research. They also aid in public health planning (e.g., determining the number of hospital beds needed) and generating more specific hypotheses around disease etiology by looking at specific risk factors.

As with the previously discussed study types, linking outcome and exposure is problematic. Although the data are collected for individuals, a person's exposure status may differ from when the disease actually began and when the study was conducted. To illustrate, if smokers tend to quit smoking and start exercising once diagnosed with lung cancer, a cross-sectional study looking at these factors would systematically underestimate the link between smoking and lung cancer, and suggest a link between exercise and lung cancer. Another problem with cross-sectional studies is that point prevalence rates are affected both by the rate at which the outcome develops and by the chronicity of the outcome. For instance, if a given disease has a longer time course in men than in women but identical incidence rates, the point prevalence rate in men would be higher than in women.

Case-control Studies

In case-control studies, subjects are selected based on whether they have the outcome (case) or not (control), and their exposures are then determined by looking backward in time. For this reason, they are also called retrospective studies, since they rely on historical records or recall. This type of study design is appropriate for rare diseases or for those with long latencies, and they can also be used to study possible risk factors. Problems with case-control studies include recall bias (which occurs if cases and controls recall past exposures differently) and difficulty in selecting controls. Ideally, one wants controls who are exactly matched to the cases in all other exposures except for the risk factor in question (Figure 61-3). Thus, controls should be matched for a variety of factors: for example, gender, socioeconomic status (SES), smoking status (unless that is what is being studied), and alcohol use. For case-control studies, an *odds ratio* is used to determine whether the outcome is more likely in those with the exposure, or in those without one, and it is an approximation of their relative incidence rates.

Cohort Studies

In a cohort study, a group of healthy individuals is identified and followed over time to see who develops the outcomes

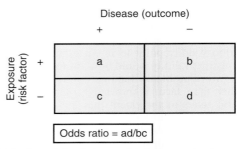

Figure 61-3. Association between risk factors and outcome in case-control and cohort studies.

(diseases) of interest and who do not. Exposures to risk factors are assessed over time, and so the sequence between exposure and outcome can be determined, as well as the relationship between different exposures and outcomes. Because neither the subjects nor the researchers know whether and who will develop which outcomes, bias in measuring exposures is avoided. Disadvantages include high cost (both in terms of manpower and time), potential for loss to follow-up, and inefficiency in studying rare diseases. In cohort studies, the association between outcome and exposure is expressed as *relative risk*, the ratio between the incidence rates in those with the risk factor and those without.

$$\text{Relative risk} = \frac{\text{Incidence rate in the group with the risk factor}}{\text{Incidence rate in the group without the risk factor}}$$

$$RR = \frac{a}{a+b} \div \frac{c}{c+d}$$

Examples of cohort studies include the Framingham Heart Study (which has followed generations of residents from Framingham, Massachusetts) and the Nurses Health Study (which has followed a national sample of nurses with annual questionnaires). One classic study in Britain followed 35,445 British physicians and found that among smokers, the incidence of lung cancer was 1.30 per 1,000, but only 0.07 for non-smokers.[3] The relative risk was therefore 1.30/0.07 = 18.6, indicating that smokers had more than 18 times the risk of developing lung cancer than non-smokers.

Randomized Controlled Trials

Randomized controlled trials (RCTs) are a type of cohort study in which the exposure is controlled by the researchers. Like standard cohort studies, a population who has yet to develop the outcome(s) of interest is defined; then, unlike standard cohort studies, the subjects are randomly assigned to different exposures. In these trials, the exposure is usually a treatment, such as a medication, or an intervention, such as counseling or a behavioral program. Those randomized to non-exposure may receive a placebo, or treatment as usual for the community. Multiple outcomes can be studied, from cessation of psychosis, reduction of depressive or anxious symptoms, to side effects or other adverse outcomes. RCTs, also known as experimental studies, are the gold standard of epidemiological research.

RCTs retain all the advantages of standard cohort studies, but because the exposure is randomized, the causal link between the exposure and the outcome is much stronger. Disadvantages are the same as for other cohort studies, but also include ethical issues around assigning subjects to treatment or non-treatment, as well as issues around adequate blinding and creation of appropriate placebo controls. Many times in psychiatric research, blinding is impossible, as with studies of psychotherapy, and defining an adequate placebo or "non-exposure" is difficult.

DEVELOPMENT OF ASSESSMENT TOOLS
Case Definition

In 1972, Cooper and colleagues[4] published a US/UK study that showed high variability in the diagnosis of psychotic disorders. It highlighted the need for having explicit operational criteria for case identification. The development of such diagnostic criteria with the publishing of the *Diagnostic and Statistical Manual of Mental Disorders*, ed 3 (DSM-III) in 1980 represented a notable step toward increasing the reliability and validity of psychiatric diagnoses.

Standardized Instruments for Case Assessment

The clinical interview is generally used to diagnose psychiatric illness. However, differences in personal styles and theoretical frameworks, among other factors, can affect the process and conclusions of a psychiatric interview. To increase inter-rater reliability, a number of standardized interview instruments have been developed. The first was the Present State Examination (PSE), initially used in the International Pilot Study of Schizophrenia sponsored by the World Health Organization (WHO). The PSE was designed for use by psychiatrists or experienced clinicians, however, so its use in larger epidemiological studies was impractical. In 1978, epidemiologists at the National Institute of Mental Health (NIMH) began developing a comprehensive diagnostic instrument for large-scale, epidemiological studies that could be administered by either lay people or clinicians. The result was the Diagnostic Interview Schedule (DIS), which used the then newly-published DSM-III (1980), and elements of other research instruments, including the PSE, the Renald Diagnostic Interview (RDI), the St. Louis criteria, and the Schedule for Affective Disorders and Schizophrenia (SADS). The DIS has been used extensively in the US and many other countries for surveys of psychiatric illness. Over time, the DIS has undergone revisions, first to incorporate DSM-III-R and then DSM-IV diagnoses. The WHO and the NIMH have also jointly developed the Composite International Diagnostic Interview (CIDI) that is structurally similar to the DIS and provides both ICD-10 and DSM-IV diagnoses. With the release of DSM-5, diagnostic instruments will need to be adapted further.

CONTEMPORARY STUDIES IN PSYCHIATRIC EPIDEMIOLOGY
The Baseline National Comorbidity Survey (NCS)[5]

The NCS, conducted between 1990 and 1992, was the first national survey of mental disorders in the US. Face-to-face structured diagnostic interviews were administered by non-clinicians to a representative sample of all people living in households within the continental US. The 8,098 NCS respondents were selected from over 1,000 neighborhoods in over 170 counties distributed over 34 states, and assessed with a modified CIDI.

The most important CIDI modifications involved the use of diagnostic stem questions, which were a small number of initial questions to assess core features of psychiatric disorders. Follow-up questions would only be asked when the subject responded positively. Another innovation of the NCS was the use of a two-phase clinical interview design for patients with evidence of schizophrenia or other non-affective psychoses. Because prior studies had shown that these types of patients could not provide reliable self-reports, they were reinterviewed

and diagnosed by experienced clinicians using a structured clinical interview.

In order to collect information on non-respondents to the study, the NCS also systematically evaluated about one-third of non-respondents using telephone interviews. Using the results of the non-response survey, the NCS study was able to adjust for the bias due to the lower rates of survey participation, especially among patients with anxiety disorders.

The NCS General Findings

DSM-III-R disorders were more prevalent than had been expected. About 48% of the sample reported at least one lifetime disorder, and 30% of respondents reported at least one disorder in the 12 months preceding the interview. The most common disorders were major depression and alcohol dependence, followed by social and simple phobias. As a group, substance use and anxiety disorders were more prevalent than affective disorders, with approximately one in four respondents meeting criteria for a substance use disorder in their lifetime, one in four for an anxiety disorder, and one in five respondents for an affective disorder (Table 61-1).

There were no differences by gender in the overall prevalence of psychiatric disorders. For individual disorders, men were more likely than women to have substance use disorders and antisocial personality disorder, whereas women were more likely than men to have anxiety and affective disorders (with the exception of mania).

NCS-Replication Survey

The NCS-Replication Survey (NCS-R) was conducted between 2001 and 2003 and involved a new sample of 10,000 respondents in the same nationally representative sampling segments as the baseline NCS. Lifetime prevalence estimates of DSM-IV disorders per the NCS-R are as follows: anxiety disorders, 28.8%, mood disorders, 20.8%, impulse-control disorders, 24.8%, substance use disorders, 14.6%, and any disorder, 46.4%. First onset of mental illness was found most often in childhood to early adulthood, with one-half of all cases starting by age 14 years and three-fourths by age 24 years.

Mental Health Services Utilization

From the NCS to the NCS-R, there was no change in the overall prevalence of mental disorders, but the rate of treatment increased in the past decade. Among patients with a psychiatric disorder, 20.3% received treatment between 1990 and 1992 compared to 32.9% between 2001 and 2003 (P < 0.001). Nevertheless, most patients with mental disorders in the NCS-R study still did not receive treatment. For those who did, there was significant delay, ranging from 6 to 8 years for mood disorders and from 9 to 23 years for anxiety disorders. The unmet need of mental health services has been greatest in traditionally underserved groups (including elderly persons, racial-ethnic minorities, residents of rural areas, and those with low incomes or without insurance).

The European Study of the Epidemiology of Mental Disorders Project

The European Study of the Epidemiology of Mental Disorders (ESEMeD) is a cross-sectional epidemiological study, conducted between January 2001 and August 2003, that assessed the psychiatric epidemiology of 212 million non-institutionalized adults from Belgium, France, Germany, Italy, the Netherlands, and Spain.[6] Individuals were assessed in-person at their homes using computer-assisted psychiatric interview (CAPI) instruments, and data from 21,425

TABLE 61-1 Lifetime and 12-Month Prevalence Estimates for Psychiatric Disorders, NCS-R Results[12-16]

	Lifetime Prevalence Estimate (%)	12-Month Prevalence Estimate (%)
Major Depressive Disorder	16.6	6.7
Bipolar disorder (I or II)	3.9	2.6
Dysthymia	2.5	1.5
Generalized anxiety disorder	5.7	3.1
Panic disorder	4.7	2.7
Social phobia	12.1	6.8
Specific phobia	12.5	8.7
Agoraphobia without panic	1.4	0.8
Alcohol abuse	13.2	3.1
Alcohol dependence	5.4	1.3
Drug abuse	7.9	1.4
Drug dependence	3.0	0.4
Antisocial personality disorder°	—	1.0
Non-affective psychosis°*	0.31	0.14

°Rates based on NCS-R screen followed by blinded clinical reappraisal interviews of a subsample of respondents.
*Non-affective psychosis: schizophrenia, schizophreniform disorder, schizoaffective disorder, delusional disorder, and atypical psychosis.
Data drawn from Kessler RC, Berglund P, Demler O, Jin R, Merikangas KR, Walters EE. Lifetime prevalence and age-of-onset distributions of DSM-IV disorders in the National Comorbidity Survey Replication. Arch Gen Psychiatry 62:593–602, 2005[12]; *Kessler RC, Birnbaum H, Demler O, et al. The prevalence and correlates of non-affective psychosis in the National Comorbidity Survey Replication (NCS-R).* Biol Psychiatry 58:668–676, 2005[13]; *Kessler RC, Chiu WT, Demler O, Walters E. Prevalence, severity, and comorbidity of 12-month DSM-IV disorders in the National Comorbidity Survey Replication.* Arch Gen Psychiatry 62:617–627, 2005[14]; *and Lenzenweger MF, Lane MC, Loranger AW, Kessler RC. DSM-IV personality disorders in the National Comorbidity Survey Replication.* Biol Psychiatry 62:553–564, 2007.[15]

respondents were collected. A stratified, multi-stage, clustered area, probability sample design was used to analyze the data.

Epidemiology

Using DSM-IV criteria, about one in four respondents reported a lifetime history of any mental disorder. MDD, specific phobia, alcohol abuse, and dysthymia were the most common mental disorders, with estimated lifetime prevalence rates of 12.8%, 7.7%, 4.1%, and 4.1%, respectively. The lifetime prevalence of other mental disorders was low (less than 3%). About 10% of respondents were diagnosed with any mental disorder in the 12 months preceding the diagnostic interview, MDD and specific phobia being the most common with prevalence estimates (3.9% and 3.5%, respectively). Only 0.7% of respondents reported a history of an alcohol abuse disorder in the preceding 12 months.

Under utilization of Health Services

The ESEMeD results suggest that the use of health services is limited among individuals with mental disorders in the European countries studied. Of the participants with a mental disorder in the preceding 12 months, only 25.7% consulted a formal health service during that period. The rates were higher for individuals with a mood disorder (36.5%) or anxiety disorder (26.1%). Among those who had used formal health services in the previous 12 months, approximately two-thirds had contacted a mental health professional. Psychotropic drug utilization was generally low (32.6%) by US standards, with only 21.2% of those diagnosed with MDD in the preceding 12 months having received antidepressants during that period.

EPIDEMIOLOGY OF MAJOR PSYCHIATRIC DISORDERS

Schizophrenia

Epidemiology

Prior to the introduction of the DSM-III, the prevalence of schizophrenia was estimated to range from 1% to 7%. In a review of recent studies, Jablensky[7] placed the prevalence rate

TABLE 61-2 Recurrence Risk* for Schizophrenia in Biological Relatives[17]

Population	Recurrence Risk
General population	1
Children of two schizophrenic parents	89
Children with a schizophrenic father	10.7
Children with a schizophrenic mother	10.3
Children with a schizophrenic full sibling	8.6
Monozygotic twin of a schizophrenic patient	50.0
First cousin of a schizophrenic patient	2.29

*Recurrence risk: the morbidity risk of the illness in a given family member of the patient compared to the risk in the general population.
Data drawn from Lichtenstein P, Björk C, Hultman CM, et al. Recurrence risks for schizophrenia in a Swedish National Cohort. Psychol Med 36:1417–1425, 2006[16] *and Tsuang MT, Tohen M, Jones PB, editors. Textbook in psychiatric epidemiology.* ed 3. Chichester, West Sussex, 2011, Wiley-Blackwell.[17]

in the range of 1.4–4.6 per thousand. This downward shift is largely due to the narrowing of the criteria for schizophrenia in nosological systems published after 1980. Based on the NCS-R, the lifetime prevalence rate for the five non-affective psychoses (schizophrenia, schizophreniform disorder, schizoaffective disorder, delusional disorder, and atypical psychoses) is 3.1 per 1000.

Risk Factors

Genetic loading is a robust risk factor for schizophrenia (Table 61-2). The prevalence of schizophrenia in a monozygotic twin of a schizophrenia patient may be as high as 50%, and 15% in a dizygotic twin. The prevalence for a child with two schizophrenic parents is 46.3%, and 12.8% for a child with one schizophrenic parent.

Other risk factors of schizophrenia include being a member of a lower social class, being unmarried, having birth complications, and being born during the winter months. The inverse relationship between social class and schizophrenia may be a result of social impairment and downward social drift rather than the cause of the illness. Studies have also shown that stressful life events, high levels of "expressed emotions" (critical and overprotective behavior and verbalizations toward the family member with schizophrenia), and substance use can precipitate psychotic episodes.

Bipolar I Disorder

Epidemiology

The NCS-R reported a lifetime prevalence of 1% for bipolar I disorder and a 12-month prevalence of 0.6%.

Risk Factors

Both Epidemiology Catchment Area (ECA) and NCS studies showed that there is no gender difference in the prevalence of bipolar disorder. Some studies conducted before 1980 showed a higher prevalence of bipolar disorder in the upper socioeconomic classes, but there has been no evidence for that in recent studies. Bipolar I disorder occurs at much higher rates in first-degree biological relatives of persons with bipolar I disorder than it does in the general population. Family, adoption, and twin studies clearly support the evidence that bipolar disorder is genetically transmitted. The concordance rate in monozygotic twins is 58%–93%, while the concordance rate in dizygotic twins is 16%–35%. The lifetime risks of suffering from bipolar disorder in relatives of bipolar probands are 2%–19% in first-degree relatives and 1.8%–2.8% in adoptive relatives. Both the ECA and the NCS studies found that there were no race differences in the prevalence of bipolar disorder.

Co-morbidities

Individuals with bipolar disorder have a high prevalence of co-morbid psychiatric disorders. In both ECA and NCS studies, about 60% of patients with bipolar disorder had co-morbid substance abuse. According to the National Epidemiologic Survey on Alcohol and Related Conditions, co-morbid alcoholism was twice as high in those with bipolar I as in those with unipolar depression,[8] and substance use was five times as high in those with bipolar I as it was in the general population.[9]

Major Depressive Disorder

Epidemiology

The NCS-R reported a 1-year prevalence for MDD of 6.8% and a lifetime prevalence of 16.9%. Studies from different nations have reported significant variations in the prevalence of major depression. However, it is not clear whether cross-national differences in the prevalence of major depression were due to variations in risk factors or to methodological differences across studies.

Risk Factors

Risk factors for MDD include being female, having a history of depressive illness in first-degree relatives, having prior episodes of major depression or other psychiatric disorders, having a 2-week period of two concurrent depressive symptoms, and being divorced.

Depression as the Cause of Disability

Depression has been shown more likely to cause disability than are other chronic medical conditions. According to the 2004 update of the Global Burden of Disease Project conducted by the WHO,[10] major depression ranked as the third leading cause of burden of disease in the world, after lower respiratory infections and diarrheal diseases.

Generalized Anxiety Disorder

Epidemiology

The NCS-R reported a 1-year prevalence for generalized anxiety disorder (GAD) of 2.7% and a lifetime risk of 5.7%.

Risk Factors

Based on the ECA study, the 1-year prevalence of GAD was significantly higher in females, African Americans, and persons under 30 years of age.

Panic Disorder

Epidemiology

The Baseline NCS reported a lifetime prevalence rate of 3.5% and 1-year prevalence rate of 2.3% for panic disorder. In the NCS-R study, respondents were assessed for DSM-IV panic attacks, as well as for panic disorder with and without agoraphobia. Lifetime prevalence estimates were 22.7% for isolated panic without agoraphobia, 0.8% for panic attack with agoraphobia but without panic disorder, 3.7% for panic disorder without agoraphobia, and 1.1% for panic disorder with agoraphobia.

Risk Factors

In general, women, persons under age 60, and non-Hispanic blacks are at higher risk of having panic. The differences among Hispanics and non-Hispanic whites are small. Panic disorder most commonly develops in young adulthood; the mean age of presentation is about 24 years, but both panic disorder and agoraphobia can develop at any age.

Social Burdens of Panic

While the major societal burden of panic is caused by panic disorder and panic disorder with agoraphobia, isolated panic attacks also have high prevalence and meaningful role impairment. Compared to patients with common chronic medical conditions (including hypertension, diabetes, heart disease, arthritis, and chronic lung problems), patients with panic disorder were found to have lower health-related quality of life.

Alcohol Abuse and Dependence

Epidemiology

The NCS-R reported a lifetime prevalence for alcohol abuse and alcohol dependence of 17.8% and 12.5%, respectively. The yearly prevalence rates for alcohol abuse and dependence were 4.7% and 3.8%, respectively. Alcoholism is one of the most common psychiatric disorders.

Risk Factors

Genetic history is an important risk factor. The risk of alcoholism in any first-degree family members of an alcoholic is at least doubled.[11] Twin studies also support genetic transmission of alcoholism; it is higher for alcohol dependence than it is for alcohol abuse. Other risk factors for dependence include male gender, younger ages, being unmarried, being white, and having a low income.

Co-morbidity

In both ECA and NCS studies, alcoholics frequently had co-morbid drug abuse and dependence, antisocial personality disorder, mania, schizophrenia, and anxiety disorders. Alcoholism is also associated with accidents, violence, cardiovascular diseases, and cirrhosis. Women who use alcohol during pregnancy may cause growth, morphologic, and neurological deficits in their offspring.

Access a list of MCQs for this chapter at https://expertconsult .inkling.com

REFERENCES

1. Hennekens CH, Buring JE. *Epidemiology in medicine*, Boston, 1987, Little, Brown, pp 73–100.
2. Teicher MH, Glod C, Cole JO. Emergence of intense suicidal preoccupation during fluoxetine treatment. *Am J Psychiatry* 147:207–210, 1990.
3. Doll R, Hill AB. Mortality in relation to smoking: ten years' observations of British doctors. *Br Med J* 1(5395):1399–1410, 1(5396):1460–1467, 1964.
4. Cooper JE, Kendell RE, Gurland BJ, et al. *Psychiatric diagnosis in New York and London*, London, 1972, Oxford University Press.
5. National Comorbidity Survey [homepage on the Internet]. c2005. Available from: <http://www.hcp.med.harvard.edu/ncs/index.php>; [cited June 26, 2013].
6. ESEMeE/MHEDEA 2000 Investigators. Prevalence of mental disorders in Europe: results from the European Study of the Epidemiology of Mental Disorders (ESEMeD) project. *Acta Psychiatr Scand* 109(Suppl 420):21–27, 2004.
7. Jablensky A. Epidemiology of schizophrenia: the global burden of disease and disability. *Eur Arch Psychiatry Clin Neurosci* 250:274–285, 2000.
8. Hasin DS, Stinson FS, Ogburn E, et al. Prevalence, correlates, disability, and comorbidity of DSM-IV alcohol abuse and dependence in the United States: results from the National Epidemiologic Survey on Alcohol and Related Conditions. *Arch Gen Psychiatry* 64:830–842, 2007.
9. Compton WM, Thomas YF, Stinson FS, et al. Prevalence, correlates, disability, and comorbidity of DSM-IV drug abuse and dependence in the United States: results from the National Epidemiologic Survey on Alcohol and Related Conditions. *Arch Gen Psychiatry* 64:566–576, 2007.
10. World Health Organization. *Global burden of disease: 2004 update*. Geneva, Switzerland, 2008, WHO Press.
11. Nurnberger JI, Wiegand R, Bucholz K, et al. A family study of alcohol dependence: coaggregation of multiple disorders in relatives of alcohol-dependent probands. *Arch Gen Psychiatry* 61(12): 1246–1256, 2004.
12. Kessler RC, Berglund P, Demler O, et al. Lifetime prevalence and age-of-onset distributions of DSM-IV disorders in the National Comorbidity Survey Replication. *Arch Gen Psychiatry* 62:593–602, 2005.
13. Kessler RC, Birnbaum H, Demler O, et al. The prevalence and correlates of non-affective psychosis in the National Comorbidity Survey Replication (NCS-R). *Biol Psychiatry* 58:668–676, 2005.
14. Kessler RC, Chiu WT, Demler O, et al. Prevalence, severity, and comorbidity of 12-month DSM-IV disorders in the National Comorbidity Survey Replication. *Arch Gen Psychiatry* 62:617–627, 2005.
15. Lenzenweger MF, Lane MC, Loranger AW, et al. DSM-IV personality disorders in the National Comorbidity Survey Replication. *Biol Psychiatry* 62:553–564, 2007.
16. Lichtenstein P, Björk C, Hultman CM, et al. Recurrence risks for schizophrenia in a Swedish National Cohort. *Psychol Med* 36: 1417–1425, 2006.
17. Tsuang MT, Tohen M, Jones PB, editors: *Textbook in psychiatric epidemiology*, ed 3, Chichester, West Sussex, 2011, Wiley-Blackwell.

62 Statistics in Psychiatric Research

Lee Baer, PhD

KEY POINTS

- Three classes of statistics are used commonly in psychiatric research: *psychometric* statistics assessing the reliability and validity of *diagnostic interviews or rating scales*; *descriptive* statistics used to describe *a group of subjects on* these clinical variables and demographic variables; and *inferential* statistics used to make probabilistic statements about *the effects of treatments or other variables on groups of subjects.*

- The more statistical tests that are performed in a study, the greater are the chances of finding one or more that will be significant, when, in fact, there is not a true effect in the population from which the sample was drawn (that is, a false-positive result).

- Researchers choose (depending on the level of measurement of their particular variables) the most appropriate statistical method to answer their particular research question. The simplest method available should be chosen to adequately answer a research question.

- Statistical power analysis determines how many subjects are needed to minimize false-negative results in inferential statistics.

THREE CLASSES OF STATISTICS IN PSYCHIATRIC RESEARCH

The word "statistics" derives from a term used for "numbers describing the *state*;" that is, the original statistics were numbers used by rulers of states to better understand their population. Thus, the first statistics were simply counts of things (such as the population of towns, or the amount of grain produced by a particular town). Today, we call these kinds of simple counts or averages "descriptive statistics," and these are used in almost every research study, to describe the demographic and clinical characteristics of the participants in a particular study.

Modern psychiatric research also involves two additional classes of statistics: psychometric statistics and inferential statistics. Most psychiatric studies will involve all three classes of statistics.

In psychiatric research, demographic variables (such as gender and height) can be measured objectively. However, most of our studies also require the measurement of variables that are not as objective (e.g., clinical diagnoses and rating scales of psychopathology). Here, we usually cannot measure directly the characteristics we are really interested in, so instead, we rely on a subject's score on either self-report or on investigator-administered scales. Psychometrics is concerned with how reproducible a subject's score is (i.e., how reliable it is), and how closely it measures the characteristic we are really interested in (i.e., how valid it is).

Psychiatric researchers study relatively small samples of subjects, usually with the intent to generalize their findings to the larger population from which their sample was drawn. This is the realm of inferential statistics, which is based on probability theory. Researchers are reporting inferential statistics when you see the tell-tale P-values and asterisks denoting statistical significance in the text and tables of the Results sections.

All three kinds of statistics (descriptive, psychometric, and inferential) are present in most published papers in psychiatric research, and are considered in a particular order, for the following reasons. First, without reliable and valid measures, neither of the other kinds of statistics will be meaningful. For example, if we rely solely on clinicians' judgments of patient improvement, but the study clinicians rarely agree on whether a particular patient has improved, any additional statistics will be meaningless. Likewise, a measure can be very reliably measured, as with a patient's cell phone number, but this measure is not reliable for any of the purposes of the study. Second, descriptive statistics are needed to summarize the many individual subjects' scores into summary statistics (such as counts, proportions, averages [or means], and standard deviations) that can then be compared between groups. Inferential statistics would be impossible without first having these summary statistics. Third, without inferential statistics and their computed probability values, the researcher cannot generalize any positive findings beyond the particular group being studied (and this is, after all, the usual goal of a research study).

Table 62-1 illustrates the characteristics of each class, as well as the order in which the classes must be considered, since each successive class rests on the foundation of the preceding class.

Concrete Examples of the Three Classes of Statistics in a Research Article

To provide a concrete example of these sometimes abstract concepts, consider a fictional study based on the simplest research design in psychiatric research: a randomized double-blind trial of a new drug versus a placebo pill for obsessive-compulsive disorder (OCD).

Figures 62-1 to 62-3 contain the annotated Method and Results sections for this fictional study, showing how the various psychometric statistics are presented in the Method section, while descriptive statistics are presented in the Method and Results sections, and inferential statistics are presented in the Results section (for definitions of terms used in these figures, refer to the section on statistical terms and their definitions).

Experiment-wise Error Rate

Researchers should test only a few carefully selected hypotheses (specified before collecting their data!) if their obtained P-values are to have any meaning. The more statistical tests you perform, the greater the chance of finding at least one significant by chance alone (i.e., a false-positive result). Table 62-2 illustrates this phenomenon.

One should not be impressed by a researcher who conducts eight t-tests, finds one significant at $P < 0.05$, and proceeds to interpret the findings as confirming his theory. Table 62-2 shows us that with eight statistical tests at $P < 0.05$, the researcher had a 33% chance of finding at least one result significant by chance alone.

TABLE 62-1 Three Classes of Statistics Used in Psychiatric Research (in Order of Applicability)

Class of Statistic	Purpose	Examples
Psychometric Statistics	Measures of reliability and validity of rating scales and other measures. Once measures are shown to have adequate reliability and validity, they can then be used as descriptive statistics.	Test-retest reliability coefficient Intra-class correlation coefficient Kappa coefficient Sensitivity Specificity
Descriptive Statistics	Statistics used to summarize the scores of many subjects in a single count or average to describe the group as a whole. After descriptive statistics have been computed for one or more samples, they can then be used to compute inferential statistics to attempt to generalize these results to the larger population from which these samples were drawn.	Mean Median Standard deviation Variance Estimates of effect size Proportions Percentages Mean differences Odds ratios
Inferential Statistics	Statistics computed to compute probability estimates used to generalize descriptive statistics to the larger population from which the samples were drawn.	t-statistic F-statistic χ^2-statistic Confidence intervals

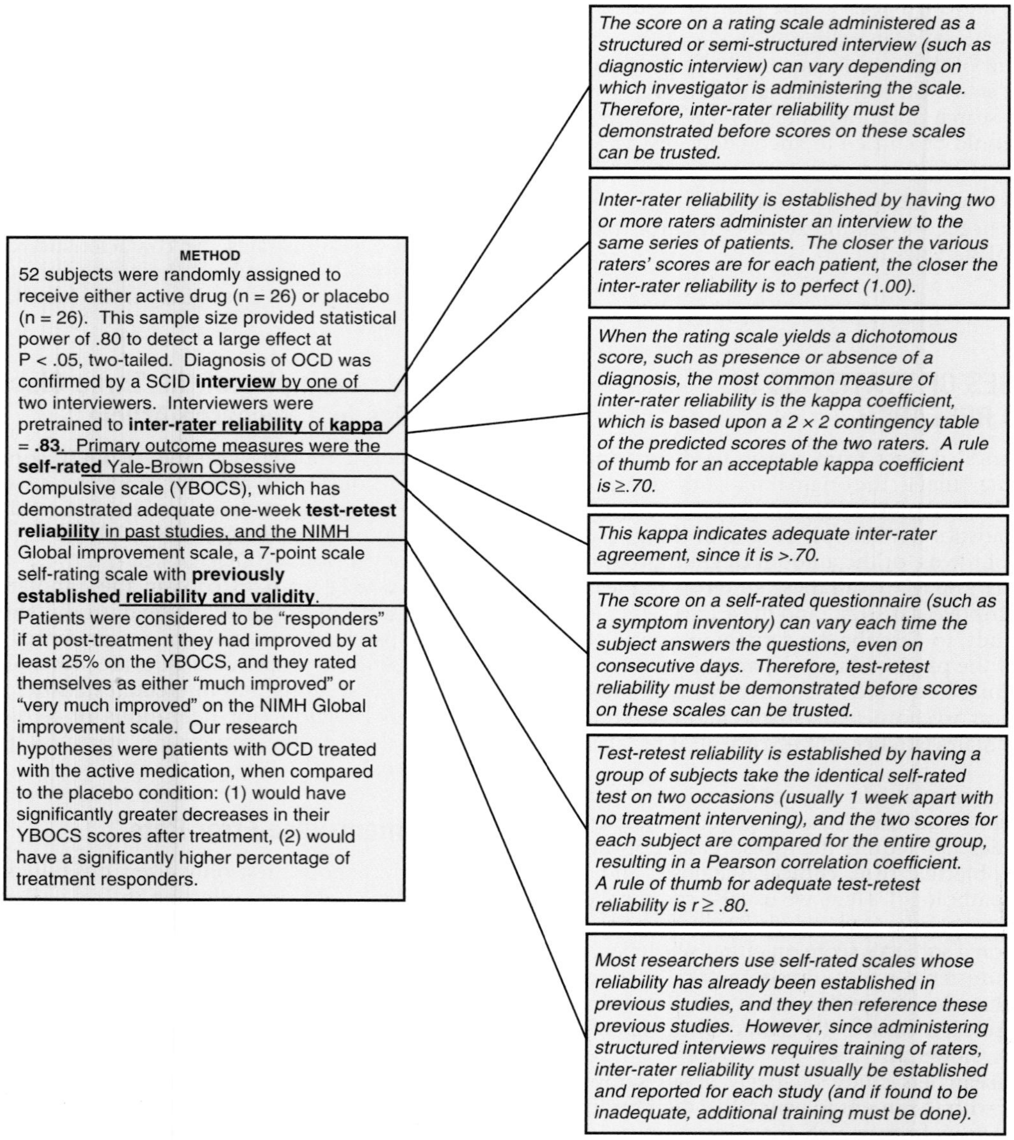

METHOD

52 subjects were randomly assigned to receive either active drug (n = 26) or placebo (n = 26). This sample size provided statistical power of .80 to detect a large effect at P < .05, two-tailed. Diagnosis of OCD was confirmed by a SCID **interview** by one of two interviewers. Interviewers were pretrained to **inter-rater reliability** of **kappa** = **.83**. Primary outcome measures were the **self-rated** Yale-Brown Obsessive Compulsive scale (YBOCS), which has demonstrated adequate one-week **test-retest reliability** in past studies, and the NIMH Global improvement scale, a 7-point scale self-rating scale with **previously established reliability and validity**.

Patients were considered to be "responders" if at post-treatment they had improved by at least 25% on the YBOCS, and they rated themselves as either "much improved" or "very much improved" on the NIMH Global improvement scale. Our research hypotheses were patients with OCD treated with the active medication, when compared to the placebo condition: (1) would have significantly greater decreases in their YBOCS scores after treatment, (2) would have a significantly higher percentage of treatment responders.

The score on a rating scale administered as a structured or semi-structured interview (such as diagnostic interview) can vary depending on which investigator is administering the scale. Therefore, inter-rater reliability must be demonstrated before scores on these scales can be trusted.

Inter-rater reliability is established by having two or more raters administer an interview to the same series of patients. The closer the various raters' scores are for each patient, the closer the inter-rater reliability is to perfect (1.00).

When the rating scale yields a dichotomous score, such as presence or absence of a diagnosis, the most common measure of inter-rater reliability is the kappa coefficient, which is based upon a 2 × 2 contingency table of the predicted scores of the two raters. A rule of thumb for an acceptable kappa coefficient is ≥.70.

This kappa indicates adequate inter-rater agreement, since it is >.70.

The score on a self-rated questionnaire (such as a symptom inventory) can vary each time the subject answers the questions, even on consecutive days. Therefore, test-retest reliability must be demonstrated before scores on these scales can be trusted.

Test-retest reliability is established by having a group of subjects take the identical self-rated test on two occasions (usually 1 week apart with no treatment intervening), and the two scores for each subject are compared for the entire group, resulting in a Pearson correlation coefficient. A rule of thumb for adequate test-retest reliability is r ≥ .80.

Most researchers use self-rated scales whose reliability has already been established in previous studies, and they then reference these previous studies. However, since administering structured interviews requires training of raters, inter-rater reliability must usually be established and reported for each study (and if found to be inadequate, additional training must be done).

Figure 62-1. Fictitious method section annotated to illustrate psychometric statistics.

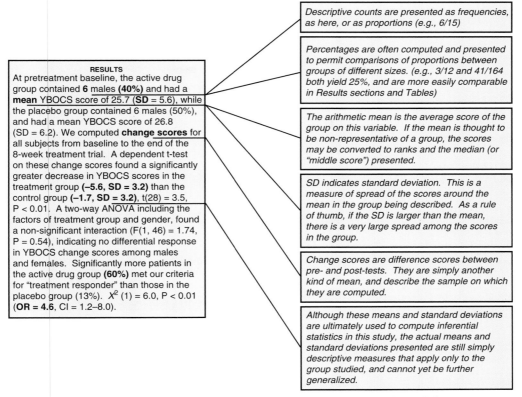

Figure 62-2. Fictitious results section annotated to illustrate descriptive statistics.

TABLE 62-2 Experiment-wise Error: Did the Researcher Find a Single Result Significant Solely by Chance?

Number of Statistical Tests Performed at P < 0.05	Probability of at Least One False-Positive Finding*
1	0.05
2	0.09
3	0.14
4	0.18
5	0.22
6	0.26
7	0.30
8	0.33
9	0.36
10	0.41
15	0.53
20	0.64
30	0.78
40	0.87
50	0.92

*Experiment-wise error rate.

Selecting an Appropriate Statistical Method

The two key determinants in choosing a statistical method are (1) your research goal, and (2) the level of measurement of your outcome (or dependent) variable(s). Table 62-3 illustrates the key characteristics of the various levels of measurement and provides examples of each.

Once the level of measurement of your outcome variable has been determined, you will decide whether your research question will require you to compare two or more different groups of subjects, or to compare variables within a single group of subjects. Tables 62-4 and 62-5 will help you choose

the appropriate statistical method once you have made these decisions. (Note that these tables consider only univariate statistical tests; multivariate tests are beyond the scope of this chapter.)

For example, if you want to conduct a study comparing a new drug to two control conditions, and your outcome measure is a continuous rating scale, Table 62-4 indicates that you would typically use the analysis of variance (ANOVA) to analyze your data. If you wanted to assess the association of two continuous measures of dissociation and anxiety in a single depressed sample, Table 62-5 indicates that you would usually select the Pearson correlation coefficient. (Note that the procedures listed for Ranked outcome measures are those typically referred to as "non-parametric tests.")

The final consideration in selecting a statistical procedure is whether subjects are measured on more than one occasion, as in the typical longitudinal clinical trial. In cases such as these, special statistical methods for "repeated measures" are used. Traditionally, a repeated measures analysis of variance has been the most-used method of analyzing a study comparing two or more treatment conditions in a longitudinal design. However, when, as is commonly the case, there are missing data due to subject dropout, the preferred analysis method is a sophisticated approach referred to as the Mixed-effect Model Repeated Measure (MMRM) model.

The Importance of Assessing Statistical Power

A non-significant P-value is meaningless if the researcher studied too few subjects, resulting in low statistical power. Tables 62-6 to 62-8 will help you estimate the number of subjects required to have a reasonable chance (usually set at 80%, or power = 0.80) of detecting a true effect (or put another way, a 20% change of a false-negative finding).

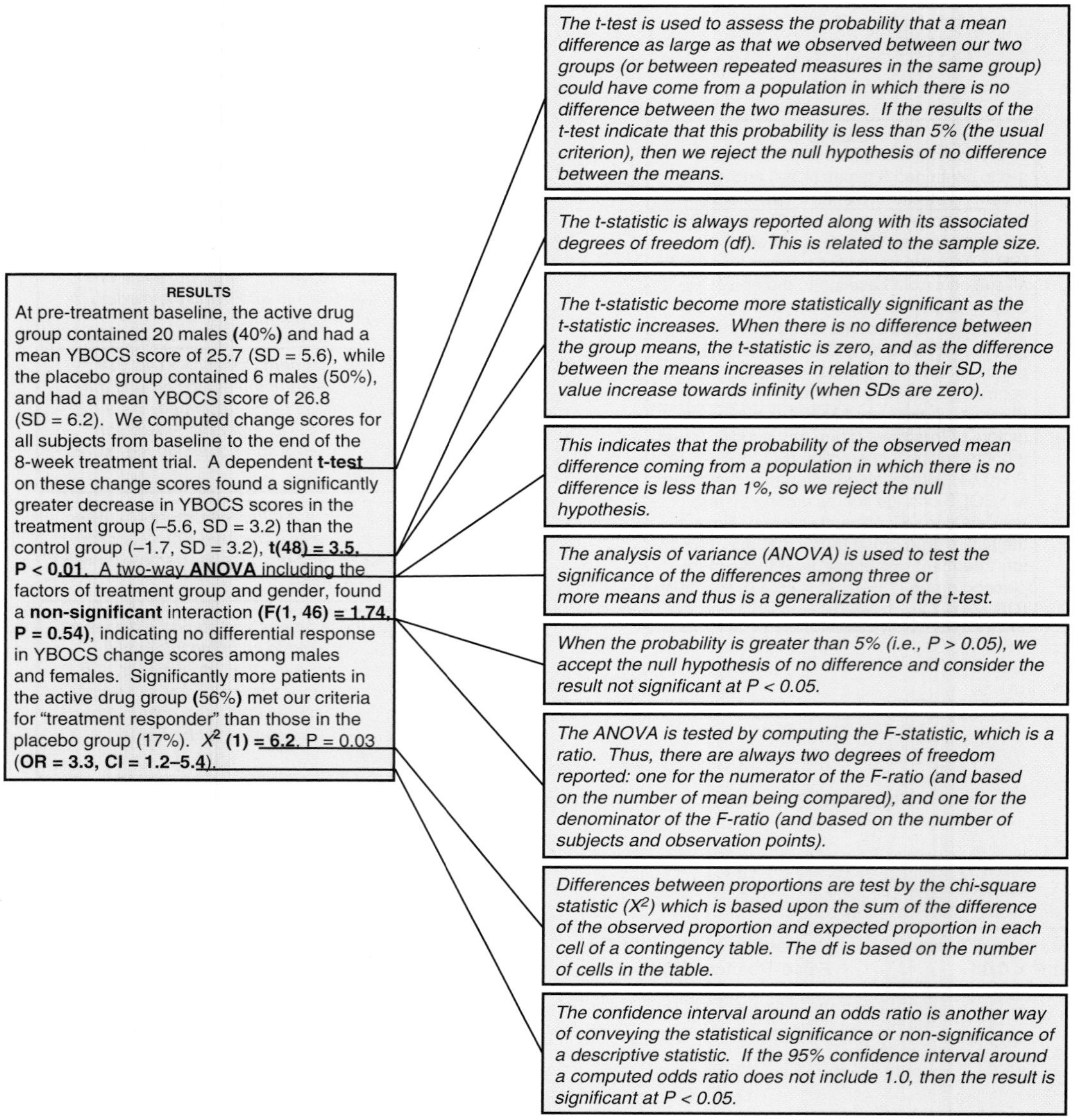

The t-test is used to assess the probability that a mean difference as large as that we observed between our two groups (or between repeated measures in the same group) could have come from a population in which there is no difference between the two measures. If the results of the t-test indicate that this probability is less than 5% (the usual criterion), then we reject the null hypothesis of no difference between the means.

The t-statistic is always reported along with its associated degrees of freedom (df). This is related to the sample size.

The t-statistic become more statistically significant as the t-statistic increases. When there is no difference between the group means, the t-statistic is zero, and as the difference between the means increases in relation to their SD, the value increase towards infinity (when SDs are zero).

This indicates that the probability of the observed mean difference coming from a population in which there is no difference is less than 1%, so we reject the null hypothesis.

The analysis of variance (ANOVA) is used to test the significance of the differences among three or more means and thus is a generalization of the t-test.

When the probability is greater than 5% (i.e., $P > 0.05$), we accept the null hypothesis of no difference and consider the result not significant at $P < 0.05$.

The ANOVA is tested by computing the F-statistic, which is a ratio. Thus, there are always two degrees of freedom reported: one for the numerator of the F-ratio (and based on the number of mean being compared), and one for the denominator of the F-ratio (and based on the number of subjects and observation points).

Differences between proportions are test by the chi-square statistic (X^2) which is based upon the sum of the difference of the observed proportion and expected proportion in each cell of a contingency table. The df is based on the number of cells in the table.

The confidence interval around an odds ratio is another way of conveying the statistical significance or non-significance of a descriptive statistic. If the 95% confidence interval around a computed odds ratio does not include 1.0, then the result is significant at $P < 0.05$.

RESULTS

At pre-treatment baseline, the active drug group contained 20 males (40%) and had a mean YBOCS score of 25.7 (SD = 5.6), while the placebo group contained 6 males (50%), and had a mean YBOCS score of 26.8 (SD = 6.2). We computed change scores for all subjects from baseline to the end of the 8-week treatment trial. A dependent **t-test** on these change scores found a significantly greater decrease in YBOCS scores in the treatment group (−5.6, SD = 3.2) than the control group (−1.7, SD = 3.2), **t(48) = 3.5, P < 0.01.** A two-way **ANOVA** including the factors of treatment group and gender, found a **non-significant** interaction (F(1, 46) = 1.74, P = 0.54), indicating no differential response in YBOCS change scores among males and females. Significantly more patients in the active drug group (56%) met our criteria for "treatment responder" than those in the placebo group (17%). X^2 (1) = 6.2, P = 0.03 (OR = 3.3, CI = 1.2–5.4).

Figure 62-3. Fictitious results section annotated to illustrate inferential statistics.

TABLE 62-3 Levels of Measurement of Variables

Level of Measurement	Description of Level	Examples
Continuous (also known as interval or ratio)	A scale on which there are approximately equal intervals between scores	Beck Depression Scale Diastolic blood pressure Age of subject
Ordinal (also known as ranks)	A scale in which scores are arranged in order, but intervals between scores may not be equal	Class ranking in school Any continuous measure that has been converted to ranks
Nominal (also known as categorical)	Scores are simply names for different groups, but the scores do not imply magnitude. Often used to define groups based on experimental treatment or diagnosis	Diagnostic category Ethnicity Zip code of residence
Dichotomous (also known as binary)	A special case of a nominal variable in which there are only two possible values	Gender (M or F) Survival (Y or N) Response (Y or N)

TABLE 62-4 Choosing an Appropriate Statistical Test to Compare Two or More Groups, Based on Your Research Goal, and the Level of Measurement of Your Outcome Measure

| Your Goal | Level of Measurement of Your Outcome Measure | | |
	Continuous	*Dichotomous*	*Ranked*
Compare two groups:	t-test of mean difference	2 × 2 contingency table of proportions tested by χ^2	Mann–Whitney U test of mean ranks
Compare three or more groups:	Analysis of variance (ANOVA)	Contingency table of proportions tested by χ^2	Kruskall–Wallis test of mean ranks
Compare two or more groups while controlling for one or more other variables measured in both groups:	Analysis of covariance (ANCOVA)	Mantel–Haenszel test (not applicable for more than two groups)	N/A
Compare two or more groups that are stratified on some other variable:	Factorial ANOVA	Mantel–Haenszel test (not applicable for more than two groups)	N/A
Compare two or more groups that are measured on repeated occasions:	Mixed (or split-plot) ANOVA or MMRM	MMRM	N/A

MMRM, mixed-effect model repeated measures design.

TABLE 62-5 Choosing an Appropriate Statistical Test for a Single Group of Subjects, Based on Your Research Goal, and the Level of Measurement of Your Outcome Measure

| Your Goal | Level of Measurement of Your Outcome Measure | | |
	Continuous	*Dichotomous*	*Ranked*
Test association of a continuous variable with:	Pearson correlation coefficient (r)	Point-biserial correlation coefficient	N/A
Test association of a dichotomous variable with:	Point-biserial correlation coefficient	Phi correlation coefficient	N/A
Test association of a ranked variable with:	N/A	N/A	Spearman rank correlation
Predict value of outcome measure from one or more continuous or dichotomous predictor variables:	Linear regression	Logistic regression	N/A
Compare two or more groups that are measured on repeated occasions:	Mixed (or split-plot) ANOVA	N/A	N/A
Compare change in an outcome variable measured on two occasions:	Dependent t-test	McNemar test	Wilcoxon test
Compare change in an outcome variable measured on three or more occasions:	One-way repeated ANOVA or MMRM	MMRM with dichotomous outcomes	Friedman test

TABLE 62-6 Statistical Power: Did the Study Have Enough Subjects to Detect a True Significant Mean Difference between Two Groups?

| Effect Size (Difference between Means) | Statistical Power | | | |
	0.50	*0.60*	*0.70*	*0.80**
0.20 SD ("small")	193	246	310	393
0.50 SD ("medium")	32	40	50	64
0.80 SD ("large")	13	16	20	26
1.20 SD	7	8	10	12

*Conventional level for acceptable statistical power.
t-Test for comparing means of two groups: N needed in each group for various levels of statistical power (two-tail test at P < 0.05).
SD, Standard deviation.
From Cohen J. Statistical power analysis for the behavioral sciences, ed 2, Hillsdale, NJ, 1988, Lawrence Erlbaum Associates, Table 2.4.1.

TABLE 62-7 Statistical Power: Did the Study Have Enough Subjects to Find a True Significant Difference in Proportions between Two Groups?

| Effect Size ("w" Statistic) | Statistical Power | | | | Examples of Values of "w" |
	0.50	*0.60*	*0.70*	*0.80**	
0.10 ("small")	384	490	617	785	45% vs. 55%
0.30 ("medium")	43	54	69	87	35% vs. 65%
0.50 ("large")	15	20	25	31	25% vs. 75%
0.70	8	10	13	16	15% vs. 85%

*Conventional level for acceptable statistical power.
2 × 2 chi-square test for comparing proportions of two groups: total N needed for various levels of statistical power (two-tail test at P < 0.05).
From Cohen J. Statistical power analysis for the behavioral sciences, ed 2, Hillsdale, NJ, 1988, Lawrence Erlbaum Associates, Table 7.4.6.

TABLE 62-8 Statistical Power: Did the Study Have Enough Subjects to Find a True Significant Correlation within a Group?

Effect Size (Pearson's r)	Statistical Power			
	0.50	0.60	0.70	0.80*
0.10 ("small")	385	490	616	783
0.30 ("medium")	42	53	67	85
0.50 ("large")	15	18	23	28
0.70	7	9	10	12

*Conventional level for acceptable statistical power.
Correlation coefficient between two variables: total N needed for various levels of statistical power (two-tail test at P < 0.05).
From Cohen J. Statistical power analysis for the behavioral sciences, ed 2, Hillsdale, NJ, 1988, Lawrence Erlbaum Associates, Table 3.4.1.

For example, a researcher reports that she has compared two groups of 12 depressed patients, and found that a new drug was not significantly better than placebo at P < 0.05, by t-test. However, this negative result is not informative, because Table 62-6 indicates that with only 12 subjects per group, this researcher had statistical power of less than 0.80 to detect even a "large" effect; that is, even if the drug were truly effective, this study had less than a 50/50 chance of finding a significant difference.

Power analysis is now required as part of virtually all grant and institutional review board (IRB) applications submitted today.

STATISTICAL TERMS AND THEIR DEFINITIONS
Analysis of Covariance

Analysis of covariance (ANCOVA) is a form of ANOVA that tests the significance of differences between group means by adjusting for initial differences among the groups on one or more covariates. As an example, a psychologist interested in studying the effectiveness of a behavioral weight loss program versus self-dieting includes pre-treatment weights as a covariate.

Analysis of Variance

This is an optimal test of significance of difference among means from three or more independent groups. As an example, if a medical researcher wants to compare the effects of three or more different drugs on a single dependent measure, he or she would compute a one-way ANOVA. The more complex, factorial ANOVA also tests for interaction effects between multiple factors. For example, if the two factors being tested were "drug/placebo" and "male/female," the ANOVA interaction test may find that the drug is more effective than the placebo in the female subjects only. The significance of the analysis of variance is tested by the F-statistic.

Analysis of Variance with Repeated Measure(s)

This is the optimal test of significance for comparing continuous variables that are obtained through repeated measurements of the same subjects (because each subject's scores are usually correlated, the regular ANOVA would give results that are "too significant"). An experimenter may select a repeated-measures design because these are generally more sensitive to treatment effects (i.e., they have high power), since score differences between subjects are ignored.

Bonferroni Correction

This is a conservative method of reducing the chances of false-positive findings by testing a set of statistical tests at a more conservative P-value. The standard Bonferroni correction divides the nominal P-value (say P < 0.05) by the total number of statistical tests being conducted. For example, with 10 t-tests

conducted, each would be tested at P < 0.005 (i.e., 0.05/10) to determine significance.

Canonical Correlation

This is a generalization of multiple regression to the case of multiple independent variables and multiple dependent variables. It is rarely used today, except in neuroimaging studies with hundreds or thousands of correlated measurements. It is considered a multivariate statistical procedure because many inter-correlated variables are analyzed simultaneously.

Chi-Square (χ^2) Test

See Contingency Table Analysis by Chi-Square.

Cluster Analysis

This is a data-reduction technique used to group subjects together into subgroups (or "clusters") based on their similarities or differences on a set of variables. This technique answers questions such as, "Do my subjects fall into subgroups?" and "What variables give a profile that distinguishes subgroups of my subjects?" A simple rule of thumb is "cluster analysis groups people, while factor analysis groups variables." It is considered a multivariate statistical procedure because many inter-correlated variables are analyzed simultaneously.

Confidence Interval

A confidence interval does more than simply report that our observed mean difference between two groups is 2.5 points, significant at P < 0.05; it is far more informative to report that the 95% confidence interval around our observed mean is 0.6 to 4.4. Since 0 (the null hypothesis value of the mean difference) is not included in the 95% confidence interval, we know at a glance that the difference is significant at P < 0.05, but we also learn of the possible values of the actual mean difference between the groups, ranging from as low as 0.6 point to a high of 4.4 points (with 95% confidence). In the case of odds ratios, a confidence interval of 0.60 to 4.40 would not be significant at P < 0.05, because the null hypothesis would state that the odds ratio is 1.00, and this is included in the computed 95% confidence interval. Many journals require the reporting of confidence intervals, instead of using only P-values.

Contingency Table Analysis by Chi-Square (χ^2)

This is a test to determine whether the frequencies in each cell of a contingency table are different from the proportions expected by chance. It is most commonly used on a 2 × 2 contingency table, represented as four cells forming a square.

A common use is to answer the following question: "Is there a difference between the occurrence of a given side effect in the drug group versus a placebo group?" In this case the table is arranged with drug versus placebo as the two rows, and side effect versus no side effect as the two columns. As the (squared) difference between the observed and expected frequencies in each cell increases, the chi-square statistic also increases, and the more significant the result becomes. If all cells contain exactly the frequencies that would be expected by chance, the chi-square statistic is zero. If the frequencies differ greatly from chance, the chi-square statistic gets larger and larger. The size of the chi-square statistic is based on the number of cells in the contingency table (since df = [# rows − 1] × [# columns − 1], a 2 × 2 table always has a single degree of freedom).

Correlation

See Pearson Correlation Coefficient.

Correlation Matrix

This is a "Table" or "Matrix" of correlation coefficients for all variables of interest.

Covariate

This is a variable that the investigator believes may influence the outcome or dependent variable and that is to be statistically adjusted for. For example, in a study of a new antidepressant, the baseline level of depression for subjects in each of the two groups may be used as a covariate.

Dependent t-Test

See t-Test for Dependent Means.

Dependent Variable

This is usually the outcome variable of interest in a study; it is also called an "end-point." In a study of a new antidepressant drug, a depression rating scale may be used as the dependent variable.

Descriptive Statistics

These are statistics used to describe a single population. Descriptive statistics used commonly to summarize the central tendency of a group are the *mean* (or arithmetic average) for continuous measures and the *median* (or "middle score") for ordinal or ranked measures. Descriptive statistics are used commonly to describe the variability within a group. These include the *variance* and its square root, the *standard deviation* for continuous measures, and the *interquartile range* for ranked measures. Researchers look at descriptive statistics first to get a "big picture" of their data (and also to look for data entry errors or obvious outliers).

Discriminant Function Analysis

This is the optimal procedure to distinguish statistically two or more groups based on a group of discriminating variables. It is an important and under-used procedure. It is considered a multivariate statistical procedure because many inter-correlated variables are analyzed simultaneously.

Effect Size

This is a measure of the practice significance of a treatment effect, as opposed to the statistical significance. For comparisons of two treatments, the most common effect size measure used is Cohen's "d" (the mean difference between the groups in standard deviation units), with values of 0.20, 0.50, and 0.80 defined by Cohen as small, medium, and large effects in the behavioral sciences. Effect sizes are essential to computing

statistical power (see Tables 62-6 to 62-8) and also form the basis of meta-analytic research.

End-point

See Dependent Variable.

Experiment-wise Error Rate

As more statistical tests are performed, you are more likely to find at least one of these tests significant by chance alone. Although you may perform each test at P < 0.05, your chance of finding one of many tests significant by chance alone is much higher than this nominal 5% level (see Table 62-2).

Factor Analysis

This is used to statistically reduce the number of variables needed to explain or to describe a larger set of original variables, based on the correlation matrix. For example, the 10 subscale scores of the Minnesota Multiphasic Personality Inventory (MMPI) personality test were derived from the 567 items that make up the questionnaire. As noted earlier, "factor analysis groups variables, while cluster analysis groups people." It is considered a multivariate statistical procedure because many inter-correlated variables are analyzed simultaneously. The most commonly used method of factor analysis today is "Principal Components Analysis" which is more empirical than the theory-driven traditional Factor Analytic Method. After factor analysis reduces the number of factors (or supervariables) needed to adequately summarize a large group of variables, the statistical method of factor rotation is conducted to make factors more interpretable.

Frequencies

See Descriptive Statistics.

Intent-to-Treat Analysis

Contrasted with a completer analysis, in which only data from subjects who complete a study are analyzed, which can introduce bias because subjects with more adverse events or lack of response are more likely to drop out and their data excluded from analysis. Traditional analytic methods of intent-to-treat analysis have used methods, such as end-point carried forward, in which a subject who drops out early has their final recorded score repeated for all subsequent assessment periods. However, recent simulation studies have found this method is prone to increased rates of false-negative and false-positive results under many conditions. As a result, the Mixed-effect Model Repeated Measure (MMRM) model is preferred.

Interaction Effect

In statistics an interaction effect occurs when the simultaneous effect of two variables on a third variable is not additive. For example, a research design for testing a new drug might include the two independent variables of Drug (Active vs. Placebo) and Subject Age (Younger vs. Older). If the active drug was found to be significantly more effective on average for younger subjects, this would be termed a significant interaction effect of Drug X Subject Age. Another way of phrasing this is that Subject Age *moderates* the effect of the Drug.

Level of Measurement

See Table 62-3.

Logistic Regression

This is an optimal procedure to predict a binary outcome variable from a set of continuous or binary predictor variables. Logistic regression yields both a probability value and an odds ratio. Often used in epidemiological studies where the outcome is occurrence/non-occurrence of a disease or survival/death. When more than one predictor variable is included, it is considered a multivariate statistical procedure because many inter-correlated variables are analyzed simultaneously.

MANCOVA

See Multivariate Analysis of Covariance.

Mann–Whitney U Test

This is the optimal non-parametric test of significance for difference between the sums of ranks from two independent groups or treatment levels.

MANOVA

See Multivariate Analysis of Variance.

Mean

See Descriptive Statistics.

Median

See Descriptive Statistics.

Mediation

In statistics, a mediation model is one in which a third explanatory variable underlies the observed relationship between an independent variable and a dependent variable. Mediation is usually tested via a set of regression models. For example, a researcher may find that a new cognitive psychotherapy reduces depression in a group of patients, and may hypothesize that this significant relationship is *mediated* by reductions in the average score on the patients' cognitive errors after treatment. An excellent discussion of mediation can be found at: http://davidakenny.net/cm/mediate.htm.

Mixed-effect Model Repeated Measure Model

This is the preferred statistical method for analyzing longitudinal clinical trials by analyzing the individual change slopes of individual subjects, including those who drop out of a study. This is preferred to commonly used intent-to-treat analysis using methods, such as end-point carried-forward because MMRM has been found through simulation studies to be less prone to both false-negative and false-positive results.

Moderation

See definition for Interaction Effect. An excellent discussion of moderation can be found at: http://davidakenny.net/cm/moderation.htm

Multiple Linear Regression

This is used to predict a single continuous outcome variable from a set of continuous or dichotomous predictor variables. It is very flexible because it allows many forms of non-linear curve-fitting, and automatically provides a measure of effect size as R^2 (this can help assess practical significance, in addition to statistical significance). When more than one predictor variable is included, it is considered a multivariate statistical procedure because many inter-correlated variables are analyzed simultaneously.

Multivariate Analysis of Variance

Multivariate analysis of variance (MANOVA) is a generalization of ANOVA when multiple dependent variables are to be assessed simultaneously. It is not used often in psychiatric research because of the difficulty that lies with its interpretation. Instead, separate ANOVAs are often computed for each dependent variable. When more than one predictor variable is included, it is considered a multivariate statistical procedure because many inter-correlated variables are analyzed simultaneously.

Multivariate Statistical Analysis

This is a statistical procedure in which multiple correlated variables are analyzed simultaneously to account for their inter-correlation. It is contrasted with univariate analyses. Examples are discriminant function analysis, factor analysis, and MANOVA. An introduction to the use of multivariate statistics in neuroimaging data is available at: http://www.jove.com/video/1988/basics-of-multivariate-analysis-in-neuroimaging-data.

Null Hypothesis

Researchers usually begin with the hypothesis that there is a zero (or "null") difference between two means, or that there is a correlation coefficient of zero (or "null") between two measures. Since statistics cannot prove a hypothesis, we usually state the null hypothesis and present data showing that it is unlikely to be true; the P-value indicates just how unlikely. Caveat: In any very large sample, the null hypothesis is likely to be rejected. That is, two groups of individuals rarely have exactly the same mean on any two characteristics; even if they only differ by, say, 0.01 mm, the null hypothesis is not true, and a sample size in the thousands could detect even a tiny difference.

Outcome Variable

See Dependent Variable. Also known as "response variable."

P-Value

This reflects the chance of a result of a statistical test being a false positive (i.e., the probability of a spurious finding). If a finding is almost certainly a spurious finding, which would not be reproducible in another sample, the P-value will be near 1.00. On the other band, if the finding almost certainly represents a "true" finding, the P-value will be near zero (small P-values are represented by several zeros after the decimal point, e.g., $P < 0.0001$—but never list a P-value as 0.00, because this is impossible, and it annoys reviewers!).

Most journals require $P < 0.05$ for significance. If many statistical tests are performed in a study, a more conservative P-value can be used to minimize experiment-wise error (see Table 62-2). Caveat: Do not be overly impressed by very low P-values. Remember that all this tells you is the chance that the difference is probably not zero. Also, remember that, given enough subjects, this is easy to prove. Thus, a very low P-value does not necessarily indicate a large clinical effect, but instead represents that it is a very reliable effect. Check the effect size (the correlation coefficient squared, or the size of the t-statistic) to get an idea of the magnitude of the difference or relation.

Most P-values cited in published research are two-tailed, or non-directional. However, when the researcher has a strong *a priori* directional hypothesis (e.g., "Drug will be more effective for reducing depression than Placebo") rather than a non-directional hypothesis (e.g., "Drug and Placebo groups will be significantly different at end-point"), a one-tailed P-value may be preferable by reducing the chances of false-negative results by increasing statistical power.

When false-negative results are more dangerous than false-positive results (as in testing for dangerous adverse events) it makes sense to test at a more liberal P-value, say $P < 0.10$, so as to minimize the risk of false-negative results due to small sample size.

Pearson Correlation Coefficient

This is the optimal measure of the association between two continuous measures. When there is no association, $r = 0$; when there is a perfect positive correlation, $r = 1.00$; and when there is a perfect negative correlation, $r = -1.00$. You can easily obtain an effect size measure by squaring r (which gives the percent of variance shared by the two variables); thus, even a correlation of $r = 0.05$ can be highly significant with thousands of Ss, however, r^2 tells us that two variables share only a trivial percent of their variance (here, <3/10 of 1%!). When researchers discuss correlation, they are almost always referring to the Pearson correlation coefficient.

Phi Correlation Coefficient

This is a special case of the Pearson correlation coefficient when two dichotomous variables are being compared. Note, however, that because the variables are not normally distributed, the maximum possible value of phi is often less than 1.00 or -1.00.

Planned Comparisons

Planned comparisons or contrasts are special kinds of t-tests for a specific subset of hypotheses involving mean comparisons that are formulated before collecting data for a study. Planned contrasts are typically performed instead of a full ANOVA.

Point-Biserial Correlation

This is a special case of the Pearson correlation coefficient when one variable is continuous and the other is dichotomous. As with the phi coefficient, the maximum value of r_{pb} often cannot achieve its limits of 1.00 or -1.00.

Power

This reflects the probability of finding a true difference or relation between two or more measures with a given sample size. It is analogous to the sensitivity of a medical test. An analogy: The power of a telescope (i.e., the magnification) is analogous to the power of a study; both indicate the ability to detect even tiny objects or changes. If a study had little chance of finding a true difference between two drugs (say, with only two subjects per group), the power of the study would be nearly zero. If the study had almost no chance of missing a true difference (say, comparing the mean height of 10,000 2-year-olds with 10,000 18-year-olds), the power of the study would be nearly 1.00. Power of 0.80 is usually the minimum required by statisticians when designing a study. Caveat: Just as any tiny difference can be found to be significant just by having enough subjects, it is possible to find all but huge differences to be

non-significant, simply by having few enough subjects! Be especially wary of false negatives in studies with few subjects (e.g., <25 per group). Several literature reviews have found that the average behavioral science study has a power of only about 40% to detect a medium-sized effect! Consult Tables 62-6 to 62-8 to estimate the statistical power of a study. For detailed power analyses download the excellent shareware program G*POWER at: www.gpower.hhu.de/en.html

r

See Pearson Correlation Coefficient.

Random Assignment

The most effective method for assigning subjects to treatment groups or conditions is randomization. Randomization ensures that there will be no systematic bias in the make-up of the groups, so that each subject has an equal opportunity to be assigned to any one of the groups. Caveat: Strictly speaking, P-values obtained when comparing two groups are only valid if subjects have been randomly assigned to the two groups!

Rank-Order Correlation

This is a special case of the Pearson correlation coefficient when assessing the association between two variables with ranked data. With only a few tied ranks, use Kendall's "tau;" with many tied ranks, use Spearman's "rho."

Regression

See Multiple Linear Regression.

Reliability

This is the dependability of a score, or the degree to which we can be certain that a measurement can be depended on (i.e., How reproducible is the score?). For self-rated scales, such as paper-and-pencil questionnaires, since there is no rater error to take into account, the main source of unreliability to assess is difference in the person's self-rating over time. For example, if a patient completes a depression questionnaire at 3 P.M., how close would his or her score be on the same questionnaire if he or she were to take the same scale at 4 P.M., assuming no change in his or her depression? If the scores were identical, and this was the case for all patients, the correlation coefficient would be a perfect 1.00 (in this case the correlation coefficient is referred to as the "reliability coefficient").

For scales or measures administered by a rater, the major question is, "Would this patient get the same score on this depression scale if Doctor A rated him, as if Doctor B rated him?" If the agreement was perfect for all patients, the reliability coefficient would be 1.00. If, on the other hand, there were a random relationship between the scores of the two raters, the inter-rater reliability would be 0.00. Reliability is necessary but not sufficient for a useful scale. Thus, a scale can be perfectly reliable, but have no validity for a particular purpose. For example, every time you ask me my phone number I will give you the same answer (perfect reliability); however, if you attempt to use my phone number to predict my anxiety level you will find a zero correlation (no validity). If a measure has no reliability (i.e., it is not reproducible), it has zero reliability. If it has perfect reliability, or repeatability, it has a reliability of 1.00.

For a continuous measure, this is assessed by the correlation coefficient, and as a rule of thumb it is generally $r = 0.80$ for adequate reliability. For a binary measure (e.g., the presence or absence of a disease), this is often assessed by the kappa coefficient, and a rule of thumb is generally $\kappa = 0.70$.

Rho

See Rank-Order Correlation.

Standard Deviation

See Descriptive Statistics.

Statistical Analysis Software

These are commercial or shareware programs used for data entry, manipulation, and statistical computations. The most commonly used commercial programs are SPSS, SAS, and Stata. The most commonly used shareware program is R (downloadable at: www.r-project.org).

Statistical Power

See Power.

Tau

See Rank-Order Correlation.

t-Test

This is the optimal test to determine whether the difference between the means of two samples of subjects is likely to be due to chance alone. If the difference between two means is zero, the t-statistic will also be zero. If all scores in both groups are the same, they both have standard deviations of zero. In this case, the t-statistic will be infinitely large.

t-Test for Dependent Means

This is the optimal test of significance for difference between means from two matched, or dependent, groups or treatment levels. As an example, a group of 30 anxious patients participated in a study of a new drug for alleviating anxiety. Anxiety levels were measured by the Hamilton Anxiety Scale at baseline and again after 3 weeks of treatment. In this test each subject's pair of scores is directly compared, and the variation between the pairs of subjects is ignored. The same test is used to compare the means of two matched pairs of subjects (whose scores are thought to be correlated).

Univariate Statistical Analysis

This analysis is used when there is only a single dependent variable to be considered in each analysis. Examples are t-test and ANOVA.

Validity

This is the degree of usefulness of a rating scale for a particular purpose. It is also the degree to which the test measures what it is supposed to be measuring. The determination of validity usually requires independent, external criteria of whatever the test is designed to measure. For example, if an investigator develops a single question that he or she purports to be a good screening instrument for clinical depression, patients' responses to this question should relate well to "gold standard" measures of clinical depression, such as structured interviews and well-established rating scales for depression. There is no real rule of thumb for validity, since there is no one measure. As a bare minimum, however, the scale should at least be significantly correlated with gold-standard measures for that characteristic.

Variance

See Descriptive Statistics.

CURRENT CONTROVERSIES AND FUTURE DIRECTIONS

- There is a movement by journals away from reporting simply P-values and toward reporting the more informative confidence interval.
- Researchers are encouraged to report effect-size statistics in addition to P-values.
- Multivariate statistical methods (such as discriminant analysis, principal components analysis, cluster analysis, and canonical correlation) are used more commonly in medical research because of the very large number of correlated variables produced by neuroimaging, genomics, and metabolomics research.
- The experiment-wise (false-positive) error rate is even more worrisome in areas of research (such as neuroimaging, genomics and metabolomics) where so many potential statistical tests are possible in a given dataset.
- MMRM analyses are preferred to end-point carried-forward approaches in analyzing longitudinal clinical trials with missing data.

Access a list of MCQs for this chapter at https://expertconsult .inkling.com

SUGGESTED READING

Altman DG. Why we need confidence intervals. *World J Surg* 29(5):554–556, 2005.

Cohen J. *Statistical power analysis for the behavioral sciences*, ed 2, Hillsdale, NJ, 1988, Lawrence Erlbaum Associates.

Cohen J, Cohen P, West SG, et al. *Applied multiple regression/correlation analysis for the behavioral sciences*, ed 3, Oxford, 2002, Routledge.

Ellis PD. *The essential guide to effect sizes: Statistical power, meta-analysis, and the interpretation of research results*, Cambridge, 2010, Cambridge University Press.

Gonick L, Smith W. *The cartoon guide to statistics*, New York, 1993, HarperCollins.

Gorsuch R. *Factor analysis*, Hillsdale, NJ, 1983, Lawrence Erlbaum Associates.

Huff D, Geis I. *How to lie with statistics*, New York, 1954, WW Norton.

Keith TZ. *Multiple regression and beyond*, Boston, 2006, Pearson Educational.

Reich D, Price AL, Patterson N. Principal component analysis of genetic data. *Nat Genet* 40(5):491–492, 2008.

Rosenthal R, Rosnow RL. *Essentials of behavioral research: methods and data analysis*, ed 3, New York, 2007, McGraw-Hill.

Siddiqui O, Hung HM, O'Neill R. MMRM vs. LOCF: A comprehensive comparison based on simulation study and 25 NDA datasets. *J Biopharm Stat* 19(2):227–246, 2009.

Tabachnick BG, Fidell LS. *Using multivariate statistics*, ed 6, 2012, Pearson.

63   Genetics and Psychiatry

Daniel H. Ebert, MD, PhD, Christine T. Finn, MD, and Jordan W. Smoller, MD, ScD

KEY POINTS

Background

- Most psychiatric disorders have a genetic component. The etiology of psychiatric disorders reflects a combination of genetic vulnerability and environmental factors

- Many psychiatric disorders can be familial and heritable due to the inheritance of genetic variations. Alternatively, psychiatric disorders can arise from *de novo* genetic mutations, mutations that are found in the offspring but not the parents or recent ancestry.

- Psychiatric disorders are highly polygenic, involving hundreds or thousands of genetic variations. Some rare variations have a large effect on disease risk, while more common risk variants have modest individual effects

History

- Genetic research will have an impact on clinical psychiatry by providing insight into the molecular basis of psychiatric disorders and identifying new targets for drug development.

Clinical and Research Challenges

- Advances in genomic science and DNA sequencing technology are starting to facilitate the identification of susceptibility genes and genetic loci that underlie psychiatric disorders. While impressive scientific progress has been made recently, our understanding of the genetic basis of a large percentage of psychiatric disorders remains limited.

- Pharmacogenetic research has begun to identify genetic variants that influence response to psychotropic medication.

Practical Pointers

- Several medical genetic syndromes have prominent psychiatric manifestations that can be relevant for differential diagnosis.

- Psychiatric genetics is providing information important for psychoeducation and genetic counseling.

OVERVIEW
Basic Organization of the Human Genome

The human genome comprises the full sequence of deoxyribonucleic acid (DNA) found in the nucleus of each nucleated human cell (mature erythrocytes and platelets lack nuclei and thus do not contain a copy of the genome). The DNA sequence is distributed over 23 pairs of chromosomes, long strands of DNA that include the 22 autosomes and two sex chromosomes. One of each pair of the autosomes and the sex chromosomes is inherited from each parent. The autosomes are numbered 1 through 22 in order of size, and most consist of two arms divided by a region called the centromere (Figure 63-1). The longer arm of a chromosome is denoted by the letter "q" and the short arm by the letter "p." Thus, the long arm of chromosome 1 is referred to as 1q. Subdivisions of chromosomes, originally identified on the basis of chromosome staining, are referred to by numbers (e.g., 1q31.2). With the sequencing of the human genome, however, references to locations on chromosomes can now be made more precisely based on their base-pair positions (e.g., a single nucleotide polymorphism at base pair 27644225 on chromosome 11).

DNA encodes the instructions for making all of the proteins in the human body. Double-stranded DNA itself is composed of a linear sequence of the nucleotides adenine (A),

cytosine (C), guanine (G), and thymine (T) (see Figure 63-1). The full genome sequence, comprising approximately 3 billion bases, was deciphered in 2001.[1,2] Genes convey the instruction for protein sequence through messenger ribonucleic acid (mRNA), which is transcribed from the gene sequence and, ultimately, translated into the amino acid sequence of a given protein (Figure 63-2). The human genome contains approximately 20,700 protein-coding genes. Protein-coding genes include protein-coding sequences (exons), intervening sequences (introns), and untranscribed regions (e.g., regulatory promoter sequences). These genes are often alternatively spliced, a process during which different combinations of exons of a gene are spliced together, resulting in different mRNAs that can potentially encode multiple protein variants from one gene. Each gene has, on average, approximately six alternatively spliced transcripts. Exons of protein-coding genes cover 2.9% of the genome. The protein-coding genes, from their start to their stop codon, including exons and introns, cover 33% of the genome.[3] Genomic sequence outside of protein-coding exons contains regulatory units that control gene expression in the different cell types in the body. The large ENCODE project recently calculated that 80% of the genome has a biochemical function, including functioning as enhancers or encoding RNA species that can regulate gene expression.[3] A significant subset of genetic mutations and variants associated with psychiatric disorders are located outside the protein-coding exons. These mutations outside of protein-coding exons may disrupt the biochemical function of that genomic locus, including the proper regulation of gene expression.

Genetic Variation and Polymorphism

Although the majority of the genomic sequence is shared identically by all humans, important variations (polymorphisms) exist across populations and individuals. Some of this variation has no effect on observable traits, while other variations influence phenotypic differences among people. A variant form of DNA sequence at a particular locus (genomic position) is referred to as an allele. Because all nucleated human cells (with the exception of the gametes) are diploid, carrying two copies of each autosome, a given allele can occur on one or both copies of a genetic locus. Variants are often described in terms of the major (more common) allele and the minor (less common) allele. Polymorphisms in which the minor allele frequency is 1% or less are referred to as mutations. Several common forms of genetic variation relevant to neuropsychiatric phenotypes are discussed below.

Microsatellites and variable number tandem repeats (VNTRs) are common forms of genetic variation involving short repeated sequences (Figure 63-3). Microsatellites typically comprise repeats of two to four nucleotides (e.g., CA repeats). These repeat sequences are typically found outside of the amino acid coding sequences, but their high degree of polymorphism has made them useful as genetic markers in genetic linkage studies. In some cases, short repeats do have functional effects.

Variable numbers of repeated three base-pair sequences, known as triplet repeats, have been shown to play a role in several neurological illnesses. For example, CAG repeats (which encode the amino acid glutamine) within the Huntingtin gene on chromosome 4 cause Huntington disease when more than 40 repeats are present (Figure 63-4). Alleles containing fewer than 35 repeats do not produce disease, but as repeat length increases, instability in replication can lead to expansion of the repeat sequence. This accounts for the phenomenon of anticipation in which the mutation "worsens" over successive generations, resulting in earlier-onset and more severe disease phenotypes. Other diseases associated with triplet repeat expansion include fragile X, spinocerebellar ataxias, and myotonic dystrophy.

Single nucleotide polymorphisms (SNPs), in which one of the four nucleotide bases is substituted for another, are the most common form of genetic variation, occurring approximately once per 1,000 base pairs (bp) of DNA sequence. Because they are so common (more than 10 million in the genome) and may have functional significance, SNPs have become the focus of genetic association analysis, the most widespread approach to identifying susceptibility genes for complex disorders (see below). SNPs may affect phenotypic variation through several mechanisms. One straightforward mechanism results when an SNP in the exon of a gene alters or disrupts the instructions for the normal amino acid sequence of the gene product. Such "non-synonymous" coding sequence SNPs can result in an abnormal or truncated protein product with aberrant or no function.[4] In addition, SNPs occurring in the regulatory regions of genes (e.g., the promoter) can induce phenotypic effects through alterations in gene expression.

Recently, the widespread occurrence of copy number variation in the genome has been reported.[4] These variations include deletions, insertions, and duplications of DNA sequence, ranging from kilobases (thousands of bases) to megabases (millions) in length, that may alter gene function or the amount of gene expression. The extent and frequency of copy number variants and their relationship to complex disease is an area of active research. Examples of copy number variation relevant to psychiatry include the 22q11 microdeletion that causes velocardiofacial/DiGeorge syndrome and is associated with psychotic illness[5] and the duplication of 15q11-13 with autism. There is a higher rate of *de novo* copy number variants (present in the offspring but not the parents) in autism and schizophrenia as compared to controls.[4]

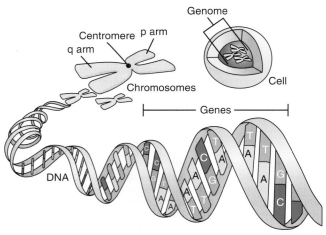

Figure 63-1. The organization of human DNA shown with increasing magnification.

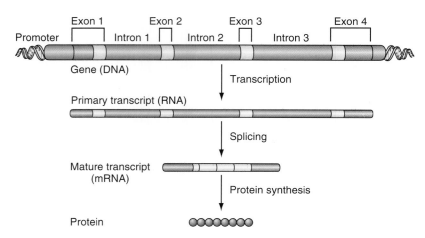

Figure 63-2. Structure of a gene and flow of information from DNA to protein. *(Re-drawn from Twyman R: Gene structure. ©Wellcome Trust, London, UK, 2003.)*

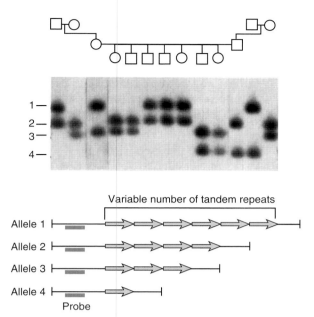

Variable number of tandem repeats

Allele 1

Allele 2

Allele 3

Allele 4

Probe

Figure 63-3. Co-dominant inheritance of an autosomal DNA polymorphism caused by a variable number of tandem repeats. Alleles 1 to 4 are related to one another by a variable number of identical (or nearly identical) short DNA sequences *(arrows)*. Size variation can be detected after restriction enzyme digestion and hybridization with a unique probe that lies outside the VNTR sequences themselves but inside the restriction sites used to define the allelic fragments. *(Courtesy of A. Bowcock, Washington University, St. Louis, Missouri.)*

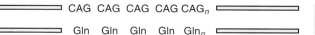

CAG CAG CAG CAG CAG$_n$

Gln Gln Gln Gln Gln$_n$

Figure 63-4. Trinucleotide repeats in exon 1 of HD gene at 4p16.3 and Huntington disease. CAG triplet repeats lead to expanding polyglutatmine tract and gene dysfunction. Clinical findings of Huntington disease are related to length of repeat expansion, with $n > 40$ associated with disease.

Linkage Disequilibrium and Haplotypes

The phenomenon of linkage disequilibrium (LD) is an important characteristic of the human genome. LD refers to the correlation or association of alleles at linked polymorphic markers. A key feature of the structure of the human genome is that it is organized into regions of high LD separated by regions of low LD. Markers that exhibit high levels of LD and that reside on the same chromosome (i.e., markers whose alleles are strongly correlated) are referred to as haplotypes. Put another way, a haplotype refers to a set of strongly associated alleles at markers along a chromosomal region that tend to be inherited together.[6] LD arises when a new variant occurs on a chromosome (e.g., through mutation). The chromosome on which the variant arises is surrounded by other alleles and so it is inherited along with those alleles in the subsequent generation. Over successive generations, recombination of chromosomes and other mutations at neighboring sites dilute the degree of correlation between the new variant allele and surrounding alleles, degrading the extent of LD between them. However, human populations are relatively young so that stretches of LD have persisted. In regions of high LD, there is limited haplotype diversity—that is, only a few haplotypes exist in the population in these regions. A major advance in cataloguing genetic variation and LD across the human genome was accomplished by the International HapMap Project.[7] A crucial dividend of the HapMap was to facilitate genome-wide association studies (described below).

Gene Expression

Gene expression refers to the process and products of gene transcription into RNA and, if applicable, translation into protein (see Figure 63-2). The regulation of gene expression involves both genetic and epigenetic factors. Genetic influences on expression include DNA sequences in regions around genes known as promoters and enhancers. These regulatory regions function in part by serving as binding sites for transcription factors that help determine where (in what tissues) or when (during which developmental periods) genes are activated or silenced. Sequence variations in regulatory regions provide another mechanism (beyond variations in protein-coding regions of genes) by which DNA sequence differences contribute to phenotypic differences among individuals and populations.[8]

Another important mechanism for modulation of gene expression involves epigenetic regulation. Epigenetics refers to the study of heritable gene expression changes that are not due to variation in DNA sequence.[9] Chromatin, the complex of DNA, histones, and associated non-histone proteins, is the primary substrate of epigenetic modulation. Histones are highly basic proteins found in the nucleus of the cell; chromatin consists primarily of DNA molecules wrapped around octomeric complexes of histones.[10] The configuration of chromatin can vary from states in which it is inactivated and condensed (also known as heterochromatin) or activated and open (also known as euchromatin).[10] Genes in regions of condensed chromatin are inaccessible to transcription factors and thus functionally repressed, while those in regions of open chromatin are available to transcriptional activation. Shifts in chromatin structure (chromatin re-modeling) may thus lead to important variations in gene expression with downstream effects on a variety of phenotypes. The chemical and molecular bases of chromatin re-modeling and epigenetic modification of gene expression include histone acetylation (which generally increases transcriptional activity), histone methylation (which can increase or decrease transcriptional activity), and DNA methylation (which generally reduces transcriptional activity). A variety of factors appear to influence epigenetic modification of chromatin and DNA, including aging, stress, diet, and various drugs and medications.[9-12] Indeed, modification of the epigenome may be a central mechanism by which environmental influences are transduced into molecular effects on gene expression and action.

A number of neuropsychiatric disorders and phenotypes have been linked to epigenetic variations, including Rett syndrome (an autism spectrum disorder caused by mutations in the transcriptional repressor *MECP2* that encodes a methylated-DNA-binding protein), depression, schizophrenia, and addiction.[10]

Finally, gene expression can also be regulated by RNA interference (RNAi) due to non-coding RNAs, including short-interfering RNA (siRNA), microRNA (miRNA), and small hairpin RNA (shRNA). These RNAs can modulate gene expression by several mechanisms, including degrading mRNAs of target genes or interfering with translation of mRNA into proteins.[13] The role of these factors in human disease is an area of active investigation.

The Complex Genetic Architecture of Psychiatric Disorders

The underlying genetic basis of psychiatric disorders is diverse and complex. Neuropsychiatric disorders may arise from mutation in one gene, variations in multiple genes that together lead to the disorder, or mutations in non-protein-coding regions of the genome.[14] A subset of psychiatric disorders has mutations in a single gene that is highly penetrant (i.e., the risk of illness in those carrying the genetic liability is high). Mutations in a single gene that causes disease with high penetrance may have classical Mendelian patterns of inheritance, including dominant, recessive, or X-linked. Dominant inheritance occurs when variations in a single copy of the relevant gene are sufficient to cause disease. In recessive inheritance, mutations in both copies of a gene, on each allele, are needed to lead to disease. In X-linked inheritance, a gene on the X-chromosome is mutated. Male offspring inherit one copy of the X-chromosome, whereas female offspring inherit two copies of the X-chromosome, one of which is inactivated in cells.

Psychiatric disorders can arise from copy number variants (CNVs). CNVs include deletions, insertions, duplications, and inversions of regions of the genome. Some of these CNVs are rare mutations in the population. There is an increased number of rare CNVs in individuals with autism and schizophrenia as compared to controls.[4]

Another subset of psychiatric disorders arise from *de novo* mutations. A *de novo* mutation is found in the individual or recent ancestry. For example, a *de novo* mutation can be found in the offspring but not in the parents. The mutation may have occurred in the sperm of the father. Increasing age of the father is a risk for autism, which may be due to increased number of mutations in the sperm of older fathers, leading to *de novo* mutations in the offspring that cause autism. Some CNVs are *de novo* alterations in the genome.[4] In schizophrenia, there is an excess rate of *de novo* CNVs.[15,16]

While some psychiatric disorders are caused by rare mutations, including rare CNVs, another subset of psychiatric disorders seem to be caused by the combination of alterations in many genes.[14] In this scenario, each gene variation contributes a small effect that, on its own, would not lead to the disorder. Only the combination of these variations in multiple genes leads to the expression of the psychiatric disorder. This hypothesis of the genetic basis of a subset of psychiatric disorders has been called the common variant, common disease model. Genome-wide association studies (GWAS), described below, can help identify these common genetic variations that can contribute to the development of a psychiatric disorder in combination with multiple other genetic variations. These multiple common variants associated with psychiatric disorders may function in convergent molecular pathways. For instance, multiple genes associated with autism spectrum disorders encode proteins that regulate synapses, the connections between neurons.[17]

At times, the underlying genetic basis crosses diagnostic boundaries defined from clinical experience. In a phenomenon named pleiotropy, a particular gene, or genetic loci, may increase the risk for developing multiple different psychiatric disorders.[18] Twin and family studies have provided evidence for genetic overlap between disorders. Using data from GWAS, variations in the calcium channel, voltage-dependent, L-type, alpha 1C subunit (CACNA1C) is associated with both bipolar disorder and schizophrenia.[19] In another example, an analysis of an extended family with a chromosomal translocation that disrupts *DISC1*, this mutation is associated with multiple mood disorders and schizophrenia.

For a subset of psychiatric disorders, environmental factors may play a key factor in whether a certain composition of genetic variations led to development of a disorder. For instance, early life stress may be an important environmental factor that contributes to the development of a psychiatric disorder in the context of certain genetic variants. One mechanism by which environmental experiences are hypothesized to contribute to the development of psychiatric disorders is by regulating gene expression in the brain through alterations in the epigenome, including by modifying methylation of DNA and post-translational modifications of histones.[10]

Approaches to the Study of Psychiatric Genetics

The goal of psychiatric genetic research is to identify and characterize the genetic basis of psychiatric disorders. This process typically involves a series of questions about familial and genetic contributions that are addressed using several study designs. In the following sections, the rationale and methodological aspects of each of these research tools will be presented, beginning with genetic epidemiological studies and then addressing molecular genetic approaches. In recent years, the advent of powerful genetic sequencing technologies has transformed the study of psychiatric genetics. These new technologies include GWAS, genome-wide studies of copy number variants, and whole-exome sequencing.

Genetic Epidemiology

Family Studies. Family studies address the question: Does the disorder run in families? A disorder that runs in families may indicate a genetic etiology. However, a disorder may run in families for non-genetic reasons, including shared environmental factors. Alternatively, a disorder may not run in families and still have a genetic etiology; an important subset of psychiatric disorders seems to be caused by *de novo* genetic mutations in which genetic mutations that lead to the disorder can be found in the offspring but not the parents.

The design of a typical family study is similar to other case-control studies. Cases (affected probands) and controls (unaffected probands) are ascertained and the lifetime prevalence of the disorder is measured among their (usually first-degree) relatives. A higher prevalence among relatives of affected probands is evidence that the disorder aggregates in families. The risk to relatives of affected probands is referred to as the "recurrence risk." One index of the strength of familiality is the "recurrence risk ratio" for first-degree relatives (λ_1), defined as the ratio of the risk of the disorder in a first-degree relative of an affected individual to the prevalence in the general population. It is important to bear in mind that the size of these risk ratios depends on both the risk to relatives (numerator) and the base rate of the disorder (denominator). Even when the relative risk of a disorder is high, the absolute risk to a first-degree relative may be relatively low if the base rate of the disorder is low. For example, siblings of probands with schizophrenia have a roughly 10-fold increased risk of the disorder compared to an individual randomly drawn from the general population ($\lambda_1 \approx 10$). However, because the population prevalence is approximately 1%, the absolute risk of the disorder for the sibling is only about 10% (with a 90% probability of being unaffected). In contrast, the lifetime prevalence of major depression is approximately 15%, so that even a two-fold increased risk to siblings would be associated with a 30% risk of being affected. Family studies can also provide information about the etiological boundaries or relatedness of different traits or diagnoses. For example, relatives of probands with Tourette syndrome have an elevated risk of obsessive-compulsive disorder (OCD), suggesting that these conditions have overlapping familial determinants (Table 63-1).

Methodological issues can influence the interpretability of family studies. Studies using the "family history method" rely on informant reports to assign diagnoses (e.g., probands may be interviewed about their relatives). Because this method can be less sensitive than direct interview methods for detecting

TABLE 63-1 Genetic Epidemiology of Some Psychiatric Disorders

Disorder	λ_1*	Estimated Concordance Rates		Estimated Heritability (Approximate)	Selected Genetic Findings[†]
		MZ	DZ		
ADHD	2–8	51%–58%	31%–33%	75%	rare CNVs, *GRM1, GRM5, GRM7, GRM8*
Autism	50–100	40%–90%	0%–30%	60%–90%	rare CNVs *de novo* CNVs, *NRXN1, NLGN3, NLGN3, NRXN1, SHANK2, SHANK3, CNTNAP2, MECP2, CHD8*
Alzheimer's disease (late onset)	2	21%	11%	60%	Early onset: presenilin-1, presenilin-2, amyloid precursor protein Late onset: ApoE (ε4), *SORL1*
Schizophrenia	10	46%	14%	70%–89%	rare CNVs *de novo* CNVs, *TCF4, NRGN, ZNF804A,* microRNA *MIR137*
Bipolar disorder	7–10	40%–45%	5%	60%–85%	*CACNA1C, ANK3, NCAN*
Major depressive disorder	3	23%–49%	16%–42%	40%	limited rigorous findings; gene–environment interactions may be key
Panic disorder	5–7	24%	11%	45%	limited rigorous findings
Phobic disorders	4	13%–26%	4%–12%	10%–39%	limited rigorous findings
Obsessive-compulsive disorder	4	Limited data	Limited data	30%–45%	*SAPAP3, SLC1A1*
Alcohol dependence	2–4	50%–58%	32%–50%	35%–60%	Alleles of *ADH* and *ADLH GABRA2,*

*λ_1, recurrence risk ratio for first-degree relatives: the risk of the disorder in a first-degree relative of an affected individual compared with the general population prevalence of the disorder.
[†]Rigorous genetic linkages and associations are beginning to be identified. Much of the genetic basis for these disorders remains not well understood.

psychopathology in relatives, the latter are considered the gold standard. The "family study method" involves direct assessment of probands and relatives, although informant reports may be incorporated to derive "best-estimate" diagnoses using all available data.

Twin Studies. The observation that a trait aggregates in families does not, in itself, establish that genes influence the phenotype. Traits and disorders may run in families for non-genetic reasons. For example, shared environmental experiences may produce the disorder in multiple family members. Twin and adoption studies can be used to assess, to a degree, the contribution of genetic and environmental causes of familial aggregation.

Twin studies compare concordance rates between monozygotic (MZ) twins (who are genetically identical) and dizygotic (DZ) twins (who share on average 50% of their alleles). A twin pair is concordant if both co-twins have the phenotype. If we can assume that environmental influences on MZ twins are not different from environmental influences on DZ twins (the "equal environments assumption"), then significantly higher concordance rates in MZ twins reflect the action of genes. Nevertheless, an MZ concordance rate that is less than 100% suggests that environmental factors influence the phenotype. Twin studies can provide an estimate of the *heritability* of the disorder, which refers to the proportion of the phenotypic differences among individuals in a population that can be attributed to genetic factors. The total variance in phenotypes (V_P) in a population can be decomposed to a genetic component (V_G) and an environmental component (V_E): that is, $V_P = V_G + V_E$. Thus, the heritability is the proportion of the total variance represented by the genetic variance: (V_G/V_P).

For quantitative traits, heritability can be estimated as $2(r_{MZ} - r_{DZ})$ where r_{MZ} refers to the co-twin phenotypic correlation for MZ twins and r_{DZ} refers to the correlation for DZ twins. For categorical traits (such as diagnosis), the concordance rate can be substituted for these correlations to obtain a rough estimate of heritability. Several caveats are important to note regarding the interpretation of heritability estimates.

- Heritability refers to the strength of genetic influences in a *population*, not a particular individual, and heritability estimates may differ depending on the population studied. A heritability of 60% says nothing about the contribution of genes to an individual's risk of a phenotype.
- Heritability refers to the additive sum of all genetic influences on a trait in a population. Thus, a heritability of 0.80 (80%) suggests that genes contribute more to trait variance in the population than does a heritability of 40%. However, heritability provides no information regarding how many genes are involved, how strong the effect of any given gene is, or how easy it will be to identify contributing genes. The number and effect of genetic influences on a trait is sometimes referred to as the "genetic architecture."
- The magnitude of heritability is not a strong predictor of the potential impact of environmental interventions. A classic illustration is the case of phenylketonuria (PKU), a recessively-inherited disorder due to a mutation in the gene-encoding phenylalanine hydroxylase that results in a toxic accumulation of phenylalanine. Untreated, PKU can result in progressive brain damage with seizures and intellectual disability. However, these devastating outcomes can be minimized by entirely environmental interventions: avoidance of dietary phenylalanine and supplementation with tyrosine.

Adoption Studies. Adoption studies can disentangle, to a degree, genetic and environmental influences on family resemblance by comparing rates of a disorder in biological family members with those in adoptive family members. For example, if an adopted child has a genetically-influenced disorder, the biological (genetic) parents should have a higher risk of the disorder than the adoptive (environmental) parents. Adoption studies provided the first convincing evidence that genes play an important role in the development of schizophrenia.

Linkage Analysis. Linkage studies address the question of where in the genome (i.e., in which chromosomal region) a disease mutation or susceptibility locus may reside. Linkage

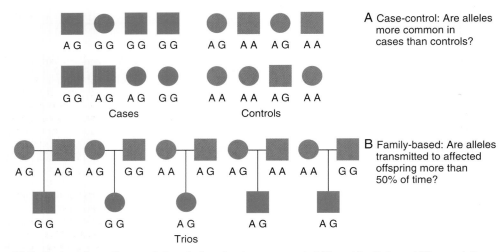

Figure 63-5. Design of genetic association studies showing case-control (A) and family-based (B) association methods.

analysis examines the degree to which alleles at two or more genetic loci are co-inherited (co-segregate) within families (thus deviating from Mendel's law of independent assortment of loci). The likelihood that two loci on a chromosome will co-segregate is inversely proportional to the distance between them. This principle is due to the phenomenon of recombination between homologous chromosomes that occurs during gamete formation (meiosis). During meiosis, the two members of each chromosomal pair (comprising a maternal and a paternal chromosome) align and undergo crossovers that result in an exchange of chromosomal segments (recombination). The closer two loci are on a chromosome, the less likely it is that they will be separated by a recombination event.

If individuals affected by a disorder within a family tend to inherit the same alleles at a marker locus, this implies that the marker locus is linked to (i.e., is physically close to) a gene that influences the disorder. In classical (parametric) linkage analysis, the strength of the evidence in favor of linkage is calculated as a *logarithm of the odds* (LOD) score. The LOD score compares the likelihood of obtaining the observed genotypes and phenotypes when linkage is present with the likelihood assuming no linkage. For classic single gene (Mendelian) disorders, a LOD score of 3 (corresponding to odds of 1,000 : 1 in favor of linkage) has been the threshold for declaring linkage; for complex disorders, such as psychiatric illnesses, higher thresholds (3.3 : 4.0) have been recommended. Traditional LOD score linkage analysis requires that a model including several parameters (mode of inheritance, disease allele frequencies, and marker allele frequencies) be specified. Thus, linkage analysis has been most successfully applied when a single major gene is involved and the mode of inheritance (e.g., dominant, recessive) is known.

The degree of genetic linkage reflects the proximity of two loci and depends on the frequency of recombination between them. The distance between two loci can be expressed as a genetic distance (in centimorgans) or a physical distance (in base pairs). Loci that are separated by recombination in 1% of meioses are 1 centimorgan (cM) apart; this corresponds roughly to a physical distance of 1 million base pairs. Even in the case of Mendelian inheritance, linkage analysis can be complicated by several phenomena that can attenuate the direct relationship between genotype and phenotype. It may be difficult to accurately classify whether an individual is affected with the disease genotype because there may be phenocopies (individuals who have the disorder for non-genetic

reasons), incomplete penetrance (individuals with the disease genotype may not manifest the phenotype), variable expression (the disease genotype may produce a spectrum of phenotypes), and genetic heterogeneity (different genes may independently produce the phenotype). All of these complicating factors are likely to apply to psychiatric phenotypes and reduce the power of linkage analysis in this setting.

Association Analysis. Whereas linkage analysis examines the co-inheritance of alleles and phenotypes *within* families, association analysis examines the co-inheritance of alleles and phenotypes *across* families (i.e., across a population of unrelated individuals) (Figure 63-5). While linkage analysis asks "where" a susceptibility gene resides, association analysis asks "which" specific genetic variants influence a phenotype. In recent years, association methods have increasingly replaced linkage methods for the study of complex diseases. This is because association methods are more powerful than linkage analysis for detecting small genetic effects. However, association between variants operates over much shorter genomic distances, so that much denser sets of genetic markers are needed.

The most common type of association study of complex traits is conceptually very similar to standard case-control epidemiological studies in which the frequency of a risk factor (e.g., smoking) is compared between cases (e.g., individuals with coronary artery disease) and unaffected controls. In the genetic context, the risk factor is an allele (or haplotype). Association is declared if the allele is significantly more common among cases than controls. However, this simple design is complicated by a number of factors.

Statistical evidence of association can result from the following: (a) direct association between a causal variant and disease; (b) indirect association between disease and a genetic variant that is in LD with the true causal variant; (c) confounded association due to population stratification (in which cases and controls differ in their population genetic backgrounds); or (d) spurious association due to chance (as often occurs due to multiple testing or the testing of variants that have low prior probability of association).

Candidate Gene Studies

Until recently, association studies have focused exclusively on *candidate genes*—that is, genes hypothesized to influence a phenotype of interest based on prior evidence. In general, two classes of candidates have been studied: biological candidates (selected based on prior evidence that the gene or pathway is involved in the biology or treatment of a disorder) and positional candidates (selected based on evidence from linkage or cytogenetic studies that a genomic region harbors susceptibility genes). In psychiatric genetics, common biological candidate genes have included those involved in monoaminergic neurotransmission (e.g., transporters, receptors, and enzymes involved in the metabolism of serotonin, dopamine, and norepinephrine [noradrenaline]).

While some candidate genes have shown evidence of association in multiple studies, findings have generally been inconsistent and non-replications are common. Candidate gene studies have commonly been underpowered. It is increasingly clear that very large sample sizes (on the order of thousands of cases and controls) are needed to detect the small effects that genes underlying complex traits are likely to exert. Thus, negative findings can be uninformative if power is inadequate.

Genome-Wide Association Studies

In recent years, advances in high-throughput genotyping technologies coupled with the extensive cataloguing of genetic variation, including SNPs, through the International HapMap Project and the 1000 Genomes Project have made genome-wide association analysis possible. These studies make use of the fact that there is extensive LD across the genome so that the alleles of many SNPs are strongly correlated. Such genotyping technology has been used to identify genes influencing common, complex disorders including psychiatric disorders. Unlike candidate gene studies, GWAS are "unbiased" in that they do not require a pre-specified hypothesis about which genes are important; as such, they offer the opportunity to uncover novel molecules and molecular pathways in the biology of these disorders.

Because of the large number of statistical tests involved, stringent statistical measures to control false-positive rates are needed. In addition, GWAS usually examine relatively common polymorphisms, so that effects of rare susceptibility variants may be missed. However, this approach has already provided conclusive evidence implicating specific genes for a wide range of common, complex medical disorders (including diabetes, heart disease, inflammatory bowel disease, macular degeneration, multiple sclerosis, rheumatoid arthritis, and a growing list of others). In addition, GWAS have identified genetic loci associated with autism, bipolar disorder, and schizophrenia, as described later in the chapter.

Copy Number Variants

Human genomes vary not only by SNPs but also by copy number variants (CNVs).[4] CNVs and structural variants include deletions, duplications, insertions, and inversions of regions of the genome. There are, on average, over 1,000 CNVs in the human genome. Some CNVs are common alleles, while others are rare. Rare CNVs have received significant scientific interest in recent years and have been associated with psychiatric disorders.[4] Cytogenetic studies have documented large chromosomal abnormalities that had association with psychiatric disorders. For instance, the deletion of 22q11.2, in velocardiofacial syndrome, has been associated with schizophrenia[5] and the duplication of 15q11-13 with autism. Genome-wide CNV studies have provided important new insight into the genetics of psychiatric disorders. For instance, there is a higher rate of *de novo* CNVs (5%–10%) in individuals with autism spectrum disorders as compared to unaffected controls.[4,20–23] Rare and large (greater than 100 kb) CNVs have been associated with schizophrenia.[24,25] In addition, there is a high rate of *de novo* CNVs in schizophrenia (5%) as compared to controls.[4,15,26]

Whole-Exome Sequencing

Facilitated by the rapidly declining cost of DNA sequencing, another new approach to psychiatric genetics is to sequence all the exons in a genome of an individual and compare cases and controls. Whole-exome sequencing can reveal rare single nucleotide variants (point mutations) that may be associated with a disorder, including mis-sense mutations (DNA mutations that result in one amino acid, of the encoded protein, being changed), nonsense mutations (DNA mutations that result in the premature stop of the protein product), and mutations that disrupt proper alternative splicing of proteins. These point mutations can be *de novo* mutations, arising in the offspring and not present in the parents. Whole-exome sequencing studies of autism have been recently published.[27–32] Whole-exome sequencing studies have found that *de novo* single nucleotide variants, particularly nonsense mutations or mutations that disrupt alternative splicing, are associated with autism.[28,29,32] Increasing age of the father and mother has been highly correlated with increased number of *de novo* single nucleotide mutations, likely from mutations in the germ cells of the parents.[28,29,33]

Gene–Environment Interaction

Genes operate in the inextricable context of environments, and the etiology of psychiatric illness is generally believed to involve additive and interactive effects of genetic susceptibility and environmental stressors. One reason for the inconsistency in genetic association findings may be that risk alleles may only have observable effects in the context of specific environmental exposures. Thus, failure to measure and incorporate environmental factors may obscure genotype–phenotype relationships.[34] More recently, the examination of gene–environment interaction has become a major focus of research, in part because genetic association methods are well-suited to examine additive and interactive effects of multiple risk factors. Ironically, it has become a simpler matter to measure genetic variation than environmental risk factors: the genome is finite but the environment is nearly unbounded. Identifying which candidate environmental factors are relevant and capturing their longitudinal effects can be difficult. In addition, the sample sizes required are likely to be very large to achieve adequate power to examine these interactions.

Intermediate Phenotypes and Endophenotypes

With the advent of high-throughput genotyping methods and the availability of large clinical cohorts, the rate-limiting step in identifying susceptibility genes for psychiatric disorders may be uncertainty about phenotype definition. While the constellations of symptoms used as diagnostic criteria in the *Diagnostic and Statistical Manual of Mental Disorders* have been useful for clinical practice, it is unlikely that they are the optimal phenotype definitions for genetic analyses. With few exceptions, these criteria are based on self-reported or observable symptoms that may be distant reflections of any underlying neurobiology that is influenced by genes. This makes the study of genetics in psychiatry even more challenging than in other areas of medicine in which direct measurements of the relevant biological phenotypes (e.g., hormone levels, histopathology) are possible. Given this, there has been great interest in identifying phenotypes related to psychiatric disorders that are closer to the genetic substrate than are clinical definitions of the disorders themselves. By more directly capturing gene effects, such "endophenotypes" or "intermediate phenotypes" could avoid the need for unfeasibly large sample sizes in genetic studies; in addition, by modeling more fundamental aspects of psychiatric illness, such phenotypes could help clarify the underlying phenotypic architecture and even inform a new nosology that would not rely exclusively on symptom checklists.

Gottesman and Gould[35] highlighted five desirable characteristics of a putative endophenotype: it is associated with illness in the population; it is heritable; it is primarily state-independent (present even when illness is not active); it co-segregates with illness within families; and the endophenotype found in affected family members is found in non-affected relatives more frequently than in the general population.

A large number of endophenotypes and intermediate phenotypes have been proposed for psychiatric disorders, though data regarding all five criteria listed above are not available for many of these. An example of an endophenotype that appears to meet most of the criteria is inhibition of the P50 evoked response to repeated auditory stimuli, a phenotype that may underlie the abnormalities in sensory gating observed in schizophrenia.[36] A deficit in P50 inhibition has been associated with schizophrenia and the phenotype appears to be heritable and to co-segregate with the illness in families.[37,38] Linkage of impaired P50 inhibition has been linked to a locus on chromosome 15q, adjacent to the alpha-7 nicotinic receptor gene,[39] and subsequent analyses provided evidence that variants in the promoter of this gene are associated with both P50 inhibition and schizophrenia.[40] A recent study identifying genetic loci associated with risk of developing Alzheimer's disease performed a GWAS using the endophenotype of elevated levels of the protein tau and phosphorylated tau in the CSF, biomarkers known to be associated with Alzheimer's disease.[41]

Neuroimaging phenotypes are attractive for genetic studies because they directly measure brain structure or function. The growing literature on imaging genetics[42] has identified several genotype–phenotype correlations involving specific genetic variants. For example, the functional promoter polymorphism in the serotonin transporter gene (5HTTLPR) has been associated with increased amygdala reactivity and reduced coupling of corticolimbic circuits, and neuroimaging phenotypes have been implicated in the biology of anxiety and depressive disorders.[43,44] Other studies have implicated functional polymorphisms in catechol O-methyltransferase (COMT) and prefrontal cortical phenotypes have been thought to underlie working memory deficits and dopaminergic dysregulation in schizophrenia.[42,45]

GENETICS OF PSYCHIATRIC DISORDERS
Genetic Aspects of Psychopathology

Evidence for a genetic component of many psychiatric disorders is growing, and molecular genetic studies have begun to provide evidence for variants in genes and genetic loci that lead these disorders (Table 63-1). Prior to the advent of new genomic technologies, many linkage and association findings have been difficult to replicate, emphasizing the need for caution in interpreting the results of those studies. Some of these findings have undoubtedly been false positives, but non-replication can also be due to inadequate power, differences in diagnosis and phenotype definition, and genetic heterogeneity (different genes acting in different samples). In recent years, the use of new genomic technologies, with large sample sizes of sufficient statistical power, have begun to provide rigorous new insight into the genetic basis of psychiatric disorders. How variations in genes and genomic loci that have

been associated with psychiatric disorders actually lead to psychopathology remains poorly understood.

Disorders of Childhood and Adolescence
Attention-Deficit/Hyperactivity Disorder

Genetic Epidemiology. Numerous family studies have demonstrated that attention-deficit/hyperactivity disorder (ADHD) runs in families. First-degree relatives (parents and siblings) of ADHD probands have a two-fold to eight-fold higher risk of the disorder than relatives of controls.[46] Family studies also suggest that ADHD and depression share familial determinants,[47] and that ADHD with conduct or bipolar disorder may be a distinct familial subtype.[48–50] Most twin studies have shown significantly higher concordance rates for MZ as compared with DZ twins. The mean heritability estimate from 20 twin studies is 76%.[46]

Molecular Genetic Studies. GWAS have failed to reveal loci associated with ADHD with genome-wide significance. Sample sizes to date may be too low for studies to have sufficient statistical power to identify loci with genome-wide significance. There is an increased burden of large and rare CNVs with ADHD patients as compared to controls.[51,52] Duplications of 16p13.11 have been associated with ADHD.[53] Rare CNVs affecting GRM1, GRM5, GRM7, and GRM8 have also been associated with an increased risk for ADHD[54]; the GRMs are metabotropic glutamate receptors that modulate excitatory synapses, suggesting an important role for glutamatergic neurotransmission in ADHD pathogenesis. A recent study, using data from GWAS, provides evidence for shared, albeit small, genetic susceptibility for ADHD and schizophrenia.[55]

Autism

Genetic Epidemiology. Autism predominantly arises from genetic mutations.[56] The risk of autism to siblings of affected children is approximately 2%–7%, which is 50 to 100 times higher than the general population prevalence.[57] When the "broader autism phenotype" (including autism spectrum disorders and milder abnormalities of social and language function) is considered, the risk to first-degree relatives may be as high as 10%–45%.[57] Concordance rates for MZ twins are markedly higher (40%–90%) than those for DZ twins (0%–30%), and the heritability has been estimated in the range of 40% to as much as 90%.[58] Advanced parental age has been associated with a modest increased risk of autism spectrum disorders among offspring.[31,33]

Molecular Genetic Studies. A significant cause of autism spectrum disorders is de novo mutations that arise in the germ line. Copy number variant (CNV) studies have revealed a high rate (10-fold higher than in controls) of de novo CNVs in autism spectrum disorders. Individuals with autism also have a higher overall number of rare CNVs as compared to controls. The molecular causes of autism are polygenic. As many as 400 to 1,000 genetic loci may be involved in autism, a figure estimated in recent studies of de novo exonic mutations in autism.[31] CNVs at 16p11.2, 15q11-13, 22q11.2, deletions of NRXN1, and duplications of 7q11.23 have reproducibly been associated with autism.[21,59] Rare mutations in NLGN4 (encoding neuroligin 4), NLGN3 (neuroligin 3), NRXN1 (neurexin 1), SHANK3, and SHANK2 have been associated with autism[59]; these proteins are involved in the assembly and function of synapses. Neuroligin 4 is a cell-adhesion molecule present post-synaptically, and neurexin 1 is a pre-synaptic binding partner for neuroligins. Rare and common variants of CNTNAP2 have been associated with autism; CNTNAP2 is another member of the neuroligin family and is a cell-adhesion molecule. *SHANK2* and *SHANK3* are post-synaptic scaffolding molecules important for the functioning of synapses. Recent exome sequencing have found *de novo* exonic mutations in *SCN2A*, *KATNAL2*, *CHD8*, *FOXP1*, *NTNG1*, *GRIN2B*, and *LAMC3*.[28,29,31,32] Together, these new genetic findings implicate the importance of synapse development and function for autism pathogenesis.[17] Autism or autistic symptoms also occur in several medical genetic disorders for which specific genes have been identified, including neurofibromatosis (the NF1, NF2 genes), tuberous sclerosis (TSC1, TSC2), fragile X (FMR1), Rett syndrome (MECP2), and Angelman syndrome (UBE3A).[17] Studies of these genetic syndromes with penetrant autism features are providing insight into molecular mechanisms that can lead to autism spectrum disorders.[17]

Tourette Syndrome

Genetic Epidemiology. Familial aggregation studies have found an approximately five-fold to 15-fold increased risk in first-degree relatives of Tourette syndrome (TS) probands compared to the general population (7% to 18% vs. 1% to 2%, respectively).[60] There is evidence for variable expression of the genetic liability for TS; for example, relatives of probands with TS have a higher risk of OCD, and chronic motor or vocal tics.[61] Concordance rates in MZ twins (50% to 70%) are significantly greater than rates in DZ twins (9%).[60] TS occurs with a male/female ratio of approximately 4 : 1.

Molecular Genetic Studies. A linkage study found genetic loci associated with TS on chromosome 2p. Cytogenetic mapping of a Tourette disorder pedigree found a rare mutation in *SLITRK1*, which may regulate dendritic growth in the striatum.[62,63] Cytogenic studies of other pedigrees reveal disruptions of *CNTNAP2* and *Neuroligin4X*, genes also implicated in autism and schizophrenia.[62] A recent GWAS of TS, using nearly 1,500 TS cases, did not find any genetic loci reaching genome-wide significance.[64] A larger number of TS cases may be needed to achieve sufficient statistical power in GWAS to detect genetic associations with TS.

Dementia
Alzheimer's Disease

Genetic Epidemiology. The familiality of early-onset (before age 60 or 65 years) Alzheimer's disease (AD) has been well established, and three specific genes influencing early-onset AD have been identified (see below). Inheritance of early-onset AD follows an autosomal dominant pattern, but the early-onset form is rare, with a prevalence under 0.1%.[65] Late-onset AD is far more common and has a more complex etiology. Having an affected first-degree relative is associated with an approximately 2.5-fold increased risk of AD.[66] Twin studies have estimated the heritability of late-onset AD at 48% to 60%.[67-69]

Molecular Genetic Studies. Mutations in three genes— *amyloid precursor protein, presenilin 1, presenilin 2*—have been shown to produce early-onset AD with an autosomal dominant mode of inheritance. Together, these genes account for roughly 13% of early-onset cases of AD.[70] *Presenilin 1* and *presenilin 2* regulate the cleavage of amyloid precursor protein. These risk genes suggest a key role for amyloid in the development of AD. The *apolipoprotein E* gene (APOE) has been associated with late-onset AD. There are three common alleles of APOE (ε2, ε3, and ε4), and it is the ε4 allele that increases risk for late-onset AD. Unlike autosomal dominant genes involved in early-onset AD, *APOE-ε4* is a susceptibility allele that acts as a risk factor for the disease but is neither a necessary nor sufficient cause. A primary effect of the ε4 allele is to reduce the age of onset of AD[71]; individuals with two copies of the allele have the earliest age of onset compared with individuals with other APOE genotypes. GWAS studies of late-onset and common AD in recent years have implicated *CLU*, *PICLAM*, *CR1*, *BIN1*, *EPHA1*, *MS4A*, *CD33*, *CD2AP*, and *ABCA7* as loci associated with risk for AD; these genes provide insight into the pathogenesis of AD.[70,72-75] Genes *CLU* and *CR1* encode regulators of the complement system, suggesting a role for inflammation, the immune system, and complement in AD. Genes *BIN1*, *PICALM*, and *CD2AP* encode proteins involved in endocytosis, a pathway important for APP processing and β-amyloid formation. Genes *APOE*, *CLU*, and *ABCA7* encode proteins involved in cholesterol and lipid metabolism. In addition, hypercholesterolemia is a risk factor for AD. These environmental and genetic risk factors suggest that cholesterol and lipid metabolism influence AD. *EPHA1* encodes a member of the ephrin receptor sub-family that is involved in axon guidance and synaptic plasticity. Additional genes are being associated with AD, including *SORL1*.[76-78] An on-line database of association studies and meta-analytic results (AlzGene) is maintained at www.alzforum.org. The high risk of AD among individuals with Down syndrome (trisomy 21) has been attributed largely to triplication of the *amyloid precursor protein* gene on chromosome 21. Onset of AD in these individuals is typically in the sixth decade of life.

Psychotic Disorders
Schizophrenia

Genetic Epidemiology. Family studies of schizophrenia have repeatedly demonstrated that the disorder is familial. Compared to the population lifetime risk of approximately 1%, first-degree relatives have an approximately 10% risk. The risk drops to about 4% for second-degree relatives and 2% for third-degree relatives.[79] There is evidence for variable expression of the genetic diathesis underlying schizophrenia. For example, schizoaffective disorder and cluster A personality disorders are more common in the relatives of schizophrenic probands. The concordance rate for MZ twins (approximately 50%) substantially exceeds that of DZ twins (approximately 15%). The heritability of schizophrenia has been estimated to be 70% to 89%.[79,80] Adoption studies have demonstrated that the prevalence of schizophrenia is significantly higher (approximately four-fold) in biological relatives than in adoptive relatives.

Molecular Genetic Studies. Recent studies have provided evidence for a role for both rare genomic structural variants and common genomic variants in the etiology of schizophrenia. Rare and large (>100 kb) CNVs have been associated with schizophrenia.[25,26] These studies show a higher overall rate of *de novo* CNVs has been associated with schizophrenia as compared to controls. The large (~3 Mb) deletion at 22q11.21 causes velocardiofacial syndrome and has long been known to significantly increase the risk for schizophrenia. CNVs encompassing *NRXN1*[81] (neurexin 1, cell-adhesion molecule present at synapses) and *VIPR2*[82] (the vasoactive intestinal peptide receptor 2, a receptor for a peptide that functions as a neurotransmitter) have been found to be associated with schizophrenia. Common genomic variants have also been associated with schizophrenia using GWAS involving many thousands of cases and controls. In this polygenic etiology, the combination of multiple common genomic variants together may lead to subset of cases of schizophrenia. More than 100 loci have reached genome-wide significance including a strong association with the major histocompatibility complex (MHC) locus (a locus with many genes and gene expression regulatory elements; the causative variation associated with schizophrenia is not clear).[83-85,245] Other genomic loci associated with schizophrenia include, among others, *TCF4* (a transcription factor involved in neurogenesis), *NRGN* (a post-synaptic protein kinase substrate involved in learning and memory), and *ZNF804A* (a transcription factor involved in regulating neuronal connectivity).[14,85-88] A GWAS for schizophrenia implicated risk variants at the microRNA *MIR137* locus, an miRNA thought to target and regulate several other genes implicated in schizophrenia.[88] Genetic findings for schizophrenia are converging on biological pathways involved in synaptic function, immune regulation, calcium channel signaling, and targets of the fragile X mental retardation protein (FMRP)

Mood Disorders

Bipolar Disorder

Genetic Epidemiology. Data from nearly 20 family studies have documented that bipolar disorder (BPD) is familial.[89] Overall, a summary estimate of familial risk indicates that the recurrence risk of BPD for first-degree relatives of bipolar probands is approximately 10% (recurrence risk ratio approximately 10), while the risk for unipolar major depressive disorder (MDD) is approximately 15% to 20% (recurrence risk ratio approximately 2 to 3). Increased familial risks have been associated with early-onset BPD. Concordance rates are substantially higher in MZ twins (approximately 40% to 45%) than in DZ twins (approximately 5%), and the heritability of BPD has been estimated to be approximately 60%–85%.[90-92] Twin studies also suggest that genetic influences on BPD overlap with those contributing to MDD, schizophrenia, and schizoaffective disorder.[91,93]

Molecular Genetic Studies. GWAS have begun to identify loci associated with BPD that reach genome-wide statistical significance.[94] These include variants in *CACNA1C* which encodes a subunit of the L-type calcium channel, suggesting an important role for calcium ion channels and calcium-dependent signaling pathways in BPD. In addition GWAS have implicated *ANK3* (encoding ankyrin 3), *NCAN* (encoding neurocan), and a locus near *ODZ4*.[87,95,96] Genetic susceptibility for BPD overlaps with susceptibility for schizophrenia,[85] and with variants in *CACNA1C*,[19] suggesting a key role for calcium-dependent signaling pathways in BPD and schizophrenia.

Major Depressive Disorder

Family Studies. A substantial body of evidence has established that MDD is a familial phenotype, with family studies estimating recurrence ratios ranging from approximately two-fold to nine-fold. A meta-analysis of family studies found that the prevalence of MDD was three-fold higher in the relatives of affected probands compared to the relatives of unaffected controls (summary OR = 2.84; 95% CI: 2.31 to 3.49).[97] Certain features of MDD in the proband have been associated with increased familial risk: early onset, recurrent episodes, chronicity, suicidality, and greater levels of impairment.[98-102] In twin studies published since 1985, the MZ concordance rates have typically fallen in the range of 30%–50% while DZ concordance rates have typically ranged from 12% to 40%, with somewhat higher rates seen in female compared with male twin pairs.[97] Combining these studies, Sullivan and colleagues[97] estimated the summary heritability at 37% (95% CI: 33% to 42%), with a larger share of the variance explained by individual-specific environment (63%, 95% CI: 58% to 67%). The absence of a significant effect of shared family environment suggests that the familial aggregation of MDD is due mostly or entirely to genetic influences. These estimates are consistent with those of the largest twin study comprising more than 15,000 Swedish twin pairs in which the heritability of MDD was estimated at 42% for women and 29% for men.[103]

Molecular Genetic Studies. A 2013 mega-analysis of GWAS for major depressive disorder (MDD), combining multiple GWAS cohorts, with over 18,000 subjects in the discovery stage and over 57,000 subjects in the replication phase, did not reveal any locus with genome-wide significance.[104] Even larger sample sizes may be required to achieve sufficient statistical power. It is possible that interaction between genes and the environment are critical for understanding the etiology of MDD. For instance, a study examining a functional polymorphism modulating the serotonin transporter (*5-HTTLPR*) showed that this genetic polymorphism was a risk factor for developing MDD only in the setting of individuals with prior stressful life events.[105] Two common alleles of the serotonin transporter exist and are distinguishable by the insertion ("long" allele) or deletion ("short" allele) of a 44 base-pair sequence. The "short" allele has been associated with reduced expression of the serotonin transporter. Subsequent reports have failed to consistently support this gene–environment interaction, however.[106-110] Evidence from functional neuroimaging studies has suggested that the "short" allele may exert its effect on negative affectivity by enhancing amygdala reactivity to threat, perhaps through reduced cortical inhibition of the amygdala.[43] Future work will be needed to determine the role of gene–environment interactions in MDD etiology. The precise genes involved in increasing risk for MDD, a disorder with high heterogeneity and lower heritability, remain unclear.[14]

Anxiety Disorders

Panic Disorder

Family Studies. In a meta-analysis of controlled family studies, Hettema and colleagues[111] estimated a five-fold increased risk of panic disorder (PD) among first-degree relatives of affected probands compared to relatives of unaffected controls. Early-onset PD appears to confer increased risk of the disorder for relatives.[112] In their meta-analysis, Hettema and colleagues[111] estimated a summary heritability of 0.43 for PD. The specificity of familial and genetic influences on PD is unclear. Family studies of PD have provided support for specific influences: that is, relatives of probands with PD appear to be at greatest risk for PD rather than other anxiety or mood disorders.[113] On the other hand, twin studies have provided evidence that genes influencing PD overlap with those influencing generalized anxiety disorder (GAD), phobic disorders, post-traumatic stress disorder (PTSD), and depression.[114-116]

Molecular Genetic Studies. Using a candidate gene approach, several genes, including catechol O-methyltransferase (*COMT*), an enzyme involved in the metabolism of catecholamines, have been suggested to associate with PD; however, these associations are not consistently replicated and may be false positives. GWAS for PD have yet to identify genomic loci associated with PD with replicable genome-wide significance.[117] Larger sample sizes are likely needed to achieve sufficient statistical power. Genetic studies of anxiety disorders are limited at this point in time, and rigorous findings are lacking.[118]

Phobic Disorders

Genetic Epidemiology. Family studies have demonstrated that phobic disorders aggregate in families, with a four-fold increased risk of having a disorder among relatives of affected probands.[111] Heritability estimates from twin studies have been in the range of 10% to 39%.[111,115] Modeling of variance components from twin data suggest that individual-specific environmental experiences appear to be the most important influence on the development of phobic disorders, a finding consistent with conditioning models of phobias.[119]

Molecular Genetics. Candidate gene studies have had mixed results and lack independent replication. Linkage and association studies are limited for phobic disorders.

Generalized Anxiety Disorder

Genetic Epidemiology. GAD has received relatively little attention from a genetic standpoint, perhaps in part because the diagnostic criteria have changed substantially since *Diagnostic and Statistical Manual of Mental Disorders*, ed 3 (DSM-III), making the diagnosis something of a "moving target." Family studies of GAD have estimated a recurrence risk ratio of approximately 6, though lower estimates have also been reported.[111,120] Twin studies indicate that GAD is modestly heritable, with a heritability range of approximately 20% to 30%.[111,115] As for the other anxiety disorders, most of the population phenotypic variance in GAD appears to be attributable to individual-specific environments. Several twin studies have suggested that the genetic determinants of GAD overlap substantially with those influencing MDD.[121,122]

Molecular Genetics. Linkage and association studies are limited for GAD. Rigorous findings that explain the genetic basis of GAD are lacking.[117]

Obsessive-Compulsive Disorder

Genetic Epidemiology. Available family studies have yielded mixed results, although the risk to first-degree relatives of OCD probands has been higher than the population prevalence of the disorder in several studies. A meta-analysis of five studies found a four-fold increased risk of the disorder among relatives of affected probands (8.0%) compared with relatives of controls (2.0%). Early-onset OCD has been associated with higher recurrence risks compared with later-onset disorder in some studies[123,124] but not others.[125] The risk of tic disorders (TS and chronic tics) is elevated in a subset of families of OCD probands, suggesting that these disorders can share genetic influences. Conversely, studies have also documented an elevated risk of OCD among relatives of probands with TS.[126] Limited twin data are available, but there is at least some evidence that obsessionality has a heritable component. In one study, heritability was estimated at 47% for obsessional symptoms.[127] A review of twin data concluded that heritability of obsessive-compulsive symptoms is moderate (45% to 65%) in children, but that further research is needed to define the heritability of adult OCD.[128]

Molecular Genetic Studies. Several studies have implicated *SLC1A1*,[129-131] which encodes a glutamate transporter, suggesting a role for glutamatergic pathways in OCD. Mouse animal models have provided insight into genetics of OCD. Genetic deletion of *Sapap3* from mice caused symptoms suggestive of OCD.[132] *Sapap3* encodes a protein located in excitatory synapses in the post-synaptic density. Based on these mouse model findings, cohorts of human patients with OCD and related disorders have been sequenced and rare *Sapap3* variants have been found in patients with OCD and grooming behaviors; this human genetic evidence is suggestive, but not determinate.[133,134] These findings suggest a role for synaptic function in OCD. Mouse models with genetic deletion of *Slirtk5* and *Hoxb8* also have OCD behaviors, suggesting that these loci may also be involved. A genome-wide association study for OCD was recently published and it found no associations of genetic loci with OCD at genome-wide significance.[135] Suggestive associations from this GWAS will require further study and replication.

Substance Use Disorders
Alcohol Abuse and Dependence

Family Studies. Family studies indicate that first-degree relatives of individuals with alcohol dependence have a two-fold to four-fold higher risk of the disorder compared with relatives of unaffected individuals.[136,137] Twin studies have demonstrated substantial genetic influence on alcoholism, with heritability estimates in the range of 35%–60%.[138-141] Adoption studies have demonstrated an increased risk of alcoholism among adoptees who have an alcoholic biological parent.[142,143]

Molecular Genetic Studies. Associations between several candidate genes and alcohol dependence have been reported, including an association between genes affecting alcohol metabolism and a reduced risk of alcohol dependence. By altering the rate of alcohol metabolism, certain alleles of the alcohol dehydrogenase (ADH) and aldehyde dehydrogenase (ALDH) genes can produce a build-up of acetaldehyde, causing an endogenous disulfiram-like flushing reaction.[144,145] By discouraging alcohol consumption, these alleles may be protective against the development of alcoholism. Genes that encode subunits of the GABA receptor, including *GABRA2*, have been associated with alcohol dependence.[144,145] Both this genetic evidence and the fact that alcohol is an agonist of the GABA receptor suggest the importance of GABA-ergic pathways in alcohol dependence. GWAS for alcohol dependence are starting to be reported; reproducibility, more statistical power, and more defined patient cases are needed. Much of the genetic basis of alcohol dependence remains unknown.

Drug Abuse and Dependence

Genetic Epidemiology. Studies have documented familial aggregation of abuse and dependence for a wide variety of illicit drugs, including cannabis, cocaine, and opiates.[146] In general, the recurrence risk ratio (λ) for these phenotypes is approximately $2 : 8$.[146,147] Twin studies have shown that drug use disorders are moderately to highly heritable, with estimates ranging from 30% to 40% for hallucinogens and stimulants to as high as 70% to 80% for cocaine and opiates.[148] Evidence also suggests that some degree of the genetic liability to addiction is shared across multiple substance use disorders—that is, there appears be an underlying genetic vulnerability to addiction that may be expressed in abuse of any of several substances.[149]

Molecular Genetic Studies. Inconsistent results have been observed in candidate gene association studies,[144] with some studies implicating variants in *OPRM1*, which encodes the *mu* opiate receptor, in opioid dependence[150] and dopaminergic genes in cocaine dependence.[151]

PHARMACOGENETICS

The use of genetic information for predicting or guiding drug response has become an area of great interest in many fields of medicine. For many drugs, there are marked inter-individual differences in response and toxicity, sometimes leading to severe adverse effects. More than three dozen drugs have been withdrawn from the market since 1990 due to safety and toxicity concerns, although in most cases only a small proportion of individuals were at risk.[152] *Pharmacogenetics* refers to "the study of the role of inheritance in inter-individual variation in drug response."[153] The related domain of pharmacogenomics is concerned with the genome as a source of drug targets or as a resource for stratifying disease for drug-response predictors. The often-stated goal of pharmacogenetic research is to inform the practice of "individualized" or "personalized" medicine,[154] in which genetic information could be used to tailor treatment to optimize therapy for an individual patient, maximizing the likelihood of response while minimizing the risk of toxicity.

Pharmacologically-relevant genes include those related to pharmacokinetics (e.g., genes involved in drug metabolism, distribution, and elimination) and those related to pharmacodynamic effects (e.g., therapeutic targets, including receptors, transporters, and intra-cellular signaling molecules). The best-studied pharmacokinetically-relevant genes are those related to hepatic metabolism. In particular, cytochrome P450 enzymes affect the metabolism of a broad range of psychotropics. It has been estimated that 2D6 is the major metabolic pathway for 25% of all prescribed drugs, and four of the most prescribed 2D6 metabolized drugs in 2003 were antidepressants.[155] In 2005, the first Food and Drug Administration (FDA)-approved genetic test became available, assaying variants of the CYP 450 2D6 and 2C19 enzymes.[156] Individual differences in 2D6 and 2C19 phenotype can result from differences in the number and activity of genes encoding these enzymes. For example, individuals with two non-functional P450 2D6 genes (approximately 7% of Caucasians, and 1%–2% of Asians and African Americans) have a "poor metabolizer" (PM) genotype that renders their 2D6 enzyme inactive. Plasma levels of drugs metabolized by 2D6 can be markedly elevated in PMs,[157] potentially increasing the risk of toxicity and drug intolerance. Limited data suggest that these genetic effects are clinically-relevant for antidepressant drugs (especially tricyclic antidepressants [TCAs]) and antipsychotic drugs for which dose-related toxicity can be a problem.[158,159] Approximately 1% to 10% of Caucasians and 2% of African Americans have an ultrarapid metabolism genotype at 2D6, resulting from duplicated or high-activity 2D6 alleles.[156] Pharmacokinetic data and case reports suggest that patients with an ultrarapid metabolizer genotype who are treated with 2D6 substrates may require higher-than-usual doses to achieve therapeutic response.[157,160] Genotype-specific antidepressant and antipsychotic guidelines for dosing or drug selection for PMs and ultra-rapid metabolizers (UMs) have been proposed.[156,157] However, because most studies that have examined drug levels or outcomes by genotype have been relatively small and vary in terms of whether single-dose or repeated dosing was used, definitive recommendations are difficult to derive at present. In addition, the effect of such dose alterations on clinical outcomes has yet to be established.

Studies of pharmacodynamically-relevant genes have also had mixed results, although several genetic variants have been implicated in multiple studies of psychotropic drug response. Because its protein product is the therapeutic target of SSRI antidepressants, the serotonin transporter gene has been the most widely studied in genetic studies of antidepressant response. In Caucasian samples, the "short" allele of the functional promoter polymorphism (5HTTLPR) has been associated with reduced or delayed therapeutic benefit and increased adverse effects with SSRI treatment.[161-164] Other examples include associations between dopamine receptor gene variants and antipsychotic response and association of variants in the serotonin 2C receptor gene with antipsychotic-induced weight gain.[165] To date, however, these associations remain uncertain and do not provide clinically useful markers.

PSYCHIATRIC ASPECTS OF MEDICAL GENETIC DISORDERS
Psychiatric Symptoms Secondary to Genetic Syndromes

In contrast to the complex genetic and multi-factorial nature of most psychiatric disorders discussed earlier in this chapter, for a limited number of psychiatric patients, the etiology of

behavioral symptoms may be a primary genetic or metabolic syndrome. Many genetic syndromes have various behavioral manifestations associated with them, and for the selected disorders reviewed here, psychiatric symptoms may be especially prominent (Table 63-2).

The presence of associated medical conditions, developmental deficits, or laboratory abnormalities in patients being evaluated for psychiatric symptoms may provide clues to the presence of an underlying genetic syndrome or inborn error of metabolism that requires further diagnostic investigation (Table 63-3). In this circumstance, correctly diagnosing the behavioral manifestations as secondary to the underlying genetic changes is essential, as treatment opportunities, need for screening or treatment for associated medical issues, and determination of risks to other family members may all depend on the primary disorder. For some patients, a psychiatrist may be the first clinician to consider the presence of such a syndrome, and it may be beneficial to supplement the standard psychiatric assessment with additional questions that target early medical and developmental history, as well as a comprehensive review of medical and psychiatric conditions present in family members. Suggested questions are depicted in Box 63-1.

Referral to colleagues in genetics for further assessment and management is appropriate when a genetic or metabolic disorder is suspected.

SELECTED GENETIC SYNDROMES WITH PSYCHIATRIC AND BEHAVIORAL SYMPTOMS (TABLE 63-2)
Disorders Due to Chromosomal Abnormalities and Microdeletions

Klinefelter Syndrome

Klinefelter syndrome refers to a group of disorders occurring in males with at least one additional X chromosome, classically 47, XXY, and secondary to failure of the sex chromosomes to separate during meiosis. The incidence of this disorder is approximately 1 per 600 live male births. Men with Klinefelter syndrome are typically tall, with long legs. In contrast to previous reports, they have a male distribution of body fat and hair, although gynecomastia may be present, and body hair may be sparse. A diagnosis of Klinefelter syndrome is often made at puberty, when hypogonadism becomes apparent. The testes and penis remain small, and secondary sexual changes fail to occur. Testosterone levels are low, and follicle-stimulating hormone (FSH) and luteinizing hormone (LH) are elevated. Men with Klinefelter syndrome may have normal sexual function, especially when treated with testosterone supplementation, but are infertile. Developmentally, boys with Klinefelter syndrome may have some minor motor and verbal delays, and increased rates of learning disorders. Individuals with Klinefelter syndrome have also been described as more shy and immature and lacking in confidence than peers. There are increased rates of ADHD in this population, and possibly depression, but major psychopathology has not been commonly reported.[166,167] Recently, increased interest in the relationship between smaller cortical brain volumes seen on magnetic resonance imaging (MRI) in Klinefelter patients and underlying cognitive deficits and psychiatric symptoms has resulted in exploration of schizophrenia-spectrum findings in these men; two studies have reported results that raise the possibility of increased rates of auditory hallucinations and other psychosis-spectrum findings.[168-170] The diagnosis of Klinefelter syndrome is made by karyotype examination of chromosomes.

TABLE 63-2 Common Symptoms Associated with Genetic Syndromes

Genetic Disorder	Commonly Associated Psychiatric Symptoms							Other Behavioral Findings
	Psychosis	Mood Symptoms	Obsessions/ Compulsions	ADHD Spectrum	PDD Spectrum	Dementia	Delirium	
Duplication 15					•			
Fragile X syndrome		•		•	•			Oppositional defiant disorder, avoidant personality disorder and traits
Huntington disease	•	•				•		Changes in personality, apathy
Klinefelter syndrome		•		•				Social immaturity
Prader-Willi syndrome	•	•	•	•	•			Hyperphagia, skin-picking, and temper tantrums
Rett syndrome					•			
Smith-Magenis syndrome		•		•				Tantrums, impulsivity, self-injurious behaviors (onychotillomania, polyembolokoilamania, skin-picking)
Tuberous sclerosis				•	•			
Turner syndrome		•		•				Anxiety, problems with social skills
Velocardiofacial syndrome	•	•	•	•	•			Oppositional defiant disorder
Williams syndrome		•	•	•	•			Anxiety, circumscribed interests, may be somatically-focused, socially-disinhibited and overly friendly

TABLE 63-3 Common Symptoms Associated with Metabolic Syndromes

Metabolic Syndromes	Psychosis	Mood Symptoms	Obsessions/ Compulsions	ADHD Spectrum	PDD Spectrum	Dementia	Delirium	Other Behavioral Findings
Acute intermittent porphyria	•	•					•	Anxiety, "histrionic" personality
Homocystinuria		•	•					
Metachromatic leukodystrophy	•					•		Late-onset form
Personality changes								
Mitochondrial disorders	•	•		•	•	•	•	
Niemann-Pick, type C	•					•		
Tay-Sachs, late onset	•	•				•		Catatonia
Wilson disease	•	•				•		Personality changes
X-linked adrenoleukodystrophy	•	•		•		•		

Turner Syndrome

Turner syndrome is a genetic condition that occurs in women, and is due to missing one copy of the X chromosome, designated as 45, X. This condition occurs in approximately 1 per 3,000 female births and is also a common cause of miscarriage. Females with this condition are short, with a broad flat chest, and may have a webbed neck (due to congenital lymphedema). Increased rates of congenital heart disease, including coarctation of the aorta and bicuspid aortic valve, are noted. Minor problems with hearing and vision are also reported, as well as renal abnormalities. Women with Turner syndrome have gonadal dysgenesis, and for this reason fail to develop secondary sexual characteristics and are infertile.

Hypothyroidism is also seen. Developmentally, intelligence is normal in more than 90% of patients, but specific learning deficits, especially in visual-spatial areas, are seen. Performance IQ may be lower than verbal IQ, and be manifest as problems in math and multitasking. ADHD is reported at increased rates in this population. Immaturity, problems reading social cues, and difficulties with peer relationships may occur.[171,172] In adults, increased rates of depression have been measured.[173] The diagnosis of Turner syndrome is made by karyotype analysis of chromosomes.

Duplication 15

Approximately 1 in 4,000 individuals are born with a marker chromosome (small amount of extra chromosomal material),

---

BOX 63-1 Sample Questions to Supplement the Standard Psychiatric Assessment

PRENATAL AND BIRTH HISTORY

Were there complications or maternal medical issues during pregnancy?

Was there maternal hypertension, toxemia, or HELLP?

Were there toxic exposures or exposure to medications during pregnancy?

Were any diagnostic tests completed during pregnancy (amniocentesis, other genetic testing)?

Were there any abnormal ultrasound findings?

What was the mode of delivery and were there associated complications?

Was there a need for urgent medical care or a neonatal intensive care unit (NICU) following birth?

Were there issues with feeding or growth during infancy or childhood, or failure to thrive?

DEVELOPMENTAL HISTORY

Were major motor and verbal milestones on track?

Was there a history of developmental regression or decline in school performance?

Was there a history of need for supplemental therapies (occupational therapy, physical therapy, speech and language)?

Was there a history of mental retardation, or a need for special educational service or education plans?

FAMILY HISTORY

What is the race and ethnicity of the family of origin?

Was there any history of consanguinity?

Was there a history of infertility, miscarriage, stillbirth, or infant deaths?

Was there a pattern of illnesses in family (it is helpful to draw a pedigree to visually depict)?

REVIEW OF SYSTEMS AND PHYSICAL EXAMINATION

Was there a history of prolonged decompensation with routine illness?

Were there co-morbid neurological findings? Do they occur at all times or on an episodic basis?

Was there facial dysmorphology?

HELLP, Hemolysis elevated liver enzymes, low platelets.

---

and 50% of these are due to extra chromosomal material from chromosome 15, which may be located within one of the chromosome 15s, or as a separate small amount of genetic material. Usually, the chromosomal material is from the long arm between bands 11 and 14, which overlaps with the Prader-Willi region (see next), and results in extra copies of genes in the duplicated region. Features of both Prader-Willi syndrome and Angelman syndrome (a disorder characterized by severe intellectual disability and developmental delay, ataxia, seizures, and unique behavioral profile of excitability and happy demeanor) may occur. The findings associated with this abnormality vary widely, from unaffected to severely affected, depending on the size of the duplicated region, and the parent of origin of the normal and abnormal chromosomes. Other features associated with this disorder include seizures (especially infantile spasms/hypsarrhythmia), hypotonia, ataxia, and genitourinary abnormalities. Developmental delays and intellectual disability are common. Pervasive developmental disorder (PDD)-spectrum symptoms are often associated with this disorder.[174,175] This chromosomal abnormality may be seen on karyotype analysis of chromosomes, but may require additional techniques to identify the exact origin of the additional material.

Prader-Willi Syndrome

Prader-Willi syndrome (PWS) is a genetic condition most often due to a microdeletion on the paternal copy of chromosome 15q11-13 (chromosome 15, long arm band 11-13). Genes in this region undergo imprinting, resulting in silencing of copies of the gene on the maternal chromosome, leaving a lack of expressed genes in this region in those with a paternal deletion. Additional genetic mechanisms, including a defect in the imprinting control region (approximately 1% to 2% of cases), and maternal uni-parental disomy (having both copies of chromosome 15 from the mother, in approximately 30% of cases), may also result in PWS. PWS is associated with prominent hypotonia in infancy, and initial failure to thrive. The characteristic hyperphagia and obesity develop in later childhood, and may be manageable with behavioral techniques. Physical findings include fair coloring, small hands and feet, and hypogonadism (Figure 63-6). Facial features include almond-shaped eyes and a small, down-turned mouth with a thin upper lip. Developmentally, PWS patients tend to show motor and verbal delays, as well as intellectual disability, usually in the mild to moderate range. Behaviorally, PWS patients often exhibit tantrums and stubbornness, and may have difficulty with change. Increased rates of obsessive-compulsive symptoms, some of which may be centered on food, and other rituals are also described. Some skin-picking is noted. Mood disorders, including BPD, are also seen, as well as increased rates of psychosis.[176-180] Testing for PWS involves a combination of methylation analysis, microsatellite profiling, and deletion testing of fluorescent *in situ* hybridization (FISH) for region and specific testing for imprinting center deletions.

Velocardiofacial Syndrome

Velocardiofacial syndrome (VCFS), which has previously been referred to as DiGeorge syndrome, and is increasingly known as 22q11 deletion syndrome (which indicates the underlying genetic abnormality of a microdeletion on chromosome 22), is due to a genetic microdeletion, most commonly 3 Mb in size. It is estimated to occur in 1 per 2,500 to 1 per 3,000 individuals in the general population, making it one of the most common genetic syndromes. VCFS is associated with a great variety of medical conditions, but most commonly conotruncal heart defects, cleft palate, or velopharyngeal insufficiency (which may manifest as hypernasal speech), immune defects, and hypoparathyroidism with hypocalcemia. A characteristic facial appearance, including facial asymmetry, a broad nasal root, bulbous nasal tip, long flat face, small and retruded jaw, and ear malformations, is seen (Figure 63-7). VCFS patients frequently have developmental delays in both motor and language ability, as well as specific learning deficits in math and reading comprehension. Verbal IQ scores may be significantly higher than performance IQ, and overall intelligence may range from normal to mild intellectual disability. VCFS has been described as a "genetic sub-type of schizophrenia"[181] and has been reported to occur in as many as 1%–2% of adults with schizophrenia and 6% of children with childhood-onset psychosis.[182-184] Certain findings related to schizophrenia, such as endophenotypes, including sensory

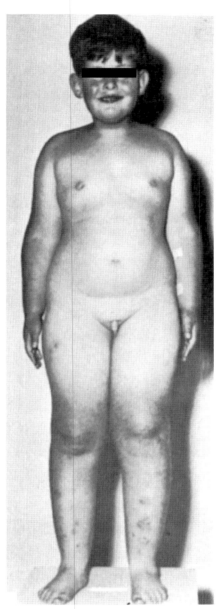

Figure 63-6. Prader-Willi syndrome. Obesity, hypogonadism, and small hands and feet in a 9.5-year-old boy who also has a short stature and developmental delay. *(From Jones KL.* Smith's recognizable patterns of human malformation, *ed 4, Philadelphia, 1988, WB Saunders, p. 173.)*

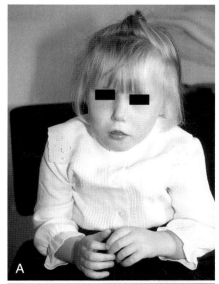

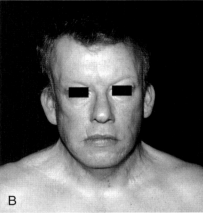

Figure 63-7. Velocardiofacial syndrome in a young girl (A) and a male adult (B). *(From Turnpenny P, Ellard S.* Emery's elements of medical genetics, *ed 12, Philadelphia, 2005, Elsevier, pp. 278, 279).*

motor gating deficits, as well as characteristic neuroimaging findings, also appear at increased rates in those with VCFS. In addition, increased rates of BPD and other mood disorders are reported, as well as anxiety, OCD, ADHD, and PDD-spectrum disorders.[182,183,185–189] The spectrum of physical and psychiatric symptoms may vary greatly in type and severity in these patients, so physicians should have a low threshold for consideration of this syndrome. Knowing that a psychiatric patient has VCFS may dictate treatment options, as there are some reports of increased rates of seizures while on atypical antipsychotics in these patients.[182] Currently, testing for VCFS employs FISH evaluation of the critical region (Figure 63-8). Of note, several genes that are considered good candidate genes for psychiatric symptoms are included in the 22q11.2 deleted region, among them, *COMT.*

Smith-Magenis Syndrome

Smith-Magenis syndrome (SMS) is another microdeletion syndrome, affecting region 17p11.2. In most patients, a deletion of approximately 4 Mb is noted, but a small number of SMS patients who lack the classic deletion have been found to have point mutations in the retinoic acid induced 1 *(RAI1)* gene, which lies within the SMS critical region.[190,191] Behavioral symptoms of SMS may be similar to pediatric-onset BPD, as prominent sleep disturbance (secondary to abnormal circadian rhythms and aberrant melatonin secretion), tantrums, impulsivity, stereotypies, aggression, and self-injurious behaviors (e.g., skin-picking and nail-pulling), as well as ADHD symptoms, are reported.[190,192–194] When happy or excited, SMS patients may give themselves a self-hug or upper body squeeze.[195] Clues to the presence of SMS include a characteristic facial appearance consisting of a broad, square-shaped face with prominent forehead, deep-set eyes, mid-face hypoplasia, short nose with full tip, relative prognathia that develops with age, and a fleshy tented upper lip (Figure 63-9). Additional findings may include skeletal abnormalities, short stature, short hands and fingers, hearing loss, hypotonia, and mild-to-moderate intellectual disability.

Williams Syndrome

Williams syndrome (WS) is due to a microdeletion at 7q11.23. Anxiety is a prominent feature of WS, and it has been proposed that the characteristic hyperverbality of those with WS may be a manifestation of generalized anxiety. Patients with WS also tend to be somewhat hypochondriacal and somatically focused, and may have circumscribed interests and obsessions. However, social anxiety is not usually present in WS individuals, and MRI findings have shown reduced activation of amygdala circuitry in response to novel faces in WS patients compared to normal controls.[196] Symptoms of mood disorders, PDD, and AHDH are also seen in these patients.[197,198] Physical clues to WS include short stature, an "elfin" facial appearance (Figure 63-10) with eye findings of a stellate appearance of the iris, and congenital heart defects (classically supravalvular aortic stenosis or pulmonary artery stenosis). Hypercalcemia is also noted. Intellectual disability in the mild-to-severe range is present, with difficulties in visuospatial tasks. Strong verbal abilities may mask the extent of underlying cognitive deficits. WS is diagnosed by FISH analysis of the critical region. The elastin gene *(ELN)*, located in the deleted region, has been implicated in the etiology of some WS symptoms, but the molecular basis of, and the genetic elements involved in, the neuropsychiatric impairments remain unclear.

Disorders Due to Single Gene Mutations

Fragile X Syndrome

Fragile X syndrome (FRX) is the most common inherited cause of intellectual disability, occurring in about 1 in 4,000 boys.

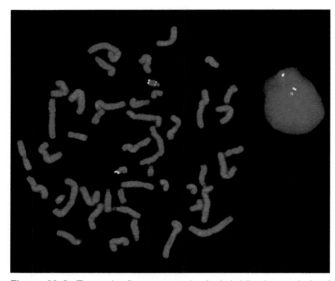

Figure 63-8. Two-color fluorescence *in situ* hybridization analysis of proband with velocardiofacial syndrome, demonstrating deletion of 22q11.2 on one homolog. Green signal is hybridization to a control probe in distal chromosome 22q. Red signal on proximal 22q is a single-copy probe for a region that is present on one chromosome 22 but deleted from the other *(arrow)*. *(Courtesy of Hutton Kearney, Duke University Medical Center.)*

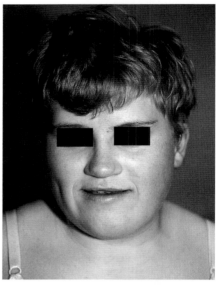

Figure 63-9. Child with Smith-Magenis syndrome. *(From Turnpenny P, Ellard S. Emery's elements of medical genetics, ed 12, Philadelphia, 2005, Elsevier, p. 280.)*

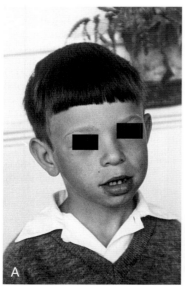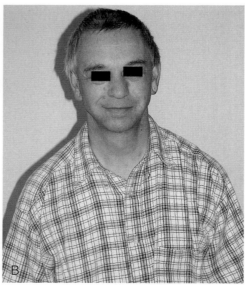

Figure 63-10. A person with Williams syndrome as a child (A) and at age 45 years (B) looking older than his chronological age. *(From Turnpenny P, Ellard S. Emery's elements of medical genetics, ed 12, Philadelphia, 2005, Elsevier, p. 279.)*

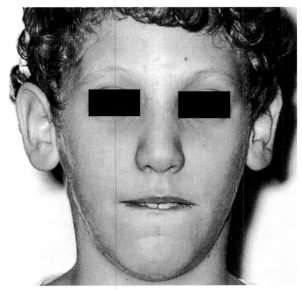

Figure 63-11. Facial view of a boy with fragile X syndrome. *(From Turnpenny P, Ellard S.* Emery's elements of medical genetics, *ed 12, Philadelphia, 2005, Elsevier, p. 283.)*

The disorder is due to mutations in the *FMR1* gene, which encodes the protein FMRP. FMRP regulates mRNA translation, near synapses and dysregulation of protein synthesis that may lead to the disorder.[176,199] This region contains an area of repetitive DNA, which involves a trinucleotide repeat, CGG. The number of repeats in the region is significant for the onset of disease. Repeat length may be normal (5 to 44 CGG repeats), intermediate (45 to 58 repeats, which are prone to expand during transmission), premutation (59 to 200 repeats, which are likely to expand to a full mutation with the next generation), and full (greater than 200 repeats). Because this disorder is X-linked, classically it has been described in males. However, females with full mutation length repeats may be unaffected, mildly affected, or as severely affected as their male counterparts. Furthermore, premutation length alleles are associated with premature ovarian failure in woman and fragile X tremor ataxia syndrome in males. Physical findings in FRX males include hypotonia, a long face with a prominent jaw and forehead, large ears, and large testicles (Figure 63-11). Of note, some changes may not be apparent until after puberty. Verbal and motor delays are common, and intellectual disability is present, which may be in the moderate-to-severe range. Seizures occur at increased rates. Psychiatric co-morbidities include ADHD and PDD-spectrum disorders.[200-203]

Huntington Disease

Huntington disease (HD) is another triplet repeat disorder, resulting from a CAG repeat in the HD gene on chromosome 4p16. Similarly, there is a normal range of repeat length (10 to 26), a premutation range that may expand to a full mutation in the next generation (27 to 35), repeat lengths that show variable penetrance (36 to 39), and full mutations (40 or greater repeats) (see Figure 63-4). Of note, psychiatric manifestations including psychosis, personality changes, and mood symptoms may be among the presenting symptoms, while motor findings (classically choreiform movements) and cognitive decline may become apparent over time.[204-206] Unfortunately, the progressive decline associated with this disorder (and lack of effective treatment to halt disease progression) has resulted in a high suicide rate among HD patients. MRI scans of the brain show involvement of the basal ganglia.

Mean age of onset is between 35 and 44 years, with the phenomenon of anticipation also contributing to onset and severity of illness. Testing for HD involves determination of the number of CAG repeats.

Rett Syndrome

Over 95% of cases of Rett syndrome (RTT) are caused by mutations in the *MECP2* gene. Located on the X-chromsome, RTT is classically described in girls. RTT is characterized by deceleration of head growth and acquired microcephaly, impaired language development, loss of social engagement, loss of purposeful hand movements, stereotyped hand movements, gait abnormalities, seizures, and respiratory abnormalities.[207] RTT has features of autism spectrum disorders and PDD. The severity of symptoms may be influenced by mutation type and pattern of X inactivation. Sequencing for *MECP2* is available on a commercial basis. *MECP2* binds to methylated DNA, recruits co-repressors (including the NCoR co-repressor complex), and represses transcription, a process that is modulated by neuronal activity.[17,208,209]

Tuberous Sclerosis

Mutations in *TSC1* and *TSC2* are associated with tuberous sclerosis. Tuberous sclerosis patients have a variety of physical findings, which may include skin abnormalities (e.g., ash leaf spots, shagreen patches, and angiofibromas) as well as tumors in multiple organ systems (CNS tubers seen on MRI, retinal hamartomas, cardiac rhabdomyomas, and renal angiomyolipomas), dental pits, and seizures. Psychiatric features that are most often associated with tuberous sclerosis are ADHD and PDD-spectrum symptoms.[210] *TSC1* and *TSC2* regulate protein synthesis; the loss of this regulation may contribute to the neuropsychiatric symptoms in tuberous sclerosis.[17]

SELECTED INBORN ERRORS OF METABOLISM WITH PSYCHIATRIC AND BEHAVIORAL SYMPTOMS (SEE TABLE 63-3)
Autosomal Dominant Disorders

Acute Intermittent Porphyria

The porphyrias are a class of metabolic disorders that result from dysfunction of enzymes in the heme biosynthetic pathway. Deficiency of the enzyme porphobilinogen deaminase (PBGD)/hydroxymethylbilane synthase (HMBS) results in acute intermittent porphyria (AIP) and is caused by mutations of the *HMBS* gene on 11q23.3. Symptoms of AIP consist of episodic "neurovisceral attacks" that are marked by abdominal (e.g., pain, distention, nausea, vomiting, diarrhea, constipation, urinary retention, and dysuria), CNS (e.g., delirium, anxiety, agitation, psychosis, and somnolence), and peripheral nervous system (e.g., peripheral neuropathy progressing to permanent nerve damage) involvement.[211-213] Symptoms are more likely to occur after puberty, and in women, but only a fraction (10%–50%) of individuals with *HMBS* mutations will go on to exhibit symptoms due to reduced penetrance in the disorder. Separate from psychiatric symptoms during acute attacks, increased rates of anxiety and depression have also been reported.[214] Onset of attacks may be triggered by agents that place demand on the affected pathway, including several medications that are commonly prescribed by psychiatrists (e.g., valproic acid, carbamazepine, benzodiazepines, and TCAs, among others). It is possible, then, for patients with undiagnosed AIP to be labeled as treatment-refractory due to the worsening of symptoms precipitated by their psychiatric medications. Diagnosis of AIP is made through measurement of urinary δ-aminolevulinic acid (ALA) and porphobilinogen (PBG), as well as enzyme levels in blood. Molecular genetic testing for disease-causing mutations in the *HMBS* gene is also available. Treatment is targeted at removal of offending agents, medications to suppress heme production, and supportive care during attacks.

Autosomal Recessive Disorders

Homocystinuria

Classic homocystinuria is a rare metabolic condition secondary to mutations in the cystathionine-β-synthase *(CBS)* gene on 21q22.3, leading to deficiency of cystathionine- β-synthase and elevated levels of homocystine, homocysteine, and methionine. Enzyme co-factor deficiencies may also result in variant forms of the disease. Screening for homocystinuria is included in the newborn panel in many states, as prompt diagnosis and initiation of proper dietary restrictions and other treatment that allows alternative excretion of pathway by-products can prevent the associated intellectual disability and physical complications associated with the disorder. Due to interference of collagen cross-linking by homocystine, affected individuals tend to have skeletal anomalies (e.g., tall with long extremities, pectus excavatum, scoliosis, and restricted range of motion at joints), and experience ectopia lentis. In addition, they are at greatly increased risk of thrombus formation secondary to disruption of the vascular endothelium by elevated homocystine levels. Originally, descriptions of these patients included increased rates of schizophrenia; recent investigation of the consequences of high homocysteine exposure and its relationship to schizophrenia have re-invigorated interest in this metabolic pathway.[215-217] Patients with homocystinuria may also exhibit symptoms of depression, OCD, learning disorders, and intellectual disability.[218] Diagnosis is made through urine nitroprusside testing for disulfides, and measurements of homocystine, homocysteine, and methionine in the blood. Mutation testing for two common alleles is clinically available, but most mutations are private and biochemical parameters are the mainstay of diagnosis and treatment monitoring.

Metachromatic Leukodystrophy (Juvenile- or Adult-onset Forms)

Dysfunction of the arylsulfatase A *(ARSA)* gene on 22q13 leads to ARSA deficiency with resultant abnormal lysosomal storage of galactosyl sulfatide (cerebroside sulfate). Deficiency of saposin B, an enzyme co-factor, may also result in metachromatic leukodystrophy (MLD). The disease occurs in three forms: infantile-, juvenile-, and adult-onset forms. Oligodendrocytes are particularly sensitive to the abnormal lysosomal storage, leading to demyelination and progressive neurological dysfunction. Physical symptoms include ataxia, optic atrophy, dysarthria, dystonia, nerve palsies, hyporeflexia progressing to hyperreflexia, cognitive decline and dementia, and ultimately a decerebrate state. Changes in personality, decline in work and school performance, and onset of psychosis are also commonly seen.[219-221] MRI imaging of the brain will show white matter changes consistent with demyelination. Diagnosis is made through measurement of elevated sulfatides in urine, and low levels of enzyme in white blood cells in blood. Molecular testing is also available. Bone marrow transplantation may slow disease progression.

Niemann-Pick, Type C

Niemann-Pick, type C (NPC) is also a disorder that is secondary to the sequelae of abnormal intra-cellular storage of lipids.

Although the disease mechanism is incompletely understood, it is thought to be related to impaired intra-cellular trafficking mediated by the protein product of the *NPC1* gene (chromosome 18q11-12). Vertical supranuclear palsy is the hallmark of this disorder, but other findings consistent with neurological dysfunction (e.g., ataxia, dysarthria, dystonia, seizures, and cognitive deficits and decline) and liver disease are also seen. Individuals affected with NPC have increased rates of psychosis and have been erroneously diagnosed with schizophrenia.[222,223] Of note, urine and blood lysosomal screens will be normal in NPC, and diagnosis requires cultured-skin fibroblasts, which show impaired cholesterol esterification and positive filipin staining. Sequencing of *NPC1* and *NPC2* (14q24.3) is also available.

Tay-Sachs, Late-onset Form

Many physicians are familiar with classic Tay-Sachs, a lysosomal storage disorder secondary to deficiency of β-hexosaminidase A, which results in GM_2 ganglioside accumulation in neurons, progressive neurodegeneration, and death, usually before age 4. Mutations in the *HEXA* gene on 15q23-24 are responsible for the enzyme dysfunction. However, a late-onset form with some preservation of enzyme activity can also be seen, with slower progression of neurological symptoms, and associated mood and psychotic symptoms.[224-227] Macular cherry red spots, a hallmark of classic Tay-Sachs, are not present in the adult-onset form.

Wilson Disease

Mutations in the *ATP7B* gene (chromosome 13q14-21), which codes for the main transporter of copper in the body, cause Wilson disease (WD). Symptoms of WD are secondary to abnormal deposition of copper in the liver and nervous system, with resultant copper-mediated oxidative damage, and include sequelae of acute, recurrent, and chronic liver dysfunction (e.g., jaundice, abnormal liver function tests, hepatitis, fulminant liver failure, and cirrhosis) and basal ganglia involvement (e.g., tremor, "wing beating," dysarthria, rigidity, parkinsonism, dyskinesia, dystonia, and chorea). Cognitive deterioration is also seen. Among the earliest symptoms of the disorder may be personality changes and disruption of mood (including pseudobulbar palsy).[228-230] The hallmark of the disorder is the golden brown Kayser-Fleischer ring, a deposition of copper in the cornea, which is visible on slit-lamp examination, and present in 90% of patients with psychiatric symptoms. Diagnosis is made through measurement of reduced bound copper and ceruloplasmin in the blood, increased urinary copper excretion, and visualization of copper deposits on liver biopsy. Treatment includes chelation therapy for copper overload, and limiting intake of copper-rich foods. Severe liver damage may require transplantation.

X-Linked Disorders

Adrenoleukodystrophy

This leukodystrophy is secondary to mutations in the *ABCD1* gene (located at Xq28), which codes for the peroxisomal enzyme lignoceroyl-CoA ligase, and results in build-up of very long-chain fatty acids (VLCFA) in the peroxisome. Symptoms are related to accumulation of VLCFA in the myelin of the CNS, in the adrenal cortex, and the Leydig cells of the testes. Adrenoleukodystrophy (X-ALD) can occur in three forms: the childhood cerebral form, adrenomyeloneuropathy (a later-onset, slowly progressive course), and Addison's disease (with adrenal findings only). In the cerebral early-onset form, the earliest symptoms are often mistaken for ADHD.[231,232] Later, symptoms of progressive cognitive impairment, vision and hearing losses, gait abnormalities, dysarthria, and dysphagia become apparent. Mood and psychotic symptoms are also frequently seen, especially in the late-onset forms.[233,234] Brain MRI scans show leukodystrophy, and are often a major clue to diagnosis. In addition, elevated levels of VLCFA can be measured in the blood of affected boys, as well as indications of adrenal dysfunction. Mutation testing is not usually performed, as the mutations are almost always unique to a particular family. Female carriers of the disorder may show symptoms as well, but these tend to be much milder than those of affected males.

Mitochondrial Disorders

Optimal mitochondrial performance requires many pathways related to energy production, including fatty acid oxidation, the electron transport chain, the Kreb cycle, and oxidative phosphorylation. In addition, disorders of carnitine (important for fatty acid transportation into the mitochondria) and pyruvate metabolism are also related to mitochondrial operation. Genes that control mitochondrial function are located both in the mitochondria's own genome and in the nuclear genome, so inheritance of these disorders may be mitochondrial or autosomal. Associated symptoms of mitochondrial dysfunction vary widely depending on which gene and pathway are involved, from specific disorders (e.g., mitochondrial encephalomyopathy with lactic acidosis and stroke-like episodes [MELAS]) to more general symptoms of energy depletion. Organ systems that are high-energy utilizers (e.g., the brain, heart, and skeletal muscle) are most likely to be affected. For this reason, multi-system involvement is often the hallmark of a mitochondrial disease. The combination of psychiatric symptoms with indications of organ dysfunction (e.g., cardiomyopathy, hypotonia, seizure, lactic acidosis, hypoglycemia, lethargy, and encephalopathy) may indicate the presence of a disorder of energy metabolism. Depending on the disorder, results of specialized metabolic studies (e.g., levels of lactate, pyruvate, urine organic acids, and plasma acylcarnitine) or molecular tests may be used for diagnostic work-up. Treatment in the form of dietary modification or supplements is offered for some disorders.

CONCLUSION

Even in aggregate, the above disorders will be responsible for a very limited number of patients with psychiatric symptoms; nonetheless, they do occur. For these individuals, making a correct diagnosis is paramount to maximize medical care and support services, and to guide psychiatric treatment. Psychiatrists should think broadly in their differential diagnosis of psychiatric symptoms, especially for patients with co-morbid medical conditions. Overall, being attentive to "red flags" that arise in the examination of patients will help identify those who require further diagnostic investigation and referral to a specialist.

CLINICAL APPLICATIONS OF PSYCHIATRIC GENETICS

The most important clinical dividend of psychiatric genetic research may be its potential to advance our understanding of the biology and treatment of neuropsychiatric disease. The genetic dissection of psychiatric illness may reveal new etiological pathways and targets for drug development, leading to novel approaches to treatment. Pharmacogenetic predictors of drug response may help optimize treatment assignment in the future. Both of these prospects await further research.

Genetic research of psychiatric disorders has provided information that is clinically relevant. As described previously, several medical genetic disorders have prominent psychiatric manifestations, and familiarity with these entities is relevant for differential diagnosis in cases where other clinical features are suggestive of a syndromic phenotype. For example, it has been estimated that 1%–2% of patients with symptoms of schizophrenia in psychiatric settings have unrecognized velo-cardiofacial syndrome, and the features of schizophrenia in patients with VCFS are not readily distinguishable from the phenotype of schizophrenia in patients without VCFS.[235] Consideration of medical genetic disorders is also highly relevant in the evaluation of children with developmental disorders and intellectual disability. As described previously, genetic testing for Mendelian disorders and chromosomal abnormalities is currently available, and referral to genetic professionals (e.g., medical geneticists and genetic counselors) is appropriate for such patients.

For common forms of psychiatric illness, specific susceptibility genes and their clinical relevance are starting to be identified. Genetic epidemiological studies provide information that may inform psychoeducation and even genetic counseling.[236] A positive family history is currently the best established risk factor for a wide range of psychiatric disorders, including psychotic, mood, and anxiety disorders.[237] Family studies provide empirical recurrence risks (risks of disorder to relatives of affected individuals), and these have been reviewed in detail elsewhere. Providing information about such risks is a key component of genetic counseling, which, according to the definition accepted by the National Society for Genetic Counselors, is "the process of helping people understand and adapt to the medical, psychological and familial implications of genetic contributions to disease. This process integrates:

- Collection and interpretation of family and medical histories to assess the chance of disease occurrence or recurrence
- Education about inheritance, testing, management, prevention, resources and research
- Counseling to promote informed choices and adaptation to the risk or condition."

Interested readers are referred to more detailed reviews of the nature, practice, and implications of psychiatric genetic counseling.[236,238]

Given the evidence that common forms of psychiatric illness are multi-factorial and polygenic and that susceptibility genes are likely to have small effects, it is not clear that clinically-useful genetic tests will be feasible for such conditions. The example of late-onset Alzheimer's disease (AD) is instructive in considering the impact of genetic testing for complex psychiatric disorders. While testing is currently available on a clinical basis in the US for autosomal dominant forms of early-onset AD, these highly penetrant mutations account for fewer than 5% of total AD cases. The best-established genetic risk factor for late-onset AD is the *APOE* *ε4* allele of the apolipoprotein E gene. However, given the lack of highly effective preventive or therapeutic interventions for AD, the potential for stigmatization and discrimination based on test results, and the fact that the APOE risk allele is neither necessary nor sufficient for the development of AD, there continues to be a consensus that APOE testing should not, at least for now, be used for predictive purposes.[239,240] Nevertheless, evidence from a randomized clinical trial suggests that demand for APOE testing might exceed available resources for counseling and testing if it were widely offered.[241] The high prevalence of several psychiatric disorders suggests that similar concerns might apply if susceptibility gene testing was offered.

With the advent of genome-wide genotyping and the prospect of affordable genome-wide sequencing in the near future, it is possible that simultaneous testing of multiple susceptibility alleles could be used to produce highly predictive genetic tests for complex diseases.[242] It is important to note that even if the scientific and statistical limitations of testing can be overcome, the complex ethical issues, coupled with the potential for adverse psychological effects that might accompany genetic testing for psychiatric disorders, would require careful consideration before such tests could be introduced.[238,243] The feasibility of testing is different from the desirability or clinical utility of testing, which may depend on the availability of effective interventions for those at increased risk, the adverse psychological and economic impact of false positives and false negatives, and other factors that are not strictly features of test performance. Nevertheless, it is likely that as advances in psychiatric genetics and genomic medicine proceed, psychiatrists may increasingly be called on to incorporate this information into clinical practice. The need for additional education in genetics for clinicians was underscored by a survey of more than 350 psychiatrists. While nearly 80% did not feel competent to convey genetic information to patients and their families, more than 80% thought that it was their role to do so, and 93% said that they discuss genetic contributions to illness with at least some of their patients.[244]

Access a list of MCQs for this chapter at https://expertconsult.inkling.com

REFERENCES

1. Venter JC, Adams MD, Myers EW, et al. The sequence of the human genome. *Science* 291(5507):1304–1351, 2001.
2. Lander ES, Linton LM, Birren B, et al. Initial sequencing and analysis of the human genome. *Nature* 409(6822):860–921, 2001.
3. Consortium EP, Dunham I, Kundaje A, et al. An integrated encyclopedia of DNA elements in the human genome. *Nature* 489(7414):57–74, 2012.
4. Malhotra D, Sebat J. CNVs: harbingers of a rare variant revolution in psychiatric genetics. *Cell* 148(6):1223–1241, 2012.
5. Murphy KC. Schizophrenia and velo-cardio-facial syndrome. *Lancet* 359(9304):426–430, 2002.
6. Morton NE. Linkage disequilibrium maps and association mapping. *J Clin Invest* 115(6):1425–1430, 2005.
7. International HapMap C. A haplotype map of the human genome. *Nature* 437(7063):1299–1320, 2005.
8. Spielman RS, Bastone LA, Burdick JT, et al. Common genetic variants account for differences in gene expression among ethnic groups. *Nat Genet* 39(2):226–231, 2007.
9. van Vliet J, Oates NA, Whitelaw E. Epigenetic mechanisms in the context of complex diseases. *Cell Mol Life Sci* 64(12):1531–1538, 2007.
10. Tsankova N, Renthal W, Kumar A, et al. Epigenetic regulation in psychiatric disorders. *Nat Rev Neurosci* 8(5):355–367, 2007.
11. Tsankova NM, Berton O, Renthal W, et al. Sustained hippocampal chromatin regulation in a mouse model of depression and antidepressant action. *Nat Neurosci* 9(4):519–525, 2006. PubMed PMID: 16501568.
12. Meaney MJ, Szyf M, Seckl JR. Epigenetic mechanisms of perinatal programming of hypothalamic-pituitary-adrenal function and health. *Trends Mol Med* 13(7):269–277, 2007. PubMed PMID: 17544850.
13. Rana TM. Illuminating the silence: understanding the structure and function of small RNAs. *Nat Rev Mol Cell Biol* 8(1):23–36, 2007. PubMed PMID: 17183358.
14. Sullivan PF, Daly MJ, O'Donovan M. Genetic architectures of psychiatric disorders: the emerging picture and its implications. *Nat Rev Genet* 13(8):537–551, 2012. PubMed PMID: 22777127.
15. Malhotra D, McCarthy S, Michaelson JJ, et al. High frequencies of de novo CNVs in bipolar disorder and schizophrenia. *Neuron* 72(6):951–963, 2011. PubMed PMID: 22196331.
16. Kirov G, Pocklington AJ, Holmans P, et al. De novo CNV analysis implicates specific abnormalities of postsynaptic signalling complexes in the pathogenesis of schizophrenia. *Mol Psychiatry* 17(2):142–153, 2012. PubMed PMID: 22083728. Pubmed Central PMCID: 3603134.
17. Ebert DH, Greenberg ME. Activity-dependent neuronal signalling and autism spectrum disorder. *Nature* 493(7432):327–337, 2013. PubMed PMID: 23325215. Pubmed Central PMCID: 3576027.
18. Solovieff N, Cotsapas C, Lee PH, et al. Pleiotropy in complex traits: challenges and strategies. *Nat Rev Genet* 14(7):483–495, 2013. PubMed PMID: 23752797.
19. Cross-Disorder Group of the Psychiatric Genomics C, Smoller JW, Craddock N, et al. Identification of risk loci with shared effects on five major psychiatric disorders: a genome-wide analysis. *Lancet* 381(9875):1371–1379, 2013. PubMed PMID: 23453885.
20. Sebat J, Lakshmi B, Malhotra D, et al. Strong association of de novo copy number mutations with autism. *Science* 316(5823):445–449, 2007. PubMed PMID: 17363630. Pubmed Central PMCID: 2993504.
21. Sanders SJ, Ercan-Sencicek AG, Hus V, et al. Multiple recurrent de novo CNVs, including duplications of the 7q11.23 Williams syndrome region, are strongly associated with autism. *Neuron* 70(5):863–885, 2011. PubMed PMID: 21658581.
22. Levy D, Ronemus M, Yamrom B, et al. Rare de novo and transmitted copy-number variation in autistic spectrum disorders. *Neuron* 70(5):886–897, 2011. PubMed PMID: 21658582.
23. Pinto D, Pagnamenta AT, Klei L, et al. Functional impact of global rare copy number variation in autism spectrum disorders. *Nature* 466(7304):368–372, 2010. PubMed PMID: 20531469. Pubmed Central PMCID: 3021798.
24. Walsh T, McClellan JM, McCarthy SE, et al. Rare structural variants disrupt multiple genes in neurodevelopmental pathways in schizophrenia. *Science* 320(5875):539–543, 2008. PubMed PMID: 18369103.
25. International Schizophrenia C. Rare chromosomal deletions and duplications increase risk of schizophrenia. *Nature* 455(7210):237–241, 2008. PubMed PMID: 18668038.
26. Xu B, Roos JL, Levy S, et al. Strong association of de novo copy number mutations with sporadic schizophrenia. *Nat Genet* 40(7):880–885, 2008. PubMed PMID: 18511947.
27. Yu TW, Chahrour MH, Coulter ME, et al. Using whole-exome sequencing to identify inherited causes of autism. *Neuron* 77(2):259–273, 2013. PubMed PMID: 23352163. Pubmed Central PMCID: 3694430.
28. Sanders SJ, Murtha MT, Gupta AR, et al. De novo mutations revealed by whole-exome sequencing are strongly associated with autism. *Nature* 485(7397):237–241, 2012. PubMed PMID: 22495306. Pubmed Central PMCID: 3667984.
29. Neale BM, Kou Y, Liu L, et al. Patterns and rates of exonic de novo mutations in autism spectrum disorders. *Nature* 485(7397):242–245, 2012. PubMed PMID: 22495311. Pubmed Central PMCID: 3613847.
30. Lim ET, Raychaudhuri S, Sanders SJ, et al. Rare complete knockouts in humans: population distribution and significant role in autism spectrum disorders. *Neuron* 77(2):235–242, 2013. PubMed PMID: 23352160. Pubmed Central PMCID: 3613849.
31. O'Roak BJ, Deriziotis P, Lee C, et al. Exome sequencing in sporadic autism spectrum disorders identifies severe de novo mutations. *Nat Genet* 43(6):585–589, 2011. PubMed PMID: 21572417. Pubmed Central PMCID: 3115696.
32. O'Roak BJ, Vives L, Girirajan S, et al. Sporadic autism exomes reveal a highly interconnected protein network of de novo mutations. *Nature* 485(7397):246–250, 2012. PubMed PMID: 22495309. Pubmed Central PMCID: 3350576.
33. Kong A, Frigge ML, Masson G, et al. Rate of de novo mutations and the importance of father's age to disease risk. *Nature* 488(7412):471–475, 2012. PubMed PMID: 22914163. Pubmed Central PMCID: 3548427.
34. Caspi A, Moffitt TE. Gene-environment interactions in psychiatry: joining forces with neuroscience. *Nat Rev Neurosci* 7(7):583–590, 2006. PubMed PMID: 16791147.
35. Gottesman II, Gould TD. The endophenotype concept in psychiatry: etymology and strategic intentions. *Am J Psychiatry* 160(4):636–645, 2003. PubMed PMID: 12668349.
36. Freedman R, Adams CE, Adler LE, et al. Inhibitory neurophysiological deficit as a phenotype for genetic investigation of

schizophrenia. *Am J Med Genet* 97(1):58–64, 2000. PubMed PMID: 10813805.

37. Hall MH, Rijsdijk F, Picchioni M, et al. et al. Substantial shared genetic influences on schizophrenia and event-related potentials. *Am J Psychiatry* 164(5):804–812, 2007. PubMed PMID: 17475740.

38. Freedman R, Adler LE, Leonard S. Alternative phenotypes for the complex genetics of schizophrenia. *Biol Psychiatry* 45(5):551–558, 1999. PubMed PMID: 10088045.

39. Leonard S, Gault J, Hopkins J, et al. Association of promoter variants in the alpha7 nicotinic acetylcholine receptor subunit gene with an inhibitory deficit found in schizophrenia. *Arch Gen Psychiatry* 59(12):1085–1096, 2002. PubMed PMID: 12470124.

40. Freedman R, Coon H, Myles-Worsley M, et al. Linkage of a neurophysiological deficit in schizophrenia to a chromosome 15 locus. *Proc Natl Acad Sci U S A* 94(2):587–592, 1997.

41. Cruchaga C, Kauwe JS, Harari O, et al. GWAS of cerebrospinal fluid tau levels identifies risk variants for Alzheimer's disease. *Neuron* 78(2):256–268, 2013. PubMed PMID: 23562540. Pubmed Central PMCID: 3664945.

42. Meyer-Lindenberg A, Weinberger DR. Intermediate phenotypes and genetic mechanisms of psychiatric disorders. *Nat Rev Neurosci* 7(10):818–827, 2006. PubMed PMID: 16988657.

43. Pezawas L, Meyer-Lindenberg A, Drabant EM, et al. 5-HTTLPR polymorphism impacts human cingulate-amygdala interactions: a genetic susceptibility mechanism for depression. *Nat Neurosci* 8(6):828–834, 2005. PubMed PMID: 15880108.

44. Hariri AR, Drabant EM, Weinberger DR. Imaging genetics: perspectives from studies of genetically driven variation in serotonin function and corticolimbic affective processing. *Biol Psychiatry* 59(10):888–897, 2006. PubMed PMID: 16442081.

45. Egan MF, Goldberg TE, Kolachana BS, et al. Effect of COMT Val108/158 Met genotype on frontal lobe function and risk for schizophrenia. *Proc Natl Acad Sci U S A* 98(12):6917–6922, 2001.

46. Faraone SV, Perlis RH, Doyle AE, et al. Molecular genetics of attention-deficit/hyperactivity disorder. *Biol Psychiatry* 57(11): 1313–1323, 2005. PubMed PMID: 15950004.

47. Biederman J, Faraone SV, Keenan K, et al. Evidence of familial association between attention deficit disorder and major affective disorders. *Arch Gen Psychiatry* 48(7):633–642, 1991. PubMed PMID: 2069494.

48. Faraone SV, Biederman J, Mennin D, et al. Familial subtypes of attention deficit hyperactivity disorder: a 4-year follow-up study of children from antisocial-ADHD families. *J Child Psychol Psychiatry* 39(7):1045–1053, 1998. PubMed PMID: 9804037.

49. Faraone SV, Biederman J, Mennin D, et al. Bipolar and antisocial disorders among relatives of ADHD children: parsing familial subtypes of illness. *Am J Med Genet* 81(1):108–116, 1998. PubMed PMID: 9514596.

50. Faraone SV, Biederman J, Jetton JG, et al. Attention deficit disorder and conduct disorder: longitudinal evidence for a familial subtype. *Psychol Med* 27(2):291–300, 1997. PubMed PMID: 9089822.

51. Williams NM, Zaharieva I, Martin A, et al. Rare chromosomal deletions and duplications in attention-deficit hyperactivity disorder: a genome-wide analysis. *Lancet* 376(9750):1401–1408, 2010. PubMed PMID: 20888040. Pubmed Central PMCID: 2965350.

52. Elia J, Gai X, Xie HM, et al. Rare structural variants found in attention-deficit hyperactivity disorder are preferentially associated with neurodevelopmental genes. *Mol Psychiatry* 15(6):637–646, 2010. PubMed PMID: 19546859. Pubmed Central PMCID: 2877197.

53. Smalley SL, Kustanovich V, Minassian SL, et al. Genetic linkage of attention-deficit/hyperactivity disorder on chromosome 16p13, in a region implicated in autism. *Am J Hum Genet* 71(4):959–963, 2002. PubMed PMID: 12187510. Pubmed Central PMCID: 378550.

54. Elia J, Glessner JT, Wang K, et al. Genome-wide copy number variation study associates metabotropic glutamate receptor gene networks with attention deficit hyperactivity disorder. *Nat Genet* 44(1):78–84, 2012. PubMed PMID: 22138692.

55. Hamshere ML, Stergiakouli E, Langley K, et al. A shared polygenic contribution between childhood ADHD and adult schizophrenia. *Br J Psychiatry* 2013. PubMed PMID: 23703318.

56. Abrahams BS, Geschwind DH. Advances in autism genetics: on the threshold of a new neurobiology. *Nat Rev Genet* 9(5):341–355, 2008. PubMed PMID: 18414403. Pubmed Central PMCID: 2756414.

57. Freitag CM. The genetics of autistic disorders and its clinical relevance: a review of the literature. *Mol Psychiatry* 12(1):2–22, 2007. PubMed PMID: 17033636.

58. Volkmar FR, Pauls D. Autism. *Lancet* 362(9390):1133–1141, 2003. PubMed PMID: 14550703.

59. State MW, Levitt P. The conundrums of understanding genetic risks for autism spectrum disorders. *Nat Neurosci* 14(12):1499–1506, 2011. PubMed PMID: 22037497.

60. Keen-Kim D, Freimer NB. Genetics and epidemiology of Tourette syndrome. *J Child Neurol* 21(8):665–671, 2006. PubMed PMID: 16970867.

61. Pauls DL, Raymond CL, Stevenson JM, et al. A family study of Gilles de la Tourette syndrome. *Am J Hum Genet* 48(1):154–163, 1991. PubMed PMID: 1985456. Pubmed Central PMCID: 1682764.

62. State MW. The genetics of Tourette disorder. *Curr Opin Genet Dev* 21(3):302–309, 2011. PubMed PMID: 21277193, Pubmed Central PMCID: 3102152.

63. Abelson JF, Kwan KY, O'Roak BJ, et al. Sequence variants in SLITRK1 are associated with Tourette's syndrome. *Science* 310(5746):317–320, 2005. PubMed PMID: 16224024.

64. Scharf JM, Yu D, Mathews CA, et al. Genome-wide association study of Tourette's syndrome. *Mol Psychiatry* 18(6):721–728, 2013. PubMed PMID: 22889924. Pubmed Central PMCID: 3605224.

65. Blennow K, de Leon MJ, Zetterberg H. Alzheimer's disease. *Lancet* 368(9533):387–403, 2006. PubMed PMID: 16876668.

66. Green RC, Cupples LA, Go R, et al. Risk of dementia among white and African American relatives of patients with Alzheimer disease. *JAMA* 287(3):329–336, 2002. PubMed PMID: 11790212.

67. Pedersen NL, Gatz M, Berg S, et al. How heritable is Alzheimer's disease late in life? Findings from Swedish twins. *Ann Neurol* 55(2):180–185, 2004. PubMed PMID: 14755721.

68. Gatz M, Reynolds CA, Fratiglioni L, et al. Role of genes and environments for explaining Alzheimer disease. *Arch Gen Psychiatry* 63(2):168–174, 2006. PubMed PMID: 16461860.

69. Bergem AL, Engedal K, Kringlen E. The role of heredity in late-onset Alzheimer disease and vascular dementia. A twin study. *Arch Gen Psychiatry* 54(3):264–270, 1997. PubMed PMID: 9075467.

70. Bettens K, Sleegers K, Van Broeckhoven C. Genetic insights in Alzheimer's disease. *Lancet Neurol* 12(1):92–104, 2013. PubMed PMID: 23237904.

71. Blacker D, Haines JL, Rodes L, et al. ApoE-4 and age at onset of Alzheimer's disease: the NIMH genetics initiative. *Neurology* 48(1):139–147, 1997. PubMed PMID: 9008509.

72. Naj AC, Jun G, Beecham GW, et al. Common variants at MS4A4/MS4A6E, CD2AP, CD33 and EPHA1 are associated with late-onset Alzheimer's disease. *Nat Genet* 43(5):436–441, 2011. PubMed PMID: 21460841. Pubmed Central PMCID: 3090745.

73. Lambert JC, Heath S, Even G, et al. Genome-wide association study identifies variants at CLU and CR1 associated with Alzheimer's disease. *Nat Genet* 41(10):1094–1099, 2009. PubMed PMID: 19734903.

74. Hollingworth P, Harold D, Sims R, et al. Common variants at ABCA7, MS4A6A/MS4A4E, EPHA1, CD33 and CD2AP are associated with Alzheimer's disease. *Nat Genet* 43(5):429–435, 2011. PubMed PMID: 21460840. Pubmed Central PMCID: 3084173.

75. Harold D, Abraham R, Hollingworth P, et al. Genome-wide association study identifies variants at CLU and PICALM associated with Alzheimer's disease. *Nat Genet* 41(10):1088–1093, 2009. PubMed PMID: 19734902. Pubmed Central PMCID: 2845877.

76. Rogaeva E, Meng Y, Lee JH, et al. The neuronal sortilin-related receptor SORL1 is genetically associated with Alzheimer disease. *Nat Genet* 39(2):168–177, 2007. PubMed PMID: 17220890. Pubmed Central PMCID: 2657343.

77. Reitz C, Cheng R, Rogaeva E, et al. Meta-analysis of the association between variants in SORL1 and Alzheimer disease. *Arch Neurol* 68(1):99–106, 2011. PubMed PMID: 21220680. Pubmed Central PMCID: 3086666.

78. Pottier C, Hannequin D, Coutant S, et al. High frequency of potentially pathogenic SORL1 mutations in autosomal dominant early-onset Alzheimer disease. *Mol Psychiatry* 17(9):875–879, 2012. PubMed PMID: 22472873.

79. Tsuang M. Schizophrenia: genes and environment. *Biol Psychiatry* 47(3):210–220, 2000. PubMed PMID: 10682218.

80. Cardno AG, Gottesman II. Twin studies of schizophrenia: from bow-and-arrow concordances to star wars Mx and functional genomics. *Am J Med Genet* 97(1):12–17, 2000. PubMed PMID: 10813800.

81. Rujescu D, Ingason A, Cichon S, et al. Disruption of the neurexin 1 gene is associated with schizophrenia. *Hum Mol Genet* 18(5):988–996, 2009. PubMed PMID: 18945720. Pubmed Central PMCID: 2695245.

82. Vacic V, McCarthy S, Malhotra D, et al. Duplications of the neuropeptide receptor gene VIPR2 confer significant risk for schizophrenia. *Nature* 471(7339):499–503, 2011. PubMed PMID: 21346763. Pubmed Central PMCID: 3351382.

83. Stefansson H, Ophoff RA, Steinberg S, et al. Common variants conferring risk of schizophrenia. *Nature* 460(7256):744–747, 2009. PubMed PMID: 19571808. Pubmed Central PMCID: 3077530.

84. Shi J, Levinson DF, Duan J, et al. Common variants on chromosome 6p22.1 are associated with schizophrenia. *Nature* 460(7256):753–757, 2009. PubMed PMID: 19571809. Pubmed Central PMCID: 2775422.

85. International Schizophrenia C, Purcell SM, Wray NR, et al. Common polygenic variation contributes to risk of schizophrenia and bipolar disorder. *Nature* 460(7256):748–752, 2009. PubMed PMID: 19571811.

86. Gejman PV, Sanders AR, Kendler KS. Genetics of schizophrenia: new findings and challenges. *Annu Rev Genomics Hum Genet* 12:121–144, 2011. PubMed PMID: 21639796.

87. O'Donovan MC, Craddock N, Norton N, et al. Identification of loci associated with schizophrenia by genome-wide association and follow-up. *Nat Genet* 40(9):1053–1055, 2008. PubMed PMID: 18677311.

88. Schizophrenia Psychiatric Genome-Wide Association Study C. Genome-wide association study identifies five new schizophrenia loci. *Nat Genet* 43(10):969–976, 2011. PubMed PMID: 21926974. Pubmed Central PMCID: 3303194.

89. Smoller JW, Finn CT. Family, twin, and adoption studies of bipolar disorder. *Am J Med Genet C Semin Med Genet* 123C(1):48–58, 2003. PubMed PMID: 14601036.

90. Mendlewicz J, Rainer JD. Adoption study supporting genetic transmission in manic–depressive illness. *Nature* 268(5618):327–329, 1977. PubMed PMID: 887159.

91. McGuffin P, Rijsdijk F, Andrew M, et al. The heritability of bipolar affective disorder and the genetic relationship to unipolar depression. *Arch Gen Psychiatry* 60(5):497–502, 2003. PubMed PMID: 12742871.

92. Kieseppa T, Partonen T, Haukka J, et al. High concordance of bipolar I disorder in a nationwide sample of twins. *Am J Psychiatry* 161(10):1814–1821, 2004. PubMed PMID: 15465978.

93. Cardno AG, Rijsdijk FV, Sham PC, et al. A twin study of genetic relationships between psychotic symptoms. *Am J Psychiatry* 159(4):539–545, 2002. PubMed PMID: 11925290.

94. Craddock N, Sklar P. Genetics of bipolar disorder. *Lancet* 381(9878):1654–1662, 2013. PubMed PMID: 23663951.

95. Ferreira MA, O'Donovan MC, Meng YA, et al. Collaborative genome-wide association analysis supports a role for ANK3 and CACNA1C in bipolar disorder. *Nat Genet* 40(9):1056–1058, 2008. PubMed PMID: 18711365. Pubmed Central PMCID: 2703780.

96. Cichon S, Muhleisen TW, Degenhardt FA, et al. Genome-wide association study identifies genetic variation in neurocan as a susceptibility factor for bipolar disorder. *Am J Hum Genet* 88(3):372–381, 2011. PubMed PMID: 21353194. Pubmed Central PMCID: 3059436.

97. Sullivan PF, Neale MC, Kendler KS. Genetic epidemiology of major depression: review and meta-analysis. *Am J Psychiatry* 157(10):1552–1562, 2000. PubMed PMID: 11007705.

98. Weissman MM, Merikangas KR, Wickramaratne P, et al. Understanding the clinical heterogeneity of major depression using family data. *Arch Gen Psychiatry* 43(5):430–434, 1986. PubMed PMID: 3964021.

99. Mondimore FM, Zandi PP, Mackinnon DF, et al. Familial aggregation of illness chronicity in recurrent, early-onset major depression pedigrees. *Am J Psychiatry* 163(9):1554–1560, 2006. PubMed PMID: 16946180.

100. Klein DN, Shankman SA, Lewinsohn PM, et al. Family study of chronic depression in a community sample of young adults. *Am J Psychiatry* 161(4):646–653, 2004. PubMed PMID: 15056510.

101. Kendler KS, Gardner CO, Prescott CA. Corrections to 2 prior published articles. *Arch Gen Psychiatry* 57(1):94–95, 2000. PubMed PMID: 10632241.

102. Kendler KS, Gardner CO, Prescott CA. Clinical characteristics of major depression that predict risk of depression in relatives. *Arch Gen Psychiatry* 56(4):322–327, 1999. PubMed PMID: 10197826.

103. Kendler KS, Gatz M, Gardner CO, et al. A Swedish national twin study of lifetime major depression. *Am J Psychiatry* 163(1):109–114, 2006. PubMed PMID: 16390897.

104. Major Depressive Disorder Working Group of the Psychiatric GC, Ripke S, Wray NR, et al. A mega-analysis of genome-wide association studies for major depressive disorder. *Mol Psychiatry* 18(4):497–511, 2013. PubMed PMID: 22472876.

105. Caspi A, Sugden K, Moffitt TE, et al. Influence of life stress on depression: moderation by a polymorphism in the 5-HTT gene. *Science* 301(5631):386–389, 2003. PubMed PMID: 12869766.

106. Uher R, McGuffin P. The moderation by the serotonin transporter gene of environmental adversity in the etiology of depression: 2009 update. *Mol Psychiatry* 15(1):18–22, 2010. PubMed PMID: 20029411.

107. Risch N, Herrell R, Lehner T, et al. Interaction between the serotonin transporter gene (5-HTTLPR), stressful life events, and risk of depression: a meta-analysis. *JAMA* 301(23):2462–2471, 2009. PubMed PMID: 19531760. Pubmed Central PMCID: 2938776.

108. Munafo MR, Durrant C, Lewis G, et al. Gene X environment interactions at the serotonin transporter locus. *Biol Psychiatry* 65(3):211–219, 2009. PubMed PMID: 18691701.

109. Karg K, Burmeister M, Shedden K, et al. The serotonin transporter promoter variant (5-HTTLPR), stress, and depression meta-analysis revisited: evidence of genetic moderation. *Arch Gen Psychiatry* 68(5):444–454, 2011. PubMed PMID: 21199959.

110. Fergusson DM, Horwood LJ, Miller AL, et al. Life stress, 5-HTTLPR and mental disorder: findings from a 30-year longitudinal study. *Br J Psychiatry* 198(2):129–135, 2011. PubMed PMID: 21282783. Pubmed Central PMCID: 3031653.

111. Hettema JM, Neale MC, Kendler KS. A review and meta-analysis of the genetic epidemiology of anxiety disorders. *Am J Psychiatry* 158(10):1568–1578, 2001. PubMed PMID: 11578982.

112. Goldstein RB, Wickramaratne PJ, Horwath E, et al. Familial aggregation and phenomenology of 'early'-onset (at or before age 20 years) panic disorder. *Arch Gen Psychiatry* 54(3):271–278, 1997. PubMed PMID: 9075468.

113. Smoller JW, Tsuang MT. Panic and phobic anxiety: defining phenotypes for genetic studies. *Am J Psychiatry* 155(9):1152–1162, 1998. PubMed PMID: 9734536.

114. Scherrer JF, True WR, Xian H, et al. Evidence for genetic influences common and specific to symptoms of generalized anxiety and panic. *J Affect Disord* 57(1–3):25–35, 2000. PubMed PMID: 10708813.

115. Hettema JM, Prescott CA, Myers JM, et al. The structure of genetic and environmental risk factors for anxiety disorders in men and women. *Arch Gen Psychiatry* 62(2):182–189, 2005. PubMed PMID: 15699295.

116. Chantarujikapong SI, Scherrer JF, Xian H, et al. A twin study of generalized anxiety disorder symptoms, panic disorder symptoms and post-traumatic stress disorder in men. *Psychiatry Res* 103(2–3):133–145, 2001. PubMed PMID: 11549402.

117. McGrath LM, Weill S, Robinson EB, et al. Bringing a developmental perspective to anxiety genetics. *Dev Psychopathol* 24(4):1179–1193, 2012. PubMed PMID: 23062290. Pubmed Central PMCID: 3721501.

118. Smoller JW. Who's afraid of anxiety genetics? *Biol Psychiatry* 69(6):506–507, 2011. PubMed PMID: 21353834.

119. Kendler KS, Neale MC, Kessler RC, et al. The genetic epidemiology of phobias in women. The interrelationship of agoraphobia, social phobia, situational phobia, and simple phobia. *Arch Gen Psychiatry* 49(4):273–281, 1992. PubMed PMID: 1558461.

120. Newman SC, Bland RC. A population-based family study of DSM-III generalized anxiety disorder. *Psychol Med* 36(9):1275–1281, 2006. PubMed PMID: 16700965.

121. Roy MA, Neale MC, Pedersen NL, et al. A twin study of generalized anxiety disorder and major depression. *Psychol Med* 25(5):1037–1049, 1995. PubMed PMID: 8588001.

122. Kendler KS, Gardner CO, Gatz M, et al. The sources of co-morbidity between major depression and generalized anxiety disorder in a Swedish national twin sample. *Psychol Med* 37(3):453–462, 2007. PubMed PMID: 17121688.

123. Hanna GL, Himle JA, Curtis GC, et al. A family study of obsessive-compulsive disorder with pediatric probands. *Am J Med Genet B Neuropsychiatr Genet* 134B(1):13–19, 2005. PubMed PMID: 15635694.

124. do Rosario-Campos MC, Leckman JF, Curi M, et al. A family study of early-onset obsessive-compulsive disorder. *Am J Med Genet B Neuropsychiatr Genet* 136B(1):92–97, 2005. PubMed PMID: 15892140.

125. Fyer AJ, Lipsitz JD, Mannuzza S, et al. A direct interview family study of obsessive-compulsive disorder. I. *Psychol Med* 35(11):1611–1621, 2005. PubMed PMID: 16219119.

126. Grados MA, Riddle MA, Samuels JF, et al. The familial phenotype of obsessive-compulsive disorder in relation to tic disorders: the Hopkins OCD family study. *Biol Psychiatry* 50(8):559–565, 2001. PubMed PMID: 11690590.

127. Clifford CA, Murray RM, Fulker DW. Genetic and environmental influences on obsessional traits and symptoms. *Psychol Med* 14(4):791–800, 1984. PubMed PMID: 6545413.

128. van Grootheest DS, Cath DC, Beekman AT, et al. Twin studies on obsessive-compulsive disorder: a review. *Twin Res Hum Genet* 8(5):450–458, 2005. PubMed PMID: 16212834.

129. Stewart SE, Fagerness JA, Platko J, et al. Association of the SLC1A1 glutamate transporter gene and obsessive-compulsive disorder. *Am J Med Genet B Neuropsychiatr Genet* 144B(8):1027–1033, 2007. PubMed PMID: 17894418.

130. Dickel DE, Veenstra-VanderWeele J, Cox NJ, et al. Association testing of the positional and functional candidate gene SLC1A1/EAAC1 in early-onset obsessive-compulsive disorder. *Arch Gen Psychiatry* 63(7):778–785, 2006. PubMed PMID: 16818867.

131. Arnold PD, Sicard T, Burroughs E, et al. Glutamate transporter gene SLC1A1 associated with obsessive-compulsive disorder. *Arch Gen Psychiatry* 63(7):769–776, 2006. PubMed PMID: 16818866.

132. Welch JM, Lu J, Rodriguiz RM, et al. Cortico-striatal synaptic defects and OCD-like behaviours in Sapap3-mutant mice. *Nature* 448(7156):894–900, 2007. PubMed PMID: 17713528. Pubmed Central PMCID: 2442572.

133. Zuchner S, Wendland JR, Ashley-Koch AE, et al. Multiple rare SAPAP3 missense variants in trichotillomania and OCD. *Mol Psychiatry* 14(1):6–9, 2009. PubMed PMID: 19096451. Pubmed Central PMCID: 2803344.

134. Bienvenu OJ, Wang Y, Shugart YY, et al. Sapap3 and pathological grooming in humans: Results from the OCD collaborative genetics study. *Am J Med Genet B Neuropsychiatr Genet* 150B(5):710–720, 2009. PubMed PMID: 19051237.

135. Stewart SE, Yu D, Scharf JM, et al. Genome-wide association study of obsessive-compulsive disorder. *Mol Psychiatry* 18(7):788–798, 2013. PubMed PMID: 22889921.

136. Nurnberger JI Jr, Wiegand R, Bucholz K, et al. A family study of alcohol dependence: coaggregation of multiple disorders in relatives of alcohol-dependent probands. *Arch Gen Psychiatry* 61(12):1246–1256, 2004. PubMed PMID: 15583116.

137. Merikangas KR, Stolar M, Stevens DE, et al. Familial transmission of substance use disorders. *Arch Gen Psychiatry* 55(11):973–979, 1998. PubMed PMID: 9819065.

138. Walters GD. The heritability of alcohol abuse and dependence: a meta-analysis of behavior genetic research. *Am J Drug Alcohol Abuse* 28(3):557–584, 2002. PubMed PMID: 12211366.

139. Liu IC, Blacker DL, Xu R, et al. Genetic and environmental contributions to the development of alcohol dependence in male twins. *Arch Gen Psychiatry* 61(9):897–903, 2004. PubMed PMID: 15351768.

140. Heath AC, Bucholz KK, Madden PA, et al. Genetic and environmental contributions to alcohol dependence risk in a national twin sample: consistency of findings in women and men. *Psychol Med* 27(6):1381–1396, 1997. PubMed PMID: 9403910.

141. Prescott CA, Kendler KS. Genetic and environmental contributions to alcohol abuse and dependence in a population-based sample of male twins. *Am J Psychiatry* 156(1):34–40, 1999. PubMed PMID: 9892295.

142. Yates WR, Cadoret RJ, Troughton E, et al. An adoption study of DSM-IIIR alcohol and drug dependence severity. *Drug Alcohol Depend* 41(1):9–15, 1996. PubMed PMID: 8793305.

143. Cadoret RJ, Yates WR, Troughton E, et al. Adoption study demonstrating two genetic pathways to drug abuse. *Arch Gen Psychiatry* 52(1):42–52, 1995. PubMed PMID: 7811161.

144. Wang JC, Kapoor M, Goate AM. The genetics of substance dependence. *Annu Rev Genomics Hum Genet* 13:241–261, 2012. PubMed PMID: 22703173. Pubmed Central PMCID: 3474605.

145. Kendler KS, Chen X, Dick D, et al. Recent advances in the genetic epidemiology and molecular genetics of substance use disorders. *Nat Neurosci* 15(2):181–189, 2012. PubMed PMID: 22281715. Pubmed Central PMCID: 3297622.

146. Agrawal A, Lynskey MT. The genetic epidemiology of cannabis use, abuse and dependence. *Addiction* 101(6):801–812, 2006. PubMed PMID: 16696624.

147. Saxon AJ, Oreskovich MR, Brkanac Z. Genetic determinants of addiction to opioids and cocaine. *Harv Rev Psychiatry* 13(4):218–232, 2005. PubMed PMID: 16126608.

148. Goldman D, Oroszi G, Ducci F. The genetics of addictions: uncovering the genes. *Nat Rev Genet* 6(7):521–532, 2005. PubMed PMID: 15995696.

149. Kendler KS, Jacobson KC, Prescott CA, et al. Specificity of genetic and environmental risk factors for use and abuse/dependence of cannabis, cocaine, hallucinogens, sedatives, stimulants, and opiates in male twins. *Am J Psychiatry* 160(4):687–695, 2003. PubMed PMID: 12668357.

150. Drakenberg K, Nikoshkov A, Horvath MC, et al. Mu opioid receptor A118G polymorphism in association with striatal opioid neuropeptide gene expression in heroin abusers. *Proc Natl Acad Sci U S A* 103(20):7883–7888, 2006.

151. Haile CN, Kosten TR, Kosten TA. Genetics of dopamine and its contribution to cocaine addiction. *Behav Genet* 37(1):119–145, 2007. PubMed PMID: 17063402.

152. Need AC, Motulsky AG, Goldstein DB. Priorities and standards in pharmacogenetic research. *Nat Genet* 37(7):671–681, 2005. PubMed PMID: 15990888.

153. Weinshilboum R, Wang L. Pharmacogenomics: bench to bedside. *Nat Rev Drug Discov* 3(9):739–748, 2004. PubMed PMID: 15340384.

154. Evans WE, Relling MV. Moving towards individualized medicine with pharmacogenomics. *Nature* 429(6990):464–468, 2004. PubMed PMID: 15164072.

155. Phillips KA, Van Bebber SL. Measuring the value of pharmacogenomics. *Nat Rev Drug Discov* 4(6):500–509, 2005. PubMed PMID: 15915153.

156. de Leon J, Armstrong SC, Cozza KL. Clinical guidelines for psychiatrists for the use of pharmacogenetic testing for CYP450 2D6 and CYP450 2C19. *Psychosomatics* 47(1):75–85, 2006. PubMed PMID: 16384813.

157. Kirchheiner J, Nickchen K, Bauer M, et al. Pharmacogenetics of antidepressants and antipsychotics: the contribution of allelic variations to the phenotype of drug response. *Mol Psychiatry* 9(5):442–473, 2004. PubMed PMID: 15037866.

158. Schenk PW, van Fessem MA, Verploegh-Van Rij S, et al. Association of graded allele-specific changes in CYP2D6 function with imipramine dose requirement in a large group of depressed patients. *Mol Psychiatry* 13(6):597–605, 2008. PubMed PMID: 17667959.

159. de Leon J, Susce MT, Pan RM, et al. The CYP2D6 poor metabolizer phenotype may be associated with risperidone adverse drug reactions and discontinuation. *J Clin Psychiatry* 66(1):15–27, 2005. PubMed PMID: 15669884.

160. Brockmoller J, Kirchheiner J, Schmider J, et al. The impact of the CYP2D6 polymorphism on haloperidol pharmacokinetics and on the outcome of haloperidol treatment. *Clin Pharmacol Ther* 72(4):438–452, 2002. PubMed PMID: 12386646.

161. Serretti A, Kato M, De Ronchi D, et al. Meta-analysis of serotonin transporter gene promoter polymorphism (5-HTTLPR) association with selective serotonin reuptake inhibitor efficacy in depressed patients. *Mol Psychiatry* 12(3):247–257, 2007. PubMed PMID: 17146470.

162. Perlis RH, Mischoulon D, Smoller JW, et al. Serotonin transporter polymorphisms and adverse effects with fluoxetine treatment. *Biol Psychiatry* 54(9):879–883, 2003. PubMed PMID: 14573314.

163. Murphy GM Jr, Hollander SB, Rodrigues HE, et al. Effects of the serotonin transporter gene promoter polymorphism on mirtazapine and paroxetine efficacy and adverse events in geriatric major depression. *Arch Gen Psychiatry* 61(11):1163–1169, 2004. PubMed PMID: 15520364.

164. Hu XZ, Rush AJ, Charney D, et al. Association between a functional serotonin transporter promoter polymorphism and citalopram treatment in adult outpatients with major depression. *Arch Gen Psychiatry* 64(7):783–792, 2007. PubMed PMID: 17606812.

165. Arranz MJ, de Leon J. Pharmacogenetics and pharmacogenomics of schizophrenia: a review of last decade of research. *Mol Psychiatry* 12(8):707–747, 2007. PubMed PMID: 17549063.

166. Mandoki MW, Sumner GS, Hoffman RP. Riconda DL. A review of Klinefelter's syndrome in children and adolescents. *J Am Acad Child Adolesc Psychiatry* 30(2):167–172, 1991. PubMed PMID: 2016217.

167. Boone KB, Swerdloff RS, Miller BL, et al. Neuropsychological profiles of adults with Klinefelter syndrome. *J Int Neuropsychol Soc* 7(4):446–456, 2001. PubMed PMID: 11396547.

168. van Rijn S, Aleman A, Swaab H, et al. Klinefelter's syndrome (karyotype 47,XXY) and schizophrenia-spectrum pathology. *Br J Psychiatry* 189:459–460, 2006. PubMed PMID: 17077438.

169. Giedd JN, Clasen LS, Wallace GL, et al. XXY (Klinefelter syndrome): a pediatric quantitative brain magnetic resonance imaging case-control study. *Pediatrics* 119(1):e232–e240, 2007. PubMed PMID: 17200249.

170. DeLisi LE, Maurizio AM, Svetina C, et al. Klinefelter's syndrome (XXY) as a genetic model for psychotic disorders. *Am J Med Genet B Neuropsychiatr Genet* 135B(1):15–23, 2005. PubMed PMID: 15729733.

171. Ross J, Zinn A, McCauley E. Neurodevelopmental and psychosocial aspects of Turner syndrome. *Ment Retard Dev Disabil Res Rev* 6(2):135–141, 2000. PubMed PMID: 10899807.

172. Lesniak-Karpiak K, Mazzocco MM, Ross JL. Behavioral assessment of social anxiety in females with Turner or fragile X syndrome. *J Autism Dev Disord* 33(1):55–67, 2003. PubMed PMID: 12708580.

173. Cardoso G, Daly R, Haq NA, et al. Current and lifetime psychiatric illness in women with Turner syndrome. *Gynecol Endocrinol* 19(6):313–319, 2004. PubMed PMID: 15726728.

174. Borgatti R, Piccinelli P, Passoni D, et al. Relationship between clinical and genetic features in "inverted duplicated chromosome 15" patients. *Pediatr Neurol* 24(2):111–116, 2001. PubMed PMID: 11275459.

175. Battaglia A. The inv dup(15) or idic(15) syndrome: a clinically recognisable neurogenetic disorder. *Brain Dev* 27(5):365–369, 2005. PubMed PMID: 16023554.

176. State MW, Dykens EM. Genetics of childhood disorders: XV. Prader-Willi syndrome: genes, brain, and behavior. *J Am Acad Child Adolesc Psychiatry* 39(6):797–800, 2000. PubMed PMID: 10846317.

177. Dykens EM, Leckman JF, Cassidy SB. Obsessions and compulsions in Prader-Willi syndrome. *J Child Psychol Psychiatry* 37(8):995–1002, 1996. PubMed PMID: 9119946.

178. Dykens E, Shah B. Psychiatric disorders in Prader-Willi syndrome: epidemiology and management. *CNS Drugs* 17(3):167–178, 2003. PubMed PMID: 12617696.

179. Clarke DJ, Boer H, Whittington J, et al. Prader-Willi syndrome, compulsive and ritualistic behaviours: the first population-based survey. *Br J Psychiatry* 180:358–362, 2002. PubMed PMID: 11925360.

180. Boer H, Holland A, Whittington J, et al. Psychotic illness in people with Prader Willi syndrome due to chromosome 15 maternal uniparental disomy. *Lancet* 359(9301):135–136, 2002. PubMed PMID: 11809260.

181. Bassett AS, Chow EW. 22q11 deletion syndrome: a genetic subtype of schizophrenia. *Biol Psychiatry* 46(7):882–891, 1999. PubMed PMID: 10509171. Pubmed Central PMCID: 3276595.

182. Sporn A, Addington A, Reiss AL, et al. 22q11 deletion syndrome in childhood onset schizophrenia: an update. *Mol Psychiatry* 9(3):225–226, 2004. PubMed PMID: 14699434.

183. Shprintzen RJ. Velo-cardio-facial syndrome: 30 Years of study. *Dev Disabil Res Rev* 14(1):3–10, 2008. PubMed PMID: 18636631. Pubmed Central PMCID: 2805186.

184. Karayiorgou M, Morris MA, Morrow B, et al. Schizophrenia susceptibility associated with interstitial deletions of chromosome 22q11. *Proc Natl Acad Sci U S A* 92(17):7612–7616, 1995.

185. Usiskin SI, Nicolson R, Krasnewich DM, et al. Velocardiofacial syndrome in childhood-onset schizophrenia. *J Am Acad Child Adolesc Psychiatry* 38(12):1536–1543, 1999. PubMed PMID: 10596254.

186. Papolos DF, Faedda GL, Veit S, et al. Bipolar spectrum disorders in patients diagnosed with velo-cardio-facial syndrome: does a hemizygous deletion of chromosome 22q11 result in bipolar affective disorder? *Am J Psychiatry* 153(12):1541–1547, 1996. PubMed PMID: 8942449.

187. Green T, Gothelf D, Glaser B, et al. Psychiatric disorders and intellectual functioning throughout development in velocardiofacial (22q11.2 deletion) syndrome. *J Am Acad Child Adolesc Psychiatry* 48(11):1060–1068, 2009. PubMed PMID: 19797984.

188. Gothelf D, Presburger G, Zohar AH, et al. Obsessive-compulsive disorder in patients with velocardiofacial (22q11 deletion) syndrome. *Am J Med Genet B Neuropsychiatr Genet* 126B(1):99–105, 2004. PubMed PMID: 15048657.

189. Bassett AS, Hodgkinson K, Chow EW, et al. 22q11 deletion syndrome in adults with schizophrenia. *Am J Med Genet* 81(4):328–337, 1998. PubMed PMID: 9674980. Pubmed Central PMCID: 3173497.

190. Elsea SH, Girirajan S. Smith-Magenis syndrome. *Eur J Hum Genet* 16(4):412–421, 2008. PubMed PMID: 18231123.

191. Bi W, Saifi GM, Shaw CJ, et al. Mutations of RAI1, a PHD-containing protein, in nondeletion patients with Smith-Magenis syndrome. *Hum Genet* 115(6):515–524, 2004. PubMed PMID: 15565467.

192. Smith AC, Dykens E, Greenberg F. Behavioral phenotype of Smith-Magenis syndrome (del 17p11.2). *Am J Med Genet* 81(2):179–185, 1998. PubMed PMID: 9613859.

193. Martin SC, Wolters PL, Smith AC. Adaptive and maladaptive behavior in children with Smith-Magenis Syndrome. *J Autism Dev Disord* 36(4):541–552, 2006. PubMed PMID: 16570214.

194. Gropman AL, Duncan WC, Smith AC. Neurologic and developmental features of the Smith-Magenis syndrome (del 17p11.2). *Pediatr Neurol* 34(5):337–350, 2006. PubMed PMID: 16647992.

195. Finucane BM, Konar D, Haas-Givler B, et al. The spasmodic upper-body squeeze: a characteristic behavior in Smith-Magenis syndrome. *Dev Med Child Neurol* 36(1):78–83, 1994. PubMed PMID: 8132119.

196. Meyer-Lindenberg A, Hariri AR, Munoz KE, et al. Neural correlates of genetically abnormal social cognition in Williams syndrome. *Nat Neurosci* 8(8):991–993, 2005. PubMed PMID: 16007084.

197. Gosch A, Pankau R. Personality characteristics and behaviour problems in individuals of different ages with Williams syndrome. *Dev Med Child Neurol* 39(8):527–533, 1997. PubMed PMID: 9295848.

198. Davies M, Udwin O, Howlin P. Adults with Williams syndrome. Preliminary study of social, emotional and behavioural difficulties. *Br J Psychiatry* 172:273–276, 1998. PubMed PMID: 9614479.

199. Bhakar AL, Dolen G, Bear MF. The pathophysiology of fragile X (and what it teaches us about synapses). *Annu Rev Neurosci* 35:417–443, 2012. PubMed PMID: 22483044.

200. Loesch DZ, Bui QM, Dissanayake C, et al. Molecular and cognitive predictors of the continuum of autistic behaviours in fragile X. *Neurosci Biobehav Rev* 31(3):315–326, 2007. PubMed PMID: 17097142, Pubmed Central PMCID: 2145511.

201. Hatton DD, Sideris J, Skinner M, et al. Autistic behavior in children with fragile X syndrome: prevalence, stability, and the impact of FMRP. *Am J Med Genet A* 140A(17):1804–1813, 2006. PubMed PMID: 16700053.

202. Goldson E, Hagerman RJ. The fragile X syndrome. *Dev Med Child Neurol* 34(9):826–832, 1992. PubMed PMID: 1526353.

203. Backes M, Genc B, Schreck J, et al. Cognitive and behavioral profile of fragile X boys: correlations to molecular data. *Am J Med Genet* 95(2):150–156, 2000. PubMed PMID: 11078566.

204. Paulsen JS, Ready RE, Hamilton JM, et al. Neuropsychiatric aspects of Huntington's disease. *J Neurol Neurosurg Psychiatry*

71(3):310–314, 2001. PubMed PMID: 11511702. Pubmed Central PMCID: 1737562.

205. Kirkwood SC, Su JL, Conneally P, et al. Progression of symptoms in the early and middle stages of Huntington disease. *Arch Neurol* 58(2):273–278, 2001. PubMed PMID: 11176966.

206. Kirkwood SC, Siemers E, Viken R, et al. Longitudinal personality changes among presymptomatic Huntington disease gene carriers. *Neuropsychiatry Neuropsychol Behav Neurol* 15(3):192–197, 2002. PubMed PMID: 12218712.

207. Chahrour M, Zoghbi HY. The story of Rett syndrome: from clinic to neurobiology. *Neuron* 56(3):422–437, 2007. PubMed PMID: 17988628.

208. Lyst MJ, Ekiert R, Ebert DH, et al. Rett syndrome mutations abolish the interaction of MeCP2 with the NCoR/SMRT co-repressor. *Nat Neurosci* 16(7):898–902, 2013. PubMed PMID: 23770565.

209. Ebert DH, Gabel HW, Robinson ND, et al. Activity-dependent phosphorylation of MeCP2 threonine 308 regulates interaction with NCoR. *Nature* 499(7458):341–345, 2013. PubMed PMID: 23770587.

210. Hunt A, Dennis J. Psychiatric disorder among children with tuberous sclerosis. *Dev Med Child Neurol* 29(2):190–198, 1987. PubMed PMID: 3582788.

211. Tishler PV, Woodward B, O'Connor J, et al. High prevalence of intermittent acute porphyria in a psychiatric patient population. *Am J Psychiatry* 142(12):1430–1436, 1985. PubMed PMID: 4073306.

212. Santosh PJ, Malhotra S. Varied psychiatric manifestations of acute intermittent porphyria. *Biol Psychiatry* 36(11):744–747, 1994. PubMed PMID: 7858070.

213. Crimlisk HL. The little imitator–porphyria: a neuropsychiatric disorder. *J Neurol Neurosurg Psychiatry* 62(4):319–328, 1997. PubMed PMID: 9120442. Pubmed Central PMCID: 1074085.

214. Millward LM, Kelly P, King A, et al. Anxiety and depression in the acute porphyrias. *J Inherit Metab Dis* 28(6):1099–1107, 2005. PubMed PMID: 16435203.

215. Picker JD, Coyle JT. Do maternal folate and homocysteine levels play a role in neurodevelopmental processes that increase risk for schizophrenia? *Harv Rev Psychiatry* 13(4):197–205, 2005. PubMed PMID: 16126606.

216. Levine J, Stahl Z, Sela BA, et al. Elevated homocysteine levels in young male patients with schizophrenia. *Am J Psychiatry* 159(10):1790–1792, 2002. PubMed PMID: 12359692.

217. Bracken P, Coll P. Homocystinuria and schizophrenia. Literature review and case report. *J Nerv Ment Dis* 173(1):51–55, 1985. PubMed PMID: 3965612.

218. Abbott MH, Folstein SE, Abbey H, et al. Psychiatric manifestations of homocystinuria due to cystathionine beta-synthase deficiency: prevalence, natural history, and relationship to neurologic impairment and vitamin B6-responsiveness. *Am J Med Genet* 26(4):959–969, 1987. PubMed PMID: 3591841.

219. Waltz G, Harik SI, Kaufman B. Adult metachromatic leukodystrophy. Value of computed tomographic scanning and magnetic resonance imaging of the brain. *Arch Neurol* 44(2):225–227, 1987. PubMed PMID: 3813937.

220. Hyde TM, Ziegler JC, Weinberger DR. Psychiatric disturbances in metachromatic leukodystrophy. Insights into the neurobiology of psychosis. *Arch Neurol* 49(4):401–406, 1992. PubMed PMID: 1532712.

221. Finelli PF. Metachromatic leukodystrophy manifesting as a schizophrenic disorder: computed tomographic correlation. *Ann Neurol* 18(1):94–95, 1985. PubMed PMID: 4037756.

222. Turpin JC, Masson M, Baumann N. Clinical aspects of Niemann-Pick type C disease in the adult. *Dev Neurosci* 13(4–5):304–306, 1991. PubMed PMID: 1817035.

223. Campo JV, Stowe R, Slomka G, et al. Psychosis as a presentation of physical disease in adolescence: a case of Niemann-Pick disease, type C. *Dev Med Child Neurol* 40(2):126–129, 1998. PubMed PMID: 9489503.

224. Streifler J, Golomb M, Gadoth N. Psychiatric features of adult GM2 gangliosidosis. *Br J Psychiatry* 155:410–413, 1989. PubMed PMID: 2611559.

225. Rosebush PI, MacQueen GM, Clarke JT, et al. Late-onset Tay-Sachs disease presenting as catatonic schizophrenia: diagnostic and treatment issues. *J Clin Psychiatry* 56(8):347–353, 1995. PubMed PMID: 7635850.

226. Navon R, Argov Z, Frisch A. Hexosaminidase A deficiency in adults. *Am J Med Genet* 24(1):179–196, 1986. PubMed PMID: 2939718.

227. MacQueen GM, Rosebush PI, Mazurek MF. Neuropsychiatric aspects of the adult variant of Tay-Sachs disease. *J Neuropsychiatry Clin Neurosci* 10(1):10–19, 1998. PubMed PMID: 9547461.

228. Dening TR, Berrios GE. Wilson's disease: a longitudinal study of psychiatric symptoms. *Biol Psychiatry* 28(3):255–265, 1990. PubMed PMID: 2378928.

229. Dening TR, Berrios GE. Wilson's disease. Psychiatric symptoms in 195 cases. *Arch Gen Psychiatry* 46(12):1126–1134, 1989. PubMed PMID: 2589927.

230. Akil M, Brewer GJ. Psychiatric and behavioral abnormalities in Wilson's disease. *Adv Neurol* 65:171–178, 1995. PubMed PMID: 7872138.

231. Kitchin W, Cohen-Cole SA, Mickel SF. Adrenoleukodystrophy: frequency of presentation as a psychiatric disorder. *Biol Psychiatry* 22(11):1375–1387, 1987. PubMed PMID: 3311181.

232. Cohen-Cole S, Kitchin W. Adrenoleukodystrophy and psychiatric disorder. *Am J Psychiatry* 142(10):1224–1225, 1985. PubMed PMID: 4037139.

233. Rosebush PI, Garside S, Levinson AJ, et al. The neuropsychiatry of adult-onset adrenoleukodystrophy. *J Neuropsychiatry Clin Neurosci* 11(3):315–327, 1999. PubMed PMID: 10440007.

234. Garside S, Rosebush PI, Levinson AJ, et al. Late-onset adrenoleukodystrophy associated with long-standing psychiatric symptoms. *J Clin Psychiatry* 60(7):460–468, 1999. PubMed PMID: 10453801.

235. Bassett AS, Chow EW, AbdelMalik P, et al. The schizophrenia phenotype in 22q11 deletion syndrome. *Am J Psychiatry* 160(9):1580–1586, 2003. PubMed PMID: 12944331, Pubmed Central PMCID: 3276594.

236. Finn CT, Smoller JW. Genetic counseling in psychiatry. *Harv Rev Psychiatry* 14(2):109–121, 2006. PubMed PMID: 16603476.

237. Merikangas KR, Risch N. Will the genomics revolution revolutionize psychiatry? *Am J Psychiatry* 160(4):625–635, 2003. PubMed PMID: 12668348.

238. Austin JC, Honer WG. The potential impact of genetic counseling for mental illness. *Clin Genet* 67(2):134–142, 2005. PubMed PMID: 15679823.

239. Relkin NR, Kwon YJ, Tsai J, et al. The National Institute on Aging/Alzheimer's Association recommendations on the application of apolipoprotein E genotyping to Alzheimer's disease. *Ann N Y Acad Sci* 802:149–176, 1996. PubMed PMID: 8993494.

240. Post SG, Whitehouse PJ, Binstock RH, et al. The clinical introduction of genetic testing for Alzheimer disease. An ethical perspective. *JAMA* 277(10):832–836, 1997. PubMed PMID: 9052715.

241. Roberts JS, Barber M, Brown TM, et al. Who seeks genetic susceptibility testing for Alzheimer's disease? Findings from a multisite, randomized clinical trial. *Genet Med* 6(4):197–203, 2004. PubMed PMID: 15266207.

242. Janssens AC, Aulchenko YS, Elefante S, et al. Predictive testing for complex diseases using multiple genes: fact or fiction? *Genet Med* 8(7):395–400, 2006. PubMed PMID: 16845271.

243. Hodgkinson KA, Murphy J, O'Neill S, et al. Genetic counselling for schizophrenia in the era of molecular genetics. *Can J Psychiatry* 46(2):123–130, 2001. PubMed PMID: 11280080. Pubmed Central PMCID: 3276586.

244. Finn CT, Wilcox MA, Korf BR, et al. Psychiatric genetics: a survey of psychiatrists' knowledge, opinions, and practice patterns. *J Clin Psychiatry* 66(7):821–830, 2005. PubMed PMID: 16013896.

245. Schizophrenia Working Group of the Psychiatric Genomics Consortium. Biological insights from 108 schizophrenia-associated genetic loci. *Nature* 511(7510):421–427, 2014. PMID: 25056061.

64 Serious Mental Illness

Oliver Freudenreich, MD, Mark Viron, MD, and Derri Shtasel, MD, MPH

KEY POINTS

- Five percent of adults in the US suffer from a serious mental illness (SMI), which is defined as a psychiatric illness that persists and is accompanied by functional disability.

- Modern, patient-centered treatment occurs in recovery-oriented community settings and includes peer support, family involvement, and chronic disease self-management.

- The treatment goal for SMI is not a cure but achieving the lowest symptom burden with the best functioning (remission) while living a healthy and meaningful life as a valued member of society (recovery).

- Patients with SMI are at risk for medical complications and societal disadvantages, driven in part by continuing stigma.

- Preventing medical morbidity and mortality (particularly cardiovascular disease) in patients with SMI is as important as addressing psychiatric problems, as medical illness is a primary contributor to the staggering 10- to 20-year premature mortality seen in this population with multimorbidity.

- Optimal rehabilitation needs to accompany optimal pharmacotherapy to prevent chronic disability as a late-stage manifestation of SMI. Optimal pharmacotherapy attempts to reduce symptoms and to prevent illness relapses, so that functional gains can accrue over time and chances for bad outcomes are minimized.

- Globally, societies struggle to create legal frameworks that balance the protection of society from dangerous patients with a respect for patient autonomy that does not inadvertently neglect suffering.

OVERVIEW

Each society has to find a solution for a vexing problem: how to deal effectively and humanely with individuals who have a serious mental illness (SMI) that might not fully respond to available treatments. This task taxes societies' allocation of resources and matters for public safety. Specific solutions are the result of historical peculiarities of time and place. In the US for example, an overly optimistic emptying of state hospitals (asylums) into poorly funded community treatment settings led to revolving door inpatient admissions but it also gave rise to recovery-oriented models of care. Encouraging

progress in many countries has led to a greater level of patient involvement in care and a great reduction in the use of long-term hospitalizations and coercive tools, like seclusion and restraints (see Community Psychiatry, Chapter 67, for details).

In this chapter, we will examine the challenges faced by physicians in caring for patients with serious mental illnesses, like schizophrenia, over the course of the long-term illness, with an emphasis on assessment and treatment goals to optimize chances for a good clinical outcome and for societal integration.

DEFINITION AND SCOPE OF THE PROBLEM

There is no agreed-upon definition of "serious mental illness" (SMI) or "severe and persistent mental illness" (SPMI), terms that have replaced the older term "chronic mental illness" to avoid its negative connotation of untreatability and life-long institutionalization in a state hospital.[1] SMI can be defined in general terms as any psychiatric illness that is characterized by (1) serious psychiatric symptoms (diagnostic criterion), (2) a long history of illness (duration criterion), and (3) poor psychosocial functioning (disability criterion).[2] Implicit in the use of the terms SMI or SPMI is the assumption that patients require ongoing and often life-long psychiatric care and societal supports. Thus defined, SMI is an umbrella term for a diagnostically heterogeneous group that is not restricted to functional psychoses. While a majority of patients have schizophrenia, others suffer from bipolar disorder, chronic depression, or severe personality disorders (Box 64-1).

Despite its heterogeneity, the term is nevertheless useful as it captures psychiatric conditions where a *restitutio ad integrum* (full restoration of health) is unlikely; and where illness management and treatment over long periods (for life in most cases) will thus be necessary, at great costs to patients, families, and society. The Substance Abuse and Mental Health Services Administration estimated that in 2011 there were 11.5 million adults aged 18 years or older with SMI living in the US, representing 5% of all adults.[3] Worldwide, neuropsychiatric disorders, including schizophrenia, contribute substantially to global disease burden and are included in the top five conditions that contribute to non-communicable disease burden.[4,5]

COMPLICATIONS OF SERIOUS MENTAL ILLNESS

One glaring consequence of having SMI is a reduced life expectancy (Box 64-2). As a group, patients with SMI live one or two decades less than comparable cohorts without mental illness.[6-8] While some of the excess mortality stems from suicide, premature death is mostly attributable to medical morbidity, particularly cardiovascular disease.[9,10] Etiological factors include a myriad of modifiable health risk factors, such as smoking and lifestyle choices; notably, both factors are also associated with poverty.[11,12] For example, the Centers for

Disease Control estimates that more than 1 in 3 adults (36%) with a mental illness smoke cigarettes, compared with about 1 in 5 adults (21%) with no mental illness. The percent of adults smoking cigarettes approaches 50% for those who live below the poverty line.[13] Iatrogenic factors contributing to cardiovascular mortality that stem from the use of psychotropics[14] and poorly coordinated care add insult to injury.[15,16] To complicate life further for patients with SMI, co-morbid substance use disorders are common. In the Clinical Antipsychotic Trials of Intervention Effectiveness (CATIE) sample, which is representative of patients with schizophrenia cared for in typical US settings, 60% of patients used substances and 37% had a current substance use disorder.[17]

Many consequences of having an SMI can be summarized under "social toxicity" (Box 64-2), which captures the pernicious, non-medical consequences of developing SMI.

A common societal complication of a serious psychiatric illness like schizophrenia is the poverty that results from illness-related challenges in attaining higher education and gainful employment.[18,19] In the CATIE sample, 73% of patients reported no employment activity in the month before the baseline assessment.[20] Patients with marginal financial resources are at risk for homelessness, and a significant number of patients with psychosis are among the homeless in Western societies.[21] In one well-characterized sample of homeless people in downtown Los Angeles, about one-third suffered from SMI.[22] If psychiatric treatment resources are insufficient, there is a risk that patients are unfairly criminalized and inappropriately cared for in the legal system, phenomena that have

been called "criminalization of the mentally ill" and "trans-institutionalization," respectively (Figure 64.1).[23-25] Finally, the likely interruption of normal adult development often precludes establishing an enduring intimate relationship, as well as sustained, meaningful social connections.

COMPREHENSIVE ASSESSMENT

A comprehensive psychiatric and medical diagnostic assessment is critical for successful treatment in order to avoid medical-psychiatric and social sequelae (Box 64-3). Often, collateral information in the form of discharge summaries from prior hospitalizations or discussions with family members will be necessary to piece together the overall illness course and psychiatric treatment history. Special attention must be given to identifying and characterizing any treatment experience with lithium, clozapine, or electroconvulsive therapy (ECT). Even in patients with significant paranoia or memory problems, a diagnostic interview that includes a life review that focuses on where and with whom the patient has lived (including periods of homelessness), traumatic life events, and achieved developmental milestones is usually possible and provides invaluable clinical information and the grounds for establishing initial rapport. Given the substantial prevalence of drug use, a detailed substance use history is key, even if substance use is distant (e.g., prior injection drug use that would increase the risk for hepatitis C or human

---

BOX 64-1 Broad Definition of Serious Mental Illness

1. Primary psychiatric diagnosis (**diagnostic criterion**)
   • Any psychiatric illness (excluding primary substance use disorders and organic disorders)
2. Prolonged illness duration and treatment needs (**duration criterion**)
   • ≥ 12 months
3. Functional disability (**disability criterion**)
   • GAF score < 60

GAF, General Assessment of Functioning.
Based on operational definition by Substance Abuse and Mental Health Services Administration (SAMHSA) in: Kessler RC et al. Screening for serious mental illness in the general population, Arch Gen Psychiatry 60(2):184–189, 2003.

BOX 64-2 Medical-psychiatric and Social Toxicities from Serious Mental Illness

MEDICAL-PSYCHIATRIC TOXICITIES
Premature death from preventable causes due to:
  Suicide
  Violence
  Medical disease (cardiovascular disease)
  Accidental drug overdose
Medical co-morbidities

SOCIAL TOXICITIES
Interrupted schooling
Loss of career
Loss of peers and friendships and families
Criminal record
Social exclusion due to stigma and self-stigma

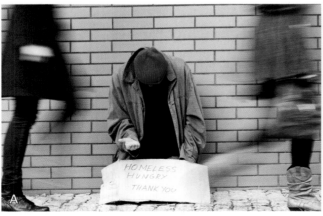
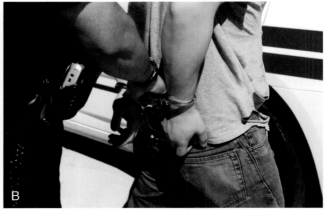

Figure 64-1. Serious mental illness increases (A) the risk for homelessness and (B) legal involvement.

immunodeficiency virus [HIV] infection). Given increased mortality from cardiac disease, risk factors for cardiovascular disease should be elicited specifically. A detailed smoking history, including an assessment of the motivation to quit, is important. Last, head trauma should be asked about as part of a comprehensive assessment of potential factors that impact neurocognition. The physical exam, enhanced by laboratory studies, needs to document the presence or absence of tardive dyskinesia and components of the metabolic syndrome (waist circumference and/or weight; blood pressure; dyslipidemia;

BOX 64-3 Comprehensive Assessment of Serious Mental Illness

Diagnostic psychiatric assessment
  Presence of psychosis
  Non-psychotic symptom clusters (negative symptoms, affective symptoms)
  Neurocognitive examination (executive function, working memory, abstraction)
  Insight into illness, including capacity to accept or reject treatment
Risk assessment: violence and suicide
  History of suicide attempts; chronic suicidality; depression and demoralization
  History of violence and legal problems; impulsivity; anger
Diagnostic medical assessment
  History of head injuries
  Iatrogenic problems from antipsychotics: neurological symptoms, metabolic syndrome
  Infectious diseases: human immunodeficiency virus, hepatitis, tuberculosis
  Risk factors for cardiovascular disease: hypertension, diabetes, dyslipidemia, smoking history
  Wellness assessment: weight (BMI), physical activity, diet
Assessment of functional capacities (strengths and weaknesses)
  Treatment motivation
  Functional ability to participate in treatment and rehabilitation
Assessment of psychosocial adjustment
  History of psychosocial adversity (homelessness; trauma; poverty)
  Work history and potential
  Relationships with family members and friends
  Estimate of financial security
  Meaningful community activities
Assessment of quality of life
  Physical pain; medical illness burden; depression and demoralization
Assessment of adherence
  Attitude towards treatment; barriers; actual adherence behavior

---

blood sugar control). No assessment is complete without a risk assessment of both suicide and violence, based on the patient's history. In addition to traditional risk factors for suicide (e.g., substance use, depression and hopelessness, medical illness, social losses), insight into the nature of illness and its ramifications for life plans should be assessed in schizophrenia as another possible risk factor.[26] Active substance use, historical incidents of violence, as well as sociopathy and a current affective state of anger are helpful factors to estimate the risk of violence in psychotic patients.[27,28] Simply asking a patient his or her self-perception of violence risk may add benefit to a risk assessment.[29] A history of legal problems can have real-world implications (e.g., ineligibility for housing or jobs). Clinicians should attempt to determine if a criminal record reflects sociopathy, an opportunity crime, drug-related activity, or the direct consequence of a mental illness.

A medical-psychiatric diagnostic assessment alone is insufficient without also considering a patient's strengths, hopes, and dreams as well as the subjective quality of life. In addition, it is necessary to assess the familial, social, and economic resources available to promote social connection, restoration of functioning, and autonomy. The appreciation of each individual patient's particular circumstances might evolve over time as particular limitations or unforeseen strengths or resources surface. Similarly, the optimal level of care in the least-restrictive setting needs to be determined on an ongoing basis.

An important area requiring continuing assessment is the patient's adherence to medication and his or her understanding and beliefs about the role of medication in his or her treatment. Adherence can be divided conceptually into a motivational-attitudinal aspect and real-world behavior. In motivated patients who fail to adhere (unintended nonadherence), it is important to determine obstacles to better adherence (e.g., cognitive difficulties, medication side effects, inability to pay for medications). In patients who deliberately decline medication (intended non-adherence), it is important to understand reasons for rejection (e.g., poor treatment efficacy with high side-effect burden, delusional beliefs about medication, denial of illness). Figure 64-2 provides examples of factors that contribute to poor treatment adherence, broken down into treatment attitude and treatment barriers. Adherence is not an all-or-nothing phenomenon but can be partial (e.g., intermittent medication adherence; acceptance of rehabilitation but not of medications).

TREATMENT AND RECOVERY GOALS

For patients with SMI, the overarching treatment goal is not necessarily a cure but rather ongoing care to mitigate the effects of having a chronic mental illness. This approach requires that a clinician look beyond symptoms and pay attention to function and quality of life. In the language of medicine, remission with regard to symptoms (i.e., sustained , with

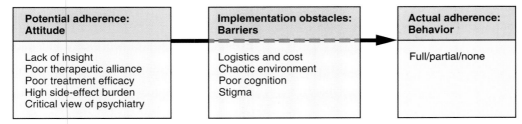

Potential adherence: Attitude	Implementation obstacles: Barriers	Actual adherence: Behavior
Lack of insight Poor therapeutic alliance Poor treatment efficacy High side-effect burden Critical view of psychiatry	Logistics and cost Chaotic environment Poor cognition Stigma	Full/partial/none

Figure 64-2. Assessment of factors contributing to poor treatment adherence. *(Based on Freudenreich O, Kontos N, Querques J. The ABCs of estimating adherence to antipsychotic medications,* Curr Psychiatry 10(6):90, 2011.)

only minimal symptoms) and function (i.e., return to previous levels of functioning) are measurable goals to strive for[30,31]; in the language of persons with lived experience, recovery (i.e., living a meaningful and healthy life despite an illness) is an attitude and process that counteracts nihilism in the face of psychiatric adversity.[32,33] Thus defined, goals of remission and recovery provide a framework for goals that patients, their families, and clinicians can negotiate and agree upon. Both setting over-ambitious goals and setting the bar too low are mistakes that cannot always be anticipated but evolve over time; value can still be found in supposed "failures" in such scenarios.[34] Extending the treatment "framework" beyond psychiatrists, nurses, and social workers, to include family, community, and peer support, is a necessary and logical step in comprehensive care for SMI.

To achieve the best outcomes, treatment needs to be optimal (with regards to timing, type, and intensity), comprehensive, and integrated (rehabilitation with medical and substance use treatment), and culturally sensitive. Not pursuing optimal treatments (e.g., clozapine for refractory schizophrenia or involuntary treatment, when warranted) can contribute to disability and impede recovery. Lengthy hospitalizations should be minimized to prevent secondary symptoms associated with institutionalization (e.g., lack of initiative), but they may be necessary for a small subset of individuals with SMI, who, despite aggressive outpatient efforts, cannot remain safely in a community setting.

Clinicians can focus treatment efforts on several broad, not mutually-exclusive categories, which follow.

Establishing a Collaborative Treatment Relationship

Current trends in the provision of care to patients with SMI focus on empowering patients to take an active role in management of their illness. Establishing shared goals is a first step to engagement with patients. Patients need to be involved in decision-making about their treatment, and treatment plans are put together in the spirit of person-centered care, with family involvement if desired.[35] Psychoeducation for families (including programs run by families themselves[36]) can be an important adjunct of psychiatric treatment as family members are given tools for how to best assist in the care of a family member with SMI. The greatest benefit of psychoeducation lies in reduced hospitalization rates, but it can also lead to better treatment satisfaction.[37] Community resources (e.g., peers, church, and recovery centers) can be used to engage patients.[38] Last, having a good working relationship with a patient has benefit: a good clinician–patient relationship is one important factor that predicts treatment adherence.[39,40] Some intrinsic aspects of illness, including cognitive limitations and negative symptoms,[41] can impede motivation for treatment; recognizing these as symptoms of illness rather than as personality flaws will create a more empathic approach to treatment engagement.

Preventing Suicide

Suicide is a major cause of premature mortality in SMI.[42] For schizophrenia, it has been estimated that 4.9% of patients die from suicide; the risk of suicide is highest in the early years of illness but it always remains higher than in the general population.[43] Psychotropics that have shown benefit for the reduction of suicidality are lithium for bipolar disorder[44] and clozapine, which is FDA-approved for the treatment of suicidality in schizophrenia spectrum conditions.[45] Specific factors that increase the suicide risk (e.g., substance use and depression or demoralization) can be targeted. Selective serotonin reuptake inhibitors (SSRIs), for example, have been shown to reduce suicidality in patients with schizophrenia.[46]

Preventing Violence

Prevention of legal problems is a legitimate treatment goal, as patients should not have to suffer legal consequences that result from suboptimally-treated mental illness. To this end, clinicians might have to pursue assisted and involuntary treatment options, such as outpatient commitment or conditional hospital discharges. Pharmacologic approaches may have direct utility in reducing the risk of violence; clozapine has been shown to have anti-aggressive efficacy that does not appear to be related to its antipsychotic properties.[27]

Preventing Late-stage Psychiatric Disease and Disability

Frequently, patients with SMI present to care in later stages of illness, where only tertiary prevention is possible. However, secondary prevention (e.g., reducing periods of untreated illness through early detection) offers hope for identifying patients in earlier stages of illness, with milder symptoms and less disability.[47] To reduce further loss of function, clear treatment goals for patients with SMI are relapse prevention and prevention of hospitalizations. Evidence-based treatments, including family-focused treatments[48] and maintenance treatment with lithium or antipsychotics, greatly reduce relapse risk for patients bipolar disorder[49] or schizophrenia,[50] respectively, so rehabilitation can occur against a background of psychiatric stability. Not offering the most effective treatments when indicated (e.g., ECT for catatonia or clozapine for refractory psychosis) are avoidable mistakes that can lead to poorly treated psychiatric illness with attendant social ramifications. Polypharmacy can be a sign of inadequate pharmacotherapy if a treatment that is more difficult to administer (e.g., clozapine or ECT) is avoided.[51]

In order to achieve the goal of preventing late stages of illness, optimal pharmacotherapy needs to be accompanied by optimal rehabilitation. Unfortunately, the latter is frequently limited by lack of non-pharmacological treatment resources (e.g., cognitive-behavioral therapy for residual psychosis). A major obstacle to favorable outcomes can be poor treatment adherence. While some adherence problems can be overcome with education, support, and persistence, a significant barrier can be lack of insight, not only into the nature of the psychiatric illness but also into the benefit from treatment or the need for treatment.[52] This anosognosia-like deficit characterizes a significant minority of patients with schizophrenia and shows little response to conventional engagement attempts.[53] Such afflicted patients often evade optimal treatment, or they receive no treatment at all. An element of coercion can become unavoidable even in recovery-oriented services.[54] Despite apparent face validity, interventions often recommended for the treatment of patients with schizophrenia when adherence is in question (e.g., the use of long-acting antipsychotics) have shown little if any benefit when studied in randomized trials.[55] Patient selection might be critical.

Preventing Medical Morbidity and Mortality

Most patients require treatment with psychotropics that can have a host of iatrogenic problems, some of which are preventable with appropriate monitoring and preventive interventions. Primary amongst these side effects are metabolic problems associated with antipsychotics. Unfortunately, guideline-concordant monitoring for antipsychotic-associated metabolic problems is frequently inadequate.[56,57] While the least medically-toxic antipsychotic medication should be used in an effort at primary prevention, it cannot be forgotten that the use of clozapine, perhaps the worst offender with respect to associated metabolic complications, is associated with the lowest risk of mortality in patients with schizophrenia compared to no treatment or treatment with other antipsychotics.[58] Patients with SMI benefit from behavioral interventions aimed to reduce weight, if those services are offered.[59] As smoking is a main cause of preventable mortality, providing maximum support for smoking cessation is one of the most critical health goals for all patients with SMI who are smokers.

The interplay between medical and psychiatric health has led to a much greater emphasis on providing better medical care for patients with SMI, including the establishment of mental (or behavioral) health homes that aim to co-locate and integrate psychiatric and primary care services.[60,61] Patients with SMI can be responsible for aspects of their general medical and psychiatric treatment (chronic disease self-management), and such approaches can empower patients and improve outcomes.[62–64]

Reducing Substance Misuse

Alcohol and illicit drug use greatly complicate treatment efforts for patients with SMI. Even low-grade use can reduce the efficacy of prescribed treatment and should be monitored and addressed if present. Stability of housing and social connections is often related to a patient's ability to engage in formal substance use treatment, particularly if there is an addiction. Effective pharmacological treatments for alcohol dependence exist (e.g., naltrexone, acamprosate, and disulfiram), and modest evidence supports the use of naltrexone and disulfiram in schizophrenia[65] and naltrexone in bipolar disorder.[66,67] However, general rates of prescriptions of anti-dipsomanic agents remain low for any patient.[68]

Improving Quality of Life

Patients can benefit greatly if clinical factors associated with poor quality of life are addressed, particularly depression and demoralization[69] and medical well-being (e.g., pain).[70] SSRIs have shown some benefit for the treatment of the subsyndromal depressive symptoms that are common in schizophrenia.[71] Quality-of-life considerations need to factor in the choice of pharmacotherapy, and sometimes less aggressive, but better tolerated, medication regimens are preferred over poorly tolerated medications with better efficacy. Non-medical, recovery-driven approaches can restore hope and purpose through the attainment of meaningful employment and relationships.

ONGOING CHALLENGES

In the US, community-based treatment has rightfully replaced institutions as the primary setting for ongoing treatment and recovery. At the same time, an under-funded mental health system complicates the delivery of services and supports known to be effective. All too often, care for patients with SMI still proceeds in a fragmented health care system with poor access to truly integrated and comprehensive services that provide timely medical, psychiatric, and substance use treatment. Moreover, instead of receiving psychiatric treatment in the psychiatric treatment setting, patients have been "trans-institutionalized" into the penal system. Rudolf Virchow was among the first modern physicians to recognize the etiopathogenic role of environmental factors for the prognosis of diseases. Psychosocial factors, such as structural violence (e.g., lack of access to treatment) more than biology determine the "natural" course of most illnesses[72] and hinder better

outcomes for patients with SMI. Untreated or delayed treatment of psychosis "damages lives," as Lieberman and Fenton put it in an editorial regarding the need for timely treatment of psychosis.[73]

Stigma is one major operative factor responsible for the current inadequacy of funding and the structural separation between mental health, substance use treatment, and primary care. Stigma is also a fundamental cause of health inequality. Despite progress on paper (e.g., health insurance parity under the federal Mental Health Parity and Addiction Equity Act), SMI remains a highly stigmatized affliction. Meaningful societal inclusion of psychiatric patients with long-term illnesses remains difficult, and psychiatric ghettos are easily created, even without state hospitals. Patients may become "institutionalized in the community" if they feel their lives are effectively limited to group home living and day program participation that is only interrupted by van trips between those two places. Frequently, not much is expected of patients, and such low expectations breed poor results.

Globally, societies struggle to create legal frameworks that balance the protection of society from dangerous patients with a respect for patient autonomy that does not inadvertently neglect suffering. There is no single agreed-upon legal framework for when involuntary treatment should be ordered or for whom it might be most effective in the long run, taking into account the patient's appraisal of the involuntary admission and corresponding view of the psychiatric profession.[74,75] Moreover, controlled trials have failed to show that involuntary admissions can be reduced by means of interventions that are often advocated (e.g., community treatment orders as a precondition for hospital discharge or joint crisis plans that were developed during a period of stability).[76,77]

Short of a cure, how to humanely and effectively care for patients with SMI will remain a vexing issue with no one best solution other than recalling an admonition ascribed to Senator Hubert Humphrey: "The moral test of government is how it treats those who are in the dawn of life, the children; those who are in the twilight of life, the aged; and those in the shadows of life, the sick, the needy and the handicapped."

Access the complete reference list and multiple choice questions (MCQs) online at https://expertconsult.inkling.com

KEY REFERENCES

1. Schinnar AP, Rothbard AB, Kanter R, et al. An empirical literature review of definitions of severe and persistent mental illness. *Am J Psychiatry* 147(12):1602–1608, 1990.
5. Murray CJ, Vos T, Lozano R, et al. Disability-adjusted life years (DALYs) for 291 diseases and injuries in 21 regions, 1990–2010: a systematic analysis for the Global Burden of Disease Study 2010. *Lancet* 380(9859):2197–2223, 2012.
6. Colton CW, Manderscheid RW. Congruencies in increased mortality rates, years of potential life lost, and causes of death among public mental health clients in eight states. *Prev Chronic Dis* 3(2):A42, 2006.
7. Crump C, Winkleby MA, Sundquist K, et al. Comorbidities and mortality in persons with schizophrenia: a Swedish national cohort study. *Am J Psychiatry* 170(3):324–333, 2013.
11. Newcomer JW, Hennekens CH. Severe mental illness and risk of cardiovascular disease. *JAMA* 298(15):1794–1796, 2007.
14. Daumit GL, Goff DC, Meyer JM, et al. Antipsychotic effects on estimated 10-year coronary heart disease risk in the CATIE schizophrenia study. *Schizophr Res* 105(1–3):175–187, 2008.
17. Swartz MS, Wagner HR, Swanson JW, et al. Substance use in persons with schizophrenia: baseline prevalence and correlates from the NIMH CATIE study. *J Nerv Mental Dis* 194(3):164–172, 2006.
18. Dohrenwend BP, Levav I, Shrout PE, et al. Socioeconomic status and psychiatric disorders: the causation-selection issue. *Science* 255(5047):946–952, 1992.

21. Fazel S, Khosla V, Doll H, et al. The prevalence of mental disorders among the homeless in western countries: systematic review and meta-regression analysis. *PLoS Med* 5(12):e225, 2008.

25. Lamb HR, Bachrach LL. Some perspectives on deinstitutionalization. *Psychiatr Serv* 52(8):1039–1045, 2001.

27. Volavka J, Citrome L. Pathways to aggression in schizophrenia affect results of treatment. *Schizophr Bull* 37(5):921–929, 2011.

28. Coid JW, Ullrich S, Kallis C, et al. The relationship between delusions and violence: findings from the East London first episode psychosis study. *JAMA Psychiatry* 70(5):465–471, 2013.

31. Emsley R, Chiliza B, Asmal L, et al. The concepts of remission and recovery in schizophrenia. *Curr Opin Psychiatry* 24(2):114–121, 2011.

35. Torrey WC, Drake RE. Practicing shared decision making in the outpatient psychiatric care of adults with severe mental illnesses: redesigning care for the future. *Community Ment Health J* 46(5):433–440, 2010.

41. Leifker FR, Bowie CR, Harvey PD. Determinants of everyday outcomes in schizophrenia: the influences of cognitive impairment, functional capacity, and symptoms. *Schizophr Res* 115(1):82–87, 2009.

43. Palmer BA, Pankratz VS, Bostwick JM. The lifetime risk of suicide in schizophrenia: a reexamination. *Arch Gen Psychiatry* 62(3):247–253, 2005.

47. McGorry PD, Nelson B, Goldstone S, et al. Clinical staging: a heuristic and practical strategy for new research and better health and social outcomes for psychotic and related mood disorders. *Can J Psychiatry* 55(8):486–497, 2010.

50. Leucht S, Tardy M, Komossa K, et al. Antipsychotic drugs versus placebo for relapse prevention in schizophrenia: a systematic review and meta-analysis. *Lancet* 379(9831):2063–2071, 2012.

54. Geller JL. Patient-centered, recovery-oriented psychiatric care and treatment are not always voluntary. *Psychiatr Serv* 63(5):493–495, 2012.

55. Rosenheck RA, Krystal JH, Lew R, et al. Long-acting risperidone and oral antipsychotics in unstable schizophrenia. *N Engl J Med* 364(9):842–851, 2011.

58. Tiihonen J, Lonnqvist J, Wahlbeck K, et al. 11-year follow-up of mortality in patients with schizophrenia: a population-based cohort study (FIN11 study). *Lancet* 374(9690):620–627, 2009.

59. Daumit GL, Dickerson FB, Wang NY, et al. A behavioral weight-loss intervention in persons with serious mental illness. *N Engl J Med* 368(17):1594–1602, 2013.

64. Goldberg RW, Dickerson F, Lucksted A, et al. Living well: an intervention to improve self-management of medical illness for individuals with serious mental illness. *Psychiatr Serv* 64(1):51–57, 2013.

70. Barnes AL, Murphy ME, Fowler CA, et al. Health-related quality of life and overall life satisfaction in people with serious mental illness. *Schizophr Res Treatment* 2012:245103, 2012.

72. Farmer PE, Nizeye B, Stulac S, et al. Structural violence and clinical medicine. *PLoS Med* 3(10):e449, 2006.

74. Fiorillo A, De Rosa C, Del Vecchio V, et al. How to improve clinical practice on involuntary hospital admissions of psychiatric patients: suggestions from the EUNOMIA study. *Eur Psychiatry* 26(4):201–207, 2011.

65 Aggression and Violence

Adrienne T. Gerken, MD, Anne F. Gross, MD, and Kathy M. Sanders, MD

KEY POINTS

Background

- The etiology of violence is multi-factorial: it has biological, environmental, and psychosocial components.
- The best predictor of violence in a patient is prior acts of violence.

History

- The initial psychiatric evaluation for all patients should include an assessment of current homicidal or aggressive thoughts as well as an assessment of past aggressive thoughts and behaviors.
- Assessment for risk factors includes a thorough history of substance use, a legal history, psychosocial stressors, exposure to violence, impulsivity, and access to firearms.

Clinical and Research Challenges

- In evaluating the acutely aggressive patient, the clinician must prioritize the safety of the patient and the clinical staff while initiating a work-up for the underlying cause(s) of the behavior.
- Treating aggressive behavior in a violent patient should begin with use of the least restrictive methods possible, while attending to the safety of both the patient and the caregivers.

Practical Pointers

- When assessing the cause of aggressive behavior in a patient, medical conditions and substance use should be ruled out before considering a psychiatric disorder.
- Medication choice should target the underlying disorder, if it is known.

OVERVIEW

Aggression and violence are complex behaviors that occur both inside and outside of the medical setting. This chapter focuses on the differential diagnosis of aggressive acts as it pertains to the medical and psychiatric setting; an exhaustive review of aggression and violence within society and its larger economic and sociocultural impact is beyond the scope of this chapter.[1,2] Although workplace violence has a significant impact on the medical and hospital environment, it is not discussed here.[3,4] Instead, this chapter will focus on understanding the complex biopsychosocial context of each patient who displays aggressive behavior.

This chapter will discuss a systematic approach to the assessment and management of patients with aggressive and violent behaviors. Care of the violent or impulsive patient poses a serious challenge to the psychiatrist, who needs to evaluate rapidly and accurately the cause of aggression while initiating treatment. In the medical setting aggressive behavior can be associated with delirium, dementia, and other medical conditions; hence, ruling out medical causes must precede the conclusion that the behavior is the consequence of psychiatric pathology.[5] The psychiatrist must have a frame of reference to adequately assess the risk of violence, as well as the skills to manage it.[6]

EPIDEMIOLOGY AND RISK FACTORS

There is debate as to whether individuals with mental illness are at greater risk for violence than are those in the general population. Current data suggest that people who suffer from mental illness commit violent acts more than twice as often as individuals without a psychiatric diagnosis.[7–11] The Bureau of Justice Statistics has reported that over 1.2 million individuals with mental health problems were confined in US jails and prisons in 2005; roughly three-quarters of these individuals had co-occurring substance use disorders.[12] In Sweden approximately 5.2% of the population's attributable risk for violent crime is due to individuals with severe mental illness, and similar rates have been found within the US.[13] The elevated rates of violent behavior are of special concern to health care providers: patients with schizophrenia who are acutely agitated are thought to account for over 20% of psychiatric emergency department visits, and more than 70% of patients with dementia who live in nursing home facilities exhibit signs of agitation.[14] Notably, however, the large majority of people with mental illness do not commit violent crimes. The MacArthur Study on violent behavior in the mentally ill population found that violence is more prevalent in this group than in the general population only if substances of abuse are involved or if the patients are not appropriately medicated, and other studies have also found substance use to be an independent risk factor for violence.[15,16] Studies also show that up to 25% of people with mental illness report that violent acts have been committed against them; this is more than 11 times greater than it is in the general public, and it is itself a risk factor for the propagation of violent behavior.[17] Therefore, while having a psychiatric diagnosis puts one at increased risk, other factors (including demographics, personal history, medical diagnoses, and psychosocial stressors) often act in an additive manner to determine an individual's likelihood of committing a violent act (Figure 65-1).

PATHOPHYSIOLOGY

Violent acts and aggression have biological, environmental, and psychological determinants.[8,18] While an "aggression center" has never been identified in the brains of humans, animal studies have implicated several brain regions that may be involved in the hierarchical control of aggressive behaviors. Some of these areas are excitatory in nature; others are inhibitory.[18–22] The anterior, lateral, ventromedial, and dorsomedial nuclei of the hypothalamus are often described as areas crucial to animal aggression and are considered to be involved in the control of aggression in humans. The limbic system (which includes the amygdala, hippocampus, septum, cingulate, and fornix) has regulatory control of aggressive behaviors in humans and animals. The prefrontal cortex modulates input from both the limbic system and the hypothalamus; it may have a role in the social context and judgmental aspects of aggression.[23,24] Cortico-limbic circuits have been identified for psychiatric disorders associated with aggression

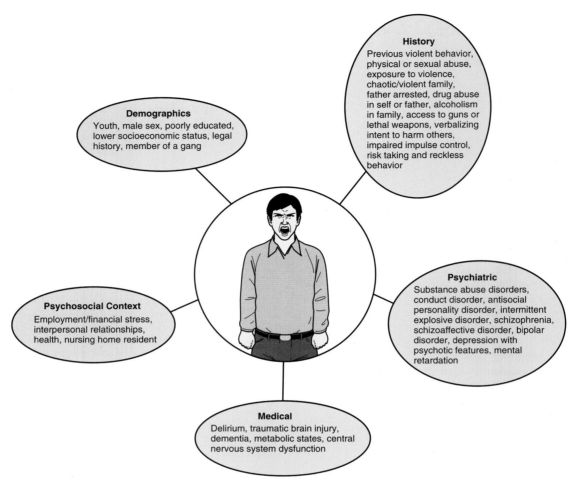

Figure 65-1. Risk factors for violent behavior.

including antisocial personality disorder and borderline personality disorder.[25]

Neuroimaging studies have found abnormalities in the prefrontal areas of individuals who exhibit violent behavior. Using magnetic resonance imaging (MRI) techniques, violent individuals have been shown to have reductions in the volume of their prefrontal gray matter. The volume of the orbitofrontal cortex has been associated with aggression in psychiatric patients.[26] Using single-photon emission computed tomography (SPECT) techniques, adolescent and adult psychiatric patients who had recently participated in an aggressive act had significantly depressed prefrontal activity when compared with control patients. Multiple positron emission tomography (PET) analyses have illustrated that violent patients have decreased prefrontal/frontal blood flow and metabolism.[27] These findings are supported by clinical evidence showing that acquired lesions within, as well as injury to, the prefrontal cortex and frontal lobe put one at increased risk for impulsive behavior and lessen executive control of emotional reactivity. Multiple SPECT and PET analyses have also found abnormalities within the temporal lobe and the subcortical structures of the medial temporal lobe in violent patients.[28]

Low central serotonin (5-HT) function has been correlated with impulsive aggression. Violent patients have been found to have a low turnover of 5-HT, as measured by its major metabolite, 5-hydroxyindoleacetic acid (5-HIAA), in the cerebrospinal fluid (CSF). Acetylcholine in the limbic system stimulates aggression in animals; cholinergic pesticides have been cited as provoking violence in humans. Gamma-aminobutyric acid

(GABA) is thought to have inhibitory effects on aggression in both humans and animals. Norepinephrine (noradrenaline) may enhance some types of aggression in animals and could play a role in impulsivity and episodic violence in humans. Dopamine increases aggressive behavior in animal models, but its effect in humans is less clear because of its psychotomimetic effects.[29-31] Hormonal influences of androgens often are cited as a major factor in aggressive behavior.[32] Some attribute a lower threshold for violence in women to lower levels of estrogen and progesterone during the menstrual cycle. Lower cholesterol levels in patients with personality disorders have been associated with aggressive and impulsive behavior[33,34] (Table 65-1).

In considering the genetics of aggressive behavior, no specific chromosomal abnormalities are yet associated with an increased risk for aggression; however, aggressive behavior has been shown to be highly heritable and can be unmasked by environmental stressors in those who are genetically prone.[35] Using twin studies, a meta-analysis that examined the etiology of aggressive behavior showed that at least 50% of the pathology could be attributable to genetics.[36] The relationship between the syndrome involving XYY and impulsivity is questionable, and the relationship remains inconclusive. Knock-out mice that lack the monoamine oxidase $(MAO)_A$ gene (which encodes for the enzyme responsible for the catabolism of serotonin, dopamine, and norepinephrine, and subsequently leads to elevated serum levels of the three neurochemicals) were shown to exhibit increased aggression in genetic studies. Within a family in the Netherlands carrying an X-linked mutation in this gene, affected members showed increased levels of aggressive

TABLE 65-1 Neurochemical Changes Associated with Increased Aggression

Neurochemical	Change in Plasma
Serotonin	Decreased
Acetylcholine	Increased
Gamma-aminobutyric acid (GABA)	Decreased
Norepinephrine	Increased
Dopamine	Increased
Testosterone	Increased
Cholesterol	Decreased

TABLE 65-2 Differential Diagnosis of Psychosis and Agitation

General Category	Cause/Diagnosis
Neurocognitive disorders	Aphasias Catatonia Delirium Dementia Frontal lobe syndrome Organic hallucinosis Organic delusional disorder Organic mood disorder (secondary mania) Seizure disorders
Drugs	Substance abuse (e.g., cocaine, opiates) Steroids Isoniazid Procarbazine hydrochloride Antibiotics Anticholinergics
Drug withdrawal	Alcohol and sedative-hypnotics (barbiturates and benzodiazepines) Clonidine Opiates
Psychotic disorders	Schizophrenia Delusional disorder Unspecified Schizophrenia Spectrum and Other Psychotic Disorders Brief reactive psychosis Schizoaffective disorder
Mood disorders	Bipolar disorder Major depression with psychotic/agitated features Catatonia
Anxiety/fear	Anxiety disorders Acute reaction to stress
Neurodevelopmental disorders	Autism-spectrum disorder Intellectual disability Attention-deficit/hyperactivity disorder
Disruptive, impulse-control, and conduct disorders	Kleptomania Pyromania Conduct disorder Intermittent explosive disorder
Personality disorders	Antisocial Borderline Paranoid Schizotypal
Discomfort	Pain Hypoxia Akathisia

behavior. Human correlates also exist for the mouse knockout studies that examined catechol O-methyltransferase (COMT) (an enzyme also responsible for the catabolism of catecholamines) gene mutations leading to increased aggression.[37] A study that examined the serotonin transporter gene (which regulates the duration of serotonin signaling) showed that a polymorphism in the promoter yielded low serotonin levels and increased aggressive behavior in children.[38] Polymorphisms of tryptophan hydroxylase may also be correlated with impulsive aggression.[39]

CLINICAL FEATURES AND DIAGNOSIS

The etiologies of aggressive and violent behavior are vast; however, if they can be identified, it is critical to do so, because the management, in both the acute and long-term setting, relies on this information. It is critical for the evaluator to assess whether the pathology is a result of major mental illness, a result of a personality disorder, or a result of a medical condition because the level of acuity, the degree of violent behavior, and the treatment approach of each type of problem will vary. When beginning the assessment of a violent patient, it is useful to generate a working differential (Table 65-2).

Medical Causes

One must first assume that there is a medical condition or a substance abuse/dependence problem that is causing aggressive behavior before considering primary psychiatric disorders. Box 65-1 lists medical causes of mental disorders.[40]

Psychiatric Causes

Most major mental disorders may manifest symptoms of violence during the course of the illness. Categories of conditions responsible for violence include psychotic states, affective disorders, disorders of impulse control, trauma-related disorders, and personality disorders.

Psychotic Disorders

The prevalence of violence in those with schizophrenia and other psychotic conditions is similar to that seen in people with bipolar disorder and major depression; of note, however, the prevalence is approximately five times higher than it is in those without a major mental illness. Paranoid individuals who suffer from delusions of persecution may interpret individuals within their immediate environment as threatening, and therefore act in a violent manner. Command hallucinations substantially increase the risk of both self-inflicted violence and violence toward others. Disorganized thought and behavior may also increase the risk of violent acts.

Affective Disorders

Affective illness is also associated with violent behavior. Unipolar depression is often associated with anger attacks (nearly half of the time).[41] Depression with psychotic features may further increase the risk of violence. Patients with bipolar disorder (whether in a manic, hypomanic, or mixed phase) are often characterized as impulsive, irritable, omnipotent, or paranoid; each can lead to violent behavior.

Disruptive, Impulse-control, and Conduct Disorders

Disorders of impulsive control, including kleptomania, pyromania, pathological gambling, trichotillomania, intermittent explosive disorder, and impulse-control disorder not otherwise specified (NOS),[42,43] are associated with violence. Individuals with these disorders are characterized by a compulsive urge to perform an act that is harmful to themselves or others; after the act is committed, they may or may not experience relief, pleasure, or gratification (see Chapter 23). People with intermittent explosive disorder experience episodes of extreme aggression that may lead to violent acts out of proportion to the precipitating event.[44,45] Unspecified disruptive, impulse-control, and

---

BOX 65-1 Medical Causes of Mental Disorders

MENTAL DISORDERS CAUSED BY A GENERAL MEDICAL CONDITION

- Delirium, dementia, and amnestic and other cognitive disorders
- Schizophrenia and other psychotic disorders
- Mood disorders
- Anxiety disorders
- Sleep disorders

CATATONIC DISORDER CAUSED BY A GENERAL MEDICAL CONDITION

Personality change (e.g., with lability, disinhibition, aggression, apathy, or paranoia) caused by a general medical condition

SPECIFIC CONSIDERATIONS

Central nervous system disorders (including HIV infection and other intracranial infections, tumors, neurodegenerative disorders [including Huntington's disease, Wilson's disease, and multiple sclerosis], and cerebrovascular disease)

Seizure-related aggression, which can occur during the ictal period (manifesting as non-purposeful, stereotypical behavior), during the post-ictal period (which is usually due to confusion), and during the inter-ictal period

Traumatic brain injury

Systemic disorders (including electrolyte abnormalities, hypoxia, uremia, metabolic abnormalities [e.g., secondary to Cushing's disease], infections, autoimmune disorders [e.g., SLE, porphyria], and toxins)

Substance-related disorders (e.g., associated with alcohol, amphetamines, caffeine, cannabis, cocaine, hallucinogens, inhalants, nicotine, opioids, PCP, sedative/hypnotics, anxiolytics)

- Substance dependence
- Substance intoxication
- Substance withdrawal
- Substance-induced mental disorders

HIV, Human immunodeficiency virus; PCP, phencyclidine; SLE, systemic lupus erythematosus.

---

conduct disorder is a category of disorders that does not meet criteria for any of the previously mentioned impulse-control disorders and includes repetitive self-mutilation, compulsive sexual behavior, and compulsive face-picking. People who perform repetitive self-mutilation often have a history of physical or sexual abuse (or both).[46]

Post-traumatic Stress Disorder

Individuals exposed to trauma may exhibit signs and symptoms of post-traumatic stress disorder (PTSD) (including hypervigilance and dissociative symptoms) that may place them at increased risk for aggressive behavior. Rates of aggression and violence are increased in veterans with severe mental illness, with traumatic brain injury, homelessness, substance use disorders, and PTSD serving as risk factors for violence.[47] Similarly, individuals who have been exposed to terrorist events or torture may be at increased risk for aggressive behavior.[48,49]

Personality and Developmental Disorders

The personality disorder most commonly associated with violence and aggressive behavior is antisocial personality disorder; affected individuals often have co-occurring substance use disorder diagnoses, which increase the likelihood of impulsive and aggressive behavior. Patients with borderline personality

disorder often act violently toward themselves, often with self-mutilatory behavior. If individuals with a paranoid personality disorder perceive a threat, they may act violently toward that threat. Developmental disorders, as well as other causes (including head trauma) of poor impulse control, may lead to violent behavior.[50–52]

Psychosocial Factors

The amount of psychosocial stress that an individual experiences directly correlates with the likelihood that an individual prone to violence will act in an impulsive and aggressive manner. For example, homelessness and a history of being a victim of violence are independently correlated with the risk of violence in individuals with major mental illness.[53] It is critical that the evaluator ask the patient about active stressors in order to understand the patient's occupational, educational, housing, economic, legal, and social context.

ASSESSMENT IN THE ACUTE SETTING

To ensure the safety of the patient and those around him or her, the evaluator must act swiftly to provide an accurate diagnosis and acute management.[54] Under more urgent conditions, the basic elements of emergency evaluation of aggressive and impulsive behavior are (1) safety, (2) diagnosis, and (3) management[6] (Figure 65-2). Safety is the first priority in the assessment of the violent patient; therefore, the clinician must first determine the level of acuity of the situation.[55] Since the initial differential diagnosis includes medical conditions, substance abuse, and psychopathology, if possible, it is important to check the patient's vital signs and medical history and to perform a visual examination of the patient.[56] It is often unsafe for the clinician to evaluate patients with cognitive impairment secondary to medical illness or to substance abuse who are actively aggressive and violent. Depending on the intensity of the violence and aggression, the patient may require use of medication and restraints in order to conduct a safe examination. Similarly, a patient with a psychotic disorder who is aggressive toward staff or other patients should receive medication to maintain behavioral calm; if this is not sufficient, use of seclusion or physical restraints should be considered.[55,57]

If violent behavior is anticipated in a patient who displays escalating tension, one or more of several techniques (including verbal de-escalation, environmental modification, and offering oral medications) should be employed.[55] It is critical, however, to attempt to determine if the patient has drug allergies or medical or physical conditions that would contraindicate a particular medication. A rudimentary examination that focuses on vital signs, evidence of head trauma, the presence of substances of abuse, and lacerations should be conducted and a basic differential formed.[56] If the patient's behavior de-escalates, a more formalized interview can begin safely; if the patient's behavior becomes more threatening, the use of seclusion, calming medications, or physical restraint should be applied. If the clinician feels there is potential for violence, but at the time of initial evaluation the clinician feels safe, the evaluation should proceed with a proper back-up plan and the presence of other staff members who are readily available to intervene if needed.[55]

The Interview

Before the examiner can interview the potentially violent patient, a safe environment must be secured. All potentially dangerous materials should be removed from the patient and from the interview room. Objects that can be used as

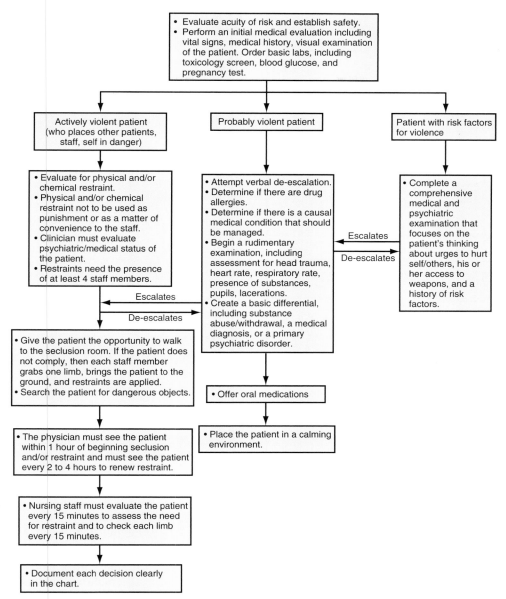

Figure 65-2. The basic elements of assessing a violent patient based on acuity.

weapons (e.g., pens, needles, phones) should be scrutinized before and during the interview. The interview room should allow for possible escape and should be highly visible to other staff members or security. The ideal room for such an interview should contain an emergency call button and the inability to lock the door from within. The physician should pay careful attention to the patient's behavior for signs of imminent danger. Behaviors that convey escalation include (1) verbal threats or gestures; (2) rapid movements, agitation, pacing, knocking over furniture, or slamming doors; and (3) invasion of personal space, clenching of the jaw, or signs of muscular tension. At this time, the examiner's interventions are designed to direct the patient to regain the locus of control. If the examiner's attempts to redirect the patient fail to decrease the patient's level of agitation and increase his or her level of self-control, tranquilization and emergency restraints may be necessary to regain control and to ensure the safety of all involved.

History

The medical history must be obtained in the initial phases of the interview process to ascertain and to treat any potentially life-threatening medical causes for the patient's agitation or aggressive behavior. The mnemonic WWHHHHIMPS can be used to quickly rule out life-threatening causes of delirium (Box 65-2); other pertinent medical history includes previous head trauma and neurological or seizure disorders (e.g., febrile childhood seizures). Past psychiatric history, including medication non-compliance, prior psychiatric hospitalizations, and current as well as past alcohol and substance abuse history, is important to obtain as these factors may increase the patient's risk of aggression, as well as guide treatment. In addition, the clinician must gather information about recent psychosocial stressors, including financial, housing, primary support, domestic violence, and legal charges. Information regarding a patient's prior violence history (including prior homicidal or

BOX 65-2 WWHHHHIMPS, a Mnemonic for Life-
threatening Causes of Delirium

Withdrawal (e.g., from benzodiazepines or barbiturates)
Wernicke's encephalopathy
Hypoxia and hypoperfusion of the brain
Hypertensive crisis
Hypoglycemia
Hyperthermia/hypothermia
Intracranial bleed/mass or infection
Meningitis/encephalitis or metabolic abnormalities
Poisoning
Seizures

Adapted from Wise MG: Delirium. In Yudofsky SC, Hales RE, editors.
Textbook of neuropsychiatry and clinical neurosciences, *Washington,
DC, 2002, American Psychiatric Publishing.*

BOX 65-3 Recommended Questions about
Violent Behavior

Determine the specifics of past violence
    At what age did violent acts begin?
    How frequently did those acts occur?
    What was the most recent act?
    How severe were the actions?
    Has there been a recurring pattern of escalation preceding
        violence?
    Have there been common precipitants surrounding the acts?
    Have any violent actions resulted in legal recourse, or
        incarceration?
    Has there been a history of recklessness, suicidality, arrests,
        or impulsivity?
    Does the patient have a family history of violence, abuse, or
        gang involvement?
Ask screening questions:
    Do you ever think of harming anyone else?
    Have you ever seriously injured another human being? (Tell
        me about the most violent thing that you have ever done.)
Ask about prior evaluations and treatments related to violent
    behavior, including medical work-ups, diagnostic tests, and
    old records.
Collect information from as many ancillary sources as possible,
    including family members, victims, court records, medical
    records, and previous treaters.

violent ideas and behaviors, specific targets of these violent acts, family history of violence, history of arson and/or harming animals, and access to weapons) is critical. Collateral history, including information from family, medical records, police documents, and prior neuropsychiatric testing, is often very helpful in assessing risk of violence.

Assessment for violence is one of the most difficult tasks for the medical and psychiatric professional. The best indicator of future violence remains a history of violence. Therefore, seeking a history of prior violence by a patient is an integral part of the interview. Given the nature of violent perpetrators, it is often difficult to elicit an accurate account. The best approach is indirect questioning for previous violent behaviors (Box 65-3).

Examination of the Violent Patient

The mental status examination of the potentially violent patient begins like a standard examination. However, as previously emphasized, careful consideration must be given to

safety. If at any time during the examination the examiner feels unsafe, the interview should cease until proper measures can be put in place to ensure safety. The initial assessment should focus on elements of the mental status (e.g., the sensorium, disordered thought, mood and affect, cognition, agitation, delusions, hallucinations, and evidence of intoxication by drugs or alcohol). Mental status abnormalities or symptoms can increase the likelihood of aggressive action and alert the physician to medical conditions that require further work-up or immediate treatment. For example, impaired judgment or impulsivity may lead to violence. The hopelessness of a depressed individual, combined with psychotic thoughts, may lead a person to attempt suicide or murder. Patients with thought disorders, psychosis with paranoid features, or command hallucinations may behave in ways that are both dangerous and difficult to predict. Just as in the evaluation of suicidal thoughts, violent thoughts toward others must be assessed in terms of a specific target, a specific plan, the lethality of the plan, and the possibility that the plan can actually be carried out. Determination of the relative risk of violence in this manner helps one develop a disposition plan (e.g., referral for inpatient versus outpatient management). Documentation of agitation through standardized rating scales, such as the Overt Agitation Severity Scale (OASS), is useful in anticipating escalating behaviors and determining when to intervene.[58] In addition, the use of risk assessment scales may lead to a reduction in aggression and the need for seclusion and restraints on inpatient psychiatric units.[59,60] There are multiple structured violence risk instruments which have been used in various settings and have been found to predict violence[61,62]; however, the future routine use of these tools will depend on whether they benefit clinical decision-making and optimize outcomes. Research evidence is lacking regarding several critical issues, including the accuracy of the violence risk assessment tools in long-term prediction of violent behavior.[62]

Physical examination is targeted to find medical causes of violence and is guided by findings in the history. Because violence is more likely in a patient with a structural or metabolic brain disorder or acute intoxication, one should focus on elements of the examination that will help identify these diagnoses, including the neurologic examination. Based on physical findings and the patient's medical history, appropriate diagnostic tests should be performed. These are not mandatory, but include the following: (1) routine chemistry tests, blood counts, and tests of serum or urine toxicology; (2) a medical work-up for dementia; (3) neuroimaging, an electroencephalogram (EEG), and other radiological tests as indicated; and, (4) neuropsychological and cognitive testing.

MANAGEMENT IN THE ACUTE SETTING

There are no medications that specifically target aggressive behavior[63]; the psychiatrist must apply general principles to guide treatment. The clinician should attempt to optimize treatment of the underlying medical or psychiatric illness, if present; if that fails, it is best to use the most benign treatments in an empirical and systematic way. Target symptoms should be well defined and monitored as specific interventions are initiated. Efficacy should be defined by parameters that can be observed and measured. The symptom checklist in the OASS is useful for documenting progress in the management of agitation and aggressive behaviors. In the acute setting, the goal in treatment of the violent patient should be to reduce the risk of harm to both the staff and the patient and to facilitate the diagnostic process. Medications that can be delivered intramuscularly and that have a rapid onset and a favorable side-effect profile should be first-line treatments. Once the patient is calm and a more thorough assessment is achieved, the psychiatrist can decide between outpatient management or hospitalization (voluntary versus involuntary). Documentation of the patient's risk for imminent violence is a critical part of the evaluation, and will help determine the appropriate level of care required for treatment and minimization of risk.

Benzodiazepines are rapid, safe, and easily administered first-line drugs for moderate to severe agitation and for cases in which the potential for escalating behavioral dyscontrol exists. A caveat concerning the use of benzodiazepines is the paradoxical reaction seen in certain character-disordered patients, individuals with traumatic brain injury or intellectual disability, or the elderly. When these medications are given in the intramuscular (IM) or oral form, they are effective sedatives in the acute care setting. Antipsychotics, particularly high-potency agents, are often effective in reducing agitation and violence in both psychotic and non-psychotic patients. Haloperidol, a high-potency typical neuroleptic, is frequently used in this setting because of its favorable side-effect profile and overall cardiopulmonary safety. Often in the acute setting a combination of medications is used because of the synergy

of the drugs' efficacy, faster onset of action, and the ability to use lower doses with a decrease in the potential for side effects. In recent years, atypical antipsychotics (e.g., clozapine, olanzapine, ziprasidone, risperidone) have gained more frequent use in the acute setting.[41,64,65] Three atypical antipsychotics are available in forms that can be used in emergency situations: olanzapine (IM and orally disintegrating), ziprasidone (IM), and risperidone (orally disintegrating).[66] In general, atypical neuroleptics are better tolerated than are conventional agents; they have fewer extrapyramidal symptoms and they are associated with better long-term adherence[67–69] (Table 65-3).

Virtually any neuroleptic may diminish aggression, but careful consideration should be given to the potency, history of response, side-effect profile of the particular medication, and the psychiatric and medical history of the patient. In the acute setting, the diagnosis may be unknown. Once a provisional diagnosis is made, medical treatment should be tailored to the underlying etiology[56] (Table 65-4). Special considerations should also be taken when working with young children, the elderly, and individuals with mental retardation

TABLE 65-3 Pharmacotherapy for Acute Management of Violent Behavior

Medication Class	Medication and Dosing	Side Effects/Considerations
Benzodiazepine	Alprazolam PO Initial dose 0.5 mg	Paradoxical reactions can be seen in character-disordered patients and can worsen symptoms in the elderly.
	Diazepam PO, IM, IV Initial dose 5 mg	Calming/sedating effect with rapid onset; however, use cautiously with elderly patients because of the drug's long half-life.
	Lorazepam PO, SL, IM, IV Initial dose 1 mg	No active metabolites; therefore, there is a small risk of drug accumulation. Metabolized only via glucuronidation; therefore, it can be used in most patients with impaired hepatic function. Drug of choice within this class due to moderately long half-life.
Typical antipsychotics	Haloperidol PO, IM, IV Initial dose 5–10 mg	High-potency neuroleptic with favorable side-effect profile and cardiopulmonary safety. IV form less likely to cause EPS. ECG monitoring needed to assess torsades de pointes or QTc prolongation.
	Perphenazine PO Initial dose 4–8 mg	Risk of NMS increases in patients who are poorly hydrated, restrained, and kept in poorly aerated rooms while given large doses of antipsychotics. Frequent vital sign checks and testing for muscular rigidity are recommended.
	Chlorpromazine PO, PR, IM Initial dose 50–100 mg	This medication is very sedating, and injections can cause pain. Can cause hypotension.
Atypical antipsychotics	Risperidone PO, orally disintegrating tablet Initial dose 1–3 mg	No IM form is available. Offers calming effect with treatment of underlying condition. Orthostatic hypotension with reflex tachycardia. Increased risk of stroke in the elderly with CVD.
	Olanzapine PO, orally disintegrating tablet, IM Initial dose 5–10 mg	Useful in patients with poor reaction to haloperidol. Calming medication with treatment of underlying disorder. Avoid IM combination with lorazepam. Increased risk of stroke in the elderly with CVD.
	Ziprasidone PO, IM Initial dose 10–20 mg	Use caution in patients with pre-existing QT prolongation. Less sedating medication; therefore, good choice if desire tranquilization without sedation.
Combinations	Haloperidol 5 mg, lorazepam 2 mg, diphenhydramine 50 mg (or substitute benztropine 1 mg for diphenhydramine)	Most commonly used in the acute setting. Young athletic men are at increased risk for dystonia. Akathisia must be considered if agitation increases after administration.
	Perphenazine 8 mg, lorazepam 2 mg, diphenhydramine 50 mg (or substitute benztropine 1 mg for diphenhydramine)	Consider if patient has had adverse reactions to haloperidol.

CVD, Cardiovascular disorder; ECG, electrocardiogram; EPS, extrapyramidal symptoms; IM, intramuscular; IV, intravenous; NMS, neuroleptic malignant syndrome; PO, per os (by mouth, orally); PR, per rectum; SL, sublingual.
Adapted from Allen M, Currier G, Carpenter D. The expert consensus guideline series: treatment of behavioral emergencies, J Psychiatr Pract 11:1–112, 2005.

TABLE 65-4 Recommended Oral and Parenteral Medications for Presumed Diagnoses

Working Diagnosis	First-line Oral Medication	First-line Parenteral Medication
Unknown	Benzodiazepine	Benzodiazepine +/– haloperidol
Medical etiology	Avoid due to concern of altering medical work-up	Haloperidol
Stimulant intoxication	Benzodiazepine	Benzodiazepine
Alcohol intoxication	Avoid unless severe agitation; benzodiazepine	Benzodiazepine
Schizophrenia	Olanzapine, risperidone +/– benzodiazepine, haloperidol + benzodiazepine	Olanzapine, ziprasidone +/– benzodiazepine, haloperidol + benzodiazepine
Mania	Olanzapine, risperidone +/– benzodiazepine, divalproex + antipsychotic, haloperidol + benzodiazepine	Olanzapine, haloperidol + benzodiazepine
Psychotic depression		Olanzapine
Personality disorder		Benzodiazepine

Adapted from Allen M, Currier G, Carpenter D. The expert consensus guideline series: treatment of behavioral emergencies, J Psychiatr Pract 11:1–112, 2005.

TABLE 65-5 Pharmacotherapy for Long-term Management of Violent Behavior

Medication Class	Patient Population	Considerations
SSRIs	Depression, anxiety, personality disorders, dementia, and mental retardation	Use with caution in bipolar affective disorder.
Lithium	Intellectual disability, conduct disorder, antisocial personality disorder, prison inmates, bipolar disorder	Medical examination must be performed before and during treatment: that is, measurement of TSH levels and renal function.
Anticonvulsants (e.g., carbamazepine, valproic acid)	Schizophrenia with or without EEG abnormalities, personality disorders, conduct disorders, seizure disorders, or bipolar disorders	Use similar dosing as in bipolar disease. There are multiple drug interactions with this class. Carbamazepine levels must be checked every month for the first 3 months and then once every 3 months after that. Valproic acid levels must be checked every week for 1–2 months and then every 2 weeks for 1 year. Monitor CBC and LFTs.
Gabapentin	Patients with co-existing anxiety and character pathology	No interactions with other anticonvulsants.
Benzodiazepines	Should have underlying component of anxiety	Must be used carefully in this population due to increased potential for abuse, dependence, and withdrawal reactions. Buspirone, a non-benzodiazepine, may have less abuse potential.
Atypical antipsychotics	Schizophrenia/psychosis, mania	Long-acting depot forms may increase compliance. Risperidone and clozapine have been shown to decrease violent behavior independently of their antipsychotic effect.
Beta-blockers	Organic brain disease including TBI, neurodegenerative disorders, and mental retardation; patients are often refractory to other medications	Propranolol can be gradually increased to 1 g/day, nadolol to 40–120 mg/day, and metoprolol to 200–300 mg/day. Propranolol is contraindicated in patients with asthma, COPD, and IDDM. Use these drugs with caution in patients with underlying hypertension.
Psychostimulants	ADD/ADHD in children and adults	Potential exists for addiction and abuse.

ADD, Attention-deficit disorder; ADHD, attention-deficit/hyperactivity disorder; CBC, complete blood count; COPD, chronic obstructive pulmonary disease; EEG, electroencephalogram; IDDM, insulin-dependent diabetes mellitus; LFT, liver function test; SSRI, selective serotonin reuptake inhibitor; TBI, traumatic brain injury; TSH, thyroid-stimulating hormone.

or developmental delay. Benzodiazepines and antipsychotics should be avoided, if possible, in both the very young and the elderly. If medication is needed to manage aggressive and violent behavior, lorazepam or risperidone is the treatment of choice for children, and the use of risperidone, olanzapine, and haloperidol is recommended for the elderly. Risperidone may be the first-line medication used to treat agitated people with developmental delay.[56]

STRATEGIES FOR LONG-TERM MANAGEMENT

The long-term management of the violent patient poses a complex challenge for the treating psychiatrist. First, one should maximize appropriate treatment of any underlying

psychiatric disorder, using both psychotherapy and pharmacotherapy. The choice of medication used should be targeted toward treating the primary diagnosis. Medications, such as selective serotonin re-uptake inhibitors (SSRIs), lithium, anticonvulsants, benzodiazepines, psychostimulants, and adrenergic blockers, have all been used successfully in specific populations. Though some studies show that atypical neuroleptics are more effective than typical neuroleptics in the management of aggressive behavior,[70-72] other studies have shown that perphenazine may be equally or more effective in reducing violence in patients with schizophrenia.[72] Regular assessment of the presence of the metabolic syndrome associated with the atypical neuroleptics in patients prescribed these medications is recommended (Table 65-5).

Psychotherapeutic approaches (e.g., behavioral techniques, cognitive-behavioral therapy, group and family therapy) have also been used to treat aggression and violence.[73] Behavioral techniques (e.g., limit-setting, contingent reinforcement, distraction and re-direction, relaxation, biofeedback) have been used in the ongoing inpatient and outpatient management of aggressive and impulsive patients, with mixed success. A trauma-informed approach to the engagement and ongoing treatment of those with aggressive behavior is recommended for successful outcomes.[74] The combination of medication and trauma-informed therapies is still the best approach to the chronic management of aggression and violence.

CURRENT CONTROVERSIES AND FUTURE CONSIDERATIONS

As our scientific knowledge of the biological component of aggressive behavior expands (including further information from genetic and neuroimaging studies), it will undoubtedly alter the way in which we as clinicians and society as a whole manage the epidemic of violence.

Access the complete reference list and multiple choice questions (MCQs) online at https://expertconsult.inkling.com

KEY REFERENCES

6. Sanders KM. Approach to the violent patient. In Stern TA, Herman JB, Slavin PL, editors: *The MGH guide to primary care psychiatry*, ed 2, New York, 2004, McGraw-Hill.
10. Swanson JW. Mental disorder, substance abuse, and community violence, an epidemiological approach. In Monahan J, Steadman HJ, editors: *Violence and mental disorder: developments in risk assessment*, Chicago, 1994, University of Chicago Press.
12. James DJ, Glaze LE. *Bureau of Justice Statistics Special Report: Mental Health Problems of Prison and Jail Inmates*, 2006, US Department of Justice, NCK 213600.
13. Fazel S, Grann M. The population impact of severe mental illness on violent crime. *Am J Psychiatry* 163:1397–1403, 2006.
14. Marder ST. A review of agitation in mental illness: treatment guidelines and current therapies. *J Clin Psychiatry* 67(Suppl. 10):13–21, 2006.
15. Steadman HJ, Mulvey EP, Monahan J, et al. Violence by people discharged from the acute psychiatric inpatient facilities and by others in the same neighborhood. *Arch Gen Psychiatry* 55:393–401, 1998.
16. Swanson JW, Swartz MS, Essock SM, et al. The social-environmental context of violent behavior in persons treated for severe mental illness. *Am J Public Health* 92:1523–1531, 2002.
17. Teplin LA, McClelland GM, Abram KA. Crime victimization in adults with severe mental illness: comparison with National Crime Victimization Survey. *Arch Gen Psychiatry* 62(8):911–921, 2005.
18. Kavoussi R, Armstead P, Coccaro E. The neurobiology of impulsive aggression. *Psychiatr Clin North Am* 20(2):395–403, 1997.
20. Volavka J. *Neurobiology of violence*, Washington, DC, 2002, American Psychiatric Publishing.
22. Oquendo MA, Mann JJ. The biology of impulsivity and suicidality. *Psychiatr Clin North Am* 23:11–25, 2000.
25. Coccaro EF, Sripada CS, Yanowitch RN. Corticolimbic function in impulsive aggressive behavior. *Biol Psychiatry* 69(12):1153–1159, 2011.
26. Gansler DA, McLaughlin NC, Iguchi L, et al. A multivariate approach to aggression and the orbitofrontal cortex in psychiatric patients. *Psychiatry Res* 171(3):145–154, 2009.
28. Bufkin J, Luttrell VR. Neuroimaging studies of aggressive behavior, current findings and implications for criminology and criminal justice. *Trauma Violence Abuse* 6:176–191, 2005.
37. Lewis DO. Adult antisocial behavior, criminality, and violence. In Sadock BJ, Sadock VA, editors: *Kaplan and Sadock's comprehensive textbook of psychiatry*, ed 8, Philadelphia, 2005, Lippincott Williams & Wilkins.
40. American Psychiatric Association. *Diagnostic and statistical manual of mental disorders, fourth edition, text revision*, Washington, DC, 2000, American Psychiatric Press.
47. Elbogen EB, Beckham JC, Butterfield MI, et al. Assessing risk of violent behavior among veterans with severe mental illness. *J Trauma Stress* 21(1):113–117, 2008.
52. Goodman M, New A. Impulsive aggression in borderline personality disorder. *Curr Psychiatry Rep* 2:56–61, 2000.
53. Swanson JW, Swartz MS, Elbogen EB. Effectiveness of atypical antipsychotic medications in reducing violent behavior among persons with schizophrenia in community-based treatment. *Schizophr Bull* 30:3–20, 2004.
55. Anderson T, Bell C, Powell T. Assessing psychiatric patients for violence. *Community Ment Health J* 40:379–399, 2004.
56. Allen M, Currier G, Carpenter D. The expert consensus guideline series: treatment of behavioral emergencies. *J Psychiatr Pract* 11:1–112, 2005.
58. Yudofsky SC, Kopecky HJ, Kunik M, et al. The Overt Agitation Severity Scale (OASS) for the objective rating of agitation. *J Neuropsychiatr Clin Neurosci* 9:541–548, 1997.
63. Fava M. Psychopharmacologic treatment of pathologic aggression. *Psychiatr Clin North Am* 20:427–451, 1997.
64. Spivak B, Mester R, Wittenberg N, et al. Reduction of aggressiveness and impulsiveness during clozapine treatment in chronic neuroleptic-resistant schizophrenic patients. *Clin Neuropharmacol* 20:442–446, 1997.
65. Schwartz TL, Masand PS. The role of atypical antipsychotics in the treatment of delirium. *Psychosomatics* 43:171–174, 2002.
66. Caine E. Clinical perspectives on atypical antipsychotics for treatment of agitation. *J Clin Psychiatry* 67(Suppl. 1):22–31, 2006.
71. Kelleher JP, Centorrino F, Albert MJ, et al. Advances in atypical antipsychotics for the treatment of schizophrenia: new formulations and new agents. *CNS Drugs* 16:249–261, 2002.
72. Swanson JW, Swartz MS, Van Dorn RA, et al. Comparison of antipsychotic medication effects on reducing violence in people with schizophrenia. *Br J Psychiatry* 193(1):37–43, 2008.
73. Alpert JE, Spellman MK. Psychotherapeutic approaches to aggressive and violent patients. *Psychiatr Clin North Am* 20:453–472, 1997.
74. National Center for Trauma-Informed Care (NCTIC). Available from <http://www.samhsa.gov/nctic/default.asp>.

66 Culture and Psychiatry

David C. Henderson, MD, Brenda Vincenzi, MD, Albert S. Yeung, MD, ScD, and Gregory L. Fricchione, MD

KEY POINTS

Background

- Cultural differences in the presentation of psychiatric illnesses exist and include most if not all psychiatric disorders, including depression and psychosis.
- Cultural aspects can play a fundamental role in the manifestation of symptoms and the appearance of syndromes that are culture specific.
- Gender, race, ethnicity, and culture may all have a tremendous impact on the diagnosis, treatment, and outcome for many individuals with psychiatric and medical problems.

History

- Recently there has been a growing interest in understanding the role of cultural differences on mental disorders and psychopharmacology.
- Exploring the ethnic variations of psychotropic responses in different ethnic populations, involving differences in pharmacokinetics and pharmacodynamics, as well as the cultural impact on diagnosis and treatment will ensure higher-quality care for ethnic minorities.

Clinical and Research Challenges

- Biological and non-biological factors have a significant impact on the use of psychotropic medications.

- The activity of cytochrome (CYP) liver enzymes is controlled genetically, although environmental factors can alter their activity.
- Understanding how pharmacokinetics and environmental factors affect different populations will help to predict side effects, blood levels, and potential drug–drug interactions.

Practical Pointers

- The DSM-5 emphasizes that clinicians must take into account an individual's racial, ethnic, and cultural context, and consider a patient's cultural identity, cultural explanations of his or her illness, the cultural impact on psychosocial function, and the impact of culture on the relationship between the patient and the clinician for effective diagnostic assessment and clinical management.
- A cultural assessment related to diagnosis and treatment should be included in one's formulation of a patient and his or her problems.
- The impact of acculturation may also lead to psychiatric symptoms.
- A physician must ask about and make an effort to understand the circumstances surrounding immigration.
- All patients receiving psychotropics should be started on low doses, so as to reduce the risk of adverse events.

OVERVIEW

Gender, race, ethnicity, and culture may all have a tremendous impact on the diagnosis, treatment, and outcome for many individuals with psychiatric and medical problems. While it is impossible to understand every culture, there are basic principles that should be used to minimize clashes of cultures and to lessen the risk of providing compromised medical care. When evaluating and treating a patient from a different culture, care must be taken when making observations or applying stereotypes. A clinician must be aware at all times of his or her own feelings, biases, and stereotypes. Additionally, the psychiatrist must assess the impact of the care environment, the attitudes of the medical and ancillary care team, and the patient's experience within the health care system. Mistrust of the health care system is common and may influence a patient's behavior, level of cooperation, and adherence with recommendations. On the other hand, disparities in health care delivery exist and are influenced by factors such as gender, race, ethnicity, and culture.[1] Understanding a patient's culture will aid in the delivery of high-quality medical and psychiatric care. However, a little knowledge may be a dangerous thing. Inter-individual variability is common; an individual may not fit into preconceived notions of his or her culture. One must probe for cultural clues while remaining flexible enough to recognize that a patient's patterns and behaviors do not necessarily match the clinician's expectations.

CULTURAL ASSESSMENT

A cultural assessment related to diagnosis and treatment should be included in one's formulation of a patient and his or her problems. The *Diagnostic and Statistical Manual of Mental Disorders*, fifth edition (DSM-5),[2] emphasizes that a clinician must take into account an individual's racial, ethnic, and cultural context for effective diagnostic assessment and clinical management. This process, called *cultural formulation*, contains several components (Boxes 66-1 and 66-2). The DSM-5 provides an updated outline for cultural formulations and presents an approach to assessment using the Cultural Formulation Interview (CFI). The CFI is a brief semi-structured interview for systematically assessing cultural factors in the clinical encounter (www.psychiatry.org/dsm5).

Determination of Cultural Identity of the Individual

Racial, ethnic, or cultural references and the degree to which individuals are involved with their culture of origin and their host culture are important. It is crucial to listen for clues about culture and to ask specific questions concerning a patient's cultural identity. For instance, an Asian American male who grew up in the southern US may exhibit patterns, behaviors, and views of the world more consistent with those of a Caucasian southerner. Attention to language abilities and

---

BOX 66-1 Treating a Patient from a Different Culture

- Care must be taken when making observations, interpretations, or stereotypes.
- Clinicians must be aware at all times of their own feelings, biases, and stereotypes.
- Significant inter-individual variability exists; individuals may not fit into the expectations of their culture.
- One should probe for cultural clues.
- One should remain flexible enough to recognize that the patient's patterns and behaviors do not necessarily match the clinician's expectations.

BOX 66-2 DSM-5 Cultural Formulation

CULTURAL IDENTITY OF THE INDIVIDUAL

The individual's racial, ethnic, or cultural references and the degree to which an individual is involved with his or her culture of origin and host culture are important.

CULTURAL CONCEPTUALIZATIONS OF DISTRESS

It is important to understand how distress or the need for support is communicated through symptoms (e.g., nerves, possessing spirits, somatic complaints, or misfortune).

PSYCHOSOCIAL STRESSORS AND CULTURAL FEATURES OF VULNERABILITY AND RESILIENCE

Cultural factors have a significant impact on the psychosocial environment and on functioning.

CULTURAL FEATURES OF THE RELATIONSHIP BETWEEN THE INDIVIDUAL AND THE CLINICIAN

Cultural features of the relationship between the individual and the clinician must be addressed.

---

preferences must also be addressed. Other clinically-relevant aspects of identity include religious affiliation, socioeconomic background, personal and family places of birth and growing up, migrant status, and sexual orientation.

Determination of Cultural Conceptualizations of Distress

How an individual understands distress or the need for support is often communicated through symptoms (e.g., nerves, possession by spirits, somatic complaints, misfortune); therefore, the meaning and severity of an illness in relation to one's culture, family, and community should be determined. This explanatory model may be helpful when developing an interpretation, a diagnosis, and a treatment plan. Many patients from non-Western cultures are unfamiliar with the concepts and terminologies used by mental health professionals, leading to misunderstanding and avoidance of mental health services. Careful elicitation of a patient's explanatory model and using it as a common platform for communication frequently facilitates disclosure of a patient's diagnosis and treatment negotiation.

Determination of Psychosocial Stressors and Cultural Features of Vulnerability and Resilience

Cultural factors can have a significant impact on the psychosocial environment and on function. It is the physician's responsibility to determine the level of functioning, disability,

and resilience in light of the individual's cultural reference group and to help the patient and his or her family adjust to role changes caused by illness.

Determination of the Cultural Features between the Individual and the Clinician

Cultural aspects of the relationship between the individual and the clinician need to be considered. Moreover, cultural differences and their impact on the treatment must not be ignored. Language difficulties, difficulties eliciting symptoms or understanding their cultural significance, difficulties negotiating the appropriate relationship, and difficulties determining whether a behavior is normal or pathological are common barriers to care. In the hospital, the psychiatrist must also attend to the environment in which the patient is receiving treatment. An intervention of this nature may improve the comfort of patients and their health care providers as well as the quality of the care provided.

IMPACT OF ETHNICITY ON PSYCHIATRIC DIAGNOSIS

In the US, race and ethnicity have a significant impact on psychiatric diagnosis and treatment.[3] In 2003 the Agency for Healthcare Research and Quality (AHRQ), a division of the US Department of Health and Human Services, issued the first National Healthcare Disparity Report (NHDR), that described differences in access, use, and patient experience of care between racial, ethnic, socioeconomic, and geographic groups. According to the 2009 NHDR, disparities in health care have increased from 2003 to 2008.[4] African Americans are frequently misdiagnosed as having schizophrenia when instead they have bipolar disorder or a psychotic depression. Depression is frequently under-recognized and under-treated among Asian Americans as they tend to under-report their affective symptoms.[5] Moreover, treatment approaches and responses often differ, depending on the diagnosis. The reasons for misdiagnosis are complicated. They include the fact that individuals from some ethnic or cultural backgrounds may not seek treatment until later in the course of their illness than do Caucasian individuals; this results in the perception of a more severe illness.[6] The late presentation may, in part, be related to mistrust of the health care system, lack of familiarity of what mental health services are about, and fear of stigma associated with mental illnesses. Physician biases also play a major role in misdiagnosis. Psychiatric diagnoses are often established by eliciting symptoms from patients that are then interpreted by the psychiatric expert. Many disorders have overlapping symptoms and can be used to support one diagnosis or to disregard another. In the case of African Americans, affective symptoms are frequently ignored and psychotic symptoms are emphasized. This pattern has also been seen in other ethnic populations, including Hispanics, some Asian populations, and the Amish (in the US). African American patients are also more likely to receive higher doses of antipsychotics, to receive depot preparations, to have higher rates of involuntary psychiatric hospitalizations, and to have significantly higher rates of seclusion and restraints while in psychiatric hospitals.[7,8] The tendency is to oversedate such patients to reduce their "risk of violence" despite, in some cases, little evidence that the patient has ever been violent. These biases in psychiatric treatment continue and must be addressed.

Differences in Presentation of Illness

Cultural differences in the presentation of psychiatric illnesses abound. For instance, a Cambodian woman may complain of dizziness, fatigue, and back pain, while she ignores other neurovegetative symptoms and is unable to describe feelings of dysphoria. American mental health care providers are generally unfamiliar with various Indo-Chinese culture-bound syndromes and with the meaning attributed to those symptoms by various cultures. For example, common American expressions such as "feeling blue" cannot be readily translated into Indo-Chinese languages. A Cambodian clinician will ask Cambodian patients if they "feel blue" by using Cambodian terms that literally translate into "heavy, overcast, gloomy." The Laotian way of describing "feeling tense" is feeling like a "balloon blown up until it is about to burst." Westermeyer,[9] in a case-controlled study in Laos, documented the general inability of Western psychiatrists to recognize the Laotian symptoms of depression. Similarly, many depressed Chinese Americans who seek help in primary care clinics complain mostly of physical symptoms, and minimize their depressed mood.

Depression may be missed by psychiatrists and by primary care physicians who search for biological and structural reasons for complaints (e.g., back pain, headaches, dizziness). Often afflicted patients are treated with meclizine for dizziness and analgesics for pain, where an antidepressant would have been more appropriate.

From a cross-cultural perspective, evaluating the meanings of bizarre delusions, hallucinations, and psychotic-like symptoms remains a clinical challenge. A non-psychotic patient may admit to hearing voices of her ancestors (a feature that is culturally appropriate in certain cultural groups). In many traditional, non-Western societies, spirits of the deceased are regarded as capable of interacting with, and possessing, those still alive. It is difficult to determine whether symptoms are bizarre enough to yield a diagnosis of schizophrenia without an adequate understanding of a patient's sociocultural and religious background. On the other hand, caution must be taken not to assume that bizarre symptoms are culturally appropriate when in fact they are a manifestation of psychosis. The use of bicultural and bilingual interpreters, along with the search for information from other sources (such as family, community leaders, or religious officials), may help to determine whether an individual's experience is culturally appropriate or acceptable.

Additionally, while a great deal of attention has been paid to the study of panic disorder in Caucasians, little empirical research within the US has looked at the phenomenology of panic disorder among minority groups. Compared to Caucasians, African Americans with panic disorder report more intense fears of dying or going crazy, more numbness and tingling in their extremities, and higher rates of co-morbid post-traumatic stress disorder (PTSD) and depression.[10] African Americans also use somewhat different coping strategies (e.g., religious practice, counting one's blessings) and endorse less self-blame. The incidence of isolated sleep paralysis is also higher in African Americans.[10]

Acculturation and Immigration

Recent immigrants or refugees arrive in the US with a host of difficulties and psychosocial problems. A physician must ask about and make an effort to understand the circumstances surrounding immigration. An individual may have been a political prisoner or a victim of trauma and torture, or may have been lost or separated from family members. Under these circumstances, the level of depression and PTSD experienced may be high. Literature on the contribution of acculturative stresses to the emergence of mental disorder is abundant.[11,12] The impact of acculturation may also lead to symptoms of depression, anxiety, and "culture shock," and even to PTSD-like symptoms.

The trauma and torture experienced by many refugees are also unfamiliar to the majority of American practitioners.[13] In spite of the numerous reports of the concentration camp experiences in Cambodia, the sexual abuse of Vietnamese boat-women, and the serious emotional distress associated with escape, refugee camps, and resettlement experiences, limited research exists on refugee trauma and trauma-related psychiatric disorders and social handicaps.

CULTURE-BOUND SYNDROMES (CULTURAL CONCEPT OF DISTRESS)

A culture-bound syndrome is a collection of signs and symptoms that is restricted to a limited number of cultures by reason of certain psychosocial features. Culture-bound syndromes are usually restricted to a specific setting, and they have a special relationship to that setting. Culture-bound syndromes are classified on the basis of common etiology (e.g., magic, evil spells, angry ancestors), so clinical pictures may vary.

According to the DSM-5 the *cultural concepts of distress* (syndromes, idioms, and explanations) are more relevant than the older formulation *culture-bound syndrome* described in the DSM-IV.[14] The current formulation acknowledges that all forms of distress are locally shaped, including the DSM disorders. The DSM-5 (Appendix, Glossary of cultural concept of distress) contains symptomatic description of nine cultural concepts of distress (Table 66-1).[2] Cultural concept of distress refers to ways that cultural groups experience, understand, and communicate suffering, behavioral problems, or troubling thoughts and emotions.

Projection is a common ego defense mechanism in many non-Western cultures. Guilt and shame are often projected into cultural beliefs and ceremonies. Guilt and shame are attributed to other individuals, to groups, or to objects, and may involve acting out, blaming others, and needing to punish others. Projection is also seen in magic and in supernatural perspectives of existence. This leads to projective ceremonies and may lead to illness when the ceremonies are not performed.

Cultural psychoses are difficult to define. In cultural syndromes, hallucinations may be viewed as normal variants. Delusions and thought disorder must be re-evaluated within a particular cultural setting. A culture may interpret abnormal behavior as relating to some kind of voodoo or anger and may regard the symptoms as normal even though symptoms are consistent with schizophrenia.

In the past, it was believed that culture-bound syndromes only occurred in the country or region of origin. However, with significant population movements and the tendency for immigrants to remain within their culture (though they have moved to a new country), culture-bound syndromes have been observed in other parts of the world. One common culture-bound syndrome is *ataque de nervios*, which is commonly known and observed in Hispanic populations. As with many culture-bound syndromes, there may be significant overlap with DSM-IV psychiatric diagnoses. In one study, 36% of Dominican and Puerto Rican subjects diagnosed with *ataque de nervios* also met the criteria for panic attacks, while the features did not necessarily occur together during the *ataque* episode.[15]

WORKING WITH INTERPRETERS

Communication problems are common even between English-speaking doctors and patients from similar socioeconomic backgrounds. Therefore, it is not difficult to imagine the challenges and obstacles that a physician faces when working with limited-English-speaking patients whose culture may be very

TABLE 66-1 Glossary of Cultural Concepts of Distress, DSM-5 (Appendix)

Cultural Concept	Description	Culture	Related Conditions in Other Cultural Contexts
Ataque de nervios ("attack of nerves")	Sense of being out of control (shouting, aggression, crying, agitation…) related to a stressful event relating to the family	Latin descent	"Indisposition" in Haiti, "blacking out" in the Southern United States, and "falling out" in the West Indies
Dhat syndrome	Severe anxiety associated with the discharge of semen	India, Sri Lanka (*sukra prameha*) and China (*shen-k'uei*)	Singapore and China
Khyâl cap ("wind attacks")	Symptoms similar to panic attack	Cambodians in the US and Cambodia	Laos, Tibet, Sri Lanka, and Korea
Kufungisisa ("thinking too much")	Ruminating on upsetting thoughts/worries	Shona of Zimbabwe	Common across many countries and ethnic groups
Maladi moun ("humanly caused illness" or "sent sickness")	Envy and malice caused people to harm their enemies by sending illnesses such as psychosis and depression	Haitian communities	Common across cultures (e.g., Spanish: *mal de ojo*; Italian: *mal'occhiu*)
Nervios	Emotional distress, somatic disturbance, inability to function	Latinos in the US and Latin America	Greeks and Sicilians in North America, white Appalachia and Newfoundland
Shenjing shuairou ("weakness of the nervous systems"/neurasthenia)	Weakness, excitement, emotions, nervous pain, and sleep symptoms clusters	Chinese	India and Japan
Susto ("fright")	The soul leaves the body causing unhappiness and sickness	Hispanics in the US, Mexico, Central America, and South America	Found globally
Taijin kyofusho "interpersonal fear disorders"	Anxiety/avoidance of interpersonal situations due to the thought, feeling, or conviction that one's appearance and actions are inadequate or can offend others (broader construct than social anxiety disorder)	Japanese	*Taein kong po* in Korea

different and unfamiliar to the doctor. Misunderstandings or a lack of comprehension about a patient's physical or psychiatric complaints may lead to misdiagnosis and result in unnecessary or inappropriate treatment. Patients, in turn, may feel frustrated, discouraged, or dissatisfied with their health care; this may lead them to refuse treatment or terminate their visits altogether.[16] Fortunately, interpreters can help bridge the communication gap between doctors and non-English-speaking patients.

Many states now have laws that require federally-funded medical facilities to provide interpreters for their non-English-speaking patients. While many interpreters are trained and certified to work with medical providers, translating for a mental health professional is very different, and it can be challenging.[17] Both interpreters and clinicians need to be aware of issues that may arise when using interpreters in psychiatric settings. Some of the issues that clinicians face when working with interpreters are listed in Box 66-3.[17]

Recommendations When Working with Interpreters

When clinicians work with interpreters, they need to know their qualifications. Do the interpreters have experience working with psychiatrists and psychologists? How much do they know about mental illness and mental health services? What are their personal views about mental illness? Interpreters who come from cultures where mental illness is highly stigmatized may bring biases or beliefs into the therapeutic process. It is well known that patients from certain cultures have been advised by their interpreters not to seek mental

---

BOX 66-3 Issues Faced by Clinicians Who Work with Interpreters

- Clinicians may feel they have less control in their work because their direct contact with the patient is decreased by the presence of the interpreter.
- Clinicians may feel uncertain about their role when working with interpreters who are more active and involved in the treatment process.
- Clinicians may have transference issues toward the interpreter.
- Conflicts may arise when clinicians and interpreters hold opposing views on a patient's diagnosis and treatment plans.
- Interpreters may find it difficult to work with clinicians of a different gender than their own.
- Clinicians may feel frustrated when they cannot verify what is being said to the patient.
- Clinicians may feel left out if the patient appears to have more of a connection with the interpreter.
- Interpreters may feel uncomfortable when asked to translate certain issues, such as sexual history or childhood abuse.

---

health services because only "crazy" people see psychiatrists and psychologists.

Clinicians should avoid using family members, friends, or clerical staff as interpreters.[17] Patients may not be able to disclose certain information in front of their spouse or child. At the same time, it may be too difficult or distressing for a young child to have to hear certain details about his or her parent.

In addition, family members have been known to omit or to alter information they feel is too embarrassing or inappropriate to reveal to the clinician. In the past, janitors and clerical staff were used as interpreters. This, of course, is strongly discouraged since cleaning and clerical staff may not have adequate medical or mental health language skills to provide accurate translations for clinicians. Unless there are no other alternatives, clinicians should avoid using family members and clerical employees as interpreters.

Trained interpreters should be treated as professional colleagues by clinicians.[17] Most interpreters are now well trained and can offer important cultural knowledge that can help promote the doctor–patient relationship. Clinicians should use the interpreters' language skills as well as their cultural expertise to help increase the clinician's understanding of the patient's culture, religion, and worldview. For some clinicians, interpreters are used only as voices to communicate with patients. They prefer word-for-word translations and do not want the interpreter to filter or alter what they say. While this allows the clinician to maintain his or her role as the primary caregiver and, to a certain extent, control what is being said to the patient, using direct translations can often lead to misunderstandings and confusions for both the patient and the clinician.

Literal translations from one language to another can be inaccurate and inappropriate. For example, "feeling blue," when translated word for word into Vietnamese, does not make any sense to the patient because it literally translates to *"cam giac xanh,"* which means "feeling color blue."[18] Certain words or concepts, such as depression and mental health, may not exist in the country of origin of the patient. Interpreters may have to explain or to describe the concept of depression to the patient, which requires much more time than the clinician might expect. Clinicians must be patient, keeping in mind that it may take 10 minutes to translate one word. In addition, certain issues may be culturally inappropriate to ask or to say to a patient. Most women from an Asian or a Hispanic background feel uncomfortable if asked directly about sensitive topics (such as sexual abuse or family discord). Interpreters can be used as cultural consultants to assist clinicians with these more complex cases. Allowing interpreters the freedom and flexibility to re-phrase or to summarize what is being said can help prevent misunderstandings and improve the exchange between the clinician and the patient.

Clinicians should meet with the interpreter briefly before each session to discuss expectations and to clarify any issues or points that the clinician would like to address during the session.[17] Patients do not get as much time with the clinicians when they have to go through interpreters. Everything has to be translated back and forth; hence, clinicians may find that they do not get as much accomplished in their session as they do with English-speaking patients. Time is a crucial factor when interpreters are involved. Thus, one should protect the patient's time by avoiding any discussions with the interpreters that can wait until after the session.

Be sure to introduce the interpreter to the patient at the start of the session if they have not met. Re-affirm issues of confidentiality.[17,18] Often, a patient may feel uneasy about revealing personal issues or conflicts to individuals from his or her own community. As most ethnic communities are small and close-knit, patients may fear that the interpreter will divulge their private information to those in the community. Patients are more likely to open up if they feel reassured that what they share with the clinician and interpreter will be kept in strict confidence. If possible, one should try to use the same interpreter to help build trust and continuity of care for the patient.[17]

During sessions, clinicians should face and speak directly to the patients instead of to the interpreters.[17] While the patient and the clinician may not be able to communicate through language, they can communicate and connect through eye contact, gestures of acknowledgment, and other non-verbal behaviors. It is helpful for the interpreter if the clinician can speak slowly and avoid using long and complicated sentences. One should stay away from technical or psychological terminology that does not translate well. In addition, it is helpful to pause often to allow the interpreter to translate, to ask for clarification if there is any confusion,[17] and avoid two-way conversations. Just as clinicians and interpreters should not engage in lengthy discussions in front of the patient, clinicians should interrupt when a patient and an interpreter are talking too long. Tension may arise when someone in the group feels left out.

After each session, it is helpful to encourage the interpreters to give their impression about the session; interpreters can often provide important observations and feedback.[17] One should ask the interpreter to clarify any issues or points that were not made clear during the session. Clinicians can use this time to learn more from the interpreter about the patient's culture. The clinician and interpreter can also provide feedback about each other's performances. Good communication and trust between clinicians and interpreters are essential to care for patients with little or limited English.

ETHNICITY AND PSYCHOPHARMACOLOGY

Emerging research on transcultural psychopharmacology ("ethnopsychopharmacology")[19-22] may aid the clinician's effective treatment of diverse populations. An understanding of ethnicity and its psychopharmacology and psychobiology is necessary to ensure quality care for ethnic minorities. Biological and non-biological issues have a significant impact on the use of psychotropic medications.

Culturally-shaped beliefs play a major role in determining whether an explanation about an illness and a treatment plan will make sense to a patient ("explanatory models"); for example, Hispanics or Asians often expect rapid relief with treatment and are cautious about potential side effects induced by Western medicine. Concerns about addictive and toxic effects of medications are extremely common among Asian Americans. Some populations continue to use a mixture of herbal medicines and typically believe that polypharmacy is more effective. The use of herbal medicines is of great concern secondary to the risk of drug interactions and the risk of medical or psychiatric side effects or toxicity. The Food and Drug Administration (FDA) has issued a number of warnings on herbal medicine products, including the most popular weight-loss products containing *Ephedra sinica (ma huang)*, which is the main plant source of ephedrine and which has been reported to cause mania, psychosis, and sudden death.

Patient compliance may be affected by incorrect dosing, medication side effects, and polypharmacy. Other factors include a poor therapeutic alliance and a lack of community support, money, or transportation; in addition, substance abuse or concerns about the addictiveness of a medication may be crucial. Communication difficulties and divergence between a patient's and a clinician's explanatory model play an important role in why a patient from an ethnic minority is significantly more likely to drop out of treatment. Exploring these beliefs will improve communication, adherence, and outcome.

Examining social support systems in each patient is vital. The ways in which a family interacts and functions has a significant impact on psychiatric treatment. For example, some Hispanics have more interactions with relatives and may become increasingly demoralized when the involvement of relatives in their treatment does not occur. Hispanics and

Asians typically have a "closed network," which consists of family members, kin, and intimate friends.

Biological Aspects of Psychopharmacology

Pharmacokinetics deal with metabolism, blood levels, absorption, distribution, and excretion of medications. However, other pharmacokinetic variables, such as conjugation, plasma-protein binding, and oxidation by the cytochrome (CYP) isoenzymes, also play a role. Pharmacokinetics may be influenced by genetics, age, gender, total body weight, environment, diet, toxins, drugs, alcohol, as well as disease states. Environmental factors include medications, drugs, herbal medicines, steroids, dietary factors, sex hormones, and use of caffeine or tobacco.

The activity of CYP liver enzymes is controlled genetically, although environmental factors can alter their activity. Understanding how pharmacokinetics and environmental factors relate to different populations will help to predict side effects, blood levels, and potential drug–drug interactions. For example, CYP 2D6 is the isoenzyme that metabolizes many antidepressants, including the tricyclic and heterocyclic antidepressants and the selective serotonin reuptake inhibitors (SSRIs); SSRIs can inhibit this enzyme, leading to accumulations of other substrates (Tables 66-2a and 66-2b). CYP 2D6 also plays a role in metabolizing antipsychotics: for example, clozapine, haloperidol, perphenazine, risperidone, thioridazine, and sertindole. While much emphasis has been placed on the CYP 2D6 metabolism of psychotropics, it is a major enzyme for the metabolism of numerous non-psychotropic medications as well. This, while often ignored clinically, can have a significant effect on the tolerability or toxicity of medications.

The incidence of "poor metabolizers" (i.e., those individuals with little enzyme activity) at the CYP 2D6 is roughly 3% to 7% in Caucasians, 0.5% to 2.4% in Asians, 4.5% in Hispanics, and approximately 1.9% in African Americans[20] (Table 66-3). Individuals from these backgrounds are at great risk for

toxicity, even when medications are used at low doses. For instance, a woman who develops hypotension and a change in mental status several days after starting 20 mg of nortriptyline may be found to have toxic blood levels and require cardiac monitoring. Table 66-3 lists drugs that are metabolized through different CYP enzyme systems.

A genetic variation of the extensive metabolizer gene that decreases activity at the CYP 2D6 enzymes by approximately 50% ("slow metabolizer") has been discovered. This group appears to have enzyme activity levels that are intermediate between poor and extensive metabolizers.[20] Approximately 18% of Mexican Americans and 37% of Asians and 33% of African Americans have this gene variation. This may explain ethnic differences in the pharmacokinetics of neuroleptics and antidepressants. While these individuals are not as likely to experience toxicity at extremely low doses (e.g., poor metabolizers) they are likely to experience significant side effects at lower doses. These individuals may quickly be classified as the "difficult patients" because they complain of side effects at unexpectedly low doses. The above information is striking considering that numerous studies, for instance, have shown that African Americans receive higher doses of antipsychotics, are more frequently treated with depot neuroleptics, and have higher rates of involuntary commitments and seclusion and restraints than do Caucasians.[19] While data on pharmacokinetics of neuroleptics have been mixed in African Americans, Asians have been shown to have a higher "area under the curve" for haloperidol.[21] Korean Americans have also been found to have higher blood levels of clozapine and to respond to lower doses of clozapine when compared to Caucasians. In fact, though sertindole, metabolized by CYP 2D6, did not make it to the US market, the phase II clinical trials included enough African Americans to determine that their sertindole blood levels were 50% higher than Caucasian subjects who took the same dose. In addition, CYP 2D6 gene can be duplicated or multiplied up to 13 copies. Subjects with these genetic mutations are called ultra-rapid metabolizers because they have more enzyme and higher enzyme activity. Therefore, they

TABLE 66-2A Cytochrome P450 Isoenzymes, Inhibitors, and Inducers

	CYP 1A2	CYP 2C9/10	CYP 2C19	CYP 2D6	CYP 2E1	CYP 3A3/4
INHIBITORS	Fluvoxamine Moclobemide Cimetidine Fluoroquinolones Ciprofloxacin/ norfloxacin Naringenin (grapefruit) Ticlopidine	Fluvoxamine Disulfiram Amiodarone Azapropazone D-propoxyphene Fluconazole Fluvastatin Miconazole Phenylbutazone Stiripentol Sulfaphenazole Zafirlukast	Fluoxetine Fluvoxamine Imipramine Moclobemide Tranylcypromine Diazepam Felbamate Phenytoin Topiramate Cimetidine Omeprazole	Bupropion Fluoxetine Fluvoxamine Hydroxy-bupropion Paroxetine Sertraline Moclobemide Fluphenazine Haloperidol Perphenazine Thioridazine Amiodarone Cimetidine Methadone Quinidine Ritonavir	Diethylthio-carbamate (Disulfiram)	Fluoxetine Fluvoxamine Nefazodone Sertraline Diltiazem Verapamil Dexamethasone Gestodene Clarithromycin Erythromycin Troleandomycin Fluconazole Itraconazole Ketoconazole Ritonavir Indinavir Amiodarone Cimetidine Mibefradil Naringenin (grapefruit) Carbamazepine
INDUCERS	Tobacco Omeprazole	Barbiturates Phenytoin Rifampin	Rifampin		Ethanol Isoniazid	Barbiturates Phenobarbital Phenytoin Dexamethasone Rifampin Troglitazone

TABLE 66-2B Cytochrome P450 Isoenzymes and Substrates

	CYP 1A2	CYP 2C9/10	CYP 2C19	CYP 2D6	CYP 2E1	CYP 3A3/4	
SUBSTRATES	Tertiary amine TCAs	THC	Citalopram	Fluoxetine	Ethanol	Carbamazepine	Amiodarone
	Clozapine	NSAIDs	Moclobemide	Mirtazapine	Acetaminophen	Alprazolam	Disopyramide
	Olanzapine	Phenytoin	Tertiary amine	Paroxetine	Chlorzoxazone	Diazepam	Lidocaine
	Caffeine	Tolbutamide	TCAs	Venlafaxine	Halothane	Midazolam	Propafenone
	Methadone	Warfarin	Diazepam	Secondary and	Isoflurane	Triazolam	Quinidine
	Tacrine	Losartan	Hexobarbital	tertiary amine	Methoxyflurane	Buspirone	Erythromycin
	Acetaminophen	Irbesartan	Mephobarbital	TCAs	Sevoflurane	Citalopram	Androgens
	Phenacetin		Omeprazole	Trazodone		Mirtazapine	Dexamethasone
	Propranolol		Lansoprazole	Clozapine		Nefazodone	Estrogens
	Theophylline		Phenytoin	Haloperidol		Reboxetine	Astemizole
	Warfarin		S-mephenytoin	Fluphenazine		Sertraline	Loratadine
			Nelfinavir	Perphenazine		Tertiary amine	Terfenadine
			Warfarin	Risperidone		TCAs	Lovastatin
				Sertindole		Sertindole	Simvastatin
				Thioridazine		Quetiapine	Atorvastatin
				Codeine		Ziprasidone	Cerivastatin
				Dextromethorphan		Diltiazem	Cyclophosphamide
				Hydrocodone		Felodipine	Tamoxifen
				Oxycodone		Nimodipine	Vincristine
				Mexiletine		Nifedipine	Vinblastine
				Propafenone		Nisoldipine	Ifosfamide
				(IC antiarrhythmics)		Nitrendipine	Cyclosporine
				β-Blockers		Verapamil	Tacrolimus
				Donepezil		Acetaminophen	Cisapride
				D & L fenfluramine		Alfentanil	Donepezil
						Codeine	

TABLE 66-3 CYP450 Enzyme Activity Levels among Various Ethnic Groups

	2D6	2C19	2C9	3A4
White	2%–7% PM 3.5% SEM	3%–5% PM		
African American/black	2.1% PM 33% IM/SM	4%–18% PM	18%–22% PM	
Asian	0.5%–2.4% PM 37% IM/SM	18%–23% PM	18%–22% PM	East Indians—reduced activity (may be diet)
Hispanic/Latino	3%–5% PM 18% IM/S			Mexicans—reduced activity (may be diet)
Other	Ethiopian 29% SEM Saudi Arabian 19% SEM Spanish 10% SEM			

IM, Intermediate metabolizer; PM, poor metabolizer; SEM, superextensive metabolizer; SM, slow metabolizer.

may not respond to the usual dose of medication and require higher dose in order to achieve therapeutic response. Ultra-rapid metabolizers are found in 29% of Ethiopians, 19% of Arabs, 19% of Spaniards, and 1% of Swedish people.[23]

The CYP 2C9 isoenzyme is involved in the metabolism of ibuprofen, naproxen, phenytoin, warfarin, and tolbutamide. Approximately 18% to 22% of Asians and African Americans are poor metabolizers of these drugs. CYP 2C19 is involved in the metabolism of diazepam, clomipramine, imipramine, and propranolol; it is inhibited by fluoxetine and sertraline. The rates of poor metabolizers of this enzyme are approximately 3% to 5% in Caucasians, 4% to 18% in African Americans, and 18% to 23% in Asians.[19–21]

Lithium appears to be a drug with significant differences in dosing and tolerability across populations. African Americans are more likely to experience lithium toxicity and delirium compared to Caucasians (likely related to a slower lithium-sodium pathway and connected to higher rates of hypertension). Some Asian populations respond to lower doses and have lower serum levels of lithium (0.4 to 0.8 mEq/L).[24]

The choice of medications, particularly atypical antipsychotics, should be tempered by an understanding of individual and population risk factors for medical morbidities (e.g., obesity, hypertension, diabetes mellitus, cardiovascular disease).[25,26] For instance, many of the reports of diabetic ketoacidosis (DKA) secondary to atypical agents have been in African Americans who are at higher risk for diabetes.[25–27]

TECHNIQUES TO MINIMIZE CULTURAL CLASHES, MISDIAGNOSIS, AND ADVERSE EVENTS

Certain techniques may be used to avoid misdiagnosis, inappropriate treatment, and cultural clashes. The first moments of an encounter are often crucial. A clinician must be respectful to all patients and address them formally (e.g., Mr., Ms., Mrs.). In some cultures, an informal introduction is considered disrespectful and may have a lasting impact on the physician–patient relationship.

The relationship will be more complex and it will take longer to develop trust and an alliance. It will also take time

---

BOX 66-4 Prescribing Recommendations

ASSESSMENT

- Invoke a cultural formulation for diagnosis and to reassess or to confirm a diagnosis

CHOICE OF MEDICATION

- Based on medical history, concurrent medications, diet and food supplements/herbal medicine combined with knowledge of enzyme activity in certain ethnic groups
- Start all patients at lower doses than in the recommended prescribing guidelines

MONITOR PATIENT

- Proceed slowly, increase the dose as tolerated, and assess for efficacy in target symptoms
- If side effects are intolerable: lower the dose, or choose a drug metabolized through a different route
- If no response: check compliance, raise the dose, and check blood levels, add inhibitors, or switch the drug

---

to assure patients about confidentiality and to educate patients about mental illness to reduce stigma that may be influenced by culture. Also, if the diagnosis is unclear or is affected by ethnicity or culture, one should consider using a structured diagnostic interview (e.g., the Structured Clinical Interview for DSM-IV [SCID]) to reduce the possibility of misdiagnosis. Finally, it is important to acknowledge the need to spend more time with a patient from a different culture. A clinician must have patience and should expect longer sessions when using an interpreter.

Psychotropic medications should be started at doses lower than what is typically recommended (Box 66-4). Medication should be titrated slowly and guided by safety and tolerability, as well as efficacy for target symptoms. Applying principles such as this will help to reduce adverse events in all populations.

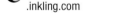 Access a list of MCQs for this chapter at https://expertconsult .inkling.com

REFERENCES

1. Shavers VL, Fagan P, Jones D, et al. The state of research on racial/ ethnic discrimination in the receipt of health care. *Am J Public Health* 102(5):953–966, 2012.
2. American Psychiatry Association. *Diagnostic and statistical manual of mental disorders*, ed 5, Washington, DC, 2013, American Psychiatry Association.
3. McGuire TG, Miranda J. New evidence regarding racial and ethnic disparities in mental health: policy implications. *Health Aff (Millwood)* 27(2):393–403, 2008.
4. AHRQ. *National Healthcare Disparities Report*. Rockville, Maryland, 2008, Services DoHaH.
5. Yeung A, Howarth S, Chan R, et al. Use of the Chinese version of the Beck Depression Inventory for screening depression in primary care. *J Nerv Ment Dis* 190(2):94–99, 2002.
6. Gonzalez JM, Alegria M, Prihoda TJ, et al. How the relationship of attitudes toward mental health treatment and service use differs by age, gender, ethnicity/race and education. *Soc Psychiatry Psychiatr Epidemiol* 46(1):45–57, 2011.
7. Hicks JW. Ethnicity, race, and forensic psychiatry: are we color-blind? *J Am Acad Psychiatry Law* 32(1):21–33, 2004.
8. Snowden LR, Hastings JF, Alvidrez J. Overrepresentation of black Americans in psychiatric inpatient care. *Psychiatr Serv* 60(6):779–785, 2009.
9. Westermeyer J. Folk concepts of mental disorder among the Lao: continuities with similar concepts in other cultures and in psychiatry. *Cult Med Psychiatry* 3(3):301–317, 1979.
10. Friedman S, Paradis C. Panic disorder in African-Americans: symptomatology and isolated sleep paralysis. *Cult Med Psychiatry* 26(2):179–198, 2002.
11. Bhugra D, Bhui K. Transcultural psychiatry: do problems persist in the second generation? *Hosp Med* 59(2):126–129, 1998.
12. Sirin SR, Ryce P, Gupta T, et al. The role of acculturative stress on mental health symptoms for immigrant adolescents: a longitudinal investigation. *Dev Psychol* 49(4):736–748, 2013.
13. Shannon P, O'Dougherty M, Mehta E. Refugees' perspectives on barriers to communication about trauma histories in primary care. *Ment Health Fam Med* 9(1):47–55, 2012.
14. American Psychiatry Association. Diagnostic and statistical manual of mental disorders. In Edition F, editor: *Text Revision 2005*, Washington, DC, 2005, American Psychiatric Press.
15. Lewis-Fernandez R, Guarnaccia PJ, Martinez IE, et al. Comparative phenomenology of ataques de nervios, panic attacks, and panic disorder. *Cult Med Psychiatry* 26(2):199–223, 2002.
16. Mirdal GM, Ryding E, Essendrop Sondej M. Traumatized refugees, their therapists, and their interpreters: three perspectives on psychological treatment. *Psychol Psychother* 85(4):436–455, 2012.
17. RRH T. *Working with interpreters in mental health*, New York, 2003, Brunner-Routledge.
18. McPhee SJ. Caring for a 70-year-old vietnamese woman. *JAMA* 287(4):495–504, 2002.
19. Herrera WL, Sramek JJ. *Cross cultural psychiatry*, New York, 1999, Wiley.
20. Lin KM. Psychopharmacology in cross-cultural psychiatry. *Mt Sinai J Med* 63(5–6):283–284, 1996.
21. Lin KM, Poland RE, Nuccio I, et al. A longitudinal assessment of haloperidol doses and serum concentrations in Asian and Caucasian schizophrenic patients. *Am J Psychiatry* 146(10):1307–1311, 1989.
22. Peterson DE, Remington PL, Kuykendall MA, et al. Behavioral risk factors of Chippewa Indians living on Wisconsin reservations. *Public Health Rep* 109(6):820–823, 1994.
23. Lin KM, Chen CH, Yu SH, et al. *Psychopharmacology: Ethnic and cultural perspectives. Psychiatry*, Chichester, 2003, John Wiley and Sons.
24. Lin TY. Psychiatry and Chinese culture. *West J Med* 139(6):862–867, 1983.
25. Henderson DC. Clinical experience with insulin resistance, diabetic ketoacidosis, and type 2 diabetes mellitus in patients treated with atypical antipsychotic agents. *J Clin Psychiatry* 62(Suppl. 27):10–14, discussion 40–41, 2001.
26. Henderson DC. Atypical antipsychotic-induced diabetes mellitus: how strong is the evidence? *CNS Drugs* 16(2):77–89, 2002.
27. Yeung A, Chang D, Gresham RL Jr, et al. Illness beliefs of depressed Chinese American patients in primary care. *J Nerv Ment Dis* 192(4):324–327, 2004.

67 Community Psychiatry

BJ Beck, MSN, MD

KEY POINTS

Background

- The four principles of community mental health are population responsibility, prevention, community-based care with citizen involvement, and continuity of care.

History

- Community psychiatry, the "third psychiatric revolution," has an undulant history of reform and neglect.

- From the military experience of World War II came three central tenets of community psychiatry: immediacy, proximity, and expectancy.

- The seamless, inclusive care system envisioned in the 1960s Community Mental Health Centers Acts was never realized.

Clinical and Research Challenges

- The historic challenge to community research or clinical care has been the need to bridge multiple sites, providers, provider types, and discontinuous systems of care with minimal resources.

- The major challenge remains to influence administrative and legislative decisions to provide incentives and adequate funding for innovative, integrative, and collaborative community care.

Practical Pointers

- The current fragmented system requires tremendous creativity to meet patients where they are, to help the most vulnerable access the services they need, and to minimize "revolving door" hospital admissions.

OVERVIEW

A broad historical context is necessary to comprehend the evolution of the complex array of discontinuous services now under the rubric of "community psychiatry." This sociopolitical system, the third psychiatric revolution[1] (the first two revolutions being moral treatment and psychoanalysis, respectively), has variously followed the doctrines of public health, prevention, population-based care, and social activism. In the US, the history of community psychiatry is a tale of decremental finances and shifting priorities (e.g., mental health for all versus focused resources for the seriously mentally ill; mainstream patients in the community versus remove and contain them in institutions) driven by surges of public outrage and activist reform, followed by ebbs of denial and neglect. The survival of community psychiatry, given the degree and rate of change in resources and mandates, has demanded a sustained and unparalleled creative effort.

TERMS AND DEFINITIONS

Because of this evolution, an appreciation for community psychiatry requires working knowledge of terms common to disciplines as disparate as sanitation and managed care. There are subtle differences in related, but not synonymous, fields

that illustrate the lack of cohesive theory and practice. Formative social and public health policies and tenets have also played an important role. Economic, political, and systemic oversight developments continue to direct the future purview and practice of community psychiatry. Beyond clinical terminology, each of these factors has its own lexicon.

Related Fields

Various and possibly confusing terms are (imprecisely) used interchangeably with the term *community psychiatry* (e.g., *social psychiatry, community mental health, public psychiatry,* and *population-based psychiatry*). The theory of social psychiatry accentuates the sociocultural aspects of mental disorders and their treatments. Research to advance this theory views psychiatry and psychological features as variables to predict, describe, and mediate the expression of social problems. Community psychiatry is a clinical application of this theory with the mandate to develop an optimal care system for a given population with finite resources. Clearly, goal achievement entails working with individuals, groups, and systems, but that is the extent of agreement (in the field and over time) on the appropriate emphasis, boundaries, core services, and guiding principles of community psychiatry.[2] The following quoted definitions hint at this lack of consensus:

> "... the body of knowledge, theories, methods and skills in research and service required by psychiatrists who participate in organized community programs for the promotion of mental health and the prevention, treatment and rehabilitation of the mental disorders in a population."[3]

> "... focusing on the detection, prevention, early treatment, and rehabilitation of emotional disorders and social deviance as they develop in the community rather than as they are encountered at large, centralized psychiatric facilities."[4]

> "... subspecialty area in which psychiatrists deliver mental health services to populations defined by a common workplace, activity, or geographical area of residence."[5]

> "... responsible for the comprehensive treatment of the severely mentally ill in the community at large. All aspects of care—from hospitalization, case management, and crisis intervention, to day treatment, and supportive living arrangements—are included."[6]

Community mental health (CMH), as defined by the Community Mental Health Center (CMHC) Acts of 1963 (Public Law 88-164) and 1965 (Public Law 89-105), was envisioned to be an inclusive, multi-disciplinary, systemic approach to publicly funded mental health services provided for all in need, residing in a given geographical locale (i.e., catchment area), without consideration of ability to pay. *Catchment* (from sanitation engineering: a cistern into which the sewage of a defined area is dumped) refers to a CMH service area with a population of 75,000 to 200,000.[7] Public psychiatry, a system of government-funded inpatient and outpatient services also initially conceived to meet the needs of all, has actually narrowed its focus on the seriously mentally ill who are unable to access appropriate services in the "private" sector (e.g., as fee-for-service, or as paid by third-party insurance). A trend to privatize (i.e., to put out to private sector bid with government oversight) the public sector services threatens to further confuse the definition and blur the public/private distinction. In population-based psychiatry, the population may be defined by geography, or by any of a number of other attributes (e.g., payer, employer, guild, or care system). However the population is defined, the system (e.g., a health maintenance organization [HMO]) is accountable for all members, as well as for an individual seeking treatment.

Social and Public Health Terms

Deinstitutionalization was a sociopolitical and economic trend to discharge long-term psychiatric inpatients to live and receive services in the community. More appropriately called de*hospitalization*[8] (or *trans*institutionalism[2]), patients were merely maintained in non-hospital institutional settings. This trend was evident, however, long before the term (and such associated terms as *policy* or *movement*) ever appeared in the psychiatric literature, which suggests the convergence of multiple precipitants, but no formal, purposeful, or driving policy.

The public health model describes three levels of prevention.[9] Primary prevention is concerned with measures to decrease the new onset (incidence) of disease (e.g., causative agent eradication, risk factor reduction, host resistance enhancement, and disease transmission disruption). Such measures, highly effective in the realms of infectious disease, toxins, deficiency states, and habit-induced chronic illnesses (e.g., lung and heart diseases), are less efficacious in the psychiatric realm where the non-intervention outcome is less predictable. Nonetheless, putative programs and clinical activities of primary prevention include anticipatory guidance (e.g., for parents with young children), enrichment and competence-building programs (e.g., Head Start, Outward Bound), social support or self-help programs for at-risk individuals (e.g., bereavement groups), and early or crisis intervention following trauma (e.g., on-site student counseling after a classmate's suicide). Secondary prevention is concerned with measures to decrease the number of disease cases in a population at a given point in time (prevalence) by early discernment (case finding) and timely treatment to shorten the course and to minimize residual disability. An educational campaign and screening for peripartum depression would be a psychiatric example of secondary prevention. Tertiary prevention is concerned with measures to decrease the prevalence and severity of residual disease-related defect or disability. Because optimal function in the setting of serious psychiatric illness is so allied with adherence to treatment, examples of tertiary prevention in psychiatry would include case management and other measures to promote continuous care and treatment.

Case, or care, managers (usually social workers or mental health clinicians) assist in the patient's negotiation of a fragmented, complex system of agencies, providers, and services, with the goal of care being continuity and coordination through better inter-provider communication.[10] Obviously, patients with more, and more complex, needs also require more intensive care management. The greater the intensity of the management needs, the fewer cases a manager can adequately handle.[11] The care manager is the member of the treatment team who follows the patient through all care levels (e.g., inpatient, aftercare, residential), types (e.g., mental health, substance use, physical health), and agencies or services (e.g., housing, welfare, public entitlements).

Terms of Managed Care

Not to be confused with care management, managed care, primarily a cost-containment strategy, manages payment for care of a population through monitoring of services allocated to members of the specified population. Prior authorization, primary care provider (PCP) specialty referral (i.e., a gate-keeper system), and concurrent (or utilization) review are strategies commonly employed to manage health care expenditure. They are also increasingly recognized as vehicles to coordinate care, to gather evidence for best practices, to promote development of alternative levels of care, and to monitor treatment outcomes. Managed care organizations (MCOs) have proliferated to provide this service for public and private insurers. Contracts between insurers and MCOs may include penalties for exceeding the service budget or financial incentives to hold service payments within a fixed budget. Health care costs have long been a concern of both providers and recipients of health care, but managed care has imposed the payer's interests into the doctor–patient relationship. While critics believe this has negatively affected the therapeutic process, proponents believe it has promoted greater transparency, standardization, and evidence-based care (and possibly paved the way for numerous pay-for-performance [P4P] initiatives[12]).

HMOs, a type of MCO, generally contract for global health care services for a specified population by paying the provider a set amount, based on a rate (i.e., cap) per member, per month (i.e., capitation). Capitation plans have spurred initiatives to develop coordinated and collaborative systems of cost-effective, high-quality care, to maintain a high standard of overall health for the entire (covered) population. However, some MCOs, including capitated plans, separate the benefit management of physical health from mental health and substance use (i.e., "behavioral health [BH]") services: that is, such plans "carve out" BH benefit management. Companies that manage only these carved-out benefits are called managed behavioral health organizations (MBHOs). The advent of carve-outs set the stage for *cost-shifting*, which is changing the care site (e.g., medical unit versus psychiatric unit) and thereby shifting the cost of care (e.g., from the physical health capitation pool to the mental health capitation pool).[13] This may or may not affect the overall quality or cost of the care, but it shifts the financial burden from (in this example) MCO to MBHO. This split-pot arrangement is antithetical to the collaborative efforts incentivized by single (i.e., global) cap programs. Cost-shifting also occurs between other care/payer systems, such as state and federal (e.g., moving patients from state-funded hospitals to the community where they are eligible for federal subsidies and entitlements), public and private (e.g., privatization shifts the risk for burgeoning BH care costs from states to MCOs or MBHOs), and mental health to physical health (e.g., when patients bypass the mental health system and seek services in the physical health care system either for their mental health problems or for vague somatic complaints). Some also argue that cost-shifting occurs from BH to correctional system because the disenfranchised (e.g., the seriously mentally ill, the dually diagnosed, and substance users) may receive consistent care only when incarcerated.[14]

A cadre of oversight and accrediting agencies has evolved to ensure that MCOs balance their focus on cost containment with quality of care. The National Committee for Quality Assurance (NCQA), the largest such accrediting body for MCOs, includes accreditation standards for MBHOs, as well as for the BH portion of non-carve-out MCOs.[15] NCQA standards address accessibility and availability of appropriate, culturally-sensitive services, coordination between BH and physical health care services, communication between all care providers, and disease management/preventive health services. Both over- and under-utilization of services must be managed to ensure that patients receive care appropriate to their needs. MCOs are also required to have a straightforward grievance and appeal process for patients when the MCO (or

BOX 67-1 Historical Development of Community Psychiatry

THE AGE OF ENLIGHTENMENT

Late eighteenth century: Pinel removes the shackles: Advent of moral treatment

Early nineteenth century: United States-funded institutions
• Dorothea Dix: village-type asylums

Late nineteenth century: Industrial Revolution: productivity and organization
• Custodial care and "scientific" somatic therapies

EARLY TWENTIETH-CENTURY AWARENESS

Adolph Meyer: mental hygiene movement

Clifford Beers: *A Mind That Found Itself*

Beers, Meyer, and William James: National Association for Mental Health

Child Guidance movement

The Great Depression

MID-TWENTIETH CENTURY

World War II

1946: The National Mental Health Act

1949: National Institute of Mental Health

1954: Chlorpromazine released

1955: Pinnacle of custodial care: expository works on poor conditions
• Mental Health Study Act: Joint Commission on Mental Illness and Health

Late 1950s: deinstitutionalization: revolving door policy
• Epidemiological studies: symptoms and impairment common

1961: Joint Commission recommendations: improve the public hospitals
• Focus on serious, persistent mentally ill

BIRTH OF UNITED STATES COMMUNITY MENTAL HEALTH MOVEMENT

1963: First ever presidential address on mental health and retardation

• Community Mental Health Center (CMHC) Acts: 1963 funds construction; 1965 funds staffing
• President Kennedy assassinated

Late 1960s: funds dwindle, few centers built, fewer staffed

Late 1970s: first grant cycle ends

1975: Congressional Act: partially revitalizes, adds services

1977: President Carter's Commission on Mental Health

1979: National Alliance for the Mentally Ill: Self-help movement in CMH

1980: Mental Health Systems Act

1981: Reagan Administration repeals 1980 Act: block grants replace categorical funding

Late Twentieth Century

Early 1980s: Privatization

1984: Epidemiologic Catchment Area Study: primary care practitioner "de facto" mental health system
• Managed care, carve-outs, cost-shifting

1992: National Comorbidity Survey (NCS)

EARLY TWENTY-FIRST CENTURY

2002: National Comorbidity Survey Replication (NCS-R)
• Depression on the rise; more being seen in mental health system
• Most who seek care in medical setting receive medication

2008: Mental Health Parity and Addiction Equity Act (MHPAE)

Current:
• Managed care networks approximating CMHC vision
• Promotion of Accountable Care Organizations (ACOs), Health Homes, and Medical Homes
• Cautious development of "Dual Eligible" programs: limited, combined funding

its MBHO) initially denies a request for care or particular services. Another form of oversight, the Federal Interim Final Rule Under the Paul Wellstone and Pete Domenici Mental Health Parity and Addiction Equity Act (MHPAE) of 2008 (Interim Final Rule on Parity) states, in general terms, that BH benefits may not be managed more restrictively than a plan's physical health benefits, "except to the extent that recognized clinically appropriate standards of care may permit a difference."[16] To the extent that NCQA appreciates the difference between BH and physical health care, entities who meet NCQA standards should also continue to meet the requirements of the Parity Law.

HISTORICAL BACKGROUND

The history of community psychiatry is a saga of alternating reform and neglect best understood within the political, economic, and sociocultural context of the times. Box 67-1 is an historical timeline of key events. Box 67-2 recaps the legislative acts that have affected the system in the US.

The Age of Enlightenment

The "first psychiatric revolution" occurred late in the eighteenth century when French alienist (i.e., psychiatrist), Philippe Pinel, endorsed physical work and fresh air to return the mentally ill to a state of mental health and well-being.[17] Moral

BOX 67-2 United States Legislation Affecting CMH

1946: The National Mental Health Act

1949: National Institute of Mental Health (NIMH)

1955: Mental Health Study Act: Joint Commission on Mental Illness and Health

1963: Community Mental Health Center (CMHC) Act: fund construction

1965: CMHC Act: fund staffing

1975: CMHC Amendments: partially revitalize, add essential services

1977: President's Commission on Mental Health

1979: National Alliance for the Mentally Ill (NAMI)

1980: Mental Health Systems Act

1981: Reagan Administration repeals Mental Health Systems Act; block grants replace categorical funding

2008: Mental Health Parity and Addiction Equity Act

treatment dawned as Pinel released the insane from their shackles.[18] By the early nineteenth century, the movement had found its way to the US, where Dorothea Dix promoted the development of village-style asylums for the mentally ill to retreat from the stresses of daily living.[19] The government-funded construction of institutions for the behaviorally deviant and mentally ill.[20]

By the end of the century, however, these institutions and asylums were hopelessly run-down and overcrowded.[21] In concert with the Industrial Revolution (focused on organization and productivity), moral treatment was replaced by custodial care and regimentation, and a wave of neglect. Even worse, however, was the onslaught of unproven, unbeneficial, and possibly harmful somatic therapies.[22,23] Among these "scientific" treatments, only two were found to have merit for select patients. Many institutionalized patients actually suffered from the general paretic form of tertiary neurosyphilis,[24] which was found to resolve with the high fevers of malaria.[25] Patients with conversion (and possibly other) disorders were helped by Freud and his disciples, who used psychological understanding in their treatment.

Early Twentieth-century Awareness

Urbanization of the Industrial Revolution spurred the preventive, public health movement, a necessity for sanitation and infection control. This was paralleled by the mental hygiene movement promoted by the writings of Adolph Meyer on prevention and the social context of mental illness. In 1908, Clifford Beers exposed the deplorable conditions inside mental institutions in his first-person account of living in one.[26] Beers joined forces with Meyer and William James to found the National Association for Mental Health, in 1909.[27,28] The mental hygiene movement advocated for smaller hospitals and the establishment of community-based outpatient evaluation clinics. These clinics (variously viewed as the forerunners or beginnings of community psychiatry[2]) were less stigmatizing than large state hospitals, and they concentrated on evaluation, prevention, and the differentiation between persistent and acute disorders. They also emphasized inter-disciplinary training, affiliation with medical schools and mainstream medicine, and the use of applied psychodynamic theory and principles.

An extension of the mental hygiene movement, the child guidance movement proposed to apply psychodynamic theory in childhood to prevent the development of adult pathology.[3] However, such assumptions proved difficult to substantiate, leading to apathy and discouragement. This wave of neglect coincided with the Great Depression. Along with dwindling funds, professional in-fighting, and long wait-lists, rigid acceptance criteria led to disillusionment and to abandonment of these programs.

Mid-twentieth Century

The confluence of military experience, pharmacological breakthroughs, and epidemiological research provided the platform for mental health legislation to both advance knowledge and improve care. During World War II, the armed services had difficulty filling the ranks as new recruits were outnumbered by those either rejected or removed from service because of psychiatric casualty. In response, military psychiatrists were urged to lower acceptance standards and to move treatment interventions to the battlefield in an effort to reduce the number of psychiatric evacuees. Coupled with the post-war optimism, three central tenets of community psychiatry were culled from this experience: immediacy, proximity, and expectancy.[29] Briefly stated: treatment should occur without delay, on site, and with the expectation of improvement/resolution. Treatment in, or near, the patient's usual environment decreased the likelihood of secondary gain and the development of avoidance. Far from being custodial, the care system was to support the concept of recovery and to promote the expectation that the patient would return to baseline function.

In 1946, at the pinnacle of custodial care, with over 550,000 state hospital inpatients, Congress passed the National Mental Health Act, approving federal funds for mental health training and research. This Act also founded the National Institute of Mental Health (NIMH) in 1949. Shortly thereafter, chlorpromazine (Thorazine)[30] was first used in the US, with a concomitant decrease in psychotic symptoms and behavioral problems in long-institutionalized state hospital patients. More patients could now be treated at home with chlorpromazine, and they had far superior outcomes (e.g., symptomatic relief, improved cognition, overall function).[31] Also in the mid- to late-1940s, several expository works[32,33] heightened recognition of the apathy and other damaging effects of prolonged institutional living (e.g., poor social function and self-care skills). The depiction of overcrowded, dehumanizing conditions in large state institutions inspired another surge of public outrage. In 1955, the Mental Health Study Act established the Joint Commission on Mental Illness and Health, providing funds to assess the nation's available treatment services for the mentally ill. By the end of the decade, deinstitutionalization was in full swing, state hospital beds had dwindled to 100,000, and the insufficiency of community resources became glaringly obvious. Long-hospitalized patients, often estranged from their families, lacked the coping and social skills to manage and advocate for themselves outside of the institution. Eighty percent were re-hospitalized within 2 years, a phenomenon called the revolving door policy.[6]

The Joint Commission reported in 1961 on its nation-wide assessment,[34] and it recommended smaller hospitals with greater resources, and funds targeted to improve services for the most severely ill patients (i.e., patients with psychosis and major mental illness). Around this time, several epidemiological studies exposed the prevalence of psychiatric symptomatology and impaired function, pervasive across rural,[35] urban,[36] and suburban populations. At least one study also demonstrated that the population in greatest need had the least access to mental health services.[37]

Birth of the American Community Mental Health Movement

By 1963, political and social optimism were ripe for the first-ever presidential address to Congress regarding mental health and retardation.[38] In this address, President Kennedy voiced his opposition to the prevailing institutional system and his conviction (in opposition to the Joint Commission recommendations) that more funding for this system would not improve the quality of care. He called for a "bold new approach," relying on new pharmacology and knowledge, to treat the mentally ill in their home communities, where they would be "returned to a useful place in society." Kennedy foresaw a "new type of health facility," the community mental health center (CMHC), as part of a comprehensive community care system, to improve quality and "return mental health care to the mainstream of American medicine." Within weeks of signing the CMHC Act, President Kennedy was assassinated.

The CMHC Acts of 1963 and 1965 provided for the funding of CMHC buildings and staff, respectively. Each CMHC was to provide five essential services: four levels of care (inpatient, outpatient, partial hospital, and emergency) and consultation/education. The goal was to use the public funds to build and staff 2,000 centers by 1980, and to have fees and private insurers fund continued services. By the late 1960s, however, both state and federal funds for health and welfare programs began to diminish. Even as a center was in construction, staff funding was decreased or withdrawn. Far from the projected number, fewer than 800 centers were built, many without adequate staff funding. This obvious failure to meet public expectations also fueled criticism and conflict about the role of community psychiatrists. Some believed psychiatrists valued social activism over the treatment needs of the mentally ill. By the mid-1970s, the imminent end of the first grant cycle funding CMHC staff, the mentally ill were generally not paying fees, insurers were also not supporting CMHC services, demand was overwhelming, and state hospital capacity was less than a fifth of what it had been. The severely mentally ill were flooding communities without adequate services in place.

Another wave of reforms and community activism followed the 1975 Congressional Act[39] to partially fund and revitalize the CMHCs (with a less idealistic mandate than Kennedy's vision), to target services for those who most perturbed the community, and to increase the essential services accordingly (i.e., to include specialized programs for children and the elderly, direct mental health screening services for the courts, follow-up care and transitional housing for the deinstitutionalized, and specialized drug and alcohol programs).[40] In 1977, President Carter established the President's Commission on Mental Health to launch another nation-wide assessment of mental health services. The self-help movement in CMH was also gaining momentum, as mothers of mentally ill children began the National Alliance for the Mentally Ill (NAMI), in 1979. In 1980, Congress passed the Mental Health Systems Act (Public Law 96-398), which included some of the Joint Commission's recommendations from their nation-wide assessment. With the intent to fund services for the most under-served populations (i.e., the old, the young, the seriously mentally ill, and minorities), the bill had provisions to build new CMHCs, to improve the coordination of total health care by linking mental and physical health care providers, and to fund essential, non-revenue-producing services (i.e., consultation, education, coordination of care, and CMHC administration).

In what can only be viewed as a major setback, 18 years of categorical federal funding for CMH disintegrated in 1981, when the Reagan Administration repealed the 1980 Mental Health Systems Act before it was implemented. The inadequate funds for substance use and mental health services were placed in block grants and left to the will of the individual states.

Late Twentieth Century

The retraction of federal funds and oversight resulted in 50 discontinuous state programs with insufficient resources to care for the most seriously mentally ill in the community. Early in the 1980s, the early 1980s privatization trend, and exemption from the Diagnosis-Related Groups (DRG) legislation, encouraged expansion of private, for-profit, psychiatric and substance use hospitals. The Epidemiologic Catchment Area (ECA) study of 1984 quantified the marked prevalence of psychiatric symptomatology and disorder in general community populations, and determined that the preponderance of symptomatic community residents never sought care in the mental health system. Rather, they accessed the general medical system, dubbed the "de facto" mental health system.[41]

Early-1990s health care cost-escalation spurred an explosion of managed care initiatives in both public and private sectors. Another epidemiological study, the National Comorbidity Survey (NCS, 1990–1992), reiterated the high life-time prevalence (50%) and 1-year incidence (30%) of mental disorder in community respondents (depression and alcoholism being most prevalent).[42] The growth of private psychiatric hospitals, and the lack of treatment guidelines, standards, or criteria for levels or types of care, made mental health an easy target. While not generally embraced by clinicians, managed care had the potential to coordinate care, gather evidence for best practices, promote development of alternative levels of care, and monitor treatment outcomes. However, it also set the stage for BH carve-outs, and the resultant cost-shifting

strategies (to benefit the bottom line of the particular MCO or MBHO) that frequently created conflict between BH and physical health providers (and payers), without adequate consideration of the patient's best interest. Carve-outs have further fragmented the health care system, as medical colleagues are not able to refer to in-house BH providers if they are not in the carve-out network (and there is clearly an inverse relationship between the difficulty and likelihood of appropriate referral). This systemic convergence of decreased federal funding and oversight, health care cost escalation, privatization, managed care, carve-outs, and cost-shifting further entrenched this complex and discontinuous system, which was increasingly difficult to access by the most vulnerable and disenfranchised (i.e., the poor, homeless, non-English-speaking, uninsured, deinstitutionalized).

Start of the Twenty-first Century

The rigorous replication of the NCS (NCS-R, 2001–2002) focused on severity, clinical significance, overall disability, and role impairment. NCS-R had several significant findings about depression, the disorder again found to be the most prevalent. First, the prevalence of depression had increased in each birth cohort since World War II. Second, slightly more than half of depressed community respondents seeking care now received that care in the mental health sector. The other significant finding, attributable to advances in pharmacotherapy and educational efforts, was that 90% of respondents treated for depression in any medical setting received medication. However, only about one in five received what current standards considered minimally-adequate treatment (and almost half of depressed community residents still received no treatment).[43]

Early in the twenty-first century, the CMH system remains substantially unchanged from that of the late 1990s. However, there is a focus on training and collaboration with PCPs to improve treatment (mostly of depression) for those who access care in the primary care sector (largely through funding mandates to federally-qualified community health centers).[44–49] This has done little to improve the quality of life or care for the more seriously mentally ill, and others beyond the expertise of PCPs. For this population, the CMH "system" remains discontinuous, and includes the revolving door policy, now often on acute, rather than state hospital, inpatient units.

UNDERLYING PRINCIPLES OF COMMUNITY MENTAL HEALTH

The principles central to CMH are summarized in Box 67-3.

Population Responsibility

President Kennedy's vision, and the initial CMHC Acts of 1963 and 1965, mandated meeting the mental health needs of an entire, geographically-defined (catchment area) population, regardless of ability to pay. No population member could be denied service. Defined catchment areas covered resident populations of 75,000 to 200,000. Population responsibility requires planning for optimal use of limited resources to develop the most favorable system to meet the population's care needs. Services developed should match the patients' needs, not be tailored to treat the masses more economically (e.g., groups offered when clinically and culturally-appropriate, not as cost-saving alternatives).

Prevention

Community psychiatry, like public health, should focus on prevention to decrease the incidence, prevalence, and

<table>
<tr><td>

BOX 67-3 Principles of Community Psychiatry

POPULATION RESPONSIBILITY
- Services for entire catchmented population
- Allocation of limited resources
- Clinically and culturally-appropriate services

PREVENTION
- Decrease incidence (primary)
- Decrease prevalence (secondary)
- Decrease residual disability (tertiary)

COMMUNITY-BASED CARE (PROXIMITY)
- Maintain family, social supports
- Avoid geographical isolation
- Promote patient's functional role in community

CITIZEN INVOLVEMENT
- Community boards: set priorities, policies
- Patient input and feedback
- Lay–provider partnerships
- Political advocacy

CONTINUITY OF CARE
- Ideal: seamless circle of care across all levels of treatment
- Reality: case managers coordinate fragmented services, facilitate communication between providers

</td></tr>
</table>

<table>
<tr><td>

BOX 67-4 Components of Community Mental Health

- Inpatient care
- Partial hospitalization
- Outpatient services
- Emergency services
- Community consultation/education
- Case management
- Homeless outreach
- Disaster or trauma response
- Evaluation and research

</td></tr>
</table>

COMPONENTS AND SERVICES OF COMMUNITY MENTAL HEALTH SYSTEMS

Components of the ideal CMH system are summarized in Box 67-4. The reality is that all of these services may not be available in a given community, and those that are, will likely span more than one agency.

Inpatient Care

Hospitalization remains a necessary resource, although reserved for the more acutely and seriously ill. Acute hospitalization is an active, intense level of evaluation, care, and safe containment, with scarce resemblance to bygone custodial care. General hospital and private psychiatric hospital beds are now more plentiful, and less stigmatizing, for brief, intense stays. Most units are now locked because most payers will only cover inpatient care when patients meet commitment standards (e.g., suicidal, homicidal, or unable to care for self on the basis of mental illness), even when patients sign in voluntarily. Financial constraints, the development of less restrictive care settings, and legal protection of the civil liberties of the mentally ill have made long-term, inpatient care largely a thing of the past. The revolving door (multiple, brief admissions) has replaced extended hospitalization for many of the seriously mentally ill.

Partial Hospitalization

For patients with stable living situations, the less restrictive partial hospital program offers a helpful step-down, or diversion, from inpatient care. Patients have the structure of the hospital-based treatment program during the day, and they return home in the evening. This gradual return to, or maintenance in, the community with continued hospital support is an attempt to combat the inevitability of the revolving door.

Outpatient Services

Extensive outpatient service options promote effective community treatment for more seriously ill patients. Such services may include, but are not limited to, those listed in Box 67-5. Besides the common modalities (e.g., medication management; individual, group, or family therapy; addictions treatment), outpatient services also encompass transitional housing (e.g., halfway houses, group homes, supervised boarding rooms), day treatment, and specialized services for children and the elderly.

Emergency Services

Twenty-four hour coverage by crisis teams, or crisis clinicians in emergency departments, allows patients to be screened

disability of mental illness or disorders. In reality, however, limited resources largely restrict the focus to tertiary prevention[29] (i.e., rehabilitation to limit disability in the seriously mentally ill).

Community-based Care

Both services and advocacy occur in the patient's home community. This proximity obviates the downfalls of geographical isolation, promotes maintenance of family and social supports, and encourages the patient's continued social role in their community. Patients with serious mental illness have been shown to retain better social and self-care skills when treated in their own communities. A variety of services have been developed to help patients access care and remain safely in the community, rather than in restrictive, long-term, custodial care.

The 1909 partnership of Beers and Meyer to form NAMI initiated lay–professional collaboration and citizen involvement in the CMH system. Community boards and BH professionals work together to establish priorities and develop policies. Involved community members also become powerful advocates to campaign for necessary continued resources.

Continuity of Care

The initially conceived CMHCs were to provide comprehensive care (i.e., across all levels and intensity of services) as well as the coordination of services across the continuum. With all levels of care (e.g., outpatient, inpatient, partial hospital, crisis stabilization, day treatment, residential) within the circle of care, the information flow would follow the patient without hindrance, and providers would have unimpeded communication to facilitate the development and consistency of comprehensive treatment plans. Unlike the current discontinuous reality, there would be no place for cost-shifting in an ideal, comprehensive system.

BOX 67-5 Outpatient Community Services

Medication Management
Therapy
   Individual
   Group
     • Psychoeducation
     • Skills training
     • Self-help
   Family
Day Treatment
Transitional Housing
   Half-way houses
   Supervised boarding rooms
   Group homes
Specialized Children's Services
Specialized Elderly Services
Alcohol and Drug Use Treatment Programs

before hospitalization for crisis intervention, assessment for level of care, and immediate access to appropriate care.

Community Consultation/Education

Such non-reimbursable activities dwindled with decreased federal funds, although partially revitalized by the primary care "gatekeeper" system. As primary care patients tend to present with somatic complaints (rather than mood, anxiety, or addiction problems), and PCPs are increasingly encouraged (e.g., by managed care, global capitation, or federal mandate) to treat the less complicated mental disorders in their practices, they look to community psychiatrists to assist with appropriate diagnosis, treatment, or referral.

Case Management

Considered essential in the conception of the seamless CMH system, case (or care) management is an absolute necessity in the current, fragmented care system. Care managers remain the liaison between care providers, though appropriate releases are now required to permit this important communication.

Homeless Outreach

The most disenfranchised, the growing numbers of the homeless mentally ill do not seek or access the services they need, for multiple reasons, including negative past experience, lack of insight, and fear. By meeting them where they are, outreach workers must be adaptable to establish credibility, work in non-traditional settings, and bring services to this disadvantaged population.

Disaster or Trauma Response

The lessons from military psychiatry, bolstered by the post-9/11 events, have prompted some agencies to develop immediate-response teams for on-site assessment and treatment of disaster victims, to mitigate post-traumatic syndromes and residual disability.

Evaluation and Research

The push to develop evidence-based treatment guidelines in psychiatry and CMH aligns with mainstream medical trends. The major impetus toward program evaluation, or "outcomes research," however, has been the need to contain cost and to identify cost-effectiveness. In the community, true cost-effectiveness research must span multiple departments, agencies, and services. Cost-offset from one program to another (e.g., improved, but more costly, BH services, decrease the overall cost by relatively larger decreases in the expense of general medical care; increased pharmacy or crisis team expense results in greatly decreased inpatient expense) is particularly difficult to identify in this diffuse system. In contrast to the cost-shifting obfuscation of carve-out BH management, the inclusive responsibility of global capitation will promote and require total systems research to identify cost-offset and cost-effectiveness.

TRENDS

Disenfranchisement

The current minimalist patchwork of community services prioritizes the most severely mentally ill. This has both increased the stigma and failed to adequately meet the needs of the targeted population. As services diminish and barriers to access increase, progressively more of the seriously mentally ill are homeless, chemically dependent, or imprisoned.

Managed Care: The "Fourth Psychiatric Revolution?"

Most MCOs have now moved beyond the initial mandate for cost containment to concerns for quality and cost-effectiveness. Early cost savings from decreased hospital days was obviously not the total means to functionally maintain this population in the community. In what might be considered convergent evolution, MCOs (or MBHOs, in the case of carve-out management) have pushed the public and private sectors to develop networks of closely affiliated services that span the levels of progressively less intensive and restrictive care, with intensive clinical managers to assist patients through these timely transitions and ensure communication between (serial and parallel) treaters. This push has included the development of alternative (previously unavailable) levels of care. These networks have been developed with much the same mandate and fiscal constraint as the 1960s CMHCs they resemble (i.e., to provide coordinated continuity of quality care, for a given population, with finite resources). Progressive MCOs solicit member and provider input through satisfaction surveys and advisory committees (similar to the CMHC community boards), to ensure relevant, culturally-appropriate programs and user-friendly service. These more inclusive networks facilitate data collection and tracking so that progressive MCOs can now use data to inform policy. In this way, they have set standards for communication with PCPs, timely access to care, coordination of services, correlation of symptoms and function to level of care, treatment planning, monitoring, and recording.

Primary Care

Once the "de facto" system, the promotion of primary care management (i.e., by gatekeeper and global capitation systems, or by federal mandate) of subsyndromal BH problems in the community has progressed to include treatment of more serious mental illness. Provider groups at financial risk for the total care of their patient population have spurred development of innovative programs to integrate and coordinate physical and mental health services.

Creative Solutions

Among the multi-disciplinary innovations to keep the seriously mentally ill functioning well in their home

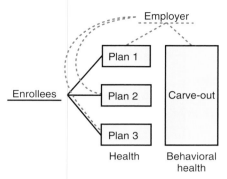

Figure 68-1. Schematic of carve-out plans. Enrollees choose among competing health plans for all services *except* carved-out behavioral health services. *(Redrawn from Frank RG, McGuire TG. Economics and mental health. In Culyer AJ, Newhouse JP. Handbook of health economics,vol 1, pt 2, 2000, Elsevier BV, p. 906.)*

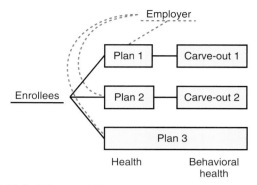

Figure 68-2. Schematic of carve-out plans. Enrollees have a choice of health plan for all services, including behavioral health services. Whether to carve-out is a business decision made at the health plan level. *(Redrawn from Frank RG, McGuire TG. Economics and mental health. In Culyer AJ, Newhouse JP: Handbook of health economics,vol 1, pt 2, 2000, Elsevier BV, p 907.)*

Cross/Blue Shield high-option plan remained the only health plan that provided generous psychiatric coverage and was severely selected against for a number of years until it was permitted to make significant cuts in benefits in 1981. This episode prompted the general perception among policymakers and insurers that broad coverage for mental health was expensive and unpredictable due to issues relating to moral hazard and adverse selection.

Managed care continued to transform MHC financing over the 1990s. With the evolution of managed care, business entities often referred to as "carve-outs" emerged to manage the delivery of MHC. Both employers and health plans increasingly contracted with care carve-out firms to manage their mental health benefits. According to a 2002 survey, about 164 million individuals with health coverage were enrolled in some type of managed behavioral health program in 2002, totaling 66% of individuals with health insurance.[20] The survey data indicated a substantial increase over the decade in enrollment in carve-outs from 70 million in 1993 to 164 million in 2002. Employers and health plans structure carve-out contracts in various ways. For example, a carve-out contract with an employer might be a risk-based or a non-risk-based contract (administrative services only); it might provide utilization review or case management services only; it might provide employee assistance program (EAP) services only; or it might contract to provide both managed behavioral health services and EAP services. Larger carve-out firms may market all of these separate services depending on the needs of a given purchaser. Figures 68-1 and 68-2 illustrate some of the more common carve-out formats.

Carve-out contracts have been touted as a strategy for improving the cost-effectiveness of behavioral health care. These firms use specialized expertise to assemble networks of mental-health specialty providers willing to accept lower reimbursement rates, to identify evidence-based treatment protocols, and to use other managed care techniques (e.g., care management and utilization review) with the promise of reducing employer expenditures without sacrificing access to needed services. Observational studies of contracting with carve-outs have consistently produced evidence of substantial reductions in mental health and substance abuse costs even in the context of benefit expansion in both the private sector[21-23] and the public sector.[21,24-27] These studies have shown that most savings result from decreases in use and spending for inpatient care. Most often, the proportion of enrollees using outpatient care increased while the number of outpatient visits decreased with adoption of carve-outs. The

evidence on how carve-outs affect quality of care is more ambiguous. To date, fewer studies have examined the effects of carve-outs on quality. Carve-outs do not appear to increase rates of re-hospitalization.[28,29] However, studies have produced mixed results on their effects on continuity of care,[28,30] adherence to treatment guidelines,[31,32] and clinical outcomes.[33]

A second rationale for contracting with carve-outs relates to employer concerns regarding the consequences of adverse selection. By "carving out" mental health benefits to a single specialty carve-out firm, an employer can eliminate the incentive among health plans to compete in avoiding enrollment of more expensive individuals with a need for mental health services. Under this arrangement, enrollees may be given a choice of health plan but are *not* given a choice of plan for the carved-out mental health services (see Figure 68-1). In this case, introduction of an employer-level carve-out can attenuate selection incentives. However, carving out will not have any impact on selection when contracting occurs at the health plan level. In this case, carve-outs are a component of a health plan's business strategy and do not affect the plan's incentives to avoid enrolling individuals with mental illness.

A common criticism of carve-outs is that these institutional arrangements fragment care in an already poorly integrated MHC delivery system. Common problems include challenges in coordinating care for patients with multiple conditions and the inability of primary care physicians to bill for providing mental health treatment when carve-outs are under contract to provide specialty mental health care services. Separate carve-out vendors and prescription drug budgets contribute to and reinforce tendencies to avoid using integrated approaches to treat patients with mental health conditions. Fragmentation may also create opportunities to shift costs. For example, carve-outs are often accused of encouraging greater use of pharmaceutical treatments that are treated as "off-budget" from a contractual standpoint. Another criticism of carve-outs is that these arrangements increase administrative costs. Estimates of increases in administrative costs due to these arrangements range from 8% to 20% of mental health benefit costs.[2]

RECENT TRENDS IN MENTAL HEALTH CARE FINANCING

This section describes statistical trends in spending on MHC from 1971 to 2001, focusing on aggregate as well as payer-specific information.

Gross Spending on Mental Health Care

Total domestic spending on MHC in the US in 2005 was $112.8 billion.[34] MHC expenditures were estimated at 6.1% of total spending on health care and 0.89% of the GDP. Frank and Glied[35] compared estimates of health care spending in 2001 with those from 1971, controlling for changes in treatment over that period. They found that in 1971 total expenditures on MHC were $8.96 billion, 11.1% of the total spending on health and nearly twice as much as in 2001. MHC spending was 0.84% of the GDP at that time.[35]

While total spending on MHC has increased slightly in terms of the GDP, relative spending on different treatment modalities has changed dramatically. Following on the heels of the CMHC movement and changes in financing, the number of institutionalized patients decreased from 433,000 people in 1971 to 170,000 in 2000. This shift in care affected financing of MHC, and the burden shifted from state governments to insurance-based mechanisms, both public and private. While the numbers of institutionalized patients fell, there was a sharp increase in MHC provided to non-institutionalized patients. The number of US citizens receiving MHC has increased by 50% since 1977.[35] Total spending on non-institutionalized patients has also increased. From 1986 to 2005, inpatient hospitalization expenditures increased from $13.3 billion to $21.7 billion, while outpatient expenditures increased from $7.6 billion to $37.2 billion.[34]

It is also important to note that many of the costs associated with long-term care of the chronically mental ill (such as housing and board) were transferred to other programs considered outside the realm of MHC. The expansion of public insurance programs, such as Supplemental Security Income (SSI), Social Security Disability Insurance (SSDI), public housing, and food stamps in the 1970s helped cover the cost of community-based living for patients.

Sources of Health Care Expenditures

Over 58% of MHC-related expenses in the US in 2005 were paid for by public funding sources.[34] Table 68-2 and Figure 68-2 describe and exhibit some of the major public funders of MHC (including Medicare, Medicaid, and non-Medicaid state-spending programs). As shown in Table 68-2, federal sources of funding (Medicaid and Medicare) increased from 16.8% of total MHC spending in 1971 to over 28% in 2005, while state spending decreased from 30.4% in 1971 to 28.9% in 2005.[34]

Private insurance was also a significant source of MHC financing in 2005, accounting for $30.4 billion, or 27% of total spending on MHC.[34] This is an increase from 1971 when it accounted for only 12.3% of expenditures. This is in contrast with "out-of-pocket" spending, which has declined as a percentage of total MHC spending from 35.6% in 1971 to 12.2% in 2005.

PARITY, EXPANSION OF COVERAGE, AND THE FUTURE OF MENTAL HEALTH CARE IN THE UNITED STATES

Insurance parity has been the stated objective of mental health advocates since differences in mental and general health coverage first arose in the early days of private health insurance.[36] Parity policies require health plans operating in the private health insurance market to provide an equivalent level of coverage for mental health and general health care. The case for parity has primarily been based on the fairness argument that insurance should not discriminate against those with mental illness.

In 1996, the United States Congress passed the Mental Health Parity Act (P.L. 104-204) prohibiting the use of annual or lifetime dollar limits on coverage for mental illnesses. This law did not apply to other kinds of benefit limits, such as special annual day or visit limits and higher cost-sharing. Companies with fewer than 50 employees and those that offered no mental health benefit were exempt from the federal parity law. Payers experiencing more than a 1% increase in premiums as a result of federal parity could apply for an exemption. Insurers found numerous ways to evade the intentions of this legislation, including limiting the number of outpatient visits and inpatient hospitalization days and charging patients higher co-pays and deductibles. Coverage of addiction services was not addressed in the Mental Health Parity Act. Employers who provided coverage as self-insured entities (i.e., who assumed the financial risk of the coverage they were providing) were exempt from the requirements.

In 2008, in an attempt to close loopholes in the Mental Health Parity Act, Congress passed the Paul Wellstone and Pete Domenici Mental Health Parity and Addiction Equity Act (MHPAEA). Implemented in 2010, the MHPAEA creates numerous standards intended to equalize coverage of mental health services with coverage of medical and surgical services. All financial requirements and treatment limits for behavioral health disorders must now equal the limits for medical and surgical care, including co-payments, deductibles, and limitations on quantities of inpatient and outpatient treatment. Treatment for substance use disorders is now mandated to

TABLE 68-2 Mental Health Spending (billions of dollars), by Payer Class, 1971, 1991, and 2001

	1971		1991		2005	
	Amount ($ billion)	**%**	**Amount ($ billion)**	**%**	**Amount ($ billion)**	**%**
Medicaid	1.28	14.2	9.2	18.8	31.1	27.6
Medicare	0.23	2.6	3.3	6.7	8.6	7.7
State (excluding Medicaid)	2.72	30.4	13.1	26.7	20.26	18.0
Private insurance	1.10	12.3	10.6	21.7	30.4	27.0
Fees/out-of-pocket spending	3.19	35.6	7.5	15.3	13.8	12.2
Total	8.96	100.0	48.9	100.0	112.8	100.0
Share of national health spending		11.1		8.4		6.1
Share of gross domestic product		0.84		0.82		0.91

Note: Numbers might not add to 100% because of the exclusion of "other" categories.
From Authors' calculations based on U.S. Department of Health and Human Services: The cost of mental illness—1971, *Washington, DC, 1975,*
U.S. Government Printing Office; Mark TL, Coffey RM, Vandivort-Warren R, et al. U.S. spending for mental health and substance abuse treatment,
1991–2001, Health Affairs Web Exclusive, *March 29, 2005; Mark TL, Levit KR, Vandivort-Warren R, Buck JA, Coffey C. Changes in US spending*
on mental health and substance abuse treatment, 1986-2005, and implications for policy, Health Affairs 30(2):284–292, 2011.

have coverage equal to that of other behavioral health disorders. Out-of-network benefits for psychiatric care must be equal to those for medical and surgical care. Self-insured employers are no longer exempt from providing equal coverage. Similar to the Mental Health Parity Act, the MHPAEA does not apply to organizations with fewer than 50 employees, nor does it apply if the organization does not offer any coverage of mental health services.

Some health insurers and employers were opposed to improving mental health insurance coverage due to the previously discussed concerns related to moral hazard and adverse selection driving up costs for mental health coverage. A recent, frequently cited review article summarizing the studies on demand-response to cost-sharing provisions for outpatient mental health services published between 2001 and 2006 noted, as did the RAND health experiment, that higher cost-sharing for psychotherapy was a necessary step to ensure efficiency.[37] These early studies contrasted with a second generation of research conducted in the late 1990s on mental health benefit expansions in the era of managed care. The second-generation studies did not find large mental health spending increases attributable to parity, and all studies that addressed risk protection identified significant decreases in consumer out-of-pocket MHC spending under managed care. The absence of quantity increases due to parity across these studies is consistent with more recent actuarial estimates of the effect of parity on premiums.

These more recent studies provide evidence that parity implemented in the context of managed care would have little impact on mental health spending and would increase risk protection for those with mental health conditions. Although the MHPAEA is too new to have produced any substantial research about its effects, studies have been done about other iterations of parity policy. A study examining parity implementation in the Federal Employees Health Benefits (FEHB) Program found that following the enactment of parity, total spending (including out-of-pocket spending) and utilization among patients with major depressive disorder and bipolar disorder was unchanged, while spending and utilization for patients with adjustment disorder declined.[38] Access to care was not compromised while patients paid less for an amount of care comparable to before the parity enactment. The introduction of parity has also seen a significant reduction in suicides.[39]

Following the implementation of mental health parity, President Barack Obama sponsored a sweeping health care bill, the Patient Protection and Affordable Care Act (ACA). Passed in 2010, the intent of this legislation was to dramatically expand health insurance coverage for uninsured Americans. This legislation imposes a mandate that most US citizens have health insurance or else pay a penalty. It also introduces low-cost health insurance through an expansion of Medicaid, largely through state-run exchanges, where insurance of varying coverage levels can be purchased for prices based on a person's income relative to the federal poverty line. In addition to numerous other changes, accountable care organizations (ACOs)—organizations of providers who attempt to meet quality thresholds in an effort to improve patient care and share in cost-savings with Medicare—were introduced.

The ACA affects mental health coverage in several ways. Plans offered through the state-run exchanges are required to cover behavioral health, resulting in expansion of access to care. The ACA's emphasis on integrated care, through ACOs and patient-centered medical homes, aims to improve the coordination of all types of care. For patients with mental illness, whose care is often fragmented and whose illnesses frequently go undiagnosed, the improved coordination of care is expected to produce improved outcomes and to set new quality benchmarks. In addition, it is hoped that payment reform—bundled payments instead of episodic—will incent large organizations to address care as continuous with an emphasis on prevention rather than simply attending to acute episodes. It has been forecasted that by 2019, as a result of the ACA, there will be 4.3 million more users of mental health services, 2.3 million through Medicaid and 2 million through private insurance.[40]

CONCLUSION

The financing of MHC continues to be a challenge for policymakers and for society. The traditional mix of state and local funding of mental hospitals has changed into a system that has focused on deinstitutionalization and an increasing level of federal support for care. Moral hazard and adverse selection concerns have led to the development of a separate industry of managed care for mental health that has been successful in limiting utilization, with unclear effects on patient outcomes. Recent legislation has suggested that the pendulum is beginning to swing in the opposite direction. Improved, stricter parity legislation combined with the expansion of Medicaid in the ACA should lead to broader distribution of MHC and, potentially, diminished stigma. Further research examining whether the intended effects of the MHPAEA and ACA are borne out will be needed to inform continued legislative refinements and future policy endeavors.

Access the complete reference list and multiple choice questions (MCQs) online at https://expertconsult.inkling.com

KEY REFERENCES

2. Frank RG, McGuire T. Economics and mental health. In Cuyler AJ, Newhouse JP, editors: *Handbook of health economics*, Amsterdam, 2000, Elsevier.
4. Grob GN. *Mental illness and American society, 1875–1940*, Princeton, NJ, 1983, Princeton University Press.
5. Grob GN. *The mad among us: a history of the care of America's mentally ill*, New York, 1994, Free Press.
6. Blumenthal D. Employer-sponsored health insurance in the United States—origins and implications. *N Engl J Med* 355(1):82–88, 2006.
7. Frank RG, Koyanagi C, McGuire T. The politics and economics of mental health parity laws. *Health Aff* 16(4):108–120, 1997.
8. Chernew ME, Hirth RA, Cutler DM. Increased spending on health care: how much can the United States afford? *Health Aff* 22(4):15–25, 2005.
10. Pauly MV. The economics of moral hazard: comment. *Am Economic Review* 58(3 pt 1):531–537, 1968.
12. McGuire TG. Financing and demand for mental health services. *J Hum Resour* 16(4):501–522, 1981.
13. Newhouse JP. *Free for all? Lessons from the RAND Health Insurance Experiment*, Cambridge, 1993, Harvard University Press.
15. Frank RG, Glazer J, McGuire TG. Adverse selection in mental health care. *J Health Economics* 19(6):829–854, 2000.
16. Tufts Managed Care Institute. A brief history of managed care, Available at: <www.thci.org/downloads/BriefHist.pdf>; 1998.
19. Hustead EC, Sharfstein SS. Utilization and cost of mental illness coverage in the Federal Employees Health Benefits Program. *Am J Psychiatry* 135:315–319, 1978.
22. Ma CA, McGuire TG. Costs and incentives in a behavioral health care carve out. *Health Aff* 17(2):53–69, 1998.
23. Grazier KL, Eselius LL, Hu TW, et al. Effects of a mental health carve-out on use, costs and payers: a four-year study. *J Behav Health Serv Res* 26(4):381–389, 1999.
24. Bloom JR, Hu TW, Wallace N, et al. Mental health costs and access under alternative capitation systems in Colorado. *Health Serv Res* 37(2):315–340, 2002.
27. Frank RG, McGuire TG. Savings from a Medicaid carve-out for mental health and substance abuse care. *Psychiatr Serv* 48(9):1147–1152, 1997.

28. Merrick E. Treatment of major depression before and after implementation of a behavioral health carve-out plan. *Psychiatr Serv* 49(11):1563–1567, 1998.

29. Sturm R. Tracking changes in behavioral health services: how have carve-outs changed care? *J Behav Health Serv Res* 26(4):360–371, 1999.

31. Busch AB, Frank RG, Lehman AF. The effect of a managed behavioral health care carve-out on quality of care for Medicaid patients diagnosed with schizophrenia. *Arch Gen Psychiatry* 61:442–448, 2004.

34. Mark TL, Levit KR, Vandivort-Warren R, et al. Changes in US spending on mental health and substance abuse treatment, 1986-2005, and implications for policy. *Health Aff* 30(2):284–292, 2011.

35. Frank R, Glied S. Changes in mental health financing since 1971: implications for policymakers and patients. *Health Aff* 25(3):601–613, 2006.

37. Trivedi AN, Swaminathan S, Mor V. Insurance parity and the use of outpatient mental health care following a psychiatric hospitalization. *JAMA* 300(24):2879–2885, 2008.

38. Busch AB, Yoon F, Barry CL, et al. The effects of mental health parity on spending and utilization for bipolar major depression, and adjustment disorders. *Am J Psychiatry* 170:180–187, 2013.

40. Garfield RL, Zuvekas SH, Lave JR, et al. The impact of national health care reform on adults with severe mental disorders. *Am J Psychiatry* 168:486–494, 2011.

69   Child and Adolescent Psychiatric Disorders

Jeff Q. Bostic, MD, EdD, Jefferson B. Prince, MD, and David C. Buxton, MD

KEY POINTS

- Psychopathology often begins and manifests, sometimes differently than in adults, in childhood and adolescence.

- Assessment of children and adolescents requires developmentally-sensitive adjustments to diagnostic criteria.

- Co-morbidities and symptoms from other disorders require consideration and sometimes targeted treatment interventions.

- Despite the resilience of children and adolescents, treatments are necessary and appropriate to minimize the effects of psychopathology on the child's development.

- Treatment planning for children and adolescents requires attention to configuring the environment to match the child's needs and existing skills, as well as consideration of biological and psychological therapies.

OVERVIEW

Children and adolescents bring diverse genetic, temperamental, perceptual, and sociological backgrounds to the environments in which they are raised. The unique constellations of these background variables match, some better and some worse, to fluctuating environmental pressures that are often outside of the control of the young person. Sometimes significant biological and/or environmental factors can stress the fit between the child and their surroundings, thereby increasing vulnerability to expressions of psychopathology. Childhood and adolescence may alter the expression of psychopathology described in adults, but young people can suffer as much as adults from psychiatric illness. Symptoms can emerge in children, particularly those who face intense stress, loss of a caregiver, chronic illness, or a personal or family history of psychiatric disorders.

Psychopathology often becomes detected as a child faces new developmental challenges. For example, children watch and emulate their caregivers as they ambulate, speak, play with others, and separate from parents to attend school. As the child faces each of these developmental hurdles, the developmental demands may exceed the child's abilities and increase the child's vulnerability for developing psychopathology. Different anxiety disorders are more prevalent at different ages; for example, separation anxiety more commonly emerges early in childhood (when the child transitions from home to school,

or to a different school, or community), while obsessive-compulsive disorder (OCD) more commonly occurs later in childhood or during adolescence. Similarly, mood disorders are diagnosed more commonly during adolescence, as the challenge to fit in among peers may prove too difficult, while loneliness and isolation increase the risk of depression (Tables 69-1 and 69-2).

A number of instruments are available to screen for the presence of psychopathology in children and adolescents (Table 69-3). Commonly employed general instruments include the Pediatric Symptom Checklist, now available in multiple languages. This and other general and specific screening tools are available online at www.schoolpsychiatry.org.

Treatments continue to evolve, and psychosocial interventions increasingly are examined to clarify which components benefit and match to certain types of symptoms and to certain types of patients. Child psychiatry has experienced proliferation of medication treatment but special considerations are required due to children's unique metabolism, possible long-term consequences, and unusual reactions[1] (Box 69-1).

DEVELOPMENTAL VARIATIONS IN PSYCHOPATHOLOGY

The diagnostic criteria from the *Diagnostic and Statistical Manual of Mental Disorders*, ed 5 (DSM-5) require developmentally-sensitive adjustments to detect symptoms in patients at different ages.[2]

CHILDHOOD ANXIETY DISORDERS

When unremitting anxiety impairs the child across multiple domains, anxiety disorders should be considered. Anxiety problems often manifest in children as somatic complaints (such as headaches, stomachaches, and nervous twitches of unknown physiological nature). Further inquiry of the child or caregivers may reveal multiple fears or incapacitating worries. Often the child has a parent with an anxiety disorder. Childhood anxiety disorders are relatively common and may persist into adult life.

Separation Anxiety

In separation anxiety, the predominant disturbance is a developmentally-inappropriate excessive anxiety on separation from familiar surroundings. A certain level of separation anxiety is an expected and healthy part of normal development that occurs in all children to varying degrees between infancy and age 6. Healthy separation anxiety is typically seen around 8 to 10 months of age, when an infant becomes anxious when meeting strangers (stranger anxiety). Children also may become mildly anxious around 18 to 24 months of

TABLE 69-1 Prevalence of Psychiatric Disorders in Children Ages 9 to 17

Psychiatric Disorder	Prevalence Past 6 Months (%)
Any psychiatric disorder	20.9
Anxiety disorders (includes generalized anxiety, separation anxiety, acute stress disorder, post-traumatic stress disorder, obsessive-compulsive disorder)	13
Disruptive behavior disorders (includes attention-deficit/hyperactivity disorder, conduct disorder, oppositional defiant disorder)	10.3
Mood disorders (includes depression, dysthymia, bipolar disorder)	6.2
Substance abuse (includes abuse or dependence with any substance, including alcohol, marijuana, opiates, stimulants)	2.0
Autism spectrum disorders (includes previous autism, Asperger's, PDD NOS)	<1%

TABLE 69-2 Other Psychiatric Disorders Usually Occurring during Childhood

Disorder	Primary Symptom(s)
Intellectual disability	Decreased intellectual function and impairments in adaptive function (e.g., self-care, independence)
Learning disorders	Achievement in reading, writing, math is below that expected based on intelligence
Motor skills disorders	Impairments in motor coordination that affect daily living
Communication disorders	Communication difficulties including expressing self, stuttering, reception of language, articulation
Autism spectrum disorder	Impairments in social interaction and communication, and restricted interests
Pica	Eating of non-nutritive substances
Rumination disorder	Repeated regurgitation, re-chewing of food after normal feeding accomplished
Avoidant/restrictive intake disorder	Eating disturbance which is based on sensory characteristics, worries about aversive events that leads to failure of nutritional needs to be met
Tourette's disorder	Multiple motor tics and one or more vocal tics
Persistent tic disorder	Motor or vocal tics
Provisional tic disorder	Single or multiple motor and/or vocal tics that for less than 1 year
Encopresis	Repeated passage of feces in inappropriate places monthly after reaching age 4 years
Enuresis	Repeated voiding of urine twice weekly while asleep or causing distress or impairing function after reaching the age of continence
Selective mutism	Persistent failure to speak in specific social situations where speaking expected, yet speaking in other situations
Reactive attachment disorder	Markedly disturbed, inappropriate social relatedness before age 5 and associated with pathological care
Stereotypic movement disorder	Driven, non-functional motor behaviors; may be self-harming

TABLE 69-3 Standardized Screening Tools and Rating Scales

General screening	Child Behavior Checklist www.aseba.org Pediatric Symptom Checklist http://psc.partners.org
Anxiety symptoms	Screen for Childhood Anxiety Related Disorders (SCARED) http://psychiatry.pitt.edu/research/tools-research/assessment-instruments Multidimensional Anxiety Scale for Children (MASC) www.mhs.com
ADHD symptoms	_ Vanderbilt ADHD Diagnostic Parent Rating Scale http://www2.massgeneral.org/schoolpsychiatry/screening_adhd.asp#Vanderbilt _ SNAP-IV Rating Scale–Revised www.adhd.net/ Connors Rating Scales–Revised www.pearsonassessments.org
Bipolar disorder/mania symptoms	Kiddie Schedule for Affective Disorders and Schizophrenia (K-SADS) http://psychiatry.pitt.edu/research/tools-research/ksads-pl
Depressive symptoms	Children's Depression Inventory www.pearsonassessments.org Reynolds Adolescent Depression Scale, Second Edition (RAD-2) www.parinc.com
Obsessive-compulsive symptoms	Children's Yale-Brown Obsessive Compulsive Scale (CY-BOCS) www.thereachinstitute.org/files/documents/cybocs.pdf
Psychosis	Kiddie Schedule for Affective Disorders and Schizophrenia (K-SADS) http://psychiatry.pitt.edu/research/tools-research/ksads-pl

age, when they are increasingly exploring their world but wanting to return to their caregiver frequently for security. In contrast, approximately 4% of children will experience separation anxiety disorder at some point with separation worries that are excessive and that overwhelm the child for even brief separations (such as leaving to go to school, going to sleep, or staying behind at home when a parent runs an errand). The child's fears usually appear to be irrational (such as a fear that the parent may suddenly die or become ill). People with separation anxiety disorder often go to great extremes to avoid being apart from their home or caregivers. They may protest against leaving a parent's side, refuse to play with friends, or complain about physical illness at the time of separating. When separation occurs or is even anticipated, the child may experience severe anxiety to the point of panic. It may develop during the preschool age, but more commonly appears in elementary-school-age children.

Treatment of Separation Anxiety

Psychosocial Treatments for Separation Anxiety. Environmental modifications are often important in the management of separation anxiety. Planned efforts to minimize the magnitude of separations (e.g., having the child transition between familiar adults [such as preferred school staff], constructing check-in notes from parents provided at various points during the preschool or school day, providing planned distracting or attractive activities as the child makes the transition) may all decrease separation fears.

Psychotherapy interventions, matched to the developmental level of the child, are often helpful. For younger children, identifying fears (that something may happen to their parent or to them, or to other adults or children) may provide clarity about the nature of the specific fear so that desensitization or successive approximations can be used to diminish anxiety. For example, for young children unable to sleep in their own rooms, sleeping on the floor, in the hall, or with a light or sibling nearby may prove viable once the child's particular distress becomes clear. Reinforcement for efforts toward sleeping alone is often needed to sustain the child's effort. Similarly, assessment of evidence that supports or negates fears, and steps to combat these fears (from relaxation techniques to keeping transitional objects, sometimes imbued with "special powers" to provide the child with strength or special skills) can replace the child's existing anxiety response. Sometimes a parent of the child with separation anxiety may similarly feel anxious around separations, so mindfulness about parent efforts and responses for separations may illuminate needs for reassurance and de-escalating acts for parents to decrease the cascade of anxiety that surrounds separations.

Pharmacotherapy for Separation Anxiety. Antidepressants and benzodiazepines are frequently used together to enable children to both separate and tolerate separations. Selective serotonin reuptake inhibitors (SSRIs) are often initiated, while benzodiazepines are simultaneously provided for several weeks until the medication exerts significant effects. Low doses of clonazepam or lorazepam may be helpful and enable the child to separate and to acclimate to the parent-absent environment. In addition, some patients require evening doses of benzodiazepines initially to counter overwhelming anxiety as they anticipate separations at bedtime or the next day.[3]

Obsessive-compulsive Disorder

Obsessive-compulsive disorder (OCD) is among the best studied of the juvenile anxiety conditions. OCD often develops early in life; nearly one-quarter of males with obsessions report the onset of their symptoms before age 10 years, and cases of the disorder have been described as early as age 3. However, 40% of patients with OCD in childhood may remit by early adulthood. OCD is characterized by persistent ideas or impulses (obsessions) that are intrusive and senseless (e.g., thoughts of having caused violence, becoming contaminated, or severely doubting oneself) that may lead to persistent repetitive, purposeful behaviors (compulsions) (e.g., handwashing, counting, checking, or touching in order to neutralize the obsessive worries). Within the medical setting, this disorder is often associated with an exaggerated, persistent, and impairing obsession with an organ, disease process, or treatment. This disorder has been estimated to affect 1%–2% of the adult population; it has been shown to be familial and associated with Tourette's syndrome (TS) and attention-deficit/hyperactivity disorder (ADHD). OCD is most effectively treated with cognitive-behavioral treatment (CBT) or an SSRI, with combined CBT + SSRI treatment yielding the best outcomes. In addition, patients who are partial responders to an SSRI alone can benefit from augmentation with CBT.

Pediatric autoimmune neuropsychiatric disorders associated with streptococcal infection (PANDAS) have also been associated with OCD/tics. Plasma exchange, intravenous (IV) immunoglobulin, and penicillin have been used to treat OCD/tics associated with PANDAS. These treatments appear to be effective only for those patients (less than 10%) whose OCD/tics were associated with streptococcal infections.[4]

Treatment of Obsessive-compulsive Disorder

Psychosocial Treatment of Obsessive-compulsive Disorder. A variety of therapies have been beneficial in the management of OCD.[5,6] CBT, both with individuals and with groups of children having OCD, have proven efficacious, including "personifying" the obsessions (e.g., "Germy"), and identifying steps to "boss back Germy," to recognize how much time the child plays with "Germy" instead of with peers (to make the obsessions more dystonic). Practicing compulsions differently to make them more uncomfortable and providing more appropriate "competing" responses to replace existing compulsions have been useful.[7]

Pharmacotherapy of Obsessive-compulsive Disorder. Pharmacotherapy with SSRI antidepressants remains the cornerstone of pharmacological treatments for OCD. Studies suggest that children with OCD respond in a fashion similar to adults, and may require doses up to four times the normal doses used to treat depression (i.e., 80 mg of fluoxetine instead of 20 mg daily).[8] The SSRI antidepressants are Food and Drug Administration (FDA)-approved for OCD in the pediatric population (e.g., sertraline [Zoloft, initiated at 12.5 to 25 mg daily and titrated to 50 to 200 mg daily], fluvoxamine [Luvox, a more sedating drug that is initiated at 25 mg at bedtime and increased to 25 to 150 mg twice per day], and fluoxetine [Prozac, initiated at 5 to 10 mg and increased to 60 mg/day]).When SSRIs cannot be tolerated, or the patient is refractory to multiple SSRIs, the tricyclic antidepressant (TCA) clomipramine (Anafranil) has also been efficacious for pediatric OCD. A variety of additional pharmacotherapy strategies have been employed to augment SSRIs in severely impaired adolescents with OCD, including: atypical antipsychotics, such as aripiprazole,[9] the amyotrophic lateral sclerosis (ALS) medication riluzole (although concerns about pancreatitis persist),[10] emantine,[11] and D-cycloserine.[12] Despite these medication treatments, augmentation of CBT appears to be particularly efficacious.[13]

Generalized Anxiety Disorder

Generalized anxiety disorder (GAD) of childhood is more frequently seen in boys than in girls. Similar to GAD in the adult patient, the essential feature is excessive worry and fear that is not focused on a specific situation or object and is not seen as a result of psychosocial stressors. Children may manifest an exaggerated or unrealistic response to the comments or criticisms of others. Less commonly, some children and adolescents experience panic attacks.

Treatment of Generalized Anxiety Disorder

Psychosocial Treatments for Generalized Anxiety Disorder. Patient education about the chronic nature of GAD and the fluctuating course of symptoms often associated with the emergence or decrease in stressors may provide reassurance to patients and decrease general stress levels. Psychotherapeutic support, using relaxation, deep breathing, and progressive muscle relaxation, may help children counter escalations of anxiety. Cognitive-behavioral techniques for appraising situations more completely and logically, and for accessing other input from others or evaluating all the evidence (e.g., the likelihood of a terrorist attack in a rural county), may enable children to control anxiety with cognitive skills.

Pharmacotherapy for Pediatric Generalized Anxiety Disorder. Treatment of GAD in children is similar to the treatment of GAD in adults; SSRIs, benzodiazepines, TCAs, and beta-blockers appear to be effective. Buspirone, a non-benzodiazepine anxiolytic without anticonvulsant, sedative, or muscle-relaxant properties, may provide some benefit alone or by using it in combination with an SSRI. The effective daily buspirone dose is estimated to range from 0.3 to 0.6 mg/kg.

Acute Stress Disorder/Post-traumatic Stress Disorder

Acute stress disorder develops within days of a traumatic event and is manifest by anxiety, dissociative symptoms, persistent re-experiencing of the trauma, and avoidance of stimuli that raise recollections of the trauma. This disorder is likely to be observed in pediatric patients or their parents after acute injuries. The severity, duration, and proximity to the trauma are factors that influence the development of acute stress disorder, and approximately 20%–50% are reported after interpersonal traumatic events, like an assault or a mass shooting. In addition to the nature (e.g., burns, self-injurious behaviors, or abuse) and extent of the injuries, pre-existing psychiatric illness increases the risk of acute stress disorder.

If the stressful symptoms surrounding the trauma last beyond 1 month, the diagnosis changes to post-traumatic stress disorder (PTSD). PTSD may occur following a traumatic event that continues to haunt a person months later, beyond the "acute" reaction to a trauma. Children, like adults, may experience nightmares months to years after a traumatic event, as well as flashbacks or distressing recollections sometimes suppressed successfully for years. Sometimes patients will not have symptoms immediately following the traumatic event, but months or years later. Events resembling a past trauma may re-kindle the trauma, culminating in anxiety symptoms, or sometimes a person will experience PTSD when reaching a developmental point related to the trauma. For example, when children reach high school or college, have their own children, or experience the loss of someone, their distress may emerge as the trauma is re-experienced from a different role (e.g., older sibling or parent instead of child). While acute stress disorder and PTSD are not genetic disorders, vulnerabilities to anxiety reactions do have genetic components; in addition, some individuals live in more dangerous or chaotic environments, as do their children, so that PTSD may occur more commonly in some families. Approximately 8.7% of Americans have been reported to experience PTSD by the age of 75 years, although susceptibility to traumatic events increases one's risk of developing PTSD.

Treatment of Acute Stress Disorder/Post-traumatic Stress Disorder

Psychosocial Treatments of Acute Stress Disorder/Post-traumatic Stress Disorder. Efforts to help children separate themselves from the traumatic event and from the victim role, are helpful. Environmental changes to reduce further risks for the child often require interventions by adults to create safety for the child. Cognitive-behavioral techniques to help the child resist traumatic recollections, and to counter recurrent distressing thoughts, to de-escalate anxiety, and to distinguish time or setting variables that surrounded the event to diminish generalization of fears can allay symptoms. Anticipatory planning with family members, if nightmares or flashbacks occur, can diminish re-traumatization during the child's recollection of past events.

Pharmacotherapy for Acute Stress Disorder/Post-traumatic Stress Disorder. Treatment has relied on multiple "off-label" agents reported to be effective for various acute stress disorder/PTSD symptoms. High-potency benzodiazepines (e.g., alprazolam 0.25 to 1 mg three times per day or clonazepam 0.25 to 1 mg three times per day) or medium-potency benzodiazepines (e.g., lorazepam 0.25 to 1 mg three times per day) can be effective.[14] While the clinical toxicity of benzodiazepines is low, higher rates of disinhibition are observed in the pediatric population than in adults. The most commonly encountered short-term adverse effects of benzodiazepines are sedation, disinhibition, and depression. With the exception of the theoretical potential risk for tolerance and dependence that appears to be low in children, no known long-term adverse effects are associated with benzodiazepines. Adverse effects of withdrawal can occur, and benzodiazepines, when being tapered, should be tapered slowly.

Long-acting benzodiazepines (such as clonazepam) may be preferable when long-term treatment with a benzodiazepine is warranted. For clonazepam, an initial dose of 0.25 to 0.5 mg can be given at bedtime. The dose can be increased by 0.5 mg every 5 to 7 days depending on the clinical response and the side effects. Typically, doses between 0.25 and 2 mg/day are effective. Clinicians should monitor for signs of disinhibition, which may manifest as either excessively silly behavior or as agitation. Children who become disinhibited on high-potency benzodiazepines may respond more favorably to the mid- or low-potency agents (such as clorazepate). Potential benefits of the longer-acting compounds are single-daily dosage and a decreased risk of withdrawal symptoms after discontinuation of treatment.

Beta-blockers, in particular propranolol, have been studied as a means of reducing arousal symptoms of PTSD. Similarly, alpha-adrenergic agents (such as clonidine or guanfacine) or prazosin may likewise reduce anxiety, hyperarousal, and impulsivity as well as improve attention.[14] In patients with dissociation, medications that enhance gamma-aminobutyric acid (GABA), such as gabapentin (Neurontin), may reduce the severity of anxiety. In patients with fear or terror, the short-term use of atypical antipsychotics in low doses may be useful.

The SSRIs have been shown to be useful in reducing symptoms of anxiety, depressed mood, rage, and obsessional thinking in adults with PTSD. The SSRIs are often used and may diminish similar target symptoms in pediatric patients with PTSD; however, SSRIs may not be helpful.[15]

TIC DISORDERS

Tics are sudden, rapid recurrent non-rhythmic motor movements or vocalizations that have the potential to make children feel ostracized or distressed. Most tics, such as eye-blinking, are mild and transient. Tics often emerge between ages 4 and 6 years, with a peak severity around 10–12 years, although tics may wax and wane particularly when the child is anxious or fatigued. DSM-5 divides tics into four categories: (1) Tourettes; (2) persistent motor or vocal; (3) provisional; or (4) unspecified. Tourette's syndrome (TS), a childhood-onset neuropsychiatric disorder afflicting up to 3–8 per 1,000 children; it involves both multiple vocal and motor tics. TS usually begins around ages 4–6 and is accompanied by other behavioral and psychological symptoms. TS is commonly associated with OCD (in about 30% of cases) and ADHD (in about 50% of cases). It is noteworthy that in many cases it is not the tics but the co-morbid disorders that are the major source of distress and disability. Some associations include the findings that ADHD appears earlier in life than tics and that stimulants may exacerbate tics. For many patients with tics and ADHD, the symptoms of ADHD appear to be associated with the most severe impairment.

Treatment of Tic Disorders
Psychosocial Treatments for Tic Disorders

Tics usually manifest at erratic and often uncomfortable times, and are usually not a planned behavior on the part of the patient, yet can be recognized and anticipated on occasion. Accordingly, behavioral interventions (such as habit reversal) may benefit patients, and warrant consideration in the treatment of tics. First, circumstances that increase stress and precipitate tics can sometimes be identified and altered. Second, premonitory urges can be recognized, so that actions can be taken to minimize expression of the tic. Third, relaxation efforts (such as deep breathing) can sometimes diminish urges. Fourth, competing responses can sometimes be identified that help allow the child to "discharge" tic-like behaviors in a less socially-distressing manner. Vocal tics, particularly, can be disruptive, so alternative vocalizations the child can use, as well as clarification to others (such as teachers) about the involuntary nature of most tics, can diminish the impact of the tics on the child's daily life. Finally, motivational practices can reinforce habit reversal and encourage patients to employ steps when urges or situations increase the risk for expression of urges.[16]

Pharmacotherapy for Tic Disorders

Alpha-agonists (such as clonidine and guanfacine) are effective in reducing the severity and frequency of tics and are first-line medications for tics and TS.[17] Clonidine is usually started at very low doses (i.e., 0.025 mg/day) to reduce the initial adverse effect of sedation, and it is increased as necessary. Comparison between clonidine and risperidone and risperidone and pimozide demonstrated similar improvements in tic severity.[18] In addition, clonidine alone and in combination with methylphenidate improved tics in patients with ADHD.[19] Compared with placebo, clonidine and methylphenidate, clonidine alone, and methylphenidate alone were associated with reductions in tic severity. Although some patients experience an exacerbation of tics during treatment with stimulants, many patients appear to benefit from treatment of their ADHD symptoms. Guanfacine, usually started at 0.5 mg twice a day, may be used if side effects (such as sedation) emerge with clonidine treatment. Both clonidine and guanfacine are now available in long-acting pill formulations to improve adherence and to diminish serum level fluctuations throughout the day.

Traditional antipsychotics (e.g., haloperidol, pimozide) have been considered the drugs of choice in TS. However, antipsychotics have limited effects on the frequently associated co-morbid disorders of ADHD and OCD, and they are associated with short-term adverse effects (e.g., extrapyramidal symptoms [EPS]) and long-term adverse effects (e.g., tardive dyskinesia [TD]). Atypical antipsychotics including ziprasidone (Geodon) initiated at 20 mg/day and increased to approximately 60 mg per/day, risperidone titrated to 3 mg/day, and aripiprazole titrated to 10 to 20 mg/day have been reported to be effective and generally well tolerated. Dysphoria and depression have been reported in some adolescents with TS who are treated with atypical antipsychotics, so monitoring of mood symptom side effects is warranted.

Alternative agents may also be useful in patients unresponsive to, or unable to tolerate, alpha-agonists or neuroleptics. The TCAs (e.g., desipramine, nortriptyline) have been found to be effective in some children with this disorder. Given concerns over cardiac safety with the TCAs, atomoxetine (ATMX) may prove to be a more attractive noradrenergic treatment for patients with ADHD and TS. Other medications have also been described and may be useful in refractory patients with TS with or without ADHD, including the selective type-B monoamine oxidase inhibitor (MAOI) L-deprenyl, the mixed $D_1/D_2/D_3$ dopamine agonist pergolide, the hypotensive agent mecamylamine, and medications that enhance cholinergic neurotransmission (e.g., donepezil, nicotine).

ATTENTION-DEFICIT/HYPERACTIVITY DISORDER

Attention-deficit/hyperactivity disorder (ADHD) is a common psychiatric condition present in 5% of children and 2.5% of adults. ADHD is characterized by the classic triad of impaired attention, impulsivity, and excessive motor activity, although up to one-third of children may only manifest the inattentive aspects of ADHD. ADHD affects children of all ages, sometimes identified as early as age 3, and it persists throughout adolescence and into adulthood. Many patients with ADHD have co-morbid disorders (such as oppositional defiant disorder in up to 70%), conduct disorder (in approximately 25%), learning disorders (in approximately 40%), anxiety disorders (in approximately 40%), and mood disorders (in approximately 33%). In addition, patients with autism spectrum disorder may be diagnosed with ADHD. Within the medical setting, ADHD needs to be differentiated from environmental stimulation, iatrogenic causes (e.g., use of beta-agonists or lead toxicity from paint ingestion), or other psychiatric disorders (such as anxiety, depression, or mania), or intoxication.

Treatment of Attention-deficit/Hyperactivity Disorder

Psychosocial Treatments of Attention-deficit/Hyperactivity Disorder

Behavioral interventions are often used to help structure the child with ADHD and minimize distractions. Parent education to prepare parents to better match the child with environments (by adjusting levels of stimulation in classrooms, within the home, and during peer activities) can reduce symptoms. Supporting parent efforts to "catch the child being good" are important to diminish the frequency of conflicts and to help parents cultivate more useful behavioral responses. Reinforcement for attention, even brief intervals, may help expand attention intervals. Coaching of patients with ADHD to help them employ planning strategies, to enact steps to impede impulsive acts, and to address frustrations more methodically can diminish the magnitude of symptoms. Evaluations of behavioral treatments, however, indicate that they remain of limited benefit in the treatment of ADHD, such that medication is often needed to optimize the child's function.[20]

Pharmacotherapy of Attention-deficit/Hyperactivity Disorder

Stimulants (and now non-stimulant medications) have been used safely and effectively in the treatment of ADHD.[21-25] Current treatment guidelines recommend starting with longer-acting preparations in most cases. Awareness of treatment-related side effects helps steer clinical practice. Contemporary research does not suggest an increased risk of cardiovascular events in patients treated with stimulants. Further discussion of these pharmacological approaches is provided in Chapter 49.

OPPOSITIONAL DEFIANT DISORDER

Oppositional defiant disorder (ODD) is characterized by hostility, defiance, and disobedience of authority figures. For diagnosis of children under the age of 5 years old the behavior should be daily for 6 months, while older children must have symptoms at least once per week for 6 months. Oppositionality must be beyond that normally seen in children of comparable age, and not attributable to mood or anxiety disorders, or intoxication. Symptoms are associated with distress in the child and others in their lives, and usually are more prominent at home initially and then spill over to school or social settings, so the clinician may not initially see the child exhibit the symptoms the parent describes. Severity of symptoms can be specified using mild (one setting), moderate (two settings) or severe (three or more settings). Patients with ODD rarely regard themselves as oppositional, but rather justify their behaviors complaining of inept or unreasonable actions of others. Children with difficult temperaments (e.g., hard-to-soothe or overly reactive to stimuli) are more likely to exert control over their environments, defy parental controls, and develop ODD, as are children with ADHD. While ODD is more common in boys at young ages, by adolescence rates between boys and girls are similar. Approximately 2% to 16% of children may develop ODD, usually before age 8. If symptoms are more severe with elements of vandalism, fire-setting, cruelty to animals or others, stealing, break-ins, truancy, running away, or other criminal behaviors exist (e.g., thefts, rape, assaults), conduct disorder may also be present and children carry both diagnosis.

Treatment of Oppositional Defiant Disorder

Psychosocial Interventions

Psychosocial treatments have become the cornerstone of treatment for ODD. Consistency in parenting practices, preparation for changes and transitions, and parenting strategies for eliciting compliance and minimizing escalations are often needed. Importantly, the patient with ODD is rarely eager to alter patterns, so psychotherapy with the child alone is often unsuccessful. Instead, efforts with parents or other caregiver adults often yield more benefit. Collaborative problem-solving has been shown to be helpful; it employs a framework in which ODD is seen as a child lacking thinking skills, thereby using manipulation, limit testing, etc., to get their needs met by caregivers. Through teaching children new skills and assisting parents in finding ways to work with children, patterns of conflict can change. Rather than presuming that parenting practices are inept, one should consider that the child with ODD may exhibit poor flexibility/adaptability, frustration tolerance, and problem-solving skill, or be unable to use these skills when they are most needed.[26] Efforts to help the child develop skills to solve problems and to adapt more flexibility replace imposition of adult rules. Collaborative problem-solving involves adults identifying a problem for both the child and the adult that *they* together need to solve. From the child's proposed solutions, the adult then tries to work so that an acceptable solution for that moment can be derived.

Pharmacotherapy of Oppositional Defiant Disorder

Medication treatments for ODD rely on addressing target symptoms treatable by medications for other disorders: that is, no medication treatment is FDA-approved for treatment of ODD. Rather, identification of co-morbid disorders, like ADHD or mood disorders, often identifies symptoms responsive to medications.[27]

MOOD DISORDERS
Depression

Children and adolescents may have various depressive disorders (including major depression, dysthymia, or mood disturbances associated with medical conditions) as a result of substance use/abuse or psychosocial problems. In the medical setting, clinicians are challenged to differentiate transient symptoms of depression from true depressive disorders. Children often manifest worry, hopelessness, and sadness as primary symptoms related to their own illness, whereas adolescents typically display anxiety, anger, or withdrawal. If the symptoms are episodic and associated with limited impairment and surround an identified event or disappointment, they are generally referred to as an adjustment disorder with depressed or anxious mood. These patients usually respond to reassurance, environmental intervention, or interpersonal or CBT. In the outpatient medical setting, children and adolescents with depression may be evaluated for a variety of medical symptoms of unclear etiology. During routine examination these patients may appear sad, withdrawn, apathetic, anxious, angry, or irritable.

The prevalence of major depression increases with age. Epidemiological studies estimate that the prevalence of major depressive disorder (MDD) is approximately 0.3% in preschoolers, 2% in children, and between 1.5% and 9% in adolescents. By the end of adolescence, the cumulative incidence of MDD has been estimated to be as high as 20%. Although the gender ratio appears to be equal in children, by age 14, girls appear to be twice as likely to experience depression as boys. Depressive disorders commonly co-occur with anxiety, ADHD, conduct disorders, and substance use disorders in older children and adolescents.

The duration of pediatric depressive episodes appears to be approximately 7 months, and in the course of a first episode, up to 40% appear to recover without specific treatment. However, patients who do not recover appear to be at high risk of chronic depression, and those who do recover have high rates of recurrence and dysthymia. Mood disorders in children tend to be chronic compared with the more episodic nature that is typical of adult mood disorders. Furthermore, children and adolescents with depression have a higher rate of conversion to bipolar disorder. In follow-up, almost half of children who initially had single-episode, non-psychotic MDD converted to bipolar disorder that lasted into their early twenties.[28] Risk factors for switching from MDD to bipolar disorder include a history of bipolar disorder in parents and grandparents and a family history of antidepressant-induced mania. Other warning signs of conversion to mania include rapid onset of depression associated with psychosis, psychomotor retardation, and hypersomnia. These patients may also be at increased risk for self-injurious behaviors or suicide.

Suicide remains the third leading cause of death (behind motor vehicle accidents and homicides) for adolescents aged 15–19 years, and the numbers of adolescent suicides increased dramatically from the 1960s to the 1990s. Overall, males are at increased risk compared with females; in particular, boys with previous suicide attempts, a mood disorder (depression or bipolar), and associated substance abuse are at higher risk. Females at greatest risk have mood disorders (depression or bipolar) and a history of previous suicidal behaviors. After a suicide attempt, patients with a history of suicidal behaviors, who continue to think about suicide, who live alone and are agitated, who are irritable and have associated MDD, and who have bipolar disorder or substance abuse are at greatest risk. In addition to medical care, these patients require close monitoring (including possible restraint, seclusion, or observation by a reliable adult). Information needs to be obtained from outside sources (e.g., family, school, therapist), and the patient must be evaluated for any underlying psychiatric disorders and treated appropriately. In outpatient settings, approximately half of children referred for depression are suicidal. For children in whom more malignant symptoms occur or in whom

there is significant impairment or suicidality, the consideration of pharmacotherapy is necessary.

Similar to adults, children with sub-syndromal depressive disorders, which are long-standing and often associated with anhedonia and negativity, may have persistent depressive disorder. Persistent depression (which replaces "Dysthymia" in DSM-5) in children and adolescents is manifest by chronically depressed mood for at least 1 year, associated with change in appetite (too little or too much), sleep disturbance (insomnia or hypersomnia), low energy, easy fatigability, low self-esteem, indecisiveness, poor concentration, and feelings of hopelessness. Juveniles with persistent depressive disorder are often self-critical and feel easily criticized or rejected. Although persistent depression is a major risk factor for future episodes of major depression, juveniles with persistent depression have fewer melancholic symptoms and suicidality.

Treatment of Depressive Disorders

Psychosocial Treatment of Juvenile Depression. Psychosocial treatments for juvenile depression require attention to other variables (e.g., regular sleep schedule, exercise, diet) that might improve depression and decrease vulnerability to subsequent episodes. Specifically, exercise patterns and diet (including addition of omega-3 agents) both deserve attention in the management of depression. Similarly, cognitive-behavioral techniques to combat depression and other psychosocial interventions (e.g., pro-social involvement with peers and participation in community or school activities) may be needed.

CBT is useful for young depressed patients; it encourages patients to increase self-awareness and challenge ideas that perpetuate depressive thoughts. Sample CBT techniques useful in all clinical encounters are provided in Table 69-4. Clinicians can encourage patients to chart their mood to detect trends, increase exercise and pleasurable activities (natural antidepressants), and expand their problem-solving repertoire to "fix" problems or mistakes rather than replay failures.

Interpersonal therapy (IPT) has also been reported helpful for juvenile depression, particularly in adolescents.[29] Techniques to help patients access and connect to others, describe their perceptions and feelings so as to cultivate empathy from others, and increase interactions with supportive peers and family members may help reduce depressive symptoms and effects.

Pharmacotherapy of Juvenile Depression. Prescription of SSRIs for children and adolescents increased approximately seven-fold during the 1990s, as these agents were perceived to be less lethal than their predecessors, the TCAs. TCAs in children and adolescents with depression demonstrated minimal advantage over placebo in multiple controlled trials. The less lethal SSRIs initially appeared to be safer, and potentially effective in pediatric patients. However, as prescriptions proliferated for SSRIs, concerns emerged that the SSRIs might not, in fact, be much more effective than TCAs, and concerns of inducing suicidality in young patients emerged (see the following discussion). Differences in study methodology may have influenced findings in SSRI trials. Specifically, diverse methodologies were employed and trials with large numbers of sites, but small samples, generally showed less benefit than studies with smaller numbers of sites, longer placebo run-in intervals, and reliance on particular instruments (Child Depression Rating Scale as compared to the Hamilton Depression Rating Scale).[30]

Fluoxetine has been approved by the FDA to treat MDD in children and adolescents between 7 and 17 years of age. In the two trials leading to this approval, patients treated with fluoxetine responded, based on standard rating scales, over

TABLE 69-4 Cognitive-Behavioral Techniques for Pediatric Depression

Cognitive-Behavioral Therapy Technique	Patient Examples	Clinician Responses
1. Evaluate the evidence for a conclusion	"I'm no good at jogging."	"What happened when you jogged? Did any good things occur? What parts of jogging go well? What parts do you wish were different?"
2. Challenge negative cognitions	"I can't go to school—people will make fun of me."	"What do students do when you arrive? What do they do that you don't like? Which students are glad to see you?"
3. Identify automatic thoughts	"I'm no fun. No one wants to be around/play with me."	"What makes you no fun? What happened that you thought this? What evidence leads you to reach such conclusions?"
4. Examine other perspectives	"I don't know what to do."	"How would Batman/your best friend/someone you admire react to this? What did your friend/classmate/parent think about your situation?"
5. Provide competing responses	"I'm afraid I'll start crying in class."	"If you start to feel sad, what can you do right before you start to cry? What can you do that makes you think about something better?"
6. Cultivate positive self-talk	"I'm bad at everything I do."	"I'm going to show up—now, I'm going to say 'Hi' to one person."
7. Practice and reinforce positive skills	"I'm too slow to finish this homework."	"I'll compare my first answers to the first few homework problems with _____ to make sure we're doing them right."

those treated with placebo (study 1: 56% fluoxetine versus 33% placebo; study 2: 65% fluoxetine versus 54% placebo), and only 30% to 40% of the fluoxetine-treated patients achieved full remission, compared with approximately 20% of placebo-treated patients.[31,32] Compared with placebo, fluoxetine treatment was associated with significantly greater improvements based on blinded-clinician perception of improvement (e.g., in study 2, 52.3% fluoxetine versus 36.8% placebo) ratings. A subsequent National Institute of Mental Health (NIMH)-supported fluoxetine and CBT trial concluded that combined medication and therapy treatment was most efficacious, and that fluoxetine alone was superior to cognitive therapy alone, and to placebo.[33]

The only other "positive" controlled SSRI trial for pediatric depression occurred with citalopram.[34] Significantly more patients treated with citalopram responded compared with placebo (36% versus 24%). Patients treated with citalopram more commonly reported nausea, influenza-like symptoms, and rhinitis. A subsequent multi-site controlled trial of escitalopram, the S-enantiomer of citalopram, did not show significant benefit on depression, although adolescents were more likely to respond than child patients.

Results of large controlled trials of other SSRIs in the treatment of pediatric depression have not shown that other SSRI antidepressants were significantly better than placebo in the treatment of pediatric depression. Sertraline, paroxetine, and the more atypical serotonergic antidepressants (venlafaxine, nefazodone, and mirtazapine) did not separate from placebo and thus are unlikely to become FDA-indicated agents for juvenile depression.

SSRI Antidepressants and Suicidality

On June 10, 2003, the British Medicines and Healthcare Products Regulatory Agency (MHRA) advised that paroxetine should not be used for the treatment of depression in patients younger than 18 years old. Although no pediatric patient completed suicide, the MHRA were concerned enough to say "the benefits of Seroxat (paroxetine) in children for the treatment of depressive illness do not outweigh the risks." The MHRA's full report and advice to prescribers is available online at www.medicines.mhra.gov.uk.

Following the MHRA, the FDA reviewed 26 controlled antidepressant trials in the treatment of juvenile depression, concluding that the risks of "suicidality" appeared to be 4% for patients receiving contemporary (non-tricyclic) antidepressants, compared to 2% of patients receiving placebo. Although no patients completed suicide in any of these studies, this potential risk led to the "black box warning" for all 34 antidepressants available in the US, and the FDA encouraged

increased monitoring of juvenile patients placed on antidepressants. Review of data in adults subsequently suggested that this risk may persist into young adults, so increased vigilance of patients up to age 25 was recommended by the FDA.

The association of SSRIs and suicidal behaviors is not new, although additional lines of evidence have emerged that question the risk: benefit profile of antidepressants in juvenile depression. However, prescriptions for antidepressants decreased approximately 20% following the black box warning, and the available evidence at the time of this writing revealed a significant increase in the suicide rate of young people for the first time since the early 1990s, after a decrease when the SSRIs became available in the US.[35] A more recent meta-analysis from 1998 to 2006 reviewing suicidal ideation/suicide attempts in children being treated for MDD, OCD, and anxiety showed SSRIs to be efficacious with benefits outweighing risks of suicide. Multiple other lines of evidence have similarly failed to suggest that antidepressants increase pediatric suicide.[36] Large database evaluations failed to show any increase in suicide rates in patients treated with SSRIs, and instead suggested that those counties where SSRI prescriptions were higher had lower suicide rates. In addition, autopsies of adolescents who completed suicide failed to show traces of antidepressants at autopsy.

Clinical Use of SSRIs

Given the likelihood of relatively similar efficacy, selection of an SSRI should take into consideration tolerability (e.g., side-effect profile), anticipated medication interactions, half-life, potential for bipolar switching, and adherence.[37] While paroxetine, fluoxetine, citalopram, escitalopram, and sertraline may be associated with agitation and increased energy, fluvoxamine appears to be more sedating and perhaps useful in children with sleep difficulties associated with their mood symptoms. SSRIs should be initiated at low doses (e.g., 5 to 10 mg fluoxetine, 12.5 to 25 mg sertraline, 5 to 10 mg citalopram, 2.5 to 5 mg escitalopram, 5 to 10 mg paroxetine, 12.5 to 25 mg fluvoxamine, and 18.75 to 37.5 mg venlafaxine) and titrated upward slowly. Fluoxetine, sertraline, paroxetine, citalopram, and escitalopram are available in liquid preparations.

Although the main pharmacodynamic effect of the SSRIs is similar, they are structurally dissimilar to each other and vary in their pharmacokinetics and drug interactions. Approximately 60% of adolescents with depression will have an adequate response to initial treatment with an SSRI and switching to another agent remains the preferred next step when the original medication is not effective. Switching to another agent and adding CBT appears more effective than just switching to a different SSRI. Venlafaxine and the newer desvenlafaxine appear similarly effective to SSRIs, but their additional noradrenergic activity appears associated with more side effects.[38]

In general, SSRIs appear to be well tolerated and to have fewer side effects than the TCAs, especially in overdose. The SSRIs have been found to inhibit specific hepatic isoenzymes and thereby increase serum levels of other compounds. Parents and clinicians should be alerted to the concern that the SSRIs may interact with various antibiotics, especially the macrolide derivatives currently used in pediatrics. Adverse effects of SSRIs include manic activation, agitation, gastrointestinal (GI) symptoms, irritability, insomnia, sexual side effects, and weight loss. Although these agents have been used for almost 25 years in juveniles without detection of significant effects on growth, clinicians should consider alternative treatments if a patient's height or weight inexplicably decelerates. In December 2012, FDA indicated that citalopram should not be given at the doses greater than 40 mg/day due to the risk of QTc prolongation, which could result in arrhythmias. Based on the current evidence and practice guidelines, vital signs, blood monitoring, and electrocardiogram (ECG) monitoring do not appear to be necessary unless there is an additional medical concern. Activation, which is distinguished from a change in mood or impulse control and may be related to akathisia, hyperactivity, or disinhibition, usually responds to lowering the dose. Signs of mania (which may include impulse dyscontrol, mood swings, grandiosity, hypersexuality, and aggression) may be observed and accompany bipolar switching. Treatment relies on pharmacologically addressing the mania. Celebration may occur in anxious children treated with SSRIs who experience relief of their anxiety, and they may seem impulsive or uninhibited. Developmental issues may be observed as patients' anxiety or depression lifts, after which additional co-morbidities become evident (e.g., ADHD or Asperger's syndrome). Frontal-lobe-type symptoms may appear and be manifest primarily by apathy. Adolescents prescribed SSRIs may experience sexual side effects, although reports of these side effects are minimal in controlled studies in this population.

Like adults, children may experience a discontinuation syndrome either as they are tapered off SSRIs after treatment or if they miss their scheduled dose. Typically this syndrome occurs in patients who are taking SSRIs with short half-lives (e.g., paroxetine or venlafaxine), although it can occur with any antidepressant. As in adults, the discontinuation syndrome is typically characterized by physical symptoms (e.g., nausea, GI disturbance, diarrhea, dizziness, insomnia, lightheadedness, headache, shakiness, sensations of mild electrical shock), cognitive symptoms (e.g., confusion, poor memory, cloudiness, forgetfulness), and emotional symptoms (e.g., increased crying, mood lability, anxiety). Patients and parents should be educated about the discontinuation syndrome and steps taken to prevent its occurrence, including using only SSRIs when necessary, encouraging adherence, tapering SSRIs gradually, and ensuring that the manufacturer stays the same throughout treatment if patients are taking a generic preparation.[39] When patients experience a discontinuation syndrome, re-introducing the medication usually provides relief, although some patients may need to be switched to an SSRI with a longer half-life (such as fluoxetine).

Disruptive Mood Dysregulation Disorder

DSM-5 provides a new diagnosis to capture a subset of children over the age of 6 who do not clearly meet criteria for bipolar disorder but who have severe recurrent temper outbursts with constant irritability in between episodes. Outbursts are inconsistent with development and are out of proportion to a stressor with physical aggression or verbal rages in two or more settings at least 3 times a week. Due to this diagnosis being new to the field, indications of treatment are limited and prevalence rates are unclear. The DSM-5 work group has advised that children that have this diagnosis should not be treated with atypical antipsychotics.

Bipolar Disorder

Growing awareness has emerged of pediatric bipolar disorder, as 50%–66% of adult bipolar patients report onset during childhood or adolescence. In children, bipolar disorder commonly manifests as an extremely irritable or explosive mood with associated poor psychosocial function often devastating to the child and family. Children with prepubertal mania appear to be much more likely to experience ultra-rapid mood changes, rather than discrete episodes of mania for several days followed by depressive symptoms for weeks to months. Rather, within a day, these children are often crying for several hours, then giddy or silly, and then explosively angry at the seemingly smallest provocation. Although the juvenile symptom complex of mania should be differentiated from ADHD, conduct disorder, depression, trauma, substance use/abuse, and psychotic disorders, these disorders commonly co-occur with childhood mania.[40] A family history of bipolar disorder increases the risk of the child developing bipolar disorder, and treatment for these co-morbidities may unmask underlying or evolving bipolar disorder. The clinical course of juvenile mania appears most frequently chronic and mixed with co-occurring manic and depressive features.

Treatment of Pediatric Bipolar Disorders

Psychosocial Treatments for Bipolar Disorder. Although bipolar disorder is usually a serious mental illness warranting medication, psychosocial interventions may reduce the frequency and intensity of symptoms. Predictable routines and responses within home and school settings may reduce mood escalations and optimize stimulation of the environment for the individual child. De-escalating strategies become important for adults to employ during the child's mood storms, including places or activities the child can use to calm down or re-direct energy, the use of calm, soft speech to interrupt mood cycles, and providing time in non-stimulating spots for the child to re-group.

Cognitive-behavioral techniques may provide the child strategies to combat distressing moods, and particularly to slow or diminish escalations of moods. Indeed, cognitive activities are often useful to help harness emotions for children with bipolar disorder, so practice in mood-charting to identify and recognize precipitants to mood episodes may reveal intervention points or opportunities. Frameworks for assessing situations, for evaluating evidence for perceptions or conclusions, using calming/relaxation statements or practices, validating perceptions with trusted others, and prioritizing wishes or expectations in a given situation may help pediatric patients with bipolar disorder to decrease mood swings and contain manic or depressive episodes. In addition, accessing helpful others, reducing stimulation, or slowing interactions or activities may all provide the child with alternative actions when distressing moods emerge.

Pharmacotherapy of Bipolar Disorder. There are no medications specifically approved to treat bipolar disorder in children younger than 10 years old. For bipolar patients between 13 and 17 years old, lithium is FDA-approved. However, investigators have noted that early-onset bipolar disorder appears to be less responsive to lithium. Therefore, children and adolescents with bipolar disorder are often treated with antipsychotic medications, anticonvulsants, or combinations of lithium, anticonvulsants, and/or atypical antipsychotic mood stabilizers. If the patient does not respond to an adequate trial (in dose and time) of a single agent or cannot tolerate the medication, subsequent trials with alternative medication(s) are recommended. In manic or mixed presentations, with psychotic symptoms, additional antipsychotic treatment is recommended. In bipolar disorder with prominent symptoms of depression, combined treatment with a mood stabilizer and an antidepressant is indicated.[41] One must be mindful of the potential destabilizing effects of SSRIs in the treatment of bipolar depression in children and adolescents.

Lithium. The use of lithium carbonate in mood disorders, particularly bipolar disorders and treatment-resistant unipolar depressions, appears to be useful; surprisingly, it has not been studied under controlled conditions. The usual starting dose of lithium ranges from 150 to 300 mg/day in divided doses, two or three times per day. Dosage guidelines for lithium in children 6–12 years old support initial total daily doses (administered three times per day) of 600 mg/day for patients weighing less than 25 kg, 900 mg for patients weighing 25–40 kg, 1,200 mg/day for patients weighing 40–50 kg, and 1,500 mg/day for patients weighing 50–60 kg. There is no known therapeutic serum lithium level in children. Based on the adult literature, serum levels of 0.8–1.5 mEq/L for acute episodes and levels of 0.4–0.8 mEq/L for maintenance therapy have been proposed.

Common short-term adverse effects of lithium include GI symptoms (e.g., nausea, vomiting), renal symptoms (e.g., polyuria, polydipsia), and central nervous system (CNS) symptoms (e.g., tremor, sleepiness, memory impairment). Short-term adverse effects associated with the use of lithium are generally dose-related. The incidence of toxicity increases directly with increased serum levels, and symptoms respond favorably to dose reduction. It is important to monitor a child's hydration status because lithium induces mild dehydration that, when more severe, may lead to toxic accumulation of lithium. Hence, it is prudent to consider withholding or reducing lithium doses in children who are dehydrated or who have experienced prolonged vomiting. The chronic administration of lithium may be associated with metabolic (e.g., substantial weight gain or decreased calcium metabolism), endocrine (e.g., decreased thyroid function), dermatological (e.g., acne), cardiac, and possibly renal dysfunction. Thus, it is necessary that children be screened for renal function (via blood urea nitrogen and creatinine), thyroid function (via thyroid-stimulating hormone [TSH]), cardiac function (via an ECG), and calcium levels before lithium treatment is started, and these tests should be repeated periodically (e.g., every 6 months). Females should undergo a pregnancy test and be educated about possible risks of lithium exposure during pregnancy. Caution should be exercised when lithium is used in patients with neurological, renal, or cardiovascular disorders.

Anticonvulsants. Alternative anti-manic medications for children and adolescents include the anticonvulsants. Valproic acid (VPA) is an anticonvulsant that is also FDA-approved for the acute and maintenance treatment of bipolar disorder in adults; therefore, it may be useful in the treatment of juvenile bipolar disorder. Kowatch and colleagues[42] compared the efficacy of lithium, carbamazepine, and VPA in 42 children and adolescents with bipolar disorder I or II. Using improvements in scores on the Clinicians Global Inventory (CGI) and Young-Mania Rating Scale (YMRS) (greater than 50% change from baseline), these investigators observed response rates of 38% with carbamazepine, 38% with lithium, and 53% with VPA.

VPA is primarily metabolized by the liver; it has a plasma half-life of 8 to 16 hours and a therapeutic plasma concentration of 50 to 100 mcg/ml. Recommended initial daily doses are 15 mg/kg/day, gradually increased to a maximum of 60 mg/kg/day, administered three times a day. Common short-term side effects include sedation, thinning of hair, anorexia, nausea, and vomiting. Idiosyncratic reactions, such as bone marrow suppression and liver toxicity, have been reported but appear to be rare. Asymptomatic elevations of liver enzymes usually resolve spontaneously. Although fatalities from hepatic dysfunction have been reported in children younger than 10 years old with monotherapy, these have occurred primarily in children younger than 2 years of age. The risk of serious hepatic involvement is increased by concomitant use of other anti-seizure medications and may be dose-related. Careful monitoring of blood counts and liver and renal function is warranted initially and during treatment.

Carbamazepine, approved for treatment of seizures and trigeminal neuralgia, is structurally related to the TCAs. Based on anecdotal reports, carbamazepine may be useful in some pediatric patients with mania. The plasma half-life after chronic administration of carbamazepine is between 13 and 17 hours. The therapeutic plasma concentration has been reported at 4 to 12 ng/ml, with recommended daily doses in children ranging from 10 to 20 mg/kg administered twice per day. Because the relationship between dose and plasma level is variable and uncertain with marked inter-individual variability, plasma level monitoring is recommended. Common short-term side effects include dizziness, drowsiness, nausea, vomiting, and blurred vision. Idiosyncratic reactions, such as bone marrow suppression, liver toxicity, and skin disorders (including Stevens-Johnson syndrome), have been reported but appear to be rare. However, given the seriousness of these reactions, careful monitoring of blood counts and liver and renal function is warranted initially and during treatment. Carbamazepine induces its own metabolism, which is usually complete after 3 to 5 weeks on the medication. Carbamazepine interacts with many medications, inducing the metabolism of substrates of 3A4 (e.g., haloperidol, phenytoin), and may reduce levels of valproic acid and increase lithium levels by reducing lithium clearance. Inhibitors of 3A4 (e.g., erythromycin) may also increase levels of carbamazepine.

Oxcarbazepine (Trileptal) has been used in place of carbamazepine recently because of reports of fewer medication interactions and adverse effects (e.g., less effect on bone marrow and skin), and because it does not require blood monitoring. Although trials are ongoing, minimal data are currently available on oxcarbazepine's safety, tolerability, and efficacy in pediatric bipolar disorder. Clinicians who prescribe it should monitor for hyponatremia and be aware that it can induce the metabolism of ethinyl estradiol.

Despite a paucity of data, several other anticonvulsants have been used in the treatment of pediatric bipolar disorder. Lamotrigine (Lamictal) is an anticonvulsant approved in the maintenance treatment of bipolar type I in adults. Lamotrigine's labeling contains a boxed warning that serious rashes, including Stevens-Johnson, occur in about 1% of patients younger than 16 years old. The risk for rash seems to increase if lamotrigine is increased too quickly, the initial dose is greater than recommended, or it is administered with VPA. However, benefits have been reported with VPA and lamotrigine combination therapy in pediatric bipolar disorder.[34]

Other anticonvulsants may also be useful, perhaps as adjunctive agents for specific or for residual symptoms, for juvenile bipolar disorder. Gabapentin (Neurontin) is approved as an adjunct therapy for seizures. It is not significantly metabolized in humans and has few medication interactions. Trials with gabapentin for bipolar disorder in adults have been negative; however, it has shown benefit in reducing anxiety, and so is used as an augmentation agent to diminish lability, particularly in patients who appear to over-react to stimuli or escalate rapidly because of anxiety.

Topiramate (Topamax) is an antiepileptic that has shown promise in treatment of bipolar disorder in adults. In trials with epilepsy, topiramate was associated with weight loss; however, it also can cause word-finding difficulties, oligohidrosis, and renal stones.

Antipsychotics for Juvenile Bipolar Disorder. The atypical antipsychotic medications, including risperidone (Risperdal), olanzapine (Zyprexa), quetiapine (Seroquel), ziprasidone (Geodon), and aripiprazole (Abilify), are often used as first-line agents in the management of pediatric bipolar disorder, and are now FDA-indicated for mania in pediatric patients. These medications differ from "typical" antipsychotics (e.g., chlorpromazine, haloperidol) in their receptor profile, reduced likelihood of causing EPS, reduced likelihood of causing hyperprolactinemia (except risperidone), and a greater benefit on the negative symptoms of psychosis and on cognition. Whenever these medications are used, patients and families should be informed about the potential for side effects (including EPS, akathisia, neuroleptic malignant syndrome, and tardive dyskinesia/dystonia [TD]). Although the risk of developing TD is lower with the atypical medications, youth remain at risk and should be monitored for symptoms with the Abnormal Involuntary Movement Scale (AIMS) examination regularly. In addition, weight gain, hypercholesterolemia, and the development of diabetes can occur with atypical antipsychotics, so labwork and weight should be monitored regularly.[43]

Risperidone has been useful in the treatment of pediatric mania, reducing manic and aggressive behaviors in pediatric bipolar patients. Common side effects include weight gain, sedation, drooling, and elevation of prolactin. Although pK studies in children are lacking, data in adults indicate that risperidone reaches peak concentrations within 1 hour, is metabolized through CYP 2D6, and has a half-life of 3 hours in extensive metabolizers and 17 hours in poor metabolizers. Risperidone is available orally as a tablet, a liquid, or a dissolvable tablet. Risperidone is usually initiated at 0.25 mg once or twice per day and titrated up to 3 to 4 mg/day in most pediatric patients, and it appears to retain its atypical properties in doses up to 6 mg/day.

Olanzapine is FDA-approved for acute and maintenance treatment of bipolar disorder. Open trials in children down to age 5 suggest that this agent may be effective for manic and possibly depressive symptoms as well. The primary side effects of olanzapine in pediatric patients appear to be sedation and weight gain (mean = 5 kg), and EPS have not been observed. In some patients the weight gain has outweighed clinical benefits and necessitated switching to an alternative treatment. Olanzapine is available in tablet and Zydis (melts-on-the-tongue) forms. Olanzapine is typically initiated at 2.5 to 5 mg and can be titrated up to 20 mg per day.

Quetiapine (Seroquel) has been used as an augmentation agent in the treatment of pediatric bipolar disorder. Patients receiving VPA plus quetiapine improved more than those treated with VPA alone.[44] The patients receiving VPA and quetiapine experienced greater sedation and weight gain, although the occurrence of EPS appears to be low. Data from adult studies indicate that quetiapine is readily absorbed from the GI tract and reaches peak concentrations 1.5 hours after ingestion.

The atypical antipsychotic ziprasidone (Geodon) may also be used in the treatment of pediatric bipolar disorder. Ziprasidone increases QTc intervals, so a baseline ECG and family history of cardiac problems (especially early-onset arrhythmia) should be pursued before this agent is initiated.[45] Co-administration of ziprasidone with medications that may also lengthen QTc (e.g., thioridazine, pimozide, droperidol, and class IA and III antiarrhythmics) should be avoided. In children and adolescents, ziprasidone is usually initiated at 10–20 mg per day or twice per day and can be increased upward to 40 to 60 mg twice per day.

Aripiprazole (Abilify) is an atypical agent that, particularly in lower doses, may be less likely to cause weight gain than other antipsychotics. Aripiprazole appears to have mixed agonist/antagonist properties and is described as a "dopamine/serotonin stabilizer." Aripiprazole has a long half-life and does not appear to cause significant interactions with other medications that are metabolized through the CYP-450 system, although aripiprazole can cause dizziness. It is usually started at 2.5 to 5 mg/day and titrated to 10 to 15 mg/day (up to 30 mg/day in adult trials).

AUTISM SPECTRUM DISORDER

Autism spectrum disorders (ASD) in DSM-5 has included previous DSM-IV diagnoses Asperger's syndrome, Rett disorder, childhood disintegrative disorder, and pervasive developmental disorder not otherwise specified under the one category of "autism." The diagnosis of an ASD implies that an affected individual will experience significant difficulty in reciprocal social interactions and communication, and exhibit repetitive or non-functional stereotyped behaviors or preoccupations. These core symptoms are now to be rated on severity (with additional specifiers of intellectual impairment, language impairment, known genetic or environmental factors and/or catatonia). Affected individuals avoid eye contact, do not develop normal social relationships appropriate for their age, do not seem to show interest in others' thoughts or feelings, and have difficulty understanding or seeing the world from the perspective of others. They may have routines that cannot be disrupted without conflict (e.g., lining up toys in a certain way), and may exhibit unusual motor behaviors (such as hand flapping, body twisting, or even head-banging).

With growing awareness, and certainly with a broader diagnostic net, the number of persons identified with ASDs has increased markedly over the past 20 years, from approximately 1 of every 4,000 to more recent epidemiological estimates of 1% of the population.[46]

No medical test is currently available for accurate detection of autism. Medical conditions that may explain ASD symptoms are found in less than 5% of cases. Rather, the diagnosis is based on the history and presence of clinical symptoms. Screening surveys, such as the Checklist for Autism in Toddlers (ChAT) are encouraged among primary care physicians working with pediatric populations to improve early identification of children with PDD. In research settings, more structured interviews are used, both to identify parent/guardian observations of the child's daily behaviors and symptoms apparent to the examiner when the patient is presented with a series of cognitive, social, and emotional tasks. These latter interviews often require several hours to administer and may still fall short of a precise diagnosis for some individuals. The etiology of ASDs remains elusive, but the variety of genetic factors that have been linked to autism support the conclusion that ASDs are heterogeneous and multi-factorial in origin. There have yet to be findings that successfully coalesced to provide a specific neurological or biochemical explanation for any of the ASD phenotypes, or to yield specific targets for existing pharmacotherapies. Moreover, the multiplicity of neurobiological findings associated with ASDs continues to suggest non-specific but perhaps common pathway phenomena (such as problems with connectivity or cerebral organization).[47]

Treatment of Autism Spectrum

Psychosocial Treatments for Autism Spectrum Disorder

While traditional psychotherapy techniques may not be appropriate for many children with ASD, psychosocial interventions remain important in the treatment of ASD. Diagnosis usually triggers additional evaluations, often through the child's school or early intervention services. Speech therapy is often very important, even in children who appear verbal, since their "pragmatic" skills for using language often lag. For children who do not speak, alternative communication approaches are initiated, usually relying on pictures the child can point to so as to signify interests or wishes. In addition, "social stories" are often constructed to prepare the child for novel experiences (such as riding on an airplane), or deviations from routines (e.g., responding to fire drills).[48]

Many children with ASDs are exquisitely sensitive to stimuli (such as touch, taste, sound, or vestibular activity). "Sensory integration" and "tactile defensiveness" are expressions often used to describe the child's difficulties responding to stimuli, usually tolerable to children of similar ages. Occupational therapy is often helpful for identifying sensory exercises or alternatives (sometimes called a "sensory diet" or "hierarchy of sensory activities" to calm or prepare the child to be ready to learn, such as swinging, sitting on special cushions, using tennis balls on chair legs, or placing partitions around the child's workspace) that a child can access when under-stimulated or over-stimulated, as well as developing motor skills in children with PDD.

The impact of ASDs varies widely, with some children having severe deficits that require substantial, if not constant, adult supervision. Clarification of the support network available to the particular child through extended family, as well as other family needs regarding other children, must be examined. Sometimes the child's network is sufficient to monitor and support the child's development, but consideration of respite needs remains important. Given elevated rates of stress and divorce in families with a child having an ASD, parent responsibilities and approaches often require ongoing attention as the child grows older, larger, and stronger.

Schools increasingly use programs that systematically evaluate a child's behavior and identify interventions tailored to each child. This systematic approach to developing a program for each child is often called *applied behavioral analysis* (ABA). The first step of ABA is to identify that the child's skill needs and strengths are identified. The next step is determining appropriate educational and treatment goals for the child. Each big-picture goal is broken down into the many individual skills needed to achieve the goal. These individual skills are then scaffolded in a step-wise manner, to facilitate successful skill-building for the child across many areas of the child's function (such as skills in academics, communication, imaginative play, social activities, and motor abilities). Programs that use ABA principles employ a variety of techniques to help children develop new skills. One technique frequently used is called *discrete trial training* (DTT). In a discrete trial, the teacher or clinician gives the child an instruction (e.g., "point to the green circle"). The adult may give the child a prompt to help the child with the task (the adult points to the green circle). If the child does not give the correct response, the adult may give the child another chance, again with prompts to assist the child. When the child provides the correct answer, the child is given a small reward, also known as a *positive reinforcement*, along with praise (as an example, the adult gives her a star

sticker and says "Great job"). Additional behavior analysis techniques are emerging, particularly those that work with behaviors already enacted by the child, so that "chains" of more complex behaviors can be "assembled" (putting on and tying shoes, cleaning up after eating, doing a real-world math problem).[49]

Pharmacotherapy of Autism Spectrum Disorder

Pharmacotherapy of patients with ASD has focused on detection of the primary emotional and behavioral target symptoms, and matching these targets with medications most likely to be helpful. Atypical neuroleptic medications appear to improve target symptoms of aggression, irritability, and hyperactivity in patients with developmental disorders. Risperidone has been approved by the FDA for treatment of aggression and irritability associated with ASD in children. Common side effects in risperidone trials of children with PDD included somnolence, headache, and weight gain (mean = 2.2 kg). Significantly more patients (69%; 34 of 49) randomized to risperidone (dose range 0.5 to 3.5 mg/day) experienced meaningful reductions in irritability compared with patients treated with placebo (12%; 6/52; P < 0.001).[50] Aripiprazole has been FDA-approved for treating irritability in children with ASD. Side effects are similar, with sedation and weight gain being problematic. Open trials with a variety of atypical antipsychotics, including olanzapine and ziprasidone, have similarly shown promise in decreasing maladaptive behaviors in patients with developmental delay.[51]

A number of alternative pharmacological agents, in addition to antipsychotics, are being employed for complications or co-morbidities of developmental disorders. Considering the relatively low toxicological profile of these drugs compared with the antipsychotics, they may be preferred in the management of these children. Beta-blockers (e.g., propranolol) may improve modulation in patients with developmental disorder, and thus reduce agitation, aggression, and self-abusive behaviors. Treatment is typically initiated at 10 mg twice per day and increased as clinically indicated. The dose range is 2 to 8 mg/kg/day. Propranolol's capacity to induce beta-adrenergic blockade can cause bradycardia, hypotension, and an increase in airway resistance. Thus, it is contraindicated in asthmatic and certain cardiac patients. In a similar manner clonidine, lofexidine, and buspirone have been used to diminish aggression in patients with developmental disorders.

For children with prominent obsessive behavior, rigidity, or compulsive rituals, recent studies indicate that the SSRIs may be helpful. Often, the full antidepressant dosage is necessary; however, children should be started with the lowest possible dose to avoid adverse effects: for example, disinhibition or agitation. Controlled trials of the SSRI antidepressants (fluoxetine and fluvoxamine) in adults with PDD have shown positive results. However, studies in children have been less robust. The long-acting benzodiazepines may also be useful as single or adjunct agents in children with prominent anxiety symptoms (e.g., difficulty when eating); however, a major adverse effect, disinhibition, may result in increased restlessness and more disturbed behavior. Antidepressant drugs and mood stabilizers may be effective in controlling affective disorders, and stimulants may improve symptoms of ADHD when these disorders co-exist.

PSYCHOTIC DISORDERS

The term *psychosis* is generally used to describe the abnormal behaviors of children with grossly impaired reality testing. The diagnosis of psychosis requires the presence of delusions, false implausible beliefs, or hallucinations or false perceptions that may be visual, auditory, or tactile. Childhood-onset schizophrenia (COS) is rare, occurring in less than 1 in 10,000 children, and less than 1% of patients with schizophrenia are diagnosed in childhood. More often, childhood psychosis is seen in pediatric patients having major depression, bipolar disorder, or severe dissociative states, such as PTSD.[52] In a recent review of COS and childhood-onset schizoaffective disorder, 99% of patients were found to have at least one co-morbid diagnosis: 84% had ADHD, 43% had ODD, 30% had depression, and 25% had separation anxiety disorder.[53] PDD, ADHD, and speech and language disorders usually have their onset before schizophrenia emerges.

Psychotic disorders in children, as in adults, can be functional or organic. Functional psychotic syndromes include schizophrenia and related disorders and the psychotic forms of mood disorders. Organic psychosis can develop secondary to CNS lesions as a consequence of medical illness, trauma, or drug use. Children may manifest psychosis for a substantial amount of time without indicating its presence to parents or caregivers. Hence, all children with major mood disorders, or those who have manifest abnormal or bizarre behaviors, should be queried for the presence of psychosis.

Children who develop schizophrenia commonly show aberrant social and cognitive development from very early stages and before the onset of psychosis. Precursors of COS include high rates of soft neurological signs, significant delays in language and motor development, and social withdrawal.

The co-morbidity and overlap between PDD and COS sometimes make these two disorders difficult to distinguish. In children with COS, up to one-third may have pervasive developmental symptomatology and perhaps 60% meet criteria for a speech and/or language disorder. Children with PDD may have more idiosyncratic peculiar thoughts, poorly formulated, and these may shift or evolve over time. Like children with COS, those with PDD may also have odd beliefs: for example, that they are able to communicate with valued inanimate toys. Phobic hallucinations usually occur in a context of anxiety, such as a child "seeing" a frightening face in the window when it is dark, and do not plague the child during the day when the anxiety is muted.

Outcome studies ranging from several years to up to 42 years after diagnosis of COS indicate that the long-term function of patients with COS is poor compared to adolescent- or adult-onset groups of schizophrenics.[54] In general, the earlier the onset of COS, the poorer the prognosis. Variables indicative of better prognoses among children with COS are higher premorbid intelligence, more positive than negative symptoms of schizophrenia, and cooperation of family in treatment.

Treatment of Childhood-onset Schizophrenia

Psychosocial Treatments for Childhood-onset Schizophrenia

Psychosocial interventions usually involve optimizing the environment to minimize stressing the patient (this increases vulnerability to psychotic episodes) and to match the level of stimulation with the patient's level of arousal. Efforts to identify precipitants surrounding episodes or deterioration can be useful in determining appropriate home and classroom expectations. Parents and other caregivers can be helpful in identifying the patient's progression toward psychosis, which may provide specific topics to "check in" with the patient about to monitor the patient's reality testing. In addition, specific strategies for addressing both positive and negative symptoms may be useful. For negative symptoms, regular interactions with others, sometimes through familiar, simple activities (such as eating lunch or listening to music), may diminish isolation. For positive symptoms, anchoring activities with others or as regular parts of the patient's daily routine may be useful. When patients with COS are more agitated, distressed, or unsure of what is and is not "real," simplifying the environment, decreasing expectations, and diminishing stimulation are needed.

Cognitive-behavioral techniques to evaluate evidence or to think through explanations surrounding patient perceptions can be helpful to alter dysfunctional behaviors. A consistent framework with similar words/techniques used at home, at school, and with friends may allow the patient to employ a regular approach to events across settings, diminishing misperceptions of daily life events and interactions.

Pharmacotherapy of Childhood-onset Schizophrenia

Available studies, as well as anecdotal clinical experience, suggest that response to antipsychotics in children with COS is less robust than in adolescents or adults with schizophrenia. Current pharmacological research for COS is focused on identifying antipsychotic agents that provide optimal efficacy without significant adverse events. Atypical antipsychotics including risperidone, olanzapine, and clozapine have all been shown in randomized clinical trials and open trials to have efficacy in the treatment of COS; however, significant side effects including weight gain, EPS, and metabolic abnormalities have occurred.[55] Clozapine has been shown to have greater efficacy than typical antipsychotic agents, such as haloperidol. Significant side effects included EPS, somnolence, weight gain, depression, and symptoms associated with hyperprolactinemia. Positive symptoms appear more responsive to antipsychotic treatment, and negative symptoms may show improvement sometimes up to a year later.[56]

Clozapine's superiority has been shown in two randomized clinical trials compared to typical and atypical antipsychotics for COS. Unfortunately, during the course of these trials clozapine was associated with serious adverse events (such as tachycardia, hypertension, cardiac and lipid abnormalities, agranulocytosis, seizure, and nocturnal enuresis).[57,58]

Pharmacological treatment for COS remains an area of active research with two large ongoing multi-site trials. First, the Early Onset Schizophrenia Study (EOSS)[59] has investigated newer atypical antipsychotic agents, and preliminary open-label data suggest that ziprasidone was beneficial in approximately 13 of 40 COS patients after 12 weeks of treatment, at a mean final dose of 118 mg/day. In this study over 1 year, 50% of patients gained weight but no significant ECG changes occurred, suggesting that ziprasidone may be useful in the treatment of COS. Second, another ongoing trial within this network (TEOSS) is comparing molindone, risperidone, and olanzapine in a double-blind trial of patients with COS.

Currently, the atypical antipsychotics (e.g., risperidone, olanzapine, quetiapine, ziprasidone, aripiprazole) are first-line agents in the pharmacotherapy of psychosis in children and adolescents. Typically, these medications are initiated at a low dose and gradually titrated up to achieve efficacy. Risperidone is started at 0.25 mg twice a day and can be increased every day or two with close observation. In patients treated over the long term with risperidone, clinicians should monitor weight, vital signs, and laboratory results (e.g., triglycerides, cholesterol, prolactin). Olanzapine and quetiapine are generally more sedating and are usually initiated at 2.5 to 5 mg/day and 25 to 50 mg/day, respectively.

If trials with two or three atypical antipsychotics are ineffective, a trial with a typical agent (e.g., chlorpromazine or haloperidol) should be considered. The usual oral dosage of antipsychotics ranges between 3 and 6 mg/kg/day for the low-potency phenothiazines (e.g., chlorpromazine) and between 0.1 and 0.5 (up to 1) mg/kg/day for the high-potency antipsychotics (e.g., haloperidol). Antipsychotic medications have a relatively long half-life, and therefore they need not be administered more than twice daily.

Common short-term adverse effects of antipsychotics are drowsiness, increased appetite, and weight gain. Anticholinergic effects (such as dry mouth, nasal congestion, and blurred vision) are more commonly seen with the low-potency phenothiazines. Short-term adverse effects of antipsychotics are generally managed with adjustments of dose and timing of administration. Excessive sedation can be avoided by using less sedating agents and by prescribing most of the daily dose at night-time. Drowsiness should not be confused with impaired cognition; it can usually be corrected by adjusting the dose and the timing of administration. In fact, there is no evidence that antipsychotics adversely affect cognition when used in low doses. Anticholinergic adverse effects can be minimized by choosing a medium- or high-potency compound.

EPS, such as acute dystonia, akathisia (motor restlessness), and parkinsonism (bradykinesia, tremor, and lack of facial expressions), are more commonly seen with the high-potency compounds (butyrophenones and thioxanthenes) and have been reported in up to 75% of children receiving these agents. The extent to which antiparkinsonian agents (e.g., anticholinergic drugs, benztropine, trihexyphenidyl, antihistamines, and the antiviral agent amantadine) should be used prophylactically when antipsychotics are introduced is controversial. Whenever possible, antiparkinsonian agents should be used only when EPS emerge. Akathisia may be particularly problematic in young patients because of under-recognition. When a child or an adolescent starts on an antipsychotic and becomes acutely agitated with an associated inability to sit still and with aggressive outbursts, the possibility of akathisia should be considered. If suspected, the dose of the antipsychotic may need to be lowered. The centrally-acting beta-adrenergic antagonist propranolol often is very helpful in treating this adverse effect.

A benign withdrawal dyskinesia and a syndrome of deteriorating behavior have been associated with the abrupt cessation of these drugs. As in adults, the long-term administration of antipsychotic drugs may be associated with TD. Although children appear to be generally less vulnerable than adults to developing TD, there is an emerging consensus that this potentially worrisome adverse effect may affect children and adolescents in 10% to 15% of cases. Prevention (appropriate use for a clear indication, clear target symptoms, periodic drug discontinuation to assess the need for drug use) and early detection (with regular monitoring) are the only effective treatments for TD.

Akathisia is a movement disorder associated with anxiety and an inability to sit still. In children and adolescents it is most often seen as a side effect of either antipsychotics or antidepressants. Akathisia may be confused with ADHD or agitation. Treatment of akathisia involves reducing the dose of the precipitating medication to the lowest effective dose and then either using benzodiazepines (0.5 to 1 mg three times per day of lorazepam) or beta-blockers. Although all beta-blockers are likely to be effective, propranolol is typically used. Propranolol should be initiated at 10 mg two times per day and the dose increased every several days to good effect.

Little is known about the potentially lethal neuroleptic malignant syndrome (NMS) in juveniles; however, preliminary evidence indicates that its presentation is similar to that in adults. This syndrome may be difficult to distinguish from primary CNS pathology, concurrent infection, or other, more benign, side effects of antipsychotic treatment, including EPS or anticholinergic toxicity. Treatment is similar to those strategies used in adults.

In patients who do not respond to trials with either first-line atypical or typical antipsychotics or who experience significant dyskinesia from these medications, consideration should be given to a trial with clozapine (Clozaril).[60] In the US and Europe, there has been a considerable experience with clozapine in adolescents. Established dose parameters are not yet available; however, in one open study of clozapine for schizophrenic youths, doses from 125 to 825 mg/day (mean = 375 mg/day) for up to 6 weeks were necessary for efficacy. Although remarkably effective in chronic treatment-resistant schizophrenia and affective psychosis, there is a dose-related risk of seizures and an increased risk of leukopenia and agranulocytosis in adolescents that is similar to the risk in adults; it requires close monitoring.

Access the complete reference list and multiple choice questions (MCQs) online at https://expertconsult.inkling.com

KEY REFERENCES

2. American Psychiatric Association. *Diagnostic and statistical manual of mental disorders*, ed 5, Washington, DC, 2013, American Psychiatric Association.
3. Connolly SD, Bernstein GA. Work Group on Quality Issues. Practice parameter for the assessment and treatment of children and adolescents with anxiety disorders. *J Am Acad Child Adolesc Psychiatry* 46:267–283, 2007.
5. Pediatric OCD Treatment (POTS) Study Team. Cognitive behavior therapy, sertraline and their combination for children and adolescent with obsessive-compulsive disorder. *JAMA* 292(16):1969–1976, 2004.
6. Franklin ME, Sapyta JS, Freeman JB, et al. Cognitive behavior therapy augmentation of pharmacotherapy in pediatric obsessive-compulsive disorder: the Pediatric OCD Treatment Study II (POTS II) randomized controlled trial. *JAMA* 306(11):1224–1232, 2011.
20. Jensen PS, Garcia JA, Glied S, et al. Cost-effectiveness of ADHD treatments: findings from the multimodal treatment study of children with ADHD. *Am J Psychiatry* 162:1628–1636, 2005.
21. Zuvekas SH, Vitiello B. Stimulant medication use in children: A 12-year perspective. *Am J Psychiatry* 169(2):160–166, 2012.
24. Cooper WO, Habel LA, Sox CM, et al. ADHD drugs and serious cardiovascular events in children and young adults. *N Engl J Med* 365(20):1896–1904, 2011.
25. MTA Cooperative Group. National Institute of Mental Health Multimodal Treatment Study of ADHD follow-up: changes in effectiveness and growth after the end of treatment. *Pediatrics* 113:762–769, 2004.
27. Steiner H, Remsing L. Work Group on Quality Issues. Practice parameter for the assessment and treatment of children and adolescents with oppositional defiant disorder. *J Am Acad Child Adolesc Psychiatry* 46:126–141, 2007.
33. March J, Silva S, Petrycki S, et al. Treatment for Adolescents with Depression Study (TADS) team. Fluoxetine, cognitive-behavioral therapy, and their combination for adolescents with depression: Treatment for Adolescents with Depression Study (TADS) randomized controlled trial. *JAMA* 292(7):807–820, 2004.
35. Bridge JA, Iyengar SI, Salary CB, et al. Clinical response and risk for reported suicidal ideation and suicide attempts in pediatric antidepressant treatment. *JAMA* 297(15):1683–1696, 2007.
41. Liu HY, Potter MP, Woodworth KY, et al. Pharmacologic treatments for pediatric bipolar disorder: A review and meta-analysis. *J Am Acad Child Adolesc Psychiatry* 50:749–762, 2011.
43. Findling RL, Drury SS, Jensen PS, et al. Practice parameters for the use of atypical medications in children and adolescents. *J Am Acad Child Adolesc Psychiatry* 49, 2011.
45. Correll CU, Manu P, Olshanskiy V, et al. Cardiometabolic risk of second-generation antipsychotic medications during first-time use in children and adolescents. *JAMA* 302(16):1765–1773, 2009.
55. Maloney AE, Yakutis LJ, Frazier JA. Empirical evidence for psychopharmacologic treatment in early-onset psychosis and schizophrenia. *Child Adolesc Psychiatric Clin N Am* 21:885–909, 2012.

70 Psychiatric and Substance Use Disorders in Transitioning Adolescents and Young Adults

Timothy E. Wilens, MD, Courtney Zulauf, BA, and Jerrold F. Rosenbaum, MD

KEY POINTS

Background

- The term transitioning adolescents and young adults (TAY) (aged 16–26 years) has been coined to categorize this development stage, which has received increased attention. Parents of TAY sustain high burdens of care, particularly for those with common unmet needs. While psychopathology and substance abuse are the leading causes of disability worldwide, they constitute 45% of the disease burden in this age range.

History

- Brain development continues into the TAY years. Psychopathology may emerge during TAY years, or may develop in childhood and persist into the TAY years.

Clinical and Research Challenges

- A disconnect in the system of care for TAY often exists. Child psychiatrists are increasingly asked to evaluate or to provide care for youth as they enter independent living settings (such as college) and adult psychiatrists are increasingly called upon to evaluate and treat TAY for psychopathology and substance abuse.

Practical Pointers

- TAY is a critical period when individuals frequently experience mental health and substance problems and manifest substantial functional impairment. Expertise in developmental psychopathology, family dynamics, and systems of care help direct and oversee the clinical care of TAY using innovative programming. Addressing cognitive, emotional, behavioral, and substance-related dysfunction in TAY necessitates a thorough evaluation and multimodal strategies for the individual and their family. The application of existing and novel therapies coupled with new treatment paradigms may enhance patient engagement and lead to better long-term outcomes.

OVERVIEW

The period of transition from childhood to adulthood known as transitioning adolescents and young adults (TAY; age 16–26 years) has received increased attention. TAY are navigating the potentially perilous developmental years while leaving childhood and entering adulthood, where more adult-like challenges are faced without having mastered much-needed tools and cognitive abilities. A number of critical developmental steps occur during this transition that reflect changing neurobiology, the tasks of separation and individuation, and the

influences of pre-existing and concurrent mental health and substance use issues. Parents with TAY sustain high burdens of care, particularly for those with common unmet needs.[1] In fact, psychopathology and substance abuse are the leading cause of disability worldwide and they constitute 45% of the disease burden in TAY.[2] A disconnect in the system of care for TAY often exists. Child psychiatrists are increasingly asked to evaluate or provide care for youth as they enter independent living settings (such as college) and adult psychiatrists are increasingly called upon to evaluate and treat adolescents and young adults for psychopathology and substance abuse. Thus, psychiatric practitioners must be prepared to address the major concerns and opportunities surrounding TAY: specifically, early recognition of the signs and symptoms, identification of risk and protective factors, and timely and effective interventions for psychopathology and substance abuse.

SALIENT NEUROBIOLOGY OF TRANSITIONING ADOLESCENTS AND YOUNG ADULTS

Brain development continues throughout adolescence and young adulthood. Developmental neurobiology offers insights into limitations in decision-making, impulsivity, risk-taking, and emotional regulation that may be related to the developing brain[3] and into behaviors manifested in TAY. Casey and colleagues[4] and Giedd and associates[3] highlighted that the limbic areas develop early in adolescence and govern reward-based drives. In contrast, areas of the frontal lobes that are related to processing, inhibiting, decision-making, and shifting continue to develop for several more years—often into TAY years.[5] The incongruity between the maturation of the limbic (emotional, reward) and executive operations (frontal, inhibition) may underpin a heightened risk for excess emotionality, reward-seeking, and poor judgment.[4] These observations may explain why TAY are particularly susceptible to the manifestation of psychopathology and substance use disorders (SUD).

Central to addiction, disruption in the normal circuitry in the reward and inhibition pathways of the brain appears operant. Disruption in signaling between the executive centers (frontal lobes, inhibition-based) and emotional/motivation centers (hippocampal formation, amygdala; reward-based) is seen with addiction, and may even pre-date some of the changes associated with addiction.[3,4,6] For instance, disruption in frontal activity dampens inhibitions, as well as a number of executive functions (planning, organization, motivation) that are critical to the functioning of TAY. Likewise, the limbic regions (the hippocampus, amygdala, and others) that develop relatively early in TAY lives are involved in reward, emotion, and risk-taking.[3] It may be that many of these regions related to addiction are affected by, or have a delay in maturation associated with specific psychiatric disorders (e.g., ADHD or bipolar disorder) known to predispose to later SUD. For instance, the lack of inhibition of limbic or emotional regions may result in disinhibited behavior, excess reward-seeking (substance use, unprotected sex), and other high-risk behaviors that may culminate in other addictive behaviors.

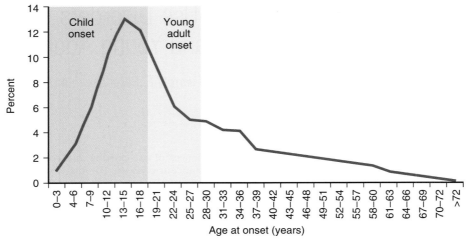

Figure 70-1. Persistent childhood-onset cases plus the new onsets of psychopathology in young adulthood encompasses the myriad of psychopathology necessitating evaluation and treatment in TAY (TAY refers to transitional aged youth). This Figure is an amalgam of the age of the onset of the following disorders: alcohol and drug use, anorexia/bulimia, anxiety, bipolar disorder, depression, obsessive-compulsive, panic, and psychosis/schizophrenia.

BOX 70-1 Common Psychiatric Disorders that Begin in Childhood or Young Adulthood

Anxiety-related disorders:
- Obsessive-compulsive disorder
- Phobias
- Generalized anxiety disorder
- Post-traumatic stress disorder

Attention-deficit/hyperactivity disorder

Autism spectrum disorders

Disruptive disorders:
- Conduct
- Oppositional defiant

Eating disorders
- Anorexia nervosa
- Bulimia nervosa
- Mixed eating disorders

Mood disorders:
- Major depression
- Bipolar disorder

Psychotic disorders:
- First-episode psychosis
- Schizophrenia

Substance use disorders:
- Drug and alcohol abuse/dependence
- Nicotine use

EPIDEMIOLOGY

Psychopathology may emerge in TAY or may be present in childhood and persist (Figure 70-1). Accumulating data suggest that a combination of the two explains the high prevalence rates of psychopathology and SUD in TAY (Box 70-1). For instance, one of the most studied childhood disorders, attention-deficit/hyperactivity disorder (ADHD), which begins in early childhood, affects 6%–9% of youth.[8,9] Childhood ADHD persists into adolescence in 75% of cases and into adulthood in approximately one-half of cases (for review see Wilens and Spencer[9]). Many of the manifestations of ADHD occur in TAY and include academic, occupational, and interpersonal dysfunction[10]—critical areas for TAY who are beginning to live independently and start working and/or attending college. Unfortunately, insufficient attention to this age range is associated with low rates of adherence to treatment, with subsequent return of ADHD symptoms, with functional impairment, and with emergence of complications/co-morbidities of the disorder (e.g., academic failure, cigarette smoking).

Anxiety and post-traumatic stress disorder (PTSD) are recognized as having their onset in childhood and young adulthood with persistence into adulthood.[11] Using data from the National Comorbidity Survey Replication that surveyed 9,282 respondents, Kessler and co-workers[12] found that the median age of onset for anxiety disorders was 11 years of age. A more recent survey, conducted by Vaingankar and associates[13] reported on 6,616 respondents and noted that the mean age of onset for generalized anxiety disorder was 20 years of age. Giaconia and colleagues[14] found that in a community sample of adolescents, 6.3% met criteria for PTSD. Furthermore, the peak period of risk for developing PTSD was 16–17 years, with almost one-third of the sample developing the disorder by age 14 years.[14] Several studies have found that early-onset anxiety disorders are associated with a greater severity and chronicity compared to adult-onset disorders.[15] Moreover, persistent childhood-onset anxiety in TAY appears to increase the likelihood for the development of subsequent psychiatric co-morbidity[16,17] and greater familial loading.[18,19]

Age of onset of obsessive-compulsive disorder (OCD) has revealed differences in the neurobiology and genetics of the disorder.[20] For example, early age of onset is associated with higher rates of co-morbid tic disorders[21] and a higher frequency of tic-like compulsions.[22] The average age of onset for OCD is in the TAY years. For example, based on a national mental health survey, Vaingankar and associates[13] found that the median age of onset for OCD was 19 years of age. Similarly, Millet and colleagues[23] collected data from 617 patients with OCD and found that the majority had their onset between the ages of 11 to 25 years. Furthermore, they found that the number of obsessions and compulsions was significantly greater in the group with an earlier age of onset (P<0.001).[23] Likewise, Delorme and co-workers[24] studied 161 patients with OCD and divided them among early-onset and late-onset OCD. The majority (88%) of their sample fell into the early-onset OCD group, mean age of onset of 11 years (SD = ± 4 years), which was correlated with a higher frequency of Tourette's syndrome and an increased family history of OCD.[24]

Mood disorders, such as dysthymia and major depressive disorder (MDD), are common and highly disabling in TAY.[11] In the National Comorbidity Survey, Kessler and colleagues[25] found that the lifetime prevalence of minor depression in 15–18 year olds was 11% and that of MDD was 14%. Zisook and colleagues[26] reported that over half of all cases of depression had their onset during childhood or TAY years. Consistent with the work of Zisook and colleagues,[26] others have shown an elevated risk for mood disorders that begins in the early teens and rises in a linear fashion throughout the TAY years, with rates of up to 25% by late adolescence.[14,27] Longitudinally-derived data indicate that having a mood disorder or prominent mood dysregulation in childhood increases the likelihood for a mood disorder in adolescence and adulthood.[26] It is not surprising then that the rates of depression reported during the TAY years approximates those in adult samples, suggesting that the peak onset of the disorders are during the TAY years.[12,28]

Mood disorders developing in TAY predict a wide variety of negative outcomes in adulthood, including unemployment, serious social and educational impairment,[29] and obesity.[30] Furthermore, early-onset mood disorders are linked with other mental health problems in adults, such as anxiety disorders and SUDs.[31,32] Of greater concern, depression in TAY is a major risk factor for suicide, a leading cause of death for this age range, with more than half of adolescent suicide victims, for instance, reporting depressive symptoms at the time of death.[33]

Despite an early belief in the absence of cyclical mood disorder during childhood, the manic behavior, poor judgment, and severe mood dysregulation of bipolar disorder can also begin in youth and worsen during TAY years.[11] Juvenile bipolar disorder affects between 1% to 4% of the pediatric population,[8,34] with up to one-fifth of psychiatrically-referred children and adolescent outpatients manifesting bipolar disorder.[35,36] Furthermore, pediatric-onset bipolar disorder is highly co-morbid with SUD, with internalizing and externalizing psychopathology, and is remarkably stable over time.[37–40]

An emerging literature has shown that the majority of adults with bipolar disorder develop their disorder in childhood and the TAY years, and at least one-third of adults with bipolar disorder have the onset of the disorder before the age of 12 years.[41] For example, Perlis and associates[42] reported on 1,469 subjects from a large multicenter systematic treatment enhancement program for bipolar disorder (STEP-BD) and found that the mean age of onset of bipolar disorder was 16.7 years. Not only are early or TAY-onset cases common but also data suggest they are more complicated in their adult form.[43,44] For example, adults with earlier-onset bipolar disorder have been reported to be at higher risk for other neuropsychiatric disorders, for more psychiatric and SUD co-morbidity, for less lithium responsiveness, and for more mixed presentations.[43]

Eating disorders are recognized as among the most complex and disabling of psychiatric disorders. Research indicates that the heterogeneous group of eating disorders (including bulimia, anorexia, binge eating) often emerge during early adolescence and show a rapid increase in incidence during the transitional years.[45] For instance, Hudson and co-workers[45] in the National Comorbidity Survey Replication (n = 2,980) reported a steep increase in the cumulative prevalence of eating disorders during the TAY years. From a prospective analysis of 8594 women, Field and colleagues[46] found that the prevalence of eating disorders increased substantially with age until early adulthood, with up to 22% of the sample manifesting an eating disorder at one point. Furthermore,

Stice and associates[47] examined the peak periods for onset of the various eating disorders. They found that peak periods for onset were between 17 and 18 years for bulimia nervosa and binge-eating disorder, and between 18 and 20 years for purging disorder. Given the prevalence and chronicity of eating disorders in TAY, these data support the importance of identifying and understanding the diagnosis and treatment of these disorders close to their onset.

Schizophrenia is recognized as one of the most debilitating psychiatric disorders, with some studies suggesting that early-onset schizophrenia (i.e., onset before age 18 years) may represent a more severe variant of the disorder,[48–51] with studies reporting lower psychosocial functioning and worse long-term outcomes.[49,52,53]

Early-onset schizophrenia has its beginning in the TAY years. In an older Swedish family study of 270 schizophrenic probands, Sham and associates[54] found that for both men and women there was a rapid increase in the onset of schizophrenia in the late teens and early twenties followed by a rapid decline in the late twenties. Similar results were found by Hafner and co-workers[55] who studied 267 schizophrenic patients and found that the onset of the disorder showed an early and steep increase in adolescents until the age of 25 years, with 47% of women and 62% of men having their first symptoms of schizophrenia before the age of 25 years.

Early identification and intervention of at-risk samples may result in a reduction of the ultimate expression of the disorder. For instance, one recent study focused on use of omega-3 as a way to prevent early psychosis in at-risk populations. A randomized, double-blind, placebo-controlled trial conducted by Amminger and associates[56] assessed 81 individuals at ultra-high risk of a psychotic disorder. Of these, 41 received 1.2 g/day of omega-3 for 12 weeks while 40 controls received placebo followed by a 40-week monitoring period. By the end of the study 2 of the 41 individuals (4.9%) in the omega-3 group and 11 of the 40 (27.5%) in the placebo group developed a psychotic disorder (P = 0.007). Omega-3 improved overall functioning compared to placebo and also reduced positive symptoms (P = 0.01), negative symptoms (P = 0.02), and general symptoms (P = 0.01).[56]

Autism spectrum disorder (ASD) consists of a group of related complex and chronic neurodevelopment disorders: autistic disorder, Asperger disorder, and pervasive developmental disorder not otherwise specified, that are generally characterized by a variable presentation of problems with socialization, communication, and behavior.[57] Symptoms of ASD can be identified in children as young as 18 months,[58] with screening recommended to begin at 24 months for all children.[59] In years past, the overall prevalence of autism was reported at 2–4 per 10,000 children[60]; however, more recent studies have indicated that 1%–2% of children and adolescents meet criteria for ASD.[61–63] Data derived from the National Survey of Children's Health (NSCH), conducted by the Centers for Disease Control and Preventions National Center for Health Statistics, found that the prevalence of ASD among children aged 6–17 increased from 1.2% in 2007 to 2.0% in 2011–2012.[63]

ASDs are typically considered a childhood diagnosis; however, most have significant functional impairment throughout their TAY and later adult years. Numerous studies have shown that ASDs are persistent, indicating that although the severity of autism may decline during the adult period, social functioning is worse than in younger adulthood.[64–67] Furthermore, the majority of the observed increase in prevalence appears to be accounted for by adolescent boys ages 14–17.[63]

Limited research on TAY with autism exists. Longitudinally, derived data in individuals with ASDs, followed from (mean) age 7 to 29 years having IQs > 50, indicated a range of outcomes: 12% were rated as "Very Good" outcome; 10% were rated as "Good" and 19% as "Fair outcome".[67] The majority was rated as having a "Poor" (46%) or "Very Poor" (12%) outcome that often required extensive family involvement and/or hospital level of care. The majority of individuals remained dependent on their families or other supports. Few had permanent jobs, lived alone, or had close friends. Stereotyped behaviors or interests frequently persisted into adulthood and their communication was generally impaired. Those with an IQ > 70 had a significantly better outcome than those with an IQ < 70.[67]

The impairments associated with ASDs in children and adolescents may be accentuated by the high rate of co-morbidity. Simonoff and co-workers[68] examined 112 children and adolescents with ASD (mean age of 11.5 years) and found that 70% had at least one co-morbid disorder and 41% had two or more. De Bruin and colleagues[69] studied 92 children with ASD (age 6–12 years) and found that 81% presented with at least one co-morbid psychiatric disorder. The children with co-morbidity showed more deficits in social communication than those with only ASD.[69]

The TAY years seem to represent a previously unrecognized but critical window for improving skills for those with ASD. Taylor and Seltzer[70] studied 242 youths who were about to exit the school system; they found that there was an overall improvement of autism symptoms and of internalizing behavior throughout the study but that the improvement slowed after they left school. Furthermore, work by Smith and associates[71] in a sample of 397 individuals with ASD showed changes in daily living skills, with skills improving during adolescence and the early 20s, peaking around the late 20s, and declining in the early 30s.[71] Due to the increased rates, early onset, lifetime persistence, and high levels of associated impairment, ASDs are currently recognized as one of the major public health issues affecting TAY.

SUBSTANCE ABUSE IN TRANSITIONING ADOLESCENTS AND YOUNG ADULTS

Substance use disorders (SUD), including drug and alcohol abuse or dependence, are now conceptualized as having their developmental roots in childhood (with the vast majority beginning during adolescence or young adulthood)[8,72–75] In support of this notion, recent epidemiological data report that 20% of youths experiment with substances before completing the 8th grade, and over 20% of high school seniors have used illicit drugs or have been drunk in the past month,[76] with other data indicating that 1-in-10 adolescents have an SUD.[8] Compton and co-workers[75] showed that in those with a drug use disorder, over half had the onset of the disorder before their 18th birthday, with roughly 80% having an onset prior to age 25. Early-onset SUD is associated with significant morbidity in multiple realms of functioning.

As with other disorders (such as depression, bipolar disorder, ADHD, or conduct disorder), the ability of TAY to manage their own emotions may be an important factor within the context of youth with SUD.[77,78] Not surprisingly, as comprehensively reviewed by Cheetham and colleagues,[78] deficits in self-monitoring and regulation of mood and anxiety frequently found in TAY (particularly with underlying psychopathology) are related to the continuation of SUD. SUD may serve as a coping mechanism for negative affect, avoidance of depression, or substance withdrawal, whereas excessive affect (such as mania or agitation) may drive SUD.[78]

Data would suggest that up to three-quarters of TAY with SUD also have psychiatric co-morbidity.[11,12,79,80] Among disorders co-morbid with SUD, conduct disorder, ADHD, mood disorder, and anxiety disorder are most frequently encountered. One of the most robust risk factors for SUD is delinquency in childhood, often referred to as conduct disorder.[81] Conduct disorder may be a result of a difficult upbringing and/or may be genetically determined. Either alone or in combination with other psychiatric disorders, conduct disorder incrementally increases the risk for cigarette smoking and SUD as well as earlier-onset SUD—as early as 10 to 12 years of age. For instance, the presence of conduct disorder has been shown to increase the risk for early-onset SUD by four- to six-fold along with a more pernicious SUD.[82]

One of the most common disorders seen in association with early-onset SUD, is ADHD. Follow-up studies of children with ADHD report their risk for SUD to be almost twice that of those without ADHD, with those with concurrent conduct disorder (delinquency) to be at highest risk.[82,83] Moreover, almost one-quarter of adults with an addiction have ADHD,[84] with higher rates in adolescent SUD.[85] The greatest time for risk for SUD in individuals with ADHD starts around the time of separation from the family (e.g., 18 years of age), although it is earlier in the context of conduct disorder or bipolar disorder.[86]

Increasingly recognized as important for long-term optimal outcome in ADHD is the use of medication treatment, including the stimulants.[9] Longitudinal data suggest that in TAY (e.g., college-aged students), pharmacotherapy may reduce the risk for cigarette smoking and SUD. For instance, a recent large study from Sweden showed in 25,656 ADHD individuals followed for over 5 years (during which approximately 50% were receiving medication), a 30%–40% reduction in criminality in general, and drug-related offenses (a proxy of drug use) in medication-treated compared to non-medication-treated ADHD youth.[87] In some studies, the reduction in SUD risk with treatment may be lost in later adulthood[88,89]; this may be related to the discontinuation of treatment for ADHD.

Long-standing interest in mood disorders in early-onset and TAY SUD exists. High rates of low-level long-standing (dysthymia) and more severe episodic depressions (MDD) are found in TAY with SUD. Longitudinal data indicate that having a depressive disorder in childhood increases the likelihood for later SUD,[90] although SUD does not appear to be the cause of a new mood disorder.[90]

Likewise, frank manic behavior, poor judgment, severe mood swings, and dysregulation indicative of bipolar disorder in youth are also highly linked with SUD. Pediatric-onset bipolar disorder occurs in 3% of youth[8] and places one at a high risk for cigarette smoking and SUD. For example, one-third of young adolescents with bipolar disorder have SUD compared to 4% of controls,[40] with the SUD rate climbing to over 50% in college-aged students with bipolar disorder.

Anxiety disorders and PTSD are increasingly recognized as being co-morbid with SUD in TAY. Anxiety in early- to mid-adolescence has been linked to the initiation and maintenance of SUD—particularly in the context of mood dysfunction.[90,91] Interestingly, SUD typically does not create the new onset of an anxiety disorder.[90,91] Rates of SUD and other psychiatric issues, are substantially higher in TAY who had a lifetime diagnosis of PTSD before the age of 18 years compared to youths who had never experienced a trauma,[14,92] and somewhat higher than youths who had experienced a trauma but did not develop PTSD. The PTSD story is further confounded in this age group as other psychopathology, such as bipolar disorder, increases the likelihood of PTSD; higher rates of SUD also aggregate in those with vs. those without PTSD with bipolar disorder.[93]

As expected, during the TAY years, one disorder may influence the emergence of, or complicate, another disorder. For instance, mood disorder, psychotic disorder, and personality disorders are linked to a two-fold increase in the likelihood of transitioning from showing substance *use* to having a substance *use disorder*.[94] Subsequently, SUD is related to current and downstream worsened psychological and health outcomes. Conversely, SUD in general, and marijuana smoking in particular, may increase the risk for other psychiatric disorders. For instance, a growing literature supports that excessive marijuana use may heighten the risk for psychosis in vulnerable youth.[95-99]

Medication Misuse in Transitioning Adolescents and Young Adults

Over the past decade, there has been an increase in the non-medical use of medications by TAY.[76,100] The data suggest that the most commonly misused medications in TAY include painkillers (opioids), sedative/hypnotics (benzodiazepines), and stimulants. For instance, up to 20% of high school youth have misused prescriptions, and from 5% to 35% of college students have misused stimulants,[101] with recent increases in the misuse of immediate-release amphetamines. Approximately three-quarters of prescription drugs arise from friends, family, and their own supplies. A higher risk for medication misuse exists in those with mental health problems.[100] Of concern, an equal number of TAY now initiate drug experimentation with prescription medications and marijuana. TAY do not appear to view prescription drug abuse as problematic (Box 70-2).

Signs and Symptoms of Prescription Drug Abuse

Parents and practitioners should be suspicious of TAY who manifest "pin-point" (constricted) pupils, slurred speech, flushing, sweating, and/or appetite changes. These individuals may also have prominent emotionality, personality changes, sleep changes, and forgetfulness. TAY who misuse or abuse prescription medication may become isolated and withdraw from their family and friends, become more secretive, socialize with a different group of friends, develop monetary issues, skip classes, and fail academically and occupationally.[102]

Practitioners and parents should communicate with TAY about the medical, psychological, addictive, and legal issues of prescription drug abuse. TAY should be advised to take their medications as prescribed and not give or sell their medications to others. Safe storage of controlled substances, such as benzodiazepines or stimulants, is important. Parents and grandparents should be instructed to safeguard their own medications, particularly controlled agents, such as to dispense of unused or old medications and to monitor active controlled prescriptions.

Treatment Issues

Child psychiatrists and developmentally-oriented adult psychiatrists are best positioned to diagnose and treat cognitive, emotional, behavioral, and substance use difficulties in TAY. While still developing their ultimate independence, TAY are often very connected to their parents, siblings, and extended families. Likewise, they are also often allied with their school, community, military branch, peers, teachers, coaches, and significant others. The current treatment system is challenged with gaps, including the discontinuity of mental health services during the transition from child to adult psychiatry services, the "special" training necessary to understand and treat mental health and SUDs in TAY, the capacity to work with systems (high school or college), the skill in including parents and/or families, negotiating reimbursement mazes, and all the

---

BOX 70-2 Barriers to Treatment

Denial/recognition:
- Patients may not recognize the signs or symptoms of their disorder
- Patients may not appreciate the effects of their disorder
- Stigma: embarrassment, feeling "defective"
- Belief system: patients may feel that it is better to overcome problems without treatment
- Cultural values

Access to care:
- Lack of expertise in TAY diagnosis and care
- Lack of services available
- Availability of practitioners
- Cost or insurance problems
- Time/flexibility of scheduling
- Transportation to/from appointments

Engagement/adherence:
- Difficulty in initially engaging TAY
- Missed appointments
- Inconsistent adherence to medications or psychotherapy

Medication:
- Unreasonable expectations; medication helps, not curative
- Uncomfortable side effects or dislike of medication effects (e.g. emotional blunting)
- Use of medication in context to substance mis(use)
- Diversion/misuse of prescribed agent

Continuity of care:
- Transient lifestyle
- Ambiguous delineation of which practitioner follows TAY
- Transition of care between child and adult systems

System work:
- Parent/family work
- College
- Occupational/military
- Peers

Special issues:
- Substance (mis)use
- Boundaries—family, college
- Confidentiality
- Legal status
- Individuation, autonomy, separation

---

sensitive, albeit less articulated, issues of confidentiality in these settings.

Recently, Massachusetts General Hospital conducted a department-wide survey assessing the care of TAY. Of the 92 participants, including psychiatrists and psychologists, the minority of who work with both children and adults, several difficulties were identified in working with TAY. The challenges thought to face TAY included the stigma surrounding mental illness, trouble accessing care, and privacy issues with parents. Respondents consistently indicated that the top three challenges involved in the care of TAY were engagement in care, adherence to treatment, and substance use.

While it is beyond the scope of this chapter to elucidate all elements of treatment, there are two areas that appear critical for good outcomes in this age group: initial engagement and adherence to the management regimen.[102] TAY frequently require complementary services given that they have not fully become independent from family and often have complicated relations with peers. The treatment of TAY involves an extended collaborative process to enhance motivation for treatment, augment self-reliance, teach skilled living, and address a range of psychiatric and social needs. Parental support, and in some cases therapy, is an important cornerstone of the treatment.

A key point is that *parent work is to be considered for all age groups within TAY*, not just those under the age of 18 years. Some programs offer parents care either as an adjunct to care with their TAY, or independently. The offer of care can be extended to the parent, even if their TAY offspring are not yet willing to engage. By engaging the parent initially, particularly in resistant situations, attitudes and changes at home may facilitate the engagement of TAY. For instance, in the program described below, almost three-quarters of the initial visits over the first month are with parents, with their TAY offspring completing three-quarters of visits in the subsequent care over the next few months.

Employing this conceptual paradigm, a program at the Massachusetts General Hospital for those 16–26 years old for addiction and mental health problems, called the Addiction Recovery Management Service (ARMS), has been developed.[102,103] The ARMS program incorporates and connects child and adult psychiatry as well as outpatient and partial substance abuse units at MGH. The core clinical faculty of ARMS is child-trained social workers, psychologists, and psychiatrists. The main areas of service delivery include consultation/evaluation, individualized treatment, family support and coaching, psychopharmacology, and care management. The evaluation process includes TAY engagement and retention, substance use and mental health services, and assessment of psychosocial, medical, and legal problems. Treatment bundles the use of traditional (cognitive and dialectic behavioral therapies, addiction coaching) as well as more contemporary and often less well tested e-technologies (e.g. texting, web-based contact, and therapies) with ongoing assessment and feedback of outcomes.[103] Programs using a similar model for TAY at the MGH include eating disorders, first-break psychosis, depression, post-traumatic stress disorders, and ASDs.

Motivational interviewing is critical as a first step to enhance TAY willingness to engage in, and remain adherent to, treatment; as well as to help parents be more effective in facilitating their offspring's treatment. One noteworthy area of TAY management is educating parents on what to expect during the early stages of symptom abatement and recovery, enhancing their skills and confidence in coping with the cycles of both partial and full remissions, and relapses, over time.

Thoughtfully working out the bounds of confidentiality can be useful in the collaborative care of TAY and their parents. While most parents recognize the need for boundaries around the care of TAY (especially those 18 years of age and older), they also want to ensure that relevant information is made available to the provider. Allowing feedback and providing access in a proactive, mutually-agreeable, manner will not only enhance safety but also facilitate treatment of TAY.

Assessing and managing cigarette smoking and substance use in TAY is essential. A number of screening instruments, such as the CRAFFT[104] or AUDIT, can be useful in determining if an addiction is present. Given the age range, practitioners should expect the use of substances in this population and have an open dialogue with TAY related to their quantity and context of substance use. An incremental strategy to help the TAY reduce their excess substance use is recommended. For TAY screened positive, or suspected of using substances excessively, discussing the potential interaction of the misused substance with the underlying mental health concern and/or treatment can be useful. Appreciating what difficulties (e.g., fights, money, occupational difficulties) the TAY may be experiencing currently that are even remotely related to the substances is often enlightening to the patient. Agreeing to brief episodes of sobriety (e.g., 15 to 30 days of being abstinent, called "sobriety sampling") is a helpful way to initiate the notion of excess substance use in this group (e.g., overcoming denial) while evaluating the ability of TAY to actually reduce

or cease their substance use. While abstinence from substances is preferred, particularly in high-risk individuals, most TAY programs employ a harm-reduction model—whereas gradual success is predicated upon lower and lower amounts of substance use over time.[102]

CONCLUSION

TAY is a critical period on which the field of psychiatry should focus, where individuals frequently experience the persistence or onset of mental health and substance problems with substantial functional impairment. Interests and expertise in developmental psychopathology, family dynamics, and systems of care are important to direct and oversee the clinical care of TAY using innovative programming. Addressing cognitive, emotional, behavioral, and substance-related dysfunction in TAY necessitates thorough evaluation and multimodal strategies for both the individuals and their families. The application of existing and novel therapies coupled with new treatment paradigms may result in improved patient engagement in treatment with better long-term outcomes.[103]

Acknowledgments

This research was supported by a NIH K24 DA016264 grant to Dr. Timothy Wilens Over the past 3 years, Dr. Wilens has received grant support from NIH (NIDA) and Shire; and has been a consultant for Euthymics and Shire. Ms. Zulauf has no conflicts of interest to report. Dr. Rosenbaum over the past 3 years has held equity in Medavante and Supernus Pharmaceuticals.

Access the complete reference list and multiple choice questions (MCQs) online at https://expertconsult.inkling.com

KEY REFERENCES

3. Giedd JN. The teen brain: insights from neuroimaging. *J Adolesc Health* 42(4):335–343, 2008.
4. Casey BJ, Getz S, Galvan A. The adolescent brain. *Dev Rev* 28(1):62–77, 2008.
9. Wilens TE, Spencer TJ. Understanding attention-deficit/hyperactivity disorder from childhood to adulthood. *Postgrad Med* 122(5):97–109, 2010.
12. Kessler RC, Berglund P, Demler O, et al. Lifetime prevalence and age-of-onset distributions of DSM-IV disorders in the National Comorbidity Survey Replication. *Arch Gen Psychiatry* 62(6):593–602, 2005.
13. Vaingankar JA, Rekhi G, Subramaniam M, et al. Age of onset of life-time mental disorders and treatment contact. *Soc Psychiatry Psychiatr Epidemiol* 48(5):835–843, 2013.
14. Giaconia R, Reinherz H, Silverman A, et al. Ages of onset of psychiatric disorders in a community population of older adolescents. *J Am Acad Child Adoles Psychiatry* 33(5):706–717, 1994.
23. Millet B, Kochman F, Gallarda T, et al. Phenomenological and comorbid features associated in obsessive-compulsive disorder: influence of age of onset. *J Affect Disord* 79(1–3):241–246, 2004.
24. Delorme R, Golmard JL, Chabane N, et al. Admixture analysis of age at onset in obsessive-compulsive disorder. *Psychol Med* 35(2):237–243, 2005.
25. Kessler RC, Walters EE. Epidemiology of DSM-III-R major depression and minor depression among adolescents and young adults in the National Comorbidity Survey. *Depress Anxiety* 7(1):3–14, 1998.
26. Zisook S, Lesser I, Stewart JW, et al. Effect of age at onset on the course of major depressive disorder. *Am J Psychiatry* 164(10):1539–1546, 2007.
42. Perlis RH, Ostacher MJ, Patel JK, et al. Predictors of recurrence in bipolar disorder: primary outcomes from the Systematic Treatment Enhancement Program for Bipolar Disorder (STEP-BD). *Am J Psychiatry* 163(2):217–224, 2006.
45. Hudson JI, Hiripi E, Pope HG Jr, et al. The prevalence and correlates of eating disorders in the National Comorbidity Survey Replication. *Biol Psychiatry* 61(3):348–358, 2007.

46. Field AE, Sonneville KR, Micali N, et al. Prospective association of common eating disorders and adverse outcomes. *Pediatrics* 130(2):e289–e295, 2012.

47. Stice E, Marti CN, Shaw H, et al. An 8-year longitudinal study of the natural history of threshold, subthreshold, and partial eating disorders from a community sample of adolescents. *J Abnorm Psychol* 118(3):587–597, 2009.

54. Sham PC, MacLean CJ, Kendler KS. A typological model of schizophrenia based on age at onset, sex and familial morbidity. *Acta Psychiatr Scand* 89(2):135–141, 1994.

55. Hafner H, Maurer K, Loffler W, et al. The influence of age and sex on the onset and early course of schizophrenia. *Br J Psychiatry* 162:80–86, 1993.

56. Amminger GP, Schafer MR, Papageorgiou K, et al. Long-chain omega-3 fatty acids for indicated prevention of psychotic disorders: a randomized, placebo-controlled trial. *Arch Gen Psychiatry* 67(2):146–154, 2010.

63. Blumberg SJ, Bramlett MD, Kogan MD, et al. Changes in prevalence of parent-reported autism spectrum disorder in school-aged U.S. children: 2007 to 2011–2012. In Statisitcs NCfH, editor: *Natl Health Stat Report*, Hyattsville, MD, 2013.

67. Howlin P, Goode S, Hutton J, et al. Adult outcome for children with autism. *J Child Psychol Psychiatry* 45(2):212–229, 2004.

68. Simonoff E, Pickles A, Charman T, et al. Psychiatric disorders in children with autism spectrum disorders: prevalence, comorbidity, and associated factors in a population-derived sample. *J Am Acad Child Adolesc Psychiatry* 47(8):921–929, 2008.

69. de Bruin EI, Ferdinand RF, Meester S, et al. High rates of psychiatric co-morbidity in PDD-NOS. *J Autism Dev Disord* 37(5):877–886, 2007.

70. Taylor JL, Seltzer MM. Changes in the autism behavioral phenotype during the transition to adulthood. *J Autism Dev Disord* 40(12):1431–1446, 2010.

71. Smith LE, Maenner MJ, Seltzer MM. Developmental trajectories in adolescents and adults with autism: the case of daily living skills. *J Am Acad Child Adolesc Psychiatry* 51(6):622–631, 2012.

75. Compton WM, Thomas YF, Stinson FS, et al. Prevalence, correlates, disability, and comorbidity of DSM-IV drug abuse and dependence in the United States: results from the national epidemiologic survey on alcohol and related conditions. *Arch Gen Psychiatry* 64(5):566–576, 2007.

78. Cheetham A, Allen NB, Yucel M, et al. The role of affective dysregulation in drug addiction. *Clin Psychol Rev* 30(6):621–634, 2010.

87. Lichtenstein P, Halldner L, Zetterqvist J, et al. Medication for attention deficit-hyperactivity disorder and criminality. *N Engl J Med* 367(21):2006–2014, 2012.

100. McCabe SE, West BT, Cranford JA, et al. Medical misuse of controlled medications among adolescents. *Arch Pediatr Adolesc Med* 165(8):729–735, 2011.

102. Wilens TE, McKowen J, Kane M. Substance abuse in transitional aged youth: It is where it is happening! *Contemp Pediatr* In Press.

104. Knight JR, Shrier LA, Bravender TD, et al. A new brief screen for adolescent substance abuse. *Arch Pediatr Adolesc Med* 153(6):591–596, 1999.

71   Geriatric Psychiatry

M. Cornelia Cremens, MD, MPH

KEY POINTS

- Depression in the elderly carries a very high risk of suicide.
- Symptoms of alcoholism and substance abuse are often confused with those of medical illness.
- The differential diagnosis of dementia is broad and the behavior problems challenging to treat.
- Delirium increases the prevalence and severity of disability, the length of hospital stay, and rates of morbidity and mortality.
- Caregivers of the elderly are at risk for depression, anxiety, and burnout.

OVERVIEW

The population older than 65 years has increased dramatically over the past several years; this trend reflects improved health, nutrition, and access to medical care. This remarkable lengthening of the average life span in the US, from 47 years in 1900 to more than 75 years at present, will continue to increase along with improvements in medicine and the health consciousness of the baby boomers.[1] Equally noteworthy has been the increase in the number of those over the age of 85 years. Older adults continue to learn and to contribute to society, despite the physiological changes associated with aging and the ever-threatening health and cognitive problems they face. Ongoing intellectual, social, and physical activity is important for the maintenance of mental health at all stages of life. Stressful life events (e.g., declining health; loss of independence; and the loss of a spouse or partner, family member, or friend) typically become more common with advancing age. However, major depression, anxiety disorders, memory loss, and unrelenting bereavement are not a part of normal aging; they should be treated when diagnosed. A host of effective interventions exist for most psychiatric disorders experienced by older adults and for many of the mental health problems associated with aging.

The prevalence of medical and psychiatric illness increases with advancing age in part due to stressful life events, the burden of co-morbid illness, and the various combinations of a bevy of medications used.[2]

The reduction in hepatic, renal, and gastric function associated with aging impairs the elder's ability to absorb and to metabolize drugs; aging also influences the enzymes that degrade these medications (Table 71-1).[1]

Disability due to mental illness in elderly individuals will increasingly become a major public health problem in the very near future. The elderly are more susceptible to disease and are more vulnerable to the side effects of prescribed drugs and other substances (be they illicit or over-the-counter substances).[3] Approximately 40% to 60% of hospitalized medical and surgical patients are over the age of 65 years; moreover, they are at greater risk for functional decline while hospitalized than are younger individuals.[4] Adequately treating older adults who have psychiatric disorders provides benefits for their overall health by improving their interest and ability to care for themselves and to follow their primary care provider's directions and advice with regard to health promotion and medication compliance. Older individuals can also benefit from advances in psychotherapy, medications, and other treatment interventions for mental disorders, when these interventions are modified for age and health status.

Barriers to access of appropriate mental health services have arisen in the organization and financing of services for the elderly. Unfortunately, numerous problems exist in the structure of Medicare, Medicaid, nursing homes, and managed care. Primary care practitioners are the critical link in identifying and addressing mental disorders in older adults. Opportunities to improve mental health and general medical outcomes are missed when mental illness is under-recognized and under-treated in primary care settings.

General themes in geriatric psychiatry include the following: the differentiation of symptoms of normal aging from the symptoms of illness in later life; the modifiability of illness in later life; the modifiability of normal aging to improve function; the capacity to change; and distinguishing differences in the manifestations of early-onset and late-onset psychiatric disorders.

An understanding of geriatric mental health relies in part on an appreciation of neurochemistry. Neurochemistry of the aging human brain is closely related to an irreversible loss of function and a decline in global abilities. Fortunately, our brain has remarkable plasticity; it allows for the well-designed compensation for neuronal loss and functional decline that is linked with an age-related loss in neurons, dendrites, enzymes, and neurotransmitters.[5] Enzymes and neurotransmitters in the brain change as we age: e.g., monoamine oxidase increases and acetylcholine and dopamine decrease.[6]

MENTAL HEALTH DISORDERS COMMON IN LATE LIFE

Late-life Depression

Depression in late life lowers life expectancy. Depression and cognitive impairment affect approximately 25% of the elderly.[1] New research confirms that the risk for post-stroke depression increases especially in the "old-old" (i.e., those over 85 years of age).[7] Depression in the elderly is not more common according to Epidemiological Catchment Area (ECA) data; however, making the diagnosis is more difficult. A higher rate of depression exists in older women as compared to older men; among those with a history of depression there is a 50% chance of a second episode (either a recurrence or a relapse).[8] Use of medications for medical problems often generates adverse effects and complicates the diagnosis of depression; moreover, medical illness may mimic depression and depression may mimic medical illness. Depression (as occurs with stroke, fractured hip, arthritis, and cardiac illness) is common in disabled elderly. Depression is also associated with both acute and chronic medical illnesses and late-onset depression is closely associated with physical illness.[9] Of note, undiagnosed medical illness can manifest as depression. Grief and loss may also contribute to depression. As many as 60% of

depressed patients have co-morbid anxiety and 40% of anxious patients have co-morbid depression.[10]

Neurological disorders also complicate the diagnosis of depression. The risk for depression in the post-stroke period is high, with 25% to 50% developing depression within 2 years of the event.[7] Alzheimer's disease (AD) carries an increased risk of depression; approximately 20%–30% (either before or at the time of diagnosis) are diagnosed with depression. Delusions are also prominent in depression associated with dementia.[11] Recent research confirms the association of depression with the increased risk of developing late-onset AD.[12] Fifty percent of patients with Parkinson's disease develop depression or have a history of depression with anxiety, dysthymia, or frontal lobe dysfunction.[13] Degeneration of the sub-cortical nuclei (especially the raphe nuclei) is related to the development of depression in Parkinson's disease.

Assessment of depression can be challenging. The Geriatric Depressions Scale (Table 71-2)[14] is a helpful tool in this regard, and often the information provided by the caregiver is crucial as elders may not be forthcoming with their symptoms.[15] However the PHQ-9 used in the primary care office is simpler to complete and therefore more readily used.[15] The criteria for diagnosing depression in the elderly are the same as they are in the general population.

Treatment of late-life depression is challenging in part because there is a decline in one's biological ability to metabolize drugs and to bind proteins (because of reduced receptor sensitivity), as well as an increased sensitivity to drug side effects. In an effort to reduce adverse consequences of medications, drugs with the fewest side effects should be started (and be used in small doses); in addition, monotherapy should be attempted[16,17] (Tables 71-3 and 71-4). In more refractory cases or with psychotic symptoms, electroconvulsive therapy (ECT) should be considered early in treatment and as an adjunct for one or more drugs.[18] Individual psychotherapy or group therapy complements somatic treatments and often leads to a swift recovery. Interpersonal therapy and cognitive-behavioral therapy (CBT) are both suited to this population as they are more focused and interactive treatments.[19]

TABLE 71-1 Metabolic Changes Associated with Aging

Function	Impact	Domain
Hepatic function	Decreased	Blood flow Affects first-pass effect
	Decreased	Enzyme activity Demethylation Hydroxylation
Absorption	Decreased	Blood flow Acidity Motility Gastrointestinal surface area
Renal excretion	Decreased	Blood flow Can lead to lithium toxicity Glomerular filtration rate Hydroxymetabolites affected Tubular excretion Benzodiazepine clearance slowed
Distribution	Increased	Volume of distribution Especially for lipophilic drugs
	Increased	Fat stores
	Decreased	Water content
	Decreased	Muscle mass
	Decreased	Cardiac output and perfusion to organs
Protein-binding	Decreased	Albumin levels (except alpha$_1$-glycoprotein)

TABLE 71-2 PHQ-9

Nine Symptom Checklist

Over the last 2 weeks, how often have you been bothered by any of the following problems?

	Not At All	Several Days	More Than Half the Days	Nearly Every Day
1. Little interest or pleasure in doing things	0	1	2	3
2. Feeling down, depressed, or hopeless	0	1	2	3
3. Trouble falling or staying asleep, or sleeping too much	0	1	2	3
4. Feeling tired or having little energy	0	1	2	3
5. Poor appetite or overeating	0	1	2	3
6. Feeling bad about yourself—or that you are a failure or have let yourself or your family down	0	1	2	3
7. Trouble concentrating on things, such as reading the newspaper or watching television	0	1	2	3
8. Moving or speaking so slowly that other people could have noticed? Or the opposite—being so fidgety or restless that you have been moving around a lot more than usual	0	1	2	3
9. Thoughts that you would be better off dead or of hurting yourself in some way	0	1	2	3

(For office coding: Total Score _____ = ___ + ___ + ___)

If you checked off any problems, how difficult have these problems made it for you to do your work, take care of things at home, or get along with other people?

Not difficult at all   Somewhat difficult   Very difficult   Extremely difficult

TABLE 71-3 Medications for Depression in the Elderly

Drugs	Dose Range	Comments
TRICYCLIC ANTIDEPRESSANTS		
Nortriptyline	10–150 mg/day	Reliable blood levels, minimal orthostasis
Desipramine	10–250 mg/day	Mildly anticholinergic
MONOAMINE OXIDASE INHIBITORS		
Tranylcypromine	10–30 mg/day	Orthostasis (possibly delayed), pedal edema, weakly anticholinergic, requires dietary restrictions
STIMULANTS		
Dextroamphetamine	2.5–40 mg/day	Agitation, mild tachycardia
Methylphenidate	2.5–60 mg/day	
Modafinil	50–200 mg/day	
SELECTIVE SEROTONIN REUPTAKE INHIBITORS		
Fluoxetine	5–60 mg/day	Akathisia, headache, agitation, gastrointestinal complaints, diarrhea/constipation
Sertraline	25–200 mg/day	
Paroxetine	5–40 mg/day	
Fluvoxamine	25–300 mg/day	
Citalopram	10–40 mg/day	
Escitalopram	2.5–20 mg/day	
SEROTONIN-NOREPINEPHRINE REUPTAKE INHIBITORS (SNRIs)		
Venlafaxine	25–300 mg/day	Increase in systolic blood pressure, confusion, light-headedness
Nefazodone	50–600 mg/day	Pedal edema, rash, hepatotoxicity (rare)
Duloxetine	20–60 mg/day	Diarrhea, dizziness
ALPHA$_2$-ANTAGONIST/SELECTIVE SEROTONIN		
Mirtazapine	15–45 mg/day	Sedation, weight gain
ATYPICAL ANTIDEPRESSANTS		
Trazodone	25–250 mg/day	Sedation, orthostasis, incontinence, hallucinations, priapism
	50–600 mg/day	Pedal edema, rash
Bupropion	75–450 mg/day	Seizures, less mania/cycling, headache, nausea

TABLE 71-4 Medications for Psychotic Symptoms in the Elderly

Drug	Dose Range	Sedation	Ach Potency	EPS/Comments
ATYPICAL ANTIPSYCHOTICS				
Clozapine	12.5–100 mg	High	High	Very low
				Check WBC count weekly; excessive drooling, hypotension
Risperidone	0.25–3 mg	Low	Low	Low
				More EPS than initially reported
Olanzapine	2.5–10.0 mg	Moderate	Moderate	Low
Quetiapine	12.5–200 mg	High	Low	Low
Ziprasidone	20–80 mg BID	Moderate	Low	Low
Aripiprazole	15–30 mg	Low	Low	Moderate

Ach, Anticholinergic; EPS, extrapyramidal symptoms; WBC, white blood cell.

Late-life Depression and Suicide

Depression with psychotic features is linked with a higher risk of suicide. The rate of suicide in those greater than 65 years is double that of the rate for the US population in general, and those with the highest suicide rates of any age group are those aged 65 years and older.[20] In 2011, suicide ranked as the 10th leading cause of death among those aged 65; this group represented 12.5% of the population, but it accounted for 15.7% of all suicides. Suicide disproportionately affects the elderly; the suicide rate among those 65 to 69 years old was 13.1 per 100,000 (N.B.: all of the following rates are per 100,000 population), and the rates increased as age increased (i.e., it was 15.2 among those between 70 and 74, it was 17.6 among those between 75 and 79, it was 22.9 between those 80 and 84, and it was 21.0 between persons 85 or older). Firearms (71%), overdose (11%), and suffocation (11%) were the three most common methods of suicide used by persons aged 65 years or older. Firearms are the most common method of suicide by both males and females, accounting for 78% of

men and 35% of women who committed suicide in that age group and cohort.[21]

Risk factors for suicide among the elderly differ from those among the young. In addition to a higher prevalence of depression, older persons are more socially isolated and they more frequently use highly lethal methods. They also make fewer attempts per completed suicide, have a higher male-to-female ratio than other groups, have frequently visited a health care provider before their suicide, and have more physical illnesses. Approximately 20% of elderly (i.e., over 65 years) persons who commit suicide have visited a physician within 24 hours of their death, 41% visited within 1 week of their suicide, and 75% were seen by a physician within 1 month of their suicide. Of every 100,000 people aged 65 and older, 14.3 died by suicide in 2004. This figure is higher than the national average of 10.9 suicides per 100,000 people in the general population. Caucasian men aged 85 or older had an even higher rate, with 17.8 suicide deaths per 100,000. Suicide rates among the elderly are highest for those who are divorced or widowed. Among men aged 75 years and older, the rate for divorced men was 3.4 times that for married men, and for widowed men it was 2.6 times that for married men. In the same age group, the suicide rate for divorced women was 2.8 times that of married women, and for widowed women it was 1.9 times the rate among married women. Several factors (including growth in the size of that population; health status; availability of, and access to, services; and attitudes about aging and suicide) relative to those over 65 years will play a role in future suicide rates among the elderly.

Suicide occurs early (often during the first 6 months) in the illness, but it can occur at any time, often in combination with other mental disorders. More than 90% of older people who commit suicide have the following risk factors: depression or other mental disorders; a substance abuse disorder or a family history of such; stressful life events, in combination with other risk factors, such as depression; a prior suicide attempt or family history of an attempt; family violence (including physical or sexual abuse); firearms in the home (the method used in more than half of suicides); incarceration; or exposure to the suicidal behavior of others, such as family members, peers, or media figures.[22] The rate of completed suicide is greater in this population than in any other age group; older adults account for 25% of all suicides. Older white males make up the highest-risk group, and rates are increasing. Isolation increases the risk for suicide, and alcoholism or substance abuse is a contributing factor to successful suicides in all populations, including older adults. Aggressive treatment with antidepressants is indicated for these individuals, and inpatient treatment is the safest venue for care.

Most of the antidepressants are equally effective for depression; however, drugs with anticholinergic effects and undue sedation should be avoided to reduce complications (such as falls, confusion, and poor compliance). However, matching the symptoms with the side effects is useful for a patient with significant weight loss and insomnia; a sedating medication that increases appetite may be beneficial. ECT early in the course of major depressive disorder (MDD) should be considered strongly as appropriate care of this high-risk population.

Alcoholism

Alcoholism, often overlooked in many patients, may go unnoticed in older adults despite a lifelong pattern of daily drinking; even if the elderly drink only small amounts, they may experience a significant and life-threatening withdrawal. Co-morbid illness (both psychiatric and medical) confounds accurate diagnosis of both the alcoholism and the medical or surgical diagnosis. Symptoms of problem-drinking include insomnia, memory loss, confusion, anxiety, and depression, as well as somatic complaints that may mimic medical illness, further delaying accurate diagnosis. Older adults who drink alcohol are at greater risk due to the fact that often they take more prescribed medications that can interact adversely with alcohol.

The prevalence of alcoholism in the ECA study was 1.5% to 3.7%. Although cross-sectional studies suggested that the percentage of alcoholism declines after age 60, longitudinal studies propose a stable pattern of lifelong alcohol abuse.[23] Women drink less than men at all ages, but older widowed women are at risk for increasing their intake. Studies note that the prevalence of alcohol problems in women is on the rise. Older adults with alcohol dependence also have a high prevalence of co-morbid nicotine dependence. Alcohol dependence can lead to liver damage, cancer, immune system disorders, and brain damage.

Depression is more common in those with alcoholism, as is grief, anxiety, psychosis, and dementia. Suicide risk is greater in elderly alcoholics; therefore, obtaining a comprehensive history from family, friends, and caretakers is essential.

Hospitalization is typically required for detoxification of the older patient.[24] Newer medications (such as naltrexone and acamprosate) and the familiar disulfiram (Antabuse) can be beneficial, but disulfiram may generate problematic side effects in older adults.[25]

Anxiety

Recently, anxiety (generally associated with normal aging and with medical, financial, and health-related hardships) has been increasingly recognized in the elderly. However, since anxiety is not a direct consequence of normal aging, the symptoms of anxiety should not be ignored. Among the most common categories of anxiety are simple phobias and generalized anxiety; if left untreated these conditions may lead to serious depression.[26] Anxiety may co-exist with many other psychiatric diagnoses (such as depression, bipolar disorder, alcoholism, and dementia). Diagnostic challenges often arise when anxiety (e.g., worry, fear, apprehension, concern, and foreboding), as well as somatic complaints (such as tachycardia, sweating, abdominal distress, dizziness, and vertigo) develop in the context of a medical illness (e.g., diabetes with hypoglycemia, hyperthyroidism, or cardiac disease with hypoxia) as it can be manifest by similar symptoms.[26] Worries, fears, and concerns are often related to finances, dependency issues, loneliness, and memory loss. Manifestations of medical illness can mimic psychiatric symptoms; certain substances or medications (e.g., caffeine, stimulants, ephedrine, and bronchodilators) produce anxiety-like symptoms. Withdrawal from a prescribed or an illicit drug can precipitate severe anxiety and panic; life-threatening withdrawal can result from sudden abstinence from alcohol, benzodiazepines, or barbiturates.

Fortunately, anxiety can be effectively managed in the elderly by use of medications, therapy, or a combination of the two.[26] Among the anxiolytics, benzodiazepines are the most frequently prescribed class of agents (especially by primary care physicians) for the elderly; however, significant side effects (such as confusion, falls, over-sedation, and paradoxical agitation) can arise.[27] Complications of long-term use include daytime somnolence, confusion, cognitive impairment, an unsteady stance or gait, paradoxical agitation, memory disturbance, depression, and respiratory depression.

Psychosis

Psychosis (manifest by hallucinations, delusions, disorganized speech, and disorganized or catatonic behavior) in the elderly has multiple etiologies (e.g., delirium, dementia, depression, mania, and schizophrenia). Not only is morbidity high with a diagnosis of delirium but also about 30% of those with delirium will die within 1 year of their illness.[28,29] (see Chapter 18). The differential diagnosis of psychosis in the elderly includes the following: various types of dementias (e.g., AD, Lewy body dementia, vascular dementia, frontal lobe dementia [Pick's disease], and Parkinson's disease), all of which can have psychotic symptoms at any point during the illness; delirium; delusional disorders; bipolar disorder; schizoaffective disorder; schizophrenia (either early-onset or late-onset); and major depression with psychotic features. Psychosis in dementia is common, and it can be episodic or persistent and can appear early or late during the disease.[30] Symptoms of psychosis (e.g., delusions, hallucinations, misconceptions, and misperceptions) are distressing to family members and to caregivers; they can be dangerous if the individual becomes frightened or energized by them. Alcoholism and substance abuse should also be considered as a possible etiology of psychosis.[25] The Charles Bonnet syndrome, with visual hallucinations beginning after a sudden loss of vision (as in

---

BOX 71-1 Activities of Daily Living (ADLs)

Feeding or eating
Bathing
Toileting
Dressing
Continence
Hygiene
Mobility or transferring

BOX 71-2 Instrumental Activities of Daily Living (IADLs)

Housework, light
Telephoning
Cooking and meal preparation
Grocery shopping
Using transportation
Managing medication
Managing finances

TABLE 71-5 Medications for Alzheimer's Disease and Other Dementias

Donepezil	5–23 mg every day
Rivastigmine	1.5–6 mg twice a day
Galantamine	4–12 mg twice a day
Memantine	5–10 mg twice a day

Nausea, diarrhea, abdominal cramps, bradycardia, and fatigue may develop.

---

macular degeneration), may be confused with a primary psychotic condition. Most individuals know that the hallucinations are not real, and they can adjust to them; however, when dementia or an anxiety disorder confounds the symptom, this may be problematic.[31]

Dementia

Many complaints of memory loss reflect the course of normal aging or the effects of a treatable condition (such as depression or delirium). Dementia is not usually diagnosed until its moderate to severe stages, as symptoms and a subtle decline in function (Boxes 71-1 and 71-2) develop over time.

The prevalence of dementia and cognitive impairment is higher in women than in men. While higher rates of AD are reported in women, higher rates of vascular dementia are reported in men.[32] AD typically affects 5%–8% of those over 65 years, 15%–20% of those over 75 years, and 25%–50% over 85 years; its course is that of a steady decline over approximately 8–10 years.

Genetics of dementia are discussed in greater detail in Chapter 63; however, the *ApoE-2* allele decreases the risk for AD (as it may have a protective effect), while patients with either sporadic or familial AD have a higher frequency of the *ApoE-4* allele than in the general population.[1]

The mechanisms by which these genetic markers confer increased risk are not completely determined. Neurobiological changes associated with normal aging include lower cortical acetylcholine levels, neuron and synaptic loss, decreased dendritic span, and decreased size and density of neurons (especially in the nucleus basalis of Meynert) and likely play a role in AD. AD is most accurately diagnosed by post-mortem examination of the brain (revealing a loss of neurons in the basal forebrain and cortical cholinergic areas, in addition to the depletion of choline acetyltransferase, the enzyme responsible for acetylcholine synthesis). The degree of this central cholinergic deficit is correlated with the severity of dementia; this has led to the "cholinergic hypothesis" of cognitive deficits in AD.[33] This hypothesis has led, in turn, to promising clinical interventions (Table 71-5). Acetylcholine is probably not the only neurotransmitter involved in AD, and numerous medication trials are underway.[34]

Vascular dementia, the second most common cause of dementia, develops as a result of multiple ischemic events or

strokes. Approximately 8% of patients develop vascular dementia after a stroke. Vascular dementia is generally manifest by an abrupt, stuttering, often stepwise, gradual decline; it commonly co-exists with AD.

Mixed dementia is a combination of AD and vascular dementia; it is common, and stroke can unmask an underlying AD.

In frontal lobe dementia, cognitive impairment may not be as noticeable as are the behavioral and personality changes. In this condition, there is a loss of personal or social awareness, a lack of insight, indifference, inappropriate and stereotyped behaviors, aggression, distraction, a loss of inhibitions, apathy, or extroverted behavior.

Early or spontaneous parkinsonism, recurrent visual hallucinations, sensitivity to antipsychotics, fluctuating cognition, falls or syncope, and a transient loss of consciousness characterize Lewy body dementia.

Mild cognitive impairment (MCI), formerly designated as age-associated memory impairment (or benign senescent forgetfulness) or age-related cognitive decline, is characterized by both subjective and objective cognitive impairment in the absence of dementia. Between 10% and 12% of persons with MCI develop AD; others remain with a stable impairment or a minimal decline, or die from other causes.[35] MCI subclassifications include an amnestic form (characterized by isolated memory impairments) and one with multiple cognitive deficits and another with a single deficit.[36]

Behavioral and Psychological Symptoms of Dementia

More than 80% of patients with dementia exhibit a variety of psychological symptoms; a majority have delusions, as well as hallucinations, paranoia, anxiety, apathy, and misidentification syndromes. Behavioral symptoms include wandering, aggression, hostility, insomnia, inappropriate eating, and abnormal sexual behaviors.[37] The caregiver burden increases with behavioral and psychological symptoms of dementia (BPSD), and the aggressive, hostile, and accusatory behaviors and psychotic symptoms often result in institutionalization. Caregivers are at risk for medical and psychiatric illness due to the stress associated with caring for such individuals. Therefore, providing treatment regimens or algorithms has the potential to improve the quality of life for both the patient and the caregiver. First-line treatment has involved non-pharmacological strategies that use environmental and behavioral interventions (such as regularly scheduled routines for meals, sleep, and bathing). Pharmacological interventions (that are not symptom-driven) are less well established. Limited studies have shown the benefit of antipsychotics, but there are significant side effects from their use; these include a neurological risk of stroke, a cardiovascular risk for metabolic syndrome, and a propensity for anticholinergic symptoms.[38] Psychotic symptoms in the elderly are best treated with antipsychotics, while the atypical agents are of benefit due to the binding affinity to both dopamine and serotonin. Agitated, hostile, and aggressive behaviors may respond to antipsychotics, anticonvulsants, or antidepressants. Patients with dementia may develop paradoxical agitation when given benzodiazepines, and they should be administered with caution. Cholinesterase inhibitors have been used for treatment of BPSD since cholinergic deficiency also appears to be involved in the development of BPSD, as well as AD.[39]

Schizophrenia

Although schizophrenia usually arises before the age of 30 years, late-onset schizophrenia is not rare. More than 20% of cases are diagnosed after age 40, and at least 0.1–0.5% of the population over 65 years has a diagnosis of schizophrenia that started late in life, with a prognosis that may be made worse by delay and avoidance of treatment.[40] Aggressive treatment of symptoms and supportive care for patients with this diagnosis is imperative.

Approximately 85% of these individuals (mostly women) live in the community. Schizophrenia remains plastic into later life, with more negative symptoms than positive symptoms. Numerous confounding factors (including cognitive decline, dementia, depression, medical co-morbidity, and use of medications for medical conditions) occur with aging. Most of the older individuals with schizophrenia have been disabled for most of their life. The side effects from typical antipsychotics, such as tardive dyskinesia or extrapyramidal symptoms, may adversely affect independent living. Lowering the dose of these medications or switching to an atypical antipsychotic may be reasonable, noting the recent evidence that atypical agents are linked with an increased risk of stroke.[38] Caregiving and community support for these individuals is the key to maintaining health and stability.

Bipolar Disorder

Bipolar disorder (BPD) may be seen for the first time in late life, and it is not uncommon in older adults; its prevalence is 0.1%–0.4%. For the majority of elderly patients the illness begins in middle-age or late-life and often has co-morbid neurological insults. The patients with co-morbid neurological diseases are more apt to have a significantly later age of onset and a family history of affective illness. Snowdon[41] reported that 25% of patients had mania after age 50, had a history of neurological disease before the onset of the mania, and had significantly lower genetic (familial) risk factors. A number of biological risk factors have been identified for BPD in the elderly, including genetic factors and medical illnesses, particularly vascular diseases.

Symptoms of mania or hypomania manifest differently in older patients, with more symptoms of anger or irritability and at times aggressive behavior, delusions, and paranoia; in addition, less grandiosity and euphoria occur, episodes of mania are longer, and cycling may be more rapid. Treatment response is inconsistent, although lithium, anticonvulsants (e.g., divalproex sodium, carbamazepine, and lamotrigine), atypical antipsychotics (e.g., olanzapine, quetiapine, and risperidone), and antidepressants have all been beneficial in the treatment of elderly patients with BPD. In the differential diagnosis of secondary mania, consideration needs to given to co-morbid illnesses. Many patients with dementia or delirium can manifest with a picture of mania secondary to their illness.[42] Although the treatment of the symptoms is similar in both cases, an accurate diagnosis is important.

Personality Disorders

Usually personality disorders in older adults have been lifelong and well articulated by family members. These disorders are distinguished from a change in personality resulting from an illness, dementia, delirium, depression, a disaster, or a catastrophic event. Neurological disorders (such as stroke, brain injury, trauma, frontal lobe syndrome, seizures, or Parkinson's disease) are examples of conditions that may precipitate a change in personality. In the differential diagnosis, although the patient may be paranoid, avoidant, or threatening, the change in personality may be related to the underlying medical or neurological disorder and not classified as a personality disorder but a change in personality due to the specific diagnosis. Major depression is commonly co-morbid with aging, ranging from 10% to 70%, most often associated with obsessive-compulsive personality disorder. Co-morbid depression and panic are also noted in older patients with somatoform disorder, specifically with hypochondriasis. The pattern of lifelong distress, social dysfunction, and exacerbation of prior symptoms or traits constitutes the diagnosis of a personality disorder. The popular thought that modification of symptoms or traits and possibly adaptation may occur through prior psychotherapy, aging, or life experiences is not evidence-based in the literature. Professionals working with older adults have noted that older adults are more vulnerable to illness, losses, and possibly forced dependency. These changes can be destabilizing and cause emergence of otherwise controlled personality symptoms. Engaging patients and caregivers in communication to allay fears and engender trust and understanding, although not an easy task in those with cluster B personalities, is the entrée to stabilization. Medications may be of benefit but their efficacy may be limited without concomitant therapy.

DISASTERS

Senior citizens comprise a sturdy, reliable generation, who has proven over the years to have the ability to survive myriad disasters (e.g., the Great Depression, world wars, threats of nuclear holocaust, terrorist attacks, and hurricanes); yet they remain proud, tough, and resilient. Older adults are a generation of survivors.[43] However, when a disaster strikes they often feel terrified, alone, and vulnerable. Older adults often need the most assistance but can mistakenly be overlooked during relief efforts. Feelings of helplessness can frighten elderly individuals; this places them at greater risk for both physical and mental health illnesses. It is important for older adults recovering from the after-effects of a disaster to talk about their feelings, to share their experiences with others, and to recognize that they are not alone. Symptoms of post-traumatic stress disorder (PTSD) can be re-ignited by war experiences or by recollections of childhood trauma. They should be encouraged to become involved in the disaster recovery process and to help others; this can be beneficial to their own recovery. Seeking assistance is a step toward recovery, and older adults should be encouraged to ask for any type of help needed (such as financial, emotional, and medical).[44]

CAREGIVER STRESS AND BURDEN

The health and well-being of the caregivers, family members, or employees of the patient need to be considered during the evaluation, because they are at risk for depression.[45] Caring for the caregiver is as important as caring for the patient. The inordinate stress and burden can place the caregiver at risk for medical and psychiatric crisis. Caregivers can become depressed or have symptoms of depression related to burnout (i.e., fatigue, loss of social contacts, lack of interest in work, inability to perform at work, weight gain or loss, feeling helpless, and using alcohol or other substances). Burnout may not present during the most stressful times in caring but emerges months later, somewhat similar to PTSD.

ELDER ABUSE

Each year thousands of elderly, who are often frail and vulnerable, are abused, neglected, or exploited by family members, caregivers, friends, and others, on whom they depend to assist them with basic needs.[46] Elder abuse may be subtle and be as simple as not providing medications, or being avoided. Family and caregivers may not intend to harm or exploit the patient but often are overwhelmed and overextended. Hotlines are available in every state (www.elderabusecenter.org) for helpful information, guidance, or reporting.

Access a list of MCQs for this chapter at https://expertconsult .inkling.com

REFERENCES

1. Sadavoy J, Jarvik LF, Grossberg GT, et al., editors: *Comprehensive textbook of geriatric psychiatry*, ed 3, New York, 2004, WW Norton.
2. Stoudemire A, Fogel BS, Greenberg DB, editors: *Psychiatric care of the medical patient*, ed 2, New York, 2000, Oxford University Press.
3. Gurwitz JH, Field TH, Harold LR, et al. Incidence and preventability of adverse drug events among older persons in the ambulatory setting. *JAMA* 289:1107–1116, 2003.
4. Lunney JR, Lynn J, Foley DJ, et al. Patterns of functional decline at the end of life. *JAMA* 289:2387–2392, 2003.
5. Cremens MC, Gottlieb GL. Acute confusional state: delirium, encephalopathy. In Sirven JI, Malamut BL, editors: *Clinical neurology of the older adult*, Philadelphia, 2002, Lippincott Williams & Wilkins.
6. Cummings JL, Mega SM. *Neuropsychiatry and behavioral neuroscience*, New York, 2003, Oxford University Press.
7. Carota A, Berney A, Aybek S, et al. A prospective study of predictors of post stroke depression. *Neurology* 64:428–433, 2005.
8. Dew MA, Whyte EM, Lenze EJ, et al. Recovery from major depression in older adults receiving augmentation of antidepressant pharmacotherapy. *Am J Psychiatry* 164:892–899, 2007.
9. Katon W, Lin EH, Kroenke K. The association of depression and anxiety with medical symptom burden in patients with chronic medical illness. *Gen Hosp Psychiatry* 29:147–155, 2007.
10. Lenze EJ, Mulsant BH, Shear MK, et al. Comorbid anxiety disorders in depressed elderly patients. *Am J Psychiatry* 157:722–728, 2000.
11. Olin JT, Katz IR, Meyers BS, et al. Provisional diagnostic criteria for depression of Alzheimer disease. *Am J Geriatr Psychiatry* 10:129–141, 2002.
12. Vilalta-Franch J, Garre-Olmo J, López-Pousa S, et al. Comparison of different clinical diagnostic criteria for depression in Alzheimer disease. *Am J Geriatr Psychiatry* 14:589–597, 2006.
13. Ravina B, Camicioli R, Como PG, et al. The impact of depressive symptoms in early Parkinson disease. *Neurology* 69:342–347, 2007.
14. Yesavage JA, Brink TL, Rose TL, et al. Development and validation of a geriatric depression rating scale: a preliminary report. *J Psychiatr Res* 17:27, 1983.
15. Richardson TM, He H, Podgorski C, et al. Screening depression aging services clients. *Am J Geriatr Psychiatry* 18:1116–1123, 2010.
16. Cremens MC. Polypharmacy in the elderly. In Ghaemi SN, editor: *Polypharmacy in psychiatry*, New York, 2002, Marcel Dekker.
17. Reynolds CF III, Dew MA, Pollock BG, et al. Maintenance treatment of major depression in old age. *N Engl J Med* 354:1130–1138, 2006.
18. Greenberg RM, Kellner CH. Electroconvulsive therapy: a selected review. *Am J Geriatr Psychiatry* 13:268–281, 2005.
19. Wei W, Sambamoorthi U, Olfson M, et al. Use of psychotherapy for depression in older adults. *Am J Psychiatry* 162:711–717, 2005.
20. Bruce ML, Ten Have TR, Reynolds CF, et al. Reducing suicidal ideation and depressive symptoms in depressed older primary care patients. *JAMA* 291:1081–1091, 2004.
21. Olin DW, Zubritsky C, Brown G, et al. Managing suicide risk in late life: access to firearms as a public health risk. *Am J Geriatr Psychiatry* 12:30–36, 2004.
22. Rowe JL, Conwell Y, Shulberg HC, et al. Social support and suicidal ideation in older adults using home healthcare services. *Am J Geriatr Psychiatry* 14:758–766, 2006.
23. Blow FC, Barry KL. Older patients with at-risk and problem drinking patterns: new developments and brief interventions. *J Geriatr Psychiatry Neurol* 13:134–140, 2000.
24. Thun MJ, Peto R, Lopez AD, et al. Alcohol consumption and mortality among middle-aged and elderly US adults. *N Engl J Med* 337:1705–1714, 1997.
25. Olin DW. Late-life alcoholism: issues relevant to the geriatric psychiatrist. *Am J Geriatr Psychiatry* 12:571–583, 2004.
26. Lenze EJ, Rogers JC, Martire LM, et al. The association of late-life depression and anxiety with physical disability: a review of the literature and prospectus for future research. *Am J Geriatr Psychiatry* 9:113–135, 2001.
27. Pinquart M, Duberstein PR. Treatment of anxiety disorders in older adults: a meta-analytic comparison of behavioral and pharmacologic interventions. *Am J Geriatr Psychiatry* 15:639–651, 2007.
28. Inouye SK, Bogardus ST, Charpentier PA, et al. A multicomponent intervention to prevent delirium in hospitalized older patients. *N Engl J Med* 340:669–676, 1999.
29. Cole MG. Delirium in elderly patients. *Am J Geriatr Psychiatry* 12:7–21, 2004.
30. Leroi I, Voulgari A, Breitner JC, et al. The epidemiology of psychosis in dementia. *Am J Geriatr Psychiatry* 11:83–91, 2003.
31. Eperjesi N, Arkbarali S. Rehabilitation in the Charles Bonnet syndrome: a review of the treatment options. *Clin Exp Optom* 87:149–152, 2004.
32. Cremens MC, Okereke OI. Alzheimer's disease and dementia. In Carlson KJ, Eisenstat SA, editors: *Primary care of women*, ed 2, St Louis, 2002, Mosby.
33. Francis PT. Neuroanatomy/pathology and the interplay of neurotransmitters in moderate to severe Alzheimer disease. *Neurology* 65:S5–S9, 2005.
34. Cummings JL. Alzheimer's disease. *N Engl J Med* 351:56–67, 2004.
35. Palmer K, Berger AK, Monastero R, et al. Predictors of progression from mild cognitive impairment to Alzheimer's disease. *Neurology* 68:1596–1602, 2007.
36. Panza F, D'Introno A, Colacicco AM, et al. Current epidemiology of mild cognitive impairment and other pre-dementia syndromes. *Am J Geriatr Psychiatry* 13:633–644, 2005.
37. Tariot PN. Treatment of agitation in dementia. *J Clin Psychiatry* 60(Suppl. 8):11–20, 1999.
38. Raivio MM, Laurila JV, Strandberg TE, et al. Neither atypical nor conventional antipsychotics increase mortality or hospital admissions among elderly patients with dementia: a two-year prospective study. *Am J Geriatr Psychiatry* 15:416–424, 2007.
39. Feldman H, Gauthier S, Hecker J, et al. Efficacy of donepezil on maintenance of activities of daily living in patients with moderate to severe Alzheimer's disease and the effect of caregiver burden. *Am J Geriatr Soc* 51:737–744, 2003.
40. Howard R, Rabins PV, Seeman MV, et al. Late-onset schizophrenia and very-late-onset schizophrenia-like psychosis: an international consensus. *Am J Psychiatry* 157:172–178, 2000.
41. Snowdon J. A retrospective case-note study of bipolar disorder in old age. *Br J Psychiatry* 158:485–490, 1991.
42. Krauthammer C, Klerman GL. Secondary mania. *Arch Gen Psychiatry* 35:1333–1339, 1978.
43. Rosenkoetter MM, Covan EK, Cobb BK, et al. Perceptions of older adults regarding evacuation in the event of a natural disaster. *Public Health Nurs* 24:160–168, 2007.
44. Borja B, Borja CS, Gade S. Psychiatric emergencies in the geriatric population. *Clin Geriatr Med* 23:391–400, 2007.
45. Steadman PL, Tremont G, Davis JD. Premorbid relationship satisfaction and caregiver burden in dementia caregivers. *J Geriatr Psychiatry Neurol* 20:115–119, 2007.
46. Kahan FS, Paris BE. Why elder abuse continues to elude the health care system. *Mt Sinai J Med* 70:62–68, 2003.

72 Neuroanatomical Systems Relevant to Neuropsychiatric Disorders

*Daphne J. Holt, MD, PhD, Dost Öngür, MD, PhD, Christopher I. Wright, MD, PhD,
Bradford C. Dickerson, MD, MMSc, Joan A. Camprodon, MD, MPH, PhD, and Scott L. Rauch, MD*

KEY POINTS

- The limbic system is composed of brain regions that participate in the comprehension of emotional meaning and the generation of emotional responses.

- The prefrontal cortex (PFC) receives and processes sensory, affective, and visceral information for the purpose of flexibly generating decisions, interpretations, social interactions, and other complex cognitions and behaviors, many of which are unique to human thought processes.

- Massive cortical input to the striatum is integrated by the striatum and the other nuclei of the basal ganglia (BG) for the purpose of selecting and executing goals that are of highest priority to the individual at a given point in time.

- The amygdala receives direct sensory inputs, as well as more processed information, to permit rapid evaluations of the emotional meaning and survival-relevance of information coming in from the environment.

- The hippocampus enables the binding together of information from unimodal and heteromodal association cortex into coherent perceptions and memories of those perceptions.

- Variations in the sequences of genes that are expressed in the brain can give rise to quantifiable variations in brain activity and in emotional and cognitive processes across individuals.

OVERVIEW

Since the mid-to-late twentieth century, neuroscience research in animals, neuroimaging experiments in humans, and studies of patients with localized brain lesions have greatly advanced our understanding of how thoughts and emotions arise in the human brain. However, the specific relationships between patterns of neuronal firing within individuals and aberrant emotional states remain poorly understood. Despite the absence of comprehensive information about the changes in brain physiology that occur in psychiatric disorders, knowledge of brain anatomy and function enhances the practice of psychiatry in several important ways. One of the gains is a philosophical one; the more we understand about how *all* human brains are organized, the more we can see that in some basic ways we are all fundamentally the same, given that the overall organization of the human brain (similar to other organs of the body) is fairly constant across individuals (over and above the inter-individual variability in the specific density of connections and neurons, chemical composition, and activity levels of some regions of the brain). This realization—of our material similarity—enhances our ability to empathize with patients and destigmatizes psychiatric illness. A second benefit is that a systems-neuroscience-based understanding of psychiatric illness can expand our theoretical models of how particular treatments work (whether the treatments are pharmacological or psychotherapeutic). This can promote more flexible and innovative clinical decision-making. Last, the exponential growth in knowledge about neural function in health and psychiatric disease will rapidly lead to the discovery of biomarkers of risk for mental illness, to new techniques for prevention, and to novel therapies for affected individuals. To keep abreast of these developments, all psychiatric practitioners must be, to some extent, fluent in the language of modern psychiatric neuroscience and the relevant neuroanatomical systems.

In this chapter, we will provide an overview of the anatomy and function of brain systems of particular relevance to the pathophysiology of psychiatric disorders—those subserving emotional and cognitive functions that are crucial to the organization of responses to the environment that promote the well-being and survival of the individual. Thus, we have focused on three neuroanatomical systems: the prefrontal cortex (PFC) (which mediates flexible control of goal-directed behaviors and regulates affective responses); the basal ganglia (BG) (which collect and integrate a wide range of sensory and affective information about the environment to direct the function of the PFC and initiate adaptive actions); and the medial temporal lobe (MTL) (which encodes, stores, and retrieves specific memories, as well as labels the emotional value of objects and situations, so that moment-to-moment interactions with the world optimally reflect knowledge gained from experience). These three systems interact with one another and with other regions of the brain to produce beliefs, decisions, emotional reactions, enduring mood states, and actions. We will also describe some of the evidence for abnormalities in these three systems in psychiatric disorders, emphasizing that it is likely that most psychiatric illnesses arise from abnormalities in the function of *networks* of brain regions, that include several regions that project to one another to serve a specific operation of the brain. For example, studies have found evidence for abnormal physiological interactions between the PFC and BG in addiction, schizophrenia, depression, and obsessive-compulsive disorder (OCD), and in the interactions of the PFC and MTL in anxiety disorders and schizophrenia. The identification of the unique pattern of functional change seen in each disorder, or a symptom or symptom cluster that arises in several disorders, is currently the subject of active investigation.

Before turning to the details of the organization of the PFC, BG, and MTL, several overall features of brain organization should be mentioned briefly. The brain tends to process incoming information from the environment in a predominantly unidirectional manner, with feedback given to previous stages of processing at many points along this input pathway. Thus, in general, sensory information is collected by the peripheral nervous system and the cranial nerves and then sent to the thalamus, which then sends information to separate territories of unimodal primary sensory cortex (i.e., visual, auditory, or somatosensory). Primary sensory information is then processed further in unimodal and polymodal association cortices, where this perceptual information is integrated and reconciled with perceptual expectations and information from other sensory modalities (in the polymodal areas), under the modulatory influence of selective attention. Thus, cortical processing proceeds from a detailed picture of a large portion of the external environment to an increasingly abstracted representation of the sensory data, such that only specific information that is required to serve the immediate needs of the individual is readily accessible. Higher-level cognitive operations in the polymodal association cortex in humans tend to be lateralized, with linguistic and computational processing occurring to a greater extent in the left hemisphere, while spatial, holistic types of processing occurring predominantly in the right hemisphere. There is evidence that emotional processing (both the evaluation of the emotional meaning of a stimulus and the expression of an emotional response), particularly of negatively-valenced emotions (such as sadness), occurs preferentially in the right hemisphere,[1,2] perhaps because emotional appraisal mechanisms are gestalt-like and holistic in nature.

Along this processing stream, the increasingly abstract representation of the outer world is integrated with sensory information sent from the internal milieu (e.g., "Am I in pain, hungry, tired, or relaxed?"); memories of past experience (e.g., "Have I seen this before?" "Who is this person?" or "Where am I?"); and current goals (e.g., "What am I trying to do now?" or "What do I want?"). This internally-generated information is collected by a loosely defined group of brain regions called the *limbic system*. This term was initially coined by the French anatomist Paul Pierre Broca in 1878,[3] who used the name the "*grand lobe limbique*," which means the lobe on the margin or rim, to refer to cortical regions on the medial edge or rim of the cortical mantle. Over subsequent decades it became clear that many of these medial cortical regions are involved in emotional function. The concept of the limbic system has subsequently undergone many revisions since it was first described in detail in the classic paper of James Papez in 1937, and expanded and popularized by Paul MacLean in the 1950s.[4] The most restrictive definition of the limbic system includes only the gyrus fornicatus (the cingulate gyrus, retrosplenial cortex, and parahippocampal gyrus), the hippocampus, and the amygdala. Based on a range of experimental data and behavioral observations gathered in animals and humans, these regions were initially deemed to represent the neural substrate of emotion. Because of the observation that emotional responses are tightly linked with endocrine and autonomic functions that are largely controlled at the central nervous system level by the hypothalamus, additional regions that have connections with the hypothalamus (including the anterior thalamus, septum, and substantia innominata) were subsequently included in the limbic system concept. Later the limbic system was expanded further to include telencephalic and mid-brain targets of the descending fibers of the medial forebrain bundle, the "limbic forebrain-mid-brain circuit," with the addition of the habenular complex, the ventral tegmental area (VTA), and dorsal raphe nuclei, among other areas.[5] Also, because the ventral striatum receives projections from the amygdala, VTA, and anterior cingulate gyrus, the ventral striatum has been referred to as the "limbic striatum." In general, a region may be deemed a member of the "limbic" system if it is part of the circuitry involved in the comprehension of the emotional meaning of information in the environment, or in the generation of emotional and related autonomic responses. However, it has been argued that many of the regions included in this designation are not primarily involved in emotion generation (e.g., the hippocampus participates in episodic memory processes and spatial navigation, but not directly in emotional responses).[6] Also, distinct networks of regions may be involved in the production of different types of emotions, such as fear, joy, or sadness. However, the general concept of the limbic system has been largely retained for the sake of convenience, in order to indicate brain regions that process emotional information and are thus involved in the planning, selection, and implementation of survival-promoting behaviors.

PREFRONTAL CORTEX

The portion of cerebral hemisphere anterior to the central sulcus is termed the *frontal lobe* (Figure 72-1). The frontal cortex is expanded significantly in primates, especially in humans. For purposes of definition, anatomists distinguish the primary motor cortex on the precentral gyrus from the rest of frontal cortex, which is termed *prefrontal cortex* (PFC) (see Figure 72-1). The nomenclature proposed by the German neuroanatomist Korbinius Brodmann is still in use, and the primary motor cortex is commonly called Brodmann's area 4 (BA4). Several PFC areas are also part of the motor system that controls striated muscle activity in the body: pre-motor cortex (BA6), supplementary motor area (medial BA6), pre-supplementary motor area (medial BA8) and frontal eye fields (BA8) on the dorsolateral surface of the frontal lobe, and cingulate motor areas on the medial surface.

The remaining PFC areas constitute a large expanse of association cortex, which defied classification and elucidation until the era of modern neuroscience. The term *association cortex* simply refers to those cortical areas that are not directly responsible either for sensory processing or for motor planning. In fact, it was recognized more than a century ago that damage to the PFC does not cause any focal abnormalities in sensory or motor function; rather, PFC lesions cause diffuse cognitive deficits and personality changes. Starting in the 1950s, advances in anatomy, physiology, and behavioral science showed that the PFC is not an amorphous association cortex that supports diffuse "higher functions"; instead, its orderly connections with other brain regions allow the PFC to subserve functions as diverse as spatial working memory, emotional vocalizations, and taste perception. In order to understand this diversity, it is best to consider three sectors within the PFC separately: the orbital PFC (often called the orbitofrontal cortex, or OFC), so-called because of its location directly superior to the orbits of the eyes; the dorsolateral PFC (DLPFC); and the medial PFC (mPFC) (which for our purposes includes the anterior cingulate cortex) (see Figure 72-1).

We will review each of these sectors in turn, while keeping in mind certain overall themes: the PFC receives significant innervation from monoaminergic systems, including dopamine and serotonin; each sector of the PFC has reciprocal relationships with a specific portion of the mediodorsal thalamic nucleus; and, like all cortical areas, PFC areas send a massive unidirectional projection to the striatum, which then

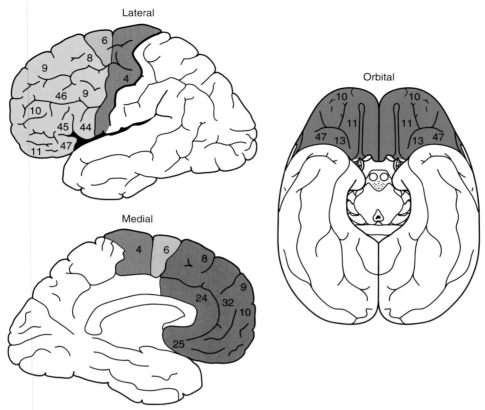

Figure 72-1. Schematic drawings of human prefrontal cortex, with the locations of Brodmann's areas (BAs) indicated with their respective BA numbers. The locations of the three main sectors of the prefrontal cortex are shown: dorsolateral prefrontal cortex (yellow), orbitofrontal cortex (blue), and medial prefrontal cortex (red). Also, on the lateral surface, the boundaries of primary motor cortex (dark green) and pre-motor cortex (light green) are shown.

funnels inputs to the pallidum and from there to the thalamus (Figure 72-2).

Orbitofrontal Cortex

The OFC is the cortex on the ventral surface of the frontal lobe. It is bounded by the insula and the basal forebrain posteriorly, the frontal pole of the brain anteriorly, the gyrus rectus medially, and the lateral frontal gyrus laterally (see Figure 72-1). There is a gradient of cortical differentiation within the OFC, with more posterior areas being more primitive agranular (i.e., lacking layer 4), five-layered cortex, while more anterior areas being well-differentiated six-layered cortex. This contrast is also reflected in the connections of the OFC, since sensory inputs from all five modalities and the viscera arrive at the posterior orbital areas, while direct sensory inputs into the anterior OFC are few. Olfactory and gustatory information reaches the posterior OFC via the primary olfactory and gustatory cortices located just posterior to the OFC, mostly within the insula. More highly-processed visual, somatosensory, and auditory information arrives in the OFC from parietal and temporal unimodal association areas devoted to each sensory modality. The somatosensory information arises from somatosensory cortex devoted to the mouth and hands, indicating a possible relationship to feeding. Finally, viscero-sensory information (denoting fullness) is relayed to the OFC from the nucleus of the solitary tract, via the ventroposterior medial thalamus and agranular insula.

Sensory inputs from each modality arrive at adjacent, but architectonically-distinct, cortical areas within the posterior

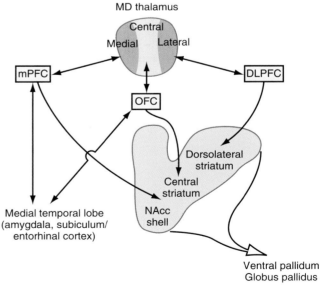

Figure 72-2. Diagram of the major connections of the prefrontal cortex. mPFC, Medial prefrontal cortex; MD, medial dorsal; OFC, orbitofrontal cortex; DLPFC, dorsolateral prefrontal cortex; NAcc, nucleus accumbens.

OFC. Each of these cortical areas then projects to more anterior OFC areas that integrate inputs from multiple modalities. Thus, there is a hierarchy of processing in the OFC, with anterior OFC areas receiving multi-modal sensory information, most of which appears to be related to appetitive or to reward-related behaviors (e.g., food and feeding-related behaviors in rats and non-human primates).[7]

No strong projections from the OFC to motor areas exist. Instead, projections from OFC areas fan out to the medial PFC (see below), and a range of sub-cortical targets (including the thalamus, striatum, MTL, hypothalamus, and brainstem). The entire PFC is reciprocally connected with the mediodorsal nucleus of the thalamus (MD), but each PFC sector appears to connect with a specific segment of the MD. The OFC receives strong projections from the central portions of the MD, and projects to the same region, creating the possibility of reverberating activity loops in this circuit (see Figure 72-2). In addition, the OFC projects to a central band in the rostral striatum, including the ventrolateral head of the caudate nucleus, dorsal nucleus accumbens, and medial putamen. This band is distinct from the striatal targets of the other PFC sectors, and projects to the ventral pallidum, which in turn innervates the MD. Thus, the OFC is embedded in a cortico-striato-pallido-thalamic loop similar to that described for the motor system.[8] The OFC also has largely reciprocal connections with the basal, accessory basal, and lateral nuclei of the amygdala, the subiculum, the entorhinal and perirhinal cortex, and the cortex of the temporal pole. Finally, the OFC sends a projection to the hypothalamus, as well as the periaqueductal gray (PAG) and other mid-brain and brainstem areas, but this projection is significantly weaker than that from the mPFC (see below). This projection also innervates the VTA and dorsal raphe nuclei, where dopaminergic and serotonergic neurons are located, respectively.

Studies in both rats and monkeys show that cells in the OFC respond not only to the sensory properties of stimuli but also to their affective significance, value, or priority. For example, the firing of neurons in the rat orbital cortex during an associative learning task codes better for the reward properties of a smell than for the identity of the smells.[9] In experiments on monkeys, neurons that fire strongly at the sight of a desirable food item while the animal is hungry have much lower response levels when the animal is satiated for the same food item. Many of these neurons are still responsive if other appetizing food items are presented. Although the OFC is part of a wider "reward" circuit (including limbic structures, the ventral striatum, and mid-brain dopamine neurons), the OFC is unique among these areas in coding for both the identity of sensory stimuli and their rewarding properties.[10]

Thus, the OFC is a cortical area that is ideally located to receive and to synthesize sensory information related to the rewarding properties of stimuli. In animals, food and feeding-related information is prominently represented in the OFC; in humans this is likely to extend to other kinds of rewarding stimuli. However, the OFC lacks the connections to prepare a motor program in response to the salient features of sensory stimuli it detects. Rather, it conveys this information to the mPFC, and to multiple brain areas involved in generating programs for action, including the striatum and hypothalamus (where fight-or-flight responses can be evoked), as well as to cell groups responsible for the release of dopamine and serotonin. In human neuroimaging studies, the OFC is activated during sensory processing of olfactory and gustatory stimuli, as well as during the determination of pleasantness and aversiveness of these stimuli.[11] Thus, it appears that the OFC is involved in the processing of appetitive and aversive aspects of sensation in humans. Also, changes in activity of this brain region have been repeatedly implicated in the

pathogenesis of anxiety and mood disorders. For instance, functional neuroimaging studies of subjects with OCD have found abnormally increased OFC metabolism at rest, as well as OFC activation during symptom provocation,[12] which may be related to elevated OFC functional connectivity in OCD.[13] In addition, subjects with bipolar disorder exhibit abnormalities in the activation of the OFC.[14] These findings indicate that the OFC likely plays a major role in the regulation of emotional activity in the brain.

Medial Prefrontal Cortex

The mPFC covers the entire medial surface of the frontal lobe, wrapping around the corpus callosum ventrally, anteriorly, and dorsally (see Figure 72-1). Similar to the OFC, there is a gradient of cortical differentiation within the mPFC where the ventroposterior mPFC areas and the anterior cingulate cortex (ACC) adjacent to the corpus callosum consist of five-layered cortex, while the more anterior areas close to the frontal pole are six-layered cortex. Here we include the ACC as part of the mPFC because of its anatomical location; however, many authors consider it phylogenetically and functionally distinct. The ACC is located on the cingulate gyrus, which wraps around the genu of the corpus callosum dorsally (the dorsal ACC is more closely related to attention and cognition) and ventrally (the subgenual ACC is implicated in mood disorders and emotional regulation).

Inputs to the mPFC arise mainly from other cortical areas: ventral mPFC areas (BA25) receive inputs from the OFC, dorsal mPFC areas (BA9) from the DLPFC, and the ACC (BA24) from other mPFC areas, as well as from the posterior cingulate cortex and parietal and temporal association cortices. The mPFC also receives relatively strong innervation from dopaminergic and serotonergic fibers. Outputs from the mPFC include projections to the medial portions of the MD thalamus, the basal nucleus of the amygdala, and lighter projections to the entorhinal cortex and subiculum. Within the mPFC, BA25 on the ventral medial wall provides the only substantial projection from all of the cerebral cortex to the shell of the nucleus accumbens.[15] BA25 and other mPFC areas also project to a ventromedial zone in the striatum (including the medial caudate nucleus, the core of the nucleus accumbens, and the ventral putamen).

There is a unique relationship between the mPFC and sub-cortical brain areas related to the autonomic nervous system. In primates, the mPFC provides the major cortical input to the hypothalamus, the PAG, and the dopaminergic, serotonergic, and noradrenergic brainstem nuclei. The mPFC projections to the hypothalamus and PAG are organized topographically. For example, the ventral mPFC (particularly BA25) projects to the ventromedial nucleus of the hypothalamus and the dorsolateral PAG, while the ACC projects to the dorsal hypothalamus and the lateral PAG. This is important because different regions within the hypothalamus and the PAG are associated with distinct functions (such as aggression, feeding, sexual behavior, thermoregulation, and anti-nociception). Such functions may occur separately, but they are often evoked together as parts of coordinated coping strategies. For example, stimulation of the lateral column of the PAG by excitatory amino acids generates tachycardia, hypertension, and analgesia as part of an overall confrontational behavioral stance.[16] Specific regions within the mPFC can therefore evoke a coordinated array of responses, and these responses will be distinct based on the part of the mPFC that is activated. This relationship between the ventral mPFC and sub-cortical autonomic areas has led some to term the ventral mPFC "visceromotor cortex" since it exerts an influence on the cardiovascular, gastric, and respiratory systems.[17]

synaptic contacts with the pallidal dendrites. The ventral pallidum, which receives projections from the ventral striatum, receives both substance P and enkephalin afferents from the ventral striatum. The GPe projects to the STN primarily via the subthalamic fasciculus.

Subthalamic Nucleus Organization

The STN is primarily composed of glutamatergic projection neurons. Many of the STN neurons have bifurcating axons that send one axon collateral to the GPi and the GPe and the other to the SNr. The STN receives massive inhibitory input from the GPe and also receives afferents from the cortex and the brainstem. The STN projects to the GPi, the SNr, and the GPe, as well as the ventral pallidum.

Substantia Nigra Organization

The SNr has a very similar organization to the GPi; the only major difference is that the SNr projects to the superior colliculus, playing an important role in the control of eye movements.

The SNc (A9) is just one of the cell groups within the midbrain dopamine neuron system, which also includes the ventral tegmental area (VTA) (A10) and the retrorubral cell group (A8). These dopamine-containing neurons can be distinguished from the overlying cells of the SNr by the fact that they contain melanin. The SNc has been divided into a dorsal and ventral tier of neurons.[40] The neurons of the dorsal tier, which includes the adjacent VTA as well as the dorsal SNc, express the calcium-binding protein calbindin, while the ventral tier neurons are calbindin-poor, express high levels of D_2 receptors and dopamine transporter, and extend their dendrites deeply into the SNr lying below the SNc. The ventral tier neurons are more vulnerable than those in the dorsal tier in Parkinson's disease.

There is a reverse dorsoventral topography in the connections between the SNc and the striatum. The dorsal tier neurons mainly project to the ventral striatum; thus, the nucleus accumbens receives its dopamine innervation almost exclusively from the VTA (which is part of the dorsal tier group). Also, the projections of the dopamine neurons to cortical regions arise primarily from the dorsal tier neurons, and the dorsal tier neurons also have reciprocal connections with the amygdala. In contrast, the ventral tier dopamine neurons largely project to the dorsal striatum.

The striato-nigro-striatal circuit has been proposed to provide one means for information exchange across the parallel cortical BG pathways. Ventral striatal regions are able to influence progressively more dorsal striatal regions by innervating portions of the mid-brain dopamine cell groups that project to larger portions of the dorsal striatum.[41] This "spiral" pattern of striato-nigro-striatal projections allows the ventral, limbic striatum to exert wide-ranging effects throughout the striatum and on cortical targets of the dopaminergic neurons.

Basal Ganglia Function

Overall

As the anatomy implies, the BG and the PFC work closely together to orchestrate goal-directed behaviors. It is assumed that each parallel BG-thalamocortical circuit performs a similar operation within its functional domain, although the exact nature of that operation remains unclear. One theory of BG function is that the massive input to the striatum from widespread areas of cortex is integrated and then used by the BG to select and to execute goals that are of high priority to the individual. Ultimately, a focused signal is sent to the PFC, via the thalamocortical projection, to execute an immediately

desired action, inhibiting less important or unwanted ones.[42] The dopamine neurons that project to the striatum exert their influence by detecting unexpected, important changes in the environment and altering their firing rates accordingly, "teaching" the striatal neurons to recognize the patterns of cortical input that signal important environmental changes. In this way, the dopamine input trains the striatum to respond to the immediate needs of the individual and to select courses of action that serve these immediate needs. Thus, although the cortex defines the individual's goals based on past and current knowledge, the BG are critical for the learning of new behaviors based on these goals, and the rapid, on-line adjustments of behavior required in the face of immediate changes in the external and internal milieu. Consistent with this model, data from experiments conducted in non-human primates suggest that the learning of rewarded associations occurs first in the BG; the BG then "teaches" the associations to the PFC, which acquires the associations more slowly.[43]

Motor

Electrophysiological recordings of neuronal activity in the striatum of monkeys have shown that neurons in the putamen increase their firing rates during both the planning and execution of movements, in a manner similar to pyramidal neurons within the motor and pre-motor cortical regions that project to the putamen. Cortical inputs to the putamen initiate movement-related activity in putamen neurons. Movement-related neurons are found throughout the BG motor circuit (motor and pre-motor cortical areas, the putamen, the GPi, and the GPe). Similarly, the oculomotor BG circuit, composed of a projection from the frontal eye fields to the central head and body of the caudate nucleus, and a projection from the caudate nucleus to the ventrolateral SNr, mediates the planning and execution of eye movements.

Cognition

The BG play an important role in unconscious, automatic forms of learning (such as procedural learning or habit formation). In humans, the striatum and cortex undergo a dramatic functional re-organization during the process of learning a repetitive sequence of movements; activity in the striatum and cortex shifts in an anterior (during initial learning of the movements) to posterior (when the movements are over-learned) direction, from more cognitively oriented (the head of the caudate nucleus and DLPFC) to motor (putamen and sensorimotor cortex) areas.[44] Abnormalities in striatal function during procedural learning have been found in patients with OCD.[45] The prefrontal-BG circuit may be selectively affected in OCD, leading to deficient routinization of cognitive processes that normally occur automatically and unconsciously (possibly giving rise to obsessions), with compensatory repetitive actions (compulsions) that take the place of normal habits of thinking and action.

Also, the prefrontal-BG circuits are involved in executive functions (such as working memory). The DLPFC, which has a central role in working memory processes as described earlier in this chapter, projects heavily onto the head of the caudate nucleus. Increased activity of the caudate nucleus during the "delay" portions of working memory tasks has been observed in both non-human primates and humans. Also, lesions of the caudate nucleus in humans and non-human primates cause working memory deficits that are similar to those produced by DLPFC lesions.[46,47] Patients with schizophrenia exhibit dysfunction of the DLPFC-caudate-nucleus circuit; the activity of the caudate nucleus and the DLPFC is abnormally increased during working memory tasks in patients with schizophrenia.[48]

Affective and Reward-Related Functions

Animal studies and neuroimaging studies in humans have shown that the dopamine neurons that project to the striatum, as well as the medium spiny projection neurons and cholinergic interneurons within the striatum, respond to reward-related stimuli (including food, pleasant odors, erotic material, pleasant pictures, and money). Studies in which monkeys are trained to associate a juice reward with a neutral cue have shown that dopaminergic neurons initially respond to the reward itself, but, after learning, the responses of these neurons shift to occur at the onset of the cue that predicts the reward.[30] The human striatum shows a similar shift following learning.[49]

Dopamine neurons are particularly sensitive to "prediction errors" or changes in reward contingencies: that is, they show increased activity when a reward is unexpected and decreased activity when a reward is expected but not delivered. Thus, when the occurrence of rewards is highly predictable, dopamine neurons stop firing. The striatum also exhibits this type of prediction-error-related activity.[50] Striatal neurons also code for reward magnitude,[51,52] and their responses are affected by internal motivational states and the relative value of a reward in a particular context. For example, the striatum and other reward-responsive regions are most active during the best outcomes in gambling tasks, regardless of the absolute value of the outcome (i.e., no loss in a high-risk situation and a large gain in a low-risk situation elicit similar levels of activity).[53] Neurons in other parts of the BG, including the GPe[54] and the ventral pallidum,[55] show reward-related responses, as well as neurons in other parts of the brain (such as the amygdala and the OFC).

Because striatal neurons also respond to aversive stimuli, such as electric shocks and aversive tastes, as well as to rewarding stimuli, it is thought that striatal neurons are tuned to the overall motivational salience of objects, regardless of whether the objects are likely to produce pleasure or cause harm.[56] Thus, given the role of the striatum in the assessment of intrinsically salient objects and experiences (such as food and pain), it is not surprising that the striatum also plays a role in complex social emotions and behaviors, such as the formation of monogamous attachments,[57] learning to trust a partner in an economic exchange,[58] and the satisfaction derived from punishing others.[59]

Psychiatric disorders (such as addiction, depression, and schizophrenia) may involve abnormalities in the reward and salience detection function of the BG. One hypothesis about addiction is that the transition from a voluntary to a compulsive, habitual use of drugs occurs when the influence of the PFC over BG activity is diminished; executive control of behavior and volitional choice give way to an automatic coupling of perception of drug-use-related cues and drug-seeking actions.[60,61]

Evidence from functional neuroimaging studies suggests that depression[62] and the negative symptoms of schizophrenia[63] are associated with deficient striatal responses to rewarding, pleasurable stimuli. Also, the hyperdopaminergic state of acute psychosis, which has been linked to increased dopaminergic neurotransmission in the striatum, may result in errors in salience detection, with misassignment of salience to non-salient stimuli, giving rise to false conclusions (delusions) and abnormal perceptions (hallucinations).[64,65]

MEDIAL TEMPORAL LOBE: AMYGDALA AND HIPPOCAMPUS

The amygdala and the hippocampus are found adjacent to one another within the medial temporal lobe (MTL); the amygdala is positioned rostral and, at more posterior levels, dorsal to the hippocampus. In the past, the proximity of these structures has led to uncertainty about their respective contributions to human behavior. However, it is now well established that the amygdala and hippocampus have different, although perhaps complementary, functions. Broadly speaking, the amygdala is central to emotional processing, while the hippocampus is dedicated to memory functions. Furthermore, these two regions are inter-connected, allowing the emotional meaning of a stimulus to influence memory, and conversely, for memory to influence the perception and expression of emotion.

Amygdala Nuclear and Cellular Structure

The amygdala is an almond-shaped group of cells located deep within the MTL (Figure 72-8). It is not a unitary structure; it is composed of several nuclei that have further sub-divisions (Figure 72-9).[66,67] The main medially located nuclei are the cortical (Co), medial (Me), and amygdalocortical transition areas (ATA; including amygdalohippocampal and amygdala pyriform transitions areas). In humans, the central nucleus of the amygdala (Ce) is centrally and dorsally located, while the lateral nucleus (La) forms the most lateral border of the amygdala. Within the basomedial nucleus (BM) and the basolateral nucleus (BL), further distinctions can be made, such as dorsal (d), intermediate (i), and ventral (v) sectors of the BL nucleus,

Coronal cross-section

Coronal T1 MRI image

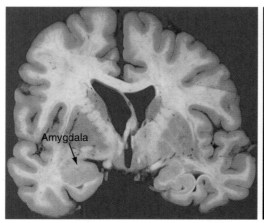
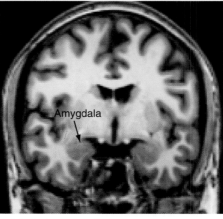

Figure 72-8. Location of the amygdala in the human brain.

which are differentiated based on cell size, with larger cells in the BLd and BLi, and smaller cells in the BLv. Dorsal and ventral parts of the BM can also be distinguished based on the presence of larger neurons in the BMd relative to the BMv.[68,69] In addition, there are a variety of other smaller nuclei, intercalated cell clusters, and structural extensions of the amygdala (i.e., the extended amygdala).

Amygdala nuclei can be grouped based on developmental, evolutionary, structural, or functional divisions. For example,

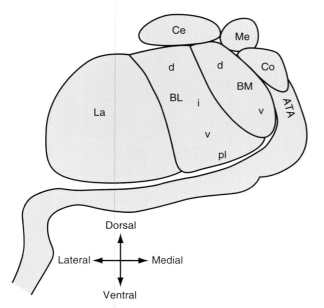

Figure 72-9. Nuclear divisions of the amygdala. La, Lateral nucleus; BL, basolateral nucleus; BM, basomedial nucleus; Ce, central nucleus; Me, medial nucleus; Co, cortical nucleus; ATA, amygdalocortical transition area; d, dorsal; i, intermediate; v, ventral; pl, paralaminar.

the cortical and medial nuclei, along with parts of the basal nuclei and piriform transition areas, may make up an evolutionarily preserved olfactory system. The central nucleus is considered to be the main output structure of the amygdala with primarily autonomic system projections, while the basolateral complex (including the lateral and basal nuclei) is particularly enlarged in primates and is closely connected to various higher-order cortical systems of the frontal and temporal lobes.

Intrinsic Amygdala Connections

Information flowing through the amygdala generally proceeds in a lateral-to-medial direction, from the lateral, basolateral, and basomedial nuclei to the central, medial, cortical, and transition areas. Thus, no nuclei project back to the lateral nucleus, but the lateral nucleus projects to essentially all other amygdala nuclei. The basolateral nucleus also projects to most other amygdala nuclei, with the exception of the lateral nucleus. Also, consistent with this lateral-to-medial organization of projections, the basomedial nucleus does not project to the basolateral or lateral nuclei, but does project to most other amygdala nuclei (including the central nucleus). In contrast, the central nucleus projects only to the medial, cortical transition area nuclei, but not back to the basomedial, basolateral, or lateral nuclei.

Extrinsic Amygdala Connections
Outputs

The amygdala heavily innervates select areas of cortex, including occipitotemporal visual cortices (including the fusiform cortex), the PFC (including the ACC and OFC), the insula, temporal pole, hippocampus, and entorhinal cortex (Figure 72-10).[68–71] Although the amygdala has weak direct projections to the DLPFC (mostly to areas 45 and 46), the ACC and the OFC receive direct connections from the amygdala and send

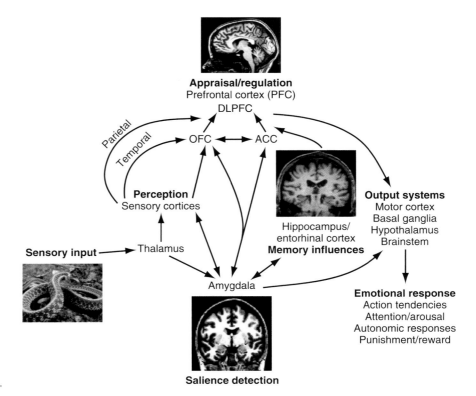

Figure 72-10. The circuitry of the amygdala.

projections to a large expanse of the DLPFC. The majority of amygdala-cortical projections come from the lateral, basolateral, and basomedial nuclei, with fewer cortical outputs emanating from central, medial, and cortical nuclei.

In addition to its cortical projections, the amygdala also projects to the hypothalamus, brainstem, basal ganglia, thalamus, and ventral forebrain structures, such as the nucleus basalis of Meynert and the bed nucleus of the stria terminalis. The lateral, basolateral, and basomedial nuclei project most prominently to the basal ganglia (including the ventral striatum) and the MD nucleus of the thalamus, allowing the amygdala to indirectly influence movement and PFC functions. The central, medial, and cortical nuclei innervate the hypothalamus, mid-line/intralaminal thalamus, pulvinar, cholinergic basal forebrain, and selected brainstem nuclei, where they may influence arousal-related, attentional, autonomic, neuroendocrine, and analgesic functions.

Inputs

The amygdala also receives substantial inputs from cortical areas, such as the occipitotemporal visual cortices, auditory cortex, PFC (including the ACC, OFC, and DLPFC), insula, piriform cortex, temporal pole, hippocampus, and entorhinal cortex. The majority of these projections are received by the lateral, basolateral, and basomedial nuclei, with fewer cortical inputs to the other amygdala nuclei. Sub-cortical projections to the amygdala come from olfactory regions, the hypothalamus, the brainstem, the thalamus, and the ventral forebrain structures. The inputs to the central nucleus of the amygdala are more varied and include many brainstem regions, such as the reticular formation, the noradrenergic locus coeruleus, the dopaminergic VTA, and the nucleus of the solitary tract, as well as the hypothalamus and the midline/intralaminar thalamus. These areas all provide the central nucleus with neuroendocrine, autonomic, visceral, and arousal-related information. The lateral, basolateral, and basomedial nuclei have inputs that are somewhat similar to those of the central nucleus, except there are fewer projections from brainstem areas, but heavier projections from the cholinergic basal forebrain.

Functions of the Amygdala

The amygdala is considered a hub for affective and social information processing in the human brain. Evidence for this comes from studies conducted in non-human primates and humans. For example, the amygdala is activated when people view human faces with neutral (Figure 72-11) or emotional expressions, individual components of emotional facial expressions, fearful bodily gestures, unpleasant scenes, and aversive olfactory and gustatory stimuli. In addition, the amygdala is engaged by positively valenced stimuli and rewards; by novel stimuli; and by movements that suggest a living organism. Not only does the amygdala respond to objects of known value, it is also instrumental in learning the value of external stimuli via the mechanisms of classical conditioning.

The Amygdala and Emotional Processing in Health and Psychiatric Disease

The amygdala mediates the rapid signaling of the biological relevance or salience of a stimulus.[6,71-78] This early signal may remain below the threshold of conscious awareness, quickly traveling to the amygdala from the thalamus, rather than taking the slower cortical route.[77,79] Rich sensory details also reach the amygdala via a relay through sensory association cortices; these cortico-amygdala pathways are thought to contribute to both non-conscious and conscious perception of the

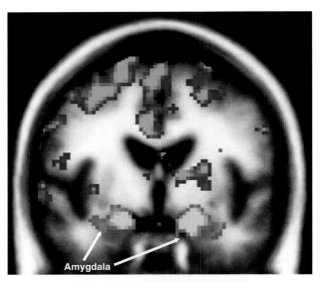

Faces > Cars   Cars > Faces

Figure 72-11. Amygdala responses to social information. A coronal view of a map of averaged functional MRI data collected from 32 young adults who viewed pictures of human faces or cars. The map shows the areas of the brain with significantly greater responses to the faces, compared to the cars (labeled in yellow-red) or the opposite comparison (labeled blue). Both the right and left amygdala are robustly activated in response to human faces, but not to cars. The significance of the activations displayed range from p = .05 to p = .0016.

emotional meaning of environmental stimuli. Directly following the initial appraisal of a stimulus, modification and regulation of the initial perception and emotional response to the stimulus ensue. This regulation process depends on communication within a network of regions including the amygdala, the hippocampus/entorhinal cortex, and various regions of the PFC, including the OFC and the ACC. The MTL memory system (entorhinal cortex/hippocampus) has a particularly important role in regulating amygdala responses, providing relevant past environmental or historical information about the stimuli of interest. The amygdala also reciprocally influences the activity of the MTL memory system, enhancing storage of emotionally salient memories. The medial PFC, including the ACC and the OFC, is also crucial for the regulation of amygdala activity, inhibiting amygdala-generated fear responses when they are no longer relevant. In addition, inputs from the diffusely projecting neurotransmitter systems from the brainstem (e.g., norepinephrine [noradrenaline] and dopamine) and basal forebrain (e.g., acetylcholine) influence amygdala activity during emotional processing and the formation of emotionally salient memories.

Variation in amygdala function is an important determinant of the individual differences in emotional processing found in healthy individuals. For example, baseline amygdala blood flow is positively correlated with self-reported levels of extroversion, and extroverts exhibit an increase in amygdala activity when exposed to pleasant or positive stimuli compared to introverts. Also, individuals with inhibited temperaments demonstrate elevated amygdala activation relative to uninhibited individuals when exposed to novel stimuli. Similarly, pessimists have greater amygdala responses to aversive visual stimuli than optimists.

Also, recent theories about the pathophysiology of psychosis, anxiety, and depressive disorders have focused on the amygdala and inter-connected structures.[75,80-84] Many functional neuroimaging studies have reported structural and functional alterations in the amygdala in schizophrenia, post-traumatic stress disorder, social anxiety disorder, generalized anxiety disorder, OCD, and depression. Also the amygdala exhibits structural and functional abnormalities in borderline personality disorder, a condition characterized by pronounced affective lability.

Genetic and Neurotransmitter Associations of the Amygdala

Recent studies have implicated specific genetic loci in the regulation of both amygdala reactivity and individual emotional responsivity. These findings may prove critical to an understanding of individual predispositions to mood and anxiety disorders. For example, several studies have documented the importance of serotonergic neurotransmission in amygdala responses to affectively laden stimuli. Human serotonin transporter and tryptophan hydroxylase gene variants are associated with increased amygdala activation to negative or emotionally evocative stimuli.[85,86] Also, the serotonin$_{1A}$ and serotonin$_{3A}$ receptor genes have been implicated in emotional processing, autonomic tone, depression, anxiety, and borderline personality disorder.

Variation in genes coding for neuromodulators other than serotonin have also been linked to variation in amygdala activity. There is evidence from animal and human studies showing that oxytocin and vasopressin receptor genes are involved in the neurobiology of affective reactivity and amygdala activity. Specifically, the balance of vasopressin and oxytocin receptor activation in the central nucleus of the amygdala may determine set-points for anxiety responses and the activation of autonomic brainstem centers by the amygdala. Also, corticotropin-releasing hormone, its receptors, and related peptides have been consistently implicated in the normal variation of amygdala responses and emotional reactivity. Future neuropsychiatric research will clarify the clinical implications of genetic variations affecting amygdala function and emotional responses.

Hippocampal and Parahippocampal Cellular Structure

The hippocampal and parahippocampal cortex are often considered together, as they make up the MTL memory system[87] and are both located in the ventromedial temporal lobe. The

parahippocampal gyrus includes the entorhinal cortex (antero-medially), perirhinal cortex (anterolaterally), and parahippocampal cortex (posteriorly) (Figure 72-12). The collateral sulcus is the major sulcal landmark that defines the lateral edge of the perirhinal cortex. The hippocampal formation lies deep to the parahippocampal cortical regions (Figure 72-13).[88] Beginning at the dorsomedial "shoulder" of the parahippocampal gyrus, there is a medial-to-lateral ordering of the parasubiculum, presubiculum, and subiculum, ending with the hippocampus proper, which all together comprise the hippocampal formation (see Figure 72-13A). The hippocampus proper includes the cornu ammonis (CA) regions CA1, CA2, CA3, and the dentate gyrus.[89]

The entorhinal, perirhinal, and parahippocampal cortex are transitional cortical regions, each with distinct cytoarchitectural features.[90] The entorhinal cortex contains layer II cell "islands," or clusters of neurons, as well as a cell-free layer IV (periallocortex). The entorhinal islands are visible grossly on the parahippocampal gyral surface as "verrucae" (warts). The perirhinal cortex, lying lateral to the entorhinal cortex, has a distinct layer IV and a patchy layer II (proisocortex). The parahippocampal cortex contains a more well-differentiated laminar structure than the entorhinal and perirhinal regions. With the transition to the subiculum, the laminar organization disappears and is replaced by three-layered cortex (allocortex). The CA fields and dentate gyrus also have only three layers, with a single pyramidal cellular layer.

Intrinsic Connections of the Medial Temporal Lobe Memory System

The classical trisynaptic circuit of the hippocampal system includes the perforant pathway (the projection from the entorhinal islands to the dentate gyrus), the mossy fibers (the projection from the dentate gyrus to CA3), and the Schaffer collaterals (the projection from CA3 to CA1). As is the case for intrinsic amygdala circuitry, the hippocampal circuit is largely unidirectional: CA3 does not project back to the dentate gyrus, nor do CA1 pyramidal cells project back to CA3. Axons from CA1 and the subiculum come together in the alveus, fimbria, and ultimately the fornix, the major output pathway of the hippocampal formation. This output pathway follows the trajectory of the ventricular system to reach the lateral septal nucleus, nucleus accumbens, neostriatum, anterior thalamus, and mammillary bodies (which project to the thalamus via the

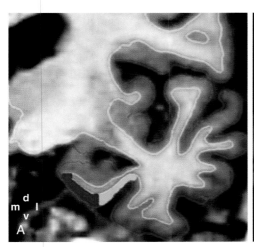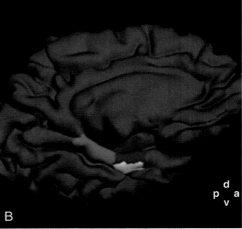

Figure 72-12. A coronal view of an MRI scan (A) and a computer-generated model of a sagittal view of the cortical surface (B) of the brain of a woman in her seventies. The cortex of the medial temporal lobe includes three major subregions: the entorhinal cortex (blue), perirhinal cortex (yellow), and posterior parahippocampal cortex (purple). m, Medial; l, lateral; d, dorsal; v, ventral; a, anterior; p, posterior.

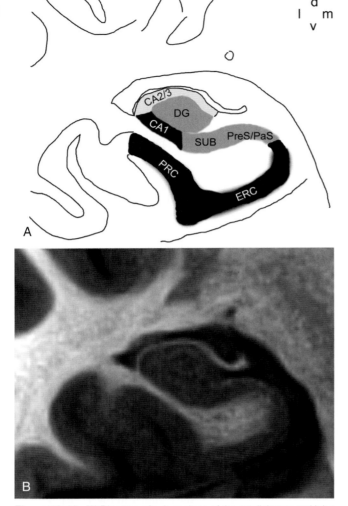

modulate signals leaving the hippocampus (via the entorhinal-to-CA1/subiculum pathway), possibly integrating these exiting signals with new input. Thus, the role of the entorhinal cortex may involve "on-line" monitoring of information processed by the hippocampus, for comparison with information newly entering the system. Projections from the entorhinal cortex to neocortical areas, such as dorsolateral and medial PFC, may allow this type of information to be used in the planning and execution of behavior in the appropriate context.[91]

Extrinsic Connections of the Medial Temporal Lobe Memory System

Visual information is sent to the MTL via two primary pathways. Visual object perception and identification are performed in the occipitotemporal (ventral, or "what") visual processing stream, which sends inputs to the lateral entorhinal cortex, which, in turn, projects to the hippocampal formation. Visuospatial and motion perception takes place in the occipitoparietal (dorsal, or "where") visual processing stream, which sends projections to the parahippocampal cortex, which, in turn, sends inputs to the medial entorhinal cortex. Processing within the hippocampal formation (particularly in CA3) is thought to enable the binding together of information coming from these two visual processing streams into one coherent perception,[92] along with the assignment of a temporal tag (a "time stamp").[93] The superior temporal gyrus, an auditory and polymodal association area, is also connected in a bidirectional manner with the entorhinal cortex.[89]

In addition to these links with sensory association cortices, there are bidirectional connections between the amygdala (primarily the lateral and basal nuclei) and the subiculum and the entorhinal cortex. In addition, multiple hypothalamic nuclei are reciprocally connected to the hippocampus, and cholinergic afferents to the hippocampus and entorhinal cortex arise from the medial septal nucleus and diagonal band of Broca. There are also hippocampal afferents arising from brainstem nuclei, including a noradrenergic projection from the locus coeruleus, and a serotonergic projection arising from the raphe nucleus, as well as some dopaminergic afferents from the VTA.

Also, prefrontal and parietal neocortical regions appear to play specific roles in memory function, which occur in part through poorly defined connections between these regions and the MTL. The PFC plays an essential role in both the encoding and retrieval of memories, but receives few direct projections from the hippocampus; instead, the MTL inputs to the PFC arise primarily from the entorhinal and medial temporal neocortex, targeting the DLPFC and mPFC. It has become increasingly clear that the medial and lateral parietal cortices, including the precuneus, posterior cingulate cortex, and retrosplenial cortex, have roles in memory that extend beyond the visuospatial processing operations that are traditionally ascribed to these parietal areas.[94] The density of connections of these parietal regions with the MTL is variable, with the posterior cingulate cortex demonstrating bidirectional connections with the entorhinal and subicular zones, while the medial parietal cortex has only sparse projections to the presubiculum.[95]

Finally, the MTL memory system, particularly the hippocampal formation, has extensive connections with the thalamus, most prominently with the anterior and medial divisions, including the anterior, medial dorsal, and intralaminar nuclei.[96] The anterior nucleus, by virtue of its inputs from the mammillothalamic tract and projections to the presubiculum, is critically involved in the encoding of new memories, and lesions of the anterior nucleus can produce dense amnesic states.

Figure 72-13. (A) Diagram of sub-regions of the medial temporal lobe memory system, including the perirhinal cortex (PRC), entorhinal cortex (ERC), parasubiculum (PaS), presubiculum (PreS), subiculum (SUB), and sectors of the hippocampus proper, including cornu ammonis 1 (CA1), CA2/3, and dentate gyrus (DG). Areas affected very early in the course of Alzheimer's disease are in black. (B) Coronal view of a high-resolution (380 μm) brain MRI, showing the medial temporal lobe of a woman in her twenties. d, Dorsal; l, lateral; m, medial; v, ventral.

mammillothalamic tract), targeting the posterior cingulate and retrosplenial cortices, as well as other neocortical regions.

In addition to the "classical" trisynaptic hippocampal pathway, which is contained within layers (or lamellae) of the hippocampus that are oriented perpendicular to its long axis, there is a projection from layer III of the entorhinal cortex directly to CA1, and a projection from CA1 and the subiculum back to deeper layers of entorhinal cortex. This second, non-classical pathway has a topographic organization; the most lateral sections of the entorhinal cortex send afferents to the most posterior zones of the hippocampus, and the most medial sections of the entorhinal cortex target the most anterior hippocampal zones. Thus, the entorhinal cortex is thought to be in a position not only to process information flowing into the hippocampus (via the trisynaptic pathway) but also to

Genetic Influences on the Medial Temporal Lobe Memory System

The expression of a large number of genes is essential for the development and normal activity of the MTL memory system. In recent years, human functional and structural neuroimaging studies have illuminated the effects of several gene variants on the MTL. Hypoactivation and reduced volume of the hippocampal formation has been demonstrated in normal young carriers of the met allele of the brain-derived neurotrophic factor (BDNF) gene.[97] Elevated prefrontal-hippocampal coupling during memory task performance has been observed in homozygous carriers of the met allele of the catechol-O-methyl transferase (COMT) gene.[98] The apolipoprotein E-4 allele is associated with altered hippocampal activation,[99] and may be related to hippocampal volume reductions in cognitively intact middle-aged individuals.[100]

These three gene variants are also associated with elevated risk for disease; certain COMT and BDNF genotypes confer increased susceptibility for schizophrenia, and the APOE genotype is related to risk for Alzheimer's disease (AD). However, it is also likely that such genetic variants explain some of the individual variability in MTL structure, function, and memory abilities throughout the life span.

The Medial Temporal Lobe Memory System in Neuropsychiatric Disorders

A number of neuropsychiatric disorders are associated with abnormalities of the MTL memory system. The most well-known disorders affecting these brain regions are AD, epilepsy, and schizophrenia, but a number of other illnesses, including depression, post-traumatic stress disorder, Korsakoff's amnesia, hypoxia, herpes encephalitis, limbic encephalitis, and some non-Alzheimer neurodegenerative diseases, are known to affect the MTL as well.[101]

Consistent with the effects of AD on memory function, it has been well established that the neuropathological process characteristic of AD targets the MTL. The layer II entorhinal islands are thought to represent a cell population that is particularly vulnerable to AD neurodegenerative pathology. These neurons undergo substantial degenerative change very early in the course of the disease, leading to disconnection of the hippocampus from the neocortex.[102] Perirhinal neurons are also devastated early in the course of AD.[90] As the disease progresses, neuropathological changes accumulate throughout the hippocampal sub-fields and MTL cortex. These abnormalities manifest at a macroscopic level detectable *in vivo* using volumetric magnetic resonance imaging (MRI)—the hippocampus and entorhinal cortex are atrophied even at early stages of AD.[103] Moreover, there appears to be a phase of MTL hyperactivation during the performance of memory tasks, detectable with functional MRI early in the course of AD,[104] similar to the physiological hyperactivity observed in animal models of the amyloid pathology of AD. Hyperactivation may reflect inefficient synaptic function within the MTL circuits. Investigation is ongoing to determine whether anticonvulsant or other medications aiming to reduce MTL hyperactivity may be useful in the treatment of prodromal AD.[105]

Complex partial seizures originating in the temporal lobe, or temporal lobe epilepsy (TLE), are associated with hippocampal sclerosis, particularly affecting CA1, an area which is particularly vulnerable to hypoxic-ischemic injury. In about two-thirds of TLE cases, hippocampal sclerosis is the only pathological change.[89] In other cases of TLE, the amygdala and other regions may be involved. Classically, the lateralization of the lesion in TLE often determines the nature of the memory deficits in these patients (i.e., left hippocampal sclerosis is often associated with more prominent verbal memory deficits, while right hippocampal sclerosis is associated with more prominent visual-spatial memory deficits).

In schizophrenia, memory deficits are present in addition to the abnormalities in executive function and other cognitive domains. Although there is no obvious neurodegenerative or pathological change in the MTL in schizophrenia, there appear to be subtle alterations in cytoarchitectural organization of several medial temporal lobe regions, including entorhinal cortex and hippocampal sub-fields.[106] Hippocampal atrophy has been observed *in vivo* in schizophrenia,[107] as has hippocampal hyperactivation.[108] As in AD, hyperactivation may reflect inefficient functioning of MTL circuits, although further study is required to clarify these observations in both disorders.

CONCLUSION

The three neural systems described in detail in this chapter are centrally involved in emotional and cognitive function in humans. Although what we know about the functions of these systems is under continuous revision, it is clear that the PFC and BG work together to guide the selection of behavioral priorities and goal-directed action, while the MTL encodes and retrieves affective and sensory experiences, which inform moment-to-moment behavioral choices. However, in addition to the three systems we have discussed, it must be emphasized that many other brain regions participate in the complex cognitive and emotional processes that are affected in psychiatric disorders. A few examples include the insular cortex (which receives sensory information from the autonomic nervous system and shows exaggerated responses to interoceptive signals in anxiety-prone individuals); medial and lateral parietal cortex (which participate in episodic and autobiographical memory); and temporoparietal cortex (including Wernicke's area, which mediates language comprehension, one of the most important social functions of the human brain). Also, the cerebellum participates in associative emotional learning and in a wide range of cognitive processes in addition to its role in extrapyramidal motor function.

Over recent decades of neuroscience research, the boundaries between "higher-order" and "lower-order" brain systems have become less well defined; for example, it has been observed that even some populations of neurons in unimodal sensory areas alter their firing rates in response to information about the emotional meaning of their inputs. Functional specialization of the brain appears to be dynamically balanced with the necessity for coordinated sets of complementary outputs (motor, cognitive, and affective) that facilitate the limited goals of the organism at each point in time. Thus, psychiatric neuroscience has increasingly focused on the detection of abnormalities in brain activity that affect coordinated networks of brain regions, which include areas that span multiple functional categories and levels of integrative processing. With an increasingly detailed and specific understanding of the normal structure and function of the components of these networks, our ability to detect relationships between human neurophysiology and conscious experience may soon lead to the development of quantitative methods to follow treatment response, and objective diagnostic tests to facilitate early detection and possibly prevention of psychiatric illness.

Access a list of MCQs for this chapter at https://expertconsult .inkling.com

REFERENCES

1. Davidson RJ, Irwin W. The functional neuroanatomy of emotion and affective style. *Trends Cogn Sci* 3:11–21, 1999.
2. Mesulam MM. Patterns in behavioral neuroanatomy: association areas, the limbic system, and hemispheric specialization. In Mesulam MM, editor: *Principles of behavioral neurology*, Philadelphia, 1985, FA Davis.
3. Broca P. Anatomie comparee des circonvolutions cerebrales. Le grand lobe limbique et la scissure limbique dans le serie des mammiferes. *Revue Anthropologique Ser 21* 21:385–498, 1978.
4. MacLean PD. Psychosomatic disease and the "visceral brain": recent developments bearing on the Papez theory of emotion. *Psychosom Med* 11:338–353, 1949.
5. Nauta WJH, Doane BK, Livingston KE. Circuitous connections linking cerebral cortex, limbic system, and corpus striatum. In *The limbic system: functional organization and clinical disorders*, New York, 1986, Raven Press.
6. LeDoux J. *The emotional brain*, New York, 1996, Touchstone.
7. Öngür D, Price JL. The organization of networks within the orbital and medial prefrontal cortex of rats, monkeys and humans. *Cereb Cortex* 10(3):206–219, 2000.
8. Haber SN, Kunishio K, Mizobuchi M, et al. The orbital and medial prefrontal circuit through the primate basal ganglia. *J Neurosci* 15(7 Pt 1):4851–4867, 1995.
9. Schoenbaum G, Eichenbaum H. Information coding in the rodent prefrontal cortex. II. Ensemble activity in orbitofrontal cortex. *J Neurophysiol* 74(2):751–762, 1995.
10. Schultz W, Tremblay L, Hollerman JR. Reward processing in primate orbitofrontal cortex and basal ganglia. *Cereb Cortex* 10(3):272–284, 2000.
11. Zald DH, Lee JT, Fluegel KW, et al. Aversive gustatory stimulation activates limbic circuits in humans. *Brain* 121(Pt 6):1143–1154, 1998.
12. Rauch SL, Jenike MA, Alpert NM, et al. Regional cerebral blood flow measured during symptom provocation in obsessive-compulsive disorder using oxygen 15-labeled carbon dioxide and positron emission tomography. *Arch Gen Psychiatry* 51(1):62–70, 1994.
13. Blumberg HP, Leung HC, Skudlarski P, et al. A functional magnetic resonance imaging study of bipolar disorder: state- and trait-related dysfunction in ventral prefrontal cortices. *Arch Gen Psychiatry* 60(6):601–609, 2003.
14. Linke J, King AV, Rietschel M, et al. Increased medial orbitofrontal and amygdala activation: evidence for a systems-level endophenotype of bipolar I disorder. *Am J Psychiatry* 169(3):316–325, 2012.
15. Ferry AT, Öngür D, An X, et al. Prefrontal cortical projections to the striatum in macaque monkeys: evidence for an organization related to prefrontal networks. *J Comp Neurol* 425(3):447–470, 2000.
16. Bandler R, Shipley MT. Columnar organization in the midbrain periaqueductal gray: modules for emotional expression? *Trends Neurosci* 17(9):379–389, 1994.
17. Frysztak RJ, Neafsey EJ. The effect of medial frontal cortex lesions on cardiovascular conditioned emotional responses in the rat. *Brain Res* 643(1–2):181–193, 1994.
18. Buckner RL, Andrews-Hanna JR, Schacter DL. The brain's default network: anatomy, function, and relevance to disease. *Ann N Y Acad Sci* 1124:1–38, 2008.
19. Etkin A, Egner T, Kalisch R. Emotional processing in anterior cingulate and medial prefrontal cortex. *Trends Cogn Sci* 15(2):85–93, 2011.
20. Carter CS, van Veen V. Anterior cingulate cortex and conflict detection: an update of theory and data. *Cogn Affect Behav Neurosci* 7(4):367–379, 2007.
21. Gusnard DA, Raichle ME. Searching for a baseline: functional imaging and the resting human brain. *Nature Rev Neurosci* 2:685–694, 2001.
22. Bush G, Luu P, Posner MI. Cognitive and emotional influences in anterior cingulate cortex. *Trends Cogn Sci* 4:215, 2000.
23. Drevets WC, Ongur D, Price JL. Neuroimaging abnormalities in the subgenual prefrontal cortex: implications for the pathophysiology of familial mood disorders. *Mol Psychiatry* 3(3):220–226, 1998.
24. Goldman-Rakic PS. Circuitry of the prefrontal cortex and the regulation of behavior by representational knowledge. In Plum F, Mountcastle V, editors: *Handbook of physiology*, vol. 5, Bethesda, 1987, American Physiological Society.
25. Miller EK, Cohen JD. An integrative theory of prefrontal cortex function. *Annu Rev Neurosci* 24:167–202, 2001.
26. Fuster JM. *The prefrontal cortex. Anatomy, physiology, and neuropsychology of the frontal lobe*, New York, 1989, Raven Press.
27. Lewis DA, Hashimoto T, Volk DW. Cortical inhibitory neurons and schizophrenia. *Nature Rev Neurosci* 6(4):312–324, 2005.
28. Nauta WJH. The problem of the frontal lobe: a reinterpretation. *J Psychiatr Res* 8:167–187, 1971.
29. Myers RE, Swett C, Miller M. Loss of social group affinity following prefrontal lesions in free-ranging macaques. *Brain Res* 64:257–269, 1973.
30. Damasio H, Grabowski T, Frank R, et al. The return of Phineas Gage: clues about the brain from the skull of a famous patient. *Science* 264(5162):1102–1105, 1994.
31. Haber SN. The primate basal ganglia: parallel and integrative networks. *J Chem Neuroanat* 26(4):317–330, 2003.
32. Schultz W, Apicella P, Ljungberg T, et al. Reward-related activity in the monkey striatum and substantia nigra. *Prog Brain Res* 99:227–235, 1993.
33. Alexander GE, Crutcher MD, DeLong MR. Basal ganglia-thalamocortical circuits: parallel substrates for motor, oculomotor, "prefrontal" and "limbic" functions. *Prog Brain Res* 85:119–146, 1990.
34. Middleton FA, Strick PL. The temporal lobe is a target of output from the basal ganglia. *Proc Natl Acad Sci U S A* 93:8683–8687, 1996.
35. Haber SN, Groenewegen HJ, Grove EA, et al. Efferent connections of the ventral pallidum: evidence of a dual striatopallidofugal pathway. *J Comp Neurol* 235:322–335, 1985.
36. Kimura M, Rajkowski J, Evarts E. Tonically discharging putamen neurons exhibit set-dependent responses. *Proc Natl Acad Sci U S A* 81:4998–5001, 1984.
37. Morris G, Arkadir D, Nevet A, et al. Coincident but distinct messages of midbrain dopamine and striatal tonically active neurons. *Neuron* 43:133–143, 2004.
38. Graybiel AM. Neurotransmitters and neuromodulators in the basal ganglia. *Trends Neurosci* 13:244–253, 1990.
39. Graybiel AM, Aosaki T, Flaherty AW, et al. The basal ganglia and adaptive motor control. *Science* 265(5180):1826–1831, 1994.
40. Meredith GE, Pattiselanno A, Groenewegen HJ, et al. Shell and core in monkey and human nucleus accumbens identified with antibodies to calbindin-D28k. *J Comp Neurol* 365(4):628–639, 1996.
41. Zahm DS, Brog JS. On the significance of subterritories in the accumbens part of the rat ventral striatum. *Neuroscience* 50:751–767, 1992.
42. Lynd-Balta E, Haber SN. The organization of midbrain projections to the striatum in the primate: sensorimotor-related striatum versus ventral striatum. *Neuroscience* 59:625–640, 1994.
43. Haber SN, Fudge JL, McFarland NR. Striatonigrostriatal pathways in primates form an ascending spiral from the shell to the dorsolateral striatum. *J Neurosci* 20:2369–2382, 2000.
44. Houk JC, Wise SP. Distributed modular architectures linking basal ganglia, cerebellum, and cerebral cortex: their role in planning and controlling action. *Cereb Cortex* 5(2):95–110, 1995.
45. Pasupathy A, Miller EK. Different time courses of learning-related activity in the prefrontal cortex and striatum. *Nature* 433:873–876, 2005.
46. Shadmehr R, Holcomb HH. Neural correlates of motor memory consolidation. *Science* 277(5327):821–825, 1997.
47. Rauch SL, Savage CR, Alpert NM, et al. Probing striatal function in obsessive-compulsive disorder: a PET study of implicit sequence learning. *J Neuropsychiatry Clin Neurosci* 9(4):568–573, 1997.
48. Battig K, Rosvold HE, Mishkin M. Comparison of the effects of frontal and caudate lesions on delayed response and alternation in monkeys. *J Comp Physiol Psychol* 53:400–404, 1960.
49. Partiot A, Verin M, Pillon B, et al. Delayed response tasks in basal ganglia lesions in man: further evidence for a striato-frontal cooperation in behavioural adaptation. *Neuropsychologia* 34:709–721, 1996.

50. Manoach DS, Gollub RL, Benson ES, et al. Schizophrenic subjects show aberrant fMRI activation of dorsolateral prefrontal cortex and basal ganglia during working memory performance. *Biol Psychiatry* 48(2):99–109, 2000.

51. O'Doherty JP, Dayan P, Friston K, et al. Temporal difference models and reward-related learning in the human brain. *Neuron* 38:329–337, 2003.

52. Pagnoni G, Zink CF, Montague PR, et al. Activity in human ventral striatum locked to errors of reward prediction. *Nat Neurosci* 5:97–98, 2002.

53. Cromwell HC, Schultz W. Effects of expectations for different reward magnitudes on neuronal activity in primate striatum. *J Neurophysiol* 89:2823–2838, 2003.

54. Delgado MR, Locke HM, Stenger VA, et al. Dorsal striatum responses to reward and punishment: effects of valence and magnitude manipulations. *Cogn Affect Behav Neurosci* 3:27–38, 2003.

55. Nieuwenhuis S, Heslenfeld DJ, von Geusau NJ, et al. Activity in human reward-sensitive brain areas is strongly context dependent. *Neuroimage* 25:1302–1309, 2005.

56. Arkadir D, Morris G, Vaadia E, et al. Independent coding of movement direction and reward prediction by single pallidal neurons. *J Neurosci* 24:10047–10056, 2004.

57. Smith KS, Berridge KC. The ventral pallidum and hedonic reward: neurochemical maps of sucrose "liking" and food intake. *J Neurosci* 25:8637–8649, 2005. 2005.

58. Zink CF, Pagnoni G, Martin ME, et al. Human striatal response to salient nonrewarding stimuli. *J Neurosci* 23:8092–8097, 2003.

59. Aragona BJ, Liu Y, Curtis JT, et al. A critical role for nucleus accumbens dopamine in partner-preference formation in male prairie voles. *J Neurosci* 23:3483–3490, 2003.

60. King-Casas B, Tomlin D, Anen C, et al. Getting to know you: reputation and trust in a two-person economic exchange. *Science* 308:78–83, 2005.

61. Tomasi D, Volkow ND. Striatocortical pathway dysfunction in addiction and obesity: differences and similarities. *Crit Rev Biochem Mol Biol* 48(1):1–19, 2013.

62. Robinson OJ, Cools R, Carlisi CO, et al. Ventral striatum response during reward and punishment reversal learning in unmedicated major depressive disorder. *Am J Psychiatry* 169(2):152–159, 2012.

63. Barch DM, Dowd EC. Goal representations and motivational drive in schizophrenia: the role of prefrontal-striatal interactions. *Schizophr Bull* 36(5):919–934, 2010.

64. de Quervain DJ, Fischbacher U, Treyer V, et al. The neural basis of altruistic punishment. *Science* 305:1254–1258, 2004.

65. Kalivas PW, Volkow ND. The neural basis of addiction: a pathology of motivation and choice. *Am J Psychiatry* 162:1403–1413, 2005.

66. Kapur S. Psychosis as a state of aberrant salience: a framework linking biology, phenomenology, and pharmacology in schizophrenia. *Am J Psychiatry* 160:13–23, 2003.

67. Holt DJ, Titone D, Long LS, et al. The misattribution of salience in delusional patients with schizophrenia. *Schizophr Res* 83:247–256, 2006.

68. De Olmos J. Amygdaloid nuclear gray complex. In Paxinos G, Mai JK, editors: *The human nervous system*, London, 2003, Academic Press.

69. Amaral DG, Price JL, Pitkanen A, et al. Anatomic organization of the primate amygdala. In Aggleton JP, editor: *The amygdala: neurobiological aspects of emotion, memory and mental dysfunction*, New York, 1992, Wiley-Liss.

70. Price J, Russchen F, Amaral D. The limbic region. II. The amygdaloid complex. In *Integrated systems of the CNS, part I, Hypothalamus, hippocampus, amygdala, retina*, vol. 4, Amsterdam, 1987, Elsevier.

71. Amaral DG, Behniea H, Kelly JL. Topographic organization of projections from the amygdala to the visual cortex in the macaque monkey. *Neuroscience* 118(4):1099–1120, 2003.

72. Weiskrantz L. Behavioral changes associated with ablation of the amygdaloid complex in monkeys. *J Comp Physiol Psychol* 49(4):381–391, 1956.

73. Calder AJ, Lawrence AD, Young AW. Neuropsychology of fear and loathing. *Nature Rev Neurosci* 2(5):352–363, 2001.

74. Phillips ML, Drevets WC, Rauch SL, et al. Neurobiology of emotion perception I: The neural basis of normal emotion perception. *Biol Psychiatry* 54(5):504–514, 2003.

75. Phillips ML, Drevets WC, Rauch SL, et al. Neurobiology of emotion perception II: Implications for major psychiatric disorders. *Biol Psychiatry* 54(5):515–528, 2003.

76. Phan KL, Wager TD, Taylor SF, et al. Functional neuroimaging studies of human emotions. *CNS Spectr* 9(4):258–266, 2004.

77. Rolls ET. *Emotion explained*, Oxford, 2005, Oxford University Press.

78. Wright CI, Wedig MM, Williams D, et al. Novel fearful faces activate the amygdala in healthy young and elderly adults. *Neurobiol Aging* 27(2):361–374, 2006.

79. Pessoa L, Japee S, Sturman D, et al. Target visibility and visual awareness modulate amygdala responses to fearful faces. *Cereb Cortex* 16(3):366–375, 2006.

80. Rauch SL, Shin LM, Wright CI. Neuroimaging studies of amygdala function in anxiety disorders. *Ann N Y Acad Sci* 985:389–410, 2003.

81. Rauch SL. Neuroimaging and neurocircuitry models pertaining to the neurosurgical treatment of psychiatric disorders. *Neurosurg Clin North Am* 14(2):213–223, vii–viii, 2003.

82. Mayberg HS. Modulating dysfunctional limbic-cortical circuits in depression: towards development of brain-based algorithms for diagnosis and optimised treatment. *Br Med Bull* 65:193–207, 2003.

83. Drevets WC. Neuroimaging abnormalities in the amygdala in mood disorders. *Ann N Y Acad Sci* 985:420–444, 2003.

84. Charney DS. Neuroanatomical circuits modulating fear and anxiety behaviors. *Acta Psychiatr Scand Suppl* 417:38–50, 2003.

85. Brown SM, Peet E, Manuck SB, et al. A regulatory variant of the human tryptophan hydroxylase-2 gene biases amygdala reactivity. *Mol Psychiatry* 10(9):884–888, 805, 2005.

86. Hariri AR, Holmes A. Genetics of emotional regulation: the role of the serotonin transporter in neural function. *Trends Cogn Sci* 10(4):182–191, 2006.

87. Squire LR, Zola-Morgan S. The medial temporal lobe memory system. *Science* 253:1380–1386, 1991.

88. Duvernoy HM. *The human hippocampus*, ed 3, Berlin, 2005, Springer-Verlag.

89. Insausti R, Amaral DG. Hippocampal formation. In Paxinos G, Mai JK, editors: *The human nervous system*, San Diego, 2004, Elsevier.

90. Van Hoesen GW, Augustinack JC, Dierking J, et al. The parahippocampal gyrus in Alzheimer's disease. Clinical and preclinical neuroanatomical correlates. *Ann N Y Acad Sci* 911:254–274, 2000.

91. Witter MP, Wouterlood FG, Naber PA, et al. Anatomical organization of the parahippocampal-hippocampal network. In Scharfman HE, Witter MP, Schwarcz R, editors: *The parahippocampal region: implications for neurological and psychiatric diseases*, vol. 911, New York, 2000, Annals of the New York Academy of Sciences.

92. Eichenbaum H. Hippocampus: cognitive processes and neural representations that underlie declarative memory. *Neuron* 44:109–120, 2004.

93. Kesner RP, Hunsaker MR, Gilbert PE. The role of CA1 in the acquisition of an object-trace-odor paired associate task. *Behav Neurosci* 119(3):781–786, 2005.

94. Wagner AD, Shannon BJ, Kahn I, et al. Parietal lobe contributions to episodic memory retrieval. *Trends Cogn Sci* 9(9):445–453, 2005.

95. Parvizi J, Van Hoesen GW, Buckwalter J, et al. Neural connections of the posteromedial cortex in the macaque. *Proc Natl Acad Sci U S A* 103(5):1563–1568, 2006.

96. Van der Werf YD, Jolles J, Witter MP, et al. Contributions of thalamic nuclei to declarative memory functioning. *Cortex* 39(4–5):1047–1062, 2003.

97. Egan MF, Kojima M, Callicott JH, et al. The BDNF val66met polymorphism affects activity-dependent secretion of BDNF and human memory and hippocampal function. *Cell* 112(2):257–269, 2003.

98. Schott BH, Seidenbecher CI, Fenker DB, et al. The dopaminergic midbrain participates in human episodic memory formation: evidence from genetic imaging. *J Neurosci* 26(5):1407–1417, 2006.

99. Bookheimer SY, Strojwas MH, Cohen MS, et al. Patterns of brain activation in people at risk for Alzheimer's disease. *N Engl J Med* 343(7):450–456, 2000.

100. Lind J, Larsson A, Persson J, et al. Reduced hippocampal volume in non-demented carriers of the apolipoprotein E epsilon4: relation to chronological age and recognition memory. *Neurosci Lett* 396(1):23–27, 2006.

101. Dickerson BC, Eichenbaum H. The episodic memory system: neurocircuitry and disorders. *Neuropsychopharmacology* 35(1):86–104, 2010.

102. Hyman BT, Van Hoesen GW, Damasio AR, et al. Alzheimer's disease: cell-specific pathology isolates the hippocampal formation. *Science* 225(4667):1168–1170, 1984.

103. Dickerson BC, Goncharova I, Sullivan MP, et al. MRI-derived entorhinal and hippocampal atrophy in incipient and very mild Alzheimer's disease. *Neurobiol Aging* 22:747–754, 2001.

104. Dickerson BC, Salat DH, Greve DN, et al. Increased hippocampal activation in mild cognitive impairment compared to normal aging and AD. *Neurology* 65(3):404–411, 2005.

105. Bakker A, Krauss GL, Albert MS, et al. Reduction of hippocampal hyperactivity improves cognition in amnestic mild cognitive impairment. *Neuron* 74(3):467–474, 2012.

106. Arnold SE. Cellular and molecular neuropathology of the parahippocampal region in schizophrenia. *Ann N Y Acad Sci* 911:275–292, 2000.

107. Weiss AP, DeWitt I, Goff D, et al. Anterior and posterior hippocampal volumes in schizophrenia. *Schizophr Res* 73:103–112, 2005.

108. Holt DJ, Kunkel L, Weiss AP, et al. Increased medial temporal lobe activation during the passive viewing of emotional and neutral facial expressions in schizophrenia. *Schizophr Res* 82:153–162, 2006.

73 The Neurological Examination

Evan D. Murray, MD, and Bruce H. Price, MD

KEY POINTS

- Cognitive impairment, behavioral changes, and psychiatric symptoms occur frequently in association with neurological conditions.
- A well-performed mental status and neurological examination are essential for the identification of medical and neurological conditions that impact cognition, behavior, and mood.
- The objective of the neurological examination is to verify the integrity of the central and peripheral nervous systems and to achieve neuroanatomical localization of signs and symptoms. Localization is a crucial step for the generation of a rational differential diagnosis.
- The neurological examination can be conceived of as being conducted along a continuum of complexity that builds on information acquired during its performance. It is fluidly adapted during its performance with components added, as needed, to clarify findings.
- The interpretation of findings requires careful and effective integration with knowledge of neuroanatomy and the clinical history.
- A well-organized and rehearsed examination promotes consistency and comprehensiveness of technique while reducing omissions of elements of the examination.

OVERVIEW

Proficiency in performing a neurological examination is advantageous to the psychiatrist. All behavior and perception occurs as a result of neural activity. Neural activity arises from brain circuitry that is developmentally sculpted through the interaction of environmental factors with human genetic potential.[1] Neural circuitry is susceptible to malfunction and damage in a host of ways; this results in many recognizable patterns of cognitive and behavioral impairments. The neurological examination is of tremendous utility for identifying these patterns and thereby allowing for recognition of neurological processes that may be treated. Neurological conditions are frequently co-morbid with psychiatric symptoms. Such symptoms may stem from the stress of illness, be a direct function of brain pathology, or result from a combination of the two. Psychiatric symptoms and behavioral changes may precede other key physical manifestations of the disorder or occur at any time during the disease course.[2] An effective and reliable neurological examination may afford opportunities for earlier detection of treatable conditions, anticipation of psychiatric manifestations, and avoidance of adverse events (e.g., neuroleptic sensitivity of patients with Lewy body dementia) in persons who are at particular risk.

By the late nineteenth century the elementary neurological examination was refined with objective, consistent, and reproducible findings.[3] The practice of the examination is consid-ered most effective when the clinician has formed a hypothesis that is based on observation and history and is prepared to fluidly adapt both the examination and the hypothesis as new information and findings appear. A well-rehearsed examination prevents omissions and ensures consistency of technique. A well-reasoned examination with an array of alternative techniques that verify findings ensures greater accuracy and confidence in those findings. The complexity of planning, performing, and interpreting the neurological examination is a challenge that persists throughout the entirety of a physician's career.

The neurological examination is performed routinely for most psychiatric admissions but is uncommonly performed in outpatient psychiatric settings. In some circumstances, a careful history alone may establish a neurological diagnosis; however, this is often not the case. The examination is helpful for corroborating the history, establishing the severity of a condition, and directing treatment. The overall assessment approach should use a reproducible methodology for obtaining and interpreting the history, performing the examination, and analyzing both. A comprehensive neurological examination is unnecessary in every patient. The clinician must learn to focus or expand the examination as needed. A good examination can be instrumental in discerning primary psychiatric illness from secondary symptoms that occur in association with a multitude of neurological conditions (such as stroke, Alzheimer's disease, Huntington's disease, Parkinson's disease, and demyelinating disease). (See Box 73-1 for a summary of major neurological findings and associated conditions that frequently manifest by psychiatric symptoms.) Malingering and conversion disorder need to be distinguished from deficits that localize to specific neuroanatomy.[4] Medication side effects, such as parkinsonism and dystonia, need to be identified, treated, and followed clinically.

General principles include:

- Assess for side-to-side symmetry during the neurological examination. One side of the body serves as a control for the other. Determine if there is focal asymmetry.
- Determine if dysfunction originates from the central nervous system (CNS), peripheral nervous system (PNS), or both.
- Consider if the finding (or findings) can be explained by a single lesion or whether a multi-focal process is required.
- Establish the lesion's location. If the process involves the CNS, clarify if it is cortical, subcortical, or multi-focal. If subcortical, clarify if it is in the white matter, basal ganglia, brainstem, cerebellum, or spinal cord.
- If the process involves the PNS, determine if it localizes to the nerve root, plexus, peripheral nerve, neuromuscular junction, muscle, skin, or if it is multi-focal.

Some of this localization, particularly to the PNS, will exceed the expertise of most psychiatrists. These principles are presented as tools to organize thinking.

There is no clear consensus among experts as to the order of performing and presenting the neurological examination. However, there is little dispute about the mental status portion being performed first followed by examination of the cranial nerves. Thereafter, there are variations in the sequence, selected components of the examination, methods of performance, terminology used to describe findings, and the interpretation

---

BOX 73-1 Neurological Abnormalities That Suggest Diseases Associated with Psychiatric Symptoms

EXAMINATION ABNORMALITIES AND THEIR POSSIBLE UNDERLYING ETIOLOGY

Vital signs
- Marked hypertension (hypertensive encephalopathy, serotonin syndrome, neuroleptic malignant syndrome, pre-eclampsia)
- Tachypnea (delirium caused by systemic infection)
- Hypoventilation (hypoxia, alcohol withdrawal, sedative intoxication)

Cranial nerves
- Hyposmia, anosmia or odor misidentification (traumatic brain injury, Alzheimer's and Parkinson's disease)
- Visual field deficit (stroke, mass, multiple sclerosis, systemic lupus erythematosus)

Pupils
- Argyll Robertson (neurosyphilis)
- Unilateral dilation (brain herniation, porphyria)
- Horner's syndrome (stroke, carotid disease, demyelinating disease)

Ophthalmoplegia
- Vertical gaze palsy (progressive supranuclear palsy)
- Mixed (Wernicke-Korsakoff syndrome, chronic basilar meningitis)

Cornea
- Kayser-Fleischer rings (Wilson's disease)

Lens
- Cataracts (chronic steroids, Down's syndrome)

Fundi
- Papilledema (intracranial mass lesion, multiple sclerosis)
- Optic pallor (multiple sclerosis, porphyria, Tay-Sachs disease)

Extrapyramidal (Parkinson's disease, Lewy body disease, Huntington's disease, stroke, Wilson's disease, numerous others)

Cerebellar (alcohol, hereditary degenerative ataxias, paraneoplastic, use of phenytoin)

Motor neuron (amyotrophic lateral sclerosis, frontotemporal dementia with motor neuron disease)

Peripheral nerve (adrenomyeloneuropathy, metachromatic leukodystrophy, vitamin B_{12} deficiency, porphyria)

Gait
- Apraxia (normal pressure hydrocephalus, frontal dementias)
- Spasticity (stroke, multiple sclerosis)
- Bradykinesia (multi-infarct dementia, Parkinson's disease, progressive supranuclear palsy, Lewy body disease)

BOX 73-2 Components of Elemental Neurological Examination

CRANIAL NERVES

Olfaction I
Vision II
- Visual fields (VF)
- Acuity
- Optic disks/vessels (performed after VF and acuity)

Pupillary reflexes II, III
Eye movements III, IV, VI
Facial sensation/jaw strength V
Facial movement VII
Hearing VIII
Palate IX, X
Speech/dysarthria IX, X, XII
Head rotation XI
Shoulder shrug XI
Tongue movement XII

MOTOR

Involuntary movements/adventitious movements
Muscle bulk
Tone
Strength
Hand drift/pronation/posturing

SENSATION

Light touch
Joint position sense
Vibration
Pinprick (pain)/temperature (pick one of these)
Romberg

COORDINATION

Finger to nose/follow the target
Fine motor movements
Rapid alternating movements
Heel to shin

GAIT

Station
Spontaneous ambulation
Toe/heel/tandem
Postural reflexes

REFLEXES

Deep tendon reflexes
Cutaneous reflexes
Plantar responses
Atavistic or primitive reflexes

---

of various findings. Clinicians should decide on a sequence, practice and become proficient at it, and then use it consistently. This improves performance and speed, provides a database of variations in responses, and reduces the likelihood of forgetting to perform aspects of the examination. A common approach and examination sequence will be offered along with some options for expanding the examination and validating findings with use of other maneuvers (Boxes 73-2, 73-3, and 73-4).

THE EXAMINATION

Patient well-being and examiner safety are important concerns from the outset. To safeguard these, assessment of the patient's receptiveness to evaluation, ability to cooperate, cultural sensitivities, and mental state should be accomplished at the earliest time. If one anticipates that the evaluation will agitate the patient or that conditions are deemed unsafe, then the evaluation should be discontinued or delayed until such a time when conditions are more favorable. The patient should be forewarned about any elements of the examination that might produce discomfort. In some cases the patient may have a heightened sensitivity to an examiner of the same or opposite gender. In such circumstances, a chaperone can provide useful reassurance during the interview and examination. Vital signs should be reviewed to assess for factors that may contribute to behavioral changes, such as very elevated blood pressure, fever, and hypoxia. Changes in blood pressure, pulse, and respirations may occur in a variety of contexts, such as with agitation, psychosis, alcohol withdrawal, complex partial seizures, and medical conditions, to name only a few. The examination begins when entering a patient's room or encountering the patient in the hallway. Initial observations are made wherever the patient is found, be it walking down the hall to meet you or lying in bed. Whether the patient is aware of being observed can be important since behavior may change when out of the physician's view.

Textbooks have been dedicated to various aspects of cognitive assessment. This section will introduce the fundamental aspects of the cognitive examination; some helpful anatomical and neuropsychiatric considerations will also be presented.

The Psychiatric Portion of the Mental Status Examination

The separation of the mental status examination into psychiatric portions and neurological portions represents a historical difference in emphasis rather than purpose; this distinction will be continued for the purpose of clarity. (See Box 73-3 for a summary of the components of the psychiatric portion of the mental status examination.)

Initial Observations of the Patient

General Appearance. Observations start with determination as to whether the patient appears morphologically normal. Consider stature, hair-line, level of ears, distance between eyes, presence of philtrum, length of neck, and body characteristics (such as gynecomastia, obesity, and digit length). These may be indicative of a genetic syndrome or a genetic disorder. Mention of these characteristics is intended as a reminder rather than a comprehensive review of this topic.

Behavioral Appearance. Hygiene, body odor, posture, demeanor, cooperativeness, motivation, spontaneity, eye contact, speed of movement, the manner of dress, social graces, and attitude toward the examiner should be noted. A patient may be anxious, inattentive, engaged, cooperative, apathetic, disinhibited, angry, hostile, or extremely courteous.

Speech. Manifestations of speech include speed, fluency, volume, and prosody. A person with a history of 4 days of speaking very quickly and being very hard to interrupt in conversation may be manic or be under the influence of drugs. Prosody describes the melodic patterns of intonation in language that convey shades of meaning. Impairment may be in the production of prosody, or in the comprehension of another person's prosody. Testing prosody is uncommonly done. If clinically indicated, appreciation of prosody can be tested by situating oneself behind the patient and saying a short sentence, such as "I'm going home now," with four different emotional tones (e.g., happy, sad, angry, and neutral). Being positioned behind the patient prevents the patient from interpreting the expression of your face. One should ask the patient to identify the emotional state of each of your theatrical renditions. Prosody production may be tested by asking the patient to repeat the same sentence in each of the emotional states previously listed. Listening for the patient's spontaneous prosody is also essential.

Mood and Affect. *Mood* is the patient's report of his or her emotional state. *Affect* is the outward expression of the patient's mood to the world. Descriptions of affect include the terms *flat, constricted, elevated, sad, expansive,* and *labile.*

A patient with a stooped posture, slow speech, and flat affect could be manifesting signs of depression. If his stated mood is "sad" or "depressed," his mood and affect are congruent. Some neurological conditions may be associated with a disassociation of mood and affect. A condition now known as *involuntary emotional expression disorder* (IEED),[5] previously named *pseudobulbar affect* or *palsy,* is characterized by episodes of involuntary or exaggerated emotional expression. This results from brain disorders affecting structures of a neural network involving the frontal lobes, limbic system, brainstem, cerebellum, or the inter-connecting white matter tracts. Extremes of emotional expression (from crying to, less often, laughing) occur without the patient actually feeling these emotions or without the patient feeling the concordant degree of the emotion expressed. IEED can occur in association with a number of neurological conditions including dementia (including Alzheimer's disease, vascular dementia, and frontotemporal dementia), amyotrophic lateral sclerosis

(ALS), multiple sclerosis, stroke, and traumatic brain injury (TBI).

Thought Process. Normal thought, as demonstrated in casual conversation and most other circumstances, is goal-directed; it does not require great effort to follow the logical progression of ideas. Some common descriptive terms include *linear thinking, loose associations, circumstantial thought, tangential ideas, flight of ideas, disorganized thinking, incoherent thought,* and *perseverative thinking.*

Thought Content. This can be derived from what the patient tells you, from what you can infer from the patient's history, and from your observations of personal interactions. A patient may be extremely guarded and careful about when, and if, to reveal his or her true beliefs. Terms that commonly refer to thought content include *preoccupations, ruminations, obsessions, paranoia, delusions, ideas of reference,* and *suicidal or homicidal ideation.* There can also be a poverty of content.

Terms such as *paranoia, thought blocking,* and *ideas of reference* may be interpreted as involving perceptions, thought process, or content.[6]

Perceptions. Hallucinations may be auditory, visual, tactile, gustatory, or olfactory. They may be simple (as in a flash of light) or complex (as in seeing panoramic scenes or feeling a kiss). The content of hallucinations and their relationship to mood are important to identify. Psychiatric disorders more often than not have mood-congruent hallucinations. Insight regarding the hallucination is an important characteristic that may aid in the differential diagnosis. For example, some persons with Lewy body dementia or an infarct to the midbrain peduncle (leading to peduncular hallucinosis) and most every person with Charles Bonnet syndrome will realize that their visual hallucinations are not real. Illusions, or perceptual distortions, may also occur.

Insight/Awareness/Concern. The level of *insight* is commonly derived from the patient's description of his or her circumstances and relates to how the patient's problems evolved and how they are understood. The patient's *comportment* (behavior and self-conduct) is an indicator of insight.

Judgment. Determination of judgment is usually derived from aspects of the history. The patient's interactions with family, friends, and health care professionals can be used to assess social appropriateness, social graces, and comportment. Disinhibition or poor judgment may be ascertained through observation or elements of the history.

The Neurological Portion of the Cognitive Mental Status Examination

The following sequence affords the opportunity to evaluate cognition in a hierarchy of increasing complexity. Subsequent performance on complex tasks requires that more basic aspects of cognition are intact. (See Box 73-4 for a more complete summary of the components of the neurological mental status examination.)

Level of Consciousness

Consciousness is most commonly viewed as being a function of the level of arousal. The lowest level of consciousness has many descriptive terms, some of which imply a pathological state, such as *coma.* A patient might appear to be comatose yet actually be in non-convulsive status epilepticus.[7] An awareness of the nuances of descriptive terms will help avoid confusion in most circumstances. One common method is to describe arousability with respect to pain, loud noise, voice, and command. The relative ease or difficulty of arousability with these stimuli is also noted.

Attention

After determination of the level of consciousness, the ability to sustain attention and the speed of task completion should be assessed. The perceived level of effort should be documented when performance is reduced. Common tasks used to assess attention and processing speed include the following:

Performance of Serial 7s. Ask the patient to subtract 7 from 100. Then ask the patient to continue subtracting 7 (and to state the results); have the patient stop when he or she reaches 65. Serial 3s from 100 or counting backwards from 20 by 1s may also be used. The patient should be able to maintain attention on task after starting without having the instructions repeated. This test must be interpreted in the context of the patient's background, education, and mathematical ability.

Spelling Tests. Have the patient spell the word "world," "march," "chair," or "radio" forward, backward, and then alphabetized. *Forward-spelling* is a test of simple attention. *Backward-spelling* requires concentration. Alphabetizing the letters is a test of concentration and verbal working memory. This testing presumes some degree of spelling ability.

Other Tests. Have the patient state the days of the week (or months) forward then backward. Digit span also tests attention. It is a test during which a patient is presented with successively longer strings of random digits starting at two or three digits and with each rendition increasing the string by one digit until the patient reaches a string between five and seven digits. Performance, to some degree, depends on age; however, there is little decay in this ability with normal aging. This test may also be performed backwards. Normal performance is seven digits forward and five digits backwards. However, recalling six digits forward and four digits backwards is probably acceptable. It is considered normal to have a difference of two between forward and backward testing.[8]

Language

Language is a term that can refer to a variety of types of thought expression that can include facial expressions, sign language, and symbolic communication, as well as written and spoken language. During a screening examination, concerns should focus on the assessment of spoken and written language. The intent is to determine whether the patient has difficulties producing language, comprehending language, or both. The examiner's answers to the following questions provide a basic screen.

Does the patient's speech sound like language? Is the speech fluent or non-fluent? Fluency has been described as speech that is flowing rapidly and effortlessly. Non-fluent speech is uttered in single words or short phrases with frequent pauses and hesitations. Fluency can usually be appreciated during conversation with the patient. The examiner should observe the patient's use of grammatical structure. Fluency can be independent of content and comprehensibility. Testing the ability to name visually presented objects screens for aphasia. A key, stapler, coin, pencil or pen, watch, clothing, and furniture are commonly used.

Comprehension. Comprehension is often easily assessed while taking the history and performing the physical examination. When there is difficulty, one can request that the patient perform a one- to three-step command. If the patient appears impaired, the examiner should start with simple questions that can be answered in a yes/no fashion. Asking a patient to point at objects or to show his or her thumb or another body part are alternatives. Bear in mind that more complex commands will require intact attention and comprehension of grammar and language. Having the patient read an instruction aloud and perform it is a brief screen of reading comprehension. Examples include "point to the window" and "close your eyes".

Repetition. Asking the patient to repeat "no ifs, ands, or buts" is a common phrase used to test repetition. If greater sensitivity is desired, the examiner can use sentences that are progressively longer, that use words of greater sophistication, that have a lower frequency of use, or that have more complex structures.[9]

Memory

Memory is associated with a collection of systems with specific neuroanatomical structures and functions. These systems support the neural processing of information in such a way as to have it available for use at a later time, with or without conscious awareness. Conceptually, memory can be divided into declarative and non-declarative systems. Declarative or explicit memory is memory for events that can be consciously recalled. Non-declarative or implicit memory is memory that is expressed as a change in behavior; it is often unconscious. Three types of declarative memory are commonly tested at the bedside: episodic, semantic, and working memory. Episodic memory refers to the memory system used to recall personal experiences (such as what you had for dinner last night or the experience of a recent walk in the park). Semantic memory systems are used to recall conceptual and factual knowledge that is not related to any specific memory of a personal experience. For example, what number of items constitutes a dozen? The working memory system refers to the ability to maintain and to manipulate information (such as retaining a phone number in your mind while searching for a pen and paper to write it down). This system is particularly dependent on attention, concentration, and short-term memory. Components of the working memory system have traditionally been referred to as the verbal, visuospatial, and executive (allocates attentional resources) systems.[10]

Memory system testing at the bedside is generally viewed as having three components. A commonly used classification divides it into immediate, short-term, and long-term recall.[11] Each of these types of recall will involve variable contributions from semantic and episodic memory systems depending on the individual patient's memory skills, natural associations with other semantic and episodic memories, and emotional valences of the particular memory items selected. Semantic and episodic memories are declarative and explicit.

Immediate Recall. This is the type of memory that is used when retaining a phone number in your mind until you can write it down. This requires intact attention to register the memory items. In the office or at the bedside it is common to choose at least three items from different categories and to have the patient repeat them after you have said them. Repetition confirms immediate registration. Then have the patient repeat the items until all of them have been registered. Then record the number of repetitions necessary before all the memory items were repeated correctly. This reflects the ability to focus attention. If an increased complexity of memory testing is desired, items of more abstract nature should be selected (such as "charity," "honesty," or "loyalty"). More sensitive assessments may use a greater number of recall items, incorporate compound nouns, or use combinations of adjectives and nouns (e.g., red bicycle). Other portions of the mental status examination can be performed after the memory items have been registered, thus serving as a distracter before

formal short-term memory recall is tested. Distraction ensures that information is encoded in a more normal fashion and then recalled rather than allowing the patient to repeat the memory items over and over, possibly allowing some degree of compensation for faulty memory systems.

Short-term Memory. Short-term memory requires the storage or encoding of information followed by the recall of information after 3 to 20 minutes. The examiner should ask the patient to recall the three (or more) memory items previously given. One should provide categorical cueing followed by multiple-choice options to aid recall if needed. An inability to recall any items, even after being provided with multiple-choice options, may be suggestive of a primary attentional problem or memory encoding impairment. When memory items can only be recalled with cueing or multiple-choice options, this may be suggestive of a memory retrieval problem.

Long-term Memory. This type of memory can be considered to include both recent and remote memory. Asking details about the patient's early life is helpful, but it requires the presence of a family member or friend to verify the information. Questions about salient historical events are often used to assess memory, but they are also subject to the patient's age, background, culture, education, and home of origin. "What happened on September 11th, 2001?" and "How did John F. Kennedy die?" are common test questions.

Visuospatial/Constructional Skills

These skills are tested at the bedside, most commonly with clock drawing. The examiner should ask the patient to draw a circle and then fill in the numbers to make it look like the face of a clock. Then one should ask the patient to set the hands to a time requiring the use of both left and right visual fields; examples include 11:10 and 10 minutes to 2. Abnormalities may include the crowding together of numbers within the circle or having the numbers, hands, or all of these on one side of the page, neglecting to put any detail on the other side. A common syndrome is that of the right parietal stroke, which may be associated with a left hemispatial neglect[12] that causes crowding of detail to the right side of the clock drawing. Attentional or executive dysfunction may cause difficulty planning the clock; the patient may write numbers in unusual locations, write the time on the clock (rather than setting the hands), or use strange hand construction or placement (Figure 73-1). Other commonly used tests include asking the patient to copy drawings provided by the examiner (such as a Greek cross, intersecting pentagons, or a three-dimensional cube). Simple handwriting may also be an indicator of visuospatial function.

Describing the Results

The patient's actual responses should be documented as clearly as possible in the medical record. Terms that are interpretive or diagnostic should be avoided.

More in-depth assessment of cognition can include tests of cortical sensory modalities, abstraction, praxis, and executive function.

Cortical Sensory or Secondary Sensory Modalities. Higher-level processing of sensory information occurs primarily in the parietal lobes.[13] This testing requires the relative preservation of primary cutaneous and proprioceptive sensory functions. Intact language function is particularly required for testing of stereognosis and graphesthesia.

Stereognosis is the recognition and interpretation of tactile sensory information. *Astereognosis* is the inability to recognize objects by touch. This can be tested by placing common

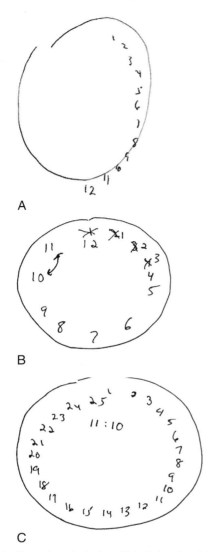

Figure 73-1. Examples of clocks. (A) Left hemispatial neglect. (B) Executive dysfunction. (C) Executive dysfunction. Note the absence of attention to detail on the left and the crowding of detail to the right in example A. Example B demonstrates poor planning and an inability to set the time properly to 10 minutes after 11. Example C demonstrates perseveration and difficulty conceptualizing a clock face and setting the time.

objects (such as coins, keys, paper clips, or closed safety pins) in the patient's hands and asking the patient to close his or her eyes and name the objects. Characteristics (such as size and shape) can be described by the patient. Often, people can identify the denomination of coins.

Graphesthesia is the ability to recognize letters or numbers written on the skin of the palm or finger pad using a sufficiently pointed object, without ink.

Double Simultaneous Stimulation. This maneuver tests for somatosensory extinction, neglect, or inattention when two simultaneous tactile stimuli are provided to opposite sides of the body. Extinction occurs when one side is not perceived. Other types of double simultaneous extinction tests involve the visual and auditory systems. Patients can be exposed to simultaneous visual stimuli in the left and right visual fields or to simultaneous auditory stimuli on both sides of the body (potentially revealing hemispatial neglect, inattention,

or extinction). The patient may perceive tactile, visual, or auditory information on the side or region of the body that demonstrates extinction when the stimulus is presented as a single stimulus without competition.

Abstraction. Asking the patient to identify three similarities between an apple and an orange can test abstraction. It is important that the patient identify the category (i.e., "fruit"). Other questions about similarities include the following: How are a bicycle and an airplane alike? How are a sculpture and a poem alike? Additional testing can include proverb interpretation.[14] One can ask the patient what a particular proverb means. Examples include the following: "People who live in glass houses shouldn't throw stones," "A shallow stream makes the most noise," "The tongue is the enemy of the throat," and "Dogs bark, and the caravan moves on." Novel proverbs are the most sensitive. Choosing a proverb with a less obvious interpretation, such as "Dogs bark, and the caravan moves on," can be useful for the assessment of the patient's range of abilities to generate novel interpretations. They may afford an opportunity to catch a glimpse of the psychodynamics of the individual, and allow subtle psychotic features to manifest in the substance of the patient's interpretation.[15] Performance, again, must be interpreted in the context of the patient's culture and education.

Praxis (Greek for "Action"). *Apraxia* is the acquired inability to perform a complex or skilled motor act in the absence of impairments of arousal, attention, language, comprehension, motivation, or sensorimotor function. More commonly described varieties include limb kinetic, buccofacial, ideomotor, and ideational apraxia. Limb kinetic apraxia is the loss of ability to make precise, coordinated fine motor movements. It has been argued that this category should not exist because its deficits are related to mild weakness secondary to a lesion in the motor pathways.[16] In buccofacial apraxia, patients are unable to perform (on request) complex acts involving the lips, mouth, and face (e.g., whistling, blowing out a match, sticking out the tongue, or coughing). Persons with ideomotor apraxia are unable to perform (on command) complex motor acts with one or all extremities. The patient may be unable to demonstrate on-command activities (such as saluting, waving goodbye, blowing a kiss, or pantomiming the brushing of teeth, combing of hair, hammering of a nail, or the use of scissors). Patients may incorrectly use their body parts as tools. Some of these patients are able to spontaneously perform these acts. The inability to perform an ideational plan consisting of a sequence of acts is referred to as an *ideational apraxia*.[17–19]

Executive Function. Executive function tasks are strongly dependent on intact frontal-subcortical circuits. Impaired performance on tasks that require attention and concentration occur in many patients with executive dysfunction. If attention and visuospatial skills are intact, clock-drawing[20] and shape-copying assess executive functions (such as planning, organization, and execution of a task).[21] Shapes that are commonly copied include those of a cube or of intersecting pentagons. Executive function deficits may include the inability to formulate goals or carry them out, deficits in abstraction and insight, impaired judgment, the inability to retrieve stored information from memory, and motor perseveration or impersistence.

Persons with executive dysfunction may have difficulty changing from one action to the next when asked to perform a repeated sequence of actions. For example, when asked to continue drawing a pattern of alternating triangles and squares, they may perseverate on one shape and keep drawing triangles. The Luria alternating hand sequencing task, in which the patient is asked to tap the table with a fist, open palm, and side of open hand and then to repeat the sequence as quickly as possible, is also useful to test for perseveration. This task is demonstrated to the patient before they are asked to perform it. The auditory Go-No-Go test assesses the ability to maintain a rule for performing a task and suppress inappropriate behaviors. In one version of this task the patient is asked to move a finger in response to one tapping sound (provided by the examiner), but must keep still in response to two tapping sounds.

Principles of Interpretation of the Mental Status Examination

The sequence of the neurological examination proceeds from elementary observations about the level of consciousness to a more in-depth assessment of specific abilities. Higher cognitive functions require prerequisite abilities that sometimes involve several domains. Each domain's performance must be interpreted in the context of function in other domains. For example, if an individual is found to be distractible, to be unable to spell "world" backward, and to make two errors on serial 7s, but has intact language, a more likely interpretation is an attention problem rather than a specific deficit in either calculation or language. If all other portions of the cognitive examination are intact yet the patient makes numerous errors on serial 7s and basic calculations, this may have significance for localization. The relationships between a patient's cognitive function, test performance, and real-life function are often complex. Test performance is rarely pathognomonic. Factors that may confound test interpretation include confusion or delirium, medication side effects, anxiety, sleep deprivation, alterations in mood or motivation, psychosis, low intellectual function, aphasia, and dyslexia. Interpretation must take into account the patient's age, gender, education, cultural background, and life accomplishments. In the event that the results of mental status testing are unclear, confounding, or insufficient to delineate the extent of the cognitive difficulty, adjunctive formal neuropsychological testing can be indispensable. Input from friends and family members may provide invaluable corroboration of history and day-to-day functioning.

CRANIAL NERVES
Olfaction (Cranial Nerve [CN] I)

This is an important sensory modality because olfactory symptoms in psychiatric and neurological patients are frequent. Unfortunately, psychiatrists rarely perform this portion of the examination and neurologists uncommonly complete it. The olfactory bulbs and tracts run along the inferior surface of the frontal lobes and project to limbic areas, as well as to regions important for memory.[22] Head trauma may be associated with loss of smell[23]; disinhibition may result from orbital frontal injury.[24] Tumors in the mid-line frontal region, known to cause apathy or abulia, may cause loss of smell. When testing is necessary, non-irritating stimuli should be used. Alcohol and ammonia may stimulate the trigeminal nerve, and the response to this stimulation may be confused with olfaction. One should bear in mind that the patient may not be able to name unfamiliar or less commonly encountered scents (such as clove or nutmeg); therefore, coffee, peppermint, wintergreen, or vanilla should be used. Each nostril should be tested individually. Abnormalities may include hyposmia, anosmia or misidentification of a smell.[25-27]

Optic Nerve (CN II)

Ocular processes (such as cataracts, old hemorrhages, and macular degeneration) should be cautiously taken into account

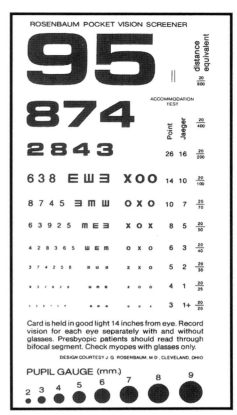

Figure 73-2. Rosenbaum visual acuity card with pupil gauge. *(Copyright © 2004–2007 Armstrong Optical Service Co. All rights reserved.)*

when interpreting eye findings. Funduscopy should be performed after portions of the examination that require vision.

Visual Acuity (CN II)

Visual acuity should be checked in each eye separately; customarily, the right eye is tested first. The most common method is to ensure that the patient is wearing whatever corrective lenses are normally worn and then to place a visual acuity card 14 inches in front of each eye while the other eye is covered (Figure 73-2). The examiner should ensure that good lighting is present in the room. Poor visual acuity can play a role in visual illusions and in hallucinations.[28]

Visual Fields (CN II)

Visual fields are tested in the clinic and at the bedside using a confrontation method. The examiner (you) should have the patient cover their left eye while situating yourself directly in front of the patient with your face 2 to 3 feet from the patient's face (Figure 73-3). The objective is to match your visual field to the patient's. Each quadrant should be tested by moving an object or by wiggling a finger into the patient's visual field from the periphery at a distance that is mid-way between you and the patient. Then the other eye should be tested. Another method is to have the patient count the number of fingers held up in each quadrant. The visual system spans from eye to occiput. The characteristics of visual field abnormalities can be very useful for localizing lesions (Figure 73-4).

Pupillary Responses (CNs II and III)

The pupils should be examined in a darkened room. The examiner should shine a penlight from below so as to illuminate both eyes just enough to compare pupillary size simultaneously. Next, the light should be shone to directly illuminate the right pupil and watch for constriction. After 1 to 2 seconds, the light should be moved to the left eye and the pupils observed for symmetry and size. Both pupils should constrict symmetrically, with a light shone in either eye. This is termed the *consensual response*. After 1 to 2 seconds, the light should be swung back to the other eye. The pupils should remain roughly symmetric in size while swinging the light from side to side. Dilation of a pupil to direct light during the swinging flashlight test is abnormal. Absence of reactivity, slow reactivity, or large pupil asymmetries are abnormal. Pupil

size in both light and darkness should be documented. Pupillary abnormalities may be seen in diseases that affect the sympathetic nervous system and in those that affect components of the visual system from the pupil, retina, optic nerve, to the brainstem. The convergence response does not involve the specific use of light (except to visualize both pupils for response). The patient should be asked to visually track your finger as you move it from a distance toward the patient in the mid-line. This will normally cause the eyes to converge and the pupils to constrict symmetrically.

Funduscopy (CN II) and the Retina

The eye is the only location in the body in which a nerve and blood vessels can be directly visualized. Optic disk swelling (papilledema) may indicate increased intracranial pressure,[29] optic disk atrophy may be present in demyelinating disease,[30] and optic disk and retinal abnormalities both may occur in vascular disease.[31]

Ocular Movements (CNs III, IV, and VI)

These three cranial nerves control eye movements and lid elevation. Any spontaneous eye movements in primary resting forward gaze should be observed. The range of conjugate gaze (tested by holding your finger about 2 feet away) should be assessed next. The finger should be moved slowly to allow for assessment of voluntary smooth pursuits in the up, down, oblique, left, and right directions (Figure 73-5). Patients with Parkinson's disease manifest "jerky" smooth pursuits.[32,33] The examiner should ask the patient to hold his or her head still. At the limits of conjugate gaze in each direction the examiner should hold gaze for several seconds and then observe for nystagmus. When present, this is referred to as *gaze-evoked nystagmus*. Barbiturates, tranquilizers, ethanol, and anticonvulsants commonly cause gaze-evoked nystagmus in both directions of gaze.[34] Normal saccades are involuntary, fast,

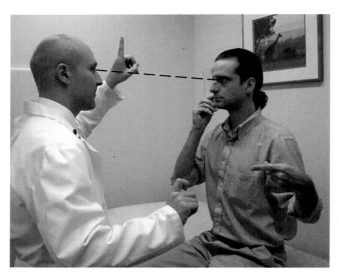

Figure 73-3. Confrontation visual field testing.

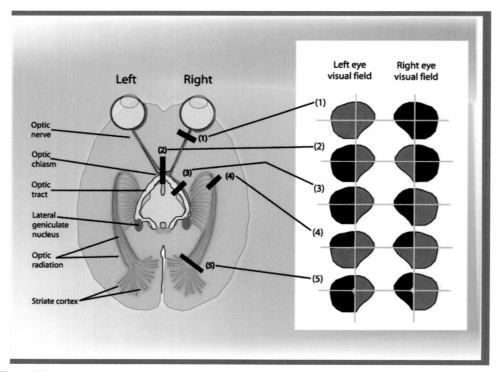

Figure 73-4. Anatomy of the visual system. Visual field defects associated with different anatomical lesions.

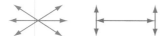

Figure 73-5. Diagram of two options for testing eye movement range.

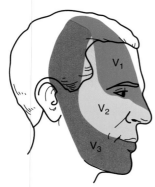

Figure 73-6. Trigeminal nerve sensory distribution. V_1, V_2, and V_3 sensory distributions in blue, yellow, and red, respectively.

conjugate changes of eye position between fixations. Saccades are tested by having the patient fixate on your nose and then look quickly toward your finger and then back to your nose. Your finger should be held in the up, down, left, and then right positions. The accuracy and speed of saccades should be assessed. The patient should be assessed for overshooting (hypermetric saccades) back to the target. Hypermetric saccades may occur in conditions with cerebellar involvement (such as the cerebellar presentation of multi-system atrophy). The patient should also be assessed for undershooting (hypometric saccades), requiring several saccades to reach the target. Patients with Parkinson's disease may manifest hypometric saccades.[35] Slowed saccades or saccadic smooth pursuits can be present in Wilson's disease.[36] Slowed vertical saccades often mark progressive supranuclear palsy.[37] Slowed and hypometric saccades may be associated with Huntington's disease,[38] and anticonvulsant toxicity.[39] These are just a few examples of neurological conditions with associated eye movement abnormalities. Ptosis of the eyelids should also be noted.

Trigeminal Nerve (CN V)

The trigeminal nerve provides sensory innervation to the face, cornea, and much of the mouth and tongue (Figure 73-6). Its motor component innervates the muscles of mastication. Unless the patient has a specific sensory complaint, it is sufficient to use light touch (tested with fingers or gauze) or temperature (tested with a cold metal tuning fork) and ask the patient if it feels the same or similar on both sides. Testing of the corneal reflex is not routinely necessary.

Muscles of Mastication

Brief observation of the jaw at rest and with movement is adequate in a patient without complaints. Having the patient move his or her chin from side to side, then open his or her mouth widely, helps assess the function of these muscles. Further testing can involve opening and closing the jaw against resistance.

Facial Nerve (CN VII)

The facial nerve provides motor innervation to the muscles of facial expression and taste to the anterior two-thirds of the tongue. The facial nerve's other motor and sensory components would uncommonly be tested. The examiner should ask the patient to raise the eyebrows, to wrinkle the forehead, to squeeze the eyes shut, and to smile (or show the teeth). One should also look for symmetry of facial markings (such as the nasolabial fold), at rest and with movement. Further testing can involve testing the strength of facial muscles by overcoming them (by trying to open the closed eyes or to pull the closed lips apart manually). Subtle facial asymmetries are common and not necessarily pathological. It is helpful to have a family member or an old photo (e.g., a driver's license) to verify the long-standing nature of a subtle asymmetry. Dysarthria can result from weakness of the orbicularis oris. Labial sounds can be tested by asking the patient to say "pa. … pa. … pa." The speed and clarity of speech should also be assessed. A central pattern of facial weakness is characterized by weakness in the lower face, with sparing of the forehead. This is due to the bilateral corticobulbar innervation of the portion of the facial nucleus subserving the forehead. A peripheral pattern of weakness is characterized by hemifacial weakness without forehead sparing. This can be caused by disruption of the facial nerve or nucleus (Figure 73-7). Taste is uncommonly tested unless there are specific indications.

Vestibulocochlear Nerve (CN VIII)

Lesions of this nerve can be associated with vertigo, hearing loss, or both. One should ensure that the external ear canal is not occluded with cerumen. Holding your fingers several inches away from the patient's ears and rubbing the fingers together softly allows for a quick, but usually adequate, assessment. Alternatively, you can ask the patient to repeat a word or numbers that you whisper into the ear while occluding the other ear. More in-depth testing can include the Rinne test, which involves the use of a vibrating tuning fork (128 to 512 Hz) applied to the mastoid bone until it can no longer be heard. It is then placed next to the ear. This comparison determines whether hearing is better with air or bone conduction. Conduction hearing loss is characterized by hearing the sound better with the tuning fork applied to the mastoid than next to the ear. In sensorineural hearing loss, the sound is better perceived next to the ear than via the mastoid bone. The Weber test uses a tuning fork placed in the mid-line at the vertex or forehead to determine on which side the sound is heard best. Sound referred to an ear with decreased acuity indicates conductive hearing loss.[40] Sound referred to the opposite (unaffected) ear occurs with sensorineural hearing loss. These tests are crude compared to audiologic testing. Hearing loss can exacerbate auditory hallucinations and paranoia.[41]

Glossopharyngeal and Vagus Nerves (CNs IX and X)

These nerves will be discussed together because of their intimately related functions. CNs IX and X serve the motor and sensory functions of the palate and vocal cords.

Speech (CNs IX and X)

Speech may be hoarse, with vocal cord weakness. An inability to swallow secretions can lead to drooling. (See CN VII.)

Palate (CNs IX and X)

This is assessed by asking the patient to say "aaah" and watching for the degree of palate elevation and symmetry. Palatal speech dysfunction can be assessed by evaluating the clarity and speed of palatal sounds such as "ga. … ga. … ga." Labial,

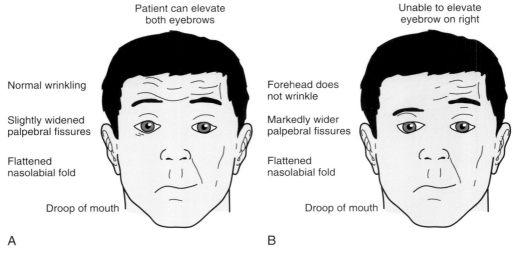

Patient can elevate both eyebrows

Normal wrinkling

Slightly widened palpebral fissures

Flattened nasolabial fold

Droop of mouth

Unable to elevate eyebrow on right

Forehead does not wrinkle

Markedly wider palpebral fissures

Flattened nasolabial fold

Droop of mouth

A   B

Figure 73-7. Depiction of (A) central facial weakness and (B) peripheral facial weakness.

lingual, and palatal sounds can be tested together by having the patient repeat "pa. … ta. … ka."

Inspection of the oral cavity is sufficient in an asymptomatic individual. The gag reflex is uncommonly tested in the screening neurological examination. When there is reasonable suspicion that swallowing is impaired, when the palate is weak, or when there are voice changes, the gag reflex should be checked. Symmetry of the response on each side should be noted.

Spinal Accessory Nerve (CN XI)

This nerve innervates the trapezius and the sternocleidomastoid (SCM) muscles. The trapezius can be assessed with a shoulder shrug against resistance. The SCM is evaluated with head rotation against resistance. The head should be fully rotated in the direction of testing, and then resistance should be applied. The right SCM turns the head to the left and the left SCM turns the head to the right. SCM muscle bulk should be inspected with the head facing forward. Asymmetry of muscle bulk can often be seen in cases of torticollis.

Hypoglossal Nerve (CN XII)

The hypoglossal nerve is involved in speech production as is CNs VII, IX, and X. The hypoglossal nerve provides motor innervation to the tongue. Gross inspection of the tongue may reveal atrophy or fasciculations in the setting of a peripheral nerve lesion. A lisp may be clinically apparent during conversation. The examiner should ask the patient to protrude his or her tongue in the mid-line and to look for deviation to one side. Lingual speech dysfunction can be evaluated by assessing the speed and clarity of lingual sounds, such as "la. … la. … la." Parkinsonian, familial, medication-induced, and thyrotoxic tremors may be apparent in the tongue.[42,43] Degenerative diseases and neuroleptic medications can induce dyskinesias of the tongue and the oromandibular region.[44]

MOTOR EXAMINATION
Muscle Bulk

The muscles should be inspected for atrophy, hypertrophy, and fasciculations. Atrophy is an important sign of lower motor neuron disease. It is not seen prominently in weakness

of CNS origin except in association with non-use. Hypertrophy can be normal when seen in the setting of weightlifting, or abnormal when seen as a feature of dystonia or selected muscular dystrophies.

Tone

Muscle tone is the residual tension present in a voluntarily relaxed muscle. This is clinically assessed by determining the degree of resistance present to passive movement of a limb or the head. Relaxation can be difficult for many patients, and distraction, such as engaging the patient in conversation or asking the patient to perform a simple activity with a contralateral limb (such as opening and closing the hand held up in the air) may be necessary. It is important to know about a variety of different tone abnormalities. Lead-pipe rigidity is characterized by a consistent and relatively stable degree of increased tone throughout the range of movement of a limb; it is not affected by velocity of movement. Cogwheel rigidity is a rhythmic increase in tone, similar to a tremor, throughout the range of movement. Spasticity is a type of hypertonicity that increases with an increase in the velocity of movement. Slow movements may reveal little abnormal tone and fast movements may result in a sudden increase in tone. *Gegenhalten* is a paratonia that manifests as an increase in resistance from the patient in proportion to the effort of the examiner. It is often reduced by distraction. *Mitgehen* is another type of paratonia that is characterized by the patient who actively assists the examiner throughout the range of motion. Both types of paratonia are thought to suggest diffuse bilateral frontal lobe disease or diffuse cerebral disease.[45]

Strength

It is beyond the scope of a screening examination in the outpatient or inpatient psychiatric setting to perform a comprehensive neuromuscular evaluation. Practical assessment of strength in an asymptomatic patient should assess the deltoid, biceps, triceps, and brachioradialis muscles, as well as grip strength and gait assessment. The patient should be able to rise independently from a sitting position without using his or her arms. A normal casual gait, toe, and heel walk in most circumstances rules out a significant motor deficit. Strength is most commonly graded using the Medical Research Council's five-level scale (Table 73-1).[46]

TABLE 73-1 Medical Research Council Scale of Muscle Strength Table

0	No contraction
1	A flicker or trace of contraction
2	Active movement with gravity eliminated
3	Active movement against gravity
4–	Active movement against gravity and slight resistance
4	Active movement against gravity and moderate resistance
4+	Active movement against gravity and strong resistance
5	Normal power

Abnormal Movements

Abnormal voluntary or involuntary movements may occur during the history and physical examination and should be described. The psychiatrist should be familiar with the following terms:

- *Tremor* is usually an involuntary, rhythmic oscillation produced by rhythmic contractions of agonist and antagonist muscles. Tremors may be present with movement, sustained postures or at rest. Tremors may affect the voice, tongue, face, head, limbs, and trunk. The frequency and amplitude of tremors are important features.
- *Myoclonus* is characterized by involuntary, non-rhythmic, brief, sometimes repetitive muscle contractions that are irregular in frequency and amplitude. They are often asynchronous and asymmetric. They may be symmetric in spinal myoclonus. They may be cortical, subcortical, or spinal in origin.
- *Clonus* is characterized by involuntary, rhythmic contractions and relaxations of a muscle or group of muscles.
- *Chorea* is manifest by involuntary, non-rhythmic, jerky, rapid movements of muscle groups.
- *Asterixis* is also known as "liver flap" or negative myoclonus. This movement is characterized by an abrupt loss of voluntary muscle tone. It is commonly elicited by asking the patient to hold his or her arms outstretched with the wrists extended. When asterixis is present, the hands, with or without the arms, may suddenly drop downward and then quickly recover, which causes an irregular and slow flapping motion.
- *Athetosis* is manifest by involuntary, slow, irregular, sinuous, snake-like writhing movements.
- *Dystonia* is an involuntary movement or sustained posture that results from abnormal tonicity of muscle. Movements may be characterized as having prolonged or repetitive muscle contractions that may result in twisting or jerking movements of the body or body part.
- *Tics* are defined in several ways. They are characterized by simple or complex coordinated movements or vocalizations that are repetitive, stereotyped, compulsive, and often abrupt, and over which the patient feels he or she has little or no control. Tics are experienced as almost irresistible impulses to perform a particular activity. Some tics can be suppressed.
- *Fasciculations* are brief, irregular twitches of a muscle. They may be localized to a muscle or limb or be diffuse, depending on the etiology. Fasciculations occur as a benign phenomenon, as well as a manifestation of various neuropathies (e.g., amyotrophic lateral sclerosis [ALS] or diabetic peripheral neuropathy), radiculopathies, and thyrotoxicosis, and they can occur in association with anticholinesterase use.

Sensory Examination

Sensory function is divided into primary and secondary modalities. The primary sensory modalities commonly tested include touch, proprioception, vibration, pain, and temperature. Secondary sensory modalities are a synthesis and interpretation of primary modality information that occurs in the parietal sensory and association cortices. Testing of secondary sensory modalities is discussed in the neurological portion of the mental status examination.

Testing for two-point discrimination is not indicated in an asymptomatic patient. Testing of light touch and either pain (sharp) or temperature sensation is usually sufficient. Having the patient close his or her eyes can increase the sensitivity of the examination and is required for proprioceptive testing. (See Figure 73-8 for an illustration of nerve and dermatomal distributions.)

Light touch can be tested by touching the patient lightly with your finger or a piece of cotton.

Proprioception can be tested by using the finger and thumb of one hand, and stabilizing the distal interphalangeal joint of a digit by holding its medial and lateral aspects. After moving the digit slightly up or down, the patient is asked to identify the direction of movement. Romberg testing is also useful for position-sense testing. One should ask the patient to stand with both feet together as closely as possible to maintain balance with the eyes open. Then one should ask the patient to close their eyes. If the patient loses his or her balance with the eyes closed (but not when the eyes are open), he or she is Romberg positive. If swaying occurs without loss of stance, this should be described in your note.

Vibration can be tested using a 128-Hz tuning fork on a distal bony prominence or distal interphalangeal joint. One should assess when the vibration fades from the patient's perception. You may use the same anatomical region on yourself for comparison.

Pain can be tested with the use of disposable sterile pins.

Temperature can be tested using a cold metal tuning fork. You may run it under cold or warm water to ensure a clear temperature change from your pocket or from room temperature.

Coordination Testing

Coordination testing is the preferred term, rather than *cerebellar testing*. The specific abilities involved in coordination testing require integration and processing of information from diverse systems that include visual, sensory, motor, basal ganglia, cortical association, and cerebellar systems.

Finger-to-nose can be assessed by positioning yourself directly in front of the patient and asking them to touch the tip of your index finger with the tip of their index finger and then touch the tip of their nose with the same finger. One can have the patient continue alternating this maneuver, ensuring that the patient's arm is extended, so as to reach for your finger. Then you should move your target finger from the patient's right side to a stationary position in front and then to a position on the left. This should be repeated with the patient's other hand. One should look for accuracy of movement, speed, and tremor. An alternative maneuver is to have the patient follow your finger as a target with their same finger (of either hand) without actually touching your finger. This should be performed within a plane equidistant from both of you while seated facing each other. Your finger should be moved around in space from left to right and up and down to various stationary positions, while the patient attempts to closely mirror your movements, dynamically following your movements to various stationary positions without touching you or drifting off target. This is a more sensitive assessment of the precision of movement.

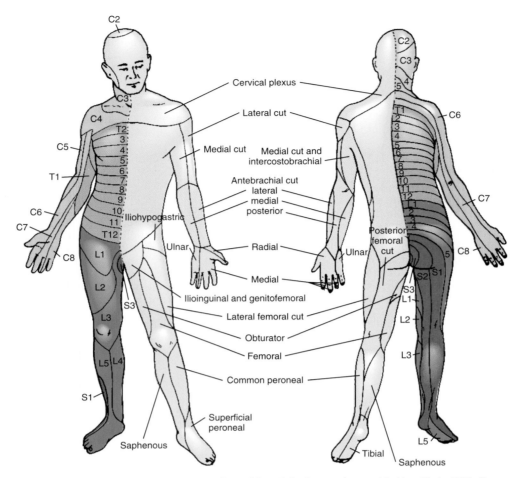

Figure 73-8. Sensory nerve distributions and dermatomes. *(From Gilroy J. Basic neurology, ed 2, New York, 1990, Pergamon Press, p. 41.)*

Rapid Alternating Movements

The most common maneuvers are finger-tapping and alternating pronation and supination of the forearm. Speed, amplitude, rhythmicity, and precision of movements are noted. Toe-tapping may be used if clinically indicated. It has been proposed that significant slowing of toe-tapping, in the absence of prominent lower limb weakness, may be a more sensitive marker for upper motor neuron dysfunction than the Babinski sign.[47]

Heel to Shin

This maneuver is optimally performed with the patient in the supine position. One should ask the patient to smoothly run their heel up and down the opposite shin along a line from below the knee to the ankle. The patient should be urged to be as accurate with the movements as possible. One should look for precision, range of motion, speed, and presence of tremor. The maneuver is then repeated on the other side.

Gait Testing

Walking is a complex form of motor coordination that requires the integrated function and synthesis of input from various systems. Some of these systems include the sensory, motor, cerebellar, basal ganglia, and vestibular systems. Gait can be affected through dysfunction in any of these components, with many characteristic manifestations. Sensory deficits may result

in a wide-based stance. Basal ganglia disorders may cause slowing of gait, reduced stride length, and festination. Gait assessment should be part of every neurological examination.

Casual stance and gait should be inspected. Posture, gait initiation, speed of gait, step height, stride length, position of legs, arm swing, and turning capabilities should be observed. Toe and heel-walking will test strength and balance. Tandem walking is useful to detect mid-line instability that is commonly seen as a result of chronic alcohol use. Postural reflexes may be assessed by asking the patient to stand with his or her feet together and eyes closed (as in the Romberg maneuver). The patient should be reassured that you will be testing the patient's balance by pushing them a bit in various directions, but you will not allow the patient to fall. (Take care to ensure that the patient does *not* fall.) At the patient's shoulder level you can variably and sequentially give the patient a nudge forward, backward, to one side, and then to the other side. Retropulsion is commonly seen in patients with parkinsonian symptoms.

REFLEX ASSESSMENT
Deep Tendon Reflexes

Deep tendon reflexes (DTRs) are also commonly called muscle stretch or proprioceptive reflexes. These reflexes are elicited by tapping the muscle's tendon or sometimes by tapping a portion of the muscle itself. Muscle stretch receptors are activated and sensory information is transmitted to the spinal cord within which a simple, monosynaptic reflex arc is generated by synapsing directly on an alpha motor neuron (causing a muscle contraction). The descending corticospinal tracts modulate this system. The activity of a DTR is judged by the latency, speed, amplitude, duration, and spread of a response. Abnormalities in DTRs can yield useful information about the integrity of the central and peripheral nervous system portions of the reflex. Commonly tested muscle stretch reflexes include the biceps, triceps, brachioradialis, quadriceps (patellar), and gastrocnemius (Achilles or ankle jerk)[48] (Table 73-2). DTRs, under normal circumstances, do not change significantly with aging.

Grading of reflexes is on a 4-point scale with 2+ usually considered to be normal (Table 73-3). It should be noted that what is normal for one person may be hypoactive or brisk when compared to another individual. There is a wide range of normal responses. Symmetry of reflexes, absence of interval changes, and absence of pathological reflexes are more important. Reflex gradients (for example, a diminished ankle reflex compared to the more proximal patella reflex) and clonus should also be assessed. In some individuals the DTRs may be diminished or apparently absent. Under such circumstances, reinforcement techniques (such as the Jendrassik maneuver)[49]

TABLE 73-2 Commonly Tested Deep Tendon Reflexes and Their Segmental Innervation

Muscle	Nerve Roots
Biceps	C5–6
Triceps	C6–7–8
Brachioradialis	C5–6
Quadriceps (knee)	L2–3–4
Gastrocnemius (ankle)	S1

TABLE 73-3 Grading Reflexes

For the purposes of documentation, most neurologists grade the deep tendon reflexes (DTRs) numerically as follows:

0	Absent
1+	Diminished
2+	Normal
3+	Increased; hyperactive; often with spread to other muscle groups
4+	Hyperactive with spread to other muscle groups and clonus; clearly abnormal

are often helpful to facilitate the reflex slightly.[50] This is a maneuver during which the reflexes are percussed while the patient flexes his or her fingers and hooks them together (palms facing each other), and attempts to pull the hands apart.

Cutaneous or Superficial Reflexes

Stroking or scratching the skin elicits these reflexes. One should use care, because a painful stimulus may cause a guarding or defensive response rather than a reflex. Examples of this reflex include the plantar reflex, abdominal reflexes, the cremasteric reflex, and anal wink.

Plantar Reflex

This reflex is the most important of the cutaneous reflexes for the psychiatrist to incorporate into the examination. It is useful for detecting corticospinal tract dysfunction. It is tested by stroking the bottom of the foot from the heel forward with only so much firmness as needed to elicit a consistent response. The normal response is plantar flexion of the foot and toes after the first 12 to 18 months of life. Disease of the corticospinal system may be associated with extension of the toes that has been described as "up-going." The up-going great toe with fanning of the other four toes is referred to as the *Babinski sign.* This may also be referred to as the *extensor plantar response.* Some authorities recommend stroking the lateral aspect of the plantar surface rather than the medial one, so as to avoid a plantar grasp response. Patients who are very ticklish may voluntarily withdraw from the stimulus and demonstrate flexion of the hip and knee (usually with plantar flexion of the foot and toes). A triple-flexion response is a spinal reflex characterized by hip and knee flexion accompanied by ankle dorsiflexion (Figure 73-9).

Primitive Reflexes or Atavistic Reflexes (Mistakenly Called "Frontal Release Signs")

These reflexes are present at birth and disappear in most people in early infancy. There is a large portion of the normal population in which a single primitive reflex persists. This is less concerning when it is a single reflex (such as a snout, glabellar, or palmomental reflex). A grasp or suck reflex is considered more worrisome. Asymmetry or multiple primitive reflexes are considered abnormal. Primitive reflexes are not

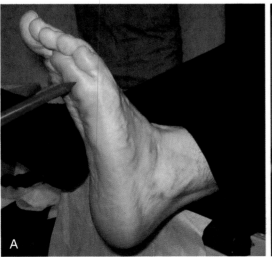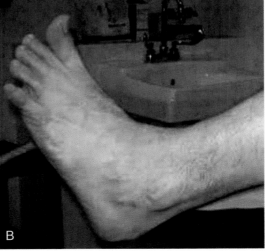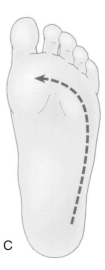

Figure 73-9. (A) Plantar reflex. (B) Babinski sign. (C) Plantar stimulus.

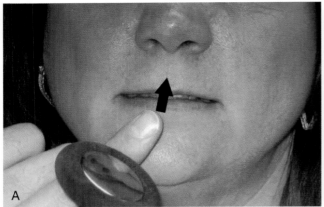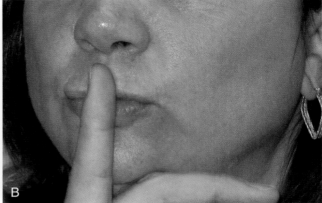

Figure 73-10. (A) Snout. (B) Snout reflex.

believed to be useful for localization purposes.[51,52] If they reappear in later life they may be suggestive of diffuse cerebral, subcortical, or bilateral frontal lobe pathology.[53-55]

The *snout reflex* can be assessed by gently tapping over the patient's upper lip. If this reflex is present, a puckering of the lips will be seen. The snout reflex is present in 30% to 50% of healthy adults over age 60 (Figure 73-10).

A *suck reflex* may also be elicited and is considered a more worrisome reflex. When present, the suck reflex is elicited by stimulation of the lips; this is followed by sucking movements of the lips, tongue, and jaw.

The *palmomental reflex* is an ipsilateral contraction of the mentalis and orbicularis oris after stimulation of the thenar region of the hand. This reflex is present in 20% to 25% of healthy adults in their thirties and forties. The *glabellar reflex* is assessed by tapping the patient's glabellar ridge between the eyes with your finger. It is best to stand to the side of or behind a seated patient so as to not cause a visual threat response. The patient should be asked not to blink. The reflex is present if there is persistence of blinking with gentle tapping.

The *grasp reflex* is elicited after first instructing the patient not to hold on to the examiner's hand, followed by stroking the palm between the thumb and forefinger of the patient's hand. This is but one version of several as to how this maneuver is accomplished. The reflex is present if the patient's fingers flex or the hand closes.

🌐 Access the complete reference list and multiple choice questions (MCQs) online at https://expertconsult.inkling.com

KEY REFERENCES

1. Legesse B, Murray ED, Price BH. Brain-behavior relations. In Ramachandran VS, editor: *Encyclopedia of human behavior*, ed 2, Waltham, MA, 2012, Academic Press.
2. Murray ED, Buttner EA, Price BH. Depression and psychosis in neurological practice. In Bradley WG, Daroff RB, Fenichel GM, et al., editors: *Neurology in clinical practice*, ed 6, Philadelphia, 2012, Butterworth-Heinemann, pp 92–116.
3. Price BH, Adams RD, Coyle JT. Neurology and psychiatry: closing the great divide. *Neurology* 54(1):8–14, 2000.
4. Hinson VK, Haren WB. Psychogenic movement disorders. *Lancet Neurol* 5(8):695–700, 2006.
5. Cummings JL, Arciniegas DB, Brooks BR, et al. Defining and diagnosing involuntary emotional expression disorder. *CNS Spectr* 11(6):1–7, 2006.
7. Bauer G, Trinka E. Nonconvulsive status epilepticus and coma. *Epilepsia* 51(2):177–190, 2010.
10. Budson AE, Price BH. Memory dysfunction. *N Engl J Med* 352(7):692–699, 2005.

12. Weintraub S, Daffner KR, Ahern GL, et al. Right sided hemispatial neglect and bilateral cerebral lesions. *J Neurol Neurosurg Psychiatry* 60(3):342–344, 1996.
13. Gottlieb J, Snyder LH. Spatial and non-spatial functions of the parietal cortex. *Curr Opin Neurobiol* 20(6):731–740, 2010.
18. Geschwind N. Disconnexion syndromes in animals and man. I and II. *Brain* 88(2):237–294, 585–644, 1965.
21. Cosentino S, Jefferson A, Chute DL, et al. Clock drawing errors in dementia: neuropsychological and neuroanatomical considerations. *Cogn Behav Neurol* 17(2):74–84, 2004.
23. Costanzo RM, Miwa T. Posttraumatic olfactory loss. *Adv Otorhinolaryngol* 63:99–107, 2006.
24. Cummings JL. Frontal-subcortical circuits and human behavior. *Arch Neurol* 50(8):873–880, 1993.
25. Serby M, Larson P, Kalstein D. The nature and course of olfactory deficits in Alzheimer's disease. *Am J Psychiatry* 148:357–360, 1991.
28. Berrios GE, Brook P. Visual hallucinations and sensory delusions in the elderly. *Br J Psychiatry* 144:662–664, 1984.
30. Balcer LJ. Clinical practice. Optic neuritis. *N Engl J Med* 354(12):1273–1280, 2006.
31. Purvin V, Kawasaki A. Neuro-ophthalmic emergencies for the neurologist. *Neurologist* 11(4):195–233, 2005.
35. Pinkhardt EH, Kassubek J. Ocular motor abnormalities in Parkinsonian syndromes. *Parkinsonism Relat Disord* 17(4):223–230, 2011.
36. Ingster-Moati I, Bui Quoc E, Pless M, et al. Ocular motility and Wilson's disease: a study on 34 patients. *J Neurol Neurosurg Psychiatry* 78(11):1199–1201, 2007.
37. Boxer AL, Garbutt S, Seeley WW, et al. Saccade abnormalities in autopsy-confirmed frontotemporal lobar degeneration and Alzheimer's disease. *Arch Neurol* 69(4):509–517, 2012.
38. Martino D, Stamelou M, Bhatia KP. The differential diagnosis of Huntington's disease-like syndromes: 'red flags' for the clinician. *J Neurol Neurosurg Psychiatry* 84(6):650–656, 2013.
39. Thurston SE, Leigh RJ, Abel LA, et al. Slow saccades and hypometria in anticonvulsant toxicity. *Neurology* 34(12):1593–1596, 1984.
41. van der Werf M, van Winkel R, van Boxtel M, et al. Evidence that the impact of hearing impairment on psychosis risk is moderated by the level of complexity of the social environment. *Schizophr Res* 122(1–3):193–198, 2010.
47. Miller TM, Johnston SC. Should the Babinski sign be part of the routine neurologic examination? *Neurology* 65(8):1165–1168, 2005.
53. van Boxtel MP, Bosma H, Jolles J, et al. Prevalence of primitive reflexes and the relationship with cognitive change in healthy adults: a report from the Maastricht Aging Study. *J Neurol* 253(7):935–941, 2006.
54. Rao R, Jackson S, Howard R. Primitive reflexes in cerebrovascular disease: a community study of older people with stroke and carotid stenosis. *Int J Geriatr Psychiatry* 14(11):964–972, 1999.
55. Bachmann S, Bottmer C, Schroder J. Neurological soft signs in first-episode schizophrenia: a follow-up study. *Am J Psychiatry* 162(12):2337–2343, 2005.

74 Neuropsychiatric Principles and Differential Diagnosis

Simon Ducharme MD MSc, Evan D. Murray MD, Bruce H. Price MD

KEY POINTS

Background

- Behavioral Neurology and Neuropsychiatry is a medical specialty that cares for patients with problems that cross traditional boundaries between neurology and psychiatry.
- Neuropsychiatric symptoms and cognitive deficits can be correlated with altered function in anatomical regions and in cerebral networks.
- A firm understanding of the main cerebral structures and networks that mediate emotions, behavior, and cognition is the foundation of a useful neuropsychiatric approach.

History

- A thorough neuropsychiatric assessment includes taking a detailed longitudinal clinical history to identify signs and symptoms that yield clues about the neuroanatomical localization and pathophysiology of the neuropsychiatric dysfunction.

Clinical and Research Challenges

- A variety of neurological diseases can produce psychiatric symptoms as part of the illness or secondary to its treatments.

- The differential diagnosis of neuropsychiatric presentations is broad, and may include rare conditions that clinicians will encounter infrequently during their careers. Each condition may carry unique implications for prognosis, treatment, and long-term management.
- Acquiring knowledge of multiple diseases with psychiatric and neurological manifestations is a major clinical challenge in behavioral neurology and neuropsychiatry.
- Integrating neurosciences into clinical practice and developing neuroimaging biomarkers for neuropsychiatric disorders is a key research challenge.

Practical Pointers

- Atypical age of onset, acute course, cognitive impairment, catatonia, and progressive clinical deterioration with seizures, alterations in level of consciousness, or abnormalities on elemental neurological exam are indicators that a behavioral syndrome could be secondary to a neurological, neuropsychiatric, or general medical process.
- The decision to obtain investigational studies should be based upon the differential diagnosis, factoring in pre-test probabilities of the suspected diseases.

GENERAL PRINCIPLES OF NEUROPSYCHIATRY

Behavioral Neurology and Neuropsychiatry is a medical subspecialty committed to understanding the link between neuroscience and behavior, and providing care to persons with conditions (e.g., Tourette disorder, frontotemporal dementia, functional neurological symptom disorder) that cross the traditional, and often arbitrary, division between psychiatry and neurology. Behavioral neurology and neuropsychiatry have historically separate, but parallel traditions.[1,2] They were recently integrated into a single subspecialty with standardized fellowship training requirements and board certification.[3,4] It requires competence beyond the scope of general psychiatry and neurology.[4] However, a basic understanding of neuropsychiatric principles and differential diagnosis should be an integral part of modern general psychiatric training.

The neuropsychiatric approach is based on the understanding that emotional and cognitive processes arise from complex electro-chemical physiological interactions within the brain's neuronal networks. Emotions and behavior occur as a result of the interplay of genetics, epigenetics, development, environment, and social influences on those neuronal networks. Abnormalities in specific networks have been documented in many major psychiatric syndromes, such as major depressive disorder (MDD)[5] and obsessive-compulsive disorder (OCD).[6] In addition, pathophysiological models have been developed for some neuropsychiatric disorders that intrinsically combine psychiatric and neurological aspects, including behavioral variant frontotemporal dementia[7] (bvFTD) and narcolepsy.[8] Although psychiatric syndromes are sometimes referred to as

being functional, due to absence of currently identified diagnostic pathology correlates, they are rooted in neurobiology. The term functional should be understood as referring to dynamic alterations in neurocircuitry, and not as the opposite of "organic", a concept that will hopefully disappear from the medical vocabulary.

Specific neuropsychiatric symptoms can be correlated with altered function in distinct neuronal networks.[5–7,9,10] Any disease, toxin, or drug that adversely impacts the function of a particular region can lead to changes in behavior that are mediated by the corresponding neural networks. For example, the Klüver-Bucy syndrome (with placidity, apathy, visual and auditory agnosia, hyperorality, and hypersexuality)[11] is secondary to medial temporal-amygdalar lesions resulting from any of multiple conditions, including herpes encephalitis,[12] traumatic brain injury (TBI), FTD, and advanced Alzheimer's disease (AD). Psychiatric symptoms (including psychosis, mania, depression, obsession/compulsion, and anxiety) can occur as a result of neurological diseases, including, but not limited to, stroke, multiple sclerosis, Parkinson's disease, and Huntington's disease.[13] These symptoms can be indistinguishable from the idiopathic form.[13–15] Consequently, a wide array of medical and neurological conditions must be considered in the differential diagnosis of any person with behavioral and emotional symptoms.

A strong neuroanatomical conceptual framework is important for lesion localization, which allows for the development of a rational differential diagnosis and plan for investigation.[16] The objective of this chapter is to provide an integrative approach towards the differential diagnosis and treatment of psychiatric symptoms arising as a result of, or in association with, neurological and general medical conditions.

COGNITIVE-BEHAVIORAL NEUROANATOMY

The neuropsychiatric approach is based on an understanding of functional brain anatomy, which is described in more detail in Chapter 72. A few key points will be reviewed.

The cerebral cortex can be subdivided into five major functional subtypes: primary sensory-motor, unimodal association, heteromodal association, paralimbic, and limbic.[17] The primary sensory areas are the point of entry for sensory information into the cortical circuitry. Processing of sensory information occurs as information moves from primary sensory areas to adjacent unimodal association areas (Figure 74-1). The complexity of processing increases as information is then transmitted to heteromodal association areas that receive input from more than one sensory modality. Further cortical processing occurs in paralimbic areas (orbitofrontal cortex, insula, temporal pole, parahippocampal cortex, and cingulate cortex), in which cognitive, emotional, and visceral inputs merge. The paralimbic structures connect to limbic structures (hippocampus, amygdala, substantia innominata, prepiriform olfactory cortex, and septal area) (Figure 74-2), which are intimately involved with emotion, memory, and motivation, as well as autonomic and endocrine functions. The highest level of cognitive processing occurs in regions referred to as

transmodal areas. These areas are composed of heteromodal, paralimbic, and limbic regions that are collectively linked, in parallel, to other transmodal regions. Inter-connections among transmodal areas allow integration of distributed perceptual processing systems, such as perceptual recognition of events becoming experiences and words taking on meaning.[17,18]

The functional organization of neuronal networks has been investigated by a variety of methods including axonal tracings in monkeys, task-based functional magnetic resonance imaging (fMRI), resting state fMRI intrinsic connectivity, and structural co-variance.[19] Cortical areas have been shown to have specialization, lateralized functions, and connections with more than one network.

Cortical Networks

At least five distributed networks govern various aspects of cognitive functions[18,19]: (1) the left temporo-perisylvian language network (which includes transmodal regions or "epicenters" in Broca's and Wernicke's areas); (2) the fronto-parietal spatial attention network (which is based on transmodal regions in the frontal eye fields, cingulate cortex, and posterior parietal area); (3) the limbic/paralimbic network for explicit memory and motivational salience (which is located in the hippocampal-entorhinal region and amygdala); (4) the prefrontal executive function and working memory network (which is based on transmodal regions in the lateral prefrontal

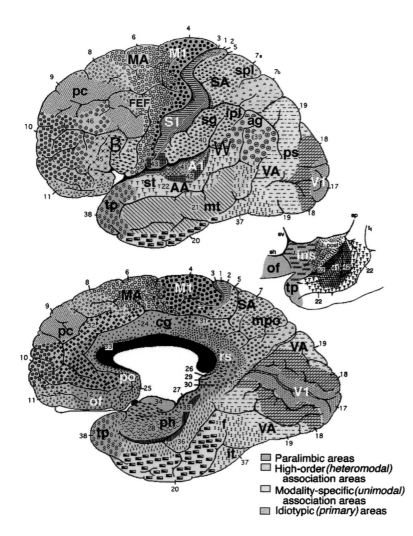

Figure 74-1. Cortical anatomy and functional subtypes (areas) in relationship to Brodmann's map of the human brain. The boundaries are not intended to be precise. Much of this information is based on experimental evidence obtained from laboratory animals and needs to be confirmed in the human brain. AA, Auditory association cortex; ag, angular gyrus; A1, primary auditory cortex; B, Broca's area; cg, cingulate cortex; f, fusiform gyrus; FEF, frontal eye fields; ins, insula; ipl, inferior parietal lobule; it, inferior temporal gyrus; MA, motor association cortex; mpo, medial parieto-occipital area; mt, middle temporal gyrus; M1, primary motor area; of, orbitofrontal region; pc, prefrontal cortex; ph, parahippocampal region; po, parolfactory area; ps, peristriate cortex; rs, retrosplenial area; SA, somatosensory association cortex; sg, marginal gyrus; spl, superior parietal lobule; st, superior temporal gyrus; S1, primary somatosensory area; tp, temporopolar cortex; VA, visual association cortex; V1, primary visual cortex; W, Wernicke's area. *(From Mesulam MM. Behavioral neuroanatomy. Large scale networks, association cortex, frontal syndromes, the limbic system and hemisphere specializations. In Mesulam MM, editor: Principles of Behavioral and Cognitive Neurology, New York, 2000, Oxford University Press, p. 13.)*

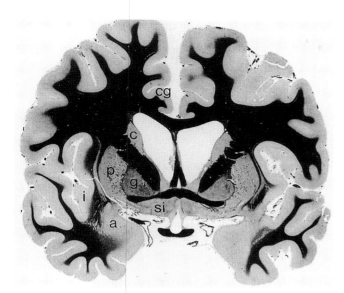

Figure 74-2. Coronal section through the basal forebrain of a 25-year-old human brain stained for myelin. The substantia innominata (si) and the amygdaloid complex (a) are located on the surface of the brain. c, Head of the caudate nucleus; cg, cingulate gyrus; g, globus pallidus; i, insula. *(From Mesulam MM. Behavioral neuroanatomy. Large scale networks, association cortex, frontal syndromes, the limbic system and hemisphere specializations. In Mesulam MM, editor:* Principles of Behavioral and Cognitive Neurology, *New York, 2000, Oxford University Press, p. 4.)*

cortex and possibly the inferior parietal cortices); and, (5) the inferotemporal face and object recognition network (which is based on temporopolar and midtemporal cortices).

Lesions of transmodal cortical areas result in global impairments (such as hemi-neglect, anosognosia, amnesia, and multi-modal anomia). Disconnection of transmodal regions from a specific unimodal input results in selective perceptual impairments (e.g., category-specific anomias, prosopagnosia, pure word deafness, and pure word blindness).[20]

The emergence of new neuroimaging technologies, such as resting state fMRI intrinsic connectivity[21] and MRI structural co-variance,[22] has facilitated the study of networks *in vivo*. Three intrinsic connectivity functional networks are particularly relevant to the understanding of emotions and behaviors: (1) the default mode network (DMN), which includes areas along the anterior and posterior mid-line (posterior cingulate, precuneus, medial prefrontal areas, anterior cingulate cortex), lateral parietal, prefrontal cortex (PFC), and medial temporal lobe, and is linked to self-referential thinking[23]; (2) the salience network, which is anchored in the fronto-insular cortex, dorsal anterior cingulate cortex (also referred to as middle cingulate cortex), has strong connections with subcortical and limbic structures, and is linked to reactions to external stimuli[24]; and (3) the executive function networks, which involve the dorsolateral prefrontal cortex and parietal neocortex, which are areas involved in working memory/sustained attention, response selection, and response inhibition.[24]

Interestingly, the characteristic pathology of neurodegenerative diseases seems to evolve along explicit networks. For example, there is evidence showing predominant initial dysfunction in the salience network in bvFTD, as opposed to the development of pathology in the DMN in AD (Figure 74-3).[25,26] The relative preservation of the salience network could explain the retained emotional warmth, sensitivity, and connectedness seen in AD, as opposed to the loss of empathy and social isolation secondary to bvFTD.[7]

Cortical networks underlie the ability to empathize with another person's psychological and physical circumstances. A system of human mirror neurons is hypothesized to be involved in comprehending the intentions and actions of others, potentially providing the basis for observational learning.[27] The parietofrontal mirror system (which includes the parietal lobe, the premotor cortex, and the caudal part of the inferior frontal gyrus) is involved in recognition of voluntary behavior. The limbic mirror system, formed by the insula and the anterior medial frontal cortex, is linked to the recognition of affective behavior. Of note, these mirror neurons do not represent self-standing neuronal networks, but rather a mechanism intrinsic to motor and limbic-related areas.[27] Dysfunction of this system may underlie deficits in theory of mind, and has been proposed as an explanation for the social deficits of autism spectrum disorders.

Frontal-Subcortical Networks

As detailed in Chapter 72, five frontal-subcortical circuits subserve cognition, behavior, and movement. Disruption of these networks at either the cortical or subcortical level can cause similar neuropsychiatric symptoms. Each of these circuits shares the same components: frontal cortex, striatum, globus pallidus, and thalamus, which then project back to frontal cortex.[28,29] There are also integrative connections to and from other subcortical and distant cortical regions related to each circuit.[6] Neurotransmitters (e.g., dopamine, glutamate, gamma-aminobutyric acid [GABA], acetylcholine, norepinephrine [noradrenaline], serotonin) are involved in various aspects of neural transmission and modulation through these circuits.

Three of the five circuits are more crucially involved in cognition and behavior: the dorsolateral prefrontal, the lateral orbitofrontal, and the anterior cingulate circuits.[6,28,30] The dorsolateral prefrontal circuit, also known as the dorsal cognitive circuit, governs executive functions (such as the ability to plan and maintain attention, problem-solve, learn, retrieve remote memories, sequence the temporal order of events, shift cognitive and behavioral sets, and generate a motor program).[31,32] Dysfunction in this network is the source of the profound executive impairments observed in subcortical dementias. The lateral orbitofrontal circuit, also known as the ventral cognitive circuit, connects frontal monitoring systems to the limbic structures. This circuit governs appropriate responses to social cues, value determination, empathy, social judgment, and interpersonal sensitivity.[33] Dysfunction in this circuit can lead to disinhibition, irritability, aggressive outbursts, and inappropriate social responses. The anterior cingulate circuit, also known as the affective circuit, is involved in motivated behavior, conflict monitoring, and potentially other complex behaviors, such as creative thought processes.[34] Lesions in this circuit may result in apathy (or akinetic mutism in its most severe form).[9] Both the lateral OFC and ACC circuits can demonstrate atrophy in bvFTD, which correlates with variable degrees of disinihibition and apathy.[7]

Of note, all the cerebral cortex shares similar features of organization, each area having neighboring, short, long, commissural (cross-hemispheric), and subcortical (striatal, thalamic, pontine) connection fibers.[35] It is important to have some knowledge of the major long association white matter tracts connecting cortical areas involved in behavior, such as the cingulum bundle and uncinate fasciculus. Lesions in these pathways can result in slowed cognitive processing and behavioral issues, such as apathy, that may occur in individuals with multiple sclerosis and subcortical strokes.

Finally, it is important to note that the cerebellum, especially the posterior lobe and posterior vermis, has been

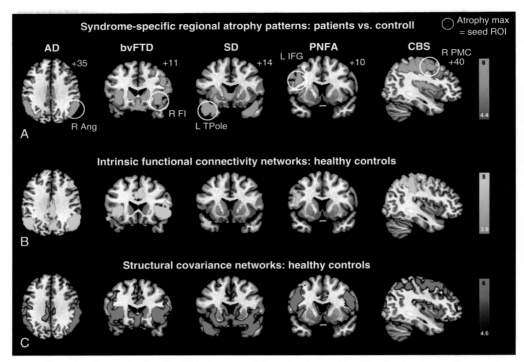

Figure 74-3. Convergent syndromic atrophy, healthy intrinsic connectivity networks, and healthy structural co-variance patterns. (A) Five distinct clinical syndromes showed dissociable atrophy patterns, whose cortical maxima (circled) provided seed regions of interest for intrinsic connectivity networks (ICN) and structural co-variance analyses. (B) ICN mapping experiments identified five distinct networks anchored by the five syndromic atrophy seeds. (C) Healthy subjects further showed gray matter volume covariance patterns that recapitulated results shown in (A) and (B). For visualization purposes, results are shown at P < 0.00001 uncorrected (A and C) and P < 0.001 corrected height and extent thresholds (B). In A–C, results are displayed on representative sections of the MNI template brain. Color bars indicate t-scores. In coronal and axial images, the left side of the image corresponds to the left side of the brain. AD, Alzheimer's disease; bvFTD, behavioral variant frontotemporal dementia; SD, semantic dementia; PNFA, progressive non-fluent aphasia; CBS, corticobasal syndrome; Ang, angular gyrus; FI, frontoinsula; TPole, temporal pole; IFG, inferior frontal gyrus, pars opercularis; PMC, premotor cortex. *(From Seeley WW, Crawford RK, Zhou J, et al. Neurodegenerative diseases target large-scale human brain networks.* Neuron 62:42–52, 2009.)

postulated to have a role in modulating executive functions, spatial cognition, language (e.g., prosody), emotion, and behavior.[36] Damage to this area may result in a cerebellar cognitive-affective syndrome.[36]

NEUROPSYCHIATRIC EVALUATION

A number of important principles must be taken into account when evaluating patients with behavioral disturbances. A few clinical key points are summarized in Box 74-1.

The medical evaluation of cognitive-behavioral disorders must be individualized based on the patient's age, gender, family history, social environment, habits, culture of origin, risk factors, and examination findings. A detailed clinical history, including collateral information from family and caregivers, is of paramount importance for precisely determining the nature and time course of symptoms, thereby aiding the diagnosis. In new-onset presentations, a careful review of the patient's medical antecedents in addition to the performance of a general physical examination with vital signs, cognitive screening, and neurological examination are necessary to assess for neurological and general medical causes of unexplained behavioral changes. Consideration should be given to checking the patient's oxygen saturation on room air, especially in the elderly, as this can be an unrecognized cause of subacute delirium.

Although it is not possible to blindly recommend hematological and biochemical tests for all symptoms, in general a basic work-up should include a complete blood cell count,

BOX 74-1 Clinical Pearls of the Neuropsychiatric Evaluation

- A normal neurological examination does not exclude neurological conditions. Lesions in the limbic, paralimbic, and prefrontal regions may cause cognitive-behavioral changes in the absence of elemental neurological abnormalities.
- Normal routine laboratory testing, brain imaging, electroencephalography, and cerebrospinal fluid are supportive of primary psychiatric disorders, but do not necessarily exclude all neurological diseases.
- New neurological complaints or behavioral changes in a person with a pre-existing psychiatric history should not be automatically assumed to be of psychiatric origin.
- The possibility of iatrogenic conditions must be taken into account. Medication side effects can complicate the clinical history and examination (e.g., hallucinations induced by dopamine agonists in Parkinson's disease). Medication side effects can also be harbingers of underlying pathology (e.g., marked parkinsonism after exposure to D_2 blocking agents can be a feature of Lewy Body Dementia before this condition has been clinically characterized).
- Treatment of psychiatric and neurological behavioral disturbances share common principles. A response to therapy does not constitute absolute evidence of a primary psychiatric disorder.

blood urea nitrogen, creatinine, electrolytes panel, serum glucose, calcium, total serum protein, liver function tests, and thyroid function assessment. Additional laboratory testing may be considered according to the clinical history and risk factors. Studies might include a toxicology panel, vitamin B_{12}, folate, HIV serology, FTA-ABS, HCV serology, Lyme serology, ANA, ESR, CRP, cortisol, prolactin, testosterone, ceruloplasmin, heavy metal screen, ammonia, homocysteine, serum paraneoplastic panel, urine copper, urine porphobilinogen, fragile X testing, whole genome microarray, number of CAG repeats for Huntington's disease, *C9ORF72* mutation, and other specialized rheumatologic, metabolic and genetic tests.[37] Regarding substance-related disorders, clinicians need to be aware that some newer designer drugs, such as "bath salts," might not be detected by current blood and urine tests.[38]

Neuroimaging

With the increased availability of MRI, obtaining brain imaging has become a common practice in psychiatry. Considerable debate continues regarding the indications for use of this technology, both in medical and economical terms. Neurological symptoms gleaned during history-taking or findings on examination that suggest central nervous system (CNS) pathology should prompt further investigation.[13] MRI is a safe method to help exclude lesions (demyelination, ischemic, neoplasm, congenital structural abnormalities) in limbic, paralimbic, and frontal regions that may not be associated with abnormalities on elemental neurological exam. It is also useful for detecting rare metabolic storage diseases than can present with a schizophrenia-like clinical picture (e.g., metachromatic leukodystrophy, Niemann-Pick type C; see Box 74-2 for complete list).[39]

At a minimum, the MRI scan should include T1 and T2/FLAIR sequences in axial and sagittal planes. When stroke or cerebral ischemia is suspected, diffusion-weighted sequences are indicated. Thin coronal cuts are helpful for close inspection of the temporal lobes in suspected cases of seizures or AD. Gradient echo or susceptibility-weighted sequences can be useful to identify remote bleeds, especially in cases of TBI. The use of contrast is recommended whenever there is a need to assess for conditions (inflammatory, autoimmune, neoplastic, traumatic and ischemic) that disrupt the blood–brain barrier. CT scanning still has some advantages in emergency settings given that it is more quickly obtained, and takes less time to complete, which is especially helpful with agitated or claustrophobic patients. CT is superior for visualizing bone and calcifications, but does not optimally visualize the posterior fossa.

Functional imaging methods include single-photon emission computed tomography (SPECT) and positron emission tomography (PET). These tests find their greatest clinical application in the differentiation of AD from FTD or from Lewy body dementia (LBD), and the localization of a seizure focus. PET ligands for amyloid have been developed recently to aid in the diagnosis of AD. Although adopted enthusiastically by some clinicians, based on limited evidence, PET and SPECT do not currently have clear clinical indications in general psychiatry outside of research settings. Details on the different neuroimaging modalities are reviewed in Chapter 75.

Electroencephalogram

An electroencephalogram (EEG) is recommended whenever the behavioral presentation suggests complex partial seizures, usually secondary to temporal and frontal lobe epilepsy.[40] Seizures should be considered in the differential diagnosis when one of the following clinical features is present: (1)

intermittent, discrete, abrupt episodes of psychiatric dysfunction (usually confusion, spells of lost time, or psychotic symptoms); (2) stereotyped hallucinations (e.g., micro/macropsia, "Alice in Wonderland" syndrome); (3) automatisms (e.g., lip-smacking, repetitive movements) during episodes of neuropsychiatric dysfunction or confusion; and, (4) acute onset of confusional or a psychotic-like state not readily explained by toxic-metabolic causes.

We recommend obtaining a baseline (routine) EEG as a first step before considering other techniques, such as sleep-deprived EEG. The sensitivity of EEG for the detection of seizure activity is highest when the patient has specific symptoms while undergoing the study. Selected cases may require 24-hour or longer EEG monitoring (outpatient or inpatient video telemetry) to capture a clinical event. EEG is a low-cost and useful screening tool that can be used whenever there is suspicion of encephalopathy or delirium, independent of its underlying cause.

Sleep Studies

Sleep disturbances are very common in primary psychiatric disorders, but can also be secondary to general medical and neurological conditions. A careful history that assesses for factors that adversely affect sleep should be conducted. Sleep apnea, restless leg syndrome, periodic limb movements of sleep (PLMS), sleep-walking, night terrors, nightmares, physical pain (e.g., musculoskeletal, headaches, neuropathy, dystonia), nocturia, and environmental factors should be reviewed, particularly in cases of treatment-refractory MDD.[41] Overnight polysomnography should be obtained for suspected cases of obstructive sleep apnea, PLMS, non-restorative sleep, excessive daytime sleepiness despite adequate sleep, fragmented sleep (which may be present in epilepsy), REM sleep behavior disorder (often associated with multiple system atrophy, Parkinson's disease, or LBD) or if other parasomnias or dyssomnias are suspected. Other tests can be considered in specific cases, such as the multiple sleep latency test for suspicion of narcolepsy or idiopathic hypersomnia.

Lumbar Puncture for Cerebrospinal Fluid Analysis

A neurological consultation to review indications for cerebrospinal fluid (CSF) testing should be obtained for any case in which an infectious, inflammatory, autoimmune, neoplastic, or paraneoplastic etiology is considered. A basic CSF analysis usually includes an opening pressure, cell counts, protein and glucose levels, oligoclonal bands (compared with serum oligoclonal bands), and sensitivity/bacterial cultures. Other tests can be performed depending on the suspected disease (e.g., CNS Lyme disease, neurosyphilis, neurosarcoid, HIV infection). Large-volume fluid collections may be useful for assessing cytology to exclude malignancy or for excluding normal pressure hydrocephalus. CSF analysis for biomarkers, including beta-amyloid (Aβ-42), phosphorylated tau, and total tau, is becoming more commonly performed in the work-up of AD.[42]

NEUROPSYCHIATRIC DIFFERENTIAL DIAGNOSIS

A variety of neurological conditions are associated with psychiatric symptoms, either secondary to the disease itself, or to its treatments.[13,15,43] Emotional and behavioral symptoms may be striking, and precede the hallmark neurological manifestations by years.[13] For example, the onset of changes in mood, personality, and OCD symptoms can precede by many years the cognitive decline and movement abnormalities in Huntington's disease.[44] While some neurological disorders do not

BOX 74-2 Neuropsychiatric Differential Diagnosis of Emotional, Behavioral, and Cognitive Symptoms

Category	Disease/Disorder	Category	Disease/Disorder
Traumatic	Traumatic brain injury and post-concussion syndrome Subdural hematoma Chronic traumatic encephalopathy	Neurodegenerative	Alzheimer's disease Frontotemporal dementia (behavioral variant, primary progressive aphasias) Lewy body dementia
Infectious	HIV infection and HIV neurocognitive disorder Opportunistic infections Neurosyphilis Viral infections/encephalitides (herpes simplex, CMV, EBV, others) Other infectious encephalitis (bacterial, fungal, parasites) CNS Whipple's disease CNS Lyme disease Prion diseases (e.g., Creutzfeldt-Jacob disease) Cerebral malaria		Progressive supranuclear palsy Corticobasal degeneration Multiple system atrophy (parkinsonian and cerebellar subtypes) Parkinson's disease Huntington's disease Idiopathic basal ganglia calcification (Fahr's disease)
		Demyelinating/ Dysmyelinating	Multiple sclerosis Acute disseminated encephalomyelitis Subacute sclerosing panencephalitis Adrenoleukodystrophy Metachromatic leukodystrophy
Inflammatory/ Autoimmune	Anti-NMDA encephalitis Anti-LGI1 (anti voltage gated potassium channel—VGKC) encephalitis Limbic encephalitis (anti-GAD and others) Systemic lupus erythematous and lupus cerebritis Sjögren's syndrome Antiphospholipid syndrome Neurosarcoidosis Hashimoto's encephalopathy Sydenham's chorea Pediatric autoimmune neuropsychiatric disorder associated with streptococcal infections (PANDAS)	Inherited metabolic	Wilson's disease Hexosaminidase deficiencies (e.g., Tay-Sachs disease, late-onset GM_2 gangliosidosis) Niemann-Pick type C Adult neuronal ceroid lipofuscinosis (Kufs' disease) Neuroacanthocytosis/McLeod syndrome Acute intermittent porphyria Other inborn errors of metabolism (e.g., urea cycle defects, MTHFR deficiency, cerebrotendinous xanthomatosis) Mitochondrial disorders
Neoplastic	Primary or secondary cerebral neoplasm Systemic neoplasm Pancreatic cancer Paraneoplastic encephalitis (anti-NMDA, anti-Hu, anti-Ma, anti-CRMP5/CV2) Pheochromocytoma Carcinoid tumors		Mitochondrial encephalopathy, lactic acidosis, and stroke-like episodes (MELAS)
		Epilepsy	Ictal, inter-ictal, or post-ictal behavioral changes (e.g., post-ictal psychosis) Changes post epilepsy surgery (e.g., forced normalization)
Endocrine/ Acquired Metabolic	Hepatic encephalopathy Renal failure and uremia Dialysis dementia Hypoglycemia Hypo/hyperthyroidism Hypo/hyperparathyroidism Addison's disease Cushing's disease Wernicke-Korsakoff encephalopathy (thiamine deficiency) Other vitamin deficiencies: vitamin B_{12}, folate, niacin, vitamin C, vitamin E Gastric-bypass associated nutritional deficiencies Celiac disease	Sleep	Obstructive sleep apnea Narcolepsy Kleine-Levin syndrome REM sleep behavior disorder
		Medications/ Drugs/Toxins	Any psychotropic medication Serotonin syndrome Neuroleptic malignant syndrome Drugs of abuse Drug withdrawal syndromes (alcohol, barbiturates, benzodiazepines, opiates) Heavy metals (e.g., lead poisoning) Inhalants Chemotherapy, interferon-alpha, anti-malarial agents
Vascular	Cerebrovascular accidents (ischemic, hemorrhagic) Vascular dementia CNS vasculitis Transient global amnesia Cerebral autosomal dominant arteriopathy with subcortical infarcts and leukoencephalopathy (CADASIL) Peduncular hallucinosis Susac's syndrome	Other	Cerebral hypoxia Normal pressure hydrocephalus Sagging brain syndrome Malignant catatonia Ionizing radiation exposure Post-radiotherapy cognitive deficits Decompression sickness

TABLE 74-1 Neurological Disorders and Associated Behavioral Features

Neurological Disorder	Behavioral Disturbances
Cerebrovascular disease	Depression, mania, apathy, rarely psychosis
Parkinson's disease	Depression, anxiety, drug-associated hallucinations, delusions (jealousy), REM sleep behavior disorder, drug-associated behavioral addictions (e.g., gambling and sexual disinhibition with dopamine agonists), apathy
Lewy body dementia	Fluctuating confusion, hallucinations (prominent visual, but also other modalities), delusions, depression, REM sleep behavior disorder
Alzheimer's disease	Depression, anxiety, irritability, apathy, delusions (persecutory, misidentification), hallucinations
Vascular dementia	Depression, apathy, psychosis
Frontotemporal dementia	Personality changes, loss of social graces, loss of empathy, impaired judgment, disinhibition, apathy, compulsions, altered food preferences, hyperorality, late-onset psychosis
Progressive supranuclear palsy	Disinhibition, apathy
Corticobasal degeneration	Depression, irritability, REM sleep behavior disorder, alien-limb syndrome
Huntington's disease	Depression, irritability, mania, obsessive-compulsive disorder, apathy, delusions, hallucinations
Traumatic brain injury	Post-concussion syndrome, depression, personality changes, disinhibition, apathy, irritability, substance abuse, psychosis uncommon
Epilepsy	Depression, psychosis (ictal, post-ictal, inter-ictal), personality changes
Multiple sclerosis	Depression, irritability, anxiety, euphoria, psychosis
Amyotrophic lateral sclerosis	Depression, disinhibition, apathy, impaired judgment, delusions

cause behavioral symptoms, they may still be highly co-morbid with psychiatric disorders. The epidemiological association between migraines and mood disorders is an example of this.[45] Table 74-1 summarizes psychiatric manifestations of common neurological and neuropsychiatric disorders. Of note, behavioral changes are linked to increased caregiver stress and to earlier placement in nursing homes for patients with neurological diseases.[46,47]

Virtually any process that affects the previously described neuroanatomical circuits can result in, or at least contribute to, the occurrence of psychiatric symptoms during the course of a condition.[48–54] Some processes are quite common (e.g., medication-induced hypothyroidism), while others are extremely rare (e.g., CNS Whipple's disease, acute intermittent porphyria). Due to the broad range of conditions that may produce behavioral changes, a systematic approach is necessary. The first step is to utilize the history and the physical examination to identify signs and symptoms. This is followed by localization of the site (or sites) of potential pathology. The differential diagnosis is then generated. Based upon these steps a work-up can be outlined. Box 74-2 categorizes (by pathophysiological processes) a number of conditions that can present with emotional, behavioral, or cognitive symptoms. Not included in this table are metabolic disorders that can lead to delirium, which is the subject of another chapter. Causes of developmental intellectual disability (e.g., fragile X syndrome, fetal alcohol syndrome, 22q11 deletion) are also not included. Detailed information regarding the evaluation, natural history, pathology, and treatment recommendations for these conditions is beyond the scope of this chapter.

CLINICAL SYMPTOMS AND SIGNS SUGGESTING NEUROLOGICAL OR GENERAL MEDICAL CONDITIONS

Given the high prevalence of disorders such as major depression, bipolar disorder, and schizophrenia, performing an extensive work-up in all patients to exclude unusual causes, such as adult neuronal ceroid lipofuscinosis, is not justifiable either from a medical or economic perspective. A more targeted and systematic approach is required.

Psychiatrists and neurologists need to be acquainted with features of the clinical history that raise one's suspicion of an underlying neurological, neuropsychiatric, or general medical condition (Box 74-3). Table 74-2 lists some key symptoms on the review of systems that can aid in creation of a differential

BOX 74-3 Clinical Features Suggesting Neurological Diseases in Patients with Psychiatric Symptoms

PRESENCE OF ATYPICAL PSYCHIATRIC FEATURES
- Late or very early age of onset
- Acute or subacute onset
- Lack of significant psychosocial stressors if expected
- Cognitive decline
- Catatonia
- Diminished comportment
- Visual hallucinations
- Altered level of consciousness
- Intractability despite adequate therapy
- Progressive symptoms

HISTORY OF PRESENT ILLNESS INCLUDES
- New or worsening headache
- Somnolence
- Incontinence
- Focal neurological complaints (e.g., weakness, sensory changes, incoordination, gait instability, falls)
- Weight loss unexplained by decreased oral intake
- Abdominal crises of unknown origin

MEDICAL HISTORY
- Risk factors for cerebrovascular disease
- Malignancy
- Immunocompromised host
- Significant traumatic brain injury
- Seizures/epilepsy
- Movement disorder
- Hepatobiliary disorders

FAMILY HISTORY
- Absence of psychiatric disorder with strong familial aggregation (e.g., bipolar I disorder)
- History of genetic diseases
- History of early-onset dementia or amyotrophic lateral sclerosis
- Biological relatives with similar unexplained complaints

UNEXPLAINED DIAGNOSTIC ABNORMALITIES
- Screening laboratories
- Endocrine
- Neuroimaging studies
- EEG
- Cerebrospinal fluid
- Hepatobiliary

TABLE 74-2 Review of Systems with Neuropsychiatric Relevance and Related Conditions

System	Related Conditions
GENERAL	
Weight loss	Neoplasia, drug or alcohol abuse, endocrine dysfunction
Decreased energy level	Multiple sclerosis, neoplasia, endocrine dysfunction
Fever/chills	Occult systemic or CNS infections
Arthritis	Vasculitis, connective tissue disease, Lyme disease
HEAD	
New-onset headaches or change in character/ severity	Many conditions
Trauma	Subdural hematoma, contusion, post-concussion syndrome, chronic traumatic encephalopathy
EYES	
Chronic visual loss	May predispose to visual hallucinations—Charles Bonnet syndrome
Episodic visual loss	Amaurosis fugax, multiple sclerosis
Diplopia	Brainstem pathology, cranial nerve lesions
EARS	
Hearing loss	May predispose to auditory hallucinations and persecutory delusions, mitochondrial disorders, Susac's syndrome
NOSE	
Anosmia	Head trauma, olfactory groove meningioma, neurodegenerative diseases
MOUTH	
Oral lesions	Nutritional deficiency, seizure, inflammatory/autoimmune diseases
NECK	
Stiffness	Meningitis
SKIN	
Rash	Vasculitis, Lyme disease, sexually-transmitted diseases
Birthmarks	Phakomatoses
CARDIOVASCULAR	
Heart disease	Ischemic cerebrovascular disease
Hypertension	Ischemic cerebrovascular disease
Cardiac arrhythmia	Cerebral emboli
GASTROINTESTINAL	
Acute abdominal pain	Acute intermittent porphyria
Diarrhea	Malabsorption, Whipple's disease
Constipation	Dysautonomia
Vomiting	Neurodegenerative disorder related dysautonomia, porphyria
MOTOR	
Focal weakness	Amyotrophic lateral sclerosis, stroke, mass lesion, post-ictal
Gait dysfunction	Hydrocephalus, cerebellar diseases, Parkinson's disease, gait apraxia, movement disorders
AUTONOMIC	
Urinary retention or incontinence	Dysautonomia, hydrocephalus, multiple system atrophy
Erectile dysfunction	Dysautonomia, multiple system atrophy
Orthostatic hypotension	Medication side effect, dysautonomia, multiple system atrophy

diagnosis. Box 73-1 in the previous chapter lists abnormalities of the elemental neurological examination associated with neurological diseases that can exhibit psychiatric features.

The presence of atypical features in major psychiatric disorders is an important factor that prompts additional investigations and consultations in clinical practice. Although there is clearly some validity to this approach, atypical symptoms should be analyzed within the clinical context.[55] It is more frequent to see atypical symptoms of a common disorder than symptoms of a rare disorder even if they are typical of the latter. For example, a clinician in a general psychiatry setting will more often encounter patients with schizophrenia having visual hallucinations (considered to be atypical) than cases of metachromatic leukodystrophy.

Late or very-early ages of onset may serve notice for consideration of a broader differential diagnosis. Acute or subacute onset of severe symptoms can suggest infectious, vascular, or autoimmune processes, among others. Although not all psychiatric disorders are associated with psychosocial stressors, the absence of any triggering factor for an acute behavioral change can raise the prospect of partial complex seizures or a rare condition, such as acute intermittent porphyria. On mental status exam, diminished comportment (blunted insight, awareness, concern, appropriateness) can suggest a neurodegenerative disease, such as bvFTD[54,56] or chronic traumatic encephalopathy.[53] Although it is most often seen in affective and psychotic disorders, catatonia[57] can be secondary to a variety of medical diseases[58] including the recently described anti-NMDA encephalitis.[49] Some level of cognitive impairment is expected with major psychiatric syndromes, such as chronic schizophrenia and bipolar disorder, but unexplained cognitive decline deserves a comprehensive neuropsychiatric assessment. The course of a disorder provides helpful diagnostic information. When intractability to treatment is present, a reconsideration of the differential diagnosis is indicated. However, a fair proportion of individuals with severe chronic diseases, such as schizophrenia, have a suboptimal response to the best available treatments. Progressive symptoms over time (including fluctuating level of consciousness, cognitive decline, seizures, onset of movement disorder, incontinence, and other motor/sensory neurological symptoms) are important factors prompting the need for further investigations. A rapid deterioration should trigger investigations along the lines of rapidly progressing dementia diagnostic algorithms.[48] As a rule of thumb, in the presence of one atypical factor, clinicians should thoroughly search for at least a second clinical feature to support the possibility of more unusual diagnoses.

Signs and symptoms should guide investigations. If necessary, a neurology and/or internal medicine consultation should be requested. Stating clear and precise reasons for consultations can help ensure effective communication between specialties, with the goal of improving patients' outcomes. Terminology that might not be familiar to consultants, such as "atypical psychiatric features," and vague requests, such as "rule-out organic causes," should be avoided. Speaking directly with the consultant regarding the nature of the concerns is advocated.

TREATMENT PRINCIPLES

Each condition has subtleties associated with its prognosis, treatment, and management that should be reviewed carefully before proceeding with a treatment plan. In general, patients with an underlying neurological condition tend to be more susceptible to the adverse reactions of psychotropic medications, particularly extrapyramidal and cognitive side effects. These adverse reactions may be minimized by initiating medications at low doses using gentle titration. When clinically indicated, second-generation antipsychotics with lower D_2 potency are often preferred over conventional antipsychotics due to lower rates of neurological adverse effects. Various types of psychotherapy can be helpful and should be considered in patients with neuropsychiatric disorders or neurological co-morbidities, unless cognitive impairment precludes meaningful participation. Specific therapies have been developed for neuropsychiatric conditions, such as habit-reversal training for Tourette disorder.[59] Electroconvulsive therapy (ECT) is a useful option for the treatment of mood disorders, catatonia, and situations where medications cannot be tolerated or are ineffective. In general, ECT can be safely performed in patients with stable neurological conditions, including Parkinson's disease, epilepsy, and non-acute cerebrovascular events.[60,61] Other options to consider for the treatment of refractory disorders, such as MDD and OCD, include rTMS,[62] vagal nerve stimulation,[63] deep brain stimulation,[64,65] and stereotactic ablative surgery.[66,67]

CONCLUSIONS

Due to advances in the basic neurosciences and the development of new imaging and other diagnostic studies, modern clinical neurology has gone from a largely phenomenological field to one characterized by focused therapy based on a rational understanding of disease mechanisms. Progress in the neurosciences of cognition, emotion, and behavior are pushing psychiatry toward similar transitional challenges, with perhaps even more complexity. However, 17th century Cartesian dualism continues to hold back both neurology and psychiatry, as reflected by the ongoing use of antagonizing terms, such as the functional versus organic dichotomy. In both disciplines, we would caution against biological oversimplification and Cartesian dualism.

The inseparability of brain and mind is the fundamental tenet of behavioral neurology and neuropsychiatry.[1] We contend that the traditional boundaries between neurology and psychiatry have become obsolete, and that an integrative neuropsychiatric framework is more scientifically valid and

promising. The future of psychiatric and neurological care, training, and research will inevitably require effective collaboration between both disciplines.[1,2] The emerging discipline of behavioral neurology and neuropsychiatry can provide leadership in this complex arena.

Access the complete reference list and multiple choice questions (MCQs) online at https://expertconsult.inkling.com

KEY REFERENCES

1. Price BH, Adams RD, Coyle JT. Neurology and psychiatry. Closing the great divide. *Neurology* 54(1):8–14, 2000.
2. Martin JB. The integration of neurology, psychiatry, and neuroscience in the 21st century. *Am J Psychiatry* 159(5):695–704, 2002.
4. Arciniegas DB, Kaufer DI. Core curriculum for training in behavioral neurology & neuropsychiatry. *J Neuropsychiatry Clin Neurosci* 18(1):6–13, 2006.
5. Price JL, Drevets WC. Neural circuits underlying the pathophysiology of mood disorders. *Trends Cogn Sci* 16(1):61–71, 2012.
6. Milad M, Rauch S. Obsessive-compulsive disorder: beyond segregated cortico-strial pathways. *Trends Cogn Sci* 16(1):43–51, 2012.
7. Seeley WW, Zhou J, Kim E-J. Frontotemporal dementia: What can the behavioral variant teach us about human brain organization? *Neuroscientist* 18(4):373–385, 2012.
13. Arciniegas DB, Topkoff JL, Held K, et al. Psychosis due to neurologic conditions. *Curr Treat Options Neurol* 3(4):347–364, 2001.
16. Marin RS. The three-dimensional approach to neuropsychiatric assessment. *J Neuropsychiatry Clin Neurosci* 24(4):384–393, 2012.
17. Mesulam M. Behavioral neuroanatomy. Large scale networks, association cortex, frontal syndromes, the limbic system and hemisphere specializations. In Mesulam M, editor: *Principles of behavioral and cognitive neurology*, ed 2, New York, 2000, Oxford University Press.
18. Mesulam M. Representation, inference, and transcendent encoding in neurocognitive networks of the human brain. *Ann Neurol* 64(4):367–378, 2008.
19. Mesulam M. The evolving landscape of human cortical connectivity: Facts and inferences. *Neuroimage* 62(4):2182–2189, 2012.
20. Catani M. The rises and falls of disconnection syndromes. *Brain* 128(10):2224–2239, 2005.
21. Damoiseaux JS, Rombouts SARB, Barkhof F, et al. Consistent resting-state networks across healthy subjects. *PNAS* 103(37):13848–13853, 2006.
25. Seeley WW, Crawford RK, Zhou J, et al. Neurodegenerative diseases target large-scale human brain networks. *Neuron* 62(1):42–52, 2009.
26. Zhou J, Gennatas ED, Kramer JH, et al. Predicting regional neurodegeneration from the healthy brain functional connectome. *Neuron* 73(6):1216–1227, 2012.
27. Cattaneo L, Rizzolatti G. The mirror neuron system. *Arch Neurology* 66(5):557–560, 2009.
30. Tekin S, Cummings J. Frontal-subcortical neuronal circuits and clinical neuropsychiatry: an update. *J Psychosom Res* 53(2):647–654, 2002.
35. Schmahmann JD, Smith EE, Eichler FS, et al. Cerebral white matter. *Ann NY Acad Sci* 1142(1):266–309, 2008.
36. Schmahmann JD. The role of the cerebellum in cognition and emotion: personal reflections since 1982 on the dysmetria of thought hypothesis, and its historical evolution from theory to therapy. *Neuropsychol Rev* 20(3):236–260, 2010.
37. Ovsiew F, Murray E, Price B. Neuropsychiatric approach to the psychiatric inpatient. In Ovsiew F, Munich R, editors: *Principles of inpatient psychiatry*, Philadelphia, PA, 2008, Wolters Kluwer Lippincott Williams & Wilkins, pp 97–124.
39. Walterfang M, Wood SJ, Velakoulis D, et al. Diseases of white matter and schizophrenia-like psychosis. *Aust N Z J Psychiatry* 39(9):746–756, 2005.
48. Paterson RW, Takada LT, Geschwind MD. Diagnosis and treatment of rapidly progressive dementias. *Neurol Clin Pract* 2(3):187–200, 2012.
49. Chapman MR, Vause HE. Anti-NMDA receptor encephalitis: diagnosis, psychiatric presentation, and treatment. *Am J Psychiatry* 168(3):245–251, 2011.

50. Anglin RE, Tarnopolsky MA, Mazurek MF, et al. The psychiatric presentation of mitochondrial disorders in adults. *J Neuropsychiatry Clin Neurosci* 24(4):394–409, 2012.

51. Kayser MS, Kohler CG, Dalmau J. Psychiatric manifestations of paraneoplastic disorders. *Am J Psychiatry* 167(9):1039–1050, 2010.

52. Sedel F, Baumann N, Turpin J-C, et al. Psychiatric manifestations revealing inborn errors of metabolism in adolescents and adults. *J Inherit Metab Dis* 30(5):631–641, 2007.

53. McKee AC, Stein TD, Nowinski CJ, et al. The spectrum of disease in chronic traumatic encephalopathy. *Brain* 136(1):43–64, 2013.

54. Galimberti D, Fenoglio C, Serpente M, et al. Autosomal dominant frontotemporal lobar degeneration due to the C9ORF72 hexanucleotide repeat expansion: late-onset psychotic clinical presentation. *Biol Psychiatry* 74(5):384–391, 2013.

55. Freudenreich O, Schulz SC, Goff DC. Initial medical work-up of first-episode psychosis: a conceptual review. *Early Interv Psychiatry* 3(1):10–18, 2009.

56. Piguet O, Hornberger M, Mioshi E, et al. Behavioural-variant frontotemporal dementia: diagnosis, clinical staging, and management. *Lancet Neurol* 10(2):162–172, 2011.

57. Fink M, Taylor MA. The catatonia syndrome forgotten but not gone. *Arch Gen Psychiatry* 66(11):1173–1177, 2009.

58. Smith JH, Smith VD, Philbrick KL, et al. Catatonic disorder due to a general medical or psychiatric condition. *J Neuropsychiatry Clin Neurosci* 24(2):198–207, 2012.

60. Ducharme S, Flaherty AW, Seiner SJ, et al. Temporary interruption of deep brain stimulation for Parkinson's disease during outpatient electroconvulsive therapy for major depression: A novel treatment strategy. *J Neuropsychiatry Clin Neurosci* 23(2):194–197, 2011.

61. Tess AV, Smetana GW. Medical evaluation of patients undergoing electroconvulsive therapy. *N Engl J Med* 360(14):1437–1444, 2009.

75 Neuroimaging in Psychiatry

Darin D. Dougherty, MD, MSc, and Scott L. Rauch, MD

KEY POINTS

- When structural neuroimaging is clinically indicated, magnetic resonance imaging (MRI) is usually the modality of choice. Computed tomography (CT) is typically recommended instead of MRI if an acute bleed is suspected.

- Guidelines for obtaining structural neuroimaging studies in patients with neuropsychiatric symptoms include patients with acute changes in mental status (including changes in affect, behavior, or personality) plus one of the following criteria: age greater than 50 years; an abnormal neurological examination (especially with focal abnormalities); a history of significant head trauma (i.e., with extended loss of consciousness, neurological sequelae, or a temporal relationship to the mental status change in question); new-onset psychosis; or new-onset delirium or dementia of an unknown cause.

- Positron emission tomography (PET) and single-photon emission computed tomography (SPECT) are functional neuroimaging modalities. They measure cerebral blood flow and cerebral glucose metabolism, both of which are tightly coupled to neuronal activity.

- In the neuropsychiatric setting, PET and SPECT are potentially useful in the evaluation of dementia and seizures.

- Many neuroimaging modalities (e.g., functional magnetic resonance imaging [fMRI] and magnetic resonance spectroscopy [MRS]) have limited clinical utility at present, but they should become more clinically useful as the field matures.

OVERVIEW

In this chapter we will review neuroimaging modalities that can be used in clinical psychiatry, including the structural neuroimaging modalities computed tomography (CT) and magnetic resonance imaging (MRI), as well as the functional neuroimaging modalities (e.g., positron emission tomography [PET] and single-photon emission computed tomography [SPECT]). We will briefly review the underlying technology for each imaging modality and then will discuss the clinical utility of each. We will conclude with a brief review regarding the use of these, and other, neuroimaging modalities in the context of research. This chapter is an extension of prior reviews we have written on these topics.[1-6]

STRUCTURAL NEUROIMAGING MODALITIES
Computed Tomography
Technology

Computed tomography (CT) uses multiple serially-acquired x-rays that are attenuated to varying degrees depending on the material through which they pass.[7,8] For example, low-attenuation materials (such as air or fluid) appear dark on a CT image, whereas high-attenuation materials (such as bone) appear white. Gradations within the spectrum of attenuation allow for the visual differentiation of brain tissue (Figure 75-1). The serially-acquired x-rays are obtained in a rotating manner and these data are then reconstructed using computerized algorithms. The spatial resolution of CT has improved over the years, reaching 1 mm or better in-plane.

Contrast

In some clinical situations CT contrast can be used. CT contrast is typically (but not always) ionic contrast that is radiopaque (i.e., very high x-ray attenuation, meaning that it appears white on the CT image). The CT contrast agent is introduced intravenously. Therefore, CT contrast is especially useful for visualization of lesions that compromise the integrity of the blood–brain barrier (e.g., cerebrovascular accidents, tumors, inflammation).[9] Non-ionic contrast is also available, but it is more expensive than ionic contrast. However, ionic contrast is associated with a greater risk of side effects.[7] With ionic contrast, idiosyncratic reactions (including nausea, flushing, hypotension, urticaria, and sometimes frank anaphylaxis) occur in approximately 5% of cases. Those at highest risk for idiosyncratic reactions include the young and the old (<1 year of age or >60 years of age) and those with a history of cerebrovascular disease, asthma, allergies, and, of course, prior contrast reactions.[10] Ionic contrast is also associated with chemotoxic reactions that can occur in the kidney and the brain. Chemotoxic reactions in the kidney include impaired renal function and renal failure. The main risk factor for renal chemotoxic reactions to ionic contrast is pre-existing renal insufficiency.[11] Chemotoxic reactions in the brain typically manifest as seizures. These occur in 1 in every 10,000 cases, unless there is a gross disruption of the blood–brain barrier[12]; this increases the complication rate to 1%–5%.

Clinical Utility

CT is particularly useful for the detection of acute bleeding (<24 to 72 hours old) or acute trauma, but (as reviewed by Park and Gonzalez[8]) it is not the modality of choice for subacute bleeding (>72 hours old) or for patients who are markedly anemic (i.e., with a hemoglobin less than 10 g/dl). MRI (described later) is superior to CT for most other clinical situations. It should also be noted that CT uses ionizing radiation; thus, it is strongly contraindicated in pregnancy and it is relatively contraindicated in children. However, CT is appropriate when MRI is contraindicated (e.g., with paramagnetic prostheses).

Magnetic Resonance Imaging
Technology

Magnetic resonance imaging (MRI) does not use radiation; instead it uses strong magnetic fields and the magnetic properties of hydrogen atoms to create structural images.[13,14] Hydrogen atoms in water act as small magnets and align themselves in the same direction when within a magnetic field. The introduction of brief radiofrequency pulses perturbs this alignment. The relaxation of the hydrogen atoms moves them back

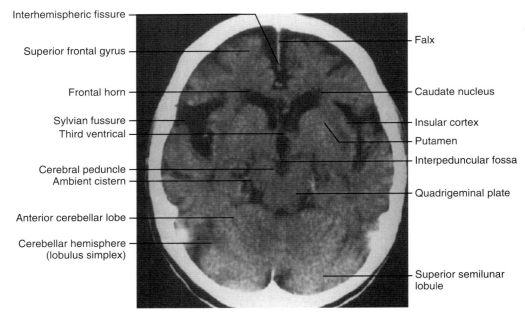

Interhemispheric fissure
Superior frontal gyrus
Frontal horn
Sylvian fussure
Third ventrical
Cerebral peduncle
Ambient cistern
Anterior cerebellar lobe
Cerebellar hemisphere
(lobulus simplex)

Falx
Caudate nucleus
Insular cortex
Putamen
Interpeduncular fossa
Quadrigeminal plate
Superior semilunar lobule

Figure 75-1. CT: normal brain. *(From Naheedy MH. Normal computed tomography and magnetic resonance imaging anatomy of the brain and the spine. In Haage JR, Lanzieri CF, Gilkeson RC, editors: CT and MRI imaging of the whole body, Philadelphia, 2003, Mosby, p. 96.)*

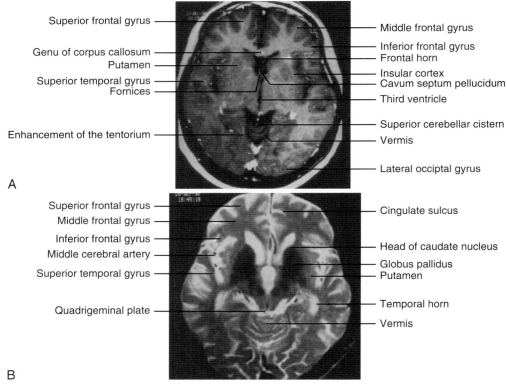

Superior frontal gyrus
Genu of corpus callosum
Putamen
Superior temporal gyrus
Fornices
Enhancement of the tentorium

Middle frontal gyrus
Inferior frontal gyrus
Frontal horn
Insular cortex
Cavum septum pellucidum
Third ventricle
Superior cerebellar cistern
Vermis
Lateral occiptal gyrus

A

Superior frontal gyrus
Middle frontal gyrus
Inferior frontal gyrus
Middle cerebral artery
Superior temporal gyrus
Quadrigeminal plate

Cingulate sulcus
Head of caudate nucleus
Globus pallidus
Putamen
Temporal horn
Vermis

B

Figure 75-2. (A) MRI T_1-weighted imaging. (B) MRI T_2-weighted imaging. *(From Naheedy MH. Normal computed tomography and magnetic resonance imaging anatomy of the brain and the spine. In Haage JR, Lanzieri CF, Gilkeson RC, editors: CT and MRI imaging of the whole body, Philadelphia, 2003, Mosby, p. 98.)*

into alignment after the radiofrequency pulse is removed; this process emits energy signals that are used to construct the images. This relaxation can occur at different rates, with each relaxation rate resulting in imaging data that may be optimal for different clinical circumstances. For example, T_1-weighted and T_2-weighted images are two commonly used MRI parameters. T_1-weighted images are best for visualizing normal anatomy, whereas T_2-weighted images are better for detecting pathology (Figure 75-2). In contrast to CT images (which can only be viewed in the axial plane), MRI images can be reconstructed in multiple planes (i.e., axial, sagittal, and coronal) for more comprehensive viewing.

Magnetic Resonance Contrast

Gadolinium is used as a contrast agent with MRI because it has paramagnetic properties that result in easy visualization.[15] Gadolinium is introduced intravenously and thus it is useful for visualizing vasculature. In turn, gadolinium is particularly useful for detecting pathology associated with disruption of the blood–brain barrier or an individual's vasculature. Gadolinium is much safer than is ionic CT contrast, and it is associated with far fewer adverse events.

Clinical Utility

Other than acute bleeds and acute trauma, for which CT is the imaging modality of choice, MRI is preferred. As reviewed by Goldstein and Price,[14] in comparison to CT, MRI provides better differentiation of white from gray matter (and thus is superior for the identification of white matter lesions) and is superior for visualizing the posterior fossa and the brainstem. MRI may soon become the imaging modality of choice for suspected acute bleeds as well. Newer magnetic resonance acquisition methods (such as diffusion weighted imaging [DWI]) are highly sensitive for the detection of acute lesions and distinguishing them from chronic infarcts.[16] DWI detects the random movement of water within tissue and quantifies this movement using an average apparent diffusion coefficient (ADC) that can be mapped onto the brain space. During an acute stroke, the ADC within brain parenchyma is markedly reduced. Over several days the ADC returns to normal and, as the lesion becomes chronic, it elevates above normal. Unfortunately, MRI is contraindicated in patients with metallic implants. The strong magnetic field used during magnetic resonance imaging may cause metallic implants to move or heat, which can cause significant injury. For patients with metallic implants, CT is often the imaging modality of choice. However, this should be considered on a case-by-case basis, with input from a radiologist, as MRI can be performed safely in some instances despite the presence of such materials in the body.

Use of Structural Neuroimaging in Psychiatry

A subset of patients with neuropsychiatric symptoms will exhibit abnormalities detectable by brain imaging. Discovery of an organic etiology for neuropsychiatric symptoms could, of course, be of tremendous value. However, the difficulty is determining which subset of patients with neuropsychiatric symptoms should undergo brain imaging. Early studies focused on CT. Across studies, approximately 12% of psychiatric patients undergoing CT imaging were found to have focal abnormalities.[6] Some factors associated with a greater likelihood of having a focal abnormality included increased age, an abnormal neurological examination (especially if focal abnormalities were noted), an altered mental status, and a history of head trauma or alcohol abuse. Therefore, Weinberger[17] proposed the following criteria for CT imaging in psychiatric populations: confusion or dementia; new-onset psychosis; movement disorder; anorexia nervosa; prolonged catatonia; and new-onset major affective disorder or personality change in those >50 years.

In the 1980s, MRI became available and the focus on neuroimaging in psychiatric populations shifted toward the use of MRI. One large study performed at McLean Hospital included 6,200 psychiatric patients who underwent MRI over a 5-year period.[5] Only 1.6% of these imaging studies revealed an unexpected and potentially treatable finding. In addition, the emergence of MRI revealed a high prevalence of white matter lesions in psychiatric populations. However, nonspecific white matter lesions are also present in 30% of normal

BOX 75-1 Guidelines for the Use of Magnetic Resonance Imaging of the Brain in Psychiatric Populations

Patients with acute changes in mental status (including changes in affect, behavior, or personality) plus one of the following criteria:

1. Age > 50 years
2. An abnormal neurological examination (especially with focal abnormalities)
3. A history of significant head trauma (i.e., with extended loss of consciousness, neurological sequelae, or a temporal relationship to the mental status change in question)
4. New-onset psychosis
5. New-onset delirium or dementia of an unknown cause

(control) subjects >60 years. Therefore, the specificity and clinical relevance of these findings is questionable.

While it is difficult to determine the exact clinical characteristics that would lead to the highest yield of potentially treatable findings on MRI, the following general guidelines have been proposed for the use of MRI (Box 75-1): patients with acute changes in mental status (including changes in affect, behavior, or personality) plus one of the following criteria: age >50 years; an abnormal neurological examination (especially with focal abnormalities); a history of significant head trauma (i.e., with extended loss of consciousness, neurological sequelae, or a temporal relationship to the mental status change in question); new-onset psychosis; or new-onset delirium or dementia of an unknown cause.[5] In addition, obtaining an MRI before undergoing a course of ECT may be advantageous in some cases as neuroimaging may reveal the presence of lesions (e.g., arteriovenous malformations, aneurysms, tumors, hydrocephalus, basal ganglia infarction) that could be associated with an adverse outcome after ECT.

FUNCTIONAL NEUROIMAGING MODALITIES
Positron Emission Tomography

As its name suggests, positron emission tomography (PET) (Figure 75-3) uses the energy emitted by positrons from radionuclides to measure brain function (as reviewed by Cherry and Phelps[18] and by Dougherty and associates[19]). Positron-emitting radionuclides are unstable isotopes that are created via particle acceleration in cyclotrons. While isotopes can be created for many atoms, because PET is used to study biological systems, isotopes for hydrogen (^{18}F), carbon (^{11}C), oxygen (^{15}O), and nitrogen (^{13}N) are typically used.

As the positively charged positrons are emitted from these unstable isotopes, they quickly make contact with negatively charged electrons. The resulting collision, termed an *annihilation event*, results in the emission of gamma rays. It is these gamma rays that the PET camera detects and uses to construct functional images. Fortunately, following an annihilation event, these gamma rays are emitted at exactly 180 degrees from each other at a specific energy. Therefore, each annihilation event results in a line of coincidence providing information regarding where the annihilation event took place within the brain.

In the clinical setting, PET is typically used to assess cerebral blood flow (CBF) (using ^{15}O) or cerebral glucose metabolism (using ^{18}F-fluorodeoxyglucose [FDG]). Both CBF and cerebral glucose metabolism are tightly coupled to neuronal activity and thus serve as powerful measures of brain function.

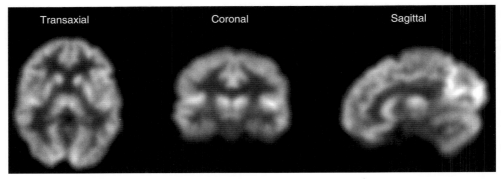

Figure 75-3. PET FDG image.

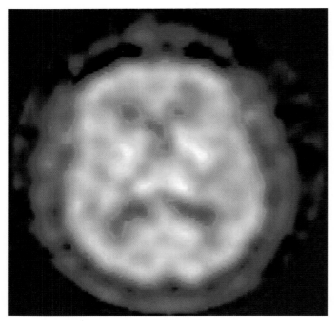

Figure 75-4. SPECT images of the brain.

PET is the "gold standard" for clinical functional neuroimaging studies, as it has excellent spatial resolution (as low as 4 mm). However, PET is also very expensive because it requires radionuclides produced by a cyclotron; the rapid decay of these isotopes makes proximity to the cyclotron critical.

Single-Photon Emission Computed Tomography

Single-photon emission computed tomography (SPECT) (as reviewed by Dougherty and colleagues[19]) (Figure 75-4) also uses radionuclides for functional brain imaging. However, SPECT cannot measure cerebral glucose metabolism. Instead, radionuclides such as ^{99m}Tc-HMPAO are used to measure CBF.[20] Instead of an annihilation event resulting in detection of dual photons (as is the case with PET), the radionuclides used for SPECT studies emit only a single photon. Therefore, lines of coincidence cannot be used to localize function within brain tissue as accurately as can be achieved with PET. Therefore, the spatial resolution of SPECT is somewhat inferior (approximately 8 mm) to that of PET. In addition, single-photon emission results in particularly inferior spatial resolution within deep brain structures. Therefore, SPECT is most useful for assessing cortical brain function. Nonetheless, SPECT does have some advantages over PET. It is more widely

available, it is typically less expensive, and it does not require an on-site cyclotron.

Use of Functional Neuroimaging in Psychiatry

The clinical applications of functional neuroimaging modalities in patients with neuropsychiatric symptoms are limited in comparison to clinical applications of structural neuroimaging modalities. However, there is some clinical utility for the assessment of dementia and seizures. Large-scale studies have demonstrated that functional neuroimaging with PET or SPECT offers better than 90% sensitivity and specificity for distinguishing Alzheimer's disease (AD) from other types of dementia.[21,22] The characteristic functional neuroimaging profile for AD is hypoperfusion or hypometabolism in bilateral temporoparietal regions. Given the advent of treatment of AD with anticholinesterase inhibitors, early and accurate diagnosis of AD could dramatically affect an individual's clinical course.

The role of functional neuroimaging in the clinical assessment of seizures is two-fold. First, seizure activity is sometimes not detected when using electroencephalography (EEG). This is because EEG is best at measuring surface cortical electrical activity. If the seizure focus is located deeper within the brain, an EEG may not detect the seizure focus. However, PET and SPECT demonstrate hyperperfusion or hypermetabolism at the seizure focus during a seizure and hypoperfusion or hypometabolism at the seizure focus during the inter-ictal period.[23,24] Therefore, PET and SPECT are often useful for the detection of seizure foci (usually during the predominant inter-ictal period) that EEG is unable to detect. Second, intractable seizures sometimes require neurosurgical intervention. PET and SPECT can be very useful for determining the precise location and extent of seizure foci in these instances.

USE OF NEUROIMAGING IN PSYCHIATRIC RESEARCH

For a detailed review of neuroimaging in psychiatric research, see Dougherty and Rauch.[25]

Structural Neuroimaging

Structural neuroimaging is predominantly used in the research setting to determine the volumes of brain structures. Specific magnetic resonance acquisition parameters are used for these morphometric MRI studies to support the most valid and reliable means of segmenting various brain components.[26] These studies allow for comparison of structural parameters between cohorts of patients with psychiatric illness and healthy volunteers. Of course, other structural parameters (such as cortical thickness) can also be assessed in this manner. A newer structural neuroimaging modality that is increasingly used in the research setting is diffusion tensor imaging (DTI).[27] DTI magnetic resonance acquisition parameters allow for measurement of white matter tract orientation and may provide indices of tract coherence or integrity. While it is still used solely in the research setting at this time, potential clinical utility may emerge in the future.

Functional Neuroimaging

In addition to their clinical utility, both PET and SPECT are commonly used in the research setting as well. Simple resting state studies comparing cohorts of patients with psychiatric illness to healthy volunteers have been tremendously useful for furthering our understanding of the pathophysiology of many psychiatric disorders. However, functional neuroimaging techniques can also be used to assess brain function during a task. A simple example would involve the collection of functional neuroimaging data during finger-tapping and then the collection of data while the fingers are at rest. If one assumes that everything else is equal between these conditions (not always a valid assumption), the difference between the two conditions should represent brain function associated with finger-tapping. Of course, more complex tasks that involve cognition or exposure to emotionally-valenced stimuli are most commonly used in the psychiatric research setting. Different activation paradigms can be used to assess function of a specific brain structure or whole brain networks. One can also use functional neuroimaging to assess brain function during symptom provocation (e.g., provoking anxiety) or symptom capture (i.e., brain function during spontaneously occurring events, such as tics or auditory hallucinations). Last, collection of functional neuroimaging data before treatment may provide information about the correlates of brain function in specific regions and subsequent clinical outcome, while collection of data before and after treatment allows for assessment of changes in brain function associated with the therapeutic intervention in question.

Functional magnetic resonance imaging (fMRI) has limited clinical utility at present.[28,29] However, like PET and SPECT, fMRI is able to measure brain function and it is used in conjunction with many of the paradigms described previously. fMRI detects changes in the local concentration of paramagnetic deoxyhemoglobin that result in a blood oxygen level dependent (BOLD) signal that is tightly correlated to neuronal activity. fMRI has better spatial resolution and much better temporal resolution than PET or SPECT. However, BOLD fMRI is only able to measure an index of change in blood flow. It cannot measure baseline or resting blood flow in an absolute sense. Therefore, the investigator does not know whether the baseline blood flow before performing a particular task was elevated or reduced. Newer magnetic resonance techniques, such as arterial spin labeling (ASL), are being developed that should help address this issue.

PET and SPECT can also be used to measure neuroreceptor binding and neurotransmitter metabolism.[30] Instead of ^{15}O or ^{18}F-FDG, isotopes are attached to molecules that bind to specific receptors or enzymes. In this manner, the amount of radionuclide binding to the receptor or enzyme can be quantified. Many receptors and enzymes, including those associated with serotonin, dopamine, gamma-aminobutyric acid (GABA), or opioids, can be studied in this manner. While receptor binding studies cannot yet be performed using magnetic resonance techniques, magnetic resonance spectroscopy (MRS) does allow for quantification of chemical concentrations within the brain.[31,32] This may include endogenous chemicals (such as *N*-acetylaspartate) or exogenous chemicals (such as fluoxetine or lithium).

CONCLUSION

Both structural and functional neuroimaging modalities have specific utility in the neuropsychiatric clinical setting. These modalities are also powerful research tools. Continued research should result in expanded uses of these technologies in clinical settings.

Access a list of MCQs for this chapter at https://expertconsult .inkling.com

REFERENCES

1. Lehrer DS, Dougherty DD, Rauch SL. Brain imaging in psychiatry. In Tasman A, Kay J, Lieberman J, et al., editors: *Psychiatry*, ed 3, London, 2008, John Wiley & Sons.
2. Dougherty DD, Rauch SL, Rosenbaum JR. *Essentials of neuroimaging for clinical practice*, Washington, DC, 2004, American Psychiatric Publishing.
3. Dougherty DD, Rauch SL. Neuroimaging in psychiatry. In Stern TA, Herman JB, editors: *MGH psychiatry update and board preparation*, ed 2, New York, 2004, McGraw-Hill.
4. Dougherty DD, Rauch SL, Luther K. Use of neuroimaging techniques. In Stern TA, Herman JB, Slavin PL, editors: *MGH guide to primary care psychiatry*, ed 2, New York, 2004, McGraw-Hill.
5. Dougherty DD, Rauch SL. Neuroimaging in psychiatry. In Stern TA, Rosenbaum JF, Fava M, et al., editors: *MGH comprehensive clinical psychiatry*, Philadelphia, 2008, Mosby Elsevier, pp 1023–1030.
6. Dougherty DD, Rauch SL. Functional neuroimaging. In Bradley WG, Daroff RB, Fenichel GM, et al., editors: *Neurology in clinical practice, principles of diagnosis and management*, ed 4, Philadelphia, 2004, Butterworth-Heinemann, pp 667–674.
7. Gibby WA, Zimmerman RA. X-ray computed tomography. In Mazziotta JC, Gilman S, editors: *Clinical brain imaging: principles and applications*, Philadelphia, 1992, FA Davis.
8. Park LT, Gonzalez RG. Computed tomography. In Dougherty DD, Rauch SL, Rosenbaum JR, editors: *Essentials of neuroimaging for clinical practice*, Washington, DC, 2004, American Psychiatric Publishing.
9. Orrison WW Jr. *Neuroimaging*, Philadelphia, 2000, WB Saunders.
10. Shehadi WH. Contrast media adverse reactions: occurrence, recurrence, and distribution patterns. *Radiology* 143:11–17, 1982.
11. Hayman LA, Evans RA, Fahr LM, et al. Renal consequences of rapid high dose contrast. *Am J Radiol* 134:553–555, 1980.
12. Witten DM, Hirsch RD, Hartman GW. Acute reactions to urographic contrast medium: incidence, clinical characteristics, and relationship to history of hypersensitivity states. *Am J Radiol* 119:832–840, 1973.
13. Horowtiz AL. *MRI physics for radiologists: a visual approach*, New York, 1992, Springer-Verlag.
14. Goldstein MA, Price BH. Magnetic resonance imaging. In Dougherty DD, Rauch SL, Rosenbaum JR, editors: *Essentials of neuroimaging for clinical practice*, Washington, DC, 2004, American Psychiatric Publishing.
15. Bradley WG, Yuh WTC, Bydder GM. Use of MR imaging contrast agents in the brain. *J Magn Reson Imaging* 3:199–218, 1993.
16. Albers GW. Diffusion-weighted MRI for evaluation of acute stroke. *Neurology* 51(Suppl. 3):S47–S49, 1998.
17. Weinberger DR. Brain disease and psychiatric illness: when should a psychiatrist order a CAT scan? *Am J Psychiatry* 141:1521–1527, 1984.
18. Cherry SR, Phelps ME. Imaging brain function with positron emission tomography. In Toga AW, Mazziotta JC, editors: *Brain mapping: the methods*, San Diego, 1996, Academic Press.
19. Dougherty DD, Rauch SL, Fischman AJ. Positron emission tomography and single photon emission computed tomography. In Dougherty DD, Rauch SL, Rosenbaum JR, editors: *Essentials of neuroimaging for clinical practice*, Washington, DC, 2004, American Psychiatric Publishing.
20. Leonard JP, Nowotnik DP, Neirinck RD. Technetium-99m-d,l-HMPAO: a new radiopharmaceutical for imaging regional brain perfusion using SPECT: a comparison with iodine-123 HIPDM. *J Nucl Med* 27:1819–1823, 1986.

21. Bonte FJ, Weiner MF, Bigio EH, et al. SPECT imaging in dementias. *J Nucl Med* 42:1131–1132, 2001.

22. Silverman DH, Small GW, Chang CY, et al. Positron emission tomography in evaluation of dementia: regional brain metabolism and long-term outcome. *JAMA* 286:2120–2127, 2001.

23. Krausz Y, Bonne O, Marciano R, et al. Brain SPECT imaging of neuropsychiatric disorders. *Eur J Radiol* 21:183–187, 1996.

24. Theodore WH, Gaillard WD. Positron emission tomography in neocortical epilepsies. *Adv Neurol* 84:435–446, 2000.

25. Dougherty DD, Rauch SL. *Psychiatric neuroimaging research: contemporary strategies*, Washington, DC, 2001, American Psychiatric Publishing.

26. Caviness VS Jr, Lange NT, Makris N, et al. MRI-based brain volumetrics: emergence of a developmental brain science. *Brain Dev* 21:289–295, 1999.

27. Taber KH, Pierpaoli C, Rose SE, et al. The future for diffusion tensor imaging in neuropsychiatry. *J Neuropsychiatry Clin Neurosci* 14:1–5, 2002.

28. Savoy RL, Gollub RL. Functional magnetic resonance imaging. In Dougherty DD, Rauch SL, Rosenbaum JR, editors: *Essentials of neuroimaging for clinical practice*, Washington, DC, 2004, American Psychiatric Publishing.

29. Jezzard P, Matthews PM, Smith SM. *Functional MRI: an introduction to methods*, Oxford, UK, 2001, Oxford University Press.

30. Dougherty DD, Alpert NM, Rauch SL, et al. In vivo neuroreceptor imaging techniques in psychiatric drug development. In Dougherty DD, Rauch SL, editors: *Psychiatric neuroimaging research: contemporary strategies*, Washington, DC, 2001, American Psychiatric Publishing.

31. Pouwels PJ, Frahm J. Regional metabolite concentrations in human brain as determined by quantitative localized proton MRS. *Magn Reson Med* 39:53–60, 1998.

32. Bolo N, Renshaw PF. Magnetic resonance spectroscopy. In Dougherty DD, Rauch SL, Rosenbaum JR, editors: *Essentials of neuroimaging for clinical practice*, Washington, DC, 2004, American Psychiatric Publishing.

show bilateral EEG slowing, but focal temporal seizures are reported. These changes resolve with successful treatment.[38,39] In limbic encephalitis, temporal slowing, epileptiform discharges or temporal seizures are variably seen.[40] In NMDAR-mediated encephalitis, the EEG is often slow. Atypical seizures may be seen clinically in this condition without obvious scalp EEG changes. A specific pattern of slowing seen in patients with limbic and NMDAR encephalitis is described, characterized by generalized rhythmic slowing with superimposed beta activity, called the "extreme delta brush".[41] Finally, patients with systemic lupus erythematosus (SLE) affecting the brain appear to have a predilection for causing left hemispheric EEG abnormalities.[42]

The Effect of Medications and Toxins on the EEG

Numerous medications that are relevant to psychiatry affect the EEG. Slowing of the EEG background is often seen with toxic levels of many psychoactive medications. Even at therapeutic doses, drugs such as carbamazepine, gabapentin, clozapine, lithium, and tricyclic anti-depressants may cause slowing of the background rhythm. Anti-cholinergic agents also cause background slowing, which may parallel a clinical delirium due to the hypocholinergic state.[43]

Background slowing is not the only EEG effect of psychoactive medications. Epileptiform EEG changes can be seen with anti-psychotic medications, most of which lower the clinical seizure threshold. The most well-known anti-psychotic to cause this is clozapine, which may be associated with EEG slowing and epileptiform discharges in more than half of patients.[44] Among the anti-depressant medications, bupropion may lead to epileptiform changes or seizures, especially at high doses and with the immediate-release formulation.[45] Lithium may produce diffuse slowing but can also enhance pre-existing epileptiform activity. Toxic levels of this medication may cause sub-clinical seizure activity that can contribute to the confusional state often seen in this clinical situation. EEG abnormalities noted in lithium toxicity include diffuse slowing, spikes, and GPDs with triphasic morphology.[46]

Sedative agents cause slowing as well but there are other associated EEG features. Benzodiazepines and barbiturates cause an increase in beta activity in the 20–25 Hz range, termed "excessive beta". The finding of excessive beta on the EEG is suggestive of drug use, and is clinically useful. Excessive beta is more pronounced in younger individuals, and with acute intake of the drug. When it is due to barbiturates, it is often predominant in the frontal leads.[47] Barbiturates, at sufficiently high doses, induce a burst suppression pattern (characterized by suppression of the EEG background interrupted by bursts of irregular EEG activity), and may even lead to complete electro-cerebral silence.[43] Withdrawal will result in generalized sharp activity and may be accompanied by withdrawal seizures. General anesthetics will induce fast frontal activity and attenuation of alpha, and, with deeper coma, a burst suppression pattern.[43] Epileptiform discharges including PLEDs have been described with toxic doses of baclofen, mercury, manganese, isoniazid, tricyclics, penicillin, and aminophylline.[48] Low-frequency (< 0.25 Hz) GPDs can be seen with ketamine and PCP intoxication.[49]

The EEG in Dementia and in Pseudodementia

With "normal aging", there may be a decrease in the frequency of the posterior dominant rhythm by up to 1 Hz or 10% of the baseline EEG obtained at a younger age. A further drop in the frequency of the posterior dominant rhythm may be a sign of a degenerative process, even if the background frequency remains in the alpha range.[50] After a dementing illnesses is established, diffuse EEG slowing is seen, with or without slowing of the posterior dominant rhythm. Alzheimer's disease (AD) often causes these non-specific findings on the EEG. At times, however, slowing may be maximal in temporal and parietal regions. The EEG in AD may also show attenuation of the beta rhythm.[51] These changes usually parallel the clinical course of the illness, but are not specific enough to allow for EEG-based case detection.[52] In multi-infarct vascular dementia, focal or multi-focal slowing may be seen. Focal temporal theta is a signature of microvascular disease. In cases where there is deep sub-cortical vascular pathology, widespread cortical pathology, or where there is mixed vascular/AD pathology, diffuse rather than focal slowing may be seen. Fronto-temporal dementias affect frontal lobes and/or the temporal lobes, often asymmetrically. EEG findings may suggest that a frontal variant of dementia if the EEG shows frontally localized slowing, but the EEG is often normal or shows diffuse slowing in this entity.[53,54] Finally, obtaining an EEG may be helpful when differentiating dementia from depression-related cognitive impairment (commonly referred to as pseudodementia), in which the EEG can be either normal or very mildly slowed. In patients with early dementia with mild cognitive complaints, the EEG may be normal or show mild abnormalities (such as slowing in the posterior dominant rhythm). However, a normal EEG in a patient with an advanced dementing illness with severe cognitive deficits is atypical and should raise doubts about the diagnosis. In contrast, the majority of patients with dementia have abnormal EEGs; in up to one-third of patients, there may be moderate or severe abnormalities.[55]

The EEG in Mood Disorders, Anxiety Disorders, and Obsessive-compulsive Disorder

The EEG plays an important role in the evaluation of patients with episodic panic and anxiety symptoms, mainly in the search of epileptiform or frankly ictal activity.[56] There are multiple case reports of patients with simple partial seizures heralded by panic and diagnosed as idiopathic panic disorder.[57,58] Furthermore, ictal and non-ictal anxiety may co-exist,[59] at times requiring an EEG to distinguish the types of anxiety episodes a given patient is experiencing. In these clinical situations, the EEG is most helpful when ictal electrographic activity is recorded during the spells of concern. An ambulatory EEG may be required to capture these spells and to increase the yield of an inter-ictal recording. Inter-ictal epileptiform discharges significantly raise the possibility of causative or co-morbid epilepsy, and support a trial of AEDs, even though they do not confer a definitive diagnosis of epilepsy. Other EEG abnormalities (including focal and asymmetric slowing) are reported in people with panic symptoms in up to 20% of cases,[60] but these abnormalities are harder to interpret. On the other hand, a normal EEG in this situation does not always rule out ictal panic (i.e. simple partial seizures causing panic symptoms) since the EEG is not infrequently negative in simple partial seizures that do not involve enough cerebral cortex that is EEG accessible. If a high degree of clinical suspicion persists, it may be reasonable to begin a therapeutic trial with or without obtaining more electrophysiologic data by such means as sphenoidal electrodes and magnetoencephalography.

The EEG has not otherwise become a routine part of clinical practice in mood and anxiety disorders. In depression, EEG abnormalities are reported in up to 20%–40% of cases,[61] but these are non-specific abnormalities and are of unclear significance. In patients with depression and cognitive impairment, a normal EEG is a good prognostic sign. In obsessive-compulsive disorder (OCD), the EEG is often unhelpful. A number of quantitative EEG findings require further investigation and carry diagnostic and prognostic promise.[62-64]

The EEG in Psychosis

An EEG is often indicated in patients with new-onset psychosis in order to rule out causes of secondary psychotic symptoms. The EEG is especially helpful in ruling out NCSE presenting with psychotic symptoms. This is particularly important in patients with known epilepsy; psychosis may be seen as an ictal, post-ictal or inter-ictal phenomenon. Obtaining a long-term video EEG can be helpful in these cases. If electrographic seizures are seen on the EEG in synchrony with psychotic episodes, psychosis is highly likely to be ictal. Post-ictal psychosis is not associated with ictal EEG activity, and is usually associated with focal or generalized slowing. In inter-ictal psychosis, the EEG does not reveal frank ictal activity, but it may manifest inter-ictal epileptic discharges.

The EEG may also be helpful in ruling out other neurological causes of secondary psychotic symptoms, including substance withdrawal and intoxication, focal brain lesions, inflammatory of infectious CNS disorders, and metabolic disorders. These disorders may show EEG abnormalities, many of which are described above in the section of EEG abnormalities in delirium.

It is otherwise controversial to routinely use an EEG in patients presenting with what seems to be a primary psychotic disorder. A body of literature describing the EEG changes in schizophrenia has accumulated since the 1950s. This literature reports EEG abnormalities and deviations from normal in 20%–60% of patients with untreated schizophrenia.[65] Such abnormalities include slowing in the background, excessive disorganized beta activity, absent PDR, "choppiness" in the EEG background, and variants of unknown significance (such as phantom spikes and the 14-and-6-Hz variant). Some studies even report epileptiform discharges in these patients.[66,67] However, the significance, consistency, and clinical utility of these EEG findings in patients with schizophrenia remains uncertain. Further work is needed in this area to overcome limitations of previous studies.[68]

There is evidence that the EEG may provide useful prognostic information in patients with psychosis. In patients with schizophrenia, a normal EEG predicts a higher likelihood of remission after 1 year of treatment.[69] A "hypernormal" EEG with hypersynchronicity and reduced reactivity to stimuli predicts a worse outcome and a poorer response to anti-psychotic medications.[70] In patients with a first psychotic break, an abnormal EEG is a negative prognostic sign, predicting a higher risk of conversion to a chronic psychotic illness.[70–73]

QUANTITATIVE EEG

Quantitative EEGs (qEEG) involve the use of computerized statistical analysis and graphical representation of EEG data. Common manipulations include spectral analysis, which involves conversion of time into a frequency domain through Fourier transformation, thus allowing for the assessment of the "power" of a frequency over a given recording; source analysis, a technique used to back-project EEG signals to derive the localization of a dipole; and electromagnetic tomography, a method of graphing statistical results onto the patient's structural neuroimaging scan (such as a magnetic resonance imaging [MRI] scan) to create a map of these results. The role of qEEG in a wide range of neuropsychiatric disorders was cast into doubt by the neurological community. The American Neuropsychiatric Association recommended cautious use of qEEG in attentional and learning disabilities of childhood, and in mood and dementing disorders.[74] However, their use is growing as a research tool, and there is already a body of literature on their potential uses as an adjunct to visual analysis of the EEG. Although most of these uses have been proven clinically, they are beyond the scope of this clinically oriented chapter; many are promising and may enter the clinical field if supported with further evidence.[75]

EVOKED POTENTIALS

Evoked potentials (EPs) can be used to test the integrity of a sensory pathway in the CNS. A sensory stimulus (visual, auditory, or somatosensory) is applied and produces a change in the EEG background. The evoked potential is the change in the EEG that is dependent on, and time-locked to, the stimulus.[76–78]

Visual evoked potentials (VEPs) are ordinarily obtained with a checkerboard stimulus that alternates black and white squares repetitively. Each eye is stimulated individually and then responses are measured from the occipital area of the scalp. The major wave measured is a large positive wave at a latency of about 100 ms (P100). In multiple sclerosis or optic neuritis, the wave is delayed.[79] Delayed or absent VEPs can be seen in many other conditions, including ocular conditions (e.g., glaucoma), compressive lesions of the optic nerve (e.g., pituitary lesions), and pathological conditions of the optic radiations or the occipital cortex.

Auditory stimulation is used to record a brainstem auditory evoked response (BAER). Stimulation with brief clicks produces six small waves in the first 10 ms. The sources of these waveforms are in serial ascending structures in the brainstem, which allows studying the integrity of the brainstem with these waves, and the test has also been used to assess "brainstem death" in cases suspected of "brain death."[80] The waves are also delayed in multiple sclerosis.

Somatosensory evoked potentials (SEPs) are the averaged electrical responses in the CNS to somatosensory stimulation. Like sensory nerve action potentials in the peripheral nervous system, most components of SEPs represent activity carried in the large sensory fibers of the dorsal column (medial lemniscus primary sensorimotor cortex pathway). SEPs can be used to test the integrity of the pathway and to test the speed of conduction in the pathway. SEPs from the upper extremity are commonly produced by stimulation of the median nerve at the wrist. The cerebral SEP in response to median nerve stimulation is best recorded from a site approximately 2 cm posterior to the contralateral central electrode. SEPs from the lower extremity are produced by stimulation of the posterior tibial nerve at the ankle or the peroneal nerve at the fibular head, and are recorded best at the vertex of the head. By stimulating leg nerves, it is possible to obtain EPs at all levels of the neuraxis, including over the spinal cord. SEPs are particularly useful in evaluation of a comatose patient. Bilaterally absent SEPs are highly predictive of poor outcome.[81]

NERVE CONDUCTION
Peripheral Nerve Conduction Studies
Sensory Nerve Conduction

The goals of sensory nerve conduction studies are to assess the number of functioning axons and to assess the state of the myelin of these axons. In the usual sensory nerve conduction study, the axons in a sensory nerve are activated with a pulse of electric current. Action potentials, termed the *sensory nerve action potentials* (SNAPs), travel along the nerve. The electric field produced by these action potentials is recorded at a site distant from the site of stimulation. Each axon makes a contribution to the amplitude of the recorded SNAP. Using the distance between the site of stimulation and the site of recording and the time between stimulation and the arrival of the action potentials at the recording site, it is possible to calculate the conduction velocity (CV), which reflects the quality of myelin of the axons.

In axonal degeneration neuropathies, the primary feature is reduced SNAP amplitudes. In demyelinating neuropathies, the primary feature is slowing of CV. In radiculopathies, SNAP amplitudes and CVs are fully normal. This is because the lesion is virtually always proximal to the dorsal root ganglion, leaving intact the continuity of the cell bodies and their peripheral axons. SNAPs, similarly, remain normal with lesions of the CNS.

Motor Nerve Conduction

To study motor nerve axons, a nerve with motor axons is stimulated along its path while recording over the muscle innervated by the nerve. Each motor axon typically innervates hundreds of muscle fibers; together they constitute a *motor unit*. When a nerve is stimulated, multiple motor units are activated, and a *compound muscle action potential* (CMAP) is recorded from over the muscle. The interval between delivery of the electrical stimulus and the onset of the muscle action potential is mainly dependent on the CV in the motor nerve and the functional integrity of the neuromuscular junction (NMJ). This interval is termed the *distal motor latency*.

In axonal degeneration neuropathies, CMAP amplitudes are reduced, although this may not be significantly abnormal until the process is moderately advanced. In demyelinating neuropathies, there will be slowing of CV and prolongation of distal motor latency. A focal lesion of a nerve will lead to slowing of conduction across the lesion, with or without a conduction block, defined as a drop in CMAP amplitude more than 30% across the lesion. Quite dramatic nerve conduction findings are seen with a focal, total lesion. The nerve is fully normal below the lesion, but electrical stimulation proximal to the lesion produces no response (similar to the patient's attempts to activate the muscle).[82]

In radiculopathy (lesion of the nerve roots), motor nerve conduction studies may be normal or may show a slight slowing of conduction velocity in direct relation to the amount of loss of large fibers. In CNS disease, there will ordinarily be no change in motor nerve conduction unless there is involvement of anterior horn cells.

Late Responses

Studying the most proximal segments of nerves is difficult, because they are deep and not easily accessible as they leave the spinal column. Processes, such as radiculopathies from disc protrusion and certain neuropathies (e.g., Guillain–Barré), predominantly affect these proximal segments. The so-called late responses, the H-reflex and the F-response, are are helpful in these situations. The H-reflex is a monosynaptic reflex response obtained from over the gastrocnemius muscle. It is similar in its pathway to that of the ankle tendon jerk. The electrical stimulus activates the I-a afferents (coming from the muscle spindles), which propagate the impulse back into the spinal cord and make excitatory monosynaptic connections to the alpha motor neurons, producing action potentials in the motor nerve that run to the muscle. Hence, action potentials travel through the proximal segment of the nerve twice during the production of the H-reflex (once in the sensory portion of the nerve and once in the motor portion).

The F-response or F-wave has an advantage over the H-reflex in that it can be found in most muscles. After a motor nerve is stimulated, an action potential runs antidromically as well as orthodromically; a small percentage of anterior horn cells that have been invaded antidromically will produce an orthodromic action potential that is responsible for the F-response. Thus, to produce an F-response, action potentials must travel twice through the proximal segment of the motor nerve.[83]

ELECTROMYOGRAPHY

EMG activity is ordinarily recorded with a needle placed into the muscle. Because the muscle fibers of a single motor unit are not packed closely together in the muscle, the EMG needle records from only about 10 fibers from each motor unit. The amplitude, duration, and configuration of the electrical activity recorded from a motor unit vary as the needle changes its orientation to the muscle fibers. Despite its variability it is possible to specify a normal range for the amplitude, duration, and configuration of motor unit action potentials (MUAPs) for each muscle and each age.

When an EMG needle is placed in a normal muscle at rest, there is no electrical activity. With weak effort, several motor units are activated. At this low level of activation, it is possible to see the individual MUAPs and evaluate their parameters. With maximal effort so many units are brought into action that individual MUAPs cannot be discerned; all that can be seen is a dense electrical pattern, called an interference pattern, which can be characterized by its density and peak-to-peak amplitude. The normal density would be either "full," if there are no gaps, or "highly mixed," if there are a few, short gaps. Some people are not willing or able to exert a maximal effort and the pattern will be less dense as a result. Hence, the degree of effort has to be taken into account when assessing the interference pattern.

Findings on the Electromyogram

Acute Partial Injury (e.g., Partial Laceration of a Nerve)

Motor axons that are injured undergo Wallerian degeneration over the course of about 5 days, leaving muscle fibers previously innervated by those axons in a denervated state. Within approximately 10 to 14 days, denervated muscle fiber action potentials are recorded by the EMG needle as fibrillations and positive sharp waves. Both are simply small, diphasic potentials beginning with a positive phase.

Chronic Partial Injury

After weeks to months, there will be collateral sprouting from surviving motor axons to innervate denervated muscle fibers. Spontaneous activity will cease. Motor units will now contain more muscle fibers than normal; hence, MUAPs will be long in duration, high in amplitude, and polyphasic. The density of the interference pattern may improve, but will probably remain less than full although the amplitude will increase.

Complete Injury

In this circumstance no voluntarily initiated motor nerve action potentials can reach the muscle due to a focal demyelinating injury. Muscle fibers will not be denervated so they will not fibrillate. EMG examination will reveal no spontaneous activity, no MUAPs, and no interference pattern. After the first days the denervated muscle fibers begin to fibrillate.

Myopathy

The simple model of myopathy is characterized by dropout of individual muscle fibers from their motor units. In active myopathies, especially polymyositis, there may be some segmental muscle necrosis. This process divides a muscle fiber into an innervated segment and an uninnervated segment. The uninnervated segment might fibrillate and, hence, result in active myopathies, some fibrillation, and positive sharp waves; most commonly spontaneous activity is lacking.

Neuromuscular Junction Studies

The most common abnormality at the neuromuscular junction is myasthenia gravis. The standard neurophysiological studies for myasthenia gravis are the repetitive nerve stimulation test and the single-fiber EMG. During the repetitive stimulation test, the nerve is stimulated with rates of stimulation of 2 to 10 Hz. In normal patients, the action potential is the same, but in those with myasthenia gravis, the amplitude of the action potentials might decline on successive stimulations. In the inverse myasthenic syndrome—Eaton–Lambert syndrome—the repetitive stimulation test shows a progressive increase in amplitude of the muscle action potential.

Single-fiber EMG is highly sensitive for the diagnosis of myasthenia gravis. In this test, a small needle is used that can detect the action potentials from single muscle fibers. The time between the firing of two muscle fibers from the same motor unit should be very stable. In myasthenia gravis, due to the slow and uncertain function of the neuromuscular junction, there may be an increase in the variability of the time between firing of these two muscle fibers; this is called "increased jitter."[84]

Access the complete reference list and multiple choice questions (MCQs) online at https://expertconsult.inkling.com

KEY REFERENCES

3. Niedermeyer E. Historical aspects. In Niedermeyer E, da Silva F, editors: *Electroencephalography: basic principles, clinical applications, and related fields*, ed 5, Philadelphia, 2005, Lippincott Williams & Wilkins.
4. Hirsch L. Continuous EEG monitoring in the intensive care unit: an overview. *J Clin Neurophysiol* 21(5):332–340, 2004.
7. Krauss G, Webber W. Digital EEG. In Niedermeyer E, da Silva F, editors: *Electroencephalography: basic principles, clinical applications, and related fields*, ed 5, Philadelphia, 2005, Lippincott Williams & Wilkins.
8. Leach J, Stephen L, Salveta C, et al. Which electroencephalography (EEG) for epilepsy? The relative usefulness of different EEG protocols in patients with possible epilepsy. *J Neurol Neurosurg Psychiatry* 77(9):1040–1042, 2006.
18. Synek V. Prognostically important EEG coma patterns in diffuse anoxic and traumatic encephalopathies in adults. *J Clin Neurophysiol* 5(2):161–174, 1988.
21. Nash B. Historical review of electroencephalography in psychiatry. In Boutros N, Galderisi S, Pogarell O, et al., editors: *Standard electroencephalography in clinical psychiatry: a practical handbook*, ed 1, 2011, John Wiley & Sons, Ltd.
22. Jacobson S, Jerrier H. EEG in delirium. *Semin Clin Neuropsychiatry* 5(2):86–92, 2000.
27. Nuwer MR. ICU EEG monitoring: nonconvulsive seizures, nomenclature, and pathophysiology. *Clin Neurophysiol* 118(8):1653–1654, 2007.
31. Van Cott AC, Brenner RP. Drug effects and toxic encephalopathies. In Ebersole JS, Pedley TA, editors: *Current practice of clinical encephalography*, ed 3, Philadelphia, 2003, Lippincott Williams & Wilkins.
35. Wieser HG, Schindler K, Zumsteg D. EEG in Creutzfeldt–Jakob disease. *Clin Neurophysiol* 117(5):935–951, 2006.
37. Gabuzda DH, Levy SR, Chiappa KH. Electroencephalography in AIDS and AIDS-related complex. *Clin Electroencephalogr* 19(1):1–6, 1988.
38. Arain A, Abou-Khalil B, Moses H. Hashimoto's encephalopathy: Documentation of mesial temporal seizure origin by ictal EEG. *Seizure* 10(6):438–441, 2001.
40. Lawn ND, Westmoreland BF, Kiely MJ, et al. Clinical, magnetic resonance imaging, and electroencephalographic findings in paraneoplastic limbic encephalitis. *Mayo Clin Proc* 78(11):1363–1368, 2003.
41. Schmitt SE, Pargeon K, Frechette ES, et al. Extreme delta brush: A unique EEG pattern in adults with anti-NMDA receptor encephalitis. *Neurology* 79(11):1094–1100, 2012.
42. Glanz BI, Laoprasert P, Schur PH, et al. Lateralized EEG findings in patients with neuropsychiatric manifestations of systemic lupus erythematosus. *Clin Electroencephalogr* 32(1):14–19, 2001.
45. Alper K, Schwartz KA, Kolts RL, et al. Seizure incidence in psychopharmacological clinical trials: an analysis of Food and Drug Administration (FDA) summary basis of approval reports. *Biol Psychiatry* 62(4):345–354, 2007.
46. Kaplan PW, Birbeck G. Lithium-induced confusional states: Nonconvulsive status epilepticus or triphasic encephalopathy? *Epilepsia* 47(12):2071–2074, 2006.
50. Jenssen S. Electroencephalogram in the dementia workup. *Am J Alzheimers Dis Other Demen* 20(3):159–166, 2005.
56. Hurley RA, Fisher R, Taber K. Sudden onset panic: Epileptic aura or panic disorder? *J Neuropsychiatry Clin Neurosci* 18(4):436–443, 2006.
65. Shelley BP, Trimble MR, Boutros NN. Electroencephalographic cerebral dysrhythmic abnormalities in the trinity of nonepileptic general population, neuropsychiatric, and neurobehavioral disorders. *J Neuropsychiatry Clin Neurosci* 20:7–22, 2008.
68. Boutros N, Galderisi S, Pogarell O, et al. EEG in psychoses, mood disorders and catatonia. In Boutros N, Galderisi S, Pogarell O, et al., editors: *Standard electroencephalography in clinical psychiatry: a practical handbook*, ed 1, London, 2011, John Wiley & Sons, Ltd.
74. Nuwer M. Assessment of digital EEG, quantitative EEG, and EEG brain mapping: report of the American Academy of Neurology and the American Clinical Neurophysiology Society. *Neurology* 49(1):277–292, 1997.
76. Chiappa KH. *Evoked potentials in clinical medicine*, ed 3, New York, 1997, Lippincott Williams & Wilkins.
79. Khoshbin S, Hallet M. Multimodality evoked potentials and blink reflex in multiple sclerosis. *Neurology* 31(2):138–144, 1981.
80. Stockard J, Pope-Stockard J, Sharbrough F. Brainstem auditory evoked potentials in neurology: methodology, interpretation and clinical applications. In Aminoff AM, editor: *Electrodiagnosis in clinical neurology*, ed 3, New York, 1992, Churchill-Livingstone.

77 Psychiatric Manifestations and Treatment of Seizure Disorders

Daniel Weisholtz, MD, and Shahram Khoshbin, MD

KEY POINTS

- Epilepsy is defined as two or more unprovoked seizures. Characterization of seizures and epilepsy syndromes is crucial in determining management and prognosis.

- Epilepsy may be caused by acquired brain damage or by genetic predisposition.

- Basic investigation of a seizure disorder includes physical examination, an electroencephalogram (EEG), and a magnetic resonance imaging (MRI) scan.

- Patients with epilepsy are at risk for multiple psychiatric co-morbidities, including affective disorders, psychosis, anxiety, and personality changes.

- Most seizures respond to medical treatment. However, patients with refractory seizures are evaluated for surgical resection or vagus nerve stimulation (VNS).

- Comprehensive care addresses the psychosocial needs of the patient with seizures.

OVERVIEW

Epilepsy is defined operationally by the International League Against Epilepsy (ILAE) as a "condition characterized by recurrent (two or more) epileptic seizures, unprovoked by any immediate identified cause." An *epileptic seizure* is "a clinical manifestation presumed to result from an abnormal and excessive discharge of a set of neurons in the brain."[1]

Epilepsy can be disabling not only due to the physical effects of seizures themselves but also due to the associated psychiatric and neuropsychological sequelae of the disease and their social stigmata. Management needs to encompass all of these domains, and is frequently challenging.

EPIDEMIOLOGY AND RISK FACTORS

Epilepsy is the most common neurological disorder after stroke. Its incidence varies widely from country to country, but it is estimated to be between 40 and 70 per 100,000 person-years in developed countries. The incidence of epilepsy is high during infancy, it decreases in adulthood, and it increases again with advancing age.[2,3]

Most structural brain lesions increase the risk for seizures and epilepsy. Known risk factors for epilepsy include head trauma, cerebrovascular diseases, brain tumors, congenital or genetic abnormalities, birth trauma, infectious diseases, alcohol/drug use, and dementia.[2,4,5]

PATHOPHYSIOLOGY
Basic Mechanism and Genetics

Epileptic seizures are caused by abnormal, repetitive firing of neurons. Although multiple etiologies may result in these discharges, it is believed that three key elements are contributory:

neuronal membrane and ion channel characteristics; reduced action of the inhibitory neurotransmitter γ-aminobutyric acid (GABA); and increased activity of excitatory circuits through glutamate or other excitatory neurotransmitters.[6,7] Absence seizures are believed to involve an abnormality in the circuitry between the thalamus and the cerebral cortex.[8]

Certain epileptic syndromes, both focal and generalized, follow single-gene Mendelian inheritance patterns. Since 1995, genetic discoveries have linked idiopathic epilepsies to mutations in genes coding for voltage-gated channels, ligand-gated ion channels, and neurotransmitter receptors, as well as genes involved in synaptic vesicle release and the development and migration of neurons.[9] Many other epilepsies with genetic predispositions are likely due to complex multiple-gene inheritance patterns, and targeted pharmacological strategies have not yet emerged from these findings.

CLASSIFICATION OF SEIZURES AND EPILEPSIES

In 2010, the ILAE revised their approach and terminology for classifying seizures and epilepsies in order to incorporate new insights about etiology and pathophysiology since the prior guidelines in 1981.[10] Seizures are classified according to their mode of onset (focal or generalized) and their associated clinical manifestations. Epilepsy is classified according to its etiology, if known, and specific electro-clinical syndromes are recognized.

Classification of Seizures

The ILAE broadly classifies epileptic seizures into two groups (Box 77-1)[10]: focal (partial) seizures (i.e., those with an initial onset in networks limited to one hemisphere of the brain); and generalized seizures (i.e., those that rapidly engage bilateral distributed networks). A third category consists of seizures that cannot be classified in these two categories.

Classification of Epilepsy by Etiology and Electro-clinical Syndrome

Epilepsy is classified according to its etiology as genetic, structural/metabolic, or unknown. Genetic epilepsies are those believed to be caused by a known or presumed genetic abnormality. These include the channelopathies (e.g., *SCN1A* mutations). Structural/metabolic causes for epilepsy include acquired lesions, such as tumors, strokes, infections, and trauma, as well as congenital malformations, some of which may be due to known genetic defects (e.g., tuberous sclerosis).

An *electro-clinical syndrome* is a specific recognizable complex of clinical features defined by age of onset, seizure types, EEG characteristics, and, at times, specific underlying etiologies (Box 77-2). Electro-clinical syndromes can be diagnosed in a minority of patients with epilepsy and are more common among the pediatric epilepsies. The most common syndromes are self-limited and/or pharmaco-responsive and include juvenile myoclonic epilepsy, childhood absence epilepsy, juvenile absence epilepsy, and benign epilepsy with centro-temporal spikes (BECTS).

CLINICAL MANIFESTATION OF SEIZURES
Generalized Seizures

Although there are multiple distinct types of generalized seizures, seizures are usually classified into three major groups: major motor seizures, absence seizures, and minor motor seizures.

Generalized tonic-clonic (GTC) seizures (also called "grand mal," generalized convulsive, or major motor seizures) are the most common type of generalized seizure; they also occur when a focal seizure evolves to become secondarily generalized. In a purely GTC seizure, the first component is a loss of consciousness. This is followed by the tonic stage, characterized by contraction of the skeletal muscles, extension of the axial musculature, upward deviation of the eyes, and paralysis of the respiratory muscles due to thoraco-abdominal contractions. Once the tonic stage ends, the patient enters the clonic phase, which is characterized by high-amplitude, low-frequency rhythmic jerking movements lasting typically less than 1 minute. Once the seizure terminates, the patient is usually conscious but confused. If after 5 minutes the patient either does not wake up or has another seizure, the diagnosis of *status epilepticus* should be considered. Once a patient regains consciousness after a GTC, he or she enters the post-ictal period in which he or she typically falls asleep for up to several hours and wakes up with a headache.

Absence ("petit mal") seizures are another form of generalized seizures. Absence seizures occur mainly during childhood and are less frequent after puberty. They are characterized by the arrest or suspension of consciousness for 5 to 10 seconds. Parents may not notice the typical brief seizures in an otherwise healthy child, but teachers will report that the child stares absently for short intervals throughout the day. Without treatment, absence seizures may occur up to 70 to 100 times a day, and such frequent blackouts can seriously impair a child's school performance. Absence seizures may sometimes be mistaken for inattention, leading to concern for ADHD. However, the physician can usually confirm the diagnosis by asking the child to hyperventilate, since this maneuver will typically precipitate an attack. Other signs include rhythmic blinking (at a rate of 3 blinks per second) and rudimentary motor behaviors, called *automatisms*, which also occur in adult temporal lobe

---

BOX 77-1 Classification of Seizure Types

Generalized seizures
  Tonic-clonic
  Absence
    Typical
    Atypical
    Myoclonic absence
    Absence with eyelid myoclonia
  Myoclonic
    Myoclonic
    Myoclonic atonic
    Myoclonic tonic
  Clonic
  Tonic
  Atonic
Focal seizures
  Without impairment of consciousness or awareness (simple)
  With impairment of consciousness or awareness (complex)
Unknown
  Epileptic spasms

BOX 77-2 Classification of Epileptic Syndromes

EPILEPTIC SYNDROMES

Electro-clinical syndromes by age of onset
Neonatal period
- Benign familial neonatal epilepsy (BFNE)
- Early myoclonic encephalopathy (EME)
- Ohtahara syndrome

Infancy
- Epilepsy of infancy with migrating focal seizures
- West syndrome
- Myoclonic epilepsy in infancy (MEI)
- Benign infantile epilepsy
- Benign familial infantile epilepsy
- Dravet syndrome
- Myoclonic encephalopathy in non-progressive disorders

Childhood
- Febrile seizures plus (FS+)
- Panayiotopoulos syndrome
- Epilepsy with myoclonic atonic seizures
- Benign epilepsy with centrotemporal spikes (BECTS)
- Autosomal-dominant nocturnal frontal lobe epilepsy (ADNFLE)
- Late-onset childhood occipital epilepsy (Gastaut type)
- Epilepsy with myoclonic absences
- Lennox-Gastaut syndrome
- Epileptic encephalopathy with continuous spike-and-wave during sleep (CSWS)
- Landau-Kleffner syndrome (LKS)
- Childhood absence epilepsy (CAE)

Adolescence–adult
- Juvenile absence epilepsy (JAE)
- Juvenile myoclonic epilepsy (JME)
- Epilepsy with generalized tonic-clonic seizures alone
- Progressive myoclonic epilepsies (PME)
- Autosomal dominant epilepsy with auditory features (ADEAF)
- Other familiar temporal lobe epilepsies

Less specific age relationship
- Familial focal epilepsy with variable foci (childhood to adult)
- Reflex epilepsies

Distinctive constellations
Mesial temporal lobe epilepsy with hippocampal sclerosis
Rasmussen syndrome
Gelastic seizures with hypothalamic hamartoma
Hemiconvulsion-hemiplegia-epilepsy
Epilepsies attributed to and organized by structural-metabolic causes
Malformations of cortical development (e.g., hemimegalencephaly, heterotopias)
Neurocutaneous syndromes (e.g., tuberous sclerosis complex, Sturge-Weber)
Tumor
Infection
Trauma
Peri-natal insults
Stroke

Adapted from Revised terminology and concepts for organization of seizures and epilepsies: report of the ILAE Commission on Classification and Terminology, 2005–2009. Epilepsia 51(4):676–685, 2010. Wiley Periodicals, Inc. © 2010 International League Against Epilepsy.

epilepsy. Absence seizures are the easiest seizure type to diagnose because of the pathognomic EEG abnormality: a 3 Hz spike-and-wave pattern that is often elicited or accentuated when the child hyperventilates. On the other hand, children with ADHD tend to have greater difficulty staying on task and completing their homework, and episodes of inattention typically do not interrupt play, and are not associated with twitches or automatisms.

Minor motor seizures most commonly involve myoclonic and atonic seizures. Although these seizures usually occur in childhood, adults may experience them. *Myoclonic seizures* are characterized by sudden, brief muscular contractions that may occur singly or repetitively. They must be distinguished from non-epileptic myoclonus. Unlike myoclonic seizures, *atonic seizures* are characterized by a loss of muscle tone.

Focal (Partial) Seizures

Focal seizures are conceptualized as beginning within discrete networks limited to one hemisphere and are frequently associated with brain lesions. Surprisingly, focal seizures may also be the result of single-gene mutations. Seizures with focal onset often propagate beyond the seizure-onset zone, and the specific symptoms reflect the functional specialization of the involved cerebral tissues. Thus, a careful history and/or observation of a seizure may provide important clues as to the seizure-onset zone as well as the pattern of propagation. Many focal seizures remain sub-clinical, detectable only with electrophysiological recordings, because they do not involve areas of cortex that produce manifestations observable to others or recognized by the patient. However, testing may reveal specific subtle deficits.[11] A focal seizure may spread to involve both hemispheres and culminate in a generalized tonic-clonic seizure, a process called secondary generalization. Focal seizures are often classified as either simple or complex, depending on whether consciousness is affected, although these terms are not favored in the 2010 ILAE classification report, which recommends the use of the term "dyscognitive" to refer to seizures that affect consciousness or other cognitive domains. Epilepsy patients whose seizures begin focally in a consistent region of the brain may be cured if the seizure-onset zone can be identified and the epileptogenic tissues surgically resected.

Focal Motor Seizures

In focal motor seizures, consciousness is maintained, because seizure activity remains localized to motor cortex. Since much of the motor cortex is devoted to controlling the face and hands, focal motor seizures most commonly affect these parts of the body. Motor movements may spread along the body, usually starting in the hands and then affecting other areas, such as the face and the upper half of the body. This is known as the "Jacksonian march" after John Hughlings Jackson, who described the phenomenon in the 1860s. There is almost never movement of the hip or trunk. Motor seizures may also occur when the lesion (particularly a tumor) affects portions of the frontal lobe anterior to the motor cortex. Turning of the head and eyes away from the side of the focus is an adversive seizure. In what is sometimes called a "fencing seizure," the arm ipsilateral to the focus flexes while the contralateral arm extends.

Experiential Seizures, Epileptic Auras, and Ictal Hallucinations. Focal seizures also include a large sub-group of sensory seizures that typically originate in parietal, temporal or occipital neocortex, and the localization may be inferred by the nature of the sensory experience. These seizures are often referred to as epileptic auras because patients may recognize these symptoms as marking the onset of a seizure. When an aura is recognized as reliably predicting progression to a more severe seizure type, it may allow the patient to take protective measures, such as getting down to the floor and/or taking sub-lingual lorazepam to abort the seizure. Sensory seizures that do not progress may be difficult to diagnose. The *vertiginous seizure*, originating in the temporal lobe, is probably the most common type of sensory seizure; as dizziness has a broad differential diagnosis, evaluation of this seizure can be challenging. *Somatosensory seizures* are usually described as a tingling feeling (paresthesia) or by a sensation of heat or water running over the affected area; this sensation may spread rapidly from one body part to another. Rarely, a patient will report pain or a burning sensation. Somatosensory seizures may mimic migraines or transient ischemic attacks (TIAs) of the middle cerebral artery. However, with careful evaluation of the patient's history, it is often possible to distinguish the three conditions clinically.

Auditory seizures are produced by discharges in the transverse temporal gyri (Heschl's convolutions) and the superior temporal convolution. The patient reports tinnitus typically in the form of hissing, buzzing, or roaring sounds. *Visual seizures,* produced by discharges from an occipital focus, take the form of flickering lights or flashing colors (usually red or white), or a brightly colored ball of light, and are distinct from the "zig-zag" pattern of light or scintillating scotoma sometimes reported by patients experiencing migraine.

Focal seizures from temporo-limbic structures (amygdala, hippocampus, parahippocampal gyrus, etc.) may produce olfactory or gustatory hallucinations (typically a noxious smell like burning rubber or a metallic taste), emotional experiences (such as fear or anxiety), or visceral sensations (such as a rising feeling in the epigastrium). Other cognitive symptoms include the feeling of familiarity known as *déjà vu* ("already seen") and, more commonly, the feeling of unfamiliarity referred to as *jamais vu* ("never seen"). Patients may not report these symptoms unless asked, but when present as part of an epileptic aura, they provide strong evidence for mesial temporal onset.

Affective symptoms, or *ictal emotions*, are a relatively common characteristic of mesial temporal lobe seizures. In some cases patients with affective symptoms do not realize they are having a seizure. Since fear and anxiety are the most common affective symptoms reported in temporal lobe epilepsy (TLE), it is always important to consider this possibility when diagnosing panic disorder. Unlike most other types of emotional experience, ictal mood changes begin and end abruptly. Pleasant ictal feelings may also occur, but they are very rare. Some females may experience orgasms; the corresponding feeling in the male genitalia is generally an uncomfortable penile sensation. Although rage reactions and aggression are sometimes associated with TLE, these behaviors are extremely rare.

Occasionally, complex visual, auditory, or somatic hallucinations may be reported that resemble those reported by patients with psychosis. For example, the patient may describe the sensation of insects crawling under the skin, a common paresthesia called *formication*. The visual phenomenon may be described not as merely flashes of lights, but true hallucinations (such as the detonation of a bomb or a display of "fireworks"). Ictal palinopsia, an experience in which an image persists or re-appears after the stimulus has disappeared, may be seen with seizures involving the posterior cerebral regions. Autoscopy, a perception in which a patient sees an image of himself, may occur with seizures involving the occipito-temporal junction. The perception that objects are getting bigger (macropsia) or smaller (micropsia) may also be reported. The British mathematician and author Lewis Carroll had TLE, and several of the events in Carroll's *Alice in Wonderland* are reminiscent of phenomena experienced by patients with TLE (e.g., things shrinking and growing, and passing through mirrors). When hallucinations are complex, the seizure generally has a broad localization involving association cortex, and when emotional salience is attached to them, limbic involvement is almost certain. Because of the high prevalence of mesial temporal lobe epilepsy and the close connectivity between mesial temporal limbic structures and the association cortices, mesial temporal onset is probable in many of the patients with complex ictal hallucinations.

The Post-ictal State

Following a seizure, there may be varying degrees of neurologic impairment, the nature and duration of which depend on the type and duration of the seizure, the amount of brain involved in the seizure, and the patient's baseline neurologic function.

There is typically no post-ictal impairment following an absence seizure, despite the apparently large region of cortex involved. Similarly, there is no appreciable post-ictal impairment following many simple partial seizures. Nevertheless, the post-ictal state is often characterized by some degree of dysfunction of the involved brain regions. On EEG, this manifests as regional attenuation and/or slow waves over the involved lobe or hemisphere.[12] This dysfunction tends to resolve gradually over the subsequent minutes to hours after seizure termination. After a focal motor seizure, there may be weakness of the limb involved in the seizure, a phenomenon referred to as Todd's paresis. In an analogous phenomenon, sensory seizures may be followed by a corresponding sensory deficit.

Following a generalized tonic-clonic seizure, a patient is typically lethargic, confused, disoriented and may briefly be difficult to arouse. The patient will gradually regain awareness of his surroundings, but may remain amnestic for a portion of the post-ictal period. The patient may go to sleep following a convulsive seizure and wake up fully recovered. However, patients should be monitored during the post-ictal period to ensure recovery of normal vital signs and gradual return to the baseline state, as persistent abnormalities may indicate ongoing sub-clinical seizure activity.

Post-ictal agitation is not uncommon, and is typically seen during the period of confusion and disorientation. Aggressive behavior is usually not purposeful. For instance, a patient might punch into the air or lash out at people attempting to restrain him, but a targeted attack is unlikely to be secondary to a seizure. Typically, post-ictal aggression can be contained by calmly interacting with the patient and re-orienting him. Wrist or ankle restraints should be avoided unless absolutely necessary due to the potential for injury if another convulsion occurs, but padded side rails may be helpful to prevent patients from getting out of bed. Rarely, small doses of haloperidol may be used to control extremely violent or agitated behavior.[13] Post-ictal confusion and occasionally aggression can be seen following focal temporal lobe seizures as well, and post-ictal wandering is common.[14]

While most patients appear to be back to baseline within a few hours after a seizure, patients often report headache, fatigue, anergia, dysphoria and lack of mental clarity for 1–2 days after a seizure. Post-ictal depressive episodes, manic episodes, and psychotic episodes are occasionally seen (see "Psychiatric disturbances in epilepsy").

SELECTED EPILEPSIES AND EPILEPTIC SYNDROMES
Mesial Temporal Lobe Epilepsy

Mesial temporal lobe epilepsy, often referred to simply as temporal lobe epilepsy (TLE), is the most common form of focal epilepsy in adults. Seizures commonly arise from the mesial temporal region: for example, from the hippocampus, the parahippocampal gyrus, or the amygdala. Such seizures may begin with an aura characterized by olfactory or gustatory hallucinations, cognitive experiences (such as *déjà vu* or *jamais vu*), emotions (such as fear or anxiety), or visceral sensations (sometimes described as nausea or "butterflies"). The auras may occur independently, but they commonly progress to involve loss of awareness, at which point they are referred to as "complex" or "dyscognitive". Staring behavior is often seen similar to that seen in absence epilepsy. However, unlike absence seizures, which last only about 6 seconds, staring episodes in complex partial seizures typically last about 1 to 3 minutes, long enough to be easily recognized, particularly if the patient is interacting with someone at the time of the seizure.

Automatisms are often observed during this portion of the seizure and may take the form of simple vegetative movements, or complex actions, such as disrobing. The most common automatisms are oral and buccal movements (e.g., lip smacking, licking, chewing), and the picking behaviors that are sometimes seen in patients with dementia. In some cases, these individuals may pick at their skin to the point of maceration. Agitated or aggressive behavior may occasionally be provoked if the patient is restrained during the automatisms.

Hippocampal sclerosis is often identified on high-resolution MRI scans in which the sclerotic hippocampus may appear atrophic with loss of the normal architecture. FLAIR or T2-weighted imaging may show hyperintensity in the hippocampus as well. Positron emission tomography (PET) scans show reduced uptake in radioactive glucose on the side of the pathology. Afflicted patients are often intractable to medical management, but can be effectively treated with surgical resection.

Idiopathic/Genetic Generalized Epilepsy

A number of specific syndromes of known or presumed genetic etiology are characterized primarily by generalized (absence, myoclonus, or tonic-clonic) seizures. Most of these patients have a characteristic EEG pattern (generalized spike-wave discharges) and an otherwise normal neurological development. Childhood absence epilepsy is common, accounting for 8%–15% of childhood epilepsies; brief absence seizures occur, at times with great frequency (up to hundreds a day), starting between ages 4 and 10. They show a characteristic 3-Hz spike-wave discharge on the EEG. They are generally well-controlled with medications. Most, but not all, patients become seizure-free, and many no longer require medications once they reach adulthood. On the other hand, juvenile absence epilepsy starts after puberty. Absences are not as frequent, GTC seizures occur more often, and patients typically require lifelong therapy. Also quite common is juvenile myoclonic epilepsy in which myoclonic and GTC seizures are the predominant seizure types. Like juvenile absence epilepsy, this syndrome also requires lifelong therapy.

Status Epilepticus

Status epilepticus is commonly defined as continuous seizure activity, or two or more seizures without full recovery of consciousness for greater than 5 minutes.[15] The mortality rate in *status epilepticus* is very high, and as such, it should be considered a true emergency. The ABCs (airway, breathing, and circulation) of emergency management should be emphasized. Immediate treatment consists of administration of intravenous (IV) lorazepam followed by a loading dose of a maintenance anti-epileptic drug (AED) available in IV form

---

BOX 77-3 Sample Protocol for the Management of Generalized Convulsive Status Epilepticus

IMMEDIATE
- Follow the ABCs
- Establish IV access
- Obtain an ECG and vital sign monitoring (HR, BP, pulse oximetry)
- Sample venous blood for glucose, electrolytes, blood urea nitrogen (BUN), toxicology screen, and levels of anticonvulsant drugs
- Administer normal saline, glucose, thiamine (not in BWH protocol)

WITHIN 5 MINUTES
- Administer lorazepam 2 mg (may repeat up to 0.1 mg/kg) at 2 mg/min

WITHIN 10 MINUTES
- Administer levetiracetam 1,000 mg OR
- Fosphenytoin 20 PE/kg (or phenytoin 20 mg/kg). If no effect, additional 10 PE/kg OR
- Valproic acid 20–30 mg/kg OR
- Lacosamide 300 mg OR
- Phenobarbital 15–20 mg/kg

WITHIN 50 MINUTES (IF SEIZURES CONTINUE OR VITAL SIGN INSTABILITY IS PRESENT)
- Intubate, transfer to ICU
- Initiate general anesthesia with
  - Propofol bolus 1–2 mg/kg, then 2–10 mg/kg/h OR
  - Midazolam bolus 0.2 mg/kg, then 0.1–0.5 mg/kg/h OR
  - Pentobarbital bolus 5–10 mg/kg, then 0.5–3 mg/kg/h

Unless the patient returns to his or her baseline mental status after convulsions stop, initiate EEG monitoring as soon as possible to evaluate for non-convulsive status epilepticus.

Adapted from protocol used at Brigham & Women's Hospital, Boston, MA.

(Box 77-3). If seizures do not cease, a second agent should be added, and preparation for intubation and subsequent administration of general anesthesia should be initiated. Neurology consultation will be required in all instances. A continuous EEG should be considered in all patients who do not recover normal consciousness after treatment for *status epilepticus* due to the high likelihood of ongoing non-convulsive seizures once convulsive movements have stopped.

Non-convulsive status epilepticus (NCSE), defined as 5 minutes or more of seizure activity with non-convulsive clinical symptoms such as alteration of mentation or behavior, has been gaining increased attention as an important clinical entity with the increasing availability of continuous EEG monitoring in the hospital setting. The clinical manifestations of *status epilepticus* are as diverse as those of brief seizures and may range from coma to mild confusion and lethargy. Very rarely, psychiatric symptoms, such as persistent hallucinations or frank psychosis, may predominate. Although there may be no obvious clinical seizure activity, the EEG shows ongoing or intermittent focal or generalized electrographic seizures. Because of the variable and sometimes non-specific clinical phenotype of NCSE, an EEG is often necessary to identify or exclude seizures as a cause of altered mental status in patients presenting with coma, delirium, or catatonia, particularly when a history of epilepsy or risk factors for seizures are present. When focal NCSE causes alterations of consciousness, it is often referred to as *complex partial status epilepticus* (CPSE)

and commonly involves seizure activity of the frontal or temporal lobes. There may be a fluctuating mental state, with strange behaviors, automatisms, and confusion. Patients with *absence status epilepticus* (ASE) typically exhibit an altered state of consciousness with cognitive slowing, verbal and motor impersistence or perseveration, but with preserved ability to respond to simple commands, withdraw from pain, eat, drink and walk.[16] The patient may exhibit clumsiness, automatic behavior, and decreased spontaneity. Amnesia for the episodes is variable. The EEG shows generalized 2–4 Hz spike-wave or poly-spike-wave discharges. ASE may be provoked by administering drugs such as carbamazepine that are known to provoke absence seizures in patients with generalized epilepsy syndromes. It can also rarely be seen *de novo* in the setting of benzodiazepine withdrawal.[16]

Epilepsia partialis continua refers to an epileptic condition characterized by continuous rhythmic muscular contractions of a part of the body due to focal seizure activity primarily involving the motor cortex and it represents a type of *simple partial status epilepticus* (SPSE) because there is no alteration of consciousness. Because of the restricted spatial extent of the seizure activity, a scalp EEG may not detect the seizure, and the condition should not be mistaken for a non-epileptic phenomenon.

EVALUATION OF A PATIENT WITH A SEIZURE
History

The history from the patient and witnesses remains the most important aspect of the evaluation. If the seizure was witnessed, a detailed description should be obtained. The physician should carefully question the patient about his or her state of consciousness at the time of the seizure. Patients invariably lose consciousness during generalized tonic-clonic seizures. However, an aura prior to loss of consciousness may suggest a focal onset and the nature of the aura may provide a clue as to the localization (see "Focal seizures" section).

Laboratory Investigations

Laboratory investigation should include screening for metabolic disorders, including hyponatremia, hypokalemia, hypocalcemia, and hypoglycemia, as well as withdrawal from alcohol or from other recreational drugs. If an infectious etiology is suspected, investigation should include blood cultures and a lumbar puncture. The patient's medications should be carefully tabulated and recent changes noted; many medications (including some antidepressants and antibiotics) may lower seizure threshold and provoke seizures in susceptible patients. Patients with epilepsy are particularly susceptible to the above-mentioned triggers. Seizures may also be precipitated when a patient misses doses of his AEDs or when AED levels are decreased as a result of an interaction with another drug that has been added or withdrawn.

Electroencephalogram

All patients with a new seizure or suspected seizure disorder should have an EEG. The sensitivity of a single EEG is relatively low (ranging from 30% to 50%) for detecting epileptiform abnormalities, but the yield may be increased (to 80%–90%) by obtaining multiple EEGs, an ambulatory 24-hour EEG, or a sleep-deprived EEG.[17–20] Hyperventilation and photic stimulation (flashing lights) during the EEG may further increase the yield of the EEG in limited circumstances.

Neuroimaging

Brain imaging is of critical importance after a first seizure, as a seizure may be the initial symptom of a brain tumor, stroke, abscess, or other treatable lesion. Magnetic resonance imaging (MRI) is the imaging modality of choice in patients with seizures. In addition to major structural abnormalities, an MRI scan may reveal more subtle lesions (such as hippocampal sclerosis), which are often seen in patients with TLE.[21] Computed tomography (CT) has a more limited role in patients suspected of having trauma, intracranial hemorrhage, increased intracranial pressure, or other similar catastrophic etiologies due to its high sensitivity for acute hemorrhage and cranial fractures and the ease with which it can often be obtained in an acute setting, but a normal CT scan does not obviate the need for an MRI, as many subtle epileptogenic lesions can be seen on MRI that are undetectable on CT.

Because of difficulties in accurately localizing focal seizures, multiple other imaging modalities are used to complement the EEG and MRI scans in patients undergoing evaluation for epilepsy surgery. These include PET,[22] single-photon emission computed tomography (SPECT),[23] and magnetoencephalography.[24]

DIFFERENTIAL DIAGNOSIS
Psychogenic Non-epileptic Seizures

Psychogenic non-epileptic seizures (PNES, also known as "pseudoseizures") represent a large and challenging subgroup of patients evaluated for a seizure disorder. They may represent up to 30% of patients with seizures refractory to traditional anti-seizure medications.[25] Most frequently, these seizures are a form of conversion disorder in which there is no apparent conscious effort or secondary gain to explain the emergence of these episodes. Patients with PNES frequently have an antecedent history of sexual or other psychological trauma,[26,27] and they are much more likely to be female.[28]

Although pre-existing risk factors and seizure descriptions (such as pelvic thrusting[28]) can be helpful in raising suspicion of PNES, conclusive diagnosis usually requires the use of video-EEG monitoring during which a typical episode is captured. A diagnosis of PNES can be made when an episode of alteration of awareness is captured with absence of an ictal EEG pattern and a preserved waking background rhythm. Hyperkinetic frontal lobe seizures may mimic psychogenic seizures,[29] and may produce dramatic and bizarre clinical semiology with little or no post-ictal state, and may be accompanied by subtle ictal EEG patterns that are often obscured by muscle artifact. This may lead to substantial difficulties in reaching the correct diagnosis in a small portion of patients even when episodes are captured on video EEG. Additionally, simple partial seizures may involve a small enough region of cortex to be undetectable on scalp EEG and should not be mistaken for PNES simply because the EEG is normal during an episode. Close communication between a psychiatrist and epileptologist is recommended when the diagnosis is in question. Despite prevailing beliefs, the number of patients with both PNES and epileptic seizures is low,[30] but it must be remembered that even once a diagnosis of PNES is made, co-morbid epilepsy cannot be fully excluded unless all of the patient's seizure types have been characterized on video EEG.

Simply communicating the diagnosis of PNES in an empathic way may lead to seizure remission in a significant proportion of patients, but relapse rate is high and additional treatment is generally needed. Co-morbid psychiatric disorders are present in 95% of patients with PNES and ought to be addressed and appropriately treated. Individual psychotherapy has been shown to lead to seizure reduction in multiple studies, but there are as yet no well-powered multi-centered randomized controlled trials to guide therapy, and there is no consensus about which forms of therapy are most effective.[31] Cognitive-behavioral therapy is commonly advocated. More than 70% of patients continue to have seizures chronically.[26,32]

Other Conditions Mimicking Seizures

A variety of other paroxysmal disorders may mimic seizures. Syncope may induce transient cerebral hypoxia and may produce seizure-like behaviors, such as myoclonic jerks, head turns, and automatisms, in more than 10% of patients.[33-35] Syncopal attacks are more often associated with feelings of light-headedness, sweating, and nausea, and are seen after prolonged periods of standing.[33] Although syncopal attacks are generally relatively benign, especially in young individuals, additional testing, including a cardiac evaluation, should be strongly considered.

Migrainous phenomena may resemble seizures; patients can experience migraine auras characterized by visual disturbances, vertigo, migrating paresthesias, and speech difficulties, all of which may also be seen with focal seizures, but the evolution tends to be slower with migraine. Some migraines may occur without headaches and, rarely, a migraine may evolve into a seizure.[36] Panic disorder may frequently mimic focal seizures from the mesial temporal lobe. However, panic attacks typically last longer than simple autonomic seizures. Some sleep disorders (such as cataplexy and hypnagogic hallucinations in narcolepsy, parasomnias with bizarre behaviors, and periodic limb movement disorders) may be mistaken for epilepsy.[30]

TREATMENT FOR SEIZURE DISORDERS
Medical Treatment

The most commonly used AEDs are summarized on Table 77-1. The modern AEDs are not believed to be more efficacious in comparison to the "classical" AEDs, but they are likely better tolerated[37]; recent evidence suggests that the modern agents may be superior in some instances,[38] while the "classical" drugs are preferable in other conditions.[39] In most instances where medications will be effective, control will be achieved by the first or second medication initiated.[40] The selection of AEDs, given the myriad of choices today, depends on multiple factors; it is not amenable to a dogmatic schema. In general, it is preferable to use a drug with broad spectrum (e.g., levetiracetam, valproic acid, zonisamide, lamotrigine, topiramate) unless it is known that the patient has a focal epilepsy syndrome. The AED choice is also guided by the side effect profiles of the various agents and the patient's co-morbidities that might be affected either positively or negatively by the AED choice.

Surgery

Surgical management of epilepsy represents the only option for a cure for the 35% of patients with epilepsy who are refractory to medications.[40] The greatest success has been achieved in patients with mesial TLE. A meta-analysis of these patients showed that two-thirds of patients were free of disabling seizures, and 85% had improved after surgery.[41] A study that randomized medically refractory-patients to medical or surgical treatment revealed that patients who underwent surgery had both better control of their seizures and a better quality of life.[42] Because of potential adverse effects on language and memory, and visual fields, in addition to the usual surgical

TABLE 77-1 Anti-epileptic Drugs (AEDs)

Medication (Brand)	Adult Starting/ Sustained Dose	Indication	Alternative Usage	Common/Serious Side Effects (Drowsiness in All)
Carbamazepine (Tegretol, Tegretol XR, Carbatrol)	100–200 mg, 600–800 mg	Partial and secondarily generalized seizures	Bipolar disorder, glossopharyngeal neuralgia, and trigeminal neuralgia	Rash, leukopenia, aplastic anemia, hyponatremia, and osteoporosis
*Oxcarbazepine (Trileptal)	300–600 mg, 600–1,200 mg	Partial and secondarily generalized seizures		Hyponatremia
Valproic acid (Depakote)	15 mg/kg/day, 10–20 mg/kg/day	Partial, absence, and generalized seizures	Mania and migraine prophylaxis	Tremor, hair thinning, weight gain, hyperammonemia, thrombocytopenia, hepatotoxicity, and teratogenicity
Phenytoin (Dilantin)	Load 18 mg/kg, 300 mg/day	Partial and GTC seizures		Rash, osteoporosis, gingival hyperplasia, cerebellar atrophy, and peripheral neuropathy
Phenobarbital	1.5–4 mg/kg	Seizures		Rash, sedation, osteoporosis, and peripheral neuropathy
Primidone (Mysoline)	125 mg/10– 20 mg/kg	Seizures		Rash, sedation, osteoporosis, and peripheral neuropathy
Ethosuximide (Zarontin)	250 mg, 750–1500 mg	Absence seizures		Nausea and drowsiness
Clonazepam (Klonopin)	0.5 mg, 1–8 mg	Seizure	Panic disorder	Drowsiness and addiction
*Gabapentin (Neurontin)	300 mg/900– 2,400 mg	Partial seizures	Post-herpetic neuralgia	Drowsiness, leg edema, and weight gain
*Pregabalin (Lyrica)	100–150 mg/150– 600 mg	Partial seizures	Diabetic neuropathy, post-herpetic neuralgia, and fibromyalgia	Drowsiness
*Lamotrigine (Lamictal)	25 mg/225– 375 mg	Partial, GTC, and primary generalized seizures	Bipolar disorder	Rash and headache
*Topiramate (Topamax)	25 mg/100– 400 mg	Partial, GTC, and primary generalized seizures	Migraine prophylaxis	Cognitive dysfunction, kidney stones, metabolic acidosis, and anorexia
*Zonisamide (Zonegran)	100 mg/100– 600 mg	Partial seizures		Cognitive dysfunction, kidney stones, and anorexia
*Levetiracetam (Keppra)	1,000 mg/1,000– 3,000 mg	Partial, GTC, and primary generalized seizures		Neurocognitive (depression and irritability)
*Tiagabine (Gabitril)	4 mg/up to 56 mg	Partial seizures		Fatigue and cognitive dysfunction
*Felbamate (Felbatol)	1,200 mg/2,400– 3,600 mg	Partial and secondarily generalized seizures		Liver failure and aplastic anemia
*Vigabatrin (Sabril)	500–1,000 mg, 2,000–3,000 mg	Seizures		Psychosis and visual field defects
*Clobazam (Onfi)	5–10 mg, 20–40 mg	Lennox-Gastaut syndrome		Sedation, cognitive impairment, physical dependence
*Rufinamide (Banzel)	400 mg, 2400–3200 mg	Lennox-Gastaut Syndrome		Dizziness, diplopia, nausea, status epilepticus, decreased QT
*Ezogabine (Potiga)	600–1200 mg	Partial seizures		Retinal abnormalities, potential vision loss
*Perampanel (Fycompa)	2 mg, 8–12 mg	Partial seizures		Dizziness, headache, irritability

*"Modern" AED.

risks, including infarcts, hemorrhages, and infections, patients are carefully and thoroughly investigated by a multi-disciplinary team (involving neurologists, neurosurgeons, radiologists, neuropsychologists, and psychiatrists). In addition to the previously stated neuroimaging studies and standard EEGs, patients often undergo neuropsychological assessment, functional MRI, an intra-carotid sodium amobarbital ("Wada") test,[43] and implantation with intra-cranial electrodes.

Vagus Nerve Stimulation

Although a relatively novel tool in the armamentarium of epileptologists, the anti-epileptic effects of vagal nerve stimulation (VNS) have been known since the nineteenth century.[44] VNS consists of a battery-powered coin-sized generator implanted in the chest that transmits pulses of electricity at regular intervals to the vagus nerve. The patient may provide additional stimulation at higher power with a hand-held magnet. Clinical trials have demonstrated that seizure frequency is reduced by at least 50% in up to one-third of patients.[45] Unlike with medications, the effectiveness of the VNS appears to increase with time.[46,47] However, few patients become seizure-free solely with VNS. Serious side effects are relatively rare, and common side effects (such as voice alterations) are well tolerated. The cognitive side effects often seen with medications are non-existent. Some studies have shown that VNS is also effective for treatment-resistant depression.[48]

PSYCHIATRIC DISTURBANCES IN EPILEPSY

The prevalence of psychiatric disorders in patients with epilepsy is high with a prevalence of 5.9%–55.5% in adults and 24%–37% in children.[49] When evaluating psychiatric symptoms in a patient with epilepsy, it is important to consider the role that the patient's epilepsy may play both from a biological and psychosocial perspective. As such, it is important to understand the nature of the patient's seizures, the frequency of seizures, the cause of seizures (if known), and the way in which a patient's lifestyle and relationships are impacted by seizures. Broadly speaking, psychiatric symptoms can be divided into those that bear no temporal relationship to the patient's seizures (inter-ictal psychiatric symptoms) and those that occur with a temporal relationship to a seizure or seizure cluster (peri-ictal or post-ictal psychiatric symptoms). For peri-ictal or post-ictal psychiatric symptoms, the primary focus is on seizure control, although short-term psychopharmacologic treatment may be indicated in some cases. Inter-ictal psychiatric symptoms, which are more common, typically require independent psychiatric treatment, and the potential positive and negative psychotropic effects of AEDs should be considered. Communication and collaboration between a neurologist and psychiatrist is often important.

Depression

Depression is the most common co-existing psychiatric disturbance in patients with epilepsy, affecting up to 30% of patients, and likely a higher percentage in those with uncontrolled epilepsy.[50,51] In patients with TLE, post-ictal depression that lasts for hours or days may occur[52] and is more likely in patients with a history of inter-ictal affective disorder. Transient post-surgical depression is seen in nearly half of patients undergoing temporal lobectomy,[53] but seems to decrease significantly after 3 months, and after 2 years, rates of depression are about half of the pre-surgical rates, suggesting that epilepsy surgery may have a beneficial effect on depression in the long run, especially if seizure freedom is achieved.[54] Depression occurs more commonly in patients with epilepsy than in neurologically normal subjects, although not necessarily more often than in persons with chronic neurological disease. More surprisingly, though, depression appears to be a risk factor for epilepsy, as studies have shown an increased incidence of depression before a first seizure.[52] The existence of depression also predicts pharmaco-resistance in epilepsy.[55] Depression and epilepsy may share common neurobiological substrates including abnormalities in various neurotransmitter systems (serotonin, norepinephrine [noradrenaline], and dopamine) and in the structure and function of fronto-limbic networks.[52,56] Treatment of co-existing depression must be included in the comprehensive treatment of a seizure disorder.

Some AEDs appear more likely than others to induce depressive symptoms. Phenobarbital has been associated with rates of depression of up to 40%, although this may occur primarily with long-term therapy. It remains a commonly used AED, but is generally no longer used as first-line therapy, given the side effect profile. Vigabatrin and tiagabine have been associated with rates of depression over 10%, but they are not commonly used. Topiramate and zonisamide are commonly used "modern" AEDs. In one study on 431 patients on topiramate, about 10% developed affective disorders, but this adverse effect may be mitigated by using a low starting dose and slow titration.[57] Mood disorders may occur in about 7% of patients taking zonisamide. However, studies have also shown potential benefit for zonisamide and topiramate for treatment of some psychiatric conditions. Levetiracetam is commonly associated with an increase in irritability and aggressive behavior. Affective symptoms occur in about 13% of patients taking levetiracetam and in as many as 25% over the long term. Most adverse psychiatric effects from levetiracetam are mild, and the rate of depression may be closer to 2%–7%, but personal and family history of psychiatric disorders seems to make patients more susceptible to psychiatric adverse effects of AEDs, and some study populations excluded patients with pre-existing psychiatric histories. Psychiatric adverse effects of levetiracetam are frequently encountered in the clinic because of the ubiquitous use of this drug, and it is a common reason for drug discontinuation. Valproate, carbamazepine, oxcarbazepine, lamotrigine, gabapentin, and pregabalin generally do not produce adverse psychiatric side effects and may have some positive effects on mood and anxiety. These agents should be preferentially considered in patients with significant psychiatric history or a history of psychiatric adverse AED effects.

When depression is severe, not attributable to AED side effects, or the AEDs can't be changed, psychiatric pharmacotherapy may be indicated. Selective serotonin re-uptake inhibitors (SSRIs) are the first-line treatment for depression in patients with epilepsy because of their low potential for lowering the seizure threshold, but interaction with the AEDs must be considered. Neither venlafaxine, a serotonin-norepinephrine re-uptake inhibitor (SNRI), nor mirtazapine, a norepinephrine agonist, appears to lower seizure threshold.[58] Amoxapine, clomipramine, and bupropion should be avoided in patients with epilepsy. Other tricyclic antidepressants (TCAs) and buspirone lower seizure threshold at higher doses.[59,60]

Psychosis

Psychosis may affect up to 7% of patients with epilepsy.[50] Psychotic symptoms may occur during the ictal, post-ictal, or inter-ictal phase,[61] and are a common co-morbidity. Ictal psychosis is a rare phenomenon. Ictal and post-ictal psychosis are infrequent; a more common form is chronic inter-ictal psychosis. It tends to occur 10–15 years after epilepsy onset and has been referred to as schizophrenia-like psychosis of epilepsy (SLPE) because of its close resemblance to schizophrenia. Disagreement exists about whether there exists a chronic inter-ictal psychosis of epilepsy that is distinguishable from schizophrenia, or whether the association of a schizophrenia-like psychosis with epilepsy reflects a co-morbidity related to shared etiologic factors. An association of inter-ictal psychosis with TLE has been suggested repeatedly, but its relationship has yet to be elucidated.

Post-ictal psychosis is most commonly seen in patients with long-standing pharmaco-resistant epilepsy and typically occurs after a cluster of convulsive or complex partial seizures. After resolution of the immediate post-ictal state there is typically a lucid interval of up to 72 hours,[62] followed by onset of psychosis, which typically lasts less than 1 week and rarely longer than two. The psychosis tends to be affect-laden, with hypomanic features in 50% of patients, and is self-limited regardless of treatment, as long as seizures are controlled. EEG should be strongly considered to evaluate for non-convulsive seizures, but scalp electrodes may be inadequate to fully exclude ictal psychosis, as ongoing focal limbic seizures may not be detectable at the scalp. This has led some to theorize that at least some cases of apparent post-ictal psychosis may actually be ictal.[63,64] Post-ictal psychosis is self-limited as long as seizures are controlled, so supportive treatment may be all that is necessary, but if the psychosis is severe enough to require pharmacological treatment, it typically responds to benzodiazepines or low-dose atypical anti-psychotic drugs.

A small number of patients may experience "alternate psychosis," a phenomenon in which periods of psychosis and seizure-freedom alternate with periods of increased seizure activity and remission of psychosis. The term "forced normalization" refers to the phenomenon described in some patients in which psychosis emerges with normalization of the scalp EEG.[65]

AED-induced psychosis occurs rarely and is most common in patients with other risk-factors for psychosis. Vigabatrin is the AED most associated with drug-induced psychosis with rates of 2.5% in double-blind placebo-controlled trials. Topiramate and zonisamide are also associated with increased rates of psychosis. Phenytoin may cause psychosis at high doses. The rate of levetiracetam-associated psychosis is approximately 1% or less[66] but may be encountered from time to time due to the frequency with which this drug is prescribed. Alternate psychosis or post-ictal psychosis occasionally may be difficult to distinguish from drug-induced psychosis if seizure cessation is associated with addition of a new AED.

Certain anti-psychotic drugs may lower the seizure threshold and even generate epileptic spikes on the EEG; these agents (including clozapine, chlorpromazine, and loxapine) should be avoided in patients with epilepsy. Haloperidol may carry the lowest risk of seizures; alternatives also include olanzapine, risperidone, and molindone.[67] Surgical treatment of patients with TLE and chronic psychosis, with subsequent control of seizures, does not exacerbate psychosis by "forced normalization."[68]

Anxiety and Panic

The prevalence of anxiety in patients with epilepsy is high (ranging from 10% to 50%), but is more difficult to assess.[69,70] Seizures emanating from the antero-mesial temporal lobe (and, in particular, the amygdala) may manifest with panic-like symptoms (e.g., fear and autonomic hyperactivity) and may sometimes need to be distinguished from panic attacks. Posing a particular challenge to the clinician is the fact that when seizures remain focal in the mesial temporal region, they may produce symptoms without being detectable on scalp EEG. Nevertheless, most patients with TLE and fear auras will, at least occasionally, experience progression of the seizure to the point of unresponsiveness and sometimes convulsions, making the diagnosis of epilepsy clear. While TLE and panic disorder may co-exist, a history of TLE makes ictal panic a likely diagnosis. When evaluating a patient for presumed panic attack or panic disorder, a history of seizures or seizure-risk factors (e.g., brain tumor or traumatic brain injury) should raise suspicion for ictal panic. Seizure is more likely to be the cause of the symptoms if there is a clear alteration of awareness, impaired recollection of the event, observed automatisms, or post-event confusion. When suspicion for seizure is high, routine EEG and possibly video EEG may be indicated. Non-epileptic panic attack is more likely if the attacks appear to be triggered primarily by specific circumstances or environments. It should be noted that some patients with epilepsy experience extreme anxiety about seizure recurrence and may avoid social activities or public places for fear of having a seizure in public.

NEUROPSYCHOLOGICAL DISTURBANCES IN EPILEPSY
Cognitive Impairments

Cognitive impairments are common in patients with epilepsy and their etiologies are multi-factorial. Deficits may be the result of the pathology underlying the epilepsy (e.g., focal or diffuse lesions, genetic or neurodevelopmental disorders), the functional effects of recurrent seizures, and inter-ictal discharges, and the effects of AEDs. Additionally, socioeconomic and educational factors may play a role. Neuropsychological profile differs among the different types of epilepsy, often reflecting focal dysfunction in the structures and circuits impacted by, and generating the seizures.[71]

In TLE, in which the hippocampus is often sclerotic and epileptogenic, particular impairment is seen episodic memory, a quintessential hippocampal function. If verbal as opposed to non-verbal memory deficits predominate, the seizure focus likely resides in the language-dominant hemisphere (typically the left). In frontal lobe epilepsy (FLE), the most common deficits involve impairments of executive functions (such as attention, working memory, response selection and inhibition, planning, and motor coordination). Among patients with IGE, and in particular, juvenile myoclonic epilepsy, which has been the most studied form of IGE, deficits resemble those seen in FLE, with a dysexecutive syndrome predominating.

Inter-ictal Personality Traits

Waxman and Geschwind[72] described the following five personality traits occurring with increased frequency in patients with TLE: hypergraphia, hyperreligiosity, hyposexuality, aggressivity, and viscosity. To some extent, this cluster of symptoms may reflect the converse of the Klüver-Bucy syndrome, which has been associated with bilateral temporal lobe damage.[73] The Russian author Fyodor Dostoyevsky is perhaps the best-known example of an epileptic with hypergraphia, which is the tendency to write prolifically. Bear and Fedio identified 18 behavioral traits that they found to occur with increased frequency in patients with TLE as compared to healthy controls and patients with neuromuscular disease.[74] Several subsequent follow-up studies have provided support for the general notion that various personality and behavioral characteristics occur with increased frequency in patients with focal epilepsy as compared to control groups, but the details have varied, and some authors have argued against a particular behavioral syndrome specific for TLE.[75] However, inter-ictal behavioral aberrations are not uncommon, and one should consider the complex interaction between the neuropsychological effects of seizure-related neural network dysfunction, the types and locations of brain lesions underlying the epilepsy, and the social and cultural impact of living with epilepsy and its physical limitations and social stigma.

SUPPORTIVE CARE AND LONG-TERM MANAGEMENT

The primary goal of enabling the patient with epilepsy to achieve or maintain a lifestyle unencumbered by the psychosocial impact of the disease is not necessarily achieved by focusing only on seizure control.[76] Quality-of-life measures specifically tailored to the patient with epilepsy have been developed,[77] and attention paid to individualized deficits in these types of measures will ultimately lead to greater patient satisfaction and medication compliance. Such comprehensive care of the patient requires a multi-disciplinary approach, which, in addition to a neurologist, may include a psychiatrist, clinical social worker, and neuropsychologist.

Access the complete reference list and multiple choice questions (MCQs) online at https://expertconsult.inkling.com

KEY REFERENCES

10. Berg AT, Berkovic SF, Brodie MJ, et al. Revised terminology and concepts for organization of seizures and epilepsies: report of the ILAE Commission on Classification and Terminology, 2005–2009. *Epilepsia* 51(4):676–685, 2010.

15. Hirsch LJ, Gaspard N. Status epilepticus. *Continuum (Minneap Minn)* 19(3 Epilepsy):767–794, 2013.

19. Salinsky M, Kanter R, Dasheiff RM. Effectiveness of multiple EEGs in supporting the diagnosis of epilepsy: an operational curve. *Epilepsia* 28(4):331–334, 1987.

26. Lancman ME, Brotherton TA, Asconape JJ, et al. Psychogenic seizures in adults: a longitudinal analysis. *Seizure* 2(4):281–286, 1993.

27. Fiszman A, Alves-Leon SV, Nunes RG, et al. Traumatic events and posttraumatic stress disorder in patients with psychogenic nonepileptic seizures: a critical review. *Epilepsy Behav* 5(6):818–825, 2004.

28. Gates JR, Ramani V, Whalen S, et al. Ictal characteristics of pseudoseizures. *Arch Neurol* 42(12):1183–1187, 1985.

29. Saygi S, Katz A, Marks DA, et al. Frontal lobe partial seizures and psychogenic seizures: comparison of clinical and ictal characteristics. *Neurology* 42(7):1274–1277, 1992.

30. Benbadis S, Agrawal V, Tatum W. How many patients with psychogenic nonepileptic seizures also have epilepsy? *Neurology* 57(5):915–917, 2001.

31. LaFrance WC Jr, Reuber M, Goldstein LH. Management of psychogenic nonepileptic seizures. *Epilepsia* 54(Suppl. 1):53–67, 2013.

33. McKeon A, Vaughan C, Delanty N. Seizure versus syncope. *Lancet Neurol* 5(2):171–180, 2006.

38. Marson AG, Al-Kharusi AM, Alwaidh M, et al. The SANAD study of effectiveness of carbamazepine, gabapentin, lamotrigine, oxcarbazepine, or topiramate for treatment of partial epilepsy: an unblinded randomised controlled trial. *Lancet* 369(9566):1000–1015, 2007.

39. Marson AG, Al-Kharusi AM, Alwaidh M, et al. The SANAD study of effectiveness of valproate, lamotrigine, or topiramate for generalised and unclassifiable epilepsy: an unblinded randomised controlled trial. *Lancet* 369(9566):1016–1026, 2007.

42. Wiebe S, Blume WT, Girvin JP, et al. A randomized, controlled trial of surgery for temporal-lobe epilepsy. *N Engl J Med* 345(5):311–318, 2001.

45. The Vagus Nerve Stimulation Study Group. A randomized controlled trial of chronic vagus nerve stimulation for treatment of medically intractable seizures. *Neurology* 45(2):224–230, 1995.

48. Rush AJ, George MS, Sackeim HA, et al. Vagus nerve stimulation (VNS) for treatment-resistant depressions: a multicenter study. *Biol Psychiatry* 47(4):276–286, 2000.

49. Hesdorffer DC, Krishnamoorthy ES. Neuropsychiatric disorders in epilepsy: epidemiology and classification. In Trimble MR, Schmitz B, editors: *The Neuropsychiatry of Epilepsy*, ed 2, Cambridge, UK, 2011, Cambridge University Press, pp 3–13.

50. Gaitatzis A, Trimble MR, Sander JW. The psychiatric comorbidity of epilepsy. *Acta Neurol Scand* 110(4):207–220, 2004.

51. Harden CL, Goldstein MA. Mood disorders in patients with epilepsy: epidemiology and management. *CNS Drugs* 16(5):291–302, 2002.

52. Hesdorffer DC, Hauser WA, Annegers JF, et al. Major depression is a risk factor for seizures in older adults. *Ann Neurol* 47(2):246–249, 2000.

56. Kanner AM, Balabanov A. Depression and epilepsy: how closely related are they? *Neurology* 58(8 Suppl. 5):S27–S39, 2002.

59. Barry J, Lembke A, Hyunh N. Affective disorders in epilepsy. In Ettinger A, Kanner A, editors: *Psychiatric Issues in Epilepsy*, Philadelphia, 2001, Lippincott Williams & Wilkins.

62. Devinsky O, Abramson H, Alper K, et al. Postictal psychosis: a case control series of 20 patients and 150 controls. *Epilepsy Res* 20(3):247–253, 1995.

65. Landolt H. Serial electroencephalographic investigations during psychotic episodes in epileptic patients and during schizophrenic attacks. In de Haas L, editor: *Lectures on Epilepsy*, Amsterdam, 1958, Elsevier.

66. Schmitz B. The effects of antiepileptic drugs on behavior. In Trimble MR, Schmitz B, editors: *The neuropsychiatry of epilepsy*, ed 2, Cambridge; New York, 2011, Cambridge University Press, pp vii–225.

67. McConnell H, Duncan D. Treatment of psychiatric comorbidity in epilepsy. In McConnell H, Synder P, editors: *Psychiatric Comorbidity in Epilepsy: Basic Mechanisms, Diagnosis and Treatment*, Washington, DC, 1998, American Psychiatric Press.

69. Manchanda R, Schaefer B, McLachlan RS, et al. Psychiatric disorders in candidates for surgery for epilepsy. *J Neurol Neurosurg Psychiatry* 61(1):82–89, 1996.

72. Waxman SG, Geschwind N. The interictal behavior syndrome of temporal lobe epilepsy. *Arch Gen Psychiatry* 32(12):1580–1586, 1975.

78 Differential Diagnosis and Treatment of Headaches

Stephen E. Nicolson, MD

KEY POINTS

Incidence/Epidemiology
- While headaches are extremely common and usually benign, there are many dangerous causes of headache. Headaches, even when benign, can be disabling.

Pathophysiology
- The pathophysiology of a headache depends on its underlying cause.

Clinical Findings
- Certain headache "red flags" may alert the clinician to dangerous causes of secondary headache.

Differential Diagnosis
- Primary headaches, such as migraines, may be differentiated from secondary headaches; a thorough headache history is crucial for this.

Treatment Options
- There are specific treatment options for each type of headache.

Complications
- Overuse of headache medications can paradoxically cause headaches.

Prognosis
- Proper treatment of headaches can significantly reduce their morbidity.

OVERVIEW

Headache is one of the most common medical complaints; up to 93% of men and 99% of women have experienced headache.[1] Although the vast majority of headaches are not life-threatening, they do cause significant disability. Among pain conditions, recurrent headache disorders account for the bulk of lost work time and disability.[2] Many headaches are self-treated, but headache is still a leading cause of emergency department (ED) and physician visits. Most people with recurrent troublesome headaches have tension-type, migraine, or cluster headaches. These are referred to as "primary headaches" in the widely used International Classification of Headache Disorders—II (Box 78-1).[3] It is vitally important, however, that clinicians rule out life-threatening causes of headaches.

EPIDEMIOLOGY AND RISK FACTORS

The lifetime prevalence of the most common of headaches, the tension-type headache, is estimated at 30%–80%,[4] though most everyone has had this type of headache at some time.

Over 28 million Americans have migraines; half remain undiagnosed.[5] Approximately 20% of women suffer from migraines, as opposed to 6% of men.[6] Worldwide prevalence studies roughly mirror the US data. Prevalence peaks during the average individual's most productive years, from ages 25 to 55. The World Health Organization considers severe migraine to be the eighth most disabling human conditions in terms of years lived with disability.[51]

Chronic daily headache, a collective term that refers to primary headaches that occur more than 14 days per month for at least 3 months, shows a stable worldwide prevalence of about 4%,[7] though there may be significant variation in the individuals who make up this group. Frequently, chronic daily headache may develop from pre-existing migraines or tension-type headaches. Less commonly, the pattern may develop *de novo* (Box 78-2).[8] Risk factors for chronic daily headache include female gender, low education level, medication overuse, a history of head or neck trauma, and cigarette smoking.[7]

Secondary headaches carry a prevalence related to the underlying condition (see Clinical Features, Diagnosis and Treatment, later in this chapter).

GENETICS

Multiple studies indicate a genetic influence in many of the primary headaches. The inheritance in migraine is likely multi-factorial, and the odds ratio may increase proportionate to the severity of migraine in the proband but does not seem to relate to the type of headache. Anticipation is noted over generations, with a tendency toward earlier age of onset. Notwithstanding, less than 50% of migraine cases are thought to exhibit genetic influences,[9] thus this is likely also a common sporadic condition.

In patients with a rare form of migraine, familial hemiplegic migraine, the responsible genetic defect results in calcium channel dysfunction (channelopathy) that is thought to explain the migraine symptoms in these patients. Familial hemiplegic migraine (FHM) has been associated with two mutations: *CACNA1A* gene on chromosome 19 is affected in FHM1 and *ATP1A2* on chromosome 1 is affected in FHM2.[10] Genetic alterations have been identified as associated with more common forms of migraines including a minor allele on chromosome 8, likely involved in the regulation of glutamate,[11] and in a potassium channel, *TRESK*, on chromosome 10.[12] Several additional gene alterations confer a higher risk for common types of migraine. However, the effect size for individual genes is small. Such genetic discoveries are likely to contribute to improved understanding of the pathophysiology of migraine.

In tension-type headache, the high prevalence confounds the detection of a genetic influence. Nonetheless, studies of several large populations suggest a complex multi-factorial mode of inheritance in favor of a sporadic condition. A genetic influence is likely in cluster headache as well, though the exact mode is unclear, possibly an autosomal dominant mode with reduced penetrance or an autosomal recessive pattern.[13]

PATHOPHYSIOLOGY

Except for the posterior fossa, which is supplied by the high cervical nerve roots, most head pain is mediated through the first division of the trigeminal nerve.[14] Nociceptive C and A-delta fibers innervate the skin, periosteum, large vessels (arteries, veins, and sinuses) and meninges[15] (Figure 78-1). Thus, pain may arise from any of these areas, yet not from the substance of the brain, which contains no nociceptive fibers. The cervical and trigeminal nociceptive information is distributed to the "trigeminocervical complex," a large ipsilateral nuclear group spanning the trigeminal nucleus caudalis (rostrally) to the high cervical dorsal horn cells (caudally). Second-order pathways then cross from there and terminate in the thalamus; third-order pathways then bring the information to the cortex. Descending endogenous inhibitory pain systems may influence the incoming signals at the juncture between the first- and second-order neurons. This simplified scheme may mediate most, if not all, head pain no matter what the cause.

As to the cause of migraine specifically, dysfunction in these brainstem systems, possibly genetically determined, is one theory of migraine generation. Also, cortical spreading depression (CSD), originally described by Leao and now thought to be the mechanism of the aura in migraine, may result in local ionic and chemical changes that might sensitize perivascular trigeminal fibers that set off a cascade of changes to produce the clinical symptomatology of migraine with aura by way of the simplified scheme above.[9] Included in this process, trigeminal neural impulses may subsequently "feedback" through various routes to the meninges, leading to local release of neuropeptides (e.g., CGRP, substance P, VIP) that can amplify and sustain the headache cascade, perhaps influencing the development of cutaneous skin hypersensitivity (allodynia) seen in some patients and perhaps also setting the stage for the development of a chronic headache pattern. Stimulation of nearby brainstem nuclei by this cascade may also explain

---

BOX 78-1 International Headache Society Classification of Headache Disorders—II

PRIMARY HEADACHES
- Migraine
- Tension-type headache
- Cluster headache and other trigeminal autonomic cephalgias
- Other primary headaches

SECONDARY HEADACHES
- Headache attributed to head and neck trauma
- Headache attributed to cranial or cervical vascular disorder
- Headache attributed to non-vascular intracranial disorder
- Headache attributed to a substance or its withdrawal
- Headache attributed to infection
- Headache attributed to disturbance of homeostasis
- Headache or facial pain attributed to disorder of cranium, neck, eyes, ears, nose, sinuses, teeth, mouth, or other facial or cranial structures
- Headache attributed to psychiatric disorder

CRANIAL NEURALGIAS, CENTRAL AND PRIMARY FACIAL PAIN, AND OTHER HEADACHES

BOX 78-2 Conditions Associated with Chronic Daily Headaches

- Medication overuse headaches (the most common cause)
- Migraine headaches
- Tension-type headaches
- Headaches associated with psychiatric conditions (especially depression and anxiety disorders)
- Headaches associated with co-morbid medical illnesses

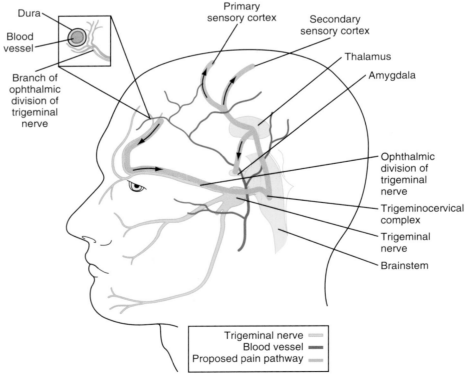

Dura
Blood vessel
Branch of ophthalmic division of trigeminal nerve
Primary sensory cortex
Secondary sensory cortex
Thalamus
Amygdala
Ophthalmic division of trigeminal nerve
Trigeminocervical complex
Trigeminal nerve
Brainstem

Trigeminal nerve
Blood vessel
Proposed pain pathway

Figure 78-1. Pain pathway showing the innervation of the meninges and cerebral vessels by the V1 division of the trigeminal nerve. The impulse moves down the trigeminal nerve to the trigeminocervical complex. Then the pathway ascends to the thalamus, before going on to the cortex—amygdala, sensory association, and primary sensory area for the head.

BOX 78-3 Clues to Dangerous Headaches

- First time to have this type of headache → investigate with diligence
- Acute onset → SAH, other thunderclap headaches (see Box 78-5)
- Chronic, progressive → rule out brain tumor, chronic SAH
- Fever → meningitis, encephalitis
- Worse when lying down → increased ICP secondary to mass (tumor or hemorrhage)
- Worse when standing up → decreased ICP secondary to LP
- Pain worse after time spent in a particular location → carbon monoxide poisoning
- Associated with N/V → mass
- Associated with localizing signs → mass
- Papilledema or increase in pain with cough or straining → mass, intracranial hypertension
- Scalp tenderness or skull fracture → subdural hematoma
- Orbital or temporal bruit → AVM, sinus thrombosis
- Nuchal pain or rigidity → acute or chronic meningitis or SAH
- Onset after age 50 or chronic and progressive → tumor, SDH

AVM, Arteriovenous malformation; ICP, intracranial pressure; LP, lumbar puncture; N/V, nausea and vomiting; SAH, subarachnoid hemorrhage.

BOX 78-4 Eliciting History: Questions to Ask Patients about Headaches

Have you ever had this type of headache before?
- Yes or no?
  Duration:
- Acute or chronic?
  Onset:
- Sudden or insidious?
  Severity:
- Dull or excruciating?
  Location:
- Orbital, temporal, occipital, or nuchal?
  Laterality:
- Unilateral or bilateral?
  Positional:
- Worse or better when lying down or standing up?
  Setting:
- Related to meals, medication, exercise, sleep, work, light, noise, or going to bathroom?
  Associated symptoms:
- Nausea, vomiting, sweating, visual or motor changes, anxiety?
  Medications:
- Which ones and how often are they used?

---

some of the associated constitutional symptoms that are commonly seen in migraine.

Tension-type headache may result from persistent peripheral nociceptive hyperstimulation and may share many of the pathophysiological features of migraine. Whether tension-type headache is ultimately viewed as a variation of migraine or as a separate pathological condition remains unsettled. Recent information suggests a central, possibly hypothalamic, cause for cluster headaches with important peripheral trigeminovascular activation as well.

The pathogenesis of a secondary headache depends on the etiology of each particular headache and will be discussed with descriptions of each condition in Clinical Features, Diagnosis, and Treatment, later in this chapter.

DIFFERENTIAL DIAGNOSIS

While most patients with dangerous headaches are treated in the ED, the psychiatrist who is familiar with the presentation of rare headache syndromes may be a life-saver. A host of conditions need to be considered when an individual complains of a headache. Differentiating among all potential causes of headaches can be daunting. The task can be made less difficult by ruling out dangerous causes of headaches (Box 78-3). Once this has been done, the clinician can match the headache history to the headache syndrome.

Because the clinical features vary for the different causes of headache, taking the headache history is the most crucial aspect of the work-up (Box 78-4).[16] The identification of life-threatening causes of a headache can usually be done with a thorough history. Elucidation of such features of the pain as timing (e.g., acute or chronic), onset (e.g., sudden or insidious), duration, severity, location (e.g., unilateral, bilateral, including the neck or eyes), associated symptoms (e.g., visual changes, motor symptoms, nausea, diaphoresis, anxiety), body position (e.g., after standing up or lying down), and setting (e.g., during sleep, at work, or after exercise) is important. The effects of medication, meals (including specific foods [such as chocolate]), substances (such as caffeine and alcohol), sleep, and exercise also offer important clues to the diagnosis. A family history of certain types of headaches may also shed

light on the etiology. For patients with more than one type of headache, a separate history should be obtained for each type.

Physical examination of a patient with headache must include a full neurological examination, a funduscopic examination, and an examination of the head. Vital signs must also be assessed (as low or high blood pressure may be contributing factors). A fever may point toward a central nervous system (CNS) infection. The neurological examination will reveal any focal findings that may indicate a stroke or multiple sclerosis (MS). The funduscopic examination will search for signs of raised intracranial pressure (ICP), manifest by papilledema (Figure 78-2).[17] Physical examination of the head will search for signs of trauma, and one should palpate for tenderness or masses, and listen over the temples and eyes for bruits that may signal the presence of an arteriovenous malformation. The neck must also be checked for rigidity.

Further testing may be indicated to evaluate etiologies suggested by the history and physical examination (Table 78-1). Imaging may be needed if a brain mass, stroke, or MS is suspected. Computed tomography (CT) scans are usually quicker and cheaper, whereas magnetic resonance imaging (MRI) is more sensitive and expensive. A lumbar puncture (LP) can help evaluate infectious etiologies, subarachnoid hemorrhage (SAH), or ICP. In an elderly person with new-onset headache, an elevated erythrocyte sedimentation rate (ESR) suggests giant cell arteritis or temporal arteritis. Electroencephalography (EEG) and evoked responses have no particular role in primary headache diagnosis but may be helpful in sorting out several of the secondary headache causes.

HEADACHE "RED FLAGS"

Historical features that may indicate a dangerous underlying cause for headache include the so-called "first and worst"

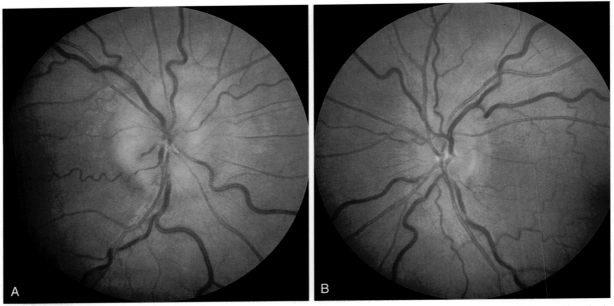

Figure 78-2. Papilledema. Asymmetric papilledema in a 54-year-old woman with constant daily headaches and transient visual loss in the right eye. She had idiopathic intracranial hypertension. *(From Friedman DI. Headache. In Schapira AHV, Byrne E, editors:* Neurology and clinical neuroscience, *Philadelphia, 2007, Mosby, Fig 61-1, p. 809.)*

TABLE 78-1 Ordering Laboratory and Other Tests

Suspected Condition	Order
Acute stroke or bleed	CT
Aneurysm	MRA or CT angiogram
CVT	MRI and MRA or CT and CT angiogram
MS	MRI
Infection	LP
Temporal arteritis	ESR, CRP
Seizures	EEG
Carbon monoxide poisoning	Carboxyhemoglobin
CNS tumor	CT
Pheochromocytoma	24-hour urine metanephrine; abdominal CT

CNS, Central nervous system; CRP, C-reactive protein; CT, computed tomography; CVT, cerebral venous thrombosis; EEG, electroencephalogram; ESR, erythrocyte sedimentation rate; LP, lumbar puncture; MRA, magnetic resonance angiogram; MRI, magnetic resonance imaging; MS, multiple sclerosis.

BOX 78-5 "Thunderclap" Headache

Only rarely is the sudden onset of a severe headache benign in origin. These patients should be assessed in the emergency department where emergent imaging is possible, cardiovascular and neurological status can be closely monitored, and urgent treatment can be administered. Rare primary causes of severe sudden headache include sexual headache, cough headache, and exertional headache. However, dangerous causes of "thunderclap" headache that must be ruled out include the following:

- Intracerebral hemorrhage
- Arterial dissection
- Cerebral venous thrombosis
- Unruptured vascular malformation
- Pituitary hemorrhagic infarct (pituitary apoplexy)
- CNS hypotension
- Acute sinusitis
- Third ventricular colloid cyst
- Hypertensive encephalopathy
- Spontaneous low-pressure headache

headache: that is, the sudden onset of a *de novo* severe headache, possibly indicating a SAH often as a result of an aneurysmal bleed. Also known as a "thunderclap headache," this pattern has been investigated in some detail, and there is a differential diagnosis beyond SAH, with both primary and secondary types described (Box 78-5). Some of these headaches are actually of benign origin with a negative evaluation; however, given the risks involved in missing an aneurysmal bleed, this pattern cannot be assumed to be benign and must be evaluated.

Headache associated with fever, chills, and change in mental status is of evident concern and not often confused with a primary headache syndrome. Similarly, a new-onset headache in a compromised individual (e.g., someone with acquired immunodeficiency syndrome [AIDS]) or in someone with a concerning past medical history (e.g., with metastatic cancer) should also prompt concern.

New-onset migraine after age 50 is unusual, and thus an evaluation (including an evaluation for temporal arteritis) is warranted, to prevent the often sudden complication of irreversible visual loss.

OTHER SECONDARY HEADACHES

Not all secondary causes of headache pose an immediate danger. Nonetheless, accurate diagnosis of such secondary causes (e.g., low-pressure headache or cervicogenic headache) should result in more targeted and productive therapy; thus, vigilance in rooting out secondary causes of headache is warranted. And, since known migraine patients may themselves develop secondary headaches, combinations of types of headache may be present in one individual, causing significant diagnostic confusion.

One particular instance of a combination of primary and secondary headache deserves mention: an individual who, in an attempt to treat a primary headache, may overuse medication and develop a secondary rebound or withdrawal headache from the overused medication—this often complicates management.

TREATMENT

Specific treatment of headache depends on the underlying cause (see next section, Headache Syndromes: Clinical Features, Diagnosis, and Treatment), but some general rules apply. Symptomatic treatment of most types of headache begins with analgesics (such as acetaminophen and non-steroidal anti-inflammatory drugs [NSAIDs]), and many medications can be used for multiple types of headaches (Table 78-2). Opiates are generally discouraged in the treatment of headaches, although for severe pain in a post-surgical setting they may be helpful in the short term. In the treatment of chronic daily headaches, opiates have been unsuccessful, with nearly three-quarters of patients either lacking marked improvement or showing problematic drug behavior, such as dose violations.[18]

HEADACHE SYNDROMES: CLINICAL FEATURES, DIAGNOSIS, AND TREATMENT
Primary Headaches

Most headaches are primary headaches: tension-type, migraine, or cluster headaches (Table 78-3). These are chronic recurring headaches for which there is no apparent structural abnormality.

TABLE 78-2 Pharmacological Treatment of Headache

Medication	Dosing	Side Effects	Headache Type
Acetaminophen	1,000 mg every 4 hours as neededto a maximum of 4,000 mg/day	Hepatotoxicity	Tension-type
Beta-blockers (e.g., propranolol)	40 mg bid, increase as HR tolerates	Dizziness, interferes with asthma treatment	Migraine, sexual, exertional, pheochromocytoma
Botulinum toxin type A	25–260 units injected every 3 months	Muscle weakness, ptosis	Chronic migraine
Calcium channel-blockers (e.g., verapamil)	40 mg tid	Hypotension, A-V block	Migraine
Carbamazepine	100 mg bid and increase until relief	Leukopenia, hepatotoxicity, weight gain, somnolence	Trigeminal neuralgia
Combination analgesics (e.g., Fiorinal)	1–2 caplets every 4 hours as needed	Somnolence, palpitations (due to caffeine), addiction	Tension-type
Dopamine blockers (e.g., prochlorperazine)	10–25 mg as needed	Sedation, dystonia, parkinsonism	Migraine (for nausea)
Ergots (e.g., ergotamine tartrate)	2 mg SL every 30 minutes (up to 6 mg/day) as needed	Dizziness. May not be used with triptans or MAOIs	Migraine, cluster
Gabapentin	900–3,600 mg daily	Dizziness, somnolence	Migraine, CDH, trigeminal neuralgia
Lithium	600–1,200 mg daily (based on therapeutic blood levels)	Renal toxicity, polyuria, polydipsia, edema, weight gain, thyroid disease, nausea, diarrhea	Cluster
NSAIDs (e.g., ibuprofen)	400–800 mg every 6 hours	Increased bleeding time, renal toxicity, GI side effects	Migraine, CDH, tension-type, sexual, exertional
Serotonin antagonists (e.g., methysergide)	2–8 mg daily	Retroperitoneal and retropleural fibrosis	Migraine
Serotonin-norepinephrine reuptake inhibitors (e.g., venlafaxine)	150 mg daily	Nausea, sexual dysfunction, hypertension	Migraine
Serotonin reuptake inhibitors (e.g., fluoxetine)	20–60 mg daily	Sexual dysfunction, nausea, somnolence	Migraine, tension-type
Steroids (e.g., methylprednisolone)	24 mg the first day and taper over 6 days	Nausea, vomiting, insomnia, anxiety	Cluster, migraine, IIH, temporal arteritis (higher doses), medication-overuse
Tizanidine	8–20 mg daily	Dry mouth, hypotension, bradycardia	Migraine, CDH
Topiramate	25–100 mg bid	Somnolence, weight loss, kidney stones	Migraine, CDH, cluster
Tricyclic antidepressants (e.g., amitriptyline)	10–150 mg at bedtime	Dry mouth, hypotension, constipation, arrhythmia, fatigue	Migraine, tension-type, cluster
Triptans (e.g., sumatriptan)	6 mg subcutaneously hourly × 2/daily as needed	Nausea. Interaction with ergots; Contraindicated in stroke, coronary artery disease[52]	Migraine, exertional, sexual
Valproic acid	500–2,000 mg/day	Nausea, somnolence, weight gain, alopecia; avoid if possible in pregnancy[53]	Migraine, trigeminal neuralgia

bid, Twice per day; CDH, chronic daily headache; GI, gastrointestinal; HR, heart rate; IIH, idiopathic intracranial hypertension; qhs, every night; SL, sublingually; tid, three times per day.

TABLE 78-3 Primary Headaches

Syndrome	Epidemiology	Symptoms	Acute Treatment	Miscellaneous
Tension-type		Band-like pain, lack of associated symptoms, not usually incapacitating, may be relieved by alcohol	NSAIDs, acetaminophen, relaxation techniques, biofeedback	Not associated with increased muscle tension
Migraine	20% of women 6% of men	Recurrent stereotyped episodes of pain; presentation varies between patients, unilateral pulsating pain in front of head, often the pain generalizes, may have multiple associated symptoms, 4–24 h	Avoid precipitating factors, NSAIDs, triptans, ergots	70% of patients have family history. 75% of women have decrease in migraines during pregnancy. Migraines tend to wane as patient enters forties
Cluster	Overall < 0.4%, vast majority are men, onset before age 25	Grouping of excruciating, sharp, pain located usually behind one eye occurring several times daily; may occur during sleep; peaks within 5–10 minutes, <3 h; associated with reddened conjunctiva, sweating, ptosis	Oxygen, lithium	May repeat in spring. Patients often smoke cigarettes and drink alcohol excessively

Tension-type Headaches

The designation may be a misnomer as recent studies have demonstrated that this type of headache is not reliably associated with increased muscle contractions or physiological tension.[19] The mechanism of the headache may be related to hyper-excitability of afferent neurons from muscle or impairments in pain inhibitory systems. Tension-type headache is somewhat more common in women than in men. Pain is the main symptom. Nausea may be a complaint as well, but vomiting is rare.[19] Patients usually describe the pain as bilateral, band-like, steady, and mild to moderate in intensity. Increased tenderness in the muscles of the head and the frontal, temporal, masseter, pterygoid, sternocleidomastoid, splenius, and trapezius muscles can sometimes be demonstrated with palpation using the second and third digits,[4] but its absence does not rule out the disorder. Most patients can continue to function with tension-type headaches.

Treatment of tension-type headaches consists of reassurance that there is no life-threatening cause and advice about treatment. Simple analgesics are used to treat individual headaches. The best evidence of effectiveness is for aspirin in doses of 500 to 1,000 mg.[20] Opioids and barbiturate-containing medications should be avoided as tolerance can develop with their use, which may lead to escalating doses and to dependence.

Evidence for non-pharmacologic options in the treatment of headaches has been mounting. A review of 94 studies of biofeedback found that for tension-type headache, biofeedback treatment yielded a medium to large effect compared with waiting-list controls and a medium effect compared with placebo, both of which were statistically significant.[21] There were also significant improvements in perceived self-efficacy, symptoms of depression and anxiety, and less medication use.

Prophylactic treatment is needed when headaches are disabling or frequent. Good evidence supports the use of amitriptyline, which is generally effective for headaches (used at doses lower than those needed to treat depression).[22] Tizanidine may also be useful.[22] Mirtazapine has also been shown to be effective.[23] Open-label studies have suggested a possible benefit for botulinum toxin injections into the head and neck, but placebo-controlled trials show no benefit.[22]

Migraine

Migraine headaches have been classified as vascular headaches, although recent evidence suggests that dysfunction of neurotransmitter systems (e.g., substance P, neurokinin A, serotonin, glutamate) are involved in the pathophysiology.[5] Migraines are more common in women (occurring in up to 20% of women). The female-to-male ratio for migraines is 3:1. These headaches tend to run in families, with 70% of patients having a family history of migraines.[5] Migraine symptomatology may be complex, but for an individual patient, headaches occur in a recurrent stereotyped manner.[19] Migraine usually causes a unilateral pulsatile pain in the frontotemporal region or around the eye. In half of patients, the pain switches sides of the head during the attack or in different attacks.[19] The pain may become dull and symmetrical, similar to that of a tension-type headache. Photophobia and phonophobia are common features. Autonomic dysfunction arises and includes slowed gastric emptying, nausea, and vomiting that can cause severe disability. The length of a headache can be greatly variable, but it usually lasts from 4 to 74 hours. Migraines may be precipitated by ingestion of certain foods (e.g., aged cheese, red wine, chocolate, nuts), by skipping meals, by too little sleep, by too much sleep, and by psychological stress. In contrast to tension-type headaches, migraines tend to begin in the morning. Often, the weekends or the start of a vacation can precipitate a migraine.[19] In women, migraines often begin at menarche and recur pre-menstrually. Contraceptive medication may worsen migraines in some women, while in others it may improve symptoms. Pregnancy offers relief from migraines in about three-fourths of women.[19] Migraine symptoms often improve when patients reach their thirties and forties. Nocturnal migraines arise during rapid eye movement (REM) sleep.[19]

Common migraines are those without an aura, while the classic migraine (which occurs in only about 25% of migraine sufferers) is preceded by an aura, usually a visual change (such as a field cut or scotoma, or flashing zig-zag lines [scintillations]).[19] Auras (any transient neurological alteration) typically evolve over several minutes and can last up to an hour. Hallucinations (e.g., visual, olfactory, auditory, or gustatory), motor deficits (e.g., hemiparesis or hemiplegia), paresthesias (e.g., of the lips and hands especially), aphasia, perceptual impairments, anxiety, and depression are varieties of migraine auras. On rare occasions an aura may not be followed by a headache and it can mimic other neurological disorders (e.g., stroke, psychosis, or intoxication).[19]

Patients who suffer from a migraine are often debilitated and attempt to avoid sensory input in an attempt to soothe sensory hypersensitivity (allodynia). They seek out dark, quiet rooms and prefer to be alone.

Several theories to account for migraines have been discussed earlier in this chapter. In addition, symptoms of aura have been shown to coincide with decreases in regional cortical blood flow corresponding to the localization of neurological symptoms.[5] Recent investigations have revealed that activated C-fibers release neuropeptides (such as substance P and neurokinin A), which then generate an inflammatory response within the meninges; this prolongs a headache.[5] Other messenger systems involving nitric oxide and calcitonin-gene-related peptide are also likely involved.[5] In addition to this peripheral sensitization, there are likely central processes at work during headaches (such as the recruitment of previously non-nociceptive neurons).[14] The painful nature of usually benign activities or stimuli (such as coughing) during a headache may be an example of this central sensitization. Migraines are associated with structural changes in the brain, including strokes[24] and white matter hyperintensities on MRI that increase with disease progression.[25]

Treatment for migraine headaches begins with avoidance of any identifiable precipitants. In order to identify potential triggers, it is helpful to obtain a headache diary in which a patient records foods, medications, and timing of menses, work/school, and headaches. Abortive therapy for mild-to-moderate migraines is similar to that of tension-type headaches. More severe migraines are effectively treated with ergotamine, dihydroergotamine, and the 5-HT$_1$ agonists (e.g., sumatriptan, naratriptan, zolmitriptan, rizatriptan, almotriptan, eletriptan, frovatriptan). If nausea precludes the use of oral medication, nasal sprays, injectable preparations, and suppositories are available. For those with frequent migraines, prophylactic medication may be necessary. Anticonvulsants (e.g., valproic acid), antidepressants (e.g., amitriptyline), beta-blockers (e.g., propranolol), calcium channel blockers (e.g., verapamil), NSAIDs, and serotonin antagonists (e.g., methysergide) have all been used effectively. In 2006, the FDA issued a warning about the possibility of serotonin syndrome in patients given triptans while concomitantly taking an SSRI or SNRI. However, the American Headache Society issued a position paper stating that evidence to support limiting the use of triptans in patients on SSRI or SNRIs is lacking.[26] For patients who suffer from status migrainosis (lasting longer than 72 hours), steroids or barbiturates are indicated. In 2010, the FDA approved onabotulinum toxin A (Botox) to prevent headaches in adult patients with chronic migraine. Multiple injections into the head and neck are given every 12 weeks.

There are also non-pharmacologic options. For prevention of migraine, the United States Headache Consortium gave Grade A recommendations (which indicated multiple well-designed randomized clinical trials yielding consistent findings) including several behavioral interventions, relaxation training, EMG biofeedback and cognitive-behavioral therapy.[27] Goals of CBT for headache management include enhancing self-efficacy and helping patients gain an internal locus of control, as opposed to an external locus of control (i.e., the belief that only the physician, medication, or medical procedures have the power to change).

Although there is no consistent association between migraine and either heart disease or hypertension, studies have shown a relationship between migraine and stroke, epilepsy, allergy and asthma, and psychiatric conditions, especially depression, bipolar disorder, panic disorder, and generalized anxiety disorder. Depression is associated with an increased risk of transformation of episodic migraine into chronic migraine.[28] Patients with migraines are at increased risk for suicide attempts and increased severity of pain is associated with an increase in suicide attempts.[29]

Chronic Daily Headache

This term describes a fairly frequent clinical syndrome arising from a number of conditions all having in common the production of headache in an individual for 15 days a month or more. This pattern may begin *de novo* (new daily persistent headache) or as an unusual primary headache (*hemicrania continua*), but it is more commonly thought to reflect a transformation (chronification) of migraine or tension-type headache.[19] Medication overuse has often contributed to the worsening of the headache. Management is a challenge, and these patients make up the bulk of referrals in most headache clinics. Often with the daily presentation the actual headache characteristics become more drab, and less dramatic and distinct, compared with the intermittent migraine pattern. Prevention of this complication is one of the goals of early aggressive headache management. Programs that combine behavioral interventions, such as patient education to improve adherence, biofeedback, and relaxation therapy, with pharmacologic treatment can improve outcomes.[30]

Psychiatric co-morbidities are not surprising in chronic daily headache since much of it may stem from migraines. Chronic daily headache is also correlated with obesity (as measured by body mass index [BMI]), female gender, and possibly with fibromyalgia.[19]

Cluster Headaches

Cluster headaches are less common than are migraine or tension-type headaches; they are estimated to have a prevalence of less than 0.4%.[16] The male-to-female ratio with cluster headaches is between 3.5 and 7 : 1.[31] Until recently, cluster headaches were not thought to have a genetic component. Risk factors include smoking and excessive alcohol intake. The onset is usually before age 25 and they may have a cyclical pattern that repeats in the spring. Cluster headaches often occur during REM sleep.[19] The syndrome is named for the grouping of headaches—one to eight times daily for several weeks—with periods of month to years without headaches. The pain peaks within 5 to 10 minutes and can last up to 3 hours. The pain is strictly unilateral, described as sharp, excruciating, and non-throbbing, located around or below one eye or temporal region. Autonomic dysfunction manifests as injected conjunctiva, profuse sweating, facial flushing, ptosis, or miosis (Figure 78-3).[19] Headaches may be triggered by the use of alcohol or tobacco.

Cluster headaches may be aborted by breathing 100% oxygen for 15 minutes.[14] Vasoconstrictive medications and triptans are also helpful. Ergotamine tartrate 2 mg sublingually (SL), repeated every 30 minutes up to 6 mg in 24 hours, is advised. A steroid burst (such as a Medrol Dosepak) can also help. Choices for prophylactic medication include verapamil and lithium. Successful dosing for lithium is based on blood levels in the therapeutic range for the treatment of bipolar disorder. Response usually takes 3 weeks. Topiramate 100 mg twice a day has also shown some efficacy.[32]

Other Primary Headache Syndromes

The IHS includes, in its categorization of primary headaches, headache syndromes that lack objective structural, metabolic, or physical causes, including headache associated with sexual activity and primary exertional headache.

Rarely, individuals develop sudden, severe headaches that begin with orgasm. Clearly, the clinician must exclude dangerous causes of secondary headaches, such as SAH or headaches due to a rise in ICP. Severe pain continues for more than 2 hours in one-fourth of patients and for as long as 24 hours in some.[33] Orgasms cause a release of vasoactive substances

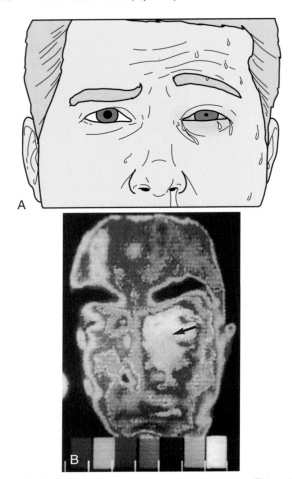

Figure 78-3. (A) Typical presentation of cluster headache. This patient has ipsilateral ptosis, injected conjunctiva, tearing, sweating, and miosis. (B) Thermogram demonstrating the areas of increased temperature in a patient with a cluster headache. *(A, Adapted from Kaufman DM, Milstein MJ. Clinical neurology for psychiatrists, ed 7, Philadelphia, 2013, WB Saunders. B, From Lance JW, Goadsby PJ. Mechanism and management of headache, ed 7, Philadelphia, 2005, Butterworth-Heinemann, Fig 12.1, p. 202.)*

(including serotonin, neurokinins, and catecholamines) that may cause vascular changes leading to pain. Treatment of orgasm-induced headaches includes long-term prophylaxis with propranolol. Triptans or indomethacin (25 to 100 mg) taken 30 minutes before initiation of sexual activity has also been effective in preventing headaches.[33]

Primary exertional headache is a pulsating headache that develops only during or after exercise. It can last 5 minutes to 48 hours.[33] As with sexual headaches, dangerous causes of headache are important to exclude. Indomethacin and triptans have been helpful in preventing these types of headaches.[33]

SECONDARY HEADACHES

Structural causes should be evaluated if the patient's headache pattern does not follow that of one of the primary headache syndromes, is accompanied by an abnormal neurological examination, is progressive, or is of acute onset. Discussed below are some of the dangerous causes of headache; they include trauma, cerebrovascular accidents, infections, and tumors. Other common causes of headache (such as trigemi-

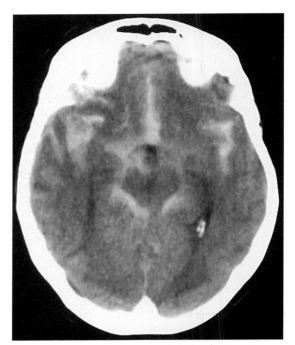

Figure 78-4. Head CT of subarachnoid hemorrhage showing blood in the Sylvian fissures and basal cisterns. *(From Lance JW, Goadsby PJ. Mechanism and management of headache, ed 7, Philadelphia, 2005, Butterworth-Heinemann, Fig 15.2, p. 293.)*

nal neuralgia, temporal arteritis, and medication overuse headaches) will be discussed below.

Post-traumatic Headache

Headache develops in over 80% of patients after head trauma.[3] Nearly half of those who have suffered a concussion have headaches that last for up to 2 months after the injury.[34] Headaches after trauma may be due to a number of factors, including acceleration and deceleration forces that can cause shear injury to neurons. Psychological, social, and medico-legal issues may also play a role. Nausea, vomiting, dizziness, vertigo, depression, and anxiety can accompany the headaches. The headaches often begin within 2 weeks of the injury and may resemble migraine or tension-type headaches.

Intracranial Hemorrhage

Cerebral bleeds are usually manifest by the sudden onset of focal neurological deficits that reflect the location and size of the bleed. Larger bleeds can cause altered mental status, headache, nausea, vomiting, loss of consciousness (LOC), and hemiplegia. Herniation and death can occur within 24 hours. The most common risk factor for intracranial hemorrhage (ICH) is chronic systemic hypertension, but trauma, anticoagulation therapy, saccular aneurysm, arteriovenous (A-V) malformation, CNS tumor, clotting disorders, angiopathy, and vasculitis are also associated with ICH.

Subarachnoid Hemorrhage

A "thunderclap" headache is the classic description of the presentation of SAH, but there are other causes of an excruciating and sudden headache (see Box 78-5). SAH is caused by rupture of the wall of a cerebral aneurysm or of a cerebrovascular malformation (Figure 78-4).[9] The fatality rate with SAH

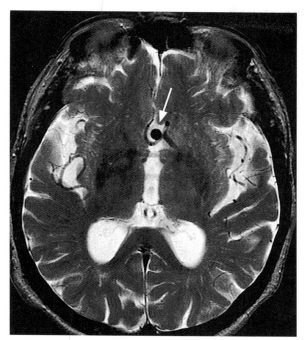

Figure 78-5. MRI of a patient with an aneurysm of the anterior communicating artery. *(From Yock DH: Magnetic resonance imaging of CNS disease: a teaching file, ed 2, St Louis, 2002, Mosby, case 726, p. 446.)*

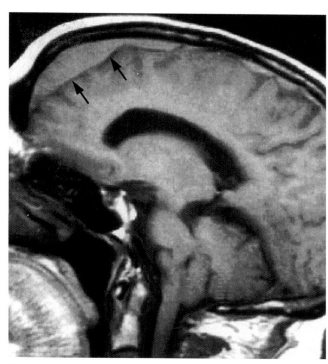

Figure 78-6. Head MRI of a 79-year-old man with chronic subdural hematoma. *(From Yock DH. Magnetic resonance imaging of CNS disease: a teaching file, ed 2, St Louis, 2002, Mosby, case 708, p. 433.)*

is nearly 50%, and half of the survivors have severe deficits.[3] The most common site of such a rupture is the circle of Willis. The sudden onset (reaching its peak within a minute) of a severe headache is the most common presentation, and it is often associated with nuchal rigidity. SAH often occurs during exertion (e.g., exercise, sexual intercourse, or straining on the toilet). Initially, there may be fever, nausea, vomiting, seizures, lethargy, and even coma. Focal neurological deficits and retinal hemorrhages point toward SAH. Diagnosis can usually be made on seeing blood on a non-contrast CT or in the cerebrospinal fluid (CSF) during an LP. Occasionally, SAH may be the result of vascular leaks from the pathological vessel, or sentinel bleeds, and the presentation is not quite as dramatic. At times no cause can be found to explain a documented SAH and in these patients the prognosis appears to be benign. Risk factors for SAH include head trauma, thrombocytopenia, use of warfarin or heparin, clotting factor deficiency, cocaine use, and ingestion of tyramine while taking a monoamine oxidase inhibitor (MAOI). Treatment of SAH and intracranial bleeds depend on their etiology, location, and symptoms. Neurosurgery consultation is indicated for larger bleeds that may cause compression and herniation. Evacuation of the bleed may be considered. Supportive care includes prevention of increases in ICP that may cause herniation, while avoiding hypotension that could cause ischemia. Use of a calcium channel blocker, nimodipine, improves outcomes in SAH.

Aneurysm

Headache, likely attributed to either sentinel bleeds or local compression, is present in 18% of those with an unruptured cerebral aneurysm[3] (Figure 78-5).[35] This can be an important and potentially life-saving warning considering the morbidity and mortality rates of SAH. The classic presentation of an enlarging posterior communicating cerebral artery aneurysm is severe posterior orbital pain associated with third nerve

palsy and a blown pupil. Between 2% and 9% of autopsies reveal berry aneurysms; half of them are detected in the circle of Willis.[36]

Intracranial Mass Lesions

Brain tumors and subdural hematomas (SDHs) may cause headaches that initially may be confused with tension-type headaches when the headache symptoms are mild, bilateral, and dull. They may worsen as ICP rises while coughing, straining, or bending over, or during REM sleep. Objective evidence of increased ICP (such as papilledema) may not be evident until late in the course. Similarly, localizing findings on neurological examination may not be apparent, though subtle cognitive and personality changes are usually seen. Chronic SDH can be a cause of a fluctuating headache accompanied by confusion and lethargy (Figure 78-6).[35] Headache is found in over 80% of those with chronic SDHs.[3] SDHs develop more commonly in the elderly, in those who are anticoagulated, and in alcoholics. Brain tumors are also seen more in those over age 50.

Ischemic Stoke

Seventeen percent to 34% of patients with ischemic stroke complain of headache.[3] The presence of focal neurological deficits helps differentiate the headache of a stroke from primary headaches. The pain is usually mild to moderate. The complaint of headache is more often seen with basilar territory than carotid strokes.

Cerebral Venous Thrombosis

Thrombosis of the cerebral veins and sinuses causes swelling of cerebral veins and reduces absorption of CSF. The increased pressure in the skull leads to infarcts and to hemorrhages. The condition can be fatal. Headache is the most common symptom of cerebral venous thrombosis, occurring in over 90% of cases, and is often the initial complaint.[37] In 90% of cases additional neurological symptoms (such as seizures, encephalopathy, papilledema, or focal deficit) develop.[3] Cerebral venous thrombosis is more likely to affect young adults and children. In adults, 75% of cases are women, and are exacerbated by use of hormonal contraception, head trauma, or ear and sinus infections.[37] Treatment usually involves anticoagulation with heparin in the hospital and oral anticoagulation for an extended period as an outpatient.

Pheochromocytoma

Fifty percent to 80% of those with pheochromocytomas have paroxysmal headache with or without elevated blood pressure.[3] The headache from pheochromocytoma can be frontal or occipital and may be constant or pulsating. The headache is associated with other symptoms of increased catecholamines: sweating, flushing, anxiety, paresthesias, and chest or abdominal pain. The episodes last less than 15 minutes in half of patients and last less than an hour in 70%.[3] The diagnosis is made with a 24-hour urine collection that measures the catecholamine breakdown product metanephrine. Treatment is usually surgical removal of the adrenal tumor. Alpha- and beta-blockers are used pre-operatively to control symptoms.

Acute and Chronic Meningitis

Acute meningitis manifests as a severe, rapid-onset headache associated with fever, neck stiffness, photophobia, and malaise. This condition often occurs as an epidemic in young adults in areas of relative confinement (such as military barracks or college dormitories). Acute meningitis is usually caused by meningococcus or pneumococcus.[19]

Chronic meningitis causes a continuous dull headache, accompanied by signs of systemic illness, typically with cognitive decline. Chronic meningitis can cause irritation and compromise cranial nerve (CN) function (creating, for example, blurred or double vision [CN III, CN IV, and CN VI], facial palsy [CN VII], or hearing impairment [CN VIII]).[19] An LP shows elevated white blood cells (WBCs), low glucose, and elevated levels of protein. Chronic meningitis is caused most often by *Cryptococcus*, but Lyme disease and fungal infections are also potential culprits. Having a compromised immune system (e.g., having AIDS, being elderly, receiving treatment with steroids) is a risk factor for the development of chronic meningitis.

Treatment of meningitis involves administration of the appropriate antibiotic and supportive care (including intravenous fluids, antipyretics, anticonvulsants, and bed rest) as needed.

Encephalitis

CNS infection causes headache through release of toxins by the infective agent, swelling of the brain, and meningeal irritation. Sporadic encephalitis is most often caused by herpes simplex virus (HSV), which has a predilection for the inferior surfaces of the frontal and temporal lobes.[38] Herpes encephalitis commonly causes fever, confusion, somnolence, and, because of its localization to the temporal lobes, partial complex seizures and amnesia.[19] An LP reveals elevated WBCs. HSV polymerase chain reaction (PCR) of CSF makes the diagnosis in 95% of cases.[3] An MRI may reveal inflammation of the inferior surfaces of the temporal and frontal lobes. Treatment is with acyclovir or valacyclovir.

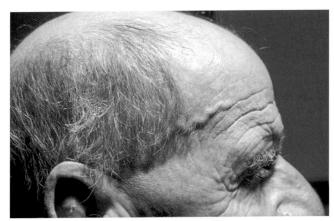

Figure 78-7. Prominent and tender temporal artery. *(From Lance JW, Goadsby PJ.* Mechanism and management of headache, *ed 7, Philadelphia, 2005, Butterworth-Heinemann, Fig 15.4, p. 296.)*

Temporal Arteritis

Temporal arteritis is seen almost exclusively in patients over age 55 years with a constant, but dull, headache over one or both temples. Jaw claudication (increasing jaw pain on chewing) is rare, but it was once considered pathognomic for the condition.[19] In advanced cases, the temporal arteries can be red and tender (Figure 78-7).[9] Often there are systemic signs (such as low-grade fever, malaise, and weight loss) and there may be joint pain or other signs of rheumatoid disease, and visual loss, including amaurosis fugax. Blindness as a result of ophthalmic artery occlusion and ischemia from cerebral artery occlusion can lead to serious and permanent complications. An ESR above 40 is present in over 90% of cases.[19] An elevation of both ESR and C-reactive protein (CRP) has a specificity of 97%.[39] A biopsy of the temporal artery that shows a focal granulomatous arteritis with giant cells is the definitive test, but is often unnecessary. Risk factors for temporal arteritis include age over 55 years and a history of polymyalgia rheumatica. Although the cause is unknown, the condition is associated with inflammation of the temporal and other medium to large cerebral and extracerebral arteries. Histologically, a focal granulatomatous arteritis with giant cells is seen. Temporal cell arteritis is treated with high-dose steroids to prevent blindness or other stroke syndromes. Prednisone (75 mg/day) should be initiated as soon as the clinical diagnosis is made.[9] When symptoms have resolved and the ESR has returned to normal, prednisone should be tapered to 10 mg/day. The patient's symptoms and ESR should be monitored closely for 1 to 2 years.

Trigeminal Neuralgia

Patients who suffer from trigeminal neuralgia, also known as tic douloureux, experience sharp pain along one of the three divisions of the trigeminal nerve, most commonly the V2 division.[19] Stimulation of the affected area often triggers the pain. This can be by brushing the teeth, eating, touching the affected area, or drinking cold water. The pain is often described as "shocks" of severe pain that last 20 to 30 seconds; shocks do not occur during sleep. The pain begins after age 60, usually the result of a blood vessel pressing against the trigeminal nerve root as it emerges from the brainstem. Tumors of the cerebellopontine angle can also produce tic douloureux. The elderly and those with MS are more likely to suffer from trigeminal neuralgia. Carbamazepine is the gold standard for

TABLE 78-4 Secondary Headaches due to Head and Neck Disturbance

Cause	Comments
Cervical spondylosis	Cervical spondylosis is seen in half of 50 year olds and 70% of 70 year olds, most often involving cervical vertebrae C6. Degenerative disease of the intervertebral discs and synovial joints may cause a compression of emerging spinal nerves. The pain can be referred to the occipital area, but it may also radiate to the front of the head. However, according to the International Headache Society (IHS), there is no association between cervical spondylosis and headache.[3]
Cold-induced headaches	Exposure of the head, or passage of a cold substance on the soft palate, can cause a sudden band of pain across the forehead that peaks within a minute. Transcranial Doppler ultrasonography has revealed decreased mean flow velocities in the middle cerebral artery in two patients experiencing the so-called "ice cream headache," compared to a control who did not experience a headache after eating ice cream.[42] Vasoconstriction is theorized to be important to the pathogenesis. Ice cream headaches stop within 2–5 minutes of removal of the cold substance. Similar headaches have been reported with cold exposure and cryosurgery.
Earache	Pain in the ear is most often the result of acute infection of the outer ear canal or the middle ear. Ear pain, however, can be referred to other areas of the head because small sensory branches from the mandibular, facial, vagus, and upper cervical nerves reach the outer ear. The epithelium of the inner ear is innervated by the glossopharyngeal and vagus nerves.
Lumbar puncture (LP) headache	The removal of CSF during an LP causes headache, perhaps due to the reduction in the brain's protective fluid. The pain is worse when sitting up or turning the head rapidly. There may be accompanying neck pain or nausea. The patient should lie down and the LP site should be checked for leakage.
Myofascial pain	Inflammation of the sternocleidomastoid and trapezius muscles can produce occipital pain, especially when tender nodules within the muscles are compressed.
Positional headaches	Orthostasis often causes headaches that occur on arising, and progressively worsen during the day; they are relieved by lying down. Accompanying complaints often include nausea, vomiting, dizziness, photophobia, tinnitus, anorexia, and malaise. Head-shaking and jugular compression often worsen the symptoms. Medication-induced orthostasis is the most common cause, but SDH, SAH (with vasospasm), third-ventricle colloid cysts, and sinus disease are other causes.[3] Patients who are taking medications (such as tricyclic antidepressants [TCAs], antipsychotic drugs, and antihypertensive medication) that block alpha$_1$-adrenergic receptors are at risk for orthostasis and for positional headaches.
Sinus disease	Maxillary sinusitis is a common cause of facial or head pain. Acute sinusitis manifests with cough, purulent nasal discharge, and sinus tenderness. A fever may be present. Acute sinusitis can manifest as a thunderclap headache.[43] If symptoms are prolonged, a chronic sinusitis may be diagnosed. For some chronic sinusitis infections, endoscopic surgery may be necessary to clear passages.

providing at least partial pain relief in 80%–90% of patients, but many other anticonvulsant medications (including gabapentin, lamotrigine, phenytoin, and pregabalin) have been effective treatments for trigeminal neuralgia.[19] Surgery may be necessary to remove a tumor that presses on the trigeminal nerve. Injection of an anesthetic at the root of the trigeminal nerve can also stop the pain.

Medication-overuse Headaches

Frequent and consistent use of medications used for the treatment of pain can lead to chronic daily headaches. Such a pattern of use may disrupt the normal pain pathways that exacerbate headache syndromes. Perturbations in normal vasoconstriction may also contribute. Implicated medications include barbiturates, benzodiazepines, ergots, triptans, narcotics, and, least likely, NSAIDs.[19] Evidence suggests that patients who overuse triptans experience medication overuse headaches faster and with lower doses than patients who use analgesics or ergots.[40] Patients who overuse triptans are more likely to have daily migraine-like symptoms, while those overusing analgesics or ergots typically have daily tension-type headaches.[40] Patients' headaches rarely respond to preventive or prophylactic measures if the patient is overusing abortive treatments. If the patient is overusing narcotics, avoidance of opiate withdrawal may play a role in the medication overuse. Substance-withdrawal and medication-overuse headaches often need to be treated by tapering the substance or medication (or a similar substance) as an inpatient or outpatient detoxification. A short course of steroids (such as 60 mg of prednisone for 5 days) may also help.[41] Up to 75% of patients improve when drug overuse is discontinued.[4]

Headaches due to Substances of Abuse

Substances of abuse are often cited as causes of headaches. Alcohol can trigger a migraine or cluster headache. Some individuals without primary headaches suffer a pulsating headache immediately after alcohol consumption. However, this is much less common than the delayed alcohol-induced headache ("hangover") that begins at least 3 hours after alcohol consumption. It is often pulsatile and is worsened by physical activity. Similar syndromes have been described after use of cocaine and marijuana. Many remedies have been proposed, but NSAIDs and acetaminophen are the standard treatments.

Headaches due to Withdrawal from Substances

Discontinuation of medication or substances can cause pain that mimics the symptoms of a tension-type headache. Common substances from which withdrawal headaches can occur include caffeine, alcohol, narcotics, NSAIDs, acetaminophen, and aspirin. Tapering the medication or substance can reduce headaches.

CONCLUSION

Headache is a common complaint that psychiatrists hear from their patients. Despite their high prevalence, headaches can be disabling. Treatment of headaches depends on their etiology. While the comprehensive headache work-up may be overwhelming, the patient can be best served by first ruling out the dangerous causes of headaches. Being familiar with the patterns of headaches will help the psychiatrist recognize and treat most headache syndromes (Table 78-4 and Table 78-5).[42–50]

TABLE 78-5 Secondary Headaches due to Systemic Illness

Cause	Comments
Carbon monoxide (CO) poisoning	CO, an odorless, colorless gas produced by the incomplete combustion of carbon-based fuel, contributes to approximately 5,000 to 6,000 accidental deaths per year. CO binds to hemoglobin with 200 times the affinity of oxygen, thus impairing cellular respiration. Exposure to CO causes cerebral vasodilation. Severe exposures are associated with tachycardia, dysrhythmias, seizures, myocardial infarction, and coma. During the winter, patients who live in poorly ventilated facilities develop mild symptoms of chronic low-level CO exposure (such as headache, nausea, and dizziness). The symptoms abate when the person is out of the house. Upper levels of normal for carboxyhemoglobin are 3% in non-smokers and 10% in smokers.[44]
Hemodialysis headache	Cerebral edema during dialysis may cause headaches usually described as a mild to moderate bilateral headache of a pressing/tightening quality that begins during hemodialysis. In some patients, the headache progresses to a more severe throbbing headache associated with symptoms of both migraine and tension-type headaches.[3] Restlessness accompanying the headache may represent what some authors have called the dialysis dysequilibrium syndrome.[45] Other features of the syndrome include nausea, emesis, blurring of vision, myoclonus, confusion, and seizures. Hemodialysis headache usually abates within 2–5 hours. Angiotensin-converting enzyme (ACE) inhibitors have been proposed as helpful. Caffeine-withdrawal headaches may be precipitated by dialysis as caffeine is removed.
Hypothyroidism	One-third of patients with hypothyroidism have headaches, though the mechanism of headache is unknown. Thyroid hormone replacement is the treatment.[46]
Idiopathic intracranial hypertension (IIH)	IIH, also known as pseudotumor cerebri or benign intracranial hypertension, is manifested by a headache in 75%–95% of patients. The pain is a dull, generalized headache that worsens with coughing or straining. Women of childbearing age are at risk for IIH; it has an annual incidence of 21 in 100,000. Irregular menses are often reported. Papilledema is out of proportion to symptoms. Typically there are no mental status or personality changes, though visual deficits and sixth nerve palsy may be seen. Persistent papilledema can lead to blindness. An LP may show elevated opening pressure. An MRI must be done to rule out other causes of increased ICP, such as a mass or SVT. Cerebral edema and decreased absorption of CHF are hypothesized to contribute to the cause of IIH. The headache of IIH responds to serial LPs. Weight reduction can also lower ICP. Medications (such as diuretics or the carbonic anhydrase inhibitor acetazolamide [starting at 200 mg bid and increasing to 1,000–1,250 mg/day]) can reduce ICP as well. Topiramate, an anticonvulsant that inhibits carbonic anhydrase, has been associated with weight loss and may be beneficial. A short course (2–6 weeks) of steroids (up to 1 mg/kg) may be necessary in severe cases. Shunt placement is reserved for refractory cases.[47]
Medication-induced headaches	Various medications may cause or exacerbate headache syndromes. Nitric oxide (NO) donors (the so-called "hot dog headache") such as isosorbide dinitrate, nitroprusside, and nitroglycerine, likely because of their vasodilating properties, can cause headaches.[3] Cytokines such as IL-2, used in the treatment of immune dysfunction and cancers, commonly cause headaches associated with other symptoms of systemic illness (e.g., malaise, irritability, and muscle aches).[48] Commonly prescribed psychiatric medications that are most often associated with headaches are atropine, buspirone, cyclosporine, disulfiram, gabapentin, lithium, naltrexone, nicotine, stimulants, selective serotonin reuptake inhibitors (SSRIs), and serotonin norepinephrine reuptake inhibitors (SNRIs).[49] Monoamine oxidase inhibitors (MAOIs) in combination with certain foods or medications can cause headaches that indicate a dangerous hypertensive crisis or cerebral hemorrhage.
Posterior reversible encephalopathy syndrome (PRES)	The most common symptoms are seizures, confusion and vision changes. Over half present with headache. MRI scans show evidence of bilateral posterior cerebral edema. PRES is associated with medical illness, including hypertensive encephalopathy, eclampsia, systemic lupus erythematosus (SLE), and treatment with immunosuppressive agents.[50]
Systemic infection	Headache is often a symptom of systemic illness, such as influenza or sepsis. There are usually other signs and symptoms of the sickness syndrome, including fatigue, fever, nausea, and cough. The headache improves as the underlying illness resolves.

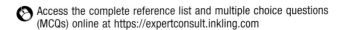 Access the complete reference list and multiple choice questions (MCQs) online at https://expertconsult.inkling.com

KEY REFERENCES

1. Dodick DW. Diagnosing headache: clinical clues and clinical rules. *Adv Stud Med* 3:S550–S555, 2003.
3. International Headache Society. The international classification of headache disorders. ed 2. *Cephalalgia* 24(Suppl. 1):1–150, 2004.
4. Welch KMA. A 47-year-old woman with tension-type headaches. *JAMA* 286(8):960–966, 2001.
7. Wiendels NJ, Knuistingh Neven A, Rosendaal FR, et al. Chronic frequent headache in the general population: prevalence and associated factors. *Cephalgia* 26:1434–1442, 2006.
8. Wiendels NJ, van Haestregt A, Knuistingh Neven A, et al. Chronic frequent headache in the general population: comorbidity and quality of life. *Cephalgia* 26:1443–1450, 2006.
9. Lance JW, Goadsby PJ. *Mechanism and management of headache*, ed 7, Philadelphia, 2005, Elsevier.
10. Low N, Singleton A. Establishing the genetic heterogeneity of familial hemiplegic migraine. *Brain* 130(2):312–313, 2007.
11. Antilla V, Stefansson H, Kella M, et al. Genome-wide association study of migraine implicates a common susceptibility variant on 8q22.1. *Nat Genet* 42:869–873, 2010.
12. Lafreniere RG, Cader MZ, Poulin JF, et al. A dominant-negative mutation in the TRESK potassium channel is linked to familial migraine with aura. *Nat Med* 16:1157–1160, 2010.
17. Friedman DI. Headache. In Schapira AHV, Byrne E, editors: *Neurology and clinical neuroscience*, Philadelphia, 2007, Mosby.
18. Saper JR, Lake AE III, Hamel RL, et al. Daily scheduled opioids for intractable head pain: long-term observations of a treatment program. *Neurology* 62:1687–1694, 2004.
19. Kaufman DM, Milstein MJ. *Clinical neurology for psychiatrists*, ed 7, Philadelphia, 2013, WB Saunders.
21. Nestoriuc Y, Martin A, Rief W, et al. Biofeedback treatment for headache disorders: a comprehensive efficacy review. *Appl Psychophysiol Biofeedback* 33:125–140, 2008.
22. Mathew NT. The prophylactic treatment of chronic daily headache. *Headache* 46(10):1552–1564, 2006.
23. Bendtsen L, Jensen R. Mirtazapine is effective in the prophylactic treatment of chronic tension-type headache. *Neurology* 62:1706–1711, 2004.
25. Palm-Meinders IH, Koppen H, Terwindt GM, et al. Structural brain changes in migraine. *JAMA* 308:1889–1897, 2012.
26. Evans RW, Tepper SJ, Shapiro RE, et al. The FDA alert on serotonin syndrome with use of triptans combined with selective serotonin reuptake inhibitors or selective serotonin-norepinephrine reuptake inhibitors: American Headache Society position paper. *Headache* 50(6):1089–1099, 2010.

27. Campbell JK, Penzien DB, Wall EM, et al. Evidence-based guidelines for migraine headache: behavioral and physical treatments. *US Headache Consortium*. Available at: <http://www.aan.com/professionals/practice/pdfs/gl0089.pdf>; 2000 [Accessed June 29, 2013].

28. Ashina S, Serrano D, Lipton RB, et al. Depression and risk of transformation of episodic to chronic migraine. *J Headache Pain* 13(8):615–624, 2012.

29. Naomi B, Schultz L. Migraine headaches and suicide attempt. *Headache* 52(5):723–731, 2012.

30. Grazzi L, Andrasik F, D'Amico D, et al. Behavioral and pharmacologic treatment of transformed migraine with analgesic overuse: outcome at three years. *Headache* 42:483–490, 2002.

31. Markley HG, Buse DC. Cluster headache: myths and the evidence. *Curr Pain Headache Rep* 10(2):137–141, 2006.

37. Stam J. Thrombosis of the cerebral veins and sinuses. *N Engl J Med* 352(17):1791–1798, 2005.

38. Aldea S, Joly LM, Roujeau T, et al. Postoperative herpes simplex virus encephalitis after neurosurgery: case report and review of the literature. *Clin Infect Dis* 36(7):96–99, 2003.

39. Eberhardt RT, Dhadly M. Giant cell arteritis: diagnosis, management, and cardiovascular implications. *Cardiol Rev* 15(2):55–61, 2007.

40. Limmroth V, Katsarava Z, Fritsche G, et al. Features of medication overuse headache following different acute headache drugs. *Neurology* 59:1011–1014, 2002.

41. Evers S, Jensen R. Treatment of medication overuse headache—guideline of the EFNS headache panel. *Eur J Neurol* 18:1115–1121, 2011.

46. Tepper DE, Tepper SJ, Sheftell FD, et al. Headache attributed to hypothyroidism. *Curr Pain Headache Rep* 11(4):304–309, 2007.

47. Skau M, Brennum J, Gjerris F, et al. What is new about idiopathic intracranial hypertension? *Cephalalgia* 26:384–399, 2005.

50. Schusse CM, Peterson AL, Caplan JP. Posterior reversible encephalopathy syndrome. *Psychosomatics* 54:205–211, 2013.

51. Vos T, Flaxman AD, Naghavi M, et al. Years lived with disability (YLDs) for 1160 sequelae of 289 diseases and injuries 1990–2010: a systematic analysis for the Global Burden of Disease Study 2010. *Lancet* 380(9859):2163–2196, 2013.

79 Pathophysiology, Psychiatric Co-morbidity, and Treatment of Pain

Ajay D. Wasan, MD, MSc, Menekse Alpay, MD, and Shamim H. Nejad, MD

KEY POINTS

- There is a high rate of psychiatric co-morbidity in patients with pain syndromes.
- Specific terminology is used to characterize pain and pain syndromes.
- Pain is transmitted in pathways involving the peripheral and central nervous systems.
- Psychiatric treatment can be effective for pain and the psychiatric co-morbidities of pain.
- Multimodal and multidisciplinary treatment facilitates provision of the highest-quality care for chronic pain.

OVERVIEW

Pain, as determined by the International Association for the Study of Pain (IASP), is "an unpleasant sensory and emotional experience associated with actual or potential tissue damage or described in terms of such damage."[1] This chapter will describe the physiological aspects of pain transmission, pain terminology, and pain assessment; discuss the major classes of medications used to relieve pain; and outline the diagnosis and treatment of psychiatric conditions that often affect patients with chronic pain.

EPIDEMIOLOGY

Psychiatric co-morbidity (e.g., anxiety, depression, personality disorders, and substance use disorders [SUDs]) afflicts those with both non-cancer-related and cancer-related pain. Epidemiological studies indicate that roughly 30% of those in the general population with chronic musculoskeletal pain also have depression or an anxiety disorder.[2] Similar rates exist in those with cancer pain.[3] In clinic populations, 50%–80% of pain patients have co-morbid psychopathology, including problematic personality traits. The personality (i.e., the characterological or temperamental) component of negative affect has been termed *neuroticism*, which may be best described as "a general personality maladjustment in which patients experience anger, disgust, sadness, anxiety, and a variety of other negative emotions."[4] Frequently, in pain clinics, maladaptive expressions of depression, anxiety, and anger are grouped together as disorders of negative affect, which have an adverse impact on the response to pain.[5]

Rates of substance dependence in chronic pain patients are also elevated relative to the general population, and several studies have found that 15%–26% of chronic pain patients have an SUD, including illicit drugs or prescription medications.[6] Prescription opiate addiction is a growing problem that affects approximately 5% of those who have been prescribed opiates for chronic pain, although good epidemiology studies are lacking. Other chapters in this textbook focus more specifically on SUDs. This chapter will concentrate on those with

affective disorders and somatoform disorders in the setting of chronic pain.

While many chronic pain patients experience somatization and have difficulty adapting to pain, a *Diagnostic and Statistical Manual of Mental Disorders*, ed 4, Text Revision (DSM-IV-TR) diagnosis of somatization disorder, *per se*, is less frequently encountered by those who treat patients with chronic pain. The DSM-IV-TR accounts for this distinction by classifying the somatoform component of a pain disorder into several categories (such as pain disorder associated with psychological factors, pain disorder associated with psychological factors and a general medical condition, and somatization disorder). With some degree of controversy, in DSM-5, some individuals with chronic pain would be diagnosed as having somatic symptom disorder, with predominant pain. For others, psychological factors affecting other medical conditions or an adjustment disorder would be more appropriate.

PATHOPHYSIOLOGY OF PAIN TRANSMISSION

Detection of noxious stimuli (i.e., nociception) starts with the activation of peripheral nociceptors (resulting in somatic pain) or with the activation of nociceptors in bodily organs (leading to visceral pain).

Tissue injury stimulates the nociceptors by the liberation of adenosine triphosphate (ATP), protons, kinins, and arachidonic acid from the injured cells; histamine, serotonin, prostaglandins, and bradykinin from the mast cells; and cytokines and nerve growth factor from the macrophages. These substances and decreased pH cause a decrease in the threshold for activation of the nociceptors, a process called *peripheral sensitization*. Subsequently, axons transmit the pain signal to the spinal cord, and to cell bodies in the dorsal root ganglia (Figure 79-1). Three different types of axons are involved in the transmission of pain from the skin to the dorsal horn. A-β fibers are the largest and most heavily myelinated fibers that transmit awareness of light touch. A-Δ fibers and C fibers are the primary nociceptive afferents. A-Δ fibers are 2 to 5 μcm in diameter and are thinly myelinated. They conduct "first pain," which is immediate, rapid, and sharp, with a velocity of 20 m/sec. C fibers are 0.2 to 1.5 μcm in diameter and are unmyelinated. They conduct "second pain," which is prolonged, burning, and unpleasant, at a speed of 0.5 m/sec.

A-Δ and C fibers enter the dorsal root and ascend or descend one to three segments before synapsing with neurons in the lateral spinothalamic tract (in the substantia gelatinosa in the gray matter) (see Figure 79-1). Second pain transmitted with C fibers is integrally related to chronic pain states. Repetitive C-fiber stimulation can result in a progressive increase of electrical discharges from second-order neurons in the spinal cord. NMDA receptors play a role when prolonged activation occurs. This pain amplification is related to a temporal summation of second pain or "wind-up." This hyperexcitability of neurons in the dorsal horn contributes to central sensitization, which can occur as an immediate or as a delayed phenomenon. In addition to wind-up, central sensitization involves several factors: activation of A-β fibers and lowered firing thresholds for spinal cord cells that modulate pain (i.e., they trigger pain

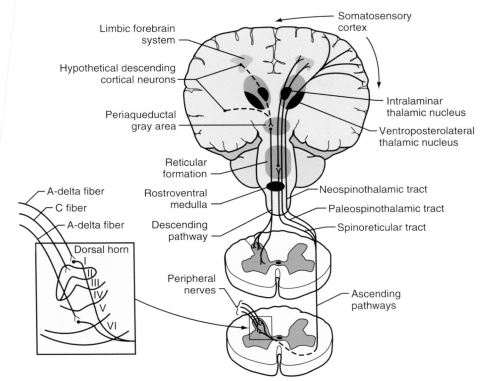

Figure 79-1. Schematic diagram of neurological pathways for pain perception. *(From Hyman SH, Cassem NH. Pain. In Rubenstein E, Fedeman DD, editors:* Scientific American medicine: current topics in medicine, *subsection II, New York, 1989, Scientific American. Originally from Stern TA, Herman JB, editors.* Psychiatry update and board preparation, *New York, 2004, McGraw-Hill.)*

more easily); neuroplasticity (a result of functional changes, including recruitment of a wide range of cells in the spinal cord so that touch or movement causes pain); convergence of cutaneous, vascular, muscle, and joint inputs (where one tissue refers pain to another); or aberrant connections (electrical short-circuits between the sympathetic and sensory nerves that produce causalgia). Inhibition of nociception in the dorsal horn is functionally quite important. Stimulation of the A-Δ fibers not only excites some neurons but also inhibits others. This inhibition of nociception through A-Δ fiber stimulation may explain the effects of acupuncture and transcutaneous electrical nerve stimulation (TENS).

The lateral spinothalamic tract crosses the midline and ascends toward the thalamus. At the level of the brainstem, more than half of this tract synapses in the reticular activating system (in an area called the spinoreticular tract), in the limbic system, and in other brainstem regions (including centers of the autonomic nervous system). Another site of projections at this level is the periaqueductal gray (PAG) (Figure 79-2), which plays an important role in the brain's system of endogenous analgesia. After synapsing in the thalamic nuclei, pain fibers project to the somatosensory cortex, located posterior to the Sylvian fissure in the parietal lobe, in Brodmann's areas 1, 2, and 3. Endogenous analgesic systems involve endogenous peptides with opioid-like activity in the central nervous system (CNS) (e.g., endorphins, enkephalins, and dynorphins). Different opioid receptors (mu, kappa, and delta receptors) are involved in different effects of opiates. The centers involved in endogenous analgesia include the PAG, the anterior cingulate cortex (ACC), the amygdala, the parabrachial plexus (in the pons), and the rostral ventromedial medulla.

The descending analgesic pain pathway starts in the PAG (which is rich in endogenous opiates), projects to the rostral

ventral medulla, and from there descends through the dorsolateral funiculus of the spinal cord to the dorsal horn. The neurons in the rostral ventral medulla use serotonin to activate endogenous analgesics (enkephalins) in the dorsal horn. This effect inhibits nociception at the level of the dorsal horn since neurons that contain enkephalins synapse with spinothalamic neurons. Additionally, there are noradrenergic neurons that project from the locus coeruleus (the main noradrenergic center in the CNS) to the dorsal horn and inhibit the response of dorsal horn neurons to nociceptive stimuli. The analgesic effect of tricyclic antidepressants (TCAs) and the serotonin-norepinephrine reuptake inhibitors (SNRIs) is thought to be related to an increase in serotonin and norepinephrine (noradrenaline) that inhibits nociception at the level of the dorsal horn, through their effects on enhancing descending pain inhibition from above.

CORTICAL SUBSTRATES FOR PAIN AND AFFECT

Advances in neuroimaging have linked the function of multiple areas in the brain with pain and affect. These areas (e.g., the ACC, the insula, and the dorsolateral prefrontal cortex [DLPFC]) form functional units through which psychiatric co-morbidity may amplify pain and disability (see Figure 79-2). These areas are part of the spinolimbic (also known as the medial) pain pathway,[7] which runs parallel to the spinothalamic tract and receives direct input from the dorsal horn of the spinal cord. The interactions among the function of these areas, pain perception, and psychiatric illness are still being investigated. The spinolimbic pathway is involved in descending pain inhibition (which includes cortical and subcortical structures), whose function may be negatively affected by the presence of psychopathology. This, in turn, could lead to heightened pain perception. Coghill and colleagues[8] have shown that differences in

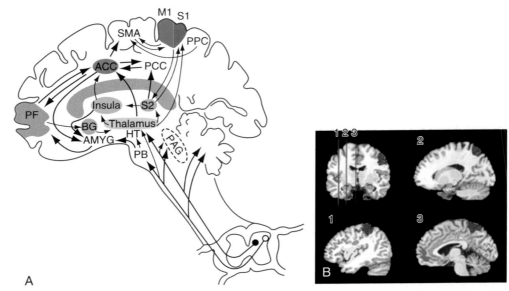

Figure 79-2. Pain processing in the brain. Locations of brain regions involved in pain perception are color-coded in a schematic A and in an example magnetic resonance imaging (MRI) scan B. (A) Schematic shows the regions, their inter-connectivity, and afferent pathways. (B) The areas corresponding to those in part A are shown in an anatomical MRI, on a coronal slice, and on three sagittal slices as indicated on the coronal slice. The six areas used in meta-analysis are primary and secondary somatosensory cortices (S1 and S2, red and orange), anterior cingulated (ACC, green), insula (blue), thalamus (yellow), and prefrontal cortex (PF, purple) Other regions indicated include primary and supplementary motor cortices (M1 and SMA), posterior parietal cortex (PPC), posterior cingulated (PCC), basal ganglia (BG, pink), hypothalamic (HT), amygdala (AMYG), parabrachial nuclei (PB), and periaqueductal gray (PAG). *(Redrawn from Apkarian AV, Bushnell MC, Treede RD, Zubieta JK. Human brain mechanisms of pain perception and regulation in health and disease, Eur J Pain 9:463–484, 2005.)*

pain sensitivity between patients can be correlated with differences in activation patterns in the ACC, the insula, and the DLPFC. The anticipation of pain is also modulated by these areas, suggesting a mechanism by which anxiety about pain can amplify pain perception. The disruption or alteration of descending pain inhibition is a mechanism of neuropathic pain, which can be described as *central sensitization* that occurs at the level of the brain, a concept supported by recent neuroimaging studies of pain processing in the brains of patients with fibromyalgia.[9] The ACC, the insula, and the DLPFC are also laden with opioid receptors, which are less responsive to endogenous opioids in pain-free subjects with high negative affect.[10] Thus, negative affect may diminish the effectiveness of endogenous and exogenous opioids through direct effects on supraspinal opioid binding.

INTERACTIONS BETWEEN PAIN AND PSYCHOPATHOLOGY

The majority of patients with chronic pain and a psychiatric condition have an organic or physical basis for their pain. However, the perception of pain is amplified by co-morbid psychiatric disorders, which predispose patients to develop a chronic pain syndrome. This is commonly referred to as the *diathesis-stress model*, in which the combination of physical, social, and psychological stresses associated with a pain syndrome induces significant psychiatric co-morbidity.[5] This can occur in patients with or without a pre-existing vulnerability to psychiatric illness (e.g., a genetic or temperamental risk factor). Regardless of the order of onset of psychopathology, patients with chronic pain and psychopathology report greater pain intensity, more pain-related disability, and a larger affective component to their pain than those without psychopathology. As a whole, studies indicate that it is not the specific qualities or symptomatology of depression, anxiety, or neuroticism, but the overall levels of psychiatric symptoms that are predictive of

poor outcome.[11] Depression, anxiety, and neuroticism are the psychiatric conditions that most often co-occur in patients with chronic pain, and those with a combination of pathologies are predisposed to the worst outcomes.

PAIN TERMINOLOGY

Acute pain is usually related to an identifiable injury or to a disease; it is self-limited, and resolves over hours to days or in a time frame that is associated with injury and healing. Acute pain is usually associated with objective autonomic features (e.g., tachycardia, hypertension, diaphoresis, mydriasis, or pallor).

Chronic pain (i.e., pain that persists beyond the normal time of healing or lasts longer than 6 months) involves different mechanisms in local, spinal, and supraspinal levels. Characteristic features include vague descriptions of pain and an inability to describe the pain's timing and localization. It is usually helpful to determine the presence of a dermatomal pattern (Figure 79-3), to determine the presence of neuropathic pain, and to assess pain behavior.

Neuropathic pain is a disorder of neuromodulation. It is caused by an injured or dysfunctional central or peripheral nervous system; it is manifest by spontaneous, sharp, shooting, or burning pain, which may be distributed along dermatomes. Deafferentation pain, phantom limb pain, complex regional pain syndrome, diabetic neuropathy, central pain syndrome, trigeminal neuralgia, and postherpetic neuralgia are examples of neuropathic pain. Qualities of neuropathic pain include hyperalgesia (an increased response to stimuli that are normally painful); hyperesthesia (an exaggerated pain response to noxious stimuli [e.g., pressure or heat]); allodynia (pain with a stimulus not normally painful [e.g., light touch or cool air]); and hyperpathia (pain from a painful stimulus with a delay and a persistence that is distributed beyond the area of stimulation). Both acute and chronic pain conditions

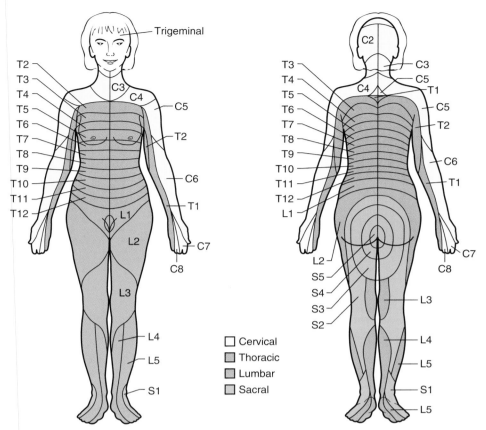

Figure 79-3. Schematic diagram of segmental neuronal innervation by dermatomes. *(From Hyman SH, Cassem NH. Pain. In Rubenstein E, Fedeman DD, editors:* Scientific American medicine: current topics in medicine, *subsection II, New York, 1989, Scientific American. Originally from Stern TA, Herman JB, editors.* Psychiatry update and board preparation, *New York, 2004, McGraw-Hill.)*

can involve neuropathic processes in addition to nociceptive causes of pain.

Idiopathic pain, previously referred to as *psychogenic pain,* is poorly understood. The presence of pain does not imply or exclude a psychological component. Typically, there is no evidence of an associated organic etiology or an anatomical pattern consistent with symptoms. Symptoms are often grossly out of proportion to an identifiable organic pathology.

Myofascial pain can arise from one or several of the following problems: hypertonic muscles, myofascial trigger points, arthralgias, and fatigue with muscle weakness. Myofascial pain is generally used to describe pain from muscles and connective tissue. Myofascial pain results from a primary diagnosis (e.g., fibromyalgia) or, as more often is the case, a co-morbid diagnosis (e.g., with vascular headache or with a psychiatric diagnosis).

ASSESSMENT OF PAIN

The evaluation of pain focuses first on five questions: (1) Is the pain intractable because of nociceptive stimuli (e.g., from the skin, bones, muscles, or blood vessels)? (2) Is the pain maintained by non-nociceptive mechanisms (i.e., have the spinal cord, brainstem, limbic system, and cortex been recruited as reverberating pain circuits)? (3) Is the complaint of pain primary (as occurs in disorders such as major depression or delusional disorder)? (4) Is there a more efficacious pharmacological treatment? (5) Have pain behavior and disability become more important than the pain itself? Answering these questions allows the mechanism(s) of the pain and suffering to be pursued. A psychiatrist's physical examination

of the pain patient typically includes examination of the painful area, muscles, and response to pinprick and light touch (Table 79-1).

The experience of pain is always subjective. However, several sensitive and reliable clinical instruments for the measurement of pain are available. These include the following:

1. The *pain drawing* involves having the patient draw the anatomical distribution of the pain as it is felt in his or her body.
2. The *Visual Analog Scale* and *Numerical Rating Scales* employ a visual analog scale from "no pain" to "pain as bad as it could possibly be" on a 10 cm baseline, or a 0 to 10 scale where the patient can rate pain on a scale of 1 to 10. It is also exquisitely sensitive to change; consequently, the patient can mark this scale once a day or even hourly during treatment trials, if desired.
3. The *Pain Intensity Scale* is a categorical rating scale that consists of three to six categories for the ranking of pain severity (e.g., no pain, mild pain, moderate pain, severe pain, very severe pain, worst pain possible).

CORE PSYCHOPATHOLOGY AND PAIN-RELATED PSYCHOLOGICAL SYMPTOMS

In patients with chronic pain, heightened emotional distress, negative affect, and elevated pain-related psychological symptoms (i.e., those that are a direct result of chronic pain, and when the pain is eliminated, the symptoms disappear) can all be considered as forms of psychopathology and psychiatric co-morbidity, since they represent impairments in mental

TABLE 79-1 General Physical Examination of Pain by the Psychiatrist

Physical Finding	Purpose of Examination
Motor deficits	Does the patient give-way when checking strength? Does the person try? Is there a pseudoparesis, astasia-abasia, or involuntary movement that suggests a somatoform disorder?
Trigger points in head, neck, shoulder, and back muscles	Are common myofascial trigger points present that suggest myofascial pain? Is there evoked pain (such as allodynia, hyperpathia, or anesthesia) that suggests neuropathic pain?
Evanescent, changeable pain, weakness, and numbness	Does the psychological complaint pre-empt the physical?
Abnormal sensory findings	Does lateral anesthesia to pinprick end sharply at the midline? Is there topographical confusion? Is there a non-dermatomal distribution of pain and sensation that suggests either a somatoform or CNS pain disorder? Is there an abnormal sensation that suggests neuropathy or CNS pain?
Sympathetic or vascular dysfunction	Is there swelling, skin discoloration, or changes in sweating or temperature that suggests a vascular or sympathetic element to the pain?
Uncooperativeness, erratic responses to the physical examination	Is there an interpersonal aspect to the pain, causing abnormal pain behavior, as in somatoform disease?

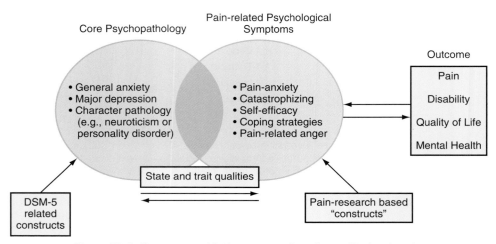

Figure 79-4. Common psychiatric symptoms in patients with chronic pain.

health and involve maladaptive psychological responses to medical illness (Figure 79-4). This approach combines methods of classification from psychiatry and behavioral medicine to describe the scope of psychiatric disturbances in patients with chronic pain. In pain patients the most common manifestations of psychiatric co-morbidity involve one or more core psychopathologies in combination with pain-related psychological symptoms. Unfortunately, not all patients and their symptoms fit precisely into DSM categories of illness.

Pain-related anxiety which includes state and trait anxiety related to pain is the form of anxiety most germane to pain.[12] Elevated levels of pain-related anxiety, such as fear of pain, also meet DSM-5 criteria for an anxiety disorder due to a general medical condition. Since anxiety is present in both domains of core psychopathology and pain-related psychological symptoms, the assessment of anxiety in a patient with chronic pain (as detailed below) must include a review of manifestations of generalized anxiety as well as pain-specific anxiety symptoms (e.g., physiological changes associated with the anticipation of pain).

Limited coping skills are often linked with pain-related psychological symptoms and behaviors including passive responses to chronic pain (e.g., remaining bed-bound), catastrophization (including cognitive distortions centered around pain and mistakenly assuming chronic pain is indicative of

ongoing tissue damage), and low self-efficacy (i.e., with a low estimate by the patient of what he or she is capable of doing).[13] Patients with decreased coping mechanisms employ few self-management strategies (such as using ice, heat, or relaxation strategies). A tendency to catastrophize often predicts poor outcome and disability, independent of other psychopathology, such as major depression. The duration of chronic pain and psychiatric co-morbidity are each an independent predictor of pain intensity and disability. High levels of anger, which tend to occur more often in men, can also explain a significant variance in pain severity.[14]

PAIN AND CO-MORBID PSYCHIATRIC CONDITIONS

Virtually all psychiatric conditions are treatable in patients with chronic pain, and the majority of patients who are provided with appropriate treatment improve significantly. Many physicians who treat pain patients often do not realize that this is the case. Of the disorders that most frequently afflict patients with chronic pain, major depression and anxiety disorders are the most common; moreover, they have the best response to medications. Whenever possible, medications that are effective for psychiatric illness and that have independent analgesic properties should be used. *Independent analgesia*

TABLE 79-3 Opioid Potencies and Special Features

Drug	Parenteral (mg equivalent)	Oral (mg)	Duration (h)	Special Features
Morphine	10	30	4	Morphine sulfate controlled release has 12-h duration
Codeine	120	200	4	Ceiling effect as dose increases, low lipophilic
Oxycodone	4.5	30	4	Every 12 h oxycontin (10, 20, 40 slow release mg)
Hydromorphone	2	8	5	Suppository 6 mg = 10 mg parenteral morphine
Levorphanol	2	4	4	Low nausea and vomiting, low lipophilic
Methadone	5	10	2–12	Cumulative effect; day 3–5 decrease respiration; equianalgesic ratio varies considerably
Meperidine	100	300	3	κ, proconvulsant metabolite, peristaltic slowing and sphincter of Oddi decrease
Fentanyl	0.1	25 μg SL	1 (patch 72 h)	50-μg patch = 30 mg/day morphine IM/IV
Sufentanil	Not recommended	15 μg SL	1	High potency with low volume of fluid
Propoxyphene	Not available	325	4	High dose leads to psychosis
Pentazocine	60	150	3	κ, σ agonist-antagonist, nasal 1 mg q1-2h
Butorphanol	2	Not available 3 (IM), 2 (NS)	μ, κ, σ, agonist-antagonist, nasal 1 mg q1-2h	
Buprenorphine	0.3	4	4–6	Partial agonist
Tramadol	Not available	150	4	μ agonist, decreased reuptake 5-HT and NE, P450 metabolism
Nalbuphine	10	Not available	3	Agonist-antagonist

5-HT, 5-hydroxytryptamine; IM, intramuscular; IV, intravenous; NE, norepinephrine; NS, nasal; SL, sublingual.

BOX 79-1 Guidelines for Opioid Maintenance

- Maintenance opioids should be considered only after other methods of pain control have been proven unsuccessful. Alternative methods (which typically include use of NSAIDs, anticonvulsants, membrane-stabilizing drugs, monoaminergic agents, local nerve blocks, and physical therapy) vary from case to case.
- Opioids should be avoided for patients with addiction disorders unless there is a new major medical illness (e.g., cancer or trauma) accompanied by severe pain. In such cases, a second opinion from another physician (a pain medicine or addiction specialist) is suggested.
- If opioids are prescribed for longer than 3 months, the patient should have a second opinion, plus a follow-up consultation at least once per year. Monitoring with a urine toxicology screen, at least yearly, is also recommended.

- One pharmacy and one prescriber should be designated as exclusive agents.
- Dosages of opioids should be defined, as should expectations of what will happen if there are deviations from it. For example, abuse will lead to rapid tapering of the drug and entry into a detoxification program. There should be no doubt that the physician will stop prescribing the drug.
- Informed consent as to the rationale, risks, benefits, and alternatives should be documented.
- The course of treatment (in particular, the ongoing indications, changes in the disease process, efficacy, and the presence of abuse, tolerance, or addictive behavior) should be documented.

---

been initiated and titrated to a satisfactory level, the analgesic effect needs to be sustained by minimizing fluctuations in blood levels and the variable effects of dosing schedules. Long-acting or controlled-release formulations are ideal for this homeostasis, because they are released more slowly than are short-acting opioids.

For the treatment of chronic pain, dosing with short-acting medications only on an as-needed basis should be avoided when possible since this makes steady relief impossible. It also predisposes the patient to drug-respondent conditioning and to subsequent behavior problems. Typically, long-acting formulations are combined with short-acting agents for breakthrough pain. In those at risk for opioid misuse or with demonstrated aberrant drug behavior, longer-acting agents

(i.e., methadone, fentanyl patch) are preferred to avoid inappropriate self-medication. Other chapters in this text discuss strategies for the prescription of opiates to those with addiction disorders. The most frequently reported side effects of opioid therapy are constipation, dry mouth, and sedation.

Treatment of Neuropathic Pain

Neuropathic pain is responsive to multiple medication classes, including TCAs, AEDs, and opioids, when used at higher doses than what is typically prescribed for chronic musculoskeletal pain. Multiple medications are often combined with physical therapy and with coping skills training for complete interdisciplinary care.

Sympathetically-Maintained Pain

Sympathetically-maintained pain is a type of neuropathic pain. Regardless of etiology (e.g., complex regional pain syndrome, inflammation, post-herpetic neuralgia, trauma, or facial pain) sympathetically-maintained or mediated pain can respond to sympathetic blockade. Medications often used in the sympathetic blockade are alpha-blocking drugs such as phentolamine, alpha-blocking antidepressants, and clonidine. Intrathecal, epidural, and systemic administration of a local anesthetic or clonidine also produces analgesia and may be useful in some types of vascular or neuropathic pain with a sympathetic component. β-Blockers are not efficacious in the treatment of sympathetically-maintained pain except in their use in the alleviation of migraine headaches. Guanethidine, bretylium, reserpine, and phentolamine have also been used to produce a chemical sympathectomy.

TREATMENT OF PAIN BEHAVIOR AND THE USE OF MULTIDISCIPLINARY PAIN CLINICS

Medicare guidelines offer a broad set of criteria to qualify for structured multidisciplinary pain management. The pain must last at least 6 months (and result in significant life disturbance and limited function), it must be attributable to a physical cause, and it must be unresponsive to the usual methods of treatment. Quality control guidelines developed by the Commission on Accreditation of Rehabilitation Facilities (CARF) have led to the certification of more than 100 multidisciplinary chronic pain management programs nationwide. Behavioral treatments are a key component of these programs and can be effective for the relief of pain and can help extinguish the behaviors associated with pain.

Inpatient or outpatient multidisciplinary pain treatment should be considered early in the course of chronic pain. This is particularly important when intensive observation is necessary (e.g., to rule out malingering); no single modality of outpatient treatment is likely to work; the patient has already obtained maximum benefit from outpatient treatments (such as NSAIDs, nerve blocks, antidepressants, and simple physical and behavioral rehabilitation); intensive daily interventions are required, usually with multiple concurrent types of therapy (such as nerve blocks, physical therapy, and behavior modification); and the patient exhibits abnormal pain behavior and agrees to the goals of improved coping, work rehabilitation, and psychiatric assessment.

REHABILITATION

Successful rehabilitation of patients who have chronic pain syndromes may require some combination of psychiatry, physiatry, and behavioral psychology. These treatments include exercise, gait training, spinal manipulation, orthoses, traction therapy, psychotherapy, and yoga. Successful rehabilitation aims to decrease symptoms, increase independence, and allow the patient to return to work. A positive, rapid return to light-normal activities and work is essential if disability is to be minimized. Psychologically, this is the key to coping with acute trauma. There is no evidence that a return to work adversely affects the course of the majority of chronic pain syndromes.

CONCLUSIONS

Pain is an exciting and burgeoning discipline for psychiatrists. Whether the psychiatrist is treating the pain or its psychological sequelae, it is critical to have a firm understanding of the physical basis for the pain complaints in conjunction with a thorough appreciation of how psychiatric co-morbidity interacts with the perceptions of pain. Patients who attend pain clinics have significant psychiatric pathology. This co-morbidity worsens their pain and disability, and this mental distress is an independent source of suffering, further reducing the quality of life. Fortunately, with the boom in psychotherapeutic medications over the past 15 years, and with more effective psychotherapies, significant improvement in pain treatment has been noted.

Access a list of MCQs for this chapter at https://expertconsult .inkling.com

REFERENCES

1. IASP Subcommittee on Taxonomy. Pain terms: a list with definitions and notes on usage. *Pain* 6(3):249–252, 1979.
2. Von Korff M, Crane P, Lane M, et al. Chronic spinal pain and physical-mental comorbidity in the United States: results from the National Comorbidity Survey Replication. *Pain* 113(3):331–339, 2005.
3. Teunissen SC, Wesker W, Kruitwagen C, et al. Symptom prevalence in patients with incurable cancer: a systematic review. *J Pain Symptom Manage* 34(1):94–104, 2007.
4. Walker EA, Keegan D, Gardner G, et al. Psychosocial factors in fibromyalgia compared with rheumatoid arthritis: II. Sexual, physical, and emotional abuse and neglect. *Psychosom Med* 59(6):572–577, 1997.
5. Fernandez E. Interactions between pain and affect. In *Anxiety, depression, and anger in pain*, Dallas, 2002, Advanced Psychological Resources.
6. Strain EC. Assessment and treatment of comorbid psychiatric disorders in opioid-dependent patients. *Clin J Pain* 18(4 Suppl.): S14–S27, 2002.
7. Sprenger T, Valet M, Boecker H, et al. Opioidergic activation in the medial pain system after heat pain. *Pain* 122:63–67, 2006.
8. Coghill RC, McHaffie JG, Yen YF. Neural correlates of interindividual differences in the subjective experience of pain. *Proc Natl Acad Sci* 100(8):8538–8542, 2003.
9. Gracely RH, Petzke F, Wolf JM, et al. Functional magnetic resonance imaging evidence of augmented pain processing in fibromyalgia. *Arthritis Rheum* 46(5):1333–1343, 2002.
10. Zubieta JK, Ketter TA, Bueller JA, et al. Regulation of human affective responses by anterior cingulate and limbic mu-opioid neurotransmission. *Arch Gen Psychiatry* 60(11):1145–1153, 2003.
11. Nelson D, Novy D. Self-report differentiation of anxiety and depression in chronic pain. *J Pers Assess* 69(2):392–407, 1997.
12. McCracken L, Gross RT, Aikens J, et al. The assessment of anxiety and fear in persons with chronic pain: a comparison of instruments. *Behav Res Ther* 34(11):927–933, 1996.
13. Keefe FJ, Rumble ME, Scipio CD, et al. Psychological aspects of persistent pain: current state of the science. *J Pain* 5(4):195–211, 2004.
14. Turk DC, Monarch ES. Biopsychosocial perspective on chronic pain. In Turk DC, Gatchel R, editors: *Psychological approaches to pain management*, New York, 2002, Guilford Press.
15. Max MB, Lynch SA, Muir J. Effects of desipramine, amitriptyline and fluoxetine on pain in diabetic neuropathy. *N Engl J Med* 326:1250–1256, 1992.
16. McHugh P, Slavney P. *The perspectives of psychiatry*, Baltimore, 1998, Johns Hopkins University Press.
17. Gallagher RM, Verma S. Managing pain and co-morbid depression: a public health challenge. *Semin Clin Neuropsych* 4(3):203–220, 1999.
18. Koenig T, Clark MR. Advances in comprehensive pain management. *Psychiatr Clin North Am* 19(3):589–611, 1996.
19. Thase ME, Entsuah AR, Rudolph RL. Remission rates during treatment with venlafaxine or selective serotonin reuptake inhibitors. *Br J Psychiatry* 178(3):234–241, 2001.
20. Goldstein DJ, Lu Y, Detke MJ, et al. Duloxetine vs. placebo in patients with painful diabetic neuropathy. *Pain* 116:109–118, 2005.
21. Barsky AJ. Patients who amplify bodily sensations. *Ann Intern Med* 91(1):63–70, 1979.
22. Sigvardsson S, von Knorring A, Bohman M. An adoption study of somatoform disorders. *Arch Gen Psychiatry* 41(9):853–859, 1984.
23. McDonald J. What are the causes of chronic gynecological pain disorders? *APS Bulletin* 5(6):20–23, 1995.

80 Psychiatric Aspects of Stroke Syndromes

Sean P. Heffernan, MD, Shamim H. Nejad, MD, Lucy A. Epstein Hutner, MD,
David M. Greer, MD, MA, FCCM, FAHA, FNCS, FAAN, and Jeff C. Huffman, MD

KEY POINTS

Clinical Findings

- *Stroke* is defined as the acute onset of a neurological deficit that is due to a cerebrovascular cause; a stroke has occurred if symptoms persist for longer than 24 hours or if a permanent lesion is detected by neuroimaging techniques.
- Strokes may be broadly described as ischemic or hemorrhagic.
- Neuropsychiatric sequelae of stroke include affective and cognitive disorders.

Prognosis

- Early intervention may improve the morbidity and mortality rates of stroke; rapid assessment is key to successful management.

OVERVIEW
Definition

An understanding of stroke is important for psychiatrists for several reasons: it is common, effective treatment is predicated on early recognition, and significant neuropsychiatric sequelae often result from injury to brain parenchyma. *Stroke* is defined as the acute onset of a neurological deficit due to a cerebrovascular cause. Strokes may be categorized as ischemic (in which the deficit is caused by blockage of an arterial feeding vessel), which results in a lack of oxygen and metabolic nutrients to the affected territory (Figure 80-1) or hemorrhagic (in which the deficit is caused by vessel rupture). Ischemic strokes occur roughly four times as often as hemorrhagic strokes. Ischemic strokes usually produce focal neurological deficits due to the cessation of blood flow to a specific territory of the brain. In contrast, hemorrhagic strokes, in addition to causing focal deficits, can cause more diffuse symptoms as a result of cerebral edema and an increase in intracranial pressure.

By convention, a stroke has occurred if the clinical deficit persists for longer than 24 hours or if a permanent deficit is seen on neuroimaging that directly correlates with the patient's syndrome. A transient ischemic attack (TIA), in contrast, involves no permanent tissue damage. Classically, it has been described as a focal deficit that lasts less than 24 hours. However, most patients with a TIA have symptoms for a shorter duration, typically less than 45 minutes. Recognition of TIAs is essential, as they may be a harbinger of stroke; 4%–20% of patients will have a stroke in the 90 days following a TIA.[1-6]

For suspected acute stroke, the time of onset and the duration of symptoms should be documented as accurately and as rapidly as possible. It is also crucial to confirm the history with a detailed neurological examination and a neuroimaging study. Time is of the essence with the diagnosis and acute management of acute stroke, as rapid treatment may reduce morbidity and mortality rates. Thus, stroke and TIA are medical emergencies that require prompt attention.

Anatomy of Cerebral Circulation

Strokes involve specific vessels of the cerebral circulation and result in focal neurological signs referable to the territory supplied by the affected vessels. Stroke syndromes can broadly be categorized into anterior (carotid) or posterior (vertebrobasilar) circulation phenomena (Figure 80-2). The anterior circulation includes branches of the internal carotid artery and the lenticulostriate arteries, which penetrate deep into the cerebral cortex. These vessels supply much of the cerebral cortex, the subcortical white matter, the basal ganglia, and the internal capsule. Symptoms of anterior circulation strokes depend on the hemisphere involved and the handedness of the patient. Manifestations include aphasia, apraxia, hemineglect, hemiparesis, sensory disturbances, and visual field defects. Specific deficits associated with the branches of the anterior circulation are listed in Table 80-1.

The posterior circulation consists of a pair of vertebral arteries and a single basilar artery with their branches, including the posterior cerebral arteries (PCAs). These vessels supply the brainstem, the cerebellum, the thalamus, and parts of the occipital and temporal lobes. Symptoms may localize to the brainstem (including coma, vertigo, nausea, cranial nerve palsies, or ataxia). Specific syndromes associated with the branches of the posterior circulation are also listed in Table 80-1.

EPIDEMIOLOGY/RISK FACTORS
Epidemiology

Stroke is the fourth most common cause of death in the US, following only heart disease, cancer, and chronic lower respiratory diseases.[7] It is the most common disabling neurological disorder. Each year in the US, over 795,000 new or recurrent strokes occur, leading to 1 in 19 deaths.[8] Furthermore, stroke is a major cause of functional impairment: 15% to 30% of stroke survivors are considered permanently disabled.[9]

Risk Factors

Several major risk factors for stroke exist. Of these, age is the most important non-modifiable risk factor; the risk of stroke more than doubles in each decade beyond age 55 years.[10] Other non-modifiable factors include gender (male > female), race (African Americans and Hispanics > European Americans), and genetic contributions.[11-16] A number of modifiable stroke risk factors have also been identified. Hypertension is one of the most important, and it is an excellent target for both primary and secondary prevention. Other risk factors include prior stroke or TIA, atrial fibrillation (AF), diabetes mellitus (DM), hyperlipidemia, metabolic syndrome, excessive alcohol use, tobacco use, and obstructive sleep apnea.[17]

Risk-profile Generation

Patients at risk for stroke may be stratified according to a variety of risk factors, including advanced age, hypertension, smoking status, DM, hypercholesterolemia, history of cardiovascular disease, and electrocardiographic evidence of left ventricular hypertrophy or AF. One risk-profile model, the Framingham

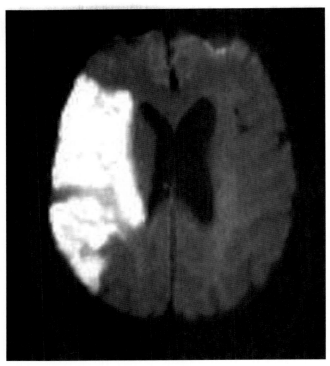

Figure 80-1. Diffusion-weighted MRI of a right middle cerebral artery territory infarct.

Stroke Profile, uses the Cox proportional-hazards method to generate an individual's 10-year, gender-specific prediction of stroke risk.[18] These and other models are important, as primary prevention efforts often focus on high-risk patients.

ISCHEMIC STROKE

Types

Several pathophysiological mechanisms lead to ischemic stroke: thrombosis, whereby a clot forms within an artery and blocks it; embolism, whereby a clot travels from a remote origin and lodges within an arterial vessel (Figure 80-3); or lipohyalinosis, whereby concentric narrowing of small penetrating arteries results in lacunar infarction. Thrombotic mechanisms cause about 20% of ischemic strokes, embolism causes about 20% of cases, and lacunar infarcts comprise an additional 25%.[19] The remainder is caused by more rare conditions or by an undetermined etiology (i.e., "cryptogenic stroke").

Given the broad array of etiologies, it is sometimes useful to categorize strokes by their anatomical basis. First, there are cerebrovascular causes of strokes. The most common is atherosclerosis of a large intracranial or extracranial artery, resulting in thrombotic stroke. Lacunar strokes are also vascular in origin, but they only affect the small branch vessels. Arterial dissection is a less common vascular cause of ischemic stroke, but it should be considered in younger patients with stroke, especially in those with a predisposing condition (such as Marfan syndrome or recent trauma to the head or neck). Use of cocaine or methamphetamine may cause stroke, likely secondary to arterial vasospasm or acute atrial dysrhythmias. Other vascular causes of stroke are rare, but include migraine, fibromuscular dysplasia, inflammation (e.g., with cerebral vasculitis), infection, and venous sinus thrombosis. Second, there are strokes related to cardiac causes, which most often result in embolic strokes. The most frequent cause of cardioembolic

Vessels dissected out: inferior view

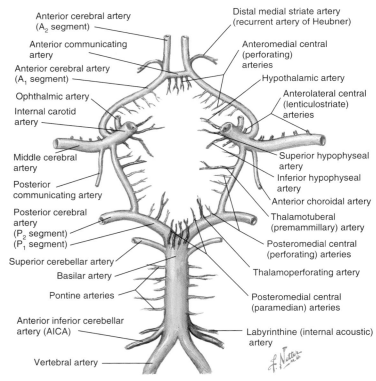

Figure 80-2. Circle of Willis showing arterial circulation of the brain. *(Reprinted from Netter Anatomy Illustration Collection, © Elsevier Inc. All rights reserved.)*

TABLE 80-1 Anterior and Posterior Circulation Stroke Syndromes

Circulation	Vessel Branch	Syndrome
Anterior	Anterior cerebral	Contralateral lower extremity paresis, mutism, apathy, pseudobulbar affect
Anterior	Middle cerebral	Contralateral hemiparesis, hemi-sensory loss, hemianopsia/quadrantanopsia, aphasia (dominant hemisphere), hemi-inattention (non-dominant hemisphere)
Posterior	Posterior cerebral	Contralateral homonymous hemianopsia, alexia without agraphia (dominant hemisphere)
Posterior	Basilar	Coma, "locked in" syndrome, cranial nerve palsies, hemiparesis/quadriparesis, ataxia
Posterior	Vertebral	Lateral medullary (Wallenburg) syndrome, appendicular or truncal ataxia

Data from Kaufman DM. Clinical neurology for psychiatrists, Philadelphia, 2001, Saunders/Elsevier, p. 275.

stroke is embolism of left atrial clot formed as a result of atrial fibrillation (AF). Other, less common, causes include cardiac mural thrombus, a clot formed at the site of a prosthetic heart valve, paradoxical embolus through a patent foramen ovale, and endocarditis. Last, strokes may be caused by blood-related disorders (such as hypercoagulability, sickle cell crisis, or elevations in blood cell counts resulting from polycythemia, leukocytosis, or thrombocytosis).

Clinical Presentation

The hallmark presentation of ischemic stroke is the abrupt onset of a focal neurological deficit. Associated symptoms, such as a seizure or headache, may occur but are less common. Thrombotic and lacunar strokes are more likely to manifest with a stuttering course of waxing and waning neurological symptoms that eventually result in a complete deficit, while embolic strokes are more likely to produce a maximal deficit at the outset.

Differential Diagnosis

The classic signs and symptoms of acute ischemic stroke are usually recognizable by physicians. However, a differential diagnosis should always be created, especially in cases with atypical features, such as a non-focal neurological examination or an impaired level of consciousness. The differential diagnosis includes intracerebral or subarachnoid hemorrhage, epidural or subdural hematoma, TIA, mass lesions (such as a tumor or abscess), seizures, migraine headaches, and metabolic causes, such as hypoglycemia.

Examination

A careful history is a crucial first step in the management of a suspected acute ischemic stroke. The exact time of onset, to the minute if possible, is an essential data point, as some therapies for the management of acute stroke (such as thrombolysis) are only available within strict time frames. If the exact time of onset is not known, or if the patient was not witnessed at the time of symptom development, the time of onset by default becomes the time at which the patient was last seen to be neurologically normal. A history of similar symptoms, which may suggest a recent TIA or even a recent stroke, should also be ascertained. Essential components of the medical history include a history of cardiac problems, hypertension, DM, hypercholesterolemia, and use of tobacco or drugs. The medication list should be reviewed, especially if the patient is taking anticoagulants or antiplatelet agents. A thorough physical examination should follow, which should include the careful assessment of vital signs (including blood pressure [BP] measured in both arms). The examiner should auscultate the carotid arteries to assess for the presence of carotid bruits. Of note, a lack of a bruit may accompany a complete or an impending occlusion. Most important, a focused neurological assessment should be done with the aim

of localizing the lesion supplied by the suspected vessel. Most stroke physicians use a standardized scale (such as the National Institutes of Health [NIH] Stroke Scale), which establishes a method of performing a rapid and focused evaluation and establishes standardized values for comparisons among stroke patients for treatment and research purposes.[20]

Diagnosis

Rapid diagnosis is critical to the management of acute ischemic stroke. Use of imaging, including computed tomography (CT) or magnetic resonance imaging (MRI), is essential. CT and MRI imaging help the clinician to distinguish ischemic strokes from intracerebral hemorrhages, to evaluate for other causes of symptoms, and to define the ischemic territory. While MRI is more sensitive to the presence of ischemia, CT is more widely available and is highly accurate in differentiating intracerebral hemorrhage from ischemic stroke. Thus, it is the first choice of imaging in most centers. It must be performed before the administration of a thrombolytic agent in order to rule out an underlying condition (such as a hemorrhage, abscess, or tumor) that would preclude its use. MRI provides superior detection of early ischemic lesions and improved visualization of lesions of the brainstem and the cerebellum. However, in order to identify pathology within the target vessel, imaging with CT angiography (CTA) or MRI angiography (MRA) is required. Laboratory testing should always include a complete blood count (CBC), metabolic panel, serum glucose, liver function tests, and a coagulation profile. These should be obtained before sending the patient for a CT scan. If clinically indicated, such as in younger patients, other laboratory tests, such as a hypercoagulability panel or toxicology screen, should be obtained. An electrocardiogram (ECG) should always be obtained to detect arrhythmias or acute myocardial ischemia. Before any neuroimaging, the patient should be stabilized from a respiratory and hemodynamic standpoint. Consideration should be given to elective intubation if the patient's airway may be compromised by his or her neurological deficit or by an impaired mental status.

A complete evaluation will include ultrasound of the carotid arteries, 24-hour cardiac monitoring, and echocardiography. In most cases, a transthoracic echocardiogram (TTE) study with an agitated saline bubble contrast study (to look for a patent foramen ovale [PFO]) will suffice. However, a transesophageal echocardiogram (TEE) may be indicated with specific conditions, such as in younger patients with a suspected PFO, valvular disease, or disease of the left atrium or aortic arch. Cerebral angiography is reserved for the investigation of unusual causes of stroke.

Treatment

Acute Management

In the acute setting, intravenous (IV) thrombolytic therapy with recombinant tissue plasminogen activator (rt-PA) may

Atrial Fibrillation

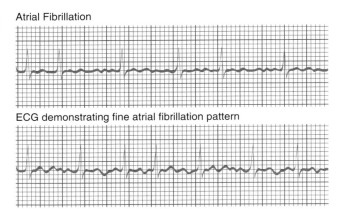

ECG demonstrating fine atrial fibrillation pattern

ECG demonstrating coarse atrial fibrillation pattern

No single mechanism causes atrial fibrillation. Small, multiple re-entrant wavelets may coalesce to form small atrial circuits. Rapid repetitive impulses generated by myocytes located in the left atrium near the pulmonary vein orifices stimulate atrial fibrillation.

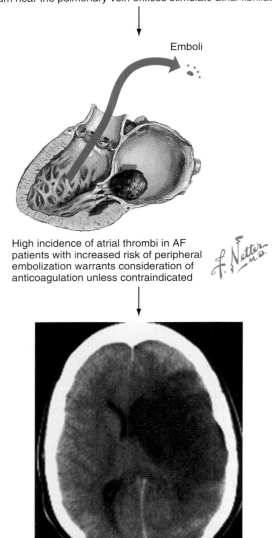

Emboli

High incidence of atrial thrombi in AF patients with increased risk of peripheral embolization warrants consideration of anticoagulation unless contraindicated

CT image of a left MCA distribution infarct

Figure 80-3. Cardioembolism leading to acute ischemic stroke. *(ECG and atrial thrombi images reprinted from Netter Anatomy Illustration Collection, © Elsevier Inc. All rights reserved.)*

significantly reduce both the short- and long-term sequelae of stroke. Rt-PA exerts its action by converting plasminogen to plasmin, which helps to dissolve fibrin-containing clots. This therapy has demonstrated a benefit to patients administered rt-PA with acute stroke less than 3 hours old; patients receiving the treatment were 30% more likely to show minimal or no disability at 3 months, with no difference in mortality rate. The main adverse event was a significantly higher percentage of symptomatic intracerebral hemorrhage in the treatment arm of the study, and this remains the most important drawback of this treatment.[21] Although some trials have indicated a potential benefit for patients who receive rt-PA within 3 to 6 hours, these patients have a higher percentage of symptomatic parenchymal hemorrhages, and thus treatment outside of the 3-hour window is not recommended.[22] Some specialized centers may perform intra-arterial (IA) thrombolysis as well. However, this is currently of limited availability, and much of the work in this area is considered investigational.[23] Another FDA-approved technique for use in acute stroke is the MERCI clot retrieval device, which allows for the mechanical retrieval of an acute thrombus within 8 hours.[24] In general, all forms of thrombolytic therapy should be delivered in a dedicated stroke center, where hemodynamic parameters and neurological status may be monitored carefully, and where neurosurgical back-up is available in the event that the patient suffers a hemorrhagic event.

Patients who are not considered candidates for thrombolysis should receive multi-modal medical management. BP in the acute setting should not be lowered aggressively. Systolic BP in the range of 150 to 160 mm Hg is often tolerated, and it may help to provide additional blood flow to ischemic, but not yet infarcted, tissue (i.e., the "ischemic penumbra"). If a patient has received IV thrombolysis, however, there is a maximum allowable BP of 185/110 mm Hg. Appropriate agents should be used emergently to lower the BP if it exceeds these values. Antiplatelet therapy has also proven beneficial both in the acute setting and for secondary prevention. Anticoagulation, with heparin or warfarin (or both), may be indicated in conditions that require ongoing anticoagulation (such as AF), but this carries the risk of hemorrhagic conversion of the ischemic infarct. The timing of anticoagulation must take into account the size and location of the stroke, the presence of any hemorrhagic conversion (even if asymptomatic), and the overall risk/benefit profile of the individual patient.

Primary Prevention

Primary prevention is the most effective means for reducing the public health burden of stroke. This includes identifying and managing modifiable risk factors, including lifestyle behaviors and co-morbid illnesses. Cigarette smoking is a well-recognized, modifiable risk factor for ischemic and hemorrhagic stroke. Compared to non-smokers, smokers have twice the risk of ischemic stroke and three times the risk for subarachnoid hemorrhage.[25,26] Physical inactivity and obesity are modifiable risk factors for stroke.[27] Abuse of alcohol and illicit substances increase the risk of both ischemic and hemorrhagic stroke.[28]

Several co-morbid conditions have been identified as important to control for prevention of stroke. Hypertension should be managed to maintain BPs at less than 140/90 mm Hg (or <130/80 mm Hg in individuals with diabetes). Thiazide-type diuretics are often recommended as the preferred initial drugs for treatment of hypertension in most patients.[29] Beta-blockers, ACE inhibitors, angiotensin II receptor antagonists (ARBs), and calcium channel blockers have all been found effective as antihypertensives in preventing stroke.[30–32] Diabetes increases the risk of stroke by nearly a factor of three.[33] Anticoagulation with warfarin can reduce the risk of stroke in atrial fibrillation by 64%.[34] However, there is no evidence that aspirin reduces the risk of stroke.[35] Last, statin therapy has lowered the risk of stroke in patients with known ischemic heart disease,[36] but its impact on patients without known cardiac disease remains under study.[37]

Secondary Prevention

Antiplatelet therapy is a key component of secondary prevention. A 1994 meta-analysis demonstrated that the use of aspirin and other antiplatelet agents (such as clopidogrel) reduced the risk of recurrent non-fatal stroke by 31%.[38] Other effective agents include aspirin and extended-release dipyridamole.[39] The use of aspirin in combination with clopidogrel is not recommended, given the lack of additional efficacy and the increased risk of bleeding.[40] Control of hypertension is another crucial component of secondary prevention. There may be a particular benefit associated with use of angiotensin-converting enzyme (ACE) inhibitors and angiotensin receptor blockers.[41,42] In non-cardioembolic stroke, warfarin has failed to prove superior to aspirin in secondary prevention. Unless contraindicated, stroke caused by AF should be treated with oral anticoagulation (OAC), with a target international normalized ratio between 2.0 and 3.0.[43] Patients should also be strongly encouraged to discontinue smoking. Lipid-lowering therapy has a proven benefit in secondary stroke prevention. A recent clinical trial demonstrated that use of statin therapy reduced the incidence of stroke and other cardiovascular events in patients with prior stroke or TIA.[44] In addition, weight loss and increased physical activity should be encouraged in all patients, and moderate alcohol intake allowed.[43] Last, carotid endarterectomy in symptomatic carotid stenosis is indicated,[45] and it may be considered for patients with severe but asymptomatic disease as well.[46] Carotid stenting is another modality that has shown promise in recent years. It is currently being studied in comparison to carotid endarterectomy and in high-risk patients who are considered unsafe for surgery.[47]

Prognosis

The extent of the deficit and the degree of functional impairment are important prognostic indicators. Negative prognostic factors also include advanced age and the presence of multiple medical co-morbidities. Approximately 80% of stroke patients achieve 1-month survival; however, only about 35% are alive 10 years after a stroke.[48]

HEMORRHAGIC STROKE
Overview

Hemorrhagic stroke refers to the acute onset of neurological dysfunction due to a ruptured cerebral vessel. Such strokes may be classified according to the location of the hemorrhage or the presumed mechanism of injury.

Intracerebral Hemorrhage

An intracerebral hemorrhage (ICH) refers to a hemorrhage into the brain parenchyma, which may extend into the ventricles or the subarachnoid space. ICH most often occurs in the cerebral cortex, basal ganglia, thalamus, pons, and cerebellum. As in other forms of stroke, lesion location predicts distinct clinical syndromes. Hypertension is the most common etiology, and it is most commonly associated with deeper hemorrhages in the basal ganglia, brainstem, or cerebellum. ICH can also be caused by amyloid angiopathy (especially in elderly patients), coagulopathy, rupture of an AVM, hemorrhagic conversion of an ischemic stroke, recreational drug use, or trauma.

These etiologies more commonly cause lobar locations of hemorrhage. ICH also has a notably high mortality rate, with only 38% of patients achieving a 1-year survival.[49]

Subarachnoid Hemorrhage

A subarachnoid hemorrhage (SAH) refers to bleeding that occurs beneath the arachnoid layer of the meninges. Non-traumatic SAH is most often due to the rupture of a previously undiagnosed saccular aneurysm. This may occur due to a developmental weakness of the vessel wall, and it may be associated with congenital disorders (such as polycystic kidney disease). Other causes of SAH include trauma, rupture of an arteriovenous malformation (AVM), hemorrhagic conversion of an ischemic stroke, primary intracerebral hemorrhage, or rupture of a mycotic aneurysm. SAH is associated with a high mortality rate: up to 45% of patients with this condition die within 30 days of the event.[50]

Subdural Hematoma/Epidural Hematoma

As these entities occur on the outer surface of the brain, strictly speaking, they are not considered cerebrovascular disorders. However, their clinical presentations may be strikingly similar to ischemic or hemorrhagic strokes. Both subdural hematoma (SDH) and epidural hematoma (EDH) usually result from trauma. SDH results from the rupture of bridging veins between the arachnoid and pia layers, and may be acute, subacute, or chronic in nature. An EDH refers to a collection of blood between the dura and the skull, often resulting from a tear in the middle meningeal artery. It is most often treated by neurosurgical evacuation.

Clinical Presentation

SAH most often manifests as the abrupt onset of a severe headache, classically described by the patient as the "worst headache of my life." This severe pain is thought to be due to an elevation in intracranial pressure, leading to distortion of pain-sensitive structures. A progressive decline in mental status often follows, which may be due to decreased cerebral blood flow in the setting of elevated intracranial pressure. These symptoms are often accompanied by nausea, vomiting, and meningismus. As free-flowing blood traverses functional territories, SAH tends to produce more diffuse neurological deficits than do ischemic strokes. Ischemia or even infarction from cerebral vasospasm may occur later in the course of SAH, resulting in more focal neurological deficits.

ICH may manifest in a similar fashion, with severe headache, nausea, and vomiting. The combination of an expanding hematoma, worsening edema, and compression of brainstem structures often leads to a progressive decline in the level of consciousness. The BP may be markedly elevated on presentation, and it may either be the cause of the hemorrhage or the effect of the concomitant massive catecholamine release.

Differential Diagnosis

The differential diagnosis of hemorrhagic stroke includes ischemic stroke, central nervous system (CNS) infections, subdural or epidural hematoma, rapidly expanding tumor or abscess (hemorrhage into a tumor or abscess is not uncommon), or drug intoxication. ICH may be particularly difficult to distinguish clinically from ischemic stroke, which underscores the importance of neuroimaging in this setting.

History/Examination

History gathering may be limited because of a patient's impaired mental status. In such a case, it is important to speak with family members or other sources of collateral information. Timing, duration, onset, and types of symptoms are all important data points. SAH in particular may be preceded by the presence of multiple "harbinger" headaches in the days to weeks leading up to the event. These may be due to aneurysmal stretching before rupture or even sentinel hemorrhages. Essential aspects of the physical examination include measurement of BP, heart rate, and temperature, as well as an examination for nuchal rigidity. A neurological examination should follow, including a careful assessment of mental status.

Diagnosis

CT scanning is the preferred imaging modality for the detection of both SAH and ICH. Approximately 5% to 10% of SAHs will be undetectable by CT, due to technical limitations. In this case, if SAH is suggested by clinical history, a lumbar puncture should be performed to detect the presence of hemoglobin breakdown products (xanthochromia), which will appear less than 12 hours after the hemorrhage. Further imaging modalities include CTA or cerebral angiography, which may help to identify the aneurysm or other vascular abnormality, and Doppler ultrasound, which can monitor for the later development of cerebral vasospasm, which typically develops 5–14 days after the SAH. Routine laboratory testing includes a CBC, metabolic panel, and coagulation parameters. An ECG should also be performed. Typical findings that may accompany SAH include diffuse peaked T waves, a prolonged QT interval, and peaked P waves.[51] A neurosurgical consultation is mandatory for further management.

Treatment

For SAH due to aneurysm rupture, current management includes neurosurgical clipping or endovascular coiling of the aneurysm to prevent re-bleeding. The optimal approach remains under study. The landmark 2002 International Subarachnoid Aneurysm Trial (ISAT) study, which randomized 2,143 SAH patients to clipping or to coiling (in cases in which either was deemed feasible), demonstrated improved disability-free survival in the coiling group at 1 year.[52] A follow-up study in 2005 of the same population demonstrated a continued survival benefit in the endovascular group for at least 7 years; however, the risk of re-bleeding was slightly higher.[53] Potential candidates for intervention may be graded according to clinical presentation, severity of hemorrhage, and estimated surgical risk.[54] For SAH due to rupture of an AVM, surgical or endovascular correction may be attempted if the anatomy is favorable.

Patients with either SAH or ICH require urgent attention for airway protection, hemodynamic management in an intensive care setting, and minimization of the sequelae of the initial hemorrhage. For SAH, interventions include bed rest with head of bed elevation to 15–20 degrees, careful use of mild sedating agents to control agitation, avoidance of hypotension, prophylactic prevention of vasospasm with calcium channel blockers, and seizure prophylaxis with antiepileptic medications for worse clinical grade patients. Any coagulopathy should be corrected. Hyponatremia due to cerebral salt wasting or the syndrome of inappropriate antidiuretic hormone (SIADH) is common, and should be investigated and treated accordingly. Fluid restriction is contraindicated in patients with cerebral vasospasm after SAH. Many patients (especially those with hydrocephalus or a depressed level of consciousness) with SAH will require extraventricular drainage (EVD). If cerebral vasospasm develops, medical management typically includes "triple H" therapy, consisting of induced hypertension, hemodilution, and hypervolemia.

With refractory vasospasm, direct intra-arterial techniques (such as direct infusion of vasodilating medications or angioplasty of severely vasospastic vessels) may be necessary.

With ICH, emergency measures (such as hyperventilation and IV mannitol) to prevent herniation and further brain injury may be required, especially for those patients who may have significant cerebral edema, brainstem compression, or severe mass effect.[55,56] Corticosteroids are not efficacious and are not indicated.[57] The optimal approach for the management of BP is controversial. Current guidelines include the use of IV antihypertensive agents for patients with a mean arterial BP $\geq$ 130 mm Hg. Neurosurgical decompression is considered in cases with low expected mortality, such as cases of cerebellar hemorrhage, young patients, or superficially-located hematomas.[56] One large randomized study (1,033 patients with spontaneous ICH) did not show overall benefit in the surgical evacuation over the conservative treatment groups.[58] Preliminary trials have indicated that stereotactic aspiration and thrombolysis of spontaneous intracerebral hemorrhage appears to be safe and effective in the reduction of ICH volume, though follow-up studies of mortality have not been done.[59,60]

Prognosis

For SAH, survival rates depend in part on the patient's age and neurological status, the time elapsed since the hemorrhage, co-morbidities, and other factors (such as degree of intracranial pressure). Approximately 50% of survivors have permanent brain injury from a ruptured aneurysm. If the SAH is due to an AVM, survival rates are in the range of 90%.[48] For ICH, the prognosis depends on the volume of the hematoma, the site of involvement, the presence of coma, the age of the patient, and the presence of intraventricular blood.[61–64]

NEUROPSYCHIATRIC SEQUELAE OF STROKE

Neuropsychiatric sequelae, including changes in affect, behavior, and cognition, are seen in more than half of post-stroke patients, and may be linked to lesion location (Table 80-2). Although the neuropsychiatric effects of stroke are wide-ranging and variable, symptoms tend to cluster into several categories and broadly can be considered acute and post-acute with regard to the timing of the manifestation of symptoms.

Acute Symptoms Following Stroke
Post-stroke Delirium

In a systematic review and meta-analysis of over 2,000 patients, delirium was found to affect 10% to 30% of patients in the acute phase of stroke.[65] These patients had less favorable clinical outcomes, including being 4.7 times more likely to die in the hospital or within the first 12 months following discharge. In addition, these patients had worse functional outcomes, were more likely to be discharged to long-term care facilities, and had an increased risk of dementia and institutionalization. The presence of delirium following a stroke may represent a diagnostic dilemma, as it can be difficult to distinguish symptoms of delirium from focal cognitive deficits that affect declarative memory. Predictors of post-stroke delirium include pre-existing neurodegenerative process, older age, impaired vision, swallowing dysfunction, and the inability to raise one's arms.[66]

Post-stroke Mania

Post-stroke mania occurs much less commonly than post-stroke depression (PSD). Signs and symptoms are generally similar to those of a primary manic episode and include pressured speech, grandiosity, an increase in goal-directed activity,

TABLE 80-2 Neuropsychiatric Syndromes and Lesion Location

Cortical Area	Potential Neuropsychiatric Symptoms
Frontal Lobes	
Orbitofrontal region	Disinhibition, personality change, irritability
Dorsolateral region	Executive dysfunction: poor planning, organizing, and sequencing
Medial region	Apathy, abulia
Left frontal lobe	Non-fluent (Broca's) aphasia, post-stroke depression (possibly)
Right frontal lobe	Motor dysprosody
Temporal Lobes	
Either side	Hallucinations (olfactory, gustatory, tactile, visual, or auditory), episodic fear, or mood changes
Left temporal lobe	Short-term memory impairment (verbal, written stimuli), fluent (Wernicke's) aphasia (left temporoparietal region)
Right temporal lobe	Short-term memory impairment (non-verbal stimuli; e.g., music), sensory dysprosody (right temporoparietal region)
Left parietal lobe	Gerstmann's syndrome (finger agnosia, right/left disorientation, acalculia, agraphia)
Right parietal lobe	Anosognosia, constructional apraxia, prosopagnosia, hemi-neglect
Occipital lobes	Anton's syndrome (cortical blindness with unawareness of visual disturbance)

and a decreased need for sleep. Symptoms may be correlated with right-sided lesions, particularly in the orbitofrontal cortex and thalamus.[67-69] Symptoms may improve with standard treatments for mania, including mood stabilizers (e.g., lithium, valproic acid, carbamazepine) and atypical antipsychotics. However, there are few randomized clinical trials to demonstrate their benefit.[69]

Post-stroke Psychosis

Post-stroke psychosis is also uncommon; it is identified in approximately 1%–2% of all post-stroke patients.[70] Temporal lobe insults may predispose to psychosis in this population. Antipsychotics may alleviate some symptoms. However, some psychotic symptoms may arise as a consequence of complex partial seizure activity arising in the temporal lobe, and anticonvulsants, such as carbamazepine, would be the medication of choice in this setting.

Other Syndromes

In addition to the psychiatric syndromes listed previously, other syndromes are seen specifically in post-stroke patients. Catastrophic reactions may affect up to 20% of post-stroke patients.[71,72] A mixture of anxiety, aggressive behavior, and compensatory boasting classically characterizes this syndrome. It may be related to lesions involving the anterior subcortical regions and left hemisphere.[72,73] Risk factors include a family history of psychiatric illness. Pseudobulbar affect, also referred to as pathological emotional behavior, is a syndrome characterized by the outward emotional expression not correlating to the affect of the situation. Selective serotonin re-uptake inhibitors (SSRIs) and tricyclic antidepressants (TCAs) may lead to some improvement in this disorder.[74,75] Last, apathy, characterized by a notable lack of feeling or interest, is noted in approximately 20% of post-stroke patients and may co-exist with depression.[76,77] It may be related to lesions in the posterior limb of the internal capsule[77] and it is notoriously difficult to treat.

Post-acute Symptoms Following Stroke
Post-stroke Depression

Post-stroke depression (PSD) is the most common neuropsychiatric disorder following stroke, with a prevalence rate ranging from 9%–34% in the initial 3–6 months to 30%–50% within the first year.[78] Risk factors for the development of PSD include prior major depression, pre-stroke functional impairment, social isolation (including living alone), and possibly female gender.[79] An untreated episode of PSD may last for 9

months to 1 year. The etiology of PSD is unclear and may be multi-factorial (e.g., related to the degree of disability or cognitive impairment, and perhaps to lesion location as well).[80] A prospective study correlating major depression within the first 4 months of the first stroke, utilizing MRI supports involvement of the limbic-cortical-striatal-pallidal-thalamic (LCSPT) circuit on the left.[81] Depression in this population may be difficult to diagnose for many reasons, including the fact that there is often an overlap of psychiatric and somatic symptoms (such as fatigue). In addition, confounding neurological symptoms (such as expressive aprosodias and aphasia) may hinder a complete evaluation.

PSD has a major impact on functional status, and thus it should be treated actively.[82] A full remission from PSD is difficult to achieve.[83] However, both SSRIs and TCAs have proven useful in improving post-stroke mood.[84-86] Additionally, low doses of stimulants possess a mild antidepressant quality that may also improve mood. However, as many stroke patients have concurrent cardiac risk factors (such as elevated BP or coronary artery disease [CAD] at baseline), these agents should be used with caution (Box 80-1). For severe depression that has not been alleviated by adequate trials of antidepressants, electroconvulsive therapy (ECT) has been used successfully and safely.[87] Non-pharmacological interventions, such as cognitive-behavioral therapy, are under investigation, but have not proven to be more effective than the use of medication in this population.[88]

The use of SSRIs has also been associated with improved recovery after stroke, even in persons without depression. Some data seem to suggest their use results in less disability, neurological impairment, along with depression and anxiety, even in non-depressed patients.[89] In a randomized, placebo-controlled in patients with ischemic stroke and moderate-to-severe motor deficit, the early prescription of fluoxetine with physical therapy improved motor recovery after 3 months.[90]

Post-stroke Anxiety

Anxiety also commonly affects the post-stroke population. More than 25% of post-stroke patients meet the criteria for a generalized anxiety disorder (GAD), which commonly co-exists with major depression.[91,92] SSRIs remain first-line treatment, as they may treat symptoms of both GAD and depression. Benzodiazepines should be used with particular caution, as they may produce disinhibition or signs of toxicity, such as ataxia and oversedation.

Post-stroke Dementia

Vascular dementia is a term that refers to a heterogeneous group of neurodegenerative processes caused by impairment

BOX 80-1 Indications for Stimulant Use in Post-stroke Depression

1. Consider possible (relative) contraindications to psychostimulant use:
   a. history of ventricular arrhythmia
   b. recent myocardial infarction
   c. congestive heart failure with reduced ejection fraction
   d. poorly controlled hypertension
   e. tachycardia
   f. concurrent treatment with MAOIs
2. Initiate treatment with morning dose of 5 mg of methylphenidate or dextroamphetamine (2.5 mg in frail elderly or medically tenuous patients).
3. Check vital signs and response to treatment in 2–4 hours (the period of peak effect).
4. If the initial dose is well-tolerated and effective throughout the day, continue with single daily morning dose.
5. If the initial dose is well-tolerated and effective for several hours, with a loss of effect in the afternoon, give the same dose twice per day (in the morning and the early afternoon).
6. If the initial dose is well-tolerated but is without significant clinical effect, increase dose by 5 mg per day until a clinical response is achieved, intolerable side effects arise, or 20 mg dose is ineffective (i.e., a failed trial).
7. Continue treatment throughout the hospitalization; stimulants can usually be discontinued at discharge.

of cerebral perfusion. These disorders fall into three broad categories and include subcortical ischemic dementia, multi-infarct dementia, and dementia secondary to focal infarctions. In a systematic review and meta-analysis of over 7,500 patients, the prevalence of post-stroke dementia in the first year after stroke ranged from around 7% in population-based studies in which pre-stroke dementia was excluded to around 40% in studies of hospital-based patients with recurrent stroke in which pre-stroke dementia was not excluded. Rates increased to about three times as high following recurrent stroke compared with first-ever stroke, and seemed to rise following each stroke event. Previous symptomatic stroke, previous asymptomatic stroke seen on imaging, several stroke lesions, aphasia, severity of stroke, hemorrhagic stroke, and location of stroke (increased with left hemisphere lesions and decreased with brainstem lesions) were all associated with the development of post-stroke dementia. Other factors seem to implicate increasing age, female sex, low education, race, diabetes, AF, leukoaraiosis, and global and medial temporal lobe atrophy.[93]

CONCLUSION

In conclusion, it is important for the psychiatrist to understand the pathophysiology, clinical presentation, evaluation, and treatment of stroke, because he or she is likely to encounter this disorder in clinical practice, and because major changes in affect, cognition, and behavior can occur as a result.

Access the complete reference list and multiple choice questions (MCQs) online at https://expertconsult.inkling.com

KEY REFERENCES

1. Kleindorfer D, Panagos P, Pancioli A, et al. Incidence and short-term prognosis of transient ischemic attack in a population-based study. *Stroke* 36:720–723, 2005.

2. Johnston SC, Gress DR, Browner WS, et al. Short-term prognosis after emergency-department diagnosis of transient ischemic attack. *JAMA* 284:2901–2906, 2000.

3. Coull AJ, Lovett JK, Rothwell PM. Population based study of early risk of stroke after transient ischaemic attack or minor stroke: implications for public education and organisation of services. *BMJ* 328:326–328, 2004.

8. Go AS, Mozaffarian D, Roger VL, et al. Heart disease and stroke statistics–2014 Update. *Circulation* 129:e28–e292, 2014.

18. Wolfe PA, D'Agostino RB, Belanger AJ, et al. Probability of stroke: a risk profile from the Framingham Study. *Stroke* 22:312–318, 1991.

19. Albers GW, Amarenco P, Easton JD, et al. Antithrombotic and thrombolytic therapy for ischemic stroke: the 7th ACCP Conference on Antithrombotic and Thrombolytic Therapy. *Chest* 126:483–512S, 2004.

26. Broderick JP, Viscoli CM, Brott T, et al. Major risk factors for aneurysmal subarachnoid hemorrhage in the young are modifiable. *Stroke* 34:1375–1381, 2003.

27. Lee CD, Folsom AR, Blair SN, et al. Physical activity and stroke risk: A meta-analysis. *Stroke* 34:2475–2481, 2003.

29. Chobanian AV, Bakris GL, Black HR, et al. The Seventh Report of the Joint National Committee on Prevention, Detection, Evaluation, and Treatment of High Blood Pressure: The JNC 7 Report. *JAMA* 289:2560–2571, 2003.

43. Sacco RL, Adams R, Albers G, et al. Guidelines for prevention of stroke in patients with ischemic stroke or transient ischemic attack: a statement for healthcare professions from the American Heart Association/American Stroke Association Council on Stroke. *Stroke* 37:577–617, 2006.

63. Vermeer SE, Algra A, Franke CL, et al. Long-term prognosis after recovery from primary intracerebral hemorrhage. *Neurology* 59:205–209, 2002.

65. Shi Q, Presutti R, Selchen D, et al. Delirium in acute stroke: A systematic review and meta-analysis. *Stroke* 43:645–649, 2012.

66. Sheng AZ, Shen Q, Cordato D, et al. Delirium within three days of stroke in a cohort of elderly patients. *J Am Geriatr Soc* 54(8):1192–1198, 2006.

67. Robinson RG, Boston JD, Starkstein SE, et al. Comparison of cortical and subcortical lesions in the production of post-stroke depression matched for size and location of lesions. *Arch Gen Psychiatry* 45:247–252, 1988.

72. Carota A, Rossetti AO, Karapanayiotides T, et al. Catastrophic reaction in acute stroke: a reflex behavior in aphasic patients. *Neurology* 57:1902–1905, 2001.

76. Starkstein SE, Fedoroff JP, Price TR, et al. Apathy following cerebrovascular lesions. *Stroke* 24(11):1625–1630, 1993.

78. Flaster M, Sharma A, Rao M. Poststroke depression: A review emphasizing the role of prophylactic treatment and synergy with treatment for motor recovery. *Top Stroke Rehabil* 20(2):139–150, 2013.

80. Whyte EM, Mulsant BH. Post-stroke depression: epidemiology, pathophysiology, and biological treatment. *Biol Psychiatry* 52:253–264, 2002.

81. Terroni L, Amaro E Jr, Iosifescu DV, et al. Stroke lesion in cortical neural circuits and post-stroke incidence of major depressive episode: a 4-month prospective study. *World J Biol Psychiatry* 12(7):539–548, 2011.

82. Robinson RG. Neuropsychiatric consequences of stroke. *Annu Rev Med* 48:217–219, 1997.

83. Hackett ML, Anderson CS, House AO. Management of depression after stroke: a systematic review of pharmacological therapies. *Stroke* 36:1092–1097, 2005.

88. Lincoln NB, Flannaghan T. Cognitive behavioral therapy for depression following stroke: a randomized controlled trial. *Stroke* 34:111–115, 2003.

89. Mead GE, Cheng-Fang H, Hackett M. Selective serotonin reuptake inhibitors for stroke recovery. *JAMA* 310(10):1066–1067, 2013.

90. Chollet F, Tardy J, Albucher JF, et al. Fluoxetine for motor recovery after acute ischaemic stroke (FLAME): a randomized placebo-controlled trial. *Lancet Neurol* 10:123–130, 2011.

93. Pendlebury ST, Rothwell PM. Prevalence, incidence, and factors associated with pre-stroke and post-stroke dementia: a systematic review and meta-analysis. *Lancet Neurol* 8:1006–1018, 2009.

81   Movement Disorders

Alice W. Flaherty, MD, PhD, and Ana Ivkovic, MD

KEY POINTS

- Movement disorders result from dysfunction of neural circuits that typically include the basal ganglia.

- Dopamine, the best-understood basal ganglia neurotransmitter, affects the drive for movements, cognitions, and emotions.

- Hypokinetic disorders, such as Parkinson's disease, may include depression and slowed cognitions.

- Hyperkinetic disorders, such as Huntington's disease or levodopa toxicity, can trigger impulse-control problems or hallucinations.

- Of movement disorders associated with psychiatric drugs, neuroleptic malignant syndrome is the most dangerous, and akathisia the most common.

- Tardive dyskinesias must be detected early to aid full resolution.

- Psychogenic movement disorders are highly prevalent, disabling, and deserve multi-disciplinary treatment that can include medication.

OVERVIEW

In movement disorders, the line between psychiatry and neurology is particularly fine. Most movement disorders can have psychiatric symptoms. The actions that movement disorders generate often hover on the border between feeling voluntary and involuntary. Even disorders with clear brain pathology have characteristics (such as being unusually affected by placebo) that suggest somatoform disorders. Moreover, many psychiatric syndromes have characteristic changes in movement, such as the hyperkinetic movements of mania or the psychomotor slowing of depression. Drugs used to treat movement disorders often have psychiatric side effects, as when dopamine agonists cause disinhibition syndromes. Further drugs used to treat psychiatric conditions frequently cause abnormal movements. Those caused by neuroleptics are covered in Chapters 42 and 55.

PATHOPHYSIOLOGY

Although movement disorders are usually classified as hypokinetic (too little action) or hyperkinetic (too much action), most contain complicated combinations of the two. This is even truer in movement disorders caused by psychiatric medications. Patients with schizoaffective disorder, for instance, may have extra movements from tardive dyskinesia (TD) yet at the same time be rigid.

Movement disorders stem from anatomic and pharmacologic changes in the basal ganglia and their associated circuits[1] (Figure 81-1). The overlap between neurologic and psychiatric symptoms in movement disorders stems from the fact that circuits controlling cognition, movement, and emotion run in parallel through the basal ganglia and interact greatly.[2] Thus, pathology in Parkinson's disease usually affects motor areas

of the mid-striatum (the putamen) but may also spread to cognitive areas in the dorsal striatum (the head of the caudate) and motivational circuits in the ventral striatum and the nucleus accumbens.

Disorders of the basal ganglia broadly affect motivation. When damage is restricted to motor circuits, it affects the initiation and cessation of movement. When damage spreads to affective circuits, it creates disorders of motivation there, too—depression and apathy on the one hand, or excessively goal-directed, manic disinhibition on the other. When a bradykinetic disorder spreads to the basal ganglia's cognitive circuits, thoughts can be slowed (bradyphrenia), and deficits in executive function may appear without the characteristic aphasia or agnosia of cortical dementias (such as Alzheimer's disease). Conversely, hyperkinetic disorders can cause wild, unregulated thought manifested by hallucinations and delusions.

Basal ganglia disorders disrupt self-generated actions more than environmentally-cued ones. Because the basal ganglia mediate motor reactions to expectations, placebo can strongly influence movement disorder symptoms. This makes it easy to misdiagnose them as purely psychiatric symptoms.

Circuitry

In basal ganglia circuitry, all of the cerebral cortex projects to the striatum (i.e., the caudate nucleus, putamen, and nucleus accumbens), which then projects to the globus pallidus (external and internal segments), the thalamus, and finally back to the cerebral cortex. Dopaminergic projections from the substantia nigra pars compacta (motor) and nearby ventral tegmental area (limbic) play an important role. Because this feedback loop ultimately affects movement through pyramidal neurons' output through the spinal cord, "extrapyramidal symptoms" (EPS) is not an entirely accurate term for basal ganglia problems. However, it is entrenched in clinical usage. The subthalamic nucleus, too, has an important modifying influence. Hypokinetic disorders usually stem from damage to the direct pathway through the internal globus pallidus; hyperkinetic movements result from damage to the indirect pathway through the external globus pallidus and subthalamic nucleus. These pathways control affect and cognition as well as movement.

Cerebellar problems, such as ataxia, and primary motor (pyramidal) symptoms, such as paralysis (complete inability to voluntarily use a muscle), paresis (partial paralysis), or spasticity are not, by convention, movement disorders, because they do not stem from damage to the basal ganglia. However, they will be covered briefly here, because their effects on movement may easily be mistaken for basal ganglia symptoms.

Pharmacology

Dopamine is the best-understood neurotransmitter related to basal ganglia function.[3] Its receptors fall into two classes: the D_1 class, of which D_1 is mostly found in the striatum and D_5 extra-striatal; and the D_2 class, of which D_2 is primarily striatal whereas D_3 and D_4 are mostly extra-striatal. Dopamine's release in the motor control areas of the striatum facilitates limb movement via D_2 receptors and inhibits movement via D_1 receptors. Medications most commonly used to affect dopamine neurotransmission are antagonists (e.g., haloperidol),

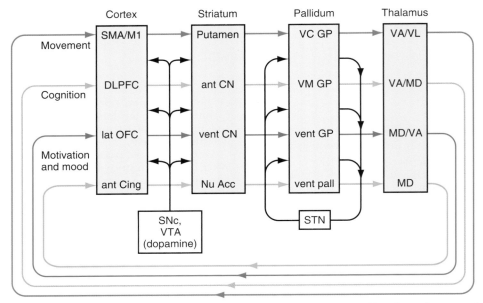

Figure 81-1. Basal ganglia circuitry. Parallel channels of information flow interact at each level of basal ganglia processing. ant, Anterior; lat, lateral; MD, mediodorsal; vent, ventral; VA, ventroanterior; VC, ventrocaudal; VM, ventromedial; VL, ventrolateral; SMA/M1, supplementary motor and motor cortex; DLPFC, dorsolateral prefrontal cortex; OFC, lateral orbitofrontal cortex; ant Cing, anterior cingulate cortex; CN, caudate nucleus; GP, globus pallidus; Nu Acc, nucleus accumbens; pall, pallidum (includes both GP and ventral pallidum); SNc, substantia nigra; STN, subthalamic nucleus; VTA, ventral tegmental area.

precursors (e.g., levodopa), receptor agonists (e.g., pramipexole), and inhibitors of dopamine metabolism (e.g., entacapone [a catechol O-methyltransferase (COMT) inhibitor] and selegiline [a monoamine oxidase-B (MAO-B) inhibitor, at least at low doses]). Acetylcholine is also important in the basal ganglia, particularly in striatal and nucleus accumbens' control of motivation and memory. To a first approximation, cholinergic effects counteract those of dopamine, making anticholinergics (e.g., benztropine) useful in the treatment of patients with drug-induced parkinsonism. Gamma-aminobutyric acid (GABA) and glutamate are the predominant neurotransmitters in basal ganglia circuitry, but their ubiquity makes them poor targets for pharmacological interventions.

Electrophysiology

In addition to the pharmacological targeting of specific neurotransmitter systems, anatomically targeted-interventions (especially deep brain stimulation [DBS][4] and repetitive transcranial magnetic stimulation [rTMS]) can powerfully affect movement disorders. DBS electrodes in the subthalamic nucleus can help Parkinson's disease. DBS in the thalamus and globus pallidus can control tremor and dystonia, respectively. Pallidal DBS may also decrease TD symptoms. DBS in the anterior cingulate and internal capsule can help treat depression and obsessive-compulsive disorder (OCD). Studies show benefit from DBS for Tourette's syndrome, eating disorders, post-traumatic coma, and drug addiction. DBS's mechanisms are complicated, but standard DBS stimulation seems to inhibit, not stimulate, gray matter around the electrode. DBS may jam normal neural transmission. The stimulator thus makes a reversible brain lesion, one whose size can be adjusted by changing electrode voltage or other parameters. Drawbacks to DBS include the risk of brain bleeds, stroke, infection, inadvertent neuropsychiatric side effects (e.g., cognitive impairment and emotional disinhibition), hardware malfunction, and the need for frequent office visits for DBS adjustments. In the future, rTMS may provide a non-invasive alternative to DBS. Studies in Parkinson's show rTMS can produce temporary subcortical dopamine release and motor benefit.[5]

CLINICAL FINDINGS

Most movement disorders are diagnosed by the history and physical examination, because blood tests and brain scans rarely show abnormalities.

Patient History

The first priority is to determine the frequency and nature of falling, as falls are the most immediate health risk. The second most immediate health risk is dysphagia causing aspiration, so it is important to ask whether the patient has had trouble swallowing pills or coughs after drinking liquids. One should ask about what daily tasks are difficult—for example, "Does the tremor interfere with using a spoon (usually an action tremor) or holding a newspaper (usually a rest tremor)?" Ask about drug use, especially neuroleptics, but also sedatives and alcohol because they can exacerbate fall risk.

Take a particularly careful history of cognitive complaints. Try to distinguish between Alzheimer's-type cortical deficits (in which there are prominent language problems and compensatory strategies) and frontal/executive, subcortical deficits (in which clues and to-do lists can help). In basal ganglia disorders, hallucinations are much more often visual than auditory. Clinicians should ask the patient about early signs of hallucinations, such as vivid dreams, seeing dust particles or a webbing over the visual field, and transiently misidentifying objects as animate.

Physical Examination

Much of the physical examination of a patient with a movement disorder can proceed through observation without direct physical contact (e.g., "Does the patient enter the room quickly or slowly?") and can thus be carried out during a psychiatric

TABLE 81-1 Symptoms, Causes, and Treatment of Movement Disorders, with a Focus on Causes Common in Adult Psychiatric Patients

	Symptom	Causes	Treatments	Differential Dx
All	All symptoms	Drugs, idiopathic, basal ganglia stroke, genetic; stress worsens all	Change offending medication; raise DA or lower ACh if hypokinetic, lower DA if hyperkinetic	Pyramidal tract damage, cerebellar, conversion disorder
Hypokinetic → Mixed → Hyperkinetic	Freezing	Parkinsonism, panic	Dopaminergics, benzodiazepines, sensory cueing	Catatonia
	Akinesia	Acute neuroleptics, parkinsonism	Anticholinergics, dopaminergics, DBS	Depressive psychomotor slowing
	Bradykinesia	Acute neuroleptics, parkinsonism	Anticholinergics, dopaminergics, DBS	Depressive psychomotor slowing, fatigue, weakness
	Rigidity	Acute neuroleptics, parkinsonism	Anticholinergics, dopaminergics, DBS	Spasticity, paratonia in dementia
	Resting tremor	Acute neuroleptics, Parkinson's	Anticholinergics, dopaminergics, DBS	Action tremor, dystonic tremor, focal seizure, myoclonus
	Action or postural tremor	Lithium, valproate, lamotrigine, SSRIs, TCAs, stimulants, thyroid	Propranolol, clonidine, gabapentin, mirtazapine, topiramate, primidone, DBS	Rest tremor, dysmetria, asterixis, focal seizure, myoclonus, alcohol withdrawal
	Restless leg syndrome	Low iron, sometimes Parkinson's prodrome	Dopaminergics, gabapentin, pregabalin	Akathisia
	Dystonia	Acute neuroleptics, excessive use syndromes	Diphenhydramine, Botox, anticholinergics, benzodiazepines, DBS	Dyskinesias, Parkinson's (especially young-onset)
	Athetosis	Huntington's, lupus, estrogens	Neuroleptics, benzodiazepines	Tardive dyskinesias, dystonia
	Chorea	Huntington's, lupus, estrogens	Neuroleptics, benzodiazepines	Tardive dyskinesias, dystonia
	Dyskinesia (drug-induced)	Chronic neuroleptics, treated Parkinson's	Clozapine, amantadine, *slow* neuroleptic wean	Non-drug causes of chorea, athetosis
	Akathisia	Acute neuroleptics, SSRIs	Propranolol, anticholinergics	Restless leg syndrome, anxiety, mania
	Tics	Tourette's, chronic neuroleptics, frontotemporal dementia	Neuroleptics, clonidine, benzodiazepines, habit-reversal	Myoclonus, obsessive-compulsive disorder
	Myoclonus	Metabolic, opiates	Clonazepam, valproate	Tics, myoclonic epilepsy
	Asterixis	Metabolic, especially liver	Treat underlying cause	Tremor, tics
	Hemiballism	Subthalamic stroke	Neuroleptics	Tremor, dyskinesias

ACh, Acetylcholine; DA, dopamine; DBS, deep brain stimulation; SSRIs, selective serotonin reuptake inhibitors; TCAs, tricyclic antidepressants.

interview. Once seated, one can assess whether the patient is restless or immobile. Facial expressiveness, if diminished, may be from parkinsonism or depression. It's helpful to remember that Parkinson's patients typically blink less often, whereas depressed patients typically blink more.

Symptoms of movement disorders are summarized in Table 81-1. They range from hypokinetic to hyperkinetic and from feeling involuntary to voluntary. Unfortunately, it is not easy to distinguish movement disorders through written descriptions of symptoms, and descriptions in this chapter are no exception. Patient videos are the best way to learn this crucial distinction. Some are available online (e.g., www.springerimages.com/Tarsy).[6] Unfortunately, many of the free web-based videos are made by patients whose deficits are actually psychogenic.

Hypokinetic Signs

Rigidity. Rigidity is the cardinal hypokinetic sign. While rigidity is characteristic of parkinsonism, it is sometimes present even in hyperkinetic conditions such as Tourette's syndrome. Rigidity produces a constant "lead pipe" resistance to movement along the whole range of the joint. It can quickly be assessed without touching the patient, by asking the patient to rapidly rotate the wrist back and forth, as if trying to screw in a light-bulb. Cogwheel rigidity is simply a tremor superimposed on rigidity, although the tremor is not always apparent visually. Patients sometimes complain of an inner tremor

not visible to others. Their complaint may be mistaken for somatization or delusion, but it is more commonly evidence for parkinsonism. Rigidity makes movements low-amplitude, and they rapidly decrease in size. Handwriting almost always demonstrates this and is another simple, non-invasive test (Figure 81-2).

Rigidity is different from spasticity, the jerky "clasp-knife" phenomenon seen after stroke-induced paralysis or paresis. The presence of hyperreflexia, muscle atrophy, flexor spasms, and toe-walking helps distinguish spasticity from rigidity.

Although patients with hypokinetic movement disorders often say they feel weak, they usually have normal muscle bulk and can exert considerable strength if given enough time to fully engage their muscles. In this, basal ganglia movement disorders differ notably from the paralytic weakness of cortical strokes or peripheral nerve injuries.

Bradykinesia. Bradykinesia (slower movements) and akinesia (fewer movements) may culminate in freezing: a sudden inability to move that most often occurs when the patient tries to initiate a movement. Freezing is related to the psychiatric syndrome of catatonia (see Chapter 55). Freezing, like many basal ganglia symptoms, is more a problem with internally motivated behaviors than with ones that are responses to environmental cues. Patients can sometimes break freezes with sensory tricks (such as stepping over a line on the floor, or hearing marching music). This can incorrectly appear to be evidence for a somatoform disorder.

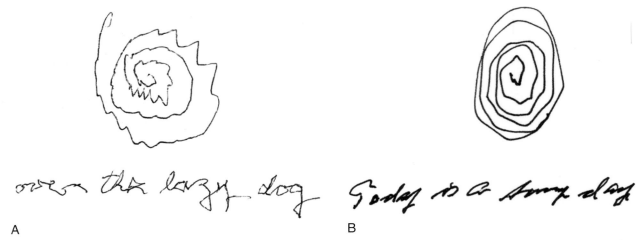

Figure 81-2. Handwriting and spiral drawing reflect tremor type. (A) The large scrawl of essential tremor. (B) Cramped, parkinsonian writing and spiral show little of the tremor—writing is an action.

Mixed Signs

Rest Tremor. Rest tremor hovers in the middle of the spectrum between hypokinetic and hyperkinetic movements. Such mixed signs often do not respond well to dopaminergic medications. Rest tremor, for instance, presents when the limb is not in use and looks hyperkinetic but is almost always associated with parkinsonism. Rest tremors are commonly coarse and low-frequency (3 to 5 Hz). Like all basal ganglia movement disorders, they disappear during sleep. Rest tremors often respond more completely to anticholinergics than to dopaminergic drugs. The archetypal rest tremor disappears with voluntary movement of the same limb, but in the real world there is sometimes a co-morbid action tremor. All tremors, rest or action, are rhythmic back-and-forth movements, in distinction to the uni-directional movements of myoclonus and asterixis or the arrhythmic movements of tics and dyskinesias. Although focal motor seizures are rhythmic, they should not vary with limb movement. A reliable way to tell a rest tremor from an action tremor is to have the patient write a sentence (not the patient's name) and draw a large spiral (see Figure 81-2).

Action Tremor. Action tremor is brought on by voluntary movement of the limb. Action tremors classically worsen with caffeine and improve with alcohol but rebound afterward. Enhanced physiological tremor, a high-frequency low-amplitude action tremor, can be present in any situation that increases epinephrine (adrenaline), including exercise, hyperthyroidism, and use of stimulants. (Note that epinephrine worsens all types of tremor.) Enhanced physiological tremor rarely interferes with tasks and generally comes to medical attention only because the patient or doctor is anxious about it. Essential tremor, also called hereditary tremor, is coarser: lower frequency and higher amplitude. Drug tremors (e.g., from lithium or valproate) may be similarly coarse when severe. Both can cause significant functional impairment and fatigue. The most important disorder to distinguish from action tremor is dysmetria—incoordination from cerebellar pathway damage. Dysmetria, sometimes rather unhelpfully called an intention tremor, gets worse the closer the hand gets to a target and is associated with other cerebellar signs (such as ataxic gait or ocular nystagmus).

Dystonia. Dystonia is characterized by abnormal trunk or limb postures produced by the simultaneous sustained contracture of both agonist and antagonist muscles. It is occasionally very painful, especially in acute drug reactions.

Such acute reactions are usually treated with diphenhydramine. Acute dystonia greatly increases the risk of later extrapyramidal complications, including TD. Task-specific dystonias (such as writer's cramp) are often labeled as psychogenic because of their oddness (e.g., being able to type, but not to play the piano); however, they respond very well to Botox injections in the affected muscle.

Hyperkinetic Signs

Chorea and Athetosis. Apart from the briefest, most ballistic movements, most hyperkinetic movements feel semipurposive, and the patient can usually suppress them for brief periods. For this reason the abnormal movements may mistakenly seem psychogenic. Athetosis, a slow, writhing, nearly dystonic movement, rarely needs to be distinguished from the quicker movements of chorea and dyskinesias, as their causes and treatment are similar. Movements typically worsen during attempted voluntary action. Although choreoathetosis is often described as dance-like, it is rarely so. Dance-like chorea was common in Charcot's day, when the most common cause was tertiary syphilis or the hysterical chorea that imitated it (Figure 81-3). Common modern causes include lupus, pregnancy, Huntington's disease, Wilson's disease, and use of oral contraceptives or neuroleptics. Typical neuroleptics (e.g., haloperidol) generally suppress choreoathetosis but may eventually cause a tardive worsening of the hyperkinesis.

Dyskinesia. The distinction between dyskinesia and chorea is largely conventional, with "dyskinesia" usually reserved for drug-related reactions. The two major types are parkinsonian dyskinesia (from the administration of dopamine agonists to patients with chronically low endogenous dopamine) and TD (from long-term exposure to dopamine antagonists). Both are probably the result of dopamine receptor hypersensitivity. Dyskinesia's large movements usually look aimless but may feel semi-voluntary, as when a bipolar patient with oro-buccal TD describes moving her tongue to rid herself of an unpleasant mouth feeling.

Akathisia. Akathisia may also be caused by use of dopamine antagonists, but it usually occurs acutely rather than after chronic exposure. Its movements both feel and look voluntary—they are low amplitude and look restless. It is similar in look and feel to the fidgetiness of mania or of boredom. It is of great clinical importance because it is triggered by a highly uncomfortable desire to move constantly, a desire that may even drive violent action. Treating akathisia often requires discontinuation of the neuroleptic. While akathisia in some ways resembles restless leg syndrome, the latter is usually not drug-induced, happens primarily when the patient relaxes before sleep, and has a more distinctly sensory trigger—such as a feeling of limb "creepiness."

Tics. Tics are more intermittent than the hyperkinetic movements described so far. They are multi-focal, usually stereotyped, and repetitive. They are typically driven by a conscious urge to move or by a premonitory sensation, and they can often be suppressed briefly. Complex tics include gestures and vocalizations that may feel meaningful and goal-directed. Complex tics exist on a continuum with the compulsive behaviors of OCD, but people with tics often report a drive toward some sensory satisfaction rather than a drive away from a feared event. Simple tics (such as winks, sniffs, and shrugs) are common in the general population. The simplest tics (e.g., arm jerks) may feel involuntary and look myoclonic.

Myoclonus. Myoclonus is an intermittent, non-rhythmic ballistic jerk caused by a single muscle group, which promptly relaxes; it is involuntary. Myoclonus during sleep is normal, and may be generated from a source outside the basal ganglia. Asterixis is negative myoclonus: that is, a sudden lapse of tone with quick recovery. Both can be seen in encephalopathy, drug intoxication (especially with opiates), and neurodegenerative diseases. Hemiballism, a repetitive flinging movement of a limb, is quite rare; it usually arises after a subthalamic nucleus lesion.

Gait

Apart from neuroleptic malignant syndrome (NMS), the most dangerous movement disorders are those that affect gait and increase the risk of falls. Gait disorders are often multi-factorial.[7]

Table 81-1 describes movement disorders common in psychiatric patients, and Table 81-2 describes types of gait disorders. Balance is often impaired by hypokinetic movement disorders, in large part because patients cannot correct their posture quickly enough when they make a mis-step. This is quite different from ataxia, the poor balance caused by cerebellar lesions or anticonvulsant toxicity. Ataxia can give a wildly swaying gait, yet it paradoxically causes fewer falls. It is often associated with spinning vertigo, distinct from the light-headedness caused by a variety of medications, anxiety, and depression. One cause of gait disorder that surgery may—occasionally—cure is normal pressure hydrocephalus (NPH). Its cardinal symptoms include a parkinsonian gait, incontinence, and, eventually, dementia. Radiographically, NPH causes dilated ventricles with normal sulci, in distinction to the global atrophy more commonly seen with dementia (Figure 81-4). By the time dementia develops, symptoms are hardly ever reversible. In the absence of parkinsonism, incontinence, and the characteristic radiographic findings, dementia is virtually never caused by NPH.

MOVEMENT DISORDERS WITH PSYCHIATRIC SYMPTOMS
Hypokinetic Syndromes
Idiopathic Parkinson's Disease

True idiopathic Parkinson's disease classically causes the triad of bradykinesia, rigidity, and tremor, although tremor is not required for the diagnosis. A strong response to levodopa is universal. Parkinson's disease also may be associated with psychiatric problems, such as depression, dementia, and

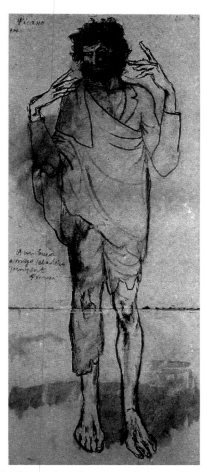

Figure 81-3. Choreoathetotic arm posturing in Picasso's Le Fol (1904). At the time of his painting, the most common causes of chorea were tertiary syphilis and hysteria. (© Succession Picasso/DACS, London 2014.)

TABLE 81-2 Types of Gait Disorder

	Description	Lesion Location	Typical Cause
Parkinsonian	Stoops, shuffles, slow, many falls	Basal ganglia	Parkinsonian syndromes, neuroleptics, NPH
Choreic	Postures, writhes, few falls	Basal ganglia	Dopaminergics, tardive dyskinesia, Huntington's
Ataxic	Wide-based, lurches, few falls	Cerebellum	Alcoholism, cerebellar stroke
Spastic	Stiff, circumducted leg, arm flexed	Corticospinal	Cortical stroke
Neuropathic	Steps high, foot slaps	Peripheral nerve	Diabetes, alcoholism, polio
Light-headedness	Sways when stands or turns quickly	Diffuse	Many drugs, ANS dysfunction, dehydration
Hysterical gait	Wild changes in balance but few falls	Frontoparietal	Conversion or somatization disorder

ANS, Autonomic nervous system; NPH, normal pressure hydrocephalus.

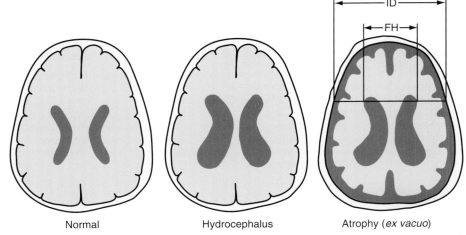

Normal   Hydrocephalus   Atrophy (*ex vacuo*)

Figure 81-4. Imaging of hydrocephalus and atrophy. In hydrocephalus, whether obstructive or normal pressure, ventricular volume increases out of proportion to volume of the sulci. The largest width of the frontal horns (FH) should be greater than half of the internal skull diameter (ID) in true hydrocephalus.

psychosis.[8] Parkinson's disease affects 3% of people over age 65 years and sometimes appears before age 40. It results from dopaminergic cell death and from Lewy body formation in the substantia nigra. People with mood disorders, especially atypical depression with its feeling of leaden paralysis, are at higher risk for Parkinson's disease.

In a patient who has been on antipsychotics, distinguishing idiopathic Parkinson's disease from drug-induced parkinsonism (from dopamine receptor blockade) is tricky. Often it is best to focus instead on which treatments can be used safely. The patient's neuroleptics should change to quetiapine, or, ideally, low-dose clozapine. The latter is under-used. Because dopamine agonists can cause hallucinations, parkinsonian patients at risk for psychosis typically receive an anticholinergic drug (e.g., benztropine) rather than a dopaminergic drug. Patients not taking neuroleptics have more options. The dopamine precursor levodopa, given with carbidopa to inhibit peripheral metabolism, is less likely to trigger hallucinations and somnolence than dopamine agonists like pramipexole, so levodopa is a better choice for patients over the age of 70. In the past, some doctors worried that levodopa can paradoxically hasten Parkinson's progression. There is little evidence for this. Long-acting dopamine agonists (such as pramipexole ER) have fewer side effects than their immediate-release formulations. Inhibitors of dopamine metabolism (e.g., entacapone and rasagiline) prolong levodopa action and typically have fewer side effects than the dopamine agonists. Rasagiline, like selegiline, is an MAO-B inhibitor. The danger of tyramine reactions or serotonin syndrome is much lower with MAO-B inhibitors than with MAO-A inhibitors (e.g., phenelzine).

"Parkinson's Personality". A personality characterized by conscientiousness, dysthymia, and a low rate of addictions may be seen in Parkinson's patients 10 to 20 years before motor symptoms are recognizable.[9] A higher rate of obsessive-compulsive personality disorder is also common. The baseline dopaminergic deficit of Parkinson's might explain the associated low novelty-seeking. High harm-avoidance has also been observed and may be secondary to a higher incidence of affective disorders.[10] Parkinson's personality is thought to be less common in early-onset patients who are more often cyclothymic.

Depression. About 30% of patients with Parkinson's disease have major depression.[11] Depressed mood is often less prominent than apathy, and patients may under-report their symptoms. Dopaminergic treatment alone may dramatically reduce depression in untreated Parkinson's disease. Although SSRIs are often prescribed, they sometimes worsen Parkinson's symptoms. Moreover, when paroxetine was compared head-to-head with nortriptyline in patients with Parkinson's disease, paroxetine had no benefit whereas nortriptyline was efficacious. Nortriptyline also helps the muscle pain common in Parkinson's patients. Bupropion can help apathy in Parkinson's depression. Mirtazapine can help with disordered sleep and anxiety, and it will not worsen tremor. In theory, the selegiline transdermal patch should help both depression and symptoms of Parkinson's disease, but it is rarely used. Electroconvulsive therapy (ECT) may improve both parkinsonian motor symptoms and depression. Some patients have pseudobulbar affect—a brainstem disinhibition of emotional expression with minimal mood changes that may be misdiagnosed as depression. It may respond to use of dextromethorphan/quinidine (Nuedexta) or selective serotonin reuptake inhibitors (SSRIs).

Treatment-induced Mood Lability and Mania. In advanced Parkinson's disease, medications wear off precipitously, and patients may need them every 2 to 3 hours. The off-phase can bring not only near-immobility, but, in some patients, panic and depressed mood. When the next dose of levodopa takes effect, the patient can become not only wildly dyskinetic but hypomanic and sometimes briefly psychotic. Longer-lasting therapies (such as pramipexole ER), reduce these fluctuations but can also cause a dopamine dysregulation syndrome (e.g., gambling, hypersexuality, binge eating).[12] Benzodiazepines may help off-state panic and sometimes decrease freezing, perhaps analogous to their effect on catatonia.

Dementia. Thirty percent of patients with true Parkinson's disease eventually demonstrate subcortical cognitive deficits including impaired attention, poor multi-tasking, and bradyphrenia (slowed thinking). Patients with subcortical cognitive problems, unlike those with the language and memory impairment of cortical dementia, can benefit from memory prompts and from strategies such as to-do lists. When cortical deficits in language and memory are present, it signals co-morbid Alzheimer's disease or Lewy body dementia. Levodopa and cholinergic agonists (e.g., rivastigmine) can help cognitive performance of both groups.

TABLE 81-5 *Somewhat* Reliable Clues That a Movement Disorder Is Psychogenic

Somewhat Reliable Clues to Somatization	Alternate Causes
HISTORY	
Abrupt onset	Stroke, Wilson's, encephalitis
Static course	Some dystonia
Many mysterious problems; "pan-yes" symptom list	SLE, Cushing's, or simply many illnesses
Presence of a model for symptoms	Hereditary, environmental, or infectious cause
Whole-body pain	Some dystonia or severe Parkinsonian rigidity
Spontaneous remissions (inconsistency over time)	Dystonias, tics, drug-induced symptoms
Precipitated by minor trauma	Post-traumatic vigilance for symptoms
Health care professional—including physicians	Coincidental
Pending litigation or compensation	Valid legal claim
Young woman	Somatization is under-diagnosed in men
EXAMINATION	
Inconsistent symptoms (amplitude, frequency, body part)	Tics, embellishment of neurological cause
Paroxysmal movement disorder	Hyperkalemic periodic paralysis, etc.
Movements decrease with distraction	Tics, some tremors, embellishment
Suggestion triggers symptoms (e.g., with tuning fork)	Dystonia, coincidental suggestibility
Self-inflicted injuries	Tourette's syndrome, Lesch-Nyhan syndrome
Functional disability out of proportion to examination findings	Dystonia
Bizarre symptoms, hard to classify	For example, Wilson's, thalamic lesions, dystonia
Over-dramatization	Dystonia, frontal disinhibition in MS
More than three stuffed animals in patient's hospital bed	Lonely chronically ill patient
Says "I have a high pain threshold" but cries at needle stick	Coincident opiate dependence or PTSD
TREATMENT RESPONSE	
Unresponsive to appropriate medications	Some tremors, dystonia
More than three odd drug "allergies" (e.g., "Tylenol causes coma")	Hypervigilance in chronically ill patient
Permanent response to placebo or suggestion	Parkinson's, dystonia have temporary response
Remission with psychotherapy	For example, decreased stress can decrease Parkinson's

MS, Multiple sclerosis; PTSD, post-traumatic stress disorder; SLE, systemic lupus erythematosus.

TABLE 81-6 MADISON Scale for Emotional Overlay

M	Multiplicity	Symptoms appear in several body parts or are of many types.
A	Authenticity	The patient is more interested in your belief that the symptom is real than he or she is in receiving a cure for it.
D	Denial	The patient denies the presence of emotional problems or paints a rosy picture in the face of chaos.
I	Interpersonal interactions	Complaints of symptoms or grimaces arise when the name of someone is mentioned; symptom changes with its interpersonal context.
S	Singularity	A patient complains of a singular and unusual symptom: "You've never seen a symptom like mine before."
O	"Only you"	"Only you can help me, Doctor." Placing the treating physician on a pedestal is an ominous sign.
N	Nothing helps	The patient typically reports that the symptom does not fluctuate from hour to hour, or day to day, or, it only worsens.

TABLE 81-7 Potential Treatments for Co-morbid Somatic and Psychosomatic Symptoms

Co-morbid Conditions		Treatment Suggestions
Pain	Depression	Duloxetine, perhaps a TCA
	Somatization	Duloxetine
	Mood lability, mania	ACDs (e.g., divalproex)
Fatigue	Medication side effects	Modafinil
	Anxiety	SNRIs (venlafaxine, duloxetine)
	Apathy	Dextroamphetamine, bupropion
	Depression + sleepiness	Bupropion, venlafaxine
	Depression + insomnia	Mirtazapine, paroxetine
Action tremor	Depression	Mirtazapine, change offending medications
	Bipolar	Change offending medications
Depression	Abulia (frontal)	Bupropion, dextroamphetamine
	Delirium, dementia	Citalopram, trazodone
	Parkinsonism	Bupropion, mirtazapine
	Seizures	SSRIs, lamotrigine
	Stroke	Citalopram
	Vertigo	Fluoxetine

ACDs, Anticonvulsant drugs; SNRIs, serotonin-norepinephrine reuptake inhibitors; SSRIs, selective serotonin reuptake inhibitors; TCA, tricyclic antidepressant.

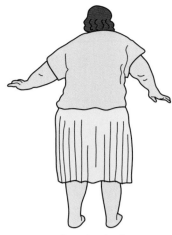

Astasia-abasia
(hysterical unsteadiness)

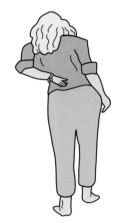

Ostentatiously antalgic gait

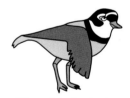

Plover feigning broken wing

Figure 81-8. Abnormal movements can be gestural communications. *(Adapted from Morris JG, et al. Psychogenic gait. In Hallett M, Fahn S, Jankovic J, et al, editors.* Psychogenic movement disorders: neurology and neuropsychology, *Philadelphia, 2006, Lippincott.)*

their symptom is not from depression—not "all in my head." Often the antidepressant failed because of a brief trial terminated by side effects. In a patient whose depression or anxiety is on the bipolar spectrum, the antidepressant may have worsened the patient's agitation. But whatever the cause of the failure, this creates a nocebo effect, in which future trials of similar treatment can fail simply because of the patient's negative expectation. One approach to circumventing this is to work hard to convince the patient to complete a long treatment trial of the new medicine, since placebo and nocebo effects are generally transient. A second approach is to present a new treatment as significantly different in kind (e.g., a patch rather than oral delivery, or for pain rather than depression), so that the patient's expectations are less negative.

Because most psychiatric medications have neurological indications as well, treatments can serve a dual function and can be presented as having a medical indication that is acceptable to the patient. Table 81-7 lists a number of drugs that may be helpful in this regard. Drugs like duloxetine can be useful for somatic anxiety as well as pain. Keep in mind, though, that bipolar patients are significantly more likely than unipolar patients to have somatic symptoms of their mood disorder. In such patients, it is better to use gabapentin or lamotrigine for pain. Fatigue is an important and often neglected aspect of many psychogenic syndromes. Patients' excessive use of caffeine may not only worsen their anxiety and cause somatic symptoms (e.g., tachycardia or tremor) but also worsen their fatigue through caffeine's rebound hypersomnolence. Modafinil can sometimes help patients wean from caffeine.

Functional imaging evidence for right frontoparietal hyperactivity in conversion disorder suggests that transcranial magnetic stimulation (TMS) over this region may help somatization. This technique is non-invasive and has few side effects. There are preliminary reports of its effectiveness for hysterical hemiparesis, PTSD, and somatization.[26] Much more investigation of these very early results is needed.

Access the complete reference list and multiple choice questions (MCQs) online at https://expertconsult.inkling.com

KEY REFERENCES

2. Nakano K, Kayahara T, Tsutsumi T, et al. Neural circuits and functional organization of the striatum. *J Neurol* 247(Suppl. 5):V1–V15, 2000.
4. Kalia SK, Sankar T, Lozano AM. Deep brain stimulation for Parkinson's disease and other movement disorders. *Curr Opin Neurol* 26(4):374–380, 2013.
7. Snijders AH, van de Warrenburg BP, Giladi N, et al. Neurological gait disorders in elderly people: clinical approach and classification. *Lancet Neurol* 6:63–74, 2007.
8. Aarsland D, Emre M, Lees A, et al. Practice parameter: evaluation and treatment of depression, psychosis, and dementia in Parkinson disease (an evidence-based review): report of the quality standards subcommittee of the American Academy of Neurology. *Neurology* 68:80, author reply 81, 2007.
11. Costa F, Rosso A, Maultasch H, et al. Depression in Parkinson's disease: diagnosis and treatment. *Arq Neuropsiquiatr* 70(8):617–620, 2012.
12. Starkstein SE, Brockman S, Hayhow BD. Psychiatric syndromes in Parkinson's disease. *Curr Opin Psychiatry* 25(6):468–472, 2012.
13. Benecke R. Diffuse Lewy body disease-a clinical syndrome or a disease entity? *J Neurol* 250(Suppl. 1):139–142, 2003.
14. Cavanna AE, Termine C. Tourette syndrome. *Adv Exp Med Biol* 724:375–383, 2012.
15. Roessner V, Schoenefeld K, Buse J, et al. Pharmacological treatment of tic disorders and Tourette Syndrome. *Neuropharmacology* 68:143–149, 2013.
16. Hu SC, Frucht SJ. Emergency treatment of movement disorders. *Curr Treat Options Neurol* 9:103–114, 2007.
17. Khan SA, Mettu K, Raja F. The restless legs syndrome: diagnosis and treatment. *Mo Med* 103:518–522, 2006.
20. Margolese HC, Chouinard G, Kolivakis TT, et al. Tardive dyskinesia in the era of typical and atypical antipsychotics. Part 2: Incidence and management strategies in patients with schizophrenia. *Can J Psychiatry* 50:703–714, 2005.
23. Stone J, Carson A, Sharpe M. Functional symptoms and signs in neurology: assessment and diagnosis. *J Neurol Neurosurg Psychiatry* 76(Suppl. 1):i2–i12, 2005.

82 Psychiatric Manifestations of Traumatic Brain Disorder

Christopher Carter, PsyD, and Kaloyan S. Tanev, MD

KEY POINTS

- Complex deficits and disorders result from brain injuries and may evolve over time.

- Most of the recovery that occurs following traumatic brain injury (TBI) is seen within the first 2 years; however, there is high interpersonal variation in the rate of recovery and some people improve even 3–5 years after TBI; rehabilitation at any time after injury can lead to further improvement.

- Assessment and diagnosis are ongoing and require cooperation from the patient and the family; multiple sources of information help the assessment of current function.

- Choice of medication rests on patient goals, target symptoms, side-effect profiles, individual tolerance, and response to treatment.

- Psychotherapy is useful to manage the psychosocial reaction to cognitive, behavioral, and psychiatric impairments that follow TBI.

- Effective treatment of behavioral and psychiatric disturbance after TBI typically involves pharmacological, psychological, educational, and environmental intervention.

- Collaboration between providers, the patient, the patient's family, and community resources is imperative to help the patient optimally rehabilitate and re-integrate into their work and social environment.

OVERVIEW

The human brain can be injured in a variety of ways. Head trauma, vascular disorders, degenerative disorders, toxic exposure, infectious processes, neoplasms, anoxia, metabolic or endocrine disorders, and nutritional deficiencies can each damage neuroanatomical structures and alter neurological function. Closed head injury (or traumatic brain injury [TBI]) is the most common source of acquired brain injury.[1]

TBI, referred to as a "silent epidemic,"[2] is one of the leading causes of death and disability in the US[3]; nearly 1.7 million head injuries occur each year[2] and of these, approximately 52,000 people die from their injuries, 275,000 require hospitalization, and 1.365 million are treated and released from the Emergency Department (ED).[2,4] An unknown number of additional patients with TBI are never seen at the hospital.[5] Injury to the brain disrupts cognitive, physical, emotional, and behavioral functioning. Long-term outcome can range from complete recovery to severe impairments and disability.[6] While the majority of individuals who sustain a TBI recover, a sizable number of individuals sustain permanent neuropsychiatric disabilities each year[2]; physical, cognitive, behavioral, and emotional impairments result in substantial disability and cause significant stress within families.[3,7] Complications (e.g., suicide, divorce, chronic unemployment, economic strain, substance abuse) develop after TBI.[5] The consulting psychiatrist plays an important role in the evaluation and treatment of patients with TBI at all stages of recovery.

EPIDEMIOLOGY AND RISK FACTORS

Among the most common causes of TBI are falls (35.2%) and motor vehicle accidents (17.3%).[2] Having the head struck by, or against, an object (16.5%), being assaulted (10%), and other or unknown causes (21%) make up the remaining cases.[2] Men sustain a TBI at a rate 1.4 times higher than women and are hospitalized almost twice as frequently.[2] TBI occurs most often in children ≤4 years of age, followed by older adolescents (15–19 years of age).[2] The highest rates of hospitalization and death following TBI are found in adults over the age of 75.[2] Falls produce the most injuries for children younger than 15 years and for adults over the age of 55.[2] Motor vehicle accidents account for the most injuries among adolescents (aged 15–19) and adults, aged 20–55.[2] Earlier research has found that 56% of adults identified as having brain injuries had an elevated blood alcohol level (BAL) at the time of injury; 49% of them had a BAL at or above the legal level. Recurrent brain injury is common; the risk of a second injury is three times higher than it is for those in the general (non-injured) population.[4] Following a second injury, the risk for a third injury becomes nearly 10 times higher than the risk for an initial injury.[4] Finally, review of data from the U.S. National Health Interview, a national database used to estimate the incidence and features of persons with brain injury, found that the highest rates of injury occurred in families with the lowest income levels (Box 82-1).[4]

PATHOPHYSIOLOGY

TBI is a spectrum disorder. Damage can occur as a result of forces exerted on the brain at the time of injury, known as the primary injury,[1,8–11] and from subsequent physiological processes (such as swelling or hypoxia) triggered by the initial insult; the latter are classified as secondary injuries.[9–11] Damage can be focal, diffuse, or both. Focal damage is typically the result of a contusion or mass lesion.[8] Most often it arises from contact injuries (such as falls or blows to the head)[8] and results in skull fractures and hematomas (extradural, subarachnoid, subdural, or intracerebral hematomas).[8] Hematomas may develop at the point of contact and at a point contralateral to the point of contact (known as *coup–contrecoup contusion*).[1] Contusions are seen more frequently in the poles of the frontal lobes, the inferior aspects of the frontal lobes, the cortex above and below the operculum of the Sylvian fissures, the temporal poles, and the lateral and inferior aspects of the temporal lobes.[8] They may develop within minutes of the injury or evolve slowly over several hours or days. The presence of these contusions contributes to neuronal necrosis and to elevated intracranial pressure (ICP).[8,9,11] In addition to contusions, contact forces can result in small or complete tears at the pontomedullary junction, damage to any of the cranial nerves, damage to the hypothalamus or pituitary gland, and damage to blood vessels.[8,9] Moreover, there can be multiple areas of focal damage.

Diffuse damage involves multiple neurological structures. It is seen more frequently in injuries that involve rapid acceleration/deceleration or rotational forces.[1] Diffuse damage can also result from disruption of vascular function and from hypoxia.[8] Diffuse axonal injury (DAI), as an example, consists of microscopic traumatic axonal damage involving the whole brain, but it is found most commonly in white matter areas (subcortical frontal and temporal white matter, the corpus callosum, and brainstem).[8,11] It disrupts cellular function and structures. While DAI is triggered by the mechanical forces of the original injury, it evolves over several hours to days.[8,11] Because this damage occurs at a microscopic level and evolves over time, DAI is often missed on computed tomography (CT) scans, particularly if it is performed in the ED.[1] It is more easily identified with magnetic resonance imaging (MRI), where the signature axonal swelling and axonal bulbs can be seen more readily, particularly if the brain is imaged several days after the injury.[1] Even with MRI, however, the absence of significant findings on radiological imaging does not mean that damage has not taken place.[9] Newer techniques, such as diffusion tensor imaging (DTI), susceptibility-weighted imagining (SWI), positron emission tomography (PET) scans, functional magnetic resonance imaging (fMRI), and high angular resolution diffusion imaging (HARDI), many of which are available only through academic research facilities, are helping to identify structural and functional changes following TBI more accurately.[12] Continued research involving the identification of characteristic biomarkers, such as elevations in cytokines, adipokines, chemokines associated with inflammation, markers of astrocyte activation, neuronal injury, or oxidative stress following injury, holds the promise of more accurate diagnosis of brain injury, particularly in the case of mild TBI.[13]

In addition to the primary injuries, further damage can occur as a result of complications associated with TBI (known as secondary injury).[1,11] Hematomas develop as a result of the hemorrhaging from torn blood vessels. Edema develops when there is an increase in inter- and/or intracellular water concentration due to direct mechanical forces or changes in cell permeability.[10,11] Since the skull of adults is fixed and unable to expand, hematomas and edema raise the intracranial pressure (ICP), which leads to further neurological damage as the surrounding (softer) structures become deformed. The pressure can push the brain through the base of the skull, with resulting damage to the brainstem.[1] When the brain's vascular system is compressed, the blood flow is restricted, resulting in ischemic damage.[10,11] Compromised cardio-pulmonary function, as either a direct result of brain damage or the structural damage sustained in the initial multi-organ trauma, can lead to hypoxic injury. Hyper-release of catecholamines following TBI can produce transient hypertension, as well as changes in glucose, cortisol, and thyroid hormones, which further disrupts neurological function.[11] Massive releases of excitatory amino acids (such as glutamate or aspartate) from injured brain cells act as cytotoxins, damaging neighboring cells, and unleashing a cascade of autodestructive events that can continue for hours or days after the original injury.[14] Inflammatory mechanisms, such as activated macrophages and microglia, may also contribute to the enlargement of the initial injury over days to weeks.[15] Focal contusions can produce seizures (that convey the severity of the injury in that

they are seen more frequently following a severe injury than with a moderate or mild injury).[11]

TBI resulting from exposure to explosions has come to be known as the signature injury for soldiers returning from Iraq and Afghanistan due to the frequent use of improvised explosive devices (IEDs) affecting 10%–20% of returning veterans. The explosion generates a blast wave that causes direct and indirect injury. Direct injury results from the pressure wave (with fluid-filled structures being the most sensitive), from objects or shrapnel propelled by the blast, from the body being thrown against solid objects, and from exposure to burns and noxious gases.[16] The above physical forces can produce skull fractures, cerebral edema, increased ICP, contusions, hemorrhages and shearing injuries to the brain. Brain injury also results indirectly from injury-generated air emboli that reach the brain[17] and from increased cerebral vasoconstriction and activation of platelets/leukocytes, which may exacerbate the primary effects of the brain injury.[18] Due to the nature of the combat theater and deployment rotations, there is a high risk of repeated exposure to subsequent blasts, particularly when the brain is still recovering from the prior exposure. Exposure to blasts during this period of increased vulnerability can result in more severe injuries.[19]

The brain's plasticity, or neuroplasticity, produces structural and organizational changes that result in recovery of function.[20] The hippocampus retains the ability to generate new neurons from progenitor cells in the dentate gyrus.[20] Surviving cortical structures take over the function of damaged areas.[20] Other adaptive and restorative processes include changes in the amount of neurotransmitters released, the number and distribution of post-synaptic receptors, the size and complexity of the dendritic trees of spared neurons, and the collateral sprouting of spared axons to innervate de-afferented neurons.[20] These processes depend on purposeful and active interactions with the environment.[20] Unfortunately, they are not well regulated, and can lead to maladaptive, as well as to beneficial, changes.[20] While they are responsible for restoring function, they can result in dysfunctional behaviors and psychiatric disorders. In the case of mild TBI, symptoms will usually resolve within 6 months of their injury.[21,22] In the case of moderate-to-severe TBI, the greatest amount of recovery typically takes place in the first 1–2 years following injury.[1] Recovery can continue, however, at an increasingly slower pace for many years following the injury.[3,6,20]

TBI is typically classified as mild, moderate, or severe (Table 82-1) based primarily on the duration of altered mental status (including the degree of responsiveness, as measured by the Glasgow Coma Scale [GCS], and the duration of disrupted memory). These terms can be misleading as they reflect the degree of damage the brain has sustained; they do not necessarily reflect the severity of the disruption in the patient's daily functioning. Individuals with a severe injury can make essentially full recovery while others with mild-to-moderate injuries can remain significantly disabled for many years. The GCS, developed by Teasdale and Jennett, assigns points for increasingly complex levels of response to three dimensions (verbal and motor response and eye opening); the ratings in each

TABLE 82-1 Classification of Traumatic Brain Injury

	Mild	Moderate	Severe
Loss of consciousness	<30 minutes*	30 minutes to 24 hours	>24 hours
Post-traumatic amnesia	<24 hours	1–24 hours	>24 hours
Glasgow Coma Scale	13–15	9–12	3–8

*Any alteration in mental state at the time of the accident.

TABLE 82-2 Glasgow Coma Scale

Category	Score
Eye Opening	
Spontaneous	4
To voice	3
To painful stimulus	2
None	1
Verbal Response	
Oriented	5
Confused	4
Inappropriate words	3
Unintelligible sounds	2
None	1
Motor Response	
Follows commands	6
Localizes pain	5
Withdraws from pain	4
Flexor response	3
Extensor response	2
None	1

TABLE 82-3 Symptoms of Mild Traumatic Brain Injury

Physical	Cognitive	Behavior
Nausea	Decreased attention	Irritability
Vomiting	Decreased concentration	Quick to anger
Dizziness	Problems with	Disinhibition
Headaches	perception	Emotional lability
Blurred vision	Problems with memory	
Increased sensitivity	Problems with speech	
to noise or light	production	
Diminished libido	Problems with speech	
Disturbed sleep	comprehension	
Quickness to fatigue	Executive dysfunction	
Lethargy		
Sensory loss		

domain are totaled to produce an overall score that can range from 3 to 15 (Table 82-2). Ratings can also be done serially to provide a measure of recovery. GCS scores have been predictive of ultimate outcome, with lower initial scores being associated with more severe injury and worse recovery.[1,4]

Mild TBI, also described as a concussion,[21,22] may not show up on a CT scan, on a conventional MRI and/or an electroencephalogram (EEG). Where there are positive radiological findings, the injury is classified as a complicated mild TBI. Performance on a routine neurological examination, which tends to focus on sensorimotor function, may be essentially normal, although performance may represent a decline relative to pre-injury performance.[21-23] Acute symptoms may persist for varying lengths of time. Physical symptoms often include nausea, vomiting, dizziness, headaches, blurred vision, an increased sensitivity to noise and light, diminished libido, disturbed sleep, quickness to fatigue, lethargy, or sensory loss (Table 82-3).[9] Cognitive deficits typically involve attention, concentration, perception, memory, speech/language, or executive functions.[9,24,25] These cognitive deficits are best identified through an in-depth neuropsychological evaluation. Behavior changes, such as irritability, quickness to anger, disinhibition, or emotional lability, may follow.[9,25] Symptoms generally resolve within 6 months of the injury. Physical, cognitive, emotional, and behavioral symptoms that cannot be accounted for by other peripheral injuries, or one's emotional state or psychological reaction to physical or emotional stressors, can persist.[23] Repeated exposure to mild TBI, such as seen in athletes with repeated concussions or soldiers with repeated blast exposures, can have a cumulative effect

and it has been associated with the development of chronic traumatic encephalopathy (CTE). CTE typically occurs after many years with varying symptoms, ranging from mild cognitive complaints to dementia, parkinsonian symptoms, and behavioral changes.[23]

While neurological damage can occur without loss of consciousness (LOC), LOC is considered a hallmark of most TBI. The duration of lost consciousness generally reflects the severity of injury. The longer the duration, the more severe the injury and more guarded the prognosis for recovery. No single pattern of recovery follows a brain injury,[3,6,20] as there are many variables involved (e.g., the location and extent of injury, the patient's age and overall health, the presence of alcohol, the medical and psychological history, concurrent processes [such as infections or seizures], availability of appropriate rehabilitation services and supports).

CLINICAL FEATURES

No single profile characterizes the presentation of TBI. A patient's profile is the result of the location, depth, and volume of focal lesions and the extent of diffuse axonal injury. Age, previous injury, use of alcohol, co-morbid conditions (such as hypoxia or hypertension) further contribute to the specific collection of deficits observed.[25] Generally speaking, cognitive deficits, personality and behavioral changes, and psychiatric disorders follow TBI. The domains of attention, memory, language, and executive function are typically affected. Since they are somewhat hierarchical, deficits in more fundamental areas (such as attention) can limit performance in higher-level tasks of executive function. Day-to-day and within-day performance can vary considerably.[26]

COGNITIVE IMPAIRMENT (TABLE 82-4)

Impaired attention is one of the most common deficits associated with TBI involving the reticular activating system and the prefrontal or connecting white matter.[25] Individuals with attentional difficulties report decreased concentration, being unable to follow conversations in a group setting (where they need to focus on the conversation in which they are interested and screen out other simultaneously occurring conversations), losing track of what they are reading, being distractible, being unable to do more than one thing at a time, and being unable to sustain attention.[1,25] Reduced speed of information processing, while not strictly an attention deficit, is the most notable consequence after mild TBI[27]; it limits the amount of information that can be processed, the ability to respond quickly, and the ability to complete tasks within traditional time frames.

Impaired memory is also common following TBI.[28] The duration of post-traumatic amnesia (PTA), the inability to recall information presented after the accident, correlates with the severity of one's injury. While some patients have a period of retrograde amnesia (i.e., the inability to recall information acquired before the trauma), problems with acquiring, storing, and retrieving new information are more common.[28] Memory is not a unitary construct; there are different forms of memory that may be affected to differing degrees depending on the nature and the location of injury.[1,28] Because different neuroanatomical structures are involved with these various forms, there is typically sparing of some forms of memory. Procedural memory (i.e., memory for motor sequences that occurs outside of conscious awareness) is typically less affected than is memory for more language-based or visual information.[1,28] This also means that there is not a specific profile of memory deficit associated with TBI. Declarative memory (i.e., the ability to recall events [episodic memory] and specific facts [semantic memory]) is more vulnerable to damage because of the active

TABLE 82-4 Cognitive Changes

Impaired Attention	Impaired Memory	Language Deficits	Executive Dysfunction
Basic arousal	Post-traumatic amnesia	Word-finding	Setting and attaining goals
Selective attention	Retrograde amnesia	Decreased fluidity	Initiating and monitoring behavior
Sustained attention	Acquisition, storage, and	Dysarthria	Inhibiting competing impulses
Divided attention	retrieval of new information	Receptive aphasia	Correcting behavior in response to feedback
Span of attention	Prospective memory	Expressive aphasia	Error recognition
Speed of processing	Working memory	Anomic aphasia	Insight and empathy
	Procedural memory	Paraphasic errors	Decision-making
	Kinesthetic memory	Circumlocution	Perseveration
	Episodic memory	Paucity of speech	Rigidity
	Declarative memory		
	Prospective memory		
	Semantic memory		
	Confabulation		

processes involved. Encoding, consolidating, and retrieving new information involve a degree of effortful, controlled, and generally conscious processing.[25] Much of this activity appears to involve the hippocampus, as well as the prefrontal, temporal, and frontal structures. The hippocampus is particularly vulnerable to damage from TBI.[28] The prefrontal and frontal areas, such as the dorsolateral prefrontal and orbitofrontal cortices, due to their anatomic location and their proximity to orbital cranial structures, are especially vulnerable to contusions and hematoma formation.[23,25] The ability to retrieve old or previously-learned information typically returns before the ability to acquire new information. For a period of time amnestic individuals may confabulate,[1] or generate false memories, which can be problematic as they can be indistinguishable from "real memories." False memories typically have elements of truth embedded within them, as people involved in the memories may actually exist or events recalled may really have happened. The memories, however, contain significant distortions. The affected individual may recall a visit the day before from a friend who has been dead for many years, or may report returning from a trip the day before that had taken place a number of years ago. Confabulation is distinguished from delusional thought in that the confabulation is often more isolated, less organized, and often more transient than delusions. It typically resolves as the patient's overall memory improves. The ability to recall new information typically takes more time to resolve and may be a persistent or permanent deficit.[25,28] Acquisition, storage, and retrieval of new information are procedures that involve attention, sensory function, language, and executive function. Deficits in any of these areas limit the acquisition of new learning. Even in individuals with mild TBI, new learning is less efficient, requiring more effort and time than was required before the injury.[25,28] This inefficiency and increased effort makes it harder for an individual to sustain performance relative to pre-injury levels.

Impaired language results from damage to frontal and temporal areas. The nature of the deficits will depend on the location and extent of the injury.[29] Disruption of language (both receptive and expressive) occurs more frequently after moderate-to-severe injuries than after mild TBI, where disturbances tend to be limited to difficulties with word-finding and with decreased fluidity when speaking. Global aphasia (total loss of both receptive and expressive language) is relatively rare. More common are specific aphasic syndromes, such as anomic aphasia (in which an individual presents with difficulty naming specific objects and proper names), paraphasic errors (in which incorrect words are substituted for the intended word), and circumlocution (in which the individual talks around the missing word describing or demonstrating the missing word). In addition to these primary language impairments, patients with TBI tend to generate less speech,

TABLE 82-5 Personality and Behavioral Changes Associated With Traumatic Brain Injury

Aggression	Need for immediate gratification
Apathy	Mood lability
Withdrawal	Erratic and difficult to predict
Lack of goal-directed activity	temper outbursts and mood swings
Lack of empathy	Abnormal jocularity
Distractible	Irritability and reduced tolerance for frustration
Difficulty learning from mistakes	Disinhibition
Impulsivity	

are less efficient in their discourse, and have more trouble managing the interpersonal pragmatics of speech (such as taking turns, maintaining a topic of conversation, taking a listener's perspective, and interpreting the non-verbal elements of communication).[25,29]

Finally, **impaired executive functions** can be seen at all levels of TBI. These skills are the functions of the frontal lobes and their projections, which are particularly prone to injury.[30] Executive function encompasses those skills needed to operate independently in the world (i.e., to identify goals, to plan, and to organize behavior to meet those goals). They involve initiating and monitoring behavior, inhibiting competing impulses or behaviors, and correcting behavior in response to feedback. They are essential for self-determination, self-direction, and self-regulation. Problems with regulation of attention, working memory, insight and empathy, verbal fluency, decision-making, perseveration, and flexibility frequently follow damage to the frontal lobes.[1,31]

PERSONALITY AND BEHAVIORAL CHANGES

In many respects the changes in behavior and personality that follow TBI, particularly when there is frontal lobe involvement, are more disabling than are the cognitive changes (Table 82-5).[1,32] They limit an individual's ability to participate in therapy. They are a source of significant stress on families and caretakers.[32] They can prevent the individual from returning home and returning to work.[33] The individual may appear to move about aimlessly, become preoccupied with seemingly trivial matters, or perseverate on topics or concerns in an obsessional manner. They may fail to be aware of, or take in, information from the environment or to alter their behavior in response to feedback. As a result they may have difficulty learning from their mistakes. Because of deficits in executive function, several tasks become difficult. Looking ahead and anticipating the implications or consequences of one's actions becomes difficult following frontal lobe damage; this can interfere with participation in therapy as the individual fails to grasp the long-term benefits of treatment in the absence of more immediate gratification. Deficits in the modulation of affect, self-awareness, and self-monitoring result in socially-inappropriate behaviors. Temper outbursts and mood swings, often dysphoric in nature, are common after temporal lobe damage.[1] Flat affect and indifference, belligerence and aggression, childishness, euphoria and abnormal jocularity, irritability and reduced tolerance for frustration, disinhibition, and lack of empathy may arise, interfering with normal social relationships.[34] Individuals have difficulty identifying and initiating activities that foster social interaction. Previously active people will be content to sit and watch television for hours on end. Individuals may begin to avoid social gatherings because the demands of selectively attending, shifting attention, self-monitoring, comprehending language, and emotive expression are overwhelming. They may become irritable and aggressive when feeling overwhelmed by these cognitive demands. All of these deficits are subject to the effects of fatigue and environmental variables (such as supportive structure, level of sensory stimulation, and degree of familiarity). Others see the individual's behavior as erratic and difficult to predict. Social isolation becomes common as friends and even family withdraw as a result of behaviors that are disruptive, embarrassing, or dangerous. The burden these behaviors place on families who are already stressed by changes in financial resources and the demands of physical care and increased dependence can be enormous.[1]

Aggressive behavior is perhaps the most disruptive of the behavioral changes observed after TBI. Agitated, combative, disinhibited behavior is common during the initial stages of post-traumatic delirium.[35] Agitated behavior at this stage tends to be reactive in nature, and often arises in response to seemingly minor or trivial stimuli. It is neither planned nor serves a purpose other than to eliminate the source of irritation. The behavior is often explosive and occurs with little build-up or warning. Brief outbursts alternate with long periods of calm. When the individual is aware of his or her behavior, he or she is often upset or embarrassed by their behavior.[36] Early agitation tends to resolve as cognition improves.

Agitated and aggressive behavior can persist beyond the acute phase of recovery; it has been observed following severe TBI in 31%–71% of cases studied and in 5%–71% of cases involving mild TBI.[35,36] Aggressive behavior has been associated with damage to the inferior orbital surface of the frontal lobes, the anterior temporal lobes, the hypothalamus, and limbic structures.[35,36] Changes in neurotransmitter levels (particularly serotonin, norepinephrine [noradrenaline], dopamine, acetylcholine, and GABA) have been associated with impulsive and aggressive behavior.[35–37] A pre-injury history of psychiatric illness, attention deficit disorder (ADD), aggressive behavior, poor social function, and alcohol and drug abuse have been identified as risk factors for aggressive behavior following TBI.[35–37]

Aggressive behavior may also occur as a result of a mood disorder, psychosis, or seizure disorder,[36,38] although aggressive behavior occurring in the context of seizure disorders can take different forms.[36] Ictal or post-ictal behavior tends to be less focused or directed and is accompanied by an altered level of consciousness. Following the outburst the individual is likely to express regret and remorse when informed about the behavior. Inter-ictal aggression tends to be more directed and less ego-dystonic. Delirium resulting from hypoxia, electrolyte imbalance, metabolic disorders, dehydration, or infection can trigger aggressive behavior.[36] Drugs and medications can produce aggressive behavior. Alcohol, barbiturates, benzodiazepines, analgesics, steroids, antidepressants, amphetamines,

---

BOX 82-2 Psychiatric Disorders Associated With Traumatic Brain Injury

Major depression
Alcohol abuse/dependence
Panic disorder
Specific phobias
Generalized anxiety
PTSD
OCD
Psychotic Disorders
Personality Disorders
  Avoidant
  Paranoid
  Schizoid

---

antipsychotics, and anticholinergic drugs can contribute to sedation and to disinhibition as well as irritability and aggression.[36] Aggressive behavior may be unwittingly reinforced by the response of others to the behavior. For instance, increased attention or the withdrawal of unpleasant demands following aggressive behaviors may increase, or maintain, aggressive behavior.

PSYCHIATRIC DISORDERS

Psychiatric disorders, particularly mood disorders, are found more frequently in individuals with TBI than they are in the general population; they are associated with longer recovery time, worse outcomes, and higher mortality rates as compared to those who have suffered a TBI, but without psychiatric disturbances.[1,39–42] Koponen and colleagues[43] found that 48% of patients developed an Axis I disorder (most commonly major depression, alcohol abuse or dependence, panic disorder, specific phobias, and psychotic disorder) after TBI (Box 82-2). Roughly one-fourth of the patients developed an Axis II personality disorder (avoidant, paranoid, or schizoid) after the injury.

Depression is the most common psychiatric disorder observed after TBI, with a frequency rate ranging from 26% to 77%.[44] Presence of depression is associated with poor psychosocial outcome, increased psychological distress, and a greater number and intensity of perceived post-injury symptoms.[45] Depression may develop acutely within the first month of the injury,[46,47] or have a delayed onset.[46] It may develop as a result of neurotransmitter changes linked with structural damage or in response to improved insight and awareness of the multiple changes and losses from the injury. Symptoms may resolve within the first 6 months[46] or may persist for many years.[48] Depression after TBI is associated with anxiety (77%), aggressive behavior (57%)[49] fatigue (29%), distractibility (28%), anger or irritability (28%) and rumination (25%).[50] Depression has not been associated with the severity of injury or with cognitive impairment. A pre-injury history of substance abuse, worse pre-morbid social function, less than a high school education, and an unstable work history predict depression post-TBI.[46,47] Individuals with TBI should be considered at greater risk for depression as a reaction to the loss of capabilities and competencies, changes in social supports, capacity for work, increased financial and medical concerns, loss of role and income, and decreased quality of life.[51] In addition to these psychosocial factors, depression is associated with the neurophysiological changes and changes in neurotransmitter levels that follow TBI. While no single structure is responsible for the development of depression, depression during the

TABLE 82-6 Risk Factors for Suicide Following Traumatic Brain Injury

Depression	Cognitive and motor disturbances
Profound feelings of hopelessness, despair, worthlessness	Emotional lability
Loss of sense of integrity	Impulsivity
Prior history of suicide attempt	Inflexibility
Male	Hyperactivity
Mid-adolescence to mid-twenties	Poor problem-solving
Lower socioeconomic level	Inability to identify alternatives
Drug or alcohol use	Heightened aggression and hostility
Cluster B personality disorder	Relationship breakdown
	Social isolation

acute stage of recovery has been closely associated with damage to left frontal and basal ganglia regions.[46]

Individuals with TBI are at higher risk for thoughts of suicide, suicide attempts, and suicide.[40,51,52] TBI and suicide share risk factors: age (mid-adolescence to mid-twenties); gender (males more than females); lower socioeconomic level; presence of drug or alcohol use; and psychological disturbance (Table 82-6).[51] Key features of TBI (such as cognitive and motor disturbances, emotional lability and impulsivity, rigidity and hyperactivity, poor problem-solving, inability to identify alternatives, heightened aggression, and hostility) increase the risk for suicide. Individuals with TBI who have attempted suicide have not differed significantly from suicide attempters without TBI in terms of age of first suicide attempt, suicidal ideation, suicidal intent, number of attempts, or maximum lethality.[40] When comparing attempters with non-attempters, Oquendo and co-workers[40] found that those who attempted suicide had higher levels of aggression and hostility, were more likely to have a substance abuse history, and were more likely to have a Cluster B personality disorder than non-attempters. Presence of profound feelings (of hopelessness, despair, worthlessness, loss of sense of integrity), relationship breakdown, and problems with isolation, contribute to the risk for suicide.[51,52]

Evaluating patients with a history of TBI for depression is complicated by the fact that the neurovegetative signs of depression (e.g., sleep disturbance, changes in appetite, anhedonia, loss of libido) occur frequently as a result of TBI. At the same time, deficits in self-awareness can interfere with an individual's ability to identify symptoms of depression.[46,53] Depression must be distinguished from an adjustment disorder, post-traumatic stress disorder (PTSD), organic apathy, and emotional lability. Pathological laughing or crying, which can occur with focal prefrontal lesions, occurs suddenly, uncontrollably, and may or may not be mood congruent, but is recognized by the individual as disproportionate to the mood or precipitating stimuli. Such an individual tends to have more anxiety, aggression, and worse social functioning than an individual without this syndrome. Apathy (marked by lack of motivation, absence of emotional reaction, and difficulty with initiation of actions) frequently follows frontal lobe damage. Apathy can co-occur with depression.[46]

The diagnosis of depression is more convincing when the psychological symptoms of depression (e.g., presence of depressed affect, irritability, ruminations, feelings of hopelessness and worthlessness, and having difficulty enjoying activities) are manifest. These factors may distinguish depressed from non-depressed patients following TBI.[47,48,54,55] Depression should be diagnosed via a semi-structured or structured psychiatric interview. Since cognitive deficits (involving awareness, memory, self-monitoring, expression, and language

comprehension) are frequently present, information from family and caretakers is invaluable.

Anxiety disorders are found at all stages of recovery: immediately following the injury, during the post-acute phase, and in those who have persistent problems. Generalized anxiety disorder (GAD), panic attacks, obsessive-compulsive disorder (OCD), simple phobias, acute stress disorder, and Post Traumatic Stress Disorder (PTSD) have all been observed following TBI.[56] For most of the disorders, the presence or severity of the anxiety disorder has not been associated with the severity of injury. The exception to this is PTSD, in which an inverse relationship has been observed (i.e., PTSD is more likely in individuals with a mild TBI than it is in individuals with severe TBI).[56] Anxiety is frequently accompanied by depression and by alcohol dependence. Anxious patients experience higher levels of functional disability and report higher levels of injury and cognitive impairment.[56,57]

Anxiety may develop in the early stages of recovery when the individual has trouble with simple, previously automatic tasks (such as dressing and bathing) or sees significant decline in areas that were particular strengths (due to the cognitive and functional changes that have taken place). The immediate environment becomes unfamiliar and unpredictable as a consequence of problems with memory and information processing. The individual loses a sense of competence and confidence in their ability to control their immediate environment. Given the sudden and traumatic nature of the injury an increased sense of vulnerability, as well as fears about further injury or increased fears about loved ones getting injured, are not uncommon. Fears arise regarding the permanence of their deficits and their ability to return to previous roles and activities. Avoidance behaviors may develop. Somatic conditions (e.g., vertigo, headaches, complex partial seizures) that frequently accompany TBI may be interpreted by the individual as symptoms of anxiety. Alcohol withdrawal may be mistaken for primary anxiety. At the same time, anxiety may develop as a result of damage to the temporal lobes, the frontal lobe pathways connecting to the caudate nucleus, the hippocampus, and the amygdala. Increases or dysregulation of circulating cortisol or catecholamines may produce primary anxiety.[57] Damage to the orbitofrontal cortex, anterior cingulate, and the caudate nucleus has been associated with the development of OCD. Orbitofrontal, cingulate, and medial temporal cortical areas, which are frequently damaged in TBI, have been associated with panic attacks.[57]

OCD occurs after TBI at rates (0.5%–7.8%) similar to those for the general population.[58] Unfortunately, research has focused on single cases or small group studies, which limits what is known about the impact of demographic variables, the severity of TBI, or co-morbidity. Fully developed OCD following TBI in the absence of pre-injury OCD is rare.[58] In diagnosing OCD following TBI, it is important to appreciate the role that cognitive dysfunction may play in the development of obsessions and compulsive or ritualistic behaviors. The rituals may be an effort to compensate for poor memory and problem-solving ability. The slowness, indecisiveness, and avoidance may reflect a realistic appraisal, based on their post-injury experiences, of the individual's ability to carry out tasks accurately and independently and to make good decisions.

PTSD following TBI often occurs in the context of a traumatic, life-threatening event (such as combat, a motor vehicle accident, or assault). While there is debate as to whether patients with amnesia for the traumatic event go on to develop PTSD (with its hallmark of re-experiencing of the original trauma), PTSD following severe TBI is well documented even in cases where the individual has no explicit or episodic memory of the event.[56,57,59] In cases where there is amnesia for the trauma, the individual may be less likely to have intrusive

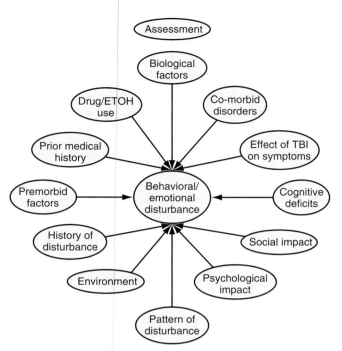

Figure 82-1. Assessment of the behavioral and emotional changes following traumatic brain injury.

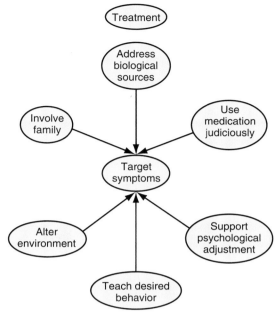

Figure 82-2. Treatment of emotional and behavioral disturbances following traumatic brain injury.

describes the behavior in objective measurable terms and the environmental response to the behavior or consequences of the behavior. This approach considers the individual's learning history (pre- and post-injury), the individual's cognitive and behavioral repertoire, the social and environmental context of the behavior, and sources of intended and unintended reinforcement for the behavior.

In the end, the psychiatric assessment aims to generate an understanding of the time-line of the development of psychiatric symptoms relative to: the nature of the TBI; changes in affect, behavior, and cognition; the contribution of pre-injury personality on post-injury behavior; and the interface between the injury and the psychiatric symptoms (Figure 82-1). The goal is not only to identify which symptoms are present but also to understand how these symptoms interact with each other and interfere with the individual's efforts to re-integrate into the world around them.

TREATMENT

The event that causes TBI usually lasts seconds, but the impact on the individual's life is lifelong. People who have sustained a TBI may have difficulties with ADLs, walking, speaking, concentrating, planning, as well as with memory, communication, and work. The goals of successful rehabilitation are to restore as much prior functioning as possible, to provide the individual with adaptive strategies and tools when full restoration of function is not possible, and to re-integrate them into their personal, family, social, and work environments. Achievement of these goals requires collaboration between multiple specialists throughout the acute and post-acute rehabilitation. The psychiatrist plays a key role in the patient's treatment. He/she will treat the patient's individual neuropsychiatric symptoms with a combination of medications and psychotherapy. By taking a careful personal, as well as a family and social history, the psychiatrist will map out the patient's life trajectory prior to the TBI, identify how this trajectory was interrupted by the TBI, and collaborate with other

rehabilitation professionals to set goals of re-integration into the work and social spheres. Setting realistic goals and providing hope that these goals are achievable is essential in helping the patient to regain the sense of competence and independence that are frequently compromised. To achieve these goals, the psychiatrist must collaborate with other professionals on the patient's team, such as physiatrists, speech-language pathologists, occupational therapists, physical therapists, neuropsychologists, social workers, vocational rehabilitation specialists, and life coaches. The psychiatrist may connect the patient with other community resources, such as volunteering opportunities, local TBI support groups, and state TBI societies. This work of setting out realistic goals and working collaboratively with others in a team fashion (whether formally or informally) constitutes most of the work in the patient's rehabilitation. Lastly, the psychiatrist will evaluate the impact of the injury and loss of function on the patient's family, and work with the family to strengthen support, adapt to the challenges of TBI, and access resources for both the patient and their family.

Medications

A limited body of well-designed randomized controlled clinical trials (RCTs) exists to guide the use of medications for the treatment of emotional and behavioral disturbances following TBI. The majority of such studies involve small groups, retrospective record reviews, or single case studies.[76,77] The general consensus of the research is that medications that are effective in treating primary psychiatric disorders are, for the most part, similarly effective in treating the symptoms of these disorders in the context of TBI.[70] Prior to introducing new medications, possible medical causes should be eliminated, the environment should be altered, and psychosocial interventions supplemented (Figure 82-2).[42,45] For example, treatment of infections, dehydration, constipation, urinary retention, and pain should be initiated. In addition, abnormalities of sodium, ammonia, or blood sugar levels should be addressed, and medications reviewed (to make sure therapeutic levels have been reached or that redundant or unnecessary drugs are stopped or reduced).[54] Headaches and chronic fatigue, which are common sequelae, need to be addressed as they can contribute to disturbances in mood and behavior. Attention should be paid to antihistaminergic and anticholinergic side effects (e.g., sedation, dry mouth, constipation, tachycardia, urinary retention, diplopia, confusion, hypotension, and impairments in memory, learning, and attention) caused by many psychotropic medications, as these will exacerbate existing problems that result from TBI. Medications that are least likely to lower seizure threshold or to cause sedation should be selected (Table 82-3). Because patients with TBI are more sensitive to the side effects of medications, a "start low and go slow" approach is recommended (Box 82-3): that is, start with doses one-half to one-third of the dose traditionally used and increase it slowly until therapeutic effects are achieved.[42,60] In general, therapeutic doses will be comparable to those used in traditional psychiatric patients.[70]

An effort should be made to determine the lowest effective dose to minimize the risk for side effects and to avoid the complications of interactions between psychoactive medications. It is not unusual to see patients prescribed an anticonvulsant to control seizures, a stimulant to improve attention and concentration, an antidepressant to address depression and anxiety, and an antipsychotic for agitation. While the overlap in medications can help to augment drug efficacy, it can also lead to potentiation and to toxic blood levels. Some medications will reduce or increase serum blood levels of other medications. Anticonvulsants can lower antidepressant levels.[45,70] Fluoxetine can raise plasma levels for phenytoin, valproic acid, and carbamazapine.[70] Anticholinergic effects can be enhanced in the presence of neuroleptics or antiparkinsonian agents.[45,70] Where possible, changes should be made one at a time to best evaluate the effects of the changes. Because of the changing nature of the recovering brain, there is an ongoing need to routinely reassess psychotropic medications. Clinical judgment and a cost/benefit analysis will be needed to determine how long medications should be continued once desired effects have been achieved.[46,70] Trial reductions or drug holidays are recommended as ways of verifying the continued need for medication[70] (Box 82-4).

BOX 82-3 Medication Side Effects of Concern for Patients with Traumatic Brain Injury

Sedation	Urinary retention
Impaired memory	Diplopia
Impaired learning	Confusion
Dry mouth	Hypotension
Constipation	Seizures
Tachycardia	

BOX 82-4 Medication Guidelines for Patients with Traumatic Brain Injury

- Eliminate biological sources first
- Alter the environment
- Treat symptoms over diagnosis
- Start low and go slow
- Target the lowest effective dose
- Make one change at a time
- Remove unnecessary medications
- Routinely review continued need for medications
- Supplement with psychotherapy

Antidepressants

No research indicates which of the available antidepressants is most effective in treating depression in the context of TBI[45,76,77] However, selective serotonin reuptake inhibitors (SSRIs) are favored, as they impact sleep regulation, headaches, sexual activity, depression, anxiety, appetite, arousal, vigilance, distractibility, neural reward systems, and working memory.[76] In addition to treating depression, the SSRIs are also effective in treating psychological distress, anger, aggression, psychomotor speed, overall cognitive efficiency, and various forms of memory problems.[45,70,76] There are indications that enhanced motor recovery may be linked with fluoxetine use following ischemic stroke.[78] The SSRIs are also effective for the treatment of anxiety disorder (including OCD, panic disorder, and PTSD).[56,57,70,78,79] The SSRIs can also reduce agitation and anxiety.[79] SSRIs are preferred over the tricyclic antidepressants (TCAs) and monoamine oxidase inhibitors (MAOIs) because of their demonstrated effectiveness, improved safety profile, and lower incidence of anticholinergic effects and orthostatic hypotension.[45] Sertraline has been used in patients with post-TBI depression, with robust response and remission rates (87% and 67%, respectively) and significant improvements in psychological distress, anger, aggression, functioning, and post-concussive symptoms.[80] Of note, however, in the single RCT, despite the significant pre- to post-treatment improvement in depression, the sertraline and placebo groups did not significantly differ from each other after treatment on the main depression outcome measure.[81] Citalopram, 20 mg–50 mg, has also been used in post-acute TBI, showing more modest response and remission rates after 6 weeks of treatment (27.7% and 24.1%, respectively; n = 54) and after 10 weeks of treatment (46.2% and 26.9%, respectively; n = 26).[82] When remitters from the above study were randomized to either same dose citalopram or placebo for 40 additional weeks of treatment, the citalopram and placebo groups did not significantly differ in either relapse rate (50% and 54.5%, respectively), or time to relapse.[83] In summary, the response rates to antidepressants in post-TBI depression are not clearly established, ranging from 46% to 87%.[80,82] Remission rates in post-TBI depression are even less well established than response rates. The results showing response and remission rates in post-TBI depression tend to have a wider spread than those in depression without TBI, where response rates are 62%–63%[84] and remission rates are 31%–55%.[84,85] This may be related to the small sample sizes in post-TBI depression trials, to the small number of studies, to TBI severity, and to other factors. Therefore, more RCTs are necessary to establish the true response and remission rates in post-TBI depression. Despite these limitations, the use of SSRIs is encouraged in post-TBI depression.

Because there are no head-to-head comparisons of the effectiveness of different SSRIs, the selection of a specific agent is typically guided by its side-effect profile and by the clinician's familiarity.[72] Caution is needed when prescribing SSRIs due to syndromes of excess serotonin and the risk of discontinuation syndromes. When high doses or multiple serotonergic agents are used there is the risk for a serotonin syndrome (including an altered mental status, neuromuscular abnormalities, disturbances in autonomic function, agitation, myoclonus, hyperflexia, diaphoresis, tremor, diarrhea, and lack of coordination). The SSRI discontinuation syndrome (including profound restlessness, bizarre ideation, headaches, nausea, lowered mood, anxiety, insomnia, lethargy, or dizziness) may occur when an SSRI is stopped abruptly.[72]

TCAs, which tend to be highly anticholinergic and antihistaminergic, can lower the seizure threshold and have a greater potential for lethal overdose.[45,46,76] Among the TCAs, nortriptyline and desipramine are used more commonly following TBI because of their more favorable side-effect profile.[45] Use of MAOIs is often problematic because of the need to comply with complex dietary restrictions.[76] Electroconvulsive therapy (ECT) is also seen as an effective treatment, particularly in cases of severe or treatment-refractory depression, though caution is urged in a population that already has problems with confusion and memory deficits.[42,45,76,77]

Anxiolytics

Benzodiazepines. While benzodiazepines are typically used to treat anxiety in non-TBI patients, their long-term use in patients with TBI is generally not recommended.[60] The short half-life of lorazepam can make it effective for acute agitation or anxiety; however, it can significantly increase sedation, further impair memory and motor function,[71] and lead to behavioral disinhibition.[56,57] Use of benzodiazepines in individuals with a history of drug or alcohol abuse or dependence should be avoided given the potential for abuse and dependence.[57,70]

Buspirone is another alternative[35,56,57] that has been found to improve depression, anxiety, somatic preoccupation, and distractability.[56,57,70] It has less impact on cognition than other anxiolytics and has less potential for abuse.[56,70] Its effects may not be seen for several weeks, which limits its usefulness for acute anxiety.[35] It can cause headaches, dizziness, and paradoxically, increased anxiety.[46,70]

Propranolol, a beta-blocker, has the best body of evidence to support its use in managing agitation and aggression following TBI.[60] It tends to reduce the intensity, but not necessarily the frequency, of agitated behavior.[60] It can lead to hypotension, bradycardia, and depression.[35]

Antiepileptic Drugs

Antiepileptic drugs (AEDs) are used to prevent seizures following TBI. Current recommendations for prophylactic use suggest that they be discontinued if no seizures have been observed after the first week following injury.[70,77] Several anticonvulsants (such as valproic acid, lamotrigine, and gabapentin) have been used to good effect to reduce agitation and aggression.[35,79] While valproic acid has been FDA-approved for treatment of acute mania and it is generally well tolerated (with fewer cognitive side effects), selection of specific anticonvulsants is typically based on side-effect profiles.[35] The more traditional anticonvulsants (phenobarbital, phenytoin, and carbamazepine) tend to sedate, and interfere with cognition. Leviteracetam can increase agitation and other problematic behaviors (including assaultiveness).[86-89] Zonisanide, pregabalin, oxcarbazepine, and topiramate are newer AEDs used as monotherapy or adjunctive agents. While the newer AEDs tend to be better tolerated, there has not been any research examining their use in TBI or to indicate that they are more effective than the older AEDs. Selection of specific agents should be guided by previous response to AED and side-effect profile.[90]

Antipsychotics

Psychosis outside of delirium is unusual after TBI. Antipsychotics are used more frequently to control aggression in patients with brain injuries.[36] Indications for such use include agitation with and without psychosis, extreme agitation or rage, and mania associated with TBI.[77,91] They, along with the short-acting benzodiazepines (such as lorazepam), are effective agents in rapidly controlling acute agitation. The use

of neuroleptics in this population is controversial. Human and animal research suggests that they may interfere with neural plasticity and the recovery process, may be associated with longer periods of post-traumatic amnesia, and may worsen outcomes.[64,70,91] Use of the typical neuroleptics risks extrapyramidal side effects and neuroleptic malignant syndrome (NMS),[91] while the more anticholinergic ones may be associated with orthostasis and may interfere with alertness and cognition.[70,91] Second-generation antipsychotics (such as quetiapine, olanzapine, and risperidone) are preferred because of their greater effectiveness in treating negative symptoms, and their lower risk of EPS, NMS, and anticholinergic effects.[60,64,91] Second-generation antipsychotics can interfere with glucose metabolism and contribute to weight gain and hyperlipidemia as part of a metabolic syndrome. It is suggested that starting doses be approximately half the standard starting dose and increased slowly, similarly to how these medications are used in geriatric patients.[64]

Stimulants

Disorders of attention and arousal can contribute to behavioral disturbances. Dopamine enhancers (such as methylphenidate and dextroamphetamine, bromocriptine, amantadine), acetylcholinesterase inhibitors (such as donepizil or rivastigmine), and the activating antidepressants (e.g., modafinil) are routinely used to improve arousal, speed of information processing, executive functioning, memory, language, attention, apathy, irritability, impulsivity, and fatigue.[70,92-95] They reduce agitation, depression, and anxiety by improving the underlying cognitive dysfunction that contributes to behavioral problems. Reductions in anger and psychopathology can occur even without improvements in cognition[95] and seem to have the additional benefit of increasing overall neuronal recovery.[70] Side effects are generally dose-dependent, occur at higher levels, and resolve with a reduction in dosage. Importantly, none of the stimulants has been found to alter the risk for seizures.[70]

ENVIRONMENTAL INTERVENTIONS

Alterations of the environmental context of the patient are crucial in managing disturbing behaviors. Anxiety, agitation, and aggression can be responses to environmental stressors or overwhelming task demands. Providing the patient with structure and routine, simplifying tasks, reducing or increasing levels of stimulation, and removing environmental distractions, irritations or triggers, can all help to reduce confusion and agitation. Providing the patient with a prosthetic environment helps to compensate for the cognitive losses that result from TBI.[34] Daily schedules, memory aids, computers, and smart phones, prompting and cuing, and pro-active collaborative problem-solving are examples of supportive interventions that reduce demand on a compromised cognitive system and increase the patient's opportunities for success and self-control. Formal training can be used to replace missing skills or increase alternative behaviors.[34] Changing antecedent conditions and the environmental response to behavior can help to decrease maladaptive or dangerous behaviors and increase safer, more adaptive behaviors.[75] These measures can be more time-consuming and labor-intensive and require more training of families or staff than the use of medications. Medication will not replace missing skills or teach more adaptive behavior. In addition, there are few negative side effects and many potential psychological benefits in terms of increasing the patient's sense of control, success, and self-confidence, as well as those of the family and caregiving team.

COGNITIVE REHABILITATION

Multiple studies support the effectiveness of cognitive rehabilitation in re-training cognitive functioning after TBI.[96–99] The Cognitive Task Force of the American College of Rehabilitation Medicine (ACRM)[100] reviewed the evidence for the effectiveness of cognitive rehabilitation approaches from 112 studies. They concluded that there is substantial evidence supporting attention training (i.e., graded exercises to stimulate attention) in post-acute TBI rehabilitation, as well as feedback, self-monitoring, self-regulation and strategy use (i.e., metacognitive strategies) to promote generalization of the cognitive rehabilitation to real-world tasks. The task force recommended the use of internalized memory strategies (e.g., visual imagery) and external memory compensations (e.g., notebooks) for mild memory impairments, specific communications interventions for social communication deficits, and therapies emphasizing meta-cognitive and emotional regulation skills to reduce cognitive and functional disability in moderate or severe TBI. Overall, the task force concluded that cognitive rehabilitation is of greater benefit than conventional rehabilitation, and that it is the best treatment for people with cognitive impairment and functional limitations after TBI.[100]

PSYCHOTHERAPY

The essential tasks of psychotherapy for patients with TBI involve maintaining a sense of hope during the recovery process, mourning the losses that have occurred, identifying remaining strengths and assets, and restoring a sense of self that incorporates the changes imposed by the brain injury.[101] Patients whose injuries are permanent will need help in resolving existential questions of identity and purpose along with re-defining their sense of purpose, their relationships, and their play.[101–103] Where the injury has interfered with normal psychosocial development, patients will likely need assistance in negotiating developmental milestones.[3] Deficits in attention, memory, awareness, self-monitoring, expressive and receptive language, impulse control, abstraction, and frustration-tolerance impact the therapeutic process.[101] Because of its focus on current problem-solving, cognitive-behavioral therapy (CBT) may be better suited to working with TBI survivors than more traditional insight-oriented therapies. Outcome research has found that CBT has been effective in enhancing emotional well-being.[104] Therapists need to take an active and directive role in therapy. Education about the impact of brain injury, the process of recovery, symptom management and the patient's role in the recovery process are important for both the patient and the patient's family and caretakers.[103,105] Cognitive limitations are addressed through the use of memory aids (such as recording sessions, taking notes, generating summaries of main themes in the session, and reviewing the last session at the start of a new session).[103,106] Sessions may be shorter and more frequent to maximize attention and avoid overloading the patient. Homework to be carried out between sessions allows opportunities to practice skills in a variety of settings to promote awareness and generalization. Positive coping, relaxation, and stress management skills are taught to reduce anxiety and frustration. The therapist engages in a practical problem-solving approach to identify and rehearse options. Language is kept concrete and the patient's comprehension is routinely assessed.[106] Family members are often included for at least a portion of sessions to verify patient experience and to provide additional feedback on performance. This is an opportunity to assess and support the patient's center of support as families and caretakers will also need education and psychological support. Families often need help in understanding the role the TBI plays in the patient's behavior. They benefit from support with emotional and practical coping with the demands of caring for the TBI survivor, addressing personal, systemic and societal barriers to accessing services, accessing peer and professional support resources (such as support groups), and individual and family counseling.[107] Unrealistic goals identified by the patient are addressed by identifying smaller short-term goals in the service of achieving more distant goals. This increases the patient's chances of success and assists in developing a more accurate sense of capabilities. A distinction is made between psychological denial and neurologically-based anosognosias. Denial protects against overwhelming affect. Lack of awareness, however, serves no psychological purpose.[101] Denial will often improve with the passage of time as the patient regains areas of competence and control, making the experience of TBI less overwhelming. The lack of awareness typically improves with improved neurological function and interaction with the real world. Resolution of denial will typically lead to improvements in depression and anxiety, whereas improved awareness can actually trigger these emotions. Both need to be approached carefully to avoid overwhelming the patient. Families who often have been traumatized by the injury and become overly protective will need support and guidance in helping the patient engage in the reasonable risk-taking needed to restore a sense of competence and independence.

In cases of co-morbid PTSD and TBI, there is evidence that CBT administered alongside cognitive rehabilitation in a residential treatment setting may be effective in improving PTSD symptoms in patients with mild, moderate, and severe TBI.[108] PTSD treatment using this approach may lead to improvement in post-concussive symptoms as well, and the decrease in PTSD and post-concussive symptoms are positively related.[109] Preliminary evidence is being collected on the effectiveness of different types of CBT in co-morbid PTSD and TBI.[110] The area of co-morbid PTSD and TBI is starting to receive increased research attention and the exact effect TBI has on the ability of patients to benefit from PTSD therapies remains to be elucidated.

CONCLUSION

Psychiatric disturbance in the context of TBI presents unique challenges to the treating psychiatrist. It requires a sophisticated appreciation for the complex etiology of the disturbance. Treatment needs to address the biological, psychological, and environmental sources of the behavior and to promote optimal independent function in addition to reducing targeted behaviors. This can best be accomplished by a team approach that includes other medical and rehabilitation professionals along with the patient and his or her family.

Access the complete reference list and multiple choice questions (MCQs) online at https://expertconsult.inkling.com

KEY REFERENCES

6. Millis SR, Rosenthal M, Novack TA, et al. Long-term neuropsychological outcome after traumatic brain injury. *J Head Trauma Rehabil* 16(4):343–355, 2001.
8. Povlishock JT, Katz DI. Update of neuropathology and neurological recovery after traumatic brain injury. *J Head Trauma Rehabil* 20:76–94, 2005.
11. Yokobori S, Bullock MR. Pathobiology of primary traumatic brain injury. In Zasler ND, Katz DI, Zafonte RD, editors: *Brain injury medicine*, 2013, Demos Medical Publishing, pp 137–147.
16. Elder GA, Cristian A. Blast-related mild traumatic brain injury: mechanisms of injury and impact on clinical care. *Mt Sinai J Med* 76:111–118, 2009.
22. McAllister TW, Arciniegas D. Evaluation and treatment of post-concussive symptoms. *Neuropsychol Rehabil* 27:265–283, 2002.

24. Rees PM. Contemporary issues in mild traumatic brain injury. *Arch Phys Med Rehabil* 84:1885–1894, 2003.

27. Frencham KA, Fox AM, Mayberry MT. Neuropsychological studies of mild traumatic brain injury: A meta-analytic review of research since 1995. *J Clin Exp Neuropsychol* 27(3):334–351, 2005.

31. Kimberg DY, D'Esposito M, Farah MJ. Frontal lobes: cognitive neuropsychological aspects. In Feinberg TE, Farah MJ, editors: *Behavioral neurology and neuropsychology*, New York, 1997, McGraw-Hill, pp 409–418.

32. Hoofien D, Gilboa A, Vakil E, et al. Traumatic brain injury (TBI) 10–20 years later: A comprehensive outcome study of psychiatric symptomatology, cognitive abilities and psychosocial functioning. *Brain Inj* 15:189–209, 2001.

34. Hart T, Jacobs HE. Rehabilitation and management of behavioral disturbances following frontal lobe injury. *J Head Trauma Rehabil* 8:1–12, 1993.

35. Kim E. Agitation, aggression, and disinhibition syndromes after traumatic brain injury. *Neuropsychol Rehabil* 17:297–310, 2002.

37. Tanteno A, Jorge R, Robinson RG. Clinical correlates of aggressive behavior after traumatic brain injury. *J Neuropsychiatry Clin Neurosci* 15:155–160, 2003.

39. Borgaro SR, Prigatano GP, Kwasnica C, et al. Cognitive and affective sequelae in complicated and uncomplicated mild traumatic brain injury. *Brain Inj* 17:189–198, 2003.

40. Oquendo MA, Friedman JH, Grunebaum MF, et al. Suicidal behavior and mild traumatic brain injury in major depression. *J Nerv Ment Dis* 192:430–434, 2004.

49. Jorge RE, Robinson RG, Moser D, et al. Major depression following traumatic brain injury. *Arch Gen Psychiatry* 61(1):42–50, 2004.

50. Seel RT, Kreutzer JS, Rosenthal M, et al. Depression after traumatic brain injury: A National Institute on Disability and Rehabilitation Research Model Systems multicenter investigation. *Arch Phys Med Rehabil* 84(2):177–184, 2003.

54. Glenn M. A differential diagnostic approach to the pharmacological treatment of cognitive, behavioral, and affective disorders after traumatic brain injury. *J Head Trauma Rehabil* 17:273–283, 2002.

56. Hiott DW, Labatte L. Anxiety disorders associated with traumatic brain injuries. *Neuropsychol Rehabil* 17:345–355, 2002.

64. McAllister TW, Ferrell RB. Evaluation and treatment of psychosis after traumatic brain injury. *Neuropsychol Rehabil* 17:357–368, 2002.

65. Arlinghaus KA, Shoaib AM, Price TR. Neuropsychiatric assessment. In Silver JM, McAllister TW, Yudofsky SC, editors: *Textbook of traumatic brain injury*, Washington, DC, 2005, American Psychiatric Publishing, pp 59–78.

75. Yody BB, Schaub C, Conway J, et al. Applied behavior management and acquired brain injury: Approaches and assessment. *J Head Trauma Rehabil* 15:1041–1060, 2000.

77. Glenn MB, Wroblewski B. Twenty years of pharmacology. *J Head Trauma Rehabil* 20:51–61, 2005.

79. Deb S, Crownshaw T. The role of pharmacotherapy in the management of behavior disorders in traumatic brain injury patients. *Brain Inj* 18:1–31, 2004.

93. Wheaton P, Mathias JL, Vink R. Impact of pharmacological treatments on cognitive and behavioral outcomes in postacute stages of adult traumatic brain injury: A meta-analysis. *J Clin Psychopharmacol* 31(6):745–757, 2011.

101. Pollack IW. Psychotherapy. In Silver JM, McAllister TW, Yudofsky SC, editors: *Textbook of traumatic brain injury*, Washington, DC, 2005, American Psychiatric Publishing, pp 641–654.

103. Ponsford J, Hsieh MY. Psychological interventions for emotional and behavioral problems following traumatic brain injury. In Zasler ND, Katz DI, Zafonte RD, editors: *Brain injury medicine*, 2013, Demos Medical Publishing, pp 1067–1085.

107. Gan C, Garago J, Brandys C, et al. Family caregiver's support needs after brain injury: A synthesis of perspectives from caregivers, programs and researchers. *Neurorehabilitation* 27:5–18, 2010.

WEBSITES

Defense and Veterans Brain Injury Center. <http://www.dvbic.org>
Brain Injury Association of America. <http://www.biausa.org>
North American Brain Injury Society. <http://www.nabis.org>

83   Intimate Partner Violence

BJ Beck, MSN, MD

KEY POINTS

Background

- Intimate partner violence (IPV) is a common, under-reported, and life-threatening public health problem that affects all segments of society.

- Societal implications of IPV include the cost of medical and psychiatric injury, chronicity and disability, as well as lost productivity, legal system costs, and generational effects and repetition.

History

- Legal systems that equate women and children with property, sociocultural and religious systems that abhor interference in the family, and the unequal status of women in many cultures and societies, have contributed to an ethos of silence, stigma, dismissal, or denial of the serious implications surrounding IPV.

- Increased recognition of male victims may demonstrate a real change or, more likely, the degree to which humiliation has historically limited self-report by men, the qualitative difference between the violence experienced by men versus women, and the use of broader definitions.

Clinical and Research Challenges

- There are many reasons victims stay in violent relationships, including the realistic fear of murder when attempting to leave.

- Fear, shame, stigma or attitudes about what constitutes violence may limit the validity of self-report in epidemiologic surveys. In smaller studies, safety concerns also favor under-reporting.

Practical Pointers

- Although not sufficient to alter outcomes, detection of IPV is necessary for any intervention. However, there is insufficient evidence to recommend routine screening.

- Clinicians should inquire about violence exposure whenever assessing a condition that may be caused or worsened by IPV, such as depression, unexplained injuries or somatic complaints. The physician's responsibilities are to detect, re-frame as unacceptable, and document IPV; to be empathic; and to refer the patient to appropriate services.

- Victims need to know that their physicians will take them seriously, respect their decisions, and continue to work with them.

OVERVIEW

The term *domestic violence* may be broadly interpreted to include child and elder abuse. Because this chapter focuses more specifically on violence in the context of an intimate relationship, the term *intimate partner violence (IPV)* will be used. Other terms for this phenomenon include *battering, spouse abuse,* and *wife-beating.* IPV is a pattern of intentionally violent, coercive, or controlling behaviors by a current or previously intimate partner. The goal of the violence is to assert and maintain power and control over the victim.[1] This behavioral pattern may encompass humiliation, emotional torment, economic control, social isolation, and sexual assault, as well as threatened and actual physical injury. Because IPV disproportionately involves male perpetrators in heterosexual relationships,[2,3] this chapter uses the convention of female pronouns for victims and male pronouns for perpetrators. This is not to imply the totality of the problem, which includes male victims and female batterers, as well as violence in same-sex relationships.

There is neither societal stratum nor civilization (past or present) exempt from IPV. This endemic affliction has grave and extensive public health implications, including physical injury, physical and mental disability, and even death. The societal costs of IPV include health care expense, lost wages, decreased or lost productivity, and the generational

implications and long-term effects on children who witness such violence.[3-5] In strictly economic terms, the World Health Organization (WHO) estimated the (2004) annual cost of IPV in the US to be 0.1% of the gross domestic product (GDP), or nearly $13 billion.[6] Studies of routine screening have shown that detection, though necessary, is not sufficient for successful intervention.[7-10] Despite improved provider awareness, attitudes, stereotypes, time constraints, a sense of futility, and lack of resources remain barriers to detection.[11,12] Victims live with shame, fear, limited (and often highly controlled) resources, and a perpetrator-distorted sense of reality, which serve as deterrents to disclosure. The danger is real. If not handled well, disclosure and detection may seriously increase the victim's risk: a victim who leaves has a 75% greater risk (than those who stay) of being murdered by her batterer.[13,14]

EPIDEMIOLOGY

Although controversy exists,[15-17] a large national survey[18] demonstrated that IPV in the US affects women six times as often as men, with approximately 4.5 million annual episodes of abuse perpetrated against women by a current or former intimate partner. A more recent US survey[3] using more inclusive definitions found that 35.6% of women (18 or older), and 28.5% of men had experienced some form of IPV (rape, physical violence, and/or stalking) within their life-time (i.e., over 42 million women and 32 million men). Annually, almost 6% of women experience one or more forms of IPV (seven million). Five percent of men report some form of IPV annually (5.6 million).[3] Most (85%) episodes of IPV involve men who abuse their female partners. In fact, women are more likely to be assaulted, raped, or murdered by a current or previous male partner than by a stranger (72.1% versus 10.6%). While US men experience more pervasive violence, they are more likely to be assaulted by a stranger (56.2%) than by a current or former intimate female partner (16.6%). The difference in the rates of IPV experienced by women versus men escalates with the severity of violence, with women being 7 to 14 times more likely to be beaten up, choked, or threatened with a firearm or drowning.[18] An estimated 30%–50% of married couples experience some instance of physical violence. The rate appears similar for same-sex couples.[19] When women are violent toward their male partners, it is often, though not always, in self-defense, and less physically injurious.[18] Men who report IPV are more often victims of physical violence or, less frequently, stalking. Sexual violence or combinations of violent actions were much less common for male victims, with the perpetrator more often being male, as well.[3] IPV has a recurrent and escalating pattern, with spousal murder accounting for approximately 1 out of 10 homicides (11%). Approximately one-third of female homicide victims are murdered by a current or former intimate partner.[20]

Abused women are prevalent in various medical settings. In the emergency department (ED), 11% of women seen for any cause are in abusive relationships,[21] although only 2% may seek treatment for abuse-related acute trauma.[22] Among women seen emergently for non-motor-vehicle trauma, the prevalence of IPV may be as high as 40%. The life-time prevalence of abuse in women seen in the ED may be over 50%.[21] For women seen in general medical settings, 14%–28% may be victims of IPV,[23,24] while 3%–17% of those seeking routine pre-natal care have been victimized.[25-27] In the pediatric setting, more than half of the mothers of abused children are themselves being abused.[28]

Psychiatrists should realize that abused women account for one-fourth of all women treated at emergency psychiatric services, one-third of all women who attempt suicide,[21,29] one-half of all women in outpatient psychiatric care, and almost two-thirds of women on inpatient psychiatric units.[30]

RISK FACTORS FOR VICTIMS AND PERPETRATORS

Psychiatrists, and other health care providers, should maintain heightened suspicion regardless of the patient's socio-economic, educational, professional, ethnic, racial, or religious affiliation. IPV, the great equalizer, respects no such boundaries.[31]

However, certain women (and couples) are at greater risk,[2,3] and deserve greater scrutiny and sensitivity. Box 83-1 lists some of these features. Young women (teens and twenties), especially if single (divorced or separated) or pregnant, are at increased risk of IPV. Filing a restraining order, especially a temporary one, further increases risk.[32] This act of independence may fuel the abuser's need to assert his domination and control. A woman may be "poor" because her abuser controls (and limits) the financial and other resources available to her. Abused women often turn to drugs or alcohol (to escape, tolerate or numb their experience of abuse). Drug or alcohol use by a woman's partner also increases her risk, as his irritability, irrationality, and disinhibition increase. An excessively jealous (controlling, easily angered) or possessive partner,[13] especially one who seems overly involved in the woman's medical visit,

***

BOX 83-1 Risk Factors for Women as Victims of Violence

- Being single, separated, or divorced
- Having recently applied for a restraining order
- Being between 17 and 28 years of age
- Being poor
- Abusing alcohol or drugs
- Having a partner who abuses alcohol or drugs
- Being pregnant or previously abused
- Having an excessively jealous or possessive partner

***

BOX 83-2 Risk Factors for Violence in Male Perpetrators

- Antisocial personality disorder
- Depression
- Youth
- Low income
- Low educational level
- Unemployment
- Intermittent employment

***

or refuses to leave the examination or interview room, should significantly raise clinical suspicion.[33]

Box 83-2 lists other traits of men at increased risk of injuring their partners.[3,34] Not surprisingly, antisocial men are overly represented among violent perpetrators. Less intuitive, young men, especially with limited finances and education, also pose increased risk, as do those suffering from depression.[35]

CLINICAL PRESENTATION OF VICTIMS

The only unifying feature of victims is the existence of a violent partner. All segments of the population are represented. No pre-victimization personality has been identified to predispose a person to be abused. However, repeated abuse predisposes a behavioral pattern that appears character-disordered. Persistent emotional badgering, physical abuse, or sexual assault may result in intense shame, an overwhelming sense of worthlessness, and incompetence. When such women seek medical attention, especially when accompanied by their batterer, they appear dependent and overly passive. They may not *look* abused, or have obvious evidence of battering. They may have vague physical or behavioral complaints, and be seen as "somatic" and emotionally unstable,[36] especially when there has been sexual violence.[37] (Such a woman may fare even less well in the legal arena.)

The victim is often entirely dependent on her abuser. Social isolation occurs as the abuser purposely severs any outside contact or support, including, and especially, from the victim's own family or friends. Humiliating economic control and deprivation further restrict her independence and increase her vulnerability. For some women, chronic fear and threats are even more detrimental than the physical abuse.[1] Despite strategies to endure, dissociate, or numb physical pain and fear, threats to her children, family, or pets[5] may be continually unbearable. Even total submission may seem reasonable to keep those she cares about safe. Such passive, dependent, and submissive behavior is the result of repeated abuse, not a predisposition. It is the goal, not the cause, of the abuse.[1]

Certain psychiatric disorders are more commonly associated with IPV.[35,38] Substance use and addiction are more common among victims. Eating disorders are also associated with IPV.[33] Depression and anxiety are frequent co-morbidities.[35] In emergency settings, women with current or past IPV are more than three times as likely to have made a suicide attempt.[21,39] Post-traumatic stress disorder (PTSD), with the associated hyperarousal, flashbacks, and nightmares, is especially common in, though not limited to, victims who have also suffered childhood abuse.[40] PTSD may go unrecognized when the patient does not volunteer the traumatic precipitant; hence the need for astute pattern-recognition skills. Chronic pain syndromes (e.g., headaches, pelvic pain, intractable abdominal pain, musculoskeletal problems) are also associated with IPV.[36,41,42]

CLINICAL PRESENTATION OF PERPETRATORS

There may be shared cultural and developmental experiences that predispose to certain personality traits, but perpetrators of IPV are not limited to any particular segment of society. Just as violence effectively shapes victim behavior and appearance, there is an identifiable pattern of behavior, experience, and style apparent in perpetrators (Box 83-3).

Perpetrator family histories frequently reveal violence in which the perpetrator was either a witness or a victim.[43]

BOX 83-3 Perpetrator Patterns of Experience, Traits, and Behaviors

EXPERIENCE
- Witnessed/experienced violence in one's family of origin
- Violence in previous relationships

TRAITS
- Being immature, needy, dependent, or non-assertive
- Having fragile self-esteem or intense feelings of inadequacy
- Being "insanely jealous" or untrusting
- Being intolerant of any victim autonomy; a need to dominate/control
- Being overly concerned with outward appearances
- Being socially congenial, or able to conceal violence from friends and professionals
- Appearing more credible/intact than the victim
- Portraying the victim as prone to exaggeration, or emotionally unstable

BEHAVIORS
- Abusing alcohol or drugs (or both)
- Minimizing/denying violence
- Blaming the victim for provoking violence

Personal histories often reveal a pattern of violence in previous relationships. Often young and poorly educated, batterers may be immature,[2,34] dependent, and needy, with an easily shattered sense of competence, worth, and self-esteem. Perpetrators tend not to be positively assertive or direct, but to feel intensely inadequate, leading to jealousy and distrust of their partners. Any suggestion of autonomy is seen as an affront and is intolerable.[13] They may rely on alcohol or drugs (or both) to bolster their sense of worth or power.[2,3,18,44–46] They may then blame intoxication for their loss of control when violence occurs (although victims often negate this association).[34]

In terms of disclosure or responsibility, perpetrators have a pattern of concealment, denial, and blaming.[47] Charming and engaging, and extremely cognizant of outward appearances, the batterer often appears grounded and reliable while portraying the victim as emotionally unbalanced and exaggerating. With their victim, perpetrators often downplay the extent, frequency, or damage of the abuse, and possibly blame intoxication. Also abusive, the perpetrator may blame their victim for provoking or deserving the abuse.

THE NATURE OF VIOLENT RELATIONSHIPS

The recognizable pattern in the development of abusive relationships is replete with overtures of caring and exceptional thoughtfulness, with no omen of what is to come. During this non-assaultive prodrome, the future perpetrator may be inordinately attentive, calling the future victim multiple times a day, accompanying her to health care appointments, dropping her off at work and waiting to pick her up afterward. He may offer financial support, spend money on her, or even provide housing. This assistance gradually leads to control over the victim's finances and outside contacts (e.g. family, friends), and even professional interactions.[48] The perpetrator's control engenders the victim's growing dependence and isolation.

Often some major life event[49] (e.g., marriage, pregnancy, birth) triggers the first violent episode. Alternatively, some form of recognition (e.g., professional advancement) of the victim may "provoke" the initial violence. Couples generally respond with shock and revulsion, followed by a firm belief and commitment that this is an isolated, never-to-be-repeated incident. However, a pattern of repetitive, often predictable, and escalating violence ensues[50] (Figure 83-1). Extreme remorse and reconciliation typically follow each episode. The perpetrator demonstrates his profuse contrition with outpourings of gifts and professions of love and affection. The victim, apologetic for the perpetrator's "pain," feels guilty for having provoked him. Both insist, and often believe, it will never happen again. This reconciliation phase is followed by a period of growing tension that ultimately concludes in another

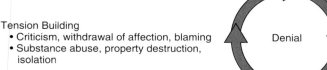

Violent Episode
- Explosive physical, verbal, sexual abuse
- Humiliation, choking, imprisonment

Tension Building
- Criticism, withdrawal of affection, blaming
- Substance abuse, property destruction, isolation

Denial

Remorse
- Apologies, promises to get help
- Declares: "It will never happen again!"

Reconciliation
- Proclamation of love, affection
- Gifts, seduction

Figure 83-1. Summary of the pattern commonly referred to as the cycle of violence.

violent eruption.[33] Some victims experience such dread and terror during this insidious tension-building phase that they choose to provoke the violence to end their mounting anticipatory anxiety. As the violence continues, it escalates in both frequency and severity. Physical acts, such as pushing and shoving, progress to punching, kicking, or burning. IPV may involve forced sexual acts or the use of drugs or alcohol. The abuse may become life-threatening, especially with the introduction of weapons (e.g., clubs, knives). The presence or use of a gun obviously poses an even greater risk of lethality.[18,20]

This physical escalation is accompanied by emotional abuse calculated to further both the perpetrator's control and dominance and the victim's dependence and submission. Emotional abuse encompasses verbal and behavioral tactics (e.g., humiliation, intimidation, threats, coercion). The abuser may purposely embarrass, berate, or humiliate the victim in front of others, including her children, family, friends, business associates, or even strangers. He may call her names and "put her down" to promote her sense of guilt and self-deprecation. He may attempt to manipulate her sense of reality to make her fear she is going crazy. Humiliating tactics also include treating her like a servant, forcing her to beg (e.g., for food, money, or access to clothing, physical needs, or bodily functions), and demanding illegal or demeaning behaviors, including sexual acts. Certain gestures or expressions may be purposefully linked to fearful consequences so that the look or gesture will in itself intimidate the victim and promote an ongoing dread of delayed consequences.[1] Other intimidating strategies include reckless driving, brandishing weapons, destroying the victim's property, or abusing her pets. Besides the threat of the violence itself, victims may be further terrorized by threats of abandonment, destitution, murder, legal action, deportation, psychiatric commitment, loss of (or harm to) their children, or harm to family. They may also be threatened with responsibility for the perpetrator's suicide if they consider leaving. These coercive tactics underscore the victim's reticence to leave what outwardly appears to be an untenable situation.

Children are both complications in, and casualties of, IPV. Suspicions of child abuse or witnessed abuse are reportable in most states, yet such reports may put the victim at increased risk. Children may be "drafted" by the perpetrator to join in the humiliation and the verbal abuse. They may be used as pawns to relay messages. Her children's safety, or her access to them (e.g., loss of custody, visitation, or kidnapping), may be used as threats to keep the victim compliant within the relationship. While the effects of child abuse are not the topic of this chapter, there are known links between IPV and child abuse that suggest they co-occur and may perpetuate the cycle of family violence.[4,5,40,51]

The nature of violent relationships hints at the myriad reasons victims stay in them. The physical and emotional damage of repetitive battering, the intermittent reinforcement of the cyclic dynamic, the true lack of resources, and the perceived and real danger keep victims from leaving. Continual berating leads to acceptance of the batterer's conviction of the victim's worthlessness. Victims come to believe they deserve their mistreatment and they should expect no better. Victims may feel not only humiliated, but also ashamed, responsible, and guilty.[49] They are isolated from family and friends, whom they may have helped drive away to quell the batterer's suspicions and jealousy, in hopes of decreasing the tensions that inevitably lead to the next episode of violence. In fact, they are isolated from all outside contacts: medical, legal, professional, social, and community. Victims are without financial resources, because such dependence gives the perpetrator ultimate control. They may have been prevented from working or made to turn all earnings, money, and other assets over to the abuser. The fear of indigence, homelessness, and inability to care for oneself or one's children is grounded in reality. A victim who has tried unsuccessfully to leave in the past will be unlikely to risk another attempt, especially if she experienced disbelief or lack of assistance from those who might have helped: family, police, medical or legal professionals, or social agencies. And finally, the remorse, affection, and avowals of reform after the explosive violence fuel the victim's hope for change. Many victims do not want the relationship to end; they want to end the abuse.[52]

EVALUATION

Although the most recent WHO Guidelines do not recommend routine screening,[53,54] they do advocate for clinician training to increase awareness, appropriate inquiry, and empathic response. They describe appropriate inquiry as gentle probing during any psychiatric or general medical assessment for conditions known to be caused or worsened by IPV (e.g., depression, PTSD, unexplained injuries, somatic complaints). Despite their reticence to volunteer such information, patients will often respond truthfully to empathic probing. However, when both men and women are asked whether they have experienced violence, either as a victim or a perpetrator, this becomes more widely recognized as part of a general survey, and patients are less likely to take offense. The guise of general screening allows for a qualifying statement, such as the following: "There are certain questions that are part of a full evaluation that I ask all patients." Asking: "Have you been hit, kicked, punched, or otherwise hurt by someone within the past year? If so, by whom?" has been shown to identify over 70% of women in violent relationships, as identified by more extensive inventories.[55] Questions about sexual assault and violence in past relationships are also important for both their effects on the patient and their predictive value. Women are at greater risk of being sexual assaulted by current partners if they have a history of assault by previous partners. This questioning should be carried out in a straightforward, non-judgmental fashion, in a private setting, and obviously not in front of the perpetrator; this would limit disclosure and endanger the victim. For non-English-speaking patients, intimates, family, or friends should never serve as interpreters.

Despite initiatives to increase provider awareness, barriers to screening and detection persist (e.g., time constraints, lack of training, inadequate resources for safety and service). There especially remains reticence to question or suspect couples who are socially well known, highly educated, professional, or of upper socioeconomic status. The qualifying statement about asking "all patients certain questions" may help ease the physician's embarrassment and the patient's sense of insult. Security, social service professionals, and interpreters are among the immediate resources to promote safe disclosure and safety planning. Increased knowledge of the reasons and dangers that prevent a victim from leaving may help dissipate the frustration medical professionals are prone to feel when they detect IPV but are unable to effect an immediate change.

The very reasons that a victim may stay in her violent relationship may dissuade her from disclosing the abuse. Persistent battering and emotional torment are correlated with shame, fear, worthlessness, hopelessness, depression, anxiety, dissociation, or numbness. She may also fear the abuser will be more violent, be more persuasive, provide counter-accusations, or be jailed, leaving her destitute and homeless.

Certain victims are even more challenged, at risk, and unlikely to disclose IPV. Victimized illegal aliens may fear legal retaliation, deportation, loss of children, or even violence or extortion to their families in other countries. There is a

neglect alone, or "reasonable grounds," is sufficient to trigger the duty to report. It is critical that physicians and other mental health providers familiarize themselves with the specific standards and requirements for mandated reporting in every jurisdiction in which they practice. For example, some physicians and mental health clinicians may feel that reporting a caregiver or a child's parents might pose difficulties in terms of the therapeutic alliance. These professionals may be tempted to try to work with these families before notifying state social services. It is important to note that doing so can leave mandated reporters vulnerable to legal prosecution for failure to file a timely report and to civil liability for failure to protect a patient from harm by delaying a mandated report.[9] Finally, many state laws grant immunity to physicians who report in good faith, thereby minimizing exposure to liability for reporting abuse and neglect.[10]

TYPES OF ABUSE AND NEGLECT

Federal and state laws describe various types of abuse and neglect for both children and the elderly. For both groups these subcategories of abuse and neglect include physical abuse, emotional (psychological) abuse, sexual abuse, and neglect. This chapter will focus on physical and emotional abuse and on neglect. The topic of sexual abuse is beyond the scope of this chapter.

CHILD ABUSE AND NEGLECT
Types of Maltreatment

The federal Child Abuse Prevention and Treatment Act (CAPTA) provides minimum standards for the definition of child abuse and neglect. Under CAPTA, which was recently amended by the federal CAPTA Reauthorization Act of 2010, *child abuse and neglect* is defined as "any recent act or failure to act on the part of a parent or caretaker, which results in death, serious physical or emotional harm, sexual abuse or exploitation, or an act or failure to act which presents an imminent risk of serious harm."[11] The federal definition in CAPTA has been the subject of many different interpretations. Specifically, there are many competing approaches to how this legislation should be applied and incorporated into state law. For example, certain states define *child abuse and neglect* as a single concept whereas others consider *abuse* and *neglect* as different entities that require separate definitions. In addition, the standard for what constitutes abuse can also vary among states. Despite these jurisdictional differences, *abuse* is most often defined by states as "harm or substantial risk of harm" or "serious threat or serious harm" to a child.[5] For example, the state of Massachusetts defines *child abuse* as "the non-accidental commission of any act by a caretaker upon a child under age 18 which causes, or creates a substantial risk of physical or emotional injury, or constitutes a sexual offense under the laws of the Commonwealth or any sexual contact between a caretaker and a child under the care of that individual."[12] As mentioned previously, each state can determine the grounds for intervention to protect a child, but there are common trends among states. For example, a "child" is generally defined as a person who is under age 18 and not an emancipated minor. Emancipation status is not available in every state, but, in the majority of states in which it is, emancipation is a legal status that allows minors to attain the rights of legal adulthood, provided certain criteria are met, before the age at which they would normally be considered adults. For example, in some states a child who is married, a parent, or in the armed forces can be considered emancipated.[13] It is important to review the relevant statutes specific to each state of practice to know which criteria apply.

Physical Abuse

Worldwide, definitions of what constitutes physical abuse vary among (1) individual country, state, or jurisdiction; (2) cultural norms; and (3) biological predispositions. When physical abuse is suspected, it is important to consider the cultural and ethnic influences that may validate different interpretations of abuse.[14,15]

In the US, Dr. C. Henry Kempe's landmark 1962 publication[16] coined the term *battered child syndrome*. Kempe described findings consistent with a pattern of abuse that included the existence of multiple bone fractures in different stages of healing that were suggestive of child maltreatment.[16] Since that time, the types of physical findings linked to non-accidental injuries have grown dramatically in scope and the methods of detection have become increasingly sophisticated. Even with increased knowledge and diagnostic abilities, one of the most common methods used to screen for the presence of physical abuse remains a discrepancy between the physical findings and the parent's or caregiver's explanation of the mechanism of injury.[17] The identification of inconsistencies between the report provided and the objective data on physical examination are important as evidence that the stories given do not reflect reality and that injuries may be sustained as the result of intentional infliction rather than by accidental means.

Emotional Abuse

Mental injury to a child can have pervasive and long-term effects on a child's development. It is important to recognize that emotional abuse may accompany physical abuse, sexual abuse, or neglect, but may also occur entirely independent of other forms of maltreatment. To date, 48 states include emotional maltreatment within their definition of child abuse.[18] (Georgia and Washington do not include emotional abuse in their statutory definitions.) Emotional abuse has been defined by a number of national organizations, including the AMA, the American Academy of Pediatrics, the United States Department of Health and Human Services, and the National Center on Child Abuse and Neglect. According to the American Academy of Pediatrics Committee on Child Abuse and Neglect, *emotional abuse* is defined as "psychological maltreatment. ... [from] a repeated pattern of damaging interactions between parent(s) and child that becomes typical of the relationship."[18,19] In some situations the pattern is chronic and pervasive, whereas in others these damaging interactions occur only in the setting of specific triggers or "potentiating factors."[20] Overall, emotional maltreatment "is a pattern of behavior that impairs a child's emotional development or sense of self-worth, [which] may include constant criticism, threats, or rejection, as well as withholding love, support or guidance."[5] Psychological maltreatment assaults a child's emotional, social, and basic human development. Gabarino and others have described forms of psychically-destructive behavior inflicted by an adult on a child and the ways these types of emotional abuses may manifest from a developmental perspective.[21,22]

Emotional abuse can be manifest in a variety of ways (Box 84-1).[23–26] The *Diagnostic and Statistical Manual of Mental Disorders, Fifth Edition* (DSM-5) is the first to include a comparable diagnosis, "childhood psychological abuse," defined as "nonaccidental verbal or symbolic acts by a child's parent or caregiver that result, or have reasonable potential to result, in significant psychological harm to the child. ... Examples. ... include berating, disparaging, or humiliating the child; threatening the child; harming/abandoning—or indicating that the alleged offender will harm/abandon—people or things the child cares about; confining the child. ... egregious

BOX 84-1 Manifestations of Emotional Abuse

CORRUPTING

A form of exploitation that encourages the development of inappropriate behaviors (e.g., aggressive, criminal, sexual, or substance-abusing behaviors).

DEGRADING

Disdainful rejection, spurning, humiliation, ridicule, or criticism that can include being shamefully singled out in public.

IGNORING

Failure to provide emotional responsiveness, or an interest or display of affect toward the child.

INCONSISTENT PARENTING

Ambivalent, contradictory, or unreliable behavior toward the child.

ISOLATING

Confining or withholding of interactions with other caregiver or peers, unreasonable limits on social interactions.

REJECTING

Avoiding the child, refusing to acknowledge or allow inclusion in activities with family or others.

TERRORIZING

Intimidating, threatening, or exposing the child to acts that make the child feel unsafe.

WITNESSING VIOLENCE OR CRUELTY

Exposure to domestic violence or destructive physical behavior by caregivers.

BOX 84-2 Full DSM-5 Diagnostic Criteria: Reactive Attachment Disorder (313.89 (F94.1))

A. A consistent pattern of inhibited, emotionally withdrawn behavior toward adult caregivers, manifested by both of the following:
1. The child rarely or minimally seeks comfort when distressed.
2. The child rarely or minimally responds to comfort when distressed.
B. A persistent social and emotional disturbance characterized by at least two of the following:
1. Minimal social and emotional responsiveness to others.
2. Limited positive affect.
3. Episodes of unexplained irritability, sadness, or fearfulness that are evident even during non-threatening interactions with adult caregivers.
C. The child has experienced a pattern of extremes of insufficient care as evidenced by at least one of the following:
1. Social neglect or deprivation in the form of persistent lack of having basic emotional needs for comfort, stimulation, and affection met by caregiving adults.
2. Repeated changes of primary caregivers that limit opportunities to form stable attachments (e.g., frequent changes in foster care).
3. Rearing in unusual settings that severely limit opportunities to form selective attachments (e.g., institutions with high child-to-caregiver ratios).
D. The care in Criterion C is presumed to be responsible for the disturbed behavior in Criterion A (e.g., the disturbances in Criterion A began following the lack of adequate care in Criterion C).
E. The criteria are not met for autism spectrum disorder.
F. The disturbance is evident before age 5 years.
G. The child has a developmental age of at least 9 months.

Specify if:

Persistent: The disorder has been present for more than 12 months.

Specify current severity:

Reactive attachment disorder is specified as **severe** when a child exhibits all symptoms of the disorder, with each symptom manifesting at relatively high levels.

Reprinted with permission from the Diagnostic and Statistical Manual of Mental Disorders, *Fifth Edition, (Copyright 2013). American Psychiatric Association.*

---

scapegoating of the child; coercing the child to inflict pain on himself or herself; and disciplining the child excessively." Another DSM-5 diagnosis that may be encountered when dealing with children who are victims of abuse and neglect is "Reactive Attachment Disorder." According to the DSM-5, this is defined as "a consistent pattern of inhibited, emotionally withdrawn behavior toward adult caregivers. ... a persistent social and emotional disturbance. ... experienced a pattern of extremes of insufficient care as evidenced by. ... social neglect or deprivation. ... repeated changes of primary caregivers. ... rearing in unusual settings that severely limit opportunities to form selective attachments."[27] (see Box 84-2 for full DSM-5 Diagnostic Criteria). Despite the fact that emotional abuse can lead to long-term harm, it is often difficult to substantiate suspicions or allegations of emotional abuse. Specifically, the damage suffered by the child may not be as apparent as can the outwardly visible signs of physical abuse. Some states therefore require that a psychiatric or psychological diagnosis be linked to the alleged emotional abuse in order to establish a causal connection between the child's disorder and the wrongful behavior by the parent or the caregiver.

Neglect

According to the most recent data report from the National Child Abuse and Neglect Data System (NCANDS), neglect is the most common form of child maltreatment reported to state protective services.[1] More children suffer from neglect than from physical and sexual abuse combined.[1] Despite the fact that neglect makes up almost four-fifths of all reported cases of child mistreatment in the US, it receives less consideration in the literature and the media as compared to physical and sexual abuse. Part of the reason that child neglect receives disproportionately less attention than abuse may be related to difficulties

in defining what constitutes neglect. In the Keeping Children and Families Safe Act of 2003, an update of CAPTA, *neglect* is defined as "any recent act or failure to act on the part of a parent or caretaker which results in death, serious physical or emotional harm, sexual abuse or exploitation; or an act or failure which presents an imminent risk of physical harm." Although the federal government, through CAPTA, provides minimum standards for child neglect, as in the case of child abuse, states have operationalized the federal standard by implementing definitions that vary widely. That being said, neglect is generally considered as an act of omission rather than one of commission and most definitions incorporate the concept of non-provision of, or inability to provide, adequate care.[1,28]

Other generalizations may be drawn from state laws about neglect. For example, neglect is typically broken down into five main categories: emotional neglect, physical neglect, medical neglect, failure to thrive (FTT), and educational neglect. Like emotional abuse, neglect is more difficult to identify than is physical abuse, because the more easily identified stigmata of scars, marks, or bruises are often not present. In the absence of demonstrable evidence of harm in settings of neglect, it is often difficult for child protective services to intervene since intervention requires such evidence.

Emotional Neglect. This form of neglect shares some similarities with emotional abuse insofar as the child's emotional requirements for development and growth are not met. A lack of affection, love, and nurturance can have devastating and lasting effects on a child's health and emotional maturation. This type of emotional deprivation can lead to a host of long-term mental health issues that include attachment disorders, behavior difficulties, emotional instability, low self-esteem, and poor social skills.[29-31]

Physical Neglect. This is defined as the failure to provide an adequate and safe environment for the child's needs. It is important to distinguish this type of neglect from environmental circumstances (e.g., due to poverty) in which a child may be living. Numerous agencies exist to assist financially challenged families in such circumstances. If a family or caregiver places a child in an environment where the child's physical needs are not met due to financial inability, the parent or caregiver has not personally engaged in neglect where he or she has exhibited adequate care under the circumstances. The mere fact that a family faces financial hardship does not constitute neglect, *per se*, but neither is it an absolute excuse for, or a defense against, claims of physical neglect.[31]

Medical Neglect. Medical neglect occurs when a child has an illness or other health concern and the parent either misuses, refuses, or fails to obtain medical attention for the child. In addition, a delay in obtaining medical care can constitute medical neglect when failure to seek the assistance of medical professionals in a timely fashion causes harm to the child. This concept is articulated by the United States Supreme Court in the case *Parham v. J.R.*, which stated that parents have "a 'high duty' to recognize symptoms of illness and to seek and follow medical advice. The law's concept of the family rests on a presumption that parents possess what a child lacks in maturity, experience, and capacity for judgment required for making life's difficult decisions."[32]

Failure to Thrive. Failure to thrive (FTT) is defined as "a significantly prolonged cessation of appropriate weight gain compared with recognized norms for age and gender after having achieved a stable pattern."[33] Inadequate provisions of nutrition and disturbed social interactions are both considered significant factors that result in the syndrome of FTT. Although FTT can be unintentional or caused by organic disease (e.g., cystic fibrosis, inborn errors of metabolism, or human immunodeficiency virus [HIV] infection), a significant number of cases are the consequence of child neglect. This neglect is often emotional, resulting from parents or caregivers who exhibit socially maladaptive "interactional behavior and less positive affective behavior" that leads to FTT in the child.[33] As such, infants, toddlers, and children with FTT are at risk for attachment disturbances. Mental health professionals should be particularly attuned to the parental or caregiver's response to the child's needs and general emotional availability when evaluating for FTT.

Educational Neglect. Generally, states require children to attend school until either a certain age or grade level. If a parent permits chronic truancy or fails to enroll a child in school, this may constitute educational neglect, especially if the caregiver has been informed of the situation but fails to correct the problem. Likewise, if a child has special educational needs and the parent or caregiver fails to follow through with providing necessary treatment or exercising diligence in obtaining educational services, a finding of educational neglect may be warranted. Some states provide avenues for legal enforcement of school attendance by truant children where parents are unable to manage the child.[34]

Epidemiology

Child maltreatment is a medical and public health problem that affects 9.3 out of every 1,000 children per year.[1] In 2009, according to the National Child Abuse and Neglect Data System (NCANDS), approximately 3 million children were alleged to have been abused or neglected. In addition, approximately 693,000 children were determined to be victims of maltreatment. In the national system that tracks child abuse and neglect, NCANDS, children are counted as victims if an investigation by a state social services agency determines the case to be either "indicated" or "substantiated" maltreatment.[1] If a case is substantiated, an allegation of risk of harm or actual abuse was founded according to individual state definition. Indicated cases of maltreatment include situations where abuse or neglect could not be substantiated, but there was reason to suspect maltreatment. Children who belong to certain age groups and ethnic groups are at heightened risk for abuse and neglect. For example, children younger than 1 year had a reported maltreatment rate of 20.6 per 1,000 compared with 5.1 per 1,000 for 16 to 17 year olds.[1] African American, American Indian, Alaskan Native, and Pacific Islander children have higher rates of maltreatment than children from other ethnic groups. Specifically, in 2009, African American children had a reported maltreatment rate of 15.1 per 1,000 children, Pacific Islander children had a rate of 11.3 per 1,000 children, and American Indian and Alaskan Native children had a reported maltreatment rate of 11.6 per 1,000 children, compared with 7.8 per 1,000 non-Hispanic white children, 8.7 per 1,000 Hispanic children, and 2.0 per 1,000 Asian children.[1]

Child death is the most significant and devastating outcome of abuse and neglect. However, the prevalence is difficult to quantify. Recent studies in Colorado and North Carolina found that deaths from child abuse and neglect were underestimated in state records by approximately 50% to 60%. This under-recording is due to many factors, including the varying state definitions of "child homicide," "abuse," and "neglect," which can result in child deaths due to maltreatment not being reported on death certificates as deaths resulting from abuse or neglect.[35-37] Child death due to maltreatment and the problem of under-recording of child deaths due to abuse and neglect occur in all nations of the world.

In 2003, the United Nations Children's Fund (UNICEF) published a report on child deaths due to mistreatment in industrialized countries.[38] The UNICEF report found that 3,500 children under age 15 die each year from abuse or neglect in 27 wealthy nations. The study also reported that "two children die from abuse and neglect every week in Germany and the United Kingdom, three a week in France, four a week in Japan, and 27 a week in the United States." Further, "five nations—Belgium, the Czech Republic, New Zealand, Hungary, and France—have levels of child maltreatment deaths that are four to six times higher than the average for the leading countries. Three countries—the United States, Mexico, and Portugal—have rates that are between 10 and 15 times higher than the average for the leading countries."[38] While child maltreatment remains a domestic and international problem, the US and international data have both shown a trend toward improvement in some areas. The US data sources show that the rate of victimization per 1,000 children in the national population dropped from 12.5 children in 2001 to 9.3 children in 2009.[1,39] Internationally, the figures for child deaths due to maltreatment appear to be on the decline in the majority of industrialized nations.[38]

Risk Factors

No child is immune from abuse, and the circumstances that lead to maltreatment are complex and only partially understood. Child abuse can be inflicted by any person who cares for a child and it can occur in many different types of settings. However, there are certain factors that place some children at higher risk for mistreatment than other children. Studies and case reports have enumerated some criteria associated with abuse and neglect. Some of the most frequently cited risk factors include child morbidity, cultural background, family violence, low socioeconomic status, parental mental or physical illness, parents who themselves were victims of abuse, and social isolation or family breakdown.[18,40-42] These risk factors are often grouped into three main categories: child-associated risk factors, family-associated risk factors, and environmental characteristics.

Child-associated Risk Factors

Many types of child-associated factors can contribute to this category of risk factors. For example, children with certain types of illnesses or deficits may be more difficult to care for and may overwhelm the abilities of caregivers to provide adequate care. Premature and disabled infants are specific categories of children that may require levels of care that exceed the abilities of caregivers to provide a safe environment for the child. That being said, even a full-term, healthy baby's persistent and inconsolable crying may provoke abuse. In addition, certain stages of childhood development may be more stressful for some parents to navigate than others and may precipitate maltreatment by exceeding the caregiver's abilities to provide for the child physically and emotionally.

Family-associated Risk Factors

Parental vulnerabilities occur in many forms. Some common examples of characteristics that are parental risk factors for abuse include mental illness, substance abuse, lack of maturity, and history of abuse. Mental illness and substance abuse can be risk factors that place a parent in a weakened state and unable to implement the necessary organizational and judgment skills to effectively parent. If a young or developmentally-delayed parent lacks the requisite maturity to care for a child, this type of deficit can lead to a child's safety being compromised. If adult members of the family have themselves been abused, they may lack the parenting skills to utilize constructive responses to their child's behaviors as a result of their own suffering as victims of abuse.[43-45]

Environmental Characteristics

Poverty and violence are critical environmental risk factors for child abuse. In 2012, government statistics indicated that 21.9% of children in the US lived below the poverty line.[46] Although the actual income varies by family size and composition, the 2012 poverty threshold for a family of four with two related children under age 18 was $23,283.[47] According to the most recent National Incidence Study of Child Abuse (NIS-4), children from poor families (defined as incomes below $15,000 per year) were 5 times more likely to be abused or neglected than other children.[48] In addition to greater stress on the individual family, community resources are most often limited in poverty-stricken communities that often have few or no social support mechanisms available for families in need.

Another risk factor for child abuse is family and community violence. Environments in which violence is more common may give the appearance that violence is a socially acceptable response to address or control child behavior. A 2001 study by the National Institute of Justice (NIJ) found that being abused or neglected as a child increased the likelihood of mental health concerns, educational problems, and arrest as a juvenile. The NIJ study also found that children who have been abused and neglected were at greater risk for criminal behavior as adults.[49]

Clinical Features of Abuse and Neglect

Physical Abuse

Child maltreatment can be deceptive and easily disguised, but for any situation in which physical abuse of a child is suspected, the AMA dictates that a thorough health assessment be conducted. The assessment should include a history, a physical examination, a developmental assessment, and related laboratory studies.[50,51] Further, several findings (e.g., abdominal injuries, bruises, burns, fractures, and lacerations or abrasions) can represent physical conditions that may be indicative of mistreatment and can assist in the overall evaluation to investigate possible child abuse (Box 84-3).

Other injuries often sustained by children who are abused involve the central nervous system (CNS). These may be in the form of subdural hematoma (which can be reflective of blunt trauma), retinal hemorrhage, and subarachnoid hemorrhage (which can be indicative of violent shaking). Although mental health practitioners may not evaluate a child with immediate injuries of this type, any of these conditions may appear as background information in the medical chart and be relevant to support the need for further investigation.[50,51]

BOX 84-3 Physical Findings That Represent Physical Conditions That May Be Indicative of Mistreatment

ABDOMINAL INJURIES

Internal injuries without external bruises or lacerations. These could be the result of having been kicked, punched, or thrown.

BRUISES

Certain patterns may be formed that indicate a particular item or article may have been used to inflict injury (e.g., a belt buckle, clothes hanger, one's hand, or an electrical cord).

BURNS

A burn pattern may indicate the agent or mode of injury (e.g., cigarettes, an iron, a coil from an electric range, or a grill), as well as immersion burns (with stocking or glove-like patterns without splash burn areas).

FRACTURES

Commonly seen are transverse or greenstick fractures (due to bending or direct impact), a spiral fracture (due to limb torsion), a metaphyseal fracture (which can result from shaking or pulling of the limb end), and other bone fractures (including fractures of the skull, ribs, and long bones).

LACERATIONS OR ABRASIONS

Cut patterns on the mouth or lips may indicate, for example, a fist mark or razor laceration; parallel linear cuts may be from a whip or switch.

Emotional Abuse

Psychological maltreatment can have devastating and long-term consequences that persist into adulthood. One definition of emotional abuse describes it as "an assault on the child's psyche, just as physical abuse is an assault on the child's body."[52-54] Although the visible signs of emotional abuse can be hidden, a number of behavioral manifestations may be exhibited and can provide clues that a child has been the victim of emotional abuse. These symptoms often include anxiety, drug abuse, eating disorders, impaired attachments, low self-esteem, mood disturbance, poor defense mechanisms, school problems, sleep disturbances, somatic complaints with no underlying medical cause, and suicidal tendencies.[18,21,55] Disturbed emotional relationships in the form of disrupted attachments can have enduring negative consequences in terms of a child's ability to function in society and possess emotional rapport with others. Attachment is a template utilized by children to explore the outside world, to develop coping styles and strategies, to regulate stress, and to use as a stepping stone to continued development and maturation. When attachment is derailed by emotional abuse, a child's ability to trust, explore, and form healthy relationships is sacrificed in place of poor defense mechanisms and the potential for psychopathology.[43,56]

Knowing that the physical signs of emotional abuse are difficult to detect heightens the importance of other indicators that may signal child abuse. From the standpoint of the child, a clinician may notice sudden changes in the child's behavior or school performance, difficulty concentrating (unattributable to other psychiatric causes), hypervigilance, excessive compliance, extreme willingness to please, a lack of desire to return home, passivity, disengagement, or withdrawal.[57]

Neglect

Features of neglect relate to the deprivation of a child's basic needs for growth and development. Victims of neglect can display similar behavioral, cognitive, or developmental signs and symptoms as can victims of emotional abuse. In addition, there are possible physical manifestations that can jeopardize the child's health, require immediate medical attention, and alert the physician or other provider of mental health services that the child may be a victim of neglect. These include malnutrition/undernutrition, poor dentition (to a degree that severe dental caries or infection may result), poor hygiene (to a point that adverse health consequences may result), and untreated medical illnesses.[58] An extreme form of neglect is abandonment. In this form of neglect, the parent or primary caretaker rejects all parental duties and relinquishes any role of responsibility for the child. Although society may consider this type of maltreatment more benign than abuse, victims of chronic neglect may subsequently suffer from an inability to form emotional bonds. There are many consequences of failure to form healthy attachments that include derangements in normal child development. One specific example is a correlation between lack of social relatedness and empathic expression and future antisocial and criminal behaviors.

Treatment

Early identification, intervention, and treatment are critical components in minimizing the long-term consequences of child maltreatment. Currently, treatment modalities take a multidimensional approach to target the problem from many angles (including parental psychopathology, child trauma and abuse issues, family dysfunction, and social/community supports). This multimodal approach to treatment is a relatively new phenomenon. Three decades of child abuse research have shifted the focus from individual pathology (which focused almost exclusively on the parent) to treatment and prevention that utilizes an expanded model of multimodal and disciplinary care. Comprehensive strategies to evaluate and address the numerous determinants of child maltreatment have been addressed by a number of theoretical models.[43,56-58] The "ecological integration" view was first introduced by Belsky in the 1980s. He proposed a shift in the treatment paradigm from a focus on the parents or caregivers to an approach that emphasizes child and environmental risk factors.[43] Wolfe, in the early 1990s, proposed a "transitional" model that moved away from the concept of an individual psychological disorder of the caregiver and analyzed child maltreatment as an escalating problem on a continuum of cultural, individual, parental, and social interactions.[56] Another theoretical model that emerged in the mid-1990s was Cicchetti and Lynch's "transactional" approach.[57,58] Cicchetti and others postulated that numerous interactions of risk factors and protective factors between the family and society occur repeatedly over time. This model described the longitudinal interplay of these variables as a way in which individual adaptation and development is shaped. For example, they showed that rates of child physical abuse were related to levels of child-reported community violence.[57,58]

These etiological models of the last 25 years have replaced the older cause-and-effect models of child maltreatment that focused on the parent/caregiver as the central factor in abuse. In following with this broader understanding of the etiology of child abuse and neglect, current treatment focuses on the multiple pathways that may lead to abuse and the contributing situational factors (placing them in a sociocultural context, specific to each case). Current treatment modalities typically take a two-pronged approach to provide treatment to the parents and the child.

Parental Treatment

Change in parental behavior through education and training in child-rearing, child development, and the basic demands of parenting is generally offered through community mental health clinics or social services agencies. It is not uncommon that a generational cycle of abuse is present in parents who themselves have abused or neglected their children. Along with training in parental competence and parenting skills, individual therapy to address a past history of abuse of the parent by his or her caregiver may be required. Psychotherapy can be used to increase insight with regard to the maltreatment, address conflicts and relational difficulties, teach coping mechanisms for stressful situations, and provide emotional support. In addition, social supports and therapeutic services (such as parental support groups and home visits) should also be implemented to provide additional support and treatment.

Child Treatment

Maltreated children can display a host of protective defenses and are at risk for many types of psychiatric disorders, disturbances of behavior and emotion, learning difficulties, and developmental delays. Because maltreated children may exhibit a variety of responses to maltreatment, a thorough assessment and an accurate diagnosis are imperative before the initiation of treatment. Specific considerations that may assist in guiding the clinician's choice of treatment include an assessment of the child's developmental level at the time of the trauma and at the time treatment begins, the child's strengths, and ongoing challenges the child is facing. Psychotherapy is frequently used to assist in relational function, to address basic trust issues, to encourage and support emotional development, and to re-work maladaptive behavioral and relationship patterns. Additional therapeutic programs may address skill-building (cognitive and social), conflict management, and promotion of positive self-esteem.

ELDER ABUSE AND NEGLECT

According to the Centers for Disease Control and Prevention (CDC), elder maltreatment "is any abuse and neglect of persons age 60 and older by a caregiver or another person in a relationship involving an expectation of trust."[59] All 50 states, the District of Columbia, Guam, Puerto Rico, and the United States Virgin Islands have laws that govern the provision of adult protective services (APS) in instances of elder mistreatment. However, the criteria used by individual states to determine whether elder abuse or neglect has occurred, and therefore there is eligibility for APS services, vary widely. Some factors that vary between jurisdictions include the age of the victim; the type of abuse; whether or not neglect, exploitation, and abandonment are included; whether reporting is mandatory or voluntary (although a mandatory reporting requirement exists for most health professionals); investigative procedures; and available remedies.

Notwithstanding the differences between states in their definitions of elder abuse, most state laws include five elements.[60] These elements are infliction of pain or injury; infliction of emotional or psychological harm; sexual assault; material or financial exploitation; and neglect. Unlike child abuse, elders may suffer from self-neglect as they age and their ability to care for themselves declines as a result of physical and mental limitations.[61] At the federal level, although laws existed to fund services and shelters for victims of child abuse and domestic violence, there were no equivalent laws providing these services for elderly victims of abuse and neglect. In addition to providing definitions of elder abuse, the 2006 update to the federal Older Americans Act (OAA) provides direct funding to states to "carry out programs for the prevention, detection, assessment, and treatment of, intervention in, investigation of, and response to elder abuse, neglect, and exploitation (including financial exploitation)."[62]

Another important concern regarding elder maltreatment is protecting the elderly who reside in long-term care facilities. The Long-Term Care Ombudsmen Program (LTCOP) is federally mandated in every state, and the federal government conditions funding for elder abuse and neglect programs on the presence of the LTCOP in every state. The purpose of this program is to advocate on behalf of individuals who reside in a long-term care facility and experience some form of maltreatment. LTCOPs are the contact agency for licensed mental health professionals who, as mandated reporters, must report cases of suspected elder abuse in long-term care facilities.[63]

Significant and sweeping changes in elder abuse reporting and collection were to have occurred with the passage of the Elder Justice Act of 2010, an amendment to the Patient Protection and Affordable Care Act. This legislation called for improved ombudsman training, funding for evaluating the effectiveness of elder abuse programs, provide funding to states for the investigation and prosecution of elder abuse, and establish the Elder Justice Coordinating Council and an Advisory Board on Elder Abuse.[64] However, despite its call for $777 million over 4 years to achieve its goals, as of 2013, only $8 million has been appropriated.[65]

Epidemiology and Risk Factors

In 2003, to facilitate research about the topic, the National Research Council proposed a two-part definition of elder maltreatment: harm to a vulnerable elder that occurs either as a result of intentional actions by a caregiver or other trusted person or as a result of a caregiver to provide for basic needs and to protect the elder from harm.[66,67] In the last decade, as awareness of the extent of the problem has increased, so has the amount of research concerning elder maltreatment.

As awareness of elder mistreatment has increased, its characterization has improved. The National Elder Mistreatment Study, conducted in 2009, sought to estimate the prevalence of elder abuse. In this sample of almost 6,000 elders, the overall 1-year prevalence of mistreatment was 11.4%; 4.6% suffered emotional abuse, 1.6% physical abuse, 0.6% sexual abuse, 5.1% potential neglect, and 5.2% financial abuse.[68] Elder abuse may occur in domestic settings and be perpetrated by family members, or it may affect individuals in institutions who are being cared for by unrelated caregivers. Elders age 80 or older are abused and neglected at two to three times their proportion of the elderly population. In addition, corroborated reports of elder mistreatment and self-neglect have been shown to be associated with shorter survival.[69]

Risk factors for elder abuse and neglect may be divided into four categories: those associated with victims of maltreatment, those associated with perpetrators of maltreatment, those associated with relationships, and those associated with environment. A 2013 review of 49 studies found 13 risk factors associated with elder maltreatment: cognitive impairment, behavioral problems, psychiatric illness or psychological problems, functional dependency, poor physical health or frailty, low income or wealth, trauma or past abuse, ethnicity (victim); caregiver stress, caregiver psychiatric illness or psychological problems (perpetrator); family disharmony, poor or conflictual relationships (relationships); and low social support (environment).[70] Elders who are depressed or cognitively impaired are more likely to suffer from self-neglect.[61] Self-neglect is associated with significantly higher rates of hospitalization, with a positive correlation as severity of self-neglect increases.[71]

Detection and Reporting

Physicians are mandatory reporters of suspected elder abuse and neglect, but may be inadequately trained to recognize elder mistreatment.[72,73] Detection of the signs and symptoms of abuse may be subtle and masked by other illness or debility. To the untrained eye, elderly victims of abuse and neglect may appear to be simply frail and sick. Since the findings may be difficult to distinguish, adequate screening in health care settings is of critical importance. In addition, for many victims of elder abuse and neglect, hospitals may be among the only sources of help, placing physicians and other members of the hospital staff in the unique and important position of recognizing and addressing suspected elder maltreatment.[74] Physicians and other providers of mental health care should familiarize themselves with reporting requirements in the jurisdictions in which they practice. Familiarity with available resources for screening and investigation in cases of suspected elder abuse is also warranted.

The AMA's Diagnostic and Treatment Guidelines on Elder Abuse and Neglect provide reference criteria to assist physicians in the recognition, diagnosis, and response to cases of elder mistreatment.[75] Elder abuse is often more difficult to detect than child abuse. Social isolation is more common among the elderly, and this can both increase the risk of maltreatment and decrease the likelihood that these individuals will come in contact with health professionals. According to the National Elder Abuse Incidence Study of 1996, approximately 25% of the elder population lives alone. Many elderly have family members as their primary contacts and may have minimal interaction with others.

Treatment

A thorough assessment should accompany the treatment of physical conditions or injuries associated with abuse or neglect. The treatment may include wound care for bedsores, provision of adequate nutrition, and assistance with hygiene. The contributing factors to the observed abuse or neglect should be assessed. It may become imperative that the elderly individual needs be removed from caretakers, family or unrelated, and protected in a safe environment. A hospital admission may be required until alternatives can be located. In other cases, provision of services in the present living situation may be enough. Overall, the data on the efficacy of interventions for elder abuse is limited and more research is needed.[76]

Also important is a determination of the elder's ability to make decisions for himself or herself. If the elder is cognitively impaired, this assessment may require the use of formal evaluations of memory and other neuropsychological functions. In cases where the elder does not possess capacity to make decisions for himself or herself, appointment of a substitute decision-maker may be required.

Access the complete reference list and multiple choice questions (MCQs) online at https://expertconsult.inkling.com

KEY REFERENCES

6. Committee on National Statistics (CNSTAT). *Elder mistreatment: abuse, neglect, and exploitation in an aging America*, Washington, DC, 2002, National Academies Press.
9. Lachs MS, Pillemer K. Abuse and neglect of elderly persons. *N Engl J Med* 332:437–443, 1995.
15. Garbarino J, Ebata A. The significance of ethnic and cultural differences in child maltreatment. *J Marriage Fam* 45:733–783, 1983.
16. Kempe CH, Silverman FN, Steele BF, et al. The battered child syndrome. *JAMA* 181:17–24, 1962.
28. Glaser D. Emotional abuse and neglect (psychological maltreatment): a conceptual framework. *Child Abuse Negl* 26:697–714, 2002.
29. Brown J, Cohen P, Johnson JG. A longitudinal analysis of the risk factors for child maltreatment: findings of a seventeen-year prospective study of officially recorded and self-reported child abuse and neglect. *Child Abuse Negl* 22:1065–1078, 1998.
33. Block RW, Krebs NF. Committee on Child Abuse and Neglect, and the Committee on Nutrition. Clinical report: failure to thrive as a manifestation of child neglect. *Pediatrics* 116(5):1234–1237, 2005.
36. Herman-Giddens ME, Brown G, Verbiest S, et al. Underascertainment of child abuse mortality in the Unites States. *JAMA* 282(5):463–467, 1999.
44. Agran PF, Anderson C, Winn D, et al. Rates of pediatric injuries by 3-month intervals for children 0 to 3 years of age. *Pediatrics* 111:e683–e692, 2003.
45. National Center on Addiction and Substance Abuse. *No safe haven: children of substance-abusing parents*, New York, 1999, Columbia University.
53. Simeon D, Gurainik O, Schmeidler J, et al. The role of childhood interpersonal trauma in depersonalization disorder. *Am J Psychiatry* 158:1027–1033, 2001.
54. Lyons-Ruth K. Attachment relationships among children with aggressive behavior problems: the role of disorganized early attachment patterns. *J Consult Clin Psych* 64:64–73, 1996.
61. Abrams RC, Lachs M, McAvay G, et al. Predictors of self-neglect in community-dwelling elders. *Am J Psychiatry* 159(10):1724–1730, 2002.
63. NORC—National Long-Term Care Ombudsman Resource Center. About ombudsmen, Available at:<http://www.ltcombudsman.org/about-ombudsmen>.
66. National Center on Elder Abuse. Statistics, research, and resources, Available at: <www.elderabusecenter.org>.
68. Acierno R, Hernandez MA, Amstadter AB, et al. Prevalence and correlates of emotional, physical, sexual, and financial abuse and potential neglect in the United States: The National Elder Mistreatment Study. *Am J Public Health* 100:292–297, 2010.
69. Lachs MS, Williams CS, O'Brien S, et al. The mortality of elder mistreatment. *JAMA* 280(5):428–432, 1998.
70. Johannsen M, LoGiudice D. Elder abuse: a systematic review of risk factors in community-dwelling elders. *Age Ageing* 42:292–298, 2013.
71. Dong X, Simon MA, Evans D. Elder self-neglect and hospitalization: findings from the Chicago Health and Aging Project. *J Am Geriatr Soc* 60:202–209, 2012.
73. Melton GB. Chronic neglect of family violence: more than a decade of reports to guide US policy. *Child Abuse Negl* 26(6–7):569–586, 2002.
75. AMA Council on Judicial and Ethical Affairs, Physicians and Domestic Violence. Ethical considerations. *JAMA* 267:113–116, 1992.

WEBSITES

Child and Adolescent

Child Trends Databank, US Department of Health and Human Services, Children's Bureau, NCANDS, Available at: <www.childtrendsdatabank.org>.

Child Welfare Information Gateway, Children's Bureau/ACYF (formerly, the National Clearinghouse on Child Abuse and Neglect Information and the National Adoption Information Clearinghouse). 2005 state statute series: definitions of child abuse and neglect (2005), Available at: <www.childrenwelfare.gov/systemwide/laws_policies/statutes/define.cfm>.

Elderly

National Center on Elder Abuse. Statistics, research, and resources, Available at: <www.elderabusecenter.org>.

85 Legal and Ethical Issues in Psychiatry I: Informed Consent, Competency, Treatment Refusal, and Civil Commitment

Ronald Schouten, MD, JD, Judith G. Edersheim, JD, MD, and José A. Hidalgo, MD

KEY POINTS

- Litigation is divided into two general categories: civil and criminal. Civil matters involve claims of injury or some other transgression that can be remedied by the payment of money (damages) or performance or cessation of certain activities (injunctive relief). Criminal matters involve acts committed in violation of a statute, for which the penalty may be a monetary fine, incarceration, or both.

- To qualify as an expert, a witness must have knowledge of the subject in question beyond that of the average layperson by virtue of education, training, and experience. Unlike fact witnesses, expert witnesses may offer opinion testimony and are generally allowed to use hearsay evidence.

- Four ethical principles form the foundation of clinical care: autonomy, beneficence, justice, and non-malfeasance.

- The patient's signature on a consent form does not constitute informed consent itself; the form is merely evidence that the informed consent process occurred.

- Only a court can declare an individual to be legally incompetent. While evaluation of a patient's decision-making capacity by a physician or a mental health professional is commonly referred to as a "competency evaluation," the evaluating clinician has no authority to change the patient's legal status.

OVERVIEW

This chapter covers four related medicolegal concepts, each of which is central to the practice of psychiatry and other mental health professions. The unifying concept for all of these topics is the ethical principle of individual autonomy, which has been made operational through various legal protections. The word *autonomy* is from the Greek "auto" = self and "nomos" = law; literally "self-rule." Autonomy is often summarized as our right to be left alone. In health care, this concept of self-rule or self-determinism gives rise to the fundamental premise that all adults have the right to make their own decisions regarding, among other things, their treatment for medical conditions, including mental illness.

In this chapter, we will examine how autonomy interests are protected, who exercises them when individuals lack the ability to do so, and under what circumstances treatment and confinement can be imposed. In this and subsequent chapters, we will describe interactions with the legal system and will use terms that may not be familiar to some readers. We will also provide an overview of the legal system as psychiatrists may encounter it.

AN INTRODUCTION TO INTERACTIONS WITH THE LEGAL SYSTEM

The American legal system is composed of parallel systems of state and federal constitutions, statutes, and courts. The United States Constitution is the controlling body of law, and any law, state or federal, that conflicts with the Constitution will be struck down if challenged. The rulings of the United States Supreme Court, which interprets the Constitution, are therefore controlling on Constitutional and federal law matters. States are free to provide greater protections of Constitutional rights than the Supreme Court interprets the Constitution as requiring, but may not provide less. On purely state law matters, including most civil matters, the decisions of state courts and state statutes are controlling.

Litigation is divided into two general categories: civil and criminal. Civil matters are those involving a dispute between parties in which one party claims to have been injured by another, or some other transgression has occurred, that can be remedied by the payment of money (damages) or performance or cessation of certain activities (injunctive relief). The purpose of civil litigation is to right the wrong that one party has inflicted on the other or otherwise correct the offensive behavior of the wrongdoer. Criminal matters are those in which a party has committed an act that has been declared illegal by a government authority, and for which the penalty may be a monetary fine, incarceration, or both. Both civil and criminal trials can be before a judge alone (bench trials) or before a judge and jury (jury trials). In a jury trial, the jury decides the issues of fact—for example, guilty or not guilty, liable or not—and the judge rules on the principles of law, such as, the admissibility of specific evidence. In a bench trial, the judge both rules on the law and is the fact-finder.

In all litigation, the party bringing the action can only prevail by supplying evidence that meets the standard of proof. That standard varies with the type of legal action involved (Box 85-1). In personal injury cases, such as malpractice claims, the plaintiff (the party claiming to have been injured) must prove his or her case by a preponderance of the evidence: that is, the plaintiff must convince the fact-finder that his or her claims are more likely true than not. This is the lowest standard of proof. At the other end is the standard used in criminal prosecutions: the prosecution must prove the defendant's guilt beyond a reasonable doubt. In other types of cases, such as civil commitment, a standard of proof between these extremes is required: clear and convincing evidence, per the United States Constitution.

There are two basic types of witnesses: fact witnesses and expert witnesses. Psychiatrists may be asked to serve in either role. Anyone who has first-hand knowledge of events and facts relevant to the case can be asked to serve as a fact witness. Fact witnesses may testify only as to first-hand knowledge; they may not introduce hearsay evidence, that is, information they have heard from others, except under certain limited circumstances. Most important, fact witnesses may not give opinion

CIVIL COMMITMENT

Civil commitment is an administrative or judicial process by which the state's power is used to identify and remove a mentally-ill individual from society and place him or her in an institutional setting. The involuntary confinement of a person due to mental illness is one of the oldest clinical interventions, if not the original clinical intervention, for the mentally ill. Throughout the ages, the purpose and justification of such confinement has cycled between protection of the rest of society and the patient's need for treatment. When the purpose is the protection of both the patient and society from the dangers associated with the illness, the state is considered to be using its *police powers*. The police powers approach focuses on the dangerousness of the patient to self or others. When the justification for commitment is the need of the patient for treatment, the state is using its *parens patriae* authority: that is, the state is acting toward the individual citizen with the same authority and responsibility as a parent toward a child. Under this rationale, the state takes a beneficent role toward its citizens and acts in their best interests to protect them from their incapacities or disabilities.[73]

With the increased focus on civil rights and autonomy in the 1970s, the best interest or *parens patriae* need for treatment approach to civil commitment was replaced by the dangerousness/police powers approach in most jurisdictions. This approach allows an individual to be involuntarily committed to a mental institution only if the individual poses a danger to himself or herself through direct injury, if there is a direct threat of physical harm to others, or if the individual is gravely disabled and unable to care for himself or herself in the community.[86,87] The definition of danger, and the level of dangerousness required for civil commitment, vary among the states.[88]

The process for civil commitment varies among jurisdictions. All states provide for an initial short-term emergency confinement without the necessity of a judicial hearing. Generally, such emergency certification requires examination by a mental health professional (such as a psychiatrist, psychologist, or psychiatric nurse), who makes the clinical findings required by the applicable commitment statute. Following the initial emergency confinement, which varies in length from 2 days to 3 weeks among the states, the facility may release the patient, convert the admission to a voluntary hospitalization, or petition a court for an order of civil commitment.[4]

Commitment hearings differ in their level of procedural safeguards. Some jurisdictions authorize administrative boards or hearing officers to conduct the proceedings, while others require a full hearing before a judge, with psychiatric examinations, witness testimony, and documentary evidence. In 1979, the United States Supreme Court ruled that the standard of evidentiary proof required for a civil commitment is clear and convincing evidence that the commitment meets statutory standards. Several states, however, have chosen to require a higher standard of proof in these proceedings (namely, proof beyond a reasonable doubt), rather than offer the Constitutional minimum.

The length of these commitments also varies by jurisdiction. Most states specify a period of confinement varying from 6 months to 1 year, with the requirement that formal re-commitment proceedings be initiated in order to extend the time period. A minority of states have no explicit commitment period and provide that the commitment terminates when the patient's clinical condition no longer meets statutory standards.

Civil Commitment of Sex Offenders

During the 1980s, a series of highly publicized and horrifying sex crimes catalyzed the enactment of state statutes providing for the civil commitment of convicted sex offenders after the completion of their prison sentences. In 1990, Washington State enacted the first sexual predator law, and now 19 states have so-called sexual predator statutes that provide for indefinite confinement in specialized treatment centers after a defendant is convicted of a sex crime and is determined to be a sexually-dangerous person.[89] Although each state has a different standard for such commitment, these statutes generally provide for the detention of offenders with broadly defined mental abnormalities or mental illnesses that predispose them to commit sex crimes.[90] A diverse array of interest groups have criticized these laws on various grounds, alleging that they violate civil rights, criminalize mental illness, depend on unreliable predictions of future behavior, and divert the focus away from longer or more effective prison sentences.[91] In addition, critics observe that these statutes confine patients based on a treatment rationale when it is not clear that effective treatment for sex offenders exists.[92]

The Supreme Court upheld the constitutionality of these laws in three cases. In *Kansas v. Hendricks*[93] the court determined that a "mental abnormality", such as pedophilia, combined with a finding of dangerousness or the likelihood of re-offense was a sufficient rationale for an indefinite civil commitment. The court also upheld the validity of sexual predator laws against a claim that the treatment is so inadequate and punitive that it is the equivalent of a second prison sentence.[94] Most recently, in *Kansas v. Crane*[95] the court lowered the threshold for the behavioral dyscontrol, requiring only proof that the offender has difficulty controlling his dangerous behavior rather than a "total or complete lack of control." In 1999 the American Psychiatric Association task force on sexually-dangerous offenders produced a report opposing the penal use of commitment statutes, concluding that they pose a threat to the integrity of psychiatric diagnosis and the therapeutic basis for other civil commitment statutes.[96] In 2006 the United States Congress, however, passed the most comprehensive sex offender law in U.S. history, the Adam Walsh Law. The law is consistent with civil commitment schemes found in the landmark sex offender cases, *Kansas v. Hendricks* and *Kansas v. Crane*, and requires the determination of a "mental abnormality" on the part of the defendant and of any volitional component to the crime.[97]

Outpatient Commitment

While involuntary hospitalization provided a treatment setting for people at imminent risk of harming themselves or others, it did not offer a treatment scheme for a significant population of chronically mentally-ill people who were unwilling or unable to comply with outpatient treatment regimens. These patients were frequently re-hospitalized, only to deteriorate immediately after discharge. In response to the problem of the "revolving door" patient and a series of highly publicized violent acts by persons with mental illness, several states decided to revitalize the seldom-used outpatient commitment statutes. These statutes, previously enacted in almost every state but rarely used, allowed judges to require patients to comply with outpatient treatment regimens or face involuntary hospitalization. Outpatient commitments could be ordered on discharge from the hospital or as an alternative to civil commitment.[98]

Outpatient commitment procedures were initially heavily criticized as a violation of Constitutional guarantees of equal protection and due process of law, and an unacceptable instrument of social control. Critics also voiced concerns that despite being ordered to comply with community mental health treatment, patients were provided with inadequate treatment in under-funded programs.[99] Some of these concerns were ameliorated by two randomized trials of outpatient commitment undertaken in New York and North Carolina.[100,101] The data from these two studies, examined in light of their methodological limitations, appear to support the use of outpatient commitment to stabilize and improve the quality of life for chronically mentally-ill people. Although the debate over the legitimacy and efficacy of outpatient commitment is still unresolved, it appears to significantly improve adherence to medication regimens and is associated with decreases in substance use, re-hospitalization, homelessness, and violent victimization among certain groups of severely mentally-ill patients.[102–104]

CONCLUSION

The topics covered in this chapter represent interactions with the legal system that are part of the day-to-day professional lives of psychiatrists, especially when working with vulnerable populations whose treatment is more likely to involve the legal issues we have discussed. Over the years, many clinicians have expressed dismay over what they perceive to be intrusions by the legal system into the care of patients, as represented by the topics covered here. In fact, some of these requirements have proven burdensome and, in some situations, have resulted in outcomes that have been unhelpful, if not overtly harmful, to specific patients. Such adverse outcomes, as well as the increased non-clinical burden on psychiatrists, are frustrating. In managing these situations, and our frustration, it may be helpful to keep in mind that these perceived intrusions are the result of our living in a system that protects the civil liberties and autonomy interests of all people, even when the ability to speak on one's own behalf has been lost. Ours is a system that balances individual rights to self-determination and autonomy of individuals against the rights of individuals to be safe, and of states to protect their citizens. As with all human endeavors, there is imperfection, and the system does not always get it right. It is a system that is open to change and input, however, and psychiatrists have an important role to play in this regard. Basic knowledge about patients' rights and the legal system, and working across disciplines is essential for providing effective care in this climate, and facilitating changes that will benefit our patients.

Access the complete reference list and multiple choice questions (MCQs) online at https://expertconsult.inkling.com

KEY REFERENCES

3. Strasburger LH, Gutheil TG, Brodsky A. On wearing two hats: role conflict in serving as both psychotherapist and expert witness. *Am J Psychiatry* 154:448–456, 1997.

4. Appelbaum PS, Gutheil TG. *Clinical handbook of psychiatry and the law*, ed 4, Philadelphia, 2006, Lippincott Williams & Wilkins.

11. Monahan J. John Stuart Mill on the liberty of the mentally ill: a historical note. *Am J Psychiatry* 134:1428–1429, 1977.

15. *Cruzan v. Director, Missouri Department of Health*, 497 U.S. 261 (1990).

24. Appelbaum PS, Lidz CW, Meisel A. *Informed consent: legal theory and clinical practice*, New York, 1987, Oxford University Press.

28. Sawicki NN. Informed consent beyond the physician-patient encounter: tort law implications of extra-clinical decision support tools. *Ann Health Law* 21:1–10, 2012.

36. Grisso T, Appelbaum PS. *Assessing competence to consent to treatment: a guide for physicians and other health professionals*, New York, 1998, Oxford University Press.

42. Appelbaum PS. Assessment of patients' competence to consent to treatment. *N Engl J Med* 357:1834–1840, 2007.

46. *Rogers v. Commissioner of Department of Mental Health*, 390 N.E.2d 489 (Mass. 1983).

55. Srebnik DS, Rutherford LT, Peto T, et al. The content and clinical utility of psychiatric advance directives. *Psychiatr Serv* 56:592–598, 2005.

59. Nicaise P, Lorant V, DuBois V. Psychiatric advance directives as a complex and multistage intervention: a realist systematic review. *Health Soc Care Community* 21(1):1–14, 2013.

61. Swanson JW, Van McCrary S, Swartz MS, et al. Superseding psychiatric advance directives: ethical and legal considerations. *J Am Acad Psychiatry Law* 34:385–394, 2006.

83. Lieberman JA, Roberts LW, Butterfield MI, et al. Ethical principles and practices for research involving human participants with mental illness. *Psychiatr Serv* 57:552–557, 2006.

96. American Psychiatric Association. *Dangerous offenders: a task force report of the American Psychiatric Association*, Washington, DC, 1999, American Psychiatric Association.

not to be held responsible for their otherwise criminal acts.[45] The concept itself, and the derivative question of what to do with individuals who are found not guilty by reason of insanity (NGRI), have been the subject of much debate and have generated fluctuating standards. Few activities of mental health professionals get as much media and public attention and spark as much controversy as testimony on these matters.

A detailed history of the evolution of the insanity defense is beyond the scope of this chapter, but interested readers may wish to consult the classic texts on the subject,[8,46,47] as well as some of the more modern and readily available treatises on the insanity defense.[48-50]

The history of the insanity defense is a chronicle of society's struggles over moral responsibility, ecclesiastical influences, historical events, the nature and level of scientific understanding of mental illness, and public attitudes about the mentally ill.[48,51] For example, the episodic mental illness of King George III is believed to have had a major influence on the attitudes of the public, and therefore the jurors of the time,[8,48] and may have benefited some criminal defendants of the period.[48] There are numerous examples of the criminal responsibility standard being tightened after the perpetrator of a notorious crime is found NGRI: for example, James Hadfield,[8] Daniel M'Naghten,[8,52] and John Hinckley.[53] The modifications tend to be such that the infamous defendant would have been found criminally responsible under the newly modified standard.

Before turning to the insanity defense itself, an overview of the basics of criminal law and related defenses is useful. In order for an individual to be convicted of a crime, there must be a guilty act (*actus reus*) and guilty intent (*mens rea*). *Mens rea* is considered in both a general and specific form. In its general form, it refers to the overall capacity of an individual to form the intent to commit the crime in question and thus his or her blameworthiness or legal liability. For example, an individual who takes someone else's automobile for his own use when directed to do so by auditory hallucinations, or who is not even aware that he is stealing a vehicle, is unlikely to be found to have had the necessary intent to be found blameworthy. In its specific or narrow form, *mens rea* is an element of a group of crimes referred to as specific intent crimes: for example, larceny of a motor vehicle (knowingly taking possession of property that is not your own, for your own use, and with the intent to deprive the true owner of its use) or murder.[54] (Under Massachusetts law, *murder* is defined as follows: "Murder committed with deliberately premeditated malice aforethought, or with extreme atrocity or cruelty, or in the commission or attempted commission of a crime punishable with death or imprisonment for life, is murder in the first degree. Murder which does not appear to be in the first degree is murder in the second degree. Petit treason shall be prosecuted and punished as murder. The degree of murder shall be found by the jury." From MGL Ch. 265 §1.)

Beyond the obvious defenses of denying that he or she committed the act, or that no crime occurred, a criminal defendant has two broad categories of defenses available: justification and excuse.[55,56] The distinction between the two categories is not always clear: for example, the difference between self-defense (justification) and duress (excuse) is often more apparent than real.[57]

Justification Defenses

Justification defenses are those in which a normally wrongful act is committed, but under circumstances that make it acceptable rather than wrongful. The justification defenses include self-defense; defense of others; defense of property; and choice of evils, that is, a choice is made to commit a criminal act that is less harmful than the available alternative act.[54-56]

Excuse Defenses

Whereas the availability of a justification defense turns on the act itself and the circumstances under which it occurred, excuse defenses look to the internal mental state of the actor. Excuse defenses have been formally debated at least since the time of Aristotle.[55] There are several related excuse defenses, including ignorance, compulsion, duress, and insanity.

Ignorance

Lack of knowledge of the crime, mistaken belief about the act, and inadvertence can all serve as complete or partial defenses under the general category of "ignorance."[54,55] There are limited roles for psychiatric testimony in such defenses, as the focus is on the knowledge of the defendant, rather than on his or her mental functioning. Where such testimony occurs, it is likely to be restricted to the cognitive abilities of the defendant.

Compulsion

Compulsion is a category of excuse defenses that focuses on the ability of a defendant to think and act rationally under the influence of external circumstances. Compulsions serve as a defense because the external force (not an internal influence, such as an impulse-control disorder, e.g., pedophilia), deprives the defendant of the ability to make choices that he or she would normally make.[55] The compulsion defenses represent the notion that it would be unfair to convict a defendant of a criminal act if the jurors, as representatives of the rest of society, would have behaved similarly under the same circumstances.[54,57] Compulsion defenses include duress, extreme emotional disturbance, and compulsion due to addiction or insanity.[55]

Duress. This defense is available where an individual (the actor) commits an act because another person has unlawfully threatened him or her with equal or more serious injury, such that the only way to avoid imminent death or serious injury is to comply with the unlawful instruction.[54,57] While duress has been held not to excuse murder, it has been found to be a valid defense to robbery, kidnapping, prison escape, possession of a weapon, and treason.[56]

Extreme Passion. Extreme emotional disturbance can also serve as a partial or complete defense. Examples include situations where an individual learns of spousal infidelity or death of a loved one at the hands of another. The defense requires that the defendant prove that he or she was under extreme emotional distress at the time of the act and that his or her action was reasonable in light of that distress.[56] New York penal law provides an affirmative defense of extreme emotional distress for assault charges, including first-degree murder: if "[t]he defendant acted under the influence of extreme emotional disturbance for which there was a reasonable explanation or excuse, the reasonableness of which is to be determined from the viewpoint of a person in the defendant's situation under the circumstances as the defendant believed them to be."[58,59] Psychiatrists may be asked to opine about the presence and level of emotional distress on the part of the defendant, but the issue of reasonableness is an issue for the jury.

Compulsion Due to Addiction or Insanity. The compulsion defense may be raised where a defendant's addiction or insanity leads him or her to criminal conduct if the actor reasonably believed he or she would suffer death or great bodily harm if he or she did not perform the criminal act. Thus, a person suffering command hallucinations may raise a compulsion defense, just as a person addicted to drugs or alcohol may raise a compulsion defense to charges of illegal use. The Supreme Court has held that it is unconstitutional to convict drug addicts of the crime of having an addiction[60] or using drugs.[61]

LACK OF CRIMINAL RESPONSIBILITY

A criminal defendant may be found to lack criminal responsibility where the defendant was impaired in his or her ability to think or to act rationally because of a mental disease or defect. The essence of this defense is that the defendant, as a result of the condition in question, has a certain status such that it would be improper to hold him or her morally blameworthy.[47,55,62] Infants, for example, are not held criminally responsible for their acts because they are not regarded as having the capacity for rational thought that would designate them as blameworthy persons in the eyes of the law.[47] Individuals who commit acts of violence due to automatisms occurring during altered states of consciousness (for example, somnambulism, complex partial seizures, and delirium tremens) may also be excused from responsibility.[63,64]

The insanity defense is the best known of the excuse defenses. As noted earlier, the essence of the insanity defense is the centuries-old recognition that certain individuals should not be held morally blameworthy and therefore are not criminally responsible for their acts.[47] Societies have drawn a line between those conditions that may relieve one of moral blameworthiness and those that do not. Like many moral issues, that line is not always clear. For example, while automatisms, as noted, may be the basis for an excuse defense, dissociative identity disorder (multiple personality disorder) has had far less success, perhaps because of skepticism about the disorder.[65] Voluntary intoxication, as a state brought on by the willful act of the defendant, is not allowed as the basis for an insanity defense.[54] However, mental conditions exacerbated by intoxication or resulting from long-term substance abuse may be used as the basis for an insanity defense.[66] In many states, voluntary intoxication can be used to argue for diminished capacity, a state of altered behavior that does not fulfill criteria for a full insanity defense but may be used to lessen the severity of the crime of which the defendant is convicted: for example, from first- to second-degree murder.[67,68]

There are a number of landmark cases that mark the development of the insanity defense in Anglo-American law. The changes in the standards mark alterations between those that are purely volitional (ability to control one's behavior), purely cognitive (knowledge of wrongfulness), combined volitional-cognitive standards, and pure *mens rea* standards. One state uses yet another approach, known as the "product" test.[48]

An early example of a volitional standard is the "Wild Beast" test, described in *Rex v. Arnold* (1723).[69] In that case, the court held that "Mad Ned" Arnold, on trial for shooting Lord Onslow, could be found NGRI only if he were completely devoid of control. The judge wrote, in part:

"It is not every kind of frantic humour, or something unaccountable in a man's actions, that points him out to be such a madman as is to be exempted from punishment: it must be a man that is totally deprived of his understanding and memory, and doth not know what he is doing, no more than an infant, than a brute or a wild beast, such a one is never the object of punishment."[69]

At the turn of that century, the insanity acquittal of James Hadfield,[70] charged with High Treason after his failed attempt to assassinate King George III, turned on the court's acceptance of defense counsel's argument that those with mental disturbances short of "Wild Beast" status were also eligible for an insanity acquittal. Lord Erskine successfully argued on Hadfield's behalf that:

"… if a total deprivation of memory was intended by these great lawyers to be taken in the literal sense of the words: if it was meant, that, to protect a man from punishment, he must be in such a state of prostrated intellect, as not to know his name, nor his condition, nor his relation towards others—that if a husband, he should not know he was married; or if a father, could not remember that he had children; nor know the road to his house, nor his property in it—then no such madness ever existed in the world."[8,48]

Hadfield was found not criminally responsible due to his illness (a delusional state that appeared to result from a sabre wound to the skull while fighting the French at the Battle of Freymar). Under the terms of the Insane Offenders' Act, passed by Parliament during the course of his trial, Hadfield was remanded to Bethlem Hospital, there to be held, "until his Majesty's pleasure be known."[8]

The next major development in the insanity defense, the M'Naghten standard,[71] has remained a major component of modern criminal responsibility standards. In 1843, M'Naghten, a Scottish wood turner, shot and killed Edward Drummond, private secretary to Prime Minister Robert Peel, after mistaking him for the Prime Minister. He was found NGRI, thanks to his skillful counsel's success in convincing the court that M'Naghten's "partial insanity" provided an adequate basis for excusing him from responsibility.[8,52]

The public was outraged by M'Naghten's acquittal, as was Queen Victoria. In response, the House of Lords posed five questions to the judges of the court and convened them to explain the rules by which criminal responsibility would be determined.[8] The Lords first wanted to know what the law was with respect to crimes:

"… committed by persons afflicted with insane delusion … : as, for instance, where at the time of the commission of the alleged crime, the accused knew he was acting contrary to law, but did the act complained of with a view, under the influence of insane delusion, of redressing or revenging some supposed grievance or injury, or of producing some supposed public benefit?"[72]

In response to this first inquiry, Lord Chief Justice Tyndal explained:

"Assuming that your Lordships' inquiries are confined to those persons who labour under such partial delusions only, and are not in other respects insane, we are of the opinion that, notwithstanding the party accused did the act complained of with a view, under the influence of insane delusion, of redressing or revenging some supposed grievance or injury, or of producing some public benefit, he is nevertheless punishable according to the nature of the crime committed, if he knew at the time of committing such crime that he was acting contrary to law."[72]

Thus, if a person suffering from a paranoid delusion killed another whom he believed was about to kill him, he could be acquitted on the basis of self-defense. However, if the delusional belief was that the victim had libeled him, he would be convicted, as libel does not justify murder.[72]

In responding to the inquiries about the proper instructions to the jury and what facts were to be considered, Lord Chief Justice Tyndal described what has come to be known as the M'Naghten Rule:

"To establish a defence on the ground of insanity, it must be clearly proved that, at the time of the committing of the act, the party accused was labouring under such a defect of reason, from disease of the mind, as not to know the nature and

quality of the act he was doing; or, if he did know it, that that he did not know he was doing what was wrong."[72]

Under this rule, for a defendant to be found not responsible, he had to be (1) mentally ill or suffering a mental defect, e.g., dementia or significant developmental disability, and either be (2) unaware of what he was doing, for example, believed he was pointing his finger when in fact he was pointing a pistol, or (3) unaware that he was committing an unlawful act, for example, believed he was defending himself against deadly attack. Notably, M'Naghten would have been convicted had this standard been applied to him.

Subsequent developments in the insanity defense, both in England and the US, tended to expand the criteria, as knowledge and attitudes regarding mental illness changed. The "irresistible impulse test," which looked to whether a defendant had the ability to conform his or her behavior to the requirements of the law, even while knowing that the act was wrongful, made its way into English and American jurisprudence by the late 1800s.[8,48] The New Hampshire Rule, which is still the standard in that state, asks the jury to find the defendant NGRI if the alleged criminal's act was the product of a mental disease or defect.[48]

In 1962, the American Law Institute's Model Penal Code introduced criteria for an insanity defense that offered alternative bases for an NGRI verdict: either the cognitive component of M'Naghten or the volitional component of the irresistible impulse test.[54] The standard is as follows:

"A person is not responsible for criminal conduct if at the time of such conduct as a result of mental disease or defect he lacks substantial capacity either to appreciate the wrongfulness of his conduct or to conform his conduct to the requirements of the law.

As used in this Article, the terms "mental disease or defect" do not include an abnormality manifested only by repeated criminal or otherwise antisocial conduct."[54]

By the early 1980s, 25 states were using the American Law Institute's Model Penal Code standard, as were the federal courts. John Hinckley's attempted assassination of President Ronald Reagan, and his subsequent acquittal on the basis of lack of criminal responsibility, changed that, however. Hinckley's acquittal, like M'Naghten's, resulted in demands to restrict, and in some cases eliminate, the insanity defense.[73] With support from the American Psychiatric Association and American Bar Association, Congress enacted a new standard for criminal responsibility in the federal courts:

"It is an affirmative defense to any prosecution under any Federal statute that, at the time of the commission of the acts constituting the offense, the defendant, as a result of a severe mental disease or defect, was unable to appreciate the nature and quality or wrongfulness of his acts."[74]

This standard essentially adopted the M'Naghten standard, completely eliminating the volitional component contained in the American Law Institute's Model Penal Code standard. It also made clear that the defendant must be unable to appreciate the wrongfulness of his or her conduct, rather than merely lacking "substantial capacity" to appreciate wrongfulness. In addition, Congress specified that the underlying disorder related to the crime must be "severe" and shifted the burden of proof to the defendant. Just as with M'Naghten, the subsequent modification of the federal standard would have likely resulted in Hinckley's conviction, had it been in place at the time of trial.

The impact of the Hinckley acquittal spread beyond the federal system to the states.[52] According to Melton and colleagues,[75] by 1995, 5 of the 25 states that had been using the Model Penal Code test in its pure form had given it up, with about half the states using a form of the M'Naghten rule. Twelve states expanded the verdicts available in cases involving mental illness by introducing "guilty but mentally ill" verdicts. In these states, a defendant may be found guilty, guilty but mentally ill, not guilty, and NGRI.[52] Three states abolished the insanity defense completely and established procedures to commit guilty but mentally ill defendants, with mixed results.[53,76,77] Changes in other jurisdictions included shifting the burden of proof from the prosecution to the defendant and tightening the definition of mental illness.[53]

As noted previously, the insanity defense is an expression of society's view that it is inappropriate to impose criminal responsibility on individuals who are not morally blameworthy. The various criminal responsibility standards are efforts by individual jurisdictions to operationalize this universal notion in a manner consistent with public attitudes. Studies of the impact of different criminal responsibility standards indicate that mock jurors using the different insanity defense standards arrive at similar verdicts in similar cases, regardless of the standard used.[78] Mock jurors given no standards, merely instructions to use their best judgment, arrived at the same verdicts as those asked to apply specific standards.[79] From these and other studies, it appears that factors other than the technical criminal responsibility standard determine whether or not a jury will find a defendant NGRI. Those factors include the nature of the crime, the nature of the illness, the nature of the act, and the consequences the jury sees attached to a guilty versus NGRI verdict.[48]

The question of what to do with insanity acquittees is an enduring one. In most jurisdictions, insanity acquittees are automatically committed to a state psychiatric facility for a defined initial period for evaluation and treatment. At the end of that initial period, a recommitment hearing is held; states are free to use lower standards of proof for commitment of insanity acquittees (preponderance of the evidence) than for noncriminal candidates for commitment (clear and convincing evidence). The Supreme Court has held that the government may automatically confine insanity acquittees, regardless of their crime, and hold them until such time as the acquittee can prove that he or she is no longer mentally ill or dangerous.[80]

Insanity acquittees who refuse treatment with antipsychotic medication may be treated against their will under the same rules that apply to other civilly committed patients in that jurisdiction. Civil standards apply because these individuals have not been convicted of any crime, and therefore can only be held in a hospital if they meet normal civil commitment standards.

EVALUATIONS OF CRIMINAL RESPONSIBILITY

Evaluations of criminal responsibility are, by necessity, retrospective determinations of the defendant's mental status at the time of the offense. The focus of criminal responsibility evaluations is assessment of the individual's mental state at that time using the current examination, a review of medical and criminal records, and information from collateral sources, and a conclusion regarding that status relative to the jurisdictional standards for criminal responsibility. Under ideal conditions, the accused is evaluated by mental health professionals as close to the occurrence of the offense as possible. In many cases, however, the forensic evaluator may not see the defendant until months or years after the crime. An excellent discussion of these evaluations is provided by Melton and associates.[75]

A number of clinical conditions can affect criminal responsibility: for example, delirium, depression, psychosis, delusions, panic and other anxiety disorders, sleep disorders, obsessive-compulsive disorder, seizures, and other neurological disorders. In light of this, the clinical evaluation should be detailed and extensive, with a full review of systems. Medical records should be examined and laboratory studies ordered to assess for the presence of other illnesses and conditions, including intoxication.

Criminal responsibility evaluations are complicated not only by the retrospective nature of the analysis, often over time, but by the fact that the sources of information are often incomplete or biased. Police reports, statements from family members, victim statements, and the defendant's self-report are also essential parts of the evaluation. And all of them are affected, to greater or lesser degrees, by their own inherent bias, which is often difficult to detect. The Model Penal Code, Section 4.05, provides an outline of what the report on a criminal defendant should contain.[54]

DEMOGRAPHICS OF THE INSANITY DEFENSE

Misperceptions of the insanity defense include the beliefs that it is frequently used, often successful, and available primarily to wealthy, educated defendants. Various studies have indicated that the insanity plea is used in 0.1% to 0.5% of felony cases,[75] except in Montana, where it was as high as 8% between 1969 and 1979.[72] Notably, Montana is one of the states that abolished the insanity defense post-*Hinckley*, although for practical purposes, the defense is still available.[77]

The success rate of the insanity defense varies across jurisdictions, but studies by Steadman and co-workers[81] and Callahan and colleagues[82] indicate that it is successful in approximately 25% of those cases where it is used. This yields an estimated successful utilization rate of approximately 0.125% nationally. The case is resolved by a mechanism such as plea bargaining, rather than a jury trial, in more than 70% of cases in which it is successful.[75]

CONCLUSION

Mental illness and the criminal justice system are inextricably intertwined. Mental illness may lead to incarceration, if only to remove mentally ill individuals from the streets in the absence of more suitable community alternatives. Psychiatrists are frequently called on to evaluate individuals involved in the criminal justice system at various points in the criminal justice process, from initial arrest to imposition of punishment. Common questions include competence to stand trial and criminal responsibility. As with all consultations and evaluations, psychiatrists who accept such assignments must be aware of the applicable standards and familiarize themselves with ethical guidelines for their participation in criminal matters. It is important for all psychiatrists to be aware of ways in which the criminal justice system may involve them and their patients.

Access the complete reference list and multiple choice questions (MCQs) online at https://expertconsult.inkling.com

KEY REFERENCES

2. American Academy of Psychiatry and the Law. *Ethics guidelines for the practice of forensic psychiatry*, Bloomfield, CT, 2006, American Academy of Psychiatry and the Law.
4. Gilligan J. The last mental hospital. *Psychiatr Q* 72:45–61, 2001.
7. Finkel NJ, Slobogin C. Insanity, justification, and culpability toward a unifying schema. *Law Hum Behav* 19:447–464, 1995.
8. Walker N. *Crime and insanity in England*, Edinburgh, 1968, University of Edinburgh Press.
10. McKenzie A. "This death some strong and stout hearted man doth choose": the practice of peine forte et dure in seventeenth- and eighteenth-century England. *Law Hist Rev* 23:279–313, 2005.
18. Grisso T. *Evaluating competencies: forensic assessments and instruments*, New York, 1986, Plenum Press.
19. Hoge SK, Poythress NG, Bonnie RJ, et al. The MacArthur adjudicative competence study: diagnosis, psychopathology, and competence-related abilities. *Behav Sci Law* 15:329–345, 1997.
24. *Jackson v. Indiana*, 406 U.S. 715 (1972).
27. *Washington v. Harper*, 494 U.S. 210 (1990).
28. *Sell v. United States*, 539 U.S. 166 (2003).
30. *Rogers v. Commissioner of Department of Mental Health*, 459 N.E.2d 308 (Mass. 1983).
35. *Ford v. Wainwright*, 477 U.S. 399 (1986).
39. American Medical Association, Council on Ethical and Judicial Affairs. *Code of medical ethics*, section 2.06: capital punishment, Chicago, 1997, American Medical Association.
40. Gutheil TG. Ethics and forensic psychiatry. In Bloch S, Chodoff P, Green SA, editors: *Psychiatric ethics*, ed 3, New York, 2007, Oxford University Press.
49. Finkel NJ, Parrott WG. *Emotions and culpability*, Washington, DC, 2006, American Psychological Association.
50. Robinson DN. Wild beasts and idle humours: the insanity defense from antiquity to the present. *J Forensic Psychiatry* 8:465–467, 1997.
53. Low PW, Jeffries JC, Bonnie RJ. *The trial of John W. Hinckley, Jr.*, Mineola, NY, 1986, Foundation Press.
55. Buchanan A. *Psychiatric aspects of justification, excuse and mitigation in Anglo-American criminal law*, London, 2000, Jessica Kingsley Publishers.
59. Kirschner SM, Galperin GJ. The defense of extreme emotional disturbance in New York County: pleas and outcomes. *Behav Sci Law* 20:47–50, 2002.
62. Moran R. The modern foundation for the insanity defense—the cases of Hadfield, James (1800) and McNaughtan, Daniel (1843). *Ann Am Acad Pol Soc Sci* 477:31–42, 1985.
66. Marlowe DB, Lambert JB, Thompson RG. Voluntary intoxication and criminal responsibility. *Behav Sci Law* 17:195–217, 1999.
73. Steadman HJ, McGreevy MA, Morrissey JP, et al. *Before and after Hinckley: evaluating insanity defense reform*, New York, 1993, Guilford Press.
75. Melton GB, Petrila J, Poythress NG, et al. Mental state at the time of the offense. In *Psychological evaluations for the courts*, ed 3, New York, 2007, Guilford Press.
79. Finkel NJ, Handel SF. Jurors and insanity: do test instructions instruct? *Forensic Reports* 1:65–79, 1988.
81. Steadman HJ, Keitner L, Braff J, et al. Factors associated with a successful insanity plea. *Am J Psychiatry* 140:401–405, 1983.
82. Callahan LA, Steadman HJ, McGreevy MA, et al. The volume and characteristics of insanity defense pleas: an eight-state study. *Bull Am Acad Psychiatry Law* 19:331–338, 1991.

87 Legal and Ethical Issues in Psychiatry II: Malpractice and Boundary Violations

Ronald Schouten, MD, JD, Rebecca Weintraub Brendel, MD, JD

KEY POINTS

- Malpractice litigation has a significant impact on the professional and personal lives of sued psychiatrists, but the evidence does not support perceptions that it is out of control.

- Liability of psychiatrists is normally limited to acts of negligence and a limited number of intentional acts that occur in the course of treatment.

- Sexual involvement with current patients and former patients is considered unethical by the American Psychiatric Association's Principles of Ethics.

- The Health Insurance Portability and Accountability Act (HIPAA) sets the minimum standard for privacy protections and does not allow for private lawsuits by patients, who may sue for breach of confidentiality under state statutes and common law.

- Good doctor–patient communication has been shown to be an effective component of malpractice risk reduction.

OVERVIEW

Of all the areas in which psychiatry and the law interact, few stimulate as much affect as does medical malpractice liability. In this chapter, we will cover some of the core concepts in personal injury law and then focus on medical malpractice in psychiatry. We will discuss specific areas of liability risk, including boundary violations.

THE MEDICAL LIABILITY CLIMATE

Approximately every 10 years, American medicine finds itself in the midst of a "malpractice crisis"[1]; the first years of the twenty-first century have been no exception. As in the past, there is debate about the nature and cause of problems related to malpractice litigation, such as rising premiums and the cost of defensive medicine, as well as what to do about them. Are there more lawsuits and higher awards? Are insurance premiums higher and, if so, why?[2–4] Calls for tort reform routinely cite the cost of defensive medicine and the impact of malpractice on rising health care costs.[5,6]

The responses of researchers and commentators to these highly charged questions are not always consistent with the most pessimistic perceptions of the medical community. Contrary to the concern that every error leads to a lawsuit, only a small percentage of cases involving injury due to medical errors actually become the basis for claims or litigation,[7–9] and defendants continue to prevail in the majority of cases that result in litigation, in part because a substantial proportion of those cases appear to lack merit.[10] From 1956 to 1990, the number of malpractice claims for all specialties rose 10-fold: from 1.5 per 100 to 15 per 100 covered physicians.[11] Overall, it appears that the median malpractice award (both jury awards and settlements) doubled in real dollars between 1990 and 2001, but it has remained essentially flat since then, albeit with variation among the states.

Psychiatrists can take some comfort from being among the physicians least likely to be sued. In their study of malpractice risk by specialty, Jena and colleagues[12] found that psychiatry had the lowest proportion of physicians facing malpractice claims annually (2.6%) from 1991 to 2005, with neurosurgery the highest at 19.1%. Even so, by the age of 65, 75% of physicians in the low-risk group, which also included family medicine and pediatrics, had been sued during the time period.

Kilgore and colleagues[13] studied the impact of various proposed tort reforms on malpractice premiums and determined that imposition of caps on malpractice damage awards resulted in significantly lower malpractice premiums. They estimated that a nation-wide cap of $250,000 on non-economic damages would result in a premium savings of $16.9 billion per year. They also found that malpractice premiums had an inverse relationship with the Dow Jones Industrial Average.[13] This observation supports the hypothesis that insurers raise premiums in order to pay their stockholders when other investments are performing less well.

It is certainly the case that malpractice premiums have increased over the years, and that multiple causes are to blame.[14] It is not at all clear, however, that malpractice premiums have increased significantly relative to other expenses. In an in-depth analysis of data from nine regions from 1970 to 2000, Rodwin and associates[15] examined actual premiums paid (as opposed to advertised rates) relative to overall physician income and expenses. They found that premiums for self-employed physicians rose from 1970 to 1986, declined from 1986 to 1996, and rose thereafter. Premiums were lower in 2000 than they were in 1986, however, and other practice expenses continued to increase while spending on malpractice premiums fell from 1986 (11% of total expenses) to 2000 (7% of total expenses).[15]

There is no end in sight to arguments over the causes of medical malpractice litigation,[7,16] the need for tort reform, and the assignment of blame for dissatisfaction with medical practice.[17,18] Whether or not there is an actual crisis, or whether premiums are a relatively smaller or a larger portion of practice expenses, there is no contesting the fact that the prospect of a lawsuit and actually being sued have a major impact on the personal and professional lives of defendant physicians, and the relationships these physicians have with their patients.[19–22] The threat of malpractice litigation is unlikely to diminish significantly, given the Institute of Medicine's 1999 estimate that 44,000 to 98,000 deaths per year are due to preventable medical errors. While the personal injury system is not without its problems, hopes for a significant decrease in medical malpractice claims appear to lie with changes in how medical care is delivered, rather than with doing away with personal injury law.[23]

Support for the argument that malpractice reforms reduce costs is mixed. In 2003, Texas adopted malpractice reforms that capped non-economic damages at $250,000 for most cases. Stewart and colleagues[24] studied the impact of the reforms on general surgery malpractice claims in an academic medical center. They found a significant drop in claims from 40 to 8 per 100,000 procedures, as well as a significant drop in litigation costs. According to Paik and colleagues,[25] this did not result in reduced spending on medical care, which would have been expected had the reforms resulted in a decrease in defensive medicine.

MALPRACTICE LIABILITY

A tort is an injury to another party that gives rise to a right on the part of the injured person to sue the party causing the injury for damages.[26] Personal injury or tort law embodies the principle that a person injured by the acts of another should receive compensation for the harm done. This concept dates back more than 2,000 years.[27] Medical malpractice is a subset of tort law that is concerned with alleged negligence by medical professionals. Medical malpractice as a concept represents the application of tort principles to the actions of professionals, and like tort law itself, is an ancient phenomenon.[27-29]

There are two types of torts, intentional and unintentional.[26] Both may be the subject of malpractice claims in psychiatry. Intentional torts are injuries that result from some intentional action on the part of the actor, also referred to as the *"tort feasor,"* who will ultimately be the defendant if a lawsuit is pursued. In psychiatric malpractice claims, typical intentional torts are battery, assault, false imprisonment, abandonment, intentional infliction of emotional distress, and undue familiarity (i.e., sexual misconduct and other boundary violations). Each of these intentional torts is discussed later in this chapter. Unintentional torts arise out of negligent acts or omissions (e.g., misdiagnosis or failure to diagnose, failure to protect the patient from self-harm or harm to others). These are also discussed later in this chapter.

Tort law serves two purposes. First, it fulfills the long-established concept that individuals who are injured by the negligent actions of others should receive compensation from the person who caused the harm for the damage they have suffered. Second, some believe that the threat of potential liability serves as a deterrent to negligent behavior.[30,31] Mello and Brennan[32] cast doubt on the deterrence idea in personal injury matters generally, and medical malpractice specifically.

Malpractice insurance also serves two purposes. First, it ensures that injured patients can receive compensation when they are harmed; second, it protects the defendant physician from having to pay damages personally, thus risking potential financial ruin.[33] Malpractice insurance is designed to insure physicians in the event that harm results from negligence (i.e., the allegedly wrongful act was inadvertent rather than intentional).

Medical treatment necessarily involves intentional actions, and liability may therefore arise from both intentional and unintentional acts and omissions that are part of the treatment. As a result, certain intentional acts are also covered by malpractice insurance. For example, a patient injured during a restraint, or hospitalized against his or her will, may sue for battery or false imprisonment, respectively, and the malpractice insurer will both defend the claim and pay any damage award. The same is not true if the psychiatrist punches the patient during a fit of anger, for example, as this action is outside the scope of psychiatric treatment and therefore has nothing to do with acts performed in the course of caring for the patient.[33] Sexual misconduct by psychiatrists raises similar questions about what actions by psychiatrists should be considered part of the scope of treatment and therefore covered by insurance, or separate from treatment and therefore not covered by malpractice insurance, as will be discussed later in this chapter.

To establish a claim of malpractice, whether the defendant's action was intentional or unintentional, a plaintiff (the party bringing the suit and claiming to have been injured) must prove four things.[26,34] (The plaintiff may be the injured party himself or herself, or a representative of the injured party, e.g., the parent of an injured child or the executor of the estate of the deceased in a wrongful death action.) First, the plaintiff must prove that the defendant owed a duty to the injured party. All individuals owe a general duty of reasonable care, such that their ordinary behavior does not result in harm to others (e.g., drivers have a general obligation not to drive recklessly). The duty to behave in a non-negligent fashion toward a specific individual or group arises when there is a special relationship.[26] Thus, while a physician does not have a specific duty to a person until a doctor–patient relationship is established, once that relationship begins the physician has a duty to perform in accordance with the standard of care of the average physician practicing in that specialty.[26]

In order to prove the existence of a duty, the plaintiff must establish that a doctor–patient relationship existed. Simply put, a doctor–patient relationship is established when the physician accepts responsibility for the patient's care by becoming involved with the treatment.[35] Curbside or informal consultations, or even more formal consultations, will not establish the existence of a relationship, so long as the consultant does not assume a treatment role.[36-39]

States differ as to whether clinicians owe a duty of care to individuals other than patients with whom they have entered into a doctor–patient relationship. Specifically, one may wonder what happens when a non-patient is injured by the actions of the clinician's patients.[40,41] This concept of duty to third parties is discussed more fully later in this chapter.

The second element of a malpractice claim is dereliction of duty, or negligence. It can be characterized as a departure from the standard of care that results from failure to exercise the level of diligence or care exercised by other physicians of that specialty. An error or injury does not constitute malpractice if it occurs in the course of treatment where the physician has exercised due diligence.[42,43]

In order to establish this element, the plaintiff must introduce evidence of the applicable standard of care. This is perhaps the most critical element in malpractice claims, as the applicable standard varies according to the situation, the type of practitioner, and the jurisdiction. Specialists, or those who claim to have special expertise, are held to a higher standard of practice than general practitioners.[26] Under the "School Rule," practitioners who belong to a defined, recognized school of practice or belief may be judged according to the standard of practice of that school,[44] although minimum standards of practice are expected of anyone who holds himself or herself out as being capable of diagnosing and treating illness.[26] In the past, the applicable standard was dependent on the community in which the physician was practicing (e.g., urban physicians were held to a higher standard than were rural physicians). That rule, known as the "Locality Rule," has gradually faded with the wide availability of journals, on-line medical resources, and educational conferences, resulting in a more uniform national standard of care.[45] While there has been a move toward a more national standard of practice, jurisdictions continue to differ as to whether residents and other trainees should be held to a standard of practice defined by others at that level of training, of general practitioners, or of specialists.[46]

The third element, causation, and the fourth element, damages, are closely tied to the first two: the plaintiff must show that the negligent behavior is the direct cause or proximate cause of actual damages.[47,48] Causation in personal injury law is assessed in two ways. First, the "but-for" test is applied:

"But-for the alleged negligence, would the injury have occurred?" Second, was there proximate or legal cause (i.e., was the injury foreseeable)? The test for forseeability is whether the claimed harm was "a natural, probable, and foreseeable consequence" of negligence on the part of the actor.[26]

Under the doctrine of "loss of chance," causation may also be established where the act or omission by the defendant-physician resulted in a lost opportunity for treatment and therefore subsequent harm.[49-51] This scenario might occur, for example, where there is a missed diagnosis, delayed referral, or delayed treatment.[52] The loss of chance rule has been rejected in professional negligence cases in some jurisdictions[53] and retained in others.[54]

Damages can be of several types. They may be economic (such as lost value of future earnings and medical expenses arising from injuries) or they may be physical (such as the loss of a bodily function). They may also be emotional (e.g., development of psychiatric disorders or pain and suffering).[55-57] Punitive damages may also be awarded, where the defendant's behavior was so reckless as to justify imposition of added damages as punishment for egregious behavior and also to serve as a means of deterring that defendant and other potential defendants who might act similarly in the future.[58]

These four elements of a malpractice claim are often referred to as the four Ds: duty, dereliction of duty, direct causation, and damages.[59] If the defendant convinces the jury, or the judge in a bench trial, that all four elements have been proved by a preponderance of the evidence (i.e., that it is more likely than not to have occurred), the defendant will be required to compensate the victim for the harm suffered.[26,59] Expert witnesses who offer their opinions on any of the four elements must testify to a "reasonable degree of medical certainty"—that is, they are confident that their opinions are more likely true than not.[60]

LIABILITY AND MANAGED CARE

Managed care has had a dramatic impact on the practice of psychiatry and the delivery of mental health services. Early on, psychiatrists recognized the potential liability associated with treatment decisions being influenced, and in some cases controlled, by insurers. One might ask, "Is the psychiatrist or inpatient unit liable if a suicidal patient is refused further insurance coverage for inpatient hospitalization, is discharged, and then succeeds in committing suicide?" In a word, yes. A psychiatrist's duty to his or her patient continues, regardless of whether the patient's insurer will continue to pay for services.[61,62]

The financial liability of employer-sponsored health plans for damages resulting from denial of health care benefits is significantly limited by the Employee Retirement Income Security Act (ERISA).[63] ERISA contains a pre-emption clause that limits the possible damages from denial of care to the value of the actual benefit or service denied, thus shielding managed care plans from liability for negligence or harm resulting from denial of care. The Supreme Court made clear in *Aetna v. Davila*[64] that ERISA applies to all covered plans, in spite of state statutes that attempt to provide state law remedies for denial of care and resultant harm. However, ERISA does not pre-empt state statutes that require independent third-party reviews of denials of service, according to the Supreme Court.[65]

The result of this federal statutory scheme is that physicians and health care institutions remain liable for harm that results from withholding or from early termination of treatment, even if the managed care organization has withdrawn funding. Injured patients have no recourse against the managed care plan other than a civil action for the value of the lost benefits.[66] They are free, however, to pursue traditional malpractice claims against providers. In order for the physician to avoid liability,

he or she must protest the denial of care, appeal it to the highest level that the insurer provides, and take other reasonable steps to ensure the patient's safety. Providers themselves may pursue administrative and civil remedies to recover the value of the care provided. However, physicians' entitlements to do so are likely to be limited by their own contracts and agreements with managed care providers.

SELECTED AREAS OF LIABILITY RISK IN PSYCHIATRY
Assault, Battery, and False Imprisonment

A *battery* is the touching of another person without consent or justification.[26] An *assault* is an action that causes fear in the victim due to the reasonable apprehension that an unpermitted touching will occur.[26] Battery and assault are intentional torts. In the setting of medical malpractice, battery claims typically arise when the clinician departs from the standard of care by providing treatment without obtaining informed consent in the absence of an emergency or other exception to informed consent.[67] That is, without consent, treatment is an unauthorized touching, which legally constitutes a battery.

False imprisonment, another intentional tort, results when the tort feasor causes the victim to have a reasonable belief that his or her movement and freedom are constrained.[26,68] This can occur with confinement to a locked ward, room seclusion, or restraints. False imprisonment does not require actual physical restraint or physical confinement. A patient who reasonably believes that the door to his or her room is locked may claim false imprisonment, even if the door is not actually secured. False imprisonment can lead to liability for violation of constitutional rights, as well as personal injury liability.[69] Conversely, failure to restrain or confine a patient who is at risk of self-harm or elopement may also give rise to liability.

In addition to claims of false imprisonment, the restraint process also may give rise to claims of assault and battery, as it necessarily involves: (1) apprehension of touching; (2) the actual touching of the patient (generally without the patient's consent); and, (3) restriction of movement. The legal aspects of restraint of patients on a medical or surgical ward vary among jurisdictions and are beyond the scope of this chapter but have been explored elsewhere.[70]

Malpractice claims based on battery or false imprisonment, whether they arise in the general hospital or in psychiatric facilities, are rarely successful. Successful defense of these claims lies in demonstrating that the restraint and seclusion were clinically reasonable, that no less restrictive alternative existed, that they were carried out and documented in a careful manner, that the techniques used complied with hospital policies and procedures, and that the restraint process occurred as required by applicable laws and regulations of the jurisdiction in which it occurred.[71-73]

Misdiagnosis

Both failure to diagnose and erroneous diagnosis can provide a basis for unintentional tort liability, if harm results.[74] As noted earlier, a medical error that results in injury does not establish negligence if it occurred in spite of practice in accordance with the standard of care, or the adverse outcome was an unavoidable result that might have occurred regardless of the treatment.

Failure to Treat

This broad category of liability risk includes the failure to treat an identified condition, or providing treatment that is unproven, not generally accepted, or disproven. In the simplest cases, the patient who suffers injury because the physician failed to treat the condition can generally recover for harm suffered as a result. Harm allegedly resulting from administering treatments that are either unproven or not yet widely accepted can also be the basis for a claim.[75-77] The quest for effective treatments for mental illnesses has included exploration of complementary and alternative treatments.[78] Psychiatrists should be aware that all of the same malpractice issues involved in other areas of psychiatry apply here. While treatment with complementary and alternative methods is a field that has not yet attracted substantial numbers of malpractice claims, significant areas of potential risk include lack of informed consent, loss of chance, failure to treat, and fraud and misrepresentation.[76-79] Psychiatry is a field in evolution, with a history of adopting apparently effective treatments that eventually declare themselves to be either unhelpful or harmful. As a result, caution must be exercised with regard to declaring certain treatments to be state-of-the-art, and the failure to provide them as constituting *prima facie* evidence of malpractice.[80,81]

Abandonment

Abandonment, as a cause of action for malpractice, is the unilateral termination of the doctor–patient relationship without justification, leading to harm to the patient.[26] In non-emergent situations, physicians are not legally obligated to treat every patient who requests care. Refusal to treat a patient on the basis of his or her race, religion, ethnic origin, or disease type (e.g., acquired immunodeficiency syndrome [AIDS]) raises ethical issues and sets the stage for liability under the Americans with Disabilities Act and state anti-discrimination statutes.[82] The obligation is ethical, as well as legal.[83] Even after the doctor–patient relationship has begun, the physician may choose to terminate the relationship and may legally do so if the method used is reasonable and does not unjustifiably put the patient at risk.[26,59] Justifiable bases for terminating the relationship can include failure to pay, threatening behavior, repeated failure to keep appointments, non-compliance with treatment, and abuse of prescribed medication.[59] Once the decision to terminate treatment has been made, the physician should notify the patient and inform him or her of available emergency services and alternative treatment options. Ideally, a specific referral can be provided. The treatment course, reasons and indications for the transfer or termination, the steps taken, and referrals provided should be documented in the record.[84]

Liability for the Acts of Others

Under the law of agency, as exemplified by the legal doctrine of *respondeat superior* (let the master answer), an employer is liable for the acts of his or her employees if they are performed within the scope of the employment. Liability arising from the master–servant/employer–employee relationship is also known as *vicarious liability*. In psychiatry, this can become an issue in several settings: for example, supervision of students and residents, supervision of non-physicians, and providing medication back-up.[85,86]

In all cases of vicarious liability, there are several key issues. The first is whether the allegedly negligent and harmful action of the supervisee was within or outside the scope of his or her employment. For example, vicarious liability could arise if the supervisee injures a patient in the course of a restraint, but not if the supervisee and the patient were to get into a fight at a hockey game. The second issue is whether the supervisor's status was that of employer or a mere advisor or consultant. In order for vicarious liability to be imposed, the alleged master must have sufficient control over the allegedly negligent actor to justify imposition of liability. Criteria include veto authority over treatment decisions, control of the amount and type of work, and hire-and-fire authority.[59,85-87] Where there is vicarious liability, both the supervisor and the supervisee may be held liable.[26,88] Supervisors may also be directly liable for harm that results from the action of their supervisees. For example, an attending physician may be held directly liable for harm to a patient where he or she fails to countermand the negligent orders of a resident.[89,90]

Confidentiality and Privilege

Psychiatrists have an ongoing ethical[91,92] and legal[93,94] duty to maintain the confidentiality of information disclosed by patients in the course of treatment, and may be held liable for unauthorized disclosure. Numerous ethical and legal exceptions exist to the requirement of confidentiality; all of these exceptions represent a balancing of the relative harms that result from maintaining or breaching confidentiality in given situations. Ethical exceptions to confidentiality tend to be permissive (e.g., "A psychiatrist may breach confidentiality. …"). These exceptions tend to be commonsense in nature, but leave the discretion to the practitioner, without imposing obligations.[95] The legal exceptions, found in case law, statutes, and regulations, tend to fall into two broad categories: immunity from liability for disclosure in good faith and required disclosures.

Whether a given exception falls into the immunity for disclosure or mandatory disclosure category depends on the nature of the exception and the jurisdiction. For example, as is discussed in depth in Chapter 84, all 50 states in the US have statutes that designate a range of professionals as mandated reporters who are obligated to report suspected child abuse or neglect to state social service agencies. Many states also require reporting of known or suspected abuse or neglect of the elderly or disabled. In recent years, a number of states have also begun requiring physicians and others to report known or suspected cases of domestic violence to law enforcement or designated agencies.[96]

Of all the exceptions to confidentiality, perhaps the best known involves the duty to protect third parties from the violent acts of patients. This duty exists in some, but not all, jurisdictions.[42,43,97] The rationale for the duty to act to protect third parties was set forth in the California Supreme Court's decision in *Tarasoff v. Board of Regents*,[98] in which the court held that psychotherapists have a duty to act to protect third parties where the therapist knows or should know that the patient poses a threat of serious risk of harm to the third party. The court addressed the balancing issue and noted, "The Court recognizes the public interest in supporting effective treatment of mental illness and in protecting the rights of patients to privacy. But this interest must be weighed against the public interest in safety from violent assault."[98]

Liability for failure to breach confidentiality resulting in harm to third parties did not originate with *Tarasoff*; preceding and subsequent cases have imposed liability on physicians for failing to disclose an individual's infectious disease status where others were subsequently infected.[99-101] Human immunodeficiency virus (HIV)/AIDS poses special problems in this regard, as some states have common law or statutory obligations to breach confidentiality to protect third parties, but also have prohibitions against disclosing HIV-positive status without written permission.[102] As with many other legal issues, the jurisdictions vary with regard to the duty to disclose HIV-positive status to a spouse.[103,104]

A substantial number of states have enacted statutes that address the duty to protect third parties.[41,105,106] Some states have eliminated the duty altogether, while others limit its scope. Those states that have statutes generally limit the situations under which the duty may arise: for example, a specific threat to an identifiable third party or a known history of violence on the part of the patient and a reasonable basis to anticipate violence. They also provide that the duty is fulfilled by taking certain steps (such as hospitalizing the patient, warning the potential victim, or notifying law enforcement). Finally, the statutes relieve the clinician of liability to the patient for good faith breaches of confidentiality, and some immunize the clinician from liability for failing to take steps to protect.

The variations among jurisdictions in the law regarding the duty to protect can lead to much confusion. Clinicians are advised, as a basic matter, to become familiar with the standards in the jurisdictions in which they practice. It is important to remember that the duty represents an exception to confidentially, which is recognized in all jurisdictions as being of paramount importance in clinical care, and that any breach of confidentiality must be justified and reasonable. It should be limited to disclosure of the minimum amount of information necessary to serve the purpose in question. Thus, even in jurisdictions in which there is a duty to protect third parties or efforts to protect are made permissible by statute, the clinician should first take steps that will protect the third party without disclosing confidential information (e.g., arranging for hospitalization). Only where absolutely necessary to prevent harm should the patient's clinical information be disclosed to the intended victim or police. The effort to prevent harm to the third party, including the decision to share information, should be regarded as a clinical intervention, with every effort made to engage the patient in the effort to avoid harm to others and the adverse consequences to himself or herself.[107]

Other exceptions to confidentiality include statutory provisions that allow disclosure of clinical information in pursuit of the civil commitment process, bill collection, and defense of malpractice claims. It is also accepted that a reasonable amount of information may be disclosed when applying to admit or transfer a patient to a hospital. For example, the Massachusetts psychotherapist patient privilege statute is typical in its exceptions to the obligation to maintain confidentiality.[108]

Passage of the Health Insurance Portability and Accountability Act (HIPAA) of 1996,[109] and its implementation in 2003, have caused considerable concern for psychiatrists. HIPAA was originally designed to ensure that individuals with pre-existing illnesses would continue to be eligible for health insurance coverage if they changed employers and to increase the ease of transmission of medical information among authorized users.[110] However, in this law, Congress went far beyond this initial purpose, enacting legislation that led to the promulgation of new rules for how health information must be managed.

HIPAA imposes a number of requirements on practitioners, health plans, and institutions, and there have been a number of misconceptions about these requirements and their impact on patient care.[111] Many psychiatrists and other mental health professionals were initially concerned that HIPAA would prohibit breaches of confidentiality that were required by state law, thus raising the specter of having to choose between a violation of HIPAA and liability under state law. In fact, there are more similarities with pre-existing confidentiality rules than differences. Even more, HIPAA expands situations in which protected health information may be released without specific consent by the patient. As with traditional rules, HIPAA calls for disclosure of the minimum amount of

information necessary to fulfill a specific need when confidentiality is to be breached, even with consent.

With regard to concerns about *Tarasoff* and related dangerousness situations, the HIPAA Privacy Rule[112] allows for disclosure of protected health information without the specific consent of patients in 13 different situations related to the good of the public. Among the 13 are disclosures required by law or public health authorities, reporting of abuse and neglect, reports to law enforcement, infectious disease reporting, and disclosures to avert serious and imminent harm to individuals. Thus, the rules regarding breaches of confidentiality for safety purposes are largely unaffected by HIPAA.[113]

Before HIPAA, in order for a physician or health care entity to release information, a patient's specific informed consent was generally obtained. In the interest of promoting efficiency in the health care system, HIPAA expressly changed this practice for covered health care providers who release information for treatment, payment, and health care operations purposes. Under HIPAA, covered entities (including physicians) may disclose a patient's protected health information for these three purposes without specific consent for the release of information provided that the patient has been notified of the new HIPAA rules through a Privacy Notice. It is important for individual providers to determine whether they are covered by HIPAA in order to bring their practices into compliance with HIPAA. In general, physicians performing "certain electronic transactions" are subject to HIPAA; the main triggering transaction is electronic billing.[111–115]

It should be noted that HIPAA sets a minimum standard for privacy protection; where state statutes and regulations provide greater protections for privacy, they override HIPAA. Finally, physicians are not subject to direct civil actions by patients under HIPAA. Enforcement of HIPAA is strictly a function of the Office of Civil Rights (OCR) of the Department of Health and Human Services. An aggrieved patient cannot file an action under HIPAA individually. However, patients are left to their long-standing civil remedies for breach of confidentiality under state statutes and common law. Violations of HIPAA can result in escalating civil and criminal penalties, depending on the nature of the violation and the frequency. In most cases, enforcement of the Privacy Rule is likely to be for corrective rather than punitive action where violations have occurred in good faith.

Among the most relevant provisions of HIPAA for psychiatrists is the distinction between general psychiatric records and psychotherapy notes. Under HIPAA, psychiatric records are generally treated the same as general medical records.[112] This approach is a departure from pre-HIPAA practices in many states. The practical implication of this change is that patients are entitled to a copy of their medical and psychiatric records. Patients are also granted the explicit right to request changes in the record. Whether or not the applicable staff member amends the contested information, the involved correspondence becomes part of the record.

HIPAA does recognize that some psychiatric records, defined as "psychotherapy notes," deserve special protection; however, the provision for these notes is narrow. Psychiatrists, under HIPAA, are given discretion regarding release of psychotherapy notes to patients. However, certain specific requirements must be followed in order for information in the medical record to qualify for the protection of psychotherapy notes. Specifically, the notes must be kept separate from the patient's medical record. Even if kept in a separate psychotherapy record, specific types of information are not subject to the psychotherapy notes exclusion; these include medications prescribed, test results, treatment plans, diagnoses, prognosis, and progress to date.[112] It should be noted, however, that psychotherapy notes are considered as part of the medical record in the event that a subpoena is received for medical records in the course of litigation.

Psychotherapist–Patient Privilege

A concept related to confidentiality is that of testimonial privilege. The distinctions between confidentiality and privilege are as follows: *confidentiality* is an ongoing obligation on the part of the clinician to maintain the privacy of information shared during the course of treatment; *privilege* is the patient's right to prohibit the treater from answering requests to share clinical information about the patient in administrative or judicial proceedings. Under English common law, an important origin of law in most jurisdictions in the US, the court was felt to be entitled to "everyman's evidence," and there were no restrictions on who could be called to testify. Over time, it came to be recognized that important societal purposes were served by preserving the confidentiality of relationships, such as attorney and client, husband and wife, priest and penitent, and doctor and patient.[116-118]

The existence of the psychotherapist–patient privilege does not serve as an absolute bar to testimony or disclosure of records by the treater. First, the patient must raise the privilege and bar the disclosure of information. While clinicians may choose to raise the privilege on behalf of the patient,[119] in most cases failure on the part of the patient to raise the privilege, and certainly the patient's request that the records and testimony be provided, leaves the clinician with no recourse. Second, there are a number of exceptions to the privilege, established by statute in most jurisdictions. The statutes in New York and Massachusetts are typical.[108,120] Chief among these is that the patient waives the privilege by putting his or her mental status into issue, for example, by claiming emotional distress damages in a civil case or raising an insanity defense in a criminal matter. In some, but not all, jurisdictions there is a "dangerous patient" exception. Under this exception, physicians may breach confidentiality and ultimately testify at criminal proceedings if the patient's statements indicate that there is a serious and imminent threat of harm that can only be avoided if the therapist discloses the information.[121] The existence of this privilege has raised concerns about continued erosion of confidentiality in the treatment of mentally ill individuals.[122]

Privilege issues can arise when patients are involved in either civil or criminal litigation. They generally begin with a subpoena that instructs a clinician to appear for a deposition or supply records or both. It is important to note that a subpoena is not a court order, with which the clinician must comply, but rather a request. The clinician must respond to the subpoena, and this is best done by passing it on to his or her attorney for analysis and appropriate response (e.g., records are confidential and require a release from the patient). As a general rule, clinicians should not reply to subpoenas without first seeking legal guidance. Even after legal consultation, no records should be sent in response to the request without first notifying the patient and giving him or her the opportunity to raise the privilege.[123]

Suicide

Although suicide is not a common occurrence, psychiatrists and other mental health clinicians are frequently and appropriately concerned about their potential liability should a patient commit suicide. While suicide is an unfortunate event, it is not grounds, *per se*, for a psychiatrist to be held liable for malpractice. As with other negative outcomes, a treater is only liable for malpractice if the bad outcome occurred due to the treater's negligence. Clinicians should familiarize themselves with principles of risk assessment for the suicidal patient and with prevailing legal requirements for managing suicidal patients in the jurisdictions in which they practice. Assessment and management of the suicidal patient is addressed in Chapter 53.

BOUNDARY VIOLATIONS

Of all the interactions between psychiatrists and patients that can lead to legal liability, boundary violations are among the most painful and damaging for patients, psychiatrists, and their families. Boundary violations are behaviors that involve an inappropriate departure from the accepted doctor and patient roles, as defined by societal and professional standards. They are the end point of a continuum of behavior that begins with the fiduciary duty of physicians to act only in the interests of the patient,[124] rather than in their own interests, and can end with the ultimate transgression, sexual involvement with a patient. Several studies involving disciplinary actions before state medical boards have demonstrated that psychiatrists are significantly more likely than other physicians to be disciplined for sexual relationships with patients.[125]

There is a large body of literature that attempts to categorize the types of boundary violations and their precipitants. In general, boundary violations are conceptualized as a progression of departures from expected roles, some of which are benign and appropriate when viewed in the treatment context and some of which lead caregivers down a "slippery slope" toward patient exploitation and abuse of trust.[126-129] On the benign end of the spectrum are so-called "boundary crossings," which are deviations from traditional psychiatric practice that do not harm the patient and are at times used to advance therapeutic purposes.[130] Examples of such deviations include offering emergency assistance to a stranded or disabled patient, or attending a wedding or other ceremony when clinically appropriate for the patient. The availability of personal information via social media and the ease of electronic communication between doctor and patient raise new issues regarding boundary crossings. In contrast to boundary crossings, "boundary violations" are deviations from a professional role that take advantage of the inherent power asymmetry in the physician–patient relationship for the gratification of the caregiver's needs.[131-133]

Whether or not a given action or event represents normative, acceptable behavior, a boundary crossing, or a boundary violation depends on its nature and its context. At one end of the spectrum are boundary violations that are egregious and clear. The American Psychiatric Association's (APA's) Annotated Principles of Medical Ethics simply and specifically states, "Sexual activity with a current or former patient is unethical."[92] Arguments for time limitations on the prohibition of physician–patient sexual relations, such that a doctor and patient could enter into a relationship after a waiting period following termination of any treatment relationship, have been rejected by the APA. As of 2002, multiple states and the District of Columbia had criminalized psychotherapist–patient sexual involvement.[135] Many non-sexual boundary transgressions are also clearly inappropriate, such as taking financial advantage of patients, employing patients in addition to treating them, or using patients to gratify narcissistic or dependency needs.[133-134]

There are, however, some situations that require flexibility with regard to the physician's role and an appreciation of the therapeutic context. For example, whereas business and social interactions with a patient are to be avoided in most contexts, the psychiatrist practicing in a rural area may have little choice but to encounter the patient at community functions or frequent the patient's retail store.[131] Similarly, while gift giving and receiving[132] are relatively common phenomena in other medical specialties, this practice has greater potential impact and meaning in psychiatry. Whether or not it constitutes "grist for the therapeutic mill" or a boundary crossing depends on how it is handled. The danger implicit in unaddressed boundary crossings is that they may lead to a more significant boundary violation.[136]

Breaching boundaries in psychiatric treatment can result in multiple sanctions and sources of liability. Patients may bring civil actions for malpractice, based on the caregiver's delivery of negligent care. In this vein, medical malpractice insurers have resisted indemnification of alleged sexual misconduct, arguing that such conduct is both intentional and unrelated to the treatment. Interpreting the language of the insurance contracts strictly, and seeking to ensure that injured patients were not left without compensation, a number of courts held that such misconduct represents negligent handling of the transference and countertransference, and was thus subject to malpractice coverage.[137,138] Under current policies, coverage for the defense of such charges is generally provided, but insurers may specify that they will not be responsible if the physician is found liable. In addition to malpractice claims, boundary violations can result in the revocation of professional licensure, expulsion from professional societies for breach of ethical codes, and even criminal prosecutions in some jurisdictions.

REDUCING MALPRACTICE RISK

In the quest to reduce malpractice risk, the clearest and most impossible solution would be to avoid all errors. Setting aside the impossibility of such an occurrence, the findings of Studdert and associates[10] that up to one-third of claimed injuries were not the result of medical error exposes the reality that even error-free practice does not completely immunize the practitioner against litigation. In addition to careful practice, a number of measures can be taken that effectively reduce malpractice risk. In-depth coverage of these measures cannot be accomplished adequately in this space, but general principles are worth noting. First, while individual practice behaviors are a key to reducing risk, it is important to recognize the impact of organizational and systemic issues on error rates.[27] Second, there is convincing evidence that physicians with poor communication skills run an increased risk of malpractice claims, while those who engage in shared decision-making, follow good informed consent practices, and represent a humanistic face run less risk of lawsuits.[139-145] Third, increasing attention has been given to the role of apology, and acknowledging error, as a means of sustaining the doctor–patient relationship in the event of an adverse outcome.[146-151] Fourth, maintaining a good clinical record, with documentation of all clinical activities (e.g., diagnosis, clinical decision-making, informed consent, medication changes, suicide risk assessment), is critical in defending any claims that may arise subsequently. The absence of a note in the record leaves the defendant clinician in the uncomfortable position of having to convince the fact-finder that he or she did, in fact, carry out the appropriate assessments and behaved in a reasonable fashion, even though there was a bad outcome.[59] Fifth, psychiatrists should avoid the tendency to "over-legalize" the doctor–patient relationship, for example, asking patients to sign waiver and consent forms for minor changes in treatment. Such actions convey the wrong message about the relationship by suggesting defensiveness on the part of the physician. Forms can be important as documentation, but do not replace the sharing of information that is so important to the therapeutic relationship. Finally, the value of consulting with colleagues when faced with clinical dilemmas cannot be

overestimated. The maxim "Never worry alone" is well worth heeding, especially in the most difficult and uncomfortable clinical dilemmas, such as potential boundary issues.[59,140,152]

CONCLUSION

Psychiatrists' risks of being sued for malpractice are small, but real. The process of being sued itself is extremely stressful and disruptive to the professional and personal life of the defendant, regardless of the outcome. The motivation to minimize the risk of a malpractice suit is uniformly strong. Yet adherence to good risk management techniques (such as sharing information with patients and families, obtaining informed consent, following and documenting good clinical practices, and maintaining clear boundaries with patients) are not consistently followed. Reducing malpractice risk does not require expertise in the law, nor does it require absolute perfection in practice. Rather, effective risk management is a function of doing what psychiatrists have been trained to do: to provide good clinical care and to serve their patients.

Access the complete reference list and multiple choice questions (MCQs) online at https://expertconsult.inkling.com

KEY REFERENCES

1. Studdert DM, Mello MM, Brennan TA. Medical malpractice. *N Engl J Med* 350:283–292, 2004.
6. Mello MM, Studdert DM, DesRoches CM, et al. Effects of a malpractice crisis on specialist supply and patient access to care. *Ann Surg* 242:621–628, 2005.
7. Localio AR, Lawthers AG, Brennan TA, et al. Relation between malpractice claims and adverse events due to negligence. Results of the Harvard Medical Practice Study III. *N Engl J Med* 325:245–251, 1991.
10. Studdert DM, Mello MM, Gawande AA, et al. Claims, errors, and compensation payments in medical malpractice litigation. *N Engl J Med* 354:2024–2033, 2006.
23. Institute of Medicine. *Crossing the quality chasm: a new health system for the twenty-first century*, Washington, DC, 2001, National Academy Press.
25. Paik M, Black BS, Hyman DA, et al. Will tort reform bend the cost curve? Evidence from Texas. *J Empir Leg Stud* 9(2):173–216, 2012.
27. Miller NP. An ancient law of care. *Whittier Law Rev* 26:3–57, 2004.
34. Gittler GJ, Goldstein EJ. The elements of medical malpractice: an overview. *Clin Infect Dis* 23:1152–1155, 1996.
46. King JH. The standard of care for residents and other medical school graduates in training. *Am Univ Law Rev* 55:683–751, 2006.
59. Gutheil TG, Appelbaum PS. *Clinical handbook of psychiatry and the law*, ed 4, Philadelphia, 2006, Lippincott Williams & Wilkins.
70. Schouten R, Brendel RW. Legal aspects of consultation. In Stern TA, Fricchione GL, Cassem EH, et al., editors: *The Massachusetts General Hospital handbook of general hospital psychiatry*, ed 5, Philadelphia, 2004, Mosby.
76. Cohen MH, Schouten R. Legal, regulatory, and ethical issues. In Lake JH, Spiegel D, editors: *Complementary and alternative treatments in mental health care*, Washington, DC, 2006, American Psychiatric Press.
86. Kachalia A, Studdert DM. Professional liability issues in graduate medical education. *JAMA* 292:1051–1056, 2004.
92. American Psychiatric Association. *The principles of medical ethics with annotations especially applicable to psychiatry*, Available at: <www.psych.org/psych_pract/ethics/medicalethics2001_42001.cfm>; 2001.
106. Soulier MF, Maislen A, Beck JC. Status of the psychiatric duty to protect, circa 2006. *J Am Acad Psychiatry Law* 38(4):457–473, 2010.
110. Brendel RW, Bryan E. HIPAA for psychiatrists. *Harv Rev Psychiatry* 12:177–183, 2004.

113. Schouten R, Brendel RW. Common pitfalls in giving medical legal advice to trainees and supervisees. *Harv Rev Psychiatry* 17(4):291–294, 2009.

115. Mermelstein HT, Wallack JJ. Confidentiality in the age of HIPAA: a challenge for psychosomatic medicine. *Psychosomatics* 49(2): 97–103, 2008.

117. Schouten R. The psychotherapist-patient privilege. *Harv Rev Psychiatry* 6:44–48, 1998.

124. Puglise SM. "Calling Dr. Love": The physician-patient sexual relationship as grounds for medical malpractice—society pays while the doctor and patient play. *J Law Health* 14:321–350, 2000.

126. Schouten R. Maintaining boundaries in the doctor-patient relationship. In Stern TA, Herman JB, Slavin PL, editors: *The MGH guide to primary care psychiatry*, ed 2, New York, 2004, McGraw-Hill.

129. Strasburger LH, Jorgenson L, Sutherland P. The prevention of psychotherapist sexual misconduct: avoiding the slippery slope. *Am J Psychother* 46:544–555, 1992.

132. Hundert EM. Looking a gift horse in the mouth: the ethics of gift-giving in psychiatry. *Harv Rev Psychiatry* 6:114–117, 1998.

143. Levinson W, Roter DL, Mullooly JP, et al. Physician-patient communication. The relationship with malpractice claims among primary care physicians and surgeons. *JAMA* 277:553–559, 1997.

145. Gutheil TG, Bursztajn H, Brodsky A. Malpractice prevention through the sharing of uncertainty. Informed consent and the therapeutic alliance. *N Engl J Med* 311:49–51, 1984.

147. Ho B, Liu E. Does sorry work? The impact of apology laws on medical malpractice. *J Risk Uncertain* 43:141–167, 2011.

88   Emergency Psychiatry

Laura M. Prager, MD, and Ana Ivkovic, MD

KEY POINTS

- The safety assessment is crucial in emergency evaluations.
- Assessment and management of acute agitation are of particular importance.
- It is critical to consider and to diagnose acute medical problems during the evaluation of a psychiatric emergency.
- Signs of intoxication and withdrawal that may herald a psychiatric emergency should be identified and treated.
- Psychiatric care plays an important role in responses to disasters.

OVERVIEW

Over the past 25 years, emergency psychiatry has developed into an independent subspecialty practice within consultation-liaison psychiatry. Although formal board certification requirements are lacking, all accredited US psychiatric residency-training programs follow training guidelines for emergency psychiatry.[1] The evolution of emergency psychiatry as a specialized practice parallels the dramatic increase in patient volume in urgent and emergency care settings over the past decade. In 2006, 4.7 million visits to US emergency departments (EDs) were for mental health-related chief complaints, more than double the number from 2001.[2] Mental health problems are the fastest-growing component of emergency medical practice; it is estimated that approximately 40% of ED patients have a diagnosable mental health or substance-related disorder. Among emergency mental health visits, substance-related disorders (30%), mood disorders (23%), anxiety disorders (21%), psychosis (10%), and suicide attempts (7%) are the most common.[3]

Psychiatric emergencies encompass a range of clinical presentations and diagnoses. Typically, such patients seek treatment in a state of crisis, unable to be contained by local support systems. Crises may be understood and addressed from a variety of perspectives, including medical, psychological, interpersonal, and social. Symptoms often consist of an overwhelming mental state that leads to increased dangerousness for that person or for others. Patients may have suicidal or homicidal (violent) ideation, overwhelming depression or anxiety, psychosis, mania, or acute cognitive or behavioral changes. A recent trend has also seen emergency services used for non-emergent conditions.[3] Increasing numbers of patients seek treatment at EDs for urgent conditions, routine conditions, or outpatient referrals because of lack of coverage for routine outpatient care, lack of community health care resources, an inability to access health care, or long waits to be seen by an outpatient mental health provider. This has led to longer lengths of stay for some psychiatric patients in the ED, especially for those with public insurance requiring transfer to another hospital.[4]

The practice of emergency psychiatry involves several core skills. In addition to the evaluation and treatment of a broad range of psychiatric conditions, practitioners of emergency psychiatry are called upon to evaluate and to manage suicidal behavior, homicidal (or otherwise violent) behavior, agitation, delirium, and substance intoxication or withdrawal. Because clinical practice lies at the interface of medicine and psychiatry, having knowledge of the assessment and treatment of medical conditions with psychiatric symptomatology is critical. More recently, emergency psychiatrists have also played important roles in responding to disasters.

The aim of this chapter is to provide a foundation for the care of psychiatric emergencies. First, an approach to the evaluation of psychiatric emergencies will be reviewed, with a particular focus on common initial symptoms. Then, special topics and the emergency treatment of children will be examined.

DEMOGRAPHICS

As of 1991, there were approximately 3,000 dedicated psychiatric emergency services (PESs) in the US.[5] Among the patients treated at these specialized services, roughly 29% are diagnosed with psychosis, 25% with substance abuse, 23% with major depression, 13% with bipolar disorder, and 22% with personality disorders.[6] Patients with co-morbid conditions (e.g., depression and substance use disorders) are frequent users of EDs and are often more difficult to treat.[2] Suicidal ideation is noted in one-third to one-half of all PES patients.[5]

Although some patients may self-refer to a PES while in crisis, others are referred by family, friends, general practitioners, medical specialists, mental health providers in the community, employees of local and state agencies, and staff at airports. Following several school shootings, teachers and school administrators have become a major source of emergency referrals for violence and for suicide assessments.[7] Police officers and representatives of the legal system also refer patients, as the PES serves as a conduit between the psychiatric system and the legal system.[8] The role of the PES is to help the police identify those individuals with psychiatric illness and to re-route them to appropriate care, while those without acute psychiatric illness are returned to the legal system.

TYPES OF DELIVERY MODELS

Two models are often used to deliver emergency psychiatric services. In one model, the PES exists as an independent service, co-located with a general emergency medical service or located separately in a stand-alone facility. In the other model, the PES functions as a service that provides consultation to primary emergency medical services. The specific model of services offered is determined by the volume of patients and the financial resources available.[9]

The primary benefit of providing emergency psychiatric services in an area that is separated from the chaos of a busy ED is safety; it provides a more secure environment (e.g., with limited access to sharp or dangerous objects, quiet surroundings to decrease stimulation, individual rooms for private interviews, and the ability to observe and rapidly initiate psychiatric treatment). The unit may also have security staff trained to understand mental health issues and who can help to maintain a safe environment. Many units also have specialized rooms for restraint and seclusion.[9]

Most states have enacted legislation that allows individuals to be held against their will if they are unable to care for themselves or if they present a danger to themselves or to others. In the PES, if there is reason to believe that a person presents a substantial risk of physical harm to him- or herself, or to others, or presents a very substantial risk of physical impairment or injury (due to inability to care for oneself), the person may be held or sequestered in the PES for further evaluation.

Another benefit of a dedicated psychiatric unit is the opportunity to staff the unit with specialized personnel who are trained in the delivery of emergency psychiatric care.[5,9] An interdisciplinary staff of psychiatric residents and attending physicians, nurses, social workers, and case managers can enhance the care of patients with acute illness, for example, by coordinating medical care with colleagues in the ED. Psychiatric nurses also play an important role in the triage of mentally ill patients within the psychiatric unit and the ED. Their ability to manage the milieu in an emergency unit, provide individual support to patients, dispense psychiatric medications, and recognize situations that require immediate nursing and physician intervention is invaluable.

Some PESs also have access to "crisis beds" or facilities that are able to provide observation for 24 to 72 hours. The ability to observe a patient whose mental state may change significantly after the initiation of antipsychotics or with a period of sobriety may decrease the need for inpatient hospitalization.[5,9,10]

A PES may also have a mobile crisis team whose role is to evaluate patients in the community, to diffuse a crisis before a patient is treated at the ED, and to decrease rates of hospitalization. As early as 1980, mobile initial response teams were described as a component of California community mental health centers and as an alternative to ED care.[11] One report from 1990 demonstrated similar hospitalization rates among hospital-based and mobile team emergency interventions,[12] whereas more recent reports have demonstrated decreased hospitalization rates when mobile teams have been employed.[13-15]

THE PSYCHIATRIC INTERVIEW

The psychiatric emergency evaluation is a concise, focused evaluation with a goal of diagnostic assessment that facilitates management of acute symptoms and disposition to the appropriate level of care. Just as a visit to an ED for a medical complaint involves an initial triage (a brief evaluation of the severity of the problem), emergency psychiatry models also depend on an initial assessment of the dangerousness of the psychiatric complaint in the context of co-morbid medical conditions. This initial, brief determination of acuity should screen for active medical issues that can cause a change in mental status, (e.g., substance intoxication or withdrawal),

---

BOX 88-1 The Emergency Psychiatric Interview and Evaluation

- Chief complaint
- History of present illness, with a focus on symptoms and the context for these symptoms; include a safety evaluation, with assessment of suicidal and homicidal ideation, plan or intent, and any associated risk factors
- Past medical history, with a focus on current problems
- Past psychiatric history, particularly symptoms or events similar to the current presentation; include diagnoses, previous hospitalizations, and suicide attempts
- Allergies and adverse reactions to medications
- Current medications, including an assessment of adherence
- Social history, particularly how it contributes to the context for the emergency visit
- Substance use history
- Family history, including symptoms or diagnoses similar to the patient's presentation
- Mental status examination
- Review of medical symptoms, particularly any medical symptoms that may account for the patient's presentation
- Vital signs
- Physical examination, if indicated
- Laboratory studies and other tests, if indicated
- Assessment, including a summary statement, a statement about the patient's level of safety, and a rationale for disposition recommendations
- Diagnoses according to DSM-5 criteria
- Plan and disposition
- Document any significant interventions (such as medication administration) and the outcome

---

suicidal or homicidal ideation, and other potentially dangerous and therefore more urgent types of psychiatric symptomatology.

The cornerstone of the initial psychiatric evaluation is a careful history that focuses on the timing and temporal development of symptoms that have led to the emergency visit, on associated signs and symptoms, and on possible precipitants and causes. In addition, a history of medical illnesses, psychiatric illnesses, medication usage, allergies, adverse reactions to medications, patterns of substance use, a family history of psychiatric illness, and a psychosocial history serve as important aspects of the initial evaluation. If available, past ED records should be reviewed. Box 88-1 describes the components of the evaluation, and Box 88-2 describes the special features of a substance abuse evaluation.

It is important to be aware of all potential information that may be included in an emergency psychiatric evaluation, and then to choose to elaborate on areas that are most relevant to the patient at hand. The interview should be a fact-gathering mission, and the elements of the history should both tell a story about the current symptoms and provide support for the disposition that the psychiatrist chooses. For example, though the developmental history may not be an important part of the evaluation for an otherwise healthy-appearing adult patient with depression, it may be very important in the assessment of a young patient with obvious cognitive deficits.

The emergency evaluation always includes an assessment of the patient's living situation and social supports, as well as a brief understanding of how he or she spends the day (e.g., at work, at school, or in a day program). This assessment helps define the patient's baseline level of function. In addition, a review of the patient's health insurance is necessary, because

BOX 88-2 The Substance Abuse Interview

For each substance used, assess the following:

- Age of first use
- Amount and frequency of use
- Method of use (e.g., drinking, smoking, intranasal, intravenous)
- Time of last use and amount used
- Medical sequelae of use
- Social sequelae (relationship problems, school or work absences, legal problems)
- Longest period of sobriety
- Previous treatment (detoxification programs, outpatient programs, partial hospitalization)
- Method of maintaining sobriety
- Participation in self-help substance abuse programs (e.g., Alcoholics Anonymous, Narcotics Anonymous)
- Risk for withdrawal syndrome
- The patient's motivation to cut down or stop substance use
- The patient's need for assistance meeting goals to cut down or stop substance use

BOX 88-3 Tests to Consider in the Medical Evaluation of Patients with Psychiatric Symptoms

- Complete blood count (CBC): to monitor for infection, blood loss
- Electrolytes, blood urea nitrogen (BUN), creatinine (metabolic changes, hyponatremia or hypernatremia, abnormal kidney function, dehydration)
- Glucose (hypoglycemia or hyperglycemia)
- Liver function tests and ammonia (liver dysfunction due to hepatitis or alcohol abuse)
- Pregnancy test
- Serum toxicology screen (ingestion, intoxication, poisoning)
- Medication levels (ingestion of medications such as lithium and tricyclic antidepressants)
- Urine toxicology screen (to identify or confirm substance use)
- Calcium, magnesium, and phosphorus (hypoparathyroidism or hyperparathyroidism, eating disorders, poor nutrition)
- Folate, thiamine (alcohol dependence, poor nutrition, depression)
- Vitamin B_{12}, methylmalonic acid, and homocysteine (cobalamin deficiency)
- Thyroid-stimulating hormone: this result may not be available immediately, but may be available during an extended observation period (hypothyroidism or hyperthyroidism)

The following tests and imaging studies may also be considered in the medical work-up:

- Lumbar puncture (infection, hemorrhage, limbic encephalitis)
- Electroencephalogram (seizure, changes due to ingestion of medications, delirium, dementia)
- Computed tomography (CT) (acute hemorrhage or trauma)
- Magnetic resonance imaging (MRI) (higher resolution than CT for potential brain masses or lesions, posterior fossa pathology, or when radiation exposure is contraindicated)

Adapted from Alpay M, Park L. Laboratory tests and diagnostic procedures. In Stern TA, Herman JB, editors: Psychiatry update and board preparation, *New York, 2000, McGraw-Hill.*

this often dictates the types of treatment programs that are available as disposition options.

Often, presentations to the PES are complicated and confusing, and patients may be unable, or unwilling, to provide an accurate history. For this reason, an important feature of the evaluation is the collection of history from multiple sources (e.g., family, friends, treaters, police, or emergency personnel who transported the patient to the ED). When several informants can be interviewed, data can be corroborated from the various sources, which can help the psychiatrist to make informed disposition decisions.

THE MEDICAL EVALUATION

For any ED patient with an altered mental status (be it a change in cognition, emotional state, or behavior), it is crucial to rule out an underlying medical condition that causes or contributes to the problem. A change in mental state may indicate a primary psychiatric condition, a primary medical condition with psychiatric symptoms (e.g., delirium [an acute and reversible condition secondary to a medical illness]), or dementia (a chronic condition associated with long-term, irreversible brain pathology). It is important to consider medical etiologies for any condition that appears psychiatric in nature because many psychiatric hospitals have limited resources to diagnose and to treat medical conditions. The ED medical evaluation may be the most comprehensive that the patient receives. A missed medical diagnosis because of an assumed psychiatric diagnosis could result in dire consequences for the patient.

A medical work-up should be considered for the new onset of psychiatric symptomatology or any significant change or exacerbation of symptoms. This initial medical work-up is often referred to as *medical clearance*, a term that generally refers to a medical evaluation aimed at ruling out underlying medical conditions that cause or contribute to a psychiatric presentation. Although much attention has been paid to defining a standard for medical clearance, there is no clear consensus regarding the required elements of the medical evaluation.[16,17]

One retrospective study of 212 consecutive patients who underwent a psychiatric evaluation in an ED demonstrated that among patients with a known psychiatric history and no medical complaints (38%), screening laboratories and radiographic results yielded no additional information; those patients could have been referred for further psychiatric evaluation with the history, the physical examination, and stable vital signs alone. Among the patients deemed to require further medical evaluation (62%), all had either reported medical complaints or their medical histories suggested that further evaluation would be necessary before psychiatric referral.[18] Another study of the medical evaluation of ED patients with new-onset psychiatric symptoms demonstrated that two-thirds had an organic cause for their psychiatric symptoms.[17] These studies suggest that careful screening is important among patients with new-onset symptoms, but additional medical tests may be of little benefit among patients with known psychiatric disorders and without physical complaints or active medical issues.

The medical evaluation should involve a thorough medical history, a general review of systems, and the assessment of vital signs, followed by a physical examination and/or laboratory tests as indicated.[19] Practitioners should be vigilant of characteristics (such as homelessness or intravenous [IV] drug abuse) which may put a patient at risk for additional medical conditions. The medical tests to consider are listed in Box 88-3.

THE SAFETY EVALUATION

The safety evaluation is a mandatory component of every emergency evaluation. It assesses the likelihood that an individual will attempt to harm him- or herself or someone else. With regard to self-harm, the intent may be to harm or to kill oneself (i.e., commit suicide). As of 2011, it is estimated that in the US alone, approximately 650,000 patients were evaluated annually for suicide attempts.[20] Despite this, evidence is limited on how best to manage suicidal ideation in the ED.[20] Of adult Medicaid beneficiaries treated in EDs for deliberate self-harm, more than 60% are discharged to the community, and many do not receive follow-up mental health care.[21] Suicide is the eighth leading cause of death in the US, and more than 90% of patients who commit suicide have at least one psychiatric diagnosis.[22] Patients aged 15–24 years and those over age 60 are in the highest-risk groups for suicide.

The psychiatrist must ask about thoughts, plans, and intent of suicide and homicide. These questions should be followed up with more specific questions about access to the means for harm, including access to firearms. If a patient has a plan or the intent to commit suicide, the lethality of the plan, as well as the patient's perception of the risk, must be assessed. A medically low-risk plan may still coincide with a strong intent to die if the patient believes that the lethality of the attempt is high. Similarly, the possibility that the patient could have been rescued if he or she had followed through on the plan should be evaluated; an impulsive ingestion of pills in front of a family member after an argument conveys less risk than a similar attempt in a remote location. If a patient has attempted suicide previously, details of that attempt may facilitate an understanding of the current risk. In addition, the clinician should assess other risk factors for suicide, which include the presence of a major mental illness, substance abuse, impulsivity, family history of suicide, recent loss (social, occupational, or financial), chronic illness, chronic pain, and access to lethal means. Although certain demographics have been associated with increased suicide risk (e.g., being elderly, Caucasian, Protestant, single), such variables should never substitute for cross-sectional clinical risk assessment that focuses on the above-mentioned risk factors. In addition, the gathering of collateral information is of paramount importance, especially in a higher-risk patient who is asking to be discharged to the community.

The assessment of violence proceeds in a fashion similar to the assessment of suicide risk. Every patient should be asked about thoughts to harm others, as well as the patient's potential plans and intent. Observation of the patient's mental status, behavior, and impulsivity during the interview provides important information. Because prior behavior is the best predictor of future behavior, if there is any suspicion of impending violence, it is important to ascertain previous violent thoughts and behaviors, triggers leading to those events, and their relationship to substance abuse. Questions about legal issues related to violence are also appropriate. In addition, the target of the violence should be assessed. Violence may lack a specific target or be directed towards a specific individual. If there is a likelihood of directed violence toward an identified person or persons, the ED psychiatrist has a duty to warn the identified target.

The safety evaluation should include contact with others who know the patient. Although civil commitment laws differ from state to state, most states have provisions for the containment of a patient who is deemed at risk for harm to oneself or others; however, in many cases, a patient with suicidal or homicidal ideation will choose voluntary hospitalization. In cases in which the patient has acknowledged suicidal or homicidal ideation, but it has resolved during the course of the ED visit, care must be taken to create a clear plan for steps that the patient should take if suicidal thoughts and feelings return. Most often, these involve contact with family members and treaters and a return to a psychiatric evaluation center or ED.

PSYCHIATRIC SYMPTOMS AND PRESENTATIONS

Diagnosis using DSM-5 criteria[23] can be difficult in the PES since patients are seen at a point in time, often in the worst crisis of their lives. Although patients will not necessarily fit the criteria exactly, a search for the most common disorders (e.g., mood disorders, psychotic disorders, anxiety disorders, substance abuse, and a change in mental status caused by a medical etiology [such as delirium]) will facilitate assessment. The following sections will outline some of the most common psychiatric presentations and patient characteristics seen in the ED.

The Depressed Patient

Depression is a common reason for seeking treatment at a PES. The severity of the depression may vary from mild to extremely severe; it may occur with or without psychosis or suicidal ideation. Anhedonia and other neurovegetative symptoms of depression are common complaints. Anxiety or anger attacks are often co-morbid with depression, and a history of mania must be assessed in every depressed patient to screen for bipolar disorder. Other medical conditions, especially hypothyroidism, must be considered. The severity of symptoms and the ability to participate in work and other routines may contribute to a diagnosis; however, the assessment of safety is essential in treatment planning.

The Anxious Patient

Although symptoms of anxiety may reflect a primary anxiety disorder, anxiety often heralds other disorders. Patients with psychosis may first describe anxiety about people who might try to harm them; patients with depression may have anxiety about financial or relationship difficulties. Psychomotor agitation, fidgeting, and pacing co-occur with anxiety but may also correlate with psychosis, alcohol withdrawal, or stimulant (e.g., cocaine, amphetamine, caffeine) intoxication. Medical problems (e.g., thyroid and parathyroid dysfunction, delirium) and medication side effects (e.g., akathisia) may also be confused with anxiety. Chest pain and shortness of breath from a possible panic attack may also prompt presentations to the ED and require a thorough medical evaluation in concert with a psychiatric evaluation. Complex partial seizures should be considered for patients with recurrent panic, especially patients at heightened risk for seizure (e.g., patients with history of head injury, other seizure disorder, or dementia).

The Psychotic Patient

Patients with psychosis suffer from disorganized thinking, hallucinations, delusions, or other forms of disordered thought (e.g., ideas of reference, thought broadcasting, or thought insertion). Patients with psychosis vary greatly in the severity of their symptoms; they may be affected by paranoia that has interfered with work or relationships, or they may suffer from loose associations, delusions, or aggressive behavior. Because some patients have lost touch with reality and may be at risk for agitation or dangerousness, the safety of staff and other patients must be maintained. Among patients with new-onset psychosis, severe anxiety is common and may be difficult to differentiate from paranoia.

or someone else. Unfortunately, controlled studies comparing the impact of methods of restraint and seclusion are lacking.[35] Recent efforts have focused on methods for reducing the need for restraint and seclusion in psychiatric settings.

All staff involved in restraint and seclusion should be well trained in the techniques for the safe management of aggressive behavior. Such management begins with the use of verbal de-escalation techniques and environmental interventions (e.g., placing the patient in a private room to decrease outside stimulation). Medication should be offered early in the course of agitation and aggression. If these interventions are not successful, and the patient remains at risk for harm to self or others, seclusion (placing the patient in a locked room alone) becomes an alternative for management. For patients who remain aggressive or at serious risk for harm, physical restraint may be the last resort to maintain their safety and the safety of those around them. Generally, it is the physician who orders restraint or seclusion, but the entire team should be clear about the reason for the restraint and the procedures involved. Each member of the team should feel responsible for maintaining the safety of the patient and the other staff.

The patient in seclusion or restraint should also be monitored at all times. In most facilities there is a limit to the time that the patient may remain in restraint; however, attempts should always be made to remove the restraints as soon as possible. Almost every patient who requires restraint or seclusion can benefit from medication to decrease the symptoms that have led to agitation.

Treatment after the Acute Crisis

The availability of outpatient treatment varies greatly by location and accessible resources in the hospital or the community. Some PESs offer prescriptions for medications on discharge and even provide follow-up while patients are awaiting referral to outpatient facilities. Other programs treat only acute problems and do not prescribe but may have access to urgent appointments or to an outpatient program with a short wait-list. Either way, after the management of the acute problem, treatment-planning is part of every disposition.

The emergency psychiatrist must have a thorough knowledge of the local mental health resources. Inpatient units, crisis stabilization units, residential treatment services, partial hospitalization programs, detoxification units, and outpatient programs serve as alternative levels of care after the PES evaluation. Admission criteria vary, and many programs depend on prior approval by insurance companies. The acuity of the patient's symptoms, the insurance coverage, and the psychosocial support system must all be weighed to determine the appropriate level of care. Decisions made with the patient, the family, and other treaters should be coordinated.

SPECIAL POPULATIONS
The Personality-Disordered Patient

Patients with borderline or antisocial personalities usually require a significant amount of time from PES staff to coordinate their care. Such patients may request services or favors that are outside of the normal routine of the unit. They may file complaints or even threaten to harm or kill themselves or others if the clinician is unwilling to provide the treatment that the patient prefers. Often these threats are statements of desperation, though each statement must be evaluated with the patient's history and current situation in mind.

Problems often occur due to splits between staff members who disagree about how the patient should be managed. The most important aspect of the treatment of these patients is for

---

BOX 88-4 Symptoms of Grief

Somatic distress
- Throat tightness
- Shortness of breath and sighing
- Muscular weakness
- Loss of appetite and abdominal discomfort or emptiness

Preoccupation with the image of the deceased
- Visualizing the deceased or hearing the voice of the deceased
- Imagining conversations with the deceased

Guilt about things done or not done
Hostility toward others
Changes in behavior
- Pacing or moving aimlessly
- Difficulty initiating the normal routine

Adapted from Lindemann E. Symptomatology and management of acute grief, Am J Psychiatry 151(6 Suppl):155–160, 1994.

---

the PES team to provide clear boundaries regarding the scope of care available, the role of individual staff members, and the goal of the emergency intervention. Outside contacts who know the patient may be able to provide insight for the purposes of the safety assessment.

The Grieving Patient

Management of acute grief (e.g., following a traumatic event or a death within the ED, the loss of a relationship, or the anniversary of a loss) is a common reason for referral to the PES. Grief is the normal response to loss. Grief can manifest in many ways, including feelings of shock, sadness, anxiety, anger, and guilt.[36] The most common symptoms are outlined in Box 88-4. A patient may exhibit any of these symptoms during the emergency evaluation. Brief periods of hearing the voice of a deceased spouse or feeling unable to participate in the routines of daily life are normal; they allow the patient time to come to terms with the loss. However, extended periods of depressed mood, anhedonia, and other neurovegetative symptoms may indicate an episode of major depression and require more immediate treatment.

The role of the psychiatrist in working with a grieving patient is to provide a supportive environment. Some patients will want to sit quietly, others will want to talk, and others will cry. If the situation is ongoing (e.g., a family member's injury is being treated in the ED), only accurate information should be provided and giving false hope should be avoided. Patients should be helped to recognize how they have handled losses in the past, and similar coping skills should be supported.

Victims of Domestic Violence and Trauma

Domestic violence (i.e., an individual's use of force to inflict emotional or physical injury on another person with whom the individual has a relationship) affects spouses, partners, children, grandparents, and siblings of all races and genders. Between 2 and 4 million women are abused each year in the US, and domestic violence has become the leading cause of injury among women between 15 and 44 years of age.[37] Men can also be victims of domestic violence.

Patients in the PES should be asked whether they have been a victim of violence or trauma, whether this contributes to their symptoms, and if they are safe in their current living environment. Symptoms of post-traumatic stress disorder should be screened for and included in treatment planning. Patients need not be asked to describe exhaustive details about past traumas. Instead, the patient can be helped to understand that the process of working through trauma should occur with a therapist who can provide long-term support, and then provide an appropriate referral.

The Homeless Patient

It is estimated that approximately 20% to 30%[38] of the patients who are treated at PESs are homeless,[6] and this characteristic adds complexity to the psychiatric evaluation. When a patient has insomnia or the fear of being harmed by others, it may be difficult to determine whether the symptoms are due to a psychiatric disturbance or to the inherent risks of homelessness. Homeless patients are at greater risk for substance abuse, tuberculosis, skin conditions, and other serious chronic medical conditions (such as diabetes, acquired immunodeficiency syndrome [AIDS], and cancer); it is especially important to provide good medical screening during the assessment. The clinician must also account for the patient's housing situation and access to meals and medical care in the course of disposition planning. A treatment plan adapted to these realities is much more likely to succeed[39]; however, despite careful disposition planning, homeless patients are more likely than other patients to have repeat visits to the PES.[38]

EMERGENCY ASSESSMENT OF CHILDREN
Demographics

It is estimated that there are about 434,000 annual pediatric visits for mental health conditions in the US, which constitutes about 1.6% of ED visits in this age group (under age 19). Adolescents between 13 and 17 years of age account for more than two-thirds of the visits, and suicide attempts account for 13% of the visits. The most common diagnoses include substance-related disorders (24%), anxiety disorders (16%), attention-deficit and disruptive disorders (11%), and psychosis (10%). Nineteen percent of ED mental health visits result in inpatient admission, compared to only 9% of non-mental-health visits in the same age group.[40] A study that analyzed data about young people (ages 7 to 24 years) treated at EDs for deliberate self-harm reported an annual rate of 225 per 100,000.[41] Among those patients, 56% were diagnosed with a mental disorder (including 15% with depression and 7% with substance use disorders), and 56% were referred for inpatient admission. Frequent precipitants for ED visits include family crises (e.g., death, divorce, financial stress, domestic abuse), disturbed or truncated peer relationships, and a recent change of school.[42-44]

Basic Principles

Few child psychiatric emergencies are life-threatening; all result from the complex interaction of psychosocial, biological, and systems issues.

The primary goal is the safety of the child, and this principle must guide all subsequent plans for treatment or disposition. The clinician must always consider the possibility of abuse or neglect as the precipitant for the visit to the ED.

The evaluation itself is based on a developmental approach. The clinician must choose age-appropriate techniques with which to conduct the assessment.

The emergency psychiatric assessment of a child is often more complicated and time-consuming than the evaluation of an adult. The clinician must be familiar with resources for children and families within the community mental health system. Thorough evaluation often requires phone calls to outside providers (including pediatricians, school administrators, guidance counselors, and outpatient mental health professionals).

The Evaluation

The initial step in the assessment of a child in the PES is identification of the child's legal guardian(s). In routine cases, the legal guardians are the biological parents who accompany the child to the hospital. In complex cases, the child's legal guardian may be court-ordered to be only one parent, another relative, a foster parent, or a representative of the state agency responsible for the care and protection of children. Custody can be split into several parts, and one guardian can have legal (or decision-making) custody while another guardian retains physical custody. Sometimes a child remains in the home of the biological parent but a state agency assumes responsibility for decisions regarding medical care. The clinician should never assume that the adult who accompanies the child is the legal guardian or that a friend or neighbor can offer consent for the assessment. Except in very rare, extenuating circumstances, the legal guardian must come to the assessment center and participate in the evaluation, because that person will be a key factor in disposition.

The clinician who evaluates children in an ED should base the method of assessment on the age of the child, although the interview may also include many standard elements of the psychiatric history as listed in Box 88-1. The *style* and *process* of the interview and mental status examination depend on the age of the child.

Pre-schoolers (1 to 5 years), many of whom may be pre-verbal, are unable to provide a coherent narrative of the events leading up to the ED visit. The clinician must interview the parent or guardian to obtain the details of the history, but should also pay careful and close attention to the interaction between the child and the caregiver, as well as to the child's hygiene. Mental status assessment should focus on the child's behavior, level of agitation, mood, affect, and ability to take direction and accept reassurance from the caregiver. Common precipitants for ED visits in this age group include impulsive or dangerous behaviors (such as running away from home or from a caregiver in a public place, fire-setting, or hitting a younger sibling).

Latency-age children (5 to 11 years) can often provide a clear description of the event that brought them to the ED but usually lack the ability to place the specific event within a larger context. It is often helpful for the clinician to interview the parent or caregiver before meeting with the child. Assessment of the mental status includes observations of the child's interaction with the caregiver, attention to speech and language, and direct questions about mood, affect, and risk for self-injurious behavior. Children who are younger than 6 years old might retain their "magical thinking" and thus not yet be able to distinguish fantasy from reality.

Adolescents (12 to 18 years) should ideally be interviewed before the clinician speaks with caregivers or other concerned adults. This approach reinforces and supports the adolescent's desire for autonomy and control. Mental status assessment involves assessment of mood, affect, thought process and content, cognition, insight, and judgment, as well as suicidal and homicidal ideation.

Finally, the evaluation must include an assessment of the social situation. Being familiar with the local communities and school systems around your hospital will help you to better understand the social context. An inner-city school with few resources is very different from a wealthy suburban school with counselors and school nurses who can identify new problems and monitor medications; knowing this will help you to make decisions about the treatment plan. It is also important to know the types of treatments that the child has accessed before. A child whose severe depression has failed to improve after several medication trials and participation in months of residential treatment programs is very different from one who seeks treatment for the first time with anxiety symptoms. The previous treatment history will inform your disposition decision.

Management

The agitated or aggressive child requires rapid diagnostic assessment and management. The differential diagnosis should focus first on organic (medical) causes of the behavior (including elevated lead levels [particularly for children under 5 years]), seizure disorders, metabolic abnormalities, medication (prescription or over-the-counter) ingestion or overdose, withdrawal from medication or recreational drugs, hypoxia, infection, and intoxication.

If an organic etiology is suspected, vital signs and laboratory studies should be obtained immediately. Laboratory studies might include a complete blood count (CBC), serum electrolytes (including blood glucose), serum and urine toxic screens,[45] and, in young women, a pregnancy test. It is usually helpful to control the environment and to decrease stimulation by placing the child in seclusion, sometimes with one family member who can be soothing and reassuring. With very young children, it can be helpful to offer food and drink.

Sometimes it is necessary to administer medication to control agitated or acutely intoxicated children, particularly if they are in danger of harming themselves or others. It is best to ask the parent or guardian which medications the child usually takes and administer either an additional dose of a standing medication or an existing as-needed (PRN) medication. Administration of an oral medication is always preferable to an IM injection, but it is not always possible if the child is unable to respond to verbal direction or limit-setting.

The choice of medication and route of administration depend on the severity of the agitation and the age of the child. Medications to consider include diphenhydramine (1.25 mg/kg/dose PO or IM if the child has no history of paradoxical excitation); clonidine (at a dose of 0.05 to 0.1 mg PO); an atypical neuroleptic (such as risperidone [0.5 to 1 mg] in oral tablet, liquid, or rapidly-dissolving form, or olanzapine [2.5 to 5 mg] in oral tablet or rapidly-dissolving form or IM preparation); benzodiazepines (particularly lorazepam [0.5 to 1 mg] PO or IM can be helpful but can also cause paradoxical excitation and disinhibition); and for an older, acutely agitated adolescent, it is appropriate to use a high-potency neuroleptic (such as haloperidol) combined with a benzodiazepine and an anticholinergic agent (diphenhydramine or benztropine).

Physical restraints (e.g., locked leather restraints) are sometimes necessary and should be placed only by trained security personnel according to guidelines established by the state department of mental health. Family members should leave the room during any form of restraint.

LEGAL RESPONSIBILITIES OF THE EMERGENCY PSYCHIATRIST

The emergency psychiatrist is responsible for knowing the legal regulations and local standards of care related to capacity evaluations, confidentiality, release of information, commitment standards, and mandatory reporting for patients with psychiatric symptoms who are treated at the PES. Although specific standards may differ, the following features may assist

with understanding these general responsibilities. In all cases, it is important to document carefully all steps involved in the decision-making process and to consult with a forensic psychiatrist or legal counsel trained in mental health law in difficult cases.

Capacity Evaluation

The capacity evaluation is often requested by other medical providers to determine whether a patient has the ability to make an informed decision about a particular medical procedure or decision. A patient is presumed to have capacity to make medical decisions until proven otherwise. The key components of this evaluation include the assessment of whether the patient can understand the relevant information, appreciate the consequences of the decision, and communicate a reasonable explanation for his/her choice. In many cases, the psychiatrist will find that the patient's ability to make a clear and rational decision is dependent on an opportunity to learn more about the specific medical procedure. Coordination with the medical or surgical team and further discussion with the patient may obviate the need for assessment of capacity.

Confidentiality and Release of Information

It is often difficult to maintain privacy in the ED setting due to architectural design flaws (semi-private rooms, open bays, curtained alcoves) and high volume with overcrowding. Nevertheless, clinicians taking the psychiatric history should make every effort to preserve confidentiality.

The care of psychiatric patients requires a strong commitment to confidentiality; in the emergency setting, all attempts are made to gain permission for any collateral contact regarding the patient's condition. However, in the care of patients who present a risk of harm to themselves or others, it is often necessary to contact outpatient providers or family members without the patient's consent. It is important to document clearly in the medical record why the contact was made and to use the contact to gain information that will assist in the safety assessment. The clinician should limit the confidential information provided to the other party.

Another situation in which a breach in confidentiality may be justified involves the duty to warn. When a clinician learns that a patient is at imminent risk to harm another individual, the clinician must inform the identified target. The standards for the clinician's duty to protect the potential victim are different in every state, but most are based on the original Tarasoff case in California in 1976.[46]

Civil Commitment

Civil commitment refers to the state's ability to hospitalize an individual involuntarily because of risk of harm due to mental illness.[46] The commitment regulations and processes vary by state. Most regulations incorporate risk of harm to self, risk of harm to others, and inability to care for self, all due to psychiatric pathology, as the basis for civil commitment. The safety evaluation described in this chapter provides the clinician with a basic outline of an assessment to determine risk and is an important component of the assessment that may lead to civil commitment.

Mandatory Reporting

Most states have regulations regarding mandatory reporting for suspected child abuse,[47] elder abuse,[48] and abuse of individuals with mental retardation. In most cases, mandatory reporters are obligated to report situations in which they suspect abuse, whether or not they have clear evidence; they are protected against claims of a breach of confidentiality under these conditions.[46] Mental health clinicians should be aware of whether they are considered mandatory reporters in their state and how to contact the appropriate agencies.

ROLE OF THE PSYCHIATRIST IN DISASTER PREPARATION

In the face of recent catastrophic events, such as terrorist attacks and large-scale natural disasters, efforts have been undertaken to prepare medical teams to manage disasters. Often, the role of psychiatry in this response is overlooked until the actual event occurs. In the midst of a disaster response, it is the ability of the psychiatrist to tolerate extreme affect that becomes immediately useful. The psychiatrist can offer aid in at least four different arenas: organizational aid and planning for disaster response; treatment of psychological reactions to stress (using pharmacological, psychotherapeutic, and interpersonal interventions), acutely and over the long term; provision of support to family members and friends of victims of the disaster; and support of medical staff who participate in disaster response (including emergency personnel, hospital staff, administrative staff, and other support personnel).[49,50]

Emergency psychiatrists are particularly well adapted to assist with disaster response. They are familiar with the medical and psychological effects of trauma, are adept at working with grieving family members, and are familiar with the resources in the community that can assist with long-term treatment. Disaster psychiatry is a growing field, and emergency psychiatrists will likely play an important role in the future of disaster-response planning.

Access a list of MCQs for this chapter at https://expertconsult .inkling.com

REFERENCES

1. Brasch J, Glick RL, Cobb TG, et al. Residency training in emergency psychiatry: a model curriculum developed by the education committee of the American Association for Emergency Psychiatry. *Acad Psychiatry* 28(2):95–103, 2004.
2. Larkin GL, Beautrais AL, Spirito A, et al. Mental health and emergency medicine: a research agenda. *Acad Emerg Med* 16(11):1110–1119, 2009.
3. Larkin GL, Claassen CA, Emond JA, et al. Trends in US emergency department visits for mental health conditions, 1992 to 2001. *Psychiatr Serv* 56:671–677, 2005.
4. Chang G, Weiss A, Kosowsky JM, et al. Characteristics of adult psychiatric patients with stays of 24 hours or more in the emergency department. *Psychiatr Serv* 63(3):283–286, 2012.
5. Allen MH. Definitive treatment in the psychiatric emergency service. *Psychiatr Q* 67:247–262, 1996.
6. Currier GW, Allen M. Organization and function of academic psychiatric emergency services. *Gen Hosp Psychiatry* 25:124–129, 2003.
7. Murakami S, Rappaport N, Penn JV. An overview of juveniles and school violence. *Psychiatr Clin North Am* 29(3):725–741, 2006.
8. Redondo RM, Currier GW. Characteristics of patients referred by police to a psychiatric emergency service. *Psychiatr Serv* 54(6):804–806, 2003.
9. Breslow RE. Structure and function of psychiatric emergency services. In Allen MH, editor: *Emergency psychiatry*, Washington, DC, 2002, American Psychiatric Publishing.
10. Breslow RE, Klinger BI, Erickson BJ. Crisis hospitalization in a psychiatric emergency service. *New Dir Ment Health Serv* 67:5–12, 1995.
11. Gaynor J, Hargreaves WA. "Emergency room" and "mobile response" models of emergency psychiatric services. *Community Ment Health J* 16(4):283–292, 1980.
12. Fisher WH, Geller JL, Wirth-Cauchon J. Empirically assessing the impact of mobile crisis capacity on state hospital admissions. *Community Ment Health J* 26(3):245–253, 1990.
13. Guo S, Biegel DE, Johnson JA, et al. Assessing the impact of community-based mobile crisis services on preventing hospitalization. *Psychiatr Serv* 52(2):223–228, 2001.
14. Hugo M, Smout M, Bannister J. A comparison in hospitalization rates between a community-based mobile emergency service and a hospital-based emergency service. *Aust N Z J Psychiatry* 36(4):504–508, 2002.
15. Merson S, Tyrer P, Carlen D, et al. The cost of treatment of psychiatry emergencies: a comparison of hospital and community services. *Psychol Med* 26(4):727–734, 1996.
16. Broderick KB, Lerner EB, McCourt JD, et al. Emergency physician practices and requirements regarding the medical screening examination of psychiatric patients. *Acad Emerg Med* 9(1):88–92, 2002.
17. Zun LS, Hernandez R, Thompson R, et al. Comparison of EP's and psychiatrists' laboratory assessment of psychiatric patients. *Am J Emerg Med* 22(3):175–180, 2004.
18. Korn CS, Currier GW, Henderson SO. "Medical clearance" of psychiatric patients without medical complaints in the emergency department. *J Emerg Med* 18(2):173–176, 2000.
19. Henneman PL, Mendoza R, Lewis RJ. Prospective evaluation of emergency department medical clearance. *Ann Emerg Med* 24:672–677, 1994.
20. Chang B, Gitlin D, Patel R. The depressed patient and suicidal patient in the emergency department: evidence-based management and treatment strategies. *Emerg Med Pract* 13(9):1–23, 2011.
21. Olfson M, Marcus SC, Bridge JA. Emergency treatment of deliberate self-harm. *Arch Gen Psychiatry* 69(1):80–88, 2012.
22. Stern TA, Perlis RH, Lagomasino IT. Suicidal patients. In Stern TA, Fricchione GL, Cassem NH, et al., editors: *Massachusetts General Hospital handbook of general hospital psychiatry*, ed 5, Philadelphia, 2004, Mosby.
23. American Psychiatric Association. *Diagnostic and statistical manual of mental disorders*, ed 5, Washington, DC, 2013, American Psychiatric Association.
24. Hopkins SA, Moodley KK, Chan D. Autoimmune limbic encephalitis presenting as relapsing psychosis. *BMJ Case Rep* 2013:2013.
25. Hyman SE. Alcohol-related emergencies. In Hyman SE, Tesar G, editors: *Manual of psychiatric emergencies*, ed 3, Boston, 1994, Little, Brown.
26. Rosenbaum CD, Carreiro SP, Babu KM. Here today, gone tomorrow … and back again? A review of herbal marijuana alternatives (K2, Spice), synthetic cathinones (bath salts), Kratom, Salvia divinorum, methoxetamine, and piperazines. *J Med Toxicol* 8(1):15–32, 2012.
27. Won S, Hong RA, Shohet RV, et al. Methamphetamine-associated cardiomyopathy. *Clin Cardiol* 36(12):737–742, 2013.
28. Weiss RD, Greenfield SF, Mirin SM. Intoxication and withdrawal syndromes. In Hyman SE, Tesar G, editors: *Manual of psychiatric emergencies*, ed 3, Boston, 1994, Little, Brown.
29. SAMHSA press office, "Report shows that bath salts" drugs were involved in nearly 23,000 emergency department visits in one year", <www.samhsa.gov/newsroom/advisories/1309160554 .aspx>; September 2013.
30. Folstein MF, Folstein SE, McHugh PR. "Mini-mental state". A practical method for grading the cognitive state of patients for the clinician. *J Psychiatr Res* 12:189–198, 1975.
31. Cassem NH, Murray GB, Lafayette JM, et al. Delirious patients. In Stern TA, Fricchione GL, Cassem NH, et al., editors: *Massachusetts General Hospital handbook of general hospital psychiatry*, ed 5, Philadelphia, 2004, Mosby.
32. Messner E. *Resilience enhancement for the resident physician*, Durant, OK, 1993, Essential Medical Information Systems.
33. Allen MH, Currier GW, Hughes DH, et al. The expert consensus guideline series. Treatment of behavioral emergencies. *Postgrad Med* (spec no):1–88, 2001.
34. Allen MH. Managing the agitated patient: a reappraisal of the evidence. *J Clin Psychiatry* 61(Suppl. 14):11–20, 2000.
35. Busch AB, Shore MF. Seclusion and restraint: a review of the recent literature. *Harv Rev Psychiatry* 8:261–270, 2000.
36. Lindemann E. Symptomatology and management of acute grief. *Am J Psychiatry* 151(6 Suppl):155–160, 1994.

90 Military Psychiatry

Gary H. Wynn, MD, James R. Rundell, MD, and David M. Benedek, MD

KEY POINTS

Background

- The discipline of military psychiatry extends psychiatric practice beyond the boundaries of traditional environments of care.
- Though resiliency is the norm, negative effects of combat exposure can persist for decades.
- Psychological casualties in chemical and biological threat scenarios may outnumber and prove more costly in terms of personnel losses than physical casualties.

History

- During World War I "gas hysteria" was common and threatened the integrity of entire military units due to psychological contagion effects. Factors that predispose to psychological contagion include rates of wounding/exposure in the unit, lack of sleep, and lack of prior experience with these phenomena/attacks.
- The psychological impact of combat has been described for millennia, under a variety of names (e.g., soldier's heart, shell shock, battle fatigue) and most often through the literature of the day.

Clinical and Research Challenges

- Psychological injury that occurs during military operations is often particularly complex given the potential for physical injury, exposure to the injury and death of others, exposure to biological or chemical

agents, and disruption of one's physical environment while deployed to a foreign country.
- Common causes of delirium in combat or in disaster settings include hypovolemia, hypoxemia, central nervous system mass effects, infection, and adverse effects of resuscitative medications.
- Situational dissociation is common in the context of any traumatic or terrorist event. Dissociation may be adaptive in the immediate aftermath of a trauma—dissociation may prevent the eruption of intolerable affect or the unleashing of potentially dangerous impulses or behaviors (e.g., fleeing the scene).

Practical Pointers

- Medications used to treat exposure to chemical warfare agents and other resuscitative medications are crucial to effective management of acutely injured patients; unfortunately, many of these can cause neuropsychiatric symptoms that mimic primary psychiatric disorders. Symptoms resulting from exposure to chemical or biological warfare agents may also mimic neuropsychiatric disorders.
- To avoid stigmatization and diminish the development of enduring psychopathology, initial management of psychiatric battlefield casualties occurs as close to the service member's area of work as safely as possible.

OVERVIEW

The discipline of military psychiatry extends psychiatric practice beyond the boundaries of traditional environments of care. The US military has established—within the US and on its bases abroad—an extensive network of community mental health clinics, combat stress centers, ambulatory care facilities, hospitals, and tertiary medical centers to address the wide range of psychiatric illnesses observed in the civilian setting. The stresses of military life—frequent moves, prolonged separations between service members and their families, repetitive deployments, and often hazardous duty in a variety of humanitarian assistance, peace-keeping, and battlefield settings—create unique challenges for the military psychiatrist.

In the theater of war, there is the terror of unanticipated injury, loss, and death. During military operations psychological injury may occur in conjunction with physical injury, exposure to the injury and death of others, potential exposure to biological or chemical agents, disruption of one's physical environment, or as a consequence of the terror and helplessness that these events combine to evoke. Therefore, the knowledge base, skills, and professional attitudes required of a military psychiatrist must include more than those associated with traditional clinic or hospital-based practice.

Negative effects of combat exposure can persist for decades, as Prigerson and colleagues[1] demonstrated in a study of 2,583 men, aged 18 to 54 years, who received standardized

psychiatric interviews in the National Comorbidity Survey. They found that combat exposure resulted in high prevalence rates of psychiatric diagnoses and psychosocial problems: 28% had post-traumatic stress disorder (PTSD); 21% engaged in spousal or partner abuse; 12% experienced job loss; 9% were currently unemployed; 8% had 12-month substance abuse problems within 1 year; 8% underwent divorce or separation; and 7% sustained major depressive disorder (MDD).

PSYCHIATRIC SYNDROMES IN THE IMMEDIATE AFTERMATH OF MILITARY OPERATIONS AND TERRORIST EVENTS

Delirium

In combat or following terrorism that leads to major illness or injuries, volume depletion and metabolic derangements as well as resuscitative efforts can cause delirium (manifest by clouded consciousness, agitation or diminished responsiveness, and disorientation) (Box 90-1). Pharmacological agents (such as neuroleptics and benzodiazepines) used to manage agitation can further complicate medical assessment and management, especially surrounding combat-related injuries. Symptomatic management of behavioral problems with sedating agents should be initially reserved to protect the life or safety of the patient and other patients or staff. Resolution

BOX 90-1 Common Psychiatric Syndromes and Phenomena in the Immediate Aftermath of Military Operations and Terrorist Events

- Delirium
- Depression
- Acute stress disorder
- Post-traumatic stress disorder
- Generalized anxiety
- Panic attacks/disorder
- Substance use disorder
- Hypochondriasis
- Unexplained physical symptoms
- Dissociation
- Dissociative disorders
- Battle fatigue
- Operational stress

of the etiology of the delirium should be the primary goal; resolution requires attention to metabolic sequelae of the injury. Common causes of delirium in combat or in disaster settings include hypovolemia, hypoxemia, central nervous system mass effects (e.g., hemorrhage, foreign bodies), infection, and adverse effects of resuscitative medications.

Depression

Depressed mood or resignation in the aftermath of combat or a terrorist event may be difficult to distinguish from the malaise and lassitude common among the prodromes to exposure to many chemical and bioterrorism agents. When depressed mood and associated depressive symptoms disrupt social and occupational function, a depressive disorder (e.g., MDD) is diagnosed.

Acute Stress Disorder and Post-traumatic Stress Disorder

Symptoms of acute stress disorder (ASD) and PTSD include intrusive re-experiencing phenomena (such as distressing dreams and flashbacks), hyperarousal, avoidance of events or situations that resemble—even symbolically—the original trauma, negative alterations in cognition and mood (such as diminished interest in significant activities), and dissociative phenomena (such as derealization or numbing).[2] When symptoms persist for more than 1 month, PTSD is diagnosed. Both ASD and PTSD have high rates of co-morbidities (see Box 90-1), the most frequent of which are MDD, other anxiety disorders (such as panic disorder), and substance use disorders. For those who suffer a concomitant physical injury during exposure to trauma, the risk of both ASD and PTSD increases.[3,4]

Somatic Symptom Disorder and Illness Anxiety Disorder (Formerly Hypochondriasis)

The fear or belief that one has a serious disease based on the misinterpretation of bodily symptoms or environmental exposure has traditionally been termed "hypochondriasis." The DSM-5 divides the symptom complex into somatic symptom disorder (fear or belief that one has serious illness accompanied by significant bodily symptoms) and illness anxiety disorder (similar fear or belief despite the lack of significant bodily symptoms).[2] In either case anxiety and fear about the somatic symptom and/or disease persist despite

normal medical evaluations and reassurance. In the chaos and uncertainty following combat or terrorist events, patients with these two disorders may have particular problems managing their anxiety and health-related beliefs. Persons without a documented diagnosis of either may seek treatment for the first time in this environment. Chronic symptoms (e.g., of at least 6 months) are typical for both of these disorders and are required for a diagnosis of illness anxiety disorder. However, subsyndromal somatic fears may be widespread following a terrorist event or potential combat-related toxic exposure. In contrast, these transient symptoms generally respond favorably to reassurance and a degree of tolerance for appointments/examination requests.

Unexplained Physical Symptoms and Conversion Symptoms

Unexplained physical symptoms are common after combat and disasters. Not all unexplained physical symptoms are conversion symptoms, although anecdotal reports of conversion are well documented after terrorist and combat events. Unfortunately, there is little scientific basis for prevention and care of unexplained physical symptoms. Nonetheless, it is important that persons with unexplained symptoms be identified in the triage process so that inappropriate and potentially harmful treatments (that could also draw resources away from victims who need treatment) are not initiated.

Use of biological or chemical agents presents a challenging differential diagnosis and contagion problem. During World War I "gas hysteria" was common and threatened the integrity of entire military units. Psychological casualties in chemical and biological threat scenarios may outnumber and prove more costly in terms of personnel losses than physical casualties. Acute symptoms of gas hysteria may mimic symptoms (e.g., dyspnea, coughing, aphonia, burning of the skin) of poison gas exposure. Patients may have air hunger and other symptoms that are consistent with anxiety and panic. The factors that predispose a patient to psychological contagion include rates of wounding/exposure in the unit, lack of sleep, and lack of prior experience with this type of phenomena/attack.[5] Therefore, it is important to know what substances a patient has *not* been exposed to. Following a faked chemical or biological agent threat, there may be a large number of individuals who fear that they have been exposed and will have realistic symptoms based on their knowledge of the alleged agent and the vital sign abnormalities produced by anxiety/fear.

Dissociation and Dissociative Disorders

The essential feature of dissociative disorders is a disruption in the usually integrated functions of consciousness, memory, identity, or perception of the environment. The centerpiece of the diagnosis, to discriminate it from situational dissociation, is the presence of significant distress, or significant disruption in social or occupational function. Situational dissociation is common in the context of any traumatic or terrorist event. Dissociation may be adaptive in the immediate aftermath of a trauma—dissociation may prevent the eruption of intolerable affect or the unleashing of potentially dangerous impulses or behaviors (e.g., fleeing the scene).

It is important not to confuse dissociation and diminished neurological responsiveness. A key role of a psychiatrist in the immediate aftermath of a disaster is to help identify dissociation. One should gently tap the patient on the shoulder, ask if there is anything the patient needs, and ask if the patient knows where he or she is and what day it is. Watching for a muted, but appropriate, response in a dissociating person should indicate his or her level of consciousness and suggest that orientation is grossly intact. Identification of otherwise uninjured disaster victims who are simply dissociating may free up medical resources for other patients.

Battle Fatigue and Operational Stress

The psychological impact of combat has been known for millennia though under a variety of names (e.g., soldier's heart, shell shock, battle fatigue) and most often through the literature of the day. Beyond traditional and historic psychiatric disorders, "battle fatigue" and "operational stress" (now termed combat operational stress reaction) are also important practical concepts in military psychiatry. Symptoms such as gastrointestinal distress, tremulousness, and transient perceptual disturbances (including depersonalization and derealization) occur in response to the traumatic exposure, to sleep deprivation, to loss of social supports, or to any combination of these stressful factors associated with military operations. Minor injury or infection, nutritional deficiencies, heat exhaustion, or cold injury may also deplete adaptive homeostatic mechanisms and contribute to operational stress symptoms.

EFFECTS OF RESUSCITATIVE MEDICATIONS

Resuscitative medications are crucial to effective management of acutely injured patients. Unfortunately, many of them can cause neuropsychiatric symptoms (Table 90-1). It is important to find out which medications an injured patient has received, in what amounts, and over what time period. Agents, such as intravenous (IV) fluids (e.g., water), epinephrine, lidocaine, atropine, sedatives, nitroglycerin, and morphine are commonly used and have significant autonomic impact or effects that can resemble symptoms of primary psychiatric disorders. For example, both atropine and epinephrine can cause a patient to have a rapid heart rate and to feel anxious or panicky while morphine can cause sedation and impair orientation and responsiveness.

TABLE 90-1 Resuscitative Medications That Can Cause or Mimic Psychiatric or Neurological Syndromes

Medications	Signs/Symptoms
Intravenous fluids (water)	Delirium/hyponatremia
Epinephrine	Blood pressure/heart rate elevations, anxiety
Lidocaine	Delirium, psychosis
Atropine	Delirium, anticholinergic effects, anxiety
Sedatives	Depressed consciousness/responsiveness
Nitroglycerin	Dizziness
Morphine	Sedation, delirium

CONFIDENCE IN A POTENTIALLY TOXIC ENVIRONMENT

Training and confidence in combat, rules of engagement, and containment/decontamination procedures following toxic exposures may be important factors in limiting psychological contagion and unexplained physical symptoms. Military experience reveals that the risk of contagion and psychiatric conditions (such as conversion disorder) is lessened when potentially exposed personnel have received effective training. This training allows personnel to feel confident in their odds of surviving a chemical or biological threat. In addition to training, the military services place a high priority on the vaccination of groups at highest risk of coming into contact with biological agents or with persons (including health care workers) exposed to them. This may also increase confidence in the ability to survive and to operate in toxic environments.

LEVELS OF CLINICAL PREVENTION AND INTERVENTION: SYMPTOMS VERSUS FUNCTION

Distress and highly emotional responses are nearly universal during combat. Therefore, initial psychiatric interventions must focus on the mobilization of effective function to allow the military mission to continue. Military psychiatric theory and doctrine have long operated on the principle that transient and near-universal symptoms (that represent normal responses) can become "medicalized" if physicians reinforce a view that these symptoms constitute a disease. Levels of clinical intervention are conceptualized and deployed according to this doctrine (Table 90-2).

Combat stress units assist in the management of clinically significant distress or psychiatric syndromes; these units are located as close to the area of operations as possible. This proximity and ease of access helps to avoid further pathologizing of the service member and possibly setting the stage for longer-term disability. Response to conservative measures, such as rest, respite, and reassurance, at such a location suggests a combat stress reaction rather than a psychiatric diagnosis. Initial use of conservative management is consistent with long-standing military doctrine (Table 90-3).[5,6] Sometimes, service members who are exposed to combat or terrorist attacks develop pathological states that require evacuation from the theater of operations. In these cases, more traditional psychiatric settings, such as outpatient clinics and inpatient psychiatric units, are called on for definitive treatment.

Other service members successfully complete their combat tours of duty and then develop mental health concerns or impaired function after returning home. In 2004 an anonymous survey[7] administered to US servicemen either before, or 3 to 4 months after, deployment to Iraq (n = 2,530) or

TABLE 90-2 Levels of Psychiatric Intervention and Care following Combat or Terrorist Attack

Intervention Level	Indication
Support during combat	Consultations with leaders to mobilize effective function, to allow the military mission to continue
Combat stress control teams	Manage distress and acute psychiatric syndromes (as closely as possible to the area of operations) to maximize chances of a rapid return to effective function; use a mobile "holding environment"
Traditional psychiatric clinics	In the theater of operations, at aeromedical evacuation staging areas, or at fixed military bases in the US, traditional psychiatric assessment and treatment can be provided at different times following one's departure from the theater of operations
Inpatient psychiatric clinics	For patients with severe psychiatric illness or those with safety issues
Consultation-liaison services	For physically-injured patients who need psychiatric care in military hospitals and rehabilitation units
Veterans administration and community medical facilities	For veterans returned to their communities with ongoing mental health needs

TABLE 90-3 Doctrinal Principles for Management of Combat-Operational Stress Reactions

PIES*		BICEPS	
Proximity	Treatment should take place as close as possible to the service member's unit	Brevity	Treatment should occur over no more than a few days
Immediacy	Treatment should take place as soon as possible	Immediacy	Treatment should take place as soon as possible
Expectancy	Treatment should be geared towards returning the service member to his/her unit	Centrality/Contact**	Higher-level mental health services should be co-located with higher-level medical/surgical care services
Simplicity	Treatment should be as simple as possible	Expectancy	Treatment should be geared towards returning the service member to his/her unit
		Proximity	Treatment should take place as close as possible to the service member's unit
		Simplicity	Treatment should be as simple as possible

*US Army doctrine until replaced by BICEPS.
**The US Marines use the term "Centrality" while the US Army uses the term "Contact".

TABLE 90-4 Factors Related to Development of Psychiatric Disorders among Service Members Exposed to Combat or Terrorist Attack

Factor Type	Observations
Neurobiological factors	Corticotropin-releasing factor release Adrenocorticotropin hormone release Peripheral catecholamine surge Amygdala activation
Predisposing factors	Women are at higher risk for post-combat PTSD, anxiety disorder, depression Men are at higher risk for substance use disorder, antisocial/violent behaviors Pre-exposure level of function Past traumatic exposure history and experience
Protective factors	Unit cohesion Unit loyalty and interpersonal trust Strong leadership
Precipitating factors	Intensity and duration of combat exposure Physical injury Witnessing death or atrocities Sexual assault
Mitigating and perpetuating factors	Safety and security of recovery environment Degree of secondary traumatization Rotation schedules Recognition and rewards Quality of medical and psychological assistance provided Psychosocial situation at home

PTSD, Post-traumatic stress disorder.

Afghanistan (n = 3,671) suggested that a significantly higher percentage met screening criteria for major depression, generalized anxiety, or PTSD (15.6%–17.1%) after deployment to Iraq than they did after duty in Afghanistan (11.2%) or before deployment (9.3%). Over one-third of Iraq war veterans accessed mental health services in the year after returning home, and 12% were diagnosed with a mental disorder. These data highlight the importance of making mental health resources available to meet the needs of returning veterans over time, and not just to those recently exposed to combat or to terrorist attack.

FACTORS RELATED TO DEVELOPMENT OF PSYCHIATRIC DISORDERS AMONG SERVICE MEMBERS EXPOSED TO COMBAT OR TERRORIST ATTACK
Neurobiological Factors

The emotional and behavioral responses to trauma are rooted in a combination of social, physiologic, and voluntary mechanisms that are increasingly being understood at the molecular level (Table 90-4). In the immediate phase, the release of corticotropin-releasing factor (CRF), the secretion of adrenocorticotropic hormone (ACTH), the surge of peripheral catecholamines, and the activation of cortical brain areas related to perception of threat accompany extremes of environmental stress. Changes in behavior and cognition correlate with these noradrenergic phenomena. The immediate impact of acute stress under most conditions is improved performance. However, as the capacity to act becomes inadequate to meet continued demands, the risk for cognitive dysfunction increases and behavior often becomes too narrowly focused. An aroused, but focused, state may result in a difficulty with shifting sets or changing plans of action (e.g., adapting). If extreme distress disrupts cognition and creates chaotic thinking, the over-focused fight-or-flight response may result in immobility.

The immediate response is followed by a cascade of neuronal and intra-cellular events that lead to elevated levels of CRF, increased synthesis of cortisol-related receptors, and activation of protein synthesis in subcortical nuclei of the amygdala that are responsible for the encoding of

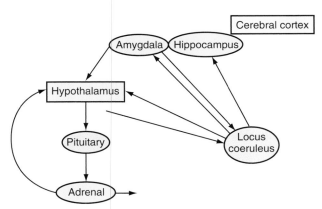

Figure 90-1. Noradrenergic circuitry in the traumatic stress response.

emotionally-laden memories and the development of conditioned responses or habits. Hypersecretion of epinephrine (adrenaline) also seems to exaggerate and consolidate fear-related memories. These changes may provide the molecular foundation for intrusive thoughts, exaggerated startle responses, and a general state of hyperarousal that is observed as clinically-significant pathology in PTSD and ASD[8] (Figure 90-1).

Predisposing Factors

The level of functional impairment in the aftermath of combat or disaster is related to pre-trauma function. Individuals who function marginally in their social or occupational roles prior to trauma are at increased risk of poor functional status after exposure to trauma. The extent to which past traumatic experiences may produce future resilience or vulnerability is unclear. If a person has successfully negotiated combat or disaster situations in the past, he or she may be less traumatized by subsequent exposures. On the other hand, if past traumatic experiences have produced PTSD or other psychiatric syndromes, further traumatic exposures may trigger exacerbations, or emergence, of new psychiatric disorders.

Protective Factors

In groups (such as exist in the military and civilian first-responders) certain factors may diminish the potential sequelae of trauma. Group loyalty and cohesion mean that individuals have ready access to social supports during the acute phase of a disaster and its aftermath. When organizations possess effective leaders, an environment embodied by strong loyalty, mutual trust, and respect is more likely to exist. Such an environment may facilitate voluntary participation in high-risk rescue/recovery or combat missions and facilitate the synchronization of individual efforts necessary for success in these types of operations.

Precipitating Factors

The high intensity and long duration of a disaster or combat situation increases the likelihood of psychiatric casualties. Specific experiences, such as physical injury, or the witnessing of grotesque deaths, torture, or other atrocities, place individuals at increased risk for adverse mental health consequences. Deployments and peace-keeping missions disrupt families and are often poorly timed with regard to other life events. Exposure to multiple simultaneous stressors and to traumatic events increases the risk of pathological outcomes.

Mitigating or Perpetuating Factors

Ongoing factors (including the security and safety of recovery environments, the extent of secondary traumatization, rotation schedules, the degree of recognition or compensation for efforts, and one's belief in the mission) all affect the rate and severity of psychiatric illness and symptoms of distress.[6] Personal attributes or behaviors (such as over-dedication to the task at hand) may further contribute to the development of dysfunction. Symptoms in civilian victims of war or the aftermath of disaster may be mitigated or exacerbated by several factors (e.g., by perceptions of community's leadership, preparedness for disaster, response to crisis, recognition of heroes, and provision of medical, financial, or emotional assistance) both immediately after the crisis and over time.

MANAGEMENT AND CARE DELIVERY
General Principles

Secondary prevention (i.e., early intervention) begins with the initial triage and treatment of victims. It is important to create a "holding environment"—a location or locations where persons demonstrating such symptoms can be observed and monitored. This area should be sufficiently removed so as not to disrupt the ongoing triage and stabilization of life-threatening physical injuries, but close enough to allow re-evaluation and further medical intervention should symptoms worsen. A holding environment may also prove to be a location where affected individuals attend to basic needs (such as food, shelter, and personal hygiene) that are critical to restoration of a sense of normalcy after engagement in prolonged or intense combat. In military psychiatry—particularly within United States Army doctrine—the Medical Detachment for Combat Stress Control (CSC) provides a mechanism for establishing just such a "mobile holding environment," which can be rapidly re-located as the battlefront moves.

The US military has attempted to decrease the incidence and severity of combat- and operations-induced psychiatric disorders through a number of mechanisms. Mental health teams are now routinely assigned to US forces in combat and are deployed in operations other than war. Each branch of the US military services has specialized rapid intervention teams to provide consultative assistance and acute treatment as necessary to units that have experienced traumatic events. These teams educate unit commanders on likely behavioral responses to stressful events and recommend leadership interventions that may reduce negative stress responses.

Therapeutic Interventions in Psychiatric Casualties

Neuropsychiatric symptoms may be manifest as an emotional response, may occur as a consequence of a neurological injury from a blast or other blunt trauma, or may occur—in the case of terrorist attack—from the neurotoxic effects of specific chemical or biological agents. Rapid identification of the underlying infectious, chemical, or physical insults to the brain will direct the treatment strategy. Regardless of etiology, delirium must be addressed rapidly, because the mortality rate from all underlying causes increases when symptoms of delirium go unaddressed.

Antipsychotics and anxiolytics used in the acute management of delirium or psychosis may alter levels of antimicrobial agents and acetylcholinesterase inhibitors used in the treatment of biological or chemical terrorist attack victims. Dose-related side effects (e.g., akathisia, somnolence) of antipsychotic agents may be mistaken for primary symptoms of an infectious, a post physical trauma, or a chemically-mediated encephalopathy. Therefore, a conservative approach that minimizes the initial use of psychotropic medications is warranted. Short-acting hypnotics may be used to restore normal sleep patterns in cases where insomnia appears to be the primary cause of dysfunction.

Psychosocial interventions have an important role in secondary prevention in military trauma victims. Group debriefing techniques and critical incident stress debriefings have been used, although there is no convincing evidence that such debriefings reduce the incidence of PTSD or hasten the recovery from a traumatic experience.[9,10] On the other hand, ongoing and frank discussions among squad members after a critical incident (such as an ambush or a raid) can open lines of communication to coordinate and evaluate the efficacy of actions, while fostering cohesion and group understanding of an event. These discussions, called "After Action Reports," "Lessons Learned," or "Historical Debriefings," may serve to sustain the performance of persons critical to the mission, decrease individual isolation, and help identify team members who require further psychiatric or other mental health attention.

Cognitive-behavioral, as well as other psychotherapeutic, approaches to anxiety, social withdrawal, depressive symptomatology, and hyperarousal can be effective; even brief interventions may reduce immediate symptoms of depression, anxiety, and PTSD and may diminish the development of long-term morbidity. Since medical resources may be quickly overwhelmed in combat situations, non-physicians, provided they are appropriately trained in the delivery of these therapies, will allow for more effective care.

MILITARY PSYCHIATRIC CARE IN PEACETIME

When not directly involved in combat operations, peace-keeping, or humanitarian relief, military psychiatric practice is in many ways similar to civilian practice. In addition to operating a medical school funded by Congress to train military medical officers for medical practice in military operational and peacetime environments, the United States Department of Defense has tertiary care hospitals and clinics throughout the world. These facilities care for military personnel and their family members, and psychiatric residency training is provided at several of the larger military medical centers. When military medical resources are over-subscribed because of operational commitments, there is a comprehensive civilian network, TRICARE, available to military medical beneficiaries. TRICARE is the tri-service (Army–Navy–Air Force) health insurance program that provides managed health care for all Department of Defense beneficiaries (active duty, family members, retirees, and survivors) by integrating available care at military treatment facilities with regional partner civilian health care providers and facilities.

Military members who develop psychiatric disorders while on active duty may be eligible for medical retirement disability pay, and continued treatment through a system of Veterans Administration hospitals. Individuals may be separated from service (without disability payment or ongoing medical care from the military) due to personality problems. Increasingly, civilian community hospitals provide ongoing psychiatric care to returning veterans, especially those in the National Guard and the Reserves. General psychiatrists must therefore understand the basic principles of military psychiatry and learn about the psychiatric disorders most prevalent in those who have been exposed to combat or man-made or natural disasters.

ETHICAL CHALLENGES

Unlike earlier US military experiences in the Persian Gulf, the current conflicts in Iraq and Afghanistan have created a significant population of detainees—prisoners of war, unlawful combatants, third-party nationals, and other persons captured on the battlefield and held for indefinite duration—for whom the US must assume responsibility for humane medical (and psychiatric) treatment under the provisions of the Geneva Conventions. Providing compassionate treatment for enemy combatants in hospital beds alongside ill or combat-injured US service members creates obvious challenges associated with dual agency for professionals (who, as they honor the requirements of their medical professional codes of conduct, must make triage decisions involving patients who may resume efforts to kill or injure US forces once released). Further, released combatants and non-combatants may have uncertain medical follow-up that is limited to the standards of the nation in which further care will be provided.

Physicians, including psychiatrists, may be asked to provide consultative assistance to persons who gather intelligence on detainees. This has created an ethical dilemma. Position statements and reports of a number of professional organizations (including the American Medical Association)[11] and the Department of Defense indicate that health care professionals who provide treatment to detainees must not assist in interrogations, and that torture, or otherwise inhumane or coercive interrogations, is not acceptable. However, disparities in these reports suggest that the degree to which health professionals *not* engaged in the treatment of detainees may apply their knowledge and skill sets to assist interrogators in safe, ethical, and humane interrogations remains unsettled.

CONCLUSION

Progress has been made in the identification of the nature of trauma-related psychological responses associated with military operations. Predisposing, exacerbating, and mitigating factors have been identified. Traumatic stress-related neuronal and hormonal events are being studied and clarified. The value of multi-disciplinary preparation and training for battlefield incident management and the need for forward-deployed outreach assessment and education programs have also been demonstrated.

Health care professionals should consider behavioral and psychiatric issues in the context of an overall medical-surgical differential diagnosis in the aftermath of combat or a terrorist event, including possible chemical and biological attacks. When psychiatric signs and symptoms confuse or co-exist with medical-surgical injuries and conditions, psychiatric consultation early in the triage and management process can ensure more timely, accurate, efficacious, and cost-effective management of combat casualties or victims of terrorism or other disasters.

Access a list of MCQs for this chapter at https://expertconsult.inkling.com

REFERENCES

1. Prigerson HG, Maciejewski PK, Rosenheck RA. Population attributable fractions of psychiatric disorders and behavioral outcomes associated with combat exposures among US men. *Am J Public Health* 92(1):59–63, 2002.
2. American Psychiatric Association. *Diagnostic and statistical manual of mental disorders, fifth edition*, Washington, DC, 2013, American Psychiatric Publishing.
3. Rundell JR, Ursano RJ. Psychiatric responses to war trauma. In Ursano RJ, Norwood AE, editors: *Emotional aftermath of the*

Persian Gulf War, Washington, DC, 1996, American Psychiatric Press.
4. Sandweiss DA, Slymen DJ, Leardman CA, et al. Preinjury psychiatric status, injury severity, and postdeployment posttraumatic stress disorder. *Arch Gen Psychiatry* 68(5):496–504, 2011.
5. Jones FD. War psychiatry. In Jones FD, editor: *Textbook of military medicine. Part I, warfare, weaponry, and the casualty*, Washington, DC, 1995, Office of the Surgeon General at TMM Publications.
6. Headquarters, Department of the Army. Combat and Operational Stress Control (FM 4-02.51). July 2006.
7. Hoge CW, Castro CA, Messer SC, et al. Combat duty in Iraq and Afghanistan, mental health problems, and barriers to care. *N Engl J Med* 351(1):13–22, 2004.

8. Krystal JH, Neumeister A. Noradrenergic and serotonergic mechanisms in the neurobiology of posttraumatic stress disorder and resilience. *Brain Res* 1293:13–23, 2009.
9. Bryant RA. Psychosocial approaches to acute stress reactions. *CNS Spectr* 10(2):116–122, 1998.
10. Adler AB, Litz BT, Castro CA, et al. A group randomized trial of critical incident stress debriefing provided to U.S. peacekeepers. *J Trauma Stress* 21(3):253–263, 2008.
11. American Medical Association. Council on Ethical and Judicial Affairs Report 10-A-06—physician participation in interrogation. June 2006.

91 Disaster Psychiatry

Elspeth Cameron Ritchie, MD, MPH, COL (Ret), Kevin M. O'Brien, EdD, MA, Marni Chanoff, MD, and Samantha Andrien Stewart, MD

KEY POINTS

- Disaster psychiatry is an evolving field that has developed in response to severe and usually unpredictable events.

- A psychiatrist has multiple potential roles in a disaster, ranging from advocating for appropriate preparation and policy to treatment of long-term effects that emerge in individuals and communities; the functions of psychiatrists shift according to the phase of the disaster.

- Disaster psychiatry involves interfacing with multiple systems.

- A variety of normal and pathological responses to disaster exist. Psychiatrists should be prepared to educate communities about normal responses, assist with triage for other health care providers, and provide treatment for individuals with pathological symptoms in response to, or in conjunction with, a disaster.

- Several treatment modalities can be employed when faced with a disaster; these include use of Psychological First Aid, psychopharmacology, and provision of individual and group psychotherapy, which should be implemented in a culturally-informed and sensitive manner with attention to pre-existing community structures and ongoing community resources and impact.

- Special populations are considered as high-risk victims of disaster and require specific attention during and after a disaster.

- Psychiatrists can help facilitate the normal recovery process and promote wellness and resiliency (on both the individual and the community level).

OVERVIEW

Disasters, especially unpredicted ones, provide fertile ground for psychiatric problems. The World Health Organization (WHO) defines disaster as "a severe disruption, ecological and psychosocial, which greatly exceeds the coping capacity of the affected community." Much as trauma can overwhelm the coping capacities of an individual, disasters overwhelm cities, systems, laws, organizations, and the smooth operation of society.[1] Mental health assessment and treatment in the face of a disaster must always consider the public health perspective and the impact that disruption of a community has on day-to-day functioning.

Disasters and their effects on the environment, populations, and individuals are often classified according to whether they are natural (e.g., hurricanes, earthquakes, floods, fires) or man-made; man-made disasters are often further classified as intentional (e.g., acts of terrorism) or accidental (e.g., an industrial accident). These classifications help shape the psychological impact of the disaster and the appropriate mental health response. In general, man-made ones cause more distress. Disaster psychiatry is a field that has emerged and continues to consolidate around the experience gained during specific disasters (i.e., with a growing body of anecdotal evidence and a lagging body of research). The field focuses on the tasks of the mental health specialists both in preparation for, and the subsequent phases of, disasters.

Disaster psychiatry includes the many interconnected psychological, emotional, cognitive, developmental, and social influences on behavior, mental health, and substance abuse, and the effect of these influences on preparedness, response, and recovery from disasters or traumatic events. Behavioral factors directly and indirectly influence individual and community risks, health, resilience, and the success of emergency response strategies and public health directives.[2]

HISTORY
Disaster Psychiatry

Although the symptoms of anxiety and depression have long been described as part of the human response to disaster, the most well-known early attempt of a psychiatrist to track such responses was by Erich Lindemann in his study of the 1942 Cocoanut Grove fire. He attempted to define in psychiatric language responses of normal grief, abnormal grief, responses to stress and loss, and the effects of witnessing a disaster.[3]

The language of traumatic response to war (e.g., nostalgia, shell shock, battle fatigue, war neurosis) began to appear in descriptions of combat trauma and disaster in the 1970s. Post-traumatic stress disorder (PTSD) first appeared as a diagnostic category under anxiety disorders in the *Diagnostic and Statistical Manual of Mental Disorders, Third Edition* (DSM-III) and as its own unique stress syndrome in DSM-IV, as a direct result of the Vietnam War. DSM-5 has just refined and expanded the diagnostic criteria.[4]

The first organized attempts to treat the mental health of people exposed to a disaster involved use of the debriefing model; developed from combat psychiatry, these efforts sought to return soldiers to full functioning for duty. Disaster psychiatry arose as a subspecialty in the late 1990s in the face of increased media coverage of large-scale disasters. The National Institute of Mental Health (NIMH) formed a "Violence and Traumatic Stress" branch in 1991. In 1993, the American Psychiatric Association (APA) recommended that branch chapters form disaster committees. Disaster psychiatry is currently a pertinent focus for psychiatry in the US in the wake of episodes of terrorism and disaster that have hit close to home, e.g., the 1995 Oklahoma bombing; the September 11, 2001, attack on the World Trade Center; Hurricane Katrina's devastation of the Louisiana and Mississippi coast; and more recently shootings in Aurora and Sandy Hook, and Hurricane Sandy, as well as the bombing at the Boston Marathon in April 2013.

A 2001 NIMH-sponsored consensus workshop on best practices established the need for a better understanding of how to facilitate research on disasters in a manner that is ethical, relevant, and capable of providing evidence-based practices (including the initial formalization of Psychological First Aid). This is difficult to do via standard research paradigms, given that disasters often come without warning and the populations to be studied are inherently vulnerable.[5]

CLINCAL AND RESEARCH CHALLENGES

Preparation for a Disaster

Successful disaster response should be flexible, creative, and have the capacity to adjust and react to an unstable and changing milieu. Disaster responses are more likely to be effective if they are organized and understand the goals of disaster psychiatry and how those goals shift according to the phase of the disaster. Tables 91-1[6] and 91-2[7] (created by the NIMH consensus) outline the organization of disaster responses, with attention to the broad scope of interventions.

Preparing for a disaster before its occurrence requires a plan that facilitates reaching the most basic and urgent goals and then expanding services as they become necessary and available. The priority should be planning for a system of communication and delegation within a team. Predicted disasters can have more comprehensive plans. These plans should be accessible.

It is important to know the functions of inter-related organizations and how to communicate with them so that efforts and resources can be distributed most effectively in the chaos of a disaster. The most effective preparation for a disaster involves familiarizing a team with the other players that will spring into action in the face of disaster. Anniversaries of disasters may be used as a reminder to rehearse or review disaster plans that are in place, at a time when participants can best understand their relevance.

TABLE 91-1[2] Key Components of Early Intervention after a Disaster

Issue Addressed	Sample Activities
Basic needs	Provide survival, safety, and security Provide food and shelter Orient survivors to the availability of services/support Communicate with family, friends, and community Assess the environment for ongoing threats
Psychological first aid	Protect survivors from further harm Reduce physiological arousal Mobilize support for those who are most distressed Keep families together and facilitate reunions with loved ones Provide information and foster communication and education Use effective risk communication techniques
Needs assessment	Assess the current status of individuals, groups, and populations and institutions/systems Ask how well needs are being addressed, what the recovery environment offers, and what additional interventions are needed
Rescue and recovery environment observation	Observe and listen to those most affected Monitor the environment for toxins and stressors Monitor past and ongoing threats Monitor services that are being provided Monitor media coverage and rumors
Outreach and information dissemination	Offer information/education and "therapy by walking around" Use established community structures Distribute flyers Host websites Conduct media interviews and programs and distribute media releases
Technical assistance, consultation, and training	Improve capacity of organizations and caregivers to provide what is needed to re-establish community structure Foster family recovery and resilience Safeguard the community Provide assistance, consultation, and training to relevant organizations, other caregivers and responders, and leaders
Fostering resilience and recovery	Foster, but do not force, social interactions Provide coping skills training Provide risk-assessment skills training Provide education on stress responses, traumatic reminders, coping, normal versus abnormal functioning, risk factors, and services Offer group and family interventions Foster natural social supports Look after the bereaved Repair the organizational fabric
Triage	Conduct clinical assessments, using valid and reliable methods Refer when indicated Identify vulnerable, high-risk individuals and groups Provide for emergency hospitalization
Treatment	Reduce or ameliorate symptoms or improve functioning via: • individual, family, and group psychotherapy • pharmacotherapy • short- or long-term hospitalization

Adapted from U.S. Department of Health and Human Services, Office of the Assistant Secretary for Preparedness and Response, Office of Policy and Planning, Division for At-Risk Individuals, Behavioral Health, and Community Resilience: Disaster Behavioral Health Concept of Operations, Washington, D.C., December 2011. Available at http://www.phe.gov/Preparedness/planning/abc/Documents/dbh-conops.pdf. Accessed July 1, 2013.

National Institute of Mental Health: Mental health and mass violence: evidence-based early psychological intervention for victims/survivors of mass violence. A workshop to reach consensus on best practices. Appendix A, 2002.

TABLE 91-2[3] Guidance for Timing of Early Interventions after a Disaster

	Phase				
	Pre-incident	**Impact (0–48 h)**	**Rescue (0–1 wk)**	**Recovery (1–4 wk)**	**Return to Life (2 wk-2 yr)**
Goals	Preparation	Survival, communication	Adjustment	Appraisal, planning	Re-integration
Behavior	Preparation versus denial	Fight/flight, freeze, surrender	Resilience versus exhaustion	Grief, reappraisal, intrusive memories, narrative formation	Adjustment versus phobias, PTSD, avoidance, depression
Role of mental health professionals	Prepare: train, gain knowledge, collaborate, inform and influence policy, set structures for rapid assistance	Basic needs Psychological first aid	Needs assessment Triage Outreach and information dissemination	Monitor the recovery environment	Treatment

Adapted from Lindemann E: Symptomatology and management of acute grief. Am J Psychiatry 101:141–149, 1944.
National Institute of Mental Health: Mental health and mass violence: evidence-based early psychological intervention for victims/survivors of mass violence. A workshop to reach consensus on best practices. Appendix B, 2002.
PTSD, Post-traumatic stress disorder.

Systems

Disaster behavioral health is an integral part of the overall public health and medical preparedness, response, and recovery system.[8] Disaster recovery is coordinated through the National Disaster Recovery Framework (NDRF), and the majority of states provide and coordinate disaster behavioral health services through a State Disaster Behavioral Health Coordinator.[9] Psychiatrists or mental health organizations interested in disaster psychiatry must prepare for disasters by familiarizing themselves with existing systems of disaster response, by building relationships with other agencies around disaster preparedness, and by forming action plans that include defined relationships within a system of disaster response (in advance of a disaster).

Perhaps the most complicated and prominent elements of disaster psychiatry involve interfacing with existing disaster response systems. The initial phases of a disaster mental health response are based on an outreach model. Mental health practitioners go out into the affected community, where they will work side-by-side with pre-existing systems within the community.

There will be formal disaster response systems already in various stages of mobilization and implementation. The mental health response occurs within a network of disaster responses that include safety, medical treatment, shelter, nutrition, transportation, distribution of clothing (and other necessities), location of individuals and families, and provision of accurate information about ongoing disaster and safety plans.

Psychiatrists can also aid in a system of disaster responses as medically-trained professionals, assisting with triage to ensure that emergency medical treatment is provided first and that identification of those individuals who have been physically injured occurs. Psychiatrists are often called on by the public to provide information about the typical and atypical psychological responses to disasters.

In addition, psychiatrists can identify first responders who appear to be suffering, because of the emotional events around them. Mental health providers can create treatment teams that include periodic checking-in to evaluate how the team/system is functioning.

In the immediate aftermath it is likely that many local systems of mental health care will be disrupted. Experience suggests that funneling resources and routines toward use of local agencies will be most productive in shifting the disaster system of care toward a long-term system of care. Disaster responders provide an emergency system while local systems find ways to resume their operation.

Staged Disaster Intervention

The phases of disaster response shift as the imminence of the disaster and the needs of the community shift. A response that is not capable of adaptation is only temporarily useful, given that the problems evolve over time.

In defining acute and traumatic stress, as well as grief reactions, the mental health field has recognized the variety of psychological responses that occur over time. A variety of short-term goals for disaster psychiatrists have been described. Common themes include the following:

- *Orienting mental health workers to the environment and to the function of the mental health team.* Practical application includes finding the existing hierarchy, making introductions, asking for their observations about needs, and defining your team's availability and capacity.
- *Observing elements of the environment.* This facilitates learning which factors interfere with stress reduction and with group and individual mental health, and effectively communicating these observations.
- *Engaging survivors in the context in which they can be found and encouraging the supportiveness of a given context.* Disaster psychiatry takes place in shelters, on the streets, in schools and hotels, in waiting rooms of housing, in health care systems, and in disaster relief centers. The outreach model appears to be the best way to engage a vulnerable population that may be resistant to mental health treatment. Providing general information and a willingness to assist in a range of activities (e.g., providing food service or clothing distribution) is often an effective way to start a conversation that touches on how a person is coping and what mental health needs he or she might have.
- *Screening survivors for risk factors and for traumatic stress reactions that suggest they need further services.* Aside from attending to blatant stress reactions, attention to risk factors can guide clinicians to individuals who may be in need of further assessment and services. Table 91-3 lists known risk factors for longer-term sequelae in response to a disaster.
- *Providing information to survivors, disaster workers, and the general public about normal and expected responses, concerning signs and symptoms, health and resilience-enhancing activities,*

TABLE 91-3 Risk Factors Associated with Adverse Mental Health Outcomes after a Disaster

Pre-disaster Factors	Within-disaster Factors	Post-disaster Factors
Female gender	Bereavement	Resource deterioration
Age: 40–60 years old	Injury	Social support deterioration
Minority groups	Severity of exposure	Social support increase
Poverty or low socioeconomic status (SES)	Panic	Marital distress
Presence of exposed children in the home	Horror	Loss of home/property finances
Psychiatric history	Life threat Relocation or displacement	Alienation and mistrust Peri-traumatic reactions Avoidance coping

From Young B. Emergency outreach: navigational and brief screening guidelines for working in large group settings following catastrophic events, NC-PTSD Clin Q 11(1):1–7, 2004.

and where to go for further help if symptoms emerge. This is best achieved by becoming familiar with the system to ensure that information is consistent and easily accessible. This goal also highlights the fact that mental health services are not limited to the survivors of the disaster.

Table 91-1 conveys the wide array of activities that are performed by a disaster psychiatrist. It is important to notice that only a small portion of the activities are listed as "treatment" in the classical sense. A large portion of the activities are devoted to restoring the ongoing function of the community of rescuers and victims. This is important because the broader the scale of the disaster, the more limited the access is to classical treatment settings. Experience during Hurricane Katrina revealed that emergency rooms and psychiatric hospitals filled up quickly and remained accessible only to the most severely disturbed.

Some tasks, such as monitoring rumors and media coverage and their impact, re-establishing community structure, fostering social interactions, and outreach, are high impact. The problem-solving abilities (meeting the challenges of individuals, groups, or families with attention, flexibility, and creativity) of mental health professionals provide preparation for provision of care in a disaster situation.

Practical Pointers
Victims of Disaster

The majority of people affected by a disaster will exhibit resilience or normal distress that responds well to the meeting of basic needs, finding or resuming familiar structures and activities, and self-regulating. A small number of disaster victims will have an acute stress response, such as severe anxiety, distress, dissociation, or psychosis. At times these responses may require immediate stabilization by medication, or stress management/relaxation techniques. Some improve rapidly while talking about what they witnessed or experienced during the disaster. Other cases recover more slowly, especially those who have been suffering for a prolonged period, e.g., living in shelters, and negotiating bureaucracies. In addition, those who have pre-existing diagnoses may have exacerbated symptoms by either a disruption in their medications or a withdrawal from medications.

Apart from those directly affected or injured by disaster, there are other, more remote victims of disaster, including witnesses, family members, and those who viewed the disaster from afar. Children and victims of prior trauma or disasters are at increased risk of remote traumatization.

When thinking about who is victimized by a disaster, individuals are often categorized by risk factors that have proven

useful in predicting a traumatic stress response for long-term psychological effects. Young[10] studied characteristics of disaster victims for their ability to predict adverse mental health outcomes; these factors were divided into post-disaster factors, within-disaster factors, and pre-disaster factors listed in Table 91-3.

Military psychiatry, Disaster Psychiatry Outreach (DPO), and the Federal Emergency Management Agency (FEMA) Crisis Counseling Assistance and Training Program (CCP) have emphasized the importance of an outreach model. Activities such as distributing information, monitoring the disaster setting, encouraging positive interactions that spontaneously develop or continue to exist, and responding to problems in their context are reliant on this model.

In practical terms this means that cell phones, adequate batteries, modes of transportation, nightly meetings to re-group and plan, good maps of the area, mobile treatment kits, and comfortable but respectful clothing and shoes are all important tools for effective psychiatry out in the field.

Responders are not exempt from the psychological sequelae of disasters. Many responders have witnessed either the immediate disaster or the devastation that resulted from it. Work, activity, and provision of aid are often healthy coping techniques. However, it is important to watch for symptoms of fatigue, burnout, and traumatization, particularly in the intermediate to late phases of a disaster. Experience has identified first responders (such as police and firefighters) as being at high risk.

More recently, "PsySTART" or Psychological Simple Triage and Rapid Treatment has been adapted as a strategy for rapid mental health triage and incident management during large-scale disasters and terrorism events. PsySTART has three components: community resilience via linkage between disaster systems of care; an evidence-based rapid triage "tag" designed for field use by responders without mental health expertise; and an information technology platform to manage the collection and analysis of triage needs in near real time. In a surge environment of many at-risk individuals, the PsySTART system uses a floating triage algorithm to prioritize those individuals who need be seen first. This allows for better management of limited acute-phase psychological resources and the prioritization of mutual aid needs based on a common evidence-based metric.

Cultural Awareness

Disasters represent a complex cultural encounter for victims, for external responders, and for the emergent and temporary disaster culture; these cultures can come into conflict.[11] This framework should be considered an overarching theme when using all of the treatment modalities described in this chapter.

Treatment needs to be culturally appropriate to both the individual and to the community in which a psychiatrist is working. If there is a cultural gap between a caregiver and a victim, it is important for the caregiver to learn about, and to understand, the rituals and healing traditions of the community, to consult with healers and leaders in that community, and to work together within the two models. If a psychiatrist tries to impose a scientifically-proven treatment that does not fit with the community's model, used for perhaps thousands of years, the community is unlikely to trust the proposed treatment.

Resiliency

Psychological resiliency has been defined as the individual's capacity for successful adaptation and competent function (despite experiencing chronic stress or adversity),[12] good outcomes in spite of serious threats to adaptation or development,[13] and the ability to maintain relatively stable and healthy levels of psychological and physical function.[14]

Trauma experts believe that most people will be able to persevere and regain full mental health without developing PTSD or other psychological disorders. To foster natural resilience, mental health workers can facilitate full use of available resources to ensure that an individual maximizes his or her social support system and community resources. Helping to maintain a schedule and a structure as soon as possible should be the goal. Re-building, getting together with family and friends, and engaging in spiritual/religious and recreational activities, are considered coping tools that can facilitate recovery and resilience. In addition, positive re-framing, or seeing the good that can come from disaster, can strengthen a sense of community and help foster resiliency at the individual and community levels.[15]

Diagnosis

Elevated rates of PTSD, depression, anxiety disorders, and substance abuse are associated with disasters (Table 91-4[16]). Individuals with pre-existing mental illness may be at heightened risk for further psychological sequelae because of their vulnerabilities or because of interrupted access to their treatment or system of care. This group includes the severely mentally ill, who may have their medication supply chain broken and hence become disruptive.

Distress should be anticipated after a disaster. Physical symptoms (e.g., startle, tension, or aches; changes in sleep, appetite, energy, libido, or bowel movements) and emotional symptoms (e.g., anger, numbing, guilt, or sadness; confusion, indecisiveness, intrusive thoughts, or worsened attention and memory) are characteristic of normal stress reactions in the days, weeks, and months that follow a disaster. Describing such symptoms as common responses to abnormal circumstances can provide relief to the majority of people who draw on resilience and coping skills to survive disasters psychologically intact. What differentiates common from abnormal reaction is whether it interferes with a person's ability to function.

General Principles of Intervention and Treatment

Medications, psychotherapy, and psychosocial interventions are all essential aspects of treatment. However, complicated logistics, system fragmentation, and lack of health care infrastructure need to be taken into consideration when creating goals and treatment plans. Psychiatrists have a unique skill set, and if used with flexibility and creativity, they are able to reach people in diverse ways.

Mental health care is commonly rejected or minimally accepted for reasons having to do with stigma, cultural biases, and unfavorable past experiences. For this reason, it can be useful to integrate mental health care into primary health care that is supported by the psychosocial, community-based effort.

Psychiatrists commonly think in terms of psychopathology, diagnosis, and the treatment of symptoms, but in the disaster setting, it is equally important to think about how to promote the natural course of recovery.

Psychopharmacology

Psychopharmacology may be an important aspect of treatment. In the early stages of recovery, many people experience difficulty sleeping because of their heightened state of arousal and adverse environmental factors in shelters and other temporary settings that can interfere with rest, such as bright lights, ambient noise, crowded spaces, and uncomfortable sleeping arrangements. Such individuals may benefit from the short-term use of sedative-hypnotics.

TABLE 91-4 DSM Diagnoses That Present after a Disaster

Diagnosis	Comments
Acute stress disorder	A stress response that interferes with function and that emerges 1 day to 1 month after a disaster.
Post-traumatic stress disorder	A stress response, with components of avoidance, re-experiencing, and excessive stress response that lasts longer than 1 month and impairs social, occupational, or other important areas of function. Previous traumatic experience is a risk factor for more severe stress response.
Anxiety disorders	Pre-existing disorders increase the risk of a pathological stress response. New anxiety disorders may emerge.
Mood disorders	Pre-existing disorders increase the risk of a pathological stress response. New depression may emerge.
Psychotic disorders	Brief psychotic reactions may be more common responses to stress in women, children, and members of non-Western cultures.
Normal bereavement	Grieving is present in most disasters, and normal grieving should be accepted with support provided as needed. Timelines vary between individuals. A key element in normal grief is an individual's ability to retain a sense of self and a sense of purpose.
Complicated grief	Complicated grief is mourning of a loss to an extent that normal life cannot be resumed.
Substance abuse	Pre-existing substance abusers and non-substance abusers alike are at high risk for using substances to cope with the stress and loss accompanying a disaster. Mental health workers should be attentive to substance-dependent individuals who may require medical detoxification to safely withdraw from a substance they do not have access to in a disaster setting. The community should be educated about the universal increased risks for using alcohol and drugs as coping mechanisms under stress.

Anxiety and somatic symptoms may include pain, weakness, dizziness, tachycardia, palpitations, or shortness of breath. These may benefit from the short-term use of long-lasting benzodiazepines. When these symptoms are only experienced episodically, shorter-acting benzodiazepines can be used on an as-needed basis. One must be careful to screen for present and past substance misuse or abuse. If there is a history of substance abuse, supervision and close follow-up should be provided whenever possible.

Screening, assessing, and treating alcohol and opiate withdrawal is essential. Alcohol withdrawal can be life-threatening and is associated with the risk of seizures, delirium tremens, and death, if not adequately treated with benzodiazepines. Opiate withdrawal, although not life-threatening, is extremely uncomfortable if not adequately treated. In addition, those who experience withdrawal are often irritable and agitated; this can be disruptive to the milieu of shelters. If formal detoxification programs are not available, benzodiazepines can be prescribed on a detailed tapering schedule to manage alcohol withdrawal. Supportive treatment for nausea, vomiting, and muscle cramping associated with opiate withdrawal is also useful.

Antidepressants (e.g., selective serotonin reuptake inhibitors [SSRIs] and serotonin norepinephrine reuptake inhibitors [SNRIs]) can be used for the treatment of acute stress disorder, depression, and generalized anxiety disorder and are commonly used to treat symptoms of PTSD.

Those with pre-existing mental illness should be maintained on their medication regimen and may require higher doses of antipsychotics, anxiolytics, and antidepressants, because stress and fear may worsen psychosis, anxiety, and depression. Often the supply chain of medications for those with chronic mental disease has been disrupted. One of the more practical roles of the psychiatrist is to re-start medications for chronic mental illness, assist in prescription writing, and help provide access to these medications.

Psychotherapy

Individual psychotherapy is another important aspect of treatment, both early on after a disaster and later in the recovery process. Immediately following a disaster, a psychiatrist can listen to victims, serving as "the calm within a storm," which allows victims to be heard and to have their needs addressed on an individual basis. This type of supportive therapy can be very helpful in giving attention to victims, reassuring them that they are safe, and normalizing their reactions, when appropriate. Supportive therapy continues to be useful after the trauma, when the necessary systems have been established, to give victims a safe and private place to be heard.

Cognitive-behavioral therapy (CBT) has been studied in randomized controlled studies and has been shown to be efficacious for the treatment of chronic PTSD.[17] CBT can focus on teaching specific strategies for coping with anxiety, hyperarousal, and avoidance.

Critical Incident Stress Debriefing

There has been extensive debate over critical incident stress debriefing, a technique adapted from procedures from the military that is used immediately or shortly after a traumatizing event. This treatment encourages people to process traumatic events, as well as their thoughts and feelings, with the hope that by sharing their experience, they will find relief from their symptoms and prevent symptoms from worsening. Because it has not been studied in randomized controlled trials and does not have evidence to support its efficacy, it is not widely recommended. In fact, many experts believe that it could be detrimental to one's recovery and may cause

re-traumatization.[18] It may still be useful, however, in first responders who have an operational debriefing as part of their routine.

Psychological First Aid

Psychological first aid, or PFA has become a critical dimension of response to the needs of those who are acutely stressed due to a disaster or emergency situation.[19,20] PFA is an approach dealing with the distress of affected populations, alongside practical assistance, information and self-help guidance, call centers and outreach.[21] There are variations of PFA taught to various responder audiences (e.g., from trained lay people to mental health specialists), and in every chapter of the Red Cross in the United States. The majority of state and local providers have adapted PFA as the primary response for the first 24 to 48 hours for disaster behavioral health. While adequate scientific evidence for psychological first aid is lacking, it is widely supported by expert opinion and rational conjecture.[22]

CONCLUSION

Disaster psychiatry is an evolving and increasingly important component of the knowledge base needed by psychiatrists. The literature is expanding; it reflects lessons learned from the terrorist attacks of September 11, 2001, tsunamis, hurricanes, shootings, and dozens of smaller disasters. Fortunately, well-accepted principles of early intervention currently exist.[23] Medical schools and residency programs should incorporate these principles into their training programs.

However, several obstacles remain. These include: being at the table with medical planners; surmounting difficulties in research; providing quality care and supervision in a disaster environment; obtaining appropriate licensing and payment; dealing with issues of cultural competency; and providing extended care to affected populations. The potential to influence the lives of thousands, or, perhaps, hundreds of thousands, cannot be ignored; energy and effort will be required to face the myriad challenges that lie ahead.

Access a list of MCQs for this chapter at https://expertconsult .inkling.com

REFERENCES

1. Garakani A, Hirschowitz J, Katz C. General disaster psychiatry. *Psychiatr Clin North Am* 27:391–406, 2004.
2. U.S. Department of Health and Human Services, Office of the Assistant Secretary for Preparedness and Response, Office of Policy and Planning, Division for At-Risk Individuals, Behavioral Health, and Community Resilience: Disaster Behavioral Health Concept of Operations, Washington, D.C., December 2011. Available at: http://www.phe.gov/preparedness/planning/abc/documents/dbh-conops.pdf. Accessed July 1, 2013.
3. Lindemann E. Symptomatology and management of acute grief. *Am J Psychiatry* 101:141–149, 1944.
4. American Psychiatric Association. *Diagnostic and statistical manual of mental disorders*, ed 5, Washington, DC, 2013, American Psychiatric Association.
5. National Institute of Mental Health. *Mental health and mass violence: evidence-based early psychological intervention for victims/survivors of mass violence. A workshop to reach consensus on best practices. NIH Publication No. 02-5138*, Washington, D.C., 2002, U.S. Government Printing Office. Available at: <http://www.nimh.nih.gov/health/publications/massviolence.pdf>; [Accessed July 1, 2013].
6. National Institute of Mental Health. *Mental health and mass violence: evidence-based early psychological intervention for victims/survivors of mass violence. A workshop to reach consensus on best practices. NIH Publication No. 02-5138*, Washington, D.C., 2002,

U.S. Government Printing Office. Appendix A. Available at: <http://www.nimh.nih.gov/health/publications/massviolence.pdf>; [Accessed July 1, 2013].

7. National Institute of Mental Health. *Mental health and mass violence: evidence-based early psychological intervention for victims/survivors of mass violence. A workshop to reach consensus on best practices. NIH Publication No. 02-5138*, Washington, D.C., 2002, U.S. Government Printing Office. Appendix B. Available at: <http://www.nimh.nih.gov/health/publications/massviolence.pdf>; [Accessed July 1, 2013].

8. 1976—Pub. L. 94–484, title IV, §407(b) (3), Oct. 12, 1976, 90 Stat. 2268, added heading "Subpart II—National Health Service Corps Program" SUBCHAPTER II > PartD> subpartii > §254d of the Public Health Service Act. Available at: <http://uscodebeta.house.gov/view.xhtml;jsessionid=dae13839dda45ad34d1a4625740a5240?req=granuleid%3ausc-prelim-title42-chapter6a-subchapter2-partd-subpart2&saved=%7cz3jhbnvszwlkolvtqy1wcmvsaw0tdgl0bgu0mi1zzwn0aw9umju0zi0x%7c%7c%7c0%7cfalse%7cprelim&edition=prelim>; [Accessed July 1, 2013].

9. U.S. Department of Health and Human Services, Office of the Assistant Secretary for Preparedness and Response, Office of Policy and Planning, Division for At-Risk Individuals, Behavioral Health, and Community Resilience: Disaster Behavioral Health Concept of Operations, Washington, D.C., 20024, December 2011. Available at: <http://www.phe.gov/preparedness/planning/abc/documents/dbh-conops.pdf>; [Accessed July 1, 2013].

10. Young B. Emergency outreach: navigational and brief screening guidelines for working in large group settings following catastrophic events. *NC-PTSD Clin Q* 11(1):1–7, 2004.

11. Marsella AJ, Christopher MA. Ethnocultural considerations in disasters: an overview of research, issues, and directions. *Psychiatr Clin North Am* 27(3):521–539, 2004.

12. Cicchetti D, Rogosch FA. The role of self-organization in the promotion of resilience in maltreated children. *Dev Psychopathol* 9:799–817, 1997.

13. Masten AS. Ordinary magic: Resilience processes in development. *Am Psychol* 56(3):227–238, 2001.

14. Bonnano GA. Loss, trauma, and human resilience: have we underestimated the human capacity to thrive after extremely aversive events? *Am Psychol* 59(1):20–28, 2004.

15. Hall RCW, Ng AT, Norwood AE: Disaster psychiatry handbook. American Psychiatric Association, Committee on Psychiatric Dimensions of Disaster. Available at: <http://www.eird.org/cd/ibis/guidelines/apadisasterhandbk.pdf>; 2004 [Accessed July 1, 2013].

16. Rousseau AW: Notes from Oklahoma City's recovery, a district branch perspective. Taken from Hall RCW, Ng AT, Norwood AE: *Disaster psychiatry handbook*. American Psychiatry Association, Committee on Psychiatric Dimensions of Disaster. Available at: <http://www.eird.org/cd/ibis/guidelines/apadisasterhandbk.pdf>; 2004 [Accessed July 1, 2013].

17. Foa EB, Keane TM, Friedman MJ, et al. *Effective treatments for posttraumatic stress disorder: Practice guidelines from the international society for traumatic stress studies*, ed 2, New York, 2009, Guilford Publications.

18. Rose SC, Bisson J, Churchill R, et al. *Psychological debriefing for preventing post traumatic stress disorder (PTSD) (2009) The Cochrane Collaboration*, 2009, John Wiley & Sons, Ltd. Available at: <http://www.thecochranelibrary.com/userfiles/ccoch/file/cd000560.pdf>; [Accessed July 1, 2013].

19. Everly GS, Flynn BW. Principles and practical procedures for acute psychological first aid training for personnel without mental health experience. *Int J Emerg Ment Health* 8(2):93–100, 2006.

20. Parker CL, Everly GS Jr, Barnett DJ, et al. Establishing evidence informed core intervention competencies in psychological first aid for public health personnel. *Int J Emerg Ment Health* 8(2):83–92, 2006.

21. Raphael B, Ma H. Mass catastrophe and disaster psychiatry. *Mol Psychiatry* 16(3):247–251, 2011.

22. Fox JH, Burkle FM Jr, Bass J, et al. Effectiveness of psychological first aid as a disaster intervention tool: research analysis of peer-reviewed literature from 1990–2010. *Dis Med Public Health Prep* 6(3):247–252, 2012.

23. Ritchie EC, Watson PJ, Friedman MJ, editors: *Interventions following mass violence and disasters: strategies for mental health practice*, New York, 2006, Guilford Press.

SUGGESTED READING

Erikson K. *Everything in its path*, New York, 1976, Simon & Schuster.

Fullerton CS, Ursano RJ, Vance K, et al. Debriefing following trauma. *Psychiatr Q* 71(3):259–276, 2000.

Horowitz MJ. Disasters and psychological responses to stress. *Psychiatr Ann* 15(3):161–167, 1985.

Hoven CW, Duarte CS, Lucas CP, et al. Psychopathology among New York City public school children 6 months after September 11. *Arch Gen Psychiatry* 62:545–552, 2005.

Lindemann E. Symptomatology and management of acute grief (reprint). *Am J Psychiatry* 101:141–149, 1944.

Norwood A, Ursano R, Fullerton C. Disaster psychiatry: principles and practice. *Psychiatry Q* 71:207–226, 2000.

Ritchie C. Assessing mental health needs following disaster. *Psychiatr Ann* 34(8):605–610, 2004.

Ritchie EC, Watson PJ, Friedman MJ, editors: *Interventions following mass violence and disasters: strategies for mental health practice*, New York, 2006, Guilford Press.

Shalev A. Biological responses to disasters. *Psychiatr Q* 71(3):277–288, 2000.

Simon A, Gorman J. Psychopharmacological possibilities in the acute disaster setting. *Psychiatr Clin North Am* 27:425–458, 2004.

Ursano R, McCaughey B, Fullerton C. *Individual and community responses to trauma and disaster*, Cambridge, UK, 1995, Cambridge University Press, pp 3–21.

World Health Organization. *Psychosocial consequences of disasters: prevention and management*, Geneva, 1992, World Health Organization.

WEBSITES

American Psychiatric Association. <http://www.psych.org/>

American Psychological Association. <www.apa.org>

American Red Cross. <www.redcross.org>

Center for the Study of Traumatic Stress. <www.usuhs.mil/csts/>

Disaster Psychiatry Outreach. <www.disasterpsych.org>

Federal Emergency Management Agency. <www.fema.gov>

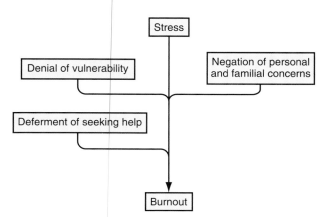

Figure 92-3. Factors contributing to self-neglect.

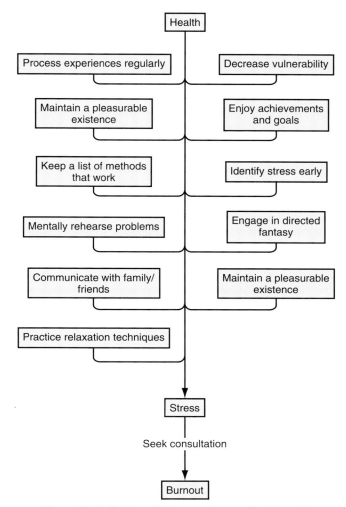

Figure 92-4. Coping with stress and preventing burnout.

patient in crisis; however, this practice can rapidly expand and soon become a pattern of working longer and sacrificing personal time. After long and stressful days, clinicians may be too emotionally exhausted for empathic listening, even-handed conversation, or recreation. As a result, clinicians may turn inward, internalizing their concerns and cutting themselves off from family and friends. This behavior compromises the strength of family and social relationships and decreases the support available for the clinician.

Deferment of Seeking Help

It is common to view seeking help for personal or family problems as a sign of frailty or personal failure. Some physicians are reluctant to seek help because of the stigma of mental illness. In general, while psychiatrists may be more open to psychotherapy for themselves, the possibility of a formal diagnosis and breaches of confidentiality, or having to report a problem to a licensing board, can make seeking help difficult. The intense pressure of a doctor's work can foster the creation of unachievable expectations. However, the physician's well-being is only undermined by this intolerance for human vulnerability.

How to Recognize Stress in Oneself

As psychiatrists, we are good at recognizing stress in others; however, recognizing stress in oneself requires a different skill set. Unrecognized and unmanaged stress can lead to anxiety or to depression and it can have long-lasting effects for clinicians, patients, and families. Signs of stress include exhaustion, apathy, anhedonia, and despair, as well as somatic manifestations, including headaches and gastrointestinal disturbances. Further warning signs include disrupted sleep, conflict in family relationships, and changes in memory, concentration, and problem-solving ability. Perhaps the most important warning sign is the suggestion from friends, family, and colleagues that help is needed.

Stress can also affect attitudes toward patients. Clinicians may develop reactive misanthropy when they frequently encounter patients' pain and suffering, especially when expressed by the patient as hostility or devaluation. Clinicians may then find that warmth and concern are replaced with apathy, or even defensiveness and contempt. This emotional detachment can progress and carry over to all patients, so that the clinician is no longer able to appreciate fulfilling patient relationships.

Stress, when prolonged or unmanaged, can progress to burnout. Signs of burnout include detachment from the

meaning of one's work, open hostility, deep-rooted cynicism, and overwhelming occupational dissatisfaction. In addition, reactive misanthropy can progress to malignant misanthropy in the burned-out clinician. In this malignant form, misanthropy extends to other relationships, including those with staff, colleagues, other health professionals, and even friends or family. The unfortunate result is then a conflict with one's social values and intentions, leading to self-punishment and feelings of guilt.

HEALING THE WOUNDED HEALER
Be Your Own Most Important Patient

Maintaining a caring and empathic attitude toward one's patients requires treating oneself with kindness and concern. While all doctors have strong coping skills (how else could physicians have made it through training?), these skills can always be expanded and refined. Anticipating and preparing for difficulty can prevent emotional overload. Some useful coping strategies are outlined here and in Figure 92-4.

Process Experiences Regularly

Talk with colleagues and supervisors regularly about difficult interactions, or reserve the commute home as a time for processing the day's events. Coping with stress on a daily basis, and processing emotions before one arrives home, can decrease the risk that one may take the strain of the day out on family or friends. Furthermore, learning important lessons from difficult events may mitigate some of the distress that they cause.

Review Your Own History and Keep a List of Methods That Work

Psychiatrists can identify useful coping strategies from the past and eliminate maladaptive ones. Since it can be difficult to recall adaptive strategies during moments of extreme distress or crisis, making a list of coping strategies that have previously helped can be beneficial. By engaging in constructive activities, such as athletics, one can discharge fury and anger, while exercise and yoga can relieve muscle tension. Even releasing emotion through tears can restore a psychic balance. It can also be helpful to identify prior manifestations of stress, so that one can recognize them early and intervene before they reach a caustic level.

Decrease Vulnerability to Stress

There are many aspects of clinical practice (such as long hours and copious amounts of paperwork) over which clinicians have no control, but there are factors (e.g., treating physical illness, eating a balanced diet, exercising, getting enough sleep) that clinicians can control and that can reduce vulnerability to emotional stress.

Doctors are frequently poor patients. Despite access to health care, many physicians rarely visit their primary care physician, even when ill. But untreated illness only compounds stress.

While hectic schedules sometimes necessitate taking meals on-the-go, or taking no meals at all, nutrition is crucial for a healthy body and a healthy mind.

Exercise releases endorphins, and it can improve mood and energy. Furthermore, exercise is an excellent way to relieve stress and reduce tension. Regular physical exercise contributes to physical health and an overall sense of well-being.

Sleeping at least 8 hours every night has benefits; fatigue can leave one vulnerable to emotional stress and to dysregulation.

Mentally Rehearse Potential Problems

When a potentially difficult meeting or conversation is anticipated, it is helpful to rehearse statements and responses to questions. Having responses in mind before a crisis makes it more likely that one will stay calm in a tense situation. This technique also fosters a sense of control over the unexpected.

Engage in Directed Fantasy

One can imagine expressing intense feelings (e.g., anger, sadness, fear) as a means of decompression. One can also imagine scenarios that are affectively intense (e.g., hitting that frustrating patient with a flaming axe, or duct-taping his mouth closed). The more outrageous these fantasies are, the more effective they will be at discharging emotion. The more unrealistic and outlandish, the easier it will be to distinguish between fantasy and a corresponding reality.

Cultivate and Maintain Professional and Personal Relationships

Healthy relationships are a key buffer against stress and burnout. Strong relationships with colleagues create a natural support network of individuals who share common challenges and stressors, and serve to decrease feelings of professional isolation. Professional insight into complex patients, difficult situations, and general work management can be shared formally and informally. Personal relationships are critical to maintain the balance between work and life, and strong connections with family and friends keep work issues in perspective. Personal relationships offer not only support and understanding but also rejuvenation and meaning to life outside of work.[15]

Communicate with Family and Friends about Anticipated Unavailability

This communication will help prepare them and lessen the likelihood that they will respond with anger and withdrawal. As one communicates about future work commitments, one can also make future social commitments. This action allows family and friends to know they are still held in high regard and it sets a framework for ongoing relationships. Above all else, open communication and a sense of togetherness should be maintained; hardship experienced as a team can deepen intimacy and mutual respect.

Enjoy Your Achievements and Your Goals

Previous triumphs, both professional and personal, should be pondered and joyful moments recalled. Original goals should be remembered, the progress made toward achieving them noted, and new professional and personal goals for the future set. Being mindful of the progress toward life goals can instill a sense of pride and mastery. The strength gathered from memories of the high points of one's life can facilitate coping with everyday stresses.

Learn and Practice Relaxation Techniques

Tension and overstimulation can make sleep difficult, and the fear of returning to work without rejuvenation only compounds this difficulty. In the midst of this pressure, one may be tempted to resort to the use of alcohol or sedatives. However, one can learn deep breathing techniques, progressive muscle relaxation, or self-hypnosis to promote tranquillity and sleep. These exercises can also be used in the middle of a hectic day or during a stressful night on call to rejuvenate an exhausted mind and body.

Maintain a Pleasurable Existence

It can be helpful to make a commitment to yourself to take a break from work each day to engage in a pleasurable experience. A pleasurable event can be having a cup of tea, taking a short walk outside, reading a favorite poem, or speaking with a friend on the telephone. Keeping balance between stress and pleasure on a daily basis prevents burnout and promotes a positive mind-set.

When to Seek Consultation

Consultation offers an objective point of view; it can be the first step in seeking help for the overwhelmed clinician. Consultation is not a sign of weakness; rather, it is the sign of a wise physician who recognizes that to help patients, one must first help oneself. Consultation should be considered for a variety of problems: symptoms of depression, disabling anxiety, self-prescribing, escalating use or abuse of alcohol, impulsive behavior, impaired clinical judgment, or inappropriate expressions of anger. Other signals that should prompt consultation include working longer hours, having trouble in significant relationships, and becoming socially isolated.

Types of Professional Help

It may not be easy for a clinician to acknowledge that he or she needs professional help. It can be extremely difficult to surrender control when one is used to being in complete control. But it may also be a wise decision, especially to halt a downward spiral.

Psychotherapy

Psychotherapy provides the psychiatrist the valuable opportunity to experience the other side of the therapeutic relationship. Psychotherapy can be a rich, life-enhancing experience, it can enhance coping skills, and it provides much-needed support for the overwhelmed clinician.

Psychopharmacology

Many physicians, and many psychiatrists, may see the need for medication as a sign of weakness or failure. However, doctors would rarely fail to use chemotherapy to treat a cancer patient or insulin to treat a patient with diabetes. So too should medication be used to treat a biologically-based psychiatric illness.

Couples Therapy

Strong family relationships are crucial for stress resilience. Ironically, family relationships are often among the first victims of vocational burnout. Couples therapy or family therapy can heal wounded relationships and restore lines of open communication, ultimately building protection against future stresses.

Group Therapy

Group therapy allows individuals to recognize that they are not alone in their suffering. Professional support groups can facilitate the sharing of common experiences and emotions, and promote connections between people who have similar strengths and difficulties. More general groups promote understanding of the difficulties inherent to all lifestyles.

Autognosis Rounds

Autognosis literally means "self-knowledge." Autognosis rounds allow psychiatrists to share common experiences and to identify individual reactions to clinical situations. This knowledge can then be used to inform diagnoses and to minimize potentially harmful reactions to patients (e.g., managing hostility toward a patient so that it will not interfere with treatment). Autognosis rounds have proven valuable for psychiatric resident groups at the Massachusetts General Hospital for the past four decades.

CONCLUSION

The practice of psychiatry, with all of its inherent stresses, is an honor and a fulfilling calling. "When we find ways to cope with. . . . conflicts, we move toward the equanimity that can enable us to serve our patients with greater effectiveness and compassion. We also progress toward greater satisfaction in this noble profession of medicine and in our personal lives as well. . . . I offer the suggestions in this [chapter] to my young and future colleagues with the hope that they will do no harm; that they will fortify and strengthen; and that they will contribute something to the glorious privilege that medical practice can be."[16]

Acknowledgment

This chapter is dedicated to Dr. Edward Messner, whose commitment to resident well-being was unparalleled. He taught us not only how to heal our patients, but how to heal ourselves.

Access a list of MCQs for this chapter at https://expertconsult .inkling.com

REFERENCES

1. Shanafelt TD, Boone S, Tan L, et al. Burnout and satisfaction with work life balance among US physicians relative to the general US population. *Arch Intern Med* 172:1377–1385, 2012.
2. Frank E, Biola H, Burnett CA. Mortality rates and causes among US physicians. *Am J Prev Med* 19:155–159, 2000.
3. Center C, Davis M, Detre T, et al. Confronting depression and suicide in physicians. *JAMA* 289:3161–3166, 2003.
4. Silverman M. Physicians and suicide. In Goldman LS, Myers M, Dickstein LI, editors: *The handbook of physician health: essential guide to understanding the health care needs of physicians*, Chicago, 2000, American Medical Association.
5. Koran L, Litt I. House staff well-being. *West J Med* 148:97–101, 1988.
6. Ruskin R, Sakinofsky I, Bagby RM, et al. Impact of patient suicide on psychiatrists and psychiatric trainees. *Acad Psychiatry* 28:104–110, 2004.
7. Chemtob CM, Hamada RS, Bauer G, et al. Patients' suicides: frequency and impact on psychiatrists. *Am J Psychiatry* 145:224–228, 1988.
8. Maltsberger J. The implications of patient suicide for the surviving psychotherapist. In Jacobs D, editor: *Suicide and clinical practice*, Washington, DC, 1992, American Psychiatric Press.
9. Hendin H, Lipschitz A, Maltsberger JT, et al. Therapists' reactions to patients' suicides. *Am J Psychiatry* 157:2022–2027, 2000.
10. Anne Alonso. Personal communication, 2005.
11. Gabbard GO. Boundary violations. In Bloch S, Chodoff P, Green S, editors: *Psychiatric ethics*, New York, 1999, Oxford University Press.
12. Norris DM, Gutheil TG, Strasburger LH. This couldn't happen to me: boundary problems and sexual misconduct in the psychotherapy relationship. *Psychiatr Serv* 54:517–522, 2003.
13. Brazeau CM. Coping with the stress of being sued. *Fam Pract Manag* 8:41–44, 2011.
14. Borritz M, Bultmann U, Rogulies R, et al. Psychosocial work characteristics as predictors for burnout: findings from 3-year follow up of the PUMA study. *J Occup Environ Med* 47:1015–1025, 2005.
15. Zwack J, Schweitzer J. If every fifth physician is affected by burnout, what about the other four? Resilience strategies of experienced physicians. *Acad Med* 88:382–389, 2013.
16. Messner E. *Resilience enhancement for the resident physician*, Durant, OK, 1993, Essential Medical Information Systems.

SUGGESTED READING

Hendin H, Haas AP, Maltsberger JT, et al. Factors contributing to therapists' distress after the suicide of a patient. *Am J Psychiatry* 161:1442–1446, 2004.
Stern TA, Prager LM, Cremens MC. Autognosis rounds for medical house staff. *Psychosomatics* 34:1–7, 1993.
Thomas NK. Resident burnout. *JAMA* 292:2880–2889, 2004.

93 Psychiatry and the Media

Cheryl K. Olson, MPH, ScD, Lawrence Kutner, PhD, and Eugene V. Beresin, MD

KEY POINTS

Background

- Portrayals of mental illness in news and entertainment media can educate the public and promote help-seeking efforts, or they can create and perpetuate stigma.

Clinical and Research Challenges

- Mass media reports of suicide can trigger imitation; following new guidelines for reporting on suicide can reduce this risk.

Practical Pointers

- Violence on television (including news programs) and in video games may promote fear or aggression in children, but its effects may depend on the context of the violence.

- Parents can gain some control over how their children access and are influenced by media content; this can be accomplished by teaching media literacy and by taking advantage of new technologies.

- Psychiatrists can use mass media to promote the public's mental health and to foster appropriate expectations of mental health treatment.

OVERVIEW

Mass media are increasingly intertwined with the lives of both adults and children. Whether subtly or overtly, media content (from children's cartoons to television news) affects the public's perceptions of mental illness and mentally ill persons, as well as the expectations patients bring to psychotherapy and other psychiatric treatments, particularly medication management. Media messages can be harmful to health by fanning fears of crime and terrorism, triggering suicide attempts, or modeling violent behavior. But the various forms of mass and targeted media also offer us new and powerful public health, educational, and psychotherapeutic tools.

This chapter addresses several issues: the role of the mass media in stigmatizing mental illness and discouraging help-seeking; the influence of media coverage of suicide; how media (especially television and video games) may affect aggression and violence among youth; the use of "media literacy" principles and new technologies to limit potential harms and increase benefits of media use for children; and how psychiatrists (through planned media campaigns or individual efforts) can use media intelligently to educate the public.

HOW THE MASS MEDIA AFFECT PUBLIC UNDERSTANDING OF MENTAL ILLNESS

Surveys in the US and elsewhere have found that many people have little understanding of what mental illness looks like (in themselves or in others), what symptoms characterize different illnesses, and what is meant by labels, such as "schizophrenia" and "mania."[1] Despite some progress in recent years, stigmatizing myths about causality persist. For example, persons with lower levels of education were more likely to blame schizophrenia or depression on a lack of willpower or an immoral lifestyle, and less likely to view medication as an effective treatment.[2] Recent studies across countries suggest that, although public understanding of the biological correlates of mental disorders has increased, this has not increased social acceptance or altered perceptions of dangerousness.[3] However, for affected individuals and their families, having a brain disease may be perceived as less stigmatizing than the "mentally ill" label.[4] Distorted views of the nature and value of psychiatric treatment persist, with some viewing it as more likely to harm than to help.[1]

National surveys (in the US) from 1998 and 2006 show increasing confidence that psychiatric medications can control symptoms, help people cope with stresses, and improve relationships, although a minority of respondents still believed that medications could interfere with everyday activities or harm the body. Despite these positive views, comparatively few respondents were willing to consider taking medication themselves for hypothetical ailments. Roughly half were very or somewhat likely to take prescribed medications for depression, whereas two-thirds might do so for more concrete symptoms (e.g., panic attacks).[5]

The stigma associated with mental illness is a major reason that many sufferers never seek treatment, do not follow treatment recommendations, or drop out of treatment prematurely (Figure 93-1).[6] Children with mental health problems (and their parents) face disdain, blame, and discrimination, in stark contrast to attitudes toward children with "physical" illnesses.[7] Research has shown that inaccurate perceptions by parents and teachers regarding children's mental health problems, and beliefs about treatment (including concerns about stigma that arises from treatment), create major barriers to receiving needed services.[8] Given that over three-quarters of children with mental health needs do not receive treatment,[9] the removal of barriers to care is a critical priority. Furthermore, since the life-time prevalence of psychiatric disorders is about 24%, and over 50% of these conditions begin in childhood, early detection and intervention may well decrease morbidity and mortality.

A number of studies point to mass media content as a major source of stigmatization and misinformation. Among people who have little first-hand experience with mental illness, beliefs about what mentally ill people are like and how they should be treated may be shaped primarily by what is read, seen, or heard in the mass media. Reviews of press coverage across many countries have found that mental illness, particularly schizophrenia, is frequently linked with violence.[10] In one US study on the reporting of mental illness by major newspapers, the focus of 39% of stories was on dangerousness or violence perpetrated by a mentally ill person; such stories also received the most prominent placement.[11] A randomized experiment found that news stories describing a mass shooting by a mentally ill perpetrator increased negative attitudes toward persons with serious mental illness.[12] This increases the desire to avoid persons with mental illnesses.[13]

Another study of US newspapers found that the word "schizophrenic" is commonly used as a metaphor in a way that perpetuates perceptions of that illness as a "split personality" (Table 93-1).[14] Moreover, hostile media reports can increase self-stigma, as well as discrimination, as perceived by people who struggle with mental illness.[15]

Entertainment media can also reinforce harmful images and beliefs. For example, a review of Disney animated films found a surprisingly high number of stigmatizing comments, including "crazy" thoughts, ideas, behaviors, or clothing, with the implication that these traits were irrational and inferior.[16] Children's cartoons often portray "twisted" or "nuts" characters as evil or funny.[17] Even video games feature negative stereotypes.[18] Mental illness is a common theme in movies (including horror films) that are popular with adolescents. These not only present persons with mental illnesses as scary and dangerous but also distort the public's perceptions of mental health professionals and their expectations about the nature and outcome of therapy (Table 93-2).[19,20] Media portrayals of electroconvulsive therapy (ECT) have been particularly distorted. ECT is routinely portrayed in films as brutal and punishing, and even as a method of torture, with no therapeutic benefit.[21,22]

HOW MASS MEDIA INTERVENTIONS CAN AFFECT STIGMA

People who are more familiar with mental illness (e.g., due to personal experience; illness of family, friends, co-workers, or neighbors; or exposure through volunteer or professional work) are less likely to want to distance themselves from people with mental illness, including those with major depression.[23] This also seems to be true after "virtual" exposure to models through educational videos.[24] Drawing on this research, and the research noted previously on the roots of stigma, the goal of many recent educational interventions has been to make the public feel comfortable with mentally ill individuals, and to refute stigmatizing ideas about the causes and treatment of mental illness.

The planning of anti-stigma initiatives has become more sophisticated, with efforts to target key attitudes or behaviors of specific populations.[25] One approach is to reach out through the mass media (using television, radio, films, and the Internet). The World Psychiatric Association's (WPA's) Programme to Reduce Stigma and Discrimination Because of Schizophrenia, begun in 1996, has programs in over 20 countries.[26] The WPA recommends a "social marketing" approach to planning outreach campaigns that includes targeting specific subgroups (e.g., criminal justice personnel), conducting needs assessments to inform the design of media messages, and pre-testing media materials before embarking on expensive campaigns.

The Royal College of Psychiatrists in Great Britain has sponsored several campaigns, including *Defeat Depression* from 1992 to 1996[27] and *Changing Minds* from 1998 to 2003.[28] Pre-post surveys for the latter found encouraging, but small, shifts

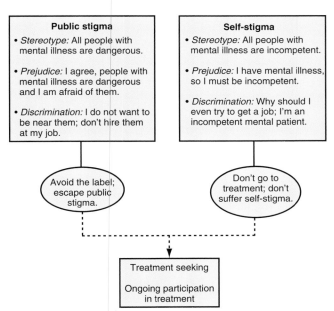

Figure 93-1. Two factors that may influence whether a person who might benefit from mental health treatment actually seeks it. *(Redrawn from Corrigan P. How stigma interferes with mental health care,* Am Psychologist *59:614–625, 2004.)*

TABLE 93-1 Types of References to Cancer and Schizophrenia in United States Newspapers

Type	Frequency (%)*	
	Cancer	**Schizophrenia**
	(N = 864)	(N = 876)
Metaphor	1.3	28.1
Obituary	24.5	0
Human interest	8.6	23.1
Medical news	14.1	13.7
Prevention education	4.4	2.4
Incidental reference	37.7	32.3
Medically-inappropriate reference	0	1
Charity	9.4	0

From Duckworth K, Halpern JH, Schutt RK, Gillespie C. Use of schizophrenia as a metaphor in U.S. newspapers. Psychiatric Services *54:1402–1404, 2003.*
X^2 = 579.12, df = 7, P < 0.001

TABLE 93-2 Schneider's Typology of Movie Psychiatrists and Psychologists

"Dr. Dippy"	**"Dr. Evil"**	**"Dr. Wonderful"**
Characteristics:	Characteristics:	Characteristics:
• Comical	• Dabbles in forbidden, dangerous experiments	• Warm, humane, modest, insightful, and caring
• Crazier or more foolish than his patients	• Performs evil deeds	• Not concerned with time
• Bizarre or impractical treatments	• Coercive in relationships with patients	• Skilled at improvisation
Sample films:	Sample films:	Sample films:
Dr. Dippy's Sanatarium (1906)	*The Cabinet of Dr. Caligari* (1919)	*The Criminal Hypnotist* (1909)
Mr. Deeds Goes to Town (1936)	*Spellbound* (1945)	*David and Lisa* (1962)
High Anxiety (1977)	*Dressed to Kill* (1980)	*Ordinary People* (1980)
Love at First Bite (1979)	*The Silence of the Lambs* (1991)	*Good Will Hunting* (1997)
Nine Months (1995)	*Batman Begins* (2005)	*The Sixth Sense* (1999)

From Schneider I. The theory and practice of movie psychiatry, Am J Psychiatry *144:996–1002, 1987.*

in attitudes (e.g., regarding perceptions of dangerousness, and whether a mentally ill person "feels different from us" or is to blame for his or her condition); these varied by type of illness. More recently, the comprehensive *Time to Change* program was linked to significant reductions in levels of discrimination reported by persons using mental health services.[29] Within this program, many prominent figures, including a member of government, came forward with their personal stories about living with mental illness.

Perhaps the most-studied anti-stigma campaign is New Zealand's *Like Minds, Like Mine*.[30,31] This research-based campaign includes strategically-placed television, radio, and cinema advertisements (some featuring nationally known and respected people who had experience with mental illness), public relations activities to support the advertising messages (including media interviews and placed articles), and more targeted locally-based education and grassroots activities. National tracking surveys found that awareness of campaign messages was high and that significant changes in attitudes and behavior were evident, as were reports of reduced stigma and discrimination.

It is critical to note that simply teaching facts about mental illness is not sufficient to dispel stigma. A review of studies shows that despite their greater knowledge, psychiatrists and other mental health professionals may hold and perpetuate stigmatizing attitudes toward the seriously mentally ill (e.g., not wanting to live near them, or believing they should not marry or have children).[32] It is also important to monitor anti-stigma efforts for the creation of unintended harmful effects. For example, it was once thought that re-casting mental illnesses as biologically-based "brain diseases" would reduce stigma. Recent research suggests that belief in biogenetic causality can actually increase the desire for social distance from mentally ill persons, especially in the case of schizophrenia.[33] Similarly, comparison of mental illness to chronic illnesses (such as diabetes and allergies), if over-emphasized, could inappropriately discount the effects of mental illness, and create new misperceptions.[34]

EFFECTS OF MASS MEDIA ON SUICIDE

A large body of multi-national research demonstrates unequivocally that exposure to media reports of suicide can increase suicide attempts and deaths. Research reviews have found that stories of both fictional and real-life suicides can lead to imitation, but the effect of news stories tends to be greater.[35] Several factors seem to increase the likelihood of imitation; these include stories of celebrities (entertainers or politicians) who commit suicide; extensive, prominent news coverage of the suicide; coverage that glamorizes or sensationalizes the suicide; and detailed descriptions of the suicide method. Imitation is decreased if the negative consequences of suicide (such as disfigurement of the body, a cult-related suicide, or suffering of, and condemnation by, the survivors) are portrayed. Adolescents, and young adults may be particularly prone to imitate suicides that are portrayed in the media, especially when the stories are of victims in their age group.[36]

A 1-year study of over 4,600 newspaper, radio, and television reports related to suicide in Australian media found a larger effect from television stories than either radio or newspapers (contrary to some earlier studies that found newspaper stories more influential).[37] A greater effect was also seen when multiple reports of suicide occurred close together, and when stories addressed completed suicides as opposed to suicide attempts or ideation.

Evidence suggests that changing the content and tone of news coverage of suicide can affect suicide rates. In Vienna, the opening of a new subway system led to an increase in subway suicides that was exacerbated by dramatic media reports. Creation of a suicide prevention media campaign, and guidelines for news reporters, led to a dramatic decrease in attempted and completed subway suicides.[38] New guidelines for media reporting on suicide suggest ways that psychiatrists can help educate the public.[39] When interviewed by reporters, it is important to stress the connection between mental illness (especially depression) and suicide, and to provide information on resources to prevent suicides and to help survivors of suicide. One should avoid weighted language, such as "committed," "failed," or "successful" when describing suicide; these words imply criminality or judgment of outcomes, which makes it difficult to put suicide into the content of mental health. It is also important not to associate suicides with simplistic explanations of causation, such as "he was fired from his job or lost his girlfriend, and committed suicide." One should take care not to be drawn into making comments on a complex clinical situation in which one has not participated. Reports of people who cope positively despite difficult circumstances and suicidal ideation may have a protective effect against suicide.[40]

EFFECTS OF MEDIA CONTENT ON CHILDREN'S BEHAVIOR

For modern American children, interacting with mass media is essentially a full-time job. A 2010 national survey of children (ages 8 to 18) about their media use found that children devote an average of 7.5 hours per day to contact with entertainment media (including print material) (Figure 93-2).[41] Due to "multi-tasking," or using multiple media at the same time, they were actually exposed to 10 hours and 45 minutes' worth of content. Despite the proliferation of new media, live

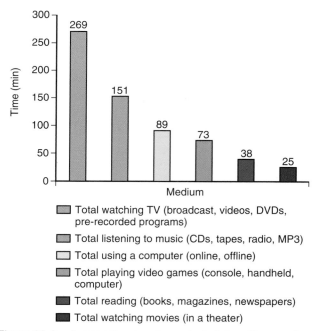

Figure 93-2. Average time spent on a typical day with recreational media by children aged 8–18. Note that 29% of media use was simultaneous (e.g., watching TV while playing a cell phone video game), so average total media use was 7 hours 38 minutes, while total media exposure was 10 hours 45 minutes. (*Redrawn from Rideout, Foehr & Roberts, Kaiser Family Foundation, 2010.*)

or time-shifted television content still claims the largest piece of media time: 4.5 hours per day. In their bedrooms at home, 71% of children had a television and one-third had Internet access. Two-thirds of children surveyed owned a cell phone in 2010, up from 39% in a 2005 survey; on average, children spent nearly an hour a day engaging with music, games, or TV programs via phone. Media time jumps in early adolescence; teens 11 to 14 are the heaviest users. While most survey respondents reported high levels of personal contentedness (e.g., got along well with parents and had lots of friends), those who were less content were more likely to be heavy media users. A variety of studies have looked at media use and relationships with parents or peers, with inconsistent results; however, heavy TV use seems particularly linked to risk of low parent attachment.[42]

The effect of media content (especially violent content) on children's behavior is a long-standing concern of psychiatrists, parents, and policymakers.[43] Unfortunately, studies of media's effects are difficult to conduct. Children cannot be randomly assigned to use or to avoid media. Longitudinal studies are hampered by problems with measures and definitions (e.g., total television viewing time used as a proxy for exposure to violence), and by the fact that media content and technology are constantly evolving.[44] Correlational studies cannot demonstrate causality, or the direction of any relationship that may exist between media content and behavior. Finally, experimental studies rarely measure effects of media exposure on actual physical violence; typical outcome measures (such as changes in attitudes or feelings measured directly after exposure) may be of limited use in the prediction of real-world violence. Thus far, research does not support a causal link between media violence and criminal violence, while strong support exists for other risk factors, such as abusive parents and family poverty.[45]

Despite these limitations, a large body of research suggests that television and other electronic media may teach violent behavior and attitudes, desensitize viewers to violence, and promote fears of becoming a victim of violence. However, the effects of violent content depend on how violence is portrayed, as well as on a child's characteristics (such as developmental stage, trait-aggression, and previous life experiences), and the social and physical context of media use. All of these affect the meaning and interpretation of the violence, and ultimately the lessons learned by viewers.[46]

The largest study of violent content to date, the National Television Violence Study,[47] involved content analyses of 10,000 hours of television programming (dramas, comedies, movies, music videos, "reality" programs, and children's shows) (Table 93-3). Content defined as "violent" included credible threats of violence, use of force intended to harm "an animate being or group of beings," and the harmful consequences of unseen violent acts.

Researchers concluded that the risk of learning aggressive behavior increases when the perpetrator of violence is attractive, the violence is seen as justified, the violence (and weapons used) are realistic, the violence is rewarded (or at least not punished), or the violence is portrayed as funny. The risk is reduced when violence is punished, or when harmful consequences of violence (such as pain) are shown.

While violent content has received the most attention, mass media also shape children's understanding of social relationships and their expectations about behavior and appearance. Television, movies, magazines, and electronic games frequently present children with unrealistic and unhealthy body images. A large prospective study of children aged 9 to 14 found that making efforts to look like same-sex media images predicted the development of weight concerns and constant dieting in girls and boys,[48] but a recent research review cautions that mass media likely play only a secondary role.[49]

TABLE 93-3 How Contextual Features Affect the Risks Associated with TV Violence

Harmful Effects of TV Violence

	Aggression	Fear	Desensitization
CONTEXTUAL FEATURES			
Attractive perpetrator	⇧	—	—
Attractive victim	—	⇧	—
Justified violence	⇧	—	—
Unjustified violence	⇩	⇧	—
Conventional weapons	⇧	—	—
Extensive/graphic violence	⇧	⇧	⇧
Realistic violence	⇧	⇧	—
Rewards	⇧	⇧	—
Punishments	⇩	⇩	—
Pain/harm cues	⇩	—	—
Humor	⇧	—	⇧

From National Television Violence Study 3.
⇧ Likely to increase outcome.
⇩ Likely to decrease outcome.
— No relationship, or inadequate research to make a prediction.

One medium of particular interest to psychiatrists is the video game, especially games with violent or sexual content (or both). The term *video game* is perhaps a misnomer, a legacy from the days of cathode ray tube displays of schematic characters and simple events. Today, the medium is far more graphically sophisticated, structurally complex, and interactive. Like other new technologies, video and computer games can seem foreign or threatening to adults who did not grow up with them.

The availability and use of interactive games have increased dramatically in recent years. On an average day, 60% of American children aged 8 to 18 play games on a console, hand-held player, or cell phone; and roughly one-third (35%) play games on a computer.[41] Game content is increasingly realistic and best-selling games are frequently violent, which raises concerns among clinicians, parents, and policymakers that exposure to such games could be a risk factor, or a trigger, for real-life aggression (Figure 93-3).

Dozens of studies have been published about the effects of electronic interactive games on children and adolescents. Until recently, most research centered on potential negative consequences on behavior, school performance, or desensitization to violence.[50] Some reviews of research on violent video games concluded that game effects are small or mixed[51,52]; others concluded that the evidence supports a large and consistent effect of violent games on aggressive thoughts, feelings, and behaviors.[53]

As with research on the effects of television, varying definitions and measures, and rapidly evolving content and technology, make it difficult to derive practical lessons from many studies of the effects of video game violence. Aggressive or hostile youths may be drawn to violent games, which might increase or decrease acting-out for an individual student; students who do poorly in school may turn to games as a way to demonstrate competence.

Some studies have looked at the effects of interactive games (both specially designed and commercially-available games) on health and well-being. Depending on the content, interactive games may promote the development of cognitive skills[54] (such as spatial representation, interpreting diagrams [iconic skills], and visual attention) and problem-solving skills.[55] Video games have shown promise as a therapeutic tool for pain management and physiotherapy, for the conveyance of

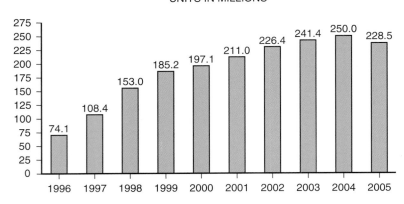

US COMPUTER AND VIDEO GAME UNIT SALES GROWTH
UNITS IN MILLIONS

Figure 93-3. Video game unit sales by year. *(Re-drawn from Entertainment Software Association: Essential facts about the computer and video game industry: 2006 sales, demographic and usage data.)*

social skills to children with disabilities (such as autism),[56] and for the treatment of post-traumatic stress disorder (PTSD) in war veterans.[57]

More research is needed on the differential effects of media on children with mental illnesses (such as depression and attention-deficit disorder). An analysis of young adolescents with clinically-elevated attention or internalizing symptoms on the Pediatric Symptom Checklist did not find a link between violent video game exposure and increased bullying or delinquent behaviors.[58] Some children with attention-deficit/hyperactivity disorder (ADHD) are adept at video games and using computers, which can provide a highly valued source of self-esteem. Judicious use of interactive games may enhance both social relationships and classroom learning for boys with ADHD.[59] Anecdotal reports also suggest that video games can facilitate therapeutic relationships, aid in assessment, and clarify conflicts during psychotherapy with children.[60]

MEDIA LITERACY: ADVISING PARENTS ON MEDIA USE

Most children age 8 and below cannot reliably tell fantasy from reality, and cannot comprehend complex motives and intentions. They focus more on how something looks than what is said about it.[61] Older children can begin to grasp more subtle aspects of program content (such as plots, themes, and historical or geographical setting), and how these combine with technical elements to affect how the program makes them feel. They can also start to question the motivations behind characters' behaviors (from sexuality to substance use) and aspects of their appearance (such as clothing or weight), and identify harmful stereotypes (such as the portrayal of "crazy people"). This analytical approach to understanding the purposes and effects of media is referred to as "media literacy."

These sorts of questions can form the underpinnings of discussions with older children as parents watch television programs or commercials with them[62]:

- Who created this message and why are they sending it? Who owns and profits from it?
- What techniques are used to attract and to hold attention?
- What lifestyles, values, and points of view are represented in this message?
- What is omitted from this message? Why was it left out?
- How might different people interpret this message?

The proliferation and ubiquity of media technologies make it difficult for parents to monitor the content available to their children. A variety of tools and resources are available to assist parents in this task. A summary of rating systems for television, films, music, and video games is available at www.parentalguide.org. This site is sponsored by entertainment industry groups; it also links to each of their sites, where frequently-asked questions about the rating systems are answered. The Federal Trade Commission's (FTC's) website also provides information, and allows parents to file complaints.[63]

New technologies make it easier to control children's use of television, computers, and video game consoles, even when parents are absent. As of January 1, 2000, the Federal Communications Commission has required all television sets larger than 13 inches to include technology that allows parents to block access to inappropriate programs. The "V-Chip" allows parents to use a "parental lock code" as a password to activate or change V-Chip settings. Programs can be blocked by age category or content label. For example, a parent may block all programs rated TV-14, or only those that contain violence (TV-14-V). The V-Chip can also block movies via Motion Picture Association of America (MPAA) ratings (such as PG-13 and R), including unedited films on premium cable channels. Unfortunately, the V-Chip can be difficult to locate and complicated to program, especially given parents' often-limited understanding of the ratings system. A 2007 survey found that only 16% of parents had ever used the V-chip, and just half were aware they had it.[64]

Cable set-top boxes or keypads come equipped with parental controls (see ControlYourTV.org). More advanced digital equipment may allow multiple options, including blocking by date, time, channel, program title, and TV or film rating (Box 93-1).[63]

Home computers are a concern in terms of access to inappropriate content (such as pornography) and release of private, identifying information. The 1998 Children's Online Privacy Protection Act (COPPA) requires that website operators post their privacy policy and obtain parental consent before collecting, using, or disclosing personal information about a child under 13. Parents may also review personal information collected on their children, and choose to revoke consent and delete it. Information on policies, as well as advice for parents, teachers, and children on safe Internet use, is available on the FTC website.[65] Perhaps of even greater concern is the use of hand-held devices, such as smart phones and tablets that offer access to children at any time of day. Texting is now the most common means of everyday communication among teens, who often exchange dozens of texts per day.[66] Far too little attention has been devoted to helping young people

---

BOX 93-1 Media Rating Systems

VOLUNTARY MOVIE RATING SYSTEM

(Motion Picture Association of America and National Association of Theatre Owners, 1968):

- G: General audiences. All ages admitted.
- PG: Parental guidance suggested. Some material may not be suitable for children.
- PG-13: Parents strongly cautioned. Some material may be inappropriate for children under 13.
- R: Restricted. Under 17 requires accompanying parent or adult guardian.
- NC-17: No one 17 and under admitted.

TV PARENTAL GUIDELINES

Designed to work with the V-Chip found in all TV sets since 2000. Parents can block programming by age-based category or content label (V, FV, S, L, D). Programs are voluntarily rated by the broadcast and cable television networks:

- TV-Y: All children; designed for young audience ages 2 to 6.
- TV-Y7: Directed to older children, age 7 and above (may include mild fantasy violence or comedic violence, or may frighten younger children)
- TV-Y7-FV: Directed to older children—fantasy violence
- TV-G: General audience. Most parents would find this suitable for all ages.
- TV-PG: Parental guidance suggested. May contain moderate violence (V), some sexual situations (S), infrequent coarse language (L), or some suggestive dialogue (D).
- TV-14: Parents strongly cautioned. Some material that many parents would find unsuitable for children under 14. Contains

intense violence (V), intense sexual situations (S), strong coarse language (L), and/or intensely suggestive dialogue (D).

MUSIC RATINGS: PARENTAL ADVISORY LABEL

(Recording Industry Association of America, 1985).

The PAL logo (Parental Advisory: Explicit Content) appears on sound recordings that contain strong language or depictions of violence, sex, or substance abuse to such an extent as to merit parental notification. The choice to use a PAL notice is made by the record label or artist, based on contemporary cultural morals and standards, the context in which the material is used, etc. Also applies to audio-visual products such as DVD music videos, concert performances, or music videos.

VIDEO AND COMPUTER GAME RATINGS: ENTERTAINMENT SOFTWARE RATING BOARD

(Self-regulatory body; established by the Entertainment Software Association, 1994):

- EC: Early childhood (may be suitable for ages 3 and older).
- E: Everyone (may be suitable for ages 6 and older).
- E10+: Everyone 10 and older
- T: Teen (may be suitable for ages 13 and older). May contain violence, suggestive themes, crude humor, minimal blood, simulated gambling, and/or infrequent use of strong language.
- M: Mature (may be suitable for persons ages 17 and older). May contain intense violence, blood and gore, sexual content, and/or strong language.
- AO: Adults only (should only be played by persons 18 years and older). May include prolonged scenes of intense violence and/or graphic sexual content and nudity.

From www.parentalguide.org.

---

appreciate the personal or even legal implications of posting inappropriate photos and comments via social media, such as Facebook or Twitter. Gorrindo and colleagues describe strategies for helping children to slow down and think before posting or texting.[67]

GetNetWise.org,[68] a website supported by a coalition of industry and advocacy groups, has an on-line safety guide that provides advice tailored to children's ages and likely activities (including chat, e-mail, instant messaging, and newsgroups). For example, as pre-teens begin to master abstract thinking and are able to explore more content on their own, it is important to talk about the credibility of web content and how to determine the quality or biases of what they find. The site also reviews the technologies available to families to restrict or monitor access to Internet content. Filtering software is controversial because it can over-block and prevent access to innocuous sites, or under-block and allow offensive material to slip through. No technology can replace parental monitoring, or discussions with children on how to handle the inevitable exposure to inappropriate or upsetting material.

Finally, parents have some ability to block inappropriate content in interactive games. Game consoles and personal computers have built-in parental controls that can prevent playing of games or DVDs based on industry ratings (e.g., all Mature-rated games). However, ratings provide little information about the context or goals of violence in a particular game; television research suggests that these factors may determine how a child is influenced by violent content. Therefore, parents may wish to play a new game with their child, or at least observe a play session, before allowing him or her to play unsupervised.

THE MEDIA AS PART OF THE PSYCHIATRIC INTERVIEW

Given the ubiquitous presence of electronic media in society, and the potential negative consequence on health, psychiatrists should themselves become more media-literate. Perhaps even more important is for a media history to be part of the psychiatric interview (see Chapter 2). Clinicians might ask parents about the media technologies and content their children have access to, especially televisions, electronic games, and Internet connections in their bedrooms, as well as how much time children spend with media each day.

Taking this history not only informs the physician about exposure to potentially vulnerable patients but also allows for an opportunity to discuss the means of controlling use of digital media. For example, one can help parents consider ways to reduce excess and unsupervised "screen time," such as not leaving the television on in the background or during meals, removing TVs from bedrooms, and using parental controls on computers and consoles. In addition, one can encourage them to learn more about the content of their children's media (e.g., by asking to learn how to play a favorite video game) and to control exposure to inappropriate content through use of ratings and parental control options. Finally, parents can be advised to use Internet resources to educate themselves and their children about cybersafety.[67]

THE USE OF MASS MEDIA TO EDUCATE AND COUNTERACT STIGMA

The most straightforward way to educate the public about mental illness is to reach out through popular channels of information. In a 2001 survey,[62] 51% of respondents said that television (especially TV news programs) was their most important source of news and information about health issues. While clinicians and researchers may recognize the power of mass media as public health and education tools for mental health promotion, primary prevention, and stigma reduction, few psychiatrists receive any formal training in how to use those tools. In addition, many are concerned that attempts to work with the media will be viewed by colleagues as self-promotion rather than public education.

To address these problems, both formal and informal media training have been incorporated into the curriculum of the Massachusetts General Hospital/McLean Hospital child and adolescent psychiatry training program. Such training includes seminars in health communication (e.g., structured practice sessions involving mock broadcasts and print interviews), and opportunities to work on media-based outreach projects. Some of the points emphasized in these sessions can be readily adapted by experienced psychiatrists who wish to explore the use of mass media as extensions of their clinical practice or research.

There are three general types of "triggers" for contact with mass media:

- *Contact by a reporter or producer about a specific story.* This is probably the most common first interaction between a physician and the press. For example, a practitioner may receive a telephone call from a journalist who is writing a news story about local children who were sexually abused, or from a journalist who is producing a television feature story on the supposed increase in autism over the past few generations.
- *Promotion of a story idea.* This includes promotion of new clinical services or a book, interpretation of research findings for the general public or for public policymakers, or even an organized mental health-related media campaign.
- *The use of natural opportunities, such as breaking national news, to help guide coverage of that news and related topics.* For example, recent concerns and publicity over the use of antidepressant medications by children provided child psychiatrists with opportunities to reach out to the press not only on that specific topic but also on the nature of childhood mood disorders, the purpose and limits of these types of studies, and the predicaments of parents who are seeking help for children who have mental illnesses.

If the story is based on newly published research, it is important to provide information that helps reporters put those findings into perspective. For example, a mention in one small study that a quarter of patients with schizophrenia carried weapons during psychotic episodes led to histrionic headlines about dangerous mental patients.[69] One should be explicit about what the data mean and what they do not tell us, and what the practical implications might be. Whenever possible, one should attempt to put the data into a real-world context. If the goal is to increase the recognition of depression, it is more compelling to state that every high school classroom has at least one student with undiagnosed depression—and to give examples of what untreated depression might mean for that child's future—than to recite statistics. Thinking in terms of examples and visual images also helps to put information into lay language (Box 93-2).

These same techniques can be used in a proactive, rather than a reactive, manner. Whether one is promoting the expansion of services at a community mental health center or working on a national stigma reduction initiative, effectiveness will increase if one starts with a detailed plan for both strategy and implementation. Key issues the plan must address include the following:

BOX 93-2   Key Points in Working with Journalists on Mental Health Stories

- Listen for, and correct, inaccurate assumptions: e.g., mental illness is a weakness, people with mental illness are violent, it's a matter of poor parenting.
- Decline to answer hypothetical questions. Stick with what you know.
- Help put data into perspective. Can one generalize from a single study? What's the difference between statistical significance and practical significance?
- Use frames of reference the general public can immediately understand: e.g., a typical school classroom contains one child who's struggling with undiagnosed and untreated depression.
- Avoid both technical jargon and overly simplistic terms. Assume that your audience is intelligent but uninformed.

- *Who is the target of the message?* One should be as specific as possible (e.g., parents of children who are making the transition to middle school). It helps to think about the types of media the members of your target audience regularly listen to, watch, or read. At times, mass media can be used effectively to influence a very small but critical group of individuals, such as using news/talk radio to reach state legislators who are about to vote on a particular bill.
- *What exactly is the message?* Media interviews do not offer time or space for complex arguments. Too often, mental health professionals focus exclusively on conveying detailed information, such as a list of symptoms. One should avoid thinking in vague terms (e.g., "My goal is to tell parents about bipolar disorder"). Writing down the message with no more than three clear points facilitates success.
- *What are the specific responses that the target audience should have once they receive the information?* How should a person feel after seeing, hearing, or reading the message? (Reassured? Empowered? Ashamed?) What specific behaviors are desired from that person? (To speak with his or her child or spouse about the topic? To call a clinic to set up an appointment?)
- *How can success of the efforts be identified?* Did readers ask for more information? Did clinical appointments increase? Was a bill passed in the legislature? Defining criteria for success ahead of time helps determine whether the information offered to the target audience leads to specific responses.

While more published studies are needed, evidence shows that reaching out to reporters with accurate background information and ideas for positive stories can improve the amount and tone of mental health coverage.[70] If psychiatrists can overcome their discomfort and develop realistic expectations and clear goals, working with the media can often be a positive experience. For clinicians, several results are evident: it provides opportunities to counter misinformation[71] and stereotypes; it removes barriers to appropriately seeking diagnosis and treatment; it improves therapeutic relationships, compliance with treatment, and treatment outcomes; and it increases social and political support for families who struggle with mental illness. It is also important to network with colleagues locally and internationally to increase knowledge of innovative and effective ways to use mass media for the benefit of the public's mental health.

Access the complete reference list and multiple choice questions (MCQs) online at https://expertconsult.inkling.com

KEY REFERENCES

1. Jorm AF. Mental health literacy: Empowering the community to take action for better mental health. *Am Psychologist* 67:231–243, 2012.

3. Schomerus G, Schwahn C, Holzinger A, et al. Evolution of public attitudes about mental illness: a systematic review and meta-analysis. *Acta Psychiatr Scand* 125:440–452, 2012.

4. Angermeyer MC, Holzinger A, Carta MG, et al. Biogenetic explanations and public acceptance of mental illness: Systematic review of population studies. *Br J Psychiatry* 199:367–372, 2011.

6. Corrigan P. How stigma interferes with mental health care. *Am Psychol* 59:614–625, 2004.

10. Pirkis J, Francis C. Mental illness in the news and information media: A critical review, Commonwealth of Australia, April 2012.<http://www.mindframe-media.info/for-media/reporting-mental-illness/evidence-and-research/evidence-about-mental-illness-in-the-media>.

14. Duckworth K, Halpern JH, Schutt RK, et al. Use of schizophrenia as a metaphor in US newspapers. *Psychiatr Serv* 54:1402–1404, 2003.

16. Lawson A, Fouts G. Mental illness in Disney animated films. *Can J Psychiatry* 49:310–314, 2004.

19. Butler JR, Hyler SE. Hollywood portrayals of child and adolescent mental health treatment: implications for clinical practice. *Child Adolesc Psychiatr Clin North Am* 14(3):509–522, 2005.

29. Henderson C, Thornicroft G. Evaluation of the Time to Change programme in England 2008–2011. *Br J Psychiatry* 202:s45–s48, 2013.

32. Wahl O, Aroesty-Cohen E. Attitudes of mental health professionals about mental illness: A review of the recent literature. *J Community Psychol* 38:49–62, 2010.

33. Angermeyer MC, Holzinger A, Carta MG, et al. Biogenetic explanations and public acceptance of mental illness: review of population studies. *Br J Psychiatry* 199:367–372, 2011.

35. Stack S. Suicide in the media: a quantitative review of studies based on nonfictional stories. *Suicide Life Threat Behav* 35:121–133, 2005.

39. World Health Organization. Preventing suicide: A resource for media professionals, 2008. Available at: <www.who.int/mental_health/prevention/suicide/resource_media.pdf>.

41. Rideout VJ, Foehr UG, Roberts DF. *Generation M²: Media in the lives of 8–18 year-olds*, Menlo Park, CA, 2010, Kaiser Family Foundation.

43. Olson CK, Kutner L, Beresin EV. Children and video games: How much do we know? *Psychiatric Times* 2007. Available at: <http://www.psychiatrictimes.com/showArticle.jhtml?articleId=202101008>.

47. Smith SL, Wilson BJ, Kunkel D, et al. Violence in television programming overall: University of California Santa Barbara study. In Federman J, editor: *National television violence study 3*, Thousand Oaks, CA, 1998, Sage.

49. Levine MP, Mumen SK. Everybody knows that mass media are/are not (pick one) a cause of eating disorders: A critical review of evidence for a causal link between media, negative body image, and disordered eating in females. *J Soc Clin Psychol* 28:9–42, 2009.

52. Ferguson CJ, Kilburn J. Much ado about nothing: The misestimation and overinterpretation of violent video game effects in Eastern and Western nations. *Psychol Bull* 136:174–178, 2010.

53. Anderson CA, Shibuya A, Ihori N, et al. Violent video game effects on aggression, empathy and prosocial behavior in Eastern and Western countries: A meta-analytic review. *Psychol Bull* 136:151–173, 2010.

55. Adachi P, Willoughby T. More than just fun and games: The longitudinal relationship between strategic video games, self-reported problem solving skills, and academic grades. *J Youth Adolescence* 42:1041–1052, 2013.

58. Ferguson CJ, Olson CK. Video game violence use among "vulnerable" populations: The impact of violent games on delinquency and bullying among children with clinically elevated depression or attention deficit symptoms. *J Youth Adolescence* 43(1):127–136, 2013.

59. Ballas P. Recent findings on the psychiatric and behavioral effects of video games on children with ADHD. *Curr Attention Disorders Rep* 1:139–141, 2009.

60. Ceranoglu TA. Video games in psychotherapy. *Rev Gen Psychiatry* 14:141–146, 2010.

65. Federal Trade Commission. Kids' online safety page. Available at: <http://www.consumer.ftc.gov/topics/kids-online-safety>; [Accessed September 28, 2013].

67. Gorrindo T, Fishel A, Beresin EV. Understanding technology use throughout development: What Erik Erikson would say about toddler tweets and Facebook friends. *Focus* 10:282–292, 2012.

71. Friedman R. The role of psychiatrists who write for popular media: Experts, commentators, or educators? *Am J Psychiatry* 166:757–759, 2009.

94 Global Mental Health in the Twenty-first Century

Richard F. Mollica, MD, MAR, Christina P.C. Borba, PhD, MPH, Jesse M. Katon, Claire E. Oppenheim, BS, Gregory L. Fricchione, MD, and David C. Henderson, MD

KEY POINTS

- Mental health is essential to general health around the world; however, there is a continuous need to educate psychiatrists in the developed world about global mental health and to build psychiatric and mental health resources to meet an expanding need.

- Mental illnesses (which are typically high-prevalence, early-onset disorders) account for 13% of the global burden of disease; yet health resources devoted to mental health are disproportionately small.

- Experience in developing countries offers lessons about how to meet these challenges (e.g., training new psychiatrists in the developing world with the help of volunteers from developed countries and the World Health Organization and training primary caregivers about mental illness).

- Recent studies have emphasized the importance of appreciating the psychological and physical suffering caused by torture; torture and degrading experiences are at least equal in their physical and mental impact on survivors.

- Special attention needs to be paid to child and adolescent mental health and to women's health related to violence.

OVERVIEW

Global health has become an area of growing interest and concern over the past several years. To quote former Director General of the World Health Organization (WHO), Dr. Gro Brundtland, "Not only how people are dying but how they are living becomes a key ingredient in any international health planning."[1] Moreover, outgoing US Surgeon General David Satcher wrote in 2001 that the time for global mental health had surely arrived.[2] One reason for this new focus was the development of an important research measure called the *disability adjusted life years* (DALYs) measure. The DALYs measure refers to the sum of years of life lost because of premature death in the population versus the years of life lost because of disability for incident cases of the health condition in question. As a health measurement, it extends the concept of potential years of life lost due to premature death to include equivalent years of healthy life lost due to disability. The DALYs measure becomes an overall global burden of disease single unit of measure that can be applied throughout the world.[3-5]

In addition to the 13% global health burden of disease accounted for by mental illnesses, there are hidden and undefined burdens to consider.[6] The "hidden burden" is reflected in social consequences that lead to unemployment, stigmatization, and human rights violations and not just in pathological findings. There is also the concept of "undefined burden," which encompasses the negative impact that social and economic effects have on the families, friends, and communities

of those who suffer from mental disorders. The potential casualties of mental illness related to disabilities include so-called social capital and community development.

In this chapter we will look at why mental illness is costly worldwide (e.g., it is prevalent) and provide an in-depth look at one part of the developing world, Ethiopia. Attempts to provide primary care mental health services in the developing world will be examined, along with the need for global mental health research. Then, we will summarize the WHO Mental Health Global Action Program, which attempts to respond to the world's needs in this area. Finally, we will describe new efforts aimed at reducing the global burden of disease secondary to mental illnesses.

THE COST OF MENTAL ILLNESS

Mental illness confers extensive disability not only in wealthy countries but also in low- and middle-income countries. In addition, recognition of mental illness appears to be on the rise throughout the world. In the WHO's 2005 report, globally, 31.7% of all years lived with disability were due to neuropsychiatric conditions. In 2004, 4.3% of all DALYs lost were due to unipolar depressive disorders.[7] In high-income countries, Alzheimer's and other dementias were the fourth leading cause of burden of disease in 2004. It is predicted that by 2030, unipolar depressive disorders will become the number one leading cause of burden of disease, with cardiovascular diseases rising to the second leading cause of burden of disease (Table 94-1).[8,9]

Mental illness has increased in importance on the world public health scene for several reasons: an increased life expectancy has led to an increase in the prevalence of dementias; societal turmoil has resulted in frayed family and social bonds and to less social support; civil wars and international strife have created more refugees and cases with post-traumatic stress disorder (PTSD); and societal shifts toward technology and commercialization may have contributed to alienation and depression. Taken together, these factors can add up to a hostile environment for mental health.

THE PREVALENCE OF MENTAL DISORDERS

In 1990, a compilation of the Diagnostic Interview Schedule adjusted for both the International Classification of Diseases and the *Diagnostic and Statistical Manual of Mental Disorders* (DSM-IV) nosologies, and diagnostic criteria called the Composite International Diagnostic Interview (CIDI) was designed. Later, in 1998, the International Consortium in Psychiatric Epidemiology was formed by the WHO to carry out cross-national comparative studies of the prevalence and correlates of mental diseases; it proceeded to use the CIDI throughout the world (in seven regions in North America, Latin America, and Europe)[10,11] (Table 94-2). Early onset of mental disorders is common, as is chronicity. This was particularly true for anxiety disorders; the median ages of onset for anxiety disorders was 15 years, while for mood disorders it was 26 years, and for substance use disorders it was 21 years. Socioeconomic measures (such as low income, little education, unemployment, and being unmarried) were all positively associated with having a mental disorder.

TABLE 94-1 Disease Burden Measured in Disability-Adjusted Life-Years (DALYs)

Estimate 2004			Projection 2030		
Rank	**Cause**	**% of total DALYs**	**Rank**	**Cause**	**% of total DALYs**
1	Lower respiratory infections	6.2	1	Unipolar major depression	6.2
2	Diarrheal diseases	4.8	2	**Ischemic heart disease**	5.5
3	**Unipolar major depression**	4.3	3	Road traffic accidents	4.9
4	Ischemic heart disease	4.1	4	Cerebrovascular disease	4.3
5	HIV/AIDS	3.8	5	Chronic obstructive pulmonary disease	3.8
6	Cerebrovascular disease	3.1	6	Lower respiratory infections	3.2
7	Prematurity and low birth weight	2.9	7	Tuberculosis	2.9
8	Birth asphyxia and birth trauma	2.7	8	Refractive errors	2.7
9	Road traffic accidents	2.7	9	HIV/AIDS	2.5
10	Neonatal infections and other	2.7	10	Diabetes mellitus	2.3

TABLE 94-2 Lifetime Prevalences* of DSM-III-R Disorders in ICPE Survey Studies

	Brazil	**Canada**	**Germany**	**Mexico**	**Holland**	**Turkey**	**United States**
Anxiety disorders	17.4	21.3	9.8	5.6	20.1	7.4	25.0
Mood disorders	15.5	10.2	17.1	9.2	18.9	7.3	19.4
Substance disorders	16.1	19.7	21.5	9.6	18.7	0.0	28.2
All study disorders	36.3	37.5	38.4	20.1	40.9	12.2	48.6

Adapted from WHO International Consortium in Psychiatric Epidemiology: Cross-national comparisons of the prevalences and correlates of mental disorders, Bull World Health Organ 78:413–426, 2000.
*Prevalences are expressed in percentages.

The International Consortium concluded that mental disorders are among the most burdensome of all disease classes. This is because of their high prevalence, chronicity, early age of onset, and resultant serious impairment. Prevention, outreach, and early intervention for people with mental disorders were recommended. The consortium called for quality assurance programs to look into the problem of inadequate treatment of mental disorders. One of these problem areas (PTSD in post-conflict societies) was investigated by de Jong and associates in 2001.[12] PTSD was found in 37.4% of those in Algeria, 28.4% of those in Cambodia, 17.8% of those in Gaza, and 15.8% of those in Ethiopia.

ETHIOPIA AND MENTAL HEALTH IN THE DEVELOPING WORLD: AN EXAMPLE OF GLOBAL MENTAL HEALTH

Ethiopia is an African country the size of Texas with a population of 75 million. Unfortunately, it has experienced a bevy of disasters (including drought, famine, human immunodeficiency virus [HIV] infection, tuberculosis, malaria, internal displacement [due to civil and border wars], abject poverty, and other stressors and traumas). Nonetheless, there are only 41 psychiatrists in the country and only one psychiatric hospital (Amanuel Hospital) with 268 beds.[13] Additionally, there are 10 government-established outpatient psychiatric clinics available throughout the country. A new general hospital is currently being built around the Kotebe area of Addis Ababa, which will contain a number of psychiatric beds. However, these services are still woefully inadequate for the large population, and largely inaccessible to the Ethiopian population living outside of the capital city.[14] In 2003, Addis Ababa University created a psychiatry residency training program which graduated its first class in 2006, significantly increasing the number of psychiatrists in the country. There are now 30 new Ethiopian-trained psychiatrists while the residency program continues to grow and develop. In addition to the psychiatrists now available in Ethiopia, there are 461 practicing psychiatric nurses.[13]

In the rural Butajira region, Awas and colleagues[15] found that the prevalence of mental distress was 17.4%. Mental distress is highest in women, in the elderly, in the illiterate, in those with low incomes, in those who abuse alcohol, and in those who are widowed or divorced. Problem drinking was found in 3.7% and use of khat (cathinone, an amphetamine-like compound found in a plant and then chewed) was found in 50%.

Using the CIDI, major mental disorders in Ethiopia have a lifetime prevalence of 31.8%. Of these, anxiety is found in 75.7%, dissociative disorders in 6.3%, mood disorders in 6.2%, somatoform disorders in 5.9%, and schizophrenia in 1.8%.[15]

In the urban Addis Ababa region, Kebede and colleagues[16] reported in 1999 that mental distress was prevalent (11.7%) in their sample of 10,203 individuals. Mental distress was most closely associated with women, the elderly, the uneducated, the unemployed, and those who had a small family. An under-reporting of mental illness in urban areas of Ethiopia may have occurred secondary to the impact of stigma, as well as governmental pressures applied at the time of the surveys. Tadesse and associates,[17] in 1999, found that the prevalence of child and adolescent disorders in the Ambo district in Ethiopia was 17.7%; this is lower than the prevalence (21%) in the US.[18]

By way of comparison, in the United States Epidemiological Catchment Area study, the lifetime prevalence of major mental disorders was 29%–38%.[19] Anxiety and somatoform disorders ranged from 10.4% to 25%, whereas MDD was in the range of 3.7%–6.7%.

No discussion of mental health in Ethiopia would be complete without reference to the acquired immunodeficiency syndrome (AIDS) epidemic; as of 2009, there were 1,116,216 people live with HIV/AIDS in the country.[20] This translates into the third largest population burden in the world. The overall adult prevalence of HIV infection in Addis is between 10% and 23%. No one has carried out a study of the psychiatric co-morbidity associated with this epidemic in Ethiopia, but the prevalence of depression alone in other cohorts of HIV-infected patients ranges from 11% to 35%.

The WHO's 2005 *Atlas of Mental Health Resources* noted that there was no mental health policy, no national mental health program, no community care in mental health, no substance abuse policy, and no applicable mental health law in Ethiopia.[21] Another obvious barrier was the low number of psychiatrists and psychiatric nurses, and lack of psychologists or social workers. However, since 2005 drastic changes and improvements have been made in the mental health system in Ethiopia. As stated previously, the number of mental health professionals has increased due to the development of various training psychiatry programs in the past few years. Additionally, according to the National Mental Health Strategy of Ethiopia,[14] the neurology program at Addis Ababa University has graduated 11 new neurologists.

PRIMARY CARE MENTAL HEALTH SERVICES IN THE DEVELOPING WORLD

In 1974, the WHO Alma-Ata Conference established several priorities in mental health (i.e., chronic mental handicaps [including mental retardation], dementia, addictions, epilepsy, and "functional" psychoses). Remarkably, every year, up to 30% of the world's population has some form of mental disorder, and at least two-thirds of those people will not receive adequate treatment.[22] In 2001, the WHO issued the *World Health Report*, which focused on mental health.[10] It suggested solutions to the problems of world mental health: providing treatment in primary care; making psychotropic medications available; giving care in the community; educating the public; involving communities, families, and consumers; establishing national policies and legislation; developing human resources; linking with other sectors; monitoring community mental health; and supporting more research efforts.

Based on a review of mental health intervention studies, it was believed that demonstration projects with rigorous evaluation and outcomes methodologies, and appropriate mental health service models should be prioritized.[23]

Psychiatrists can advance the cause of mental health around the world by contributing to the education of non-psychiatrists (i.e., primary care physicians, nurses, health officers, and caregivers [who are most likely to provide mental health care in the developing world]). Through education, consultation, and supervision of patient care, the scarce number of psychiatrists available can have their impact felt. A number of evidence-based studies have demonstrated that professionals in the primary health system, with the proper training, assistance and supervision, can identify, diagnose and treat those suffering from mental disorders. For this reason, practitioners of psychosomatic medicine, who commonly teach about psychiatric diagnoses and management to non-psychiatrists and provide clinical consultations, are ideal ambassadors for global psychiatry.

The 2007 *Lancet* series identified key barriers to the advancement of global mental health goals, accompanied by various strategies to help overcome these barriers. Among the most frequently mentioned strategies was the integration of mental health care into general health care. Treating psychiatric disorders in primary care settings is a proven and critical way to increase both access to, and quality of, comprehensive health care, as physical and mental distress are highly related. Psychiatric and neurological illnesses are frequently co-morbid with chronic physical illnesses, such as heart disease and stroke, diabetes, chronic respiratory disease, cancer, and HIV/AIDS. In the US, recent statistics from the US National Comorbidity Survey showed that 68% of individuals diagnosed with mental health disorders developed at least one physical disorder. The failure to treat co-morbid mental health issues both increases overall health care costs, while simultaneously impeding their efficacy. Furthermore, because of the stigmatization of mental illness in many cultures, those affected tend to describe mental distress somatically, and, therefore, if treatment is sought, it is often within primary care.

The 2007 *Lancet* series further described guidelines for innovative models that would successfully integrate mental health and primary care systems. These guidelines call for low-cost human resources, a specific mental health budget within primary health care, and the appointment and training of mental health professionals to oversee and support the primary health care staff.[22] Since 2007, there has been some progress in developing countries towards the integration of mental health and primary care systems. Political leaders and decision-makers in some countries have increased the funding for mental health in recent years. Additionally, there has been some movement towards health care decentralization and the reorganization of mental health care into primary health care by providing primary care doctors with mental health training in conjunction with improving the availability and accessibility of psychotropic medications.[24]

THE ETHIOPIAN PUBLIC HEALTH TRAINING INITIATIVE

In 1997, the Ethiopian government, with the help of the Carter Center, established the Ethiopian Public Health Training Initiative (EPHTI), which emerged from discussion between former US President Jimmy Carter and then Ethiopian Prime Minister Meles Zenawi. The initiative had two major objectives: to strengthen the teaching capacities of the public health colleges in Ethiopia through education of their teaching staff and to collaborate with Ethiopians to develop materials specifically created to meet the learning needs of health center personnel.

Modules (e.g., on malaria, diarrhea, dehydration, pneumonia, measles, HIV infection, AIDS, syphilis, tuberculosis, trachoma, ascariasis, malnutrition, intestinal roundworms, breastfeeding, immunization, acute febrile illnesses, anemia, and family planning) have been produced to educate public health care workers, and in May 2002, the Ethiopian Council approved a program to train health care workers about mental health in Ethiopia.

This training module is used in public health colleges in Ethiopia. Interactions with primary care take place at the unit level since patients come to these health units seeking general care. Psychiatric nurses and health care workers are charged with educating primary care physicians, nurses, and health care workers about mental health. Today, more than 26,000 EPHTI-trained health care professionals serve 90% of Ethiopia's population.

The Ethiopian story is important for international psychiatry. Providing good mental services in developing countries requires a bimodal approach like that adopted by Ethiopia. Establishing an in-country psychiatry residency is also an important step. It offers a modicum of protection against the "brain drain" that often occurs when doctors train overseas, and it provides much-needed manpower and professional expertise. This model could be replicated elsewhere in the developing world. For example, in 2007 the EPHTI Replication Conference gave ministries, leaders, and workers of mental health from 10 African governments the opportunity to learn about the strategies utilized in the EPHTI model, and to discuss how these strategies could help improve the shortages of mental health professionals in their own countries. Since there will never be enough psychiatrists in countries such as Ethiopia, it is important to train other mental health professionals. In late 2010, as part of the original agreement, the

Carter Center-assisted EPHTI was officially moved to Ethiopia's Federal Ministries of Health and Education.

CHILD AND ADOLESCENT PSYCHIATRY

Knowledge of child and adolescent mental health problems throughout the world will be an important educational goal in the twenty-first century.[25] Although there is limited research on child and adolescent mental health, it is known that about 10%–20% of children worldwide are affected by mental health problems.[26] Appreciating the stresses on children and adolescents in areas engulfed by conflict and learning about the nature of their responses provides the opportunity to learn more about resiliency and about what must be done to develop more effective programs. Even in developed countries the likelihood that a psychiatrist will see a child, adolescent, or family from a different culture has significantly increased (as a result of increased immigration and migration). Cross-cultural sensitivity is crucial to recognize differences in presentation, compliance, and acceptable interventions.

Overcoming a lack of trained child and adolescent psychiatrists in developing countries requires innovative approaches for teaching and providing clinical care. Packages and manuals to guide training programs for managing childhood mental disorders are now found in low- and middle-income countries. However, extensive future research needs to be conducted in the low- and middle-income countries as the vast majority (90%) of children and adolescents of the world live in these countries. Furthermore, it is essential to integrate and form partnerships between child and adolescent mental health care and agencies outside of the health sector, such as the criminal justice, education, and social care systems.[26]

Although some interventions have been developed and even successfully attempted in a variety of high-, middle-, and low-income countries, there are still many gaps and limitations imbedded within these particular interventions. Though child and adolescent-specific interventions are needed, it must also be recognized that maternal mental health is inextricable from child and adolescent mental health, as well as from cognitive and motor development. The effects of maternal mental disorders on child development have been studied less extensively in low- and middle-income countries than in developed countries where for example post-partum depression is known to affect 10% to 15% of women and is linked to adverse consequences in the child's development. Though less studied in low- and middle-income countries, the prevalence of maternal depression seems to be somewhat higher in these countries, which implies an even more significant impact on child and adolescent mental health. Child and adolescent psychiatry is an important area of specialization; however, effective and comprehensive child and adolescent care must also include the mental health of the entire family unit.[7] Much can be learned by developed countries from the way in which less developed countries have supported families and individuals with mental disorders.

PSYCHIATRY IN AREAS OF CONFLICT

The psychological damage caused by violence, terror, torture, and rape during war and violent conflicts has not been adequately addressed or been made a priority in the field of psychiatric medicine.[27] Not surprisingly, substantial research now demonstrates that mental health is a serious problem among post-conflict populations.[28] More evidence-based research is needed to maximize the benefits of interventions (e.g., psychiatric programs and activities) for societies affected by disruptive conflicts.

Individuals (including refugees, asylum-seekers, internally-displaced persons [IDPs], and illegal immigrants) directly affected by war, civil conflict, and terrorism struggle to piece their lives together after enduring unimaginable cruelty and violence. The cruel and violent acts witnessed and experienced by these individuals come in many forms; one of the most common of these is *torture*. In its most recent annual report, Amnesty International concluded that in 112 countries, comprising 70% of the world, citizens are tortured. The report also states that, although there has been many successful human rights movements in the last decade, there is still "distortion of sovereignty," meaning millions of people continue to be left behind and remain in danger.[29] The following sections describe and define torture (as elaborated by major existing international conventions), elucidate the major physical and psychiatric effects of torture (with an emphasis on the mental health consequences of the torture experience), and present a scientifically-based and culturally-valid model for the identification and treatment of torture survivors in the health care sector.

DEFINITIONS OF TORTURE

Though the word "torture" is commonly used without restraint in everyday language, its use should be clearly differentiated from words for inhumane and degrading actions that fail to match the true definition of "torture." One of the most frequently cited definitions of torture is the World Medical Association's (WMA's) 1975 Declaration of Tokyo[30]: "The deliberate, systematic, or wanton infliction of physical or mental suffering by one or more persons acting alone or on the orders of any authority, to force another person to yield information, to make a confession, or for any other reason."

The other frequently-cited definition comes from the 1984 United Nations Convention Against Torture that expands on this definition, distinguishing the legal and political components typically associated with torture[31]: "Any act by which severe pain or suffering, whether physical or mental, is intentionally inflicted on a person for such purposes as obtaining from him or a third person information or a confession, punishing him for an act he or a third person has committed or is suspected of having committed, or intimidating or coercing him or a third person, or for any reason based on discrimination of any kind, when such pain or suffering is inflicted by or at the instigation of or with the consent or acquiescence of a public official or other person acting in an official capacity."

These internationally-accepted definitions of torture share two basic elements: individuals are placed in captivity and subjected to extreme mental and physical suffering, and the capturers have a political goal or agenda.

Health care providers (including primary care practitioners and mental health specialists) often do not have these international covenants in mind. However, remaining cognizant of the two central features of torture can help identify those who may have been tortured and who may not be asking for medical and psychiatric care related to torture. The majority of afflicted individuals are aware that cruel and inhumane acts have been perpetrated against them, but they cannot contextualize these actions as torture with regard to the international covenants. At times, health care practitioners are the first civilian authorities to tell the patient what is obvious: that is, that he or she has been tortured.

Types and Purpose of Torture

The most common types of torture are summarized in Box 94-1. Torturers use these techniques to achieve several goals.

BOX 94-1   Most Common Forms of Torture

- Beating, kicking, striking with objects
- Beating to the head
- Threats, humiliation
- Being chained or tied to others
- Exposure to heat, sun, strong light
- Exposure to rain, body immersion, cold
- Being placed in a sack, box, or very small space
- Drowning, submersion of head in water
- Suffocation
- Overexertion, hard labor
- Exposure to unhygienic conditions conducive to infections and other diseases
- Blindfolding
- Isolation, solitary confinement
- Mock execution
- Being made to witness others being tortured
- Starvation
- Sleep deprivation
- Suspension from a rod by hands and/or feet
- Rape, mutilation of genitalia
- Sexual humiliation
- Burning
- Beating to the soles of feet with rods
- Blows to the ears
- Forced standing
- Having urine or feces thrown at one or being made to throw urine or feces at other prisoners
- (Non-therapeutic) administration of medicine
- Insertion of needles under toenails and fingernails
- Being forced to write confessions numerous times
- Being shocked repeatedly by electrical instrument

From Mollica RF, Caspi-Yavin Y, Lavelle J, et al. The Harvard Trauma Questionnaire (HTQ) manual: Cambodian, Laotian, and Vietnamese versions, Torture (Suppl 1):19–42, 1996.

The major goal of torture is to break down an individual both physically and mentally to render the victim, his or her family, and his or her community politically, socially, and militarily impotent. As Mollica[32] discussed in *Healing Invisible Wounds: Paths to Hope and Recovery in a Violent World*, humiliation is a major instrument of torture. Second, torturers seek to spread fear throughout the community or culture in which the victim lives. A single act of torture can have a devastating effect on an entire community (e.g., the systematic rape of women during the civil war in Bosnia).

Medical and Psychiatric Effects of Torture

The medical and psychiatric impact of torture has been extensively described.[33-35] As the famous Norwegian epidemiologist Leo Eitinger reported in his large-scale epidemiological study of Norwegian and Jewish Holocaust survivors, every organ system of the body is affected by extreme violence.[36,37] The health and mental health care practitioner, by learning about the type of torture experienced, will have a preliminary idea of the physical stigmata of torture that might be found. For example, beating to the soles of the feet with rods (called *falanga* in Latin America) can result in major orthopedic problems. Since sexual violence is a common form of torture, its effects (including an increased risk for cervical cancer, HIV infection and AIDS, and a range of sexual dysfunction, including impotence) must be identified and treated by medical

professionals. Studies have shown that many victims of torture have persistent and pervasive sensory and memory deficits, cognitive impairment, chronic pain, and certain forms of motor impairment (as serious as paraplegia). Other, more specific, physical symptoms include headaches, impaired hearing, gastrointestinal distress, and joint pain. Scars on the skin and bone dislocations and fractures are also typically observed.[36,38]

Until very recently, the psychiatric effects of torture remained largely invisible, due to difficulty assessing mental symptoms in culturally-diverse populations, unsuccessfully searching for a unique "torture syndrome," and a misconception held in some medical circles that extreme violence almost always leads to PTSD.[35,39,40]

Two decades of work on the identification of medical and psychiatric sequelae of torture have demonstrated that there is no "torture syndrome" and that PTSD and depression can be readily identified in all cultures. In addition, while physical complaints in torture survivors are common, usually these bodily complaints are signs of emotional stress related to torture and they do not prevent survivors from revealing the nature of their torture and the impact these experiences had on their body and mind.

Recent studies have emphasized the importance of appreciating the psychological and physical suffering caused by torture; torture and degrading experiences are at least equal in their physical and mental impact on survivors.[41]

In addition, studies by Mollica and colleagues[42] confirmed the 1965 findings of Eitinger[36] regarding the overlap of physical and psychological distress from extreme violence. Gronvik and Lonnum, in Strom's series of articles that examined Norwegian concentration camp survivors, linked the concentration camp syndrome to cerebral changes.[43] Thygesen and associates,[44] in their study of 1,000 concentration camp survivors living in Denmark, demonstrated significant neurological and psychiatric morbidity in their study population associated with the most commonly reported torture, "blows and kicks to the head." Research on the aftermath of war's mental health impact on American prisoner of war (POW) torture survivors and refugee populations exposed to mass violence has suggested similar conclusions to earlier pioneering studies. Extensive evidence on the extreme abuse associated with the POW experience of World War II, Korea, and Vietnam is associated with decline in the POW's neurocognitive status.[45-50] Clinical case studies have documented chronic neuropsychiatric findings (including abnormal neurological examination and cerebral atrophy) in torture survivors.[51,52] Rasmussen,[34] in his examination of 200 torture survivors, found that 64% had neurological impairments, two-thirds of whom had experienced a head injury. Other studies of torture survivors have revealed similar associations between the presence of neuropsychiatric symptoms and traumatic brain injury (TBI).[53]

In numerous studies Mollica and co-workers[42,54] demonstrated the long-term effects of mass violence. Mollica and colleagues[55-58] found many examples in which Cambodian survivors of mass violence and Vietnamese political detainees had been subjected to TBI as a common form of torture, which was subsequently highly associated with PTSD, depression, and post-concussive syndrome. All of these studies point in the direction of Eitinger's[37] original hypothesis, that extreme violence has both a psychological component (due to the degradation and humiliation of extreme traumatic events) and the resulting TBI. In effect, this means that PTSD and depression (which have been shown to be many times more common in torture survivors with TBI as compared to those with a head injury) might be masking a more serious underlying brain injury.[42,59,60]

Medical and Psychiatric Treatment for Torture Survivors

Torture survivors from all cultures primarily seek care for their physical and mental health problems from spiritual leaders, elders, traditional healers, and general medical doctors. Rarely do torture survivors initially present to psychiatric practitioners[33,61]; this is due to the stigma associated with psychiatric care in most societies and also to the fact that most torture survivors are unaware that their medical and psychiatric problems are related to the torture experience. Usually torture survivors seek care from all of their community healers simultaneously, hoping that at least one approach will provide relief from suffering. Management by health and mental health care practitioners, as described here, will not describe the valuable role of complementary approaches.

In general, health and mental health care providers often avoid the identification of torture as a cause of medical and psychiatric illness, in large part because they do not feel that they have the tools or the knowledge to help torture survivors even if they elicit their trauma stories. Therefore, the trauma history of the patient is often overlooked. As a result, torture survivors and clinicians create a doctor–patient relationship founded on the avoidance of discussions about torture.

Over the last 10 years, the Harvard Program in Refugee Trauma has developed an 11-point model (i.e., as stated in *Healing the Wounds of Mass Violence*) for the identification and treatment of the physical and psychiatric problems of torture survivors; it has been successfully implemented in the trainings of health and mental health care providers in the US, and in post-conflict countries (such as Peru, Uganda, Rwanda, Cambodia, Afghanistan, and Iraq) (Box 94-2). A discussion of the 11-point program follows.

Ask about the Patient's Trauma Story

At the core of the physical and psychological problems of torture survivors is the patients' "trauma story."[31,61,62] Many torture survivors readily tell their trauma story to their health and mental care practitioners regardless of their gender, ethnic background, or the severity of the torture—if they are asked about it by the health care provider. Not uncommonly, torture survivors do not tell their trauma story within the medical setting, because they do not believe that their doctor's office is an appropriate place for the trauma story to be revealed. Therefore, health and mental health care providers must specifically ask the patient about his or her torture experience. Many health care providers are afraid of doing this because they are afraid of opening up a Pandora's box (filled with emotional upset) that cannot be closed within a brief doctor's visit. However, this fear is unfounded. Patients will use their time, no matter how limited it is, to give a brief account of

---

BOX 94-2 An 11-Point Toolkit Model for the Recognition and Management of Reactions to Trauma

1. ASK the question! Open conversation with questions such as: "Many of my patients feel that their experiences of mass violence or trauma have had a major impact on their health and well-being. Has this been the case for you?" Listen to the answer and acknowledge the patient's trauma story. This simple act is usually healing in itself. Use words such as "I see," or "I can understand how that would upset you."

2. IDENTIFY any concrete physical or mental effects that are due to the results or continued threat of violence or torture. For example, is the patient complaining of headaches, stomach upset, back pain, or sleep disturbances? Does the patient exhibit feelings of anxiety and depression? Have medical or psychiatric disorders *worsened*?

3. DIAGNOSE AND TREAT. Most patients will *not* suffer from serious mental illness. The majority of patients will benefit from your attention to their grief, generalized anxiety, depression, PTSD, and insomnia. Use HPRT's Simple Screen to decide (see HPRT's website at www.hprt-cambridge.org).

4. REFER screened cases of serious mental illness (i.e., danger to self and others, complicated grief, severe forms of PTSD and/or depression, physical and social disability) to a mental health practitioner.

5. REINFORCE AND TEACH positive behaviors and coping techniques during the patient visit. Remind the patient to build physical, spiritual, and mental strength. Use phrases such as: "I want you to keep up the good work—it's good for you and will help you cope." Encourage exercise, relaxation, and anti-anxiety techniques.

6. RECOMMEND altruism, work, and spiritual activities. Use phrases such as: "I strongly recommend that you work and keep busy, try to help others, and consult with your clergy or engage in spiritual activities such as meditation or prayer."

7. REDUCE high-risk behaviors (such as smoking, drinking, drug use, and unprotected sex). Ask questions such as: "Have you started to use or increased your use of cigarettes, drugs, or alcohol? Are you having unprotected sex?"

8. BE CULTURALLY ATTUNED to differences in meaning and interpretations of emotional upset between cultures. Different cultures have different conceptions of the causes of illness. Pay close attention to dosage strength and side effects as they relate to ethnically influenced factors (such as tolerance levels and body weight). Be aware of a patient's pre-existing "sustained threshold" for trauma or difficult circumstances (i.e., previous trauma, domestic or economic hardship, domestic or community violence). Some patients may have a narrower capacity for additional trauma or anxiety in their lives.

9. PRESCRIBE psychotropic drugs if necessary. Psychotropic medication prescriptions should be tailored to the racial and ethnic background of the patient, since there are well-documented differences in drug metabolism and response to treatment according to race/ethnicity. For simple and detailed guides about the drugs most commonly used to treat grief reactions, generalized anxiety, depression, PTSD, and insomnia, see HPRT's psychopharmacology pamphlet.

10. CLOSE AND SCHEDULE follow-up visits. Add the physical and emotional symptoms to the problem list. Use phrases such as: "Thank you for telling me about these upsetting events. You have helped me to understand your situation better." Then ask the patient: "How would you like me to help you?" Make a plan with the patient that includes follow-up visits. Just having an additional conversation with the patient at a later date can be very beneficial in strengthening the patient's mental health.

11. PREVENT BURNOUT by discussing with your colleagues. Dealing with these issues can be stressful for doctors. We recommend that you regularly discuss these cases and your reactions with at least one colleague to prevent burnout.

HPRT, Harvard Program in Refugee Trauma.

their trauma experience, and in fact, may benefit from a well-circumscribed medical visit, because it places boundaries around their emotional distress. In other words, the patient believes that he or she cannot lose control during a brief medical visit. Medical practitioners do not need to collect the entire trauma story within a single visit. In fact, it is beneficial to the patient for the story to be collected over time. Simple questions can be used by the medical and psychiatric practitioner (see Box 94-2).

Identify Concrete Physical and Mental Effects

The trauma history, when obtained, is an essential component of the history of the present illness. Knowing what actually happened to the patient allows the practitioner to discover the physical and mental sequelae associated with torture. The medical and psychiatric practitioner must distinguish between symptoms of emotional distress that are cultural expressions of suffering and more specific symptoms of disease and illness. It is useful for the health and mental health care practitioner to review Amnesty International's (AI's) description of the most common torture events in the patient's country of origin (found at AI's website: www.amnesty.org), and to learn about the symptoms of emotional distress that are significant within the patient's culture. This review will help build a therapeutic alliance with the patient and spare the practitioner from pursuing somatic complaints associated with major medical disorders.

In addition, the medical and psychiatric practitioner must always be on the lookout for the chronic physical and psychological effects of sexual violence and head injury (i.e., the two most common forms of torture).

Diagnose and Treat

Most torture survivors do not suffer from serious mental illness; however, they may have emotional suffering that affects their well-being. Despair, hopelessness, revenge, and hatred are the most common emotions associated with the humiliation of torture. Many individuals fall shy of meeting diagnostic criteria for depression and PTSD. Nevertheless, health and mental health practitioners should treat symptoms (e.g., demoralization, despair, intrusive memories of torture, nightmares, and insomnia). Many others meet full diagnostic criteria for complex grief reaction, generalized anxiety disorder (GAD), MDD, PTSD, and chronic insomnia.[35,63] MDD is the most common psychiatric disorder in torture survivors and is often co-morbid with PTSD. It is also important that an underlying TBI be assessed.

Use of Screening Instruments for Treatment of Psychiatric Diagnosis. Two instruments that have been successfully used over the past two decades are the Hopkins Symptom Checklist 25 and the Harvard Trauma Questionnaire (HTQ). These instruments have been translated into over 30 languages, and their psychometric properties are valid across cultures.[64]

In the early 1980s, the Harvard Program in Refugee Trauma (HPRT) was told that the Hopkins Symptom Checklist 25 (HSCL-25) could help facilitate a psychiatric interview with refugee patients.[65] The Hopkins Symptom Checklist (HSCL) is a well-known and widely used screening instrument whose history dates from the 1950s.[66] Since its inception, it has been refined, resulting in its most common version, the SCL-90.[67] Developers of the HSCL, Rickels and colleagues demonstrated the usefulness of a 25-item version of the HSCL in a family practice or a family planning service.[68,69] Remarkably, when Indochinese versions of the HSCL-25 were used, patients were able to provide their symptoms with little distress.

The Harvard Trauma Questionnaire (HTQ) further revealed that these same patients could provide answers to lists of trauma events and symptoms without becoming re-traumatized. In fact, patients were grateful that the health worker knew about their trauma and interviewed them about it.

Two major lessons have been learned from the use of these simple checklists with trauma survivors: the checklist acknowledges the traumatic life experiences of the survivors and *de facto* gives them permission to elaborate on the details of their trauma; and the checklist helps survivors "put words around" events and symptoms that might be overwhelming in an open-ended interview.

Nonetheless, checklists can never replace a mental health professional; these instruments should be administered by health care workers under the supervision of a psychiatrist, medical doctor, or nurse. Further information regarding the application of these screening tools can be found in *Measuring Trauma, Measuring Torture.*[70]

Psychiatric Treatment. Evidence for the treatment of torture survivors has supported the use of selective serotonin reuptake inhibitors (SSRIs), general supportive psychotherapy, and cognitive-behavioral therapy (CBT).

Care of torture survivors using these modalities in randomized clinical trials has been slow in coming because of the ethical dilemmas that arise in the treatment of torture survivors. However, in a recent study of PTSD, using prolonged exposure therapy (a therapy that enhances emotional processing of traumatic events by helping patients face trauma memories and situations associated with them) was more effective treatment for women veterans and active duty personnel than was standard psychotherapy; exposure therapy itself has not been studied in the care of torture survivors.[71]

A recent study by Danish investigators showed that the remission rate of mental health problems in torture survivors using a multidisciplinary treatment approach has been limited.[32] The treatment of PTSD and depression in torture survivors is less effective than it is in non-traumatized patients with PTSD and depression.[72]

Furthermore, specific clinical trials using psychotropic drugs in the treatment of torture survivors have only been studied in other traumatized populations (such as combat victims and survivors of criminal violence and accidents).

Refer

Health care practitioners who do not have specialized training in psychiatry need to learn how to identify and refer to psychiatric professionals. If generic approaches to the treatment of torture survivors (such as psychotherapy and use of psychotropics) fail, the health care provider needs to consider that a more specific treatment approach may bring the patient into remission.

Reinforce and Teach

It is important for health and mental health care providers to build on coping techniques that the patient is already using to deal with his or her suffering secondary to torture. It is extremely important for the health and mental health care practitioner to point out the inherent self-healing capacity to torture survivors.

Recommend Work, Altruism, and Spirituality

Numerous studies have identified methods of self-healing commonly used by torture survivors and other victims of extreme violence (e.g., altruism, work, and spiritual activities).[73] Torture survivors should be encouraged to participate in activities where they help others, engage in productive economic activities, and pursue spiritual and existential beliefs. Torture survivors and other survivors of extreme violence have an intrinsic desire—despite a general scarcity of resources—to "help others"; by helping others they in effect are helping themselves.

Reduce High-risk Behaviors

High-risk behaviors (such as smoking, drinking, using drugs, and having unprotected sex) are more prevalent after torture.

Be Culturally Attuned in Communicating and Prescribing

In some cultural settings, psychotropic drugs are viewed as a sign of weakness or failure or as a sign that individuals cannot overcome their own problems. Many others fear they will become addicted to medications. Cultural beliefs related to compliance with medication must be explored.

Patients from different cultures, age groups, and social classes interpret trauma and responses to trauma differently (e.g., disgrace associated with sexual violence can exacerbate painful feelings of humiliation experienced by the torture survivor). Western diagnoses and treatment plans involving medication may seem ominous and highly stigmatizing. As folk diagnoses are common within particular cultures, the literal translation of the doctor's questions or diagnosis may be meaningless. Use of medical interpreters whose native background matches the patient's can help develop a supportive and culturally-appropriate therapeutic alliance with the patient.

Prescribe

Several basic principles for treatment of patients from varied cultural and ethnic backgrounds should be followed to ensure safety in prescribing psychotropic medications.[74–76]

Identify Target Symptoms. Identify target symptoms that interfere with function or cause significant distress. Torture survivors may experience a combination of depression, PTSD, GAD, other types of anxiety disorders, or substance abuse problems.

Pay Attention to the Patient's "Explanatory Model." The experience of the illness and the meaning around the use of a psychotropic medication are important for the patient.

Use Counseling. Counseling can help determine the causes of poor compliance, as well as remove financial and psychosocial barriers to the use of medication.

Keep the Medication Regimen Simple. Keeping the medication regimen simple will help improve compliance.

Pay Attention to Ethnic Differences in Metabolism of, and Response to, Medication. Research has shown that Asians, in general, respond to lower doses of antidepressants, and usually require starting doses and maintenance doses at half of the standard dosage.

Certain ethnic populations respond differently to psychotropic medications; thus, patients may experience side effects at unexpected doses due to biological differences in metabolism of the medication.

Schedule Follow-up Visits

Health care practitioners, in particular, usually have short visits with their medical patients on a regular basis over time; this is often presented by medical staff as a barrier to the management of the torture survivor. However, the brief medical setting is an ideal setting for those who have been highly traumatized. The caveat must be "a little bit, a lot, over a long period of time."

Prevent Burnout

Individuals working with torture survivors are exposed to unique stresses related to the intensity of suffering experienced by the torture survivor; these result in burnout and stress-induced illnesses.

Risk factors for burnout include excessive demands from self, others, and the work situation; lack of resources, personnel, and time to complete a job; excessive time in the same job; unrealistic expectations around recovery of patients; and lack of clinical/personal support in the workplace.[77] Care providers for survivors of torture may even experience other stress-related illnesses as serious as vicarious traumatization, depression, or PTSD.[78]

Protective factors (e.g., personal attributes that promote resiliency, self-esteem, resourcefulness, a strong physical or psychological constitution, or simply the desire and ability to help others) in the care provider should be enhanced. These protective factors may lower the likelihood of stress-related illness.

Evaluation

Numerous outcome measures have been established related to the medical and psychiatric care of torture survivors. These measures focus not only on symptom relief but also on the self-perception of health and the social function of the patient.

The self-perception of health status is a simple measure that provides a general overview of the patient's health and well-being, and is extremely sensitive to the progress of treatment.

PSYCHIATRIC RESEARCH IN THE DEVELOPING WORLD

According to Kleinman and Han,[79] research is essential to improve the health of populations, to address the global burden of disease, to organize and fund appropriate systems of mental health care, to prove outcomes, and to reduce disability.[28] Increasingly, there is recognition that important imbalances exist in health research output when population densities and disease burden are taken into account.[80] When the burden imposed by psychiatric diseases is considered, it is clear that research on mental health is an under-supported area around the world. High-income countries (with only 15% of the world's population) contribute 94% of the mental health articles, whereas low- and middle-income countries with more than 85% of the world's people contributed only 6% of the literature. Even though there has been a rise in pilot studies worldwide, there is rarely any follow-up or scaling up of these studies even if they had been well researched and had produced positive results. This lack of scaling up is mostly due to absence of funding needed to implement larger research endeavors.[24] Psychiatry needs to continue to do a better job of studying mental illness around the world.[81]

Multidisciplinary ethnographic studies on how stigma emerges must also be done. These studies should also include anthropological and epidemiological perspectives. For example, a detailed database could be made on approximately 100,000 people in population laboratories, complete with epidemiological surveillance, pertinent clinical research, sociological surveys, and anthropological ethnographies. In these laboratories, demonstration projects and different cultural contexts (using comparable psychiatric diagnostic criteria, a treatment process focus, and blind assessment of psychiatric outcomes) could be done. This is needed for extrapolating intervention programs. However, the successful implementation of the World Psychiatric Association's Global Program Against Stigma and Discrimination Because of Schizophrenia in more than 20 countries around the world has demonstrated that the reduction of stigma and mental health discrimination is an attainable goal.[82]

Gender studies are needed to examine the effects of poverty, refugee status, and exposure to violence and infectious disease on the mental health of women and the production of depression. Special focus should be placed on post-partum depression, given its potential public health implications and its inter-generational effects. Studies should also focus on men and the effects of alcoholism and violence. Attention should also be paid to neuropsychiatric and psychosocial aspects of HIV infection and AIDS and to multi-drug-resistant tuberculosis. Issues of compliance, depression, and course of illness are of special importance in these epidemics. Political violence and refugee trauma resulting in "invisible wounds"[83] are important areas for research around the world.

Suicide should be another area of special interest. Although there has been some suicide research in countries such as China where the suicide rate is very high despite being greatly under-reported,[84] further extensive research needs to be done in other areas of the world, where suicide is under-reported by as much as 100%.[71] Mental health services research (looking at primary care models, including both public and private sectors) is also needed. The recognition and treatment of common mental disorders through integration of mental health services into primary care is obligatory. It will require high-level training, best psychiatric practices research, and global ethical norms.

International collaborative centers for research should continue to be developed to achieve these goals. These collaborative centers should be multi-disciplinary.

Given the burden of disease secondary to mental illnesses around the world, interest in the promotion of mental health and prevention of mental illnesses has emerged. In December 2000, the Inaugural World Conference on the Promotion of Mental Health and the Prevention of Mental and Behavioral Disorders: The Coming Together of Science, Policy, and Programs Across Cultures was held at the Carter Center in Atlanta, Georgia.[85] Subsequent meetings have taken palace in London, Auckland, Oslo, Melbourne, Washington DC, and Perth. Moreover, a strategy for worldwide action to promote mental health and to prevent mental and behavioral disorders has been established and the Perth Charter was established in 2012. Considerable progress has been recognized in several areas; randomized control trials, time-series studies, and quasi-experimental community trials have demonstrated the significant success of programs in reducing risk factors and problematic behaviors.[85] For example, child abuse, pre-term deliveries, low birth weight, and insecure attachments can be decreased through interventions made during the pre-natal, infant, and toddler years.

In addition, aggressive behavior and violence can be decreased through parental training, good-behavior-focused interventions in elementary schools, and comprehensive mental health promotion programs in primary and middle schools. The initiation of smoking in 14 year olds can be lowered through early elementary school year interventions. By the same token, in twelfth-graders, drug use can be decreased through life-skills training during the middle school years. Adolescent unprotected sexual encounters can be reduced through behavioral-skills training during high school.

Teenage pregnancies can be reduced and negative marital communication styles and divorce can be decreased through education and skills training in young couples.

Research trials have also revealed that the onset of some specific mental disorders can be prevented, at least in the short term, through cognitive-behavioral approaches. Such findings have been reported in MDD in adolescents at high risk, in GAD (in children aged 7–14 years who are anxious), and in PTSD in victims of motorcycle and industrial accidents. These early studies are promising and suggest that research in prevention should become more of a priority.

More recently, there has been heightened research in the global crisis of human rights violations. The crisis is truly global as findings show people with mental disabilities experiencing human rights violations across the globe. In one such study, Drew and colleagues,[86] interviewed people who live with mental and psychosocial disabilities in low- and middle-income countries. They asked participants about what human rights violations they have experienced; the context in which the violations occurred; and what they believe needs to be done in order to improve the human rights violation crisis. Participants reported a wide range of human rights violations, including civil, cultural, social, political, and economic. Due to the continuing crisis, it is essential to continue research on the violation of human rights so that progress can be monitored both on the state and global levels.

WORLD HEALTH ORGANIZATION MENTAL HEALTH GLOBAL ACTION PROGRAM

Despite the presence of many barriers (including centralization of services in large institutions, a lack of awareness among health care workers and policymakers, poor service organization and financing, poor quality assurance, a lack of availability of psychotropic medications, and stigma), in 2001 the WHO defined a Mental Health Global Action Program to address many of the needs outlined earlier in this chapter. Through its updated 2011 Project Atlas,[87] the WHO collected information from 184 countries. This analysis showed that 60% of countries have a mental health policy as of 2011; 71% possess a mental health plan; and 59% report having dedicated mental health legislation. Higher-income countries typically have more facilities and higher admission and utilization rates. The global median number of facilities per 100,000 peoples is 0.61 for outpatient facilities, 0.05 for day treatment facilities, 0.01 for community residential facilities, and 0.04 for mental hospitals. The rate of available psychiatrists throughout the world is extremely varied, ranging from 0.05 per 100,000 people in low-income countries to 8.59 per 100,000 people in high-income countries.

The Mental Health Global Action Program initiative seeks to support WHO member states in the enhancement of their capacity to reduce the stigma and the burden of mental disorders. The initiative focuses on the burden of six conditions: depression, schizophrenia, substance use disorders and dependence, dementia, epilepsy, and suicide. Information concerning the magnitude, burden, determinants, and treatment of mental disorders is disseminated to enhance awareness. It is hoped that dissemination of information will lead to advocacy against stigma and discrimination and encourage better policy decisions. A broad-based "university" for research in mental health is envisioned, making use of the worldwide network of WHO collaborating centers and mental health experts to set up local and regional fellowships in mental health research and evaluation. This will lead to promotion of local research capacity, contributing to the development of culturally-relevant mental health information. This should increase WHO's ability to understand, and to respond to, changing trends in priority areas of inquiry.

CONCLUSION

International psychiatry has a new urgency now that the burden of disease secondary to mental illnesses around the world has been recognized as a public health crisis. Information about the epidemiology and burden of mental illnesses needs to be disseminated so that a ground-swell of support for development of mental health policy and legislation will follow in countries where they do not presently exist. With the coming of policy improvements, services may receive a higher priority. In order for services and resources to be used efficiently and effectively, better psychiatric outcomes research and practical psychiatric demonstration projects are necessities.

Models such as the one being built in Ethiopia (that use layered caregiving with co-location of primary care services and mental health services at the health unit level with health care workers seeing patients together) are promising, but will need to be studied vis-à-vis outcomes. The supervision of health care workers by psychiatric nurses and supervision of psychiatric nurses and health care workers by visiting psychiatrists makes most efficient use of the resources available. Co-location of mental health caregivers should aid in the education of primary care doctors and nurses. Psychiatrists working in the developing world should have well-developed consultation skills because they will be called on to consult on patients and then to supervise others, often from afar. In addition, given the high prevalence of HIV infection, tuberculosis, malaria, and other neuromedical illnesses, international psychiatrists must be well trained in neuropsychiatry and psychosomatic illness.

The best way to realize the goals of international education, clinical care, service improvement, and research is to develop an international psychiatry research and training center. By so doing, such centers can help revolutionize the development and apportionment of state-of-the-art psychiatry adapted for use in areas of the world with scarce resources.[88,89] Such an enterprise could help develop mental health policies, mental health service resources, mental health research, and the implementation of services in an evidence-based and compassionate fashion in the developing world.

Access the complete reference list and multiple choice questions (MCQs) online at https://expertconsult.inkling.com

KEY REFERENCES

13. Toronto Addis Ababa Academic Collaboration. Available at: <http://www.missbdesign.com/clients/TAAAC/programs_Psychiatry.html>.
14. Federal Democratic Republic of Ethiopia Ministry of Health. *National Mental Health Strategy*, Addis Ababa, 2012, Ethiopian Ministry of Health.
20. Malaju MT, Alene GD. Assessment of utilization of provider-initiated HIV testing and counseling as an intervention for prevention of mother to child transmission of HIV and associated factors among pregnant women in Gondar town, North West Ethiopia. *BMC Public Health* 12:226, 2012.
22. Lancet Global Mental Health Group, Chisholm D, Flisher AJ, et al. Scale up services for mental disorders: a call for action. *Lancet* 370(9594):1241–1252, 2007.
26. Kieling C, Baker-Hennigham H, Belfer M, et al. Child and adolescent mental health worldwide: evidence for action. *Lancet* 378(9801):1515–1525, 2011.
29. Amnesty International. *Amnesty International Annual Report 2013*, London, 2013, International Amnesty.
54. Mollica RF, Brooks R, Tor S, et al. The enduring mental health impact of mass violence: A community comparison study of Cambodian civilians living in Cambodia and Thailand. *Int J Soc Psychiatry* 60(1):6–20, 2014.
82. Sartorius N. Stigma and mental health. *Lancet* 370(9590):810–811, 2007.
84. Zhang J, Li Z. The association between depression and suicide when hopelessness is controlled for. *Compr Psychiatry* 2013.
86. Drew N, Funk M, Tang S, et al. Human rights violations of people with mental and psychosocial disabilities: an unresolved global crisis. *Lancet* 378(9803):1664–1675, 2011.
87. World Health Organization. *Mental health atlas 2011*, Geneva, 2011, World Health Organization.

Index

Page numbers followed by "f" indicate figures, "t" indicate tables, and "b" indicate boxes.

T

Tacrolimus (Prograf, FK 506), side effects of, 642t
Tactile hallucinations, 314b
Tadalafil, for erectile dysfunction, 408t
Taijin kyofusho ("interpersonal fear disorders"), 721t
Tamoxifen, for cancer, 625
TANs. see Tonically active neurons (TANs)
Tardive dyskinesia (TD), 480–481, 574b, 879
Task vigilance, 85t
TAT. see Thematic Apperception Test (TAT)
TAY. see Transitioning adolescents and young adults (TAY)
Tay-Sachs syndrome, late-onset form, 689t, 694
TBI. see Traumatic brain injury (TBI)
TCAs. see Tricyclic antidepressants (TCAs)
TCM. see Three-component model (TCM)
TD. see Tardive dyskinesia (TD)
Teleconsultation, 648t
Telegraphic speech, 952t
"Telepsychiatry", 958
Television, parental advice on use of, 986
Tellegen Absorption Scale, 147b, 148
Temazepam, for insomnia, 235t
Temperament, 433–434
  in infancy, 52, 52t
Temperature, test for, 801
Temporal arteritis, 848, 848f
Temporal lobe epilepsy (TLE), 624, 832
  MTL and, 787
Temporo-perisylvian language network, 806–807
Tension-type headache, 844, 844t
Termination phase, of planned brief psychotherapy, 118
Tertiary amine, in tricyclic antidepressants, 562t, 563
TESD. see Treatment-emergent sexual dysfunction (TESD)
Test categories, 74–80, 75t
Test development, 73–74
Testosterone test, 26t
Test-retest reliability, 73–74
Texting, parental advice on, 986–987
Thalamocortical circuits ("loops"), in basal ganglia, 779
Thalamus, 450–451, 451f, 772
Thalidomide, side effects of, 620b
Thematic Apperception Test (TAT), 80
Theophylline, 562t
Theory
  attachment, and psychiatric interview, 8–9
  integration, example of, 135–136
  of mind, 56
Therapeutic relationship, use of, in interpersonal therapy, 105b
Therapist, active, 117–118, 117b
"Therapy of the absurd", 130
Thiamine
  for alcohol withdrawal delirium, 275
  deficiency of, 215t, 216, 217f
  for Wernicke's encephalopathy, 275–276
Thiazide diuretics, sexual dysfunction and, 404t
Thioridazine, 562t
  change in QTc and, 181t
  sexual dysfunction and, 404t
Thorazine. see Chlorpromazine
Thought content, of patient, in neurological examination, 794
Thought content disorders, 16b
Thought process, of patient, in neurological examination, 794

Thoughts, in somatic symptom disorder, 257
Three Essays on the Theory of Sexuality, 47
Three-component model (TCM), in collaborative care, 648t, 649
Threshold of responsiveness, of temperament, 52t
Thrombosis
  cerebral venous, 847–848
  stroke and, 864
"Thunderclap" headache, 841–842, 842b, 846–847
Thyroid dysfunction, 218, 218f
Thyroid-stimulating hormone test, 26t
Thyroxine (T$_4$) test, 26t
TIA. see Transient ischemic attack (TIA)
Tiagabine, 536, 835t
  for generalized anxiety disorder, 468
Tic disorders, 745–746
  ADHD plus, 548
  treatment of, 745–746
Tic douloureux, 848–849
Tics, 745, 801, 873t, 875, 878t
Time to Change, 983–984
Tizanidine, for headache, 843t
TLE. see Temporal lobe epilepsy (TLE)
Tobacco, insomnia-inducing, 234t
Todd's paresis, 832
Tolmentin, properties of, 860t
Tonic neck reflex, 52
Tonically active neurons (TANs), rewarding information and, 779–780
Topiramate, 835t, 893
  for binge-eating disorder, 425t
  for bipolar disorder, 536, 751
  for bulimia nervosa, 425t
  depressive symptoms and, 836
  for headache, 843t
  side effects of, 579–580
  for trichotillomania, 253
Torsades de pointes ventricular arrhythmia, 575f
"Tort feasor", 930
Tort law, 913, 930
Torture, 993
  definitions of, 993–997
  evaluation, 997
  medical effects of, 994
  psychiatric effects of, 994
  purpose of, 993–994
  treatment for survivors, 995–997, 995b
    ask about patient's trauma story, 995–996
    be culturally attuned in communicating and prescribing, 997
    diagnosis and treatment, 996
    identify concrete physical and mental effects, 996
    prescribe, 997
    prevent burnout, 997
    psychiatric treatment, 996
    recommend work, altruism, and spirituality, 996–997
    refer, 996
    reinforce and teach, 996
    schedule follow-up visits, 997
    use of screening instruments, 996
  types of, 993–994, 994b
Tourette syndrome (TS), 742t, 745, 877
  genetic epidemiology of, 685
  molecular genetic studies of, 685
Tower tasks, 86
Toxic leukoencephalopathy, 625
Toxic reaction, delirium and, 943t

Toxins
  laboratory tests/diagnostic procedures for, 31, 32t
  mental disorders due to another medical conditions and, 221–222
Toxoplasmosis, cerebral, 633, 633f
Trail-Making Test, 86
Trait hypnotizability, 148
Tramadol, for pain management, 860, 861t
Tranquilization, 478
Transcranial magnetic stimulation, 521–524
  coils of, 522–523
  with deep brain stimulation, 523
  depth of, 522
  parameters of, 522b
  randomized clinical trial for, 523
  repetitive, 521
  safety profile of, 523
Transgenerational approaches, couples therapy, 107b
Transient ischemic attack (TIA), 863
Transinstitutionalism, 727
"Transinstitutionalization", 704
Transitioning adolescents and young adults (TAY), 755
  medication misuse in, 759, 759b
  prescription drug abuse in, 759
  psychiatric disorders in, 755–761
    treatment issues in, 759–760
  salient neurobiology of, 755
  substance abuse in, 758–760
    treatment issues in, 759–760
Transmodal areas, 806
Transplant centers, 639–640
Transplant recipients, 638
Transvestic disorder, 406t
Tranylcypromine, 466, 492, 503, 570
  for social anxiety disorder, 470
Trastuzumab, side effects of, 620b
Trauma, 380–394
  11-point toolkit model for recognition and management of reactions to, 995b
  acute stress disorder, 383, 384b
  delirium and, 177t
  mental disorders due to another medical conditions and, 225, 225f–226f
  PTSD. See Posttraumatic stress disorder
Trauma-related disorders, DSM-5 for, 168t, 169
Traumatic anxiety, 388
Traumatic brain disorder, psychiatric manifestations of, 883–895
Traumatic brain injury (TBI), 883
  aggression and, 887
  alcohol abuse and, 889
  anticonvulsants for, 892–893
  antidepressant for, 892–893
  antiepileptic drugs for, 893
  antipsychotics for, 893
  anxiolytics for, 893
  attention impairment, 885
  behavioral changes after, 886–887, 886t
  behavioral disturbances in, 811t
  benzodiazepines for, 893
  classification of, 884–885, 884t
  clinical features of, 885
  cognitive impairments, 885–886, 886t
  cognitive rehabilitation for, 894
  depression after, 887–888
  diagnosis of, 889–890, 889t
  environmental interventions for, 893
  epidemiology of, 883
  evaluation of, 890–891, 891f
  executive function impairments, 886
  language impairments, 886